Primary Care Medicine

THIRD EDITION

ALLAN H. GOROLL, M.D.
Associate Physician
Massachusetts General Hospital
Associate Professor of Medicine
Harvard Medical School
Boston, Massachusetts

LAWRENCE A. MAY, M.D.
Assistant Clinical Professor of Medicine
University of California, Los Angeles
Los Angeles, California

ALBERT G. MULLEY, JR., M.D., M.P.P.
Chief, General Internal Medicine Unit
Massachusetts General Hospital
Harvard Medical School
Boston, Massachusetts

With 60 contributors

Primary Care Medicine

Office Evaluation and Management of the Adult Patient

J.B. LIPPINCOTT COMPANY
Philadelphia

Acquisitions Editor: Richard Winters
Project Editor: Amy P. Jirsa
Indexer: Victoria Boyle
Art Director: Susan Hermansen
Interior Designer: Holly Reid McLaughlin
Production Manager: Helen Ewan
Production Coordinators: Maura C. Murphy, Robert Randall
Compositor: Compset, Inc.
Printer/Binder: Courier Book Company/Westford

Third Edition

6 5 4 3 2

Library of Congress Cataloging-in-Publication Data

Primary care medicine : office evaluation and management of the adult patient / [edited by] Allan H. Goroll, Lawrence A. May, Albert G. Mulley, Jr. ; with 60 contributors. — 3rd ed.
p. cm.
Rev. ed. of: Primary care medicine : office evaluation and management of the adult patient / Allan H. Goroll, Lawrence A. May, Albert G. Mulley, Jr. ; with 60 contributors. 2nd ed. c1987.
Includes bibliographical references and index.
ISBN 0-397-51130-2
1. Family medicine. I. Goroll, Allan H. II. May, Lawrence A. III. Mulley, Albert G. IV. Goroll, Allan H. Primary care medicine.
[DNLM: 1. Primary Health Care. 2. Ambulatory Care. W 84.6 P94916 1995]
RC46.G56 1995
616—dc20
DNLM/DLC
for Library of Congress 94-18815
CIP

The authors and publisher have exerted every effort to ensure that drug selection and dosage set forth in this text are in accord with current recommendations and practice at the time of publication. However, in view of ongoing research, changes in government regulations, and the constant flow of information relating to drug therapy and drug reactions, the reader is urged to check the package insert for each drug for any change in indications and dosage and for added warnings and precautions. This is particularly important when the recommended agent is a new or infrequently employed drug.

To JOHN D. STOECKLE, M.D., pioneer, mentor, and friend

Contributors

Michael J. Barry, M.D.
Assistant Professor
Harvard Medical School
Director, Primary Care Program
Massachusetts General Hospital
Boston, Massachusetts

Arthur J. Barsky, III, M.D.
Associate Professor of Psychiatry
Harvard Medical School
Director of Psychosomatic Research
Brigham and Women's Hospital
Boston, Massachusetts

Stephen L. Boswell, M.D.
Instructor in Medicine
Harvard Medical School
Medical Director
Fenway Community Health Center
The MGH AIDS Clinical Trials Group
Boston, Massachusetts

Robert J. Boyd, M.D.
Assistant Clinical Professor of Orthopaedic Surgery
Harvard Medical School
Visiting Orthopedic Surgeon
Massachusetts General Hospital
Boston, Massachusetts

David C. Brewster, M.D.
Associate Clinical Professor of Surgery
Massachusetts General Hospital
Harvard Medical School
Boston, Massachusetts

Elaine M. Carlson, M.D.
Clinical Instructor
Brown University School of Medicine
Director, Women's Health Associates
Rhode Island Hospital
Providence, Rhode Island

Gregory D. Curfman, M.D.
Deputy Editor
New England Journal of Medicine
Assistant Professor
Harvard Medical School
Assistant in Medicine
Massachusetts General Hospital
Boston, Massachusetts

Jules L. Dienstag, M.D.
Associate Professor of Medicine
Harvard Medical School
Physician
Massachusetts General Hospital
Boston, Masschusetts

Linda L. Emanuel, M.D., Ph.D.
Assistant Director
Division of Medical Ethics
Assistant Professor of Medicine and Social Medicine
Harvard Medical School
Boston, Massachusetts

Leslie Shu-Tung Fang, M.D., Ph.D.
Chief
Bauer Firm Medical Services
Massachusetts General Hospital
Boston, Massachusetts

Mason W. Freeman, M.D.
Assistant Professor of Medicine
Harvard Medical School
Associate Physician
Massachusetts General Hospital
Boston, Massachusetts

Lawrence S. Friedman, M.D.
Associate Professor of Medicine
Harvard Medical School
Massachusetts General Hospital
Boston, Massachusetts

Stephen J. Friedman, M.D.
Clinical Assistant Professor
Division of Dermatology
University of California, Los Angeles
School of Medicine
Los Angeles, California

Nancy J. Gagliano, M.D.
Instructor
Harvard Medical School
Clinical Director of Women's Health Associates
Massachusetts General Hospital
Boston, Massachusetts

Jeffrey E. Galpin, M.D.
Associate Clinical Professor of Medicine
University of Southern California
Chairman
Shared Medical Research Foundation
Tarzana, California

Ellie J.C. Goldstein, M.D.
Director, H.M. Alden Research Laboratory
Santa Monica Hospital Medical Center
Santa Monica, California
Clinical Professor of Medicine
University of California, Los Angeles
School of Medicine
Los Angeles, California

John D. Goodson, M.D.
Assistant Professor of Medicine
Harvard Medical School
Associate Physician
Massachusetts General Hospital
Boston, Massachusetts

Allan H. Goroll, M.D.
Associate Physician
Massachusetts General Hospital
Associate Professor of Medicine
Harvard Medical School
Boston, Massachusetts

David A. Greenberg, O.D., M.P.H.
Vice President for Academic Affairs/Dean
Illinois College of Optometry
Chicago, Illinois

Aina Julianna Gulya, M.D.
Associate Professor of Otolaryngology-Head and Neck Surgery
Georgetown University
Georgetown University Hospital
Washington, DC

Eleanor Z. Hanna, Ph.D.
Special Expert
National Institute of Health
National Institute on Alcohol Abuse and Alcoholism
Bethesda, Maryland
Instructor
Harvard Medical School
Psychologist
Massachusetts General Hospital
Boston, Massachusetts

Gale S. Haydock, M.D.
Instructor in Medicine
Harvard Medical School
Assistant Physician
Massachusetts General Hospital
Boston, Massachusetts

Carolyn Crimmins Hintlian, M.P.H., R.D.
Associate in Ambulatory Care and Prevention
Harvard Medical School
Boston, Massachusetts
Business Manager/Nutritionist
Massachusetts General Hospital East
Charlestown, Massachusetts

Robert A. Hughes, M.D.
Instructor
Harvard Medical School
Associate Physician
Massachusetts General Hospital
Boston, Massachusetts

Steven E. Hyman, M.D.
Associate Professor of Psychiatry
Director of the Division on Addictions
Harvard Medical School
Massachusetts General Hospital
Boston, Massachusetts

Michael A. Jenike, M.D.
Associate Professor of Psychiatry
Harvard Medical School
Associate Chief of Psychiatry for Research
Massachusetts General Hospital
Boston, Massachusetts

Jennifer Jeremiah, M.D.
Clinical Instructor in Medicine
Brown University School of Medicine
Division of General Internal Medicine
Rhode Island Hospital
Providence, Rhode Island

Jesse B. Jupiter, M.D.
Visiting Orthopaedic Surgeon
Chief, Orthopaedic Trauma Service
Massachusetts General Hospital
Associate Professor of Orthopaedic Surgery
Harvard Medical School
Boston, Massachusetts

John P. Kelly, D.M.D., M.D.
Associate Professor of Oral and Maxillofacial Surgery
Harvard School of Dental Medicine
Visiting Oral and Maxillofacial Surgery
Massachusetts General Hospital
Boston, Massachusetts

Eric Kortz, M.D.
Private Practice
Englewood, California

Richard R. Liberthson, M.D.
Associate Professor of Pediatrics
Harvard Medical School
Pediatrician
Associate Physician
Massachusetts General Hospital
Boston, Massachusetts

Nicholas J. Lowe, M.D.
Professor of Dermatology
UCLA School of Medicine
Director
Skin Research Foundation of California
Santa Monica, California

Michael N. Margolies, M.D.
Associate Professor of Surgery
Harvard Medical School
Visiting Surgeon
Massachusetts General Hospital
Boston, Massachusetts

Lawrence A. May, M.D.
Assistant Clinical Professor of Medicine
University of California, Los Angeles
Los Angeles, California

Charles J. McCabe, M.D.
Associate Professor of Surgery
Harvard Medical School
Associate Chief
Emergency Services
Massachusetts General Hospital
Boston, Massachusetts

Karyn Montgomery, M.D.
Instructor
Harvard Medical School
Associate Physician
Massachusetts General Hospital
Boston, Massachusetts

Anne W. Moulton, M.D.
Associate Professor
Brown University School of Medicine
Associate Physician
Division of General Medicine
Rhode Island Hospital
Providence, Rhode Island

Albert G. Mulley, Jr., M.D., M.P.P.
Associate Professor of Medicine
Harvard Medical School
Chief, General Internal Medicine Unit
Massachusetts General Hospital
Boston, Massachusetts

Samuel R. Nussbaum, M.D.
Associate Professor of Medicine
Harvard Medical School
Associate Physician
Massachusetts General Hospital
Boston, Massachusetts

L. Christine Oliver, M.D., M.S., M.P.H.
Assistant Professor of Medicine
Harvard Medical School
Associate Physician
Massachusetts General Hospital
Boston, Massachusetts

Richard D. Presavento, M.D.
Clinical Assistant in Ophthalmology
Harvard Medical School
Assistant Clinical Professor
Tufts Medical School
Active Staff
Massachusetts Eye and Ear Infirmary
New England Medical Center
Boston, Massachusetts

Amy A. Pruitt, M.D.
Assistant Professor of Neurology
University of Pennsylvania
School of Medicine
Attending Neurologist
Hospital of the University of Pennsylvania
Philadelphia, Pennsylvania

Scott L. Rauch, M.D.
Assistant Professor of Psychiatry
Harvard Medical School
Massachusetts General Hospital
Boston, Massachusetts

Ronald M. Reisner, M.D.
Professor of Medicine/Dermatology
University of California, Los Angeles
School of Medicine
Chief, Dermatology Service
West Los Angeles, VA Medical Center
Los Angeles, California

Claudia U. Richter, M.D.
Clinical Assistant in Ophthalmology
Harvard Medical School
Assistant Surgeon in Ophthalmology
Massachusetts Eye and Ear Infirmary
Boston, Massachusetts

James M. Richter, M.D.
Assistant Professor of Medicine
Harvard Medical School
Physician
Massachusetts General Hospital
Boston, Massachusetts

Nancy A. Rigotti, M.D.
Assistant Professor
Medicine and Ambulatory Care and Prevention
Harvard Medical School
Director, Quit Smoking Service
Massachusetts General Hospital
Boston, Massachusetts

Jerrold F. Rosenbaum, M.D.
Assistant Professor Psychiatry
Harvard Medical School
Director of Patient Psychiatry Division
Chief, Clinical Psychopharmacology Unit
Massachusetts General Hospital
Boston, Massachusetts

Frederick W. Ruymann, M.D.
Clinical Instructor of Medicine
Harvard Medical School
Gastroenterologist
Harvard Community Health Plan
Brigham and Women's Hospital
Boston, Massachusetts

Linda C. Shafer, M.D.
Instructor in Psychiatry
Harvard Medical School
Assistant Psychiatrist
Massachusetts General Hospital
Boston, Massachusetts

William V.R. Shellow, M.D.
Associate Professor of Dermatology
University of California, Los Angeles School of Medicine
Chief, Inpatient and Consultation Dermatology
VA Medical Center
West Los Angeles, California

Harvey B. Simon, M.D.
Associate Professor of Medicine
Harvard Medical School
Physician
Massachusetts General Hospital
Boston, Massachusetts

Arthur J. Sober, M.D.
Associate Professor of Dermatology
Harvard Medical School
Associate Chief of Dermatology
Massachusetts General Hospital
Boston, Massachusetts

Roger F. Steinert, M.D.
Assistant Clinical Professor
Harvard Medical School
Associate Surgeon
Massachusetts Eye and Ear Infirmary
Boston, Massachusetts

John D. Stoeckle, M.D.
Professor of Medicine
Harvard Medical School
Physician
Massachusetts General Hospital
Boston, Massachusetts

Katharine K. Treadway, M.D.
Instructor
Harvard Medical School
Associate Physician
Massachusetts General Hospital
Boston, Massachusetts

Flora Treger, M.D.
Division of Internal Medicine
Women's Health Associates
Rhode Island Hospital
Providence, Rhode Island

Jeffrey B. Weilberg, M.D.
Assistant Professor of Psychiatry
Harvard Medical School
Clinical Associate in Psychiatry
Massachusetts General Hospital
Boston, Massachusetts

Debra F. Weinstein, M.D.
Instructor in Medicine
Harvard Medical School
Associate Chief of Medicine
Director of Residency Training
Massachusetts General Hospital
Boston, Massachusetts

William R. Wilson, M.D.
Professor of Surgery (Otolaryngology)
George Washington University Medical Center
Washington, D.C.

Jerry Younger, M.D.
Instructor
Harvard Medical School
Associate Physician
Massachusetts General Hospital
Boston, Massachusetts

Foreword to the First Edition

Physicians have traditionally provided direct, initial, comprehensive care for patients as well as continuity of care. In the past two decades the growing proportion of specialist physicians has endangered this traditional role of the physician. The development of highly technologic, tertiary, inpatient medical care has preoccupied the attention of our teaching institutions. Coping with the increased armamentarium of diagnostic and therapeutic interventions has distracted some physicians from traditional roles in patient care. The primary care movement has been a national response to this situation aimed at providing more physicians skilled in dealing wisely and humanely with illness in their patients and providing the overall supervision and continuity of medical care that we expect of good generalists. It encourages these physicians to know their patients as human and social beings as well as bearers of organ pathology. Promotion of prevention as well as the practice of curing is an important part of primary care.

The concerns which have led to renewed attention of the medical profession to primary care medicine have had a very salutary effect on our teaching institutions. There has been a resurgence of training in the ambulatory setting. Medical students and residents have learned that many illnesses formerly thought to require hospitalization can be effectively managed in the ambulatory setting. As usual, this is not an original discovery; rather, it is a return to the emphasis that was very much a part of training programs in the earlier decades of this century.

Primary Care Medicine has grown out of the experiences of a group of young physicians who have pioneered in the rebirth of primary care medicine within the Harvard medical community. They have organized primary care practices which have served as training sites for other physicians and health workers. They have examined their own practices, as well as the published experience of others, in order to provide within this text a synthesis of the best available information for ambulatory management of adult medical patients. Their discussions are brief and practical rather than exhaustive, but the interested reader is provided with a key annotated bibliography which directs him to further sources of information. This book is not meant to compete with the traditional exhaustive textbook of Medicine. Rather, its brief, clear discussions and analyses of current knowledge are prepared for the busy practitioner who daily encounters many problems for which he needs to quickly know the best available answers.

To whom is the book addressed? To the primary care physician, of course. It will be his bible—a valuable source of guidance and of solace in innumerable management situations. But it is becoming increasingly evident that the medical subspecialist devotes a considerable portion of his practice time to the provision of first contact and continuous care of the medical needs of his patients. This book will, therefore, find a welcome place on the desk of both the medical subspecialist and the medical generalist and is addressed to everyone engaged in the clinical practice of adult Medicine.

Alexander Leaf, M.D.
Jackson Professor of Medicine
Harvard Medical School; and
Chief, Medical Services
Massachusetts General Hospital
Boston, Massachusetts
April 1981

Preface

Since publication of the first edition of *Primary Care Medicine* in 1981, the field of primary care has moved from the periphery to the center of American medicine. The shift reflects recognition of the critical role played by primary physicians in the provision of comprehensive, personalized, affordable medical care. The third edition of *Primary Care Medicine* is designed to help clinicians and students meet the increasingly complex demands of the primary care role. These include efficient, cost-effective approaches to screening, diagnosis, and treatment and enhanced involvement of the patient in clinical decision-making.

While retaining the terse, problem-oriented, practical style of previous editions, the third edition has been expanded and almost every chapter thoroughly rewritten to incorporate the wealth of new information emerging from the literature, as evidenced by more than 2,500 new papers reviewed in the annotated bibliographies. New approaches to screening and diagnosis are critically examined (eg, MRI for back pain, tilt-table testing for syncope, PSA testing for prostatic carcinoma, CA 125 and vaginal ultrasound for ovarian cancer). Major advances in treatment are incorporated (eg, for hypertension, hypercholesterolemia, diabetes, depression, smoking cessation, osteoporosis). New approaches to difficult problems are underscored by several new chapters and new sections of chapters, including those on refractory peptic ulcer disease, chronic fatigue syndrome, HIV infection, substance abuse, fibromyalgia syndrome, sleep apnea, Lyme disease, multiple sclerosis, hepatitis C, and chlamydial infection. The unique clinical requirements of the elderly, pregnant patients, postmenopausal women, and other important subpopulations are extensively and specifically addressed in the context of each clinical problem.

As the manager of care, the primary physician faces increased responsibility to contain costs, ensure quality, and counsel the patient, both in health and illness. To help in these tasks, the third edition includes new chapters on estimating and communicating risk and prognosis, interpreting evidence of therapeutic efficacy, and helping patients to formulate a "living will" and other advance directives. New cost-effectiveness and relative-cost data are extensively cited.

The third edition is designed to be an efficient source of critical information pertinent to clinical decision-making, to be used as much during an office visit as afterward. The book remains problem-based to effectively focus on the clinical questions encountered in practice. The index and chapters are carefully organized, subtitled, and cross-referenced to facilitate quick location of all needed information; tables are used extensively; and specific management recommendations are provided. Though the emphasis is on practical decision-making, the relevant pathophysiology and clinical study data are cited whenever possible to provide the scientific basis for the recommendations made.

We have been deeply moved by the enthusiastic response to the first two editions of *Primary Care Medicine*. The third edition has taken several years to prepare. We think it is the best one yet and hope you will find it useful in the care of your patients.

Allan H. Goroll, M.D.
Lawrence A. May, M.D.
Albert G. Mulley, Jr., M.D., M.P.P.

Acknowledgments

Although *Primary Care Medicine* is written predominantly by primary physicians for primary physicians, it depends heavily on and benefits greatly from the contributions of our valued subspecialty colleagues. Many serve as authors of specific chapters. Others have graciously reviewed manuscript and made excellent recommendations. Some did both. Special thanks are due to William Shellow, Associate Professor of Medicine (Dermatology) at UCLA, and Jerry Younger, Associate Physician (Oncology) at Massachusetts General Hospital, who were instrumental in preparation of the dermatology and oncology sections respectively. Much-appreciated manuscript review and critique of chapters written by east coast authors were provided by our west coast colleagues, including Richard Ress, Associate Professor of Medicine (Rheumatology) at UCLA; Michael Burnam, Assistant Professor of Medicine (Cardiology) at UCLA; Stephen Levinson, Assistant Professor of Medicine (Gastroenterology) at UCLA; and Stephen Pine (Obstetrics and Gynecology). Such review is invaluable to providing the book with a national perspective.

There are a number of contributors to previous editions whose efforts deserve recognition, because their work contributed to the success of prior editions and facilitated the preparation of this one. They include Drs. Jacob J. Lokich of The Cancer Center of Boston, and Mark S. Huberman of The New England Deaconness Hospital, who authored most of the oncology chapters of the second edition; Dr. Robert T. Schooley, who while a member of the Infectious Disease unit at Massachusetts General Hospital authored *Primary Care Medicine*'s first chapter on AIDS, which appeared in the second edition; Drs. Lynn Butterly and Alan Smith, who as fellows in gastroenterology at Massachusetts General contributed to the chapters on abdominal pain, indigestion, and gastroesophageal reflux for the second edition; the late Dr. Anne Barnes of the Gynecology Service at the Massachusetts General Hospital, whose chapters in the second edition on female sexual dysfunction and unwanted pregnancy were among her very last writings before her untimely death from cancer; Dr. Wayne L. Peters, now of Denver, Colorado, who while at Massachusetts General authored the second edition's chapters on screening and management of hyperlipidemia; and Dr. Daniel S. Singer of the General Medicine Unit of Massachusetts General Hospital who authored the second edition's chapters on acute monoarticular arthritis and polyarticular arthritis. We are grateful to them for their contributions.

The dedication of our publishing colleagues at J.B. Lippincott Co. was exemplary, especially that of Mr. Richard Winters, the publishing editor, whose professionalism, support, and commitment to this book were extraordinary. Also noteworthy were the dedicated and exacting editorial and administrative efforts of Ms. Amy Jirsa and Ms. Jody Schott; their hard work was essential to ensuring the book's editorial quality. Finally, our special thanks to Lippincott's Mr. J. Stuart Freeman, who came to us in 1975, wondering what primary care was about and offering us the opportunity to help define it.

To our families, we cannot say enough of the love, patience, and support they provided during the several years it took to prepare the third edition. Without them, this book would never have been written.

Contents

Primary Care Medicine

Primary Care Medicine: Office Evaluation and Management of the Adult Patient, 3rd edition, edited by Allan H. Goroll, Lawrence A. May, and Albert G. Mulley, Jr. J.B. Lippincott Company, Philadelphia

1 Principles of Primary Care

1 Tasks of Primary Care

JOHN D. STOECKLE, M.D.

DEFINITION OF PRIMARY CARE

Primary care is coordinated, comprehensive, and personal care, available on both a first-contact and a continuous basis. It incorporates several tasks: medical diagnosis and treatment, psychological assessment and management, personal support, communication of information about illness, prevention, and health maintenance.

This book addresses the clinical problems encountered by primary care physicians in office practice of adult medicine. In this setting, the physician's responsibilities and tasks extend beyond the narrow technological confines of medical diagnosis and treatment. Although a great deal of effort must be focused on accurate diagnosis and technically sound therapy, the other clinical tasks that complete the very definition of primary care also assume major importance.

Alongside this clinical definition of primary care stands a plethora of other definitions; these derive from organizational, functional, professional, and academic perspectives. For example, policy planners have defined primary care as a *level of medical services,* one that is provided outside the hospital. Presumably, primary care (community-based services) is, then, a less technical practice compared with secondary care (consultant or specialty services) and tertiary care (hospital services). This organizational definition provides a scheme for the allocation of public resources among these health services, each of which has a distinct professional, economic, institutional, and political structure. For another definition, Alpert and Charney have looked at important *patient care functions* of doctors, namely, to provide access, continuity, and integration. Although this view is useful in describing the functions performed by practitioners for their patients within organized health services, it does not define the content of their clinical work. From the standpoint of professionalism, primary care has been defined as a *specialty* concentrating on humanistic medicine practiced outside the hospital but devoid of the special procedures and technology that typically characterize medical specialization. This definition has been useful in organizing a segment of the profession (eg, family practice) and in providing a new curriculum for the education and training of doctors. From the university comes still another definition of primary care as an *academic discipline* concerned with the expansion of knowledge unique to primary practice and to personal care, a definition that contains the promise of a departmental position for primary care in the medical school.

Although each of these definitions presents a particular perspective about primary care and serves some special purpose, none explains the primary care physician's day-to-day work with patients.

By taking the perspective of the doctor's practice, primary care can be defined by several tasks: 1) medical diagnosis and treatment; 2) psychological diagnosis and treatment; 3) personal support of patients of all backgrounds, in all stages of illness; 4) communication of information about diagnosis, treatment, prevention, and prognosis; 5) maintenance of patients with chronic illness; 6) prevention of disability and disease through detection, education, behavioral change, and preventive treatment. These tasks comprise the clinical work of doctors providing primary care. They not only restate medicine's central mandate of patient care, but also constitute a clinical definition of primary care to which the information in this text is applied.

THE TASKS AND THEIR RATIONALES

Except for medical diagnosis and treatment, the tasks that define primary care may seem merely vocational, that is, practical but not scientifically based. However, social science research has provided a logical and rational basis for the clinical work of primary care. The data derived from these studies concern the patient's illness rather than the doctor's definition of disease; they are contained in the cognitive, communicative, and behavioral processes by which the patient defines being ill; and they are found in the clinical and social science literature on such topics as the patient's emotional reactions, personality, expectations, requests, attributions, views of treatment, and social networks, to mention but a few. Knowledge concerning such aspects of care in conjunction with statistical thinking contributes a rational framework for the tasks of primary care.

Medical Diagnosis and Treatment remain central tasks, although they are by no means the end point of care. As the patient's first contact with medical services, the primary doctor not only must be knowledgeable about disease but must exercise critical judgment in determining the scope, site, and pace of the medical workup and management. In organizing diagnosis and management, the physician needs to know the clinical presentation and natural history of illness, the uses and limits of the laboratory, and the indications for and shortcomings of invasive tests and therapeutic measures. In continuing care, the issues are the same. The doctor's critical attitude toward the use of technology and the referral of patients for special therapies or diagnostic techniques remains essential. Chapter 2 considers methods developed in clinical epidemiology and decision analysis, which promise to help the clinician rationally choose among a sometimes bewildering array of diagnostic and therapeutic options.

Psychological Diagnosis and Treatment and Personal Support complement the medical components of care. Studies documenting the relationship between emotional reactions and illness, coupled with surveys showing a high frequency of such reactions in office practice, underscore their importance in patients seeking medical help. Recognition of anxiety, depression, sexual dysfunction, personality disturbance, and psychosis is necessary for the interpretation of bodily complaints, the communication of personal feelings, and the joint decision of doctor and patient on acceptable and effective treatment plans.

Recognition of emotional reactions alone is insufficient. The doctor's response to the normal patient's psychological defenses is essential to securing cooperation and relieving anxiety. Understanding the patient's defenses and personality style allows the clinician to provide meaningful support and to respond appropriately to the patient's emotional needs. The care rendered is then likely to be perceived as personal and psychologically acceptable. Much of this analysis of the psychological aspects of clinical practice derives from classic case studies by Kahana and Bibring, Lipsett, Balaint, and Zaborenko on the emotional reactions and personality traits among patients with medical disorders. More recent qualitative surveys of medical practice populations document the importance of emotional states, especially depression, in the outcome of treatment.

Eliciting and Addressing Patient Expectations and Requests are also important. *Expectations* often play a major part in seeking help, complying with treatment, and feeling satisfied with care. In their studies of illness behavior and patients' use of doctors, Zola and Mechanic viewed expectations as explanations of patients' decisions to go to see the doctor. If attention was not paid to the patient's reason for coming, the corollary was clear: The patient would not stay in treatment. In health centers in Israel, Shuval found specific expectations of visits to doctors: status enhancement in seeing socially important professionals; catharsis of grief, anger, and despair; sanctioning of failure to cope; and understanding and control of illness through medical "scientific" explanations. This brief list is by no means complete, for along with these so-called latent expectations are traditional or "real" medical ones—for example, that the doctor is a healer of disease and possesses techniques for its control, relief, or cure. Such expectations not only explain the decision to seek medical care but are, in fact, elements of the clinical tasks of personal support and communication of information about illness.

Newer clinical studies by Lazare and colleagues have separated *requests* from expectations. Requests are specific and concrete helping actions and behaviors identified by patients. These studies identified some 14 requests and demonstrated that their prompt recognition and negotiation benefited both patient and doctor. The doctor's interest in ascertaining what treatment the patient wants indicates a reciprocity that is associated with greater satisfaction and adherence to medical advice. These efforts are part of the task of personal support and management. Still other elements of the management task, such as decisions about continued care, referral, and discharge, are also realized through an understanding of requests; thus, physicians need both to elicit and to respond to them.

Communication of Information About Illness. The need to inform, explain, reassure, and advise patients is essential to primary care. This task is often dependent on a knowledge of the patient's *attributions* (ie, what the patient thinks is the cause of illness). If the patient's attributions differ from the doctor's and are not uncovered, his anxieties may not be relieved, nor will the doctor's explanation be accepted. Knowing how and what to tell the patient about his illness is often difficult, especially if the patient's interpretation of the illness has not been elicited.

Mechanic, for example, suggests that patients with bodily complaints may go to the primary care doctor not for relief of physical discomfort but rather to learn what causes their complaints and sometimes to obtain reassurance that their complaints have less serious causes than they thought. Such confirmation or correction of the patient's attributions is a kind of "attribution therapy." From a broader perspective, Kleinman assigns to attributions a major function in all medical care systems, namely, the control of illness through the explanation of its cause. In effect, the doctor's clinical or scientific explanations of illness provide labels, names, and models so that the patient feels his illness can be understood and controlled, regardless of its technical treatment. In essence, the patient's beliefs about illness need to be elicited so that they can be used in explanation, education, and reassurance. (See Appendix I.)

Maintenance of the Chronically Ill requires continuous, long-term treatment and is a distinct task of primary care. Here, obtaining patient compliance is essential because most long-term treatment now takes place without daily medical supervision, and most of that treatment requires the self-administration of drugs. To improve adherence to therapy, it has become increasingly important to learn about the *patient's views of treatment* and actual self-treatment. So far the record on adherence to treatment has not been good. A wide discrepancy between what is prescribed and what is done typifies the literature of "following the doctor's orders," and the problem seems to be as much the doctor's as the patient's.

Knowledge about patients' views and behaviors can be used to design more effective therapeutic regimens and to alter therapeutic directions. Moreover, the act of eliciting information may improve communication between doctor and patient, thus strengthening their relationship and further promoting therapeutic efforts. More studies of patient views of treatment and of the dynamics of the doctor–patient relationship should provide new knowledge that can be used to enhance compliance.

Prevention of Disease and Disability, an essential task of primary care, emphasizes screening and the assessment of risk and function. With early intervention through health education, behavioral change, and preventive treatment, some of the expected morbidity, disability, and mortality may be delayed—if not prevented—and costly technologic interventions and therapies avoided. The primary physician needs to know which conditions and risk factors are worth screening for and how best to detect and effectively manage them. (See Chapter 3.)

A less commonly considered but no less important aspect of prevention involves attention to the patient's *social network,* because illness is often precipitated by disruption of interpersonal relationships. For example, Parkes and others have noted an increased mortality and morbidity among recent widows, while Zola has reported that interpersonal crises were among the most frequent of five common circumstances that spurred the individual to come for medical attention. Knowledge of patients' social situations can help in prevention of illness and visits to the doctor by focusing attention on stresses that might be precipitants. Attention to social networks is important for personal treatment. If significant loss or separation occurs, a major part of treatment can involve helping the patient reestablish his social network, thus lessening dependence on professional help from the doctor, nurse, or social worker. Patient illness narratives and doctors' clinical experiences illustrate that much of the work of care is done by patients themselves, their families, and their informal networks. Helping patients to share the preventive work with others can be of major benefit.

THE PROMISE OF PRIMARY CARE MEDICINE

So far the clinical tasks of primary care have been proposed as a perspective from which readers might view the information in this text. In addition, the tasks also promise changes in our ideas about standards of treatment, the doctor–patient relationship, professional relations, organization, prevention, clinical excellence, and clinical effectiveness.

Treatment. The ideal of personal treatment is revived and reemphasized. Though it is not entirely dead, the increasing size, specialization, and organization of practice often make personal, patient-oriented treatment a luxury rather than a medical care necessity. Patient-centered treatment also means that specific therapeutic regimens not only must be technically correct, but must be designed to be acceptable to patients, especially because more patients than ever are being cared for on an outpatient basis.

Doctor–Patient Relationship. Patient-centered treatment in primary care practice implies a doctor–patient relationship in which the doctor acts out several behaviors that will enhance the patient's participation in care and treatment:

1. Making the relationship more democratic by eliciting and responding to patients' preferences in decisions about the scope of diagnosis and alternatives of treatment.
2. Developing patient participation by transmitting appropriate information so that patients can make intelligent choices.
3. Attending to patients' feelings about illness and treatment with regard, genuine concern, and empathy.
4. Providing helping actions that are person-centered by eliciting, acknowledging, and responding to patients' own perspectives of their illness and care.
5. Responding by negotiation to the patients' choices, decisions, and requests; similarly, acknowledging and negotiating conflict even if in the relationship itself.
6. Promoting health education, self-help, and preventive behaviors by communicating information about diagnosis, treatment, and prevention.
7. Conveying respect for the person of the patient without regard to the patient's gender, race, ethnicity, age, or social class.

Professional Relations. The primary physician's responsibility for accessible, integrated, and continuous care is enhanced and made central. One consequence is that decision making is now collaborative, coordinated by the generalist; so often in the past it was not.

Organization. The ambulatory practice organizations outside the hospital (offices, health centers, group practices, HMOs) have become essential sites for delivery of primary care services. Because the goals of primary care include not only cure but also prevention and health maintenance, the ambulatory setting emerges as the major organizational locus for delivery of primary care services. The move to outpatient care has been greatly facilitated by the direct availability to the primary physician of the major technologies for screening, diagnosis, and treatment. Even the management of chronic illness, one of society's major health problems, is now largely conducted in the outpatient setting.

The form of ambulatory practice organization is also changing, with the practices becoming more corporatized and the physician working more as an employee. Divided loyalties—the organization versus the patient—may develop, confronting the primary care physician with new pressures to maintain the professional ethos as the patient's advocate.

Prevention. The ideal of prevention in practice has been to deal with the individual patient seeking help. Primary care medicine also examines the epidemiology of the entire practice, and perhaps even its community base, to institute a program of effective preventive intervention.

Clinical Excellence and Ethics. Skills in medical diagnosis and treatment have often been the only measure of clinical excellence. The ideal of excellence is now expanded to include *all* the tasks of primary care, the communicative as well as the technical. In decision making about the use of technologies, new ethical considerations are also required. For public accountability of medical practice, the primary physician must support professional group efforts that scientifically examine the appropriate use of medical technologies for practice. These are now being conducted as outcome, clinical effectiveness, and technology assessment studies. For the care of the individual, the primary physician must continue to elicit preferences and exercise discretionary decisions for the personal needs and benefit of the patient.

Clinical Effectiveness. The usual objective criteria for efficacy of diagnosis and treatment have been derived from the standards of clinical science. Consideration of subjective parameters such as patient acceptance and a sense of well-being is mandatory in the primary care setting and must be added to the assessment of clinical efficacy.

These themes on the clinical tasks and promises of primary care run through the chapters that follow, sometimes explicitly, sometimes latently; but they are always central to providing personalized care to patients.

ANNOTATED BIBLIOGRAPHY

Alpert JJ, Charney E. The Education of Physicians for Primary Care. DHEW Publication No 74–31B. US Government Printing Office, 1975. (*Functional definition of primary care.*)

Balaint M. The Doctor, the Patient and the Illness. New York, International Universities Press, 1957. (*A classic study of the British general practitioner's negotiations with patients about diagnosis and treatment.*)

Kahana RJ, Bibring GL. Personality types in medical management. In Zinberg NE (ed): Psychiatry and Medical Practice in a General Hospital, pp 108–123. New York; International Universities Press, 1965. (*Discusses the use of defense mechanisms derived from personality assessment in treatment.*)

Kasl SV, Cobb S. Health behavior, illness behavior and sick role behavior. I: Health and illness. Arch Environ Health 1966; 12:245. (*A thorough review of sociological and psychiatric studies on the factors that lead to a decision to seek help.*)

Kleinman AM. Toward a comparative study of medical systems: An integrated approach to the study of the relationship of medicine and culture. Sci Med Man 1973;1:55. (*A study that examines the specific and general significance of attributions.*)

Lazare A, Cohen F, Mignone R et al. The walk-in patient as a customer: A key dimension in evaluation and treatment. Am J Orthopsychiatry 1972;42:872.

Lazare A, Eisenthal S, Frank A et al. Studies on a negotiated approach to patienthood. The doctor–patient relation. In Gallagher E (ed): Fogarty International Center Series on the Teaching of Preventive Medicine, Vol 4. Washington DC, US Department of Health, Education, and Welfare, 1977. (*Two studies that systematically examine requests of patients in a psychiatric clinic.*)

Lindemann E. Symptomatology and management of acute grief. Am J Psychiatry 1944;101:141. (*A classic paper on the symptoms in medical patients.*)

Lipsett D. Medical and psychological characteristics of "crocks." Psychiatr Med 1970;15:293. (*Describes the patient who needs to have bodily complaints and suggests management taking this need into account.*)

McDill MS. Structure of social systems determining attitudes, knowledge and behavior toward disease. In Enelow AJ, Henderson JB (eds): Applying Behavioral Sciences to Cardiovascular Risk. New York, American Heart Association, 1975. (*Reviews the potential use of networks in prevention of heart disease.*)

McKinlay JB. Social networks, lay consultation and help-seeking behavior. Social Forces 1973;51:275. (*Uses networks to explain differences in help-seeking behavior.*)

McWhinney IR. General practice as an academic discipline. Lancet 1966;1:419. (*Defines primary care from an academic perspective.*)

Mechanic D. Medical Sociology. New York, Free Press, 1968. (*A classic text detailing the interaction of social factors and illness.*)

Mechanic D. Social psychologic factors affecting the presentation of bodily complaints. N Engl J Med 1972;286:1132. (*A sociological study that examines the factors influencing the patient's decision to seek medical help.*)

Parkes CM. Effects of bereavement on physical and mental health—A study of medical records of widows. Br Med J 1964;2:274. (*One of a number of studies documenting increased morbidity and mortality among widows shortly after the death of their husbands.*)

Mulley AG. Applying effectiveness and outcomes research to clinical practice. In Heitoff HA, Lohr KM (eds): Effectiveness and Outcomes in Health Care. Washington, DC: National Academy Press, 1990. (*A very useful overview.*)

Shuval JT, Antonovsky A, Davies AM. Social Function of Medical Practice: Doctor–Patient Relationship in Israel. San Francisco, Jossey-Bass, 1970. (*An analysis of the rates and reasons for medical visits; provides a typology of the uses of medical visits.*)

Stewart AL, Greenfield S, Hays RD et al. Functional studies and well-being of patients with chronic conditions. JAMA 1989; 262:907. (*A demonstration of the usefulness of expanded outcomes measures that include emotional and functional elements.*)

Stoeckle JD. Reflections on modern doctoring. Milbank Q 1988; 66:79. (*A discussion of some of the organizational, professional, and ethical issues involved in the contemporary practice of medicine.*)

Stoeckle JD, Zola IK, Davidson GE. On going to see the doctor. The contributions of the patient to the decision to seek medical aid. J Chronic Dis 1963;16:975. (*An analysis of patients' expectations in medical practice.*)

Stoeckle JD, Zola IK, Davidson GE. The quality and significance of psychological distress in medical patients. J Chronic Dis 1964;17:959. (*A review of studies on the psychological distress found in medical patients.*)

Waitzkin H, Stoeckle JD. The communication of information about illness: Clinical, sociological and methodological considerations. In Lipowski ZJ (ed): Advances in Psychosomatic Medicine: Psychosocial Aspects of Physical Illness, Vol 8, pp 180–216. Basel, S Karger, 1972. (*The role of communication in the patient–doctor relationship and a review of the research on communication in medical practice.*)

Zaborenko RN, Zaborenko L, Hengea RA. The psychodynamics of physicianhood. Psychiatry 1970;33:102. (*An illustration of the importance of understanding patients' defenses and personalities and the uses this knowledge may have in the treatment relationship.*)

Zola IK. Studying the decision to see a doctor. In Lipowski ZJ (ed): Advances in Psychosomatic Medicine: Psychosocial Aspects of Physical Illness, Vol 8, pp 216–236. Basel, S Karger, 1972. (*Describes the typology of decisions and their dynamics.*)

Appendix I: Approaches to Encouraging Compliance

John D. Stoeckle, M.D.

That 20 percent to 80 percent of patients do not comply with medical advice is repeatedly quoted. Such dismal statistics are derived from a rigid definition of compliance as patients' all-or-nothing adherence to medical instructions, whereas their treatment behaviors are far more variable, ranging from the optimal cooperative response to the ritualistic, retreatist, and innovative. Regardless of the extent and variability of noncompliance, patients' adherence to medication regimens is critical in effectively treating medical disorders, as is their adoption and learning of appropriate behaviors (in eating, exercise, smoking, drinking, relaxation, and drug use) for preventing disease.

Explanations and theories of noncompliance have focused on patients' beliefs, attitudes, expectations, and feelings that interfere with their "taking pills" or "changing habits." Even if such factors do interfere, they can be changed. Compliance can be improved by practitioner–patient communication that responds to patient views and develops the patient's ability to adhere to medical advice through education and the learning of new behaviors. Fostering compliance is a major goal of patient education.

Specific Strategies

The educational/communication strategies and techniques helpful in facilitating compliance begin with the doctor–patient relationship. A positive, mutually respectful doctor–patient relationship is important for making the patient "ready" to receive patient education and to negotiate the goals and means of treatment. Moreover, the physician's explanations and educational efforts, in turn, contribute to that relationship. Specific strategies utilize persuasion, medical advice, feedback, and monitoring.

Persuasion, or Why Do It?

1. Describe immediate and long-term treatment benefits with health risk and cost. If possible, present treatment options and acknowledge if rationale differs from view of patient.
2. Assist patients in clarifying their priorities (requests) for treatment (eg, patients presenting with pain may request explanation rather than medication).
3. Use your expertise, experience, and relationship to assert your own expectations that the patient should comply, in supporting the patient's treatment choice and capacity to carry it out.

The Medical Advice, or What to Do

1. Adapt instruction to the patient's language and knowledge level, responding to any misconceptions about treatment.
2. Make directions explicit, simple, personalized, and operational (how many, what kind, and when to take "pills"; organizing "pill taking" into the routine of the patient's everyday life).
3. Use multiple modes of communication, both verbal and written instructions and, where available, audiovisual materials that reinforce general knowledge about treatment. Enlist other members of the clinical team in providing instructions; also recruit family in the educational process.

Feedback, or What Advice Was Negotiated?

1. Have the patient repeat the medical advice given and the rationale for it.
2. Have the patient rehearse how medical advice will be carried out.
3. Jointly plan return visits, phone calls, and additional reviews with clinical team (nurse practitioners, physician assistants), if needed.

Monitoring Compliance, or What Have You Done?

1. At return visits, review the patient's compliance by direct questioning, again eliciting the rationale along with the problems the patient experienced in treatment.
2. Use information to reexplain or redesign treatment, reinforce behaviors, and reward the patient.
3. Encourage and organize the patient's self-monitoring of treatment (eg, blood pressure measurements).

In general, these educational strategies and tactics are not systematically carried out in practitioner–patient communication. Their use in patient education should result in greater compliance with medical advice.

ANNOTATED BIBLIOGRAPHY

DiMatteo MR, Nicola DD. Achieving Patient Compliance. New York, Pergamon Press, 1982. (*Another thoughtful review with emphasis on what to do.*)

Harris L et al. Americans and Their Doctors. New York, Pfizer Pharmaceuticals, 1985. (*More on the relationship.*)

Mumford E. The responses patients have to medical advice. In Understanding Human Behavior in Health and Illness. Baltimore, Williams & Wilkins, 1985. (*Responses range from the ritualistic to the innovative.*)

Sackett DL, Snow JC. The magnitude of compliance and noncompliance. In Haynes R, Sackett D (eds): Compliance in Health Care. Baltimore, Johns Hopkins University Press, 1979. (*One of many useful chapters in this book devoted to both academic and practical aspects of the compliance issue.*)

Stimson GV. Obeying the doctor's orders: A view from the other side. Soc Sci Med 1974;8:97. (*A study that details what patients think after they have left the doctor's office.*)

Swarstad BL. Patient–practitioner relationships and compliance with prescribed medical regimens. In Aiken LH, Mechanic D (eds): Applications of Social Science to Clinical Medicine and Health Policy. New Brunswick, NJ: Rutgers University Press, 1986. (*Emphasis on the relationship to facilitate compliance.*)

Appendix II: Approaches to Common Ethical and Legal Issues in Primary Care Practice

Linda L. Emanuel, M.D., Ph.D.

Confidentiality

Trust—the *sine qua non* of the patient–doctor relationship—requires that patients' confidences be kept by the physician. This precept is well articulated in the Hippocratic Oath. It is also honored in the law as part of the constitutional right to privacy. Physicians should be able to reassure the patient who is concerned about confidentiality of the primacy and privacy of the patient–doctor relationship. However, there are some limits to this confidentiality, and these should be clarified and discussed with the patient at the earliest relevant moment.

Limits to Confidentiality. Confidentiality is limited by the imperative *to protect third parties from harm,* such as may occur when a patient reveals to a psychiatrist a plan to murder someone. In everyday primary care practice, balancing obligations to the patient with obligations to a third party depends on an assessment of relative harms. This can be a difficult judgment. One such example is the reporting of a venereal disease or AIDS to the patient's sexual contact(s). State requirements vary. Persuading the patient to reveal the information directly to the third party often discharges all obligations to the third party with minimal damage to the patient–doctor alliance. Occasionally, confidentiality must be breached when it is *in the best interests of the patient,* although this rule should be used sparingly. The physician should reveal the minimum that is necessary in such situations.

Sometimes, the *physician's role* or *responsibility* limits the ability to keep a patient's confidence. A physician employed by a company, school, military unit, or court has split allegiances, which the patient must be made aware of at the outset. Reporting of medical information to insurance companies must be done but requires the consent of the patient before it can occur. More subtle constraints on confidentiality occur where *medical records* are readily accessed by other employees, such as those in a billing office. Policies and procedures for affording extra protection to patients who may be known to employees are indicated. Physicians may receive *court subpoenas,* in response to which they must appear in court with the appropriate information. The patient's privilege to bar the physician from testifying may be invoked but certainly can be overruled by the court.

Sharing of Information Within the Limits of Confidentiality. Sharing of information about a patient among members of the health care team is rarely problematic. However, the risk of losing sight of the confidential nature of the relationship with the patient rises as the number of individuals included in the health care team increases; this is a problem that needs to be guarded against. Patient information used for public teaching rounds or publication should be carefully edited to remove any identifying features.

Involving family or friends in the patient's care is often in the best interests of the patient, but sharing patient information with them must be preceded by the patient's explicit permission. When family members reveal information relevant to the patient that they ask the physician to withhold from the patient, the request cannot be honored, and the family should be made aware of this obligation ahead of time if possible. Resolution of the conflict may be achieved by persuading the family of the inadvisability of such secrecy.

Improperly Motivated Requests for Confidentiality. Such requests may be encountered from seductive, suicidal, hostile, or criminal patients. The physician should immediately involve another colleague, either as chaperone or consultant, and document the encounter. These steps will serve to protect the physician from such charges as sexual misconduct, harboring a fugitive, or facilitating a suicide. They also help to preserve good judgment and justified levels of confidentiality and they free the physician from the intimidating nature of the secret.

Informed Consent

Informed consent is much more than a legal document. In fact, a signed document in the absence of valid discussion with the physician is unlikely to be of legal benefit. Informed consent is a continuing part of the patient–physician relationship and involves information giving, interpretation, deliberation, and joint decision making. As such, informed consent represents an integral part of the continuing therapeutic alliance.

It is required for most non-emergency decisions, routine or major.

Required Components of Information Giving and Consent. Laws and legal opinions have defined the following required components of information giving: The patient must receive a description of the *nature of the treatment,* its *risks* (both the major and the frequent), and their expected time of occurrence. It is neither reasonable nor appropriate for the physician to furnish an exhaustive catalog of risks; the physician's role here is to provide relevant information and judgment. The *expected benefits* and *alternative treatments* should also be reviewed relative to the recommended action.

Each component of informed consent can be pursued to varying levels of intensity. The courts initially adopted a *"standard of practice"* criterion in which the physician is expected to provide information according to the standards of current practice in the community. Later the criterion shifted toward providing what a hypothetically *"reasonable person"* would want to know. Presently, a mixed standard is in general use. In practice, valid consent is most likely to occur when information giving is tailored to suit the needs of the individual patient.

Consent also has required components. First, there must be *understanding of the information* by the patient. A practical means of assessing understanding is to ask the patient about concerns and expectations; the responses can guide further information giving. Second, the decision must be *voluntary.* However, persuasion is fully appropriate, and the physician need not feel constrained from expressing his or her best medical judgment.

Consent to Research. Consent by a patient to participate in a research protocol requires particular attention to the patient's sense of volunteerism and understanding. The design of the study protocol must be fully understood. Randomized controlled trials require patients to take the chance of receiving the standard treatment instead of what may be the desired treatment. In some trials, patients also take the chance of receiving placebo treatment, and in double-blind studies the patient's physician will not know which treatment the patient is receiving. Benefit to patients in the control arm may be limited to improved monitoring.

Patients must understand that there may be conflicting interests for the physician. For example, there may be gain in collegiality, career advancement, or even material benefit. Many of these interests are inevitable and acceptable, but they must be fully disclosed and discussed with the patient. Reassurance of a true primary commitment by the physician to the patient should be possible. Lack of such a primary commitment to the patient should result in transferring the patient's care or forgoing participation in the research protocol.

Advance Directives for Health Care: Living Wills, Proxy Decision Makers, and Comprehensive Directives

The term *"advance directives"* refers to provisions made by patients to direct their health care in case of future incompetence. Advance directives are written statements and can include a living will and designation of a proxy decision maker (sometimes referred to as durable power of attorney for health care). Ideally, advance directives combine both modalities. They are inactive until such time as incompetence occurs.

The Office Discussion. For the sake of clear communication, advance directives should be completed in the context of a discussion with the patient and witnessed by the person who will be the designated proxy decision maker. Outpatients have been found to be very receptive to advance planning, often expecting physicians to take the initiative. When structured around completion of an advance directive document, the initial discussion can be expected to take about 15 to 30 minutes. Interval follow-up discussions are appropriate and particularly relevant at times of significant change in the patient's health or personal circumstances. While it is common to perform advance planning for the elderly and seriously ill, planning for the young and healthy can be quite worthwhile. Planning discussions can be regarded as a good investment of time in that they can make subsequent difficult decisions more efficient.

Choosing the Document. Using a standardized document or outline of a document can be very helpful. Many facilities have recommended documents available. In addition, there are generic documents designed to be binding in all states. Usually, there are separate documents for a written statement of preferences and for proxy designation, although more efficient documents combining the two are increasingly available. If a patient has a document already drawn up, the physician should review it with the patient. If scenarios are used in the document, they should cover a range of prognoses, so that the patient's threshold for withholding or withdrawing treatment can be ascertained. Patients should be advised that advance directives can elect for intervention as well as withdrawal or withholding of treatment, depending on the situation. Treatment decisions should be as specific as possible, and linked to statements regarding the goals of intervention. Statements of values for health care can complement specific instructions.

Legal Considerations. Federal law requires that patients be informed of hospital policy regarding living wills at the time of admission and be asked whether they have any advance directives already drawn up. This information must be entered into the medical record. Advance directives must be honored under constitutional law as a statement of the patient's autonomous wishes. Rarely, there may be a conflict between a patient's wishes and local statutes. For example, some states restrict withdrawal of nutrition and hydration to terminally ill patients, potentially preventing withdrawal from hopelessly but not terminally ill patients, such as those in a persistent vegetative state. The patient should be informed of the potential conflict. Any conflict due to differences in values between patient and physician should be discussed fully so that it might be resolved before problematic decisions arise. Inability to resolve the conflict is cause for asking the patient to agree to transfer of care should the circumstances in question arise.

The Patient Who Refuses Care

Many treatment refusals arise from fear, perceived loss of control, distrust, or anger. Discussing patient concerns in a receptive, respectful manner that also gives the patient some choices and a sense of control may often suffice to reverse the refusal. Treatment refusal may be a result of patient incompetence, but other refusals may be well reasoned and valid.

The Right to Refuse Treatment. The right to refuse medical care is strongly endorsed by the law as part of a constitutional right to privacy. The Supreme Court has affirmed that this right exists for competent patients, incompetent patients with explicit preferences, and even incompetent patients without explicit preferences (although the right is more difficult to implement in this circumstance). Treatments that have been determined in case law to be terminable range from mechanical respiration to artificial nutrition and hydration. The Patient Self-determination Act of 1990 requires that patients be reminded upon enrollment in or admission to a health care facility of their right to accept or refuse medical treatment.

However, the right to refuse care is *not absolute*. It can be limited by opposing interests. Some states invoke their interest in preserving life to restrict withholding or withdrawing of life-sustaining treatments from incompetent patients unless they are terminally ill or, in some states, in a hopeless or persistent vegetative state. Protection of minors may cause limitations on a competent patient's right to refuse treatment.

Declaring and Determining Incompetence. If a patient's refusal of care appears related to mental or psychological incompetence(s), he can be declared incompetent and the refusal can be overridden. Incompetence is commonly declared by the physician, sometimes with the help of a consulting psychiatrist. Review by an institutional ethics committee or even the judiciary should be considered if 1) there is a question about who should be the surrogate decision maker for the patient; 2) there is current or anticipated legal action; or 3) the case involves termination of life-sustaining treatment in the absence of a valid advance directive to that effect.

Determining incompetence involves assessing inability to make the individual decision at hand. Competence is not an all-or-nothing state. A patient may be competent for some decisions but incompetent for others. There are four minimum standards of competence: the patient must 1) be able to *communicate a choice;* 2) have adequate *factual understanding* of information relevant to the decision (eg, be able to paraphrase the information); 3) have an *appreciation of the implications* of the decision; and 4) have the ability to *rationally manipulate relevant information.* Rational manipulation refers to the ability to understand not only, for example, that nontreatment of a gangrenous limb may result in death, but also that death means the end of his or her life.

If incompetence is determined, a proxy decision maker should be appointed promptly. Generally, this person should be someone other than the physician and will be responsible for speaking with the physician on behalf of the patient.

ANNOTATED BIBLIOGRAPHY

Applebaum PS, Lidz CW, Meisel A. Informed Consent: Legal Theory and Clinical Practice. New York, Oxford University Press, 1987. (*An excellent resource for the theory, relevant case law, and clinical guidance on informed consent.*)

Emanuel LL, Barry MJ, Stoeckle JD et al. Advance directives for medical care: A case for greater use. N Engl J Med 1991; 324:889. (*Scenario-based advance planning in a reasonable amount of office time.*)

Emanuel EJ. A review of the ethical and legal aspects of terminating medical care. Am J Med 1988;84:291. (*Discusses issues of competence, use of advance directives, and types of care terminated.*)

Reiser SJ, Dyck AJ, Curran WJ (eds). Ethics in Medicine: Historical Perspectives and Contemporary Concerns. Cambridge, MIT Press, 1977. (*Useful selection of essays and a good resource for the general ethics reader.*)

2
The Selection and Interpretation of Diagnostic Tests

Primary Care Medicine: Office Evaluation and Management of the Adult Patient, 3rd edition, edited by Allan H. Goroll, Lawrence A. May, and Albert G. Mulley, Jr. J.B. Lippincott Company, Philadelphia

Laboratory investigations are often essential to patient care. Although the history and physical examination remain the foundation of a clinical database and sometimes suffice, the limits to what we can know about a patient are continually expanding with the addition of new diagnostic tests. These tests have many uses: to make a diagnosis in a patient known to be sick; to provide prognostic information for a patient with known disease; to identify an individual with subclinical disease or at risk for subsequent development of disease; and to monitor ongoing therapy. The ultimate objective is to reduce patient morbidity and mortality and improve satisfaction and sense of well-being. If the physician and patient are to reach these objectives, they must avoid some pitfalls along the way that may result from misuse or misinterpretation of laboratory tests.

Pitfalls are more likely to be avoided if the physician appreciates the inherent uncertainty and probabilistic nature of the diagnostic process and understands the relationship between the characteristics of a diagnostic test and those of the patient(s) being tested. Sometimes a diagnosis is evident when a patient presents with a pathognomonic constellation of signs and symptoms. In most cases, however, presenting signs or symptoms are not specific. Rather, they can be explained by a number of diagnoses, each with distinctly different implications for the patient's health. On completion of the history and physical examination, the clinician considers a list of conditions, referred to as the *differential diagnosis,* that might explain the findings. The diagnoses may then be ranked, reflecting an implicit assignment of probabilities to each. Such a ranking can be thought of as the physician's index of suspicion for each condition, based on knowledge and past experience with similar patients. The purpose of subsequent laboratory testing is to refine the initial probability estimates and, in the process, to revise the differential diagnosis. The probability of any particular disease on the revised list will depend on its probability of being present before testing and the validity of the information provided by test results.

THE VOCABULARY OF DIAGNOSTIC TEST INTERPRETATION

Terminology is important in diagnostic test interpretation. Clinical pathologists often focus on a test's accuracy and precision. *Accuracy* is the degree of closeness of the measurement made to the true value, measured by some alternative "gold standard" or definitive test. *Precision* is the test's ability to give nearly the same result in repeated determinations. Clinicians are more concerned with the ability of a test result to discriminate between persons with and persons without a given disease or condition; this discriminating ability can be characterized by a test's sensitivity and specificity. *Sensitivity* is the probability that a test will be positive when it is applied to a person who actually has the disease. *Specificity* is the probability that a test will be negative when it is applied to a person who actually does not have the disease. A perfectly sensitive test can rule out disease if the result is negative. A perfectly specific test can rule in disease if the result is positive. Because most tests are neither perfectly sensitive nor perfectly specific, the result must be interpreted probabilistically rather than categorically.

Although sensitivity and specificity are important considerations in selecting a test, the probabilities they measure are not in themselves what ordinarily concern the physician and the patient after the test result has returned. Both are concerned with the following questions: If the result is positive, what is the probability that disease is present? If the result is negative, what is the probability that the patient is indeed disease-free? These probabilities are known respectively as the *predictive value positive* and the *predictive value nega-*

		Disease		
		Present	Absent	
Test	Positive	*a*	*b*	$a + b$
	Negative	*c*	*d*	$c + d$
		$a + c$	$b + d$	$a + b + c + d$

Definitions

Sensitivity:	$\frac{a}{a+c}$	False negative rate:	$\frac{c}{a+c}$
Specificity:	$\frac{d}{b+d}$	False positive rate:	$\frac{b}{b+d}$
Predictive value positive:	$\frac{a}{a+b}$	False alarm rate:	$\frac{b}{a+b}$
Predictive value negative:	$\frac{d}{c+d}$	False reassurance rate:	$\frac{c}{c+d}$

Figure 2-1. The two-by-two table clarifies relationships between test characteristics (sensitivity and specificity) and predictive values of positive and negative test results. The clinician, interpreting a diagnostic test, can fill in the table if he is aware of the test's sensitivity and specificity and the patient's (population's) pretest probability (prevalence) of disease. Pretest probability is $(a + c)$ and (1 − the pretest probability) is $(b + d)$. Multiplying $(a + c)$ by the sensitivity provides the value for *a,* and multiplying $(b + d)$ by the specificity provides the value for *d.* Values for cell *c* and cell *b* can be determined by simple subtraction. With the cells filled in, the predictive value of a negative or positive test can be calculated easily. It is worth noting that this calculation method is precisely equivalent to Bayes' theorem of conditional probability.

tive. They are determined not only by the sensitivity and specificity of the test, but also by the probability of the disease being present before the test was ordered.

Relationships between sensitivity and specificity and positive and negative predictive values can be better understood by referring to a two-by-two table (Fig. 2–1). The two columns indicate the presence or absence of disease (note that a gold standard of diagnosis is assumed), and the two rows indicate positive or negative test results. Any given patient with a test result could be included in one of the four cells labeled *a, b, c,* or *d.* Definitions of sensitivity, specificity, predictive value positive, and predictive value negative can be restated using these labels. It is important to note that each of these four ratios has a complement. The complement of sensitivity (1 − sensitivity) is referred to as the *false-negative rate,* while the complement of specificity (1 − specificity) is referred to as the *false-positive rate.* These terms are often used ambiguously in the medical literature: the false-negative rate is confused with the complement of the predictive value negative which is termed the *false-reassurance rate;* the false-positive rate is confused with the complement of the predictive value positive, the *false-alarm rate.* The terms false-reassurance rate and false-alarm rate have been designated to help avoid ambiguity.

INTERPRETING TESTS: REVISING DIAGNOSTIC PROBABILITIES

When the clinician interprets a test result, he usually processes the information informally. Rarely is a pad and pencil or calculator used to explicitly revise probability estimates. But sometimes the revision of diagnostic probabilities is counterintuitive; for instance, it has been shown that most clinicians rely too heavily on positive test results when the pretest probability or disease prevalence is low.

Attention to the two-by-two table indicates why predictive values are crucially dependent on disease prevalence. This is particularly true when one is using a test to screen for a rare disease. If a disease is rare, even a very small false-positive rate (remember, that is the complement of specificity) is multiplied by a very large relative number—that is, $(b + d) \times (a + c)$. Therefore, b will be surprisingly large relative to a, and the predictive value positive will be counterintuitively low. Examples of this effect are evident in Table 2–1.

Consider the example of a noninvasive test to detect coronary disease applied to a 40-year-old man with a history of atypical chest pain. Based on test evaluations reported in the literature, the sensitivity and specificity of the test can be estimated at 80 percent and 90 percent, respectively. Based on symptoms and risk factors, the clinician estimates that the patient's pretest probability of coronary disease is 0.20. (This is the same as saying that the prevalence of coronary disease in a population of similar patients would be 20%.)

Referring to Figure 2–1, with a pretest probability of 0.20, $a + c = 0.20$ and $b + d = 0.80$. Multiplying 0.20×0.8 (the sensitivity) gives us a value of 0.16 for *a* (subtraction gives us a value of 0.04 for *c*). Multiplying 0.80×0.9 (the specificity) gives us a value of 0.72 for *d* (again, subtraction gives us 0.08 for *b*). The predictive value positive, then, is 0.16/0.24, or 0.66. The predictive value negative is 0.72/0.76, or 0.95.

The clinician can use another method to quickly revise probabilities to test his or her intuition. It requires an understanding of *odds* as well as probability. If *P* is the probability that a particular disease is present, the ratio of *P* to (1 − *P*), or *P*/(1 − *P*), is called the odds favoring that disease. The odds against that disease being present are represented by (1

Table 2-1. Effect of Prior Probability (Prevalence) on Predictive Value of Positive Test Results

PRIOR PROBABILITY (PREVALENCE), %	PREDICTIVE VALUE OF POSITIVE TEST, %		
	Sensitivity 90%/ Specificity 90%	*Sensitivity 95%/ Specificity 95%*	*Sensitivity 99%/ Specificity 99%*
0.1	0.9	1.9	9.0
1	8.3	16.1	50.0
2	15.5	27.9	66.9
5	32.1	50.0	83.9
50	90.0	95.0	99.0

− *P*)/*P*. Just as one can estimate the pretest probability of disease before diagnostic tests are performed, one can express that estimate as the pretest odds.

Pretest odds can be revised simply by multiplying a ratio called the *likelihood ratio,* which is the relative occurrence of the test result among persons with and without disease—that is, the probability of the result (either positive or negative or a particular range of values) given the presence of disease divided by the probability of that result given the absence of disease. Note that the positive likelihood ratio is nothing more (or less) than the ratio of sensitivity to the false-positive rate (ie, 1 − specificity). The negative likelihood ratio is the ratio of the false-negative rate (ie, 1 − the sensitivity) to the specificity. Likelihood ratios therefore include all the information contained in estimates of sensitivity and specificity. When the pretest odds of a disease are multiplied by the likelihood ratio, the result—sometimes termed the posttest odds—represents the odds favoring disease given the test result.

Returning to the example, the patient with atypical chest pain could have his chances of having coronary disease expressed as odds rather than a probability. A probability of 0.20 is equivalent to odds of 1/4 (0.20/0.80). The likelihood ratio for a test with a sensitivity of 0.8 and a specificity of 0.9 is 8 (0.8/[1 − 0.9]). The pretest odds can be converted to posttest odds following a positive test simply by multiplying by the positive likelihood ratio: 1/4 × 8 = 2. Note that the posttest odds ratio of 2:1 is equivalent to the posttest probability of 0.66.

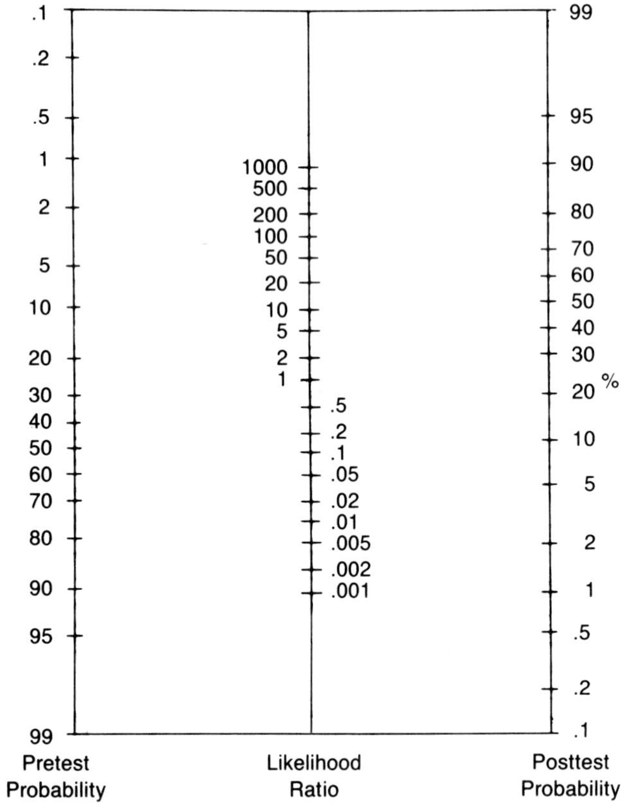

Figure 2-2. A nomogram for applying likelihood ratios. Adapted from Fagan TJ: Nomogram for Bayes' theorem. N Engl J Med [Letter] 293:257, 1975. (Sackett DL, Haynes RB, Tugwell P: Clinical Epidemiology, 1985.)

For some, it is easier to revise probabilities in the clinical setting by using likelihood ratios. A nomogram can be helpful until one gets used to converting from probabilities to odds and back again (Fig. 2–2). Likelihood ratios also have the advantage of capturing more clinical data from the patient's particular test results. Whereas estimates of sensitivity and specificity usually rely on a dichotomous positive-negative result threshold, different likelihood ratios can be determined for different ranges of test results. For example, a very high creatine phosphokinase (CPK) will have a higher positive likelihood ratio than a moderate elevation. The degree of elevation will then be reflected in the revised probability of myocardial infarction.

WHERE DOES THE INFORMATION COME FROM?

One of the reasons clinicians are reluctant to take a quantitative approach to diagnostic test interpretation is that such an approach suggests a precision that belies our uncertainty about pretest probabilities and about sensitivity and specificity of even commonly used tests. Estimation of pretest probability hinges on epidemiologic information about the incidence and prevalence of various diseases, modified on the basis of patient characteristics and presenting symptoms. This kind of information is all too rarely presented in the medical literature. Estimates are necessarily uncertain.

There is also uncertainty about the sensitivity and specificity of tests. Rarely are these values presented in medical texts, and test evaluations in the medical literature can sometimes be misleading. The clinician should be familiar with some of the reasons that a test rarely performs as well in general use as it does during the evaluation study that appears in the medical journal.

The False-Positive Rate and Pretest Probability: Overestimating Predictive Values

The importance of the pretest probability of disease in an individual patient (or the prevalence of disease in a population of such patients) for determining the predictive values of a test is often not fully appreciated and may lead to disappointment in the clinical performance of the test. Consider how, during its evaluation, the sensitivity and specificity of a test are estimated. Two groups of patients are assembled. One consists of patients known to have the disease in question as defined by some gold standard (represented by $a + c$ in Fig. 2–1). The other consists of persons without disease based on the same gold standard (represented by $b + d$). The test being evaluated is then applied to both populations. The proportion of those with disease who have a positive result ($a/[a + c]$) provides us with an estimate of the test's sensitivity. The proportion of those without the disease who have a negative test ($d/[b + d]$) gives us an estimate of the test's specificity. Our confidence that these estimates of sensitivity and specificity are accurate increases with the number of people in each group tested. The investigator can most efficiently maximize confidence in the estimates of both sensitivity and specificity by applying the test to disease and nondisease groups of equal size. It is not surprising, therefore, that tests are often evaluated by applying them to populations in which disease and nondisease occur with equal frequency, or nearly so.

If sensitivity, specificity, and predictive values are sufficiently high in such an evaluation study, the test is proposed for general use. What happens when the test is adopted and applied in a general population in which the disease is much less likely to occur than nondisease? The sensitivity and specificity should remain the same, but the predictive value positive will necessarily fall, and its complement, the false-alarm rate, will necessarily increase. This phenomenon is most important when the disease in question is rare, as is evident in Table 2–1.

Defining Disease for Diagnostic Test Evaluation: The Gold Standard Problem

To evaluate a diagnostic test, an investigator must be able to distinguish between persons with and without disease by some alternative method. Often this gold standard test is more invasive or more expensive than the newer, proposed test being evaluated. (The newer test would not be worth evaluating, if it did not confer some advantage for patient or clinician.) Sometimes a gold standard is not readily available. If the disease is one with a short, predictable natural history (eg, pancreatic cancer), an investigator may resort to follow-up, defining the absence of disease by morbidity-free survival over a specified period. But if the disease has a highly variable natural history (eg, coronary disease or most rheumatologic disorders), the follow-up approach becomes impractical. Instead, the investigator must rely on more arbitrary and often more subjective criteria to define disease, including combinations of tests, signs, or symptoms. Herein lies a potential pitfall that can affect the accuracy of the estimates of sensitivity and specificity. If the diagnostic criteria are not assessed independently of the test being evaluated, the sensitivity, specificity, or both will be overestimated.

The problem occurs in its most obvious form when a positive test result leads the investigator to a more extensive search for disease than was applied to those with a negative test. A related problem occurs when the test and the diagnostic criteria are very similar biologic measures. An example of this problem is the estimation of the sensitivity and specificity of isoenzymes for myocardial infarction. In the absence of a ready gold standard, investigators have used various criteria to define acute myocardial infarction. Some have included total enzyme levels among the criteria when evaluating the diagnostic value of isoenzymes. This will result in too optimistic estimates of sensitivity and specificity. To the extent that false-negative isoenzyme results are correlated with false-negative total enzyme results, the sensitivity of the isoenzyme test will be overestimated. To the extent that false-positive isoenzyme results are correlated with false-positive total enzyme results, the specificity of the new test will be overestimated.

The Narrow Spectrum Problem: Overestimating Sensitivity When the "Disease" Group Is Too Sick

When an investigator assembles a group known to have the disease in question by means of some gold standard, he may choose patients with unequivocal diagnostic (gold standard) findings. In doing so, the investigator may select a severely ill group that is not representative of the disease in the general population; that is, he will focus on too narrow a spectrum of disease.

Consider the investigator evaluating a noninvasive test for coronary artery disease such as an electrocardiographically monitored exercise tolerance test. To be sure that he is dealing with true coronary disease, he includes only people with unequivocal prior myocardial infarction or with classic angina symptoms. Using his chosen criteria for a positive test, he determines that the sensitivity of the test is 90 percent. What he (and the readers of his report) may not realize is that the test is more sensitive when coronary disease is extensive (two- or three-vessel rather than single vessel) or severe (99% stenosis rather than 80% stenosis) and that his gold standard criteria have selected for patients with extensive or severe disease. When the test is used to detect less extensive disease, producing more equivocal symptoms in the general population, its sensitivity will prove disappointing. Recognize that the sensitivity estimate provided by the evaluation is accurate for the narrow spectrum of disease severity found in the test population. The disappointment comes when that estimate is generalized inappropriately to include those with less severe disease.

An important historic example of the spectrum problem is the evaluation of carcinoembryonic antigen (CEA) as a test for colon cancer. Early studies, documenting very high sensitivity, were conducted in patients with extensive colon cancer. Enthusiasm for CEA as a screening test heightened (despite the low predictive value positive made inevitable by the disease's relatively low prevalence among asymptomatic persons). Later studies, however, proved the sensitivity of the test to be substantially lower among those with early limited disease, that is, among those most likely to benefit from early detection by a screening program.

The Comorbidity Problem: Overestimating Specificity When the "No-Disease" Group Is Too Well

In the same way that an investigator can assemble a "disease" group that is sicker than the population to which the test will eventually be applied, he can assemble a "no disease" group that is too healthy. Many tests will perform better when asked to discriminate between "disease A" and "no disease" than when asked to discriminate between disease A, on the one hand, and diseases B through Z, on the other. Consider the fledgling investigator who wishes to estimate the sensitivity and specificity of guaiac testing as a screening test for colonic cancer. He knows about the spectrum problem and has included in his "disease" group people with early cancers. For his "no disease" group, he has selected medical school students. It should be clear that this choice of controls will provide an estimate of specificity that is higher than could be expected when the test is generally applied to a population including older individuals more likely to have a nonmalignant source of occult bleeding. Obviously the controls should not have the target disease (ie, colon cancer). But if the investigator also excludes from the control population all comorbid conditions that the test might confuse with the disease (eg, peptic ulcer disease, diverticular disease), his estimate of specificity will be too optimistic.

Investigators can guard against such disappointments by drawing their "disease" and "no disease" populations from the target population in which the test will eventually be used. The spectrum of disease that should be detected in the target population should be represented in the "disease" group. Comorbid conditions that might be confused with that disease should be included in the "no disease" control group. Such an effectiveness evaluation of a diagnostic test might be preceded by a simpler study comparing very sick with completely well individuals. If it cannot discriminate between the very sick and the very well in such an efficacy study, the more difficult effectiveness trial need not be undertaken. The clinician can guard against being misled by reports of a test's efficacy by carefully considering the populations in which a test has been evaluated and not generalizing the results inappropriately to larger, more heterogenous groups.

How Does the Test Compare With Others?

A final reason for disappointment with the application of apparently promising tests is failure to consider adequately the test's potential role in the constellation of tests that is already available. Does the new test provide new information? Does it obviate the need for more invasive or more expensive tests? If the answer to these questions is no, the worth of the test and its evaluation are in obvious doubt.

WHICH TESTS SHOULD WE USE?

Perfect tests are rare. Clinicians must choose among tests with imperfect sensitivity and specificity. The physician frequently has some choice about the sensitivity and specificity of a test. Obviously, alternative tests—usually those that are more costly or invasive—may be more sensitive and more specific. A new technology or an improved skill in interpretation may improve both measures. Often, however, the physician can increase specificity only by accepting a decrease in sensitivity. The most graphic examples of this principle involve tests that provide quantitative results, such as the measurement of serum prostate-specific antigen when considering the diagnosis of prostate cancer. The general case is illustrated in Figure 2–3. Note that all too often the "normal" values for the test results are derived from frequency distributions of results among apparently well individuals; the potential trade-off between sensitivity and specificity is not considered.

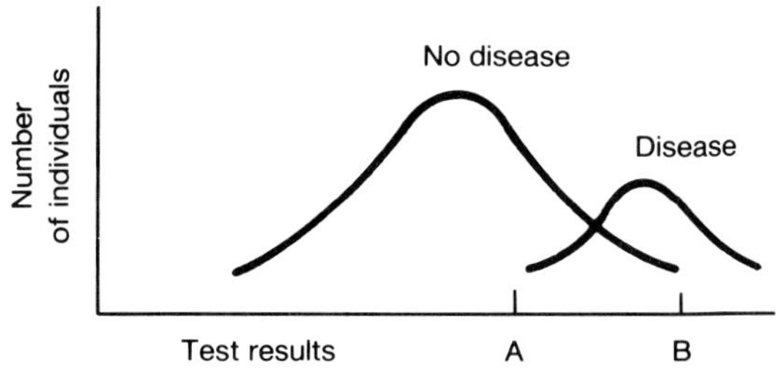

Figure 2-3. Hypothetical distribution of test results among patients with disease and without disease. Because the distributions overlap, the test is far from perfect. If all patients with values to the right of **A** are said to have "positive" results, the test will be 100 percent sensitive but will have a low specificity. If only those patients with values to the right of **B** are said to have "positive" results, the test will be 100 percent specific but will have a low sensitivity. The choice of a cutoff value between **A** and **B** should depend on the relative importance of true and false, positive and negative results.

Which is more important, sensitivity or specificity? In general, the answer depends on the cost—including patient inconvenience, morbidity, and mortality as well as dollars—of false-negative results compared with that of false-positive results, and the benefits of true negative and of true positive results. Sensitive tests or less stringent criteria for disease and the resulting low false-negative rate should be favored when effective treatment for the condition exists and the cost of lost opportunity is great. High specificity or more stringent criteria for disease and the resulting low false-positive rate are most important when a positive diagnosis does not significantly influence therapy or outcome but may be a burden for the patient.

The clinician who is mindful of the purpose of making a particular diagnosis, who considers the natural history of disease as well as prognostic and therapeutic implications of the diagnosis, is likely to make efficient use of the laboratory while maximizing health benefits for his or her patients.

A.G.M.

ANNOTATED BIBLIOGRAPHY

Department of Clinical Epidemiology and Biostatistics, McMaster University Health Sciences Centre. How to read clinical journals. II: To learn about a diagnostic test. Can Med Assoc J 1981;124:703. (*Part of a superb series that distills principles of clinical epidemiology for the practitioner.*)

Griner PF, Mayewski RJ, Mushlin AI et al. Selection and interpretation of diagnostic tests and procedures: Principles and applications. Ann Intern Med 1981;94(4 Pt 2):557. (*A very well presented primer with many good examples.*)

Griner PF, Panzer RJ, Greenland P. Diagnostic Strategies for Common Medical Problems. Philadelphia, American College of Physicians, 1991. (*A superb resource. Information about prior probabilities, sensitivity and specificity of tests, and well-reasoned recommended strategies.*)

Ransohoff DF, Feinstein AR. Problems of spectrum and bias in evaluating the efficacy of diagnostic tests. N Engl J Med 1975;299:926. (*Reviews problems in disease definition and population selection that may affect evaluations of diagnostic tests.*)

Sox HC Jr. Common Diagnostic Tests: Use and Interpretation, 2nd ed. Philadelphia, American College of Physicians, 1990. (*An excellent volume with introductory chapters on diagnostic reasoning and probability theory followed by 16 chapters on specific tests.*)

Vecchio TJ. Predictive value of a single diagnostic test in unselected populations. N Engl J Med 1966;274:1171. (*Early paper pointing out the importance of prevalence to predictive value.*)

Primary Care Medicine: Office Evaluation and Management of the Adult Patient, 3rd edition, edited by Allan H. Goroll, Lawrence A. May, and Albert G. Mulley, Jr. J.B. Lippincott Company, Philadelphia

3
Health Maintenance and the Role of Screening

Public interest in health maintenance or, more positively, health enhancement has grown dramatically in recent years. Many Americans have demonstrated their interest in exercise, good dietary habits, maintenance of appropriate body weight, and stress reduction. Increased enthusiasm stems from growing awareness of associations between elements of lifestyle and health. Despite reliable evidence and public acceptance of these associations, however, many people continue to indulge in self-destructive habits such as smoking, overeating, and alcohol abuse. Efforts to alter such behavior are often frustratingly ineffective. Patients who seek reassurance from physician visits that include routine screening procedures often persist in behavior that greatly increases their risk of morbidity.

Physicians must acknowledge their primary role in prevention as that of educators. Accurate information regarding risk factors is most likely to reinforce health-enhancing behavior and alter self-destructive behavior. The physician must appreciate the potential for behavior modification and familiarize himself with local resources. Routine screening for specific diseases, the health maintenance activity most closely identified with the physician, should be performed selectively. The limits of screening tests as well as their potential health benefits should be clearly understood by every primary physician.

Specific risk factors and screening tests are discussed in subsequent chapters. This chapter will focus on the question, "What makes a disease or risk factor worth screening for?" The relationship between prevalence and predictive value of a test is particularly important in the screening situation (see Chapter 2). Because the physician is more interested in improving health outcomes for patients than in simply providing them with diagnoses, elements of the natural history of the disease and of the effectiveness of therapy are critically important.

CRITERIA FOR SCREENING

Whether or not a screening policy results in improved health outcomes depends on the characteristics of the disease(s), of the test(s), and of the patient population. These are summarized in Table 3–1.

NATURAL HISTORY OF THE DISEASE AND EFFECTIVENESS OF THERAPY

Screening tests are performed to identify asymptomatic disease. The alternative is to wait until the patient presents with symptoms and then make a diagnosis. The question then is, "What makes a disease worth diagnosing early?" The practical objective of screening is prevention of morbidity and mortality—not simply early diagnosis. There is little benefit to the patient, and perhaps considerable harm, in advancing the time of diagnosis of a disease for which earlier treatment does not influence outcome.

The importance of the natural history of the disease and effectiveness of therapy can be illustrated by considering Figure 3–1. As it shows schematically, some variable time after the biological onset of a disease, a diagnosis is possible using a screening test. This is followed by another variable time period during which the patient has no symptoms. Usually, a short time after symptoms appear, the clinical diagnosis is made. Eventually, after the course of therapy has been selected and completed, there is an identifiable clinical outcome that can range from cure and complete health to death.

Often, outcome depends somewhat on the point during the natural history of the disease at which therapy is initiated. This is most clear in the case of localized versus metastatic cancer. Many tumors can be readily excised, and the patient cured of the disease, during early stages. The opportunity for cure is often lost when tumor spread makes excision or other local therapy impractical. The "escape from cure" may not be as dramatic as the point of tumor metastasis; a disease may simply become more refractory to therapy, increasing the likelihood of morbid complications. The practical purpose of screening is to advance the time of the diagnosis to a point in the natural history of the disease when a relative or absolute "escape from cure" is less likely to have occurred.

While the natural history of any disease varies a great deal among individuals afflicted, some generalizations are worthwhile. If an "escape from cure" generally occurs at point A in Figure 3–1 or at any point before available screening tests can detect the disease in question, the value of screening must be questioned. The most common result will be bad news sooner for the patient but no difference in outcome. If "escape from cure" routinely occurs after symptoms appear (eg, at point C), screening may be valuable but could likely be supplanted by patient and professional education programs aimed at ensuring early presentation and prompt diagnosis. Diseases in which "escape from cure" generally occurs after the disease is detectable but while it remains asymptomatic (eg, at point B) are the most appropriate targets of screening efforts.

Several points about the evaluation of screening programs can also be made with reference to Figure 3–1. Critics of indiscriminate screening point out that the benefits of a screening program can easily be overestimated if the relationship between time of diagnosis and natural history is not understood. One fallacy results from neglecting the importance of *lead time* when evaluating the effect of screening on subsequent survival. Because screening has the potential to advance the time of diagnosis from one point in the natural

Table 3-1. Criteria for Screening

Characteristics of the Disease
Significant effect on the quality or length of life
Prevalence sufficiently high to justify costs
Acceptable methods of treatment available
Asymptomatic period during which detection and treatment significantly reduce morbidity and/or mortality
Treatment in the asymptomatic phase yields a better therapeutic result than treatment delayed until symptoms appear
Characteristics of the Test
Sufficiently sensitive to detect disease during the asymptomatic period
Sufficiently specific to provide acceptable predictive value positive
Acceptable to patients
Characteristics of the Population Screened
Sufficiently high disease prevalence
Accessibility
Compliance with subsequent diagnostic tests and necessary therapy

history to another and because survival is, by necessity, measured from the time of diagnosis rather than the time of onset, the survival of patients whose diseases are detected by screening should be expected to be longer than that of patients who present symptomatically. Extensive follow-up data on many patients allow approximation of the average length of time by which the diagnosis is advanced by screening. This illusory gain in survival, the lead time, can then be subtracted from any measured difference in survival duration to learn the true benefits of the screening program.

The second fallacy that can lead to overestimation of screening benefits depends on the variability in natural history among individual cases of the same disease. Individuals who have less aggressive disease and thereby spend more time in a detectable but asymptomatic stage are, other things being equal, more likely to be detected by a screening test than are patients with more aggressive disease. If patients with indolent asymptomatic disease are more likely to have an indolent clinical course after diagnosis, patients diagnosed by screening should be expected to have longer survival rates than patients who present symptomatically. Arguments about the impact of such biological determinism versus that of advancing the time of diagnosis have most frequently been raised with regard to breast and prostate cancers but they apply generally to all screening. This potential bias toward prolonged survival among patients detected by screening tests has been called *time-linked bias sampling*.

Neither of these arguments is meant to deny the value of screening for treatable disease. They simply advise caution in interpreting apparently favorable results based on unsophisticated measures of effectiveness.

VALIDITY OF AVAILABLE SCREENING TESTS AND POPULATIONS SCREENED

Diseases worth identifying usually have a relatively low prevalence in the asymptomatic population. As a result, the specificity of the diagnostic test used is the principal determinant of the predictive value positive of the test. Tests that may be very useful in diagnosis when the prior probability of disease is 10 percent or 20 percent may produce an unacceptable number of false-positive results when used in a screening situation. Such nonspecificity has been referred to as the *cost* of a screening test. The costs, including morbidity and patient concern, of diagnostic evaluations among patients with false-positive screens can far outweigh other costs of a screening program. The sensitivity and specificity of the screening test, costs, and patient acceptability are critical considerations in the decision to screen for disease.

The importance of disease prevalence in determining the predictive value positive is one basis for the use of risk factors in screening policy. By limiting screening to a high-risk population, the physician in effect increases the prevalence of the disease in the population tested (and alternatively increases the prior probability of the disease in any individual), thereby increasing the predictive value positive and decreasing the false-alarm rate and the number of false-positive results.

HEALTH MAINTENANCE—WHAT IS APPROPRIATE?

Periodic health evaluation has been recommended with varying degrees of enthusiasm throughout the 20th century. Many patients believe in its value; the majority of Americans feel that more health resources should be expended on preventive efforts. However, the value of periodic examinations and specific preventive measures has been questioned. Evidence regarding the effectiveness of periodic examinations,

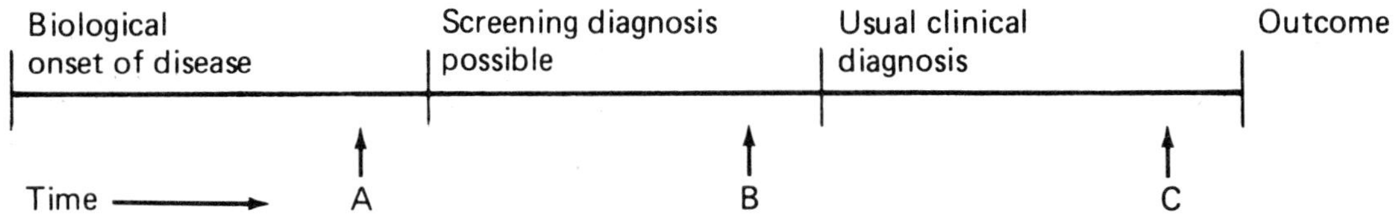

"Escape from cure" at point A: Screening may not affect outcome

"Escape from cure" at point B: High priority for screening

"Escape from cure" at point C: Education and improved access to care may be more efficient than screening tests

Figure 3-1. Relationships between screening and natural history of disease.

Table 3-2. Conditions That Warrant Periodic Evaluation in All Patients of Appropriate Age and Gender

DISEASE	COMMENTS
Hypertension	See Chapters 14, 19, and 26
Hyperlipidemia	See Chapters 5 and 27
Smoking	See Chapter 54
Colon cancer	See Chapter 56
Breast cancer	See Chapter 106
Cervical cancer	See Chapter 107
Alcoholism	See Chapter 228

measured in terms of decreased morbidity and mortality, is fragmentary. Supporters of periodic evaluation argue that the additional benefits of regular physician contact result in a greater sense of well-being. Such contact provides opportunities for appropriate patient education.

Routine examinations should be tailored to the individual patient. Although the importance of characteristics of the patient, the diseases, and the test in determining appropriate prevention strategies must be recognized, summary recommendations can be useful. A number of reviews, each applying the criteria discussed in this chapter, have offered recommendations for preventive health care. The recom-

Table 3-3. Conditions That Warrant Periodic Evaluation in Selected Patients

CONDITION	RISK FACTORS	COMMENTS
Rubella susceptibility	Anticipated pregnancy Occupation (health care worker)	See Chapter 6
Human immunodeficiency virus infection	Anticipated pregnancy and risk-group membership	See Chapter 7
Endocarditis susceptibility	Valvular heart disease	See Chapter 16
Rheumatic fever susceptibility	Rheumatic fever history	See Chapter 17
Tuberculosis (PPD reactivity)	Occupation Exposure	See Chapters 38 and 49
Occupational lung disease	Occupational exposure	See Chapter 39
Susceptibility to hepatitis B virus	Homosexual male Exposure Occupation (health care worker)	See Chapter 57
Anemia	Pregnancy	See Chapter 77
Sickle cell trait	African American of childbearing age	Genetic counseling must be acceptable; see Chapter 78
Thyroid cancer	Radiation of head and neck	See Chapter 94
Diabetes	Pregnancy	See Chapter 93
Endometrial cancer	Exogenous estrogens	See Chapter 109
Vaginal cancer	In utero diethylstilbestrol exposure	See Chapter 110
Syphilis	Homosexual male Pregnancy Other sexually transmitted disease	See Chapter 124
Chlamydial genitourinary infection	Other sexually transmitted disease Woman of childbearing age	See Chapter 125
Bacteriuria	Pregnancy Kidney stones	See Chapter 127
Lower urinary tract cancer	Occupational exposure to aromatic amines (eg, dyestuffs, leather tanning, rubber)	See Chapter 128
Testicular cancer	Cryptorchidism	See Chapters 131 and 143
Osteoporosis	Early menopause	See Chapter 144
Cerebrovascular disease	Advanced age, TIA history	See Chapter 171
Skin cancer	Fair skin, sun exposure Family history	See Chapter 177
Glaucoma	Family history Advanced age	See Chapter 198
Oral cancer	Alcohol Tobacco	See Chapter 211
Decreased hearing	Advanced age, excessive noise	See Chapter 212

mendations of the American Cancer Society, the American College of Physicians, the Canadian Task Force on the Periodic Health Examination, and the US Preventive Services Task Force have received the most attention. Relatively few conditions have received general endorsement as targets for screening among *asymptomatic* persons *without* specific *risk factors*. These are summarized in Table 3–2. The rationales for these recommendations are presented in the subsequent chapters noted in the table.

Table 3–3 provides a summary of recommendations that have been made for other preventive services that are warranted in selected patients. Again, the rationales for these recommendations are presented in subsequent chapters. It should be noted that uncertainty about both the natural history and the effectiveness of therapy, the importance of specific risk factors, and the sensitivity and specificity of potential screening tests rarely, if ever, allow proof of the effectiveness of a screening procedure. Some conclusions and recommendations, necessarily based on speculative data, remain controversial. The clinician must also be mindful of the potential to help patients avoid preventable morbidity and early death by taking the time to provide advice and counsel about behavior and lifestyle. Patients often need specific advice, not only about use of alcohol, tobacco, and harmful substances, but also about diet, exercise, sexual practices, and injury prevention. Such discussions have the potential to have far greater impact on health and longevity than specific screening tests and procedures.

A.G.M.

ANNOTATED BIBLIOGRAPHY

American Cancer Society. Report on the cancer-related health check-up. Cancer 1980;30:194 240. (*A superb review of screening principles followed by detailed presentation and defense of current recommendations.*)

Canadian Taskforce on the Periodic Health Examination. The periodic health examination, 1984 update. Can Med Assoc J 1979;121:1193. (*This 60-page initial report has been updated in recent years at 2-year intervals.*)

Feinleb M, Zelen M. Some pitfalls in the evaluation of screening programs. Arch Environ Health 1969;19:412. (*Reviews problems with predictive value positive, lead time, and time-linked bias sampling.*)

Frame PS, Carlson SJ. A critical review of periodic health screening using specific screening criteria. J Fam Pract 1975;2:29. (*Highly influential early review that considers 36 diseases. Screening recommended for only a few based on specific criteria.*)

Frame PS. A critical review of adult health maintenance. J Fam Pract 1986;22:341. (*Valuable update.*)

Hayward RS, Steinberg EP, Ford DE et al. Preventive care guidelines: 1991. Ann Intern Med 1991;114:758. (*Reviews the history of preventive care guidelines as well as explanations for the different recommendations from different consensus groups. Includes encyclopaedic comparisons of recommendations—made by the ACP, both Canadian and American Task Forces, and others—for many conditions and procedures including immunization and chemoprophylaxis.*)

Medical Practice Committee, American College of Physicians. Periodic health examination: A guide for designing individualized preventive health care in the asymptomatic patient. Ann Intern Med 1981;95:729. (*Succinct summary of recommendations.*)

Spitzer WO, Brown BP. Unanswered questions about the periodic health examination. Ann Intern Med 1975;83:257. (*Reviews the issue in terms of impact on health and effect on the doctor–patient relationship.*)

US Preventive Services Task Force. Guide to Clinical Preventive Services. Washington, DC: US Department of Health and Human Services, 1989. (*Superb summary of evidence for 100 selected conditions. Strong emphasis on counseling patients about harmful or risky behavior.*)

4
Estimating and Communicating Risk and Prognosis

Primary Care Medicine: Office Evaluation and Management of the Adult Patient, 3rd edition, edited by Allan H. Goroll, Lawrence A. May, and Albert G. Mulley, Jr. J.B. Lippincott Company, Philadelphia

Diagnosis is a process of classification. A constellation of symptoms, signs, and test results is given a label, and the patient who presents with those characteristics is implicitly grouped with other patients who have presented with similar findings. What makes the classification process and the resulting label so significant for both patient and clinician is what it implies about the future. Will symptoms persist, get worse, or resolve spontaneously? What other health outcomes can be expected? Will therapeutic interventions improve chances for a good outcome?

Similar questions arise when a patient is found to have a risk factor that increases the likelihood of future disease. How great is the risk? What are the chances of avoiding the anticipated bad outcome, either because of efforts to lower risk or by good fortune? To answer such questions, the primary care physician must understand the methods by which valid information about prognosis and risk is derived from the experience of previous patients. Doctor–patient dialogues about the future implications of an illness or risk factor are often momentous for patients. Information about an uncertain future must be communicated with clarity, compassion, and an appreciation for the uniqueness of each patient's needs.

RISK AND PROGNOSIS: PREDICTING THE PATIENT'S FUTURE

The source for information about the future of any particular patient is the collective experience of previous patients with the same condition. The accuracy of the information so derived depends on the manner in which that experience is collected and recorded and on the degree of similarity between the patient at hand and past patients who have been followed over time.

Theoretically, the best mechanism for studying prognosis would be to carefully characterize patients at the time of diagnosis (or when a risk factor is identified) with regard to disease stage and severity, presence or absence of any comorbid conditions, and other factors that could be expected to have an impact on outcome. Because such factors are often systematically influenced by the pattern of patient referral, the setting in which patients are seen and the manner in which they happened to be there would be described. All patients would be examined with the same level of scrutiny at the time they entered the *cohort* and during subsequent follow-up examinations. Relevant outcomes, and criteria by which they would be measured, would be specified in advance. Those conducting follow-up examinations would be unaware of baseline differences among patients so as not to be influenced by expected associations between these variables and outcomes. All patients would be followed, and their status with regard to outcomes would be known at the time the experience was analyzed. The impact of different baseline characteristics on relevant outcomes would be examined by reporting experience for different subgroups or developing statistical models. The predictive validity of these models would be tested in separate samples of patients.

Rarely, if ever, is it possible to meet all of these methodological objectives. As a result, much of the research that clinicians rely upon for information about risk and prognosis is potentially misleading. To avoid being misled, and misleading patients, clinicians must understand the biases that can be introduced when suboptimal methods are used to gather information to help predict the future.

When the outcomes of interest are rare events, it may not be feasible to assemble a cohort large enough, and follow it long enough, to accumulate sufficient experience to provide useful estimates of prognosis or risk. Alternatively, patients who have already experienced the outcome may be identified as *cases,* and their past histories examined to identify events or *exposures* that may have conferred risk and be of prognostic value. *Control* patients without the outcome of interest may also be questioned about the same exposures. Comparison of the rates of exposure among cases and controls can produce an estimate of the degree of risk associated with the exposure. The *odds ratio* is an estimate of the *relative risk* that is very accurate when the disease or outcome in question is rare. This retrospective case–control approach places a heavy burden on the investigator and sources of information to assure that similar degrees of scrutiny are applied to the histories of cases and controls. Selective recollection of the past, often with greater vigilance stimulated by the outcome of interest, can produce misleading estimates of risk and prognosis.

Even if patients with a particular risk factor or diagnosis are identified prospectively and followed forward in time, biases that can lead to faulty conclusions may be introduced. Perhaps the most important bias for primary care physicians to recognize has been termed *referral filter bias*. It occurs frequently as a result of the fact that patients in many published reports have been described *because* they have been referred to academic centers. Such patients often have complicating characteristics and exhibit a worse prognosis than patients who are drawn from an entire population or a representative sample of a population. Similar problems arise when patients are selected for study based on particular test results. Patients with more worrisome signs and symptoms may be more likely to be tested and may be more likely to fare poorly over time. Alternatively, patients who are tested may have better access to medical care and fare better than average as a result.

Differences in the ways patients are followed over time can also introduce important biases. Patients lost to follow-up may be different from those who remain in the cohort. A conservative approach to estimating prognosis when some patients are lost to follow-up before the relevant outcome has occurred is to assume that all lost patients experienced the outcome, and then to assume that no lost patients experienced it. The first assumption produces an upper *bound estimate* with lost patients included in both numerator and denominator; the second produces a *lower bound estimate* with lost patients included only in the denominator.

Even when patients are successfully followed over time, biases may be introduced by the selective use of tests and other outcome measures or by the expectations of clinicians who are aware of patient characteristics that may or may not have real prognostic significance. Statistical models that have not been validated on independent samples may mistake random variation among characteristics and outcomes for important prognostic associations.

DESCRIBING RISK OF FUTURE DISEASE

People are generally very interested in risk of untoward events and ways to reduce risks. Despite the high level of interest, there is a great deal of confusion about the meaning of quantitative expressions of risk. This confusion often carries over to conversations between doctors and patients. An important source of confusion is the distinction between *relative* and *absolute* risk. The effect of risk factors is usually expressed as a relative risk or risk ratio, that is, the incidence of disease among people with the risk factor divided by the incidence without the factor (often estimated as the odds ratio from a case control study). However, for the individual patient with the risk factor, the incidence of disease, the absolute risk of the outcome, may be more useful. For example, a patient may have a 20- or 30-fold increased risk of a rare disease, but still face less than a 1 percent absolute risk of developing that disease in his or her lifetime. Another way of conveying the implications of a risk factor is to cite the attributable risk, which is the difference between the incidence among exposed people and those who are not exposed.

Such distinctions are also important when weighing the harms and benefits of interventions designed to reduce risk. Treatment of hypertension may well reduce risk of stroke by 40 percent (the relative risk reduction). But doctor and patient should also understand that baseline risk of stroke over the next 10 years may be as low as 1 percent for some patients with mild hypertension. This means that the risk-reduction benefit, or the risk difference attributable to the untreated mild hypertension, is the difference between 1.0 percent and 0.6 percent, or 0.4 percent. Another approach to summarizing this kind of data is to cite the number of patients one would need to treat to have the desired effect in a single patient. Returning to the hypertension example, treating 1000 patients would reduce the number of stokes from 10 to 6, so 250 people with mild hypertension would have to be treated to avoid one stroke.

DESCRIBING OUTCOMES DURING AN UNCERTAIN FUTURE

The diagnosis of a particular condition is generally much more predictive of future outcomes than identification of risk factors. Outcomes are more frequent and are often described as simple rates. The proportion of people with a particular condition who eventually die of that disease is the *case-fatality rate*. Some indication of the duration of survival may be included by describing survival at a point in time after diagnosis (eg, the 5-year survival rate). Simple rates have the advantage of being easy to remember and communicate. But valuable information is lost when prognosis, the distribution of uncertain events over time, is summarized by a single rate. The more complete picture of prognosis is captured in a *survival curve*. Survival curves are often used to display the proportion of a cohort surviving over time, but the same technique can be used to display the occurrence, or lack thereof, of other events such as onset of symptoms or recurrence of disease. Survival curves are constructed by plotting sequentially calculated probabilities of survival (or freedom from events) over time. The decrease in the height of the curve at any time period depends on the proportion of the remaining cohort who experience the event during that period, with patients lost to follow-up excluded from the denominator. Sometimes the proportion of people who experience events, rather than the proportion who are event-free, is plotted on the vertical axis. Such cumulative incidence curves convey the same information.

It is important to remember that survival curves display serial estimates that are based on the experience of fewer and fewer people as events and loss to follow-up deplete the denominator. Therefore, the clinician can be more confident in the estimates displayed on the left-hand part of the curve than the right. The distant future is more uncertain than the near term. But when a new diagnosis of serious disease is made, it is often the near term that is of greatest interest to the patient. A cumulative recurrence risk of 30 percent may be frightening to the woman with early stage breast cancer, and this may be a case where use of the simple rate to express prognosis may be a disservice. The more complete picture presented by a survival curve, including attention to the low annual incidence of recurrence in the near term, may be more helpful to the patient.

THE UNIQUENESS OF EACH PATIENT

Descriptions of risk and prognosis should be provided to patients with an appreciation for the uniqueness of each person and her or his predicament. Different people respond differently to the same risk. A 1 percent risk of stroke over a 5- or 10-year period may be threatening to some but inconsequential to others. This may be explained by the very real competing risks that different people face due to other medical conditions or the environment in which they live. Similarly, different people have different attitudes about tradeoffs between the present or near-term future and the distant future. Putting up with side effects or inconvenience now for some *possible* benefit in the future makes good sense to some but little sense to others. Again, competing risks explain some of these differences. Another important difference among patients is in their desire for information about the future. Many demand such information. Others would rather not know details about prognosis even when that means that they must defer to the clinician for important decisions. As in other aspects of patient education, respect for the patient's autonomy and personal values during communication of information about illness and its implications for the future requires a negotiated approach to patient care.

A.G.M.

ANNOTATED BIBLIOGRAPHY

Concato J, Feinstein AR, Holford TR. The risk of determining risk with multivariable models. Ann Intern Med 1993;118:201. (*Reviews principles and standards for application of multivariable statistical methods in general medical literature.*)

Fletcher, RH, Fletcher SW, Wagner EH. Clinical Epidemiology: The Essentials, 2nd ed. Baltimore, Williams and Wilkins, 1988. (*A good general reference with careful treatment of risk and prognosis in chapters 5 and 6.*)

Forrow L, Taylor WC, Arnold RM. Absolutely relative: How research results are summarized can affect treatment decisions. Am J Med 1992;92:121. (*Examines the impact of reporting methods on perceptions of risk or treatment effectiveness.*)

Laupacis A, Sackett DL, Roberts RS. An assessment of clinically useful measures of the consequences of treatment. N Engl J Med 1988;318:1728. (*An analysis of alternative approaches to summarizing effectiveness data, including the number needed to treat, or NNT.*)

Rose G. Sick individuals and sick populations. Int J Epidemiol 1985;14:32. (*Describes relative importance of risk factors and condition-specific prognoses in predicting future outcomes.*)

Sackett DL, Haynes RB, Tugwell P. Clinical Epidemiology: A Basic Science for Clinical Medicine. Boston, Little, Brown and Co, 1985. (*Very well written from the perspective of the clinician who wants to be a critical appraiser of published experience relevant to prognosis.*)

Wasson JH, Sox HC, Neff RK, Goldman L. Clinical prediction rules: Applications and methodological standards. N Engl J Med 1985;313:793. (*Provides a checklist for methodological standards for studies that purport to define prognostic variables.*)

Primary Care Medicine: Office Evaluation and Management of the Adult Patient, 3rd edition, edited by Allan H. Goroll, Lawrence A. May, and Albert G. Mulley, Jr. J.B. Lippincott Company, Philadelphia

5
Choosing Among Treatment Options

Although discerning diagnosis and accurate prognosis are essential to effective patient care, the process of choosing among treatment options can have the greatest impact on relief of suffering and prolongation of life. The right choice depends on accurate information about the effects of alternative treatment strategies on health outcomes. Will symptoms be relieved or at least reduced? Will serious complications of disease be averted by timely intervention, or will treatment side effects or complications decrease the quality or length of life? Treatment choices also depend on the patients' preferences for different possible health outcomes and on their attitudes toward risks or their willingness to endure morbidity now for some possible future benefit. And, as noted in Chapter 4, different patients have different preferences and attitudes toward risks and time trade-offs. Effective therapeutic decision making therefore requires both a strong clinical knowledge base and the communication skills necessary to gain empathic understanding of the individual patient's wants and needs.

WHAT WE KNOW ABOUT TREATMENT EFFECTIVENESS

The cumulative knowledge base about the effectiveness of treatments of human disease is prodigious. And yet the use of the vast majority of therapeutic interventions in clinical practice is not supported by evidence derived from clinical trials. Clinicians often rely on their own experience with similar patients supplemented by published case series to estimate the likelihood of relevant health outcomes with alternative treatments. This less than rigorous approach produces different opinions about treatment effectiveness that lead to wide variations in clinical practices for ostensibly similar patients. Because of less stringent regulatory control, the knowledge gaps are generally greater with devices and surgical procedures than with drugs. For example, diskectomy for lumbar disk disease was first described in 1934. Yet the first and only randomized trial was published in 1983 and included only 60 surgical patients. The collective experience of the millions of patients who have undergone diskectomy worldwide contributes relatively little to our knowledge. Similarly, transurethral prostatectomy represented the standard of care for benign prostatic hyperplasia for 40 years before publication of a clinical trial.

RANDOMIZED CLINICAL TRIALS AND TREATMENT EFFECTIVENESS

Even when randomized trials are done, uncertainty remains about the effectiveness of treatment for a specific patient. This in part reflects the methods used in clinical trials to measure the isolated effects of the experimental treatment. Explicit inclusion and exclusion criteria are applied to assure that the study population is homogeneous, thereby minimizing the impact of patient-specific variables on outcomes. Patients with severe disease or important comorbid conditions are often excluded. Others may be excluded because of age or gender. Patients who meet criteria are then randomized to one of two or more carefully defined alternative treatment strategies. Barriers are erected to discourage patients from switching from one treatment to another, and other steps are taken to preserve the integrity of the treatments.

The course of patients in randomized trials is carefully monitored, with equal attention to patients regardless of treatment, and their outcomes are determined using explicit, predefined measures. Ideally, both patients and those who measure outcomes will be unaware of the treatment assignment, even if this requires the use of placebos or sham procedures. Otherwise, expectations may have a real effect on perceived treatment outcomes and be interpreted as specific effects of treatment.

All of these steps serve to protect the validity of the trial as a test of the hypothesis that the alternative treatments in the trial have different effects on outcome. But these same steps often limit the applicability, or generalizability, of the study findings to patients for whom the study treatment might be considered. The clinician must be concerned both about the internal validity of the trial as a test of the effectiveness hypothesis, and about its external validity, that is, the extent to which results are applicable to the different patients seen in practice.

OTHER STUDIES OF TREATMENT EFFECTIVENESS

Randomized trials are not always necessary. When a new treatment has unprecedented or dramatic effects, such as penicillin for pneumococcal pneumonia or pacemaker insertion for life-threatening bradycardia, a trial is neither possible nor desirable. When results of trials would be helpful because treatment effects are more equivocal, they are often not available. Randomized trials are costly, time-consuming, and poorly accepted by many clinicians and patients. Sometimes a trial is obsolete before it is completed because the experimental treatment is modified or replaced altogether by a newer approach or technology.

For all these reasons, clinicians must rely on data from observational studies as well as randomized trial results. But great caution must be used when applying conclusions of observational studies to patient care. Differences in patient characteristics among alternative treatment groups may lead to erroneous conclusions about treatment effectiveness. While there have been important advances in the use of statistical methods to control for such different prognostic factors in an attempt to isolate the treatment effect, the investigator can only control for those factors that are anticipated and measured. Observational studies complement randomized trials. They can be used to design efficient and targeted trials and to assess generalizability of trial results. However, the clinician should be mindful of the quality of evidence when making treatment choices, and there is no substitute for a well-conducted randomized trial.

TREATMENT CHOICE AND PATIENT VALUES

Even if the probabilities of outcomes contingent on alternative treatment choices can be estimated precisely, there is still much work to be done to assure a wise treatment choice for a particular patient. Consider the predicament of the 75-year-old male who is bothered by nocturia and urinary frequency due to benign prostatic hyperplasia. He can live with his symptoms, but this means accepting a diminished quality of life. He may choose to try a medical approach, such as finasteride or an alpha-blocker, with hope of modest relief of symptoms. Alternatively, surgical therapy offers a good chance of more dramatic symptom relief but also confers small but real risk of a catastrophic event that could result in death. Surgery also puts the patient at risk for complications such as incontinence or impotence that may diminish the quality of life as much or more than the nocturia and frequency.

The probabilities of these outcomes are critically important to the decision. But equally important is how the man feels about the outcomes. Different men feel differently about trade-offs between urinary function and sexual function, and they have different attitudes toward the small risk of perioperative death. These personal value judgments are as important in determining the "right" choice as are the probabilities that are derived from clinical research. The right choice, therefore requires careful communication between clinician and patient about what the possible outcomes will mean for that patient's quality of life.

A.G.M.

ANNOTATED BIBLIOGRAPHY

Department of Clinical Epidemiology and Biostatistics, McMaster University. How to read clinical journals. V: To distinguish useful from useless or even harmful therapy. Can Med Assoc J 1981;124:1156. (*A classic in the series of "critical appraisal articles" that provides a thoughtful checklist for the clinician who turns to the literature to learn about therapeutic effectiveness.*)

Guyatt G, Sackett D, Taylor DW, et al. Determining optimal therapy—randomized trials in individual patients. N Engl J Med 1986;314:889. (*Persuasive argument for blinded, placebo-controlled, crossover trials in individual patients to more critically evaluate the specific effects of medical treatments.*)

Fletcher RH, Fletcher SW, Wagner EH. Clinical Epidemiology: The Essentials, 2nd ed. Baltimore: Williams and Wilkins, 1988. (*Concise and clear chapter on treatment effectiveness.*)

Mulley AG. Assessing patients' utilities: Can the ends justify the means? Med Care 1989;27:S269. (*A somewhat technical discussion of the role of patients' preferences and their measurement in clinical decision making.*)

6
Immunization

HARVEY B. SIMON, M.D.

Primary Care Medicine: Office Evaluation and Management of the Adult Patient, 3rd edition, edited by Allan H. Goroll, Lawrence A. May, and Albert G. Mulley, Jr. J.B. Lippincott Company, Philadelphia

Immunizations are an effective and important means of controlling many communicable diseases through primary prevention. The power of immunization programs is nowhere more evident than in the case of smallpox, which has been eradicated as a result of an aggressive worldwide vaccination program. But if smallpox vaccine has been rendered obsolete through its own effectiveness, the other immunizing agents have not. An appalling number of Americans have not received their recommended immunizations. In large part, this is a failure of public education and of access to health care delivery. But while the pediatrician has been traditionally effective in immunizing individual patients, the primary care internist too often overlooks the importance of immunization. Evidence continues to mount on the efficacy of immunizing both the elderly and the high-risk patient.

Except for travelers, patients usually do not request immunizations. It is up to the primary care physician, then, to initiate consideration of immunization. The first step is to take a detailed immunization history. In addition, a history of prior adverse reactions (being careful to distinguish patient attributions—"the vaccine gave me the flu"—from true adverse reactions to vaccines) and of egg allergy should be sought. Finally, it is important to be aware of the current prevalence of infectious diseases in the local community and, in the case of the traveler, in other parts of the world.

GENERAL PRINCIPLES OF IMMUNIZATION

Types of Vaccines, Their Uses, and Contraindications. In general, *live attenuated vaccines* (Table 6–1) provide more complete and longer lasting immunity than inactivated agents. However, because live vaccines can produce serious disseminated disease in the immunosuppressed host, these preparations should be avoided in patients who are immunologically deficient (eg, those with human immunodeficiency virus [HIV] infection, leukemia, lymphoma, steroid or cancer chemotherapy, or agammaglobulinemia). In addition, the oral polio vaccine should not be given to individuals sharing a household with an immunocompromised patient, because the virus can be transmitted person-to-person. An exception is the measles-mumps-rubella (MMR) vaccine, which should be administered to all HIV-infected children. *Inactivated vaccines* (see Table 6–1) are safe in these patients.

Two inactivated vaccines can be given simultaneously at separate injection sites, as can an inactivated vaccine and a live vaccine. However, if significant local or systemic reactions are anticipated, as is often the case with cholera or typhoid vaccines, for example, it may be best to administer the vaccines on separate days. On theoretical grounds, it is desirable to separate vaccinations with live virus vaccines

Table 6-1. Immunizing Agents

Live Attenuated Vaccines
1. Viral
   a. Polio
   b. Measles
   c. Rubella
   d. Mumps
   e. Yellow fever
2. Bacterial
   a. BCG
   b. Typhoid

Inactivated Agents
1. Viral
   a. Influenza
   b. Rabies
   c. Polio
   d. Hepatitis B
   e. Rabies
   f. Japanese encephalitis
2. Bacterial
   a. *Pneumococcus*
   b. *Meningococcus*
   c. *Haemophilus influenzae* type B
   d. Diphtheria (toxoid)
   e. Tetanus (toxoid)
   f. Pertussis
   g. Typhoid
   h. Cholera

Vaccines Prepared from Egg Media
1. Influenza
2. Rabies
3. Rocky Mountain spotted fever
4. Typhus
5. Yellow fever

Immunoglobulin Preparations for Passive Immunization
1. Human
   a. Immune globulin
   b. Tetanus immune globulin
   c. Measles immune globulin
   d. Hepatitis B immune globulin
   e. Rabies immune globulin
   f. Varicella-zoster immune globulin
2. Equine
   a. Diphtheria antitoxin
   b. Botulism antitoxin

by at least 1 month. However, studies have shown that a combination of measles, mumps, and rubella vaccines can be given to children along with the trivalent oral polio vaccine without adverse reactions or loss of effectiveness.

Mixing passive and active immunization can sometimes be problematic. Passive immunity can *interfere* with active immunity, but such interference is of little practical importance with inactivated vaccines, which can therefore be administered any time after the use of immune globulin. However, with live attenuated vaccines, it is best to defer immunizations until 3 months have elapsed following administration of immune globulin, blood, or plasma. If immune globulin becomes necessary after vaccination and the interval between the live attenuated vaccine and the immune globulin is less than 14 days, the vaccine doses should be repeated in about 3 months, unless serologic testing demonstrates that antibody has been produced. Travelers requiring both vaccines and immune globulin should receive the immune globulin 2 weeks after completing the vaccinations, if possible.

Patients who have exhibited *hypersensitivity reactions* to a vaccine should not receive that product again. Individuals with egg allergies should not be given vaccines prepared in egg cultures (see Table 6–1). If multiple-dose immunization schedules are delayed or interrupted, they should be resumed without administering extra doses, no matter how long the interval between doses.

In general, immunization should be postponed only during significant febrile illnesses. The decision to immunize must include consideration of the frequency of the condition, chances of exposure, risks and benefits of immunization, and cost.

Vaccination in Pregnancy. In pregnancy and in women likely to become pregnant within 3 months after vaccination, live attenuated-virus vaccines should not be given. In particular, the *MMR vaccine* is *absolutely contraindicated* because of its potential teratogenicity. All pregnant women should be evaluated for immunity to rubella, and those who are negative need to be immunized promptly after delivery. In general, other live-virus vaccines should be avoided in pregnancy unless the risk of exposure and illness clearly outweighs the possible risks of the vaccine itself (for example, oral polio vaccine can be given to pregnant women in the setting of an epidemic outbreak). *Inactivated vaccines* and toxoids are generally considered *safe* in pregnancy. Passive immunization with immune globulin does not harm the fetus. It is recommended that all pregnant women be tested for hepatitis B infection so that infants born to mothers who test positive can be treated with hepatitis B immune globulin and receive hepatitis B vaccine.

Common Misconceptions About Immunization. Many physicians mistakenly believe that certain conditions are contraindications to routine immunization, including concurrent antimicrobial therapy, convalescent phase of an illness, pregnancy in the household, breast-feeding, history of nonspecific allergies, recent exposure to an infectious disease, mild acute illness with low-grade fever, and allergy to duck feathers or penicillin. (No vaccines in the United States contain penicillin, though MMR vaccine does contain a very small amount of neomycin, and oral polio vaccine contains streptomycin.)

Immunizations in Patients with HIV Infection. As noted above, live viral and bacterial vaccines can cause disseminated infection in the immunocompromised HIV-infected patient. Patients with HIV infection should not receive live viral (oral polio and smallpox) or bacterial (BCG) vaccines. An exception is HIV-infected children. Severe measles has been reported in such patients; because there have not been reports of unusual side effects of MMR vaccination in these children, MMR vaccination should be administered to HIV-infected children. Because of vaccine failures, all HIV-infected children who are exposed to measles should receive immune globulin within 6 days. Inactivated vaccines, including inactivated polio vaccine, should be administered according to routine schedules. As in other immunosuppressed patients, *influenza vaccine* should be administered annually, and *pneumococcal vaccine* should be given on a one-time basis as soon as the diagnosis of HIV infection is made. Patients with HIV infection have been shown to mount antibody responses to both vaccines if the vaccines are administered early in the course of HIV disease, especially during the asymptomatic phase. Delay in immunization may result in a lost opportunity, because antibody responses clearly decline as HIV disease progresses.

Record Keeping. The National Childhood Vaccine Injury Act of 1988 requires all health care providers who administer certain vaccines to maintain careful records of vaccinations (including the lot number of the vaccine used) and to notify the Centers for Disease Control and Prevention (CDC) of the Food and Drug Administration if an adverse reaction occurs. The vaccines covered by the Act include diphtheria-pertussis-tetanus (DPT); pertussis (P); diphtheria-tetanus (DT); MMR; either singly or in combination, and both live and inactivated polio vaccines.

SPECIFIC IMMUNIZING AGENTS

Diphtheria and Tetanus Toxoid and Pertussis Vaccine

Although both diphtheria and tetanus are now uncommon in the United States, all individuals should receive the excellent protection afforded by the toxoids that are prepared by formaldehyde treatment of the bacterial toxins. Pertussis vaccine is indicated in all children younger than 6 years of age, but older individuals are not nearly as susceptible to pertussis and should not receive the vaccine. Children between 6 weeks and 6 years of age should be given the combined DPT product. For patients first receiving immunization after age 6, three tetanus-diphtheria (Td) injections should be administered, with the second dose given 1 to 2 months after the initial dose and the third dose 6 to 12 months later. A booster should be administered every 10 years.

Tetanus-diphtheria immunization is the only immunization universally indicated in adults (Table 6–2), but it is frequently overlooked. Immigrants and elderly individuals, particularly women and men who have not served in the military, are especially likely never to have been immunized.

If a patient has received a full primary tetanus series and boosters at regular 10-year intervals, additional boosters are not necessary at the time of injury. Other individuals should receive tetanus-diphtheria toxoids for minor wounds and both tetanus-diphtheria toxoids and tetanus immune globulin (TIG) for more serious wounds (Table 6–3).

Polio Vaccine

Although all children should receive polio vaccine, the very low incidence of poliomyelitis in the United States makes the routine immunization of adults unnecessary. Previously immunized travelers who are anticipating visits to rural areas of developing countries should receive a single *booster dose* of oral polio vaccine (TOPV), as should certain health care and laboratory workers who may be exposed to polio virus. An *enhanced inactivated vaccine (eIPV)* is available for use in immunosuppressed patients. Previously *un*immunized adults who may be exposed to polio virus (through travel, occupation, etc.) should be given eIPV because of the slight risk of vaccine-associated paralysis following OPV; three doses should be given at intervals of 1 to 2 months, with a fourth dose given 6 to 12 months later. Some authorities recommend two doses of eIPV for unimmunized parents of infants who are to be given TOPV.

Table 6-2. Indications for Immunization in Adults

Primary Immunization or Booster in All Adults
Tetanus-diphtheria
Immunization in Selected, Vulnerable Individuals
Influenza (the elderly and debilitated, HIV, cardiopulmonary disease, diabetes, and other chronic disease)
Pneumococcus (sickle cell disease, splenectomy, elderly, debilitated HIV, chronic disease, diabetes)
Rubella (women of childbearing age who are antibody negative; must avoid pregnancy for 3 months)
Meningococcus (splenectomy)
? *Haemophilus influenzae* type B (splenectomy)
Measles (individuals born after 1956 who have received fewer than two doses of measles vaccine)
Immunizations in Certain Epidemiologic Situations
Hepatitis B vaccine (for certain high-risk individuals including selected medical and dental personnel, dialysis patients, recipients of frequent transfusions, residents and staff of institutions for the retarded, sexual contacts of HbsAg carriers, and male homosexuals)
Meningococcus (epidemics; possibly household contacts; only types A and C available)
Immune globulin (for household exposure to hepatitis A and possibly non-A, non-B hepatitis)
Hepatitis B immune globulin (hepatitis B-negative patients who have acute intensive exposure to hepatitis B as in needle sticks)
BCG (selected tuberculin-negative individuals expecting intense exposure to tuberculosis)
Immunizations for International Travel (Depending on Area)
Typhoid
Cholera (within 2 months of departure)
Yellow fever (Africa, South America)
Polio (tropical or developing areas; booster or primary series if never immunized)
Plague (rural Vietnam, Cambodia, Laos)
Typhus (rarely necessary)
Immune globulin (for hepatitis A)
Passive Immunizations After Exposure
Rabies immune globulin (plus vaccine)
Tetanus immune globulin (plus toxoid)
Diphtheria antitoxin (plux toxoid)
Botulism antitoxin
Immune globulin (for hepatitis A)
Hepatitis B immune globulin (for hepatitis B—acute intense exposure)
Varicella-zoster immune globulin (for certain vulnerable individuals after exposure)
Measles immune globulin (for certain vulnerable individuals after exposure)

Table 6-3. Summary Guide to Tetanus Prophylaxis in Routine Wound Management—United States

HISTORY OF ADSORBED TETANUS TOXOID (DOSES)	CLEAN, MINOR WOUNDS		ALL OTHER WOUNDS*	
	Td†	*TIG*	*Td*†	*TIG*
Unknown or < three	Yes	No	Yes	Yes
≥ Three‡	No§	No	No‖	No

*Such as, but not limited to, wounds contaminated with dirt, feces, soil, saliva, etc.; puncture wounds; avulsions; and wounds resulting from missiles, crushing, burns, and frostbite.

†For children under 7 years old, DTP (DT, if pertussis vaccine is contraindicated) is preferred to tetanus toxoid alone. For persons 7 years old and older, Td is preferred to tetanus toxoid alone.

‡If only three doses of *fluid* toxoid have been received, a fourth dose of toxoid, preferably an adsorbed toxoid, should be given.

§Yes, if more than 10 years since last dose.

‖Yes, if more than 5 years since last dose. (More frequent boosters are not needed and can accentuate side effects.)

(Source: MMWR Morbid Mortal Wkly Rep 34:405, 1986.)

Measles, Mumps, and Rubella Vaccines

These three live attenuated virus vaccines are available in a combined preparation for use in children at age 15 months or older.

Mumps vaccine is rarely indicated in adults. Nonimmune adult males are at risk of mumps orchitis. However, susceptibility is difficult to predict, as many adults with no history of clinical mumps are immune and the skin test is not a reliable predictor of immunity. Hence, routine mumps vaccination of adult males cannot be recommended. Immune globulin is not of proven value in postexposure prophylaxis.

Rubella vaccine is recommended for adolescent and adult women if serologic tests for rubella antibody are negative and if they are able to avoid pregnancy for 3 months following immunization. The most common side effects of rubella vaccination are arthralgias. Rubella vaccine has not been demonstrated to cause congenital rubella syndrome or teratogenicity, though there is a theoretical risk in using a live attenuated virus in this setting.

An inactivated *measles vaccine* was introduced in 1963, but was replaced by a much more effective live attenuated vaccine in 1967. Persons born before 1956 can be considered immune by virtue of natural infection. However, measles vaccine should be administered to persons born after 1956 unless documentation of vaccination with two doses of attenuated vaccine after 1 year of age is available. *Measles revaccination* is particularly important for susceptible college students, health care workers, and international travelers. Immunization of previously immune individuals is not harmful. Combined MMR vaccine is recommended for revaccination. As noted, female recipients must avoid pregnancy for 3 months following vaccination (see rubella vaccine).

Smallpox

Universal smallpox immunization in the United States was abandoned in 1971 because of the disappearance of the disease. Vaccination is no longer recommended for travelers. The vaccine is now recommended only for laboratory personnel exposed to orthopoxviruses. Smallpox vaccine is available to civilians in the United States only through the CDC.

Influenza Vaccine

Influenza remains a major worldwide problem because of frequent antigenic shifts in the virus. New vaccines are prepared in anticipation of the viral strains that are expected to prevail during the winter flu season. Indications for vaccination vary from year to year, depending on vaccine availability, the likelihood of influenza epidemics, and vaccine toxicity. In general, the elderly and debilitated, particularly those with cardiopulmonary disease, should receive influenza vaccine during the autumn prior to the flu season. Other vulnerable individuals who are candidates for the vaccine include nursing home residents and those with renal disease, sickle cell anemia, or diabetes; HIV-infected individuals and other immunosuppressed hosts should also receive the vaccine. Health care workers who have extensive contact with high-risk patients should consider annual vaccination.

Many elderly patients refuse influenza vaccination, citing fear of "getting sick from the shot." The observed risk of a flu-like adverse reaction is actually very small, in the range of 4 percent to 5 percent.

Unlike other viral infections, a chemical agent, *amantadine*, is available to prevent clinical disease in patients exposed to influenza A. Although not a substitute for vaccination, the agent is effective both for prophylaxis and treatment. Amantadine is particularly useful in elderly patients directly exposed to the flu, as in nursing home outbreaks. Adjunctive administration to previously immunized high-risk persons enhances the vaccine's protective effect. When used therapeutically within 48 hours of the onset of symptoms, amantadine can substantially shorten the illness and reduce symptoms.

Meningococcus Vaccine

A quadrivalent vaccine containing 50 mg each of cell wall polysaccharides from meningococcal types A, C, Y, and W-135 is available. It is not recommended for general use but is indicated for control of epidemics (as in the military) and for travelers to areas experiencing outbreaks of meningococcal meningitis. Meningococcal vaccine may be of some benefit in household contacts of patients with meningococcal disease. Meningococcal vaccine is immunogenic for splenectomized patients (except those who have received chemotherapy or radiotherapy for lymphoma); asplenic individuals should receive the vaccine.

Pneumococcus Vaccine

Despite the use of penicillin and other antibiotics, pneumococcal pneumonia has remained a major cause of morbidity and mortality in the United States, with an estimated 500,000 cases annually and a case fatality rate of 5 percent to 10 percent. A vaccine released in 1977 contained 14 polysaccharide types, responsible for about 80 percent of pneumococcal disease. An enhanced vaccine released in 1983 contains 23 polysaccharide types, responsible for about 90 percent of pneumococcal disease, and has replaced the

14-valent preparation. The vaccine appears to be at least 70 percent effective in preventing pneumonia caused by these serotypes, and has been safe and well tolerated. Pneumococcal vaccine is indicated in individuals with increased susceptibility to pneumococcal infection, including those with HIV infection, splenectomy, sickle cell disease, nephrotic syndrome, cirrhosis, diabetes, and chronic cardiopulmonary disease. Because mortality from pneumococcal pneumonia increases with age, vaccination should be considered for all people over age 65. Antibody response to pneumococcal vaccine has been poor in children younger than 2 years of age.

Vaccination produces adequate antibody levels in patients with sickle cell anemia, nephrosis, uremia, diabetes, and asplenia, but vaccine failures have been reported in these groups as well as in normals. Because patients with Hodgkin's disease respond poorly after splenectomy plus chemotherapy and radiotherapy, it seems wise to administer vaccine to these patients as soon after diagnosis as possible. Early immunization has also been urged in HIV-positive patients (see Chapter 13). Although only 30 percent of myeloma patients respond serologically, vaccination seems reasonable in these high-risk patients.

Pneumococcal vaccine is safe. Side effects consist mainly of pain and erythema at the injection site and occasional mild fever. Local side effects appear to be increased following revaccination; protective levels of antibody persist for years, and revaccination is not recommended. Patients who have previously received the 14-valent vaccine in use from 1977 through 1983 should not receive the newer 23-valent vaccine, as the risk of local reactions does not seem to warrant the slight additional protection. The safety of pneumococcal vaccine for pregnant women has not been evaluated.

Pneumococcal vaccine and influenza vaccine can be administered simultaneously at separate sites without impairing efficacy or increasing toxicity.

Haemophilus influenzae Type B

H. influenzae type B is a major bacterial pathogen in childhood, causing meningitis, bacteremia, epiglottitis, pneumonia, and other invasive infections. Other strains of *H. influenzae,* however, are more likely to cause otitis media. In the United States, the risk of developing *H. influenzae* type B invasive disease during the first 5 years of life is about 1 in 200. The risk is even higher in Native Americans, African-Americans, individuals with asplenia, sickle cell disease, Hodgkin's disease, or antibody deficiencies, and children who attend day care centers.

A vaccine prepared from *H. influenzae* type B capsular polysaccharide was licensed in 1985. Improved vaccines in which the polysaccharide is conjugated to proteins are even more effective. Vaccinations are recommended for all children, with the series beginning at 2 months of age.

At present, there are not enough data to recommend the use of this vaccine in older individuals, but it may merit consideration for those who are especially vulnerable to *H. influenzae* type B (such as those with splenectomy).

Rabies Vaccine and Rabies Immune Globulin

Although human rabies is rare in the United States (zero to five cases per year), thousands of people are at risk because of animal bites and scratches. Approximately 25,000 persons receive prophylaxis in the United States each year. Rabies in domestic animals has become very uncommon, but wildlife (especially skunks, foxes, raccoons, and bats) still pose a risk. Fortunately, rabies prophylaxis has become much less toxic with the availability of a human diploid cell rabies vaccine (HDCV) and an inactivated vaccine derived from rhesus monkey cells (RVA). HDCV and RVA appear equally safe and effective. Both are administered into the deltoid muscle (anterolateral thigh in infants). Dosage and administration schedules for the two vaccines are identical (except that RVA should not be administered intradermally for preexposure immunization).

Preexposure rabies vaccination is recommended only for people with occupational exposure to rabies virus. Both active immunization with vaccine and passive immunization with rabies immune globulin may be indicated after animal bites or scratches. Table 6–4 presents the U.S. Public Health Service guidelines for postexposure prophylaxis.

Further information about rabies prophylaxis can be obtained from the CDC (telephone number: 404-639-3111 weekdays and 404-639-2888 at other times).

BCG Vaccine

Bacillus Calmette-Guérin (BCG) vaccine is a live, attenuated strain of *Mycobacterium bovis,* which was introduced in 1922. Seniority notwithstanding, the efficacy of BCG is unknown. Earlier European trials showed up to 80 percent protection, but recent Indian trials showed little value. Despite the increase in cases of primary tuberculosis in the United States, BCG is still recommended only in selected tuberculin-negative individuals with unavoidable intense exposure to tuberculosis, such as children of mothers with active tuberculosis (see also Chapter 49). BCG may be useful in travelers anticipating close contact with people infected with tuberculosis, but an alternative approach is tuberculin skin-testing before and after travel, with administration of isoniazid in the event of skin-test conversion (see Chapter 49).

Viral Hepatitis

Hepatitis A. Commercially available *pooled human gamma globulin* is of proven benefit in preventing or clinically modifying type A hepatitis (infectious hepatitis), particularly if it is given within 2 weeks of exposure to the virus. Individuals closely exposed to patients with hepatitis should be given gamma globulin, especially household contacts of patients. The recommended dosage is 0.02 mL per kilogram of body weight, or about 2 mL in adults. Immune globulin is also useful in preventing hepatitis A in travelers to underdeveloped areas where hepatitis is endemic; the dosage is 2 mL for brief travel, and 5 mL for travel of longer than 3 months, with repeat doses every 4 to 6 months if needed (see also Chapter 57).

Hepatitis B. *Passive Immunization.* Two globulin products are currently available in the United States. *Immune globulin* is prepared from normal donors; although pre-1972 lots of immune globulin had low anti-HBs titers, current lots have titers between 1:100 and 1:1000. *Hepatitis B immune*

Table 6-4. Guide to Postexposure Rabies Prophylaxis*

ANIMAL SPECIES	CONDITION OF ANIMAL AT TIME OF ATTACK	TREATMENT OF EXPOSED HUMAN
Wild:		
Skunk Fox Coyote Raccoon Bat Bobcat Other carnivores	Regard as rabid unless proven negative by laboratory tests (the animal should be killed and tested at once; observation not recommended).	RIG† + HDCV or RVA‡
Domestic:		
Cat or dog	Healthy and available 10 days of observation	None
	Unknown (escaped)	Consult public health officials; if treatment is indicated, give RIG and HDCV or RVA
Other	Rabid or suspected	RIG† + HDCV or RVA‡ Consider individually

*These recommendations are only a guide. They should be applied in conjunction with knowledge of the animal species involved, circumstances of the bite or other exposure, vaccination status of the animal, the presence of rabies in the region. Public health officials should be consulted if questions arise.

†RIG (rabies immune globulin, human) is administered only once, at the beginning of therapy. Dose is 20 IU/kg, one-half intramuscularly (IM) in the buttocks and one-half thoroughly infiltrated around the wound. Equine antirabies serum should be used only if RIG is not available. *All wounds should be thoroughly cleansed with soap and water.*

‡HDCV (human diploid cell vaccine) and Rabies Vaccine, absorbed (RVA) appear equally effective. One mL of vaccine should be given IM into the deltoid muscle (anterolateral thigh in infants) on day 0, 3, 7, 14, 28. (WHO currently recommends a sixth dose 90 days after the first dose.) HDCV and RVA are so effective that serologic testing of recipients is no longer recommended.

globulin (HBIG) is prepared from high-titer donors and has titers of at least 1:100,000. Immune globulin is of *no* proven efficacy in preventing hepatitis B, though it may have some value in chronic low-dose exposure (travelers, closed institutions, family contacts).

HBIG will prevent or modify some cases of hepatitis B following exposure. HBIG is indicated for hepatitis B antigen- and antibody-negative individuals with an *acute intense exposure* to hepatitis B (needle stick, sexual partner, oral ingestion). HBIG should be given in a dose of 0.06 mL/kg (5 mL for adults) as soon as possible. (See Tables 6–5 and 6–6.) HBIG is very expensive.

Active Immunization. Active immunization utilizing a *recombinant DNA vaccine* is recommended for high-risk individuals including medical, dental, and laboratory personnel exposed to blood products and other bodily fluids; intimate contact with hepatitis B patients; institution residents and staff; hemodialysis patients and their families; male homosexuals; and travelers to endemic areas.

The recombinant vaccine has mostly replaced the *plasma-derived hepatitis B vaccine,* which failed to gain patient acceptance due to the unfounded fear of contracting acquired immunodeficiency syndrome (AIDS) from its administration. This led to the marked underutilization of this inactivated vaccine which was derived from the plasma of patients whose plasma contained surface antigen. The newer vaccine utilizes recombinant DNA technology to produced hepatitis B surface antigen. No infectious particles are present in the preparation, but the hepatitis B surface antigen in the vaccine induces an immune response in vaccine recipients, with

Table 6-5. Hepatitis B Virus Postexposure Recommendations

	HBIG		VACCINE*	
EXPOSURE	***Dose***	***Recommended Timing***	***Dose***	***Recommended Timing***
Perinatal	0.5 mL IM	Within 12 h of birth	0.5 mL (10 μg)IM	Within 7 d, repeat at 1 and 6 mo
Percutaneous†				
Sexual	0.6 mL/kg IM or 5 mL for adults	Within 14 d of sexual contact	1.0 mL (20 μg)IM§	Within 2 wk of sexual contact; repeat at 1 and 6 mo

*The first dose can be given at the same time as the HBIG dose but at a separate site.

†See Table 6-6.

§Vaccine is recommended for homosexually active males and for regular sexual contacts of chronic HBV carriers but optional for heterosexuals with a limited exposure.

(Source: US Department of Health and Human Services/Public Health Service: Post-exposure prophylaxis of hepatitis B. MMWR Morbid Mortal Wkly Rep 33:286, 1984.)

Table 6-6. Recommendations for Hepatitis B Prophylaxis Following Percutaneous Exposure

SOURCE	EXPOSED PERSON	
	Unvaccinated	*Vaccinated*
HBsAg-positive	1. HBIG × 1 immediately* 2. Initiate HB vaccine† series	1. Test exposed person for anti-HBs‡ 2. If inadequate antibody,§ HBIG (×1) immediately plus HB vaccine booster dose
Known source High risk HBsAg-positive	1. Initiate HB vaccine series 2. Test source for HBsAg; if positive, HBIG × 1	1. Test source for HBsAg only if exposed is vaccine nonresponder; if source is HBsAg-positive, give HBIG × 1 immediately plus HB vaccine booster dose
Low risk HBsAg-positive	Initiate HB vaccine series.	Nothing required
Unknown source	Initiate HB vaccine series	Nothing required

*HPIG dose 0.06 mL/kg IM.

†HB vaccine dose 20 μg IM for adults; 10 μg IM for infants or children under 10 years of age. First dose within 1 wk; second and third dose, 1 and 6 mo later.

‡See text for details.

§Less than 10 SRU by RIA, negative by EIA.

(Source: MMWR Morbid Mortal Wkly Rep 34:331, 1985.)

the production of protective antibody. Excellent antibody titers and safety have been reported.

Two 20-μg doses of the recombinant DNA vaccine are administered 1 month apart, and a third dose is administered 6 months after the first. A dose of 40 μg is recommended for immunosuppressed patients and for those on hemodialysis. The common practice in patients with a hepatitis B exposure of administering HBIG with the first dose of hepatitis B vaccine does not interfere with immunization.

The recombinant DNA hepatitis B vaccine was licensed for clinical use in the United States in 1986. Because of poor delivery of hepatitis B vaccine to vulnerable adults, the U.S. Public Health Service Immunization Practices Advisory Committee has recommended that hepatitis B vaccine be administered to all children at the time of DTP and OPV immunizations.

Hepatitis C. At present there is no definitive immunization available for prophylaxis against hepatitis C. Immune globulin has not proven of value, but it may be a reasonable precaution for intimately exposed individuals (eg, needle stick, oral ingestion, sexual contact) in a dose of 0.06 mL/kg within 1 week of exposure. Now that the hepatitis C virus has been identified, a vaccine should be forthcoming.

Typhoid Fever Vaccine

Although typhoid vaccination is not required, it is recommended for people traveling to parts of Africa, Asia, and Central and South America where the disease is endemic. Two vaccines are available. The older, inactivated vaccine immunization series consists of two subcutaneous injections separated by at least 1 month, with boosters every 3 years if needed for additional travel. Febrile reactions to the vaccine are relatively common. The newer oral live attenuated vaccine is given in four doses on alternate days. The oral vaccine is better tolerated and appears as effective as the parenteral one. Typhoid vaccine is only about 70 percent effective in preventing infection with *Salmonella typhi;* travelers should maintain vigilance with regard to food and water.

Cholera Vaccine

Although cholera vaccine is incompletely effective and the risk of cholera in Americans traveling abroad is low, cholera vaccination is required for travel to certain countries. One injection of vaccine prior to departure is sufficient for travel certification; a full primary series for individuals traveling to areas in which the disease is endemic includes a second injection at least 1 week after the first, with a booster every 6 months if indicated.

Yellow Fever Vaccine

This live, attenuated viral vaccine is available only at designated yellow fever vaccination centers. Yellow fever is endemic in parts of tropical South America and Africa, and vaccination is required for travelers to these areas.

Typhus and Plague Vaccines

These vaccines are seldom indicated in American travelers, except for the occasional individual anticipating prolonged exposure in rural areas of Southeast Asia and other scattered remote regions.

Additional Prophylactic Measures for International Travel

In addition to ascertaining and obtaining appropriate immunizations, the traveler faces a number of potential health problems. All travelers should be evaluated medically before a long or difficult trip and should be fully informed about their medical status. The patient with chronic illness may find it useful to take along medical summaries and copies of electrocardiograms. An adequate supply of medication is essential. Patients with potentially serious illnesses might best be advised to avoid medically unsophisticated areas of the world.

Malaria. Travelers to areas where malaria transmission might occur should be advised to take *malaria prophylaxis*. The standard drug has been *chloroquine phosphate*, which is administered once weekly beginning at least 1 week prior to departure and continuing for 6 weeks after return. The drug is generally well tolerated, and serious toxicity on this schedule is rare, even if it is continued for prolonged periods. The dose of chloroquine is 5 mg per kilogram of body weight up to the full adult dose of 300 mg base (500 mg of chloroquine phosphate).

The prophylaxis of *chloroquine-resistant Plasmodium falciparum* malaria is a difficult problem. Chloroquine-resistant strains are increasing in frequency and are found in parts of Southeast Asia, Central America (including Panama), northern South America, and Africa. Chloroquine-resistant *P. falciparum* malaria remains a difficult problem for travelers. At present, *mefloquine* is recommended for prophylaxis. The dose is 250 mg weekly, beginning 1 week prior to travel and continuing for 4 weeks after return. *Pyrimethamine-sulfadoxine* (Fansidar) is also effective for prophylaxis of chloroquine-resistant malaria but has been associated with severe and fatal cutaneous and hepatic reactions. Mefloquine is preferred. Malaria prophylaxis is imperfect; additional measures are important and are reflected in the following guidelines.

1. Travelers must be informed that malaria may occur up to 1 year after departure from an endemic area no matter which prophylactic regimen is used. The symptoms should be explained, and travelers should be prepared to seek medical care if symptoms arise.
2. Travelers should avoid contact with mosquitoes, especially between dusk and dawn, when most malaria transmission occurs. Screening and nets, clothing that covers most of the body, insect repellents (ideally containing *N,N*-diethyl-m-toulamide [DEET]), and insect spray (containing pyrethrum) are all important measures.
3. The CDC maintains a telephone hot line for up-to-date advice about malaria and its prophylaxis: 404-332-4555.

Traveler's Diarrhea. *Prevention* is essential. Travelers to tropical and underdeveloped areas should be cautioned to avoid potentially contaminated water and ice. Carbonated beverages, boiled water, and tea and coffee made with boiled water are generally safe. Chemical treatment of water with chlorine or iodine is also helpful, but while most pathogenic viruses and bacteria are killed, cysts capable of causing amebiasis or giardiasis may survive. Foods must also be selected with care. Most well-cooked hot food is safe, but raw fruits and vegetables should be avoided, and dairy products should be consumed only if hygienic preparation and proper refrigeration are ensured.

Although a number of antibiotic regimens are effective for *prophylaxis* (eg, one tablet a day of either double-strength trimethoprim-sulfamethoxazole, doxycycline [100 mg], trimethoprim [200 mg], or ciprofloxacin [500 mg]), they are usually not recommended because of the potential for adverse effects and the self-limited nature of most cases of traveler's diarrhea. For example, doxycycline (a tetracycline) can cause photosensitivity, and trimethoprim-sulfa can cause hypersensitivity skin rashes and marrow suppression. *Bismuth subsalicylate* (Pepto-Bismol) is the least problematic for prophylactic use but requires that two tablets be taken faithfully with each meal and before bed.

Treatment is imperfect, largely empirical, and symptomatic. Mild self-limited diarrhea should remain untreated, except for appropriate fluid replacement (with high glucose solutions). Potent obstipating agents such as Lomotil may actually prolong the course of a bacterial diarrhea, which is the etiology of many cases of traveler's diarrhea. Enteropathogenic strains of *Escherichia coli* are often responsible. *Loperamide* (Imodium), a nonprescription synthetic opioid, can be used to provide a modicum of diarrhea control. Starting dose is 4 mg, followed by 2 mg at the time of each diarrheal stool (up to a maximum of 16 mg/d). Duration and severity of symptoms can be lessened by adding an antibiotic, either *ciprofloxacin* (500 mg bid) or *trimethoprim-sulfa* (one double-strength tablet bid) for up to 3 days. Travelers should be advised to seek medical attention if they develop severe or protracted diarrhea, especially if accompanied by passage of blood or mucus, or if high fever is present. Physicians faced with this problem should call the CDC for the latest recommendations. (See also Chapter 64.)

Japanese Encephalitis. Japanese encephalitis is the most common form of epidemic viral encephalitis in the world. The virus is mosquito-borne and can lead to fatal or crippling disease. The disease occurs in annual epidemics in Asia during the rainy season (June to September). Northern Thailand has experienced particularly severe outbreaks among children. Military personnel and travelers have also been at risk. Prevention involves mosquito avoidance and vaccination. The *inactivated vaccine* is effective and safe when given in two doses 1 to 4 weeks apart. Availability of the vaccine in the United States for civilian use has been limited but is improving.

FURTHER INFORMATION

An authoritative source of additional information on vaccinations and travel is the Centers for Disease Control and Prevention, 1600 Clifton Road, N.E., Atlanta, GA 30333. Useful publications include the *Morbidity and Mortality Weekly Reports*, which is available for a modest subscription fee from the *New England Journal of Medicine*. The annual *Health Information for International Travel* can be obtained from the superintendent of Documents, U.S. Government Printing Office, Washington DC 20402.

ANNOTATED BIBLIOGRAPHY

Committee on Immunization, American College of Physicians. Guide for Adult Immunization, 2nd ed. Ann Intern Med

1990;112:1. (*A definitive review of the evidence and specific recommendations.*)

Butler JC, Breiman RF, Campbell JF, et al. Pneumococcal polysaccharide vaccine efficacy. JAMA 1993;270; 1826. (*An evaluation of current recommendations.*)

Centers for Disease Control. Recommendations for the prevention of malaria among travelers. JAMA 1990;263; 2729. (*Mefloquine recommended.*)

Centers for Disease Control, Immunization Practices Advisory Committee. General recommendations on immunization. Ann Intern Med 1989;111:133. (*Excellent summary of recommendations as well as useful sections on vaccination during pregnancy and misconceptions concerning contraindications to immunization.*)

Centers for Disease Control, Immunization Practices Advisory Committee. Pneumococcal polysaccharide vaccine. MMWR Morbid Mortal Wkly Rep 1989;38:64 and JAMA 1989; 261:1265. (*Recommends use in all adults over age 65 as well as those with debilitating illness, including HIV infection.*)

Centers for Disease Control, Immunization Practices Advisory Committee. Rubella prevention. MMWR Morbid Mortal Wkly Rep 1990;39:15. (*Recommends testing in young women and those who have just delivered so that they can be immunized, provided pregnancy can be avoided for 3 months after vaccination.*)

Centers for Disease Control, Immunization Practices Advisory Committee. Haemophilus B conjugate vaccines. MMWR Morbid Mortal Wkly Rep 1991;40:1. (*Indicated predominantly for infants, but may be useful in compromised hosts, such as those undergoing splenectomy.*)

Douglas RG. Prophylaxis and treatment of influenza. N Engl J Med 1990;322:443. (*A comprehensive review of the literature, with 93 refs.*)

Hibberd PL, Rubin RH. Immunization strategies for the immunocompromised host: The need for immunoadjuvants. Ann Intern Med 1989;110:955. (*An editorial summarizing the status of this important problem, arguing that adjuvants are needed to improve the immunogenicity of available vaccines, because many fail in immunocompromised hosts.*)

Hill DR, Pearson RD. Health advice for international travel. Ann Intern Med 1988;108:839. (*Its detailed discussion on malaria prophylaxis is particularly useful, as is the section on traveler's diarrhea.*)

LaForce, Eickoff TC. Pneumococcal vaccine: An emerging consensus. Ann Intern Med 1988;108:757. (*An editorial summarizing the evidence for the efficacy of the pneumococcal vaccine, especially in the elderly, and arguing for routine administration as early as age 55, before age-related increases in pneumococcal infection and debilitating diseases set in.*)

Margolis KL, Poland GA, Nichol KL et al. Frequency of adverse reactions after influenza vaccination. Am J Med 1990;88:27. (*Absolute risk of flu-like illness 1 week after vaccination was only 5.5%.*)

Mostow SR. Prevention, management, and control of influenza: Role for amantadine. Am J Med 1987;82(suppl 6A):35. (*Amantadine recommended for use in high-risk persons who are caught in an outbreak of influenza A.*)

Petrocelli BP, Murphy GS, Sanchez JL, et al. Treatment of traveller's diarrhea with ciprofloxacin-loperamide. J Infect Dis 1992;165:557. (*An effective treatment regimen.*)

Poland GA, Love KR, Hughes CE. Routine immunization of the HIV-positive asymptomatic patient. J Gen Intern Med 1990; 5:147. (*A review of the literature and discussion arguing that immunization should indeed be carried out and as soon as possible after the diagnosis of HIV infection, because antibody response is likely to become blunted as the disease progresses; 59 refs.*)

Primary Care Medicine: Office Evaluation and Management of the Adult Patient, 3rd edition, edited by Allan H. Goroll, Lawrence A. May, and Albert G. Mulley, Jr. J.B. Lippincott Company, Philadelphia

2

Systemic Problems

7

Screening for HIV Infection

STEPHEN L. BOSWELL, M.D.

Knowledge of human immunodeficiency virus (HIV) infection status in the asymptomatic period permits infected persons to seek potentially beneficial medical treatment in a timely fashion, including antiviral agents and medications that decrease the risk of developing opportunistic infection (see Chapter 13). These measures may delay the onset of acquired immunodeficiency syndrome (AIDS) in infected persons and prolong survival. In addition, early identification can increase the effectiveness of tuberculin skin testing and thus improve tuberculosis screening and prophylaxis (see Chapter 49). Appropriate counseling, an essential part of screening for HIV infection, may help some individuals prevent HIV transmission by modifying their behavior. However, unselective testing, especially in patients at very low risk for HIV infection, raises the chance of a false-positive result and its attendant psychosocial morbidity. The primary physician needs to know how best to advise the patient who asks about HIV testing and whom to recommend for testing.

EPIDEMIOLOGY, RISK FACTORS, AND HIV-POSITIVE STATUS AS A RISK FACTOR FOR AIDS

In the United States, those at highest risk of infection are men with a history of *homosexual* or *bisexual* activity; *intravenous drug users* and their sexual contacts; the *sexual contacts* of homosexual or bisexual men; persons who received blood and *blood products before 1985;* and *children* born to infected women. The risk of directly acquiring HIV infection through processed blood or selected blood products (plasma and clotting factor concentrates) has dramatically decreased since 1985 as a consequence of the widespread screening of those who donate blood and plasma, the use of serologic tests for HIV, and the viral inactivation of various plasma products.

A knowledge of the epidemiology of HIV infection is necessary to estimate the pretest probability of HIV infection in the person being considered for screening. Consideration of the pretest probability estimate is critical to the decision to screen. A common mistake is to place too much weight on the high sensitivity and specificity of HIV antibody testing and ignore pretest probability (see Chapters 2 and 3).

Prevalence estimates are very dynamic numbers that are changing all the time and are dependent not only on the population in question but also on geographic location. For example, among recent prevalence estimates for HIV infection are figures of 50 percent for intravenous drug abusers in New York City and gay men in Los Angeles; 10 percent for sexual partners of hemophiliacs and intravenous drug abusers in San Francisco; 1 percent for military recruits in Washington, D.C., and for African-American women bearing children; 0.1 percent for military recruits nationally and blood donors in New York City; and 0.01 percent for blood donors nationally and white women bearing children. The numbers are changing but they can help in estimating pretest probability of HIV infection for the person in question.

Most evidence suggests that all patients who are HIV-positive go on to develop AIDS (see Chapter 13). Exceptions are being sought, but their numbers are likely to be small.

EFFECTIVENESS OF TREATMENT

A growing body of evidence from U.S. studies has suggested that treatment with zidovudine (AZT) of the asymptomatic patient with a CD4 count less than 500 could delay onset of AIDS and might prolong survival (though some European data contradict this view). Asymptomatic patients with CD4 counts less than 500 appear to benefit from prophylactic efforts against pneumocystis pneumonia and perhaps toxoplasmosis. Responses to pneumococcal, influenza, and hepatitis vaccines are enhanced if immunization occurs before counts fall. Results from tuberculin skin testing and treatment are improved if management takes place early in the course HIV infection (see Chapters 13 and 49).

TESTING FOR HIV INFECTION

Viral and Immunologic Response to HIV

After transmission of HIV, there is usually a 2- to 4-week period before the acute retroviral syndrome develops (Fig.

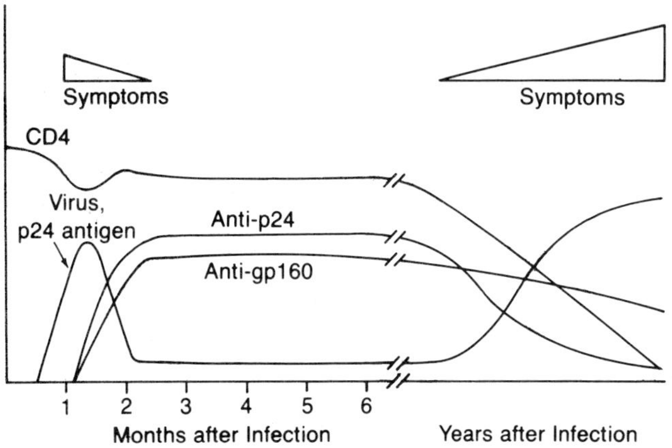

Figure 7-1. Natural history of HIV-1 infection. Adapted from Clark SJ, Saag MS, Decker WD et al. N Engl J Med 324:951.

7–1). This flu-like illness is experienced by 40 percent to 60 percent of infected individuals, lasts 1 to 2 weeks, and resolves spontaneously. Coincident with the acute illness, high-grade viremia develops, usually measured by p24 antigen. Within 2 to 3 weeks from the onset of symptoms, antibodies to envelope glycoproteins and p24 begin to appear. Approximately 50 percent of infected individuals will develop detectable antibody within 2 months, with 95 percent developing antibody within 6 months of initial infection. At about the same time as the appearance of antibody, p24 antigen rapidly declines, usually to undetectable levels. Serum antigen usually remains undetectable until much later in the disease when it reemerges, often in association with signs and symptoms of immune dysfunction. In the vast majority of persons, antibody will remain detectable for life.

Enzyme-Linked Immunosorbent Assay (ELISA or EIA)

ELISA is the screening test of choice in the United States for HIV disease. It has a reported sensitivity in excess of 99.5 percent and a specificity of 99.85 percent. It detects total serum antibodies directed against epitopes of HIV-1. There is also a variant that detects antibodies against HIV-2 proteins. The ELISA uses viral antigens coated onto beads, microwells, or dipsticks to adsorb antibody and trigger an enzyme-linked colorimetric reaction that is proportional to the amount of antibody present. Although the test is easily automated, inexpensive, and well suited for testing large numbers of samples, it has a tendency to nonspecifically bind antibodies and produce excessive *false-positives* in patients exposed to *multiple infections* or *vaccines*. In addition, antibodies to impurities in the antigen preparation can lead to cross-reactions and repeated false-positive tests. This potential to produce false-positive reactions necessitates use of a confirmatory or supplementary test of added specificity.

Western Blot

Patients with a positive ELISA test are candidates for confirmation by Western blot testing. Relative to ELISA, the Western blot is slower, more labor-intensive, and much more expensive, but it is able to measure specific HIV antibodies and enhance the specificity of testing. It detects antibodies directed at specific HIV-1 proteins (core, envelope, polymerase) after their separation by gel electrophoresis. Definition of a positive test relies on the demonstration of bands of antibody from two or three major antigen groups: *gag* (p55,p24,p18), *pol* (p66,p51,p31), and *env* (gp160,gp120, gp41). Although there is no universally accepted definition of a positive Western blot, the Centers for Disease Control and Prevention have established widely accepted criteria for confirming HIV-1 infection using the Western blot:

Positive: at least two of the bands p24,gp51,gp120/160
Negative: no HIV-related bands
Indeterminate: any HIV-related band(s) not meeting the criteria for a positive result.

Other Tests

In addition to ELISA and Western blot testing, there are several other techniques available to test for HIV infection: antibody assays, tests for virus or viral components, and surrogate marker tests. *Rapid antibody screening* tests have been developed for use in endemic areas, but accuracy in low prevalence populations has yet to be established.

Tests for virus or viral components include *virus culture*, *p24 antigen* assay, and *polymerase chain reaction* assays. Culture is time-consuming, costly, difficult to standardize, and relatively insensitive. Assays for p24 antigen are hampered by the low prevalence of the antigen during the asymptomatic phase of HIV infection. Polymerase assays have a high false-positive rate, being very sensitive to the slightest degree of contamination of reagents or test specimen.

Surrogate markers do not test directly for virus or antibody. The most common is the *CD4 count*, which is useful for assessing prognosis and therapeutic decision making (see Chapter 13), but it should not be used as an indirect method of determining whether a patient is HIV-infected. *Beta$_2$-microglobulin* and *neopterin* are other surrogate markers.

Test Interpretation—Minimizing False-Positives and False-Negatives

When testing for the presence of HIV antibodies and interpreting the results, it is necessary to consider the *timing of antibody responses* to HIV infection (see Fig. 7–1), the *sensitivity and specificity* of the ELISA and Western blot tests, and the *pretest probability* of the person being tested. For example, a negative ELISA test in a patient with a pretest probability of 0.1 percent (1 in 1000) virtually rules out the diagnosis of HIV infection. However, the same test result in a person with a 50 percent pretest probability of HIV infection does not drop the posttest probability to zero (in biologic terms, testing might be occurring before appearance of antibody). Conversely, a positive ELISA test result in a person with a low pretest probability (0.1%) produces a posttest probability of only 40 percent, necessitating confirmatory testing.

A major objective is to limit the risk of a *false-positive result* and its potentially adverse psychological and social consequences. *Pretest counseling* is especially important for the low-risk person who needs to be informed of the risk of a false-positive result. It is often advisable to *repeat* a positive ELISA if it occurs in an individual with no identifiable risk factor or from a site that performs anonymous testing. There is always the finite possibility of laboratory error or sample mislabeling. *Confirmatory testing* with the Western blot test is essential and a standard procedure in most laboratories.

A negative Western blot result in the setting of a positive ELISA and a small pretest probability of HIV rules out HIV infection. A positive Western blot following a positive ELISA virtually rules in the diagnosis of HIV infection, even among persons with a low pretest probability, but an "indeterminate" result can be problematic.

Despite the enhanced specificity afforded by adding the Western blot to the testing sequence, a small but important proportion (10%–13%) of individuals with a positive ELISA result will test *"indeterminate."* The most frequent cause of an indeterminate Western blot result is the presence of a single band of antibody, usually against p24. In high-risk individuals, this may reflect ongoing seroconversion. Low-risk persons with this result are virtually never infected. *Repeat testing* should take place within 2 to 6 months of the initial indeterminate result. If the individual is HIV-infected, a positive ELISA will usually be accompanied by two or more positive bands on the Western blot. Among low-risk persons, the single band will frequently persist. In general, low-risk individuals with indeterminate test results should be reassured that HIV infection is extremely unlikely.

False-negative test results most frequently occur when testing occurs during the "window period"—usually 2 to 6 months after viral transmission. Data suggesting high false-negative rates have not been confirmed. Alternative methods of identifying HIV infection are available in cases where further clarification is desirable. These include polymerase chain reaction, viral culture, and detection of p24 antigen. These tests should not be used in place of antibody testing, but occasionally they may be useful as an adjunct.

Repeat Screening

Repeated screening at 6- to 12-month intervals is indicated for those who continue to practice high-risk behavior. An essential part of HIV testing is the provision of HIV counseling. Careful instruction should be given to *all* persons in how to minimize the risk of HIV transmission.

RECOMMENDATIONS

- Patients at high risk for HIV disease should be screened (Table 7–1).
- High-risk patients who are negative but continue high-risk behavior should be rescreened every 6 to 12 months.
- Patients at low risk who are donors of blood, semen, or organs should also be screened.
- Low-risk donors and low-risk persons who desire to know their HIV status should be counseled about the possibility of a false-positive result, especially about an indeterminate Western blot after a positive ELISA.
- Test result interpretation must take into account pretest probability, sensitivity and specificity of testing methods, and timing of the testing in relation to time of possible infection.

Table 7-1. Centers for Disease Control Recommendations for HIV Serologic Testing*

- Persons who have sexually transmitted diseases.
- High-risk individuals: intravenous drug users, sexually active gay and bisexual men, hemophiliacs, regular sexual partners of persons in these categories and persons with known HIV infection; lower incidence groups include prostitutes and persons who received transfusions during 1978–1985.
- Persons who consider themselves at risk or request the test.
- Women at risk who are of child-bearing age or who are pregnant. Women at increased risk include IV drug users; prostitutes; women who have had male sexual partners who are IV drug users, bisexual, or HIV infected; women living in communities or born in countries with a high prevalence in women; and women who received blood transfusion between 1978 and 1985.
- Individuals with clinical or laboratory findings suggesting HIV infection. These include generalized lymphadenopathy; unexplained dementia; chronic, unexplained fever or diarrhea; unexplained weight loss; or diseases that commonly complicate HIV such as chronic or generalized herpes, thrush, and recurrent or refractory vaginal candidiasis, oral hairy leukplakia, and "opportunistic" tumors including Kaposi's sarcoma and B-cell lymphoma.
- Patients with active tuberculosis.
- Recipient and source of blood and body fluid exposures. Body fluids besides blood considered at risk include semen, vaginal secretions, cerebrospinal fluid, synovial fluid, pleural fluid, peritoneal fluid, pericardial fluid, amniotic fluid, and any blood body fluid. Body fluids not considered at risk are feces, nasal secretions, sputum, saliva, sweat, tears, urine, and vomitus unless they contain visible blood.
- Health care workers who perform exposure-prone invasive procedures.
- Patients who are 15–55 years of age and who are admitted to a hospital at which the seroprevalence rate is ≥ 1% or where AIDS patients account for ≥ 1/1000 of discharges.
- Donors of blood, semen, and organs.

*From MMWR Morbid Mortal Wkly Rep 1993: 42(RR-2)1.

- Patient education regarding HIV transmission should be part of every screening effort.

A.H.G.

ANNOTATED BIBLIOGRAPHY

Clark SJ et al. High titers of cytopathic virus in plasma of patients with symptomatic primary HIV-1 infection. N Engl J Med 1991;324:954. (*Natural history of infection.*)

False-positive serologic tests for human T-cell lymphotropic virus type I among blood donors following influenza vaccination, 1992. MMWR Morbid Mortal Wkly Rep 1993;42:173. (*Vaccination increases risk of false-positive ELISA.*)

Higgins DL et al. Evidence for the effects of HIV antibody counseling and testing on risk behaviors. JAMA 1991;266:2419. (*Behavior improves.*)

Horsburgh CRJ et al. Duration of human immunodeficiency virus infection before detection of antibody. Lancet 1989;2:637. (*Window period defined.*)

Jackson JB et al. Absence of HIV infection in blood donors with indeterminate Western blot tests for antibody to HIV-1. N Engl J Med 1990;322:217. (*The meaning of an indeterminate result.*)

Kessler HA et al. Diagnosis of human immunodeficiency virus infection in seronegative homosexuals presenting with an acute viral syndrome. JAMA 1987;258:1196. (*May be seronegative in early phase of illness. Repeat testing is usually positive.*)

O'Gorman MR et al. Interpretive criteria of the Western blot assay for serodiagnosis of human immunodeficiency virus type 1 infection. Arch Pathol Lab Med 1991;115:26. (*Criteria for positive, negative, and indeterminate results; published erratum appears in Arch Pathol Lab Med 1991;115:783.*)

Pan LZ et al. Lack of detection of human immunodeficiency virus in persistently seronegative homosexual men with high or medium risks for infection. J Infect Dis 1991;164:962. (*Refutes false-negative fear.*)

Public Health Service guidelines for counseling and antibody testing to prevent HIV infection and AIDS. MMWR Morbid Mortal Wkly Rep 1987;36:509. (*Recommends testing high-risk persons and identifies groups.*)

Quinn TC. Screening for HIV infection—benefits and costs. N Engl J Med 1992;327:486. (*An editorial focusing on testing patients at time of hospital admission.*)

Recommendations for HIV testing services for inpatients and outpatients in acute-care hospital settings. Centers for Disease Control and Prevention. MMWR Morbid Mortal Wkly Rep 1993;42(RR-2):1. (*Delineates the responsibilities of hospitals toward HIV testing.*)

Technical guidance on HIV counseling. Centers for Disease Control and Prevention. MMWR Morbid Mortal Wkly Rep 1993; 42(RR-2):11. (*Best available information.*)

Update: Universal precautions for prevention of transmission of human immunodeficiency virus, hepatitis B virus, and other bloodborne pathogens in health-care settings. MMWR Morbid Mortal Wkly Rep 1988;37:3771. (*Best advice on preventive measures in health care settings.*)

8
Evaluation of Chronic Fatigue

Primary Care Medicine: Office Evaluation and Management of the Adult Patient, 3rd edition, edited by Allan H. Goroll, Lawrence A. May, and Albert G. Mulley, Jr. J.B. Lippincott Company, Philadelphia

Chronic fatigue ranks as one of the most common complaints in primary care practice, with a reported frequency in excess of 20 percent. It can also be one of the more frustrating problems to assess, because it is a sensitive but nonspecific indicator of underlying medical and/or psychological pathology. Regardless of cause, the patient typically reports a lack of energy, listlessness, and being too tired to participate in family, work, or even leisure activities. Many speculate that they have a vitamin or mineral deficiency and self-treat accordingly before coming for evaluation. Others fear an underlying malignancy, endocrine disorder, or serious infection (eg, human immunodeficiency virus [HIV], tuberculosis, hepatitis, "chronic mono") and request extensive testing.

Most patients bothered by chronic fatigue come to the primary physician looking for an organic cause, especially those with a rather abrupt onset of symptoms. Although most studies of chronic fatigue find the vast majority of cases have a psychological basis (eg, depression), few patients initially report psychological symptoms, and if they do, they view such symptoms as secondary to a medical illness. Attempts by the physician to address psychological issues may be misinterpreted by the patient as not being taken seriously. Thus, the primary physician has the difficult tasks of sorting through a vast number of potential etiologies and patient concerns, determining what proportion of the problem is physiological and what part is psychological, and helping the patient to understand and deal with his illness.

PATHOPHYSIOLOGY AND CLINICAL PRESENTATIONS

Almost all illnesses are capable of causing fatigue; however, a few are noteworthy for the prominence of the symptom in the clinical presentation.

Psychological Etiologies. As just noted, fatigue is an important somatic symptom of *depression,* often coexisting with early morning awakening, appetite and sexual disturbances, and multiple bodily complaints. Abnormalities of central nervous system neurotransmitter metabolism and function are believed to play a major role in the pathogenesis of depression (see Chapter 227). *Chronic anxiety* may result in generalized fatigue, due in part to difficulty in obtaining adequate physical and psychological rest. Patients report trouble falling asleep and a host of associated bodily complaints. Many maintain their neck muscles in constantly tensed states, giving rise to occipital-nuchal headaches. Seemingly unprovoked episodes of palpitations, difficulty breathing, and chest tightness may occur, especially in those whose anxiety is accompanied by a panic disorder (see Chapter 226).

Patients who somatize because of an underlying *personality disorder* may complain of chronic fatigue, often accompanied by a host of other refractory symptoms. Such individuals have a lifelong history of bodily complaints that elude diagnosis and treatment. Their symptoms are a cross they bear in a crude attempt at achieving a modicum of self-esteem (see Chapter 230).

Medications. Many of the medications used to treat anxiety, depression, and insomnia have substantial sedating effects. When used in excess, they may actually worsen the patient's symptoms and sense of fatigue rather than alleviate them. Of the antidepressants, *amitriptyline, doxepin,* and *trazodone* are among the more sedating, which makes them useful when agitation is a problem, but they can also lead to a feeling of being "knocked out" (see Chapter 227). Chronic use of *hypnotics* and withdrawal from them may exacerbate difficulty falling asleep (see Chapter 232). Excessive use of *minor tranquilizers* can cause tiredness, especially when daily doses are sufficient to produce high serum levels of the drug and its active metabolites (see Chapter 226).

Antihypertensives that penetrate the central nervous system (eg, *reserpine, methyldopa, clonidine, propranolol*) may precipitate depression or fatigue. Reserpine can cause depression when used in doses exceeding 0.5 mg per day, especially in patients with a prior history of depression. The same is true for beta-blockers, though fatigue is the more common side effect (see Chapter 26) and a major reason for discontinuing the medication. *Antihistamines* used for allergic rhinitis are another common pharmacologic precipitant of fatigue, especially those that penetrate the central nervous system (eg, *diphenhydramine, chlorpheniramine*).

Endocrine Disturbances are important, treatable precipitants. Dysfunction of the thyroid, adrenal, pituitary, parathyroid, or endocrine pancreas can be subtle in onset, starting out inconspicuously as fatigue, perhaps accompanied by more specific symptoms. For example, *hypothyroidism* may present as fatigue, perhaps in association with weight gain, dry skin, mild hoarseness, or cold intolerance (see Chapter 104). In the elderly, hyperthyroidism may take an atypical form (*apathetic hyperthyroidism*), characterized by fatigue, marked weight loss, apathy, and otherwise unexplained atrial fibrillation (see Chapter 103).

Patients with *Addison's disease* manifest insidious onset of fatigue in conjunction with weight loss, vague gastrointestinal upset, postural hypotension, and eventually, hyperpigmentation. *Panhypopituitarism* from postpartum hemorrhage or a tumor of the sellar region can cause fatigue. The postpartum patient fails to lactate or resume menstruation; lassitude, decreased libido, and loss of axillary and pubic hair ensue. Later, symptoms of hypothyroidism may develop. The patient with a pituitary tumor may note galactorrhea and amenorrhea (see Chapter 100).

Poorly controlled *diabetes mellitus* may present as fatigue accompanied by polyuria when glycosuria is severe enough to produce caloric wasting and volume depletion (see Chapter 102). Similarly, fatigue may be the initial symptom of *hyperparathyroidism* and other causes of hypercalcemia.

Metabolic Disturbances. *Chronic renal failure* may present inconspicuously with fatigue and few localizing symptoms or signs aside from laboratory findings of azotemia, mild anemia, impaired renal concentrating ability, and an abnormal urinary sediment (see Chapter 142). *Hepatocellular failure* is an important source of lassitude. Jaundice, ascites, petechiae, asterixis, spider angiomata, and other signs of hepatic insufficiency usually contribute to the clinical picture. However, in anicteric hepatitis and mild forms of chronic hepatitis, jaundice may be minimal or absent while fatigue is prominent; the same holds for the prodromal phase of acute viral hepatitis (see Chapters 70 and 71).

Hematologic and Oncologic Etiologies. *Iron deficiency* is often blamed for fatigue, although the correlation between iron deficiency anemia and fatigue is poor, especially when the anemia is mild (see Chapter 79). In a double-blind study of menstruating women with mild anemia due to iron deficiency, there was no significant difference between the effects of iron and of placebo on fatigue. The relation between severe anemia (hematocrit < 20) and fatigue is more direct. Lassitude prevails, at times in association with exertional dyspnea or with postural hypotension when blood loss is acute.

Occult malignancy is a much feared etiology. Although fatigue and lassitude accompany most cancers, *pancreatic carcinoma* is the archetypical example of a tumor that may present initially as marked fatigue with few localizing symptoms. Severe weight loss, depression, and apathy may also dominate the clinical picture before other manifestations of the malignancy become evident. Malignancies causing hypercalcemia (eg, breast cancer, myeloma) may present with fatigue, though usually the hypercalcemia is a late development.

Cardiopulmonary Disease. The hallmark of fatigue due to cardiopulmonary disease is a history of exertional dyspnea. Fatigue sometimes dominates the clinical presentation of patients with *chronic congestive heart failure* or *chronic lung disease,* especially when patients with heart failure are treated aggressively for symptoms of pulmonary congestion (see Chapters 32 and 47). Chronic fatigue from disturbed sleep due to *sleep apnea* is an often overlooked etiology. Daytime sleepiness, excessive snoring, irregular breathing, disturbed sleep, and hemoglobin desaturation are characteristic. If untreated, it may progress to pulmonary hypertension (see Chapter 46).

Infectious Diseases. Profound fatigue, low-grade fever, and lymphadenopathy are the hallmarks of a number of much feared infectious etiologies, including *mononucleosis, viral hepatitis,* and *HIV* disease. Other viral illnesses, such as *cytomegalovirus* infection, and the possibly virus-triggered *chronic fatigue syndrome* (see below) may also present in this way. *Tuberculosis* and *subacute bacterial endocarditis* are important infectious etiologies of fatigue in which there may be few localizing symptoms. A history of cough, night sweats, HIV infection, or exposure is sometimes elicited from the patient with tuberculosis (see Chapter 49). Recent dental work, heart murmur and intravenous drug abuse are risk factors for subacute bacterial endocarditis.

Lyme disease is noteworthy for fatigue accompanied by joint complaints, headache, and low-grade fever (see Chapter 160).

Connective Tissue Disease and Other Forms of Immune Dysfunction. Marked fatigue may dominate the initial clinical presentation of most *rheumatoid diseases,* before joint or skin manifestations become evident (see Chapter 156). Symmetrical arthralgias typically involving the metacarpal-phalangeal joints or wrists is another early manifestation.

Chronic fatigue syndrome (CFS) is characterized by abrupt onset of disabling fatigue that persists for at least 6 months in a patient without a prior history of such fatigue. Also reported are low-grade fever, arthralgias, myalgias, sore throat, headache, lymphadenopathy, postexertional malaise, depression, cognitive defects, and disordered sleep. The current Centers for Disease Control and Prevention (CDC) definition of CFS requires eight of these associated symptoms in addition to the new onset of persistent disabling fatigue that reduces functional capacity by 50 percent in a patient who demonstrates no other etiology after thorough investigation. The initial presentation is flu-like, but symptoms persist.

CFS accounts for less than 5 percent of patients presenting with chronic fatigue and predominantly involves patients 20 to 40 years of age. Initial studies of selected patients suggested reactivation of chronic Epstein-Barr virus (EBV) infection, and for a time the condition was referred to in the lay press as "the chronic mononucleosis syndrome." However, further viral, immunologic, and clinical investigations—including those using drugs active against the virus and viral isolation studies—failed to confirm the EBV hypothesis or reveal another infectious agent. Chronic candidiasis had been invoked as an etiology but without substantiation when rigorously investigated.

An association with *fibromyalgia* has been noted, but it is unclear whether it is due to a common pathophysiology or overlapping diagnostic criteria. (See also Chapter 159.)

Though its etiology remains unknown, CFS involves marked activation of the immune system, with high circulating levels of immune complexes, immunoglobulins, activated T cells, macrophages, and atypical lymphocytes. Some view CFS as predominantly a psychiatric condition, given the high prevalence of concurrent psychiatric disease, particularly somatization disorder, found in CFS patients subjected to detailed psychiatric study (range 20%–70%). There is also a trend toward an increased risk of suicidality and a high prevalence of major depression, but no higher than that found in patients with other chronic disabling disease. In addition, the physical manifestations noted above are atypical for such psychiatric disorders as depression or anxiety, and there is little of the anhedonia, guilt, or low motivation that characterizes depression. In fact, these patients are highly motivated and work hard to deal with their illness. A unifying hypothesis allows a wide range of triggering stressors (ranging from psychiatric disease to infection) to produce an exaggerated immunologic response that leads to symptoms. This view leads some to label the condition the "chronic fatigue immune dysfunction syndrome (CFIDS)."

DIFFERENTIAL DIAGNOSIS

Although the list of conditions that may present with fatigue is extensive, most cases have a strong overlay of anxiety and/or depression, even when the cause is medical. Fatigue, of course, may accompany any illness, but those listed in Table 8–1 are notable for the prominence of lassitude in the clinical presentation. In a series of 300 cases of fatigue evaluated at the Lahey Clinic prior to the CFS era, 80 percent were found due to an emotional problem, 4 percent to chronic infection, 3 percent to heart disease, 2 percent to anemia, and 1 percent to nephritis. In a more recent study, CFS has been infrequent among patients with symptoms of persistent fatigue subjected to comprehensive medical and psychological evaluation. It accounted for only 5 percent, with active psychiatric disease accounting for 67 percent, medical disorders for 3 percent, and 25 percent remained indeterminate but not meeting criteria for CFS.

WORKUP

In most instances, the evaluation of fatigue can be conveniently performed in the office. Two or three visits may be

Table 8-1. Some Conditions Presenting as Chronic Fatigue

1. Psychological
   a. Depression
   b. Anxiety
   c. Somatization disorder
2. Pharmacologic
   a. Hypnotics
   b. Antihypertensives
   c. Antidepressants
   d. Tranquilizers
   e. Drug abuse and drug withdrawal
3. Endocrine–Metabolic
   a. Hypothyroidism
   b. Diabetes mellitus
   c. Apathetic hyperthyroidism of the elderly
   d. Pituitary insufficiency
   e. Hyperparathyroidism or hypercalcemia of any origin
   f. Addison's disease
   g. Chronic renal failure
   h. Hepatocellular failure
4. Neoplastic–Hematologic
   a. Occult malignancy (eg, pancreatic cancer)
   b. Severe anemia
5. Infectious
   a. Endocarditis
   b. Tuberculosis
   c. Mononucleosis
   d. Hepatitis
   e. Parasitic disease
   f. HIV infection
   g. Cytomegalovirus
6. Cardiopulmonary
   a. Chronic congestive heart failure
   b. Chronic obstructive pulmonary disease
7. Connective Tissue Disease–Immune Hyperreactivity
   a. Rheumatoid disease
   b. Chronic Fatigue syndrome
8. Disturbed sleep
   a. Sleep apnea
   b. Esophageal reflux
   c. Allergic rhinitis
   d. Psychological etiologies (see above)

needed to establish the underlying etiology; at times the patient may insist that medical illness be ruled out before agreeing to discuss psychosocial matters.

History should begin with a thorough *description of the fatigue* to be sure that the patient is not confusing focal neuromuscular disease with generalized lassitude. Because *depression* underlies many cases of fatigue, it is essential to check for its somatic manifestations, such as early morning awakening, alteration of appetite, and multisystem functional complaints. It is also important to ask about significant losses, low self-esteem, and occurrence of crying spells and suicidal thoughts. *Anxiety* is suggested by unresolved conflict, persistent nervousness, recurrent bouts of excessive uneasiness, and trouble falling asleep. A lifelong history of *refractory bodily complaints* that defy diagnosis and treatment should raise suspicion of a personality disturbance.

Any abuse of *hypnotics* or *tranquilizers* needs to be ascertained and considered as a cause of disturbed sleep and resultant fatigue. Fatigue in the elderly patient should not be ascribed to age; an underlying psychogenic or medical illness is likely.

A history of *fever, sweats, weight loss,* and *adenopathy* points toward smoldering infection and occult neoplasm. Symptoms suggesting a metabolic or endocrinologic cause include *polyuria,* polydipsia, changes in skin pigmentation and texture, hoarseness, *cold intolerance,* nausea, and *abnormal menses.* Symmetrical *joint pain* and morning stiffness are clues to underlying rheumatoid disease.

Checking into factors that might disturb sleep can lead to detection of treatable etiologies such as *sleep apnea* (see Chapter 46); *esophageal reflux* (see Chapter 61); and *allergic rhinitis* (see Chapter 222).

The *past medical history* should be investigated for anemia, rheumatic fever, mononucleosis, heart murmur, recurrent urinary tract infection, proteinuria, liver disease, alcohol and drug abuse, and depression. *Epidemiologic considerations* ought to include exposure to tuberculosis, mononucleosis, and hepatitis; any risk factors for acquired immunodeficiency syndrome (AIDS) are important to note (see Chapter 13). *Travel* to areas where parasitic infections are endemic, work in meat-packing industries or on a farm, and sudden common-source outbreak of illness are other potentially important epidemiologic clues.

A full listing of all the patient's *medications* should be obtained. Often overlooked are over-the-counter antihistamines that patients use for sleep, allergies, and colds. Most centrally acting antihypertensive agents are capable of causing fatigue, and their use should be noted, as should that of all psychotropic agents.

Physical Examination often provides important evidence and needs to be thorough. Vital signs should include *postural pulse and blood pressure* determinations, rectal temperature, and *weight.* If there is no fever on examination in the office but it is suggested by history, then a 10 PM reading at home is indicated. *Skin* is assessed for change in pigmentation, purpura, dryness, rash, jaundice, and pallor. Endocarditis may first be suggested by the finding of splinter hemorrhages or petechiae. *Funduscopic examination* may reveal Roth's spots, diabetic retinopathy, or even, in rare instances, a tuberculoma. The *sclerae* are observed for icterus. If examination of the *pharynx* reveals petechiae at the junction of the hard and soft palate, mononucleosis ought to be considered. The *thyroid* is checked for goiter.

Careful examination of all *lymph nodes* is essential; size, degree of tenderness, and distribution should be noted. Diffuse adenopathy suggests malignancy and infection and is sometimes a sign of the HIV infection (see Chapter 12). *Breasts* should be checked for masses, as breast cancer and its attendant hypercalcemia may present as fatigue. The *lungs* are examined for rales, consolidation, and effusion, and the *heart* for murmurs, rubs, gallops, and rhythm disturbances. Unexplained atrial fibrillation in the elderly may be a manifestation of apathetic hyperthyroidism.

The *abdomen* is palpated for organomegaly, masses, ascites, and hepatic tenderness. *Rectal examination* includes a look for masses, prostatic pathology, and occult blood. *Genitalia* should be checked for masses suggestive of malignancy and tenderness indicative of infection. *Joints* are assessed for signs of inflammation. A complete *neurologic examination* is necessary to be sure that the patient's fatigue is not really a manifestation of neuromuscular disease. Any tenderness, atrophy, focal weakness, or fasciculations in the muscles is noted. Deep tendon reflexes that have a slow relaxation phase are suggestive of hypothyroidism. Even visual field testing is important, for a pituitary lesion may produce a bitemporal hemianopsia. *Mental status assessment* is critical, including observation of affect, thinking, judgment, and memory. Formal testing for suicidality is indicated (see Chapter 227) because of the high prevalence of depression in this patient population.

Laboratory Studies. In the overtly depressed patient with an otherwise completely normal history and physical examination, there is no need to proceed with an extensive laboratory workup for occult medical illness. A *complete blood count* (CBC) and *erythrocyte sedimentation rate* (ESR) are often ordered for screening purposes. The CBC, particularly if accompanied by a look at the peripheral smear and differential, may provide important clues to underlying infection, inflammatory disease, hepatocellular failure, or malignancy. Unfortunately, the ESR has not proven to be sensitive or specific enough to help in detecting or ruling out occult illness. Consequently, many physicians no longer order the ESR, while others continue to use it with the intent of acting on it only if the result is markedly elevated (eg, > 75mm/h).

A particularly difficult situation is the patient with no evidence of depression as a primary cause and an unrevealing history and physical. Here, a few extra serum chemistries (*calcium, albumin, blood urea nitrogen* [*BUN*], *creatinine, glucose,* and *transaminase-aminotransferase*) are warranted to help rule out clinically subtle conditions that may present as fatigue, such as hypercalcemia, mild renal failure, early diabetes mellitus, and anicteric hepatitis. A *thyrotropin (TSH)* test is worth considering, because thyroid disease represents a very treatable cause that can have a very subtle presentation, and the improved TSH assay is very sensitive for detection of most forms of hyper- and hypothyroidism. The elderly fatigued patient with weight loss and unexplained atrial fibrillation is a prime candidate for a TSH determination. Other thyroid indices add little and should not be obtained unless the TSH is abnormal (see Chapters 103 and 104).

Patients with recent onset of persisting fatigue and adenopathy should undergo a *heterophile* test for acute mononucleosis. However, *viral antibody titers* (with the exception of testing for the *viral hepatitis* and *HIV infection*) are of no known utility in patients with undiagnosed chronic fatigue. Testing for viral hepatitis is clearly indicated in those with a transaminase elevation, and HIV testing is appropriate when there is diffuse adenopathy or a history of high-risk behavior.

Ordering a battery of viral antibody titers was popular when CFS was thought to be caused by chronic EBV infection. Lacking an etiologic role for viruses in CFS, viral titers proved to be useless and sometimes misleading, especially when they were "positive" in a patient with severe depression who refused to accept a psychiatric diagnosis. The same holds true for *Candida* and *fungal testing*. *Lyme titers* are also of little use in the absence of other evidence suggestive of Lyme disease, such as polyarthritis, history of tick bite, or erythema chronicum migrans (see Chapter 160).

Diagnosis of Chronic Fatigue Syndrome. There is no diagnostic test for CFS. A CDC working case definition has been developed by consensus to provide a more uniform basis for studying patients with unexplained chronic fatigue. The definition is also used by clinicians, although this was not the original intent, because the definition is somewhat arbitrary in the absence of a known etiology. It is based on clinical findings and the ruling out of other causes of chronic fatigue. Patients must fulfill two major criteria, plus either six symptom criteria and two physical criteria or eight symptom criteria (Table 8–2). Some have argued that such criteria, with their large emphasis on multiple bodily complaints, inadvertently select for patients with somatization disorders. Others note that the definition precludes a concurrent illness in patients with preexisting psychiatric disease. Until the etiology of CFS is better understood, these shortcomings will have to be taken into consideration when using the working definition for diagnostic purposes. (The reader is urged to watch the literature closely for further developments.)

PATIENT EDUCATION

It is often useful to find out the patient's view of his illness before proceeding with patient education so that the explanation will address patient concerns and perspectives. Patients who have a medical view of their condition are more receptive to a biologic explanation for their symptoms, even if the cause is psychogenic. However, one must be careful not to evoke a misleading medical explanation, such as "viral infection," especially in the setting of a suspected psychogenic origin, because this might cause the patient to delay or refuse psychiatric intervention. Patients with evidence of underlying psychogenic disease need an especially thorough review of the evidence for their diagnosis and a careful explanation of their symptoms, because many come to the physician thinking they have a medical problem. For example, reviewing the diagnostic criteria for depression and describing the neurochemical mechanisms by which depression leads to fatigue (see Chapter 227) can be helpful.

The attention given to CFS in the lay press often necessitates addressing the issue of its likelihood and some of its purported, though unfounded, causes (eg, EBV, yeast, vitamin deficiency). Many patients prefer to cling to this diagnosis as an acceptable explanation of their psychophysiologic symptoms rather than face a diagnosis of depression, anxiety, or somatization disorder. In addition to a careful workup, a respectful, sympathetic, open-minded approach is essential (see Chapter 230).

Approach to the CFS Patient. In addition to the measures noted above, the physician should emphasize the legitimacy of the patient's symptoms and summarize the workup, its

Table 8-2. Criteria for Diagnosis of Chronic Fatigue Syndrome
CDC Working Class Definition*

Major Criteria (must meet both)
1. New onset of persistent, relapsing, or debilitating fatigue that impairs daily activity to below 50% of the premorbid level for at least 6 months
2. Exclusion of other physical and psychiatric conditions that could produce similar symptoms

Minor Criteria–Symptoms (must have at least 6 + 2 physical findings or 8 of 11 symptoms)
1. Mild fever
2. Sore throat
3. Painful lymph nodes
4. Unexplained muscle weakness
5. Myalgias
6. Arthralgias
7. Prolonged fatigue after exercise
8. Headaches
9. Neuropsychiatric complaints
10. Sleep disturbance
11. Rapid onset of main symptom complex

Minor Criteria–Physical Findings (must have 2 or 8 of 11 symptoms)
1. Low-grade fever
2. Nonexudative pharyngitis
3. Palpable or tender anterior or posterior cervical or axillary lymph nodes documented by a physician

*Adapted from Holmes GP, Kaplan JE, Gantz NM et al: Chronic fatigue syndrome: A working definition. Ann Intern Med 108:387, 1988.

rationale, and findings. Also useful is a review of the idiopathic nature of the illness (its possible immune mechanism), its nonprogressive nature, and its gradually improving clinical course, with an excellent chance of full recovery.

SYMPTOMATIC RELIEF

When the cause of fatigue is endocrinologic, metabolic, or infectious, treatment needs to be specific and aimed at the underlying condition. Malignancy is often accompanied by a reactive depression that can be helped by development of a strong, supportive *doctor–patient relationship* (see Chapter 87). The fatigue of endogenous depression can be treated with support and tricyclic *antidepressants;* imipramine may be less sedating than amitriptyline (starting dose is 25–50 mg at bedtime, increased by 25–50 mg at a time). The sleep disorder caused by depression may respond well to small doses, with the fatigue dissipating as the patient gets a good night's sleep. Affective changes may not occur at low doses (see Chapter 227).

Anxiety-related fatigue can be difficult to treat. Prescribing antianxiety agents can lead to excessive use and worsening of symptoms (see Chapter 226); however, a brief and limited trial of *benzodiazepine* therapy at bedtime is worth an attempt. For example, 5 mg of chlordiazepoxide can help the patient to fall asleep and get much-needed rest. There is no evidence that any one benzodiazepine is superior to any other for sleep, although flurazepam is widely promoted and prescribed, often in conjunction with another benzodiazepine. (This can sometimes lead to excessive benzodiazepine intake.) Once symptomatic control of anxiety is accomplished, work can begin on helping the patient to deal with his or her problems.

If fatigue results from disturbed sleep due to sleep apnea, reflux, or allergic rhinitis, then treatment should be directed toward the underlying pathophysiology (see Chapters 46, 61, and 222).

Chronic Fatigue Syndrome. There are no therapies that provide prompt relief from symptoms. A gentle *exercise program* combined with *low-dose antidepressant therapy* (amitriptyline 25 mg qhs or doxepin 10–20 mg qhs) seems to help some patients, especially those bothered by disordered sleep. Higher doses do not appear to confer better results. Experience with fluoxetine (Prozac) and sertraline (Zoloft) is limited, though low doses appear to be best. *Nonsteroidal anti-inflammatory agents* provide symptomatic relief in patients bothered by myalgias, arthralgias, or headache.

A host of enthusiastic reports from uncontrolled studies has appeared claiming marked benefit from liver extract, antifungal therapy, antiviral drugs, vitamins, immunoglobulin infusions, fatty acids, and so on. Most of these observations are not confirmed when such therapies are subjected to randomized, double-blind, placebo-controlled study. The initially favorable results appear secondary to a marked placebo response. Definitive therapy will have to await a better understanding of the condition's etiology and pathophysiology. Fortunately, it appears that symptoms are self-limited, usually clearing within 12 to 18 months. A strong *patient–doctor alliance* is essential, not only for providing support, but also for protecting the patient from unnecessary testing and unproven therapies.

A.H.G.

ANNOTATED BIBLIOGRAPHY

Aurbach G, Mallette L, Patten B et al. Hyperparathyroidism: Recent studies. NIH conference. Ann Intern Med 1973;79:566. (*Fatigue headed the list of symptoms reported in 57 cases of primary hyperparathyroidism; 24 percent reported the problem.*)

Croog SH, Levine S, Testa A et al. The effects of antihypertensive therapy on the quality of life. N Engl J Med 1986;314:1657. (*Methyldopa and propranolol were associated with fatigue and lethargy in about 5 percent of patients.*)

Dismukes WE, Wade JS, Lee JY et al. A randomized, double-blind trial of nystatin therapy for the candidiasis hypersensitivity syndrome. N Engl J Med 1990;323:1717. (*Strong evidence against yeast infection as the cause for the chronic fatigue syndrome.*)

Gold D, Bowden R, Sixbey J et al. Chronic fatigue: A prospective clinical and virologic study. JAMA 1990;264:48. (*Isolation of EBV was no more frequent from patients with chronic fatigue than it was from healthy controls, and improvement in chronic fatigue patients was not associated with any change in EBV levels.*)

Goldenberg DL, Simms RW, Geiger A, Komaroff AL. High frequency of fibromyalgia in patients with chronic fatigue syndrome seen in a primary care practice. Arthritis Rheum 1990;33:381. (*An interesting association, but significance unclear.*)

Holmes GP, Kaplan JE, Gantz NM et al. Chronic fatigue syndrome: A working case definition. Ann Intern Med 1988;108:387. (*An important consensus paper on diagnostic criteria for chronic fatigue syndrome in the absence of a definitive diagnostic test.*)

Kales A, Bixler E, Tan T et al. Chronic hypnotic use: Ineffectiveness, drug withdrawal, insomnia, and hypnotic drug dependence. JAMA 1974;227:513. (*Chronic hypnotic use may actually worsen the problem of sleeplessness and fatigue.*)

Kaslow JE, Rucker L, Onishi R. Liver extract-folic acid-cyanocobalamin vs placebo for chronic fatigue syndrome. Arch Intern Med 1989;149:2501. (*A double-blind, placebo-controlled, crossover study showing no benefit.*)

Katon W, Russo J. Chronic fatigue syndrome criteria: A critique of the requirement for multiple physical complaints. Arch Intern Med 1992;152:1604. (*A study of 285 patients, finding a high prevalence of patients with lifetime psychiatric illness inadvertently selected by requiring multiple bodily complaints in the working CDC definition.*)

Kendell RE. Chronic fatigue, viruses, and depression. Lancet 1991;337:160. (*An editorial summing up the evidence. Favors the view that most have depression and a few might have some kind of post-viral syndrome.*)

Khan AS, Heneine WM, Chapman LE et al. Assessment of a retrovirus sequence and other possible risk factors for the chronic fatigue syndrome in adults. Ann Intern Med 1993;118:241. (*Evidence ruling-out retrovirus infection or HIV-type risk factors as causative.*)

Kroenke K, Wood DR, Mangelsdorff et al. Chronic fatigue in primary care. JAMA 1988;260:929. (*Documents a high prevalence, persistence, and functional impairment.*)

Komaroff AL, Buchwald D. Symptoms and signs of chronic fatigue syndrome. Rev Infect Dis 1991;13(suppl 1):8S. (*Best summary of clinical presentation.*)

Manu P, Lane TJ, Matthews DA. The frequency of the chronic fatigue syndrome in patients with symptoms of persistent fatigue. Ann Intern Med 1988;109:554. (*The prevalence was only 5 percent, indicating the condition is actually quite uncommon among those presenting with fatigue.*)

Sox HC, Liang MH. The erythrocyte sedimentation rate. Ann Intern Med 1986;104:515. (*A critical review arguing the test is not a useful screening procedure.*)

Strauss SE. Defining the chronic fatigue syndrome. Arch Intern Med 1992;152:1569. (*An editorial discussing problems with the current definition of CFS.*)

Straus SE. History of chronic fatigue syndrome. Rev Infect Dis 1991;13(suppl 1):S2. (*Nice historical review, indicating this is not a new condition.*)

Straus SE, Dale JK, Tobi M et al. Acyclovir treatment of the chronic fatigue syndrome: Lack of efficacy in a placebo-controlled trial. N Engl J Med 1988;319:1692. (*Acyclovir did not work; strong evidence against EBV infection as the cause of the syndrome.*)

Thomas F, Mazzaferri E, Skillman T. Apathetic thyrotoxicosis: A distinctive clinical and laboratory entity. Ann Intern Med 1970;72:679. (*A classic paper identifying the condition; patients are typically elderly, depressed, and exhibit marked weight loss and otherwise unexplained atrial fibrillation.*)

Wood M, Elwood P. Symptoms of iron deficiency anemia: A community survey. Br J Prev Soc Med 1966;20:117. (*Correlation between hemoglobin concentration and symptoms was poor; iron therapy produced no statistically significant improvement in symptoms.*)

9
Evaluation of Weight Loss

Primary Care Medicine: Office Evaluation and Management of the Adult Patient, 3rd edition, edited by Allan H. Goroll, Lawrence A. May, and Albert G. Mulley, Jr. J.B. Lippincott Company, Philadelphia

Involuntary weight loss is a sensitive, though nonspecific, symptom; it often suggests the presence of serious pathology, yet a substantial fraction of patients turn out to be free of organic illness. For example, in a series of patients with involuntary weight loss followed for 1 year, 50 percent either died or deteriorated over the course of the study; however, another 35 percent were well at the time of follow-up. Involuntary weight loss in excess of 2.5 kg is usually considered a reasonable threshold for evaluation, as more than 95 percent of patients with an organic etiology will have lost at least that much weight. However, unless extreme, the amount of weight loss is not predictive of an organic etiology. In many cases of weight loss, accompanying symptoms readily suggest the cause, but when a marked fall in weight is the sole or predominant complaint, the assessment can be difficult. The primary physician needs to determine at the time of initial presentation who requires an extensive medical evaluation and who can be followed expectantly.

PATHOPHYSIOLOGY AND CLINICAL PRESENTATION

When the number of calories available for utilization falls below daily needs, weight is lost; 1 lb of fat is consumed for every 3500-calorie deficit. The principal mechanisms resulting in caloric deficits are reduced food intake, malabsorption, excess nutrient loss, and increased caloric requirements. Loss of fluid will also register as a fall in weight, with about 1 kg (2.2 lb) lost for every liter removed. Although more than one mechanism may be operating in a given case, each mechanism has a few characteristic clinical features. Anorexia or disinterest in food typifies causes of *reduced intake*. Foul-smelling, bulky, greasy stools are seen in the later stages of *malabsorption;* subtle changes in stool consistency and frequency are noted earlier (see Chapter 64). Recurrent vomiting, profuse diarrhea, polyuria, or fistulous drainage can lead to *excessive loss*. Increased food intake, hyperactivity, and fever are prominent in cases of *increased demand*.

Many conditions associated with weight loss are clinically obvious and require little discussion, but others may be subtle in presentation, with few obvious manifestations beyond a substantial fall in weight. Anorexia nervosa, carcinoma of the pancreas, early malabsorption, apathetic hyperthyroidism of the elderly, and diabetes are examples of illnesses that sometimes fall into the latter category and deserve further elaboration. In addition, acquired immunodeficiency syndrome (AIDS) presents a new set of challenges in the evaluation of involuntary weight loss.

In the elderly, a host of social and psychological issues may be operative yet defy identification unless examined for specifically.

The patient suffering from *anorexia nervosa* may deny any disturbance of appetite yet persist in restricting food intake to the point of cachexia. The condition occurs predominantly among adolescent girls and young women. They decide to diet to an extreme degree, are preoccupied with a phobic concern about being fat, and are motivated by a relentless pursuit of thinness. Dieting persists because its psychological gratifications outweigh those derived from the intake of food. Paradoxically, the patient often reports feeling well and initially appears bright and undisturbed by the weight loss; anorexia is usually denied. At times, a few specific foods are the only ones consumed (eg, vegetable juices). Amenorrhea is invariable and appears shortly after weight loss begins. A variant of anorexia nervosa consists of surreptitiously induced vomiting following engorgement with food; hypokalemic alkalosis results (see Chapter 234).

Carcinoma of the pancreas is the prototypical neoplasm associated with dramatic weight loss. Mean age of onset is 55; males outnumber females 2 to 1. There are about 9.5 cases per 100,000 population. Weight loss is found in 79 percent to 90 percent at time of diagnosis and averages 15 to 20 lb. The degree of weight loss does not seem to correlate with size, location, or extent of disease. For example, in a series of 100 cases, eight patients had resectable tumors; of the eight, two had weight losses of 25 and 40 lb, respectively.

Aversion to food is more typical of this malignancy than is true anorexia. In many instances, weight loss precedes all other symptoms; once jaundice and abdominal pain supervene, the tumor is usually far advanced. Many other gastrointestinal (GI) malignancies follow a similar clinical course.

In addition to occult malignancy, a host of other conditions may present predominantly with weight loss due to an appetite disturbance; these are described elsewhere: depression (see Chapter 227), alcoholism (see Chapter 228), the prodrome of viral hepatitis (see Chapter 70), hypercalcemia (see Chapter 96), uremia (see Chapter 142), hypokalemia, and digitalis excess (see Chapter 32).

Most patients with *human immunodeficiency virus (HIV) infection* come to experience weight loss; the spectrum of etiologies is wide. The cause may be inadequate intake due to dysphagia, depression, or medication. Early satiety is another mechanism that may result from GI invasion by lymphoma, Kaposi's sarcoma, or *Mycobacterium avium-intracellulare* (MAI). Weight loss in the setting of adequate caloric intake suggests disseminated infection by MAI or *cytomegalovirus* as well as occult malignancy. Often, the later stages of *AIDS* are characterized by a *wasting syndrome,* which includes loss of more than 10 percent of baseline weight, recurrent fever, and persistent diarrhea in the absence of alternative explanations (see Chapter 13).

Marked weight loss is a late sign of *malabsorption,* but modest reductions can occur in the early stages of illness when stools are noted to be a bit softer and more frequent than usual. Steatorrhea, abdominal discomfort, bloating, and pain accompany more dramatic falls in weight when disease is farther advanced. Early *Crohn's disease* in adolescents has been noted on occasion to begin inconspicuously with anorexia predominating. For example, in a small series of 11 adolescent girls labeled as having anorexia nervosa, three were shown to have Crohn's disease when barium studies were obtained. *Blind loop syndrome* and *giardiasis* may also have indolent presentations with weight loss and vague abdominal discomfort; however, changes in stools are usually present as well, with patients reporting mushy, foul-smelling bowel movements (see Chapter 58).

Increased caloric demand due to hyperthyroidism is usually obvious; however, *apathetic hyperthyroidism* of the elderly may be mistaken for malignancy because weight loss is profound and the patient appears listless. The typical symptoms of excess thyroid hormone are absent, and unexplained atrial fibrillation is often present (see Chapter 103).

Although *diabetes mellitus* is commonly found in overweight adults, it may be the cause of weight loss when there is substantial wasting of calories due to a poorly controlled glycosuria. Young male insulin-dependent diabetics are sometimes plagued by diarrhea, which exacerbates fluid and nutrient losses; true malabsorption has been noted in a few (see Chapter 102).

In the elderly, cancer is most often feared, but psychosocial factors leading to inadequate intake are more likely. Bereavement, social isolation, poverty, and dementia can be important etiologies, as can immobility, poor dentition, side effects of medication, and decrease in sense of taste.

Patients with an underlying medical cause for their weight loss usually present with symptoms and signs that strongly suggest organic illness. In a Veterans Administration (VA) medical center study of 91 patients with involuntary weight loss, the overwhelming majority were readily diagnosed on the basis of initial history and physical examination; only one patient had a truly occult malignancy (see below).

DIFFERENTIAL DIAGNOSIS

The extensive number of causes of weight loss can be grouped pathophysiologically. Decreased intake, impaired absorption, increased loss, and excess demand are the principal mechanisms around which the differential can be organized (Table 9–1). Almost any illness can cause involuntary weight loss; the table emphasizes those conditions seen in the ambulatory setting that may present as unexplained loss of weight. Data are scarce on the frequency of etiologies. The VA study of 91 patients with weight loss included both hospitalized and ambulatory patients. Cancer was the most common cause (19%); GI disease ranked second (14%); psychiatric and cardiac problems, third (9%); nutritional/alcoholic, fourth (8%); followed by pulmonary, endocrine, and infectious causes. After a full medical evaluation and 1 year

Table 9-1. Some Important Causes of Weight Loss

A. Decreased intake
   1. HIV infection, AIDS
   2. Depression, bereavement
   3. Anxiety
   4. Poor dentition, loss of taste
   5. Esophageal disease
   6. Gastrointestinal disease worsened by food (eg, peptic ulcer)
   7. Drugs (eg, digitalis excess, Quinidine, amphetamines, NSAIDs, antitumor agents)
   8. Hypercalcemia
   9. Alcoholism
   10. Prodrome of viral hepatitis
   11. Hypokalemia
   12. Uremia
   13. Malignancy
   14. Chronic congestive heart failure
   15. Chronic inflammatory disease
   16. Anorexia nervosa
   17. Social isolation, poverty
   18. Dementia
B. Impaired absorption
   1. Cholestasis
   2. Pancreatic insufficiency
   3. Postgastrectomy
   4. Small bowel disease
   5. Parasitic infection (eg, giardiasis)
   6. Blind loop syndrome
   7. Drugs (eg, cholestyramine, cathartics)
   8. AIDS
C. Increased nutrient loss
   1. Uncontrolled diabetes mellitus
   2. Persistent diarrhea
   3. Recurrent vomiting
   4. Drainage from a fistulous tract
D. Excess demand
   1. Hyperthyroidism
   2. Fever
   3. Malignancy
   4. Emotional states (eg, manic disease)
   5. Amphetamine abuse

of follow-up, 26 percent were listed as having no apparent physical cause.

In a study of 45 patients with involuntary weight loss from seven primary care practices, depression was the most common cause (18%), followed by cancer (16%) and noncancerous GI disease (11%). Of note, 24 percent remained undiagnosed after 2 years of extensive medical evaluation and follow-up. Psychosocial factors are believed to contribute to many such cases.

WORKUP

Because the workup of weight loss can be arduous, it is helpful, when possible, to first identify those patients *likely to have a medical etiology* and spare the remainder a major medical evaluation. The VA group developed a decision rule using the data available from the initial history and physical examination to help select those patients for whom further investigation is warranted.

In their study they found that out of 123 clinical attributes tested, 6 proved to be independent diagnostic predictors of a medical cause for weight loss. These predictors included *nausea or vomiting*, a *cough* that had recently changed, and an *abnormal physical examination* (cachexia, abdominal mass, adenopathy, thyromegaly, etc.). Conversely, patients who proved to have a relatively benign etiology had fewer than 20 pack-years of smoking, no decrease in activities due to fatigue, no nausea or vomiting, normal physical examination, no recent change in appetite, and no history of cough that had recently changed. Screening laboratory studies were only weak predictors.

A discriminant rule was developed using these predictors. Its error rate was 12 percent; it misclassified 9 of 32 patients who proved not to have a physical etiology and 2 of 59 with a medical cause for weight loss. Thus, a good estimate of the probability of a serious underlying etiology was made on the basis of a careful initial history and physical examination. It is important to note that this decision rule was developed and tested in a VA medical center setting, where most of the patients are male and many were inpatients. The decision rule might not be as valid among other outpatient populations. Nevertheless, the study suggests that patients with no evidence of a physical etiology by history and physical examination are likely to have a good prognosis. They might be more profitably evaluated first for a psychiatric cause or poor caloric intake, rather than be subjected to extensive diagnostic testing in search of an occult malignancy or other serious medical pathology.

History

The first task is to document that weight loss has indeed occurred and to determine its extent. In the VA report, almost half of the patients considered for study did not prove to have weight loss when available records were checked. In the absence of recorded weights, meaningful historical data include change in clothing size, ability to give exact weight change, and confirmation of history by a family member.

History can be used to help identify the mechanism(s) responsible for the decline in weight by obtaining the details of daily food intake (including calorie count) and inquiring into the presence of any appetite disturbance, dysphagia, odynophagia, steatorrhea, diarrhea, vomiting, polyuria, or symptoms of a hypermetabolic state.

When *decreased intake* is suspected, one needs to inquire into somatic symptoms of depression (see Chapter 227), excessive use of alcohol (see Chapter 228), poor dentition, fever, oral candidiasis, aphthous ulcers, discomfort induced by eating, early satiety, drug use, history of renal disease, symptoms of heart failure, melena, abdominal pain, anxiety, and exposure to hepatitis. If the patient is a young woman, anorexia nervosa should be considered, and inquiry into eating habits, self-image, and attitudes about weight is worthwhile. Family members should be questioned as well. Review of HIV status and attendant risk factors and associated symptoms should be carried out (see Chapter 13).

In the elderly, questions about social isolation, bereavement, physical impairment, poor dentition, and poverty can be of critical importance to identifying impediments to adequate food intake. Review of drug use in the elderly is also essential because of the large number of medications prescribed and their potential for inducing anorexia and GI upset. Loss of taste is sometimes responsible for poor intake in the elderly and should be checked for.

When *impairment of absorption* is suspected, inquiries are made into previous GI surgery, the character of the stools, jaundice, history of pancreatitis, travel to an area known for giardiasis or other parasites, symptoms of inflammatory bowel disease (see Chapter 73), easy bruising, paresthesias, and sore tongue. Increased nutrient loss is assessed historically by ascertaining the quality and quantity of material lost as well as the frequency and duration of the condition. Of major importance is checking for symptoms of diabetic enteropathy (diarrhea in conjunction with polyuria and polydipsia).

When *excess demand* is under consideration, the patient needs to be questioned about fever, malignancy, symptoms of hyperthyroidism, amphetamine abuse (see Chapter 235), chronic anxiety (see Chapter 226), manic states, and HIV disease (see Chapter 13).

Physical Examination

The examination should begin with an accurate weight determination, followed by noting any wasting, apathetic appearance, fever, tachycardia, pallor, ecchymoses, jaundice, stigmata of hyperthyroidism or hepatocellular failure, or signs of Kaposi's sarcoma. Next, the head and neck are examined for glossitis, stomatitis, poor dentition, goiter, and lymphadenopathy. The lungs and heart are examined for crackles, wheezes, consolidation, effusion, cardiomegaly, murmur, and S3. The abdomen is studied for surgical scars, organomegaly, hyperactive bowel sounds, focal tenderness, distention, ascites, and masses. The rectum is examined for masses, tenderness, discharge, blood, and the appearance of the stool. The neurologic examination includes a check for signs of vitamin B_{12} deficiency suggestive of terminal ileal disease (see Chapter 79) as well as any tremor, manic or depressive affect, or signs of dementia.

Laboratory Testing

Because the number of potential investigations is enormous, laboratory testing should be selective to avoid being wasteful, burdensome, and misleading. History and physical examination will usually identify the basic mechanism(s) of weight loss and suggest specific causes that can be confirmed or ruled out by further investigation. Patients with a perfectly normal physical examination and a history devoid of any symptoms suggestive of serious underlying medical illness are at low risk. It is reasonable to watch them for a month and not immediately initiate an extensive laboratory workup. They should be given nutritional advice and a follow-up appointment for 4 weeks and asked to keep a diary of food intake and weight.

Decreased Intake. When the precise cause of decreased intake remains obscure, it is worth obtaining a *complete blood count* and *smear* (for evidence of a nutritional anemia); a few selected serum chemistries (*calcium, albumin, potassium, transaminase, blood urea nitrogen* [*BUN*], and *creatinine*); and a serum *drug level* if the patient is taking a digitalis preparation, quinidine, or other drug that can cause GI upset if serum levels become markedly elevated. In the aforementioned study of the elderly, esophagogastroduodenoscopy (EGD) and upper GI series were of surprisingly high yield in patients presenting with unexplained weight loss. A number of silent benign peptic ulcers were discovered in this fashion. In the HIV-infected patient, EGD may be necessary to document upper GI mucosal erosion.

Impaired Absorption. Stool should be obtained for gross and microscopic examination and guaiac testing performed. A *qualitative stool fat* examination, in which fecal material is stained for neutral fat, is a basic step in the workup of suspected malabsorption. If doubt persists, a 72-hour stool collection for *quantitative stool fat* provides more precise information, with less than 8 g per day ruling out malabsorption. *Serum carotene* level is another useful marker of fat absorption. Its absorption is independent of pancreatic function, so that a normal level in the setting of malabsorption suggests pancreatic dysfunction. Similarly, the D-*xylose* test can help distinguish pancreatic dysfunction from small bowel disease, because D-xylose absorption also does not require pancreatic enzyme activity (see Chapter 74). An elevated *serum amylase* or radiologic demonstration of *pancreatic calcification* indicate pancreatitis (see Chapter 72), but a *secretin stimulation test* may be necessary to better assess pancreatic exocrine function. Sprue and blind loop syndrome are the most common forms of small bowel pathology responsible for malabsorption. A small bowel radiologic *contrast study* might be suggestive, but a *small bowel biopsy* is necessary for the diagnosis of sprue; an abnormal *C14 glycolate breath test* will help document bacterial overgrowth, though usually the test is unnecessary.

For diagnosis of *giardiasis*, a *stool sample for ova and parasites* suffices in many instances. Because parasites are passed intermittently, three or more stools on alternate days should be examined. Because the cysts are hardy, a fresh stool specimen is not required. Trophozoites are more likely to be found in acute cases. Examination of a duodenal aspirate or jejunal biopsy is resorted to when suspicion is high but stools are negative. Although these tests are more productive, they are cumbersome; some clinicians instead advocate a diagnostic trial of an antigiardial drug such as metronidazole.

Increased Nutrient Loss. Laboratory assessment should include testing for significant glycosuria.

Excess Demand. Suspicion of hyperthyroidism necessitates *thyrotropin (TSH)* determination, especially in the elderly apathetic patient with unexplained atrial fibrillation and weight loss (see Chapter 103). In the febrile HIV patient with adequate caloric intake, the weight loss is likely due to excessive demand, necessitating *cultures* of blood and stool for *acid-fast bacilli* and of blood and urine for *cytomegalovirus*.

One of the most difficult diagnostic issues encountered in the workup of weight loss concerns the possibility of *occult malignancy*. Deciding when to embark on a search for tumor requires an estimate not only of the likelihood of finding a malignancy but also of the chances that it will be treatable. Unfortunately, by the time weight loss has occurred, most GI malignancies are rather far advanced. When weight loss is the only symptom, pancreatic carcinoma may still be resectable if no other symptoms have appeared. *Abdominal ultrasonography* and *computed tomography (CT) scanning* have improved case detection in some settings but not in others. Impact on survival remains to be realized (see Chapter 76). In the primary care study of elderly patients with undiagnosed weight loss, CT scanning was of very low yield in the absence of clinical evidence of an underlying lesion.

SYMPTOMATIC THERAPY

The first task is to be sure food is available to the patient, particularly the elderly person who may be too isolated, impoverished, infirm, or depressed to take in adequate calories. It is estimated that 10 percent to 15 percent of elderly persons take in less than 1000 kcal/day. Ensuring at least one hot meal per day is essential and can usually be arranged with the help of local social service agencies.

Most medical causes of weight loss require correction of the etiology and cannot be readily treated symptomatically. However, there are important exceptions to this generalization. Sometimes the severe anorexia associated with malignancy or use of antitumor agents can be overcome by pharmacologic means (see Chapter 91). The poor intake seen with hepatitis can be improved by providing small, frequent feedings, especially in the morning when nausea is less severe (see Chapter 70). Appetite disturbances associated with depression are often amenable to tricyclic therapy (see Chapter 227). Maldigestion due to pancreatic insufficiency can be compensated for by use of oral pancreatic enzyme preparations (see Chapter 72). The bacterial overgrowth of blind loop syndrome responds to oral broad-spectrum antibiotic therapy (eg, tetracycline 250 mg qid or amoxicillin 250 mg tid) for multiple 10-day courses or for 3 or 4 days each week indefinitely. Caloric supplements in the form of medium-chain triglyceride and dextrose preparations can provide marked improvement when there is severe fat and carbohydrate maldigestion or malabsorption. Initially, 3 ounces are given with each meal; gradually this is increased to 6 ounces, including supplements between meals. If sprue is suspected, a gluten-free diet can be tried empirically.

Fat-soluble vitamin supplements are also needed in cases of malabsorption to prevent malnutrition, even though caloric intake may be replenished. The fat-soluble vitamins A, D, and K are the most likely to be depleted. Dosage requirements in such cases are 25,000 units to 50,000 units per day for vitamin A, 30,000 units for vitamin D, and 4 mg to 12 mg for oral vitamin K. Monthly vitamin B_{12} injections of 1000 g are needed for terminal ileal disease presenting with megaloblastic anemia (see Chapter 82). Control of excessive vomiting and diarrhea is discussed in Chapters 59 and 64, respectively.

INDICATIONS FOR REFERRAL AND ADMISSION

Anyone with a weight loss in excess of 15 kg is likely to have a life-threatening condition and requires prompt hospitalization. The AIDS patient with unexplained weight loss may also benefit from some form of inpatient care while undergoing further evaluation. Any person with substantial weight loss suspected of having anorexia nervosa should be hospitalized and seen by a psychiatrist experienced in dealing with anorectics, because this too may be a life-threatening condition (see Chapter 234). When malabsorption is documented by 72-hour stool fat assessment, consultation with a gastroenterologist should coincide with proceeding to further assessment. The HIV patient with weight loss can certainly be evaluated by the primary care physician provided he is familiar with the evaluation of such patients. Otherwise, referral is indicated.

A.H.G.

ANNOTATED BIBLIOGRAPHY

Bach MC, Howell DA, Valenti AJ. Aphthous ulceration of the gastrointestinal tract in patients with AIDS. Ann Intern Med 1990;112:465. (*An important cause of decreased intake from odynophagia and dysphagia.*)

DeWys W. Management of cancer cachexia. Semin Oncol 1985; 313:84. (*A useful approach to the evaluation and management of persistent weight loss in the cancer patient.*)

Greene JB. Clinical approach to weight loss in the patient with AIDS. Gastroenterol Clin North Am 1988;17:573. (*A very useful algorithm for guiding the potentially complex workup in the AIDS patient.*)

King CE, Toskes PP. Breath tests in the diagnosis of small intestine bacterial overgrowth. Crit Rev Clin Lab Sci 1984;21;269. (*A critical review of breath tests, their indications, and limitations.*)

Kotler DP. Intestinal and hepatic manifestations of AIDS. Adv Intern Med 1989;34;43. (*A detailed review of the many gastrointestinal problems that might result in weight loss in the AIDS patient; extensive list of references.*)

Marton KI, Sox HC, Krupp JR. Involuntary weight loss: Diagnostic and prognostic significance. Ann Intern Med 1981;5: 568. (*A prospective study attempting to identify predictors of serious pathology and poor prognosis.*)

Morley JE, Silver AJ, Fiatarone M et al. Nutrition and the elderly. J Am Geriatr Soc 1986;34:823. (*A review of critical factors that are often overlooked.*)

Ryan ME, Olsen WA. A diagnostic approach to malabsorption syndromes. Clin Gastroenterol 1983;12:533. (*A pathophysiologic approach.*)

Schiffman SS, Warwick ZS. Flavor enhancement of foods for the elderly can reverse anorexia. Neurobiol Aging 1988;9:24. (*A very practical idea.*)

Schwabe AD, Lippe BM, Chang RJ et al. Anorexia nervosa. Ann Intern Med 1981;94:371. (*A comprehensive review.*)

Thomas FB, Massaferri EL, Skillman TG. Apathetic thyrotoxicosis: A distinctive clinical and laboratory entity. Ann Intern Med 1970;72:679. (*Classic article describing this syndrome, which is characterized by marked weight loss, apathy, and unexplained atrial fibrillation in the elderly.*)

Thompson MP, Morris LK. Unexplained weight loss in the ambulatory elderly. J Am Geriatr Soc 1991;39:497. (*A study of patients from seven primary care centers; depression the most common cause; malignancy next; many cases remained undiagnosed; CT scan low in yield.*)

10
Evaluation of Excessive Weight Gain and Obesity

CAROLYN J. CRIMMINS HINTLIAN, M.P.H., R.D.

Primary Care Medicine: Office Evaluation and Management of the Adult Patient, 3rd edition, edited by Allan H. Goroll, Lawrence A. May, and Albert G. Mulley, Jr. J.B. Lippincott Company, Philadelphia

Excess weight and excessive weight gain are nearly universal afflictions of modern life. When weight seems out of proportion to a patient's perceived food intake, the patient comes in wondering about an underlying medical cause. In the vast majority of patients, the observed weight gain is a consequence of consuming too many calories. Nevertheless, the primary physician needs to be skilled in the evaluation of weight gain and obesity, because effective management requires a careful understanding of what is driving the patient's food intake and metabolism. In addition, the assessment needs to address the potentially serious complications of being too fat.

Obesity is a pathologic state characterized by the accumulation of fat in excess of that necessary for optimal body function. The condition is a major public health problem, with an estimated 34 million Americans aged 20 to 74 being 20 percent or more above their "ideal" weight as defined by insurance company actuarial studies. Of those identified as obese, 90 percent are characterized as *mildly obese* (20%–40% above ideal weight), 9 percent are *moderately obese* (40%–100% above ideal weight), and 0.5 percent or 1.7 million American adults are *morbidly obese* (> 100% or > 100 lbs. overweight). The prevalence of obesity is higher with advancing age and with decreasing socioeconomic status. Recent statistics indicate that the average weight of the general U.S. population, particularly that of men of the same height, has been increasing over the last few decades.

Obesity costs billions of dollars annually when medical complications, lost wages, and expenditures for weight reduction efforts are taken into account. Obese persons may or may not be fat for psychological reasons, but their obesity can be the cause of untold psychic pain and physical discomfort. Morbid obesity is a health hazard with 12-fold increase in mortality for persons aged 25 to 34. The earlier the onset of overweight in adult life (eg, ages 20–29), the more pronounced an effect it has on mortality later in life. The most important medical complication of obesity is an increase in mortality from coronary artery disease, due to the development or exacerbation of such cardiac risk factors as adult-onset diabetes, hypertension, and hyperlipidemia. The Framingham heart study illustrated that obesity is a significant *independent* predictor of cardiovascular disease. The Nurses' Health Study also concluded that obesity is a strong risk factor for coronary heart disease in middle-aged women. Obesity is associated with increased incidences of impaired pulmonary function (including sleep apnea), surgical risk, osteoarthritis, gallbladder disease, and cancer mortality.

The severe health consequences and high prevalence of obesity place considerable responsibility on the primary physician to effectively evaluate and manage the patient who presents with excessive weight or marked weight gain. This chapter focuses on the diagnostic evaluation; see Chapter 233 for the approach to treatment.

PATHOPHYSIOLOGY AND CLINICAL PRESENTATION

In the simplest sense, obesity results when intake of food exceeds caloric needs. Why this happens is usually far from clear, inasmuch as the mechanisms responsible for alteration of appetite and caloric needs and stimulation of excessive food intake are still not well understood. The hypothalamus plays a role in the regulation of appetite. Destructive lesions of the ventromedial nucleus lead to appetite arousal, including hyperphagia. A lateral but less well-defined region of the hypothalamus seems to be responsible for integration of food-selecting behavior: injury to this region can result in aphagia and inactivity in other spheres.

A small fraction of obese patients have an identifiable genetic, neurologic, or endocrinologic disorder. More often, psychological, developmental, dietary, exertional, socio-occupational, and pharmacologic factors operate and interact in a complex fashion to precipitate weight gain.

Psychological Factors. Emotional problems frequently contribute to the onset and perpetuation of obesity. In many, obesity results from overeating as a pattern of coping with emotional turmoil during important events. *Loss* often prompts overeating, be it loss of a significant person, body part, or function. Sometimes it is not the loss itself that causes the problem but merely the threat of separation or rejection. Another major setting for "compensatory" eating is *frustration,* such as that due to anger at a spouse in the context of a dependent-hostile relationship. In either loss or frustration, eating becomes a *defense* to ward off the pangs of anxiety, depression, or even self-destruction. Other people lose their appetite when they are angry, tense, or "blue." There is no known explanation of why some people develop reactive hyperphagia while others react to stress with anorexia. Indeed, considerable research has been unable to determine any particular personality organization or cluster of psychologic defense mechanisms clearly linked to obesity.

Developmental obesity refers to excessive weight gain that begins in childhood as a result of prenatal influences, constitutional and environmental factors, and, probably most important, rearing practices. The prognosis for reversal of childhood-onset obesity is generally poor. Eighty percent of overweight children become overweight adults. There is a 70 percent to 75 percent likelihood of becoming obese if both parents are obese; there is a 40 percent chance of obesity if one parent is obese and the other lean; and if both parents are lean there is a 10 percent chance of obesity. Although fat children can in themselves pose many problems for their parents, most often it is the parents who have deep-seated psychological conflicts long antedating the child's overeating and overweight. Obesity that begins in early childhood is associated with changes in fat cell numbers and composition, body image distortion, and refractoriness to later weight reduction (often because of a striking depression that accompanies weight loss).

Despite the negative medical and societal responses to obesity and the poor self-image associated with it, many obese people have *difficulty keeping weight off.* Often this is because of emotional problems that arise during such efforts. Weight reduction can *precipitate severe depression* or even psychosis, especially in people with a history of childhood-onset obesity or weight loss-induced depression. Those with the *night-eating syndrome,* characterized by insomnia, massive late-evening "refrigerator raids," and morning anorexia, also experience particular emotional distress when trying to reform their eating behaviors. Usually there are coinciding social stresses as well. Indeed, because of the rigors of weight reduction, people undergoing considerable situational distress should be advised to defer weight reduction programs until the psychosocial situation has stabilized.

Having survived the pitfalls and potential *complications* of weight reduction, the formerly obese person faces new problems. Many now find that previously unsatisfactory, though stable, relationships begin to fall apart when their morbid image is shed. Moreover, *new sexual demands* may be encountered by people who previously had avoided such demands by remaining fat and physically unattractive. Some obese women have prominent fantasies of promiscuity and fear they would "act out" sexually should they lose weight and become physically attractive. In sum, loss of obesity poses new psychological and interpersonal challenges that may be resisted and that compromise efforts for change.

Biologic Factors. *Altered thermogenesis* has been postulated. Animal experiments on thermogenesis by brown fat suggest that this tissue might serve as an energy buffer. Brown adipose tissue dissipates substantial amounts of energy in the form of heat during eating and during exposure to cold. It is hypothesized that obese people might be more susceptible to weight gain because they have a disturbance in normal *energy release* that occurs at time of food intake. Too little energy dissipation would result in greater preservation of calories and, eventually, in obesity, even under conditions of modest food intake that might not lead to obesity in a person with normal brown fat thermogenesis. The findings are intriguing and might help to at least partially explain why some people eat unrestrictedly and never gain weight while others become obese in spite of strenuous efforts to limit intake.

The *fat cell theory* holds that hyperplastically obese people (a small subset of the total obese population) are likely to be very heavy because of their large number of fat cells and very efficient lipoprotein lipase, which facilitates accumulation of energy and results in a lower caloric requirement for weight maintenance and gain.

Autonomic activity has been found to decrease with increase in weight. While autonomic dysfunction may not be the cause of obesity, it may contribute to it, affect responses to therapy, and predict the development of such complications as hypertension.

The *set point theory* views each person as having an ideal biologic weight that is maintained by internal physiologic and psychological signals. The body resists being displaced from this set point weight by adjusting rates of energy expenditure. After weight loss, the number of calories needed for weight maintenance is reduced because of this marked decrease in the rate of energy expenditure. The set point is defended by control of both the ingestion of food and its rate of energy expenditure. Exercise, not dieting, lowers the set point. Of interest, patients who report being "refractory" to dietary programs have been found to overestimate their energy expenditures and underestimate their caloric intake, suggesting a possible defect in the self-monitoring mechanisms.

Neurochemical research has provided new insights into appetite regulation. The neurotransmitter *serotonin* may influence regulation of food choice, specifically the ability to choose a desired proportion of carbohydrates in the diet. Common abnormalities in eating behavior, such as *carbohydrate craving,* may be related to disturbances in serotonin-mediated neurotransmission.

Some patients seem to have an unwise preference for foods high in fat and calories. It has been shown that these people may have a *biologic predisposition* to consume foods high in energy density. In our society this problem is more pronounced because not only are these "fattening" foods readily available, but their consumption is often encouraged. Another factor in dietary obesity involves the *timing of food intake*. There is some evidence that those who eat once daily, particularly before going to bed, may be prone to accumulate adipose tissue.

The contribution of *decreased physical activity* to the initiation, propagation, and maintenance of obesity is unclear, but available evidence suggests a role. It has been noted that obese people exercise and move about less than nonobese people. Also they tend to overestimate the amount of exercise they engage in. The question of whether inactivity precedes or follows obesity is unanswered. The athlete who stops running a mile a day and does not reduce his caloric intake can gain 11 to 22 pounds a year.

Pharmacologic agents prescribed for clinical conditions other than obesity may cause weight gain. *Beta-blockers* and central sympatholytics (eg, *clonidine*), can decrease metabolic rate and energy expenditure. *Glucocorticosteroids* cause hypertrophic obesity in a characteristic truncal pattern. *Tricyclic* antidepressants and some antihistamines (eg, cyproheptadine) act as appetite stimulants. Weight gain is common with oral contraceptive use.

Endocrine disturbances are more often the result rather than the cause of excess weight. However, *hypothyroidism* (see Chapter 104) has been found to account for up to 5 percent of cases in some series. *Cushing's syndrome* is a rare cause and is usually accompanied by characteristic features of truncal obesity and peripheral muscle wasting. *Stein-Leventhal syndrome*—polycystic ovaries, absent menses, and moderate hirsutism (see Chapter 112)—often goes unrecognized as an endocrinologic form of obesity; the precise mechanism of the obesity is unknown. *Eunuchism* and *hyperinsulin states* may also be associated with obesity.

Neurologic causes of obesity are usually not cryptic; they mostly result from *hypothalamic injury,* as occurs with craniopharyngiomas, encephalitis, or trauma. Visual field defects or headaches are usually present. Two rare types of neurologic disease without obvious CNS symptoms have been described. Kleine-Levin syndrome consists of periodic hyperphagia and hypersomnia. A second syndrome is characterized by preoccupation with food and accompanying electroencephalographic abnormalities that respond to phenytoin.

The importance of *genetic influences* in determining human fatness was underscored in a large-scale Danish study of adopted subjects. There was a strong relation between weight class of adoptees and their biologic parents, but none between adoptees and their adopted parents. A large American twin study reaffirmed the premise that obesity is under substantial genetic control. Recent studies indicate that many obese people are predisposed from birth to be overweight and have a tougher time than most losing and keeping weight off.

Socio-occupational obesity is commonplace. Excess weight occurs far more frequently among people in lower socioeconomic classes (1 in 3) than among those in upper socioeconomic classes (1 in 20). Whether this difference represents dietary preference, socially motivated behavior, or interactional factors is unclear. In certain occupations, such as wrestling, obesity is a help, not a hindrance. In former times, corpulence was a sign of prosperity and was cultivated by bankers and businessmen.

DIFFERENTIAL DIAGNOSIS

The causes of obesity can be divided into primary and secondary, with the latter being medical conditions that re-

Table 10-1. Important Causes of Obesity

Primary	
Psychological Factors	
	Depression
	Anxiety
	Frustration
Biologic Factors	
	Reduced thermogenesis
	Increased fat cell mass
	Autonomic dysfunction
	Altered hypothalamic set point
	Single large daily meal taken before bedtime
	Decreased energy expenditure
	Drugs (eg, tricyclic antidepressants, oral contraceptives, corticosteroids, phenothiazines)
Genetic Influences	
	Familial obesity
Socio-Occupational Factors	
	Lower socioeconomic class
	Social/occupational situation
Secondary	
Endocrine Disease	
	Hypothyroidism
	Stein-Leventhal syndrome
	Cushing's syndrome
Neurologic Disease	
	Hypothalamic injury (eg, trauma, encephalitis, craniopharyngioma)

sult in obesity. Some forms of secondary weight gain are due to salt retention and fluid overload rather than increase in fat cell mass. Among the important causes of sodium retention are congestive heart failure, severe hepatocellular disease, and renal failure (see Chapters 32, 71, and 142). Primary forms of obesity can be classified by their underlying pathophysiology. The vast majority of cases are primary in nature. An etiologic/pathophysiologic diagnosis is essential to design of an effective management program. (See Table 10–1.)

WORKUP

Determination of Obesity. To establish whether an individual is obese requires first a measurement of body fat. It is then necessary to relate body fatness to some standard or range of acceptable degrees of fat for the particular population under study. The distribution of fat also appears to be important. Health risks appear to correlate more closely with distribution of body fat than with total amount. Women generally have been observed to have more subcutaneous fat than men, but men appear to suffer a greater cardiovascular risk from a given degree of fat than women. Distribution may be an indicator of this difference.

A host of standards is used for determination of obesity. The *"eyeball test"* for obesity still holds true: If a person looks fat, he is fat. In fact, recent studies suggest that health risks associated with obesity are more closely correlated with the distribution of body fat than with the total body fat, making observation particularly useful. However, the most widely used quantitative indices used to identify obesity are the *anthropometric measurements* of height; weight; circumferences of chest, waist, hips, or extremities; and skinfold thickness. These measurements correlate well with the more sophisticated methods used in research studies of obesity, such as total body radioactive potassium-40 densitometry.

A simple quantitative determination of adiposity is measurement of *skinfold thickness*. Use of suitable skinfold calipers on triceps and subscapular skinfolds provides a reasonable index of an individual's fatness. However, reliability can be a problem when using skinfolds as a measure of fatness, because body fat increases with age, grossly obese patients are difficult to measure, and results vary among providers using the calipers.

The ratio of waist or *abdominal circumference* to the *hip or gluteal circumferences* provides a quantitative index of regional fat distribution. The circumference of the waist is obtained at the narrowest area above the umbilicus. The hip circumference is at the maximal gluteal protrusion. As noted earlier, distribution of body fat correlates with risk. Individuals with excess upper body fat *(android obesity)* are at higher risk for diabetes, atherosclerosis, and stroke than those who have more adipose tissue in the hips, buttocks, and thighs (gynoid obesity). In quantitative terms, individuals with waist:hip ratios greater than 0.8 for women and 1.0 for men have an increased risk of coronary disease.

Bioelectric impedance analysis (BIA) is a relatively inexpensive means of measuring body fat. Impedance is proportional to the aqueous composition of the body; results provide reasonably good estimates of body fat composition. Electrodes are applied to one arm and leg, and the impedance is measured. Formulas are used to estimate the percentage of fat in the body. BIA is less useful as a means of measuring fat loss.

Height and weight tables have the advantage of simplicity. However, there are serious limitations to their use. Standard charts typically list "ideal" or desired weights based on actuarial data, yet it is not weight per se that minimizes morbidity or incidence of disease. The person having a significant percentage of lean body mass, such as a physical laborer, may well exceed "ideal" body weight yet not be obese. On the other hand, some individuals may be within the ideal range but have noninsulin-dependent diabetes mellitus, hypertension, or other conditions that would benefit from weight reduction.

The Metropolitan Life Insurance Company has published revised reference weights in an attempt to isolate the effect of weight alone on longevity; individuals with major diseases, such as cancer, diabetes, or heart disease, were omitted from the study (see Table 10–2). While the consensus of the American Heart Association and the National Institutes of Health is to recommend continued use of Metropolitan Life tables, basing tables only on mortality ignores possible nonfatal risks of increased weight.

Body Mass Index (BMI = [body weight in kilograms] divided by [height in meters]^2) is based on the Metropolitan Life tables. Ratios of weight to height estimate total body mass rather than fat mass, but they correlate highly with amount of body fat. The BMI range of 20 to 24.9, classified as normal, correlates well with mortality rates derived from life insurance tables. Mortality begins to increase at BMI ratios above 25, and it is here that health professionals should be concerned. The major weakness of the BMI is that some very muscular individuals may be classified as obese when they are not. The National Institutes of Health Consensus Development Conference on the Health Implications of Obesity recommended that health professionals adopt this as an index for evaluating obesity (Fig. 10–1).

A *height–weight formula* provides a quick and easy way for determining a patient's ideal body weight as well as estimating the degree of overweight.

Female:
Allow 100 lb for first 5 feet of height plus 5 lb for each additional inch.
Male:
Allow 106 lb for first 5 feet of height plus 6 lb for each additional inch.

Appropriate weight goals for patients can be determined only by a thorough analysis of the medical history and physical findings, supplemented by appropriate laboratory evaluation.

Weight and Diet History. An extensive weight history should include age of onset of obesity, identifiable circumstances associated with the onset of obesity, and highest and lowest adult weight. The patient's past dieting attempts, duration of the effort, and the weight loss attained and maintained should be noted, as well as physical activity patterns. A careful review of ongoing psychological and situational stress is also essential. This information may provide some idea of underlying mechanisms.

Table 10-2. Optimal Weights,* in Pounds, for Adults Aged 25 and Over (Light Clothing)

HEIGHT (IN SHOES)	SMALL FRAME	MEDIUM FRAME	LARGE FRAME
Men			
5 ft 2 in	112–120	118–129	126–141
5 3	115–123	121–133	129–144
5 4	118–126	124–136	132–148
5 5	121–129	127–139	135–152
5 6	124–133	130–143	138–156
5 7	128–137	134–147	142–161
5 8	132–141	138–152	147–166
5 9	136–145	142–156	151–170
5 10	140–150	146–160	155–174
5 11	144–154	150–165	159–179
6 0	148–158	154–170	164–184
6 1	152–162	158–175	168–189
6 2	156–167	162–180	173–194
6 3	160–171	167–185	178–199
6 4	164–175	172–190	182–204
Women			
4 10	92–98	96–107	104–119
4 11	94–101	98–110	106–122
5 0	96–104	101–113	109–125
5 1	99–107	104–116	112–128
5 2	102–110	107–119	115–131
5 3	105–113	110–122	118–134
5 4	108–116	113–126	121–138
5 5	111–119	116–130	125–142
5 6	114–123	120–135	129–146
5 7	118–127	124–139	133–150
5 8	122–131	128–143	137–154
5 9	126–135	132–147	141–158
5 10	130–140	136–151	145–163
5 11	134–144	140–155	149–168
6 0	138–148	144–159	153–173

*Weights associated with the lowest mortality rates (derived from actuarial data, Metropolitan Life Insurance Company).

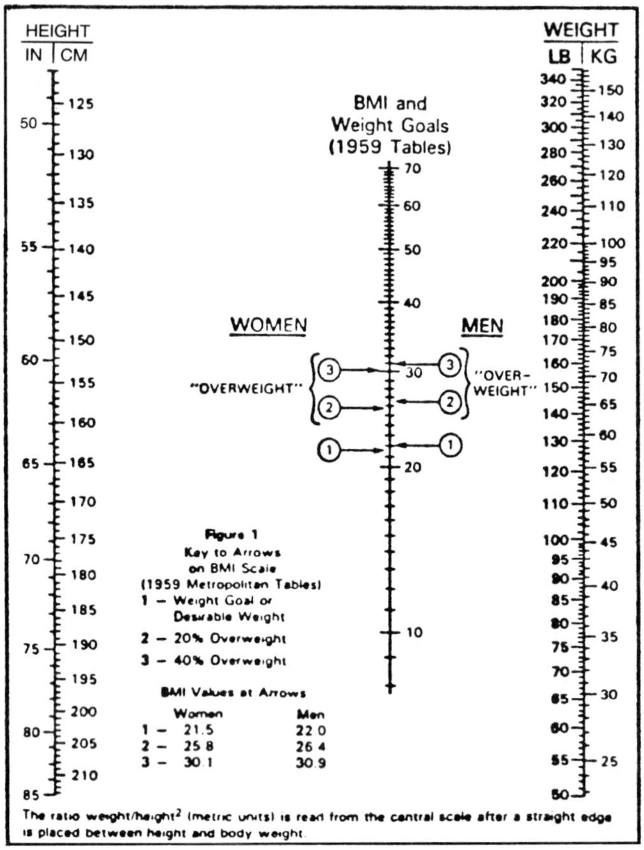

Figure 10-1. Nomogram for body mass index (kg/m²). Weights and heights are without clothing. With clothes, add 5 lb (2.3 kg) for men and 3 lb (1.4 kg) for women and 1 in (2.5 cm) in height for shoes. (J Am Diet Assoc 85:1119, 1985. New weight standards for men and women. Stat Bull Metrop Life Ins Co 40:1, 1959.)

Workup for an Underlying Medical Etiology. Even in a patient without obvious medical pathology, a workup that screens for underlying endocrinologic and neurologic disease is essential, as is a check for drug-induced etiologies and concurrent cardiovascular risk factors. Regardless of the cause of obesity, the medical evaluation should include a careful examination for common consequences of obesity (eg, hypertension, diabetes, sleep apnea, degenerative joint disease).

History requires a thorough neuroendocrine review of symptoms: fatigue, unexplained weight gain, cold intolerance, hoarseness, change in skin and hair texture, amenorrhea, hirsutism, easy bruising, weakness, visual disturbances, and headache. It is also important to ask about hypertension, disturbed sleep, excessive snoring, daytime sleepiness, polyuria, polydipsia, claudication, leg edema, and knee and hip pain.

Physical examination is checked for such etiologic clues as moon facies, hirsutism, dry and thickened skin, coarse hair, truncal obesity, pigmented striae, goiter, adnexal masses, lack of secondary sex characteristics, delayed relaxation of ankle jerks, and visual field deficits. The physical should include examining for blood pressure elevation, peripheral vascular disease, upper airway soft tissue obstruction, and degenerative changes in the hips and knees (see Chapters 151 and 152). Although many morbidly obese patients have sleep apnea, most sleep apneic patients are not classically "pickwickian" in appearance (see Chapter 46).

Laboratory testing has two components: diagnosis of an underlying medical etiology and detection of metabolic consequences. A strategy of routinely testing for all possible medical etiologies in the absence of suggestive clinical findings is fraught with increased risk of generating a high percentage of false-positive results (see Chapter 2). Nonetheless, some clinicians routinely screen for hypothyroidism with a *thyrotropin (TSH)* determination because testing is sensitive, the condition has a relatively high frequency, and its clinical presentation can be very subtle (see Chapter 104).

The laboratory evaluation is most productive when directed at causes suggested by history and physical examination. For example, the obese patient suspected of Cushing's syndrome because of truncal obesity, peripheral wasting, and pigmented striae is a reasonable candidate for an overnight *1 mg dexamethasone suppression test*. If there are headaches accompanied by a visual field disturbance, then a *computed tomography (CT) scan* of the sella turcica is needed to check for the possibility of a pituitary tumor (see Chapter 100).

Testing for the metabolic consequences of obesity is straightforward and includes a random serum glucose, lipid profile (see Chapter 15), and uric acid. These results help determine overall cardiovascular risk. Patients bothered by daytime sleepiness and a history of excessive snoring and disturbed sleep due to irregular breathing should be considered for evaluation of sleep apnea (see Chapter 46). At the present time, measures of energy expenditure, thermogenesis, autonomic function, fat cell count, and set point are relegated to the research laboratory, but, in time, they may become part of the clinical evaluation.

Symptomatic Therapy and Indications for Referral The management of obesity is discussed in detail in Chapter 233. Patients who are morbidly obese and demonstrate such adverse sequelae as marked respiratory compromise, disabling arthritis, or symptomatic coronary disease require consultation for consideration of a very–low-calorie diet under the supervision of persons experienced in its implementation (see Chapter 233). Obstructive sleep apnea occurring in patients with mild to moderate obesity may not require such extreme measures, but pulmonary consultation in conjunction with a weight loss program is indicated (see Chapter 46). The patient with symptomatic degenerative disease of weight-bearing joints may also derive substantial benefit from a program of modest weight reduction (see Chapter 157).

ANNOTATED BIBLIOGRAPHY

Bogardus C, Lillioja S, Ravussin E et al. Familial dependence of the resting metabolic rate. N Engl J Med 1986;315:96. (*The rate was a familial trait in this study of Native Americans, though its contribution to familial predisposition to obesity was unsettled.*)

Danforth E Jr, Sims EAH. Obesity and efforts to lose weight. N Engl J Med 1992;327:1947. (*An editorial reviewing mechanisms of obesity.*)

Harrison GG. Height-weight tables. Ann Intern Med 1985;103: 989. (*A critical review of the major tables; 42 refs.*)

Himms-Hagen J. Thermogenesis in brown adipose tissue as an energy buffer. N Engl J Med 1984;311:1549. (*An intriguing theory of energy regulation and its implications for obesity and weight control.*)

Hubert HB, Feinleib M, McNamara PM et al. Obesity as an independent risk factor for cardiovascular disease: A 26-year follow-up of participants in the Framingham Heart Study. Circulation 1983;67:968. (*Found to be an independent cardiovascular risk factor; benefits of weight reduction and harmful effects of weight gain also detailed.*)

Lichtman SW, Pisarska K, Berman ER et al. Discrepancy between self-reported and actual caloric intake and exercise in obese subjects. N Engl J Med 1992;327:1893. (*Obese patients who were "resistant" to dietary measures had normal energy expenditure but underreported food intake and overreported physical activity.*)

Liebel RL, Hirsch J. Metabolic characterization of obesity. Ann Intern Med 1985;103:1002. (*Terse review of regulatory mechanisms of body composition.*)

Manson JE, Colditz GA, Stampfer MJ et al. A prospective study of obesity and risk of coronary heart disease in women. N Engl J Med 1990;322:882. (*Striking report from the Nurses' Health Study, a prospective 8-year study of women 30–55; 40 percent of coronary events were attributable to excessive body weight.*)

National Institutes of Health Consensus Development Conference. Health implications of obesity. Ann Intern Med 1985; 103:977. (*A definitive review of the issue; finds obesity is a major contributor to morbidity and mortality; essential reading for all primary physicians.*)

Peiris AN, Sothmann MS, Hoffman RG et al. Adiposity, fat distribution, and cardiovascular risk. Ann Intern Med 1989;110: 867. (*Intra-abdominal fat deposition proved to be a greater cardiovascular risk than obesity alone, perhaps due to the hyperinsulinemia associated with it.*)

Peterson HR, Rothschild M, Weinberg CR et al. Body fat and the activity of the autonomic nervous system. N Engl J Med 1988;318:1077. (*Evidence that changes in autonomic activity correlate with body fat composition, though the etiologic significance of this finding remains to be determined.*)

Ravussin E, Lillioja S, Knowler WC et al. Reduced rate of energy expenditure as a risk factor for body-weight gain. N Engl J Med 1988;318;467. (*Evidence supporting the low-energy expenditure hypothesis.*)

Rodenstein DO, Stanescu DC. The soft palate and breathing. Am Rev Respir Dis 1986;134:311. (*Upper airway obstruction in moderately obese patients can cause sleep apnea.*)

Senie RT, Rosen PP, Rhodes P et al. Obesity at diagnosis of breast carcinoma influences duration of disease-free interval. Ann Intern Med 1992;116:26. (*Obesity reduced rate of disease-free survival by more than 25 percent.*)

Smith PL, Gold AR, Meyers DA et al. Weight loss in mildly to moderately obese patients with obstructive sleep apnea. Ann Intern Med 1985;103:850. (*Moderate weight loss can alleviate sleep apnea.*)

Williamson DF, Kahn HS, Remington PL et al. The 10-year incidence of overweight and major weight gain in US adults. JAMA 1990;150:665. (*The incidence of a major weight gain was greatest among people in their early 20s, especially among already overweight women.*)

11
Evaluation of Fever

HARVEY B. SIMON, M.D.

Primary Care Medicine: Office Evaluation and Management of the Adult Patient, 3rd edition, edited by Allan H. Goroll, Lawrence A. May, and Albert G. Mulley, Jr. J.B. Lippincott Company, Philadelphia

Since antiquity, fever has been recognized as a cardinal manifestation of disease. Indeed, people identify fever as a sign of illness more readily than they recognize the importance of most other symptoms. In addition to causing concern, the presence of fever usually raises high therapeutic expectations. Even in the preantibiotic era, John Milton observed that "the fever is to the Physitians, the eternal reproach" (1641). In the popular mind today, fever is equated with infection, and infections are expected to respond to the administration of "wonder drugs." As a result, the physician is faced with the challenge of defining the cause of the fever, instituting appropriate therapy, and explaining the reasons for limiting antibiotic usage to bacterial infections.

PATHOPHYSIOLOGY AND CLINICAL PRESENTATION

"Normal" Body Temperature. Popular lore notwithstanding, 98.6°F (37°C) is *not* normal body temperature. In fact, there is no single normal value; like so many other biological functions, body temperature displays a circadian rhythm. In healthy individuals, mean rectal temperatures vary from a low of about 97°F (36.1°C) in early morning to a high of about 99.3°F (37.4°C) in late afternoon. In children, the normal range may be even greater. Moreover, physiologic factors such as exercise and the menstrual cycle can further alter body temperature. In practical terms, understanding the diurnal rhythm of body temperature is important for two reasons. First, many patients have been unnecessarily subjected to extensive workups and even psychologically incapacitated in the erroneous quest of a cause for deviation from the mythical "normal" of 98.6°F. Second, the fever of disease states is superimposed on the normal cycle, so that fevers are generally highest in the evenings and lowest in the mornings. As a result, frequent temperature recordings throughout the day are required to monitor fever in sick patients. The absence of fever in a single office visit does not exclude a febrile illness.

Clinical Manifestations of Fever. The presenting complaints of the febrile patient may be explained by the underlying disease process or by the fever itself. The signs and symptoms of fever vary tremendously. Some patients are asymptomatic; more often there is a sensation of warmth or flushing. Malaise and fatigue are common. The hypothalamus, acting through somatic efferent nerves, increases muscle tone in order to generate heat and raise body temperature; many febrile patients experience *myalgias* as a result.

These same factors account for one of the most dramatic manifestations of fever: the *shaking chill* or *rigor.* It is taught that rigor is a manifestation of bacteremia, but in fact any stimulus that raises the hypothalamic set point rapidly may produce a rigor. Patients experiencing a rigor exhibit uncontrolled violent shaking and trembling, and they characteristically heap themselves with blankets even as their temperatures are shooting up. This phenomenon also has a physiologic basis. Despite the high central or core temperature, these patients subjectively feel cold because surface temperature is reduced. In order to generate fever in response to hypothalamic stimuli, cutaneous vasoconstriction occurs, skin temperature falls, and cold receptors in the skin sense this as cold. Quite the reverse occurs during defervescence; body temperature falls in response to cutaneous vasodilation, and drenching sweats typically terminate an episode of fever.

Other manifestations of temperature elevation include central nervous system symptoms ranging from a mild inability to concentrate to *confusion, delirium,* or even stupor, especially in the elderly or debilitated patient. High fevers (104°F–106°F) may produce *convulsions* in infants and young children without any primary neurologic disorder. Increased cardiac output is an invariable consequence of fever, and *tachycardia* typically accompanies fever. Tachycardia is so usual that its absence should lead one to suspect uncommon problems such as typhoid fever, in which relative bradycardia is typical (for unknown reasons), drug fever, and factitious fever. Patients with underlying heart disease may respond to the high output stress of fever with angina or heart failure.

Another sign of fever is the so-called fever blister—*labial herpes simplex*. The problem is probably not precipitated by fever per se, for it is much more common in some infections, such as pneumococcal pneumonia and meningococcal meningitis, than in other febrile states.

Because fever accompanies infection so frequently, numerous investigators have tried to determine if fever has any protective or beneficial role. There are a few circumstances, such as central nervous system syphilis, in which elevations of body temperature may exceed the thermal tolerance of the infectious agent. In fact, induced fever was once a form of therapy for syphilis. In several animal models, fever enhances recovery from experimental infections; however, there is no such proven clinical benefit from fever in humans.

Consequences of Fever. Is fever detrimental? Most otherwise healthy individuals can tolerate temperatures up to

105°F (40.5°C) without ill effects, although even in these individuals symptoms often warrant therapy. In children, high fevers should be suppressed because convulsions may occur. Patients with heart disease should also receive antipyretic therapy. Each 1°F of temperature increases the basal metabolic rate by 7 percent, resulting in increased demands on the heart, which may precipitate myocardial ischemia, failure, or even shock. In addition, extreme hyperthermia beyond 108°F (42.1°C) may cause direct cellular damage. Vascular endothelium seems particularly susceptible to such damage, and disseminated intravascular coagulation frequently accompanies extreme hyperthermia. Other structures that may be directly damaged are brain, muscle, and heart. Finally, metabolic derangements such as hypoxia, acidosis, and sometimes hyperkalemia can result from extreme pyrexia and, in turn, further contribute to coma, seizures, arrhythmias, or hypotension, which could be lethal. Nevertheless, patients have survived temperatures of up to 108°F without demonstrable organ damage, but mortality in this temperature range is appreciable. Body temperatures as high as 113°F have been demonstrated in humans, but these have been uniformly lethal.

DIFFERENTIAL DIAGNOSIS

Many inflammatory, infectious, neoplastic, and hypersensitivity processes may produce fever. Most acute fevers encountered in the office setting are of obvious cause and due to upper respiratory or urinary tract infection. Viral illnesses, drug allergy (especially to antibiotics), and connective tissue disease are other important precipitants.

Unexplained persistent fever can be a major diagnostic challenge. Table 11–1 lists causes of "fevers of unknown origin (FUOs)," defined as those persisting for 3 weeks, exceeding temperatures of 101°F, and eluding 1 week of intensive diagnostic study. Infections, both localized and systemic, neoplasms, and collagen-vascular diseases account for 75 percent of cases. The spectrum of FUO disease has evolved in recent years, with a greater proportion being due to collagen-vascular or granulomatous disease (polymyalgia, cranial arteritis, sarcoidosis) and fewer resulting from undiagnosed tumor (presumably due to enhanced diagnostic techniques). Human immunodeficiency virus (HIV) infection raises a whole new set of diagnostic possibilities (see Chapter 13).

WORKUP

The acutely febrile patient presents a common but demanding problem in differential diagnosis. In most cases, a careful history and physical examination will reveal the diagnostic clues, so that laboratory studies can be used selectively. The evaluation of persistent fever can be more demanding. The initial office evaluation should help determine the proper pace of diagnostic testing and need for therapeutic intervention. If the illness is insidious in onset and only slowly progressive, or if the patient is nontoxic and clinically stable, one may proceed with the workup in a deliberate manner on an ambulatory basis, utilizing serial clinical observations and time as key diagnostic tools. On the other hand, if the patient is a compromised host, or if he is acutely ill and toxic, several immediate diagnostic studies are mandatory, and treatment may even be required before all the results are available; hospitalization is usually necessary in such cases. Table 11–2 lists some factors that should prompt an aggressive approach to diagnosis and therapy.

Febrile illnesses are most commonly acute processes that are either readily diagnosed and treated (common bacterial infections) or self-limited despite the lack of a specific diagnosis (viral infections, allergic reactions). However, patients will occasionally present with undiagnosed fevers, fulfilling the classic criterion for FUO. In both situations, the keys to diagnosis are a careful history and a meticulous physical examination.

History

The infectious disease history should stress several items not routinely emphasized: 1) host factors, 2) epidemiology, 3) symptomatology, and 4) drug history.

Host Factors. One should determine if the patient is basically healthy or if he has an underlying disease that may render him unusually susceptible to infection. Patients with hematologic and other *malignancies, HIV infection, diabetes mellitus, neutropenia,* or *sickle cell anemia* may become infected with unusual opportunistic pathogens or may fail to respond normally to common infectious agents. Patients taking *corticosteroids* or other *immunosuppressive agents* are especially vulnerable to infection. Individuals with implanted *prosthetic devices,* such as artificial heart valves or hip prostheses, are also at increased risk of serious infection. Finally, patients with a *past history* of certain infectious processes, such as pyelonephritis, may be prone to relapses or recurrences of similar problems.

Epidemiology. It is important to ask about *high-risk sexual activity* in screening for HIV infection and about *travel* for exposure to infections such as typhoid fever or malaria. Less obvious factors, such as exposure to *animals,* may be of great importance. Vectors of infection may be found even among household pets, such as cats (eg, cat-scratch disease and *Pasteurella multocida* cellulitis from bites or scratches, toxoplasmosis from fecal contamination), parakeets (psittacosis), and turtles (salmonellosis). A history of *bites* by stray dogs, skunks, or bats may suggest the possibility of rabies.

An inquiry into what is "going around" in the *community* may be helpful. A very localized outbreak of a flu-like illness or atypical pneumonia may be a clue to *Legionella* infection (see Chapter 52). Being exposed to or part of a *population with a high incidence* of tuberculosis (see Chapter 49), HIV infection (see Chapter 13), or viral hepatitis (see Chapter 70) raises the risk of having contracted the infection. Intravenous drug abusers are notoriously high-risk for such conditions as well as bacterial endocarditis. The patient's *occupation* is sometimes revealing as well. For example, abattoir workers may be exposed to brucellosis, leather workers to anthrax, and gardeners to sporotrichosis. Patients with underlying chronic disease, especially of the liver, or who eat raw oysters or have skin wounds exposed to seawater are at increased risk for contracting *Vibrio vulnificus,* a newly appreciated pathogen that is halophilic (thrives in the setting of high iron levels) and found predominantly in warm (> 20°C) seawater. The vibrio infection can produce a febrile illness that ranges from mild temperature elevation and wound cellulitis to chills, high-grade fever, bullous skin lesions, and shock, especially in those who ingest the organism.

Symptomatology may serve to pinpoint the site of infection. *Localizing symptoms* should be sought. They include rash, headache, cranial tenderness, sinus discomfort, ear pain, toothache, sore throat, tender thyroid gland, breast mass or tenderness, pleuritic chest pain, cough, dyspnea, abdominal pain, flank pain, dysuria, vaginal discharge, pelvic pain, anorectal or perineal discomfort, testicular pain, bone pain, joint swelling, joint stiffness or pain, calf or vein tenderness, neck stiffness, focal neurologic deficit, and alteration in consciousness.

Medications. A full review of all drug use and any substance abuse (see Chapter 235) is essential. Is the patient taking any medications that may be responsible for fever as a manifestation of hypersensitivity? Does the patient have any drug allergies? Has the patient been taking antibiotics, which may alter his susceptibility to infection by favoring drug-resistant organisms or mask infection by rendering him culture-negative? Is there an underlying problem (eg, renal failure) that may alter the choice of therapeutic agents and lead to the use of a less common agent?

Physical Examination

Vital signs should be determined in all cases. Fever is an important but nonspecific sign of infection; some patients with infections are afebrile, whereas others may have a fever resulting from noninfectious causes, such as hypersensitivity states and lymphoreticular malignancies. The shaking chill or rigor may suggest bacteremia, but it is also not specific. In the neonate or in occasional adults with overwhelming sepsis, hypothermia may be present. Respiratory distress may signal pulmonary infection or septic shock, and hypotension may be the presenting finding leading to a diagnosis of sepsis.

The *skin and mucous membranes* may provide crucial information. To cite a few examples: Petechial eruptions on the skin suggest meningococcemia or Rocky Mountain spotted fever, and those at the junction of the hard and soft palate occur with infectious mononucleosis. Pustular lesions raise the question of gonococcemia (see Chapter 137) or staphylococcal endocarditis. Splinter hemorrhages and conjunctival petechiae herald endocarditis. Ecthyma gangrenosa is a hallmark of *Pseudomonas* septicemia. Macular or vesicular eruptions occur with viral infections, bullae with *Vibrio vulnificus*. Erythema chronicum migrans is an important sign of Lyme disease.

The *sinuses* should be percussed for tenderness and transilluminated for evidence of sinusitis. In the elderly, the *scalp* is palpated for the tender arteries of cranial arteritis. The optic *fundi* are examined for the retinopathy of connective tissue disease (see Chapter 146), the Roth spots of endocarditis, and the choroidal tubercles of miliary tuberculosis and *Candida* septicemia. The *tympanic membranes* should be examined for effusion and erythema, and the *oral cavity* for tonsillar pathology, tooth abscess, and salivary gland tenderness. The *neck* is checked for thyroid gland tenderness and local adenopathy. Careful examination of all the *lymph nodes* for enlargement may provide a very important clue to etiology, as might the distribution of the adenopathy (see Chapter 12).

The *breasts* are examined for masses, tenderness, and nipple discharge. The *chest* is noted for rubs and signs of consolidation and effusion. A careful *heart* examination for murmurs and rubs is essential. The *abdomen* is checked for organomegaly, masses, tenderness, guarding, rebound, and tenderness of the costovertebral angle.

The *genitorectal area* is all too frequently overlooked, yet it is often a source of key information. The woman without an obvious source of fever must have a careful pelvic examination looking for cervical discharge, adnexal tenderness, and mass lesions (see Chapter 114). In men, the prostate and testicles need to be gently checked for tenderness and masses and the penis for discharge and rash (see Chapter 136). Rectal examination should include evaluation for discharge, tenderness, and masses (see Chapter 66), and the stool is tested for occult blood.

Musculoskeletal examination may suggest inflammation or infection of the bone or joints if there is swelling, increased warmth, or tenderness. The *lower extremities* are examined for evidence of phlebitis (asymmetrical swelling, calf tenderness, palpable cord). The *neurologic evaluation* should include a look for signs of meningeal irritation, the presence of focal deficits, and disturbances in mentation.

Laboratory Studies

If the history and physical examination provide strong indications of an infectious process, laboratory studies can be used selectively to confirm or refute the clinical diagnosis. For example, in the patient with an obvious viral upper respiratory infection, no studies are necessary. In patients with bronchitis, a sputum smear and culture may be all that is required, but if pneumonia is a possibility, a chest radiograph and complete blood count (CBC) are minimal additional requirements (see Chapter 52). In the patient with probable lower urinary tract infection, a urinalysis and perhaps a culture may suffice, but if there is concern about upper tract infection, especially as a complication of obstruction, then renal function tests, blood cultures, renal ultrasonography, and/or intravenous pyelography deserve serious consideration (see Chapter 133).

In other patients, however, more extensive tests are needed to establish a diagnosis when the cause of fever remains unknown. Although such studies must be individualized, the approach to diagnosis of an obscure fever should include the following.

Complete Blood Count, Differential, and Sedimentation Rate. Leukocytosis and a "shift to the left" suggest but do not prove bacterial infection. Toxic granulations, Döhle bodies, and vacuoles in polymorphonuclear leukocytes are suggestive of bacterial sepsis but are not entirely specific. In most instances, the erythrocyte sedimentation rate (ESR) lacks the sensitivity and specificity needed for it to serve as an adequate means of detecting or ruling out such causes of fever as tumor, connective tissue disease, and infection. Although a very elevated ESR is an invitation to additional testing and may be a clue to a specific process such as temporal arteritis (see Chapter 161), many elevations are due to trivial conditions unrelated to the cause of fever. The ESR should be ordered and interpreted cautiously and not viewed as a screening test for "disease."

Urinalysis. Pyuria strongly suggests urinary tract infection. Gram stain of the unspun urine specimen can be diagnostic (see Chapter 127). Isolated hematuria may be a clue to an underlying glomerular disease or urinary tract malignancy such as hypernephroma, which is notoriously difficult to diagnose early and a classic FUO etiology.

Radiographic Studies. Chest radiographs may detect infiltrates, effusions, masses, or nodes even in the absence of abnormalities on physical examination, while kidney-ureter-bladder (KUB) and upright abdominal films can disclose air–fluid levels in the bowel. Ultrasound or computed tomography (CT) study may be needed if there is suspicion of a mass lesion, such as an abscess or tumor (see below).

Blood Chemistries. The blood sugar determination is helpful in search of previously unsuspected diabetes mellitus. The test is also important in evaluating the significance of the sugar concentration in various body fluids. Liver function tests are useful in helping to define obscure sources of fever. For example, transaminase elevation suggests hepatitis, and isolated rises in alkaline phosphatase point to infiltration of the liver.

Examination of Body Fluids. If there is any possibility of meningitis, a lumbar puncture is mandatory. Aspiration and study of pleural effusions, ascitic fluid, or joint effusions may be diagnostic. Such specimens should be examined directly by cell counts and stains (see below). Sugar and protein determinations help differentiate etiologies; in general, bacterial, mycobacterial, and fungal infections produce low sugar and high protein levels in body fluid.

Cultures. If the patient has a heart murmur or a prosthetic heart valve or appears seriously ill, cultures of blood should be obtained. (Having at least two blood cultures from separate venipunctures is preferred.) Most patients should have cultures taken of urine (clean catch or catheterized specimen) and sputum. If other body fluids are obtainable, they should likewise be cultured. Special mycobacterial and fungal media are required if these agents are suspected, especially if the patient is a compromised host. Anaerobic cultures are important when one is dealing with a possible abscess or other infection of the pulmonary, gastrointestinal, or pelvic regions.

Microscopic Evaluation. Any body fluid that can be obtained should be examined by the Gram stain technique. Sputum, urine, wound exudates, cerebrospinal fluid, pleural fluid, ascitic fluid, and joint fluid often reveal the cause of infection on Gram stain. Even Gram stains of the stool may be helpful in certain specific situations, such as acute diarrhea (see Chapter 64). The presence of bacteria in a specimen of body fluid that is normally sterile is presumptive evidence of infection. This is particularly true when one is examining the spun sediment obtained from cerebrospinal fluid. Likewise, bacteria are not found in normal ascitic, joint, or pleural fluid. Bacteria in unspun urine correlates well with the presence of a significant urinary tract infection. However, Gram stains must be examined and interpreted with a certain amount of caution. For example, if one sees epithelial cells in a sputum specimen, one can be certain that the specimen contains mouth organisms and is not representative of conditions in the tracheobronchial tree. In such instances, one should obtain a better sputum sample. In the presence of bacterial pneumonia, the sputum usually contains many polymorphonuclear leukocytes and a large number of bacteria. Acid-fast stains are required to visualize mycobacteria (see Chapter 49), and specially stained wet mounts of body fluids can be useful in uncovering numerous types of fungal infections.

Immunologic Studies. In selected instances, serologic testing for evidence of infection can be of great help. Examples include suspected HIV infection (ELISA and Western Blot testing—see Chapter 13), rheumatic fever and other streptococcal infections (antistreptolysin O [ASLO] titers), infectious mononucleosis (heterophile test), and salmonella (Widal titers). Skin tests (especially the tuberculin test) can provide confirmatory evidence and need to be considered when clinical findings are suggestive. Testing for antinuclear antibody and rheumatoid factor may help in the diagnosis of a suspected vasculitis or rheumatoid disease. The presence of rheumatoid factor or immune complexes can be clues to "culture-negative" endocarditis or underlying connective tissue disease (see Chapter 146). In the diagnosis of obscure fevers, it is often useful to freeze and save an "acute phase serum" for later comparison with a "convalescent serum."

The Undiagnosed Febrile Patient

Although an enormous number of studies are available for the evaluation of undiagnosed febrile illnesses, it is important to proceed with these in a logical, step-by-step fashion instead of subjecting the patient to a random series of expensive, time-consuming, uncomfortable, or even hazardous studies. The first step in the subsequent workup is to *document fever* by measuring rectal temperatures every 4 hours. If fever is documented, further testing should be directed to the most common causes of FUO, as listed in Table 11–1. Obviously, the order of testing should be determined by clues present in the individual patient, beginning with the simplest, least expensive studies.

Radiographic and Invasive Studies may be revealing, but they require careful selection. At times a contrast study or radionuclide scan will reveal a source of fever. *Ultrasonography* is useful for noninvasively identifying pathology in the liver, gall bladder, pancreas, kidneys, and pelvis. *Abdominal CT* helps visualize a suspected fever source in the retroperitoneum (eg, lymphoma), upper abdomen (eg, pancreatic or

Table 11-1. Causes of Fever of Undetermined Origin

"The Big Three"

I. Infections: 20%–40%
  A. Systemic
    1. Tuberculosis (miliary)
    2. Infective endocarditis (subacute)
    3. Miscellaneous infections: cytomegalovirus infection, toxoplasmosis, brucellosis, psittacosis, gonococcemia, chronic meningococcemia, disseminated mycoses
  B. Localized
    1. Hepatic infections (liver abscess, cholangitis)
    2. Other visceral infections (pancreatic, tubo-ovarian, and pericholecystic abscesses, and empyemia of gallbladder)
    3. Intraperitoneal infections (subhepatic, subphrenic, paracolic, appendiceal, pelvic, and other abscesses)
    4. Urinary tract infections (pyelonephritis, renal carbuncle, perinephric abscess, prostatic abscess)

II. Neoplasms: 7%–20%. Especially lymphomas, leukemias, renal cell carcinoma, atrial myomas, and cancers metastatic to bone or liver

III. Collagen-vascular and other multisystem disease: 15%–25%. Including temporal arteritis and juvenile rheumatoid arthritis as well as systemic lupus erythematosus, rheumatoid arthritis, polyarteritis nodosa, Wegener's granulomatosis, mixed connective tissue disease, sarcoidosis

Less Common Causes: 5%–15%

I. Noninfectious granulomatous diseases (eg, granulomatous hepatitis)
II. Inflammatory bowel disease
III. Pulmonary embolization
IV. Drug fever
V. Factitious fever
VI. Hepatic cirrhosis with active hepatocellular necrosis
VII. Miscellaneous uncommon diseases (familial Mediterranean fever, Whipple's disease, etc.)
VII. Undiagnosed

(Modified from Jacoby GA, Swartz MN: Fever of unknown origin. N Engl J Med 289:1407, 1973.)

liver cancer), and large bowel (eg, diverticular abscess). *Bone scan* may localize an abscess or malignancy that has invaded bone, though a normal study does not always rule out such disease. *Bone marrow* or *liver biopsy* may detect a granulomatous or neoplastic process. A *lumbar puncture* is unlikely to help unless nuchal rigidity or neurologic abnormalities are present. A blind *laparotomy* is not performed unless there are clear-cut clues to intra-abdominal abnormalities that cannot be evaluated with less invasive procedures.

Therapeutic Trials. Only in the acutely ill toxic patient is it necessary to begin broad antibiotic coverage before the diagnosis is established. It is essential, though commonly forgotten, to obtain cultures of blood, urine, and other pertinent fluids prior to initiating treatment, so that rational decisions can be made later concerning therapy. In the nontoxic patient with an acute febrile illness and in the person with a true FUO, blind therapeutic trials are rarely helpful and are often confusing or even harmful. In this context, it is useful to remember one definition of empiric therapy: that which the ignorant do to the helpless. In occasional patients with FUO, therapeutic trials may be necessary, including intravenous antibiotics for suspected culture-negative endocarditis, combined chemotherapy for occult tuberculosis, or salicylates or steroids for noninfectious inflammatory disease. Such trials should always be conducted with a specific end point or time limit in mind, carefully planned observations, patient consent, and a mixture of humility and trepidation.

The Second Look. Despite the array of sophisticated technology available for the study of febrile illnesses, the history and physical examination remain the keys to diagnosis in most cases. Time can be a most valuable diagnostic tool. Unless the patient is progressively deteriorating, it may be advisable to interrupt the workup for a period of clinical observation, possibly with the aid of symptomatic therapy such as antipyretics. A second look, beginning with the history and physical examination, may then be fruitful.

SYMPTOMATIC THERAPY

The best therapy is obviously to treat the underlying cause. However, antipyretic therapy may provide comfort and prevent complications. The first issue, of course, is to determine if fever should be treated. Elevated temperature itself does not necessarily call for therapy. But if unpleasant symptoms are present, if the patient has limited cardiac reserve, or if the complications of fever are imminent, antipyretics should be administered.

Antipyretic therapy depends on the use of both chemical agents and physical methods. The most effective antipyretic drugs are the *salicylates* and *acetaminophen;* both appear to act on the hypothalamus to lower the thermal set point. Although parenteral salicylates are available, oral or rectal administration of either aspirin or acetaminophen is preferable. Doses of up to 1.2 g of either drug may be given to adults to initiate antipyretic therapy. In addition to intrinsic toxicities, it must be remembered that both aspirin and acetaminophen occasionally produce an overresponse, with hypothermia and even dangerous hypotension. Patients with typhoid fever or Hodgkin's disease and the elderly and debilitated seem to be at somewhat greater risk for this uncommon complication.

Physical cooling is also extremely effective. At the simplest level, undressing the patient and exposing him to a cool ambient temperature will allow cooling by radiation; a bedside fan will promote cooling by convection, as well. Sponging with cool water or alcohol is also helpful, promoting evaporation. With extreme elevations (greater than 106°F), more drastic measures are necessary and hospitalization is urgent. *Immersion in an ice water bath* is the most efficient of these methods and may be indicated in hyperthermic emergencies such as heat stroke. All methods of physical cooling present the risk of hypothermic overresponse and should, therefore, be discontinued when the body temperature begins to fall below critical levels.

Hyperthermic emergencies are rare, but fever is common and most often presents as an unpleasant symptom rather than a medical crisis. It seems appropriate, therefore, to con-

Table 11-2. Febrile Patients Who Require Special Attention

1. Vulnerable Hosts
   a. Age (very young or very old)
   b. Corticosteroid or immunosuppressive therapy
   c. Serious underlying diseases (neutropenia, sickle cell anemia, diabetes, cirrhosis, advanced COPD, renal failure, malignancies, AIDS)
   d. Implanted prosthetic devices (heart valves, joint prostheses, etc.)
   e. Intravenous drug abuse
2. Toxic Patients
   a. Rigors, prostration, extreme pyrexia
   b. Hypotension, oliguria
   c. CNS abnormalities
   d. Cardiorespiratory compromise
   e. New significant cardiac murmurs
   f. Petechial eruption
   g. Marked leukocytosis or leukopenia

clude with a comment about patient comfort. Although fever causes discomfort in most patients, use of physical cooling produces discomfort in virtually all individuals; often the treatment is remembered as far worse than the illness itself. As a result, these measures should be employed only when fever itself presents medical problems. The same is true to a lesser extent of aspirin and acetaminophen. In particular, many patients find rapid rises and falls of temperature very distressing; therefore, administering antipyretics every 4 hours for the first day or two of treatment may be preferable to waiting for the height of the fever spike.

INDICATIONS FOR ADMISSION

The very toxic or vulnerable patient (see Table 11–2) should be admitted promptly for aggressive study, monitoring, and consideration of means to lower temperature. With weight loss and debilitation, early hospitalization should also be considered. Moreover, when fever remains elevated beyond 101°F for weeks and ambulatory diagnostic efforts have been unsuccessful, it is often beneficial to bring the patient into the hospital for closer evaluation and documentation of fever; the advice of an infectious disease consultant can be helpful.

PATIENT EDUCATION

Whenever fever is suspected in the ambulatory setting, the patient should be instructed to keep a record of temperatures, preferably rectal, taken each evening, when elevations are most likely to occur. The patient needs to be assured that there is nothing abnormal about temperatures in the range of 97.0°F to 99.3°F.

ANNOTATED BIBLIOGRAPHY

Dinarello CA, Cannon JG, Wolff SM. New concepts on the pathogenesis of fever. Rev Infect Dis 1986;10:168. (*A basic science review of the mechanisms of fever.*)

DiNubile MJ. Acute fevers of unknown origin. Arch Intern Med 1993;153:2525. (*A plea for restraint in empiric use of antibiotics when etiology is unknown.*)

Hirschman JV. Normal body temperature. JAMA 1992;267:414. (*A discussion of the patient who claims his normal temperature is less than 98.6°F.*)

Jacoby GA, Swartz MN. Fever of undetermined origin. N Engl J Med 1973;289:1407. (*A slightly dated but useful review of the etiologies that should be considered in the patient with fever of unknown origin.*)

Klontz KC, Lieb S, Schreiber M et al. Syndromes of *Vibrio vulnificus* infections. Ann Intern Med 1988;109:318. (*A previously unrecognized and potentially important cause of fever and infection.*)

Knockaert DC, Vanneste LJ, Vanneste SB et al. Fever of unknown origin in the 1980s. Arch Intern Med 1992;152:51. (*An update of the diagnostic spectrum, including HIV-related diseases.*)

Kumar KL, Reuler JB. Drug fever. West J Med 1986;144:753. (*Superb review of drug fever, especially of clinical presentations.*)

Larson EB, Featherstone HJ, Petersdorf RG. Fever of undetermined origin: Diagnosis and follow-up of 105 cases. Medicine (Baltimore) 1982;61:269. (*Major review; cancer was the leading cause.*)

Marantz PR, Linzer M, Feiner CJ et al. Inability to predict diagnosis in febrile intravenous drug-abusers. Ann Intern Med 1987;106:823. (*Initially difficult to determine risk of serious underlying illness.*)

Petersdorf RG. Fever of unknown origin: An old friend revisited. Arch Intern Med 1992;154:21. (*An editorial commenting on the changing pattern of etiologies cited in the Knockaert study.*)

Petersdorf RG, Beeson PB. Fever of unexplained origin: Report on 100 cases. Medicine (Baltimore) 1961;40:1. (*A classic paper that details a logical diagnostic approach which is still useful today.*)

Simon HB. Current concepts: hyperthermia. N Engl J Med 1993; 329:483. (*Review of non-infectious causes of fever.*)

Sox HC, Liang MH. The erythrocyte sedimentation rate. Ann Intern Med 1986;104:515. (*A critical review of the test, arguing that it is not a useful screening procedure.*)

Styrt B, Sugarman B. Antipyresis and fever. Arch Intern Med 1990;150:1589. (*A thoughtful review of the evidence on need to treat temperature elevations.*)

Young EJ, Fainstein V, Musher DM. Drug-induced fever. Rev Infect Dis 1982;4:69. (*Antibiotics were responsible for most cases.*)

12
Evaluation of Lymphadenopathy

HARVEY B. SIMON, M.D.

Primary Care Medicine: Office Evaluation and Management of the Adult Patient, 3rd edition, edited by Allan H. Goroll, Lawrence A. May, and Albert G. Mulley, Jr. J.B. Lippincott Company, Philadelphia

Of the nearly 600 lymph nodes throughout the body, only a few are normally palpable, including small nodes in the submandibular, axillary, and inguinal regions. Nevertheless, lymphadenopathy is a very common presenting symptom. Most often, adenopathy indicates benign, self-limited disease; this is particularly true in children and young adults, who are more prone to reactive lymphatic hyperplasia. Despite this, patient concern is often substantial, due to worry about serious infectious processes (eg, acquired immunodeficiency syndrome [AIDS]) on the one hand and neoplastic diseases on the other. A systematic evaluation of lymphadenopathy will provide reassurance as well as a correct diagnosis. A critical decision for the primary physician is when to refer the patient for lymph node biopsy.

PATHOPHYSIOLOGY AND CLINICAL PRESENTATION

Localized Adenopathy. Small lymph nodes in the neck, axilla, and groin may be palpable in normal individuals. Palpable nodes in other regions or any node exceeding 1 cm in size should be regarded as potentially abnormal. Inflammation and infiltration are responsible for pathologic enlargement. Although size alone is not itself diagnostic, nodes *larger than 3 cm* suggest neoplastic disease. Localized lymphadenopathy may represent spread of disease from an area of drainage. Of particular importance are palpable supraclavicular nodes. The left one, which is sometimes referred to as the *"sentinel"* node, is in contact with the thoracic duct, which drains much of the abdominal cavity. The right supraclavicular node drains the mediastinum, lungs, and esophagus.

Hilar Adenopathy. Bilateral hilar adenopathy encountered as an incidental finding on chest radiograph in an otherwise asymptomatic patient is likely to be due to *sarcoidosis*. In about 80 percent of such cases, the adenopathy will resolve spontaneously. In areas endemic for fungal infection, asymptomatic bilateral hilar adenopathy may result from exposure to *coccidiomycosis* or *histoplasmosis*. *Lymphoma* and *bronchogenic carcinoma* can cause bilateral hilar adenopathy, but the patient is rarely asymptomatic at the time of presentation. The same pertains, though to a lesser degree, to primary *tuberculosis (TB)*.

Unilateral hilar adenopathy is most often a manifestation of lymphoma or bronchogenic carcinoma, although granulomatous diseases may also present in this fashion.

Generalized Lymphadenopathy results from systemic processes, such as infection, malignancy, hypersensitivity, and sometimes even metabolic disease with node infiltration. The adenopathy associated with human immunodeficiency virus (HIV) infection may be due to the disease itself or to secondary infection (eg, cytomegalovirus). The finding of generalized adenopathy in an otherwise asymptomatic HIV-infected patient still indicates a high risk of progression to AIDS (see Chapter 13).

Other Lymphatic Abnormalities. In addition to lymphadenopathy, abnormalities of the lymphatic system may present in other ways. *Lymphangitis,* appearing as red, warm streaks along the course of superficial lymphatic networks, suggests an acute inflammatory response to pyogenic infection in the drainage area; staphylococci and streptococci are frequently responsible. *Lymphadenitis,* presenting as a tender, warm, soft, rapidly enlarging node, has similar significance and often reflects acute pyogenic infection of the node itself. *Lymphedema* results from interruption of lymphatic drainage; surgical node dissection, radiotherapy, or fibrosis due to chronic infections, such as filariasis or lymphogranuloma venereum, are causes of lymphedema.

DIFFERENTIAL DIAGNOSIS

The causes of lymphadenopathy can be conveniently considered in terms of location of the enlarged nodes (Table 12–1). In children and young adults, most adenopathy is due to reactive hyperplasia and is less likely to represent serious pathology than is its occurrence in adults. Under the age of 30, the cause proves to be benign in 80 percent of cases; over age 50, the rate of benign disease falls to 40 percent.

WORKUP

History and Physical Examination

A number of basic questions arise in the evaluation of lymphadenopathy that can be readily addressed by a careful history and physical examination:

1. Is the palpable mass indeed a lymph node? A variety of other structures, including enlarged parotid glands, cervical hygromas, thyroglossal and branchial cysts, hemangiomas, abscesses, lipomas, and other tumors, may on occasion be confused with lymphadenopathy.
2. Is the lymphadenopathy acute or chronic? Clearly, lymph node enlargement due to acute viral or pyogenic infection becomes less likely as the days and weeks pass, and granulomatous inflammation (sarcoidosis, TB, fungal infection) and neoplastic disease become greater worries. Even so, chronicity alone is not always a harbinger of serious disease, for on occasion reactive hyperplasia can persist for many months.
3. What is the character of the enlarged node itself? Tender, mobile nodes most often reflect lymphadenitis or lymphatic hyperplasia in response to acute inflammation. Firm, rubbery, nontender nodes may be found in lym-

Table 12-1. Important Causes of Lymphadenopathy

GENERALIZED LYMPHADENOPATHY	LOCALIZED LYMPHADENOPATHY
Infections	***Anterior Auricular***
Mononucleosis	Viral conjunctivitis
AIDS	Trachoma, posterior auricular
AIDS-related complex (ARC)	Rubella
Toxoplasmosis	Scalp infection
Secondary syphilis	***Submandibular or Cervical (Unilateral)***
Hypersensitivity Reactions	Buccal cavity infection
Serum sickness	Pharyngitis (can be bilateral)
Phenytoin and other drugs	Nasopharyngeal tumor
Vasculitis (lupus, rheum. arthritis)	Thyroid malignancy
Metabolic Disease	***Cervical Bilateral***
Hyperthyroidism	Mononucleosis
Lipidoses	Sarcoidosis
Neoplasia	Toxoplasmosis
Leukemia	Pharyngitis
Hodgkin's disease (advanced stages)	***Supraclavicular, Right***
Non-Hodgkin's lymphoma	Pulmonary malignancy
	Mediastinal malignancy
	Esophageal malignancy
	Supraclavicular, Left
	Intra-abdominal malignancy
	Renal malignancy
	Testicular or ovarian malignancy
	Axillary
	Breast malignancy or infection
	Upper extremity infection
	Epitrochlear
	Syphilis (bilateral)
	Hand infection (unilateral)
	Inguinal
	Syphilis
	Genital herpes
	Lymphogranuloma venereum
	Chancroid
	Lower extremity or local infection
	Any Region
	Cat-scratch fever
	Hodgkin's disease
	Non-Hodgkin's lymphoma
	Leukemia
	Metastatic cancer
	Sarcoidosis
	Granulomatous infections
	Hilar Adenopathy, Bilateral
	Sarcoidosis
	Fungal infection (histoplasmosis, coccidioidomycosis)
	Lymphoma
	Bronchogenic carcinoma
	Tuberculosis
	Hilar Adenopathy, Unilateral
	Lymphoma
	Bronchogenic carcinoma
	Tuberculosis
	Sarcoidosis

phoma. Painless, stone-hard, fixed, matted nodes suggest metastatic carcinoma.

4. Is the adenopathy localized or generalized? Numerous systemic processes, including *infections* (eg, infectious mononucleosis and other viral infections, toxoplasmosis, secondary syphilis); *hypersensitivity reactions* (serum sickness, reactions to phenytoin [Dilantin] and other drugs, and vasculitis, including systemic lupus erythematosus and rheumatoid arthritis); *metabolic diseases* (hyperthyroidism and various lipidoses), and *neoplasia* (especially leukemia) can produce generalized lymphadenopathy. However, Hodgkin's disease is usually unicen-

tric in origin and spreads to contiguous regional nodes, so that generalized adenopathy is rare except in very advanced disease. While certain non-Hodgkin's lymphomas may be multicentric, generalized adenopathy is also a late finding and is usually asymmetric, unlike the earlier and more symmetric adenopathy of some leukemias, such as chronic lymphocytic leukemia.

Generalized adenopathy, particularly if accompanied by weight loss, fever, or other constitutional symptoms, should raise the question of *AIDS* or HIV infection. Male homosexuals, intravenous drug abusers, hemophiliacs and other multiply transfused individuals, and Haitians are at particular risk (see Chapter 13).

Localized adenopathy should raise additional possibilities, depending on the area involved. For example, *submandibular* lymphadenopathy, which is perhaps the most common type of adenopathy, frequently results from pharyngitis (viral, streptococcal, gonococcal) or head and neck or intraoral infection. While these benign processes vastly predominate, it should be remembered that patients with Hodgkin's disease most often present with cervical lymphadenopathy. *Preauricular* adenopathy may be a component of "occuloglandular fevers" due to adenoviral conjunctivitis, sarcoidosis, tularemia, cat-scratch disease, and other processes. *Posterior auricular* or *posterior cervical* adenopathy frequently reflects infections of the scalp but may also be prominent in systemic processes, such as rubella or toxoplasmosis.

While *anterior cervical* lymphadenopathy often results from head and neck infections, isolated supraclavicular node enlargement is more indicative of metastatic malignancy; the *right supraclavicular* nodes drain the mediastinum, esophagus, and thorax, while *left supraclavicular* adenopathy (Virchow's node) is suggestive of primary intra-abdominal neoplasia. *Axillary* nodes become enlarged in response to upper extremity infection, but breast cancer must be considered as well. Although enlarged *epitrochlear* nodes are traditionally associated with secondary syphilis, this finding reflects generalized lymphadenopathy in lues; epitrochlear lymphadenopathy can be seen in many other systemic processes, as well as in response to hand infections. *Inguinal* lymphadenopathy is much more common. Inguinal nodes are palpable in most normal individuals, but they can enlarge substantially in infections of the genitalia or perineum, as well as in lower extremity infections.

Bilateral hilar adenopathy in an asymptomatic patient raises the possibilities of sarcoidosis and fungal exposure. *Unilateral hilar disease* suggests lymphoma, cancer, and granulomatous disease, as does bilateral disease in a symptomatic patient or one with an abnormal physical examination.

5. Are there associated systemic or localizing symptoms or signs? Fever, rash, weight loss, sore throat, dental pain, genital inflammation, and infections of the extremities are clues that may be particularly helpful. Of these symptoms, night sweats and weight loss are suggestive of granulomatous and neoplastic disease. Ear, nose, and throat symptoms suggest reactive lymphatic hyperplasia secondary to viral or localized bacterial infection.

   A careful examination of the skin for a primary inoculation site may provide the clue to a diagnosis of cat-scratch disease or tularemia. Checking for scalp infections, dermatophytes, and scabies is also needed. The liver and spleen are carefully examined; finding organomegaly may be an important clue for mononucleosis, sarcoidosis, or malignancy. Sternal tenderness may be present in leukemia.
6. Are there unusual epidemiologic clues? To cite a few examples, patients exposed to cats may develop cat-scratch disease or toxoplasmosis, which may also result from eating poorly cooked meat. Travel to the southwest United States may suggest the possibility of plague. An appropriate travel history or exposure to bird droppings may suggest fungal infection, as may lacerations sustained while gardening, in the case of sporotrichosis. Contact with wild rodents may result in tularemia, as may tick bites. A history of exposure to TB may be an important clue to scrofula. More commonly, community outbreaks may provide clues to the diagnosis of streptococcal pharyngitis or rubella, while a history of sexual exposure may raise the question of gonorrhea, syphilis, genital herpes, or lymphogranuloma.

Laboratory Studies

Laboratory studies need not be very elaborate. A *complete blood count* with *differential* often provides useful information and is almost always indicated. For example, atypical lymphocytosis suggests mononucleosis, other viral infections, and toxoplasmosis; granulocytosis is indicative of pyogenic infection; eosinophilia raises the question of a hypersensitivity reaction; pancytopenia is consistent with marrow suppression by tumor and HIV infection.

Other studies are based on the clinical presentation of the lymphadenopathy. A variety of blood chemistries may help in selected cases. Elevations of *uric acid* may reflect lymphoma or other hematologic malignancies. *Liver function tests* (especially the *alkaline phosphatase*) provide an objective parameter to follow. While such abnormalities are nonspecific, they do suggest liver involvement, which can be further evaluated by biopsy.

Localized Adenopathy. If pharyngitis and cervical or submandibular adenopathy are present, a *throat culture* is mandatory. It should be remembered that while these are routinely processed for streptococci, special Thayer-Martin medium must be used as well if gonococci are suspected. *Urethral* or *cervical cultures* and smears should also be obtained if gonorrhea is a potential cause of inguinal lymphadenopathy. *Blood cultures* are indicated in the rare cases of suspected plague, tularemia, or brucellosis or if the clinical picture suggests staphylococcal or streptococcal lymphadenitis. Biopsy may be necessary to rule out lymphoma and Hodgkin's disease if the adenopathy is progressive and the remainder of the workup is unrevealing (see below).

On occasion, lymphomatous retroperitoneal or intra-abdominal nodes may enlarge enough to present as an abdominal mass. When lymphoma is a serious possibility, or when staging is necessary in known lymphoma or Hodgkin's disease, *abdominal computed tomography (CT) scanning* can be used to detect enlargement of the retroperitoneal nodes; *bone marrow biopsy* may provide a tissue diagnosis (see Chapter 84).

Generalized Adenopathy. Serologic tests may be of great value. The *heterophile test* and *serologic tests for syphilis* are obvious examples. In addition, a serum sample from the acute phase of the illness can be frozen to be submitted with a later convalescent phase serum specimen for antibody titers against viruses, fungi, and toxoplasmosis. Brucellosis may also be diagnosed serologically. Serologic tests, including *antinuclear antibodies* and *rheumatoid factor,* may suggest a noninfectious process, such as collagen-vascular disease.

Hilar Adenopathy. *Tuberculin skin testing (PPD)* and the *angiotensin converting enzyme (ACE)* determination can facilitate the assessment. If both are negative and the patient is Caucasian, then bronchoscopy and mediastinoscopy may be necessary to rule out lymphoma. If the patient is ACE+/PPD-, then the probability is very high that sarcoidosis is the cause and there is little need for further evaluation. If the patient is ACE-/PPD+, then primary TB is likely. Reliable skin tests are also available for coccidioidomycosis and tularemia. On the other hand, cutaneous anergy may suggest sarcoidosis or lymphoma, but this is a nonspecific finding. Skin testing may be very helpful in the diagnosis of cat-scratch disease, but, as with the Kveim test, the necessary antigen is available only on a research basis in selected centers.

Among radiologic studies, the *chest radiograph* is particularly valuable, because hilar adenopathy may be present in patients with enlargement of peripheral nodes. Hilar adenopathy may also be detected on chest radiograph in the absence of peripheral lymphadenopathy. Sarcoidosis, lymphoma, fungal infection, TB, or metastatic carcinoma (particularly from a lung primary) should be among the diagnostic considerations. *CT scanning* can provide additional definition. *Mediastinoscopy* may be required for tissue diagnosis, though not in asymptomatic patients with bilateral hilar adenopathy and clear lung fields, who most likely have sarcoidosis or a fungal exposure.

Lymph Node Biopsy should be considered as the most direct approach to the diagnosis of lymphadenopathy. Although the majority of such procedures are technically easy and can be accomplished under local anesthesia, this is an invasive test and it can sometimes prove nondiagnostic. It should be employed only when simpler approaches have failed to give a diagnosis and suspicion of a therapeutically important cause remains (eg, TB, lymphoma, cancer, sarcoidosis, cat-scratch disease). Sometimes, careful *observation* over a period of time may be diagnostically useful before resorting to biopsy. In many cases of benign lymphadenopathy, the nodes will regress spontaneously even if no etiologic diagnosis has been made. However, some lymphomas may regress transiently and simulate a more benign etiology.

If undiagnosed adenopathy persists over a period of weeks to months, especially if the nodes are enlarging or if neoplastic disease remains a concern, then consideration of node biopsy is indicated. In one retrospective study, weight loss, night sweats, nodes larger than 2 cm, and abnormal chest radiograph were the strongest prebiopsy predictors of important disease. In the case of fluctuant nodes, *needle aspiration* can be used to diagnose infectious processes in some cases.

The node to be biopsied should be selected with care; if generalized adenopathy is present, it is best to avoid inguinal or axillary nodes if possible, because reactive hyperplasia in these areas may make interpretation difficult. In general, enlarged *supraclavicular nodes* have the highest diagnostic yield. When possible, *excisional biopsy* is preferred. At the time of biopsy, tissue should be submitted for appropriate bacteriologic smears and cultures, as well as for histologic study. Touch preps may be useful. Special stains for bacteria, mycobacteria, and fungi may be helpful, as may specific stains for unusual processes, such as periodic acid-Schiff (PAS) stains for Whipple's disease or lipidosis and Congo red stains for amyloid. Interpretation of lymph node pathology can be quite difficult and requires careful study by experienced observers. With such study, benign processes such as toxoplasmosis or cat-scratch disease can be suspected histologically, and detailed analysis of serial sections may reveal lymphomas that are not diagnosed with less intensive pathologic study. Finally, if pathologic study reveals reactive hyperplasia or is nondiagnostic, patients should be followed carefully, as up to 25 percent may eventually exhibit an illness responsible for the lymphadenopathy, most often lymphoma.

Evaluation of Lymphadenopathy in the HIV-Infected Patient. In most patients who are HIV-positive, the lymphadenopathy represents follicular hyperplasia in response to HIV infection. However, the list of possible causes includes lymphoma, mycobacterial and viral infections, Kaposi's sarcoma, and other cancers (see Chapter 13). The principles for evaluation and biopsy are similar to those for the non-HIV patient, with the proviso that the probability of serious underlying pathology is increased. Suggested criteria for lymph node biopsy in these patients include size greater than 2 cm in diameter, rapidly enlarging or asymmetric adenopathy, constitutional symptoms, and intrathoracic adenopathy on chest radiograph. Using these rather restrictive criteria and needle aspiration as the mode of biopsy, yields of less than 50 percent have been reported, with most having follicular hyperplasia.

INDICATIONS FOR REFERRAL

Any patient suspected of harboring a malignancy should have a consultation with an oncologist or oncologic surgeon to further consider the need for biopsy and to determine the best approach to obtaining a tissue diagnosis. Simply arranging for the biopsy of an accessible node may fail to achieve a diagnosis and subject the patient to an unnecessary invasive procedure. Consultation may also be useful if one is thinking about a period of observation and wants to be sure that this represents a reasonable approach.

ANNOTATED BIBLIOGRAPHY

Greenfield S, Jordan MC. The clinical investigation of lymphadenopathy in primary care practice. JAMA 1978;240:1388. (*A still useful algorithm for workup of peripheral lymphadenopathy in the ambulatory setting.*)

Saltzstern SL. The fate of patients with nondiagnostic lymph node biopsies. Surgery 1965;58:659. (*A retrospective study of lymph node biopsies in 177 adult males. In 68 patients, the indication for biopsy was lymphadenopathy; 52 percent of these were nondiagnostic, but 17 percent of patients with nondiagnostic biopsies subsequently developed lymphoma. Supraclavicular node biopsies had the highest diagnostic yield.*)

Schroer KR, Fransilla KO. Atypical hyperplasia of lymph nodes: A follow-up study. Cancer 1979;44:115. (*Of patients with nondiagnostic lymph node biopsies, 25 percent to 6 percent were found within a few months to have lymphoma, cancer, connective tissue disease, or infection. Emphasizes importance of follow-up.*)

Sinclair S, Beckman E, Ellman L. Biopsy of enlarged superficial lymph nodes. JAMA 1974;228:602. (*A retrospective pathologic study of 135 lymph node biopsies performed because of undiagnosed lymphadenopathy. Sixty-three percent of the biopsies were diagnostic; 50 patients had lymphoma, 14 carcinoma, 6 tuberculosis, 1 histoplasmosis, 7 acute lymphadenitis, and 1 Dilantin sensitivity. Of the 50 patients with nondiagnostic biopsies, 25 percent developed a disease related to the indications for biopsy, which was most often lymphoma, and which usually occurred within 8 months of the initial biopsy.*)

Slap GB, Brooks JSJ, Schwartz JS. When to perform biopsies of enlarged peripheral lymph nodes in young patients. JAMA 1984;252:1321. (*A retrospective study of 123 patients up to the age of 25 who underwent lymph node biopsy. A predictive model was developed to determine before biopsy which patients were likely to have "treatable" causes of adenopathy.*)

Slap GB, Connor JL, Wigton RS et al. Validation of a model to identify young patients for lymph node biopsy. JAMA 1986; 255:2768. (*Model found useful for detection of treatable causes.*)

13
Approach to the Patient with HIV Infection

STEPHEN L. BOSWELL, M.D.

Primary Care Medicine: Office Evaluation and Management of the Adult Patient, 3rd edition, edited by Allan H. Goroll, Lawrence A. May, and Albert G. Mulley, Jr. J.B. Lippincott Company, Philadelphia

Despite the fact that a cure remains elusive, the management of the person infected with human immunodeficiency virus (HIV) has improved. Most care is now conducted in the outpatient setting, even for patients with acquired immunodeficiency syndrome (AIDS). Intervention in the asymptomatic period, new therapies, and innovative strategies to prevent secondary infections have significantly decreased morbidity and in some instances increased survival. With the shift in management to the outpatient setting, primary care physicians have assumed an increasingly central role in the comprehensive care of the HIV-infected patient; they are responsible for initial diagnosis, counseling, prevention of spread, initiation of antiviral and prophylactic therapies, outpatient treatment of secondary infection, determination of need for hospitalization, and provision of supportive care in the late stages of illness. This requires that the primary care physician be knowledgeable about HIV risk behaviors, disease manifestations, laboratory techniques, current therapy, and prophylaxis strategies.

CASE DEFINITION AND EPIDEMIOLOGY OF HIV INFECTION AND AIDS

Case Definition. The Centers for Disease Control and Prevention (CDC) criteria for *HIV infection* in patients older than 13 years of age include the following:

- repeatedly reactive screening tests for HIV antibody with specific antibody identified by the use of supplemental tests, *or*
- direct identification of virus in host tissues by virus isolation, *or*
- HIV antigen detection, *or*
- a positive result on any other highly specific licensed test for HIV.

In 1993, the CDC revised the criteria for the *definition of AIDS* to incorporate clinical presentations in women and heterosexuals and advances in understanding the significance of counts of CD4+ T lymphocytes (known as helper T lymphocytes or CD4 cells). This CDC surveillance definition of AIDS requires the following:

- a CD4+ T-lymphocyte count < 200 cells/mm^3 and laboratory evidence of HIV infection *or*
- presence of an AIDS-indicator disease *or*
- presence of pulmonary tuberculosis (TB), recurrent pneumonia, or invasive cervical cancer in a patient with laboratory evidence of HIV infection; *and*
- absence of another reason for immune impairment.

Epidemiology. It is estimated that 1.0 to 1.5 million Americans are now infected with HIV, and the numbers continue to rise. AIDS has become the second-leading cause of death among men 25 to 44 years of age and is rising among women of the same age group. The National Commission on AIDS predicts AIDS will "clearly outstrip all other diseases in lost human potential." The problem is worldwide, with outbreaks of epidemic proportion in Africa and Thailand. In the United States, the African-American and Hispanic communities are particularly affected, accounting for more than 4 percent of AIDS cases during the first decade of the epidemic. This overrepresentation is likely to increase as the epidemic continues to spread among intravenous drug users, their sexual partners, and their children. The epidemic appears to have peaked in the gay population, helped by educational efforts.

In the United States, those at highest risk of infection are men with a history of *homosexual* or *bisexual* activity; *intravenous drug users* and their sexual contacts; the *sexual contacts* of homosexual or bisexual men; persons who received blood and *blood products prior to 1985;* and *children* born to infected women. The risk of directly acquiring HIV infection through processed blood or selected blood products (plasma and clotting factor concentrates) has dramatically decreased since 1985 as a consequence of the widespread screening of those who donate blood and plasma, the use of serologic tests for HIV, and the viral inactivation of various plasma products.

AIDS is only part of the much larger epidemic of HIV infection. For every person who is living with AIDS in the United States, there are 10 to 20 individuals who are HIV-infected with minimal or no symptoms. They often present to health care providers for problems related to high-risk activity (eg, intravenous drug use), unaware they are carrying HIV. These encounters provide a critical opportunity to teach about HIV infection.

PATHOPHYSIOLOGY, CLINICAL PRESENTATION, AND COURSE

Pathophysiology

The *human immunodeficiency virus* is an RNA retrovirus that includes a core protein (p24), a reverse transcriptase, and envelope glycoproteins. Isolates of HIV differ genetically and antigenically, particularly in regard to envelope proteins (a feature that has complicated development of an effective vaccine).

HIV is transmitted through *sexual contact, parenteral exposure* to blood and selected blood products, and *maternal transmission* (via breast milk and perinatal transmission). Once the virus enters the body, it attaches to the surface of *CD4+ T lymphocytes*. These helper T lymphocytes are the target of HIV, by virtue of the virus's affinity for receptors on their surface. Once attached, the virus enters the lymphocyte and uncoats. Its RNA is transcribed to DNA by reverse transcriptase. The DNA may remain in the cytoplasm or become integrated into the host cell genome, where it remains latent until some stimulus (as yet undefined) triggers replication of virus. In addition to intracellular viral multiplication, transmission of virus to macrophages that fuse with HIV-infected CD4 cells occurs.

HIV entry into a cell followed by replication is often *cytotoxic,* leading to destruction of the involved cells. CD4 cells are most susceptible to cell death; *macrophages* appear to be largely spared. It is believed that macrophages are the principal reservoir of virus and the vehicle for transport to other areas of the body, including the central nervous system (CNS). Pathogenicity of HIV appears to be a function of destruction and disruption of CD4 cells, which are central to maintenance of immunocompetency. With damage to the CD4 cell population, opportunistic infection and malignancy may follow. Antibodies to HIV begin to appear within 6 to 12 weeks of infection, though some patients may not manifest detectable titers for several months.

Clinical Presentations and Course

HIV infection in humans is a continuum that can be crudely broken into four phases: 1) primary HIV infection; 2) asymptomatic HIV-seropositive; 3) symptomatic (pre-AIDS) HIV-seropositive; and 4) AIDS. The most recent CDC classification designates three categories: category A encompasses phases 1 and 2; category B, phase 3; and category C, phase 4.

Primary Infection. This first phase of the illness is brief and consists of a *mononucleosis-like syndrome*. In the initial years of the epidemic, the syndrome was not recognized, but after the development of serologic tests, it became possible to link HIV to this clinical syndrome. The syndrome consists of fever, sweats, lethargy, malaise, myalgias, arthralgias, headaches, photophobia, diarrhea, sore throat, lymphadenopathy, and a truncal maculopapular rash. It is of sudden onset and lasts 3 to 14 days. More than 50 percent of individuals infected with HIV experience one or more of these symptoms. Less frequently, neurologic signs and symptoms occur, such as those of meningoencephalitis, myelopathy, peripheral neuropathy, and Guillain-Barré syndrome. The most common neurologic symptoms in primary HIV infection are headache and photophobia. The symptoms that most markedly differentiate seroconversion subjects from control subjects are *swollen lymph nodes,* truncal or generalized *rash, depression,* irritability, anorexia, *weight loss,* and *retroorbital pain*.

Asymptomatic Seropositivity. This second phase of HIV infection is the longest of the four phases and is also the most variable. This phase typically lasts *3 to 6 years* and is distinguished by the lack of overt evidence of HIV infection. Approximately 500,000 individuals fall into this category in the United States.

Symptomatic Seropositivity (Pre-AIDS). The onset of the third phase of HIV infection ushers in the first physical evidence of immune system dysfunction. *Persistent generalized lymphadenopathy* is often an early sign of this phase. *Localized fungal infections* of the toes, fingernails, and mouth frequently occur. Among women, recalcitrant *vaginal yeast* and *trichomonal infections* often recur. *Oral hairy leukoplakia,* one of the most commonly missed signs of HIV infection, is very prevalent and typically found on the tongue. Cutaneous manifestations of this phase of illness include widespread *warts, molluscum contagiosum,* exacerbations of *psoriasis,* and *seborrheic dermatitis*. Multidermatomal *herpes zoster* and an increased severity or frequency of *herpes simplex* infections can occur. Constitutional symptoms including *night sweats, weight loss,* and *diarrhea* are often seen. The duration of this phase is approximately *3 to 5 years*.

AIDS is the fourth phase of HIV infection, characterized by development of disseminated opportunistic infections and unusual malignancies. Pulmonary, gastrointestinal, neurologic, and systemic symptoms are common.

Pneumocystis carinii pneumonia (PCP) is among the most common infections in AIDS patients, with an attack rate of almost 80 percent in patients not receiving primary prophylaxis (see below). Fever, night sweats, malaise, and weight loss typically precede onset of pulmonary symptoms by days to weeks. A dry cough may be the first pulmonary manifestation, followed by shortness of breath. Diffuse infiltrates on chest radiograph, widening alveolar-arteriolar oxygen gradient (> 30 mm Hg), and a low PO_2 (< 50 mm Hg) are associated with reduced survival.

Pulmonary and disseminated forms of invasive fungal infection with *Cryptococcus neoformans, Histoplasma capsulatum,* and *Coccidioides immitis* are other hallmarks of AIDS. Cryptococcal infection occurs throughout the United States and often presents subtly, with headache, fever, and malaise. Altered mentation and stiff neck are absent in most cases. At times, pulmonary complaints dominate the clinical picture of cryptococcal infection. Pulmonary and systemic complaints are prominent in patients with histoplasmosis or coccidiomycosis. Infiltrates on chest film of a patient living in an endemic area suggest the diagnosis; splenomegaly can be marked in histoplasmosis.

Mycobacterial infections, both pulmonary and disseminated, are consequences of falling CD4 cell counts. HIV-positive patients with latent TB infection are at increased risk of reactivation and dissemination. Meningeal involvement is the most common form of disseminated disease. Many strains isolated from AIDS patients demonstrate multiple-drug resistance (see Chapter 49). *Mycobacterium avium-intracellulare* infection is an accompaniment of very advanced disease. The clinical presentation is one of wasting, fever, sweats, diarrhea, and weight loss. Blood cultures are often positive.

Recurrent bacterial pneumonia (two or more episodes per year) is a more recently appreciated manifestation of AIDS. The presentations and organisms are typical of those for bacterial pneumonia, with positive sputum cultures and infiltrates on chest radiograph. Such pneumonias are 20 times more common in HIV patients with low CD4 cell counts (< $200/mm^3$) than in those with normal counts. The recurrent development of such pneumonias represents significant immunosuppression.

Cytomegalovirus (CMV) infection, often due to reactivation of latent disease, is common in AIDS. *Retinitis,* presenting as unilateral visual loss or floaters and, if untreated, progressing to bilateral disease and blindness, afflicts about 5 percent to 10 percent of AIDS patients. Exudates and hemorrhages are noted on funduscopic examination. Esophagitis, gastritis, and colitis also may develop.

Enteric infections cause much morbidity for AIDS patients and typically present as weight loss, cramping pain, and large volume diarrhea. *Salmonella, Shigella,* and *Campylobacter* are the leading causes, with the latter two more characteristically presenting with bloody diarrhea and leukocytes on Wright's stain of a fecal smear. *Cryptosporidia,* a protozoa, is an important cause of diarrheal illness in AIDS patients in undeveloped areas.

HIV wasting syndrome is characterized by profound involuntary loss of more than 10 percent of body weight in conjunction with either chronic diarrhea (2 or more stools/day for more than 1 month) or fever and persistent weakness for a similar period in the absence of another cause.

Neurologic injury from HIV infection ranges from mild *peripheral neuropathy* causing paresthesias to *encephalopathy* with debilitating dementia. The virus appears to be neurotropic, causing significant neurologic injury in up to 30 percent of AIDS patients. *AIDS dementia complex* results from direct injury to neurons from HIV invasion of the CNS. Early on, there may be only minor impairment of cognitive or motor function, but in later stages, frank dementia and disabling motor disturbances ensue. Neuroimaging studies show diffuse atrophic changes.

Opportunistic CNS infections also occur. *Toxoplasmosis* is an important one. Most toxoplasmal disease represents reactivation of latent infection. About one-third of those who are IgG-seropositive experience reactivation. CNS involvement can cause symptoms both of a mass lesion (discrete deficits, headache) and those of encephalitis (fever, altered mental status). The images on scanning by computed tomography (CT) or magnetic resonance imaging (MRI) are characteristic: multiple (> 3) contrast-enhanced mass lesions in the basal ganglia and subcortical white matter.

Syphilis is of increased likelihood in HIV patients with a history of high-risk sexual behavior, and it may take an atypical or accelerated course, including CNS spread.

Malignancies are a consequence of the reduction in cellular immunity. Kaposi's sarcoma, non-Hodgkin's lymphoma, and primary CNS lymphoma occur with greatly increased frequency in the setting of HIV infection and serve to define the onset of AIDS. *Kaposi's sarcoma* is characterized by raised violaceous nonblanching plaques or nodules on the skin or mucus membranes. Visceral involvement may occur, presenting as hematemesis, melena, or hematochezia. A mass lesion on neuroimaging study may represent a *primary CNS lymphoma,* especially in a patient free of the encephalopathic findings that occur with toxoplasmosis of the CNS. Such lymphomas are rare except in the context of HIV infection. There is a 10-fold increase in the incidence of *cervical dysplasia* in HIV-positive women. The development of *invasive cervical cancer* is indicative of severe immune compromise.

Skin problems in addition to Kaposi's sarcoma are an important source of morbidity. They range from cellulitis to drug eruptions and increase in frequency with worsening of immune function. Drug reactions are particularly common, with trimethoprim-sulfamethoxazole, dapsone-trimethoprim, and aminopenicillins most often implicated.

Prognosis. Prognosis closely parallels CD4 cell count. Asymptomatic HIV-positive patients with CD4 cell counts greater than 500 may remain otherwise healthy for years. On the other hand, those with CD4 cell counts lower than 200 are now considered to have AIDS. Once diagnosed with AIDS, survival is usually 1 to 3 years. Most frequently, death is caused by opportunistic infection or malignancy. Earlier intervention in HIV infection postpones the onset of AIDS and improves overall survival and quality of life (see below).

DIAGNOSIS

The diagnosis of *HIV infection* is usually made serologically, by presence of persistent HIV antibody positivity. Alternative diagnostic methods include virus isolation and HIV antigen detection. The very sensitive *ELISA* method (enzyme-linked immunosorbent assay) is used for HIV antibody screening, with positive tests subjected to the more specific *Western blot analysis* for confirmation. Sensitivity and specificity of the ELISA are in the range of 99 percent for patients at high risk, but the predictive value of a positive test falls in patients at low risk. Occasionally, it is necessary to attempt isolation of the virus or the provirus when clinical suspicion is high but standard screening tests are normal.

The *diagnosis of AIDS* has predominantly been a clinical one, based on the identification of an indicator condition. However, the original AIDS definition emphasized conditions seen in HIV-infected gay men and omitted attention to CD4 cell count and to presentations in other populations, such as women and heterosexuals. These shortcomings have been addressed in the new CDC surveillance definition of AIDS (see above), which expands the list of indicator conditions to include pulmonary TB, invasive cervical cancer, and recurrent pneumonia in patients who are HIV-positive. In addition, the importance of immunocompetence is acknowledged in the new diagnostic criteria, with HIV-positive patients having a CD4 cell count lower than 200 now included among those considered to have AIDS.

WORKUP

Once a diagnosis of HIV infection is made, the goals of the workup are to identify the stage of illness, determine prognosis, and promptly identify complications of immunoincompetence. Progression to full-blown AIDS is a major concern. Patients with falling CD4 cell counts are at particularly high risk and should be examined frequently and closely.

History

The initial interview of the HIV-infected patient should seek information about *infections, malignancies,* and *exposures* that may indicate ongoing immune dysfunction or the potential for future difficulty.

Past Medical History is carefully reviewed for a previous diagnosis of herpetic infections; aseptic meningitis; recurrent sinusitis; skin problems such as folliculitis, staphylococcal infections, psoriasis, molluscum contagiosum, warts, persistent tinea, or seborrhea; recurrent bacterial pneumonia due to encapsulated organisms (*Haemophilus influenzae,* pneumococci); 1301 and vaginal candidiasis; abnormal Papanicolaou smear results; sexually transmitted diseases (if there is a history of syphilis, the details of treatment and serologic titers should be carefully documented); hepatitis B infection or vaccination; hepatitis C infection; TB (including history of skin testing, exposures, chest radiographs, vaccination, prophylaxis, and treatment); and gastrointestinal infections with parasitic organisms or more common bacterial pathogens. A travel history is useful to assess risk of exposure to histoplasmosis and coccidiomycosis.

Review of Systems. Since HIV infection is usually a multisystem disease, the review of systems takes on particular importance. It begins with inquiry into *systemic symptoms* (fever, chills, drenching night sweats, fatigue, weight loss), which may be manifestations of acute infection or more advanced disease. *Skin* complaints should be reviewed, particularly reports of violaceous nodules or plaques, pustules, petechiae, groin rashes, or herpetic lesions. Moving to the *HEENT* review, it is important to ask about sinus pain and any purulent drainage, sore throat, coated tongue, and white patches in the pharynx. Inquiry into *lymphadenopathy* may prove informative. The *pulmonary* review includes a check for dyspnea, persistent dry or productive cough, and hemoptysis.

A nonproductive cough of recent onset in conjunction with dyspnea on exertion should raise suspicion for pneumocystis pneumonia. Patients should be asked about *gastrointestinal* symptoms, especially odynophagia (painful swallowing suggestive of fungal esophagitis), abdominal pain, nausea, vomiting, diarrhea, melena, hematochezia, hematemesis, tenesmus, and perianal pain. Diarrhea and tenesmus suggest large bowel pathology. Cramping periumbilical pain, diarrhea, and increased flatus point to a small bowel process. Early satiety, anorexia, and weight loss may be manifestations of gastrointestinal lymphoma. Genitourinary involvement is screened by inquiry into abnormal vaginal bleeding or discharge, dyspareunia, urinary frequency, dysuria, and hematuria.

The *neurologic* review is critical. Unilateral headache becoming more generalized in conjunction with a stiff neck suggests spread of a parameningeal focus of infection into the CNS. New onset of lateralized weakness or numbness, especially if accompanied by a worsening unilateral headache, raises the question of a mass lesion (lymphoma, toxoplasmosis, brain abscess). Monocular visual field disturbances and floaters are characteristic complaints in patients with CMV retinitis. Diplopia and homonymous hemianopsia may indicate a CNS infection or malignancy. Numbness or tingling in the fingers or toes points to a peripheral neuropathy or myelopathy.

Neuropsychiatric difficulties raise the question of AIDS dementia complex. Suggestive symptoms include cognitive problems, difficulty with concentration, memory loss, insomnia, apathy, social isolation, and alterations in mood, especially depression. When accompanied by fever and delirium, they are more likely to be the consequence of an encephalopathy, but such difficulties may also occur as a consequence of a reactive depression. Distinguishing among these conditions can sometimes be difficult and may require neuropsychiatric testing and other diagnostic tests.

Physical Examination

The physical is directed toward signs of immunocompromise and its consequences. It includes a careful inspection of the skin, sinuses, eyes, oral cavity, lymph nodes, chest, abdomen, pelvis, and central and peripheral nervous systems. In addition, vital signs should be obtained and carefully recorded. Subtle but persistent unintended weight loss occurs frequently in HIV infection and can be one of the earliest manifestations of disease progression, secondary infection, or malignancy.

Skin is one of the most frequently affected organs. Kaposi's sarcoma (especially prevalent in gay men), warts, molluscum contagiosum, psoriasis, seborrheic dermatitis, and fungal infections of the toes and nails are especially common. A painless, persistent, raised purple lesion, especially if there is more than one such lesion, may be Kaposi's sarcoma and warrants biopsy. Facial seborrhea, scars from recurrent herpetic infections, and premature graying are among the more subtle signs of immunocompromise.

HEENT. The sinuses are noted for tenderness, failure to transilluminate, and purulent discharge. Funduscopic examination may reveal retinal exudates, hemorrhages, or cotton-wool spots suggestive of CMV infection. The exudate is typically pale and with associated hemorrhage; it usually begins peripherally and may be difficult to visualize during routine funduscopic examination.

Careful examination of the oral cavity is essential, looking for signs of oral hairy leukoplakia, thrush, mucosal petechiae, stomatitis, gingivitis, and Kaposi's sarcoma. Thrush is an important indicator of disease progression. The most common form is *pseudomembranous candidiasis*, removable white plaques on any oral mucosal surface. *Atrophic oral candidiasis* appears as smooth red patches on the hard or soft palate, buccal mucosa, or dorsal surface of the tongue. These may be easily missed without careful inspection. Rarely, candidiasis can occur in a leukoplakia-like form consisting of white lesions that cannot be wiped off but regress with prolonged antifungal therapy. This form of *Candida* infection can easily be confused with oral hairy leukoplakia and is distinguished primarily by its response to therapy (biopsy is rarely warranted). *Angular cheilitis* caused by *Candida* can appear as erythema, cracks, and fissures at the corner of the mouth. This may require the addition of a topical antifungal cream for adequate treatment. Mucosal petechiae can be the sole evidence of HIV-associated thrombocytopenia. *Kaposi's sarcoma* often produces oral lesions on the hard and soft palate and gingiva. Aphthous stomatitis may be easily confused with stomatitis due to herpes simplex or CMV infections. Biopsy may be required to distinguish them. Lymphoma may appear as a mass or ulcer(s), most commonly seen in the peritonsillar region.

Lymph nodes are checked periodically, as adenopathy may be an important sign of disease progression. If lymphadenopathy occurs in two or more noncontiguous extrainguinal sites, persists for longer than 3 months, and no cause other than HIV can be found, it is referred to as *persistent generalized lymphadenopathy (PGL)*. Occasionally, *splenomegaly* may be found in association with PGL. Asymmetric, large, firm, tender nodes may be evidence of malignancy or secondary infection and often require biopsy.

Chest, Abdomen, Rectum, and Genitalia. The lungs are examined for signs of consolidation, pleural inflammation, and effusion. The heart is checked for murmurs and rubs. The abdomen is noted for enlargement of the liver or spleen and for localized tenderness. Genital and rectal examinations are essential in all patients. Although evidence suggests that Papanicolaou test sensitivity may be reduced among HIV-infected women, it is currently recommended that it be performed semiannually, because of the greatly increased risk of invasive cervical cancer. Lymphoma, squamous cell carcinoma, CMV infection, and acyclovir-resistant herpes simplex infections are examples of unresponsive anorectal lesions that may require biopsy for diagnosis. Anoscopy or sigmoidoscopy may be necessary to diagnose rectal or colonic lesions or diarrhea.

Neurologic Examination should be conducted regularly and include a careful assessment for meningeal irritation, focal neurologic deficits, and changes in mental status. Evidence for peripheral neuropathy, myelopathy, and myopathy should be sought, since these are common and often treatable abnormalities. A detailed mental status examination may aid in the early detection of AIDS dementia complex.

Laboratory Testing

Laboratory testing plays an essential role, not only in workup and monitoring, but also in deciding on the nature and timing of therapy. Testing is used to identify those patients who might benefit from special interventions (eg, hepatitis B vaccine for those who are negative for both HBsAb and HBcAb). In other instances, it may reveal hidden medical problems that can be treated (eg, interferon-α for the treatment of chronic hepatitis C infection). Decisions regarding the initiation of antiretroviral therapy and PCP prophylaxis are largely based on laboratory tests, especially the CD4 cell count (see below). Increasingly, the effectiveness of antiretroviral therapy is being measured by such tests.

Initial Testing of the HIV-Positive Patient. *Complete blood count* and *platelet count* are essential (Table 13–1). Anemia of chronic disease, lymphopenia, and thrombocytopenia are common among HIV-infected patients, especially those patients with advanced disease. Idiopathic thrombocytopenia is sometimes seen in the acute phase of HIV infection. Macrocytic anemia occurs in patients receiving zidovudine. Marrow suppression with pancytopenia may develop in the context of invasion by lymphoma or disseminated fungal infection. Proper workup may require measurement of serum iron, ferritin, folate, and vitamin B_{12} concentrations (see Chapter 79). When assessing the cause of anemia, it should be recognized that the measurement of mean corpuscular volume (MCV) may be confounded by the macrocytosis that commonly occurs when patients are taking zidovudine.

Before initiating any drug therapies (many of which are toxic), baseline *serum chemistries* (electrolytes, blood urea nitrogen [BUN], creatinine, transaminase, alkaline phosphatase) are worth obtaining to help in monitoring.

Serologic testing for syphilis is essential because of its high prevalence among HIV-infected individuals. The natu-

Table 13-1. Initial Laboratory Evaluation of the HIV-Positive Patient

Complete blood count with differential, including platelet count
T-cell subsets; particularly CD4 count and CD4 percentage
Chemistries (electrolytes, liver function tests, creatinine, BUN)
Urinalysis
Syphilis serology (STS, RPR, FTAabs)
Hepatitis serology (HBsAg, HBcAb, HBsAb, anti-HCV antibody)
PA and lateral chest radiograph
PPD (modified Mantoux) with anergy control
Serum *T. gondii* IgG antibody titer

ral history of syphilis may be altered by HIV infection, and therefore careful attention to a past history and treatment for syphilis is essential. If a prior history of syphilis cannot be documented, further workup including a lumbar puncture is advocated by many physicians (see Chapters 124 and 141).

Toxoplasma gondii IgG serology may be helpful in identifying those individuals who might benefit from chemoprophylaxis to prevent reactivation. Studies are currently underway to determine the utility of this concept. Antibody testing helps select the encephalitis patient who might respond to antitoxoplasmal therapy.

CMV culturing has little role in managing the HIV-seropositive asymptomatic patient. However, *CMV serology* should be obtained prior to nonemergent transfusion. Patients who are CMV-seronegative should be given CMV-negative cellular blood products only. Whether CMV-positive cellular blood products should be given to CMV-seropositive, HIV-seropositive patients remains unclear.

All HIV-seropositive patients should have an *intermediate strength purified protein derivative (PPD)* tuberculin skin test unless they have previously been documented to be PPD-positive, have a history of TB, or have received the bacillus Calmette-Guérin (BCG) vaccine. This test should be interpreted as positive if the area of induration is *greater than 5 mm* (modified Mantoux test).

Screening for hepatitis B (see Chapter 57) should be performed to determine the need for immunization. *Hepatitis C screening* may help to identify patients who might benefit from interferon therapy.

A *chest radiograph* should be obtained at baseline and when cardiopulmonary symptoms develop. Periodic screening of *vitamin* B_{12} levels should be conducted, because vitamin B_{12} deficiency is extremely common, especially among those patients with advanced HIV disease and chronic diarrhea.

Formal *neuropsychiatric testing* may be needed to document AIDS dementia complex and is best conducted by a technician experienced in the assessment of HIV-infected patients.

Assessing Degree of Immunocompromise and Prognosis. The *CD4 cell count* is the best single indicator of disease progression and suffices in most instances for decision making. Approximately 30 percent of patients with a CD4 cell count lower than 200 develop AIDS within 1 year. Fifty percent of patients with a count between 200 and 400 develop AIDS within 3 years. Individuals with CD4 cell counts greater than 400 have a 15 percent chance of developing AIDS within 3 years. CD4 cell count is now used to determine when to initiate antiretroviral therapy and PCP prophylaxis. It is one of the most important laboratory tests in HIV care. Table 13–2 categorizes CD4 cell counts according to their current therapeutic implications.

The percentage of CD4 cells to total lymphocytes, also referred to as the *CD4 percentage,* is believed to be less subject to variation than the absolute CD4 cell count, but fewer data correlating it to prognosis are available. Nonetheless, a CD4 cell count greater than 500 is believed equivalent to a CD4 percentage greater than 29; a count between 200 and 499 is equivalent to a percentage of 14 to 28, and a count lower than 200 is equivalent to a percentage lower than 14.

A host of other tests have been studied for value in assessing prognosis: ratio of CD4 to CD8 lymphocytes, beta$_2$-microglobulin, neopterin, and HIV p24 antigen. None has proven as useful as the CD4.

Diagnosis of Conditions Indicative of AIDS. As noted earlier, the diagnosis of AIDS depends principally on the identification of an indicator condition or on finding in an HIV-positive patient a CD4 cell count lower than 200. Although clinical findings help in making a presumptive diagnosis of an indicator condition, definitive diagnosis depends on laboratory confirmation. Diagnostic modalities include histologic or cytologic study, culturing, serologic study, neuroimaging, and endoscopy.

A few comments are warranted. Candidiasis is diagnosed by direct observation or microscopy, not from culture, since *Candida* is a common contaminant. The diagnosis of HIV encephalopathy is one of exclusion, requiring examination of cerebrospinal fluid and neuroimaging to rule out other causes. HIV wasting syndrome is another diagnosis of exclusion, necessitating a search for cancer, TB, cryptosporidiosis, and other specific forms of enteritis before concluding it is the cause.

PRINCIPLES OF MANAGEMENT

The major components of therapy are vaccination, antiretroviral agents, prophylaxis and treatment of opportunistic infections, and counseling. Each plays a major role. Although the disease remains invariably fatal pending development of curative therapy, a comprehensive and humanely administered treatment program can do much to preserve quality of life and reduce suffering.

Vaccination

An HIV-seropositive adult (especially if the CD4 cell count is greater than 200) should be vaccinated to the degree possible. However, no live-virus vaccines should be used, because the patient may already be immunocompromised. All HIV-seropositive individuals should receive the *pneumococcal polysaccharide* vaccine, the *influenza vaccine,* the *hepatitis B vaccine* (if not already antibody-positive), and

Table 13-2. CD4 Cell Count and HIV Disease Management

CELL COUNT (CELLS PER MM³)	RECOMMENDATIONS
> 500	Benefits of antiretroviral therapy and PCP prophylaxis uncertain
200–500	Antiretroviral therapy; PCP prophylaxis beneficial in some patients
50–200	Antiretroviral therapy; PCP prophylaxis beneficial; prophylaxis of other opportunistic infections (eg, *Mycobacterium avium* complex, *Toxoplasma gondii, Cryptococcus neoformans*) currently under investigation
< 50	Risk of mortality increases significantly; PCP prophylaxis beneficial; prophylaxis of other opportunistic infections under investigation

the *H. flu vaccine*. In addition, a *tetanus-diphtheria booster* should be given if one has not been received within the last 10 years. The immunogenicity of these vaccines in HIV patients has been called into question, especially as disease progresses. Consequently, vaccination should be conducted as early in HIV infection as possible (Table 13–3).

Antiretroviral Therapy

Antiretroviral therapy is changing frequently, with a trend toward earlier use and multidrug regimens. The finding that early use helps delay onset of clinical disease has stimulated initiation of treatment in relatively asymptomatic patients, based largely on CD4 cell counts (see Table 13–2).

Zidovudine (AZT, azidothymidine, Retrovir), the first drug to receive Food and Drug Administration (FDA) approval for the treatment of HIV infection, is recommended for any HIV-infected patient whose *CD4 cell count* is *lower than 500,* regardless of whether symptoms of HIV infection are present or not. It inhibits viral replication, postpones the development of AIDS, improves quality of life, and extends

Table 13-3. Recommended Immunizations for HIV-Seropositive Adults

VACCINE	RECOMMENDATIONS
DPT	All patients: booster every 10 years
IPV (polio)	Inactivated vaccine only; *live vaccine contraindicated*; persons who have never been immunized: three doses of enhanced potency *inactivated* vaccine; persons previously immunized traveling to a developing country: 1 dose of inactivated vaccine
MMR	Persons born after 1956 who (1) have not been immunized or (2) were immunized before 1980 and who have neither serologic evidence of infection nor a history of physician-diagnosed measles
Haemophilus B	All patients: single dose early in HIV infection
Pneumococcal	All patients: single dose early in HIV infection
Influenza	All patients: yearly
Hepatitis B	Patients who do not demonstrate antibody or antigen: series of three injections
Typhoid	Patients traveling to developing countries: inactivated parenteral typhoid vaccine, booster doses every 3 years
Meningococcus	Patients traveling to areas with recognized epidemics or to regions where such disease is endemic, especially if prolonged contact with the populace is anticipated
Plague	Patients traveling to areas where there is a high probability of exposure
Japanese encephalitis	Patients traveling to endemic or epidemic areas
Cholera	Rarely indicated for patients traveling to developing countries, but may be required by destination country
Rabies	Patients anticipating contact with uncommon wild animals or living for prolonged times in areas where rabies is prevalent
Yellow fever	Contraindicated; vaccine is a live preparation
BCG	Contraindicated; vaccine is a live preparation
Typhoid	Contraindicated; vaccine is a live preparation
Live oral polio	Contraindicated

survival among those patients with advanced disease. Data are conflicting as to whether zidovudine therapy improves survival when given to patients with early disease. Studies are currently underway to determine whether benefit accrues to those with CD4 cell counts greater than 500.

Average-sized adults should be given 500 to 600 mg of zidovudine per day. FDA dosing recommendations state that zidovudine should be taken every 4 hours. However, the relatively long intracellular half-life of phosphorylated zidovudine has led several centers to study 8-hour dosing with encouraging results. This dosing scheme may have the added advantage of improved compliance. Lower daily dosages of zidovudine cannot be routinely recommended on the basis of currently available data.

Other Antiretroviral Agents. Currently, two additional drugs are approved for the treatment of HIV infection: *dideoxyinosine* (ddI, didanosine, Videx) and *dideoxycytidine* (ddC, zalcitabine, HIVID). Didanosine is indicated for patients with advanced HIV infection who are either intolerant to zidovudine therapy or who have exhibited significant clinical or immunologic deterioration during zidovudine therapy. Recent data suggest that HIV-infected individuals who have taken zidovudine for at least 4 months may benefit by switching from zidovudine to didanosine provided they do not have AIDS. Studies are currently underway to assess the relative effectiveness of zidovudine versus didanosine for those patients who have never taken antiretroviral therapy.

Zalcitabine is approved for treatment of HIV infection in combination *with zidovudine* for adult patients whose CD4 cell counts are *lower than 300* and who have demonstrated significant clinical or immunologic deterioration. Zalcitabine does not appear to be as effective as zidovudine when used as initial monotherapy. At the current time, zalcitabine, alone, should not be used to treat HIV infection unless given in the context of a clinical trial. The approval of the combination zalcitabine/zidovudine was based on data that demonstrated a significantly larger and more sustained rise in CD4 cell counts than that seen with zidovudine alone (similar data have recently been reported for the combination didanosine/zidovudine). Superior clinical benefit in this combination has not yet been reported.

Failure of Antiviral Therapy. The recommendations for the use of didanosine and zalcitabine/zidovudine do not explicitly state what constitutes failure. This is left to the judgment of the treating physician. A persistent drop in CD4 cell count (usually to half that which was present at the initiation of therapy) and the development of a serious new opportunistic infection in a patient who has been taking zidovudine for at least 6 months have been used by some to define failure and deterioration, respectively.

Infection Prophylaxis and Treatment

Prophylaxis and prompt treatment of opportunistic infection can significantly lessen disease morbidity and need for hospitalization. The infections of greatest concern are PCP, TB, toxoplasmosis, and candidiasis.

Pneumocystis Carinii Pneumonia is the most common infection in HIV-infected adults. Adults with CD4 cell counts lower than 200 (or < 20% of total lymphocytes) should receive PCP prophylaxis (see Table 13–3). Several prophylaxis regimens are available. *Trimethoprim-sulfamethoxazole (TMS)* (one double-strength tablet per day) is the most effective and least expensive regimen. For most patients, it is well tolerated, but a substantial proportion of patients experience adverse reactions necessitating consideration of an alternative means of PCP prophylaxis.

Aerosolized pentamidine (300 mg once every 4 weeks via a Respirgard II nebulizer) has also been shown to be effective in preventing PCP, though not quite to the same degree as TMS. When breakthroughs occur, they may have an upper lobe predominance. The dissemination of *Pneumocystis carinii* to other tissues has been reported. Individuals with active TB should not receive aerosolized pentamidine, as this greatly increases the risk of TB among health care providers giving the therapy.

Growing evidence suggests *dapsone* (50–100 mg once daily) is an effective prophylactic agent for PCP. This is a very inexpensive drug with a long half-life. Less frequent dosing may be effective, but such dosing schemes may decrease overall compliance.

Workup for an HIV patient with a CD4 cell count lower than 200 and new respiratory symptoms includes a *chest radiograph* and an *induced sputum*. The sputum should be sent for *Gram stain*, routine *culture*, *mycobacterial stain and culture*, *fungal wet prep* and *culture*, and *immunofluorescent stain* for *Pneumocystis carinii*. *Arterial blood gases* may provide additional information. If the radiograph reveals a bilateral interstitial infiltrate and the sputum Gram stain is not diagnostic of a specific etiology, the patient should be treated presumptively for PCP while awaiting immunofluorescent stains. If the patient appears clinically stable and is not in respiratory distress, treatment can be initiated on an outpatient basis. Careful follow-up is essential.

Effective *oral therapies* for PCP include *dapsone-trimethoprim*, *TMS*, and *clindamycin-primaquine*. The most easily tolerated of these regimens is dapsone (75–100 mg/d in an average-sized adult) combined with trimethoprim (15 mg/kg/d in three or four divided doses). TMS (15 mg/kg/d by trimethoprim content, in three or four divided doses) is effective, but causes more adverse reactions than dapsone-trimethoprim. Glucose-6-phosphate dehydrogenase (G6PD) deficient patients should not receive dapsone. Clindamycin-primaquine may be used in patients who are unable to tolerate dapsone-trimethoprim or TMS. Effective intravenous therapies include TMS and *pentamidine* (3–4 mg/kg/d).

Oral corticosteroid therapy is useful in patients with PCP who demonstrate a significant alveolar-arterial oxygen gradient (> 30 mm Hg), provided it is started early (within the first 72 hours). Later therapy has not been shown to improve outcome. If a patient is in respiratory distress or has a significant A-a gradient, then hospitalization of the patient should be considered.

Tuberculosis and Atypical Mycobacteria. All seropositive individuals whose PPD status is unknown should have a *5 TU PPD* planted. HIV individuals are judged positive if there is *5 mm or more of induration* (see Chapter 38). All such patients should receive a 1-year course of *isoniazid* (INH) prophylaxis if they have not been previously treated. Many authorities suggest that an anergic individual with a history of positive PPD also should receive a course of isoniazid.

As noted above, the use of aerosolized pentamidine may induce coughing and thereby facilitate transmission of undiagnosed pulmonary TB from HIV-infected patients to persons sharing the same breathing space during or after treatment. The potential for transmission of TB depends on the prevalence of TB infection in the HIV-infected population being served and on such factors as room ventilation, the number of infectious droplet nuclei generated by the patient, and duration of exposure. Aerosolized pentamidine should not be given in the home setting. Specially ventilated facilities are required to deliver the drug safely.

The development of *active TB* in the HIV patient is a potentially serious matter, because of the associated risk of *multidrug-resistant strains*. Such patients require very careful handling (see Chapter 49).

The organism is resistant to most antimycobacterial drugs, often necessitating use of complex, multidrug parenteral regimens. *Clarithromycin,* which can be administered orally, has demonstrated considerable efficacy against *M. avium*. Because this is an infection of very late or end-stage disease, decisions regarding its treatment should be made taking into account the overall condition of the patient and the likelihood of improved quality of life with successful treatment.

Toxoplasmosis. Dapsone-pyrimethamine appears to provide effective chemoprophylaxis in patients seropositive for *T. gondii* who have CD4 cell counts lower than 200. However, rash, fever, and hemolytic anemia are common adverse effects, often necessitating cessation of therapy. For those individuals who are not seropositive, the thorough cooking of meat and careful hand washing after contact with raw meat should be emphasized. Further, cat owners should clean litter boxes daily while wearing gloves and practice careful hand washing afterward or have another person perform this chore. If the individual is a gardener, he or she should be encouraged to use gloves while enjoying this pastime. Patients with encephalitis require hospitalization for initiation of sulfadiazine, pyrimethamine, and leukovorin.

Candidiasis occurs frequently in HIV-infected individuals. Topical agents for prophylaxis of *oral candidiasis* are effective and well tolerated. One 10-mg *clotrimazole troche* held in the mouth for 15 to 30 minutes three times each day is effective. *Chlorhexidine gluconate* may be useful, especially among patients with significant gingivitis and periodontitis. *Nystatin* is available in either an oral suspension or a pastille. Nystatin oral pastilles (200,000 U), one pastille taken three times each day, or nystatin suspension (100,000 U/mL), 15 mL swish-and-swallow six times per day, can also be used.

Vulvovaginal candidiasis is a common problem for HIV-infected women. It tends to occur earlier in HIV infection than does oral candidiasis. Again, there are several agents available for *prophylaxis: clotrimazole* or *nystatin suppositories,* and *miconazole* or *clotrimazole cream.* Although controlled trials are lacking, the use of one of these agents several times each week may decrease the frequency of vulvovaginal candidiasis.

Cytomegalovirus. Ganciclovir and foscarnet are the drugs approved for treatment of CMV retinitis. *Foscarnet* has been shown superior to ganciclovir in patients with normal renal function and also appears to have the added benefit of acting synergistically with zidovudine against HIV. For patients with impaired renal function, *ganciclovir* is preferred. However, granulocyte counts have to be monitored closely because both cause granulocytopenia.

Approach to Occupational Exposure

Risk of seroconversion is very low. In a survey of 1103 health care workers with documented percutaneous exposure, only 4 (0.36%) had seroconverted, and none of those with nonintact skin or mucus membrane exposure had seroconverted. About one-third of exposed persons took AZT after exposure; one seroconverted despite AZT prophylaxis. There are no placebo-controlled, randomized trial data available. In their absence, a consensus treatment protocol has been established as part of a multicenter open study. Data are pending.

In the absence of definitive data, the decision to administer AZT prophylaxis must be individualized and shared with the patient. In counseling the patient, one should take into account the severity of the exposure, the very low risk of seroconversion, the fact that AZT does not provide absolute protection, the high incidence of drug side effects, and the need for biweekly monitoring of blood counts. It must be emphasized that AZT treatment is not of proven benefit and that one can stop therapy at any time one chooses.

Counseling

Counseling the HIV-infected patient involves many aspects, including personal, psychosocial, and financial issues. Assisting the patient in understanding and accepting the changes in his or her sense of self and in life plans and goals is essential to successful care. It is particularly important to educate the individual as much as possible about the disease and its treatment; this helps one to regain some sense of control. It is particularly helpful to focus on what the patient can do, rather than on what is out of one's control. Giving accurate information on current estimates of *prognosis* is essential but can and should be done without destroying hope.

The *risk of suicide* is increased 30- to 60-fold in HIV patients, especially early in the illness when the diagnosis is first known and in the very late stages of the disease when delirium may be present. Most patients who eventually commit suicide talk of it beforehand to friends and health care workers. Prevention through careful patient preparation at the time of diagnosis and screening for suicidality (see Chapter 227) should be an intrinsic part of the counseling and supportive effort.

It is essential to review *safe-sex measures* with HIV-seropositive individuals and their partners. These steps are useful in preventing transmission of not only HIV but also other sexually transmitted diseases. This is extremely important for the HIV-infected individual.

Understanding the patient's existing *support network* and helping the patient develop additional supports can be very important. It is often helpful if the patient can link up with infected peers to share experiences and concerns; this helps to minimize isolation, loneliness, and fear.

In many cities there now exist special *community resources* to aid HIV-infected patients with legal, social, and financial issues pertaining to the infection. It is important for every physician who cares for these individuals to identify these resources.

Finally, it is essential to *discuss death and dying* with each patient in an open manner. Often these issues are shunned by others in the patient's support network. The value of being able to get honest and direct answers about death and dying from one's physician cannot be underestimated. During these discussions, the physician and patient should strive to come to a common understanding of the patient's wishes regarding this very important issue.

INDICATIONS FOR ADMISSION AND CONSULTATION

Although outpatient care is preferred for many elements of HIV management, there are several instances in which prompt hospitalization is essential. The patient with signs or symptoms suggestive of pulmonary, CNS, or disseminated infection (especially that which may be due to *Pneumocystis,* tuberculosis, atypical mycobacteria, syphilis, toxoplasmosis, histoplasmosis, coccidiomycosis, cryptococcus, or CMV) requires prompt hospital admission for parenteral therapy and infectious disease consultation. Outpatient treatment may be possible later, even for administration of parenteral therapy, but treatment should be initiated in the hospital. Also requiring immediate hospitalization is the suicidal patient, particularly one who admits to having made specific plans for suicide. Urgent psychiatric consultation is essential. Toward the final stages of disease, referral for *hospice care* should be considered. Best is care that can be arranged at home, provided the home environment is appropriate. At this stage of illness, hospital admissions should be kept to a minimum except as needed for purposes of providing comfort.

ANNOTATED BIBLIOGRAPHY

Anastos K, Palleja SM. Caring for women at risk of HIV infection. J Gen Intern Med 1991;6(1S):S40. (*Many issues often overlooked.*)

Buehler JW, Ward JW. A new definition for AIDS surveillance. Ann Intern Med 1993;118:390. (*An editorial on the implications of the expanded surveillance definition.*)

Bourgoignie JJ, Pardo V. HIV-associated nephropathies. N Engl J Med 1992;327:729. (*A useful editorial summarizing renal impairments.*)

Centers for Disease Control and Prevention. 1993 Revised classification system for HIV infection and expanded surveillance case definition for AIDS among adolescents and adults. MMWR Morbid Mortal Wkly Rep 1992;41(RR–17):1. (*Current CDC criteria for diagnosis and classification of HIV infection and AIDS.*)

Centers for Disease Control and Prevention. Recommendations for prophylaxis against *Pneumocystis carinii* pneumonia for adults and adolescents infected with human immunodeficiency virus. MMWR Morbid Mortal Wkly Rep 1992;41(RR–4):1. (*Recommends TMS prophylaxis, with aerosolized pentamidine for those who cannot tolerate TMS.*)

Coopman SA, Johnson RA, Platt R et al. Cutaneous disease and drug reactions in HIV infection. N Engl J Med 1993;328:1670. (*Very high incidence of cutaneous reactions noted, especially drug reactions, and these increase as immune function worsens.*)

Fahey JL, Taylor JMG, Detels R et al. The prognostic value of cellular and serologic markers in infection with human immunodeficiency virus type 1. N Engl J Med 1990;322:166. (*CD4 was most predictive, followed by CD4:CD8; the others added little.*)

Frieden TR, Sterling T, Pablos-Mendez et al. The emergence of drug-resistant tuberculosis in New York City. N Engl J Med 1993;328:521. (*A 33 percent incidence of drug-resistant strains noted; many among HIV patients; 19 percent resistant to both INH and rifampin.*)

Gerberding J. Is antiretroviral treatment after percutaneous HIV exposure justified? Ann Intern Med 1993;118:979. (*An editorial; concludes that evidence is insufficient to recommend its routine use.*)

Girard PM, Landman R, Gaudebout C et al. Dapsone-pyrimethamine compared with aerosolized pentamidine as primary prophylaxis against *Pneumocystis carinii* and toxoplasmosis in HIV infection. N Engl J Med 1993;328:1514. (*Found as effective as pentamidine, but not as well tolerated; however, also effective for toxoplasmosis.*)

Hirsch MS, D'Aquila RT. Therapy for human immunodeficiency virus infection. N Engl J Med 1993;328:1686. (*Excellent review of available agents, mechanisms of action, and treatment strategies; 134 refs.*)

Hirsch MS. The treatment of cytomegalovirus in AIDS—more than meets the eye. N Engl J Med 1992;326:264. (*An editorial; foscarnet preferred in patients with normal renal function; synergy with AZT noted.*)

Hollander H. Neurologic and psychiatric manifestations of HIV disease. J Gen Intern Med 1991;6(1S):S24. (*Helpful summary and review.*)

Jacobson MA, Mills J. Serious CMV disease in AIDS, clinical findings, diagnosis, and treatment. Ann Intern Med 1988; 108:585. (*Comprehensive review of this important complication.*)

Levine AM. Epidemiology, clinical characteristics, and management of AIDS-related lymphoma. Hematol Oncol Clin North Am 1991;5:331. (*Lymphoma is a serious malignant complication; useful review.*)

Malone JL et al. Sources of variability in repeated T-helper lymphocyte counts from human immunodeficiency virus type 1-infected patients: Total lymphocyte count fluctuations and diurnal cycle are important. J Acquir Immune Defic Syndr 1990;3:144. (*Documents variability and its causes.*)

Navia BA, Jordan BD, Price RW. The AIDS dementia complex. I: Clinical features. Ann Neurol 1986;19:517. (*An important and debilitating accompaniment of advanced disease that must be distinguished from more treatable forms of CNS deterioration.*)

Pantaleo G, Graziosi C, Fauci AS. The immunopathogenesis of human immunodeficiency virus infection. N Engl J Med 1993;328:327. (*Best review of pathophysiology; essential basic science reading.*)

Perry SW, Markowitz JC. Counseling for HIV testing. Hosp Community Psychiatry 1988;39:731. (*Excellent approach to working with the patient.*)

Powderly WC, Saag MS, Cloud GA et al. A controlled trial of fluconazole or amphotericin B to prevent relapse of cryptococcal meningitis in patients with the acquired immunodeficiency syndrome. N Engl J Med 1992;326:793. (*Fluconazole orally was superior to weekly intravenous amphotericin.*)

Schafer A, Friedman W, Mielke M et al. The increased frequency of cervical dysplasia–neoplasia in women infected with the human immunodeficiency virus is related to the degree of immunosuppression. Am J Obstet Gynecol 1991;164:593. (*An example of a unique presentation of AIDS in women and its relation to CD4 counts.*)

Schneider MME et al. Controlled trial of aerosolized pentamidine or trimethoprim-sulfamethoxazole as primary prophylaxis against *Pneumocystis carnii* pneumonia in patients with human immunodeficiency virus infection. N Engl J Med 1992; 327:1836. (*TMS proved superior, but not always well tolerated.*)

Soave R, Johnson WD Jr. *Cryptosporidium* and *Isosporabelli* infections. J Infect Disease 1988;157:225. (*Review of this cause of diarrhea in AIDS patient.*)

Studies of Ocular Complications of AIDS Research Group, in collaboration with the AIDS Clinical Trials Group. Mortality in patients with the acquired immunodeficiency syndrome treated with either foscarnet or ganciclovir for cytomegalovirus retinitis. N Engl J Med 1992;326:213. (*Foscarnet more effective but not as well tolerated.*)

Tokars JI, Marcus R, Culver DH et al. Surveillance of HIV infection and zidovudine use among health care workers after occupational exposure to HIV-infected blood. Ann Intern Med 1993;118:913. (*Risk of seroconversion for percutaneous exposure was 0.36 percent, for mucus membrane exposure was 0.0 percent, and for skin exposure was 0.0 percent; use of zidovudine was not fully protective.*)

The AIDS Clinical Trials Group. The safety and efficacy of zidovudine (AZT) in the treatment of subjects with mildly symptomatic human immunodeficiency virus type 1 (HIV) infection. A double-blind, placebo-controlled trial. Ann Intern Med 1990;112:727. (*Benefit and safety documented in this well designed trial.*)

The National Institutes of Health/University of California Expert Panel for Corticosteroids as Adjunctive Therapy for *Pneumocystis* Pneumonia. Consensus statement on the use of corticosteroids as adjunctive therapy for *Pneumocystis* pneumonia in the acquired immunodeficiency syndrome. N Engl J Med 1990;323:1500. (*Worthwhile if used within the first 72 hours.*)

Volberding PA et al. Zidovudine in asymptomatic human immunodeficiency virus infection. A controlled trial in persons with fewer than 500 CD4-positive cells per cubic millimeter. N Engl J Med 1990;322:941. (*Found safe and effective, though effect on survival not addressed.*)

Primary Care Medicine: Office Evaluation and Management of the Adult Patient, 3rd edition, edited by Allan H. Goroll, Lawrence A. May, and Albert G. Mulley, Jr. J.B. Lippincott Company, Philadelphia

3
Cardiovascular Problems

14
Screening for Hypertension
KATHARINE K. TREADWAY, M.D.

Hypertension can justifiably be considered the most significant condition the practitioner concerned with health maintenance will meet in clinical practice. The size of the affected population is staggering—20 percent of adults in the United States have systolic pressures greater than 160 mm Hg or diastolic pressures greater than 95 mm Hg. Among the elderly, the prevalence is even greater. Excess morbidity and mortality caused by hypertension have been well documented. Nevertheless, despite improvement in hypertension management in recent years, many who should be treated remain either unaware of their elevated blood pressure, not treated, or not controlled.

Evaluation and management of the identified hypertensive patient are presented in Chapters 19 and 26. This chapter reviews the epidemiology of high blood pressure, its importance as a risk factor, its measurement, and the evidence for the effectiveness of therapy.

EPIDEMIOLOGY AND RISK FACTORS

Depending on the definition of hypertension used, 15 percent to 25 percent of the U.S. population is considered hypertensive. Of those who are hypertensive, approximately 70 percent fall into the so-called stage I or "mild" category (see below). Most estimates of the prevalence of hypertension derive from the National Health and Nutrition Examination Surveys of the early 1960s and late 1970s. Subsequent smaller surveys have both substantiated its prevalence and confirmed that prevalence is significantly affected by age, race, and sex.

Age. Systolic and diastolic blood pressures rise steadily with age into the fifth and sixth decades, when the increase levels off. By then, the prevalence of hypertension approaches 50 percent. The complication risk also rises steadily with age. The prevalence of hypertension (using the rather stringent definition of systolic $\geqslant$ 60 mm Hg or diastolic $\geqslant$ 95 mm Hg) among persons aged 25 to 34 is approximately 5 percent. By age 55 to 64, it has risen to 35 percent to 40 percent.

Gender. Males in all age groups have a higher prevalence of hypertension than females. In the third and fourth decades, it is more than twice as common among men as among women. The ratio decreases with advancing age, so that by age 60 there is only a slight male predominance. Men have substantially higher complication rates than women. The Framingham Study demonstrated that for all the major complications, risk in mildly hypertensive women equals that of normotensive men. The postulated mechanisms for this reduced risk in women include lower peripheral resistance and higher cardiac output. The phenomenon begins to disappear with the onset of menopause. By age 70, the incidences of stroke and coronary disease in women approach those of men.

Race. There is a marked *increase* in prevalence of hypertension among *African-Americans*. Compared to whites, the overall prevalence ratio is 2:1. It is higher in young adults and lower in the elderly. The hypertension tends to be more severe and the complication rate greater for any given blood pressure. For example, severe hypertension is nearly five times more common in African-Americans than in whites. Although some racial differences in physiology have been identified, inadequate access to health care emerges as an important causative factor.

Obesity. Prevalence increases in obese patients, as do the risks of hyperlipidemia and type II diabetes mellitus. The association of these three conditions has been attributed to the presence of relative insulin resistance, which may cause hypertension in some patients (see Chapter 19).

Other Risk Factors. Hypertension is more likely in patients with a *positive family history. Increased salt intake* correlates with increased prevalence in large populations, though not in individuals. This suggests differing individual susceptibilities to the effects of high salt intake. An individual's prior or current salt intake, per se, is not a predictor of blood pressure level. *Alcohol* intake in excess of 2 ounces per day is linked to hypertension. Although the mechanism is not well understood, there appears to be both a direct effect on blood pressure and an indirect effect associated with the sympathetic stimulation of withdrawal. The role of *psychological stress* and its concomitant sympathetic stimulation appears to be variable and possibly a function of underlying differences in susceptibility. *Cigarette smoking,* an important risk factor in its own right, is not positively associated with increased blood pressure, but hypertensive smokers are at significantly greater risk to develop cardiovascular complications than are hypertensive nonsmokers.

HYPERTENSION AS A RISK FACTOR FOR CARDIOVASCULAR MORBIDITY AND MORTALITY

The complications of hypertension may be divided into *hypertensive risks*—those that result directly from the presence of high blood pressure—and *atherosclerotic risks*—those that ensue from the increased risk of atherosclerosis, for which hypertension is one of several risk factors. The major hypertensive complications are *stroke, congestive heart failure,* and *renal failure.* The atherosclerotic complications are *coronary artery disease* and *peripheral vascular disease.* While the risk of all these complications rises gradually over all levels of blood pressure, increasing by about 30 percent for every 10 mm Hg rise in pressure, the risk in a given individual for developing atherosclerotic complications varies enormously, depending on what other risk factors are present. The risk of hypertensive complications correlates most closely with systolic blood pressure, especially the risks of hemorrhagic and nonhemorrhagic stroke in both men and women. Hypertensives show a fourfold increase in risk of cerebral infarction. Even *isolated systolic hypertension* in the elderly is associated with an increased risk of stroke.

Although hypertension remains one of the principal atherosclerotic risk factors for development of coronary artery disease, the additive effects from smoking, hypercholesterolemia, glucose intolerance, and left ventricular hypertrophy are also extremely important (see Chapters 15, 54, and 93). For example, the chance of a 40-year-old male with moderate hypertension alone developing ischemic heart disease over an 8-year period is about 5 percent, but it rises to 70 percent if all coronary risk factors are present. The Framingham study has also shown hypertension to be the dominant predictor of congestive heart failure, with a sixfold increase in incidence among hypertensives.

NATURAL HISTORY OF HYPERTENSION AND EFFECTIVENESS OF THERAPY

Natural History. With rare exceptions, hypertension is an *asymptomatic* disease. The natural history is one of *insidious* damage that is most often clinically silent for a decade or more. Consequently, it is a more ominous finding and, in particular, a potent predictor of coronary disease in younger age groups.

The natural history of hypertension is not uniformly dismal. Most patients with hypertension fall into the *stage I* or *"mild"* range (diastolic pressure 90–104 mm Hg). Of these, some 20 percent to 30 percent will progress to higher pressures if untreated, while about the same number will revert spontaneously to normotension. At present, there is *no way to predict* the course for an individual patient. In addition, some mild hypertensives will not suffer complications related to their blood pressure elevation. As noted above, risk is a function not only of hypertension severity but also of presence of other coronary risk factors. While it is clear that hypertension carries significant risks, a substantial proportion of patients with mild disease may not suffer complications. This leaves the clinician with the difficult tasks of deciding if and when to initiate therapy (see Chapter 26).

Effectiveness of Treatment. Convincing evidence for vigorous *early treatment* of hypertension began to appear 25 years ago with publication of the landmark Veterans Administration Cooperative Study, the first large-scale, placebo-controlled, randomized prospective study. It involved patients with moderate to severe hypertension and found that rates of major nonfatal events and cardiovascular death fell with treatment more than 10-fold among those with severe hypertension and three-fold among those with moderate pressure elevations. Treatment was most effective in reducing risks of stroke and congestive heart failure. Those with mild hypertension showed no significant benefit from treatment, particularly if younger than 50 years of age and free of preexisting cardiovascular disease. However, the study was limited to men, and there were only limited data on patients with mild hypertension.

Later randomized studies expanded these initial findings, and meta-analyses of such studies confirmed the efficacy of treatment. Meta-analytic study of 14 major randomized treatment trials found that a treatment-induced mean pressure reduction of 5 to 6 mm Hg was associated with a 42 percent reduction in rate of stroke and a 14 percent reduction in incidence of coronary events. Because the reduction in coronary risk was less than that for stroke, the question arose of a possible adverse drug effect on cardiovascular risk. A companion meta-analysis using epidemiologic data to estimate expected reductions in cardiovascular risk calculated an expected reduction of 34 percent for stroke and 21 percent for coronary disease, suggesting that some antihypertensive agents might also contribute to coronary risk (see Chapter 26).

Findings from other studies indicate that 1) benefit from blood pressure reduction increases with severity of blood pressure elevation; 2) African-Americans and those older than 50 years of age benefit most; 3) young white women benefit least; and 4) treatment of mild hypertension produces a marked reduction (38%) in stroke but only a modest reduction (8%) in coronary events. As regards treatment of systolic hypertension in the elderly, a lowering of isolated systolic hypertension produces results similar to those for mild hypertension (ie, a substantial reduction in risk of stroke, a minor reduction in coronary events).

While the benefits of treating hypertension appear clear, it is interesting to note that mildly hypertensive patients whose blood pressure spontaneously reverts to normal seem to do even better than those whose pressure is brought down by medication. This finding was first noted in a landmark Australian study of mild hypertensives, in which almost half of the placebo group became spontaneously normotensive over the 5-year period of the study. Such patients had fewer complications than those who achieved a similar level of blood pressure with medication.

In sum, the benefit of lowering blood pressure is real and particularly important as regards incidence of stroke. Reduction in rate of coronary events is also achieved, though to a lesser extent. Treatment of mild hypertension can reduce the complication rate, but many patients must be treated in order to benefit a few. In the Hypertension Detection and Follow-up Program, which demonstrated a 26 percent decline in cardiovascular mortality, it was calculated that 100 patients would have to be treated for 1 year to prevent 1 death. In most studies, the *benefit* from treatment of hypertension appears *within 2 to 3 years of initiation of therapy.*

The Decision to Treat. The decision to initiate pharmacologic therapy is based on an estimate of *overall cardiovascular risk.* Such an estimate requires consideration not only of blood pressure but also of age, race, sex, smoking, hypercholesterolemia, diabetes, and family history of hypertensive or cardiac complications. The costs from medical therapy are weighed against the expected benefits, an especially important determination in young patients with mild, uncomplicated disease (see Chapter 26). The current trend toward lowering the threshold for treatment should continue with further improvements in the efficacy, safety, convenience, and cost of antihypertensive therapy.

SCREENING METHODS

Although the process of identifying patients with hypertension seems relatively straightforward, there are numerous pitfalls and chances for error in measuring the blood pressure. Reliable equipment is important. Mercury bulb manometers are best. Aneroid manometers, if used, should be checked and recalibrated regularly. Note should be made if the patient is cold, anxious, has a full bladder, or has recently exercised, smoked, or had caffeine, since any of these factors may transiently elevate pressure.

Proper technique is essential. All personnel responsible for recording blood pressures should be aware of sources of measurement error, such as inappropriate cuff size and improper positioning. The pressure should be taken in both arms while the patient is seated comfortably. The cuff should be placed as high up the arm as possible and the arm supported and positioned at *heart level* while the pressure is taken. Although most auscultate using the diaphragm of the stethoscope, the *bell* is recommended for its superior transmission of the low-pitched sounds that characterize the last of the Korotkoff sounds (see Chapter 19).

Systolic pressure is defined as the point at which sound is first heard (Korotkoff 1). *Diastolic pressure* is taken at the point at which sound *disappears* (Korotkoff 5) rather than when it changes in quality (Korotkoff 4). *Cuff size* must be adequate to avoid falsely elevated readings. The *width* of the cuff's inflatable bladder should be greater than *two-thirds* the arm *width* and its *length* greater than two-thirds the arm *circumference.* Using a standard size cuff in a muscular or obese adult will result in a reading that is as much as 10 mm Hg higher than the true blood pressure. To avoid this error, a large adult size cuff should be used in such patients.

The *averages* of two successive measurements in each arm are recorded. Variability of blood pressure may be related to recent physical activity, emotional state, or body position. Although such factors must be kept in mind, the predictive value of the "casual" blood pressure determination has been validated. Nonetheless, the diagnosis of hypertension must never be made on the basis of a single reading, but rather should be based on multiple determinations taken over several visits. A check of the blood pressure should be a routine component of every patient visit, regardless of the presenting complaint.

CONCLUSIONS AND RECOMMENDATIONS

Hypertension is an extremely common condition and the strongest predictor of subsequent cardiovascular and cerebrovascular morbidity and mortality. It is usually asymptomatic, with insidious damage to target organs occurring. A large segment of the hypertensive population will benefit from treatment, showing significant reductions in rates of stroke and coronary disease. Detection is simple, reliable, and inexpensive. All adults should be screened for hypertension. Its detection and treatment are among the foremost responsibilities of the primary care physician (see also Chapters 19 and 26).

ANNOTATED BIBLIOGRAPHY

Collin R, Peto R, MacMahon S et al. Blood pressure, stroke, and coronary disease. Part 2: Short-term reductions in blood pressure: Overview of randomized drug trials in their epidemiological context. Lancet 1990;335:827. (*Important meta-analysis of randomized trials demonstrating significant reductions in risk of stroke and coronary disease.*)

Fifth Report of the Joint National Committee on Detection, Evaluation, and Treatment of High Blood Pressure. Arch Intern Med 1993;153:154. (*An important consensus report.*)

Freis ED. Should mild hypertension be treated? N Engl J Med 1982;307:306. (*Reviews the evidence and recommends treatment for patients with borderline or mild hypertension and other risk factors, but withholding of drug therapy from those without other risk factors.*)

Frohlich ED, Grim C, Labarthe DR et al. Report of a special task force appointed by the Steering Committee, American Heart Association: Recommendations for human blood pressure determinations by sphygmomanometers. Hypertension 1988;11:209A. (*Consensus panel recommendations on technique.*)

Hypertension Detection Follow-Up Program Cooperative Group. The effect of treatment on mortality in "mild" hypertension. N Engl J Med 1982;307:976. (*Twenty percent lower 5-year mortality was found in patients with diastolic blood pressures between 90 and 104 mm Hg who were treated intensively with stepped care compared with similar patients who were simply referred to their usual source of care for treatment.*)

Kannel WB, Wolf PA, McGee DL. Systolic blood pressure, arterial rigidity, and risk of stroke. JAMA 1981;245:1225. (*Classic paper. Subjects with isolated systolic hypertension experienced two to four times as many strokes as did normotensive persons in the Framingham study.*)

Lerman CE, Brody DS, Hui T et al. The white-coat hypertension response: Prevalence and predictors. J Gen Intern Med 1989;4:226. (*Prevalence was 39% and most common in the elderly and those on more medication.*)

MacMahon S, Peto R, Cutler J et al. Blood pressure, stroke, and coronary heart disease. Part 1: Prolonged differences in blood pressure: Prospective observational studies corrected for the regression dilution bias. Lancet 1990;335:765. (*Major meta-analysis documenting that risk of stroke and coronary disease correlate closely with level of blood pressure over the range of 70–110 mm Hg diastolic.)*

Maxwell MH et al. Error in blood pressure measurement due to incorrect cuff size in obese patients. Lancet 1982;2:8288. (*The standard adult size cuff results in readings of about 10 mm Hg in excess of the true pressure in obese patients. A large cuff is needed.*)

Medical Research Council Working Party. MRC trial of treatment of mild hypertension: Principal results. BMJ 1985;291:97. (*Documents reduction in strokes by treatment of patients with mild disease.*)

Messerli FH, Garavaglia GE. Disparate cardiovascular findings in men and women with essential hypertension. Ann Intern Med 1987;107:158. (*Best documentation of the differences.*)

Systolic Hypertension in the Elderly Program (SHEP) Cooperative Research Group. Prevention of stroke by antihypertensive drug treatment in older persons with isolated systolic hypertension. JAMA 1991;265:3255. (*Treatment of isolated systolic hypertension reduced risk of stroke in the elderly.*)

Veterans Administration Cooperative Study Group on Antihypertensive Agents. Effects of treatment on morbidity in hypertension. I: Results in patients with diastolic blood pressures averaging 115 through 129 mm Hg. JAMA 1967;202:1028.

Veterans Administration Cooperative Study Group on Antihypertensive Agents. Effects of treatment on morbidity in hypertension. II: Results in patients with diastolic blood pressure averaging 90 through 114 mm Hg. JAMA 1970;213:1143.

Veterans Administration Cooperative Study Group on Antihypertensive Agents. Effects of treatment on morbidity in hypertension. III: Influence of age, diastolic pressure, and prior cardiovascular disease. Further analysis of side effects. Circulation 1972;45:901. (*The classic studies documenting efficacy of treatment.*)

Primary Care Medicine: Office Evaluation and Management of the Adult Patient, 3rd edition, edited by Allan H. Goroll, Lawrence A. May, and Albert G. Mulley, Jr. J.B. Lippincott Company, Philadelphia

15
Screening for Hyperlipidemia

GALE S. HAYDOCK, M.D. AND
MASON W. FREEMAN, M.D.

The epidemic of hypercholesterolemia in the United States continues to be a major risk factor for development of coronary heart disease (CHD). Twenty percent of all adults older than 20 years of age have a total serum cholesterol concentration in excess of 240 mg/dL, a level associated with an accelerating risk of CHD. Fifty percent of the population have total cholesterol levels exceeding 200 mg/dL, the level considered desirable.

Correction of hyperlipidemia by diet, exercise, weight reduction, and medication can reduce CHD risk. Patient and professional awareness of the importance of hypercholesterolemia has contributed to a modest (8%) reduction in mean total cholesterol over the past 15 years, but the problem remains widespread. Screening for hyperlipidemia is a key element in the primary and secondary prevention of CHD. Proper screening requires attention to several questions: Which lipid abnormalities truly increase coronary risk? To what degree will lowering them reduce such risk? How are they best measured? At what age should screening be initiated and for how long?

RISK FACTORS FOR HYPERLIPIDEMIA

Age. Cholesterol levels increase with age. Total cholesterol increases, on the average, more than 2 mg/dL per year during early adulthood and continues increasing but at a lesser rate until age 65, after which it declines slightly.

Gender. Men have higher total cholesterol levels than women until age 50. Women carry a higher proportion of cholesterol in the form of high-density lipoprotein (HDL) cholesterol (primarily HDL_2). At the onset of menopause, women lose the protective effect of estrogen, resulting in a net increase in cholesterol and an increased risk of CHD that approaches the risk in men.

Genetic Factors. Primary disorders inherited by means of a *monogenic* mechanism account at present for only a small fraction of patients with hyperlipidemia. However, there is suspicion that increased concentrations of lipoprotein(a) (a possible CHD risk factor) may be controlled by a single gene. *Polygenic* hypercholesterolemia is far more common, estimated to affect 5 percent of the general population.

Diet. A diet high in *saturated fatty acids* raises total and low-density lipoprotein (LDL) cholesterol. Total and LDL cholesterol are also increased by dietary *cholesterol*, but the effect is smaller than that of saturated fatty acids. *Caloric excess* resulting in obesity has more of an effect on triglycerides than on cholesterol. *Alcohol* has little effect on total cholesterol levels, but it can cause an acute rise in triglycerides among people with hypertriglyceridemia. Moderate alcohol ingestion also causes a rise in HDL levels, but not in the "protective" HDL_2 subfraction.

Medications. Antihypertensive agents that adversely affect lipid levels can compromise the effort to reduce CHD risk. *Thiazides* increase LDL cholesterol, at least temporarily, when taken in full doses. The effect is hypothesized to account for the shortfall in reduction in mortality found among hypertensives treated with thiazides (see Chapter 26). *Beta-blockers* cause modest reductions in HDL cholesterol. *Exogenous estrogens* increase HDL_2 and can cause extreme triglyceride increases in patients with hypertriglyceridemia.

Exercise, Weight, Smoking, and Concurrent Diseases. Activity increases HDL cholesterol; inactivity and obesity appear to decrease it. A reduction in HDL cholesterol occurs with *smoking*. *Diabetes* is associated with elevations in triglycerides, LDL, and total cholesterol. *Hypothyroidism, nephrotic syndrome,* and *liver disease* are important causes of secondary hypercholesterolemia, characterized by increases in total and LDL cholesterol levels.

HYPERLIPIDEMIA AS A RISK FACTOR FOR CORONARY HEART DISEASE

Total Cholesterol. Epidemiologic and prospective studies have demonstrated that hypercholesterolemia is an independent risk factor for the development of CHD in persons younger than 65 years of age. Coronary risk has been shown to increase curvilinearly with increasing total cholesterol levels, even within the "normal" range. Over the usually encountered range of total cholesterol values (180–300 mg/dL), risk increases by an average of four- to fivefold. Risk begins to accelerate when the total cholesterol level exceeds 240 mg/dL. Levels lower than 200 mg/dL are considered desirable.

Low-Density Lipoprotein (LDL) Cholesterol. The positive relationship between total cholesterol and CHD risk derives mainly from the atherogenic LDL cholesterol component. Because the LDL cholesterol accounts for about two-thirds of the total cholesterol in the typical patient, the total cholesterol concentration is generally used as a proxy for LDL cholesterol. LDL cholesterol serum levels in excess of 160 mg/dL are associated with significant increases in CHD risk.

Recent studies suggest that *lipoprotein(a),* which can bind to LDL receptors and inhibit tissue plasminogen activator, may also be an independent determinant of CHD risk and account for some forms of familial CHD. Whether lipoprotein(a) is an important risk factor in all age groups and across all ethnic backgrounds has yet to be determined.

High-Density Lipoprotein (HDL) Cholesterol. The relation of the HDL cholesterol level to CHD risk is an inverse one. HDL cholesterol exerts a protective effect that is at least as strong as the atherogenic effect of LDL. For every 10 mg/dL increment in HDL cholesterol concentration, there is a 50 percent decrease in coronary risk. An HDL cholesterol level lower than 35 mg/dL has come to be recognized as a major independent risk factor for CHD. A level in excess of 60 mg/dL is considered a "negative" risk factor (see Chapter 27). A low HDL cholesterol increases CHD risk across the full range of total and LDL cholesterol concentrations. A patient with a low total cholesterol level is still at increased risk of CHD if HDL cholesterol is low. Conversely, it is possible for a person with an elevated total cholesterol to be at low risk for CHD by virtue of having a very high HDL cholesterol (60–100 mg/dL). The determination of a *total-to-HDL cholesterol ratio* helps to distinguish such low-risk individuals from others with elevated total cholesterol. The Framingham Study showed that the ratio was a strong predictor of risk. A ratio of 5 approximates the average or standard risk, with ratios of 10 and 20 denoting double and triple the risk. A ratio of *4.5* or less is considered desirable.

Subfractions of HDL (eg, HDL_2, HDL_3) and subcomponents (eg, *apolipoprotein A-1*) also appear protective and inversely predictive of CHD risk. However, they are difficult to measure, and their contribution to estimation of CHD risk does not appear additive to that provided by the ratio of total to HDL cholesterol.

Effect of Other CHD Risk Factors on Cholesterol-Related Risk. Presence of other CHD risk factors (glucose intolerance, smoking, hypertension), or a history of prior CHD or other atherosclerotic disease markedly raise the risk of future coronary events.

Triglycerides. The observed statistical contribution of *hypertriglyceridemia* to cardiovascular risk is not an independent one, but an elevated triglyceride level may connote the presence of associated CHD risk factors, such as diabetes or low HDL.

Lipid-Related CHD Risk Among the Young and the Elderly. The importance of hypercholesterolemia as a predictor of coronary disease is best established in middle-aged men and postmenopausal women. In the young and the elderly, the relationship is less well established due to a paucity of data.

For young men (under age 35) and premenopausal women, elevated total and LDL cholesterol levels increase *long-term risk* of developing CHD. However, *short-term* CHD risk among those with even moderately high LDL cholesterol levels (160–220 mg/dL) but no other CHD risk factors remains relatively low. However, presence of additional CHD risk factors, particularly diabetes or family history of early CHD, appears to increase short-term risk, as does development of a very high LDL cholesterol level (> 220 mg/dL).

CHD risk due to hypercholesterolemia in the *elderly* is also incompletely defined. The relative risk of CHD observed in men 60 to 79 years of age with marked hypercholesterolemia is about 1.5. This relative risk is lower than that in comparably hypercholesterolemic patients younger than 60 years of age. The difference is believed related to the high prevalence of already established CHD, hypertension, and diabetes in this age group. Among hyperlipidemic elderly patients with established CHD, the relative risk of a new coronary event is just as high as in younger patients.

EFFECTIVENESS OF TREATMENT

Nonpharmacologic Measures. Decreases in intake of cholesterol and saturated fat in controlled settings can *reduce total and LDL cholesterol* levels by up to 30 percent. The reduction averages 10 percent when reasonably intensive diets are used in the outpatient setting. Dietary measures may also produce a small (approximately 5%) reduction in HDL cholesterol concentration, though the overall total-to-HDL ratio still improves. Weight loss (if obese), aerobic exercise, and smoking cessation can raise the HDL cholesterol level and facilitate the dietary lowering of LDL cholesterol. These measures also reduce CHD risk by decreasing blood pressure and glucose intolerance. Caloric and fat restrictions and control of diabetes lower triglyceride levels, an effect added to by prohibition of alcohol. Reductions in CHD risk follow from cholesterol lowering and amelioration of other risk factors.

Addition of Pharmacologic Measures. Adding drug therapy to a diet and exercise program enhances the lipid-lowering effort. Reductions two to three times greater than those achieved by dietary measures alone are attainable and associated with a further lowering of CHD risk. The reduction is most evident among patients with established CHD—a *secondary prevention* effect. Pharmacologic therapy for patients without clinically evident coronary disease (so-called *primary prevention*) also reduces CHD risk, but to a lesser degree. A halt to plaque progression and a modest amount of *plaque regression* have been demonstrated in patients with established CHD treated aggressively with medical therapy.

Yet to be demonstrated for pharmacologic therapy is a reduction in *all-cause mortality*. Data are still very sparse, but a meta-analysis of available trials was conducted to examine the morbidity and mortality associated with lipid-lowering therapy. It found a significant reduction in *nonfatal cardiac events* (odds ratio, 0.74), a more modest decrease in *cardiac deaths* (odds ratio, 0.90), and an increase in *noncardiac deaths* (odds ratio, 1.19). No increase in noncardiac deaths has been found among patients treated by nonpharmacologic measures alone. The increase in noncardiac deaths remains unexplained, with no consistent pattern of noncardiac deaths emerging from the studies examined. The finding may be an artifact of the limited data available, or it may represent an adverse effect of some forms of pharmacologic therapy. Its significance remains unclear. The reader should watch for additional data.

SCREENING METHODS

Determinations of total cholesterol, LDL cholesterol, and HDL cholesterol levels would allow reasonable estimates of CHD risk. Decisions about which test(s) to order in screening a particular patient require consideration of test accuracy, cost, availability, significance, and presence of other CHD risk factors.

Measurement of Cholesterol and Choice of Method. The total blood cholesterol is the sum of the cholesterol concentrations contained in the three major circulating lipoproteins (HDL, LDL, and very low-density lipoproteins [VLDL]). Thus, total cholesterol = LDL cholesterol + HDL cholesterol + VLDL cholesterol. Most laboratories measure total cholesterol and HDL cholesterol directly, calculate the VLDL concentration by dividing the triglyceride concentration by 5 (as long as triglyceride is less than 400), and then mathematically derive the LDL cholesterol concentration.

The accuracy of determinations of total cholesterol and its fractions can vary considerably. The popular *finger-stick method* using a capillary tube and *desktop analyzer* has demonstrated false-negative rates ranging from 12 percent to 47 percent for detection of lipid elevations, though measurements of nonfasting total cholesterol most closely approximate those obtained by *venous sampling* and *laboratory processing* (which average 3%–5% higher). However, finger-stick determinations of HDL cholesterol concentration may underestimate the true serum HDL cholesterol level by as much as 40 percent. If an HDL cholesterol concentration is desired, it should be measured by laboratory methods. Calculation of the LDL cholesterol level from finger-stick results can identify patients with LDL cholesterol elevations, but the estimate of CHD risk is no better than that obtained from measuring total cholesterol alone.

Not all laboratories assure accuracy of results. Acceptable laboratories are those with instruments calibrated to the standards of the Centers for Disease Control and Prevention, with a margin of error of 3 percent for total cholesterol. If finger-stick screening methods reveal a total cholesterol elevation, the determination should be repeated by a proper laboratory before deciding to initiate lipid-lowering therapy (see Chapter 27).

Fasting is unnecessary when screening for measurement of the total cholesterol level, because it is not markedly affected by immediate food intake. However, chronic stress or serious illness might cause the level to gradually fall by as much as 20 percent but not at the time of acute onset. A significant drop in total cholesterol and triglyceride levels has been demonstrated when a patient assumes a recumbent position, usually within 5 minutes, and it reaches a maximum of 10 percent to 12 percent within 20 to 30 minutes.

Selection of Persons for Screening. The best patients to screen for hypercholesterolemia are those at *highest CHD risk* (multiple CHD *risk factors, established CHD,* or *other atheromatous disease*), because they benefit most from treatment. Moderate-risk populations (men > 45 years of age, postmenopausal women, persons with > two CHD risk factors) also benefit from preventive therapy and warrant screening. The importance of cholesterol screening in populations at *low risk* (eg, otherwise healthy *young men* < 35 years of age, *premenopausal women*) is less well established. Those with CHD risk factors (particularly a family history of premature CHD or concurrent diabetes) should be considered for screening because of their increased CHD risk. However, there are no prospective data on the benefits and risks of treating such persons, especially as regards pharmacologic therapy. Expanding the screening effort to healthy young persons could be argued on the basis of stimulating good health habits, such as dietary modification, exercise, and weight control. Whether early detection and treatment alter outcomes in such low-risk persons is unknown.

The issue of cholesterol screening in the *elderly* also remains somewhat unsettled. It is clearly indicated for those at high risk for CHD (multiple CHD risk factors, established CHD, other clinically evident atherosclerotic disease) who remain intact. Screening otherwise healthy persons older than 70 years of age is of unknown value but likely to be beneficial, given the high prevalence of CHD in the population. More data are needed.

What to Screen. A nonfasting total cholesterol measurement is sufficient for patients with no other cardiovascular risk factors. For those with CHD or other CHD risk factors, determination of both total cholesterol and HDL cholesterol is a reasonable screening combination, so long as a laboratory that can accurately measure HDL is available. A growing appreciation for the importance of a low HDL cholesterol level to CHD risk has led some to recommend that all persons be screened for it. A person's HDL cholesterol status helps guide risk assessment and selection of drug therapy in hypercholesterolemic patients (see Chapter 27). Whether it influences treatment decisions in patients with an isolated low HDL cholesterol level will have to await data from prospective studies.

LDL cholesterol, triglycerides, VLDL cholesterol, and lipoprotein electrophoresis are not indicated for screening purposes, though they are often part of the lipid evaluation in patients found to be hypercholesterolemic (see Chapter 27). The literature should be followed for developments regarding measurement of lipoprotein(a) for lipid screening.

CONCLUSIONS AND RECOMMENDATIONS

- Hypercholesterolemia is a problem of epidemic proportions in the United States and a major risk factor for CHD.
- Elevations in levels of total cholesterol and LDL cholesterol and reduction in HDL cholesterol are strongly positive independent risk factors for the development of CHD in persons younger than 65 years of age.
- Diet, exercise, smoking cessation, and drug therapy can effectively reduce total and LDL cholesterols and raise HDL cholesterol.
- Reductions in CHD morbidity and CHD mortality have been demonstrated with treatment, particularly in such high-risk hyperlipidemic patients as those with established CHD. However, a reduction in all-cause mortality has not yet been demonstrated.
- A random serum total cholesterol measurement should be performed at least every 5 years in persons older than 20 years of age. Those at increased risk of CHD, other symptomatic atheromatous disease, or other CHD risk factors (smoking, diabetes, hypertension, family history of premature CHD) require more frequent screening.
- Elderly persons are reasonable candidates for cholesterol screening, provided their overall clinical condition would warrant treatment of hypercholesterolemia.
- The total serum cholesterol determination is the preferred screening test. A random determination is sufficient, and it may be performed by the finger-stick method.
- An HDL determination should be part of the screening profile, provided the technology for performing the measurement is available. Results from desktop analyzers using finger-stick blood samples are often erroneous.
- The ratio of total cholesterol to HDL cholesterol should be calculated. A ratio lower than 4.5 is desirable.
- Determination of LDL cholesterol level is not necessary for screening purposes.
- Neither a triglyceride determination nor a lipoprotein electrophoresis is indicated for screening.
- The value of measuring biologically important risk factors such as lipoprotein(a) and certain apolipoproteins is yet to be demonstrated.
- If the screening serum total cholesterol is greater than 200 mg/dL, then a repeat determination using venipuncture and laboratory techniques is indicated for confirmation. Further testing and treatment are based on the patient's age and risk-factor profile (see Chapter 27).

ANNOTATED BIBLIOGRAPHY

Bachorik PS, Cloey TA, Finney CA, et al. Lipoprotein-cholesterol analysis during screening: Accuracy and reliability. Ann Intern Med 1991;114:741. (*Total cholesterol by fingerstick screening methods was accurate, but HDL-cholesterol was grossly underestimated, and LDL cholesterol calculations added little to screening accuracy.*)

Brensike JF, Levy RI, Kelsey SF, et al. Effects of therapy with cholestyramine on progression of coronary arteriosclerosis: Results of the NHLBI Type II Coronary Intervention Study. Circulation 1984;69:313. (*Cholestyramine treatment retards the progression of coronary heart disease as assessed by angiography in patients with Type II hyperlipoproteinemia [primary hypercholesterolemia].*)

Brown G, et al. Regression of coronary artery disease as a result of intensive lipid-lowering therapy. N Engl J Med 1990; 323:1289. (*Significant plaque regression is documented in coronary arteries in this angiographic study of intensive therapy.*)

Canadian Task Force on the Periodic Health Examination: 1993 Update. 2: Lowering the blood total cholesterol level to prevent coronary heart disease. Can Med Assoc J 1993;148:521. (*Meta-analysis of outcomes data; also recommends screening with a total cholesterol determination for men ages 30–59.*)

Criqui MH. Cholesterol, primary and secondary prevention, and all-cause mortality. Ann Intern Med 1991;115:973. (*A provocative article addressing the question of why all-cause mortality is not reduced. Could there be an increased non-cardiac risk from treatment?*)

Criqui MH, Heiss G, Cohn R et al. Plasma triglyceride level and mortality from coronary heart disease. N Engl J Med 1993; 328:1220. (*No independent association with CHD risk found.*)

Expert Panel on Detection, Evaluation, and Treatment of High Blood Cholesterol in Adults: Summary of the Second Report. JAMA 1993;269:3015. (*Major consensus panel recommendations, revising those of 1988 report; more emphasis on total CHD risk, on importance of HDL.*)

Grundy SM, Bilheimer D, Blackburn H et al. Rationale of the diet-heart statement of the American Heart Association: Report of the nutrition committee. Circulation 1982;65:839A. (*A detailed review of the evidence for a diet–coronary heart disease relationship and the rationale for the American Heart Association dietary recommendations.*)

Holme I. An analysis of randomized trials evaluating the effects of cholesterol reduction on total mortality and coronary heart disease incidence. Circulation 1990;82:1916. (*A meta-analysis study pooling data from the major randomized studies.*)

Hunninghake DB, Stein EA, Dujovne CA et al. The efficacy of intensive dietary therapy alone or combined with lovastatin in outpatients with hypercholesterolemia. N Engl J Med 1993; 328:1213. (*Diet alone provided only a 5 percent LDL reduction; medication added another 27 percent.*)

Kannel WB. High-density lipoproteins: Epidemiologic profile and risks of coronary artery disease. Am J Cardiol 1983;52:9B. (*Specifically profiles the contribution of the individual values and ratios of total cholesterol, HDL cholesterol, and LDL cholesterol toward predicting cardiovascular risk.*)

Klag KJ, Ford DE, Mead LA et al. Serum cholesterol in young men and subsequent cardiovascular disease. N Engl J Med 1993;328:313. (*Strong association found between serum cholesterol level in early life and CHD in midlife.*)

Krauss RM. Regulation of high density lipoprotein levels. Med Clin North Am 1982; 66:403 (*Reviews the current concepts of the structure, metabolism, and factors influencing the levels of HDL in humans.*)

Lipid Research Clinics Program: The Lipid Research Clinics Coronary Primary Prevention Trial. JAMA 1984;251:351. (*A significant reduction was observed in the incidence of coronary heart disease by lowering the total cholesterol and LDL cholesterol in asymptomatic middle-aged men with primary hypercholesterolemia.*)

National Cholesterol Education Program Adult Treatment Panel. Prevalence of high blood cholesterol among US adults. JAMA

1993;269:3009. (*20 percent of Americans have cholesterol > 240 mg/dL; 50 percent > 200 mg/dL; best available epidemiologic data.*)

National Cholesterol Education Program. Report of the expert panel on detection, evaluation, treatment of high blood cholesterol in adults. Arch Intern Med 1988;148:36. (*Consensus panel report; urges screening all adults for total cholesterol every 5 years.*)

Pooling Project Research Group: Relationship of blood pressure, serum cholesterol, smoking, relative weight and ECG abnormalities to incidence of major coronary events. J Chronic Dis 1978;31:201. (*A concerted epidemiologic evaluation of cardiac risk factors.*)

Rubin SM, Sidney S, Black DM. High blood cholesterol in elderly men and the excess risk for coronary heart disease. Ann Intern Med 1990;113:916. (*Relative risk was 1.5, indicating that cholesterol is an independent risk factor for cardiovascular mortality.*)

Sox HC Jr. Screening for lipid disorders under health system reform. N Engl J Med 1993;328:1269. (*An editorial reviewing recommendations for screening from a cost-effectiveness perspective.*)

Stampfer MJ, Sacks FM, Salvini S, et al. A prospective study of cholesterol, apolipoproteins, and the risk of myocardial infarction. N Engl J Med 1991;325:373. (*HDL cholesterol was important in predicting risk for myocardial infarction; the ratio of total to HDL cholesterol was especially useful. A one unit change in the ratio was associated with a 53 percent change in risk.*)

16
Bacterial Endocarditis Prophylaxis

Primary Care Medicine: Office Evaluation and Management of the Adult Patient, 3rd edition, edited by Allan H. Goroll, Lawrence A. May, and Albert G. Mulley, Jr. J.B. Lippincott Company, Philadelphia

Once universally fatal, bacterial endocarditis remains a serious disease, with a mortality rate of about 25 percent. Despite the now widespread availability of antibiotics, the incidence of this infection has not changed dramatically. Although controlled data are lacking, logic and the pathogenesis of endocarditis argue that individual infections might be prevented by judicious use of prophylactic antibiotics. The primary care provider must be able to assess risks in individual patients. In addition, an understanding of the basis for prophylaxis recommendations is necessary if individuals likely to benefit from preventive measures are to be instructed effectively.

EPIDEMIOLOGY AND RISK FACTORS

Over the past several decades, there has been a shift in the incidence of endocarditis to older age groups; the current mean age is about 50. Males predominate among patients older than 50 years of age, but the sex ratio is more nearly equal among those younger than 50.

The risk of endocarditis in an individual patient is partially a function of the predisposing cardiac lesion and of the occurrence of procedures likely to induce bacteremia. However, as many as 30 percent to 40 percent of cases of endocarditis occur in the absence of underlying heart disease, and transient bacteremia is common. Additionally, the intensity of bacteremia, the characteristics of the blood-borne organisms, and host factors all play important roles. Since these additional determinants cannot readily be estimated, individual risk must be based on the diagnosis of predisposing lesions and the likelihood of bacteremia.

In the preantibiotic era, chronic rheumatic heart disease was the underlying lesion in 80 percent to 90 percent of cases of endocarditis. Currently, rheumatic heart disease is present in approximately 40 percent of patients with endocarditis. Congenital heart disease, undiagnosed murmurs, and atherosclerotic disease each account for 10 percent of underlying lesions. The remaining 30 percent to 40 percent of infections occur without known predisposing cardiac disease. In one series of 25 autopsies, 8 patients had no underlying heart disease.

Clearly, all individuals have some finite risk of developing endocarditis. Relative risks cannot be accurately estimated for specific heart lesions because of a lack of epidemiologic data. Because approximately 40 percent of endocarditis cases occur in the presence of *rheumatic heart disease* (which has a prevalence of slightly more than 1 percent in the adult population) and another 40 percent occur in the absence of heart disease, the risk of endocarditis is increased 100-fold in the rheumatic heart as opposed to the normal heart.

Risk in *congenital heart disease* seems comparable. Patent ductus arteriosus, ventricular septal defect, and tetralogy of Fallot are the congenital lesions most commonly associated with endocarditis. Pulmonary and aortic stenoses constitute lesser risks. Atrial septal defect is very rarely responsible for endocarditis. Prophylaxis is not recommended for the patient with an isolated secundum atrial defect.

Hypertrophic cardiomyopathy confers significant risk of endocarditis. In a series of 126 patients with hypertrophic cardiomyopathy followed for varying periods up to 12 years, there were three definite cases and three suspected cases. Nine cases were reported in three other series, with a combined total of 158 patients followed for varying periods.

Mitral valve prolapse is also associated with increased risk of endocarditis. One natural history study reported five cases of endocarditis in 855 patient-years of follow-up, an incidence higher than in patients free of valvular heart disease. A case–control study estimated that mitral valve prolapse confers an eightfold increase in endocarditis risk. Although this risk is substantially lower than that associated with rheumatic or other acquired valvular disease, the public health consequences are great because of the high prevalence of mitral valve prolapse. In one series of apparent failures of endocarditis prophylaxis, mitral valve prolapse was the most common underlying cardiac lesion.

Prosthetic valves involve special risks. Prosthetic valve endocarditis has been divided into two groups: 1) early, as-

Table 16-1. Cardiac Risk Factors for Endocarditis

1. High Risk
   a. Prosthetic heart valve(s)
   b. History of endocarditis
2. Moderate Risk
   a. Rheumatic or other acquired valvular disease
   b. Congenital heart disease (excluding atrial septal defect of the secundum type)
   c. Idiopathic hypertrophic subaortic stenosis
3. Probable Moderate Risk
   a. Mitral valve prolapse
   b. Undiagnosed murmurs

sociated with surgery and most often involving nosocomial pathogens such as staphylococci; and 2) late, often following procedures that induce bacteremia and frequently associated with bacteria of low virulence. Late prosthetic valve endocarditis deserves special attention for two reasons: 1) organisms that are rarely able to infect damaged natural valves are more apt to infect prosthetic valves; and 2) when one deals with prosthetic valve endocarditis, the stakes are higher; treatment often involves valve replacement, and even with medical and surgical treatment, overall mortality is significantly higher. Prophylaxis is not recommended following coronary artery bypass graft surgery or placement of pacemakers or implanted defibrillators.

Another particularly high-risk group includes those who have *previously had endocarditis*. Recurrence rates as high as 10 percent have been cited, and third infections have been reported in some individuals. Table 16–1 summarizes known predisposing lesions in approximate order of risk. It must be kept in mind that the absolute risk of endocarditis, even for the patient at high risk, is extremely low, fewer than 1 case per 1000 tooth extractions.

The association of bacteremia with various events is shown in Table 16–2. Leading the list are dental procedures, rigid bronchoscopy, and genitourinary (GU) manipulations in the presence of urinary infection.

Table 16-2. Events Predisposing to Bacteremia

EVENT	PERCENTAGE OF INSTANCES IN WHICH BACTEREMIA OCCURS (%)
Dental extraction	75
Tooth brushing, flossing or irrigation	
Normal gingiva	20
Gingivitis	50
Bronchoscopy	
Fiberoptic	Less than 1
Rigid	15
Fiberoptic endoscopy	10
Sigmoidoscopy	5
Barium enema	10
Liver biopsy	5
Transurethral resection of prostate	
Sterile urine	10
Infected urine	50

NATURAL HISTORY OF ENDOCARDITIS AND EFFECTIVENESS OF THERAPY

Untreated endocarditis is uniformly fatal. Current mortality rates are about 10 percent with natural valves and 25 percent to 65 percent with prosthetic valves. Death often follows congestive heart failure, arterial emboli, myocardial infarction, myocardial abscesses, or other complications.

The efficacy of antibiotics used prophylactically has not been demonstrated in prospective trials. The large number of patients needed for such a study and the difficulties in identifying patients at risk and diagnosing episodes of potential bacteremia practically preclude such proof. Estimates of protective efficacy of antibiotic therapy derived from case-control studies range from 91 percent in a small study with 8 eligible cases to 49 percent in a larger study with 48 cases. Recommendations for prophylactic antibiotic regimens are based primarily on experience with experimental animal models.

RISK OF PROPHYLACTIC THERAPY

In the absence of previous sensitivity, the risk of serious reaction to penicillin prophylaxis is very small. No deaths were associated with the administration of benzathine penicillin G to over 300,000 Navy recruits for rheumatic fever prophylaxis. In a more recent study, more than 32,000 injections of benzathine penicillin G in 11 countries resulted in four cases of anaphylaxis, one of which was fatal. This falls within the reported range of serious reactions to penicillin among patients without prior allergy and without a history of rheumatic fever, which is 1 to 4 per 100,000. The risk of death due to serious penicillin reaction has been estimated at 1 to 2 per 100,000 patients receiving the drug.

Less information is available concerning risks associated with other prophylactic antibiotics, including amoxicillin, which is now recommended because it is better absorbed from the gastrointestinal (GI) tract and provides higher and more sustained serum levels. Surveys have identified very few serious reactions to other oral regimens, including clindamycin. Even with parenteral regimens including aminoglycosides, there is little toxicity when the drug is given for the brief period necessary for adequate prophylaxis.

IDENTIFYING PATIENTS AT RISK

As discussed previously, a rough estimate of risk can be made by identifying the underlying heart disease and estimating the likelihood that bacteremia will occur. Predisposing cardiac disease is detected by history and physical examination. A history of congenital or rheumatic heart disease and presence of a murmur indicate substantial risk. Documentation of hypertrophic cardiomyopathy or the presence of valve calcification can also be considered an indication for prophylaxis. All individuals with diastolic murmurs should be considered to be at risk.

Difficulty arises when the patient is at *probable* moderate risk. This is the case for most patients with mitral valve prolapse or with an isolated systolic murmur without a helpful history or other cardiac findings (see Chapter 21). Bacterial endocarditis prophylaxis for this group is controversial. The results of two independent risk–benefit analyses suggest that expected morbidity and mortality associated with penicillin therapy outweigh the benefits of prevention. Nevertheless, many clinicians continue to recommend prophylaxis. The American Heart Association currently recommends prophylaxis for patients with mitral valve prolapse only if there is evidence of valvular regurgitation.

CONCLUSIONS AND RECOMMENDATIONS

- Clinical effectiveness of endocarditis prophylaxis is difficult to demonstrate definitively. However, when the extreme degress of morbidity and mortality associated with the disease are weighed against the small risk associated with prophylaxis, vigorous preventive efforts are justified. It is estimated that about half of cases occur in patients with known predisposing heart disease following an anticipated episode of bacteremia.
- Identifiable risk varies with the type of heart abnormality and the event responsible for bacteremia, as summarized in Tables 16–1 and 16–2.
- Because patients with prosthetic valves are especially susceptible, they should be carefully counseled about the need for prophylaxis with any procedure—oral, GU, or GI—known to cause bacteremia. Similar advice should be given to patients with a history of endocarditis.

Specific Recommendations for High-Risk Patients

For dental procedures or surgery of the respiratory tract:

Standard regimen for high-risk patients:

Amoxicillin, 3.0 g orally 1 h before procedure, then 1.5 g 6 h after the initial dose.

For high-risk patients not considered candidates for standard regimen:

Ampicillin, 2.0 g IM/IV, plus gentamicin, 1.5 mg/kg (not to exceed 80 mg), 30 min before the procedure; then either the same regimen 8 h after the initial dose or amoxicillin, 1.5 g orally 6 h after the initial dose.

For high-risk patients allergic to ampicillin/amoxicillin/penicillin:

Vancomycin, 1 g IV infused over 1 h, starting 1 h before the procedure; no repeated dose necessary.

For GU or GI tract procedures:

Standard regimen for high-risk patients:

Ampicillin, 2.0 g IM/IV, plus gentamicin, 1.5 mg/kg (not to exceed 80 mg), 30 min before the procedure; then either the same regimen 8 h after initial dose or amoxicillin, 1.5 g orally 6 h after the initial dose.

For high-risk patients allergic to ampicillin/amoxicillin/penicillin:

Vancomycin, 1 g IV infused over 1 h, plus gentamicin, 1.5 mg/kg (not to exceed 80 mg), 1 h before the procedure; may be repeated once 8 h after initial dose.

- Patients with congenital or acquired valvular disease or with undiagnosed murmurs thought to reflect an anatomic abnormality should receive prophylaxis for all dental and upper respiratory tract procedures known to induce gingival or mucosal bleeding, including professional cleaning. Genitourinary and gastrointestinal procedures associated with a high frequency of bacteremia (including GU procedures in the presence of infected urine or prostate) should be done with antibiotic coverage. Examples of common procedures for which prophylaxis is recommended include incision and drainage of infected tissue, rigid bronchoscopy, gallbladder surgery, esophageal dilatation or sclerotherapy, vaginal hysterectomy, and cystoscopy. Endoscopy, barium enema, sigmoidoscopy, dilation and curettage, cesarean section, and insertion of an intrauterine device (IUD) do not require antibiotic coverage.

Specific Recommendations for Patients Not at High Risk Include the Following:

For dental procedures or surgery of the respiratory tract:

Standard regimen for patients not at high risk:

Amoxicillin, 3.0 g orally 1 h before procedure, then 1.5 g 6 h after the initial dose.

For patients not at high risk who are allergic to ampicillin/amoxicillin/penicillin:

Erythromycin ethylsuccinate, 800 mg, or erythromycin stearate, 1.0 g orally 2 h before procedure, then half the dose 6 h after initial dose, or clindamycin, 300 mg orally 1 h before procedure and 150 mg 6 h after initial dose.

For patients not at high risk who are unable to take oral medications:

Ampicillin, 2.0 IV or IM 30 min before procedure; then 1.0 g 6 h after initial dose.

For patients not at high risk who are allergic to ampicillin/amoxicillin/penicillin and unable to take oral medications:

Clindamycin, 300 mg IV 30 min before procedure; then 150 mg IV 6 h after initial dose.

For GU or GI tract procedures:

Standard Regimen for patients not at high risk

Ampicillin, 2.0 g ampicillin IM/IV, plus gentamicin, 1.5 mg/kg (not to exceed 80 mg), 30 minutes before the procedure; then either the same regimen 8 h after initial dose or amoxicillin, 1.5 g orally 6 h after the initial dose.

For low-risk patients allergic to ampicillin/amoxicillin/penicillin:

Vancomycin, 1 g IV infused over 1 h, plus gentamicin, 1.5 mg/kg (not to exceed 80 mg), 1 h before the procedure; may be repeated once 8 h after initial dose.

Alternative regimen for low-risk patients:

Amoxicillin, 3.0 g orally 1 h before procedure; then 1.5 g 6 h after initial dose.

- As in all preventive efforts, patient education is extremely important. All patients with identifiable risk should be urged to maintain a high level of oral health to minimize the potential for recurrent bacteremia. Patients receiving rheumatic fever prophylaxis must understand that their continuous therapy will *not* protect them from endocarditis.

A.G.M.

ANNOTATED BIBLIOGRAPHY

Allen HA, Leatham A et al. Significance and prognosis of an isolated late systolic murmur: A 9- to 22-year follow-up. Br Heart J 1974;36:525. (*Sixty-two patients with isolated late systolic murmur [33 also had a click] were followed for minimum of 9 years [mean 13.8]. Bacterial endocarditis occurred in 5 patients.*)

Bor DH, Himmelstein DU. Endocarditis prophylaxis in patients with mitral valve prolapse. Am J Med 1984;76:711. (*An analytic review of the risks of endocarditis and drug prophylaxis concluding that no prophylaxis or prophylaxis with erythromycin is preferable to prophylaxis with a penicillin.*)

Clemens JD, Horwitz RI, Jaffe CC et al. A controlled evaluation of the risk of bacterial endocarditis in persons with mitral valve prolapse. N Engl J Med 1982;307:776. (*A case-control study estimating a substantially higher risk—odds ratio of 8.2—of endocarditis for people with mitral valve prolapse than for those without it.*)

Clemens JD, Ransohoff DF. A quantitative assessment of predental antibiotic prophylaxis for patients with mitral valve prolapse. J Chron Dis 1984;37:531. (*A cost-effectiveness analysis concluding that the risk of postdental endocarditis in mitral valve prolapse may be outweighed by the risk of fatal reactions to parenteral penicillin prophylaxis.*)

Dajani AS, Bisno AL, Chung KJ et al. Prevention of bacterial endocarditis. Recommendations of the American Heart Association. JAMA 1990;264:2919. (*Recommendations moving toward greater emphasis on oral therapy, summarized in this chapter.*)

Doyle EF, Spagnuolo M, Taranta A et al. The risk of bacterial endocarditis during antirheumatic prophylaxis. JAMA 1967; 201:807. (*Sixteen cases of endocarditis were reported during 3615 patient-years of antirheumatic prophylaxis. No controls, but calculated incidence was not statistically different from that in historical control group. Four of the 16 organisms were penicillin-resistant.*)

Durack DT, Kaplan EL, Bisno AL. Apparent failures of endocarditis prophylaxis. JAMA 1983;250:2318. (*Summary of 52 cases submitted to the National AHA Registry. Mitral valve prolapse was the most common underlying cardiac lesion; only 6 of 52 endocarditis patients received recommended antibiotic regimens.*)

Epstein EJ, Coulshed N. Bacterial endocarditis in idiopathic hypertrophic subaortic stenosis. Cardiologia 1969;54:30. (*This paper reviews reported cases of endocarditis in a combined series of 158 patients with IHSS.*)

Everett ED, Hirschman JV. Transient bacteremia and endocarditis prophylaxis. A review. Medicine (Baltimore) 1977;56:61. (*Incidence data for bacteremia associated with relevant clinical procedures gathered from the literature are reviewed.*)

Imperiale TF, Horwitz RI. Does prophylaxis prevent postdental infective endocarditis? A controlled evaluation of protective efficacy. Am J Med 1990;88:131. (*Authors of this case-control study, with 8 cases and 24 controls, estimate a 91% protective efficacy for antibiotic prophylaxis.*)

Ivert TS, Dismukes WE, Cobbs CG et al. Prosthetic valve endocarditis. Circulation 1984;69:223. (*Documents the high risk of both early and late endocarditis among people with prosthetic valves; the highest risk were for those with prior native valve endocarditis and mechanical rather than biological prostheses.*)

Kaye D. Prohylaxis for infective endocarditis: An update. Ann Intern Med 1986;104:419. (*Somewhat dated by the new AHA recommendations, but still a valuable review.*)

Madlon-Kay DJ. Endocarditis prophylaxis in a primary care clinic. J Fam Pract 1991;32:504. (*One of many studies that document poor compliance with AHA recommendations.*)

Van der Meer JT, Van Wijk W, Thompson J et al. Efficacy of antibiotic prophylaxis for prevention of native-valve endocarditis. Lancet 1992;339:135. (*Based on a case-control study with 48 cases and 200 controls, authors estimate a 49 percent protective efficacy for prophylaxis.*)

Primary Care Medicine: Office Evaluation and Management of the Adult Patient, 3rd edition, edited by Allan H. Goroll, Lawrence A. May, and Albert G. Mulley, Jr. J.B. Lippincott Company, Philadelphia

17
Rheumatic Fever Prophylaxis

Despite a decline in incidence that began before the availability of antibiotics, rheumatic fever and rheumatic heart disease remain significant causes of preventable morbidity. Primary prevention depends on appropriate diagnosis and effective treatment of group A streptococcal pharyngitis, discussed in Chapter 220. Vaccination against streptococcal infection may be possible in the future, but current preventive measures depend on discriminating antibiotic use.

The prophylactic use of antibiotics has been shown to be effective for primary prevention during epidemics among closed populations. The major role of antibiotic prophylaxis, however, is in prevention of second attacks. The risk of recurrence following streptococcal infection is especially high in patients with evidence of carditis. Continuous streptococcal prophylaxis in patients with prior rheumatic fever is the major means of preventing the cardiac sequelae of rheumatic fever recurrences. It is the task of the primary physician to identify patients who would benefit from such prophylaxis and to provide the instruction necessary for long-term compliance.

EPIDEMIOLOGY AND RISK FACTORS

The epidemiology of rheumatic fever parallels that of streptococcal infection. Rare in children younger than 5 years of age, it is most common in older children and adolescents. Incidence decreases after adolescence; cases after age 40 are very rare. There is no clear predilection for either sex.

Although a genetic predisposition has not been proven, an association between certain HLA antigens and rheumatic diseases has been identified, at least among white patients. Heterogeneity in the immune response to a specific streptococcal cell-wall antigen, the group A carbohydrate, has been demonstrated, but predictors of the hyperimmune response associated with the clinical sequelae of rheumatic fever have not been identified.

Racial differences in the incidence of rheumatic fever exist but disappear when socioeconomic status is considered; crowded living conditions is an important variable. Crowding may also explain the high incidence in cold climates and during winter months in temperate climates.

All demographic risk factors are heavily outweighed by a previous history of rheumatic fever. The likelihood of an attack following streptococcal infection is at least five times higher among individuals with previous rheumatic fever.

NATURAL HISTORY OF RHEUMATIC FEVER AND EFFECTIVENESS OF THERAPY

Rheumatic fever follows between 0.5 percent and 3.0 percent of ineffectively treated cases of group A streptococcal upper respiratory infections. Diagnosis and appropriate antibiotic therapy will prevent rheumatic fever in the individual case, but such efforts cannot be expected to eliminate rheumatic disease because of the high proportion of streptococcal infections that are subclinical. Approximately one-third of patients with primary rheumatic fever have no history of preceding respiratory infections. Another one-third have symptoms but do not seek medical care. The remainder are ineffectively diagnosed or treated.

Among all patients with group A streptococcal infection and a history of previous rheumatic fever, the recurrence rate is 15 percent. More specific rates can be estimated for subgroups depending on 1) the number of previous rheumatic attacks; 2) the interval since the last attack; and 3) whether or not there was evidence of carditis. Specific attack rates are summarized in Table 17–1.

Because of these high secondary attack rates and the ubiquity of the streptococcus, *continuous* antibiotic prophylaxis of streptococcal infection is the only feasible method of preventing rheumatic fever recurrences. Three antibiotic regimens have gained general acceptance:

1. Benzathine penicillin G, 1,200,000 units IM every 4 weeks
2. Sulfadiazine, 1 g PO qd (500 mg for patients weighing less than 60 lb)
3. Penicillin G, 250 mg PO bid

Although the effectiveness of erythromycin (250 mg PO bid) has not been studied, it is recommended for the rare patient allergic to both penicillin and sulfonamides. The classic study comparing the effectiveness of these three regimens in preventing streptococcal infection and rheumatic fever is summarized in Table 17–2.

There are no firm guidelines regarding the duration of continuous antibiotic prophylaxis following an episode of rheumatic fever. Factors that influence the likelihood of rheumatic recurrence following infection have already been reviewed. Within limits, the physician can estimate the risk of exposure of a particular patient to streptococcal infection. For example, parents of young children, teachers and other school personnel, health care providers, and military personnel are at high risk.

Table 17-1. Risk of Recurrent Rheumatic Fever After Group A Streptococcal Infection

	PERCENTAGE OF RECURRENCES OF STREPTOCOCCAL INFECTION
Interval Since Onset of Last Rheumatic Episode	
Up to 2 years	28
2–5 years	15
5 years and over	10
Number of Previous Attacks of Rheumatic Fever	
2 or more	27
1	14
Rheumatic Heart Disease	
Not present	13
Present	26

(Modified from Spagnuolo M, Pasternack B, Taranta A et al. Risk of rheumatic fever recurrences after streptococcal infections. N Engl J Med 285:641, 1971.)

RISKS OF ANTIBIOTIC PROPHYLAXIS

The risks of penicillin administration are discussed in Chapter 16 on endocarditis prophylaxis. It should be emphasized that, in a large series, reactions following parenteral administration were no more common than those following oral therapy.

CONCLUSIONS AND RECOMMENDATIONS

- Primary prevention of rheumatic fever depends on accurate diagnosis and treatment of symptomatic streptococcal upper respiratory infections. Prevention of rheumatic fever recurrences depends on continuous streptococcal prophylaxis of the patients at risk.
- Monthly injections of benzathine penicillin G (1,200,000 units IM) provide the most effective prophylaxis and are recommended in patients with a high risk of both streptococcal exposure and a rheumatic recurrence after infection. Acceptable oral regimens in patients at lower risk include the following:

  Sulfadiazine, 1 g PO qd, *or*
  Penicillin G, 250 mg PO bid, *or*
  Erythromycin, 250 mg PO bid (in patients allergic to both penicillin and sulfa drugs)

- The duration of prophylaxis should be based on the risk incurred by the particular patient.
- All patients with rheumatic fever should be treated until age 25 or for 5 years after an episode (whichever is longer). In those with two or more previous attacks or with rheumatic heart disease, therapy should be continued until age 40 or for 10 years after the last episode. Prophylaxis in patients with rheumatic heart disease at high risk of streptococcal exposure should be continued indefinitely.

A.G.M.

Table 17-2. Prophylaxis and Attack Rates of Streptococcal Infection and Rheumatic Fever Recurrences

	ORAL SULFADIAZINE (1 G DAILY)	ORAL PENICILLIN G (200,000 UNITS DAILY)	IM BENZATHINE PENICILLIN G (1.2 MILLION UNITS EVERY 4 WEEKS)
Number of patient-years	576	545	560
Number of streptococcal infections (rate/100 patient-years)	138 (24.0)	113 (20.7)	34 (6.1)
Number of rheumatic fever recurrences (rate/100 patient-years)	16 (2.8)	30 (5.5)	2 (0.4)

(Modified from Wood H, Feinstein AR, Tarant A et al. Rheumatic fever in children and adolescents III: Comparative effectiveness of three prophylaxis regimens in preventing streptococcal infections and rheumatic recurrences. Ann Intern Med 60:31, 1964.)

ANNOTATED BIBLIOGRAPHY

International Rheumatic Fever Study Group. Allergic reactions to long-term benzathine penicillin prophylaxis for rheumatic fever. Lancet 1991;337:1308. (*Risk found to be very low.*)

Ayoub EM. The search for host determinants of susceptibility to rheumatic fever: The missing link. Circulation 1984;69:197. (*Reviews evidence for genetic markers and immune hyperresponsiveness to streptococcal antigens among people predisposed to rheumatic fever.*)

Berrios X, del Campo E, Guzman B, Bisno AL. Discontinuing rheumatic fever prophylaxis in selected adolescents and young adults. A prospective study. Ann Intern Med 1993; 118:401. (*Documents relatively low risk of recurrence, 0.7 cases per 100 person-years when prophylaxis was discontinued in selected patients in Chile.*)

Breese BB, Disney FA. Penicillin in the treatment of streptococcal infections. A comparison of effectiveness of five different oral and one parenteral form. N Engl J Med 1958;259:57. (*No difference was found in reaction rates between IM and PO use.*)

Holmberg SD, Faich GA. Streptococcal pharyngitis and acute rheumatic fever in Rhode Island. JAMA 1983;250:2307. (*Of patients receiving throat cultures, nearly 90 percent were given antibiotic therapy before the culture results were known, and nearly 40 percent continued antibiotic therapy for 10 days regardless of results. Only three definite cases of rheumatic fever were identified during a 5-year period.*)

Kaplan EL, Bisno A, Derrick W et al. Prevention of rheumatic fever: AHA Committee Report. Circulation 1977;55:1. (*Summary of argument for prophylaxis with recommendations.*)

Land MA, Bisno AL. Acute rheumatic fever: A vanishing disease in suburbia. JAMA 1983;249:895. (*A retrospective analysis in Memphis–Shelby County detecting a 0.64 case per 100,000 population annual incidence of acute rheumatic fever. An accompanying editorial ponders explanations for the dramatic fall in acute rheumatic fever incidence in the United States.*)

McFarland RB. Reactions to benzathine penicillin. N Engl J Med 1958;259:62. (*Reaction rate of 1.3 percent following single injection in 12,858 naval recruits.*)

Schwartz RH, Wientzen RL, Pedreira F et al. Penicillin V for group A pharyngeal tonsilitis. JAMA 1981;246:1790. (*A randomized-control trial demonstrating a treatment failure rate of 31 percent for patients treated for 7 days compared with 18 percent for those treated for 10 days.*)

Sellers TF. An epidemiologic view of rheumatic fever. Prog Cardiovasc Dis 1973;16:303. (*Reviews epidemiology.*)

Spagnuolo M, Pasternack B, Taranta A. Risk of rheumatic fever recurrences after streptococcal infections. N Engl J Med 1971;285:641. (*Data are reviewed in Table 17–1.*)

Stollerman GH. Variation in group A streptococci and the prevalence of rheumatic fever: A half-century vigil. Ann Intern Med 1993;118:467. (*Editorial that provides historical perspective on RF and its prevention.*)

Wood HF, Feinstein AR, Taranta A et al. Rheumatic fever in children and adolescents. III: Comparative effectiveness of three prophylaxis regimens in preventing streptococcal infections and rheumatic recurrences. Ann Intern Med 1964;60:31. (*Data are reviewed in Table 17–2.*)

Primary Care Medicine: Office Evaluation and Management of the Adult Patient, 3rd edition, edited by Allan H. Goroll, Lawrence A. May, and Albert G. Mulley, Jr. J.B. Lippincott Company, Philadelphia © 1995

18
Exercise and Prevention of Cardiovascular Disease

HARVEY B. SIMON, M.D.

Exercise has become a central part of the lifestyle of many Americans. An estimated 20 million to 40 million Americans jog regularly, making it the most popular participant sport. In addition, other active sports, such as tennis, racquetball, cross-country skiing, and bicycling, have grown in popularity. Unlike other recreational activities, these sports attract participants not only for their intrinsic pleasures, but because they are widely believed to be beneficial to health. In the case of jogging, the public has been exposed to conflicting claims ranging from the hypothesis that marathon running helps prevent myocardial infarctions to warnings that long distance running is a health hazard. Because of these controversies, the primary care physician is increasingly called on to advise his patients about the effects of exercise on health and to prescribe an effective and safe exercise program.

PHYSIOLOGY AND CLINICAL EFFECTS OF EXERCISE

Physiology

Physical work may involve either aerobic or anaerobic metabolism, and it may rely on either isotonic or isometric muscular activity. The concept of *aerobic* exercise provides the foundation for endurance training. The total amount of stored energy available to muscle groups in the form of preformed adenosine triphosphate (ATP) and phosphocreatine is sufficient to sustain less than 10 seconds of maximal exertion. Clearly, energy must be generated continuously during exercise, and the majority of this energy comes from the metabolism of muscle glycogen. The availability of oxygen determines whether this metabolism will be aerobic or anaerobic. When oxygen supply is adequate, metabolism is aerobic and glycogen is completely metabolized to pyruvate and then to water and CO_2 through the Krebs cycle.

With increasing exercise intensity, the ability of the lungs to take up oxygen and of the heart and blood vessels to deliver it to muscle cells is exceeded, and metabolism becomes *anaerobic*. The costs of anaerobic metabolism are substantial. Anaerobic metabolism is inefficient; it generates only one-third as much energy from each gram of glycogen, and it increases production of lactic acid, resulting in muscle cramps, fatigue, and dyspnea. Lactic acid is buffered by bicarbonate, resulting in increased CO_2 production and hyperventilation. Clinically, an abrupt rise in respiratory rate indicates that the anaerobic threshold has been crossed. Endurance training can be expected to increase the anaerobic threshold, thus allowing more work to be performed under favorable aerobic conditions.

Aerobic and Anaerobic Exercise. The goal of training is to improve cardiovascular function and muscular efficiency. The type of exercise is critical. While maximal exertion or anaerobic training is beneficial to certain competitive athletes, the cornerstone of training for fitness is endurance or *aerobic exercise* using large muscle groups in continuous rhythmic activity for prolonged periods. *Jogging* and *brisk walking* are ideal for this. Other good training activities include *bicycling, swimming, cross-country skiing, rowing,* and *rope jumping*. These activities provide *isotonic exercise* whereby skeletal muscle fibers shorten in length with little change in tension. Heart rate and cardiac output increase, but peripheral vascular resistance falls. In contrast, sports depending on very brief bursts of intense activity, such as weight lifting, provide *isometric exercise* in which muscle tension increases with little change in fiber length. Such exercise produces a marked increase in peripheral vascular resistance and blood pressure with little increase in cardiac output. Aerobic power does not increase with isometric exercising, and the hypertensive response can be hazardous to patients with cardiovascular disease. Because arm work has a greater tendency to produce tachycardia and hypertension than does an equivalent degree of leg work, it is particularly important to limit the resistance level in arm exercises for patients with hypertension or heart disease.

Sports that allow prolonged periods of inactivity, such as baseball or golf, are poor for cardiopulmonary conditioning. Similarly, although activities providing sustained but gentle muscular effort, such as yoga, can be important parts of a fitness program because they are excellent for promoting flexibility and strength, they are poor tools for attaining cardiopulmonary fitness.

Effects of Exercise

The effects of regular exercise can be classified in terms of cardiovascular, musculoskeletal, metabolic, and psychological functions. Regular endurance-type exercise improves cardiovascular performance and tends to lower blood pressure, body fat, weight, and serum triglycerides while elevating serum high-density lipoproteins. Physical fitness may also assist in the psychological response to stress.

Cardiovascular. The most thoroughly documented results of aerobic exercise concern changes in cardiovascular performance. Exercise requires an increase in the body's oxygen consumption, which is made possible by increased oxygen uptake by pulmonary ventilation, increased oxygen delivery by the heart and the peripheral circulation, and increased oxygen extraction by muscle. Endurance training enhances the efficiency of these processes by both central and peripheral mechanisms. At rest and at submaximal work loads, the fit individual has a slower heart rate than does the untrained person. Stroke volume is increased so that cardiac output for a given work load is unchanged. While the achievable maximum heart rate is not increased by training, the maximum cardiac output and maximum oxygen consumption are greatly enhanced so that the well-trained individuals can both attain higher work loads and sustain them for longer periods before becoming exhausted.

Although there is little firm evidence that exercise increases myocardial oxygen supply or produces collateral vascularization in humans, *myocardial oxygen demand* for a given work load *decreases*. This diminution in myocardial oxygen consumption is made possible by the lower heart rate (HR) and lower systolic blood pressure (BP) that accompany exercise in the fit individual. This can be of particular benefit to the patient with angina, as this "double product" of HR × BP determines the angina threshold (see Chapter 30). In addition, animal studies have demonstrated increased coronary artery cross-sectional area, increased myocardial capillary density, and myocardial hypertrophy in rats and dogs forced to exercise.

The peripheral effects of exercise are also of great importance in endurance training. *Capillary blood flow* to muscle is increased. Muscle fibers increase in volume, and muscle strength and endurance are enhanced. Muscle mitochondria increase in size and number, and respiratory enzymes increase. As a result, muscle oxygen extraction is improved. Training also improves neuromuscular coordination and musculoskeletal efficiency.

Another important cardiovascular effect of exercise is on the *blood pressure*. Systolic pressure normally rises during aerobic exercise, but this rise tends to be slightly less in the fit individual. More important, total peripheral resistance falls as a result of improved muscle blood flow and decreased circulating catecholamine levels. The net result in trained individuals is lower blood pressure, both during exercise and at rest. Because this effect is actually more prominent in hypertensive subjects, endurance training can be an important nonpharmacologic treatment for the control of mild to moderate hypertension (see Chapter 26).

Less well-established cardiovascular benefits of exercise training include a possible *diminution of arrhythmias,* perhaps because of lower catecholamine levels. In addition, exercise increases *fibrinolytic activity* and decreases platelet adhesiveness; these hematologic effects may, to some degree, protect against atherogenesis. In these areas, too, the data are preliminary.

Metabolic. The metabolic benefits of exercise are well documented. *Weight control* is an important motivating factor for many runners. An average jogger can be expected to consume about 600 calories in an hour of running. Other endurance activities have similar effects (Table 18–1). While exercise alone will produce only a slow reduction in total body weight, the percentage of body fat falls more rapidly, resulting in visible increases in muscle tone. Perhaps most important, fit people often become motivated to adhere to dietary patterns that will permit sustained weight control.

Another metabolic effect of great interest is that of regular exercise on the blood lipids. In many runners, serum *triglyceride* levels fall dramatically without changes in the dietary intake of fats or carbohydrates. The total *cholesterol* level changes less predictably, but *high-density lipoprotein* levels are reliably increased by aerobic exercise, and these higher levels correlate with a lower risk for coronary artery disease (see Chapter 15).

Psychological. Most individuals who engage in regular exercise develop an *improved self-image.* This can be of great importance in the rehabilitation of patients with ischemic heart disease (see Chapter 31) and can also be used to help motivate healthy individuals to modify other risk factors by following a prudent diet and discontinuing smoking. The recreational aspects of exercise tend to lessen anxiety and depression. Running is being studied as a tool for the treatment of depression, and early results in small groups of patients are encouraging. Nevertheless, the so-called runner's high proves elusive or illusionary for many joggers. Although exercise has many psychological benefits, it is hardly a panacea. Patients can be encouraged to exercise for both psychological and physical gains, but they must have realistic expectations.

Survival. Because of its amelioration of many cardiovascular risk factors, it would seem reasonable to expect regular exercise to reduce risk of cardiovascular morbidity and mortality. Although there are data suggesting this, they derive from epidemiologic and observational studies. As one critical appraisal points out, there are no data from prospective, randomized, controlled studies to allow a reliable conclusion about cause and effect.

In further evaluating observational studies of exercise, it must be remembered that attention to inactivity as a risk factor is relatively recent, with most work being done in the last two to three decades. In addition, there is the potential bias introduced by self-selection: if healthier people tend to exercise more, then improved mortality in active people may relate to underlying factors rather than to exercise per se. Problems in quantifying exercise, small sample sizes, and confounding variables, such as psychosocial factors, diet, alcohol consumption, smoking, genetic background, body build, lipid levels, and blood pressure further limit the conclusions that can be drawn from these studies.

Despite such limitations, the vast majority of investigations suggest that regular physical activity does indeed have a favorable effect on morbidity and mortality from cardiovascular disease. Perhaps the best known studies in this

Table 18-1. Approximate Metabolic Expenditures Associated with Selected Activities*

AVERAGE ENERGY OUTPUT	ACTIVITY
1 met	Rest
1½–2 mets 2–2½ kcal/min	Desk work Standing Strolling (1 mile/h)
2–3 mets 2½–4 kcal/min	Level walking (2 miles/h) Level biking (5 miles/h) Golf (power cart)
3–4 mets 4–5 kcal/min	Walking (3 miles/h) Bicycling (6 miles/h) Badminton Housework
4–5 mets 5–6 kcal/min	Golf (carrying clubs) Dancing Tennis (doubles) Raking leaves Calisthenics
5–6 mets 6–7 kcal/min	Walking (4 miles/h) Bicycling (10 miles/h) Skating Shoveling garden soil Average sexual activity
6–7 mets 7–8 kcal/min	Brisk walking (5 miles/h) Tennis (singles) Snow shoveling Downhill skiing Water skiing
7–8 mets 8–10 kcal/min	Jogging (5 miles/h) Bicycling (12 miles/h) Basketball Canoeing Mountain climbing Ditch digging Touch football
8–9 mets 10–11 kcal/min	Jogging (6 miles/h) Cross-country skiing Squash or handball (recreational)
Over 10 mets Over 11 kcal/min	Squash or handball (competitive) Running 6 miles/h: 10 mets 8 miles/h: 13½ mets 10 miles/hd: 17 mets

*Energy outputs are expressed in mets. One met is the energy expended at rest, and equals 3.5 ml O_2/kg body weight/minute. (Calorie consumption values are a 70-kg person.)

(Modified from Fox SM, Naughty JP, Gorman DA. Physical activity and cardiovascular health. III: The exercise prescription; frequency and type of activity. Mod Concepts Cardiovasc Dis 41:6, 1972.)

country are those of Paffenbarger and his coworkers (see Annotated Bibliography).

Although most investigations concentrate on men, an evaluation of 3120 women and 10,224 men demonstrated that exercise is equally beneficial to both sexes. The least fit individuals were eight times more likely to die of cardiovascular disease than those who were most fit.

A meta-analysis of 27 cohorts evaluating the relationship between physical activity and coronary artery disease found that sedentary living imposes a relative risk of dying from coronary artery disease of 1.9. The magnitude of this excess relative risk approaches that of smoking (2.5), elevated cholesterol (2.4), and hypertension (2.1). Because sedentary living is to two to three times more prevalent than any of these other risk factors, it can be argued that physical inactivity is the single largest contributor to the epidemic of coronary artery disease.

While these studies concentrate on the role of exercise in the primary prevention of cardiovascular disease, attention is also being directed to the role of physical training in the treatment of patients with established atherosclerotic heart disease (secondary prevention). A meta-analysis of 22 prospective trials of exercise in the treatment of coronary artery disease demonstrated a 20 percent decrease in overall mortality in the exercise group; fatal reinfarction and total cardiovascular deaths were also significantly reduced in the exercise group, but nonfatal reinfarctions were no different in the exercise and control groups.

Other Benefits. Although the greatest protective effect of exercise is on the cardiovascular system, there are other important benefits of habitual exercise. Women who begin exercising in early adulthood experience nearly a 50 percent reduction in their lifetime risk of *breast* and *reproductive cancer.* Physically active men have a significantly lower risk of *colon cancer.* Exercise increases bone density, helping to prevent *osteoporosis.* Patients with *chronic obstructive lung disease* and *peripheral vascular disease* report symptomatic and functional improvements.

MEDICAL SCREENING OF POTENTIAL EXERCISERS

The physician can and should play a central role in promoting physical fitness. An important goal is to provide patient motivation through education: A clear understanding of the benefits and techniques of endurance training enhances compliance. Medical screening of the prospective participant and prescription of an appropriate exercise program are essential for the person who has been inactive.

History. The first step in medical screening is obtaining a detailed personal and family history. Each patient should be carefully questioned about symptoms that suggest cardiovascular disease, including chest pain, palpitations, dyspnea, undue fatigue, syncope, and claudication. It is very important to review health habits in detail, with special attention to previous exercise patterns, smoking, diet, and the use of oral contraceptive agents. Of particular importance in the family history is the presence of coronary heart disease, peripheral vascular disease, hypertension, stroke, diabetes, or sudden death.

Physical Examination. A complete physical examination is also vital to the medical screening of the prospective exerciser. Height and weight should be recorded, and it may be useful to calculate the body mass index or to measure the percent body fat (see Chapter 10). The blood pressure is taken at rest with the patient supine and standing, and the heart rate and pressure are recorded after mild exercise (stair climbing or sit-ups are satisfactory for this purpose). The chest is examined for rales, wheezes, and rhonchi, and the heart for cardiomegaly, gallops, murmurs, and rhythm disturbances. The peripheral pulses and abdomen should be palpated to exclude atherosclerotic disease and an aortic aneurysm. The musculoskeletal system should be evaluated both to exclude significant pathology and to determine whether specific flexibility or strengthening exercises are required as part of the training program.

Laboratory Studies. Several laboratory studies are helpful in the screening process. Most patients ought to have a complete blood count, urinalysis, and determinations of blood sugar, creatinine, and cholesterol. For patients older than 40 years of age, a *resting electrocardiogram* is helpful to check for ischemia, left ventricular hypertrophy, and disturbances of rate and rhythm.

If any of these screening procedures discloses evidence of overt cardiovascular or pulmonary disease, then *exercise stress testing* is mandatory before an exercise program is initiated. Even if preliminary screening is negative, stress testing may be helpful for high-risk patients, including those with hypertension, diabetes, hyperlipidemia, or positive family history of coronary disease. Obesity, cigarette smoking, and a previous sedentary lifestyle are further indications for considering stress testing. Heavy exertion can trigger an acute myocardial infarction, especially in persons who are sedentary. Exercise training is protective. Because atherosclerotic heart disease is so prevalent in our society, stress testing may be a prudent precursor to a vigorous exercise program in males older than 50 and females older than 60 years of age, even if they are asymptomatic and apparently healthy. An evaluation of exercise electrocardiographic stress testing in 3617 asymptomatic hypercholesterolemic men between 35 and 59 years of age found that the test had a sensitivity of only 18 percent in predicting exercise-induced cardiac events, even though specificity was 92 percent. These findings cast doubt on the ability of the electrocardiographic stress test to identify underlying coronary disease in asymptomatic patients. Whether thallium stress testing would be more sensitive remains to be determined (see Chapter 36). Stress testing may be useful for uncovering exercise-induced arrhythmias and hypotension, evaluating the individual's exercise capacity, and establishing the maximal and target heart rates for use in the exercise prescription.

In special cases, additional studies may be desirable, such as forced expiratory volume (FEV_1), vital capacity, and arterial blood gases in patients with subjective dyspnea or suspected pulmonary disease. Specialized ergometric testing can determine maximal oxygen consumption, total work capacity, and other physiologic parameters. Another powerful tool is 24-hour ambulatory *Holter monitoring* for arrhythmias. Finally, telemetry enables constant monitoring of rate and rhythm during actual jogging.

Medical screening and exercise testing allow the physician to assign each patient to one of three categories:

1. Individuals with normal studies who can undertake an exercise program without medical supervision. Even in these healthy people, individualized exercise prescriptions and guidance regarding training techniques and safety precautions will be of great value.
2. Patients with ischemic heart disease, moderate hypertension, or moderate chronic obstructive lung disease will benefit from graded exercise programs, but they should be referred to a specialized exercise rehabilitation program that can provide medical supervision and facilities for emergency treatment. People taking digitalis, nitrates, or beta-blocking agents should be included in this supervised exercise group. However, if structured rehabilitation is not available, milder forms of exercise can still be recommended (eg, walking, stationary bicycling) with appropriate precautions.
3. Physical exertion is contraindicated in the presence of congestive heart failure, ventricular irritability, uncontrolled hypertension, unstable diabetes, or uncontrolled epilepsy, although patients with these conditions can sometimes be enrolled in supervised programs if they respond to medical therapy. Patients with A-V block, sick sinus syndrome, left ventricular or aortic aneurysms, or aortic valve disease should be excluded from exercise programs.

THE EXERCISE PRESCRIPTION

The fitness program depends on three elements: frequency, intensity, and duration of exercise. Three exercise sessions per week are required to develop and maintain fitness, and five sessions per week probably provide near maximum benefit. Hence, the exercise prescription should call for at least three workouts each week. Many individuals prefer a routine of daily activity; this is an excellent program, but it is advisable to schedule easier and harder workouts on alternate days to prevent injuries and allow the muscles to recover.

The *intensity* and *duration* of training are intimately related. Equal degrees of fitness can be attained through less intense exercise sustained over a longer period or through more vigorous effort for shorter periods. Maximum cardiopulmonary fitness can be attained by 15 to 60 minutes of continuous aerobic exercises that are strenuous enough to raise the heart rate to 60 percent to 80 percent of maximum or the oxygen uptake to 50 percent to 85 percent of maximum.

Optimal fitness goals must be attained very slowly and gradually, and the physician's exercise prescription should provide a practical means of attaining them. Both the starting point and the rate of progression depend on the health, age, and fitness of the participant. As a rule of thumb, the beginner should plan to exercise aerobically for 10 to 12 minutes at a pace sufficient to increase heart rate to 60 percent to 80 percent of maximum without producing breathlessness.

Each running session begins with a 5- to 10-minute *warm-up period*. At the beginning of exercise, even the well-conditioned athlete experiences some degree of dyspnea due to anaerobic metabolism. It takes 45 to 90 seconds for cardiac output to increase enough to meet the new work load and provide the "second wind." A warm-up period will minimize this initial anaerobic period and also allow muscles to loosen and stretch out, which prevents many injuries. For the runner, the warm-up period should consist of stretching exercise, calisthenics, and a gradual progression from walking to slow jogging to running.

The actual *training period* should initially consist of a total of 10 to 12 minutes of exercise. At first, it is best to alternate periods of effort with periods of recovery. This is easily accomplished by alternately walking and jogging. For example, an unfit or older individual might alternate 1 minute of jogging with 1 minute of walking, repeating this cycle 10 to 12 times during each training day. When this can be accomplished with comfort—perhaps at the end of 10 to 20 sessions over 2 to 3 weeks—the schedule can be advanced to 2 minutes of jogging alternating with 2 minutes of walking, with six cycles in each session. After this is mastered, the jogging ritual can be extended to 3 or 4 minutes with only 1 or 2 minutes of rest for three or four cycles, and then to two 6-minute runs with 1 or 2 minutes of walking in between. By the end of 1 or 2 months, most individuals can expect to be able to jog for 10 to 20 minutes continuously and to cover 1 to 2 miles during this period. Similar schedules can be used for other aerobic fitness activities.

Although the young and athletic person will progress more rapidly than the older or unfit one, it is important to urge restraint. One of the most common causes of orthopedic injuries is attempting too much too quickly. Once a base of 10 to 20 minutes of exercise is well established, further progress can be encouraged. It is reasonable to increase time or distance by a rate of about 10 percent per week. This can be accomplished by extending one or two sessions while preserving some short-distance days, or by gradually extending each session. At the end of 4 to 6 months, 3 to 4 miles of jogging or equivalent exercise 3 to 5 days per week will provide maximum conditioning. This level must be maintained to sustain the cardiopulmonary benefits of exercise. Feelings of accomplishment and well-being usually provide motivation for sustained participation, often at even higher levels. As little as 20 minutes of aerobic exercise three times per week is beneficial, but 3 to 4 hours of exercise per week provides the maximum longevity benefits.

In addition to the duration of exercise, the *intensity* or *pace* of exercise requires consideration. The most precise readily available measure of intensity is the *heart rate*. Patients should jog at a pace sufficient to raise the pulse to 60 percent to 80 percent of maximum. If exercise testing has been performed, an observed maximal heart rate can be used for this calculation. In the absence of such data, the maximal heart rate can be estimated for healthy individuals by subtracting the age from 220. As a rough guide, the target of 60 percent to 80 percent of this maximum translates to 130 to 150 beats per minute for younger persons and to 110 to 125 beats per minute for older ones. The patient can be taught to take his carotid or radial pulse just before and immediately after exercise and to adjust his pace to attain and maintain the target heart rate. It can be very helpful to have the patient keep a daily record of these figures together with the time and approximate distance covered. As training progresses, a more rapid pace will be required to achieve the target heart rate.

Many people find it difficult or unpleasant to take their pulse. For such persons, intensity of effort can be roughly gauged by the "talking" pace—the intensity sufficient to feel one is working hard while still able to talk to a companion without feeling dyspneic.

The *cool-down period* completes the exercise prescription. A period of 5 to 10 minutes of walking and stretching exercises is desirable. This prevents the marked vasodilatation for dissipation of heat from causing hypotension and hypoperfusion. Very hot or very cold showers should be avoided.

PATIENT EDUCATION

Many patients do not know that next to smoking, hypertension, and hypercholesterolemia, inactivity is one of the most important treatable cardiac risk factors. Furthermore, they do not appreciate that exercise not only can help them to look, feel, and work better, but it can reduce overall mortality. These advantages should provide sufficient justification for the physician to encourage endurance-type exercise.

However, exercise is not without potential adverse effects, and patients need to be educated about them as well. There is no question that exercise can precipitate cardiac arrhythmias and myocardial ischemia in persons with coronary artery disease. Sudden death is a tragic, though infrequent, complication of exercise. Careful medical screening of potential exercisers, an individualized exercise prescription, and meticulous supervision of high-risk individuals can minimize complications. Closely controlled conditioning programs have enabled survivors of myocardial infarctions to engage safely in aerobic exercise, even marathon running. Some runners encounter exercise-induced asthma, particularly during cold weather. Advising use of a face mask that warms inspired air often suffices; sometimes pre-exercise treatment with inhaled cromolyn or albuterol is necessary. Extreme environmental conditions may also produce thermal stress ranging from frostbite to heat stroke. Here too, prevention is the best therapy. The physician should be able to advise the runner about appropriate fluid intake, clothing, acclimatization, and safe duration of exposure and exercise. Similar advice prevents dehydration and electrolyte depletion.

Musculoskeletal injuries are very common and result from overuse, inflexibility, and muscle imbalance (see Chapters 152 and 154). Overuse is prevented by gradual increases in exercise; inflexibility and imbalance are avoided by stretching and strengthening (see below). Providing advice about equipment and technique can also help lessen the risk of injury.

PRACTICAL ADVICE FOR THE BEGINNING EXERCISER

Food and Fluid Intake. It is best to avoid exercise within 2 hours of a substantial meal. Despite many claims to the contrary, no specific dietary programs are required for running. The obese person should restrict calories to reduce, while the lean individual may require increased caloric intake to maintain weight. Competitive athletes feel that increased carbohydrate intake during the 3 days prior to a race helps increase endurance, and there is some experimental evidence suggesting that such "carbohydrate loading" does increase muscle glycogen content. Adequate fluid intake is essential, particularly in warm weather. Although thirst will dictate the need for fluid replacement, it is best to begin drinking small amounts before thirst becomes overt, so that large volumes will not be needed at any one time. Water is excellent, though some runners prefer balanced electrolyte solutions or even carbonated beverages.

Climate. Thermal stress presents a potentially serious threat. When confronted with an abrupt change in climate, the exerciser should sharply reduce distance and speed for several days until acclimatization is achieved. In warm, humid weather, outdoor exercise should be confined to early morning or evening hours or shady locations, distances and speed should be reduced, fluids should be taken at frequent intervals during the run, and clothing should be light colored and lightweight. Environmental temperatures between 50°F and 60°F are ideal for exercising in shorts and T-shirts. Between 40°F and 50°F, a warm-up suit is generally sufficient; below 40°F, gloves or mittens and a hat are important. Multiple layers of thin, flexible clothing are better than a single bulky garment. Woolen fabrics are ideal, but a soft cotton layer should be next to the skin. An extra layer of thermal underwear is vital for temperatures below 30°F, and if winds are strong or temperatures drop below 15°F, an additional layer such as a turtleneck, extra shorts, and possibly a ski mask are required. Again, distances should be reduced in bitter cold, and it is particularly important to avoid wet conditions, which can lead to frostbite, especially of the feet.

Air Pollutants may cause irritation of the upper and lower respiratory tract, and carbon monoxide can impair oxygenation and precipitate angina. One should avoid running on heavily traveled roads, during rush hours, and on days when temperature inversions increase air pollution.

Safety is of utmost importance. The runner should run facing the flow of cars. Sidewalks are preferred when possible. Although country roads are ideal, it is desirable to run with a companion in isolated areas in case of injury. Daytime running is safer both because the runner is more visible to cars and because he can see road hazards more easily. Bright-colored clothing should be encouraged, and at night reflectorized vests are mandatory. Dogs are best avoided by means of an impromptu detour, but if this is not possible they can generally be intimidated by a firm command to "go home" or by the threat of a stick or stone.

Equipment. One of the advantages of running is that elaborate equipment is not required. However, good running shoes are essential. Many excellent shoes are available; the choice should be dictated by fit, comfort, and support rather than by endorsements or ratings. The toe box should provide enough room for dorsiflexion during takeoff, the sole should be flexible and provide adequate cushioning, and the heel should be fairly snug without exerting pressure on the Achilles tendon. Most good running shoes are costly but can be expected to last for up to 500 miles. Shoes are important, but other items ranging from stopwatches to designer sweat suits are optional to say the least. Good shoes will help prevent musculoskeletal injuries. In addition, a relatively soft running surface is helpful; grass and turf are best if they are smooth and level; asphalt is preferable to concrete.

Orthotics and other orthopedic devices are sometimes helpful for refractory problems. Patients with overuse injuries who fail to limit their activity may require a splint or cast to enforce inactivity, even if immobilization is not actually necessary for healing. The use of such devices requires referral to an orthopedist or podiatrist skilled in treating runners' musculoskeletal problems.

Stretching. Regular running produces asymmetric muscular development. The calf, hamstring, and Achilles can become overdeveloped and/or shortened and tight. Hill running and sprinting may produce similar effects on the quadriceps and hip flexors. A regular program of stretching exercises is essential to promote flexibility and balanced muscular development. These exercises are ideal for the warm-up and cool-down periods before and after running.

Stretching routines are almost as numerous and varied as runners themselves. Four exercises are of particular value: the Achilles and soleus stretch (Fig. 18–1), the hamstring stretch (Fig. 18–2), the quadriceps stretch (Fig. 18–3), and the hip and side stretch (Fig. 18–4).

With increased running, more stretching will be necessary. In addition to flexibility, balanced muscular strength can be important. Bent knee sit-ups are particularly valuable in strengthening abdominal muscles and preventing "side-stitches." Upper extremity strength is surprisingly important for runners. Push-ups are the simplest upper extremity exercise, but advanced runners often include limited weight lifting or isometrics as well.

Running is not a panacea, but it has many cardiopulmonary, metabolic, and psychological benefits. The physician has a crucial role in the medical screening of potential runners, and he can prevent most problems with simple instructions. Periodic return visits may be necessary for dealing with various running-related problems. These visits afford the opportunity for the physician to counsel patience and persistence. Joggers who get through the difficult 2 or 3 months at the beginning of training are likely to develop running habits that are both enjoyable and healthful.

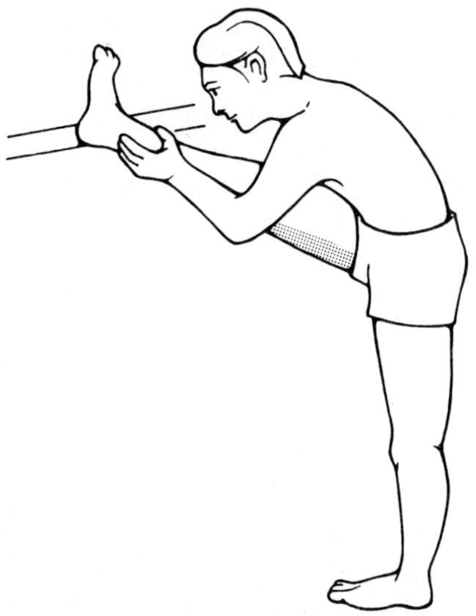

Figure 18-2. Hamstring stretch. Rest one leg on a sturdy table or desk. Keeping both legs straight, slowly bend forward at the waist so that you feel the hamstring stretch. Hold for 30 seconds. Repeat with the other leg up.

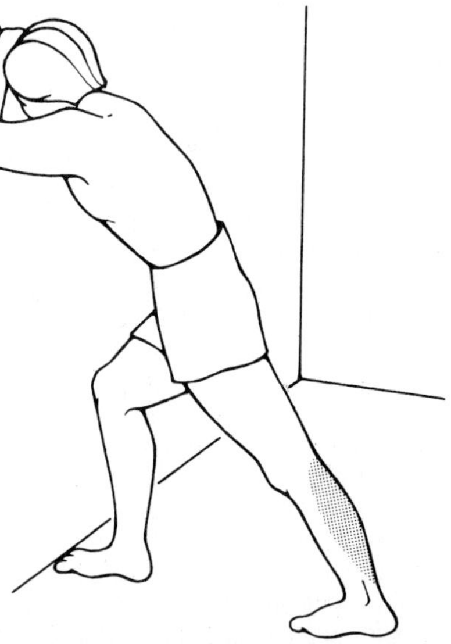

Figure 18-1. Calf, Achilles, and soleus stretch. Stand 3 feet from a wall with one foot forward, leaning forward to support your upper body by resting your forearms against the wall. Bend the forward leg at the knee. Keep the rear leg straight with the heel on the floor, and slowly press your hips forward until you feel the calf stretch. Hold for 15 seconds. Relax and then repeat with the rear knee slightly bent so that you feel the Achilles stretch. Repeat with the other leg forward.

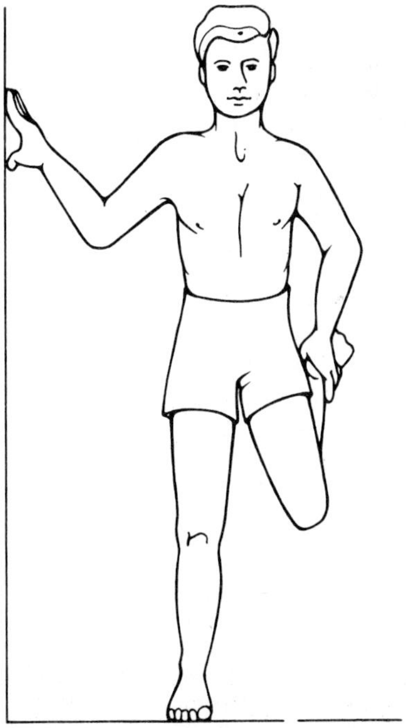

Figure 18-3. Quadriceps stretch. Stand at arm's length from a wall with your feet parallel to the wall. Rest your hand on the wall for support. Hold your ankle in your free hand, and pull the foot back and up until the heel touches the buttocks, while leaning slightly forward from the waist. Repeat with the other leg.

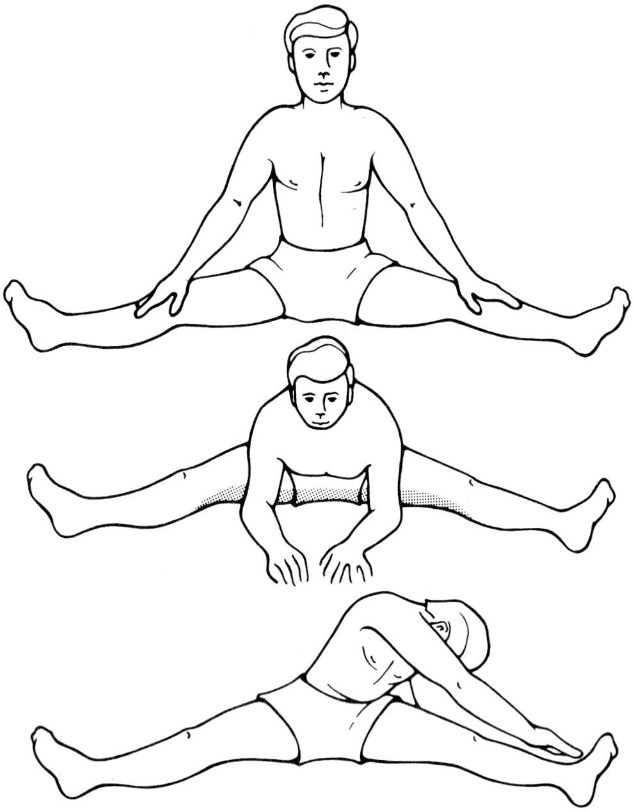

Figure 18-4. Hip and side stretch. Sit on the floor and spread your legs as far apart as possible. With your legs and back straight, bend forward from the waist until you feel a stretch at the inner thighs. Hold for 20 seconds. Relax, then twist at the waist, and lean to touch your right hand to your left foot. Hold for 20 seconds. Repeat on the other side.

ANNOTATED BIBLIOGRAPHY

Books and Reviews

(*These four works provide comprehensive overviews of cardiovascular and metabolic aspects of exercise.*)

Astrand PO, Rodhal K. Textbook of Work Physiology, 3rd ed. New York, McGraw-Hill, 1986.

Bouchard C, Shephard RJ, Stephens T et al (eds). Exercise, Fitness and Health: A Consensus of Current Knowledge. Champaign, IL, Human Kinetics Books, 1990.

Fletcher GL. Exercise in the Practice of Medicine. Mt. Kisco, NY, Future Press, 1988.

Simon HB, Levisohn SR. The Athlete From Within: A Personal Guide to Total Fitness. Boston, Little, Brown, 1987.

Individual Papers

Berlin JA, Colditz GA. A meta-analysis of physical activity in the prevention of coronary heart disease. Am J Epidemiol 1990; 132:612. (*Sedentary living increases the risk of coronary artery disease; relative risk 1.9.*)

Blair SN, Kohl HW, Paffenfarger RS et al. Physical fitness and all-cause mortality: A prospective study of healthy men and women. JAMA 1989;262:2395. (*Exercise reduces mortality from CAD, cancer, and all causes; even modest exercise exerts a protective effect.*)

Blumenthal JA, Emery CF, Madden DJ et al. Effects of exercise training on cardiorespiratory function in men and women > 60 years of age. Am J Cardiol 1991;67:633. (*Documents cardiorespiratory benefit from regular aerobic training in elderly patients.*)

Cooper KH, Pollock ML, Martin RP et al. Physical fitness levels vs. selected coronary risk factors. A cross-sectional study. JAMA 1976;236:116. (*A classic prevalence study of nearly 3000 men showing an inverse relationship between physical fitness and resting heart rate, blood pressure, body weight, percent body fat, and serum levels of cholesterol, triglycerides, and glucose.*)

Curfman GD. Is exercise beneficial—or hazardous—to your health. N Engl J Med 1993;329:1730. (*The answer is "both."*)

Curfman GD. The health benefits of exercise: A critical reappraisal. N Engl J Med 1993;328:574. (*An editorial examining the quality of the data supporting the health benefits of exercise; notes most data are observational.*)

Curfman GD, Thomas GS, Paffenbarger RS Jr. Physical activity and primary prevention of cardiovascular disease. Cardiol Clin 1985;3:203. (*Part of a superb symposium on preventive cardiology.*)

Gibbons LW, Blair SN, Cooper KH et al. Association between coronary heart disease, risk factors and fitness in healthy adult women. Circulation 1983;67:977. (*A study of 3000 subjects demonstrating an inverse relationship between risk factors and physical fitness in women.*)

Kelemen MH, Effron MB, Valenti SA et al. Exercise training combined with antihypertensive drug therapy. JAMA 1990; 263:2766. (*A prospective randomized trial of 52 hypertensive men demonstrating that exercise training can control moderate hypertension as effectively as propranolol or diltiazem.*)

Lane NA, Bloch DA, Hubert HB et al. Running, osteoarthritis, and bone density: Initial 2-year longitudinal study. Am J Med 1990;88:452. (*Running increases bone density without producing osteoarthritis.*)

Mittleman MA, MacClure M, Tofler GH, et al. Triggering of acute myocardial infarction by heavy exertion: Protection against triggering by regular exertion. N Engl J Med 1993;329:1677. (*The title summarizes the findings.*)

Paffenbarger RS Jr, Hyde RT, Wing AL et al. The association of changes in physical activity level and other life-style characteristics with mortality among men. N Engl J Med 1993; 328:538. (*Beginning moderately vigorous sports activity independently lowered all-cause and CHD mortality.*)

Sandvik L, Erikssen J, Thaulow E et al. Physical fitness as a predictor of mortality among healthy, middle-aged Norwegian men. N Engl J Med 1993;328:533. (*A high level of fitness was associated with lower all-cause mortality; fitness was an independent predictor of cardiovascular mortality.*)

Siscovick DS, Ekelund LG, Johnson JL et al. Sensitivity of exercise electrocardiography for acute cardiac events during moderate and strenuous physical activity. Arch Intern Med 1991;151:325. (*A submaximal electrocardiographic exercise stress test was not sensitive in asymptomatic hypercholesterolemic men.*)

Primary Care Medicine: Office Evaluation and Management of the Adult Patient, 3rd edition, edited by Allan H. Goroll, Lawrence A. May, and Albert G. Mulley, Jr. J.B. Lippincott Company, Philadelphia

19
Evaluation of Hypertension

KATHARINE K. TREADWAY, M.D.

High blood pressure, if unrecognized or untreated, significantly increases the risks of coronary disease, heart failure, renal failure, and stroke. Risk further increases dramatically in the presence of smoking, glucose intolerance, hyperlipidemia, left ventricular hypertrophy (LVH), male gender, African-American race, or increasing age. Treatment of hypertension—even if only partial—can greatly reduce its morbidity and mortality.

The workup of the hypertensive patient has three major functions. First is to rule out any secondary causes. Although about 95 percent of patients have primary disease (no clearly definable underlying cause), a search for a secondary etiology is important, because if such a cause is present, treatment will need to be etiologic if it is to be effective. Second is to assess the severity of disease, because risk and type of treatment program derive from the degree of pressure elevation and amount of end-organ damage. Third is to identify any concurrent cardiovascular risk factors, because their presence will affect the threshold for initiating therapy as well as the nature of the treatment program. As of yet, attempts to determine the principal underlying pathophysiology have proven elusive, though when it becomes feasible to do so, the results should facilitate diagnosis and further rationalize treatment.

DEFINITION AND CLASSIFICATION OF HYPERTENSION

Definition of hypertension is arbitrary (it even varies from country to country). Actuarial data have shown that morbidity and mortality related to complications of hypertension increase linearly with increasing levels of either systolic or diastolic blood pressure. Hence, no critical level of blood pressure exists beyond which risk becomes highly magnified. Most definitions of hypertension refer to a level of blood pressure associated with a substantial risk of complications. A major consensus report, The Fifth Report of the Joint National Committee on Detection, Evaluation, and Treatment of High Blood Pressure, recommends a *systolic blood pressure (SBP) greater than or equal to 140 mm Hg* and a *diastolic pressure (DBP) of 90 mm Hg or more* for the definition of hypertension.

The definition of hypertension must be *individualized* for each patient. The diagnosis derives not only from the absolute level of blood pressure, but also from the presence or absence of other *cardiovascular risk factors*. Factors besides hypertension identified by the Framingham study as significant contributors to cardiovascular risk include cigarette smoking, elevated serum cholesterol, glucose intolerance, and electrocardiographic evidence of LVH with strain. In addition, African-American race, male gender, and age greater than 50 need to be taken into account. The patient with borderline hypertension, a moderately elevated serum cholesterol level, and a history of smoking has a fivefold higher risk of incurring cardiovascular disease than the patient with borderline hypertension alone.

The National Committee recommended that the traditional designations of *"mild," "moderate,"* and *"severe"* hypertension be eliminated to avoid the misleading notion than mild hypertension is not a significant health risk. Instead, they designate four *stages: I* (DBP 90–99, SBP 140–159); *II* (DBP 100–109, SBP 160–179); *III* (DBP 110–119, SBP 180–209), and *IV* (DBP > 119, SBP > 209). (See Table 19–1).

PATHOPHYSIOLOGY AND CLINICAL PRESENTATION

Pathophysiology

Control of blood pressure and the pathophysiology of hypertension are still incompletely understood. Blood pressure most certainly represents the complex interaction of multiple mechanisms playing varyingly significant roles in particular patients. Because there is a strong familial predisposition to hypertension, much of the pathophysiology is likely to be an expression of inherited defects in the regulation of blood pressure. There are probably several mechanistic subtypes of so-called "primary" hypertension. As of yet, it is usually not possible to identify specific etiologic mechanisms in a given case. Nonetheless, several elements deserve elaboration and help provide a rational basis for workup and therapy.

Primary Determinants of Blood Pressure are the *cardiac output* and *peripheral resistance*. Each of these is affected by a variety of factors, which, in turn, have multiple points of control (Fig. 19–1).

Sodium. Several lines of evidence continue to implicate sodium as a major factor in the pathogenesis of hypertension. Studies of large populations demonstrate the relationship of high blood pressure to high sodium intake. In cultures where salt intake is low, hypertension is exceedingly rare. When members of those same cultures migrate into cultures in which salt intake is high, approximately 25 percent to 30 percent will develop hypertension. Sodium restriction, as well as use of diuretics, has long been known to reduce blood pressure in a subset of hypertensives. However, sodium intake is a poor predictor of hypertension in a given individual, suggesting that susceptibility is dependent on many other factors, probably genetic and environmental. It is postulated that many hypertensives have an inherited defect in the ability of the kidney to excrete excess sodium. This leads to an increase in intravascular volume that is corrected by an as yet unidentified factor—the putative "natriuretic hormone"—which inhibits the Na^+–K^+ pump. The net result is an increase in intracellular sodium, which raises *free intracellular calcium*. The rise in intracellular calcium heightens vascular tone and elevates blood pressure. Natriuresis is ef-

Table 19-1. Classification of Blood Pressure for Adults Aged 18 Years and Older*

CATEGORY	SYSTOLIC, MM HG	DIASTOLIC, MM HG
Normal†	<130	<85
High normal	130–139	85–89
Hypertension‡		
Stage 1 (mild)	140–159	90–99
Stage 2 (moderate)	160–179	100–109
Stage 3 (severe)	180–209	110–119
Stage 4 (very severe)	≥210	≥120

*Not taking antihypertensive drugs and not acutely ill. When systolic and diastolic pressures fall into different categories, the higher category should be selected to classify the individual's blood pressure status. For instance, 160/92 mm Hg should be classified as stage 2, and 180/120 mm Hg should be classified as stage 4. Isolated systolic hypertension is defined as a systolic blood pressure of 140 mm Hg or more and a diastolic blood pressure of less than 90 mm Hg and staged appropriately (eg, 170/85 mm Hg is defined as stage 2 isolated systolic hypertension).

In addition to classifying stages of hypertension on the basis of average blood pressure levels, the clinician should specify presence or absence of target-organ disease and additional risk factors. For example, a patient with diabetes and a blood pressure of 142/94 mm Hg, plus left ventricular hypertrophy should be classified as having "stage 1 hypertension with target-organ disease (left ventricular hypertrophy) and with another major risk factor (diabetes)." This specificity is important for risk classification and management.

†Optimal blood pressure with respect to cardiovascular risk is less than 120 mm Hg systolic and less than 80 mm Hg diastolic. However, unusually low readings should be evaluated for clinical significance.

‡Based on the average of two or more readings taken at each of two or more visits after an initial screening.

From: Fifth Report of the Joint National Committee on Detection, Evaluation, and Treatment of High Blood Pressure. Arch Intern Med 153:154, 1993.

fected at the cost of a higher resting pressure. Additionally, in salt-sensitive patients, a high sodium intake has been associated with higher levels of norepinephrine and an increased responsiveness to norepinephrine.

Catecholamines. Catecholamines affect blood pressure regulation both centrally via the vasomotor centers in the brain and peripherally through the action of the sympathetic nervous system. Catecholamines elevate blood pressure both by increasing peripheral resistance and increasing cardiac output. Sympathetic hyperactivity has been suggested as playing a primary role in the development of hypertension in some patients. *Pheochromocytoma* provides a model for secondary hypertension based on excessive catecholamines. Studies on patients with borderline hypertension have allowed clear identification of subgroups in which a defect in autonomic nervous system controls exists, resulting in excessive sympathetic and reduced parasympathetic activity. An exaggerated pressor response to external stressful stimuli has been demonstrated in some hypertensive patients as well as in their normotensive offspring. Also described are "hyperkinetic" hypertensives, who are generally young and present with tachycardia and elevated cardiac output. Their hypertension may reflect the interaction of an underlying predisposition and various environmental stimuli.

Renin–Angiotensin System. Renin is secreted by the juxtaglomerular apparatus in response to a number of stimuli, including a decrease in intravascular volume, decreased perfusion pressure, beta-adrenergic stimulation, and hypokalemia. Renin acts on angiotensinogen (a decapeptide produced in the liver) to form *angiotensin I,* a substance with no known biologic activity. Angiotensin I is converted in the lung to *angiotensin II* by *angiotensin converting enzyme.* Angiotensin II is a potent vasoconstrictor that also acts on the adrenal cortex to release *aldosterone,* which increases sodium and water reabsorption in the distal tubule of the nephron. Renin production is inversely proportional to effective blood volume: Anything that increases effective blood volume suppresses renin; anything that decreases effective blood volume stimulates renin. For example, in *primary hyperaldosteronism,* autonomous production of the salt-retaining hormone aldosterone by an adrenal adenoma results in intravascular volume expansion and renin suppression. Con-

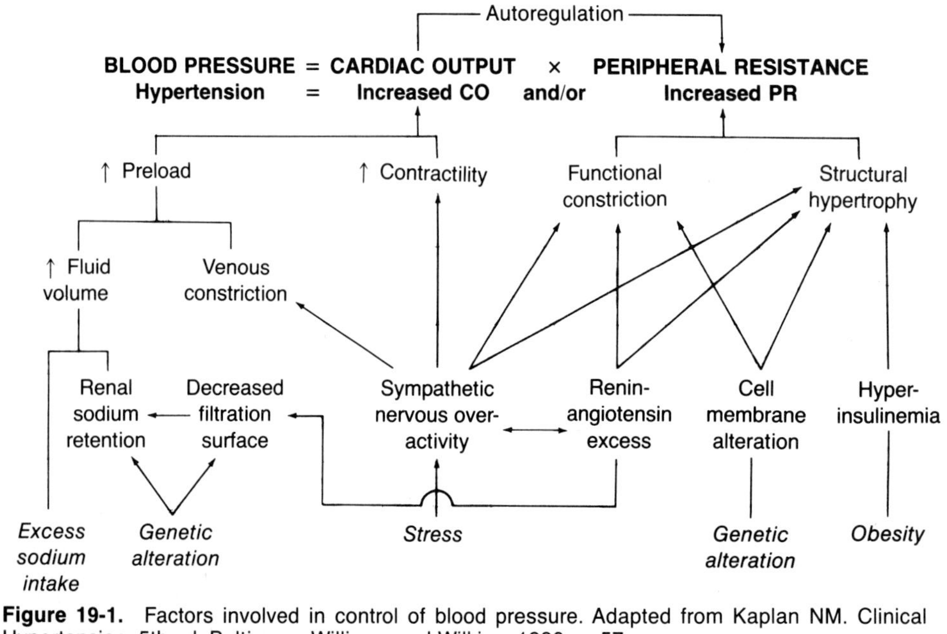

Figure 19-1. Factors involved in control of blood pressure. Adapted from Kaplan NM. Clinical Hypertension, 5th ed. Baltimore, Williams and Wilkins, 1990, p. 57.

versely, in *renal artery stenosis,* decreased renal perfusion on the affected side is perceived by that kidney as decreased effective blood volume. In renin studies of patients with primary hypertension, about 15 percent have a high renin, the remainder showing normal or low levels. It is still not clear how much of a role this system plays in the pathogenesis of primary hypertension. One theory suggests that in patients with hypertension, a "normal" renin may in fact be inappropriately high due to a relative insensitivity to the adrenal cortical effects of angiotensin II.

Insulin. The increased frequency of hypertension in patients with type II diabetes has stimulated search for a common mechanistic link. Elevations in serum insulin have been found capable of increasing plasma catecholamines and stimulating sodium reabsorption, both of which are capable of raising blood pressure. In addition, insulin serves as a potent growth factor for vascular smooth muscle, which could lead to hypertrophy and increased peripheral resistance. Insulin levels are higher in obese nondiabetic hypertensives than in their normotensive counterparts, suggesting a mechanism linking obesity with hypertension.

Calcium. Increased intracellular calcium appears to increase vascular tone. Alteration in calcium binding at the cellular level may lead to increased levels of free intracellular calcium with a resultant increase in vascular tone.

Clinical Presentations

Primary or "Essential" Hypertension accounts for about 95 percent of cases. Onset is usually between ages 30 and 50, except for *isolated systolic hypertension,* which is typically a disease of the elderly. Often, a family history of hypertension can be elicited. For 80 percent of patients, the onset is gradual and the severity mild. Patients with uncomplicated disease are asymptomatic. While some patients report fatigue, headache, light-headedness, flushing, or epistaxis, the correlation between symptoms and blood pressure is poor, except in patients with dangerous elevations in pressure. The rare syndrome of *hypertensive encephalopathy* occurs in the setting of malignant hypertension, where DBP rises rapidly above 130 mm Hg, accompanied by symptoms and signs of increased intracranial pressure (restlessness, confusion, somnolence, blurred vision, nausea, vomiting, blurred disc margins, retinal hemorrhages) and heart failure (dyspnea, rales, third heart sound).

Most patients remain asymptomatic unless end-organ damage develops, causing symptoms of congestive failure, renal failure, cerebrovascular insufficiency, peripheral vascular disease, or ischemic heart disease.

Labile Hypertension is blood pressure that intermittently rises above the normal levels for each given age group and sex. Established hypertension has been shown to develop more commonly in such patients.

"White-Coat Hypertension" is a term used to describe blood pressure elevations that occur in the doctor's office but not in the home or work environment. The condition is seen in both hypertensive and normotensive patients. Persons who manifest this condition typically have systolic and diastolic pressures at least 10 mm Hg greater in the office than at home but do not have greater blood pressure reactivity in the ambulatory setting. They tend to be older and are more likely to receive more antihypertensive medication than their peers, because they seem to be refractory.

Pseudorefractory Hypertension. A form of apparently refractory disease has been described in patients who manifest a marked vasoconstrictor response to blood pressure determinations performed with an arm cuff. Their predominant elevation is in DBP, compared with the white-coat hypertensive, who responds with a rise in SBP. Such patients are apt to be mistaken for truly refractory hypertensives because pressures may remain elevated both in the office and at home. The tip-off to this condition is the absence of end-organ damage (eg, normal fundi, normal cardiac ultrasound) despite apparent persistence of hypertension.

Secondary Hypertension has a definable etiology (Table 19–2), occurs within a wide age range, and is often abrupt in onset and severe in magnitude; family history is commonly negative. Certain forms of secondary hypertension may be heralded by specific symptoms. For example, leg claudication may be a manifestation of *coarctation* of the aorta causing lower extremity ischemia. The patient with *Cushing's syndrome* may complain of hirsutism or easy bruising. The patient with *pheochromocytoma* may experience excessive perspiration, severe paroxysmal headaches, or palpitations. Hypokalemia ensues from *primary aldosteronism* and may trigger muscle cramps, weakness, and polyuria.

DIFFERENTIAL DIAGNOSIS

About 95 percent of new hypertensive patients encountered in primary care practice have primary or "essential" disease. Secondary causes account for the remainder, with one large study showing renal failure accounting for 2.4 percent, renovascular disease for 1.0 percent, primary aldosteronism for 1.0 percent, drugs for 0.8 percent, pheochromocytoma for 0.2 percent, and Cushing's syndrome for 0.1 percent. Coarctation of the aorta is usually detected earlier in life and rarely presents as unexplained adult-onset hypertension (Table 19–2).

WORKUP

As noted earlier, the goals of the evaluation include firmly establishing the diagnosis, ruling out secondary causes, and determining the severity of pressure elevation, the degree of end-organ damage, and the presence of associated risk factors.

Establishing the Diagnosis. Use of proper technique for measurement of the blood pressure is essential (see Chapter 14 and below). Except in patients with severely elevated blood pressure, the diagnosis of hypertension should almost always be based on *multiple determinations* of blood pressure, preferably not only on different visits but by different personnel and in different settings. As noted above, there is a tendency for blood pressures to be higher when taken by a physician than when taken by a nurse or other medical worker. Studies comparing the correlation of LVH with pressures obtained in the physician's office, at home, and at work show that work-site readings are the most meaningful.

Table 19-2. Primary versus Secondary Hypertension: Specific Screening Protocols

CAUSE (PREVALENCE, %)*	SCREEN	CONFIRMATION
Coarctation (NA)	Arm and leg BPs, chest radiograph	Angiography
Cushing's syndrome (0.1)	Cushingoid appearance; 1-mg dexamethasone suppression test	High-dose dexamethasone suppression test, etc.
Drug-induced hypertension (0.8)	History: amphetamines, oral contraceptives, estrogens, corticosteroids, licorice, thyroid hormone	
↑ Intracranial pressure (NA)	Neurologic evaluation	
Pheochromocytoma (0.2)	History of paroxysmal hypertension, headache, perspiration, palpitations *or* fixed diastolic ≥130 mm Hg; 24-hour urinary metanephrine or VMA	Catecholamine levels, angiography, CT scan
Primary aldosteronism (Conn's or idiopathic) (0.1)	Serum K^+, urine K^+, stimulated PRA	Aldosterone levels, venography with differential level, CT scan
Renal disease (2.4)	History of congenital disease, diabetes, proteinuria, pyelonephritis, obstruction; urinalysis; BUN or creatinine	Creatinine clearance, IVP, ultrasound, biopsy
Renovascular disease (1.0)	Suspect in young female or elderly patient with atherosclerosis, especially if abrupt in onset, negative family history, and abdominal bruit present; captopril renal scan	Angiography and differential renal vein renins

*(Danielson M, Dammstrom B. The prevalence of secondary and curable hypertension. Acta Med Scand 209:451, 1981.)

Teaching the patient to take his or her own pressure at home and at work can greatly facilitate diagnosis and management, but it should be viewed as an adjunct, not as a replacement for office-based measurements.

If *home determinations* are to be undertaken, the patient's technique and equipment should be checked and calibrated during an office visit, comparing their readings taken in the office with those obtained by the physician using a mercury bulb manometer. In general, the mechanical aneroid manometers are simple, inexpensive, and accurate but need to be checked frequently. When there is a marked discrepancy between home and office pressures or a wide variation in pressures obtained throughout the day, *24-hour ambulatory monitoring* may be useful, though usually it is unnecessary and quite expensive. Often, evidence of end-organ effects suffices to settle discrepancies (see below).

History. It is best to begin by eliciting the patient's hypertensive history: date of onset or last previously normal blood pressure, level at time of onset, medications taken if any, response to therapy. Such information facilitates determination of etiology and helps guide workup. For example, sudden onset at a young age, very high pressure, no family history, and refractoriness to treatment suggest a secondary cause (see below). In addition, the history is checked for contributing factors, such as prior *renal disease, salt* and *alcohol* excess, and recent *weight* gain. Noting any associated modifiable cardiovascular risk factors (*smoking, hypercholesterolemia, diabetes*) facilitates assessment of total coronary risk. Evidence of cardiovascular and neurologic *complications* (angina, dyspnea, syncope, claudication, stroke, transient ischemic attack) should be sought. Inquiry into use of *drugs* and substances is often rewarding (eg, alcohol, cocaine, amphetamines, oral estrogens, corticosteroids, thyroid hormone, over-the-counter sympathomimetic decongestants, even large quantities of licorice).

Awareness of the *symptoms* associated with *secondary etiologies* is essential. Complaints such as hirsutism, easy bruising, paroxysms of palpitations and sweats, weakness, muscle cramps, and leg claudication should all suggest a secondary form of hypertension. Other clues to a secondary cause—especially renovascular disease—are onset at the extremes of age, rapid and severe course, and refractoriness to medication.

Physical Examination. Blood pressure is properly measured in *both arms* while the patient is seated comfortably. The cuff should be placed on the bared upper arm, which is supported at heart level. The Korotkoff sounds are best listened for by using the stethoscope *bell* rather than the diaphragm; the bell better transmits the low-pitched sounds of diastole. The average of two successive measurements in each arm is recorded. *Diastolic pressure* is taken at the point at which *sound disappears* (Korotkoff 5) rather than when it changes in quality (Korotkoff 4). *Cuff size* must be adequate to avoid falsely elevated readings (cuff width greater than two-thirds of arm width, length of inflatable portion greater than two-thirds of arm circumference). Coffee intake and smoking should be halted at least 30 minutes prior to taking the pressure.

The remainder of the examination focuses on *weight* and *pulse* measurements; the *skin* for stigmata of Cushing's syndrome, chronic renal failure, or neurofibromatosis; *funduscopy* for arteriolar narrowing, increased vascular tortuosity, A-V nicking, or hemorrhages; the *thyroid* for enlargement or nodularity; *carotid pulses* for bruits or diminution of pulse; *lungs* for signs of heart failure; *heart* for left ventricular lift and S_4 and S_3 heart sounds; *peripheral vasculature* for pulses, bruits, and abnormalities in bilateral arm and leg pressure measurements and simultaneous radial and femoral pulse palpation; *abdomen* for masses and bruits; and the *neurologic exam* for focal deficits.

Basic Laboratory Studies. The laboratory evaluation of high blood pressure has three purposes: 1) to ascertain the degree of end-organ damage resulting from hypertension; 2) to identify patients at high risk for the development of cardiovascular complications; and 3) to screen for secondary, possibly reversible forms of the disease. Despite the wide array of sophisticated diagnostic techniques now readily available, there is increasing evidence that the diagnosis of secondary hypertension can be made accurately and economically by the alert physician on the basis of a careful history, a physical examination, and only a few simple diagnostic tests. Extensive laboratory evaluation of patients with high blood pressure is unwarranted.

The basic laboratory investigation of hypertension for detection of both secondary causes and end-organ damage need to include little more than a complete blood count, *urinalysis, blood urea nitrogen (BUN)* or serum *creatinine,* serum *potassium,* fasting *blood sugar,* serum *cholesterol,* and *electrocardiogram* (ECG). The urinalysis provides evidence of primary renal disease. The extent of renal compromise due to renal disease or secondary to the hypertension itself is indicated by the BUN or creatinine. Fasting blood sugar, serum cholesterol, and ECG supply data regarding cardiovascular risk and presence of left atrial enlargement and ventricular hypertrophy. Serum potassium is a valuable screening test for primary aldosteronism and should be known before diuretic therapy is instituted. Total cost of these determinations is reasonable. In most patients, evaluation can and should stop here.

More extensive routine laboratory evaluation of patients with high blood pressure has come under a great deal of criticism. The yield in the absence of clinical evidence for a secondary cause is low, and such testing is not cost-effective. It was hoped that *renin profiling* would help identify the underlying pathophysiology in patients with primary disease, guide workup for secondary causes, and rationalize selection of therapy. However, the renin assay continues to suffer from difficulties with accuracy and reliability, except in certain research laboratories. Moreover, the vast majority of hypertensives have normal renin levels, undermining the value of widespread testing. Finally, when renin profiling has been used to guide choice of therapy, benefit has been hard to demonstrate.

Echocardiography for detection of LVH has been useful in research studies, with presence of LVH associated with an increased risk of cardiovascular complications. However, its routine use rarely adds much to the assessment, except in the setting of refractory hypertension where definitive evidence of end-organ hypertrophy helps one distinguish between true and apparent refractoriness to therapy (see Chapter 26). When the need to search for LVH is less pressing (eg, in the patient with newly encountered blood pressure elevation), the ECG can provide a reasonable though less sensitive estimate.

Evaluation of the Patient Suspected of Having Secondary Hypertension. Patients at somewhat higher risk for *secondary hypertension* include 1) those younger than 35 years of age; 2) those with rapid onset of elevated blood pressure and a negative family history; 3) those with severe hypertension; and 4) those who have failed to respond to empirical therapy despite compliance. Fortunately, in a majority of patients at high risk for secondary hypertension, a specific diagnosis will be suggested by history and physical examination, supplemented by a few simple laboratory studies. Thus, the patient with *Cushing's syndrome* should be easily identified by *appearance;* the patient with *coarctation* can be diagnosed by measurement of *arm and leg blood pressures* and simultaneous radial femoral pulse palpation.

About half of patients with *pheochromocytoma* will give a story indicative of *paroxysmal sympathetic discharge* (sweats, palpitations, tachycardia). The remainder will have fixed hypertension and no such symptoms. The *24-hour urine* assay for *catecholamines, VMA,* or *metanephrines* is a sensitive screening test for pheochromocytoma, especially when collected the same day that the patient reports symptoms. Two normal 24-hour urines performed while the patient is symptomatic virtually rules out the diagnosis. Two positive urines have a high predictive value for the presence of pheochromocytoma. Methyldopa can falsely elevate metanephrines. Although combination studies are often ordered (ie, urinary catecholamines plus metanephrines or VMA), each alone has about the same sensitivity and specificity. In one study, combination determinations were found to be no better than singular determinations in screening for pheochromocytoma. Computed tomography scan of the adrenals should never be used as a screening test for pheochromocytoma, because innocent adrenal masses having nothing to do with hypertension are common.

Primary hyperaldosteronism is almost always apparent by otherwise unexplained *hypokalemia. Renovascular disease* is most common in young patients and in older ones in whom onset of hypertension is abrupt and refractory. A *two-component bruit* in the right upper or left upper quadrant of the abdomen is very suggestive, especially in the setting of diffuse vascular disease.

When a specific form of secondary hypertension is suspected on the basis of the initial assessment, further workup is indicated (see Table 19–1). For example, the Cushing's syndrome evaluation begins with an overnight 1 mg *dexamethasone suppression test.* If urinary screening for pheochromocytoma is positive, then one can proceed to *CT scan of the adrenal glands*—sensitivity is about 90 percent for lesions larger than 1 cm in diameter. A *chest radiograph* to search for rib notching is indicated if coarctation is under consideration. For primary aldosteronism, a *stimulated plasma renin* and *urinary* $K+/Na+$ are excellent initial studies, followed by serum *aldosterone* levels if results are suggestive.

Considerable controversy remains regarding the best way to screen for *renovascular hypertension.* The gold standard remains selective *renal arteriography* in combination with *renal vein renins.* In patients in whom there is a high clinical suspicion based on the factors outlined above—young female or elderly patient with atherosclerosis, abrupt onset of hypertension, negative family history, rapid deterioration of renal function on angiotensin converting enzyme inhibitor therapy, abdominal bruit—it is reasonable to proceed directly to invasive evaluation.

For patients in whom the clinical evidence for renal vascular disease is less compelling, there are a number of noninvasive options, none of which is completely satisfactory for screening. The options include hypertensive intravenous pyelogram (IVP), renal scan, and captopril renal scan. Work is also being done to assess the utility of a vascular magnetic resonance imaging, but cost may be an issue.

Renin profiling is fraught with the assay difficulties mentioned above as well as wide scattering of values among patients with proven renovascular disease. The use of *captopril* before sampling increases test sensitivity but does not improve results enough to recommend it. One may consider a *hypertensive IVP* in the evaluation, although its false-negative rate is as high as 40 percent. The *renal scan* is more sensitive but less specific. Performing a *renal scan* 1 hour after oral administration of *captopril* enhances differences in glomerular filtration between normal and hypoperfused kidneys. At present the captopril renal scan is probably the most useful screening test for patients for whom the possibility of renovascular disease is raised but suspicion is not high enough to warrant immediate angiography.

ANNOTATED BIBLIOGRAPHY

American College of Physicians. Automated ambulatory blood pressure and self-measured blood pressure monitoring devices: Their role in the diagnosis and management of hypertension. Ann Intern Med 1993;118:889. (*A position paper suggesting these methods have an adjunctive role in selected situations but cannot be recommended for widespread use.*)

Duncan MW, Compton P, Lazarus L. Measurement of norepinephrine and 3,4-dihydroxyphenylglycol in urine and plasma for the diagnosis of pheochromocytoma. N Engl J Med 1988;319:136. (*Measurement of urinary epinephrine had a sensitivity of 100 percent and a specificity of 98 percent; adding the DHPG improved specificity.*)

Feldman JM. Diagnosis and management of pheochromocytoma. Hosp Prac 1989;1:145. (*An excellent review for the practitioner by the recognized authority on the subject.*)

Ferguson RK. Cost and yield of the hypertensive evaluation: Experience of a community-based referral clinic. Ann Intern Med 1975;82:761. (*Emphasizes that secondary hypertension can be detected on the basis of a careful examination and only a few simple diagnostic tests.*)

Ferrannini E, Hoffner SM, Stern MP. Essential hypertension: An insulin resistant state. J Cardiovasc Pharmacol 1990;15(suppl 5):518. (*Details the growing evidence linking hypertension and insulin resistance.*)

Fifth Report of the Joint National Committee on Detection, Evaluation, and Treatment of High Blood Pressure. Arch Intern Med 1993;153:154. (*Major consensus report.*)

Frohlich ED, Grim C, Labarthe DR et al. Report of a special task force appointed by the Steering Committee, American Heart Association. Recommendations for human blood pressure determinations by sphygmomanometers. Hypertension 1988;11: 209A. (*The most critical review of technique.*)

Goldenberg K, Snyder DK. Screening for primary aldosteronism. J Gen Intern Med 1986;1:368. (*An examination of the serum potassium's utility as a screening test for this condition.*)

Lerman CE, Brody DS, Hui T et al. The white-coat hypertension response: Prevalence and predictors. J Gen Intern Med 1987;4:226. (*Thirty-nine percent of the study sample was found to manifest this response; the elderly and those with the least hostility on psychological testing were most likely to show it.*)

Mejia AD, Egan BM, Schork NJ et al. Artifacts in measurement of blood pressure and lack of target organ involvement in the assessment of patients with treatment-resistant hypertension. Ann Intern Med 1990;112:270. (*Identifies three types of artifacts in the measurement of blood pressure in patients who appear refractory to treatment.*)

Weiss NS. Relation of high blood pressure to headache, epistaxis, and selected other symptoms. N Engl J Med 1972;287:631. (*No clear relation was shown between these symptoms and the level of blood pressure; emphasizes that all but malignant hypertension is usually asymptomatic.*)

Working Group on Renovascular Hypertension. Detection, evaluation, and treatment of renovascular hypertension. Arch Intern Med 1987;147:820. (*A consensus panel's recommendations regarding this difficult problem.*)

Young WF, Hogan MJ, Klee GC. Primary aldosteronism: Diagnosis and treatment. Mayo Clin Proc 1990;65:96. (*Useful review and practical approach to evaluation.*)

20
Evaluation of Chest Pain

Primary Care Medicine: Office Evaluation and Management of the Adult Patient, 3rd edition, edited by Allan H. Goroll, Lawrence A. May, and Albert G. Mulley, Jr. J.B. Lippincott Company, Philadelphia

In the outpatient setting, the patient who presents with chest pain poses a diagnostic challenge. Concerns about serious heart and lung disease intermix with depression, anxiety, esophageal dysfunction, and musculoskeletal disease. Although most chest pains prove to be harmless, the primary physician must be skilled in quickly and accurately recognizing the patient with serious underlying cardiovascular or pulmonary pathology. In the office setting, the evaluation is predominantly a clinical one, based on data available from the history, physical examination, electrocardiogram (ECG), and perhaps chest radiography. Of particular challenge is the assessment of the patient with atypical chest pain.

PATHOPHYSIOLOGY AND CLINICAL PRESENTATION

Most structures within and about the thorax are capable of producing chest pain, as is psychopathology.

Chest Wall. Pain originating in the chest wall is usually due to musculoskeletal pathology, though occasionally nerve injury is responsible. Typically, the pain can be pinpointed by the patient, being somatic in nature. It is aggravated by deep inspiration, cough, direct palpation, and movement. Common sites of involvement are the costochondral and chondrosternal junctions. Duration ranges from a few seconds to several days, and quality from sharp to dull or aching. Sometimes the patient complains of tightness. Vigorous and unaccustomed exertion can lead to muscular and ligamentous strain, which may account for some cases. Others are due to *costochondritis* (Tietze's syndrome), which is an inflammatory condition that causes localized swelling, erythema, warmth, and tenderness at the costochondral or chondrosternal junction. *Rib fracture* may produce a similar picture, though location is different, and there is a history of antecedent trauma or metastatic cancer. Of interest, there is an increased frequency of musculoskeletal pain in patients with angina, which makes for a potentially confusing clinical presentation.

Nerve injury due to a recrudescence of *Herpes zoster* infection can be very painful, with a dermatomal distribution being characteristic. The pain may precede the typical rash (prosaically described as "dew drops on a rose petal"—see Chapter 193) by 3 to 5 days. The neurologic complaints range from hypoesthesia to dysesthesia and hyperesthesia. In the elderly, the pain may persist for months, long after the rash resolves.

Nerve injury from *cervical root compression* (see Chapter 148) due to cervical spine disease or a *thoracic outlet syndrome* can produce pain in the chest and upper arm, superficially resembling angina. In the outlet syndrome, a cervical rib may compress part of the brachial plexus, resulting in motor and sensory deficits in an ulnar distribution at the same time that there is discomfort in the chest and upper arm (see Chapter 167).

Lungs and Pleura. *Inflammation or distention of the pleura* produces true "pleuritic pain," which is worsened by deep inspiration and cough but relatively unaffected by movement or palpation. A host of causes can trigger the inflammatory process, including infection, pulmonary infarction, neoplasm, uremia, and connective tissue disease. The more florid the inflammation, the greater the pain. An infectious origin is more likely to cause pain than is a low-grade serositis associated with connective tissue disease. Stretching of the pleura after a *spontaneous pneumothorax* results in acute onset of pleuritic pain and dyspnea. The condition occurs in young persons and those with emphysema, in which there can be rupture of a bleb. If the pneumothorax is large, deviation of the trachea may be observed.

Pleurodynia is a self-limited source of pleuritic pain, most common in children and young adults and associated with a respiratory viral infection, such as that due to coxsackievirus B. A typical viral syndrome precedes the acute onset of chest pain. Chest pain in the setting of a viral upper respiratory infection may also occur from cough-initiated injury to the chest wall or from bronchospasm. Young, healthy persons sometimes note a sudden sharp pleuritic episode relieved by taking a deep breath, referred to as the *precordial-catch syndrome*. Its mechanism is unclear, but a transient folding of the pleura on itself is hypothesized.

Most diseases of the *pulmonary parenchyma* do not cause chest pain unless they extend to a pain-sensitive structure (eg, vessel wall, pleura). Consequently, the chest pain occurring in the context of *pneumonia,* pulmonary *tuberculosis,* or *pulmonary embolization* will be pleuritic and represent extensive disease. It is estimated that fewer than 10 percent of embolic episodes trigger chest pain. The most common manifestations of embolization are dyspnea, tachypnea, and tachycardia, which are nearly universal but may be short-lived. Pleural rub, effusion, fever, and hemoptysis suggests the presence of pulmonary infarction and pleural reaction.

Heart and Pericardium. *Coronary artery disease* impairing myocardial blood supply and presenting as *angina pectoris* is the most important cardiac source of chest pain. Coronary perfusion may be similarly compromised by critical *aortic stenosis* leading to angina (see Chapter 33). The classic hallmarks of angina are its sudden onset with exertion, emotional stress, or eating (usually a very large meal) and its relief within minutes by rest or nitroglycerin. Patients usually describe their chest pain as a squeezing, heaviness, or pressure, though it may be burning or sharp. The quality of the pain is not diagnostic, and many patients state the sensation is more a "discomfort" than a true pain. Radiation to the jaw, neck, shoulder, arm, back, or upper abdomen is common and may present in the absence of chest symptoms. At times, the arm is reported to feel numb. Autonomic epiphenomena such as diaphoresis and nausea may accompany the episode, as may dyspnea if there is transient pump failure or marked anxiety. Episodes last 2 to 20 minutes. Prompt response to nitroglycerin is characteristic; relief is usually obtained within 5 minutes. Ischemic pain persisting longer suggests *acute coronary insufficiency* or myocardial infarction. Fleeting pains of a few seconds' duration are not anginal in origin, nor are prolonged periods of constant chest tightness that last for days.

Other forms of angina include *nocturnal angina,* in which the patient awakens from sleep experiencing his typical angina pain. The cause is unclear, but nocturnal adrenergic hyperactivity and pump failure are postulated. *Variant angina,* as originally described by Prinzmetal, refers to anginal pain occurring exclusively at rest in conjunction with transient ST segment elevation on ECG. Classically, this syndrome was associated with coronary artery spasm at the site of high-grade proximal fixed stenosis. However, other forms of coronary disease may produce a similar clinical picture, and coronary vasospasm may present in ways other than Prinzmetal's description. *Cocaine abuse* can trigger ischemia by precipitating coronary vasoconstriction, increasing myocardial oxygen demand, and enhancing platelet aggregation.

Atypical angina (atypical chest pain) is a nonspecific term used to denote chest pain that differs in location, quality, or other characteristics from more typical angina yet is still suggestive by virtue of similar precipitants, timing, or other features. As many as 50 percent of such patients who come to angiography prove to have coronary disease. Among the remainder, there appear to be increased incidences of panic disorder, major depression, esophageal disease, and coronary microcirculatory dysfunction.

The mechanisms for many of these causes are not well understood, but recent interest has focused on the coronary microcirculation. *Coronary microvascular dysfunction* has been noted, characterized by abnormal responses to autonomic and biochemical stimuli. Normally, vasodilatory endothelial stimuli such as acetylcholine fail to lower arterial resistance. These patients exhibit increased microvascular resistance and reductions in perfusion. Such microvascular dysfunction has been found with increased frequency among patients with atypical angina who exhibit an ischemic response to exercise stress testing yet have entirely normal coronary angiograms. The terms *"microvascular angina"* and *"syndrome X"* have been applied to such persons. The significance of these findings is still is unclear and requires much more study, but they suggest a possible explanation for the chest pain of patients with *hypertrophic cardiomyopathy.*

Mitral valve prolapse is notorious for its association with atypical chest pain. The commonly held view of a link between the two has been challenged by recent studies controlling more stringently for selection bias. Some argue the apparent association is due to an increased frequency of underlying psychopathology, such as panic disorder (see below), that may trigger chest pain. Symptoms of autonomic dysfunction (eg, palpitations, sweating, dizziness) may sometimes accompany the chest pain and simulate an ischemic attack.

Pericarditis may present with pleuritic pain, resulting from spread of the inflammatory process from the relatively insensitive pericardium to the adjacent pain-sensitive parietal pleura. The pain is sharp, aggravated by respiratory activity, and sometimes precipitated by swallowing if the posterior aspect of the heart is involved. When the diaphragmatic surface of the pericardium is involved, pain will be referred to the tip of the shoulder. Change in position may alter the pain. Patients often note lessening of pain on sitting up and leaning forward. Pericarditis can also produce a second type of pain that mimics angina. Its most diagnostic physical finding is a two- or three-component friction rub.

A vexing pericardial problem is the development of chest pain after coronary bypass surgery. The return of typical angina raises the spectre of graft occlusion, but pleuritic pain suggests the *postpericardiotomy syndrome*.

Aorta. *Aortic dissection* is a must-not-miss cause of chest pain. Almost invariably, it begins with sudden onset of severe chest pain, maximal from the start, tearing or ripping in quality, and radiating to the interscapular region. Associated symptoms include neurologic deficits from cutoff of blood supply to the brain, spinal cord, or limb. Loss or diminution of a major peripheral pulse is a key physical finding, as are new onset of aortic insufficiency and pericardial tamponade due to dissection into the aortic root.

Esophagus and Other GI Tract Sources. *Esophageal motor dysfunction* (see Chapter 60) is the great mimicker of anginal chest pain, producing chest discomfort that can resemble angina in quality, location, radiation, and even precipitants (eg, exposure to cold, exertion). "Spasm" may occur spontaneously or in the context of meals or acid reflux. Unlike angina, it is more likely to persist as a dull sensation for several hours after an acute attack and may occur with swallowing. Some patients report *dysphagia* as an accompanying symptom. Nitrates and calcium channel blockers provide relief, as they do for angina. Some patients with atypical chest pain and normal coronary angiograms manifest both esophageal spasm and microcirculatory dysfunction, raising the intriguing possibility of a generalized disorder of smooth muscle reactivity.

Esophageal reflux gives a rather characteristic retrosternal burning sensation that may be brought on by a large meal, lying down, or bending over and may be relieved by antacids. The pain sometimes radiates to the interscapular region. An attack of acute *cholecystitis* may resemble angina by producing substernal discomfort that responds to nitrates, which reduce cystic duct spasm. On rare occasions, *pancreatitis* or *peptic ulcer* disease produces substernal chest pain. Even a patient with gaseous distention of the bowel in the area of the splenic flexure may complain of precordial discomfort.

Psyche. Dramatic chest pain presentations are common among patients with underlying psychopathology. In addition to presentations that may be clinically indistinguishable from angina, patients with *anxiety* or *depression* often describe feelings of chest heaviness or tightness that can last for hours to days, unrelated to exertion and unrelieved by rest. In patients with anxiety disorders, this sensation may be accompanied by a feeling of inability to take in a deep breath. When there is associated hyperventilation, the resulting hypocapnia leaves the patient light-headed and the extremities tingling.

Cardiac neurosis may lead to reports of chest pain mimicking angina. At other times, the patient misinterprets a noncardiac chest sensation. Patients with a *personality disorder* and *somatization* may describe almost any form of chest pain, including some suggestive of angina. A lifelong pattern of multiple refractory bodily complaints is characteristic (see Chapter 230). *Malingering* represents a conscious effort to feign illness for secondary gain. The hallmark is inconsistency of the story. Although other forms of psychogenic chest pain may bring secondary benefits to the patient, there is no premeditated attempt to deceive.

Patients with atypical chest pain related to an underlying depression or panic disorder tend to be younger, more often female, more apt to have a higher number of accompanying autonomic symptoms, more bothered by phobias, and more likely to describe an atypical form of chest pain than those with chest pain and a positive coronary angiogram.

DIFFERENTIAL DIAGNOSIS

The differential diagnosis of chest pain can be organized along anatomic lines, as outlined in Table 20–1. Must-not-miss diagnoses include coronary heart disease (CHD), critical aortic stenosis, aortic dissection, pneumothorax, cholecystitis, pericarditis, and pleuritis from pneumonia, embolization, or cancer.

WORKUP

Faced with a patient complaining of chest pain, there is the temptation to proceed directly to the plethora of sophisticated diagnostic studies for detection of coronary artery disease. However, the cost and the false-positive rate of such premature testing are likely to be unacceptably high because of the low pretest probability of CHD in unselected patients (see Chapter 2). More useful is a workup strategy that attempts to determine and stratify CHD risk on the basis of an initial history, physical examination, and ECG. Recent studies suggest this is quite attainable. However, many clinicians are strongly influenced by the patient's style of presentation, which may override its content and alter diagnostic approach.

History

Estimating Probability of Coronary Disease by History. A careful chest pain description is critical. The prevalence of angiographically confirmed CHD approaches 90 percent in persons with a classic story for angina (see above). Preva-

Table 20-1. Differential Diagnosis of Chest Pain

I. Chest Wall
  A. Muscular disorders
    1. Muscle spasm (precordial-catch syndrome)
    2. Pleurodynia
    3. Muscle strain
  B. Skeletal disorders
    1. Costochondritis (Tietze's syndrome)
    2. Rib fracture
    3. Metastatic disease of bone
    4. Cervical or thoracic spine disease
  C. Neurologic disorders
    1. Herpes zoster infection or post-herpetic pain
    2. Nerve root compression
II. Cardiopulmonary
  A. Cardiac disorders
    1. Pericarditis
    2. Myocardial ischemia
    3. Prolapsed mitral valve
  B. Pleuropulmonary disorders
    1. Pleurisy of any origin
    2. Pneumothorax
    3. Pulmonary embolization with infarction
    4. Pneumonitis
    5. Bronchospasm
III. Aortic
  A. Dissecting aortic aneurysm
IV. Gastrointestinal
  A. Esophageal disorders
    1. Reflux
    2. Spasm
  B. Others
    1. Cholecystitis
    2. Peptic ulcer disease
    3. Pancreatitis
    4. Splenic flexure gas
V. Psychogenic
  A. Anxiety (with or without hyperventilation)
  B. Cardiac neurosis
  C. Malingering
  D. Depression

lence declines to less than 15 percent in those coming to catheterization who have nonanginal chest pain. In the Framingham Study, patients presenting with new onset of definite angina had a relative risk of a coronary event over 2 years of 3.7 for men and 5.9 for women. Relative risk fell for those with possible angina to 3.0 for men and 2.9 for women, and to 1.3 for men and 0.8 for women with nonanginal chest pain.

Among the features of the chest pain description with the greatest discriminant value are its *timing* in relation to *precipitating* and *alleviating factors*. Quality, location, radiation, and intensity of pain are notoriously nonspecific. Precordial pain radiating down the left arm can occur with almost any cause of chest pain. A common pitfall in taking the history is to provide classic descriptions of chest pain to the patient who cannot give a quick, crisp account of his chest pain. Under the duress of the physician's interrogation, the patient may agree to one of these neat descriptions, leading to a false-positive diagnosis. The initial vagueness may have been more useful. No accommodations for racial differences in clinical presentation need be made, because the acute chest pain presentations are similar among whites and African-Americans.

Note is taken of patient's *age* and *gender,* and past medical history is reviewed for major *cardiac risk factors* (eg, hypertension, diabetes, smoking, hypercholesterolemia). *Family history* is checked for *premature coronary disease.*

Assessment of History for Other Important Causes. Some elements of the history suggestive of coronary disease are also important for the other causes they suggest:

Pain brought on by exertion and relieved by rest is certainly indicative of angina, but psychogenic disease and esophageal spasm may behave in similar fashion. A check for anxiety, depression, panic episodes, headache, lightheadedness, nervousness, weakness, fatigue, and lifelong history of other bodily complaints may suggest a psychogenic origin. Heartburn, dysphagia, and an absence of CHD risk factors raise the possibility of esophageal disease. Episodes that last hours to days provide further evidence of a noncardiac origin.

Prompt response to nitroglycerin is another characteristic feature of CHD, but esophageal spasm, coronary microvascular disease, cystic duct spasm, and even some psychogenic etiologies may also respond to nitrates.

Chest pain brought on by eating may be due to angina, but in the absence of other risk factors for CHD, one needs to consider gastroesophageal or pancreaticobiliary pathology. As noted earlier, response to nitroglycerin is not necessarily helpful in differentiating.

Some chest pain patterns not indicative of CHD also have an important differential:

Pain worsened by deep inspiration or cough is a hallmark of pleural irritation, but it is suggestive of pericarditis and chest wall pathology as well. Focal chest wall tenderness worsened by movement quickly narrows the differential to a chest wall origin. In the absence of focal chest wall pain, one needs to search promptly for evidence of intrathoracic pathology. Inquiry is needed into fever, cough, sputum production, tuberculosis exposure, hemoptysis, smoking, HIV exposure or high-risk behavior, unilateral leg edema, calf tenderness, shortness of breath, past history of embolization, recent orthopedic surgery, and oral contraceptive use. Pneumothorax should come to mind when pleuritic pain is sudden in onset and accompanied by dyspnea in a young patient with a previous history of pneumothorax or when the patient has long-standing bullous emphysema. Precordial-catch syndrome is suggested by brief, self-limited episodes in an otherwise healthy young person. Pleuritic pain worsened by turning but relieved by sitting up and leaning forward is indicative of pericarditis, which can be further assessed by physical examination. Pleuritic pain in the setting of an epidemic of minor viral respiratory disease suggests pleurodynia.

Sudden onset of maximally severe pain is a worrisome presentation, necessitating consideration of aortic dissection. Although such patients do not usually present to the office, they may call and require telephone triage. If the episode is accompanied by a new neurologic deficit or a syncopal episode, then urgent hospitalization is indicated. History of blunt trauma, known aortic disease, and radiation to the interscapular region provide additional support for the diagnosis. However, many less serious conditions can cause chest pain that radiates into the back, with esophageal pathology being the most common. Physical examination helps differentiate the two, as does the more indolent course of esophageal spasm and its absence of associated neurologic or vascular deficits.

Attention to *the context* of the patient's chest pain often suggests the differential. For example, onset of "pleuritic" pain in a person with known metastatic cancer may be due to a pathologic fracture or pleural metastasis. The same pain in an otherwise healthy young person with new onset of a dry cough, low-grade fever, and myalgias is consistent with viral-induced pleurodynia and muscle soreness from coughing.

Physical Examination

There is no standard physical examination for the patient with chest pain. The appropriate examination is based on the hypotheses suggested by the history, though checking for a few must-not-miss items is always in order. *General appearance* and *vital signs* can be telling. An anxious, sighing, hyperventilating individual who complains of constant chest tightness is likely to be suffering from an anxiety disorder, whereas tachypnea and tachycardia in a person with pleuritic pain are indicative of pulmonary embolization. Blood pressure needs to be noted as an important risk factor for CHD and taken in both arms in the patient with a suspected aortic dissection. The *skin* is noted for cyanosis, herpetic rash, pallor, jaundice, and xanthomata. Examination of the *fundi* may provide evidence of atherosclerotic, diabetic, or hypertensive disease. The *carotid pulse* is palpated for delay in upstroke, suggesting hemodynamically significant aortic stenosis, and checked for its loss in the person with possible disease of the aorta. The *jugular venous pressure* is noted; it may be transiently elevated during an ischemic episode.

The *chest wall* is examined carefully in the person reporting "pleuritic" pain, beginning with inspection for signs of trauma and the rash of *herpes zoster* and palpation for swelling and focal tenderness. If pain is elicited, it is important to be sure the pain on palpation is identical to the patient's presenting complaint. One should next listen to the *lungs* for a pleural friction rub during inspiration and expiration and note any signs of consolidation or effusion. Hyperresonance, absent breath sounds, and tracheal deviation suggest a significant pneumothorax that requires immediate attention. Checking for rales (crackles) in the patient with possible angina assesses the possibility of ischemic left ventricular dysfunction.

On examination of the *heart,* the left ventricular impulse is observed and noted for signs of hypertrophy (indicative of significant aortic stenosis or a hypertrophic cardiomyopathy). Signs of ischemic myocardial dysfunction, such as loss of physiologic splitting of the second heart sound and development of a fourth heart sound, are sought; they may be transient, occurring only during chest pain. Listening for the systolic ejection murmur of aortic stenosis should not be forgotten in the patient with angina. If the chest pain is pleuritic, then carefully listening for the two- to three-component pericardial friction rub is indicated. Though the relation between mitral valve prolapse and chest pain is questionable, listening briefly for a mid-systolic click and late systolic murmur help complete the examination.

The *abdomen* is checked for epigastric and right upper quadrant tenderness and masses (including an abdominal aneurysm). The *legs* require careful examination for unilateral edema and other signs of phlebitis (see Chapter 22), a potential source of pulmonary embolization in the person presenting with pleuritic pain. All *peripheral pulses* are checked, noting any absences and evidence of acute ischemia, which might occur with an aortic dissection. The *spine* is palpated for areas of tenderness along the cervical and thoracic segments, and the *neurologic* examination needs to include a check for new focal deficits, another possible clue to dissection.

Laboratory Studies

Test selection for the workup of chest pain should always be based on the working differential suggested by the history and physical examination. Repeated studies have documented the validity of clinical data for assessing the likelihood of cardiac risk in patients who present with chest pain. As noted earlier, unselective testing greatly accelerates the cost of evaluation and increases the risk of generating a false-positive diagnosis, a potentially serious but preventible outcome for the patient with chest pain.

Suspected Coronary Heart Disease. *Clinically High Risk.* The patient with a classic angina history, CHD risk factors, a positive family history, a few crackles, a fourth heart sound, and loss of physiologic splitting has such a high probability of CHD that diagnostic testing will add little except cost (assuming aortic stenosis has already been clinically ruled out). One can proceed directly to management (see Chapter 30).

Clinically Low Risk. The patient with clearly nonanginal chest pain, no CHD risk factors or family history, and a normal cardiac examination has such a low probability of CHD that testing for it is likely to generate only negative or false-positive results and excessive medical bills. Even a CHD test with high sensitivity and specificity (eg, thallium stress testing) will perform poorly and produce an excessive proportion of false-positive results if applied to a person with a very low pretest probability of CHD (see Chapter 2). Occasionally, a *resting ECG* is obtained to reassure the low-risk, high-concern patient. Performing the low-cost test has been found to speed resumption of normal activity in the overly concerned patient, but there is always the risk of a false-positive, and the approach ought not be used unless there is strong patient need for such "objective" reassurance.

Clinically Intermediate Risk. The patient most in need of a CHD workup is the one who clinically appears intermediate in risk (eg, atypical chest pain, a single cardiac risk factor, questionable fourth heart sound). In such persons, a positive or negative test result is likely to have a significant effect on the posttest probability of CHD, and careful design of an evaluation program is indicated.

Suspected Esophageal Disease. Laboratory studies for esophageal dysfunction are usually not necessary if the clinical presentation is strongly suggestive, coronary disease has been ruled out, and the patient responds symptomatically to measures that reduce reflux and spasm. Attention usually turns to testing for esophageal disease when the patient at intermediate risk of CHD (eg, atypical chest pain plus a few risk factors) has a negative stress test and a decision about proceeding to angiography is pending. As many as 20 percent of patients with pain suspicious enough to warrant coronary angiography have been shown to have esophageal disorders. A convincing diagnosis of esophageal disease might save the patient a cardiac catheterization.

Chest pain due to a disorder of esophageal motility is not easy to document. A trial of antacids or H_1-blocker therapy is a helpful empiric measure but not likely to be convincing unless all pain episodes cease. This leads to consideration of esophageal manometry, acid perfusion testing, and 24-hour pH monitoring. Although potentially diagnostic, *manometry* often gives indeterminate data. Many patients suspected of achalasia or esophageal spasm fail to show typical manometric findings at the time of testing. Furthermore, others who are symptom-free may demonstrate abnormalities when tested. Still others end up being placed in a category of nonspecific motility disease. Nevertheless, many authorities insist on manometric data before concluding a patient has esophageal spasm or a related motor disorder.

Provocative testing is more useful. It provides a ready means in the office of identifying an esophageal origin for atypical chest pain, though it does not specify a mechanism. The objective is to reproduce the patient's exact symptoms. Two tests have proven most useful: the acid perfusion (Bernstein) test and edrophonium (Tensilon) infusion. The *Bernstein test* consists of instilling a small amount of acid through a nasogastric tube placed in the esophagus. A positive test (reproduction of pain on acid instillation) has identified an esophageal origin for atypical chest pain in 10 percent to 25 percent of noncardiac cases.

Edrophonium testing grew out of a desire to find a safe and well tolerated means of stimulating esophageal contractions. Edrophonium (a relatively gentle muscarinic agonist) has proven superior to acid perfusion and other provocative agents in reproducing atypical chest pain complaints, with 24 percent to 34 percent of noncardiac patients having a positive test (reproduction of pain during wet swallows). As with the Bernstein test, edrophonium only identifies an esophageal origin for the pain, it does not specify the mechanism (correlation between response to edrophonium and manometric findings is poor). Side effects from a rapid bolus of intravenous edrophonium (80 mcg/kg body weight) included mild degrees of light-headedness, nausea, and abdominal cramps but no adverse cardiac effects.

Ambulatory monitoring of intraesophageal pH and pressures is becoming increasingly available and may prove useful, especially in cases that defy explanation despite provocative testing. Esophageal pH monitoring over 24 hours has emerged as a very useful tool in the evaluation of noncardiac chest pain, providing an opportunity to correlate acid reflux with occurrence of symptoms. In a study comparing manometric and provocative esophageal tests with 24-hour pH monitoring, the latter proved superior in providing an explanatory correlation in 46 percent of instances of chest pain versus 19 percent for both edrophonium and Bernstein testing. A single manometric study was of little use. Because abnormal motor activity may be difficult to detect at the time of a particular study or may be induced by the study and have little to do with the patient's problem, round-the-clock monitoring opens up new avenues of evaluation. The precise indications for such testing remain to be defined; studies are ongoing. Because there is no gold standard, determinations of sensitivity and specificity for esophageal testing methods are not possible.

Pleuritic Chest Pain. *Suspected Pulmonary Embolization.* Patients with pleuritic pain should have a *chest radiograph.* In a study of 97 young patients (ages 18 to 40) with pleuritic chest pain, the combination of history, physical examination, and chest film identified 95 percent of cases of proven embolization. The most frequent radiographic finding in cases of embolization was a unilateral effusion. When history and physical findings were used alone, the detection rate for embolization was 80 percent. When *lung scan* was added after the chest radiograph, there was only a 5 percent improvement in detection rate, but the scan did substantially reduce the number of false-positive diagnoses from 39 percent after history, physical, and chest radiograph to 16 percent after scan. Other studies have shown that a normal scan virtually rules out the diagnosis of clinically significant embolism, but high false-positive rates have been reported, especially in those with preexisting lung disease and in the elderly. The addition of ventilation scanning has not resolved the problem. *Arterial blood gases* are insensitive and are often no help in identifying patients with pulmonary emboli.

In sum, history, physical examination, and chest radiography can be used to identify patients who might have an embolism and require further assessment. If the patient is young and free of underlying lung disease, a scan can reduce the number of false-positive diagnoses. If the patient is elderly or has underlying lung disease, the scan is unlikely to be sufficiently specific; angiography without prior scanning is urged by some experts, especially if the considerable risk of anticoagulant therapy is high and a definitive diagnosis is needed before commencing treatment. The utility of an ECG in patients with suspected embolus is marginal. The electrocardiographic findings of acute right heart strain, $S_1Q_3T_3$, are helpful if present, but sensitivity is low and a normal ECG certainly does not rule out the diagnosis. Likewise, serum enzymes are insensitive and of little use.

Suspected Infection. The chest radiograph may also reveal pneumonitis. Pneumococcal pneumonia and tuberculosis often present with acute pleuritic chest pain and may be mistaken clinically for pulmonary embolism. Consequently, any patient with pleuritic pain and sputum production should have both *Gram*'s and *acid-fast stains* made. A pleural effusion may also be detected on chest film. Any nonloculated pleural effusion of unknown etiology should be tapped, Gram-stained, cultured, examined microscopically, and sent for cell count, glucose, lactic dehydrogenase (LDH), and protein determinations (see Chapter 43).

Suspicion of pneumothorax is an indication for a chest film, but if radiography is not immediately available and the patient is in respiratory distress, decompression should not be delayed. Chest radiography is sometimes of use in aortic dissection, but if dissection is truly suspected, emergency admission for aortic angiography is indicated. Delaying admission to obtain a chest film is foolish. A computed tomography (CT) scan with contrast is useful when the aortogram is negative but clinical suspicion remains high.

When *pericarditis* is under consideration, an *ECG* is essential. However, the ECG changes of early repolarization, a harmless finding seen in young men, may closely resemble those of acute pericarditis. The presence of concave ST segment elevations in both limb and precordial leads and the presence of PR segment depressions in the precordial leads, if they occur in the limb leads, distinguish pericarditis from early repolarization. *Cardiac ultrasonography* may reveal a pericardial effusion. An antinuclear antibody (ANA), blood urea nitrogen (BUN), and tuberculin skin test are indicated when the cause of pericarditis is not readily evident.

Other Conditions. Only a few *musculoskeletal* disorders require chest radiography: suspected rib fractures and cervical or thoracic spine disease. If a *gastrointestinal* cause is suspected, a contrast study may be in order. The ECG may show T wave depression in cholecystitis and pancreatitis and may mistakenly be interpreted as evidence of coronary disease.

The anxious patient with *psychogenic* pain may find a chest radiograph and/or ECG reassuring. In most instances, however, a thorough history and careful physical examination combined with a detailed explanation should suffice. Repeating tests "just to be sure" may begin to undermine the patient's confidence in the physician's explanation and even heighten anxiety, especially if there are repeat studies.

It is important to realize that as many as 10 percent to 15 percent of cases remain undiagnosed, even after careful and thorough evaluation. Nevertheless, in such instances it is still possible to rule out the presence of an acutely serious etiology. Most patients with chest pain that initially eludes diagnosis can be followed expectantly for the time being.

SYMPTOMATIC RELIEF

Relief of pain must be based on an etiologic diagnosis. To simply suppress the pain with analgesics or sedatives before a diagnosis is made may hide important clues. However, musculoskeletal forms of chest pain may require analgesia. When the diagnosis of costochondritis is certain, local injection with lidocaine into the point of maximal tenderness can provide dramatic relief. An antacid regimen or H_2-blocker therapy in conjunction with other antireflux and acid-reducing measures are helpful in patients with esophagitis. Nitrates and calcium channel blockers are sometimes of benefit to patients with esophageal spasm (see Chapter 61). Patients with depression or panic disorder require specific therapy directed at the underlying psychopathology. Failure to treat etiologically may result in prolonged, refractory disability from the chest pain (see Chapters 226 and 227).

PATIENT EDUCATION AND INDICATIONS FOR REFERRAL

A careful and thorough explanation is essential to avoid precipitating a cardiac neurosis or unnecessary visits to several physicians for evaluation of chest pain. Patients making many visits usually harbor unexplored concerns that have not been adequately addressed in an open and detailed explanation. Discussion of concerns can be extremely reassuring and comforting to the patient and family; this must not be overlooked when workup reveals a benign etiology. When evaluation reveals chest pain in the setting of cocaine use, serious counseling efforts are required (see Chapter 235), as well as strong warning about the cardiac risks involved, even with so-called "recreational use." Urgent referral to the nearest emergency room is indicated for the patient with severe anginal chest pain lasting over 30 minutes, especially of accompanied by Q waves or ST and T wave changes on ECG not known to be old. Similarly, the patient with suspected pulmonary embolization, pneumothorax, or aortic dissection requires immediate hospitalization. The patient with panic disorder or depression severe enough to cause disabling symptoms deserves consideration for psychiatric referral (see Chapters 226 and 227).

A.H.G.

ANNOTATED BIBLIOGRAPHY

Beitman BD, Kushner MG, Bash I et al. Follow-up status of patients with angiographically normal coronary arteries and panic disorder. JAMA 1991;265:1545. (*Increased disability in patients with panic disorder.*)

Beller GA, Gibson RS. Sensitivity, specificity, and prognostic significance of noninvasive testing for occult or known coronary disease. Prog Cardiovasc Dis 1987;29:241. (*Comprehensive data on stress testing and other diagnostic modalities for coronary disease.*)

Birdwell BG, Herbers JE, Kroenke K. Evaluating chest pain: The patient's presentation style alters the physician's diagnostic approach. Arch Intern Med 1993;153:1991. (*The effect of style was marked in the videotape-review study.*)

Branch WT, McNeil BJ. Analysis of the differential diagnosis and assessment of pleuritic chest pain in young adults. Am J Med 1983;75:671. (*Analysis of previously published series of 97 patients with pleuritic chest pain with recommended diagnostic approach.*)

Cannon RO. Chest pain with normal coronary angiograms. N Engl J Med 1993;328:1706. (*A brief discussion of the evidence for microvascular disease.*)

Cannon RO, Cattau EL, Yakshe PN et al. Coronary flow reserve, esophageal motility, and chest pain in patients with angiographically normal coronary arteries. Am J Med 1991;88:217. (*More than 80 percent of angiographically normal patients in this series had evidence of microvascular and/or esophageal spasm, suggesting a common underlying disorder of smooth muscle.*)

Carney RM, Freedland KE, Ludbrook PA. Major depression, panic disorder, and mitral valve prolapse in patients who complain of chest pain. Am J Med 1990;89:757. (*Eighty percent of chest pain patients without angiographic evidence of coronary disease who had mitral valve prolapse had either depression or panic disorder, suggesting these disorders may be the cause of the pain.*)

Daton W, Hall ML, Russo J. Chest pain: Relationship of psychiatric illness to coronary arteriographic results. Am J Med 1988;84:1. (*Greatly increased incidence of major depression and panic disorder in patients with angiographically negative chest pain.*)

DeSanctis RW, Dorochazi RB, Austen WG et al. Aortic dissection. N Engl J Med 1987;317:1060. (*An authoritative review, with emphasis on clinical features; 83 refs.*)

Diamond GA, Forrester JS. Analysis of probability as an aid in the clinical diagnosis of coronary artery disease. N Engl J

Med 1979;300:1350. (*A now classic paper on probability of coronary disease by history and laboratory studies.*)

Egashira K, Inou T, Hirooka Y et al. Evidence of impaired endothelium-dependent coronary vasodilatation in patients with angina pectoris and normal coronary angiograms. N Engl J Med 1993;328:1659. (*Evidence for microvascular dysfunction in patients with angina and normal angiography.*)

Epstein SE, Gerber LH, Borer JS. Chest wall syndrome. JAMA 1979;241:2793. (*A detailed description of 12 patients seen at the NIH, including a description of the physical maneuvers that might elicit the pain of chest wall syndrome.*)

Feldman RL. Ambulatory electrocardiographic monitoring: The test for ischemia? Ann Intern Med 1988;109:608. (*An editorial urging caution in the use of the technology for detection of ischemia, pointing out the many problems in interpreting ST segment depression on Holter monitoring.*)

Goldman L, Lee TH. Noninvasive tests for diagnosing the presence and extent of coronary artery disease. J Gen Intern Med 1986;1:258. (*A rigorous analytic review of exercise electrocardiography, thallium scintigraphy, and radionuclide ventriculography.*)

Hewson EG, Sinclair JW, Dalton CB. Twenty-four-hour esophageal pH monitoring: The most useful test for evaluating noncardiac chest pain. Am J Med 1991;90:576. (*Had the highest yield when correlated with symptoms.*)

Isner JM, Mark Estes NA, Thompson PD et al. Acute cardiac events temporally related to cocaine abuse. N Engl J Med 1986;315:1438. (*Documents this serious cause of cardiac chest pain in young patients.*)

Johnson PA, Lee TH, Cook EF et al. Effect of race on the presentation and management of patients with acute chest pain. Ann Intern Med 1993;118:593. (*No racial difference in presentation found.*)

Kayser HL. Tietze's syndrome—A literature review. Am J Med 1956;21:982. (*Points out the often epidemic nature of the illness; still the best review.*)

Kirshenbaum HD, Ockene IS, Alpert JS et al. The spectrum of coronary artery spasm. JAMA 1981;246:354. (*Emphasizes the variability of clinical presentation of coronary artery spasm and the difficulty of diagnosis.*)

Lasky WK. Assessment of cardiovascular risk: A return to basics. Ann Intern Med 1993;118:149. (*An editorial on the validity of clinical assessment in determining CHD risk.*)

Murabito JM, Anderson KM, Kannel WB et al. Risk of coronary heart disease in subjects with chest discomfort: The Framingham Heart Study. Am J Med 1990;89:297. (*The chest pain history was an independent and powerful predictor of diagnosis and prognosis.*)

Pryor DB, Shaw L, McCants CB et al. Value of the history and physical in identifying patients at increased risk of coronary disease. Ann Intern Med 1993;118:81. (*Clinical assessment effectively predicted CHD risk and need for further study.*)

Richter JE, Bradley LA, Castell DO. Esophageal chest pain: Current controversies in pathogenesis, diagnosis, and therapy. Ann Intern Med 1989;110:66. (*Excellent review; 119 refs.*)

Robin ED. Overdiagnosis and overtreatment of pulmonary embolism. Ann Intern Med 1977;87:775. (*A critical discussion of the shortcomings of methods of diagnosis of pulmonary embolism; argues that lung scan should be limited to ruling out embolism in young patients and that arterial blood gases are of no help.*)

Rustgi AK, Chopra S. Chest pain of esophageal origin. J Gen Intern Med 1988;4:151. (*A comprehensive review that includes a detailed discussion of clinical presentations and diagnostic approaches; 89 refs.*)

Sox HC, Kickam DH, Lee TH et al. Using the patient's history to estimate the probability of coronary artery disease: A comparison of primary care and referral practices. Am J Med 1990;89:7. (*The predictive value of the chest pain history is reduced if the prevalence of coronary disease is low, as is likely in the primary care setting.*)

Spodnick DH. Differential characteristics of the electrocardiogram in early repolarization and acute pericarditis. N Engl J Med 1976;295:523. (*Presents data suggesting that one can differentiate between the two based on location and occurrence of ST and PR segment changes.*)

Primary Care Medicine: Office Evaluation and Management of the Adult Patient, 3rd edition, edited by Allan H. Goroll, Lawrence A. May, and Albert G. Mulley, Jr. J.B. Lippincott Company, Philadelphia

21
Evaluation of the Asymptomatic Systolic Murmur

Systolic murmurs are often noted incidentally in otherwise asymptomatic patients. Although many such murmurs result from harmless conditions, it is important to recognize those which may represent more serious pathology. In many instances, early detection can improve outcomes (see Chapter 33). The primary physician should be able to conduct a very reasonable clinical assessment in the office setting. Routinely ordering a cardiac ultrasound examination on every patient discovered to have a heart murmur is both expensive and unnecessary.

PATHOPHYSIOLOGY AND CLINICAL PRESENTATION

Systolic murmurs can be divided into two broad categories: ejection and regurgitant. *Ejection murmurs* result from turbulent flow of blood across the ventricular outflow tracts during systole. They are characteristically crescendo–decrescendo, medium- to low-pitched, and heard best at the base of the heart, beginning after the first heart sound and ending before the second. *Regurgitation murmurs* represent backflow of blood due to incompetence of the mitral or tricuspid valve or the ventricular septum. They are typically higher in pitch, heard best at the apex or midsternal border, and holosystolic or mid- to late-systolic in timing. Ejection murmurs are common and do not always indicate underlying heart disease. Regurgitant murmurs are associated with some abnormality of the mitral or tricuspid valves or septum, but the underlying lesion may be mild or transient and of no clinical significance.

Ejection Murmurs

"Physiologic" murmurs occur when there is increased ejection velocity across a normal valve creating turbulence.

Causes of increased velocity include fever, anemia, pregnancy, hyperthyroidism, exercise, and conditions associated with a large stroke volume (eg, aortic regurgitation, bradycardia, atrial septal defect). Dilation of the aorta, as in hypertension or aging, may also produce a flow murmur by causing turbulent flow in the dilated segment.

"Innocent" murmurs occur in normal hearts under resting conditions. The origin of such murmurs is a subject of debate, with recent evidence pointing to the aortic root. Since there is no obstruction in the outflow tract, the murmur reflects the normal ejection pattern of blood from the ventricles and is early systolic and crescendo–decrescendo. Because chamber pressures are normal, there is normal splitting of heart sounds. Valves are normal; there are no adventitious sounds or other murmurs.

Early *aortic* and *pulmonic valve disease* may produce murmurs identical to physiologic ones, except that the former are often accompanied by an early systolic *ejection click*. In *pulmonic stenosis*, the murmur increases with inspiration, and the pulmonic component of the second sound is delayed as disease progresses. With increasing stenosis, ejection murmurs usually become louder and more prolonged, with peak intensity occurring later in systole. In hemodynamically significant aortic stenosis, a sustained left ventricular heave develops, and the carotid upstroke becomes delayed.

The physical findings in elderly persons with hemodynamically significant *calcific aortic stenosis* may be deceptively subtle and atypical. The murmur tends to be softer, higher pitched, and louder at the apex than at the base. The left ventricular lift may be less prominent due to myocardial decompensation, and the carotid upstroke may be normal if the artery has lost its compliance. The degree of valve calcification noted on echocardiography often corresponds to the severity of stenosis.

Hypertrophic cardiomyopathy produces an ejection quality murmur by dynamically obstructing the left ventricular outflow tract. Displacement of the mitral valve may also occur dynamically and cause regurgitation. The ejection murmur is affected by the size of the left ventricular cavity and contractility. Maneuvers that decrease cavity size (eg, Valsalva) increase obstruction and intensify the murmur. When there is marked obstruction, the murmur lasts through most of systole and its peak is delayed beyond mid-systole. Some patients are prone to tachyarrhythmias. The electrocardiogram (ECG) shows high voltage.

Atrial septal defects (ASD) produce physiologic murmurs due to increased right ventricular stroke volume. However, unlike other physiologic murmurs, there is often wide and fixed splitting of the second sound due to left-to-right shunting of blood and a delay in right ventricular ejection.

Patients with physiologic or innocent murmurs are generally asymptomatic from a cardiac standpoint and usually have no previous history of heart disease. Patients with mild varieties of aortic or pulmonic stenosis, hypertrophic cardiomyopathy, or a small ASD may be asymptomatic as well. In patients with aortic stenosis, onset of symptoms (eg, angina, dyspnea, postural light-headedness) is usually a late development indicating advanced disease (see Chapter 33).

Regurgitant Murmurs

Holosystolic murmurs and hemodynamically significant regurgitation are usually associated with *rheumatic heart disease*, dilated valve rings secondary to dilated *cardiomyopathy*, or dysfunction of the valve apparatus due to *myxomatous degeneration* of a chordae tendineae or *infarction* of a papillary muscle. A *ventricular septal defect (VSD)* may also explain a holosystolic murmur.

Far more common is *mitral valve prolapse (MVP)* with its late systolic murmur, most often preceded by a click; the redundant mitral valve leaflets prolapse into the atrium during late systole. Most patients with MVP have no other signs or symptoms of heart disease, though an important minority experience atypical chest pain, dysrhythmias, or dyspnea. In a few instances, hemodynamically significant mitral regurgitation occurs. MVP is common and more frequent in women than in men. In the Framingham Study, the prevalence was as high as 17 percent among young women, 4 percent among young men. Overall, 5 percent of the population had echocardiographic evidence of MVP, with 4 percent manifesting a murmur of grade 2/6 or louder. Asthenic builds in both men and women have been associated with MVP, as has small breast size in women. Nonspecific T-wave changes, particularly inferior lead T-wave inversion, have been described. Diagnosis is confirmed by finding prominent late systolic prolapse on M-mode echocardiography or definite prolapse on the mitral valve leaflets in the parasternal long-axis view on two-dimensional ultrasound study.

DIFFERENTIAL DIAGNOSIS

The differential diagnosis can be listed according to the underlying pathophysiology. Thus, systolic ejection murmurs can be classified as innocent, physiologic, aortic, and pulmonic. Regurgitant murmurs may be caused by incompetence of the mitral or tricuspid valves or by a VSD (Table 21–1).

WORKUP

Differentiating Regurgitant from Ejection Murmur. Making this differentiation early in the evaluation helps focus the workup and narrow the differential diagnosis (see Table 21–1). Timing, quality, and location are the most helpful features. As noted earlier, ejection quality murmurs are crescendo–decrescendo, harsh, best heard with the bell, usually loudest at the base, and radiate into the neck and down to the apex. In elderly patients with calcific aortic stenosis, the murmur may be higher-pitched and maximal at the apex, mimicking mitral regurgitation. The *systolic regurgitant murmurs* of mitral and tricuspid regurgitation are characteristically high-pitched, well localized to the apex or left sternal border (unless very loud), and pansystolic or late systolic (and sometimes preceded by a click).

A few additional characteristics and responses to *maneuvers* help in the differentiation. Ejection murmurs change in intensity with *heart rate* and length of the cardiac cycle, becoming softer with increases in rate and louder as rate decreases. Regurgitant murmurs change little if at all with heart

Table 21-1. Differential Diagnosis of Systolic Ejection Murmur

1. Innocent Murmurs
2. Physiologic Murmurs
   a. Exercise or emotion
   b. Fever
   c. Anemia
   d. Hyperthyroidism
   e. Conditions with large stroke volumes: atrial septal defect, aortic regurgitation, bradycardia
   f. Pregnancy
3. Aortic Murmurs
   a. Aortic stenosis
   b. Hypertrophic cardiomyopathy
   c. Sub- and supravalvular fixed stenoses
4. Pulmonic Murmurs
   a. Pulmonic stenosis
5. Mitral Regurgitation Murmurs
   a. Rheumatic mitral insufficiency
   b. Mitral valve prolapse syndrome
   c. Congenital mitral valve disease
   d. Rupture of chordae tendineae
   e. Papillary muscle dysfunction
   f. Left atrial myxoma
   g. Dilated mitral valve ring
6. Tricuspid Regurgitation Murmurs
   a. Rheumatic tricuspid insufficiency
   b. Dilated tricuspid valve ring
7. Ventricular Septal Defect

rate. *Handgrip* markedly augments the intensity of the regurgitant murmurs of mitral regurgitation and VSD. Right-sided heart murmurs can be differentiated from left-sided ones by the augmentation in intensity that occurs with *inspiration*.

Systolic Ejection Murmurs. Here, one must separate innocent and physiologic ejection murmurs from those caused by significant aortic and pulmonic outflow tract obstructions and ASDs. *Innocent and physiologic murmurs* are usually midrange in frequency, less than 3/6 in intensity, peak in early systole, stop long before S_2, are heard best at the base, and can radiate to neck and apex. Valsalva maneuvers and standing decrease their intensity. The second sound is normally split; there are no clicks, heaves, S_3S_4, or other murmurs. The ECG and chest radiograph are normal. Signs of anemia, fever, hyperthyroidism, and anxiety should be sought.

The murmurs resulting from ASD and hemodynamically insignificant aortic and pulmonic stenoses may resemble physiologic murmurs. However, in most cases of *atrial septal defect* there is widened and fixed splitting of S_2, and in more than 90 percent of cases there is a conduction defect of the right bundle branch type, producing a QRS and lead V_1 with an RSR′ configuration. A normal ECG and normal splitting of S_2 make an ASD unlikely. When one is in doubt, an echocardiogram can be used to look for abnormal septal motion and right ventricular enlargement; a normal study rules out the diagnosis.

Mild aortic stenosis in the young patient may be impossible to distinguish from a physiologic murmur; the presence of an ejection click is an important clue to the former. As stenosis progresses and becomes more hemodynamically significant, the murmur typically gets louder and peaks later in systole, a left ventricular lift develops, a thrill may be palpable, and the carotid upstroke becomes delayed. Evidence of left ventricular hypertrophy may appear on ECG (eg, increased voltage, strain pattern), though the test is not a sensitive indicator.

A high index of suspicion is necessary both for the detection of *aortic stenosis in the elderly* and the estimation of its severity. One needs to remember to listen at the apex as well as at the base and not to be lulled into a false sense of security by the softness of the murmur, the absence of a vigorous left ventricular heave, or the normality of the carotid upstroke. Its presentation as a medium- to high-pitched murmur, heard best at the apex, may lead to confusion with mitral regurgitation.

Several characteristics which help differentiate the systolic ejection murmur of *hypertrophic cardiomyopathy* from other ejection murmurs should be checked for. Most distinctive are the murmur's responses to Valsalva and squatting. The murmur uniquely *increases* markedly with *Valsalva* (due to decrease in left ventricular chamber size and increase in outflow obstruction) and *decreases* on going from standing to *squatting* (which increases chamber size and lessens outflow obstruction). In addition, the murmur peaks around mid-systole, which helps distinguish it from an innocent murmur, which peaks early in systole. Moreover, it is usually heard most clearly along the left sternal border and associated with a *carotid upstroke* that is brisk and sometimes *bisferiens* (bifid) in quality.

Confirmation of suspected valvular and subvalvular obstruction to left ventricular outflow and accurate estimation of its severity can be accomplished noninvasively by *cardiac ultrasound* performed in conjunction with a continuous wave *Doppler study*. For aortic stenosis, reasonably accurate estimates can often be obtained of valve area and pressure gradient across the valve. The test is also diagnostic of hypertrophic cardiomyopathy and essential to estimation of its severity.

Hemodynamically significant pulmonic stenosis is suggested by wide splitting or absence of the pulmonic component of the second heart sound, an ejection click that decreases with inspiration, a prolonged and loud murmur (greater than 3/6) that characteristically increases with inspiration, a right ventricular lift, evidence of pulmonary artery dilation on chest film, and prominent R wave in V_1 indicative of right ventricular hypertrophy. A normal ECG and an early systolic murmur rule out significant pulmonic stenosis. Mild, hemodynamically insignificant pulmonic stenosis may be indistinguishable from an innocent murmur, but usually no therapy is indicated and therefore misdiagnosis is of little consequence.

In summary, the key components of the initial evaluation of the systolic ejection murmur in the asymptomatic patient include attention to carotid upstroke, left and right ventricular impulses, second heart sound, clicks, the quality, timing, intensity, and location of the murmur, and the effects of such provocative maneuvers as change in position, respiration, and Valsalva. ECG and chest radiograph may be helpful. Cardiac ultrasound examination, in conjunction with Doppler study, are indicated if there is clinical suspicion of hemodynamically significant disease or the diagnosis remains in doubt and there are adverse consequences to not identifying the lesion.

Regurgitant Murmurs. Here, duration and timing during systole are helpful distinguishing characteristics. A *holosystolic murmur* suggests rheumatic or cardiomyopathic mitral insufficiency, tricuspid insufficiency, or a VSD. The murmur of classic *mitral insufficiency* is best heard at the apex and radiates laterally into the axilla; it varies little with cycle length or with respiration but increases markedly with hand grip. With chronic increase in volume load, there is likely to be palpable enlargement of the left ventricle. Because multivalve involvement is the rule and heart failure may occur, a careful listening for other murmurs and a check for signs of heart failure (eg, rales, third heart sound) are in order. However, a third heart sound is quite common in mitral regurgitation and not as predictive of systolic dysfunction as it is in other forms of heart disease.

The murmur of *tricuspid insufficiency* is usually loudest at the lower left sternal border, but when the right ventricle is very large, it may be heard at the apex. It does not radiate well to the axilla. Intensity is strongly influenced by respiration, increasing at the beginning of inspiration and fading during early expiration. *Hepatojugular reflux* is very suggestive and should be checked for.

The holosystolic murmur of *ventricular septal defect* can be heard best at the sternal border and does not radiate to the axilla. Intensity does not vary with respiration. It often has some mid-systolic accentuation and may be confused with an ejection murmur. Like mitral regurgitation, intensity of the murmur increases markedly with hand grip.

The presence of a *mid- to late-systolic regurgitant murmur* suggests *MVP*. Some forms of *papillary muscle dysfunction* will also result in a mitral regurgitant murmur of similar timing, usually in the setting of anteroseptal ischemia. Suspicion of MVP is reinforced by hearing a mid-systolic click, which tends to move toward the first heart sound with standing (a maneuver that reduces left ventricular volume and softens the murmur). The MVP murmur may occur in the absence of a click. The intensity of the suspected MVP murmur should be noted. The louder the murmur, the more hemodynamically significant the regurgitation, and the greater the risks of endocarditis and other cardiovascular complications.

An *echocardiogram* can confirm MVP when uncertainty persists. Minor degrees of valve prolapse are normal. One should insist that ultrasound criteria are met before giving the patient a diagnosis of MVP. The major criterion is *systolic displacement* of one or both valve leaflets into the left atrium beyond the plane of the mitral annulus in the parasternal long-axis view on two-dimensional ultrasound study. *Valve thickening* and *redundancy* are other features, but a *nonclassic form of MVP* has been described in which there is no thickening, little risk for endocarditis, and little hemodynamically significant regurgitation. Ultrasound can differentiate the two and thus may help with cardiac risk stratification, though a very small risk of embolic stroke is similar in both forms.

Indiscriminate use of echocardiography is to be avoided. Searching for "silent" MVP in the patient with vague chest pains and an entirely normal cardiac examination is of no value. Use of ultrasound in suspected MVP can facilitate diagnosis, but the contribution to outcome remains to be demonstrated. In most instances, the change in management engendered involves initiation of endocarditis prophylaxis (see Chapter 16). However, Doppler echocardiographic studies suggest that audible, and especially loud, systolic regurgitant murmurs are very likely to represent hemodynamically significant disease. An ultrasound examination is indicated when such a murmur is encountered.

PATIENT EDUCATION AND INDICATIONS FOR REFERRAL

In general, when the murmur is determined to be innocent or hemodynamically insignificant after careful evaluation, it is essential to provide detailed explanation as part of the delivery of meaningful reassurance. Marked concern and even distrust may be precipitated by a perfunctory explanation that "it's harmless and nothing serious," especially if detailed auscultation continues to be conducted on subsequent visits. Concern about a murmur that is left incompletely explained can lead to unnecessary self-restriction of activity. Reassurance should include a discussion of the cause of the murmur, its significance, and prognosis. Informing the patient of other possible causes considered and ruled out is particularly helpful to the well educated or medically curious patient. The patient with a harmless murmur should be specifically told there is no need to restrict activity or undergo further evaluation at the present time.

Asymptomatic persons found to have aortic stenosis (especially the elderly) should be informed of the symptoms of hemodynamically significant disease (eg, marked postural light-headedness, angina, exertional dyspnea) and instructed to report them immediately should they occur. Prompt evaluation in conjunction with cardiac consultation is indicated (see Chapter 33). Worsening exertional dyspnea in the patient with rheumatic, ischemic, or cardiomyopathic mitral regurgitation is also an indication for further evaluation and cardiac consultation (see Chapter 33).The same pertains to the patient with tricuspid regurgitation and worsening hepatojugular reflux and other signs of right-sided failure.

Counseling is particularly important for the patient with *MVP*. Patients should be informed that MVP is a heterogeneous condition, with most at no increased risk for cardiac complications. Those with readily audible MVP regurgitant murmurs should be advised about the need for endocarditis prophylaxis (see Chapter 16). Those with particularly loud murmurs suggestive of hemodynamically significant disease should be referred for cardiac consultation after undergoing ultrasound examination for confirmation. The vast majority can be reassured that they are at no increased risk and that progression to more serious disease is very rare. Prompt referral is indicated for the rare MVP patient with complex ventricular irritability, prolonged QT intervals, a family history of sudden death, or a transient ischemic event.

A.H.G.

ANNOTATED BIBLIOGRAPHY

Coughlin HC. Mitral valve prolapse: Is echocardiography yielding too little or too much information to the practicing physician?

Am J Med 1989;87:367. *(A strong plea for viewing MVP as a heterogeneous disorder and using ultrasound selectively.)*

Craige E. Should auscultation be rehabilitated? N Engl J Med 1988;318:1611. *(An editorial urging reemphasis on physical diagnosis.)*

Devereaux RB, Kramer-Fox R, Kligfield P. Mitral valve prolapse: Causes, clinical manifestations, and management. Ann Intern Med 1989;111:305. *(Comprehensive review; 172 refs.)*

Finegam RE, Gianelly RD, Harrison DC. Aortic stenosis in the elderly: Relevance of age to diagnosis and treatment. N Engl J Med 1969;281:1261. *(Physical findings such as carotid upstroke and quality and location of the murmur may be misleading in assessing aortic stenosis in the elderly.)*

Folland ED, Kriegel BJ, Henderson WG et al. Implications of third heart sounds in patients with valvular heart disease. N Engl J Med 1992;327:458. *(Indicative of failure in aortic stenosis, but not in mitral regurgitation.)*

Heckerling PS, Wiener SL, Moses VK et al. Accuracy of precordial percussion in detecting cardiomegaly. Am J Med 1991; 91:328. *(Not often performed, but found surprisingly useful.)*

Hershman WY, Moskowitz MA, Marton KI et al. Utility of echocardiography in patients with suspected mitral valve prolapse. Am J Med 1989;87:371. *(Diagnosis changed in 56 percent, treatment in 27 percent, but significance unclear.)*

Lembo NJ, Dell'Italia LJ, Crawford MH et al. Bedside diagnosis of systolic murmurs. N Engl J Med 1988;318:1572. *(One of the few studies providing sensitivity and specificity data on diagnostic maneuvers.)*

Lombard TJ, Selzer A. Valvular aortic stenosis. Ann Intern Med 1987;106:292. *(Clinical presentations of 397 patients, with emphasis on disease in the elderly.)*

Maisel AS, Atwood JE, Goldberger AL. Hepatojugular reflux: Useful in the bedside diagnosis of tricuspid regurgitation. Ann Intern Med 1984;101:781. *(Specificity 100 percent, sensitivity of 66 percent in detecting tricuspid regurgitation; increase in murmur intensity with deep inspiration was as specific and more sensitive.)*

Maron BJ, Bonow RO, Cannon RO 3rd et al. Hypertrophic cardiomyopathy: Interrelations of clinical manifestations, pathophysiology, and therapy; parts 1 and 2. N Engl J Med 1987; 316:844. *(Best discussion of correlations between pathophysiology and clinical findings.)*

Nishimura RA, McGoon MD, Shub C et al. Echocardiographically documented mitral valve prolapse: Long-term follow-up of 237 patients. N Engl J Med 1985;313:1305. *(Identifies a low-risk subgroup.)*

Popp RL. Echocardiography. N Engl J Med 1990;323:101. *(Comprehensive review; over 100 refs.)*

Rothman A, Goldberger AL. Aids to cardiac auscultation. Ann Intern Med 1983;99:346. *(Critical review of maneuvers.)*

Stein PD, Sabbah H. Aortic origin of innocent murmur. Am J Cardiol 1977;39:665. *(Presents extensive data for an aortic origin.)*

Tavel ME. The systolic murmur—innocent or guilty. Am J Cardiol 1977;39:757. *(An editorial arguing that much of the evaluation can be done clinically.)*

Primary Care Medicine: Office Evaluation and Management of the Adult Patient, 3rd edition, edited by Allan H. Goroll, Lawrence A. May, and Albert G. Mulley, Jr. J.B. Lippincott Company, Philadelphia

22
Evaluation of Leg Edema

Leg edema can be a bothersome complaint as well as an initial symptom of important underlying disease. The problem is particularly common in the elderly and usually a manifestation of chronic venous insufficiency, though at times it can be mistaken for congestive heart failure. When acute in onset, the most worrisome concern is deep vein thrombophlebitis. Accurate determination of etiology is essential to prompt recognition of important underlying pathology and initiation of effective treatment. Noninvasive methods have greatly facilitated evaluation, and the primary physician needs to be knowledgeable in their use.

PATHOPHYSIOLOGY AND CLINICAL PRESENTATION

Edema is defined as an increase in extracellular volume. It develops if hydrostatic pressure exceeds colloid oncotic pressure, capillary permeability increases, or lymphatic drainage becomes impaired. Hydrostatic pressure is a function of intravascular volume, blood pressure, and venous outflow. Colloid oncotic pressure is dependent on the serum albumin concentration.

Decreased oncotic pressure is usually due to *hypoalbuminemia,* which can occur secondary to malnutrition, hepatocellular failure, or excess renal or gastrointestinal loss of albumin. The resultant fall in intravascular volume from excessive transudation of fluid stimulates salt retention. This compensatory effort to maintain adequate intravascular volume leads to further edema formation because the underlying oncotic deficit remains. Edema sets in when the serum albumin concentration falls below 2.5g/100mL. Leg swelling due to hypoalbuminemia is typically bilateral, pitting, and sometimes accompanied by edema of the face and eyelids (especially on awakening).

Increased hydrostatic pressure may result from excessive *fluid retention* (such as is seen with congestive heart failure) or *impairment of venous outflow.* A localized increase in hydrostatic pressure develops in the legs during prolonged standing, especially if the valves in the leg veins are incompetent. Increased hydrostatic pressure due to fluid retention produces bilaterally symmetrical edema, whereas swelling due to venous insufficiency may be asymmetrical and accompanied by varicosities and such other signs of venous disease as stasis dermatitis.

Deep vein thrombophlebitis (DVT) may have a very subtle presentation, with acute onset of *unilateral or asymmetric leg edema* as the only manifestation. Such textbook findings as calf tenderness, palpable cord, and positive Homan's sign are often absent. Most clots due to thrombophlebitis form in the small veins of the calf; 20 percent to 30 percent propagate proximally into the popliteal and femoral veins of the knee and thigh. Clot below the knee poses little risk of pulmonary embolization, but extension above the knee markedly increases its chances. Unilateral lower leg edema can also result from venous compression by a *popliteal (Bak-*

er's) cyst. A stroke that causes paresis in one leg may result in unilateral edema due to reductions in vascular tone and venous and lymphatic drainage; thrombophlebitis may ensue.

Increased capillary permeability is another mechanism of leg edema associated with immunologic injury, infection, inflammation, or trauma. A permeability defect is also believed to be responsible for *idiopathic edema,* a poorly understood but common problem seen almost exclusively in women. Although some patients report a periodicity to the problem that seems to parallel the menstrual cycle, careful studies have failed to find sufficient evidence to warrant the label *"cyclic edema."* The condition is especially aggravated by hot weather and standing, more so than occurs with venous insufficiency. Transient abdominal distention is common, and weight may fluctuate several pounds over the course of the day. The disorder is not progressive, but it can cause considerable discomfort. It is often accompanied by headache, fatigue, anxiety, and other functional symptoms. Some patients are bothered by nocturia.

Lymphatic obstruction hinders reabsorption of interstitial fluid. The swelling usually starts in the feet and progresses upward; often the problem is unilateral. The edema of lymphatic obstruction tends to have a brawny quality and evidences little pitting, except in its early stages. Recumbency provides only minor relief compared with edema from other causes.

Table 22-1. Important Causes of Leg Edema

- I. Unilateral or Asymmetric Swelling
  - A. Increased hydrostatic pressure
    1. Deep vein thrombophlebitis
    2. Venous insufficiency
    3. Popliteal (Baker's) cyst
  - B. Increased capillary permeability
    1. Cellulitis
    2. Trauma
  - C. Lymphatic obstruction (local)
- II. Bilateral Swelling
  - A. Decreased oncotic pressure
    1. Malnutrition
    2. Hepatocellular failure
    3. Nephrotic syndrome
    4. Protein-losing enteropathy
  - B. Increased hydrostatic pressure
    1. Congestive heart failure
    2. Renal failure
    3. Use of salt-retaining drugs (eg, corticosteroids, estrogens)
    4. Venous insufficiency
    5. Menstruation
    6. Pregnancy
  - C. Increased capillary permeability
    1. Systemic vasculitis
    2. Idiopathic edema
    3. Allergic reactions
  - D. Lymphatic obstruction (retroperitoneal or generalized)

DIFFERENTIAL DIAGNOSIS

The differential diagnosis of edema can be organized according to clinical presentations and pathophysiologic mechanisms (Table 22–1). Certain infiltrative conditions may be mistaken for edema, such as pretibial myxedema and lipedema (a familial, bilateral deposition of excess fat).

WORKUP

History. The distribution of the swelling should be ascertained from the patient. If edema is predominantly unilateral, the patient ought to be questioned about risk factors for thrombophlebitis such as use of oral contraceptives, recent surgery, previous phlebitis, and prolonged inactivity. Inquiry into recent injury, redness, tenderness, or fever may prove productive. If the edema is bilateral, it is important to check for a history of dyspnea on exertion, orthopnea, ascites, jaundice, proteinuria, chronic kidney disease, malnutrition, varicose veins, chronic diarrhea, rash, and use of salt-retaining drugs such as corticosteroids and estrogens. Antihypertensive drugs, including methyldopa and nifedipine, and nonsteroidal anti-inflammatory drugs, especially ibuprofen, have also been associated with dependent edema. A report of acute facial swelling suggests an allergic reaction or hypoalbuminemia if the swelling is more chronic.

Physical Examination should be used to detail the extent of the edema. Careful measurements of calf and thigh diameters can be very helpful. If the swelling is predominantly limited to one leg, the limb ought to be examined for tenderness, redness, increased warmth, varicosities, and a palpable thrombosed vein. Unfortunately, the utility of the physical examination for detection of deep vein phlebitis is limited. The often-mentioned signs of deep venous thrombosis—calf tenderness, palpable cord, positive Homan's sign—have not proved to be very sensitive or specific; unilateral edema may be the only clue aside from a suggestive history. It is important to check for pitting; if edema is prominent but pitting is only minimal, it suggests that lymphatic obstruction might be the cause.

The patient with bilateral leg edema should have the blood pressure measured for elevation, especially if there is a history of kidney problems; new onset of hypertension may be a sign of renal failure. The skin is checked for signs of hepatocellular failure (jaundice, spider angiomata, ecchymoses), the jugular veins for distention, the chest for rales and evidence of a pleural effusion, the heart for a third heart sound indicative of failure, the abdomen for masses, ascites, and other manifestations of portal hypertension, and the pelvis for masses. Any lymphadenopathy should be noted.

Laboratory Studies. The patient with a question of DVT—including those with acute onset of unexplained unilateral or asymmetric leg edema—requires vascular testing, because clinical findings are a notoriously unreliable basis for initiating anticoagulant therapy. Only 20 percent to 50 percent of patients thought to have DVT on clinical grounds prove to have clot on further testing. Particularly important is detection of DVT above the knee, because clot here is associated with a high risk of pulmonary embolization. Ruling out clot above the knee is a major objective of testing in the patient with unexplained leg edema. High test sensitivity and specificity are required in this setting, not only to rule out DVT, but also to provide sufficient positive predictive value to justify initiation of anticoagulant therapy.

The definitive test for the detection of acute deep vein occlusion has been the *venogram*. When performed and interpreted by an experienced radiologist, it is nearly 100 percent sensitive and specific. However, it is invasive, expensive, often painful, requires considerable expertise to perform and interpret, and includes a small (2%–3%) risk of inducing thrombosis or a hypersensitivity reaction to the contrast medium. Moreover, as many as 25 percent of patients who are candidates for venography have unsuccessful studies. These disadvantages plus the advent of noninvasive methods have relegated venography to a back-up role in the evaluation for DVT.

A number of excellent noninvasive methods have been developed and are becoming more widely available. The combination of B-mode or two-dimensional *ultrasonography* and color-flow *Doppler* ultrasound (so-called triplex scanning) has proven practical and highly sensitive and specific. Failure of the vein to compress during ultrasound scanning is highly correlated with DVT. At times direct visualization of clot is possible. Doppler measures blood flow, helping to identify the vein and any reduction in flow due to clot. Doppler alone is highly technician-dependent. Computerized color enhancement of Doppler data facilitates test performance and interpretation. For detection of thrombophlebitis above the knee, sensitivity and specificity of triplex scanning range from 97 percent to 99 percent. For thrombophlebitis below the knee, sensitivity and specificity fall to 80 percent, because as many as 40 percent of calf vein studies are technically unsuccessful due to poor sound penetration. Successful below-the-knee studies have the same sensitivity and specificity as those above the knee. Duplex ultrasound (triplex minus the color enhancement) is becoming the minimum standard for noninvasive testing for DVT. A technically satisfactory study that is negative for clot above the knee virtually rules out the diagnosis of worrisome DVT. A positive study has a very high predictive value, sufficient to warrant initiating anticoagulation.

Impedance plethysmography remains a widely used noninvasive approach to the diagnosis of DVT. It detects changes in leg volume that follow respiration and inflation and deflation of a thigh blood pressure cuff. In DVT, the normal pattern is altered and detectable by plethysmography. Most reports of test sensitivity range from 83 percent to 93 percent and specificity from 83 percent to 97 percent, but some figures are in the 65 percent to 70 percent range for tests performed in outpatients. The test is somewhat technician-dependent, accounting for some of the variation in test performance figures reported. Calf-vein and nonobstructing thrombi are not well detected. Sensitivity can be enhanced by serial studies, which are obtained if there is suspicion of propagation. The test is useful for detection of recurrent thrombophlebitis, because an abnormal test usually reverts to normal 3 months after initiation of anticoagulant therapy. When specificity in a particular laboratory is less than 90 percent, then the predictive value of a positive test for DVT in a patient with unilateral leg edema will be in the range of 75 percent to 80 percent, not high enough to justify anticoagulation without further confirmatory testing. A negative test in a patient suspected on clinical grounds to have DVT should be followed either by a venogram or by serial plethysmography studies 2 and 4 days after the initial study.

Prior to the onslaught of human immunodeficiency virus (HIV) disease, *^{125}I fibrinogen uptake* scanning held some promise. But because it is made from pooled fibrinogen, its HIV risk is deemed too great, and use of the test has greatly declined. The availability of safer, more accurate tests, and the 24 to 48 hours needed to obtain fibrinogen scan results have all but removed the test from active use.

In the case of suspected lymphedema, venography is the test of first choice for detecting a cause of lymphatic obstruction and should be obtained before *lymphangiography* is attempted. Severe lymphatic obstruction may interfere with attaining a satisfactory lymphangiogram.

The patient with more generalized edema involving both legs should have a *chest film* in search of heart failure and pleural fluid, a *urinalysis* for detection of albuminuria, a check of the serum *albumin*, and determinations of the serum *creatinine* and *blood urea nitrogen (BUN)* for evidence of renal insufficiency. If the serum albumin is low, then measurements of the prothrombin time and liver function testing are indicated for further documentation of hepatocellular failure (see Chapter 71). If the serum albumin is low and protein is detected in the urine, a *24-hour urine* collection for albumin and creatinine is indicated (see Chapter 130).

PATIENT EDUCATION AND SYMPTOMATIC THERAPY

When edema is due to increased hydrostatic pressure or decreased oncotic pressure, a number of simple measures can provide the patient some symptomatic relief. The patient should be advised to *restrict salt* intake, avoid prolonged standing or prolonged sitting with the legs dependent, elevate the legs whenever possible, and avoid wearing garments that might restrict venous return (eg, garters and girdles). Proper *support stockings* might provide some added benefit. If possible, use of salt-retaining drugs should be discontinued or minimized. Severe edema may require *diuretic* therapy. (See Chapter 35 for details on therapy of venous insufficiency.) Lymphatic obstruction and increased capillary permeability do not respond well to these measures.

Patients with idiopathic edema are sometimes helped by salt restriction, support hose, elevation, and diuretic use in the early evening. In addition to diuretics, other drugs have been reported to be useful; these include propranolol and captopril. It is important to reassure the patient with this condition that the edema poses no threat to health. Furthermore, idiopathic edema often runs a self-limited course, subsiding spontaneously over a few months to several years.

Patients with chronic leg edema should be instructed to call the physician at the first sign of unilateral increase in swelling or pain, because they are at increased risk of thrombophlebitis.

A.H.G.

ANNOTATED BIBLIOGRAPHY

Anderson DR, Lensing AWA, Wells PS et al. Limitations of impedance plethysmography in the diagnosis of clinically suspected deep-vein thrombosis. Ann Intern Med 1993;118:25. *(A study in outpatients; reports lower sensitivity than widely quoted.)*

Bettmann MA, Robbins A, Braun SD et al. Contrast venography of the leg: Diagnostic efficacy, tolerance, and complication rates with ionic and nonionic contrast media. Radiology 1987;165:113. *(Critical review of the methodology.)*

Cranley JJ, Canos AJ, Sull WJ. The diagnosis of deep vein thrombosis, fallibility of clinical symptoms and signs. Arch Surg 1976;111:34. *(Classic signs of deep vein thrombosis occurred with approximately equal frequency in people with and without deep vein thrombosis.)*

Huisman MV, Buller HR, Tencate JW et al. Serial impedance plethysmography for suspected deep venous thrombosis in outpatients. N Engl J Med 1986;314:823. *(Sensitivity enhanced by serial studies; especially useful for detection of propagating clot.)*

Lensing AWA, Prandoni P, Brandjes D et al. Detection of deep-vein thrombosis by real-time B-mode ultrasonography. N Engl J Med 1989;320:342. *(Sensitivity 100 percent, specificity 99 percent for clot above the knee; both fall to 80 percent for clot below the knee.)*

Philbrick JT, Becker DM. Calf deep venous thrombosis. A wolf in sheep's clothing? Arch Intern Med 1988;148:2131. *(Twenty percent to 30 percent of patients with calf-vein thrombosis have proximal propagation.)*

Rose SC, Zwiebel WJ, Nelson BD et al. Symptomatic lower extremity deep venous thrombosis: Accuracy, limitations, and role of color duplex flow imaging in diagnosis. Radiology 1990;175:639. *(Accuracy 99 percent for DVT above the knee, but only 81 percent below the knee.)*

Streeten DHP. Idiopathic edema: Pathogenesis, clinical futures and treatment. Metabolism 1978;27:353. *(Comprehensive review; concludes that upright posture is an important contributor to excess transudation of fluid in more than 30 percent.)*

White RH, McGahan JP, Daschbach MM et al. Diagnosis of deep-vein thrombosis using duplex ultrasound. Ann Intern Med 1989;111:297. *(A review of available studies; combined figures for sensitivity and specificity in the range of 95 percent for DVT above the knee; 51 refs.)*

23
Evaluation of Arterial Insufficiency of the Lower Extremities

DAVID C. BREWSTER, M.D.

Primary Care Medicine: Office Evaluation and Management of the Adult Patient, 3rd edition, edited by Allan H. Goroll, Lawrence A. May, and Albert G. Mulley, Jr. J.B. Lippincott Company, Philadelphia

Vascular occlusive disease of the lower extremities is seen with greater frequency as patients continue to live longer and their atherosclerosis progresses. Arteriosclerotic occlusive disease is by far the most common cause of arterial insufficiency, although lower extremity ischemia may also be caused by embolism, arterial dissection, trauma, thrombosis of an aneurysm, or other unusual conditions. It is more common in men and increases in prevalence with age. Approximately 5 percent of patients older than 70 years of age have symptomatic disease.

Proper clinical management requires the physician first to recognize the manifestations of ischemic disease and carefully evaluate its severity. Many patients with mild to moderate vascular insufficiency can be managed conservatively, whereas others with acute ischemia or more severe chronic ischemia that threatens to cause tissue necrosis require more intensive investigation and often surgery (see Chapter 34).

The primary physician must be able to differentiate between patients with arterial insufficiency and those with exertional limb pain due to other causes. Moreover, one needs to know the indications for and limitations of the newer noninvasive techniques for evaluating blood flow and the indications for arteriography and surgical referral.

PATHOPHYSIOLOGY AND CLINICAL PRESENTATION

Occlusive disease generally becomes symptomatic by gradual reduction of blood flow to the involved extremity or organ. Symptoms finally occur when a critical arterial stenosis is reached. Pressure and blood flow are not significantly diminished until at least 75 percent of the cross-sectional area of the vessel lumen is obliterated by the disease process. This is approximately equivalent to a 50 percent reduction in lumen diameter. More severe stenoses or even total occlusions may remain essentially asymptomatic as long as collateral circulation maintains sufficient blood flow around a lesion to satisfy the metabolic demands of the distal limb at rest and during exercise. Development of ischemic symptoms in the leg implies either inadequate collateral circulation or additional occlusive disease distal to the particular collateral bed. Thus, lesions in the aortoiliac segment may cause little difficulty unless, as is commonly the case, there is associated disease in the femoropopliteal arterial territory.

Arteriosclerotic plaques producing stenosis or occlusion of the arterial lumen are often segmentally distributed, with a predilection for arterial bifurcations. The infrarenal abdominal aorta and aortic bifurcation are common sites of disease, as are the iliac and femoral artery bifurcations. Diabetic patients seem prone to onset of arteriosclerosis at an earlier age and often have a more distal distribution of occlusive arterial lesions.

The earliest manifestation of impaired arterial circulation is usually *intermittent claudication*, or muscular pain in the leg brought on by exercise and relieved within several minutes by rest. Blood flow is adequate for local metabolic demands at rest but cannot increase sufficiently to meet the increased oxygen demands of the muscle mass resulting from exercise, a situation quite analogous to the pain of angina pectoris. The relatively high resistance across collateral vessel beds limits the required threefold to fourfold increase of blood flow to the exercising leg.

As the severity of the occlusive process worsens, blood flow becomes inadequate for tissue needs even at rest, resulting in the manifestations of more severe arterial insufficiency: *ischemic rest pain* and tissue *necrosis* (ischemic ulceration or gangrene). Rest pain typically occurs at night from leg elevation associated with lying in bed. Patients complain of diffuse foot discomfort on the affected side. Ischemic ulcers are painful and appear as punched out lesions on the dorsum or lateral aspect of the foot.

Peripheral arterial insufficiency has three basic anatomic variations, though any number many be present in a given patient. Aortoiliac disease is most common in patients who smoke or have hypercholesterolemia. Claudication in the buttock or thigh is characteristic. The femoral pulses are absent or diminished, but pedal pulses may be intact. *Femoropopliteal disease* accounts for two-thirds of cases and presents as calf pain with exertion. Femoral pulses may be preserved, but popliteal and pedal pulses are absent or diminished. *Tibioperoneal occlusion* is a disease of diabetics and older patients. Skin ulcers and atrophic skin changes are common.

The *clinical course* is quite variable and often favorable. In the Framingham study population, only one-third of those developing claudication went on to have persistent symptoms; the remainder experienced remission or transient symptoms. However, 15 percent of those presenting with severe disease required amputation over the ensuing 2 years. Persistent smokers and diabetics have the worst prognoses.

DIFFERENTIAL DIAGNOSIS

Lower extremity ischemia may also be caused by arterial embolism, dissection, trauma, thrombosis of an aneurysm, or thromboangiitis obliterans (Buerger's disease). Other nonvascular conditions may mimic the symptoms of claudication or ischemic rest pain. Pain in the hip, thigh, or knee region with walking is frequently a result of *degenerative disc disease*, *osteoarthritis* of the hip or knee, or *Paget's disease*. Sciatic or other radicular pain may cause confusion. Various other neurologic or musculoskeletal disorders may be at fault. *Cauda equina compression* by disc, tumor, or spinal canal stenosis produces a well-known *"pseudoclaudication"* syndrome. Such nonvascular causes of pain may be suspected when pain is not clearly related to a predictable amount of exercise and is not promptly relieved by cessation of activity. *Nocturnal leg cramps* are commonly mistaken for ischemic pain, being localized to the calf but differing in that they are exclusively a nighttime phenomenon.

Diabetic neuropathy can be difficult to differentiate from ischemic rest pain, particularly in a patient with diminished or absent pulses. In both conditions, a burning constant ache is often present in the forefoot and toes. The presence of paresthesias in addition to pain suggests a neurologic source. True ischemic rest pain is usually worse with elevation and frequently is relieved somewhat by dependency of the limb. Such features may be used in differentiation. In all such instances, noninvasive studies during exercise may be of substantial help in the differential diagnosis.

WORKUP

The diagnosis of peripheral vascular disease and an accurate assessment of its level and severity may be made by a careful history and physical examination to an extent not usually possible in many other disease states. The availability of effective treatment for peripheral vascular disease makes it mandatory that early and accurate diagnosis be established before end-stage problems develop and threaten limb loss.

History. *Intermittent claudication* is the hallmark of vascular insufficiency, and a reliable history can be diagnostic. The pain of claudication is usually described as a cramp or ache in the *calf* or *thigh* muscles after walking a predictable distance. The location of the pain may help to localize the occlusive process. In some instances of proximal disease, the pain may be located principally in the hip or buttock region, causing confusion with other neuro-orthopedic conditions. The pain should be reproducible by *walking* a certain distance and should be relieved within minutes of stopping. If the walking distance required to produce the pain varies considerably from day to day, or if the patient must sit or lie down for more than several minutes to obtain relief, the physician should suspect a nonvascular cause, such as spinal stenosis. Weight bearing and other activities that extend the lumbar spine will aggravate the pain of spinal stenosis. Similarly, the pain should involve the same areas consistently and not different portions of the leg from day to day. Crampy pain occurring in the calf at rest, particularly at night, rarely signifies a vascular problem.

Complaints of *pain at rest* as well as with exercise suggests more advanced ischemia. A history of prior claudication is almost always obtained in such patients unless the distribution of the occlusive process is quite distal or in small vessels only. Ischemic rest pain typically involves the toes or forefoot, not the calf or thigh. It is usually improved with dependency of the limb and therefore is worse at night. Pain that is not confined to the distal foot, that is better with elevation, or that occurs in a patient without intermittent claudication should alert the physician to look for other possible causes, such as diabetic neuropathy or a neuro-orthopedic problem.

Symptoms of tissue necrosis will usually be quite apparent. Peripheral gangrene without prior symptoms should raise the possibility of embolic disease or small vessel occlusions due to conditions other than chronic arteriosclerosis. In patients with leg ulceration, historical clues suggesting a traumatic, dermatologic, or venous origin should also be sought; many leg and foot ulcers are not ischemic in origin.

A complete history should include questioning for sexual difficulties; erectile *impotence*, long associated with severe aortoiliac occlusive disease, has been termed the *Leriche syndrome* after the French surgeon who first reported its significance in 1923. Finally, it is of utmost importance to note the existence of known risk factors for arteriosclerosis (eg, family history, smoking, diabetes mellitus, hypertension, lipid disorders) as well as related problems in the coronary and cerebrovascular systems indicative of the systemic nature of the atherosclerosis. There is a high prevalence of coronary disease, stroke, and congestive failure in patients with peripheral arterial disease.

Physical Examination can help confirm, localize, and establish the severity of the arterial lesion. *Palpation of peripheral pulses* is the keystone of the examination. Palpation of the abdomen for the aortic pulsation, and of both extremities for femoral, popliteal, posterior tibial, and dorsalis pedis pulses should be routine in all patients. Reduced or absent pulses in the symptomatic region are characteristic of arterial insufficiency. In one study, the absence of the posterior tibial pulse was the best predictor of peripheral arterial disease. Local factors such as edema or marked obesity may hinder palpation. Abnormally prominent pulsations suggest aneurysmal disease. *Auscultation* of the aortic and groin regions should also be performed, with the finding of *bruits* further supporting the possible existence of arterial occlusive disease. Simple exercise of the patient at the bedside may greatly intensify femoral bruits, and this is occasionally a useful maneuver. The absence of a bruit, however, has little meaning, since marked reduction of flow in a severely stenotic or occluded vessel will not produce a bruit.

Other useful findings are abnormal pallor on elevation of the legs, *rubor on dependency,* and *prolonged capillary filling time* (especially when one leg is compared with the other). Temperature differences and atrophic skin and nail changes are less reliable indicators of chronic arterial insufficiency. Careful spine, hip, knee, and neurologic examinations are important to rule out nonvascular causes of exertional lower extremity pain.

History and physical examination are usually sufficient to establish the diagnosis and provide a rough estimate of severity. In patients with mild to moderate disease and without limb-threatening ischemia or unacceptable activity limitations, no further investigation is necessary other than evaluation for potential *risk factors* such as smoking, diabetes, hypertension, and hyperlipidemia (see Chapters 14, 15, 54, and 93). Blood sugar determination may detect a previously undiagnosed diabetic, but there is still no firm evidence that tight control of the serum glucose level prevents or ameliorates vascular disease (see Chapter 102).

In patients with premature atherosclerotic disease but no evident precipitants, the possibility of *hyperhomocysteinemia* deserves consideration. The relation between this inborn error of metabolism and vascular disease has now been established. Diagnosis is suggested by elevated serum homocysteine levels after overnight methionine-loading.

Noninvasive Vascular Laboratory Studies are indicated if the diagnosis or degree of impairment is uncertain, or if the disease is severe enough to warrant consideration of surgical correction. A wide variety of noninvasive testing methods is available, ranging from segmental blood pressure measurements to Doppler and two-dimensional ultrasound techniques. These methods are becoming widely available and are relatively simple to use, inexpensive compared to angiography, and without risk or discomfort to the patient. Such tests may be extremely helpful in establishing a vascular etiology for complaints of pain in the leg and in quantifying clinical impressions, which are often somewhat imprecise. Because they can be used repeatedly, such tests are also particularly helpful in evaluating improvement or deterioration of the patient's condition over time and in assessing the benefit of various forms of treatment or operation.

Segmental blood pressure measurements are taken at the arm, upper thigh, above and below the knee, and above the ankle with the patient supine. A Doppler device measures systolic pressure in each location. Normally there is an increase in pressure as the pressure wave moves distally. A reduction in pressure suggests arterial occlusion. Sensitivity and specificity are maximized by using the ratio of ankle to brachial systolic pressures. An ankle/brachial ratio or "index" of less than 0.9 has a 95 percent sensitivity in patients with angiographically proven disease and a 100 percent specificity in normals. Segmental pressures can be used as a screening test for further evaluation and in gauging severity. A ratio of less than 0.8 correlates with moderate disease, 0.6 with severe or multilevel disease, and less than 0.4 with severe disease and a high risk of complications. The test is not reliable in patients with calcified vessels (eg, diabetics).

Pulse-volume recordings are particularly useful for assessment of distal vascular disease, especially in patients with stiff vessels. Doppler and plethysmographic methods are used. The patient with stiff vessels and distal disease may have a normal ankle pressure, but the normally sharp pulse-volume wave form becomes blunted with obstruction. Sensitivity is improved when treadmill exercise is added to the examination. Diabetics, who tend to have stiff vessels and distal disease, are good candidates for pulse-volume recording.

Duplex ultrasonic scanning combines two-dimensional (B-mode) real-time ultrasound with pulsed Doppler to provide more precise anatomic and flow data than are available from other methods. The ultrasound probe is placed over specific vessels to measure velocity of flow. B-mode ultrasound identifies the site and nature of the stenosis. Adding *color-flow enhancement* (triplex scanning) improves test performance. Triplex scanning has a sensitivity of 88 percent and a specificity of 95 percent; the figures for duplex scanning are 82 percent and 92 percent, respectively. Although such examinations are somewhat time-consuming and require an experienced examiner, they are likely to play an increasing role in noninvasively assessing peripheral vascular disease.

It should be emphasized that these methods are not meant to replace or lessen the value of a good history and physical examination but rather to supplement them and provide such additional information as site and severity of stenosis.

Arteriography has little place in the diagnostic evaluation of arterial insufficiency. However, once a decision has been reached for surgical intervention (see Chapter 34), arteriography is indicated. The procedure is generally regarded as indispensable to the surgeon for precise localization of the disease process and proper selection of the most appropriate invasive procedure.

INDICATIONS FOR REFERRAL AND ADMISSION

Patients with rest pain or a nonhealing ischemic ulcer require consideration for surgery and ought to be referred to an experienced vascular surgeon. Patients with severe intermittent claudication that interferes with daily activity may also benefit from a surgical consultation but often can be managed conservatively (see Chapter 34). Patients with gangrenous lesions of the lower extremities or an infected ischemic ulcer require prompt hospital admission, particularly if they are diabetic.

ANNOTATED BIBLIOGRAPHY

Baker JD. The vascular laboratory. In Moore WUS (ed): Vascular Surgery: A Comprehensive Review, 3rd ed, pp 168–185. Philadelphia, WB Saunders, 1991. *(A thorough discussion of the use of the vascular laboratory in the care of patients with peripheral vascular disease; excellent reference list.)*

Clarke R, Daly L, Robinson K et al. Hyperhomocysteinemia: An independent risk factor for vascular disease. N Engl J Med 1991;324:1149. *(Documents this condition to be an independent and important risk factor for premature vascular disease.)*

Criqui MH, Fronek A, Klauber MR et al. The sensitivity, specificity, and predictive value of traditional clinical evaluation of peripheral arterial disease: Results from noninvasive testing in a defined population. Circulation 1985;71:240. *(Lack of a posterior tibial pulse was the single best predictor of peripheral vascular disease.)*

Goodreau JK, Creasy JK, Flanigan DP et al. Rational approach to the differentiation of vascular and neurogenic claudication. Surgery 1979;84:749. *(Helpful discussion of diagnostic approach useful in differentiating vascular and nonvascular exercise-related pain.)*

Kohler TR, Nance DR, Cramer MM et al. Duplex scanning for diagnosis of aortoiliac and femoropopliteal disease: A prospective study. Circulation 1987;76;1074. *(Well designed study showing a favorable comparison between duplex scanning and conventional arteriography in the diagnosis of peripheral vascular disease.)*

Lynch T, Hobson RW, Wright CB et al. Interpretation of Doppler segmental pressure in peripheral vascular occlusive disease. Arch Surg 1984;119:465. *(Useful discussion of the method and its sensitivity and specificity.)*

Polack JF, Karmel MI, Mannick JA et al. Determination of the extent of lower-extremity peripheral arterial disease with color-assisted duplex sonography: Comparison with angiography. AJR Am J Roentgenol 1990;1550:1085. *(Description of the methodology; sensitivity 88 percent, specificity 95 percent.)*

Strandness DE Jr, Langlois YE, Roederer GO. Noninvasive evaluation of vascular disease. In Haimovici H (ed): Vascular Surgery: Principles and Techniques, 3rd ed, pp 17–38. Norwalk, Appleton & Lange, 1989. *(Good review of noninvasive techniques to assess peripheral vascular disorders.)*

Primary Care Medicine: Office Evaluation and Management of the Adult Patient, 3rd edition, edited by Allan H. Goroll, Lawrence A. May, and Albert G. Mulley, Jr. J.B. Lippincott Company, Philadelphia

24
Evaluation of Syncope

Syncope and near-syncope are among the most difficult of conditions to evaluate, especially when recurrent and not accompanied by readily identifiable precipitants. Often contributing to the diagnostic difficulty are vague descriptions of the event, an unrevealing physical examination, and initial laboratory studies that are unremarkable. When confronted with a report of loss of consciousness, the primary physician first needs to check for an underlying cardiovascular or seizure disorder, for these may require prompt attention. In about 50 percent of cases, the cause of syncope will not be evident on initial evaluation, necessitating consideration of a more extensive workup. A detailed knowledge of important clinical clues and a thorough understanding of the indications for and limitations of available testing modalities are essential for a cost-effective evaluation of this difficult problem.

PATHOPHYSIOLOGY AND CLINICAL PRESENTATIONS

Syncope may ensue from inadequate cerebral perfusion, seizure activity, severe metabolic derangement, or psychological disturbance. The pathophysiologic common denominator of many cases is inadequate cerebral perfusion. Contributing mechanisms include sudden decrease in peripheral vascular resistance, inadequate cardiac output, failure of vasoconstrictive reflexes, and functional or anatomic cerebral vascular occlusion. Any number may be operative in a given case. Metabolic disturbances, such as hypoglycemia, hypocarbia, and hypoxia, usually do not result in syncope unless profound, though they may alter consciousness. Generalized seizure activity that spreads to the brainstem will rapidly lead to loss of consciousness. Most psychogenic precipitants of syncope operate by the neurocardiovascular mechanisms noted above, with the exception of hysteria, in which there may not be a true loss of consciousness.

Neurocardiogenic Syncope, previously referred to as "vasodepressor" or "vasovagal" syncope, accounts for a large number of cases, especially those occurring in otherwise healthy young persons. Although the precise mechanistic details are still being elucidated, its hallmarks are inappropriate bradycardia and vasodilation. The normal compensatory responses to standing up are vasoconstriction, tachycardia, withdrawal of vagal tone, and release of vasoconstricting and volume-retaining hormones (renin and vasopressin). In persons with neurocardiogenic syncope, there is interruption of these sympathetic reflex responses and an increase in vagal activity. The result is *bradycardia, vasodilation,* and marked falls in systemic blood pressure and cerebral perfusion. Among the explanations advanced to account for the phenomenon are excessive vagal tone, excessive initial sympathetic stimulation producing very vigorous contractions that overstimulate intracardiac parasympathetic mechanoreceptors, and hypersensitivity of these receptors. Beta-blockers and disopyramide have been found helpful. The myocardium and conduction system are normal—an important reason why prognosis is excellent.

Clinical presentations range from the common "simple faint" associated with emotional distress to the near-syncopal episode of a trained athlete in the midst of competition. Distention of a viscus (as occurs in performing an esophagoscopy, pleural tap, or bladder puncture) may also trigger an episode.

The patient experiences *premonitory symptoms* of sweating, epigastric queasiness, light-headedness, and pallor. Dilation of the pupils, blurring of vision, yawning and sighing, or hyperventilation may occur. The patient feels restless and unable to concentrate. At the outset, the heart rate may be rapid, but it slows markedly as the process unfolds. The onset of premonitory symptoms usually helps prevent a drop attack and resultant injury. After several minutes, full consciousness is regained, though weakness, sweatiness, and nausea may persist. Control of bladder and bowels is never lost.

The presence of *pallor* and *diaphoresis* is paradoxical, but both may be prominent and reflect the high circulating levels of epinephrine found in this state of otherwise marked sympathetic inhibition. Such features make for a very distressing clinical presentation, mimicking serious cardiovascular disease.

Sometimes the hypotension and hypoperfusion that occur are so profound that cerebral hypoxia and seizure activity (*convulsive syncope*) ensue. This convulsive syncope is distinct from loss of consciousness that accompanies a generalized seizure disorder and does not respond to antiseizure medication.

Tilt-table study can reproduce the symptoms in susceptible persons. Many patients report a prodrome of blurred vision, vertigo, tinnitus, and nausea when tested on a tilt table (see below).

Autonomic Insufficiency is another cause of reduced cerebral perfusion pressure, and it is particularly important in the setting of a fall in intravascular volume from dehydration or acute blood loss. On standing, the patient experiences *orthostatic hypotension*, because reflex vasoconstriction and increase in heart rate fail to occur. Hypotension progresses over seconds to a few minutes, until perfusion is inadequate for maintenance of consciousness. During the presyncopal period, there is no increase in heart rate or other signs of autonomic response, such as pallor, nausea, or sweating. The period of syncope is brief, and consciousness returns promptly. Near-syncope is common among these patients, as are impotence and bladder and bowel disturbances.

Carotid Sinus Hypersensitivity can cause marked *reflex bradycardia* and a fall in arterial resistance. Most patients with this condition are elderly and have underlying atherosclerotic heart disease manifested by ischemic changes on electrocardiogram (ECG). Massage of the carotid sinus often results in long asystolic pauses. Digitalis administration seems to aggravate the condition. Carotid sinus syncope may also cause a vasodepressor form of syncope in which heart rate remains unchanged. Minor events can trigger symptoms; wearing a tight collar, turning the head, or shaving may cause light-headedness, sweating, pallor, and nausea, followed by fainting. When the predominant mechanism is asystole, the loss of consciousness can be precipitous.

Posttussive Syncope is characterized by loss of consciousness that follows a prolonged bout of forceful coughing. Men with chronic bronchitis are most often affected. The mechanism is believed to involve decreased cardiac output due to decreased venous return, increased cerebral vascular resistance secondary to hypocapnia, and compression of cerebral vessels by an increase in cerebrospinal fluid pressure. Prolonged Valsalva maneuvers have a similar effect; the increase in intrathoracic pressure impedes venous return and decreases cardiac output.

Postmicturition Syncope takes place in the context of emptying a distended bladder. The typical setting involves a male who has gotten up at night to urinate after consuming considerable amounts of alcohol. Consciousness is lost without much warning. Drainage of ascitic fluid or a distended bladder may produce a similar effect. The mechanism is unknown. Valsalva maneuver and reflex vasodilation have been implicated. Valsalva plays an important role in *postdefecation syncope*, in which straining decreases venous return and consequently cardiac output.

Cerebrovascular Disease leads to syncope if there is vertebrobasilar insufficiency of the midbrain affecting the reticular activating system or in the rare instance of total or near-total occlusion of the major vessels supplying the brain. Lesser degrees of obstruction may contribute to minor light-headedness on standing and can be aggravated by use of antihypertensive agents and volume depletion. Patients with substantial cerebrovascular disease often have evidence of previous strokes manifested by focal neurologic deficits. A *transient ischemic attack* involving the vertebrobasilar circulation may lead to syncope by temporarily depriving the brainstem's reticular activating system of adequate perfusion. Brainstem neurologic deficits typically accompany or precede the loss of consciousness.

The Subclavian Steal Syndrome results from occlusion of the proximal subclavian artery, leading to reversal of flow in the adjacent vertebral artery. When vascular resistance in the arm falls, for example, during exercise, flow is redirected away from the brain and ischemic symptoms may ensue.

Effort Syncope occurs in the setting of underlying *valvular heart disease*. Exercise induces peripheral vasodilation, but cardiac output cannot be increased adequately and syncope results. *Severe aortic stenosis* and marked *hypertrophic cardiomyopathy* obstruct the ventricular outflow tract to a degree sufficient to limit cardiac response to exercise (see Chapter 33). Total blockade of the mitral orifice from an *atrial myxoma* and *pulmonary hypertension* can have similar consequences. Loss of consciousness comes with little warning.

Cardiac Dysrhythmias may precipitate sudden loss of consciousness with none of the premonitory manifestations of neurocardiogenic syncope. Important dysrhythmias associated with syncope include *complete heart block* (Stokes-Adams attacks) and *ventricular tachycardia* (see Chapter 29). Occasionally, a supraventricular tachycardia with a very rapid ventricular response rate will sufficiently compromise cardiac output to result in near-syncope (see Chapter 28). Once effective systoles have ceased, fewer than 5 seconds of consciousness remain. Palpitations are sometimes reported, and loss of consciousness can occur while the patient is supine. Common precipitants of these dysrhythmias include acute ischemia, sick sinus syndrome, digitalis toxicity, and the preexcitation syndromes. Patients with chronic bifascicular and trifascicular block are more likely to have syncopal attacks, but those with syncope have not been found to have an increased risk of sudden death.

Seizures differ from other causes of syncope in that aura, postictal symptoms, incontinence, and tonic–clonic movements often dominate the clinical picture. However, akinetic petit mal attacks have few of these features, though normal blood pressure and pulse help distinguish them from seizures having cardiovascular causes (see Chapter 170). As noted above, convulsions may occur in the setting of vagally mediated cerebral hypoperfusion in the absence of an underlying seizure disorder.

Hysteria produces syncope characterized by graceful fainting to the floor or couch, frequent presence of an audience, normal pulse, skin color, and blood pressure, and an emotionally detached description of the episode.

Metabolic Factors (eg, hypoxia, hypocarbia, hypoglycemia) are more likely to alter consciousness than to cause actual syncope. Restlessness, confusion, and anxiety are prominent and precede loss of consciousness. When hyperventilation is responsible, the patient first complains of a smothering or suffocating feeling in conjunction with paresthesias in the limbs and circumorally (see Chapter 226). Syncope may take place while the patient is sitting or lying down. Hypoglycemia rarely causes loss of consciousness (see Chapter 97).

Table 24-1. Important Causes of Syncope

1. Cardiac
   a. Arrhythmias (sick sinus syndrome, ventricular tachycardia, very rapid supraventricular tachycardia)
   b. Heart block (Stokes-Adams attacks)
   c. Aortic stenosis, severe
   d. Asymmetric septal hypertrophy, severe
   e. Primary pulmonary hypertension
   f. Atrial myxoma
   g. Prolapsed mitral valve
2. Vascular-Reflex
   a. Neurocardiogenic (vasovagal, vasodepressor)
   b. Orthostatic hypotension (ganglionic blocking agents, diabetes, old age, prolonged bed rest)
   c. Carotid sinus hypersensitivity
   d. Cerebral vascular disease, severe
   e. Subclavian steal syndrome
   f. Post-tussive syncope
   g. Valsalva syncope
   h. Postmicturition syncope (emptying distended bladder)
3. Psychologic–Neurologic
   a. Seizures
   b. Hysteria
4. Metabolic
   a. Hyperventilation
   b. Hypoxia
   c. Hypoglycemia (rarely)

DIFFERENTIAL DIAGNOSIS

Important causes of syncope are listed in Table 24–1. In a series of 176 ambulatory patients evaluated for syncope, 9 percent had a cardiac etiology, 45 percent had some form of vasomotor instability, 1 percent had seizures, 6 percent had other causes, and 39 percent were unexplained. In the elderly, the prevalence of cardiac disease among patients presenting with syncope increases to about 33 percent. Of those cases that remain unexplained after initial evaluation, many will remain undiagnosed even after extensive investigation, though growing appreciation of neurocardiogenic syncope is likely to reduce this number (see below).

The prognosis for syncope due to underlying cardiac disease is much worse (1-year mortality rates of 18%–33%) than that for noncardiac or unexplained syncope (1-year mortality rates of 6%–12%). In the elderly with unexplained syncope, the mortality rate nearly doubles. However, recurrence rates are similar for both categories (about 33%), and recurrence is not a risk factor for adverse outcome.

WORKUP

The principal task is to differentiate between cardiac and noncardiac etiologies, since prognosis is poorest for those with underlying heart disease. History, physical findings, and the resting 12-lead ECG are the most valuable elements of the initial evaluation of syncope. These alone provide a diagnosis in 60 percent to 85 percent of cases in which a diagnosis is eventually made. The physician and patient should appreciate that exhaustive laboratory evaluation often fails to identify a cause for syncope and, in many instances, is wasteful. Fortunately, the prognosis for patients with a single unexplained episode of syncope is excellent. Nonetheless, a detailed search for underlying heart disease is essential and a major priority in the evaluation. Detection of a seizure disorder with its potential for associated neuropathology ranks as another important priority.

History

The differentiation of cardiac and neurologic disease from less worrisome etiologies begins with a *thorough description* of the syncopal event and its surrounding circumstances. The absence of premonitory symptoms in the presyncopal period is consistent with a sudden fall in cardiac output or the abrupt onset of generalized seizure activity. Nausea, diaphoresis, pallor, and light-headedness are more typical of reflex and vascular causes. If recall of premonitory details is sketchy, one should be careful about interrogating the patient too vigorously with leading questions, for the absence of associated or prodromal symptoms may have important diagnostic meaning. Although a seizure disorder may present with sudden loss of consciousness and no warning, more typically there are some vague premonitory symptoms as well as the characteristic tonic–clonic movements and sphincter incontinence.

Identification of precipitants requires asking about emotional upsets, crowded hot surroundings, sudden standing, prolonged and forceful coughing, Valsalva maneuvers, micturition, vigorous exercise, hyperventilation, and symptoms of acute blood loss. Effort syncope suggests hemodynamically significant ventricular outflow tract obstruction. Exertional chest pain is another important clue of underlying organic heart disease. Position just prior to syncope is worth noting, because loss of consciousness while recumbent argues against a reflex or vascular mechanism.

The *past medical history* should be searched for prior infarction, heart murmur, and use of cardioactive medications. A history of diabetes, stroke, use of antihypertensive agents, prolonged bed rest, impotence, and bladder and bowel incontinence should be checked for when the patient reports light-headedness or syncope on standing.

Reports from *witnesses* should be sought whenever possible. Activity, position, complaints, and appearance prior to syncope as well as duration of the episode, associated motor activity, and behavior on regaining consciousness deserve attention. Some observers will even be able to report pulse and respirations.

A seizure disorder is usually not difficult to distinguish from cardiac syncope because of the preceding aura, motor activity, incontinence, and postictal symptoms of confusion, drowsiness, and paresis. However, when there are no motor manifestations, as in akinetic petit mal seizures, the differentiation may be impossible to make by history alone.

It is important not to mistake other conditions for true loss of consciousness. Vertigo (see Chapter 166), neuroglycopenic symptoms (see Chapter 97), and the light-headedness associated with an anxiety attack (see Chapter 226) are sometimes confused with syncope.

Physical Examination

The emphasis is again on the cardiovascular system. *Postural signs* provide essential information. *Blood pressure* and *pulse* are first measured in both arms with the patient lying supine for about 5 minutes and again on standing up. Most patients who demonstrate a postural fall in blood pressure will do so within 30 to 60 seconds of assuming the standing position. However, it may be necessary to wait as long as 5 minutes. Recent studies have found that 95 percent of cases with postural hypotension will be detected within 2 minutes of standing and most within 30 to 60 seconds. The skin is checked for pallor and ecchymoses (the latter, a sign of trauma from a seizure). Torso and head, including the tongue, require scrutiny for signs of trauma sustained during a motor seizure.

Carotid pulses are auscultated for bruits and gently palpated for volume and carotid upstroke (see Chapter 33). If there is no evidence of carotid artery disease, one can massage the carotid and observe for reflex bradycardia and hypotension. The maneuver is indicated when a hypersensitive carotid sinus reflex is suspected, as in elderly patients with unexplained falls. However, because it may also cut off blood supply and cause syncope when there is severe cerebral occlusive disease, it should not be attempted in such patients.

The neck veins are noted for distention and the chest for rales and rhonchi. The *heart* is palpated for heaves and thrills and is auscultated for clicks and murmurs with the patient in the supine, decubitus, and sitting positions. Systolic murmurs should be evaluated for evidence of aortic stenosis, asymmetric septal hypertrophy (ASH), and mitral valve prolapse (see Chapter 21). A variable diastolic murmur raises the question of atrial myxoma. Neurologic assessment includes a search for focal deficits indicative of prior stroke.

Provocative maneuvers are particularly helpful in identifying conditions that alter consciousness but do not cause syncope. Asking the patient to voluntarily hyperventilate or spin around may reproduce symptoms and confirm a clinical suspicion. Exercising the arm is worthwhile if subclavian steal syndrome is suspected.

Laboratory Studies

Unselective use of the wide array of available laboratory studies for evaluation of the patient with syncope of is very cost-ineffective. Though one wants to be sure not to miss the patient with underlying cardiovascular disease, test selection should be based on an assessment of the pretest probability of the condition in question. Yield in patients with very low pretest probabilities is extremely low, and risk of false-positives is high (see Chapter 2).

Electrocardiogram. Most patients should have an ECG performed at the time of initial evaluation, since detection of underlying heart disease remains a major priority of the diagnostic workup. One needs to check not only for ischemic changes, heart block, and tachyarrhythmias, but also for subtle clues such as a short PR interval, delta waves, or new onset of bundle branch block. However, neither an ECG nor other laboratory studies is necessary when the history strongly suggests a harmless faint brought on by emotional factors, the physical examination is normal, and the patient has no risk factors for organic heart disease.

Holter Monitoring. If the ECG is unrevealing but an arrhythmia, transient heart block, or other form of underlying heart disease is still suspected on clinical grounds (eg, sudden loss of consciousness without warning, effort syncope, chest pain), then a *24-hour ambulatory ECG recording (Holter monitor)* deserves consideration. Holter monitoring has become an almost routine part of the syncope workup, especially in patients who remain undiagnosed after initial history, physical examination, and resting ECG. Yet, the correlation between findings on Holter monitoring and symptoms is poor. In a study of more than 1500 patients referred for Holter studies because of syncope, arrhythmia-related symptoms occurred in only 2 percent Syncope or, more commonly, presyncope occurred without an associated arrhythmia in 15 percent.

Though the correlation between symptoms and Holter findings is not strong, Holter findings do provide an independent assessment of risk for underlying heart disease and sudden death. Syncopal patients with frequent premature ventricular contractions (>10/h), repetitive premature ventricular contractions (≥2 in a row), or sinus pauses (>2 sec) on Holter monitoring were found in a major 2-year study to be at increased risk of sudden death and overall mortality. The risk was independent of other factors, and patients with these findings constituted a high-risk subgroup that deserved further cardiac evaluation. There may be an increase in yield of arrhythmias detected if Holter monitoring is extended to 48 hours, but many are asymptomatic and of unclear significance.

Longer-term monitoring for symptomatic arrhythmias is made feasible with *patient-activated intermittent recorders*. By virtue to their continuous loop technology, these recorders can capture the previous several minutes of cardiac rhythm and detect a symptom-producing dysrhythmia shortly after it has occurred, provided the patient is capable of activating the unit. Continuous loop recorders can be useful in patients with recurrent episodes of unexplained syncope.

Exercise Stress Testing may bring out arrhythmias not found during Holter monitoring, but even more useful is the test's sensitivity for the diagnosis of ischemic heart disease (see Chapter 36). Patients who report chest pain prior to syncope or have an abnormal resting ECG suggestive of ischemic disease are prime candidates for stress testing, especially if performed with thallium imaging. However, those with effort syncope should not be subjected to stress testing until tight aortic stenosis and other forms of critical ventricular outflow tract obstruction have been excluded, since there is the risk of sudden death.

Echocardiography can provide diagnostic information in patients suspected of valvular or structural heart disease because of effort syncope, chest pain, palpitations, or an abnormal carotid upstroke, murmur, or click on physical examination (see Chapters 21 and 33). It is also the noninvasive test of choice if a left atrial myxoma is suspected.

Intracardiac Electrophysiologic Study (EPS) has been advocated to detect arrhythmogenic causes of syncope, because of the limited specificity of Holter monitoring results described above. EPS's value in the assessment of patients with structural heart disease and fixed conduction defects is well documented, but its sensitivity and specificity for identifying transient rhythm disturbances, especially bradyarrhythmias, in patients with unexplained syncope has been disappointing. To improve on EPS performance, criteria for better patient selection have been sought. In the largest study to date, patients with evidence of underlying organic heart disease and frequent premature ventricular contractions on resting ECG were at increased risk for sustained ventricular tachycardia during EPS. Those with first-degree AV block, bundle branch block, or sinus bradycardia on resting ECG were at increased risk of a hemodynamically significant bradyarrhythmia during EPS. Overall, 87 percent of those with at least one of these clinical risk factors had an important outcome on EPS, whereas the EPS was normal in 95 percent of those with none of these risk factors. Holter findings may also prove predictive, but data is limited. Patients with unexplained syncope but no evidence of structural heart disease and a normal ECG are not likely to benefit from EPS.

Upright Tilt-Testing. The growing appreciation of neurocardiogenic mechanisms of syncope has stimulated interest in provocative maneuvers such as upright tilt-testing. Potential candidates are patients who experience syncope while upright yet remain undiagnosed despite careful evaluation for cardiac, central nervous system, and metabolic disease. The test is predicated on the hypothesis that in susceptible persons the decrease in venous return from placement on a tilt table will trigger the potent reflex responses that lead to neurocardiogenic syncope (see above). Criteria for a positive test vary, but reproduction of symptoms is the *sine qua non*.

Some have advocated infusion of isoproterenol (which increases contractility) to enhance test sensitivity and shorten study time (which can be up to 1 hour). In some older patients, sensitivity does appear to improve with isoproterenol administration, but in many others it increases the rate of false-positive responses. Most authorities recommend first performing the tilt-test without isoproterenol infusion, reserving it for repeat testing in patients with a negative study. In older patients, tilt-testing with isoproterenol can be conducted with safety, even in those with underlying heart disease, provided they have no evidence for arrhythmias or ongoing ischemia and are carefully monitored.

The tilt-test used to be reserved for patients who remained undiagnosed after exhaustive workup (eg, after a negative EPS). However, growing experience with its diagnostic utility and potential for obviating more invasive study argue for its being employed earlier in the evaluation of the syncopal patient. It appears helpful for determining response to therapy for neurocardiogenic disease. Additional data are needed for more precise guidelines to use of tilt-testing.

Other Studies *Electroencephalogram (EEG).* The EEG has repeatedly been shown to be of little use in evaluating syncope in the absence of either a history suggestive of seizure or neurologic deficits. Even when a seizure disorder is present, the routine EEG has a sensitivity of only 50 percent. Sleep studies and photic stimulation may improve sensitivity to 80 percent (see Chapter 170). Similarly, neuroimaging studies (CT, MRI) should generally be reserved for patients with focal seizures or defects on neurologic examination (in one study, 7 of 20 patients with and none of 17 patients without such findings had abnormalities detected on CT scan).

Serum Chemistries. Random *blood sugar* determinations are of little use in documenting hypoglycemia; a blood sugar at the time of symptoms is better (see Chapter 97). Arterial *blood gases* will reveal hypocarbia when hyperventilation is suspected and hypoxia when it is felt to be the cause.

The Patient with Unexplained Syncope. When the above evaluation ends without an answer other than the absence of evidence for serious underlying pathology, then a period of watchful waiting is indicated. Patients with a fully negative evaluation are at low risk for an occult, life-threatening etiology and sudden death. Those with a rare event can be reassured and followed expectantly. Those with recurrent episodes require careful follow-up and reassessment by careful history and physical examination at the time of recurrences. *Hospitalization* to observe the patient with frequent episodes is sometimes worth consideration and may help direct the evaluation.

SYMPTOMATIC THERAPY AND PATIENT EDUCATION

All drugs capable of causing hypotension should be carefully reviewed, especially in elderly patients, and consideration given to dose reduction or discontinuation. Patients with confirmed neurocardiogenic disease may be candidates for a trial of a beta-blocker (eg, metoprolol) or disopyramide. The patient bothered by orthostatic hypotension needs to avoid abrupt postural changes by sitting on the edge of the bed in the morning before getting up. Loosening the collar is sometimes helpful for the person with a hypersensitive carotid sinus reflex.

Patients with chronic orthostatic hypotension due to autonomic dysfunction experience not only hypotension on standing but hypertension when supine. To minimize the latter, elevation of the head at night is useful. Girdles, garters, and other constricting garments should not be worn if they decrease venous return, but elastic stockings may be helpful. One can advise the patient to avoid prolonged standing and to contract the calf muscles when standing to increase venous blood flow. Liberalization of salt intake is useful; fludrocortisone may be necessary. It may be necessary to discontinue or alter dosages of drugs that contribute to postural hypotension, particularly diuretics, antihypertensive agents, and hypnotics.

A demand pacemaker is indicated only when heart block or severe bradycardia has been proven responsible for syncope. It is of no use in neurocardiogenic disease nor as an empiric therapy in patients with undiagnosed recurrent episodes.

The patient without evidence of underlying cardiac or neurologic disease can be reassured even if syncopal episodes continue. Mortality does not increase with recurrent episodes, as long as there continues to be no evidence of underlying cardiac or neurologic disease. The value of a thoughtful workup in conjunction with thorough explanation should not be underestimated in helping patients with unexplained syncope to remain active.

INDICATIONS FOR ADMISSION

Pending further study, it is safest to hospitalize patients with syncope suspected to be of cardiac origin or caused by a seizure disorder of recent onset. If serious heart and neurologic diseases have been ruled out, further evaluation can safely proceed on an outpatient basis even though the cause may remain undetermined. Family members should be instructed to make careful note of all events surrounding the syncopal period, including appearance, position, activity, complaints, and behavior. They might be taught to palpate the radial or femoral pulse to provide data on heart rate and rhythm during the episode. Admission to the hospital for observation of the obscure case is a difficult decision but, as noted above, is most useful if episodes are frequent.

A.H.G.

ANNOTATED BIBLIOGRAPHY

Abboud FM. Neurocardiogenic syncope. N Engl J Med 1993;328:1117. *(A very concise and excellent summary of pathophysiology, plus an editorial on the clinical implications.)*

Almquist A, Goldenberg IF, Milstein S et al. Provocation of bradycardia and hypotension by isoproterenol and upright posture in patients with unexplained syncope. N Engl J Med 1989;320:346. *(Tilt-testing and isoproterenol reproduced symptoms in patients who otherwise had unexplained syncope after exhaustive evaluation.)*

Atkins D, Hanusa B, Sefcik T, Kapoor W. Syncope and orthostatic hypotension. Am J Med 1991;91:179. *(Orthostatic hypotension was found to be very common in patients with syncope, and present in most within 2 minutes of standing; those with greater degrees of orthostasis tended to have fewer syncopal recurrences.)*

Barron SA, Rogovski Z, Hemli Y. Vagal cardiovascular reflexes in young persons with syncope. Ann Intern Med 1993;118:943. *(High level of vagal tone found.)*

Calkins H, Byrne M, El-Atassi R, et al. The economic burden of unrecognized vasopressor syncope. Am J Med 1993;95:473. *(Much unnecessary testing.)*

Eagle KA, Black HR, Cook EF et al. Evaluation of prognostic classification of patients with syncope. Am J Med 1985;79:455. *(An outpatient study with 176 patients finding 8.5 percent with cardiac etiologies, 44.9 percent with vasomotor instability, 1.1 percent with seizures, 6 percent with others, and 39 percent unexplained.)*

Fujimura O, Yee R, Klein GJ. The diagnostic sensitivity of electrophysiologic testing in patients with syncope caused by transient bradycardia. N Engl J Med 1989;321:1703. *(Sensitivity and specificity were disappointingly low in patients with proven bradyarrhythmic syncope.)*

Gibson TC, Heitzman MR. Diagnostic efficacy of 24-hour electrocardiographic monitoring for syncope. Am J Cardiol 1984;53:1013. *(Of 1512 patients referred for Holter monitoring because of syncope, 15 had an episode of syncope, of which seven were related to an arrhythmia, and 241 reported presyncope, of which 24 were arrhythmia-related.)*

Grubb BP, Temesy-Armos P, Hahn H et al. Utility of upright tilt-table testing in the evaluation and management of syncope of unknown origin. Am J Med 1991;90:6. *(The test proved valuable in a highly selected group of patients with unexplained syncope; false-positive rate was zero in six control subjects. Treatment halted episodes in those who were positive.)*

Kapoor WN, Brant N. Evaluation of syncope by upright tilt testing with isoproterenol. Ann Intern Med 1992;116:358. *(A controlled study in young persons showing the test had a low specificity, with high rates of positive responses in both syncopal patients and controls; dampens enthusiasm for the test.)*

Kapoor WN, Karpf M, Wieand S et al. A prospective evaluation and follow-up of patients with syncope. N Engl J Med 1983;309:197. *(Patients with a cardiovascular cause for syncope face much higher risk than those with noncardiovascular or unknown causes.)*

Kapoor W, Karpf M, Levy GS. Issues in evaluating patients with syncope. Ann Intern Med 1984;100:755. *(An editorial describing emphasis on meticulous history, physical examination, and electrocardiogram with discriminating use of additional tests in evaluation of patients with syncope.)*

Kapoor WN. Evaluation and management of the patient with syncope. JAMA 1992;268:2553. *(Very useful review, especially for its critical look at yields of laboratory studies; 74 refs.)*

Kapoor W, Cha R, Peterson JR et al. Prolonged electrocardiographic monitoring in patients with syncope. Am J Med 1987;82:20. *(Patients with syncope and frequent or repetitive ventricular premature beats or sinus pauses had an increased risk of overall mortality and sudden death.)*

Kapoor W, Snustad D, Peterson J et al. Syncope in the elderly. Am J Med 1989;80:419. *(They have an increased risk of underlying heart disease and overall mortality.)*

Kapoor WN, Peterson J, Wieand HS et al. Diagnostic and prognostic implications of recurrences in patients with syncope. Am J Med 1987;83:700. *(Recurrences are common but not a predictor of mortality, sudden death, or etiology.)*

Kwoh CK, Beck JR, Pauker SG. Repeated syncope with negative diagnostic evaluation. Med Decis Making 1984;4:351. *(A sophisticated decision analysis approach to the question of whether or not to pace, including a well-structured review of the literature.)*

Lee RT, Cook EF, Day SC et al. Long-term survival after transient loss of consciousness. J Gen Intern Med 1988;3:337. *(Patients with a cardiac, neurologic, drug, or metabolic etiology had a worse prognosis; 7-year follow-up.)*

Linzer M, Prystowsky EN, Divine GW et al. Predicting outcomes of electrophysiologic studies of patients with unexplained syncope. J Gen Intern Med 1991;6:113. *(Identifies predictors of a positive EPS study and thus selection criteria for those who should be studied.)*

Lipsitz LA. Syncope in the elderly. Ann Intern Med 1983;99:92. *(An extensive clinical review stressing the selective use of diagnostic tests in evaluating syncope as well as attention to drug effects and treatment of symptomatic abnormalities.)*

McIntosh SJ, Lawson J, Henry RA. Clinical characteristics of vasodepressor, cardioinhibitory, and mixed carotid sinus syndrome in the elderly. Am J Med 1993;95:203. *(A cause of unexplained falls in the elderly.)*

Onrot J, Goldenberg MR, Hollister AS et al. Management of chronic orthostatic hypotension. Am J Med 1986;80:454. *(An excellent review of therapeutic measures based on an etiologic formulation; 71 refs.)*

Silverstein MD, Singer DE, Mulley AG et al. Patients with syncope admitted to medical intensive care units. JAMA 1982; 248:1185. *(Among this ICU population, those with cardiovascular syncope had a 19 percent 1-year mortality rate while those with noncardiovascular or unexplained syncope had a 6 percent rate. The authors conclude that patients discharged with unexplained syncope do not face increased risk of death during the subsequent year.)*

Primary Care Medicine: Office Evaluation and Management of the Adult Patient, 3rd edition, edited by Allan H. Goroll, Lawrence A. May, and Albert G. Mulley, Jr. J.B. Lippincott Company, Philadelphia

25 Evaluation of Palpitations

Palpitations are disconcerting and often incite fear of serious heart disease, although the majority of cases seen in the office occur among the worried well. The patient with palpitations reports a disquieting awareness of his or her heartbeat, which may be described as a pounding, racing, skipping, flopping, or fluttering sensation. The primary physician must be able to diagnose and treat important dysrhythmias and provide convincing reassurance to the anxious person with no underlying heart disease. Ambulatory monitoring techniques have improved detection of arrhythmias; their indications and limitations need to be understood.

PATHOPHYSIOLOGY AND CLINICAL PRESENTATION

Most healthy individuals are unaware of their resting heartbeat. Increase in stroke volume or contractility, sudden change in rate or rhythm, or unusual cardiac movement within the thorax may cause a perceptible beat. Isolated palpitations are noted when *premature atrial or ventricular contractions* are followed by a long pause; the prolonged filling time leads to an increase in stroke volume and the vigorous ejection of a large volume of blood on the next beat. A constant pounding is felt at rest by patients with *hyperkinetic states* (eg, fever, severe anemia, hyperthyroidism, anxiety); the rate is rapid and the rhythm is regular. A regular rhythm is also noted in those with large stroke volumes due to *aortic regurgitation* and other forms of valvular heart disease.

Excess adrenergic stimulation results in increased contractility and sinus tachycardia, which may present as palpitations. High levels of circulating catecholamines may trigger atrial and ventricular premature beats as well as atrial fibrillation, especially in someone with underlying organic heart disease. *Anxiety* is a common cause of such catecholamine-induced palpitations; symptoms are most pronounced in patients with a *panic attack* disorder (see Chapter 226). A heightened awareness of bodily sensations often compounds the problem and is particularly troublesome in patients with *depression*. The normally perceptible heartbeat that occurs with exercise is not unpleasant unless one is preoccupied with worries about health. *Hyperthyroidism* may have a presentation similar to anxiety (see Chapter 103).

In rare instances, the source of adrenergic outpouring is a *pheochromocytoma*. Its incidence is less than 0.1 percent, with about half of cases presenting as paroxysms of palpitations, hypertension, perspiration, tremor, nervousness, and other signs of adrenergic stimulation. Episodes are often spontaneous in origin but may be triggered by emotion and thus mimic an anxiety attack. An *insulin reaction* can produce a similar clinical picture (see Chapter 102). Onset of palpitations from adrenergic stimulation can be abrupt; resolution is usually more gradual.

Any sudden change in rate or rhythm may be perceptible. Attacks of palpitations that are regular in rhythm and rapid in rate are not unique to catecholamine excess; paroxysms of *supraventricular tachycardia (SVT)*, often referred to as *paroxysmal atrial tachycardia (PAT)*, are an important cause. SVT occurs in a wide variety of patients, including those with normal hearts, sick sinus syndrome, mitral valve prolapse and other forms of valvular disease, coronary artery disease, cardiomyopathy, and the preexcitation syndromes (eg, *Wolff-Parkinson-White [WPW] syndrome*). Onset of SVT is characteristically sudden and may be precipitated by excess *coffee, alcohol* consumption, emotional upset, or strenuous exertion. Often there is no obvious precipitant. Resolution is typically abrupt. A reentrant mechanism is postulated to account for SVT. Pathways that have been implicated involve the AV node, atria, and accessory conduction fibers. The dysrhythmia seems to be initiated by the occurrence of premature beats that alter conduction in the normal pathway. Paroxysms cease when the conducting properties of the reentrant circuit are disturbed by changes in vagal tone.

Some of the conditions associated with SVT are responsible for other dysrhythmias as well. For example, almost half of patients with *sick sinus syndrome* experience *heart block* or marked *bradycardia* in addition to bouts of SVT.

Sudden onset of palpitations with an irregular rhythm and rapid rate typifies *paroxysmal atrial fibrillation (PAF)* and may also be seen if there are runs of *multifocal atrial tachycardia (MAT)*. PAF occurs in a host of settings including alcohol excess, infection, and acute worsening of congestive heart failure; the condition is also found among otherwise healthy young people. MAT takes place in the context of severe pulmonary disease, particularly when there is an acute fall in PO_2 or pH. Frequent *atrial* or *ventricular premature contractions* can lead to a similarly irregular rhythm and rapid rate. Most chronic tachyarrhythmias do not produce palpitations.

Abnormal motion of the heart may be felt as a "turning over" or "flopping." The sensations are isolated and can occur with premature beats, the beat after a compensatory pause, or the beat after a blocked beat.

When there is serious preexisting cardiac pathology, palpitations are usually not the major or sole symptom. Syncope, near-syncope, chest pain, or dyspnea often results when a hemodynamically significant arrhythmia occurs in the setting of underlying heart disease. Most worrisome are runs of nonsustained and sustained *ventricular tachycardia*, which have a very high mortality risk and are usually associated with ischemic injury or scarring of the myocardium (see Chapter 29). Sometimes they produce little more than weakness and a rapid heartbeat, but sudden onset of near-syncope or drop attacks are other possible presentations. Drop attacks or near-syncope might also be the principal manifestation of *complete heart block* in a patient with an inadequate ventricular escape mechanism. *Very rapid SVT* may seriously compromise cardiac output in a patient with significant coronary or valvular disease and present as palpitations followed quickly by chest pain, dyspnea, profound weakness, or even loss of consciousness.

Table 25-1. Important Causes of Palpitations

1. Isolated Single Palpitations
   a. Premature atrial or ventricular beats
   b. The beat following a blocked beat
   c. The beat after a compensatory pause
2. Paroxysmal Episodes with Abrupt Onset and Resolution (Rate Usually Rapid)
   a. Rhythm irregular
      1. Paroxysmal atrial fibrillation
      2. Paroxysmal atrial tachycardia with variable block
      3. Frequent atrial or ventricular premature beats
      4. Multifocal atrial tachycardia
   b. Rhythm regular
      1. Supraventricular tachycardias with constant block or 1:1 conduction
3. Paroxysmal Episodes with Less Abrupt Onset or Resolution (Rhythm Usually Regular, Rate Rapid)
   a. Exertion
   b. Emotion
   c. Drug side effect (eg, sympathomimetics, theophylline compounds)
   d. Stimulant use (coffee, tea, tobacco)
   e. Insulin reaction
   f. Pheochromocytoma
4. Persistent Palpitations at Rest with Regular Rhythm (Rate Normal, Slow, or Rapid)
   a. Aortic or mitral regurgitation
   b. Large ventricular septal defect
   c. Bradycardia
   d. Severe anemia
   e. Hyperthyroidism (may also cause atrial fibrillation)
   f. Pregnancy
   g. Fever
   h. Marked volume depletion
   i. Anxiety neurosis

DIFFERENTIAL DIAGNOSIS

The causes of palpitations can be listed in terms of their clinical presentation (Table 25–1).

WORKUP

History. The first priority is the *detection of underlying heart disease*. Inquiries into dyspnea, chest pain, and syncopal or near-syncopal episodes are essential. Additionally useful are questions about risk factors for coronary disease (smoking, diabetes, hypertension, hyperlipidemia, positive family history) and prior cardiac history (heart murmur, rheumatic fever, myocardial infarction, other forms of cardiac illness). A costly error is to mistake symptoms of anxiety, such as chest tightness and air hunger at rest, for evidence of organic heart disease. Use of all cardiotonic drugs should be detailed, including digitalis preparations, theophylline compounds, sympathomimetics, and anticholinergics, including tricyclic antidepressants (see Chapter 227). Many over-the-counter decongestants and diet pills contain catecholamines or theophylline derivatives; their abuse may be responsible for symptoms. The history should include inquiry into alcohol abuse (see Chapter 228), a common precipitant of paroxysmal SVT.

A careful *description* of the palpitations in terms of onset, frequency, rate, rhythm, and pattern of resolution can sometimes be of help in diagnosis (see Table 25–1). Unfortunately, many patients are unable to give an accurate or detailed account of their symptoms. The relation of the onset of symptoms to exertion can aid in separating the anxious individual, whose symptoms may occur at rest and are usually not worsened by exertion, from the patient with heart disease and impaired exercise tolerance. Identification of precipitants such as emotional upset, stimulant intake, fever, pregnancy, volume depletion, and severe anemia is essential, for their recognition can contribute to design of proper therapy. Inquiry into symptoms of an insulin reaction (see Chapter 102) and hyperthyroidism (see Chapter 103) may also prove productive.

Physical Examination. At the beginning of the physical examination, one should look for evidence of excessive anxiety, such as tremor, sighing, and nervous mannerisms. Other important observations include determination of the blood pressure for elevation, marked postural change, and widened pulse pressure. The apical pulse is noted for rate and rhythm disturbances; relying on the peripheral pulse may be misleading when there is a pulse deficit, as occurs in atrial fibrillation or premature beats. The temperature should be recorded. The skin is examined for pallor and signs of hyperthyroidism; eyes for exophthalmos; neck for goiter; carotid pulse for upstroke; jugular venous pulse for distention and cannon waves; chest for rales, rhonchi, wheezes, and dullness; heart for heaves, thrills, clicks, murmurs, rubs, and third heart sound; and extremities for edema and calf tenderness. In addition to possibly providing important diagnostic information, the careful, unhurried physical examination can be of considerable use in reassuring the worried patient.

Laboratory Studies. Hematologic and chemistry studies are limited and rather straightforward. Patients with signs of a hyperkinetic state require a *hemoglobin* determination to rule out a significant anemia and a *thyrotropin (TSH)* test to rule out hyperthyroidism. Patients with underlying heart disease should have a check of the serum *potassium* and *calcium*, especially if taking a digitalis preparation; a *serum digoxin* or *digitoxin* level is essential in patients on cardiac glycoside therapy. A finger-stick *blood glucose* can be diagnostic in the setting of a suspected insulin reaction (see Chapter 102).

Patients with paroxysms of palpitations in conjunction with labile hypertension probably deserve to be screened for pheochromocytoma, although the oft-considered condition is actually quite rare. The best screening tests remain the *24-hour urine* collections, checking for either *catecholamines* plus *vanillylmandelic acid (VMA)* or catecholamines plus *metanephrines*. Two normal 24-hour urines collected when the patient is symptomatic rule out the diagnosis with more than 95 percent certainty. If urine testing is clearly positive (two separate determinations are abnormally elevated), then a *plasma catecholamine* determination followed by *computed tomography (CT) scanning* of the adrenals is indicated. CT scanning should never be done unless urine and serum testing are positive, because there are many harmless adrenal masses that might be mistaken for a pheochromocytoma. Plasma catecholamine testing requires only a single venipuncture, but the patient needs to be supine for 30 minutes prior to the venipuncture, and other causes of catecholamine elevation (eg, stress, use of sympathomimetics) need to be eliminated.

Most patients with palpitations should have a resting 12-lead *electrocardiogram (ECG)*. Even if physical examination is completely normal and no disturbances of rate or rhythm are noted, one might detect evidence of conduction system disease (eg, bundle branch block or preexcitation), ischemia, chamber enlargement, or other forms of organic heart disease. In particular, the ECG needs to be studied for axis shift, QRS widening, short PR interval (<0.12 sec), prolonged QT interval, delta waves, abnormal P-wave morphology, and ST- and T-wave changes. If a dysrhythmia is noted, it is worth obtaining a 2-minute rhythm strip to better characterize the rhythm disturbance. The anxiety-laden person often insists on having an ECG and finds comfort in a normal result; unfortunately, in many cases the reassurance is only transient.

Ambulatory Electrocardiographic Monitoring provides the opportunity to examine the relationship between symptoms and rhythm disturbances, especially when history, physical examination, and resting ECG have not yielded a definitive diagnosis. Patients who have palpitations accompanied by findings suggestive of underlying heart disease are among the best candidates for ambulatory monitoring, because they are at increased risk of having a clinically significant arrhythmia. So long as they are not experiencing syncope, near-syncope, heart failure, or angina in association with their palpitations, they can undergo an outpatient evaluation that includes ambulatory monitoring. The utility of ambulatory monitoring in otherwise healthy patients who complain solely of palpitations remains less clear, though the reassurance value can be considerable if typical episodes occur in the presence of a normal ECG recording.

The most commonly utilized method of ambulatory monitoring is the *Holter* technique, in which a portable 2-lead electrocardiographic recording system is attached to the patient to provide a 24- or 48-hour ECG record. The yield from Holter monitoring is greatest in patients with daily symptoms. Patients are asked to keep a diary in order to ascertain the relationship between symptoms and rhythm disturbances. Atrial and ventricular premature beats and short runs of SVT are common in normal asymptomatic patients. A positive test requires a clear-cut correlation between symptoms and ECG findings. Most studies show a very high incidence of recorded "abnormalities" but a very poor correlation between ECG findings and reported symptoms. The patient who experiences his typical symptoms but no concurrent rhythm disturbances during the Holter monitoring can be reassured. The patient who fails to have a symptomatic episode during Holter monitoring—a common occurrence—may be scheduled for a repeat study; however, yield is low in patients whose initial Holter study is normal and frequency of episodes is low. The cost of repeat Holter monitoring can be high.

Patients with infrequent but worrisome or bothersome episodes might benefit from use of an *intermittent ECG recorder*. Intermittent recorders are typically patient-activated at the time of symptoms. Although monitoring may be continuous, preservation of the ECG record is usually limited to a few minutes about the time of activation. Most units utilize continuous loop recording technology, though more advanced storage technologies are under development. Some permit telephone transmission of the rhythm disturbance. Intermittent ECG recorders allow prolonged monitoring at reasonable cost in patients with relatively infrequent episodes of palpitations. A major limitation is the need for patient activation, which can be problematic if the arrhythmia disables the patient.

Exercise Stress Testing. Palpitations precipitated by exertion—especially if accompanied by angina-like chest pain—suggests an ischemic mechanism. In this setting, exercise stress testing deserves consideration, both for diagnosis of coronary artery disease (see Chapters 20 and 36) and perhaps for detection of exercise-induced arrhythmias. In a study comparing the stress test to Holter monitoring for detection of ischemia-induced arrhythmias in patients with known coronary disease, Holter monitoring was found to be the more sensitive test, especially for ventricular irritability. Nevertheless, there were instances in which ventricular tachycardia occurred on stress testing but did not appear on monitoring, suggesting that the studies might be complementary. Ambulatory monitoring has been disappointing as a method for detecting ischemia. If underlying ischemia is suspected, then a stress test is the study of choice.

One of the more disconcerting findings is a wide QRS tachycardia. At issue is whether it represents a rather harmless *SVT with aberrancy* or a more ominous *ventricular tachycardia*. Findings associated with a ventricular origin include a history of heart disease; evidence of an old myocardial infarction on a resting ECG; AV dissociation (which is often absent but can be diagnostic if present); a QRS duration of >160 ms if there is a right bundle branch pattern or >140 ms if the pattern is left bundle; a combination of left bundle branch block and right axis deviation; extreme left axis deviation ($<-90°$ to $+180°$); and a different QRS pattern during tachycardia than on resting ECG in patients with preexisting bundle branch block. The combination of these findings provides reasonable sensitivity and specificity; most single findings are relatively weak discriminants.

Electrophysiologic Study. Palpitations leading to syncope or near-syncope raise the question of a major rhythm disturbance (eg, very rapid SVT, ventricular tachycardia, complete heart block). When occurring in the context of underlying organic heart disease, such arrhythmias have an especially poor prognosis (see Chapter 28 and 29). As noted above, patients reporting syncope in conjunction with palpitations need a careful assessment for evidence of organic heart disease. If such evidence is found, then consideration of intracardiac *EPS* is warranted in the search for a malignant arrhythmogenic cause of syncope. Its value in syncopal patients who have significant organic heart disease is well documented, but sensitivity and specificity for identifying important arrhythmias or conduction system disturbances in syncopal patients without signs of underlying heart disease have been disappointing. EPS remains an important diagnostic modality in the evaluation of patients with suspected ventricular tachycardia or documented heart block. Careful patient selection is essential (see Chapters 24 and 29). EPS is very expensive and not without risk, as it includes induction of potentially dangerous dysrhythmias. The study requires cardiac catheterization, sophisticated equipment, and a highly trained and experienced staff.

SYMPTOMATIC RELIEF

When palpitations are a manifestation of neurotic concern, efforts should be addressed toward providing reassurance. Hasty words of comfort are worthless. A careful history and physical examination, combined with eliciting and responding to patient concerns, views, and requests, must take place before the patient can be told the palpitations are harmless. Such reassurance may be all that is needed, especially when combined with advice to increase physical activity and cut down on alcohol, smoking, and stress. Exercise stress testing may have a role in helping to reassure the anxious patient. If the palpitations persist and are bothersome, a trial of beta-blocker therapy may be beneficial. Often as little as 50 mg of atenolol or the equivalent per day decreases the frequency of symptoms to the point where they are tolerable. Use of a minor tranquilizer or tricyclic antidepressant is also worth incorporating into the program if a panic attack disorder is the cause of episodes (see Chapter 226). All nonessential drugs capable of causing palpitations should be stopped.

The role of *caffeine* in precipitating cardiac arrhythmias and the usefulness of restricting its intake in symptomatic patients has been debated for decades. A single electrophysiologic study showed a tendency toward increased susceptibility to provoked arrhythmias. In an epidemiologic study, patients consuming more than nine cups of coffee per day demonstrated an increased incidence of ventricular ectopy. However, several placebo-controlled clinical studies examining the effects of up to 500 mg of caffeine per day (five to six cups of coffee) on the frequency and severity of atrial or ventricular arrhythmias revealed no increase in normals, patients with known coronary disease, or those with ventricular ectopy. There seems to be little reason for restricting coffee and tea use so long as long as excessive intake (>five cups/day) is avoided and the patient does not complain of caffeine-induced symptoms.

Detailed discussion of treatment for SVT is presented in Chapter 28. A few highlights of symptomatic management are included here. Vagal maneuvers are often effective in halting SVT. Valsalva and carotid sinus massage (in the absence of carotid disease) can be taught to the patient and suggested as the first line of therapy after the onset of an attack. Digitalis, propranolol, and verapamil are effective in terminating SVT, but when SVT is due to a preexcitation syndrome (eg, WPW syndrome), propranolol is preferred because digitalis may only prolong the problem by enhancing conduction in the accessory pathway. Prophylaxis of SVT attacks can be accomplished by avoiding known precipitants, such as alcohol and stimulants, and by using digitalis or propranolol; sometimes quinidine proves helpful by reducing the frequency of premature beats (the agent should usually be used in conjunction with digitalis, because of its vagolytic effects). Digitalis is the drug of choice for PAF. If

SVT or PAF is accompanied by ischemia or failure, admission is urgent.

Treatment of MAT requires correction of the underlying pulmonary problem rather than use of antiarrhythmic drugs. Improvement in oxygenation and pH status is essential. The approach to ventricular irritability depends on the setting in which it occurs (see Chapter 29). Correction of severe anemia, volume depletion, hyperthyroidism (see Chapter 103), fever (see Chapter 11), or congestive failure (see Chapter 32) is of prime importance to attaining symptomatic relief. Patients with hypoglycemic episodes need an adjustment in their insulin regimen and/or dietary program (see Chapter 102).

INDICATIONS FOR REFERRAL AND ADMISSION

Patients with a history of palpitations that lead to syncope, near-syncope, angina-like chest pain, or disabling dyspnea are candidates for referral and inpatient evaluation, especially if they have evidence of underlying organic heart disease or show complex ventricular ectopy or sinus pauses on Holter monitoring. Immediate hospitalization is indicated if a patient with known coronary disease demonstrates runs of ventricular tachycardia, even if these are not sustained or hemodynamically compromising; mortality risk is high. Patients with SVT who manifest hemodynamic compromise (eg, fall in blood pressure, dyspnea, angina, near-syncope) also need prompt hospital admission.

A.H.G.

ANNOTATED BIBLIOGRAPHY

Akhtar M, Shenasa, Jazayeri M et al. Wide QRS complex tachycardia. Ann Intern Med 1988;109:905. *(The vast majority proved to be ventricular in origin; good discussion of criteria for distinguishing between supraventricular and ventricular sources.)*

Barnett PA, Peter CT, Swan HJC et al. The frequency and prognostic significance of electrocardiographic abnormalities in linically normal individuals. Prog Cardiovasc Dis 1981;23:299. *(Normals have a high incidence of arrhythmias; provocative discussion on what constitutes "normal.")*

Brown AP, Dawkins KD, Davies JG. Detection of arrhythmias: Use of a patient-activated ambulatory electrocardiogram device with a solid-state memory loop. Br Heart J 1987;58:251. *(Description of intermittent recording technology in patients with infrequent episodes.)*

Cohen EJ, Klatsky AL, Armstrong MA. Alcohol use and supraventricular arrhythmia. Am J Cardiol 1988;62:971. *(Alcohol excess precipitates a host of SVTs.)*

DiMarco JP, Philbrick JT. Use of ambulatory electrocardiographic (Holter) monitoring. Ann Intern Med 1990;113:53. *(A comprehensive and critical review focusing on advantages and limitations of Holter monitoring; 139 refs.)*

Feldman JM. Diagnosis and management of pheochromocytomas. Hosp Prac 1989;1:145. *(An authoritative yet terse and practical discussion for the practitioner.)*

Fugimura O, Yee R, Klein GJ. The diagnostic sensitivity of electrophysiologic testing in patients with syncope caused by transient bradycardia. N Engl J Med 1989;321:1703. *(Sensitivity and specificity were disappointingly low in patients with proven bradyarrhythmic syncope.)*

Kapoor WN, Cha R, Peterseon JR et al. Prolonged electrocardiographic monitoring in patients with syncope. Am J Med 1987;82:20. *(Patients with syncope and frequent or repetitive ventricular premature beats or sinus pauses had an increased risk of overall mortality.)*

Krol RB, Morady F, Flaker S et al. Electrophysiologic testing in patients with unexplained syncope: Clinical and noninvasive predictors of outcome. J Am Coll Cardiol 1987;10:358. *(Predictors include previous MI, low ejection fraction, and conduction abnormalities on ECG.)*

Lowenstein SR, Gabow PA, Cramer J et al. The role of alcohol in new onset atrial fibrillation. Arch Intern Med 1983;143:1882. *(Among 40 cases of new onset atrial fibrillation, alcohol caused or contributed to approximately two-thirds; 90 percent of these converted spontaneously to sinus rhythm within 24 hours.)*

Myers MG. Caffeine and cardiac arrhythmias. Ann Intern Med 1991;114:147. *(Reviews the evidence for and against a causative role; moderate intake appears to have little effect, even in patients with heart disease.)*

Narula OS. Wolff-Parkinson-White syndrome: A review. Circulation 1973;47:872. *(A still useful and detailed description of the syndrome; 38 refs.)*

Rubenstein JJ, Schulman CL, Yurchak PM et al. Clinical spectrum of the sick sinus syndrome. Circulation 1972;46:5. *(Classic article reporting on a series of 56 patients; over 60 percent of patients had bradycardia and SVT.)*

Ryan M, Lown B, Horn H. Comparison of ventricular ectopic activity during 24-hour monitoring and exercise testing in patients with coronary heart disease. N Engl J Med 1975;292:224. *(Monitoring proved better in exposing ventricular irritability, but there were instances when ectopic activity was detected only by stress testing.)*

Shen WK, Holmes DR, Hammill SC. Transtelephonic monitoring: Documentation of transient cardiac rhythm disturbances. Mayo Clin Proc 1987;62:109. *(Another method for capturing infrequent, but potentially important episodes.)*

Appendix: Evaluation of Atrial Fibrillation in the Outpatient Setting

Atrial fibrillation (AF) is one of several dysrhythmias that can produce an irregularly irregular heartbeat. It is often a manifestation of underlying heart disease but sometimes is discovered in a patient with no overt cardiac pathology. Many patients tolerate the arrhythmia well and can be evaluated thoroughly and safely in the outpatient setting. Cases that present without other signs of underlying heart disease are particularly challenging; some are harmless, but others are resistant to standard therapy and associated with potentially serious conditions that may elude diagnosis unless specifically sought. The primary care physician needs to determine if it is safe to conduct the assessment in the office setting and how to carry out a cost-efficient evaluation.

PATHOPHYSIOLOGY

The postulated electrophysiologic mechanisms of AF include focal automaticity and a complex form of reentry. Factors that may precipitate or perpetuate AF include increased atrial size, increased atrial pressure, varying repolarization times of neighboring areas of atrial myocardium, and occurrence of atrial premature beats during the vulnerable period of an atrial cycle. Increases in circulating catecholamines may precipitate atrial premature beats and AF. Ischemia and disease of the sinoatrial nodes also predispose to atrial dysrhythmias by suppressing the SA node and allowing other atrial foci to fire. Epidemiologic data from the Framingham study reveal that heart failure and rheumatic heart disease are the most powerful predictors of AF and hypertension the most commonly associated condition, suggesting that myocardial damage and left atrial dilatation are important precursors of the condition.

CLINICAL PRESENTATIONS

The hallmarks of AF are the characteristic electrocardiographic findings of an irregularly irregular ventricular rhythm and atrial fibrillatory waves. The fibrillatory waves range in appearance from fine irregular undulations of the baseline to very coarse waves. The QRS duration is usually normal but may widen with aberrant conduction and simulate ventricular tachyarrhythmias. The ST segments and T waves may be abnormal in appearance if there is rapid ventricular response, underlying heart disease, or use of digitalis.

AF can present as a paroxysmal or chronic dysrhythmia, both with and without evidence of underlying heart disease. Its incidence in the Framingham study was 2 percent over 20 years. The overwhelming majority of AF patients in that study had evidence of underlying heart disease at the time of the arrhythmia's onset. AF was often a sign of advanced heart disease complicated by congestive failure; the onset was associated with a twofold increase in mortality.

Some patients with incidentally discovered AF are asymptomatic; however, if the AF is paroxysmal or the ventricular rate is very rapid, palpitations may be reported. If cardiac output falls precipitously, symptoms of heart failure may occur. Rapid rate may also lead to myocardial ischemia in patients with underlying coronary artery disease. Systemic embolization may be the first sign of AF and present as an acute neurologic or peripheral vascular event.

A number of acute noncardiac conditions can precipitate AF in the absence of clinically apparent heart disease; these include acute alcohol intoxication, decompensated chronic obstructive lung disease, pneumonia, and pulmonary embolization. However, AF does not always occur in the context of overt heart disease or an acute event such as sudden pulmonary decompensation. The entities associated with seemingly isolated bouts of AF deserve particular attention because detection is sometimes difficult and therapy is different from that for most other causes of AF (see Chapter 28).

Lone Atrial Fibrillation is a term used to denote AF in patients without clinically evident heart disease. In about two-thirds of cases, the condition presents as isolated or recurrent episodes of paroxysmal AF; in the remainder, the AF is chronic. Studies of military recruits found its prevalence to be about one in 10,000. Lone AF is a harmless condition in young people; they characteristically experience episodes precipitated by emotional stress, alcohol, use of stimulants, or smoking. Detailed investigations have failed to reveal underlying heart disease, chamber enlargement, or risk of embolization. The prognosis in young patients is excellent. In the Framingham study, elderly patients carrying the diagnosis of lone AF had a worse prognosis (see Chapter 29), but there is some suspicion that many had subclinical heart disease, since 30 percent had concurrent hypertension. Some older patients are inappropriately diagnosed as "lone fibrillators" when the actual cause may be one of the less clinically apparent conditions such as early alcoholic or hypertensive cardiomyopathy, sick sinus syndrome, Wolff-Parkinson-White syndrome, or apathetic hyperthyroidism.

Alcoholic Cardiomyopathy. The early stages of alcoholic cardiomyopathy may present as paroxysms of AF triggered by binge drinking. The distinction between this condition and "lone fibrillation" triggered by alcohol (*"holiday heart"*) may be difficult but is suggested by the finding of cardiomegaly even in the absence of heart failure. Abstinence can halt or even reverse the condition, but continued drinking leads to progression and, in some, chronic AF.

Tachycardia–Bradycardia Syndrome *(sick sinus syndrome)* is an important and sometimes subtle cause of AF. The exact cause of this condition is unknown but is believed to be related to diffuse degeneration of conducting system tissue. Patients exhibit sinus node dysfunction, often in conjunction with AV nodal disease and lack of an adequate escape mechanism. Atrial tachyarrhythmias may alternate with symptomatic bradycardia and sinus arrest. Clinical presentations include palpitations, light-headedness, and syncope. At times, the first manifestation may be a paroxysm of AF. Identification is most important, because treatment directed only toward the AF may worsen the bradyarrhythmia (see Chapter 28). Paroxysmal AF due to sick sinus syndrome is associated with an increased risk of thromboembolism.

Wolff-Parkinson-White Syndrome (WPW) is a preexcitation syndrome that produces a host of supraventricular and ventricular dysrhythmias, particularly paroxysms of AF associated with a very rapid ventricular response rate. In fact, a ventricular rate greater than 200 beats per minute in the absence of another cause for AF should make one suspicious of WPW. The condition is believed to be at least partially congenital in nature and characterized by rapid atrioventricular conduction over an accessory pathway (the Kent bundle). This anomalous conduction pathway bypasses the AV node and produces preexcitation, manifested by the characteristic baseline ECG findings of a shortened PR interval (<0.12 sec) and delta waves. Some WPW patients have normal baseline ECGs and show anomalous conduction only during tachyarrhythmias, making diagnosis difficult. During rapid AF, there may be a widening of the QRS, mimicking ventricular fibrillation. The reported incidence of AF among patients with WPW ranges from 11 percent to 39 percent. WPW is an important cause of AF to recognize, because the

AF may actually worsen with digitalis therapy (see Chapter 28) and has the potential to degenerate into ventricular tachycardia and fibrillation.

Apathetic Hyperthyroidism of the Elderly is another cause of AF that may appear to occur without evidence of underlying heart disease. These patients characteristically manifest marked apathy that may be mistaken for severe depression and impressive weight loss that may simulate occult malignancy (see Chapter 103). Sometimes, AF is the predominant manifestation of the condition. The usual signs and symptoms of thyrotoxicosis are absent. The AF is difficult to control with standard modes of therapy for AF but usually reverts to sinus rhythm with correction of the hyperthyroid state (see Chapter 28).

DIFFERENTIAL DIAGNOSIS

Atrial fibrillation is only one of a number of dysrhythmias that present as an irregularly irregular pulse. Frequent atrial premature beats, multifocal atrial tachycardia (MAT), paroxysmal atrial tachycardia (PAT) or atrial flutter with variable block, sinus arrhythmia, and frequent ventricular premature beats all may produce an irregularly irregular rhythm.

The most common cause of AF in the community setting is hypertensive heart disease; however, only those hypertensive patients with evidence of left ventricular hypertrophy are likely to develop AF. The major causes of AF are listed in Table 25–2.

WORKUP

The diagnosis of AF is based on the characteristic *ECG findings* of an irregularly irregular ventricular response and atrial fibrillatory waves. These fibrillatory waves range from barely perceptible irregular undulations of the ECG baseline to very coarse waves. The standard lead best suited for detection of atrial activity is lead V_1, followed by leads II, III, and aVF. Occasionally, the routine 12-lead ECG will show no atrial activity; in such instances, one can check lead V_{3R} for evidence of atrial activity or infer the diagnosis of AF based on the characteristic ventricular response pattern and a QRS of normal duration. MAT, PAT, or atrial flutter with variable block, frequent atrial premature beats, and sinus arrhythmia all produce rhythms that can resemble AF, but the presence of P waves or flutter waves on ECG separate them from AF. If the ventricular response rate is too rapid to reveal atrial activity, vagal maneuvers and gentle carotid sinus massage can be attempted (provided there is no evidence of carotid artery disease) to slow the rate and uncover any hidden fibrillatory or P waves.

Once the diagnosis of AF is established, one needs to determine if workup can proceed on an outpatient basis. Prompt hospital admission is needed for the patient with evidence of acute congestive heart failure, ischemia, embolization, hypotension, or a very rapid ventricular response rate (>150–170 beats/min). If there is no hemodynamic compromise, an outpatient workup can commence. A retrospective study of 97 patients with new onset AF who were admitted to the hospital as a routine procedure found that 98 percent had an uncomplicated course. The authors concluded that hospitalization is unnecessary for new onset of uncomplicated AF.

Table 25-2. Important Causes of Atrial Fibrillation

Paroxysmal Atrial Fibrillation
"Lone fibrillation"
Acute ischemia
Alcohol intoxication and early alcoholic cardiomyopathy
Sick sinus syndrome
Wolff-Parkinson-White syndrome
Acute pulmonary embolization
Acute pericarditis
Acute pulmonary decompensation
Acute heart failure
Any cause of chronic AF
Sustained Atrial Fibrillation
Advanced rheumatic mitral valve disease
Chronic congestive heart failure
Advanced aortic valve disease
Advanced hypertensive heart disease
Coronary artery disease
Advanced cardiomyopathy
Congenital heart disease
Apathetic hyperthyroidism of the elderly
Sick sinus syndrome
"Lone" fibrillation
Constrictive pericarditis
Digitalis toxicity (rarely)

History. The young patient with a paroxysm of AF should be questioned about a prior history of such episodes, excess intake of stimulants and alcohol, emotional stress, fever, heart murmur, and chest pain. Older patients should be queried about preexisting heart disease, hypertension, chest pain, dyspnea, cough, calf pain, leg edema, fever, light-headedness, near-syncope, loss of consciousness, weight loss, depression, history of heart murmur or rheumatic fever, and any prior attacks of palpitations. A careful drug history should be taken with emphasis on alcohol abuse (see Chapter 228). Any use of digitalis should be noted; however, digitalis toxicity only rarely results in AF. A long-standing history of attacks dating from young adulthood suggests WPW syndrome. The presence of marked weight loss and depression in an elderly patient with unexplained AF points to apathetic hyperthyroidism. The older patient with episodes of altered consciousness may suffer from sick sinus syndrome.

Physical Examination. In addition to noting heart rate, blood pressure, respiratory rate, jugular venous pulse, and other signs of hemodynamic status, the patient should be checked for apathetic appearance, evidence of marked weight loss, cyanosis, goiter, wheezes, friction rub, heart murmur, calf tenderness, asymmetrical leg edema, and signs of alcohol intoxication. The most common cause of "silent" mitral valve disease is failure to listen specifically for the murmurs of mitral stenosis and mitral regurgitation. Placing the patient in the left lateral decubitus position may be necessary to appreciate the murmurs. Only in rare instances are the murmurs of mitral valve disease truly inaudible (see Chapter 33).

Laboratory Studies. The *electrocardiogram* often provides useful information beyond identification of the arrhythmia. A ventricular response rate greater than 200 beats/min suggests WPW syndrome, as does a widened QRS due to aberrant conduction; delta waves may be seen within some of the aberrantly conducted beats. The appearance of the fibrillatory waves on ECG provides some hints of etiology. Coarse fibrillatory waves are most typical of AF resulting from rheumatic heart disease and other causes of marked left atrial enlargement, whereas fine fibrillatory waves are more common in cases due to atherosclerotic and hypertensive heart diseases. The ST and T wave segments should be checked for evidence of ischemia, strain, digitalis effect, and pericarditis (see Chapter 20). Advanced valvular and hypertensive forms of heart disease are suggested by finding ECG evidence of left ventricular hypertrophy.

A cardiogram taken after return to sinus rhythm should be checked for a shortened PR interval and delta waves diagnostic of WPW syndrome. Occasionally, preexcitation is concealed on the resting ECG, so that the ECG of some WPW patients appears normal; in such instances, the diagnosis of WPW syndrome can be difficult. Other clues to WPW syndrome include a ventricular response rate during AF of greater than 200 beats/min and delta waves distorting the QRS complex.

A rhythm strip sometimes reveals sinus node disease, but often a 24-hour *Holter monitor* will be needed to detect the episodes of bradycardia and tachycardia that characterize the sick sinus syndrome. *Chest radiograph* is the best simple test for determining heart failure, cardiomegaly, and intrapulmonary pathology. Cardiomegaly may be the only evidence of an underlying cardiomyopathy. *Echocardiogram* provides an excellent noninvasive means of further evaluating suspected valvular, congenital, cardiomyopathic, and pericardial forms of heart disease. However, the cost-effectiveness of ordering an echocardiogram routinely in the workup of AF to search for an occult, high-risk cause such as mitral stenosis remains a subject of debate. The elderly, apathetic patient with unexplained AF requires measurement of the *thyrotropin (TSH)* to rule out hyperthyroidism (see Chapter 103). Although AF is a very uncommon manifestation of digitalis toxicity, a serum *digoxin level* is probably worth checking when no other cause is apparent and the patient is known to be taking the drug.

In summary, the evaluation can be performed on an outpatient basis if the patient is tolerating the rhythm well and there is no evidence of failure, ischemia, or embolization. A careful history and physical examination, supplemented by ECG, chest radiograph, and in selected instances, an echocardiogram, complete the evaluation in most patients. Patients with AF of unknown cause should be studied further for evidence of sick sinus syndrome, apathetic hyperthyroidism, alcoholic cardiomyopathy, and WPW syndrome.

A.H.G.

ANNOTATED BIBLIOGRAPHY

Brand FN, Abbott RD, Kannel WB et al. Characteristics and prognosis of lone atrial fibrillation: 30-year follow-up in the Framingham Study. JAMA 1985;254:3449. *(A fourfold increase in stroke risk was noted, but patients were older and had more cardiovascular risk factors than patients in other studies of lone AF.)*

Campbell RWF, Smith RA, Gallagher JJ et al. Atrial fibrillation in the preexcitation syndrome. Am J Cardiol 1977;40:514. *(AF due to preexcitation syndromes can cause very rapid and aberrantly conducted ventricular responses; ventricular dysrhythmias can sometimes result.)*

Culler MR, Boone JA, Gazes PC. Fibrillatory wave size as a clue to etiologic diagnosis. Am Heart J 1983;66:425. *(Coarse atrial fibrillatory waves found most frequently in patients with mitral valve disease and left atrial enlargement; also noted in "lone" AF and hyperthyroidism.)*

Desbiens NA. Should all patients with atrial fibrillation be screened with echocardiography? J Gen Intern Med 1992;7:131. *(A decision-analysis study on the efficacy of routinely screening AF patients by echocardiography for unrecognized mitral stenosis; the benefit was small and screening was not recommended.)*

Engel TR, Luck JC. Effect of whiskey on atrial vulnerability and "holiday heart." J Am Coll Cardiol 1983;1:816. *(Alcohol enhanced vulnerability to atrial fibrillation in patients without clinical evidence of cardiomyopathy or heart failure.)*

Ettinger PO, Wu DF, De La Cruz C Jr et al. Arrhythmias and the "holiday heart": Alcohol-associated cardiac rhythm disorders. Am Heart J 1978;895:955. *(Paroxysmal AF may be a sign of early alcoholic cardiomyopathy and be induced by binge drinking.)*

Forfar JC, Miller HC, Toft AD. Occult thyrotoxicosis: A correctable cause of "idiopathic" atrial fibrillation. Am J Cardiol 1979;44:9. *(Ten of 75 patients presenting with AF of unknown cause were hyperthyroid.)*

Hanson HH et al. Auricular fibrillation in normal hearts. N Engl J Med 1949;240:947. *(Classic paper describing the entity of "lone fibrillation.")*

Kannel WB, Abbott RD, Savage DD et al. Epidemiologic features of chronic atrial fibrillation: The Framingham Study. N Engl J Med 1982;306:1018. *(A major epidemiologic study; heart failure and rheumatic heart disease were the most powerful predictive precursors of chronic AF; chronic AF was associated with a doubling of overall and cardiovascular mortality.)*

Kopecky SL, Gersh BJ, McGoon MD et al. The natural history of lone atrial fibrillation: A population-based study over three decades. N Engl J Med 1987;317:669. *(A retrospective study of patients under the age of 60 showing that lone AF was associated with a very low risk of stroke.)*

Shlofmitz RA, Hirsch BE, Meyer BR. New onset atrial fibrillation. J Gen Intern Med 1986;1:139. *(A retrospective study showing that urgent hospitalization is rarely necessary.)*

Primary Care Medicine: Office Evaluation and Management of the Adult Patient, 3rd edition, edited by Allan H. Goroll, Lawrence A. May, and Albert G. Mulley, Jr. J.B. Lippincott Company, Philadelphia

26
Management of Hypertension

KATHARINE K. TREADWAY, M.D.

Hypertension is one of the few conditions in medicine that can be readily detected and effectively treated in the asymptomatic period before irreparable harm is done. It ranks as a leading risk factor for cardiovascular disease and as a major reason for office visits and prescription of medication. Cardiovascular disease is the leading cause of death in the United States. Of these deaths, 83 percent are caused by myocardial infarction, and 17 percent are from stroke. There has been a steady decline in cardiovascular death over the last 3 decades, at least some of which is attributable to the lowering of blood pressure in the general population. The frequency and importance of hypertension demand that the primary physician be expert in its management and capable of designing a regimen that is safe, effective, and well tolerated.

PRINCIPLES OF THERAPY

Confirming the Diagnosis and Determining Overall Cardiovascular Risk

Because treatment of hypertension is likely to be lifelong, it is essential that the diagnosis be well established before committing the patient to therapy (see Chapters 14 and 19). Initiation of antihypertensive treatment should be preceded by a careful evaluation that includes ruling out secondary causes, identifying additional cardiovascular risk factors, and assessing degree of target-organ damage (see Chapter 19).

Once the tasks of the initial evaluation are accomplished, attention can shift to design of a treatment program, which usually entails both pharmacologic and nonpharmacologic measures. The program is *individualized*, based on an assessment of *total cardiovascular risk*. (See Appendix.) This assessment is critical to guiding the decision to treat, because there is *no numerical blood pressure threshold* above which the risks of stroke and coronary disease greatly accelerate. Risk increases in a nearly linear fashion along the continuum of blood pressure (see Chapter 14) and is exacerbated by *smoking*, *diabetes*, *hypercholesterolemia*, *advancing age*, *male sex*, *African ancestry*, and evidence of *target-organ disease* (eg, left ventricular hypertrophy, retinopathy, nephrosclerosis—see Chapter 14).

Attention to total cardiovascular risk is particularly important in managing patients with stage I ("mild") hypertension (diastolic blood pressure 90–99 mm Hg, systolic blood pressure 140–159 mm Hg). They represent almost 80 percent of all hypertensives and account for nearly 60 percent of the excess cardiovascular morbidity and mortality attributable to hypertension; yet, as a group, they benefit least from antihypertensive therapy when compared to their more severely hypertensive counterparts (see Chapter 14). In these patients (whose numbers make them an important public health problem), deciding when and how to treat is strongly influenced by the degree of total cardiovascular risk (see below).

Nonpharmacologic Measures

The principal nonpharmacologic measures for treatment of hypertension include *salt restriction*, *reduction of excess weight* (see Chapter 223), and *exercise* (see Chapter 18). They should be the foundation of every treatment program and also serve as an excellent means of primary prevention. Behavioral therapies and calcium and potassium supplementation have been suggested, but more essential are the other nonpharmacologic measures that help to limit overall cardiovascular risk (eg, *cessation of smoking*—see Chapter 54, *reduction of fat and cholesterol* intake—see Chapter 27). All nonpharmacologic measures should continue even if drug therapy needs to be instituted, because they enhance its effectiveness and allow for use of fewer medications at lower doses.

Salt Restriction ranks as one of the mainstays of nonpharmacologic therapy for all hypertensive patients, regardless of underlying pathophysiology. The response to salt restriction is particularly marked in patients with low-renin/volume-expanded hypertension (eg, African-Americans and the elderly). Patients should be instructed in either a *no-added-salt diet* (4 g sodium/d) or a *low-sodium (2 g/d) diet*, depending on their volume status. Not only may salt restriction alone provide adequate control in some mild cases, but it can profoundly affect the efficacy of pharmacologic therapy. Patients receiving diuretics who had an unrestricted salt intake showed a blood pressure reduction of 4 percent compared to a 15 percent reduction for those restricting their sodium intake.

Weight Reduction achieves significant decreases in blood pressure, even if ideal weight is not reached. The effect is independent of salt intake. All patients who are more than 15 percent above their ideal body weight should be urged to lose weight. In addition, weight loss is important in patients with central adiposity (hip to waist ratio >0.85 in women and >0.95 in men). Such patients have a higher incidence of hypertension, diabetes, and hyperlipidemia and a higher risk of cardiovascular disease. The relation between obesity and blood pressure is particularly strong among young to middle-aged adults.

Reduction in Excess Alcohol Consumption. Epidemiologic data indicate a relationship between excess alcohol consumption and risk of hypertension. More than 2 oz of alcohol per day significantly increases the risk of becoming hypertensive. Small-scale studies suggest that a daily alcohol intake of less than 1 oz may result in a modest decrease in blood pressure. Excessive alcohol intake is a frequent cause of "refractory" hypertension.

Exercise of the aerobic variety helps to reduce weight, improves cardiovascular conditioning and lipid profile, and may help in patients with mild, uncomplicated hypertension (see Chapter 18). Patients with mild hypertension given an exercise program of aerobic and circuit weight training three times per week for 10 weeks showed pressure reductions comparable to those achieved with beta-blocker or calcium channel blocker therapy and obviated the need for chronic drug treatment. Candidates for an exercise program should be stress-tested before engaging in any vigorous exercise program (see Chapter 18).

Behavioral Therapies such as *relaxation* techniques and *biofeedback* programs have gained popularity in recent years. Small-scale studies suggested a modest benefit, especially in those with mild pressure elevations, but a rigorous meta-analysis of available studies found little specific benefit. Although behavioral techniques were superior to no therapy, they provided no more benefit than self-monitoring or sham techniques and should not be prescribed in lieu of more proven nonpharmacologic and pharmacologic treatments.

Potassium and Calcium Supplements have been touted as capable of reducing blood pressure. Correction of *diuretic-induced hypokalemia* can produce impressive short-term decreases in pressure, but chronic potassium supplementation fails to achieve sustained pressure reductions in patients consuming a low-sodium diet. Although potassium supplements are useful in hypokalemic patients, they are not sufficient to obviate need for drug therapy in normokalemic patients.

Intracellular *calcium* is important in blood pressure regulation, and an inverse relationship has been demonstrated between calcium intake and blood pressure. However, the overall effect of calcium supplementation is small and unpredictable. Routine calcium supplementation cannot be recommended at present, but maintenance of adequate calcium intake is reasonable.

Pharmacologic Therapy—Basics Issues

When to Initiate Medication. There are no definitively established exact guidelines for initiation of pharmacologic therapy, decisions regarding when and how to add drug therapy must be individualized and based again on total cardiovascular risk. An obese, 35-year-old African-American male with a blood pressure of 158/98, a markedly elevated cholesterol, and a two-pack/day smoking habit is a far more appropriate candidate for early pharmacologic intervention than is a slim, 35-year-old white female with the same blood pressure but no other cardiovascular risk factors. In fact, such young white women appear to have the same risk as normotensive men and benefit least from pharmacologic treatment. (Some argue these women may not require treatment, though more data are needed to clarify the issue.)

The consensus view is that stage I patients with no other cardiovascular risk factors should begin nonpharmacologic measures, be followed expectantly, and undergo reassessment in 6 months, while those with risk factors should be started on medication much sooner if they fail to respond fully to nonpharmacologic measures over 3 to 6 months (Fig. 26–1).

Definition of and indications for treatment of *isolated systolic hypertension* have been a source of uncertainty but are becoming clearer. The problem is particularly common in the *elderly*. Although epidemiologic data have long shown increased cardiovascular risk with isolated systolic elevations in pressure (*>160 mm Hg*), only recently has treatment demonstrated efficacy in reducing such risk. The Systolic Hypertension in the Elderly Program (SHEP) found a significant reduction in fatal and nonfatal strokes and a lesser reduction in fatal and nonfatal myocardial infarction when the systolic pressure was lowered to *less than 160 mm Hg*. Data in younger patients are scarce, but isolated systolic hypertension is less of a problem in younger age groups.

The decision to start antihypertensive medication entails a risk–benefit estimate. The estimate is particularly important to the asymptomatic hypertensive patient because of the likelihood for prolonged treatment and the possibility of adverse effects from taking medication. Fortunately, the newer antihypertensive agents offer the prospect of excellent blood pressure control with little impairment of quality of life.

Goals, Efficacy, and Duration of Treatment. The principal objective of antihypertensive therapy is to lower overall cardiovascular risk and prevent heart attack and stroke. As noted earlier, this requires not only reducing blood pressure but also attending to the other cardiovascular risk factors amenable to treatment (smoking, lipids, etc). The importance of addressing *all* cardiovascular risk factors is underscored by the fact that medication-induced pressure reductions noted with some agents produce only 50 percent of the expected reduction in coronary events. If a drug lowers blood pressure but exacerbates other cardiovascular risk factors or they are ignored, then the accomplishment of pressure reduction may be only a Pyrrhic victory.

The degree to which blood pressure should be lowered remains a matter of debate. Some argue that 85 mm Hg is the appropriate diastolic endpoint. The view is based on the *"J-curve" phenomenon*, in which diastolic pressures below 85 mm Hg appear to be associated with an increased risk of cardiovascular events. While this phenomenon does appear to be present among patients with preexisting coronary disease, it does not appear in those without coronary disease. Pending more data, it seems reasonable to set a goal of 85 mm Hg in those who have preexisting coronary disease and to aim for less than 85 mm Hg in all other patients. The specific goal should be individualized for each patient according to pretreatment pressure, overall cardiovascular risk, impact on coexisting conditions, and the effects of treatment on quality of life and functional status. Whatever pressure target is set, it should be achieved gradually, except in the setting of malignant hypertension (see below).

Because there is no cure for essential hypertension, drug treatment has often been viewed as lifelong. Some patients with very mild hypertension may be able to stop medication, provided they continue nonpharmacologic measures and successfully control other risk factors. Even patients with substantial hypertension who require multidrug regimens

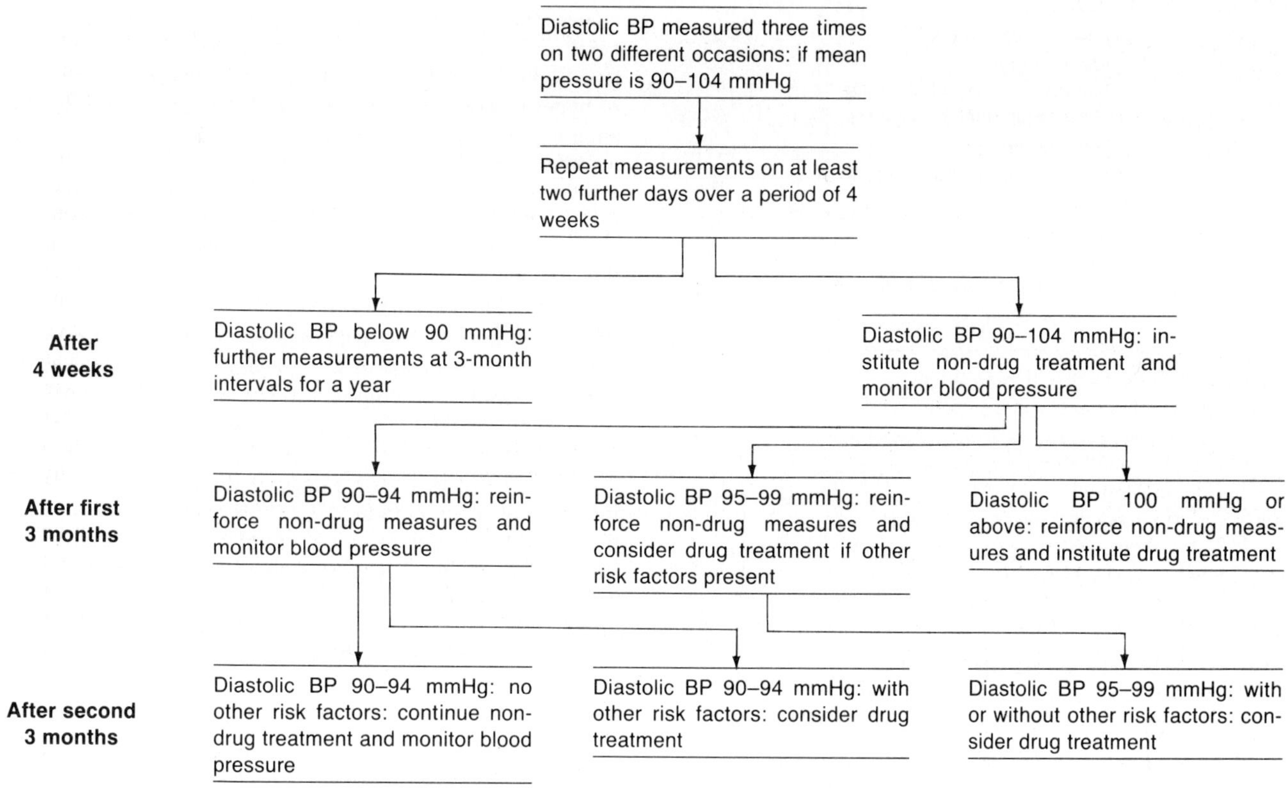

Figure 26-1. Approach to the patient with Stage I ("mild") hypertension. Adapted from World Health Organization/International Society of Hypertension. J Hypertens 1989;7:689.

may be candidates for a reduction in drug therapy. An observational study using multivariate analysis identified drug-treated patients prescribed a high-intensity program (the equivalent of two or more agents) for a prolonged period (mean 5.5 y) as those most likely to successfully tolerate a reduction in drug therapy (diastolic blood pressure remaining <95 mm Hg). However, systolic pressure did rise in these patients by an average of 8.8 mm Hg, and discontinuation of therapy was not possible.

Selection and Sequencing of Drugs. The pharmacologic armamentarium has changed considerably over the past decade, though *thiazides* and *beta-blockers* still remain mainstays of therapy because of their proven ability to reduce cardiovascular morbidity and mortality, a benefit yet to be demonstrated for many other agents. Sometimes the reduction in coronary events is less than that predicted, raising concern about their having adverse metabolic effects (see below).

There has been a gradual reduction in use of many *centrally acting sympatholytics*, *ganglionic blockers*, and *older peripheral vasodilators* in favor of the newer agents that are more effective and better tolerated, such as the *angiotensin converting enzyme (ACE) inhibitors*, *calcium channel blockers*, and the *newer beta-blockers* and *alpha-blockers*.

The traditional "stepped-care" approach of adding pharmacologic agents has been supplanted by a modification in which a first-line agent is started and increased in dose as tolerated to achieve adequate control. If no response is achieved, then switching to another first-line agent of a different class is recommended, rather than adding a second agent. Monotherapy suffices in about 60 percent to 80 percent of cases and may even be phased out over time in patients with stage I (mild) hypertension if other risk factors are brought under good control. If there is only a partial response, then the choice is either to further increase dose or to add a low dose of another first-line drug from a different class—often a thiazide diuretic which enhances the efficacy of most other agents (Fig. 26–2).

The initial choice of agent is often dictated by the clinical context as well as the suspected underlying mechanism of hypertension. Regardless of medical regimen selected, all nonpharmacologic measures should be continued, because they enhance the effectiveness of therapy and allow for use of fewer medications at lower doses.

Pharmacologic Therapy—First-Line Agents

Thiazide diuretics remain the most commonly used drugs for both initiation and maintenance of antihypertensive drug therapy. They block the reabsorption of sodium, leading to decreases in intravascular volume, intracellular sodium, and peripheral resistance. One shortcoming is that they do not reverse left ventricular hypertrophy. When used at low doses in properly selected patients, thiazides remain a safe, well-tolerated, inexpensive, and effective means of treatment (Table 26–1). Thiazides are particularly useful in those with sodium retention and volume expansion (eg, African-Americans and the elderly). Modest doses (eg, hydrochlorothia-

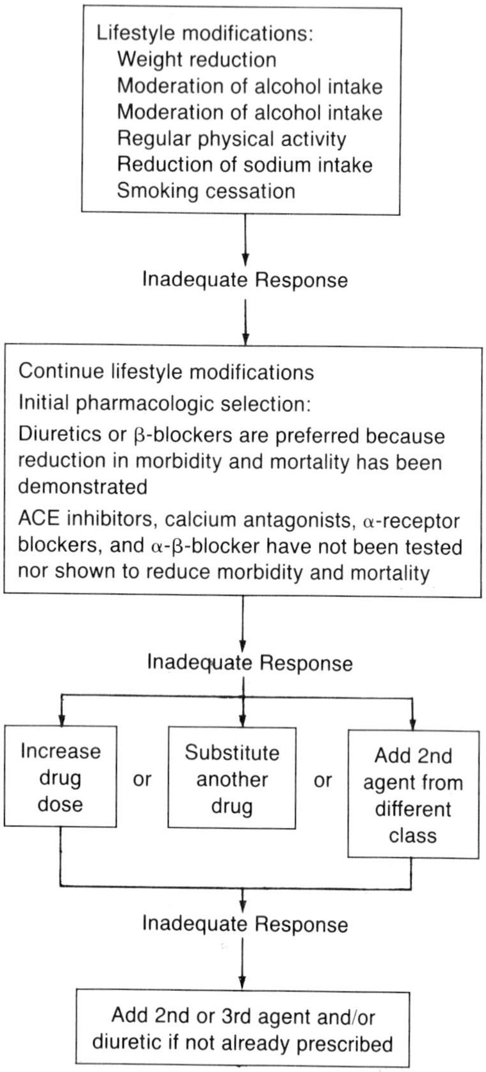

Figure 26-2. Treatment algorithm for pharmacologic therapy of high blood pressure. Adapted from the Fifth Report of the Joint Committee on Detection, Evaluation, and Management of High Blood Pressure. Arch Intern Med 1995;155:15.

zide 25–50 mg/d) will often suffice in mild hypertension. Larger doses are associated with an increase in adverse metabolic consequences (see below) without significant improvement in pressure reduction. Low thiazide doses (12.5–25 mg/d of hydrochlorothiazide) enhance the efficacy of other front-line antihypertensive agents (eg, ACE inhibitors, beta-blockers). As a result, thiazides have also become an important adjunct in patients whose pressure does not respond to monotherapy.

Adverse Effects. Recent revelations about the potentially adverse metabolic effects of thiazides have tempered enthusiasm for their use. The Multiple Risk Factor Intervention Trial (MRFIT) study found an increased rate of cardiac sudden death in thiazide-treated patients with baseline electrocardiogram (ECG) abnormalities. In addition, an appreciation that the metabolic side effects of thiazides (*hypokalemia*, *increase in low-density lipoprotein* [*LDL*] *cholesterol*, increased *insulin resistance* leading to *hyperglycemia*, and *hyperuricemia*) may adversely affect cardiovascular and stroke risks have led to a reassessment of their traditional role as the drug class of first choice for treatment of hypertension. Fortunately, the degree of glucose intolerance associated with thiazide use is usually mild, even in diabetics (see Chapter 102). However, new findings linking insulin resistance to the development of hypertension (see Chapter 19) make any worsening of glucose intolerance a potentially undesirable side effect. (The literature should be followed closely for new data on this important issue).

Mild hyperuricemia occurs in as many as 60 percent of patients; however, only if the patient develops recurrent attacks of gouty arthritis or kidney stones is treatment of the hyperuricemia or discontinuation of the diuretic necessary (see Chapter 155).

While the risks attributable to thiazide use remain to be more fully defined, it still appears that the benefits outweigh the risks. A major meta-analytic study that took into account the cholesterol-raising action of thiazides found thiazides second only to generic propranolol as the most cost-effective monotherapy for hypertension in terms of reduction in cardiovascular morbidity and mortality. Such analyses suggest that thiazides not be abandoned as first-line therapy but that care be taken in patient selection and monitoring and that doses not exceed the equivalent of 25 to 50 mg/d of hydrochlorothiazide.

Patient Selection. Optimal candidates are those likely to have volume-expansion hypertension (ie, African-Americans and the elderly—see Chapter 19). Patients with rhythm and conduction system disturbances, left ventricular hypertrophy, underlying ischemic heart disease, or digitalis use might best be served by an alternative antihypertensive agent. The same is true if there is severe hyperlipidemia, poorly controlled diabetes, or symptomatic gout.

Monitoring. If thiazides are used, monitoring for hypokalemia, LDL cholesterol elevation, rhythm disturbances, and hyperglycemia are essential, especially if the patient is elderly. Thiazide patients who take a digitalis preparation are very susceptible to developing dysrhythmias in the setting of hypokalemia (see Chapter 32). Regular monitoring of the serum potassium and correction of even mild hypokalemia are essential if there is underlying heart disease. Hypokalemia can be prevented by concomitant salt restriction, increased dietary potassium, and when necessary, the addition of potassium-sparing agents or supplements (see Chapter 32). Modest degrees of hypokalemia (3.0–3.5 mg/dL) in patients free of cardiac problems are probably harmless, but many hypertensive patients may harbor undiagnosed coronary disease, necessitating careful monitoring and correction in most patients. Severe degrees of hypokalemia may cause muscle weakness.

Beta-Blockers are highly effective, proven in long-term prospective randomized studies to reduce rates of stroke and cardiovascular morbidity and mortality. They decrease contractility, decrease renin release, and possibly reduce central sympathetic output. Left ventricular hypertrophy recedes. Acutely, peripheral resistance rises, but it quickly returns to normal.

Adverse Effects. Adverse effects include *bradycardia*, exacerbation of congestive *heart failure*, *fatigue*, *impotence*,

Table 26-1. Antihypertensive Drugs

CLASS	DRUG	TRADE NAME	INITIAL/MAXIMUM DOSE (mg/day)	FREQUENCY OF DOSAGE	RELATIVE COST (dose in mg)
Diuretics	Thiazides				
	Chlorothiazide	Diuril	125/500	qd/bid	1.3 (25)
	Hydrochlorothiazide	Hydrodiuril	12.5/50	qd/bid	1.00 (25)
	Phthalimidine derivatives				
	Chlorthalidone	Hygroton	12.5/50	qd	0.9 (25)
	Metolazone	Zaroxolyn	1/10	qd	11.0 (25)
	Chlorobenzamide				
	Indapamide	Lozol	2.5	qd	19 (2.5)
	Side Effects ↓ K^+; alkalosis; ↓ Mg^+; insulin resistance; hyperglycemia; ↓ Na^+; ↓ Ca^{++}; ↑ total cholesterol, LDL, triglycerides; impotence; fatigue; photosensitivity; rash; plts; WBC; ↑ PRA; ↓ GFR; pancreatitis, hepatic toxicity (rare)				
	Distal tubular diuretics				
	Spironolactone	Aldactone	25/100	tid	1.0 (25)
	Triamterene	Dyrenium	100/300	qd	11.0 (100)
	Side Effects ↑ K^+, rash, hyperpigmentation, megaloblastic anemia (triamterene), ↑ PRA, ↓ GFR, nausea, vomiting, diarrhea, menstrual irregularities and gynecomastia (spironolactone), impotence, drowsiness, ataxia				
	Combination drugs				
	Spironolactone and hydrochlorothiazide	Aldactazide	1/4 tablets	bid	4.2
	Triamterene and hydrochlorothiazide	Dyazide	1/2 tablets	qd/bid	10.5
		Maxide	1/2 tablets	qd	10.5
	Amiloride and hydrochlorothiazide	Moduretic	1/2 tablets	qd	13.8
	Side Effects Same as for the constituent agents, except less ↑ K^+ or ↓ K^+				
Sympatholytics (centrally acting)	Methyldopa	Aldomet	250/3000	tid or qd	6.0 (250)
	Side Effects Drowsiness (usually transient), sedation, depression, impotence, fluid retention, orthostatic hypotension, positive direct Coombs' test (usually without clinical hemolysis), transaminase elevation, ↓ PRA, GFR unchanged				
	Clonidine	Catapres	0.1/2.4	bid or qd	8.5 (0.2)
	Side Effects Same as for methyldopa, plus weakly positive Coombs' test (without clinical hemolysis), sudden rebound hypertension with abrupt discontinuation of drug, bradycardia or heart block, impaired glucose tolerance				
	Guanabenz	Wytensin	8/64	bid	32 (8)
	Side Effects Similar to clonidine				
Sympatholytics (beta-blocking agents)	Acebutolol	Sectral	400/800	qd	6 (400)
	Side Effects Similar to propranolol, except lupus-like syndrome, less risk of bronchospasm, little orthostatic hypotension or bradycardia ($beta_1$ selective and alpha agonist), intrinsic sympathomimetic activity				
	Atenolol	Tenormin	25/100	qd	5 (50)
	Side Effects Similar to propranolol, except less risk of bronchospasm and fewer CNS effects ($beta_1$ selective; low lipid solubility)				
	Labetalol	Trandate Normodyne	200/2400	bid	6 (400)
	Side Effects Similar to propranolol except increased risks of orthostatic hypotension and impotence (nonselective beta blocker, selective $alpha_1$ blocker)				
	Metoprolol	Lopressor	100/400	qd or bid	3 (100)
	Side Effects Similar to propranolol except for less risk of bronchospasm ($beta_1$ selective)				

(*continued*)

Table 26-1. (Continued)

CLASS	DRUG	TRADE NAME	INITIAL/MAXIMUM DOSE (mg/day)	FREQUENCY OF DOSAGE	RELATIVE COST (dose in mg)
	Nadolol	Corgard	40/320	qd	5 (40)
	Side Effects Similar to propranolol (nonselective beta blocker)				
	Pindolol	Visken	10/80	bid	5 (10)
	Side Effects Similar to propranolol except less resting bradycardia (nonselective beta blocker; some agonist activity)				
	Propranolol	Inderal	40/2000	qid or bid	1 (80)
	Side Effects Bradycardia, congestive heart failure, bronchospasm, insomnia, depression, paresthesias, claudication, masking of hypoglycemia, impotence, sedation, possible precipitation of angina with abrupt discontinuation of drug, ↓ PRA, ↓ GFR, ↑ K^+, GI disturbances				
	Timolol	Blocadren	10/60	bid	6 (10)
	Side Effects Similar to propranolol but less risk of CNS effects (nonselective beta blocker; low lipid solubility)				
	Propranolol LA	Inderal LA	60–120g	qd	15 (60)
Sympatholytics (peripherally acting)	Reserpine	Raudixin Serpasil Sandril	100/300 0.1/0.5	qd	0.4 (0.25)
	Side Effects Drowsiness, nasal congestion, increased appetite, bradycardia, depression (can be severe), nightmares, ↑ gastric acidity (may be ulcerogenic), parkinsonian rigidity, galactorrhea, postural hypotension (rare), impotence (rare), ?breast cancer (may promote development of preexisting disease)				
Sympatholytics (alpha-blocking agents)	Prazosin Teraxocin Doxazosin	Minipress Hytrin Cardura	3.0/20 1/20 1/16	tid qd qd	2 (2) 6 (1) 6 (1)
	Side Effects Dizziness, drowsiness, headache, weakness, depression, palpitations, tachycardia, orthostatic hypotension, syncope (may occur suddenly after first dose), nausea, diarrhea, constipation, edema, dyspnea, rash, pruritus, dry mouth, blurred vision, impotence, urinary frequency, hallucinosis, ↓ PRA				
Vasodilators	Hydralazine	Apresoline	40/400	qid or bid	1.2 (40)
	Side Effects Headache, tachycardia, palpitations, fever, weight gain, edema, lupus erythematosus-like syndrome (rare if dosage <200 mg/day), exacerbation of coronary insufficiency, ↑ PRA, ↑ or − GFR				
	Minoxidil	Loniten	2.5/40	qd–qid	20 (2.5)
	Side Effects Sodium retention, peripheral edema, hirsutism, pericardial effusion; GFR unaffected				
Angiotensin Converting Enzymes	Captopril	Capoten	25/75	bid/tid	8.5 (50)
	Side Effects Cough, orthostatic hypotension, dysguesia, angioedema, leukopenia, agranulocytosis, pancytopenia, renal failure in patients with bilateral renal artery stenosis, renal damage in patients with renal disease				
	Enalapril	Vasotec	5/40	qd/bid	6 (5)
	Side Effects Similar to captopril				
	Lisinopril	Prinivil Vasotec	5/40	qd	5.5 (5)
	Side Effects Similar to captopril				
	Ramipril	Altace	2.5/20	qd	5.5 (2.5)
	Side Effects Similar to captopril				
	Fosinopril	Monopril	10/40g	qd	5.5 (10)
	Side Effects Similar to captopril				

Table 26-1. (Continued)

CLASS	DRUG	TRADE NAME	INITIAL/MAXIMUM DOSE (mg/day)	FREQUENCY OF DOSAGE	RELATIVE COST (dose in mg)
	Quinapril	Accupril	10/40	qd	5.5 (10)
	Side Effects Similar to captopril				
Calcium Channel Blockers	Nifedipine	Procardia	30/120	tid/qid	8 (40)
	Nicardipine	Cardene	60/120	tid	8 (60)
	Isradine	Dynacire	5/20	bid	7 (5)
	Verapamil	Isoptin	120/480	tid	4 (240)
		Calan	120/480		4 (240)
		Verelan	120/480		4 (240)
	Diltiazem	Cardizem	90/240	tid	8 (90)
Calcium Channel Blockers (long-acting)	Nifedipine	Procardia XL	30/120	qd	8 (30)
	Felodipine	Plendil	5/20	qd	6.5 (5)
		Cardizem CD	180/300	qd	8 (180)
	Diltiazem	Cardizem SR	120/240	bid	10 (120)
	Diltiazem	Calan SR	180/240	qd	7.5 (240)
	Verapamil	Verclan SR			8 (240)
	Verapamil	Isoptin SR			7.5 (240)
	Side Effects Verapamil decreases AV conduction, repairs inotrope, constipation, nausea. Diltiazem similar but less AV note effects and less negative intropy. Nifedipine, nicardipine, isradine, felodipine have no AV nodal effects, + flushing, HA, pedal edema, nausea, less constipation compared with verapamil.				

depression, decreased exercise tolerance, nightmares, and *increased airway resistance.* As such, these agents should not be used in patients with asthma, heart failure, severe chronic obstructive pulmonary disease (COPD), or serious depression. They also increase insulin resistance and decrease high-density lipoprotein (HDL) cholesterol, both to a mild degree. These adverse effects do not seem to cancel their beneficial effects on hypertension and its associated risks.

Preparations. All appear to be equally effective for treatment of hypertension, though differences in their cardioselectivity, lipid solubility, and intrinsic sympathomimetic activity can be utilized to advantage. *Cardioselectivity* is characterized by greater effect on $beta_1$-adrenoreceptors of the heart than on the $beta_2$-receptors of blood vessels and bronchi. A cardioselective preparation is useful in patients with COPD because it reduces the chances of inducing bronchospasm. However, cardioselectivity is a relative quality that declines as dose increases. Furthermore, even cardioselective beta-blockers are not well tolerated in asthmatics and COPD patients with active bronchospasm. *Atenolol* and *metoprolol* are examples of the commonly used cardioselective beta-blockers.

Another difference is in degree of *lipid solubility*, which theoretically predicts the degree of central nervous system (CNS) penetration and the likelihood of neuropsychiatric side effects, such as depression, lethargy, sexual dysfunction, and nightmares. The elderly are particularly susceptible to such side effects. Atenolol and nadolol are the most lipid-insoluble, while *propranolol* and *metoprolol* are among the most *lipid-soluble*. Studies of drug-induced sedation have produced similar results for both lipophilic and lipophobic preparations. However, sexual dysfunction and depression appear to be more common with lipophilic agents than lipophobic ones, though still occurring on occasion with use of the latter.

Some beta-blockers have *intrinsic sympathomimetic activity (ISA).* Those with ISA tend to cause less bradycardia and less disruption of lipid and carbohydrate metabolism. They help maintain cardiac output with exercise, allowing for cardiac conditioning. They are comparable to non-ISA beta-blockers in ability to lower blood pressure. Examples include *pindolol* and *acebutolol.*

One beta-blocker, *labetalol*, is unique in that it has both *alpha- and beta-blocking* actions, with about one-fourth the potency of propranolol and one-sixth the potency of phentolamine, the archetypical alpha-blocker. Its rapid onset of action has made it useful for use in hypertensive emergencies—especially when given parenterally—but its chronic oral use has been limited by tendencies to cause orthostatic hypotension, sexual dysfunction, and hepatocellular injury.

Patient Selection. In general, beta-blockers are well tolerated at low doses and may be used as initial monotherapy in most patients. Concerns about their effects on quality of life and sexual function have lessened with additional experience in their proper selection and use. Their cardioprotective effect makes them a drug of choice in hypertensive patients with underlying coronary artery disease. In meta-analytic study, generic propranolol was the most cost-effective of all major antihypertensive agents. At times they may cause some minor fluid retention. Adding a small dose of thiazide can greatly enhance efficacy.

Alpha-Blockers act peripherally at vascular postsynaptic alpha-adrenergic receptors, causing arteriolar and venous dilation. Because they affect both the arterial and venous systems, they cause less reflex tachycardia than pure arterial vasodilators (see below). With some of the older alpha-blockers (eg, *prazosin, terazosin*), profound *postural hypotension* leading to *syncope* occurred 1 to 3 hours after the initial dose, especially in elderly patients and those taking diuretics. This can be avoided by starting with a low dose at bedtime and instructing the patient to stay supine for at least 3 hours. The newer preparations such as *doxazosin* are longer-acting and appear less likely to cause first-dose syncope. Postural light-headedness is still a problem, affecting about one-fifth of patients and more likely as dose is increased above 1 mg per day. These drugs have no adverse effects on lipids; in fact, they *mildly raise HDL* cholesterol and *slightly reduce LDL* (both on the order of 3%–5%). In addition, they reverse left ventricular hypertrophy. They can temporarily *relieve* the *obstructive symptoms* of prostatic hypertrophy, which improves their desirability in elderly men. The newer alpha-blockers now qualify as first-line agents for treatment of hypertension and may be attractive for use in patients with concomitant hyperlipidemia or symptomatic prostatism.

Angiotensin Converting Enzyme (ACE) Inhibitors, such as *captopril, enalapril, lisinopril*, and others, block the conversion of renin-activated angiotensin I to angiotensin II, an extremely potent vasoconstrictor that also stimulates the production of aldosterone. By their blocking action, ACE inhibitors reduce aldosterone levels and blunt the volume retention caused by other vasodilators. There may be other mechanisms of action as well. At recommended doses, these drugs are safe and very effective. They have become first-line agents for treatment of hypertension, being well tolerated and free of the fatigue and lethargy so common to many other antihypertensive medications. In diabetic patients, ACE inhibitors help to reduce proteinuria and preserve renal function, presumably through dilation of efferent arterioles and reduction in intraglomerular pressure. Cardiac output improves in patients with impaired left ventricular systolic function.

Adverse Effects. The most troublesome side effect is an annoying *dry cough* that occurs in about 10 percent of patients. It is mostly nocturnal and is described as an irritation in the throat. About half of patients who experience the cough find it severe enough to warrant discontinuation of the medication. Switching to another ACE inhibitor rarely solves the problem. Uncommon side effects include rash and taste disturbances.

Because the ACE inhibitors block the production of aldosterone, they can lead to dangerous degrees of *hyperkalemia* when used in conjunction with a potassium-sparing diuretic or potassium supplementation. Potentially fatal hyperkalemia has been reported in diabetic patients with hyporenin/hypoaldosterone hypertension. Close monitoring of the serum potassium is indicated in such situations, but not when an ACE inhibitor is used alone. There are no adverse effects on lipids.

In the setting of large doses and underlying kidney disease, *renal failure* has been noted, such as with significant bilateral renal artery stenosis. The originally reported *glomerular injury* and *agranulocytosis* are very rare, except at the *extremely high doses* used in early clinical trials. However, patients with renal failure are still at risk for glomerular injury when large doses are used, necessitating careful monitoring of renal function.

Preparations. There are a large number of ACE inhibitors on the market, differing predominantly in cost and duration of action. An interesting quality-of-life study noted that only captopril of the ACE inhibitors studied conferred an enhanced sense of well-being, raising the question of its having a beneficial central effect. Cost should decrease as the patent protection of captopril and other preparations expires.

Patient Selection. When used as monotherapy in moderate doses (eg, <150 mg of captopril per day), the ACE inhibitors are effective and well tolerated. In a double-blind study comparing captopril to methyldopa and propranolol, captopril produced fewer side effects and less impairment of the patient's sense of well-being. Except for their high cost, these agents have broad appeal and particular advantages for patients with diabetes, left-sided heart failure, volume overload, depression, or poor tolerance for the CNS effects of other antihypertensive drugs. The ACE inhibitors may be used alone or in combination with a *diuretic* or a *beta-blocker*, which enhance their effectiveness.

Calcium Channel Blockers impede the intracellular entry of calcium in heart and vascular smooth muscle. The resultant decrease in cellular calcium concentration reduces vascular smooth muscle contraction and lowers peripheral resistance. These agents also have a mild natriuretic effect, making them potentially useful in patients with sodium retention (eg, the elderly and African-Americans). None adversely effects lipids or insulin sensitivity, and all reduce left ventricular hypertrophy.

Preparations and Adverse Effects. There is considerable variation in action and side effects among the major calcium channel blockers (nifedipine, diltiazem, and verapamil—see Table 26–1). *Nifedipine* and its congeners (*nicardipine, isradipine*, and *felodipine)* are the most potent *vasodilators* and produce the most *reflex tachycardia* but the least net reduction in inotropy. Their main drawback is *peripheral edema*, secondary to venodilating effects. Occasionally, headache and flushing may be troublesome. *Verapamil's* main disadvantages are *negative inotropy* and *conduction system disturbances* leading to AV nodal block and bradycardia; the drug should not be used in patients with heart failure or suspected conduction system disease. Leg edema is usually not a problem unless heart failure worsens, but *constipation*, headache, and dizziness can be problematic. *Diltiazem* falls between nifedipine and verapamil, having mildly negative effects on inotropy and conduction but less likely than nifedipine to cause leg edema. Efficacy is enhanced by addition of a small dose of thiazide diuretic. The introduction of long-acting formulations has increased patient acceptance.

Patient Selection. The efficacy, relatively mild side-effect profile, lack of adverse metabolic effects, and once-daily dosage of these agents make them broadly appealing. However, they are expensive, though generic formulations are forthcoming. Use in hypertensive patients with concurrent coronary artery disease is popular because they can provide symptomatic relief of angina; but, unlike beta-blockers, they have yet to demonstrate cardioprotectivity. As noted above, these agents are suitable for use in the elderly, blacks, and others with evidence of volume overload.

Second-Line Agents

Second-line agents are generally reserved for patients who are refractory to combinations of first-line agents or who have special underlying conditions such as renal failure. They include loop diuretics, distal tubular diuretics, centrally acting sympatholytics, and the older peripheral vasodilators.

Loop and Potassium-Sparing Diuretics. *Loop diuretics* (furosemide, ethacrynic acid, and bumetanide) are reserved for patients with evidence of *renal insufficiency* (creatinine clearance <30% of normal) or with allergy to thiazides. They are typically used in conjunction with *minoxidil* (see below).

Distal tubular diuretics (spironolactone, triamterene, amiloride) are weak antihypertensive agents, used predominantly in combination with thiazides to *spare potassium loss*. The combination preparations are widely promoted, but it is best to avoid starting with such a fixed combination until the necessary thiazide dose has been established. Hypertensive patients who must avoid hypokalemia (eg, those taking digitalis, experiencing ventricular irritability, or suffering from organic heart disease) are the best candidates. Other indications are mineralocorticoid hypertension, thiazide hypersensitivity, and severe gout. These drugs must be used with extreme *caution* in patients with renal insufficiency, ACE inhibitor use, or insulin-dependent diabetes with renin deficiency, where risk of serious *hyperkalemia* is great. The tendency of spironolactone to cause gynecomastia limits its use in hypertension is usually limited to patients with Conn's syndrome.

Centrally Acting Sympatholytics. *Alpha-methyldopa, clonidine*, and *guanabenz* are *the centrally acting sympatholytics* that reduce blood pressure by stimulating central alpha-receptors, which in turn reduce sympathetic outflow to the heart and vasculature. Because they cause secondary *sodium retention* and generally require the use of a diuretic, they should be considered *second-line* agents. Although all these agents frequently cause drowsiness, fatigue, and impotence, lower doses are often quite well tolerated, even in the elderly. Alpha-methyldopa occasionally causes fever, acute or chronic hepatitis, and a Coomb's-positive hemolytic anemia. *Clonidine* (and sometimes methyldopa) are more likely to cause sedation, dry mouth, and *rebound hypertension* with abrupt cessation of therapy. A slow-release transdermal clonidine patch is available and convenient but very expensive and commonly irritating to the skin. Low-dose clonidine (0.1 mg) given as a once-daily dose before bed is well tolerated in the elderly. Guanabenz and guanfacine are similar to clonidine in action and side effects.

Reserpine is one of the oldest antihypertensive agents, acting as a postganglionic adrenergic neuron antagonist. Its advantages are low cost, good efficacy, and once-daily dose. Significant side effects include *severe depression*, nightmares, drowsiness, nasal congestion, gastrointestinal disturbances, and bradycardia. Its use continues to decrease.

Older Arterial Vasodilators. The older arterial vasodilators (eg, *hydralazine, minoxidil*) act directly to relax arterial smooth muscle, thus causing a reflex tachycardia and sodium and water retention. *Hydralazine* is typically used as a third-line agent in combination with a beta-blocker and a diuretic agent. Four-times-a-day dosing often limits compliance. It typically causes headache, dizziness, and a lupus-like syndrome, especially in doses exceeding 200 mg/d. Reflex tachycardia may exacerbate angina. *Minoxidil* is an extremely potent vasodilator that should be used only in patients with moderately severe hypertension uncontrolled by other medications (see below). Both a beta-blocker and a loop diuretic must be used. Salt and water retention may be marked, requiring high doses of furosemide. Hypertrichosis is common and has led to the drug's topical use for hair loss. Minoxidil has been rarely associated with pericardial effusion and even more rarely with cardiac tamponade.

Cost

The high cost of treatment is a major reason for poor compliance. The advent of ACE inhibitors, calcium channel blockers, and the newer alpha- and beta-blockers has greatly improved efficacy and convenience and reduced side effects and adverse reactions. However, these drugs are expensive. Until cost is reduced by market pressures and expiration of patent protection, expense is likely to remain a barrier to proper use. Physicians need to consider the patient's financial status and insurance coverage in the design of the modern antihypertensive regimen. Thiazides and generic beta-blockers (eg, propranolol) are effective, relatively inexpensive drugs that provide a very reasonable alternative to the more expensive antihypertensive preparations. Side effects are somewhat more frequent and dosing less convenient but possibly worth the difference in cost to the patient. Others may be willing to pay more for a better tolerated program that does not compromise quality of life.

Additional approaches to minimizing cost include use of a *generic* preparation when available, substituting a *sustained-release form* if it is less expensive than a multidose regimen, staying with a less expensive older antihypertensive agent if reasonably effective and well tolerated, and attempting to reduce dose to the minimum necessary. If a second agent must be added, one might consider prescribing a *thiazide* diuretic in low dose, which may greatly enhance efficacy at very little additional cost. If the patient has concurrent coronary disease, use of a beta-blocker or calcium channel blocker might suffice for both. In addition, purchase of prescription-benefit insurance could be beneficial, if available.

TREATMENT RECOMMENDATIONS

For All Patients:

- Prescribe a sodium-restricted diet (2–4 g/d).
- Advise weight reduction (especially if >15 percent above ideal weight).
- Limit alcohol intake to less than 2 oz/d.
- Insist on complete smoking cessation (see Chapter 54).
- Prescribe an exercise program (see Chapter 18).

For Patients With Stage I (mild) Hypertension (Diastolic Pressure 90–99 mm Hg, Systolic Pressure 140–159 mm Hg), *No* Additional Cardiovascular Risk Factors, and *No* Signs of Target-Organ Disease:

- Institute the above-mentioned nonpharmacologic measures.
- Repeat blood pressure determinations regularly over the next 6 months
- If improvement noted (diastolic <90, systolic <140), then

continue nonpharmacologic measures indefinitely and monitor blood pressure at least every 6 months.

- If no improvement after 6 months of nonpharmacologic therapy or if it fails to lower the blood pressure to <140 mm Hg systolic or <90 mm Hg diastolic, then *add* a first-line antihypertensive agent to the nonpharmacologic program.

For Patients With Stage I Hypertension *Plus* Additional Cardiovascular Risk Factors or Signs of Target-Organ Disease:

- Immediately institute a full nonpharmacologic program.
- Repeat blood pressure determinations regularly over 3 months.
- If blood pressure not normalized after 3 months, then *add* a first-line antihypertensive agent to the nonpharmacologic program.

For Patients With Stage II Hypertension (Diastolic 100–109 mm Hg, Systolic 160–179 mm Hg):

- Same as above for patients with stage I disease with additional risk factors or target-organ disease.

For Patients With Stage III Disease (Diastolic 110–119 mm Hg, Systolic 180–209 mm Hg):

- Immediately institute full doses of a first-line agent and consider early use of two first-line agents.
- If pressure improved but not normalized within 1 week, add the second first-line agent.
- If no response within a few days, begin a first-line agent from a different class at full doses and consider adding a second drug at the same time.
- Prescribe a full nonpharmacologic program.
- Follow closely.

For Patients With Stage IV Disease (Diastolic >120 mm Hg, Systolic >210 mm Hg):

- Consider immediate hospitalization, especially if there is evidence of target-organ disease (eg, papilledema, retinal hemorrhages, heart failure, altered mental status).
- Patients with a similarly elevated pressure but no evidence of target-organ involvement can be given sublingual nifedipine in the office to acutely reduce pressure, started on a two- or three-drug regimen, and followed up in a few days.

Initiation and Advancement of Pharmacologic Therapy:

- Begin pharmacologic therapy with a first-line agent.
- Choose agent based on consideration of patient's overall clinical situation (see below) and start with a modest dose (see Table 26–1).
- If pressure does not improve within 1 month of initiating drug therapy, increase dose and recheck in 4 weeks.
- If there is no response despite increasing dose, then switch to another first-line drug from a different class.
- If there is only a partial response, then the choice is either to further increase dose or to add a low dose of another first-line drug from a different class (eg, add hydrochlorothiazide, 12.5–25 mg/d).
- Once pressure normalizes, recheck blood pressure at 3- to 6-month intervals.
- If a two-drug regimen utilizing two first-line agents from different classes does not suffice, select a third drug from a new class. A particularly effective three-drug regimen is an ACE inhibitor or calcium channel blocker, a thiazide diuretic, and a beta-blocker.
- For patients who are truly refractory but without an underlying cause, consider minoxidil, usually in combination with a loop diuretic (eg, furosemide) and a beta-blocker (see below).
- Consider a sustained-release formulation if it is likely to increase compliance and reduce cost of a daily dose.

First-Line Agents and Indications for Their Use:

- ACE Inhibitors: appropriate for a wide spectrum of patients, including those with volume overload, sexual dysfunction, depression, hypercholesterolemia, glucose intolerance, heart failure, and left ventricular hypertrophy; *contraindicated in pregnancy* and in bilateral renal artery stenosis. Monitor renal function and serum potassium. Least expensive preparation: captopril.
- Beta-blockers: class of choice for those with concurrent coronary artery disease or high cardiovascular risk; most cost-effective; relatively cardioselective preparations with low CNS penetration (eg, atenolol) preferred. Avoid in patients with preexisting depression or sexual dysfunction. Prescribe generic formulations (eg, propranolol, atenolol) to keep costs low. Avoid in patients with bronchospasm or nonischemic heart failure.
- Calcium channel blockers: useful in patients with volume overload hypertension (eg, elderly, blacks) and those with angina (though not proven cardioprotective). Use cautiously in patients with heart failure or conduction defects, especially if already taking a beta-blocker. Avoid in patients bothered by peripheral edema. Prescribe a sustained-release preparation (except in patients with concurrent coronary disease) to reduce cost.
- Thiazide diuretics: effective, low-cost therapy for those with volume overload hypertension (eg, the elderly, blacks, those with nocturia or leg edema). Avoid in patients with marked hypercholesterolemia, poorly controlled diabetes, symptomatic gout, cardiac arrhythmias, or severe underlying coronary disease. Use low doses (eg, 12.5–25 mg/d of hydrochlorothiazide) to enhance effect of beta-blocker, calcium channel blocker, or ACE inhibitor. For monotherapy, use no more than moderate doses (eg, 50 mg/d of hydrochlorothiazide). Monitor potassium, glucose, LDL cholesterol.
- Alpha-blockers: excellent initial drug for patients with marked hyperlipidemia or prostatism. Avoid in elderly patients bothered by falls or postural hypotension. Doxazosin or one of the other newer long-acting preparations preferred.

Special Situations

Refractory Hypertension. Patients are considered "refractory" if they fail to achieve target blood pressure reductions despite full doses of a three-drug regimen. The most common causes are *poor compliance*, *alcohol excess*, and *overweight*. Worrisome etiologies include *renal failure*, *renovascular disease*, and other secondary causes of hypertension (see Chapter 19). Use of over-the-counter decongestants containing *sympathomimetics*, *nonsteroidal anti-in-*

flammatory agents, and *exogenous estrogens* are among the pharmacologic causes. At times, the cause is a treatment regimen that contains an irrational combination, such as two agents within the same class, or an *inadequate amount of diuretic* for the degree of salt intake and sodium retention present. Occasionally, the *anxiety* of the office visit results in pseudo-refractoriness, so-called "white-coat" hypertension (see Chapter 19).

The assessment should begin with a check for medication compliance, weight gain, salt and alcohol excess, and use of other drugs. Pill counts are the best compliance check. A history of nocturia or ankle edema is suggestive of volume overload, either from excessive salt intake or deterioration of renal function. Physical examination is performed to check for signs of secondary etiologies (see Chapter 19), target-organ damage, and volume overload. If "white-coat" hypertension is suspected, blood pressures should be taken by the patient at home and at work, after checking patient technique in the office. *Continuous ambulatory monitoring* may also be of use in this situation (see Chapter 19).

If there is no evidence of a secondary cause, then a check of the serum sodium, potassium, blood urea nitrogen (BUN), and creatinine should suffice. The *echocardiogram*, a sensitive measure of target-organ disease, can help differentiate between true refractoriness and pseudorefractoriness.

If workup fails to reveal a definite cause, the patient should be placed on a 2 g/d sodium/reduced-calorie diet, restricted to 1 oz of alcohol per day, prescribed an exercise program, continued on a maximal three-drug regimen (including an adequate diuretic dose), instructed to monitor pressure at home, and followed closely. If these measures fail, then before escalating the medication program, one should consider consultation with a hypertension specialist for further consideration of possible causes (eg, renal artery stenosis—see Chapter 19). Patients who are truly refractory yet free of a serious underlying etiology often respond to the combination of *minoxidil*, a *loop diuretic*, and a *beta-blocker*.

Hypertension Associated with Estrogen Use. Elevation of systolic and diastolic blood pressure occurs in most patients receiving estrogen therapy over prolonged periods. Five percent of patients become hypertensive, and approximately one-half of these remain hypertensive after hormonal therapy has been discontinued. Factors that predispose to the development of hypertension include family history or past history of high blood pressure, chronic renal disease, and hypertension with a previous pregnancy. A patient should be started on oral contraceptive or estrogen replacement therapy only after a careful history has excluded these predisposing factors. Once therapy has begun, continued blood pressure monitoring is required for the duration of treatment. The development of hypertension should prompt cessation of therapy.

Hypertension and Pregnancy. Hypertension that develops during pregnancy may represent either preeclampsia or preexisting hypertension. Pressure elevations that appear before 20 weeks are almost certainly caused by preexisting disease. Some preexisting hypertension improves during pregnancy because of the hemodynamic changes that occur. Such patients may terminate therapy for the duration of their pregnancy, but pressures should be followed closely. Others require continuation of treatment. The goal of lowering blood pressure in those with preexisting disease is the safety of the mother. There is no fetal benefit to blood pressure reduction; antihypertensive drugs do not cure or reverse preeclampsia.

The usual threshold for initiating antihypertensive medication is a diastolic pressure exceeding 100 mm Hg. For diastolic pressures between 90 and 100 mg Hg, *modest sodium restriction* and increased *rest* often suffice. If they do not, and the blood pressure continues to rise, then beginning *methyldopa* or *hydralazine* is safe and effective. *Beta-blockers* should be avoided in the first trimester due to risk of growth retardation, but they may be used in low doses later. *ACE inhibitors* are *contraindicated* due to the dependence of placental blood flow on intrauterine renin–angiotensin. *Diuretics* taken prior to pregnancy may be continued, as may *alpha-blockers* and *calcium channel blockers*, though recommendations regarding their use remain to be fully formulated.

Preeclampsia is characterized by a blood pressure of 140/90 mm Hg or higher, *edema*, and *proteinuria*, all of which appear in the *third trimester*. The typical patient is a very young primagravida. Multiple births, diabetes, or hydatidiform mole are common associated factors. At 17 to 20 weeks of gestation, a resting blood pressure higher than 110/75 mm Hg while the patient is sitting, or higher than 100/65 mm Hg while the patient is in the left lateral decubitus position, suggests increased risk of preeclampsia (normally the pressure is lower at this time of pregnancy). Once diastolic blood pressure rises above 90 mm Hg, *bed rest* and, if necessary, hospitalization are initiated.

Most medications which have been safely used in pregnancy to control chronic hypertension are appropriate for treatment of preeclampsia. Nitroprusside is given in severe cases that require hospitalization. The use of volume expansion remains controversial. *Diuretics and salt restriction* are to be *avoided*, as these patients usually are intravascularly volume-constricted. Such treatment might aggravate the condition by further stimulating the renin–angiotensin–aldosterone axis. *Magnesium sulfate* is still the treatment of choice for prevention of seizures in patients who are at high risk for developing eclampsia.

The Elderly Patient. Epidemiologic data indicate that in patients older than 65 years of age, isolated systolic hypertension (>160 mm Hg) as well as diastolic hypertension (>90 mm Hg) increases the risks of cardiovascular and stroke-related morbidity and mortality. In fact, systolic pressure is the most predictive (see Chapter 14). Treatment lowers these risks. The goals of therapy are to reduce systolic pressure to less than 160 mm Hg and diastolic pressure to less than 90 mm Hg.

The elderly tend to have low-renin/volume-overload hypertension and exhibit considerable sensitivity to salt intake. For those with very modest pressure elevations, one can begin with *salt restriction*, a gentle exercise program, and *weight reduction*, if overweight. Many elderly patients respond well to a 2 g/d low-sodium diet. Reduction of excess *alcohol* intake to no more than 1 oz/d is also important and occasionally overlooked. Nonpharmacologic measures can lower pressure by as much as 10 mm Hg.

When drug treatment is necessary, the starting dose should be *one-half the usual starting dose* of a first-line agent (eg, *thiazide, ACE inhibitor, calcium channel blocker, or beta-blocker*). Increases in dose ought to be small to allow pressure to decrease gradually; rapid lowering is to be avoided. In general, the elderly do not tolerate aggressive diuretic therapy or sympathetic inhibition as well as younger patients. Drugs likely to cause marked postural hypotension (eg, alpha-blockers) or daytime sedation (centrally acting sympatholytic agents such as methyldopa and clonidine) are also less desirable.

A low dose of a thiazide diuretic (eg, hydrochlorothiazide, 12.5–25 mg/d) is usually well tolerated, inexpensive, and may be all that is needed, though the caveats regarding thiazide use in patients with underlying organic heart disease (see above) should be kept in mind and serum potassium monitored. Calcium channel blockers are also well tolerated in the elderly, having a slight diuretic effect in addition to a vasodilating one. Theoretically, beta-blockers and ACE inhibitors should be less effective, but they too work quite well as first-line drugs and may be especially useful if there is concurrent coronary disease or heart failure, respectively.

The African-American Patient. Hypertension is more prevalent in African-Americans (38.2%), more commonly of the low-renin/salt-sensitive variety, and more likely to be accompanied by target-organ damage than in whites. The high prevalence of obesity, smoking, and salt excess contribute, as does decreased access to medical care. African-Americans show twice the risk of developing renal insufficiency, even when treated. They respond particularly well to *thiazides*, *sodium restriction*, *weight loss*, and *smoking cessation*. The metabolically adverse effects of thiazides and their inability to reverse left ventricular hypertrophy make them less than ideal agents. *Calcium channel blockers* have shown very promising results, though their use greatly increases cost of treatment, which, in turn, might compromise long-term compliance. *ACE inhibitors* and *beta-blockers* are somewhat less effective, perhaps because of the low-renin physiology prevalent in this population.

The Diabetic Patient. Control of hypertension is particularly important in diabetics to reduce the already high risks of stroke, cardiovascular disease, and renal failure. *ACE inhibitors* are the drugs of choice, because they decrease proteinuria and may slow the progression of diabetic nephropathy. *Calcium channel blockers* also may be protective of the kidney and are tolerated and effective. Although *thiazide* diuretics may worsen glucose intolerance and hyperlipidemia, these adverse effects can be minimized by using small doses (eg, 12.5–25 mg/d of hydrochlorothiazide). If the patient is taking insulin but a *beta-blocker* is deemed desirable, then a relatively cardioselective preparation (eg, atenolol or metoprolol) is preferred, since it is less likely to mask catecholamine-induced hypoglycemic symptoms.

The Patient with Renal Failure. Hypertension can lead to renal injury as well as exacerbate it. Its control is essential in the setting of renal parenchymal disease. A *reduced-protein* (40–45 g/d), *low-salt diet* is central to preservation of renal function and control of blood pressure in patients with azotemia. When the serum creatinine rises above 2.5 mg/dL, sodium retention occurs, which can lead to exacerbation of blood pressure. *Furosemide*, *metolazone*, and other potent diuretics may be needed to counter the sodium retention and reduce pressure. *ACE inhibitors* reduce proteinuria and often can be helpful in the setting of renal failure, unless the cause is renal artery stenosis, in which case they may aggravate renal dysfunction. *Beta-blockers, vasodilators*, and *calcium channel blockers* are also effective. *Minoxidil*, in combination with a loop diuretic and a beta-blocker, may be necessary in refractory cases.

The Stroke Patient. Control of hypertension reduces the risk of recurrent stroke. The main pitfall of treatment is too rapid and too vigorous a reduction in blood pressure. Gradual, gentle pressure reduction that preserves CNS perfusion and avoids postural hypotension is the goal.

PATIENT EDUCATION: ENSURING COMPLIANCE

Being a silent condition, hypertension does not always command the full attention of patients. High cost of medication, high frequency of doses, and drug side effects further compromise compliance. Nonetheless, some educational and behavioral efforts can enhance patient cooperation. Educationally, one needs to *review the cardiovascular consequences* of untreated hypertension as well as the *efficacy of treatment*. Knowledge of the *importance of nonpharmacologic measures* is also critical and reassuring to many. That weight reduction, smoking cessation, and decrease in sodium intake may allow reduction or even elimination of antihypertensive medication can serve as a powerful motivating force.

One of the best behavioral methods is to give the patient an active role in monitoring. Teaching the patient to perform *home blood pressure determinations* can foster considerable interest in blood pressure control and greatly stimulate compliance. Effective home monitoring may even decrease the need for some office visits.

Medication side effects need to be addressed. *Sexual dysfunction*, *fatigue*, and *depression* have long bothered hypertensive patients who require drug therapy and led patients to stopping their medication, often without notifying the physician. It is essential to specifically inquire about symptoms of sexual dysfunction (see Chapter 229) and depression (see Chapter 227) before as well as after initiation of a medical regimen and to incorporate the findings into design of the patient's program. Patients may be reluctant to raise these issues themselves. Use of a medication that does not interfere with sexual capacity or mental function (eg, captopril) may be indicated (see above).

INDICATIONS FOR REFERRAL AND ADMISSION

Immediate hospitalization is indicated for patients with evidence of *malignant hypertension* (diastolic pressure >130 mm Hg, retinal hemorrhages, bulging discs, mental status changes, heart failure). Referral is indicated for patients with refractory hypertension (see above), a suspected secondary cause, or worsening renal failure in the setting of adequate control.

ANNOTATED BIBLIOGRAPHY

Anastos K, Charney P, Charon RA et al. Hypertension in women: What is really known. Ann Intern Med 1991;115:287. *(Many of the generalizations about treatment of hypertension might not apply to women; reviews available data and emphasizes the large knowledge gaps.)*

Cappuccio FP, Markandu ND, Saganella GA, et al. Acute and sustained changes in sodium balance during nifedipine treatment in essential hypertension. Am J Med 1991;91:233. *(Natriuretic effect found.)*

Christlieb AR. Treatment selection considerations for the hypertensive diabetic patient. Arch Intern Med 1990;150:1167. *(ACE inhibitors and calcium channel blockers are the drugs of choice; 78 refs.)*

Collins R, Peto R, MacMahon S et al. Blood pressure, stroke, and coronary disease. Part II: Short-term reductions in blood pressure. Lancet 1990;335:827. *(A major meta-analysis documenting efficacy of blood pressure reduction in reducing risk, especially of stroke but also of coronary disease.)*

Croog SH, Levine S, Testa MA et al. The effects of antihypertensive therapy on the quality of life. N Engl J Med 1986;314:1657. *(A multicenter randomized double-blind study showing that ACE inhibitors were the best tolerated.)*

Cunningham FG, Lindheimer MD. Hypertension in pregnancy. N Engl J Med 1992;326:927. *(An excellent review; 61 refs.)*

Dimsdale JE, Newton RP, Joist T. Neuropsychological side effects of beta-blockers. Arch Intern Med 1989;149:514. *(A review of 55 studies on the issue, concluding that there is little evidence for a difference in CNS effects of the lipophilic and lipophobic preparations.)*

Dzau VJ. Renin and myocardial infarction in hypertension. N Engl J Med 1991;324:1128. *(An editorial summarizing the uses and problems with renin profiling, especially as it regards predicting risk of infarction.)*

Edelson JT, Weinstein MC, Tosteson AN et al. Long-term cost-effectiveness of various initial monotherapies for mild to moderate hypertension. JAMA 1990;263:407. *(Propranolol was best, followed by hydrochlorothiazide, nifedipine, prazosin, and captopril.)*

Eisenberg DM, Delbanco TL, Berkey CS et al. Cognitive behavioral techniques for hypertension: Are they effective? Ann Intern Med 1993;118:964. *(A meta-analysis incorporating data from the limited number of available well-designed studies; found no benefit over placebo.)*

Eisenberg DM, Landsberg L, Allred EN et al. Inability to demonstrate physiologic correlates of subjective improvement among patients taught the relaxation response. J Gen Intern Med 1991;6:64. *(Blood pressure did not go down in this study of patients with borderline or labile hypertension.)*

Farnett L, Mulrow CD, Linn WD et al. The J-curve phenomenon and the treatment of hypertension. JAMA 1991;265:489. *(An analysis of 13 major studies; diastolic reduction below 85 mm Hg increased risk of an adverse cardiac event, though stroke risk continued to decline.)*

Fifth Report of the Joint National Committee on Detection, Evaluation, and Treatment of High Blood Pressure. Arch Intern Med 1993;153:154. *(Major consensus report; 117 refs.)*

Fletcher AE, Bulpitt CJ. How far should blood pressure be lowered. N Engl J Med 1992;326:251. *(Argues that the J-curve phenomenon is the consequence, not the cause of coronary disease.)*

Freis ED et al. Veterans Administration cooperative study group on antihypertensive agents. I: Effects of treatment on morbidity in hypertension: Results in patients with diastolic blood pressures averaging 115 through 129 mm Hg. JAMA 1967;202:1028. II: Results in patients with diastolic blood pressure averaging 90 through 114 mm Hg. JAMA 1970; 213:1143. *(The classic studies demonstrating that treatment of hypertension reduced morbidity and mortality from heart failure, renal failure, and stroke.)*

Grimm RH, Neaton JD, Elmer PJ et al. The influence of oral potassium chloride on blood pressure in hypertensive men on a low-sodium diet. N Engl J Med 1990;322:569. *(Supplemental potassium was not sufficient to eliminate the need for antihypertensive therapy in men on a sodium-restricted diet.)*

Houston MC. New insights and new approaches for the treatment of essential hypertension: Selection of therapy based on coronary heart disease risk factor analysis, hemodynamic profiles, quality of life, and subsets of hypertension. Am Heart J 1989;117:911. *(Excellent discussion of the factors that should guide design of the treatment program.)*

Kannel WB, Wolf PA, McGee DL. Systolic blood pressure, arterial rigidity, and risk of stroke. JAMA 1981;245:1225. *(The classic paper from the Framingham Study on increased risk of stroke with isolated systolic hypertension.)*

Kaplan NM. Maximally reducing cardiovascular risk in the treatment of hypertension. Ann Intern Med 1988;109:36. *(Redirects attention from level of blood pressure to overall cardiovascular risk; recommends ACE inhibitors, calcium channel blockers, and alpha-blockers from this perspective.)*

Kelemen MH, Effron MB, Valenti SA et al. Exercise training combined with antihypertensive drug therapy. JAMA 1990; 263:2766. *(Exercise was just as effective as drug therapy and obviated the need for medication in mildly hypertensive patients.)*

Langdon CG. Doxazosin: A study in a cohort of patients with hypertension in general practice. Am Heart J 1991;121:268. *(This new alpha-blocker was remarkably well tolerated and improved the lipid profile of hyperlipidemic hypertensive patients.)*

MacMahon SW, Norton RN. Alcohol and hypertension. Ann Intern Med 1986;105:124. *(An editorial summarizing the evidence linking the two conditions and recommending a limit of less than 2 oz per day.)*

MacMahon SW, Peto R, Cutler J et al. Blood pressure, stroke, and coronary heart disease. Part 1: Prolonged differences in blood pressure; prospective observational studies corrected for the regression dilution bias. Lancet 1990;335:765. *(A meta-analysis of data from nine population-based studies showing a continuous relation between blood pressures between 70 and 110 mm Hg and risks of stroke and coronary disease.)*

Medical Research Council Working Party. Stroke and coronary heart disease in mild hypertension: Risk factors and value of treatment. Br Medical J 1988;296:1565. *(Excellent benefit analysis of treating mild hypertension; concludes that treatment is worthwhile.)*

Mejia AD, Egan BM, Schork NJ et al. Artifacts in measurement of blood pressure and lack of target organ involvement in the assessment of patients with treatment-resistant hypertension. Ann Intern Med 1990;112:270. *(Identifies artifactual causes of elevated office blood pressure in patients who seem refractory to three-drug therapy.)*

National Heart Foundation of Australia Study. Treatment of mild hypertension in the elderly. Med J Aust 1981;2:398. *(Elderly patients with diastolic pressures greater than 95 mm Hg benefitted from therapy.)*

National High Blood Pressure Education Program Working Group. Report on Primary Prevention of Hypertension. Arch

Intern Med 1993;153;186. *(Major review of nonpharmacologic measures; 327 refs.)*

National High Blood Pressure Education Program Working Group. Report on High Blood Pressure in Pregnancy. Am J Obstet Gynecol 1990;163:1689. *(Comprehensive consensus report and excellent review of the issue.)*

Neaton JD, Grimm RH, Prineas RJ, et al. Treatment of mild hypertension study: Final results. JAMA 1993;270:713. *(Drugs plus nonpharmacologic measures better than nonpharmacologic measures alone.)*

Oberman A, Wassertheil-Smoller S, Langford HG et al. Pharmacologic and nutritional treatment of mild hypertension: Changes in cardiovascular risk status. Ann Intern Med 1990;112:89. *(Diet can greatly enhance the lowering of cardiovascular risk.)*

Oparil S. Antihypertensive therapy—Efficacy and quality of life. N Engl J Med 1993;328:959. *(An editorial reviewing the importance of this issue to the successful treatment of hypertension.)*

Pettinger WA. Minoxidil and the treatment of severe hypertension. N Engl J Med 1980;303:922. *(Reviews its pharmacology and clinical use.)*

Psaty BM, Koepsell TD, LoGerfo JP et al. Beta-blockers and primary prevention of coronary heart disease patients with high blood pressure. JAMA 1989;261:2087. *(A case-control study showing that hypertensive patients taking beta-blocker therapy had a 38 percent reduction in risk of coronary disease.)*

Radack K, Deck C. Do nonsteroidal anti-inflammatory drugs interfere with blood pressure control in hypertensive patients? J Gen Intern Med 1987;2:108. *(A critical review of available studies, concluding there is some evidence of impairment, but better data are needed.)*

Rutan G, Kuller LHJ, Wentworth DN, et al. Mortality associated with diastolic hypertension and isolated systolic hypertension among men screened for the Multiple Risk Factor Intervention Trial. Circulation 1988;77:504. *(The MRFIT study showing increased risk of sudden cardiovascular death in thiazide-treated patients with baseline ECG abnormalities.)*

Saunders E, Weir MR, Kong BW et al. A comparison of the efficacy and safety of a beta-blocker, a calcium-channel blocker, and an ACE inhibitor in hypertensive blacks. Arch Intern Med 1990;150:1707. *(The calcium channel blocker was the most effective, but response rates to the others exceeded 50 percent; all were well tolerated.)*

Schmieder RE, Rockstroh JK, Messerli FZ. Antihypertensive therapy: To stop or not to stop? JAMA 1991;265:1566. *(A review of the evidence for cessation of therapy; 80 refs.)*

Schoenberger JA, Testa M, Ross AD et al. Efficacy, safety, and quality of life assessment of captopril antihypertensive therapy in clinical practice. Arch Intern Med 1990;150:301. *(Reports the experience in 30,000 patients, with mean pressure reduction of 15 mm Hg, efficacy across all age and racial groups, few side effects and no adverse effects on quality of life.)*

Steiner JF, Fihn SD, Koepsell TD et al. Clinical predictors of treatment reduction in hypertensive patients. J Gen Intern Med 1990;203. *(More than 5.5 years of therapy with the equivalent of two or more agents correlated with likelihood of successful reduction in therapy.)*

Stewart EM, Deckro JP, Mamish ME et al. Non-pharmacologic treatment of the elderly hypertensive patients. Circulation 1989;80(suppl II):189. *(Nondrug therapies lowered pressures by an average of 9.0 mm Hg; salt restriction was especially effective.)*

Systolic Hypertension in the Elderly Cooperative Research Group. Prevention of stroke by antihypertensive drug treatment in older persons with isolated systolic hypertension. JAMA 1991;265:3255. *(Treatment of isolated systolic hypertension does indeed significantly reduce risk of stroke.)*

Testa MA, Anderson RB, Nackley JF et al. Quality of life and antihypertensive therapy in men—A comparison of captopril with enalapril. N Engl J Med 1993;328:907. *(Captopril was the better tolerated.)*

The Working Group on Hypertension in Diabetes. Statement on hypertension in diabetes mellitus. Arch Intern Med 1987; 147:830. *(A consensus panel approach to treatment.)*

Townsend RR, Holland OB. Combination of converting enzyme inhibitor with diuretic for the treatment of hypertension. Arch Intern Med 1990;150:1175. *(The case for an ACE inhibitor plus low-dose diuretic.)*

Wassertheil-Smoller S, Blaufox D, Oberman A et al. Effect of antihypertensives on sexual function and quality of life: The TAIM study. Ann Intern Med 1991;114:613. *(Treatment with low-dose thiazide or atenolol did not to impair quality of life; sexual function problems occurred only in thiazide-treated patients.)*

Williams GH. Converting-enzyme inhibitors in the treatment of hypertension. N Engl J Med 1988;319:1517. *(Comprehensive review; 102 refs.)*

Working Group on Management of Patients with Hypertension and High Blood Cholesterol. National Education Programs Working Group Report on the Management of Patients With Hypertension and High Blood Cholesterol. Ann Intern Med 1991;114:224. *(Provides an integrated approach to treating these major risk factors when they occur concurrently.)*

World Health Organization. Recommendations for management of mild hypertension. J Hypertens 1989;7:689. *(Important consensus view of treatment goals for mild disease.)*

Appendix: Coronary Heart Disease Risk Factor Prediction Chart — American Heart Association

1. Find Points For Each Risk Factor

Age (If Female)				Age (If Male)				HDL-Cholesterol		Total-Cholesterol		Systolic Blood Pressure			
Age	Pts.	Age	Pts.	Age	Pts.	Age	Pts.	HDL-C	Pts.	Total-C	Pts.	SBP	Pts.	Other	Pts.
30	−12	47–48	5	30	−2	57–59	13	25–26	7	139–151	−3	98–104	−2	Cigarettes	4
31	−11	49–50	6	31	−1	60–61	14	27–29	6	152–166	−2	105–112	−1	Diabetic-male	3
32	−9	51–52	7	32–33	0	62–64	15	30–32	5	167–182	−1	113–120	0	Diabetic-female	6
33	−8	53–55	8	34	1	65–67	16	33–35	4	183–199	0	121–129	1	ECG-LVH	9
34	−6	56–60	9	35–36	2	68–70	17	36–38	3	200–219	1	130–139	2		
35	−5	61–67	10	37–38	3	71–73	18	39–42	2	220–239	2	140–149	3	0 pts for each NO	
36	−4	68–74	11	39	4	74	19	43–46	1	240–262	3	150–160	4		
37	−3			40–41	5			47–50	0	263–288	4	161–172	5		
38	−2			42–43	6			51–55	−1	289–315	5	173–185	6		
39	−1			44–45	7			56–60	−2	316–330	6				
40	0			46–47	8			61–66	−3						
41	1			48–49	9			67–73	−4						
42–43	2			50–51	10			74–80	−5						
44	3			52–54	11			81–87	−6						
45–46	4			55–56	12			88–96	−7						

2. Sum Points For All Risk Factors

_____ + _____ + _____ + _____ + _____ + _____ + _____ = _____

Age + HDL-C + Total-C + SBP + Smoker + Diabetes + ECG-LVH = Point Total

NOTE: *Minus Points Subtract From Total.*

3. Look Up Risk Corresponding To Point Total

Probability			Probability			Probability			Probability		
Pts.	5 Yr.	10 Yr.	Pts.	5 Yr.	10 Yr.	Pts.	5 Yr.	10 Yr.	Pts.	5 Yr.	10 Yr.
≤1	<1%	<2%	10	2%	6%	19	8%	16%	28	19%	33%
2	1%	2%	11	3%	6%	20	8%	18%	29	20%	36%
3	1%	2%	12	3%	7%	21	9%	19%	30	22%	38%
4	1%	2%	13	3%	8%	22	11%	21%	31	24%	40%
5	1%	3%	14	4%	9%	23	12%	23%	32	25%	42%
6	1%	3%	15	5%	10%	24	13%	25%			
7	1%	4%	16	5%	12%	25	14%	27%			
8	2%	4%	17	6%	13%	26	16%	29%			
9	2%	5%	18	7%	14%	27	17%	31%			

4. Compare To Average 10 Year Risk

Probability		
Age	Women	Men
30–34	<1%	3%
35–39	<1%	5%
40–44	2%	6%
45–49	5%	10%
50–54	8%	14%
55–59	12%	16%
60–64	13%	21%
65–69	9%	30%
70–74	12%	24%

These charts were prepared with the help of William B. Kannel, M.D., Professor of Medicine and Public Health and Ralph D'Agostino, Ph.D., Head, Department of Mathematics, both at Boston University; Keaven Anderson, Ph.D., Statistician, NHLBI, Framingham Study; Daniel McGee, Ph.D., Associate Professor, University of Arizona.

Framingham Heart Study

Primary Care Medicine: Office Evaluation and Management of the Adult Patient, 3rd edition, edited by Allan H. Goroll, Lawrence A. May, and Albert G. Mulley, Jr. J.B. Lippincott Company, Philadelphia © 1995

27

Approach to the Patient With Hypercholesterolemia

MASON W. FREEMAN, M.D.

Over the last several years, evidence has accumulated demonstrating that treatment of hypercholesterolemia can reduce atherosclerosis and its attendant cardiovascular complications (see Chapter 15). These findings have heightened physician and patient awareness of the importance of hypercholesterolemia. The primary care physician needs to be capable of evaluating hypercholesterolemia and of designing and implementing a treatment program that effectively utilizes dietary treatment, exercise, weight loss, and, when necessary, cholesterol-lowering drugs.

PATHOPHYSIOLOGY

The production of atherogenic lipoproteins and lipoprotein-induced formation of atheromatous plaques involve distinct pathways. The mere presence of an elevated serum cholesterol level does not guarantee the development of advanced plaques any more than a normal cholesterol concentration ensures plaque-free coronary arteries. A host of factors besides cholesterol elevation interact in a complex fashion to determine plaque formation. Such factors include genetic variations in lipoprotein structures, receptors, and metabolic enzymes, as well as the complex interactions between lipids and cellular constituents of the vessel wall.

Lipoproteins

An understanding of lipoproteins is essential for understanding the approach to evaluation and treatment. In order to circulate in the aqueous environment of the blood, lipids such as cholesterol and triglyceride are complexed with proteins and the more polar phospholipids into spheres called *lipoproteins*. The protein components of the lipoproteins are known as *apoproteins*; they play both a structural and functional role in metabolism of the particles. Genetic alterations in apoproteins can have clinical consequences. The lipoproteins are usually divided into four major classes based on density, which is a reflection of their relative protein and lipid

Table 27-1. Lipoprotein Composition

LIPOPROTEIN	PROTEIN%	CHOL%	CHOL ESTER%	PL*%	TG%
VLDL	10.4	5.8	13.9	15.2	53.4
IDL	17.8	6.5	22.5	21.7	31.4
LDL	25.0	8.6	41.9	20.9	3.5
HDL2	42.6	5.2	20.3	30.1	2.2
HDL3	54.9	2.6	16.1	25.0	1.4
Chylomicrons	1–2	1–3	2–4	3–8	80–95

*PL = Phospholipid
values are % composition by weight

content: 1) chylomicrons; 2) very low density lipoproteins (VLDL); 3) low density lipoproteins (LDL); and 4) high density lipoproteins (HDL). There are also subdivisions and minor classes of lipoproteins (Table 27–1).

Chylomicrons derive from dietary fat and carry triglycerides throughout the body. They have the lowest density of all lipoproteins and will float to the top of a plasma specimen left in the refrigerator overnight. The chylomicron itself is probably not atherogenic, but the role of the triglyceride-depleted chylomicron remnant remains uncertain. Triglyceride makes up most of the chylomicron and is removed by the action of lipoprotein lipase. Patients deficient in this enzyme or its cofactors (insulin and apo C-II) have very high serum triglyceride levels and increased risk of acute pancreatitis.

Very Low Density Lipoproteins are also triglyceride-rich and are acted on by lipoprotein lipase. Their function is to carry triglycerides synthesized in the liver and intestines to capillary beds in adipose tissue and muscle, where they are hydrolyzed. After removal of their triglyceride, VLDL remnants can be further metabolized to LDL. Native VLDL is not known to have any role in atherogenesis. VLDLs serve as acceptors of cholesterol transferred from HDL, possibly accounting in part for the inverse relation between HDL cholesterol and VLDL triglyceride. The process is mediated by the enzyme cholesterol ester transfer protein (CETP).

Low Density Lipoproteins are the major carriers of cholesterol in humans, responsible for supplying cholesterol to the tissues, and most clearly implicated in atherogenesis. LDL levels are increased in persons who consume large amounts of saturated fat and/or cholesterol, have defects in the LDL receptor (familial hypercholesterolemia), have defects in the structure of LDL apoprotein apo B, or have a polygenic form of increased LDL. When serum LDLs exceed a certain threshold concentration, they traverse the endothelial wall and can become trapped in the arterial intima. There, they may undergo oxidation or other modification, be taken up by macrophages, and stimulate atherogenesis. The association of serum cholesterol with coronary heart disease (CHD) is predominantly a reflection of the role of LDL.

High Density Lipoproteins are believed to function in peripheral tissues as an acceptor of free cholesterol which has passively diffused out of cellular membranes. The cholesterol is esterified and stored in the central core of the HDL, and may be further metabolized. This reverse transport system may explain why patients with very high HDL levels have a reduced risk of developing CHD, even if their LDL levels are elevated. *Apo A-I* is the major apoprotein of HDL, and its level also inversely correlates with the risk of CHD. Women have higher levels of HDL cholesterol than men, in part because of their higher estrogen levels. Exercise increases HDL, while obesity, hypertriglyceridemia, and smoking lower HDL. The HDL cholesterol concentration is the single most powerful predictor of CHD risk. A ratio of total cholesterol to HDL cholesterol of less than 4.5 indicates low CHD risk.

Dietary Influences

Dietary fat and cholesterol have a substantial influence on serum cholesterol and LDL, with saturated fat by far the most important. For each increase in percentage of total calories contributed by saturated fats, serum cholesterol increases by a factor of 2.16, whereas the serum cholesterol increase is only .068 for each percentage increase in dietary cholesterol. This relationship is summarized in the equation of Hegsted:

$$\text{Change in total cholesterol} = 2.16 \text{ delta S} - 1.65 \text{ delta P} + 0.068 \text{ delta C}$$

where delta S, delta P, and delta C are the changes in the percentage of total calories contributed by saturated fats, polyunsaturated fats, and cholesterol, respectively. Fats are characterized by their constituent fatty acid composition. The fatty acids are characterized as saturated, polyunsaturated, or monounsaturated. The state of saturation refers to the number of carbon–carbon double bonds contained in the fatty acid.

Saturated Fatty Acids *can raise LDL cholesterol*, in part by altering the LDL receptor's catabolic activity. The long-chain saturated fatty acids common to the American diet—lauric (12 carbons), myristic (14 carbons), palmitic (16 carbons), and stearic (18 carbons)—have no double bonds and are not essential for human growth and development. *Not all* saturated fatty acids trigger rises in LDL cholesterol. For example, stearic acid and some shorter chain fatty acids (caproic and caprylic) do not. In the typical American diet, about one-third of the saturated fat content of the diet derives from *meat* and meat products, while another third comes from *dairy products* and eggs, and 10 percent from baked goods. Vegetable oils also may contain saturated fat (see Appendix I), especially the so-called *"tropical oils"* (coconut and palm) and cocoa butter, which are commonly used in commercial food preparation. Even when unsaturated oils (see below) are used in processed foods, they usually undergo partial "hydrogenation" (conversion of double bonds to single ones). This saturation process is performed to make them more solid at room temperature, but it also makes them more hypercholesterolemic.

Monounsaturated Fatty Acids are present in all animal and vegetable fats. The most common dietary form is oleic acid, plentiful in peanuts, almonds, olives, and avocados. Oils derived from these sources *neither raise nor lower LDL cholesterol* by themselves, though cholesterol will fall if they are used as a substitute for a saturated fat.

Polyunsaturated Fatty Acids (PUFAs), unlike saturated and monounsaturated fatty acids, are not synthesized by the body. They must be present in the diet and are referred to as essential fatty acids. The location of the first double bond from the methyl end of the molecule determines the nomenclature of the PUFAs. The major dietary fatty acids contain either an n-6 or n-3 first double bond. Linoleic and arachidonic acids are the common n-6 PUFAs, found in considerable quantities in *liquid vegetable oils* (sunflower, safflower, corn, and soybean). The n-3 fatty acids are represented by linoleic acid (found in canola oil and leafy vegetables) and the omega-3 *fish oils* (eicosapentanoic and docosahexanoic acids). They attracted considerable interest when epidemiologic studies found a link between their consumption and reduced rates of CHD, but prospective clinical trials of diets high in n-3 fatty acids have yet to demonstrate an ability to reduce coronary mortality.

The double bonds of polyunsaturated fatty acids are normally in the "trans" configuration, which is atherogenically favorable. Commercial hydrogenation can convert PUFA double bonds from the trans configuration to the less favorable "cis" configuration.

Cholesterol. As the Hegsted formula indicates, dietary cholesterol has a much smaller effect than saturated fatty acids on raising total cholesterol. For every additional 100 mg of dietary cholesterol consumed per day, the serum cholesterol will rise by about 8 to 10 mg/dL. However, *organ meats* (eg, brain, kidney, heart, sweetbreads) and *egg yolks* are concentrated sources of dietary cholesterol (see Appendix II) and can have a substantial impact on serum cholesterol levels. Although *shellfish* contain moderate amounts of cholesterol, they have relatively small amounts of saturated fat and are sources of n-3 PUFAs. Cholesterol is absent from food derived from plants.

Other Dietary Factors. There is no evidence that either dietary *carbohydrate* (whether simple sugars or complex ones) or *protein* significantly affects LDL cholesterol. Increased total caloric intake associated with obesity may induce overproduction of VLDL triglycerides. HDL levels are reduced in obese individuals. The *fiber* content of food has generated much interest. *Insoluble fiber* (typically cellulose found in wheat bran) has no cholesterol-lowering effect, though it is beneficial for lowering the risk of diverticular disease and colon cancer (see Chapter 65). *Soluble fiber* (pectins, certain gums, psyllium) have received much attention in the lay press stimulated by claims about *oat bran*, which contains the gum beta-glycan. Initial studies were encouraging, but subsequent data suggested the cholesterol decreases observed were no greater than those found with use of insoluble fiber and probably resulted from replacement of dietary fat in the diet, rather than from a direct effect on lipid metabolism. When studied in patients already taking a low-fat diet, high soluble fiber intake appeared to lower serum cholesterol by a modest amount (3–7%).

WORKUP

Diagnosis. The diagnosis of hypercholesterolemia should always be based on *repeat measurements* of serum lipids, because combined analytic and biologic variations in serum lipids range from 10 percent to 20 percent. A single measurement should never be viewed as sufficient for a diagnosis of hypercholesterolemia. A *venous sample* processed in a laboratory meeting Centers for Disease Control and Prevention standards for cholesterol determination (see Chapter 15) is essential for confirmation.

Once an elevated (>200 mg/dL) total cholesterol level is confirmed, then follow-up and further investigation are based on degree of elevation and presence of other CHD risk factors. Patients considered appropriate for lipoprotein analysis are those with a *total cholesterol level higher than 240 mg/dL*, or a total cholesterol level of 200 to 239 mg/dL plus established CHD or two other CHD risk factors (Table 27–2). In such individuals, a fasting venous sample for determination of serum cholesterol, *HDL cholesterol*, and *triglycerides* is necessary for characterization of the lipid disorder and design of therapy.

Some patients present with HDL cholesterol having already been measured as part of the lipid-screening effort.

Table 27-2. Initial Classification and Recommended Follow-Up Based on Total Cholesterol*

Classification, mg/dL	
<200	Desirable blood cholesterol
200 to 239	Borderline-high blood cholesterol
≥240	High blood cholesterol
Recommended followup	
Total cholesterol, <200 mg/dL	Repeat within five years
Total cholesterol, 200–239 mg/dL	
Without definite CHD or two other CHD risk factors (one of which can be male sex)	Dietary information and recheck annually
With definite CHD or two other CHD risk factors (one of which can be male sex)	Lipoprotein analysis; further action based on LDL-cholesterol level
Total cholesterol ≥240 mg/dL	Lipoprotein analysis; further action based on LDL-cholesterol level

*CHD indicates coronary heart disease; LDL, low density lipoprotein.

From: Report of the National Cholesterol Education Program. Expert Panel on Detection, Evaluation, and Treatment of High Blood Cholesterol in Adults. Arch Intern Med 1988;148:36.

The growing appreciation of a low HDL cholesterol (<35 mg/dL) as a CHD risk factor has led to recommendations for including it in lipid screening (see Chapter 15). Only if the measurement was performed in a manner assuring its accuracy (see Chapter 15) should it be used in the initial determination of CHD risk. Otherwise, it is best to wait until the HDL cholesterol is remeasured as part of the formal lipoprotein evaluation.

With measurement of total and HDL cholesterol and triglyceride levels, it is possible to *estimate the VLDL* level and *calculate* the *LDL cholesterol* concentration using the Friedwald formula:

LDL cholesterol = total cholesterol − [HDL cholesterol + triglyceride/5]

The triglyceride/5 factor represents a close estimate of VLDL cholesterol and derives from the observation that VLDL cholesterol is usually 20 percent of the serum triglyceride value. The validity of this formula for estimating LDL cholesterol has been confirmed by direct LDL cholesterol measurement and remains fairly accurate so long as the total triglyceride is less than 400 mg/dL. A *fasting* sample is required for best results, since triglyceride levels can change acutely with eating. If the triglyceride level is greater than 400 mg/dL, the LDL cholesterol can be determined accurately only by methods available to a lipid research laboratory.

Excluding Secondary Causes. Before embarking on a treatment plan, one must exclude conditions that might secondarily lead to hyperlipidemia. The most important are *hypothyroidism, nephrotic syndrome,* and diabetes (Table 27–3), best screened for by a serum TSH, urine dipstick for protein, and serum glucose, respectively (see Chapters 93, 104, and 130). Drugs can affect lipid levels as well, with LDL elevations occurring with *thiazide* use and, to a lesser extent, with *beta-blockers*; postmenopausal *estrogen replacement* increases HDL and lowers LDL.

Classification. The original classification scheme of Fredrickson is of limited utility now that a better understanding of the genetics of these diseases has emerged. However, no unified classification of comparable simplicity has replaced it. For most clinical purposes, it is probably simplest to separate patients into three broad categories: those with 1) elevated cholesterol, 2) elevated cholesterol and triglyceride, or 3) elevated triglyceride only. Table 27–3 summarizes the likely diagnoses under these broad categories. The possibility of a genetic disorder should be considered if extremes of any lipoprotein-cholesterol level are encountered or if there is a history of premature CHD in the patient or family. Classification by risk stratification is also helpful for both patient and physician (see below and Tables 27–4 and 27–5).

Table 27-3. Classification of Lipoprotein Disorders

NAME	PRIMARY DISORDER	SECONDARY DISORDER	LIPOPROTEIN INVOLVED	XANTHOMAS
		Increased Triglycerides and Cholesterol		
Combined hyperlidemia	Unknown	Hypothyroidism	VDL and VLDL	None
Remnant hyperlipidemia	Familial dysbetalipoproteinemia	Hypothyroidism SLE	IDL	Tuberous tuberoeruptive
		Increased Cholesterol		
Familial hypercholesterolemia	LDL receptor defects		LDL	Tendon
Combined hyperlipidemia	Unknown	Hypothyroidism Nephrotic syndrome	LDL	
Polygenic hypercholesterolemia	Unknown	Hypothyroidism	LDL	
Familial hyperalphalipoproteinemia	Unknown		HDL	
		Increased Triglycerides		
Exogenous hypertriglyceridemia	Lipoprotein (LPL) Lipase deficiency Apo C-II deficiency LPL inhibition	SLE	Chylomicrons	Eruptive
Endogenous hypertriglyceridemia	Familial hyper TG	Diabetes Dysglobulinemia Uremia Nephrotic syndrome Lipodystrophies Steroids Alcohol Estrogen Hypothyroidism	VLDL	Usually none
Mixed hypertriglyceridemia	Familial hyperTG LPL deficiency Apo C-II deficiency	(same as for endogenous hypertriglyceridemia)	VLDL and Chylomicrons	Eruptive

Table 27-4. CHD Risk Associated with Lipoprotein Cholesterol Abnormalities*

LIPOPROTEIN-CHOLESTEROL	LEVEL (MG/DL)	ESTIMATED CHD RISK
LDL-cholesterol	<130	Low
	130–159	Moderate
	>160	High
HDL-cholesterol	>65 (and total cholesterol/HDL ratio <4.5)	Low
	<35 (and total cholesterol/HDL ratio >4.5)	Moderate-high
VLDL-cholesterol	50–100 (or fasting triglycerides 250–500)	Low
	>100 (or fasting triglycerides >500)	?

*Presence of additional CHD risk factors greatly increases risk for any level of lipoprotein cholesterol.

PRINCIPLES OF MANAGEMENT

The goals are to reduce coronary morbidity and mortality. Both *primary prevention* (reducing risk of having a first coronary event) and *secondary prevention* (reducing risk of a new coronary event in a person with established CHD) are sought. The most impressive reductions in risk are achieved in patients at greatest risk (see below).

The growing appreciation for the importance of lipid abnormalities and for the efficacy of treatment have stimulated the National Institutes of Health to sponsor a National Cholesterol Education Program (NCEP). It convened an expert panel, which has formulated consensus treatment recommendations, many of which are included below. The approach to treatment of hyperlipidemia is guided by an assessment of total CHD risk, not just the lipid abnormality. For a given degree of LDL cholesterol elevation, the threshold for initiation of therapy decreases and the intensity of therapy increases with increasing CHD risk. Dietary modification, complemented by exercise and weight reduction, is the core of the lipid treatment program, with pharmacologic therapy reserved for those at highest risk.

Table 27-5. CHD Risk Factors and CHD Risk Status

Risk Factors Other Than Elevated LDL Cholesterol Level

Age >45 for male; >55 or premature menopause for female without estrogen replacement

Family history of premature CHD (definite MI or sudden death in first-degree male relative before age 55 or before 65 in female first-degree relative)

Current cigarette smoking

Hypertension (systolic >140 or diastolic >90)

Low HDL cholesterol (<35 mg/dL)

Diabetes mellitus

CHD Risk Status

Highest

Clinically evident CHD or other atherosclerotic disease (peripheral arterial insufficiency, symptomatic carotid artery disease)

No CHD but two or more CHD risk factors in addition to hypercholesterolemia

No CHD and fewer than two other CHD risk factors in addition to hypercholesterolemia

No CHD, no risk factors

Lowest

Adapted from: Summary of the Second Report of the National Cholesterol Education Program Expert Panel on Detection, Evaluation, and Treatment of High Blood Cholesterol in Adults. JAMA 1993;269:3015.

Risk Assessment as a Guide to Selection of Therapy

With benefit from treatment of hypercholesterolemia closely linked to the degree of pretreatment CHD risk, a careful assessment of that risk is imperative to deciding whom to treat, when to treat, and how aggressively to treat. The CHD risk assessment should be a *comprehensive* one, extending beyond lipid levels to include consideration of blood pressure, smoking, diabetes, family history of premature CHD, age, sex, and presence of established CHD or other atherosclerotic disease. The increasing awareness of elevated *HDL cholesterol* as a factor in reducing CHD risk has led to its designation as a *"negative risk factor."* Conversely, an HDL serum level of less than 35 mg/dL comes onto the list of positive risk factors (see Table 27–5).

A *gradient of CHD risk* has been defined by the NCEP expert panel, taking into account degree of LDL elevation and presence of other CHD risk factors (see Tables 27–4 and 27–5). For a given elevation in LDL cholesterol level, patients considered at highest risk are those with *established CHD* or other atherosclerotic disease (eg, peripheral arterial insufficiency, symptomatic carotid disease), followed by patients without CHD who have *two or more CHD risk factors*, and concluding with those having no CHD and *fewer than two CHD risk factors*.

The NCEP *treatment recommendations* follow directly from the degree of estimated *CHD risk*. Dietary modification is the sole mode of therapy for patients at the lower end of the CHD risk spectrum, while pharmacologic measures are reserved for patients at higher risk or for those who fail dietary intervention (Table 27–6). Additional considerations include possible adverse effects of long-term pharmacologic therapy (an issue when dealing with young persons) and appropriateness of the patient for treatment (an issue in the frail elderly and seriously ill).

Dietary Modification

Dietary modification remains the cornerstone of treatment, effective for both treatment and prevention of hypercholesterolemia. As suggested by the Hegsted equation (see

Table 27-6. Treatment Recommendations

PATIENT CATEGORY	INITIAL LDL LEVEL (mg/dL)	LDL GOAL (mg/dL)
	Dietary Therapy	
No CHD, <2 risk factors	>160	<160
No CHD, ≥2 risk factors	>130	<130
With CHD	>100	<100
	Add Drug Treatment	
No CHD, <2 risk factors	>190	<160
No CHD, ≥2 risk factors	>160	<130
With CHD	>130	<100

Adapted from: Summary of the Second Report of the National Cholesterol Education Program Expert Panel on Detection, Evaluation, and Treatment of High Blood Cholesterol in Adults. JAMA 1993;269:3015.

above), the greatest contributor to hypercholesterolemia is the consumption of saturated fat, with excess cholesterol taking second place. *Reductions* in *total fat*, *saturated fat*, and dietary *cholesterol* are recommended for all adults.

In conjunction with exercise and weight loss (which enhance the efficacy of dietary LDL cholesterol reduction and ameliorate other cardiac risk factors), dietary modification provides an excellent nonpharmacologic means of improving the patient's lipid profile and reducing CHD risk. The adverse effects are nil, making it the safest of treatments for hypercholesterolemia and especially well suited for persons with only a modest increase in CHD risk (eg, hypercholesterolemic young men and premenopausal women with no other CHD risk factors). Even for high-risk patients, diet is central to the treatment program, having an additive effect.

Efficacy. Decreases in intake of cholesterol and saturated fat in controlled settings can reduce total and LDL cholesterol by up to 30 percent, but the reductions average about 10 percent when similarly intensive dietary programs are prescribed for outpatient use. Dietary measures may also produce a small (approximately 5%) reduction in HDL cholesterol, though the overall total-to-HDL cholesterol ratio still improves. Weight loss (if obese), aerobic exercise, and smoking cessation can increase HDL and contribute to the dietary lowering of LDL and CHD risk. They also reduce CHD risk by decreasing blood pressure and glucose intolerance. Caloric and fat restrictions and control of diabetes are also effective in lowering triglyceride levels, an effect enhanced by prohibition of alcohol. Reductions in CHD risk parallel the degree of cholesterol lowering and reduction of other risk factors.

Response to dietary modification is determined to some extent by the etiology of the hypercholesterolemia. When the Phase I diet is prescribed for outpatient use in patients with non-monogenic hypercholesterolemia, the total and LDL cholesterol levels fall by 5 percent to 15 percent. The total serum cholesterol level will fall to 140 to 160 mg/dL in normal individuals consuming a very low fat (5%–10% of total calories) diet. More modest but still useful reductions can be expected from less stringent diets. Patients with severe monogenic hypercholesterolemias rarely respond to diet alone, whereas other individuals consuming a high-fat diet may demonstrate marked benefit.

Phased Approach to Dietary Modification. The phased approach, as exemplified by the American Heart Association's three-phase dietary plan, maximizes adherence. Total fat, saturated fat, and cholesterol intake are gradually reduced with partial replacement by polyunsaturated fats (which by the Hegsted equation have a modest cholesterol-lowering effect). Excess dietary fat is supplanted by use of complex carbohydrates (fruits, vegetables, cereals, pasta, grains, and legumes). It is recommended that all Americans adopt the *Phase I diet*, in which 1) *total fat* as a percentage of total calories is *reduced* from an average 40 percent to 45 percent to 30 percent; 2) *saturated fat* is *reduced* to 10 percent of total calories; 3) *polyunsaturated fat* is *increased* to 10 percent of calories; and 4) *dietary cholesterol* intake *reduced* from 500 mg per day to 300 mg per day. Protein is held constant (Table 27–7). The n-6 polyunsaturated fatty acids found in vegetable oils should not exceed 10 percent of calories, because they may lower HDL cholesterol.

The Phase I diet usually does not require a dramatic alteration in one's eating habits and can be readily adopted by most persons. The *Phase II diet* entails more effort, since it goes beyond eliminating the obvious sources of fat and cholesterol. It is indicated for patients already utilizing a Phase I diet at the time of diagnosis, those who do not achieve adequate results with Phase I, and patients at highest CHD risk (eg, established CHD).

If just the Phase I dietary interventions were widely implemented, the overall rate of CHD would be likely to drop significantly. These percentages must be translated into real menus and food recommendations. The help of a dietician is often beneficial, particularly if a Phase II diet is indicated, but a good working knowledge of the fat content of common foods is essential for patient, family, and health care team (see Appendix III). A number of "heart healthy" cookbooks are on the market to help patients in their food choices and preparation, though cholesterol fad books are also present and should be discouraged. Many restaurants offer low-fat items, and patients should be encouraged to select them.

Exercise and Weight Loss. The Second Report of the National Cholesterol Education Program places renewed emphasis on exercise and weight reduction as complements to dietary therapy and essential components of a comprehensive nonpharmacologic program. They are helpful not only in correcting lipid abnormalities but also in reducing other CHD risk factors. For example, exercise will raise the level of HDL cholesterol, decrease blood pressure, and increase efficiency of peripheral oxygen extraction (see Chapter 18). Weight loss efforts can lower fat intake, reduce risk of diabetes mellitus, and decrease myocardial work.

Non-Prescription Dietary Supplements. Non-prescription dietary supplements are no substitute for dietary reduction in total fat, saturated fat, and cholesterol. Nonetheless they are popular with patients, even though they can be expensive. Preliminary data from prospective studies of *omega-3 fish oil* supplements are encouraging, but they are too limited to serve as the basis for dietary recommendations. Impairment of clotting has been noted with use of high doses.

Anti-oxidant vitamins (E, C, and beta-carotene) do not lower cholesterol levels, but they may increase LDL resistance to oxidative change and thus reduce risk of arterial wall injury. Prospective data are needed, but daily doses of 400 IU of vitamin E, 0.5 to 1.0 g of vitamin C, and 25 mg of beta-carotene appear safe and perhaps may prove helpful.

Garlic supplements (half to 1 clove/d) can produce a modest (5–10%) reduction in serum cholesterol, as can taking *psyllium* (10 g/d).

Drug Therapy

Dietary modification is not uniformly effective in achieving target reductions in LDL cholesterol or desired increases in HDL cholesterol. Addition of drug therapy to a diet-and-exercise program should be considered in high-risk patients whose lipid abnormalities remain inadequately controlled despite intensive dietary efforts. More widespread application of drug therapy remains controversial, with concerns persisting as to its cost-effectiveness and risk–benefit ratio in patients at the lower end of the risk spectrum.

Effectiveness and Safety of Drug Therapy. The addition of drug therapy to a diet-and-exercise program can markedly enhance lipid-lowering results and lead to significant reductions in CHD risk. The best responses have been noted in patients with established atherosclerotic disease, who experience significant reductions in coronary morbidity and mortality. Patients with moderate CHD risk also benefit from addition of pharmacologic therapy, but to a lesser degree than those at highest risk. A halt to *plaque progression* and a small amount of *plaque regression* have been demonstrated with use of intensive drug therapy. Not yet demonstrated is a reduction in *all-cause mortality*. Data from appropriately designed studies remain sparse.

Meta-analytic study of six investigations reporting morbidity and mortality data for lipid-lowering therapy revealed a significant reduction in *nonfatal cardiac events* (odds ratio, 0.74), a more modest decrease in *cardiac deaths* (odds ratio, 0.90), but an increase in *noncardiac deaths* (odds ratio, 1.19). The net result was no significant change in all-cause mortality. The increase in noncardiac deaths remains unexplained, with no consistent pattern emerging from the studies examined. No increase in noncardiac deaths has been found among patients treated only with dietary modification.

The observed increase in noncardiac deaths needs to be confirmed, links to particular drugs ascertained, and overall significance determined. Until then, caution and good clinical judgment are indicated when considering use and selection of lipid-lowering medications (see below). Weighing the possible risks (eg, increase in noncardiac death) against the expected benefits (reductions in cardiac morbidity and mortality) is essential.

There is no evidence that lipid-lowering medication reduces *risk of stroke*. However, presence of carotid atherosclerosis increases the likelihood of CHD and need for lipid-lowering therapy.

Candidacy for Pharmacologic Therapy. The risk–benefit ratio for pharmacologic therapy appears most favorable in patients at greatest CHD risk and least favorable in those at lowest risk. Because most data derive from studies involving *middle-aged men* and *postmenopausal women* with established CHD or multiple CHD risk factors, one must extrapolate to estimate effects in other populations. Until outcomes data on pharmacologic treatment of elderly patients, young men, and premenopausal women emerge, clinical judgment will have to suffice, taking into account patient preferences, drug costs, and side effects as well as expected benefits.

In the *elderly*, high CHD risk is common. One might reasonably expect the benefit noted in high-risk middle-aged patients to accrue also to elderly persons at similar risk. Duration of therapy is less likely to be very prolonged, lessening risk of an adverse effect from long-term effect. These expectations remain to be proven.

Young men (age <35) and *premenopausal women* with no CHD risk factors other than hypercholesterolemia are best considered for nonpharmacologic therapy, because their short-term risk of CHD is low and the safety of long-term drug therapy is not established. For young persons at greater

Table 27-7. American Heart Association Three-Phase Dietary Plan

	AVERAGE U.S. DIET	PHASE I	PHASE II	PHASE III
Total fat (as % total calories)	40–45	30	25	20
Saturated	17	10	~6	~3
Monounsaturated	18	10	~9	~7
Polyunsaturated	7	10	~10	~10
Protein (as % total calories)	15–20	15	15	15
Carbohydrate (as % total calories)	40–45	55	60	65
Dietary cholesterol	500 mg	300 mg	200–250 mg	100–150 mg

CHD risk (eg, LDL cholesterol >220 mg/dL, potent CHD risk factors such as diabetes mellitus or strong family history of premature CHD), the potential gain from use of lipid-lowering medication may outweigh the risk, but there are no outcomes data yet available to confirm this. Again, the exercise of good clinical judgment is essential.

Selection of Drug Therapy and Available Agents. Design of a pharmacologic regimen must take into account the patient's degree of *CHD risk*, the nature of the *lipoprotein abnormality*, and the drugs' *mechanisms of action* and *side effects*. The best program is one that addresses and fits well into the patient's overall clinical state. A large degree of individualization is necessary. The range of available drugs is extensive, varying greatly in cost, effect on cholesterol fractions, efficacy, and side effects (Table 27–8).

Niacin. This agent is an effective and inexpensive first-line, cholesterol-lowering drug. Its exact mechanism of action remains unknown, though it does affect fatty acid mobilization, *lowers LDL* and VLDL levels, and *raises HDL* levels. These changes can be dramatic, though the average LDL reduction is about 15 percent to 20 percent. Data from the Coronary Drug Project demonstrated decreased rates of new infarction and mortality in niacin-treated men with a prior myocardial infarction. Also, reduction in all-cause mortality appears to result from use in patients with established CHD. The combination of niacin plus colestipol has produced documented regression of atheromatous plaque in coronary arteries. Being a B complex vitamin (nicotinic acid), niacin is available over-the-counter in non-prescription form.

Its principal disadvantages include a litany of side effects, reflecting the *large doses* required. Niacin can exacerbate *gout* and *diabetes*, elevate *liver enzymes*, and produce *rashes*, *nausea*, and *vomiting*. It also triggers acute prostaglandin-mediated vasodilation that can result in *flushing* and even postural light-headedness. Pretreatment with aspirin mitigates this reaction. Dry skin and occasionally acanthosis nigricans may accompany niacin use. Lanolin cream helps the former, and prompt cessation clears the latter. Side effects can be minimized by starting with a dose of 100 mg three times daily, taken with meals, and gradually increasing the dose. Doses of 1.5 to 6.0 g/d may be needed to achieve the desired results. Niacin is available in regular and *time-release* preparations, with the latter more expensive but much more convenient and better tolerated except for a higher incidence of *hepatic toxicity*. One should find a brand of niacin that is inexpensive and reliable, and suggest that patients take only that form. Transaminases (aminotransferases) should be monitored regularly, as well as glucose and uric acid levels.

HMG-CoA Reductase Inhibitors (Lovastatin, Simvastatin, Pravastatin). The "statins," as they are sometimes called, have been second-line agents to date, but their effectiveness, patient acceptability, and increasingly favorable safety record are likely to soon place them into the first-line category of lipid-lowering drugs. They block the rate-limiting enzyme for cholesterol synthesis, HMG-CoA reductase. This inhibition decreases intracellular cholesterol and increases clearance of *LDL*. Serum LDL levels fall by 20 percent to 45 percent, depending on dose, and there is emerging evidence of ability to affect plaque regression, even when used alone. HDL levels generally stay the same or increase slightly.

Lovastatin was the first of these agents. Simvastatin and pravastatin followed. Simvastatin is more potent on a weight basis compared to lovastatin and pravastatin. Pravastatin is equipotent to lovastatin. Starting dose for lovastatin and pravastatin is 20 mg/d and for simvastatin, 10 mg/d. The maximum recommended lovastatin dose is 80 mg/d, and 40 mg/d for simvistatin and pravastatin. Lovastatin works best if taken at night. Equipotent doses of these three agents pro-

Table 27-8. Drugs Used To Treat Hyperlipidemia

NAME	INDICATIONS	EFFECTS	DOSAGE	SIDE EFFECTS	RELATIVE COST (PER YEAR)
Bile acid sequestrants (cholestyramine, colestipol)	↑ LDL	↓ LDL ↓ or no change HDL	cholest 8–24 g/d colestipol 10–30 g/d	Constipation, heartburn, bloating	cholest: 14.2 colest: 12.3
HMG-CoA Reductase Inhibitors (Lovastatin, simvastatin, pravastatin)	↑ LDL	↓ LDL ↑ HDL (minor) ↓ VLDL (minor)	Lov: 20–80 mg Simva: 10–40 Prava: 20–40	↑ transaminases, myositis	Lov: 9.0 Simva: 8.1 Prava: 7.7
Niacin (nicotinic acid)	↑ LDL ↓ HDL, VLDL	↓ LDL ↑ HDL ↓ VLDL	1.5–8 g/d	Flushing, pruritus, PUD, hyperglycemia, rashes	1.0
Gemfibrozil	↑ VLDL	↓ VLDL ↑ HDL ↑ LDL (if triglycerides high)	600–1200 mg/d	? + gallstones potentiates warfarin	4.3
Probucol	↑ LDL	↓ LDL ↓ ↓ HDL	500 mg bid	↓ ↓ HDL, diarrhea	9.6
Fish oils (N-3 fatty acids)	↑ VLDL	↓ VLDL ↑ ↓ LDL	? 2–3 g or more of N-3 fatty acids/d	Platelet inhibition	0.5

duce similar results. Selection can be based on price. These agents are best taken at night, the time of peak cholesterol synthesis.

The predominant adverse reaction is an increase in serum levels of liver *transaminases*. The elevation is usually modest and asymptomatic, but it can be substantial enough to warrant discontinuation of the drug. Early animal evidence of an increased rate of cataract formation has not appeared in humans, and the initial Food and Drug Administration (FDA) recommendation of a slit lamp examination has been dropped. However, transaminase monitoring is strongly recommended, every month or two during the initial phases of therapy, and every 3 to 6 months thereafter. Minor, harmless elevations are sometimes seen, but in the setting of concurrent gemfibrozil use, severe *myositis* leading to *rhabdomyolysis* has occurred. The two agents should not be used together. The major drawbacks to the reductase inhibitors are their cost and lack of data on long-term safety. However, when cost is considered as a function of LDL-lowering capacity, only niacin is more cost-effective.

Bile Acid Sequestrants (Cholestyramine and Colestipol). These nonabsorbable agents have been first-line pharmacologic therapy for many years, with an established record of safety. They are very useful for patients who are not at great CHD risk but in whom diet alone fails to lower LDL cholesterol to target levels. Though not as cost-effective as the reductase inhibitors or niacin, they are very effective when used in combination with them to treat high-risk patients with severe hypercholesterolemia. They bind bile acids in the gut and interrupt their normal enterohepatic circulation. The resultant shunting of cholesterol in the liver to bile acid production leads to a fall in total and LDL cholesterols. The bile sequestrants are nonabsorbable resins whose major side effects are gastrointestinal—*constipation*, *bloating*, *heartburn*, and *nausea*. A high-fiber diet or psyllium supplement and use of these agents just before a meal will usually ameliorate the gastrointestinal upset. The potential to *impede absorption* of certain drugs (eg, digoxin, thyroxine, warfarin, tetracycline, phenobarbital) necessitates that bile sequestrants not be taken until at least 1 hour after or 4 hours before these other drugs. In rare instances, steatorrhea and malabsorption of the fat-soluble vitamins (A, D, E, and K) can occur. The usual starting dose is one scoop of the powdered form of the drug (4 g of cholestyramine, 5 g of colestipol) in a large glass of water twice a day. Dose can be increased to a total of three scoops twice daily.

Estrogens. In postmenopausal women, estrogen replacement therapy is effective in *lowering* the levels of *LDL* cholesterol and *raising* those of *HDL* cholesterol, with attendant reductions in CHD risk. Because of the risk of endometrial cancer associated with unopposed estrogen use (see Chapter 118), a progestin is usually prescribed as well. The addition of progestin does not appear to significantly reduce the CHD benefit of estrogen replacement therapy, but confirmation by prospective randomized trial is needed.

Fibrates (Gemfibrozil and Clofibrate). Because these drugs do not substantially lower LDL cholesterol, they are not considered major drugs for treatment of hypercholesterolemia, though they do have specific uses. They *decrease VLDL synthesis* and enhance its clearance. Clofibrate's role in cholesterol treatment has dramatically decreased in recent years because of reports of *increased mortality* associated with its use. It has largely been superseded by gemfibrozil, which has not been linked to such risk. The fibrates are the most potent of triglyceride-lowering agents due to their effect on VLDL. Gemfibrozil also *raises HDL* levels, but it appears to be most efficacious *only* in those who have *concomitant triglyceride elevations* that respond to the drug. The effect on LDL is variable. Gemfibrozil is generally well tolerated, though it may potentiate the effect of oral anticoagulants and increase bile cholesterol content, raising the risk of gallstone formation. The FDA has issued a warning about its use in combination with lovastatin (see above).

Probucol. This agent is also not listed as a major drug for treatment of hypercholesterolemia. It *lowers LDL* cholesterol about 15 percent but frequently *decreases HDL* by 20 percent to 30 percent. The net effect is a more atherogenic lipid profile. However, probucol is an effective *LDL antioxidant* and decreases LDL uptake by macrophages, which theoretically could inhibit atherogenesis independent of any effect on LDL concentration.

Treatment Goals and Monitoring

The ultimate *treatment goal* is reduction in CHD risk; the immediate one is reduction of LDL cholesterol level. *For primary prevention* (no established CHD), the *target LDL cholesterol* level is *less than 160 mg/dL* for those with no other CHD risk factors, and *less than 130 mg/dL* for those with *two or more CHD risk factors*. For *secondary prevention* (established CHD), the goal is an LDL cholesterol level of *less than 100 mg/dL*. Such targets are considered minimums.

Monitoring is performed by measurement of the LDL cholesterol level, beginning about 6 weeks after initiation of therapy and then every 3 to 4 months until control is established. Afterward, every 6 to 12 months is usually sufficient. More frequent monitoring for development of abnormalities in serum chemistries is indicated when using certain pharmacologic agents (see below).

THERAPEUTIC RECOMMENDATIONS

Effective reduction of CHD risk requires identifying and aggressively treating *all CHD risk factors* responsive to medical intervention, including smoking, hypertension, diabetes, and obesity (see Chapters 26, 54, 102, and 233). Focusing on hyperlipidemia alone is insufficient. In treating hypercholesterolemia, one should determine total CHD risk (see Tables 27–4 and 27–5) and treat accordingly (see Table 27–6).

High Risk (Established CHD; LDL >160 mg/dL Plus ≥2 Risk Factors; or LDL >190 mg/dL and ≤2 CHD Risk Factors): Attempts to markedly reduce intake of saturated fat and cholesterol should be maximized in these patients, even though the addition of drug therapy is usually necessary. Sometimes, highly motivated individuals can avoid the need for lifelong medication by strict adherence to *Phase II* or *Phase III* programs, achieving LDL reductions of 40 to 80 mg/dL. Four to six months should be allowed for implementation of these significant dietary lifestyle changes. Even if dietary change does not bring LDL cholesterol down to desired levels, diet will enhance the effect from lipid-lowering therapy.

Drug therapy is indicated for most high-risk cases. The best agents are *niacin* (average dose 3 g/d), the *HMG-CoA reductase inhibitors* such as *lovastatin* (20–80 mg/d), and the *bile sequestrants cholestyramine* and *colestipol* (1–2 scoops bid). Niacin and the reductase inhibitors are the most cost-effective and should be tried first. *Combination therapy* with a bile resin plus a reductase inhibitor or niacin has shown considerable promise in patients at greatest risk (known coronary disease, high-risk lipid profile) who fail to adequately respond to diet plus a single agent. Such regimens have demonstrated significant reductions in CAD morbidity and mortality as well as plaque regression. However, the combination of a statin plus gemfibrozil is generally to be avoided (risk of rhabdomyolysis), and risk of myositis may be increased when a statin and niacin are used together.

As noted above, the minimum goal for LDL cholesterol is less than 100 mg/dL for those with established CHD, less than 130 mg/dL for those with no CHD but two or more CHD risk factors, and less than 160 mg/dL for those with no CHD and fewer than two risk factors.

Moderate Risk (LDL Cholesterol 130–159 mg/d Plus ≥2 CHD Risk Factors; or LDL 160–189 and No Other CHD Risk Factors): In some patients, especially those with large intakes of saturated fat and cholesterol, the *Phase I diet* can produce reductions in cholesterol of 20 to 40 mg/dL. More aggressive dietary fat restriction (*Phase II diet*) may be needed in those who do not respond adequately. Polyunsaturated fatty acids should be increased moderately, but to no more than 10 percent of total calories. The minimum goal is a reduction of LDL cholesterol to less than 130 mg/dL in those with two or more CHD risk factors, and to well under 160 mg/dL in those with fewer than two risk factors. Drug therapy is usually not necessary.

Isolated Low HDL Cholesterol Level (<35 mg/dL). HDL cholesterol can be increased by a host of nonpharmacologic measures, including *aerobic exercise*, *smoking cessation*, and *weight loss* if obese. Such actions can increase HDL by 5 to 15 mg/dL. Dramatic diet-induced reductions in total cholesterol are sometimes accompanied by moderate reductions in HDL cholesterol. There is no evidence that such reductions are harmful, perhaps because the important ratio of total cholesterol to HDL cholesterol usually decreases to a more favorable number.

Although epidemiologic data show a strong inverse relation between HDL level and CHD risk, there are no data yet from randomized prospective clinical trials showing that drug treatment that increases HDL cholesterol reduces CHD risk. As a result, it is too soon to recommend drug treatment for an isolated low HDL cholesterol level. However, the HDL cholesterol level should be taken into account during drug selection when a pharmacologic program is deemed necessary because of LDL cholesterol elevation. Of currently available drugs which can substantially raise HDL cholesterol and lower LDL cholesterol, *niacin* and post-menopausal *estrogen* replacement are the most prominent.

Elevated Triglycerides (Fasting Triglycerides >250 mg/dL). Serum triglycerides are not an independent risk factor for CHD, and no consensus exists on the need for treating elevations. However, many believe that the treatment of an elevated triglyceride value is warranted in the presence of a low HDL cholesterol level (<35 mg/dL), as the latter may rise substantially with use of a triglyceride-lowering drugs. *Gemfibrozil* (600 mg bid) is the best of the triglyceride-lowering agents and has been used to reduce the risk of pancreatitis in patients with very high triglyceride levels (>800 mg/dL).

Treatment in the Elderly

Prevalence of hypercholesterolemia is greatest in those older than 65 years of age. As in other age groups, elevations in total cholesterol and LDL cholesterol are predictive of increased cardiovascular risk. However, the statistical risk relationship is not as strong as in younger patients, due in part to the frequent occurrence of other important risk factors in the elderly (eg, diabetes, hypertension). Elderly patients may have other advanced diseases, making prevention of coronary disease appear irrelevant to their overall quality of life.

Several factors favor treatment. The coronary disease of women may be less advanced than that of men due to the protective effects of estrogens prior to menopause or due to use of postmenopausal estrogen replacement therapy. In addition, the benefits from secondary prevention of coronary disease by lowering of cholesterol exceed even the benefits of primary prevention. With the advent of better tolerated cholesterol-lowering medication, the risks of adverse effects and their negative impact on quality of life are declining. All of these factors combine to recommend treatment of hypercholesterolemia in *high-risk* elderly patients.

Dietary Measures, as detailed above, are the first step, though they are not likely to suffice by themselves. Modifications of the usual low-saturated fat diet are needed to insure adequate calcium intake for prevention of osteoporosis. Use of skim milk and low-fat and non-fat yogurts are examples of ways to *maintain calcium* intake while cutting down on saturated fat. Maintaining *adequate protein intake* is also essential, meaning that lean cuts of red meat ought to be allowed in addition to fish and skinless chicken to assure palatability of the diet. As noted earlier, the n-6 polyunsaturated fatty acids found in vegetable oils should not exceed 10 percent of calories. *High fiber* is essential for good bowel function and cannot hurt the cholesterol-lowering effort.

Pharmacologic Therapy. Because dietary therapy alone frequently fails to achieve the goal of an LDL cholesterol lower than 130 mg/dL, medical therapy must often be considered. *Bile sequestrants* are safe but can cause considerable gastrointestinal upset, especially constipation. This may be helped by increasing fiber. Because sequestrants can impair drug absorption, their use in elderly patients must include instruction to take other medications at least 1 hour before or 4 hours after sequestrant use. Among the drugs that might be affected by sequestrants are warfarin, propranolol, digitalis preparations, thyroxine, and antibiotics. Low-dose sequestrants are a reasonable first choice for pharmacologic therapy.

The *HMG-CoA reductase inhibitors* are indicated when more aggressive lowering of LDL cholesterol is needed. These drugs are well tolerated in the elderly, with minor diarrhea and occasional sleep disturbances being the most common problems. Minor transaminase elevations are common; they are usually asymptomatic and not a cause for discontinuation unless they reach three times normal. However, regular transaminase monitoring is required throughout the course of therapy. The initial concern about an increased risk of cataract formation has not been borne out by follow-up study. These agents will probably become the drug class of choice if they prove safe for prolonged use.

Nicotinic acid is effective, though not always well tolerated. Its advantages over HMG-CoA reductase inhibitors are its ability to also raise HDL and its low cost. The incidence of side effects in the elderly is high, with flushing, gastrointestinal upset, dry mouth, and dry eyes being particularly annoying. The drug may exacerbate peptic ulcer disease, elevate transaminases, and trigger arrhythmias and hypotension. Multiple daily doses are usually required.

PATIENT EDUCATION

The importance of patient education in the management of hyperlipidemia cannot be overemphasized, because treatment consists essentially of changing one's eating and exercise habits (see Chapters 233 and 18). The first step in therapy should be a careful review of the rationale for treating hypercholesterolemia, followed by a discussion of basic dietary principles for lowering cholesterol. Many patients are surprised to learn that dietary fat is more atherogenic than dietary cholesterol itself (witness the patient who eats his cholesterol-free potato chips with abandon). Reviewing the saturated fat content of foods regularly consumed by the patient is quite worthwhile. At times, simply removing a few grossly offending foods from the diet (eg, processed snack foods, cheese, grossly fatty meats, cold cuts, fried food) will ensure a good start to a change in eating habits. More comprehensive diet planning can be aided by discussion with the nurse or dietician, facilitated by written material such as that produced by the American Heart Association. Periodic visits to check diet, weight, and cholesterol are excellent, though often overlooked, means of facilitating compliance and providing reinforcement.

INDICATIONS FOR REFERRAL

Patients with high-risk profiles who do not respond to diet plus one or two first-line drugs should be referred for consultation to a physician familiar with drug treatment of lipid disorders. Some genetic disorders are among the most refractory and should be considered if extremes of any lipoprotein cholesterol level are encountered or there is a family history of premature coronary disease (onset before the age of 55). Lipid research laboratories can often categorize the specific genetic abnormalities by directly measuring LDL cholesterol with ultracentrifugation and precisely determining apolipoproteins, HDL subfractions, and various enzyme or receptor systems. However, therapy in most instances is still the same—dietary and behavioral interventions followed by drug therapy as necessary. Screening of other family members for hypercholesterolemia is recommended.

ANNOTATED BIBLIOGRAPHY

Bradford RH, Shear CL, Chremos AN, et al. Expanded clinical evaluation of lovastatin (EXCEL) study results. Arch Intern Med 1991;151:43. *(Detailed data on efficacy and safety; found to be highly effective and safe, especially when used in low doses in combination with a dietary program.)*

Canadian Task Force of the Periodic Health Examination. 1993 update: 2. Lowering the blood total cholesterol level to prevent coronary heart disease. Can Med Assoc J 1993;148:521. *(Includes a meta-analysis of available data; marked reduction in CAD events; modest reduction in CAD mortality; but no reduction in all-cause mortality.)*

Carlson LA, Rosenhamer G. Reduction of mortality in the Stockholm Ischaemic Study by combined treatment with clofibrate and nicotinic acid. Acta Med Scand 1988;223:405. *(Combined therapy reduced mortality in high risk patients.)*

Cashin-Hemphill L, Mack WJ, Pogoda JM, et al. Beneficial effects of colestipol niacin on coronary atherosclerosis: a 4-year follow-up. JAMA 1990;264:3013. *(A report from the Cholesterol Lowering Atherosclerosis Study [CLAS] documenting decreased progression and increased regression of coronary atherosclerosis.)*

Criqui MH, Heiss G, Cohn R, et al. Plasma triglyceride level and mortality from coronary heart disease. N Engl J Med 1993; 328:1220. *(No independent association with CHD risk found, but relation to low HDL noted.)*

Denke MA, Grundy SM. Hypercholesterolemia in the elderly: resolving the treatment dilemma. Ann Intern Med 1990;112: 780. *(A detailed review of the risks and benefits; favors treatment of high-risk patients; 83 refs.)*

Expert Panel on Detection, Evaluation, and Treatment of High Blood Cholesterol in Adults. Report of the National Cholesterol Education Program. Arch Intern Med 1988;148:36. *(The first report of this major consensus panel's recommendations.)*

Expert Panel on Detection, Evaluation, and Treatment of High Blood Cholesterol in Adults. Summary of the Second Report of the National Cholesterol Education Program. JAMA 1993;269:3015. *(Latest report from this major consensus panel.)*

Goldman L, Weinstein MC, Goldman PA, et al. Cost-effectiveness of HMG-CoA reductase inhibition for primary and secondary prevention of coronary heart disease. JAMA 1991; 265:1145. *(Lovastatin found very cost-effective for secondary prevention, less so for primary prevention, except in very-high-risk groups.)*

Henkin Y, Oberman A, Hurst DC, et al. Niacin revisited: clinical observations on an important but underutilized drug. Am J Med 1991;91:239. *(Makes the case for more use of this effective, inexpensive drug; but notes dose-related toxicities.)*

Hunninghake DB, Stein EA, Dujovne CA, et al. The efficacy of intensive dietary therapy alone or combined with lovastatin in outpatients with hypercholesterolemia. N Engl J Med 1993;328:1213. *(Diet alone provided only a 5 percent LDL reduction; medication added another 27 percent.)*

Jain AK, Vargas R, Gotzkowsky S, et al. Can garlic reduce levels of serum lipids? A controlled clinical trial. Am J Med 1993; 94:632. *(Yes, and by about 5–10%.)*

Jenkins DJA, Uolever TMS, Venketshwer R, et al. Effect on blood lipids of very high intakes of fiber in diets low in saturated fat and cholesterol. N Engl J Med 1993;329:21. *(Foods rich in soluble fiber can lower cholesterol.)*

Kreisberg RA. Low high-density lipoprotein cholesterol: What does it mean, what can we do about it, and what should we do about it? Am J Med 1993;94:1. *(Very thoughtful editorial comments on these questions.)*

Klag KJ, Ford DE, Mead LA, et al. Serum cholesterol in young men and subsequent cardiovascular disease. N Engl J Med 1993;328:313. *(Strong association found between serum cholesterol level in early life and CHD in midlife.)*

Martin KA, Freeman MW. Postmenopausal hormone-replacement therapy. N Engl J Med 1993;328:1115. *(An editorial recommending replacement therapy from the perspective of its favorable effects on lipids and CHD risk.)*

Mensink RP, Katan M. Effect of dietary trans fatty acids on high-density and low-density lipoprotein cholesterol levels in healthy subjects. N Engl J Med 1991;323:439. *(Distressing data indicating that the partially hydrogenated unsaturated fatty acids found in processed foods are just as atherogenic as saturated fatty acids.)*

Nabulsi AA, Folsom AR, White A, et al. Association of hormone-replacement therapy with various cardiovascular risk factors in postmenopausal women. N Engl J Med 1993;328:1069. *(An epidemiologic study showing estrogen plus progestin to be associated with a beneficial effect on lipids, similar to estrogen alone.)*

Peason TA, Patel RV. The quest for a cholesterol-decreasing diet. Should we subtract, substitute, or supplement. Ann Intern Med 1993;119:627. *(An editorial arguing for reduction in fat intake as the primary therapy; good review of dietary supplements.)*

Pierce LR, Wysowski DK, Gross TP. Myopathy and rhabdomyolysis associated with lovastatin-gemfibrozil combination therapy. JAMA 1990;264:71. *(Documents this serious complication; the combination is to be avoided.)*

Rossouw JE, Lewis B, Rifkind BM. The value of lowering cho-

Appendix I Fatty Acid Composition of Commonly Consumed Foods (as percentage of total fatty acids)

FOOD	SATURATED	MONOUNSATURATED	POLYUNSATURATED
Butter, cream, milk	65	30	5
Beef	46	48	6
Bacon and pork	38	50	12
Lard	42	45	13
Chicken	33	39	28
Fish	29	31	40
Coconut oil	92	6	2
Palm kernel oil	86	12	2
Cocoa butter	63	34	3
Olive oil	15	76	9
Peanut oil	20	48	32
Cottonseed oil	27	20	53
Soybean oil	16	24	60
Corn oil	13	26	61
Sunflower seed oil	11	22	67
Safflower seed oil	10	13	77

Appendix II Cholesterol Content of Common Foods

FOOD	AMOUNT OF FOOD	CHOLESTEROL CONTENT (MG)	FOOD	AMOUNT OF FOOD	CHOLESTEROL CONTENT (MG)
Brains	3.5 oz (100 g)	>2000			
Liver, chicken	3.5 oz	555	Beef	3.5 oz	65
Kidney	3.5 oz	375	Pork	3.5 oz	62
Liver, beef	3.5 oz	300	Clams	3.5 oz	50
Caviar	1 tbsp	>300	Flounder	3.5 oz	50
Egg yolk	1	252	Oysters	3.5 oz	50
Shrimp	3.5 oz	150	Ice cream (regular)	1 cup	40
Crab	3.5 oz	100	Butter	1 tbsp	35
Mackerel	3.5 oz	95	Scallops	3.5 oz	35
Lobster (cooked)	3.5 oz	85	Milk, whole	1 cup	14
Cheese, cheddar	3.5 oz	84	Milk, 2%	1 cup	9
Veal	3.5 oz	70	Milk, skim	1 cup	2
Chicken, breast	3.5 oz	67	Margarine	1 tbsp	0

lesterol after myocardial infarction. N Engl J Med 1990; 323:1112. *(The case for secondary prevention is reviewed and found to be powerful; 64 refs.)*

Schulman KA, Kinosian B, Jacobson TA, et al. Reducing high blood cholesterol level with drugs: cost-effectiveness of pharmacologic management. JAMA 1990;264:3025. *(Niacin and lovastatin were the most cost-effective for lowering LDL cholesterol and reducing cardiovascular risk.)*

Sprecher DL, Harris BV, Goldberg AC, et al. Efficacy of psyllium in reducing serum cholesterol levels in hypercholesterolemic patients on high- or low-fat diets. Ann Intern Med 1993; 119:545. *(A 5–10% lowering achieved in both groups.)*

Appendix III Fat Content of Meats, Poultry, Fish, and Other Protein Sources, 3-Ounce Portions

	TOTAL FAT (g)	SATURATED FAT (g)	CALORIES	CHOLESTEROL (mg)
Red Meat				
Veal top round (roasted)	2.9	1.0	127	88
Pork tenderloin (roasted)	4.1	1.4	133	67
Beef top round (broiled)	4.2	1.4	153	71
Beef eye of round (roasted)	4.2	1.5	143	59
Pork sirloin chop, boneless (broiled)	5.7	1.5	156	78
Pork loin roast, boneless (roasted)	6.4	2.4	160	66
Lamb leg (roasted)	6.6	2.3	162	78
Pork loin chop, bone in (broiled)	6.9	2.5	165	70
Beef tenderloin (broiled)	8.5	3.2	179	71
Frankfurter, beef and pork (boiled)	24.8	9.1	272	42
Pork sausage, country-style (cooked)	26.5	9.2	314	71
Poultry				
Turkey breast, skinless (roasted)	2.7	0.9	133	59
Chicken breast, skinless (roasted)	3.0	0.9	140	72
Turkey thigh, skinless (roasted)	6.1	2.1	159	72
Chicken thigh, skinless (roasted)	9.3	2.6	178	81
Chicken breast, skin on (fried)	11.2	3.0	221	72
Duck, skin on (roasted)	24.1	8.2	286	71
Fish and Seafood				
Lobster meat (cooked)	0.5	<0.1	83	61
Scallops, bay or sea (raw)	0.6	<0.1	75	28
Cod (broiled)	0.7	0.1	89	47
Shrimp (moist heat cooked)	0.9	0.2	84	166
Flounder (broiled)	1.3	0.3	99	58
Crab, Alaska king (steamed)	1.3	0.1	82	45
Oysters (eastern, raw)	2.1	0.5	59	47
Tuna, white (canned in water)	2.1	0.6	116	36
Trout, rainbow (broiled)	3.7	0.7	128	62
Tuna, light (canned in oil)	7.0	1.3	168	15
Salmon, sockeye (broiled)	9.3	1.6	184	74
Other				
Tofu/bean curd	4.1	0.6	65	0
Eggs (hard-boiled)	9.5	2.8	134	466
American cheese food (pasteurized process)	20.9	13.1	279	54
Cheddar cheese	28.2	17.9	343	89
Peanuts (roasted in shell)	41.4	7.3	495	0
Peanut butter	43.5	7.2	502	0

Sources: United States Department of Agriculture, Composition of Foods, Handbooks 8–1, 8–5, 8–7, 8–10, 8–12, 8–13, 8–15, 8–16, 8–17; HVH–CWRI Nutrient Data Base.

28
Management of Atrial Fibrillation and Other Supraventricular Tachycardias

Primary Care Medicine: Office Evaluation and Management of the Adult Patient, 3rd edition, edited by Allan H. Goroll, Lawrence A. May, and Albert G. Mulley, Jr. J.B. Lippincott Company, Philadelphia

Atrial Fibrillation

Atrial fibrillation (AF) discovered in the office setting can usually be managed on an outpatient basis by the primary care physician, provided the ventricular response rate is not dangerously fast and there is no evidence of heart failure, ischemia, hypotension, or embolization. Thus, the first priority is to quickly assess the patient's hemodynamic state and determine the need for urgent hospitalization. Only then should diagnosis (see Chapter 25) and management commence. Regardless of etiology, the first therapeutic objective is to control the ventricular response rate. A second priority is to assess the risk of embolization and determine the need for anticoagulation. Patients who do not revert to sinus rhythm need consideration of elective cardioversion.

CLINICAL PRESENTATION AND COURSE

AF may be paroxysmal or chronic. Paroxysms typically occur in patients with lone atrial fibrillation, sick sinus syndrome, or Wolff-Parkinson-White (WPW) syndrome, as well as during exacerbations of cardiomyopathic, valvular, and ischemic forms of organic heart disease. Advanced forms of these conditions often result in chronic AF. In the elderly, AF may also be triggered by hyperthyroidism (see below). Although chronic fibrillation may be a manifestation of serious organic heart disease and represent an increase in overall risk, chronicity is not the prime determinant of embolic risk; the prime determinant is the presence of underlying heart disease.

Lone Atrial Fibrillation is characterized by the occurrence of atrial fibrillation in the absence clinically evident heart disease. In about two-thirds of cases, the condition presents as isolated or recurrent episodes of paroxysmal AF; in the remainder, the AF is chronic. Lone AF may be annoying and sometimes frightening; the key question has been the risk of embolization. In a long-term, community-based study of patients with lone AF who were younger than 60 years of age (mean age 44), investigators from the Mayo Clinic found survival to be no different than that of a population of similar age; moreover, the risk of embolic stroke was negligible (1.3% in 15 y). Survival rates and stroke risks were similar regardless of whether the AF episodes were paroxysmal or chronic. Data from the Framingham study were more worrisome. A fourfold increase in incidence of stroke was noted, but most patients were elderly (mean age 64) and had other cardiovascular risk factors (30% had hypertension). Risk of stroke was greatest early in the course of AF. Taken together, these studies suggest that lone AF appears to pose little risk, but only if the patient is young and has no other cardiovascular risk factors.

Apathetic Hyperthyroidism of the Elderly may be mistaken for lone AF, because not only might there be little evidence of organic heart disease, but the typical symptoms and signs of hyperthyroidism can also be absent. The clinical presentation more closely resembles depression or occult malignancy, with significant weight loss, marked apathy, and unexplained AF dominating the clinical picture. Diagnosis is made by ruling out underlying organic heart disease and finding the thyrotropin (TSH) to be undetectable and the free thyroxine (T_4) index or total triiodothyronine (T_3) substantially elevated (see Chapters 8 and 103). Treatment directed at the hyperthyroidism usually terminates the AF. Although uncommon, this eminently treatable form of AF should not be missed. Stroke risk is minimal if there is no accompanying organic heart disease.

Underlying Heart Disease. Patients with AF in the context of underlying heart disease have a much more serious problem. Not only is the risk of embolization significantly increased, but the AF may also lead to hemodynamic compromise. Chronic atrial fibrillation in such patients usually reflects serious cardiac pathology. In the Framingham study, onset of atrial fibrillation and *heart failure* were closely linked. Furthermore, the development of chronic AF corresponded with a doubling of cardiovascular mortality.

Some conditions that cause AF also manifest concurrent disease of the conducting system, further increasing risk. For example, patients with the *tachycardia–bradycardia (sick sinus) syndrome* have sinus node dysfunction, often in conjunction with AV nodal disease and lack of an adequate escape mechanism. Characteristic presentations include episodes of atrial fibrillation with a slow ventricular response rate and bouts of severe bradycardia leading to syncope or near syncope.

Paroxysms of rapid AF and other supraventricular tachycardias are characteristic of *Wolff-Parkinson-White syndrome*. In this condition, an accessory connection between the atrium and the ventricle (eg, the Kent bundle) leads to preexcitation (short PR interval, delta waves) and a host of supraventricular dysrhythmias. The AF may be associated with a very fast ventricular response rate facilitated by rapid antegrade conduction over the accessory conduction pathway. There may be a widening of the QRS, mimicking ventricular fibrillation. In rare instances, the rapid ventricular response can degenerate into true ventricular fibrillation and sudden death. Fortunately, the risk of such serious ventricular dysrhythmias is very low in previously asymptomatic WPW patients, in part because the accessory pathways tend to lose antegrade conductivity over time.

An episode of AF in a patient with preexisting heart disease may be precipitated by such factors as *acute heart failure*, *ischemia*, *fever*, *infection*, *hypoxia*, or *hypovolemia*.

Correction of the precipitant often results in at least a temporary return to sinus rhythm. If there is a *valvular*, *cardiomyopathic*, or *ischemic* process that continues unabated, the paroxysms of AF may become more frequent and prolonged, culminating in chronic AF. AF is particularly common in patients with *mitral valve disease*, due to rather early onset of increased left atrial pressure and size. AF is much less common in disease of the aortic valve; when it does occur, it signifies very severe, advanced disease (see Chapter 33).

Alcohol has been implicated as a major precipitant of AF. Binge drinking may induce paroxysms of AF as well as ventricular dysrhythmias (so-called *"holiday heart"* disease). Although there may be no overt evidence of underlying heart disease, there is some debate as to just how normal the hearts really are of patients who experience alcohol-induced arrhythmias. Chronic alcohol abuse can lead to *alcoholic cardiomyopathy*, which may present as paroxysmal AF during binge drinking. As drinking continues, the cardiomyopathy progresses and the AF becomes more established. The condition is potentially reversible with total abstinence.

Systemic Embolization leading to *stroke* and other forms of serious ischemic injury is among the most dangerous complications of AF. Both prospective and retrospective studies have documented an increased risk of embolization in patients with AF. It used to be thought that such risk applied only to patients with AF caused by *rheumatic mitral valve disease*. However, data from the Framingham study and elsewhere document significant increases in the risk of stroke for *all* patients with AF and *underlying heart disease*. Moreover, as noted above, risk might even be increased for elderly patients with no apparent heart disease. Nevertheless, the risk of stroke in mitral disease is still three times that of patients with other cardiac etiologies and as much as seventeen times that of patients without atrial fibrillation. The risk from AF is statistically independent of other risk factors, such as heart failure and coronary artery disease.

Data from the Framingham study suggest that risk of stroke is greatest at the onset of AF, with more than 25 percent of AF-associated strokes occurring at the time of onset. In addition, patients with AF have twice the likelihood of having a recurrence of stroke within the first 6 months compared to patients with stroke and no AF.

WORKUP

See Chapter 25.

PRINCIPLES OF MANAGEMENT

The first priority is to control the ventricular response rate and prevent hemodynamic compromise. The second is to identify and specifically treat any underlying precipitants. Third, one must assess the risk of systemic embolization and initiate oral anticoagulant therapy where risk is high. Finally, candidacy for cardioversion needs to be assessed. (See Chapter 25.)

Rate Control

Heart rate is an important determinant of hemodynamic state and myocardial oxygen demand. If there is any evidence of significant hemodynamic compromise (eg, hypotension, congestive heart failure, ischemia), the patient must be immediately hospitalized. Patients exhibiting no such compromise can be treated as outpatients, especially if the ventricular rate is less than 150 beats/min. The goal is a resting heart rate of less than 85 at rest and less than 110 after mild exercise (eg, 10 sit-ups or 10 stand-ups from a chair). Heart rate may appear well controlled at rest, when there is little adrenergic stimulation, but rise markedly with mild effort; one needs to evaluate control both at rest and on exertion.

Digoxin, verapamil, and beta-blockers are the principal drugs used for rate control in the outpatient, nonemergency setting. AF patients who present with a slow ventricular response rate (<80 beats/min even with exertion) probably have coexisting conduction system disease and should not be treated with drugs that slow ventricular response rate.

Digoxin remains an excellent drug for control of the ventricular response rate in the setting of *chronic AF*, especially when there is systolic dysfunction. By increasing the responsiveness of AV nodal tissue to vagal stimuli, directly decreasing conduction in AV nodal tissue, and enhancing contractility, the cardiac glycoside both directly and indirectly blocks AV conduction, effectively slows the ventricular response rate, and improves cardiac output. *Paroxysmal AF* resulting from an exacerbation of heart failure also responds well to digoxin and may revert to sinus rhythm.

Although still very useful in properly selected patients, digoxin should not be considered the sole cornerstone of AF therapy, because the drug has several important shortcomings. It tends to be *less effective* in slowing heart rate when vagal tone is low and adrenergic stimulation is high, such as during *exercise*. Control may be fine at rest but less so with activity. Performance has also been disappointing when digoxin is used to maintain *sinus rhythm* or reduce the frequency and severity of *paroxysmal AF*. This lack of efficacy is believed related to the drug's dependence on *vagal tone* for full effect and the high level of adrenergic stimulation common to situations that trigger paroxysms of AF. Another drawback is that, in the absence of heart failure, digoxin *does not restore sinus rhythm*. Electrophysiologic studies show the drug actually shortens the atrial refractory period and may contribute to persistence of AF. Finally, digoxin may exacerbate AF due to WPW syndrome by facilitating conduction through the bypass tract and shortening its refractory period. Careful case selection is critical to effective digoxin use.

Digoxin therapy can be initiated safely in the outpatient setting if the patient is tolerating the AF well. Treatment can be started with a *maintenance dose* if the ventricular rate is *less than 120* beats/min. About 5 days are required to achieve standard therapeutic serum levels, though the best measure of adequate dose is heart rate. If the ventricular rate is *between 120 and 150* and still well tolerated, outpatient management remains reasonable, though more rapid digitalization is indicated. An *oral loading dose* of digoxin is given over the first 24 hours. Heart rate is monitored to assess need for further immediate doses in the loading phase and to determine appropriate maintenance doses.

Patients who appear *refractory to digoxin* therapy for rate control require evaluation for factors which might be aggravating the rhythm disturbance. The rapid rate may be a physiologic response to heart failure, fever, hypovolemia, or hypoxia, or it may be a manifestation of an underlying condition, such as hyperthyroidism, alcoholic cardiomyopathy, or WPW syndrome. Treatment should be directed at precipitants and underlying etiologies (see below). Poor compliance is another possible cause of inadequate rate control; measurement of a serum digoxin level will help determine if this is the case.

The clinician using digoxin for AF needs to be alert to the subtle manifestations of *digitalis toxicity* in this setting. AF patients on digoxin who manifest a *regularization* of their rhythm may not have converted to sinus rhythm but rather entered into a *junctional rhythm*, which signifies digitalis excess. The underlying irregularity of rhythm in AF may obscure another important manifestation of digitalis toxicity—*ventricular premature beats*. Such beats should not be confused with the widened QRS complexes caused by the Ashmann phenomenon (prolonged relative refractory period in the beat following a long R-R interval). Careful monitoring is essential. Although the AF rate provides a "bioassay" of digitalis effect and makes frequent sampling of digoxin levels unnecessary, watching for changes in rhythm can be very informative. Whenever there is suspicion of digitalis toxicity, digoxin should be held and a serum level checked.

Verapamil and Beta-blockers. If adequate doses of digoxin prove insufficient to control AF, or if digoxin is deemed inappropriate for the situation (no systolic dysfunction, high adrenergic stimulation, low vagal tone), then adding or switching to a calcium channel blocker or a beta-blocker deserves consideration. Controlled studies have shown both agents to be effective adjuncts as well as alternatives to digoxin therapy in properly selected patients.

Verapamil is the calcium channel blocker of choice for AF, because it has a direct effect on the AV node, prolonging its refractory period and conduction time. These qualities have made the drug an important alternative to digoxin for establishing rate control in AF. Unlike digoxin, it does not require vagal tone to be maximally effective and consequently demonstrates the ability to terminate or control AF under circumstances that ordinarily would be refractory to digoxin. Verapamil may be used alone or in conjunction with digoxin. If used in conjunction with digoxin, careful monitoring of the serum digoxin level is required, because verapamil slows digoxin clearance and may increase its serum concentration. Verapamil does have some negative inotropic effect and must be used with care in patients with heart failure—digoxin would be a better alternative. Caution is also required in patients with underlying conduction system disease (eg, sick sinus syndrome), because verapamil may exacerbate heart block. The drug is contraindicated in WPW syndrome, due to its ability to enhance conduction through the accessory pathway (see below). Diltiazem, another calcium-channel blocker, also is effective.

Beta-blockers (eg, propranolol, atenolol) work by increasing the refractoriness of the AV node and blocking the beta-adrenergic effect of catecholamines on heart rate. They are particularly useful in AF triggered by situational stress, hyperthyroidism, or ischemia, and they are relatively contraindicated in the presence of heart failure (see Chapter 32), where digoxin might be a better choice. Small doses (40–80 mg/d of propranolol, 25–50 mg/d of atenolol) may enhance the efficacy of digoxin in situations where sympathetic stimulation is high.

Other Agents. *Clonidine*, the centrally acting antihypertensive agent, has been studied for control of ventricular rate in patients with rapid AF who are hemodynamically stable. Its ability to decrease sympathetic outflow makes it a good candidate for reducing the high sympathetic tone believed responsible for triggering and sustaining AF. A controlled study of small oral doses (0.075 mg at baseline and repeated after 2 h) showed clonidine to be effective and safe in both slowing and terminating rapid AF. Further study is needed before it can be widely recommended.

Special Situations. Patients with *WPW syndrome* require special mention because of the small but important risk of hemodynamic compromise. Patients with occasional bouts of AF that are well tolerated and self-limited require no treatment so long as the shortest R-R interval during an attack is greater than 180 milliseconds—a shorter interval is associated with an increased risk of ventricular fibrillation. No restrictions on activity are necessary. Patients with very rapid ventricular rates and hemodynamic deterioration during an attack of AF should be hospitalized and treated with urgent *electrical cardioversion. Digoxin and verapamil should not be used*, because they encourage conduction through the accessory pathway by blocking conduction through the AV node. Future episodes of AF are prevented by the use of *quinidine*, *procainamide*, or *disopyramide*. Inpatient electrophysiologic testing is used to help judge which agent is most likely to provide optimal control of ventricular rate during AF. *Propranolol* is sometimes helpful in protecting against recurrent episodes of AF but should also be subjected to electrophysiologic study before being used in patients with potentially serious attacks of AF. Cardiac consultation is essential.

Patients with the tachycardia–bradycardia form of *sick sinus syndrome* pose a therapeutic dilemma: although their AF usually responds well to digoxin, verapamil, or beta-blockade, these therapies may seriously exacerbate episodes of bradycardia by further suppressing conduction through the AV node. Consequently, pacemaker implantation is often necessary for patients with symptomatic tachycardia–bradycardia syndrome.

AF caused by *hyperthyroidism* responds best to beta-blockade, though definitive treatment of the underlying thyroid disease (see Chapter 103) is essential to successful prevention of future episodes of AF. At times, elective cardioversion (see below) is necessary to restore sinus rhythm after successful treatment of the hyperthyroidism.

Search for the Underlying Etiology

Evaluation to identify underlying precipitants and etiologies is discussed in Chapter 25.

Prevention of Systemic Embolization and Stroke

Prevention of systemic embolization and stroke is the next most important therapeutic priority after establishment of rate control. Epidemiologic data from the Framingham study suggested that the risk of stroke from AF extended to all AF patients with underlying heart disease and was not limited to those with rheumatic valvular disease. Relative risk was about 5 for patients with nonrheumatic AF and 13 for those with rheumatic AF. An additional finding was that strokes appeared to cluster about the time of onset of AF, suggesting that patients with recent onset of AF and those with paroxysms of the arrhythmia are at particularly high risk.

Warfarin Anticoagulation. Several prospective, randomized, multi-center, controlled trials have now demonstrated convincingly that warfarin anticoagulation can significantly reduce the risk of systemic embolization and stroke due to nonrheumatic AF. Moreover, so-called "low-dose" therapy (prothrombin time 1.2–1.4 times control) has been shown to be as effective and less likely to cause bleeding complications in patients with nonrheumatic AF than the traditional practice of prolonging the prothrombin time to 1.5 to 1.8 times control (see Chapter 83).

The physician reluctant to begin warfarin therapy for stroke prophylaxis because of relative contraindications to oral anticoagulation (see Chapter 83) should be sure the risk of anticoagulation exceeds that of stroke. AF patients at especially high risk for stroke include those with prior embolic stroke, left atrial mural thrombus, tight mitral stenosis, left atrial enlargement, or poor cardiac output.

Transesophageal echocardiography is the most sensitive indirect means of detecting left atrial thrombus. Although expensive and requiring skilled operators, the study may be worth performing to better estimate embolic risk in the patient with a relative contraindication to anticoagulation.

Aspirin has been suggested as a possible alternative to warfarin for patients not deemed candidates for warfarin, but prospective, randomized, controlled study of its utility for stroke prophylaxis remains to be conducted.

A related question is whether to anticoagulate prior to *elective cardioversion.* The concern is that fresh atrial thrombus which has not had sufficient time to organize may be dislodged with resumption of vigorous and coordinated atrial contraction. There are no definitive randomized, prospective studies to resolve the issue. One reviewer pooled data from all available retrospective studies to see if any trends were evident. Pooling produced a heterogeneous population of approximately 1650 AF patients who were not prophylactically anticoagulated prior to cardioversion. In this diverse group, the frequency of embolic events was 1.7 percent. The same pooled data show a rate of 0.7 percent for the 450 patients who were anticoagulated. The difference in frequency of embolization was not statistically significant. Since the etiology and nature of the AF in most of these patients was never specified, the data cannot be used to identify high-risk subgroups. Although there is some suspicion that patients with rheumatic heart disease, cardiomegaly, left atrial enlargement, or a history of embolization are at increased risk of embolization from elective cardioversion, the available data are inadequate to substantiate this view. Preliminary data from studies utilizing transesophageal echocardiography suggest that in the absence of detectable left atrial thrombus, embolic risk is very low and that one can proceed directly to cardioversion without prior anticoagulation. Prospective randomized studies are needed.

If prophylactic anticoagulation is to be undertaken, it should be initiated 3 to 4 weeks before elective cardioversion (to allow existing thrombi to endothelialize) and continued for a few weeks after cardioversion, because of the risk of late embolization due to atrial instability. Embolic episodes have been documented to occur as late as several days after cardioversion; this correlates with the time noted for resumption of full atrial mechanical function.

Cardioversion. Patients who cannot tolerate the fall in cardiac output or the increase in myocardial oxygen demand associated with AF are prime candidates for *urgent cardioversion,* especially if there is acute heart failure or myocardial ischemia. Indications for *elective cardioversion* include reduced exercise tolerance, symptomatic palpitations, persistence of AF after effective treatment of the underlying etiology, angina with onset of AF, and systemic embolization from left atrial stasis.

Elective cardioversion is contraindicated if there is digitalis toxicity (ventricular arrhythmias may ensue), a slow ventricular response rate in the absence of digitalis (may lead to sinus arrest after cardioversion), or inability to tolerate quinidine and other agents used to maintain sinus rhythm after cardioversion.

Maintenance of sinus rhythm for more than 6 months after cardioversion is most likely in patients with recent onset of AF, coarse fibrillatory waves on ECG, and a left atrium that is within normal size limits. Conversely, those with chronic AF, left atrial enlargement, advanced mitral stenosis, or chronic congestive heart failure are least likely to attain long-term benefit from elective cardioversion; AF almost always returns within a short period of time.

Electrical cardioversion is the procedure of choice for urgently converting AF to sinus rhythm. For elective cardioversion, pretreatment with quinidine and its continuation for 3 to 6 months after cardioversion enhance the probability of maintaining sinus rhythm. Digoxin is withheld for 2 days prior to cardioversion, because there is an increased risk of ventricular dysrhythmias when the heart is countershocked in the presence of high digoxin levels. As noted above, the risk of embolization is small but can be lessened by use of prophylactic anticoagulation (see above).

Pharmacologic cardioversion using *quinidine* or procainamide is an alternative approach used by some cardiologists before resorting to electrical cardioversion. It too requires hospital admission because high doses are required and monitoring is necessary to assure safety. Pro-arrhythmic effects sometimes occur, including ventricular torsade de pointe.

PATIENT EDUCATION

The young patient with paroxysmal AF who is free of underlying heart disease needs to be fully reassured to prevent cardiac neurosis and the unnecessary restriction of activity. Such patients should be instructed to quit smoking, avoid sleep deprivation, and limit use of alcohol and stimulants. They often will benefit from use of relaxation techniques (see Chapter 226) at times of stress. WPW patients whose episodes of AF are brief, infrequent, and well tolerated can also be reassured and encouraged to remain fully active. Patients with AF secondary to alcohol abuse and evolving cardiomyopathy need to be informed of the risk of alcoholic cardiomyopathy and strongly urged to abstain from alcohol. In addition, patients at risk for AF from any other cause should be advised to use caution in their social drinking, since excess intake may increase vulnerability to AF (see Chapters 25 and 228).

It is important to teach AF patients and family members to watch for signs of hemodynamic compromise, such as rapid heart rate, unexplained weight gain, worsening dyspnea on exertion, and decreased exercise tolerance. Patients often fear that long-term digoxin therapy will be habit-forming or injurious to the heart; reassurance and education about its use are often much appreciated. However, they need to be aware of the symptoms and signs of digitalis toxicity (see Chapter 32) so that correction of the problem is not unnecessarily delayed.

INDICATIONS FOR ADMISSION AND REFERRAL

Patients unable to tolerate their AF due to congestive heart failure or ischemia should be immediately hospitalized. The same is true if the ventricular response rate is extremely rapid (>170 beats/min). Electrical cardioversion may be urgent. Hospitalization is also indicated for patients refractory to medical therapy and those with new onset of embolization. Patients who are candidates for elective cardioversion need at least a temporary stay, even if only for the day.

Referral is indicated for patients with refractory AF, suspicion of WPW syndrome, sick sinus syndrome, or AF resulting in hemodynamic compromise. Patients deemed possible candidates for elective cardioversion also should be referred for cardiac consultation.

THERAPEUTIC RECOMMENDATIONS

- If there is no evidence of congestive failure, ischemia, or embolization and the ventricular response rate is less than 150 beats/min, outpatient management can be undertaken, provided the patient is reliable and the home environment is supportive.
- The first priority is to slow ventricular rate. Digoxin is the drug of choice, although it is contraindicated in cases of AF due to preexcitation syndromes such as WPW syndrome.
- If heart rate is between 100 and 120 and well tolerated, begin therapy with a maintenance dose of digoxin (.25–.375 mg/d). Control should be achieved within 5 days, the time it takes to reach a therapeutic serum level.
- If the rate is between 120 and 150 and well tolerated, begin therapy with an oral loading dose of digoxin (1.0–1.25 mg over 24 h in divided doses) to achieve rate control more rapidly. Ventricular rate is monitored to determine daily dose.
- The goal of rate control should be a heart rate of less than 85 at rest and less than 110 after modest exercise (eg, 10 stand-ups). Rate must be checked after exercise because it may rise markedly, even though it appears well controlled at rest.
- If rate control is difficult to achieve, check for failure, ischemia, fever, hypovolemia, hypoxia, recurrent pulmonary embolization, hyperthyroidism, and WPW syndrome. Treatment should be directed at the underlying condition. Hospitalize if the AF is not well tolerated.
- Patients who are well controlled at rest, but have rates which rise unacceptably with exertion (>120) might benefit from a cautious trial of adding a beta-blocking agent (eg, timolol 10 mg bid) or verapamil (80 mg tid) to the digoxin regimen. Do not use in patients with heart failure or preexcitation syndrome. Monitor serum digoxin level regularly if verapamil is used, since it may rise.
- Young patients with brief and infrequent bouts of AF due to WPW need not be treated if episodes are well tolerated and the shortest R-R interval is greater than 180 milliseconds. All others require prompt referral to a cardiologist. Do not treat with digitalis.
- Patients with sick sinus syndrome may be very susceptible to bradycardia; use digoxin with care and only if there is no history of symptomatic bradycardia; obtain cardiac consultation if symptomatic bradycardia occurs.
- Begin oral anticoagulant therapy as early as possible in all AF patients with underlying heart disease, unless there is a serious contraindication to warfarin therapy (see Chapter 83). Patients with mitral valve disease, prior embolization, heart failure, left atrial thrombus, left atrial dilation, or low cardiac output are at particularly high risk for systemic embolization.
- Refer for consideration of elective cardioversion patients with AF that persists after definitive treatment of its underlying etiology, rapid ventricular rate refractory to medical therapy, symptomatic palpitations, or systemic embolization thought to arise from the left atrium.
- The need for prophylactic anticoagulation prior to elective cardioversion remains unproven. If it is to be employed, it should be started 3 to 4 weeks before cardioversion and continued for at least 2 to 3 weeks after the procedure, because there may be some residual atrial instability.
- Admit for urgent cardioversion the patient with hemodynamic deterioration, ischemia, or extremely rapid rates (eg, >200).
- Continue quinidine for 6 months to prevent relapse. Patients least likely to hold in sinus rhythm after cardioversion are those with chronic AF, advanced mitral stenosis, chronic congestive heart failure, or other causes of marked left atrial dilation.
- Advise patients with paroxysms of AF from whatever cause to use alcohol only in moderation and avoid bouts of acute intoxication, since such bouts increase vulnerabilitly for AF.

Management of Paroxysmal Supraventricular Tachycardias

Paroxysmal supraventricular tachycardia describes a heterogeneous group of arrhythmias characterized electrocardiographically by a regular rhythm, rapid rate, and narrow

QRS complex. These arrhythmias can occur in young people with no apparent heart disease and in older patients with severe coronary, valvular, or myocardial disease. Electrophysiologic studies have identified several mechanisms.

Pathophysiology and Clinical Presentation. *Reentry* accounts for most cases and has been localized with greatest frequency to the AV node. Less common sites of reentry are the AV nodal bypass tract (as in Wolff-Parkinson-White syndrome), the sinus node, and the atria. The tachycardia is initiated by premature beats that dissociate refractoriness between conduction pathways and permit circulating electrical activity. The tachycardia ceases when conductivity in the reentrant circuit is altered. A separate form of supraventricular tachycardia, paroxysmal atrial tachycardia with block, is characteristic of digitalis intoxication and is caused by *increased automaticity* in atrial tissues as well as block at the AV junction.

There are some useful guidelines to help the clinician distinguish between reentry and increased automaticity. The rhythm disturbance is more likely to be reentrant if it is initiated by a premature beat, is perfectly regular (usually without defined P waves), and can be halted by vagal maneuvers such as Valsalva. Characteristics of increased automaticity include no initiating premature beat, a gradual increase in rate (the "warm-up" phenomenon), and no response to vagal maneuvers.

Principles of Management. In theory, selection of treatment modality can be based on the underlying pathophysiology. For reentrant cases, agents which can block the reentrant circuit should be more effective; these include digitalis, beta-blockers, and the calcium channel blockers verapamil and diltiazem. Agents which stabilize the membrane (eg, quinidine, procainamide, disopyramide) are preferred for episodes caused by increased automaticity.

In reality, there is much overlap, and it is sometimes very difficult on clinical or even electrophysiologic grounds to predict which type of agent will work best. For example, the calcium channel blocker verapamil has been found to be extremely effective in cases of multifocal atrial tachycardia, a condition characterized by increased automaticity. While it is not useful to be dogmatic about drug selection, an attempt at determination of the underlying mechanism can help in initial choice of therapy.

Treatment of both the acute tachyarrhythmia and prevention of recurrent episodes has been greatly enhanced by the advent of *calcium channel blockers*. These agents prolong AV nodal refractoriness, which helps terminate reciprocating AV tachycardias that involve the AV node. When used intravenously, they are among the most effective agents for terminating an acute attack. When used orally for chronic prophylaxis, they have proven to be safe and extremely beneficial, markedly reducing the frequency and severity of attacks without significant side effects or complications. Studies using diltiazem have produced similar results. The effective verapamil dose for prophylaxis is 240 to 480 mg/d (usually given as 80–160 mg tid).

Need for *prophylactic therapy* is based on the frequency and severity of attacks as well as their effect on the patient's cardiac status. A young person may find the episodes annoying, but an elderly patient with coronary disease may develop myocardial compromise from the tachycardia. For patients with reentrant physiology who experience only one or two attacks per year and tolerate them without difficulty, it is best to teach them vagal maneuvers such as Valsalva and carotid sinus massage. These can be carried out at the onset of an attack. For patients with more frequent episodes and/or limited myocardial reserve, chronic therapy with a calcium channel blocker, beta-blocker, or digitalis is worth a try. Patients with increased automaticity may benefit from one of the membrane-stabilizing antiarrhythmic agents, although verapamil has proven effective even in this setting.

A.H.G.

ANNOTATED BIBLIOGRAPHY

Boston Area Anticoagulation Trial for Atrial Fibrillation Investigators. The effect of low-dose warfarin on the risk of stroke in patients with nonrheumatic atrial fibrillation. N Engl J Med 1990;323:1505. *(One of several randomized trials demonstrating benefit in patients with chronic or paroxysmal AF; also shows efficacy of low-intensity therapy.)*

Brand FN, Abbott RD, Kannel WB, et al. Characteristics and prognosis of lone atrial fibrillation: 30-year follow-up in the Framingham Study. JAMA 1985;254:3449. *(A fourfold increase in stroke risk was noted, but patients were older and had more cardiovascular risk factors than patients in other studies of lone AF.)*

Daniel WG. Should transesophageal echocardiography be used to guide cardioversion? N Engl J Med 1993;328:803. *(A cautiously optimistic editorial, but argues it is too early to incorporate the technology into routine decision making.)*

Engel TR, Luck JC. Effect of whiskey on atrial vulnerability and "holiday heart." J Am Col Cardiol 1983;1:816. *(Alcohol enhanced vulnerability to AF in patients without clinical evidence of cardiomyopathy or heart failure.)*

Ezekowitz MD, Bridgers SL, James KE, et al. Warfarin in the prevention of stroke associated with nonrheumatic atrial fibrillation. N Engl J Med 1992;327:1406. *(Data from the VA study further confirming that low-intensity therapy reduces risk; extends documentation of benefit to patients over 70.)*

Falk RH. Proarrhythmia in patients treated for atrial fibrillation or flutter. Ann Intern Med 1992;117:141. *(A review of the potential for dysrhythmias from drugs used to treat AF.)*

Falk RH, Leavitt JI. Digoxin for atrial fibrillation: a drug whose time has gone? Ann Intern Med 1991;114:573. *(A review critical of digoxin that emphasizes its shortcomings in the treatment of AF; 22 refs.)*

Kannel WB, Abbott RD, Savage DD, et al. Epidemiologic features of chronic atrial fibrillation: the Framingham Study. N Engl J Med 1982;306:1018. *(A major epidemiologic study; heart failure and rheumatic heart disease were the most powerful predictive precursors of chronic AF; chronic AF was associated with a doubling of overall and cardiovascular mortality.)*

Kopecky SL, Gersh BJ, McGoon MD, et al. The natural history of lone atrial fibrillation: a population-based study over three decades. N Engl J Med 1987;317:669. *(A retrospective study of patients under the age of 60 showing that lone AF was associated with a very low risk of stroke.)*

Manning WJ, Silverman DI, Gordon SPF, et al. Cardioversion from atrial fibrillation without prolonged anticoagulation with use of transesophageal echocardiography to exclude presence of atrial thrombi. N Engl J Med 1993;328:750. *(Preliminary data suggesting this technology may make possible early cardioversion in many patients.)*

Mauritson DR, Winniform MD, Walker WS, et al. Oral verapamil for paroxysmal supraventricular tachycardia. Ann Intern Med 1982;96:409. *(A long-term double-blind randomized trial demonstrating that verapamil is both safe and effective for prophylaxis of this arrhythmia.)*

Meyers DG, Gonzalez ER, Nelson WP. The role of prophylactic anticoagulation in cardioversion of atrial fibrillation. Cardiovasc Rev Reports 1985;6:647. *(A critical review of the available evidence presented in pooled form. Argues that few conclusions can be drawn from available data and that prospective randomized studies are needed.)*

Panidis JP, Morganroth J, Baessler C. Effectiveness and safety of oral verapamil to control exercise-induced tachycardia in patients with atrial fibrillation receiving digitalis. Am J Cardiol 1983;52:1197. *(A double-blind controlled study; oral verapamil plus digoxin was safe and superior to digoxin alone; digoxin serum levels increased with verapamil use.)*

Rawles JM, Metcalfe MJ, Jennings K. Time occurrence, duration and ventricular rate of paroxysmal atrial fibrillation: the effect of digoxin. Br Heart J 1990;63:225. *(Digoxin was observed in this Holter monitoring study to have little effect on preventing recurrences, slowing rate at the onset of a paroxysm, or terminating episodes.)*

Roth A, Felner S, Keller K, et al. Clonidine for patients with rapid atrial fibrillation. Ann Intern Med 1992;116:388. *(A small-scale randomized controlled study in which low-dose oral therapy proved effective in hemodynamically stable patients; a promising finding.)*

Singer DE. Randomized trials of warfarin for atrial fibrillation. N Engl J Med 1992;327:1451. *(A fine editorial tersely summarizing the known and unknown.)*

The Stroke Prevention in Atrial Fibrillation Investigators. Predictors of thromboembolism in atrial fibrillation. Ann Intern Med 1992;116:1,6. *(A two-part study; recent CHF, hypertension, previous embolism, LV dysfunction, and left atrial enlargement were independent predictors of stroke risk.)*

Wolf PA, Kannel WB, McGee DL, et al. Duration of atrial fibrillation and imminence of stroke: The Framingham Study. Stroke 1983;14:664. *(Important epidemiology data; risk of embolic stroke found to be maximal at onset of AF, independent of other risk factors for stroke, and substantial, even in AF patients without rheumatic mitral disease; recurrence was twice as likely in patients with AF.)*

29
Management of Ventricular Irritability in the Ambulatory Setting

Primary Care Medicine: Office Evaluation and Management of the Adult Patient, 3rd edition, edited by Allan H. Goroll, Lawrence A. May, and Albert G. Mulley, Jr. J.B. Lippincott Company, Philadelphia

The discovery of ventricular ectopy in the outpatient setting poses difficult questions for the primary care physician. At issue are how much risk the onset of ventricular irritability poses and whether the benefit from suppressing the ectopy outweighs the adverse effects associated with treatment. The growing recognition of the proarrhythmic potential of many antiarrhythmic drugs and the attendant risks incurred by attempting to suppress ventricular irritability have dampened enthusiasm for drug therapy, especially for asymptomatic patients. The primary care physician's tasks in the management of ventricular irritability are to identify the high-risk patient, help counsel the patient on treatment options, and monitor therapy. Determining the need for and selecting a safe and effective treatment program require close consultation with a cardiologist experienced in treating ventricular dysrhythmias. Knowledge of the commonly used antiarrhythmics and approaches to monitoring therapy are essential for effective long-term follow-up by the primary physician.

CLINICAL PRESENTATION AND COURSE

Premature ventricular contractions (PVCs) are ubiquitous and commonly found among patients both with and without underlying heart disease. In studies of the general population, at least one PVC per routine electrocardiogram (ECG) was found in 1 percent of Air Force recruits, 4 percent of life insurance applicants, 7 percent of men older than 34 years of age, and 40 percent to 75 percent of normal persons subjected to 24 to 48 hours of continuous ambulatory (Holter) monitoring. The incidence and prevalence of PVCs increase with age and with exercise.

In the ambulatory setting, ventricular irritability usually presents in one of several ways: 1) as an incidental finding on routine examination or ECG; 2) as an ECG finding in a patient being evaluated for palpitations, dizziness, or syncope; 3) as a complication of underlying heart disease noted on resting ECG, exercise stress test, or Holter monitoring. Prognosis is a function of the complexity of the ectopic activity and the presence and severity of underlying heart disease.

Benign Ventricular Arrhythmias

Initially, prospective studies of large populations of ambulatory men were thought to have shown a correlation between PVCs on routine ECG and subsequent sudden death; however, when these results were reexamined controlling for other cardiac risk factors, PVCs were not found to be an independent determinant of cardiac death in the general population. A long-term study of 73 *asymptomatic, healthy* subjects with frequent and complex ventricular ectopy (>60 beats/h plus multiforms, repetitive forms, bigeminy, or R on T) showed *no increased mortality* after a mean follow-up of 6.5 years. Regardless of the presence and persistence of worrisome ventricular irritability, these patients had prognoses no different from those of other healthy people; there was no increased risk of cardiac death.

Other natural history surveys have also emphasized that in the absence of hypertension, angina, history of myocardial infarction, cardiomegaly on chest x-ray, or ECG signs of ischemia, left ventricular (LV) hypertrophy, or bundle branch block, people with PVCs are at no greater risk for cardiac death than the general population.

Potentially Adverse Ventricular Arrhythmias

In comparison to patients free of underlying heart disease, the situation is more worrisome for patients with a variety of cardiac problems, such as those recovering from a *recent myocardial infarction*. In the Coronary Drug Project study of over 2000 survivors of myocardial infarction, the occurrence of even a *single PVC* on a routine ECG taken 3 months or more after the infarct was associated with a *doubling* of the *mortality* rate during the 3-year follow-up period. Numerous studies have revealed that the features most predictive of mortality are *high frequency* of PVCs (>30/h over a 24-h period) and presence of *complex* ventricular ectopy, especially repetitive beats (≥3 consecutive complexes). Prognosis is particularly poor in the setting of a *failing left ventricle* (ejection fraction <0.4).

In patients with a history of *remote myocardial infarction*, the frequency and complexity of PVCs also influence prognosis. For example, in a 5-year study of 1739 male survivors of acute myocardial infarction, the absence of ventricular irritability on a 1-hour ECG recording performed 3 to 9 months postinfarction was associated with a 6 percent risk of sudden cardiac death over 5 years. Risk was 12 percent in patients with unifocal PVCs and 25 percent in those with complex ventricular ectopy. Multivariate analysis showed that *complex* ventricular ectopy had the strongest influence on risk for sudden cardiac death.

The situation is similar for patients with *other forms of heart disease* that cause myocardial scarring and abnormal wall motion. Patients with hypertrophic or congestive cardiomyopathy, hemodynamically significant valvular disease, congenital heart disease with ventricular hypertrophy, hypertensive left ventricular hypertrophy, and revascularization or valve surgery have been found to be at significantly increased risk of sudden death if experiencing frequent or complex PVCs, especially in the context of a *reduced ejection fraction*. The ventricular ectopy is not merely a manifestation of the underlying heart disease but an independent predictor of prognosis.

Malignant Ventricular Arrhythmias

Nonsustained ventricular tachycardia is a worrisome arrhythmia characterized by runs of ventricular tachycardia (VT) that spontaneously revert to sinus rhythm within several beats. In the context of chronic coronary artery disease and left ventricular dysfunction, it represents a malignant form of electrical instability that is an independent risk factor for sudden death. It has a more benign form, found in young patients with no demonstrable heart disease and characterized by resolution with exercise, no associated symptoms, and a regular, relatively slow rate (<150 beats/min) with uniform cycle length and QRS morphology.

Recurrent sustained ventricular tachycardia is a very dangerous ventricular arrhythmia, especially when it occurs in the context of left ventricular dysfunction. The arrhythmia is characterized by repeated episodes of ventricular tachycardia, some of which may persist for up to several hours. Many patients become symptomatic due to a fall in cardiac output. Coronary artery disease and cardiomyopathy account for almost 90 percent of cases. About 1 percent of postinfarction patients experience this arrhythmia during the first year of follow-up. Untreated, the 1-year mortality rate is about 40 percent. Prognosis is poorest in symptomatic patients with compromised left ventricular function.

Torsade de pointes is a rapid, polymorphic ventricular tachycardia that often deteriorates into ventricular fibrillation. Its characteristics are a QRS axis that twists about the ECG baseline, going from positive to negative and back again, and an association with a prolonged QT interval. This is a very malignant ventricular dysrhythmia seen in patients with electrolyte abnormalities (especially hypokalemia) and use of drugs that prolong the QT interval, including many antiarrhythmics (procainamide, quinidine, disopyramide).

In sum, the main determinants of prognosis in patients with ventricular ectopy are the complexity of the rhythm disturbance, the presence of underlying heart disease, and the health of the left ventricle. Each of these factors is an independent predictor of survival. Patients with organic heart disease who manifest symptomatic VT and LV failure are at significant risk of sudden death.

As long as the asymptomatic patient with PVCs has no evidence of underlying heart disease, the prognosis appears fine, but what is the *probability of occult heart disease* in an otherwise apparently healthy patient presenting with PVCs? In a study of 25 such patients presenting with frequent and complex PVCs and subjected to coronary catheterization and angiography, only six were found to have significant coronary artery disease (>50% luminal narrowing). The characteristics of the ventricular ectopy did not differentiate those with from coronary disease from those without it. These asymptomatic patients were treated with modest doses of beta-blocking agents and had no decrease in survival at 5 years into follow-up.

PRINCIPLES OF MANAGEMENT

Candidates for Antiarrhythmic Treatment

Despite the demonstration of increased risk in patients with complex ventricular irritability, only the most *symptomatic* of patients (syncope, out-of-hospital cardiac resuscitation) with the most *malignant* forms of ventricular irritability (recurrent sustained VT) and *poor LV function* (ejection fraction <.40) appear to *benefit* from prophylactic antiarrhythmic therapy. Survival in patients experiencing an out-of-hospital cardiac arrest can be improved 10-fold if an effective antiarrhythmic agent can be identified. In most others, improved survival remains an elusive goal.

Controlled trials of antiarrhythmic therapy for complex ventricular irritability in minimally symptomatic post-myocardial infarction patients with reduced ejection fractions actually show *increased* rates of arrhythmic death in those treated. For example, in the Cardiac Arrhythmia Suppression Trial (CAST)—a large multicenter randomized, placebo-controlled study—asymptomatic postinfarction patients with complex ventricular ectopy who were treated with flecainide or encainide (two potent antiarrhythmics that suppressed ectopy) experienced an increase rather than the expected decrease in incidence of sudden death compared to those randomized to placebo. In other studies, up to 10 percent of patients experienced a proarrhythmic effect and a worsening of ventricular irritability when treated with antiarrhythmic drugs—a response that is idiosyncratic, unpredictable, and associated with all classes of antiarrhythmics.

The realization of the risk associated with antiarrhythmic therapy has greatly increased the threshold for treatment. Now, only patients with underlying heart disease, poor LV function, and symptomatic sustained VT are considered definite candidates for antiarrhythmic therapy. No longer should one embark on an empiric trial of antiarrhythmic therapy "to clean up the ECG" in asymptomatic or mildly symptomatic patients with preserved LV function, no matter how complex the ventricular ectopy. The risk of doing more harm than good is too great.

Selection and Initiation of Therapy

At present, there is no means of predicting what effect a particular antiarrhythmic agent will have on a given patient. No single agent appears distinctly superior, and, with rare exception, no particular arrhythmia appears to warrant a particular antiarrhythmic agent. Selection of an agent is somewhat arbitrary, often based more on side effects and interactions with other agents and other clinical problems than on electrophysiologic principles. To be practical for chronic outpatient use, an antiarrhythmic must be available in an oral form and have an effective half-life of at least 6 hours. Initial choice of an agent is an educated guess based on its reported efficacy, safety, duration of action, and severity and frequency of side effects. Grouping agents by cellular electrophysiologic effects may be useful for classification, but current knowledge of the electrophysiology of most ventricular arrhythmias and drugs is still too fragmentary to allow matching an antiarrhythmic drug with a corresponding arrhythmia.

The largely arbitrary nature of drug selection and the risks of treatment necessitate testing for efficacy before committing a patient to long-term prophylactic drug therapy. With a heightened appreciation for the risks of both the arrhythmias and their therapy comes an increase in the *standards* for antiarrhythmic efficacy. Complete suppression of VT and a marked reduction in other forms of ventricular ectopy are the most accessible and immediate criteria; improved survival is the most meaningful. At issue is the most valid method for demonstrating suppression.

A heated debate continues among authorities as to the relative merits of *invasive testing (electrophysiologic study [EPS] with programmed stimulation)* versus *noninvasive study (Holter monitoring and exercise stress testing)* for predicting efficacy of prophylactic antiarrhythmic therapy. Typical *noninvasive study criteria* are total elimination of VT on Holter monitoring and stress testing, 90 percent reduction in other complex forms of ventricular ectopy, and 50 percent reduction in frequency of unifocal PVCs. The principal *invasive study criterion* is ability to fully suppress induction of VT during EPS.

EPS is an invasive procedure, requiring formal cardiac catheterization and an experienced staff. Arrhythmia inducibility correlates well with clinical findings. Close to 95 percent of coronary disease patients with episodes of sustained VT and 70 percent of patients with noncoronary heart disease and VT demonstrate inducible VT on EPS. Proponents of EPS argue that antiarrhythmic suppression of EPS-induced VT best predicts clinical outcome. In one of the only randomized studies comparing noninvasive testing with invasive testing of arrhythmia suppression, the EPS approach required more hospital days and more drug trials but identified therapy that was significantly more effective in suppressing VT. There were no significant differences in patient survival, but numbers were small. Anecdotal evidence cited against the adequacy of noninvasive testing include reports of high-risk patients who have died arrhythmic deaths while exhibiting drug-induced suppression judged adequate by noninvasive standards. For these reasons, the invasive approach has prevailed in recent years, though randomized studies large enough to evaluate any differences in survival are sorely needed. The literature should be followed closely for such data, since it may alter the approach to initiating therapy.

Pending more definitive data, the standard of care is to subject patients deemed candidates for antiarrhythmic therapy to inpatient EPS testing, both before and during initiation of pharmacologic therapy. Starting therapy empirically on an outpatient basis and evaluating efficacy by noninvasive means is not considered sufficient, though noninvasive testing may be an excellent means of monitoring therapy (see below) and a complement to invasive study during initial evaluation. As a general rule, only those drugs demonstrating ability to suppress the target arrhythmia (usually VT) during programmed stimulation deserve consideration for long-term use.

For patients who survive an *out-of-hospital cardiac arrest*, antiarrhythmics demonstrating suppression of VT during programmed stimulation achieve a 95 percent survival rate at 18 months, compared to 50 percent survival in the absence of effective therapy. When no agent is judged sufficient by EPS criteria, an exception is made to EPS criteria and *empiric amiodarone* therapy is sometimes prescribed for cardiac arrest survivors, because it has been shown capable of reducing mortality from 50 percent to 20 percent at two years.

Antiarrhythmic Agents

The most commonly prescribed agents for outpatient treatment of ventricular irritability remain the *Class IA agents*: quinidine, procainamide, and disopyramide. The orally effective *Class IB drugs,* mexiletine and tocainide, are second-line drugs sometimes used alone or as supplements to Class IA therapy. The potent *Class IC* agents such as encainide and flecainide effectively suppress VT, but they caused excess mortality in the CAST study of minimally symptomatic patients. They are reserved for the most refractory of cases, as is the orally administered *Class III* agent amiodarone. Beta-blocking agents—sometimes referred to as *Class II* antiarrhythmics—are safe and useful when the ventricular dysrhythmia is caused by underlying ischemic heart disease. They are among the few drugs proven to reduce coronary disease mortality (see Chapter 30).

Quinidine remains a first-line drug for outpatient treatment of chronic ventricular irritability, being among the most effective agents for suppression of a wide range of ventricular arrhythmias. Quinidine is available as a sulfate salt and in gluconated form; there are also sustained-release preparations. The 200 mg sulfate preparation has the same amount of quinidine base as the 325 mg gluconate tablet. Quinidine is almost fully absorbed from the gastrointestinal (GI) tract and has an elimination half-life of 7 to 10 hours, being metabolized by the liver and partially excreted unchanged by the kidneys. Renal failure does not appreciably increase serum levels. Peak serum levels are reached within 1 to 2 hours of taking quinidine sulfate and 4 hours after a dose of quinidine gluconate. Quinidine *reduces the clearance of digoxin* and can double its serum concentration, necessitating reduction in digoxin dose when both are used simultaneously.

The most common side effects of quinidine and the ones most often responsible for discontinuation of the drug are nausea, vomiting, and diarrhea. Sometimes switching from the sulfate to the gluconate form can lessen the GI side effects. Other common side effects include tinnitus and vertigo. Hypersensitivity reactions are occasionally encountered; rash, thrombocytopenia, hepatitis, or hemolytic anemia may result. The most potentially serious side effect is marked *prolongation of the QT interval*, usually a result of excessive dose but occasionally an idiosyncratic reaction to a single dose. Although some degree of QT prolongation is seen normally as therapeutic levels are achieved, marked prolongation is abnormal and increases the risk of serious VT (especially *torsade de pointes*), which can lead to ventricular fibrillation.

"Quinidine syncope" is probably a manifestation of torsade de pointes.

Several long-acting quinidine preparations are available (Table 29–1), allowing administration as infrequently as every 8 hours. The percentage of actual quinidine alkaloid in each preparation ranges from 60 percent to 82 percent, making dose adjustment important to insure that a full dose of quinidine is provided when switching from quinidine sulfate (which is 82% quinidine) to a long-acting preparation. A common error is to forget to make the dose adjustment and inadvertently cut down on the patient's daily dose. Although long-acting preparations might help improve compliance and provide more even serum levels of the antiarrhythmic, they are considerably more expensive than generic quinidine sulfate.

Disopyramide has many of the same electrophysiologic properties as quinidine and is also useful in the outpatient treatment of chronic ventricular irritability. It is well absorbed; about 60 percent is excreted unchanged by the kidney, while the remainder is metabolized by the liver. The dose and frequency of administration need to be reduced in the setting of renal or hepatic failure. Serum half-life ranges from 5 to 9 hours, making administration every 6 hours feasible. Disopyramide also comes in a sustained-release preparation that allows administration every 12 hours and actually saves the patient money over the regular brand name formulation; however, the availability of generic disopyramide eliminates this cost advantage.

Unlike quinidine, disopyramide has a rather pronounced *negative inotropic effect*, limiting its usefulness in patients with heart failure and low ejection fraction. This negative inotropic effect is especially significant when the drug is used in conjunction with a beta-blocking agent. Although disopyramide does not cause the often troublesome gastrointestinal side effects associated with quinidine, it does have substantial *anticholinergic activity*, which commonly produces urinary retention, constipation, blurred vision, and dry mouth.

Procainamide is similar in antiarrhythmic effect to quinidine and disopyramide. One major drawback to its use in the outpatient setting is its short serum half-life (3–4 h), necessitating frequent administration. Sustained release preparations are on the market, making administration every 6 to 8 hours possible and providing more steady plasma concentrations. Cost to the patient is increased considerably when switching from generic procainamide to a sustained release preparation. The drug is well absorbed and excreted renally; in renal failure one needs to reduce the frequency of administration. Like quinidine and disopyramide, procainamide can cause *AV block* and should not be used in patients with high-grade heart block. Chronic use of procainamide is associated with appearance of antinuclear antibodies in about 80 percent of patients; 20 percent of these patients develop a *lupus-like syndrome*. Rate of development of this syndrome is a function of acetylator phenotype; patients who slowly acetylate the drug are at greater risk. Concurrent use of amiodarone, ranitidine, or trimethoprim can increase the serum procainamide level.

Table 29-1. Long-Acting Preparations of Common Antiarrhythmics

PARENT DRUG	QUINIDINE			PROCAINAMIDE	DISOPYRAMIDE
Preparation	*Quinidex Extentabs*	*Duraquin/ Quinaglute*	*Cardioquin*	*Pronestyl SR Procan SR*	*Norpace CR*
Compound	Sulfate	Gluconate	Polygalacturonate	HCl	Phosphate
Amount of active drug (%)	82	62	60		
Duration of action (h)	8	8	8	6–8	12
Relative cost of using long-acting preparation*	1.68	1.39	1.89	1.60	0.77

*Costs are based on Redbook; they compare the wholesale price of a long-acting compound with the equivalent total daily dose of its generic preparation.

Mexiletine and Tocainide are orally effective *analogues of xylocaine* that resemble the parent drug in activity against ventricular arrhythmias. Unlike quinidine, procainamide, and disopyramide, these agents do not prolong the PR, QRS, or QT intervals; as such they are theoretically very attractive for treatment of ventricular irritability. Although they can suppress ventricular dysrhythmias refractory to previously available agents, their antiarrhythmic potency in crossover studies is about the same as quinidine and, like other agents, they occasionally worsen ventricular irritability. Response to parenteral xylocaine is a good predictor of response to these drugs. The relatively long half-lives of these agents (8–12 h) makes possible dosage schedules that are practical for chronic outpatient use (ie, bid and tid). These agents can be used in conjunction with quinidine or other antiarrhythmics for added efficacy, and they are even well tolerated in the presence of heart failure, having little negative inotropic effect. Of the two, mexiletine is the more negatively inotropic and also has modest suppressive effect on AV nodal conduction.

Side effects are mostly of the central nervous system (CNS) and GI variety (tremor, ataxia, confusion, dizziness, nausea, anorexia); the GI upset can often be prevented by taking the medication with meals. Side effects are dose-related and resolve with discontinuation of the drug. About 15 percent of patients are unable to tolerate these agents due to CNS or GI side effects. Tocainide causes bone marrow suppression, with *agranulocytosis* reported in 0.2 percent. Rare instances of pulmonary fibrosis and pneumonitis have occurred. These serious adverse effects have limited tocainide's role to symptomatic patients who fail other therapies.

Amiodarone is a very potent antiarrhythmic drug that belongs to the same class as the parenteral agent bretylium. Its role is in the treatment of refractory, life-threatening ventricular dysrhythmias, particularly recurrent sustained VT and out-of-hospital VF cardiac arrest. Often, the drug's effect on VT cannot be predicted from response to programmed electrophysiologic study, leading to empiric use in some instances.

Amiodarone has several worrisome side effects that are predominantly dose-related. The most dangerous is pulmonary fibrosis that is preceded by a reversible patchy pneumonitis. Another complication is corneal deposits; these usually do not interfere with vision and disappear with discontinuation of the drug. GI upset is common, and clinical hepatitis occurs in 4 percent of patients. Ataxia and tremor also occur. The drug contains an iodinated segment that can interfere with thyroid metabolism. Amiodarone prolongs the QT interval and has a modestly negative inotropic effect. Interactions with other drugs are substantial: amiodarone increases the serum levels of digoxin, quinidine, and procainamide and potentiates the effect of warfarin. Dose adjustments are necessary when amiodarone is used. In spite of all these side effects, the drug is reasonably well tolerated when used carefully by experienced clinicians.

Beta-blocking Agents are useful for suppression of ventricular irritability related to underlying ischemic disease, digitalis toxicity, exercise, emotional stress, prolonged QT interval syndromes, and tricyclic antidepressants. Although these drugs are not particularly effective in directly suppressing life-threatening ventricular irritability, they are the only agents to date that are known to prolong survival in patients who have suffered a myocardial infarction and are the first choice for treating coronary patients with complex ventricular irritability that is not life-threatening (eg, nonsustained VT, multifocal PVCs, frequent unifocal PVCs). Many of these agents have negative inotropic effects and can worsen heart block; they should be used with caution in patients with heart failure and conduction disturbances (see Chapter 30).

Investigational Agents. Flecainide, encainide, and moricizine were promising oral Class I (local anesthetic-type) antiarrhythmic agents capable of suppressing sustained ventricular arrhythmias in patients who had experienced a myocardial infarction. However, randomized, prospective, controlled clinical trials (CAST I and II) found these agents increased the rate of arrhythmic deaths. These findings underscore the point that *suppression of ventricular arrhythmias does not predict increased survival*, at least in patients with prior myocardial infarction. The clinician should keep this fact in mind when reviewing claims of efficacy for antiarrhythmic drugs.

Nonpharmacologic Measures

Not all symptomatic patients with sustained VT are candidates for drug therapy. About half of those with inducible VT on programmed stimulation fail to suppress with drug therapy. Others with an inadequate response include patients with noncoronary heart disease and those with noninducible VT on programmed stimulation. Patients suffering an out-of-hospital cardiac arrest on antiarrhythmic therapy are also poor candidates for continued attempts at pharmacologic therapy. Such patients with refractory life-threatening arrhythmias are potential candidates for an *automatic implantable cardioverter defibrillator* or *ablative therapy*. Implantable defibrillator therapy has shown considerable promise, but long-term follow-up data on safety, patient acceptability, and survival are not yet available. For ablative therapy, the objective is to sever, remove, or destroy the anatomic substrate of the arrhythmia. Surgical cure rates of 70 percent to 80 percent have been reported. Among the 20 percent to 30 percent who do not obtain a surgical cure, about half become more responsive postoperatively to pharmacologic therapy than they were before surgery. However, operative mortality is high (10%–15%); these are very high-risk patients with serious underlying heart disease.

There is no evidence that moderate intake of *caffeinated beverages* is harmful to patients with serious ventricular irritability.

Monitoring Therapy

As discussed earlier, the current standard for assessing drug efficacy is its ability to *suppress programmed stimulation of VT* during electrophysiologic study. This has proven superior to *Holter monitoring* and *exercise stress testing* for predicting recurrence of VT, though not necessarily for predicting survival. Noninvasive methods still have important roles, especially in monitoring therapy and in testing drugs in patients who are poor candidates for EPS or who do not have inducible VT on EPS. Exercise stress testing is especially useful for monitoring patients with exercise-induced VT. Holter monitoring provides important information in patients with recurrent syncope (see Chapter 24).

Unfortunately, the correlation between ability to suppress VT and survival is not perfect. In the CAST study, antiarrhythmics that achieved suppression of VT actually increased the risk of sudden death. Ability to suppress VT represents an imperfect standard and not one that automatically translates to improved survival. The reader is urged to watch the literature for survival data from prospective, controlled clinical trials.

Even though treatment of ventricular irritability is still largely problematic, the primary physician can do much to ensure the safety of antiarrhythmic therapy and minimize iatrogenic complications. Monitoring *serum potassium* and maintaining normokalemia are of major importance in limiting the risk of a proarrhythmic effect from antiarrhythmic therapy. When a digitalis preparation is used, it too needs careful monitoring in the setting of antiarrhythmic use. Renal and hepatic function determinations *(blood urea nitrogen [BUN], creatinine, transaminase)* bear watching, since they represent the principal routes of antiarrhythmic excretion. Drugs with potential for bone marrow suppression (eg, tocainide) necessitate periodic checking of the *complete blood count.*

Monitoring the *ECG* for evidence of excessive dose and idiosyncratic reactions is also essential. Quinidine, procainamide, and disopyramide can substantially *prolong the PR, QRS, and QT intervals* when serum levels are in the toxic range. Modest QT interval prolongation is to be expected and is a sign of therapeutic effect, but marked prolongation is an important sign of excessive dose and a need to withhold further medication. Marked prolongation of the QT interval also can occur idiosyncratically in some patients at the very onset of therapy; it should be watched for.

Measurement of *serum drug levels* is an important aid to safe use of these antiarrhythmic agents (Table 29–2). Proper interpretation of the data requires that levels be drawn long enough after the last dose so that one is not mistaking a peak serum level for a steady state one.

INDICATIONS FOR REFERRAL AND ADMISSION

Any symptomatic patient found to have sustained ventricular tachycardia in the setting of underlying heart disease and left ventricular dysfunction should be promptly admitted and referred to a cardiologist skilled in performing electriphysiologic study and treating life-threatening ventricular irritability. The primary care physician should never attempt to institute antiarrhythmic therapy for an episode of sustained VT on an empiric, outpatient basis, even if the patient is asymptomatic.

Asymptomatic patients with normal LV function who manifest complex ventricular ectopy other than nonsustained VT are not candidates for antiarrhythmic therapy and do not require admission. While cardiac consultation may be reassuring to such patients and their primary care physicians, it is unlikely that antiarrhythmic therapy would be recommended beyond the addition of a beta-blocker in patients with underlying coronary disease.

PATIENT EDUCATION

Patients with worrisome ventricular irritability pose a problem in patient education. On the one hand, the physician is reluctant to scare the patient who may be relatively asymptomatic, yet without full knowledge of the significance of the problem, compliance and monitoring of one's condition might suffer. Most patients and their families benefit from knowing the prognostic meaning of the ventricular arrhythmia and appreciate the frankness. Fear can be lessened by informing them of the efficacy of therapy for the most serious forms of ventricular irritability. Full disclosure improves compliance by reinforcing the importance of therapy; patients are also more willing to put up with annoying side effects from the drugs.

Patient education is also crucial to patients with harmless forms of ventricular irritability. Knowing that the palpitations and abnormal ECG have no implications for long-term survival is tremendously reassuring and can prevent development of a cardiac neurosis and unnecessary restriction of activity.

Table 29-2. Commonly Used Agents for Outpatient Treatment of Ventricular Irritability

DRUG	HALF-LIFE (HRS)	THERAPEUTIC SERUM CONC/mL	ELIMINATION	ECG	ADVERSE EFFECTS
Quinidine	5–12	2–5 μm/mL	liver	QT, PR, QRS	GI, hypotension, heart block, syncope
Disopyramide	6–8	2–8	renal/liver	same	GI, CHF, anticholinergic
Procainamide	3–6	4–10	renal	same	GI, lupus, CNS
Tocainide	9–20	5–12	renal/liver	none	GI, CNS, marrow
Mediastina	10–13	1–2	liver	none	GI, CNS
Propranolol	4–6	not estab.	liver	PR QT	heart block, CHF bronchospasm
Amiodarone	25+ days	1–2	?	QT	pulm. fibrosis, corneal deposits, neurologic, GI, drug–drug effects, thyroid

CONCLUSIONS AND THERAPEUTIC RECOMMENDATIONS

- No antiarrhythmic treatment is needed for patients with infrequent unifocal PVCs (<30/h), regardless of whether there is underlying heart disease or not. The risks of therapy outweigh any potential benefit. If there is underlying coronary disease, beta-blocker therapy may be added (see Chapter 30).
- No antiarrhythmic treatment is indicated for patients with ventricular ectopy who are free of underlying heart disease, even though they may have frequent PVCs (>30 beats/h) and/or complex PVCs (repetitive beats, R on T, bigeminy, multiform, or nonsustained VT). These patients are at no increased risk of sudden cardiac death. However, a careful search for underlying heart disease and LV dysfunction should be made before concluding there is no heart disease (see Chapters 20, 24, and 32).
- Asymptomatic or minimally symptomatic patients with underlying heart disease and nonsustained VT or other forms of frequent and/or complex PVCs pose an unresolved dilemma regarding need for antiarrhythmic treatment. Although they are clearly at increased risk of sudden death, the risks of available antiarrhythmic therapy appear to outweigh the benefits of treatment. Treatment is best directed at the underlying heart disease (eg, beta-blockade for coronary disease).
- Patients with underlying heart disease, LV dysfunction, and sustained VT are at very high risk of sudden death and require prompt admission and cardiac consultation, especially if they experience arrhythmia-induced symptoms of hemodynamic compromise. Antiarrhythmic therapy is indicated for these patients and is best initiated in the inpatient setting, in collaboration with a cardiologist skilled in treating malignant ventricular arrhythmias.
- Drug selection is largely empirical, but should not be done without cardiac consultation, due to the risk of proarrhythmic effects. No antiarrhythmic agent should be prescribed without its demonstrating an ability to fully suppress VT. The best approach at present is to individualize therapy and treat only with an agent that has proven effective by objective testing for the patient in question.
- Whether invasive testing (electrophysiologic study) or noninvasive assessment (Holter monitoring plus exercise stress testing) is the best means of judging drug efficacy remains to be determined.
- When VT cannot be induced during testing, drug selection is more problematic. Options include empiric use of amiodarone—especially useful in patients surviving out-of-hospital cardiac arrest—and consideration of nonpharmacologic therapies.
- Nonpharmacologic therapy is indicated when high-risk patients clinically fail drug therapy (recurrent symptomatic episodes) and when no effective antiarrhythmic drug can be identified during testing. Implantable defibrillators and ablation of the irritant focus are the leading nonpharmacologic options.
- Once the appropriate agent and effective daily dose are established, one can consider switching to a long-acting preparation, provided that adjustment is made to ensure equivalent dose of active ingredient and the patient is able to afford the incremental cost of using a long-acting preparation.
- Monitor serum drug levels in all patients on chronic antiarrhythmic therapy; have sample drawn sufficiently after last oral dose (usually 4–6 h) to avoid measurement of peak serum levels. Also monitor ventricular rate and PR and QT intervals on ECG, and serum concentrations of potassium, BUN, creatinine, and digoxin (if in concurrent use). Patients on drugs that have effects on bone marrow and liver function need to have checks of the complete blood count, transaminases, and prothrombin time.
- Definition of therapeutic end point remains somewhat arbitrary, though complete suppression of VT remains the "gold standard" at present, whether assessed by invasive or noninvasive testing.

A.H.G.

ANNOTATED BIBLIOGRAPHY

Bigger JT. Definition of benign versus malignant ventricular arrhythmias. Am J Cardiol 1983;52(6):47C. *(A excellent review of the various forms of ventricular irritability and the degree of risk associated with each of them.)*

Bikkina M, Larson MG, Levy D. Prognostic implications of asymptomatic ventricular arrhythmias: The Framingham Heart Study. Ann Intern Med 1992;117:990. *(Increased risk of myocardial infarction or death from coronary disease.)*

Buxton AE. Antiarrhythmic drugs: good for premature ventricular complexes but bad for patients? Ann Intern Med 1992;116:420. *(An editorial; reviews the disappointing results with Class IC antiarrhythmics; more proarrhythmic than suppressive; good discussion of the implications.)*

Cardiac Arrhythmia Suppression Trial II Investigators. Effect of the antiarrhythmic agent moricizine on survival after myocardial infarction. N Engl J Med 1992;327:227. *(The CAST II results with moricizine were as disappointing as for flecainide and encainide—see next ref; all had proarrhythmic effects and increased mortality.)*

Echt DS, Liebson PR, Mitchell B, et al. Mortality and morbidity in patients receiving encainide, flecainide, or placebo: the Cardiac Arrhythmia Suppression Trial. N Engl J Med 1991;324:781. *(A major randomized controlled study of antiarrhythmic therapy in mildly symptomatic patients with complex ventricular ectopy, coronary artery disease, and reduced ejection fraction; demonstrates an excessive incidence of arrhythmic deaths in patients randomized to antiarrhythmic therapy.)*

Kennedy HL, Pescarmona J, Bouchard RJ, Goldberg RJ. Coronary artery status of apparently healthy subjects with frequent and complex ventricular ectopy. Ann Intern Med 1980;92:179. *(One quarter of apparently healthy patients being followed for complex and frequent VEA were found to have significant coronary stenosis; no clinical features of the ectopy that differentiated them.)*

Kennedy HL, Whitlock JA, Sprague MK. Long-term follow-up of asymptomatic healthy subjects with frequent and complex ventricular ectopy. N Engl J Med 1985;312:1983. *(Important study; regardless of the presence of frequent and complex ventricular irritability, there was no increase in mortality among these healthy patients; mean follow-up: 6.5 years.)*

Marchlinski FE. Treatment of sustained ventricular arrhythmias: Which therapy to use? Ann Intern Med 1988;109:522. *(An editorial providing a thoughtful approach to selection of ther-*

apy, including pharmacologic and nonpharmacologic measures.)

Mason JW, et al. A comparison of electrophysiologic testing with Holter monitoring to predict arrhythmic drug efficacy for ventricular tachycardias. N Engl J Med 1993;329:445. (*Holter monitoring was more predictive of efficacy in this first large prospective randomized trial of the two methods. However, very narrow spectrum of patients, making generalizations difficult.*)

McLenachan JM, Henderson E, Morris KI, et al. Ventricular arrhythmias in patients with hypertensive left ventricular hypertrophy. N Engl J Med 1987;317:787. *(Documents increased frequency of complex ventricular irritability in such patients.)*

Meinertz T, et al. Significance of ventricular arrhythmias in idiopathic dilated cardiomyopathy. Am J Cardiol 1981;53:902. *(Ventricular irritability was a determinant of increased risk in these patients.)*

Meyers MG. Caffeine and cardiac arrhythmias. Ann Intern Med 1991;114:147. *(Critical literature review; no evidence that moderate intake of caffeine increases the frequency or severity of dysrhythmias in normals or those with heart disease, even those with preexisting, serious VEA.)*

Miller JM, Kienzle MG, Harken AH, et al. Subendocardial resection for ventricular tachycardia: predictors of surgical success. Circulation 1984;70:624. *(The surgical approach to VT, with useful clinical criteria for case selection.)*

Minardo JD, Heger JJ, Miles WM, et al. Clinical characteristics of patients with ventricular fibrillation during antiarrhythmic drug therapy. N Engl J Med 1988;319:257. *(VF occurred early and was most likely in patients with LV dysfunction and concomitant digitalis and diuretic therapy.)*

Powell AC, Gold MR, Brooks R, et al. Electrophysiologic response to moricizine in patients with sustained ventricular arrhythmias. Ann Intern Med 1992;116:382. *(Another of the promising Class IC antiarrhythmics proves ineffective in suppressing VT and manifests proarrhythmic activity; failure of suppressibility to predict outcome.)*

Ruberman W, et al. Ventricular premature complexes and sudden death after myocardial infarction. Circulation 1981; 64:297. *(Frequent and complex ventricular irritability in post-MI patients was associated with increased risk of sudden death.)*

Ruskin J. Ventricular extrasystoles in healthy subjects. N Engl J Med 1985;312:238. *(An editorial summarizing current knowledge and pinpointing areas of continued uncertainty.)*

Stanton MS, Prystowsky EN, Fineberg NS, et al. Arrhythmogenic effects of antiarrhythmic drugs. J Am Coll Cardiol. 1989;14:209. *(A review of over 1000 drug trials; risk was highest in patients with a low ejection fraction and a history of VT.)*

Tchou PJ, Kadri N, Anderson J, et al. Automatic implantable cardioverter defibrillators and survival of patients with left ventricular dysfunction and malignant ventricular arrhythmias. Ann Intern Med 1988;109:529. *(Use of an important nonpharmacologic alternative in very high-risk patients.)*

Ward DE, Camm AJ. Dangerous ventricular arrhythmias—can we predict drug efficacy? N Engl J Med 1993;329:498. (*A lucid and critical discussion of EPS versus Holter.*)

Primary Care Medicine: Office Evaluation and Management of the Adult Patient, 3rd edition, edited by Allan H. Goroll, Lawrence A. May, and Albert G. Mulley, Jr. J.B. Lippincott Company, Philadelphia

30
Management of Chronic Stable Angina

Several million Americans suffer from coronary heart disease (CHD), and more than 600,000 die each year from the condition and its complications. Even for patients with chronic stable angina—the form of the disease most commonly encountered in the outpatient setting—the risk of death is high (2–12% annually). The array of treatment modalities is extensive, ranging from nitrates, beta-blocking agents, and calcium channel blockers to aspirin, angioplasty, and coronary bypass surgery. These medical and surgical approaches are complemented by exercise programs (see Chapters 18 and 31), stress reduction efforts, and control of cardiovascular risk factors such as hypertension (see Chapter 26), hyperlipidemia (see Chapter 27), and smoking (see Chapter 54). Patients with angina secondary to aortic stenosis are candidates for valve replacement (see Chapter 33).

One must understand the limitations as well as the indications for this vast array of therapeutic options. Design of the basic medical regimen and ascertaining possible need for interventional measures are among the important responsibilities of the primary care physician. Patients with coronary heart disease often request cardiac consultation, and knowing when such a consultation is indicated is essential. However, long-term management of the patient with stable angina usually falls to the primary physician. The goals include symptom relief, improved exercise capacity, prevention of infarction, and ultimately, improved survival.

PATHOPHYSIOLOGY

Angina is a symptomatic manifestation of *myocardial ischemia*. In the setting of stable coronary disease, angina occurs when oxygen demand exceeds available vascular supply. Coronary artery occlusion due to *atherosclerotic disease* is by far the most common etiology. The emerging view of its pathophysiology involves cholesterol deposition and reactive endothelial injury leading to episodes of acute *thrombosis*. Activated *platelets* and other elements of the clotting system appear to play major roles. A series of stepwise thrombotic events is believed to account for much of the atherosclerotic occlusion that occurs in the large epicardial arteries. Many, if not most, episodes of *acute coronary insufficiency* and *infarction* are associated with acute thrombosis, often occurring at an ulcerated, eccentrically located, or ruptured plaque, not necessarily at a site of severe stenosis.

Restriction of coronary blood supply may also ensue from *coronary vasospasm*, believed related to loss of normal endothelial vasoregulatory activity. The coronary endothelium appears to cease production of vasoactive peptides and prostaglandins, leaving vascular smooth muscle unopposed and susceptible to spasm. It has been documented in patients both with and without underlying atherosclerotic disease and sometimes presents as *variant angina* (rest pain, ST-segment elevation). Prevalence is about 3 percent in patients undergoing coronary angiography with ergonovine stimulation, but the true prevalence is estimated to be far greater. Spasm is suspected of playing a role in acute myocardial infarction, as well as triggering anginal episodes. Cigarette smoking and hyperlipidemia appear to interfere with normal endothelial activity. Precipitants include stress, cold, alpha-adrenergic stimulation in the setting of beta-blockade, abrupt nitrate withdrawal, ergonovine, cocaine use, and direct mechanical irritation from cardiac catheterization.

Aortic stenosis can lead to angina when hemodynamically significant valvular stenosis or calcific obstruction of a coronary ostia results in inadequate coronary perfusion (see Chapter 33).

Coronary microvascular dysfunction, characterized by inappropriately vasoconstrictive responses to autonomic and biochemical stimuli, can increase total resistance and reduce myocardial perfusion. The significance of these findings is still unclear, but they have been found with increased frequency among patients with the combination of atypical angina, an ischemic response to exercise stress testing, and a normal coronary angiogram. The terms *"microvascular angina"* and *"syndrome X"* have been applied to such persons. More study is needed, but the findings suggest a possible explanation for the ischemic chest pain of patients with *hypertrophic cardiomyopathy*. Diabetics with hyperinsulinism may also be at increased risk for microvascular disease.

There is a growing appreciation for the frequency and importance of *silent myocardial ischemia*, defined as objectively documented ischemia occurring in the absence of symptoms. On the basis of results from exercise stress testing and ambulatory monitoring, it is estimated that more than half of patients with chronic stable angina experience episodes of silent ischemia. Contrary to common belief, controlled studies find that the incidence in diabetics is no greater than in nondiabetics. Mechanism remains a subject of investigation, but it does not appear to be the result of less severe or less extensive ischemia.

Regardless of etiology, ischemic episodes are often triggered or aggravated by conditions that increase myocardial oxygen demand (eg, *hyperthyroidism*, *fever*) or decrease oxygen supply (eg, *severe anemia*, *respiratory insufficiency*). A *circadian susceptibility* to ischemic events has been identified, with the morning hours being the time of greatest risk. Mechanism(s) remain unknown, but the phenomenon can be blocked by beta-blockers or aspirin.

NATURAL HISTORY

Although the clinical course of some patients may extend over 15 to 20 years, most patients with chronic stable angina are at considerably increased risk of cardiovascular death. Among the factors strongly affecting prognosis are the *number* and *location* of *stenoses*. Combined angiographic data obtained prior to widespread use of bypass surgery reveal that patients with significant disease in one vessel have a mean annual mortality rate of 2.2 percent. This increases to a rate of 4.5 percent to 7.0 percent if the lesion involves the *left main* coronary artery. High-grade, proximal stenosis of the left anterior descending artery has a prognosis similar to that of left-main disease, and is sometimes referred to as a "left-main equivalent" lesion. With stenosis of two vessels, the mean annual mortality rate is 6.8 percent; the rate rises to 11.4 percent for *three-vessel disease*.

Prognosis also closely correlates with *severity of ischemia*, as measured by thallium images and electrocardiographic changes during exercise stress testing (see Chapter 36), regardless of whether the disease is symptomatic or silent. Other major independent determinants of increased risk are *left ventricular (LV) dysfunction* (see Chapter 32), ventricular ectopy (see Chapter 29), an intercurrent ischemic event within the last 6 months, and cigarette smoking. The onset of angina in a patient with hemodynamically significant aortic stenosis reduces mean survival to about 2 to 3 years (see Chapter 33).

Many *CHD risk factors* are powerful, independent determinants of prognosis. Smoking, hypertension, hypercholesterolemia, low HDL cholesterol, and age (>45 y in men, >55 y in women) are well documented prognostic determinants in patients with stable angina due to atherosclerotic coronary artery disease.

The natural history of *coronary artery spasm* is highly variable, reflecting the heterogeneity of patients with this condition. An important variable is the presence of underlying atherosclerotic disease. If spasm occurs in the absence of fixed stenoses, the prognosis is relatively good (eg, no mortality, 39% remission over 6 years). Some investigators even suggest that spasm may be a temporary condition; however, myocardial infarction, heart block, and malignant arrhythmias have been documented. The prognosis of patients with spasm in the setting of underlying coronary stenosis is a function of the coronary anatomy; patients with multivessel disease are at greatest risk. Whether risk is significantly enhanced by the presence of spasm is not yet known.

PRINCIPLES OF MANAGEMENT

The ultimate goals are to reduce the risks of infarction and death. In patients with CHD, identification and aggressive treatment of atherosclerotic risk factors—*hypertension* (see Chapter 26), *hypercholesterolemia* (see Chapter 27), *smoking* (see Chapter 54), and perhaps *diabetes* (see Chapter 102)—can reduce cardiovascular morbidity and mortality. The magnitude of risk reduction from such *secondary prevention* efforts can be impressive, exceeding that associated with primary prevention, though such efforts are often overlooked or mistakenly viewed as not productive. Beta-blockers and bypass surgery also provide effective secondary prevention in high-risk individuals, as does aspirin (see below).

The more immediate objectives are to control symptoms and enhance exercise capacity, which entail *improving blood supply* and *reducing oxygen demand*. Although drug therapy and interventional methods are the most heavily utilized treatment modalities (see below), attention also needs to be paid to conditions that increase oxygen demand and reduce oxygen availability. Among the former are heart failure (see Chapter 32), severe anemia (see Chapter 82), and hyperthyroidism (see Chapter 103). The latter include severe anemia (see Chapter 82), chronic obstructive pulmonary disease (see Chapter 47), and interstitial lung disease (see Chapter 46). An exercise program helps reduce peripheral oxygen demand (see Chapters 18 and 31). For patients with angina caused by hemodynamically significant aortic stenosis, *correction of the outflow tract obstruction* is indicated (see Chapter 33).

Only a program that addresses the full spectrum of issues affecting myocardial ischemia is likely to succeed. As important as medical and interventional therapies are, they must not be prescribed in a vacuum. On the other hand, their skillful use is essential to maximizing quality of life, if not survival.

Nitrates

Nitrates continue to be one of the cornerstones of therapy for angina, and for many patients with mild predictable episodes of angina, they are sufficient for control of symptoms. These agents are *smooth muscle relaxants* that cause vascular dilation, predominantly of the venous *capacitance vessels*, though they have a lesser effect on the arterial bed. Nitrates have no proven direct chronotropic or inotropic effects but are believed to decrease myocardial oxygen demand predominantly by *reducing left ventricular filling pressure* (preload) and *end-diastolic volume*. Nitrates also have a modest effect on systemic blood pressure (afterload). A *reflex tachycardia* results from the reduction in systemic blood pressure. There is some suggestion that regional myocardial perfusion may be improved by the ability of nitrates to *dilate epicardial coronary arteries*, but total coronary blood flow is not increased. Nitrates are moderately effective in lessening coronary vasospasm. *Tolerance* to nitrates can develop if dosing intervals are too short (see below). Nitrates and beta-adrenergic blocking agents have complementary effects on myocardial oxygen demand and are often used together (see below).

Sublingual Nitroglycerin (TNG) provides short-term (up to 30 min) relief of anginal pain and improvement in exercise tolerance when taken prophylactically. Advantages include low cost, rapid onset of action (30 sec to 3 min), safety, and proven efficacy for symptomatic relief. The drawback is its short duration of action. TNG must be taken sublingually because oral doses are denitrified and hepatically inactivated on the first pass through the portal circulation. Since the drug is volatile, it is best kept in a tightly capped amber vial, stored in a cool place. Once a bottle of TNG is opened, the contents remain maximally effective for up to 6 months. After that, it is best to assume the TNG has lost some of its potency and to prescribe a fresh bottle. Often, the patient using old TNG will notice less benefit and fewer of the usual side effects accompanying use of TNG (headache, burning under the tongue). Before concluding that a patient's failure to respond to TNG is due to disease progression or nitrate resistance (see below), it is important to be sure that "fresh" TNG is being used.

An *aerosolized TNG* spray preparation is available. Each spray from a metered-dose aerosol cannister delivers 0.4 mg of TNG to the surface of the tongue, from which it is absorbed transmucosally. Onset and duration of action and efficacy of a single dose are similar to those of a 0.4 mg sublingual TNG tablet. Each canister contains about 200 doses. Canister-stored TNG will retain efficacy for up to 3 years. Cost per dose is substantially greater than for TNG tablets, but prolonged shelf life helps to reduce total cost to the patient. The spray is a reasonable alternative in patients who wear dentures or have dry mucus membranes. Proper use requires holding the canister close to the tongue, directing the spray at the tongue, not inhaling the spray, and closing the mouth after each dose.

Isosorbide Dinitrate is the best studied of the oral nitrates, developed to provide more sustained nitrate activity and better *anginal prophylaxis*. Single oral doses of 20 to 40 mg significantly improve hemodynamic parameters and exercise tolerance, and the effect persists up to 4 hours. A sustained-release form of isosorbide with a 12-hour serum half-life is available but not recommended because of highly variable intestinal absorption and risk of nitrate tolerance (unless used only once daily—see below). Onset of action is 15 to 30 minutes; clinical duration of action, 4 to 8 hours. The optimal *dosage schedule* is two or three times a day, with an *eccentric pattern* (eg, early morning, mid-afternoon) to minimize risk of nitrate tolerance (see below). Such eccentric schedules appear to strike the best balance between avoidance of tolerance and control of angina.

Both *chewable* and *sublingual* isosorbide preparations are available and provide a more rapid onset of action (5–15 min), but duration of action falls to about 2 hours. It remains to be seen whether the faster-onset, shorter-acting forms of isosorbide are so much better than sublingual TNG as to warrant their added expense.

A once-a-day preparation, *isosorbide mononitrate,* offers no significant advantage over generic isosorbide dinitrate for control of chronic stable angina, except convenience. The mononitrate costs 10 times more per day than the generic dinitrate preparation. There is little development of nitrate tolerance with mononitrate (see below).

Nitroglycerin Ointment has been rediscovered as an effective method for providing long-acting anginal prophylaxis. Improved exercise tolerance and hemodynamic effects persist for up to 6 hours. Because the ointment can be messy and irritating to the skin if applied to the same area around-the-clock, it is best suited for nocturnal use.

Transdermal nitroglycerin patches The patch can deliver nitroglycerin for 24 hours in a convenient-to-use form. Serum nitrate levels approach the peak level obtained with sublingual nitroglycerin. Initial round-the-clock improvements in symptoms and exercise tolerance decline after 7 to 10 days of continuous patch use, because the sustained, high nitrate levels lead to *nitrate tolerance* (see below). Proper use requires a 10- to 12-hour period of *nitrate washout*, having the stable angina patient put the patch on in the morning and remove it in the evening. Continued use of the patch is reasonable in those patients who show definite clinical benefit. If there is none, then the patch should be discontinued. In patients who have been using patches for months to years, termination is best conducted in a tapering fashion to avoid precipitation of a nitrate withdrawal syndrome.

Nitrate Tolerance refers to the loss of hemodynamic benefit associated with continuous nitrate use over prolonged periods. It is believed linked to sulfhydryl depletion in vascular endothelial cells. Tolerance is both dose- and time-dependent. In the outpatient setting, nitrate tolerance is seen after 7 to 10 days of continuous 5 mg transdermal TNG patch use and with as little as 30 mg of isosorbide given four times daily. The common denominator is insufficient time for adequate nitrate washout. Onset can be as rapid as 12 to 24 hours with use of intravenous TNG. Tolerance develops to both the peripheral and coronary vasodilator effects of nitrates. Prevention of tolerance appears to require a regimen that provides for rapid increases and decreases in nitrate levels over the course of the day as well as a daily nitrate-free period. A daily period of 10 to 12 hours off nitrate therapy is recommended to minimize the risk of nitrate tolerance. Patients who do not attain sufficient anginal prophylaxis with such a schedule will need the addition of a second agent (see below).

Initiation of Nitrate Therapy. Determining the *proper dose* of a long-acting nitrate is achieved by monitoring the effect of the agent on heart rate, blood pressure, and exercise tolerance. Long-acting nitrate therapy should be introduced gradually; starting with too large a dose produces severe vascular headaches that force many patients to stop their medication. Beginning with a low-dose program (eg, 5 mg of isosorbide tid) and advancing it slowly over 1 to 2 weeks, one can achieve substantial nitrate doses without significant headache. Patients with migraine headaches may be very intolerant of nitrates; combining nitrate therapy with a beta-blocking agent can often overcome this difficulty, especially if the beta-blocker is started first.

Dosage is increased until 1) customary activity can be undertaken without pain; 2) the heart rate at rest rises by 10 to 15 beats per minute; or 3) the blood pressure falls to the point of causing postural light-headedness. The development of headache is not a reliable therapeutic end point, because this side effect usually disappears with continuation of therapy.

There is little question as to the efficacy of nitrates for relief of anginal pain and improvement in exercise tolerance in patients with stable coronary artery disease. In addition, nitrates remain the drug of first choice in patients with variant angina due to coronary vasospasm. However, the effect of nitrates on prognosis remains unknown. Most studies of survival involve multiple-drug regimens combining nitrates with beta-blocking agents; such studies do document improved survival in postinfarction patients.

Beta-Adrenergic Blocking Agents

Beta-blockers decrease myocardial oxygen consumption by *reducing contractility*, *blood pressure*, and *heart rate*. As such, they are particularly beneficial for treatment of exertional angina. The reduction in heart rate also allows more time for myocardial perfusion, which occurs during diastole. Beta-blockers have demonstrated efficacy in prophylaxis of angina, improvement in exercise tolerance, and *prolongation of survival* in patients surviving myocardial infarction—45 percent reduction in sudden death reported. Comparable trials in anginal patients without prior infarction are yet to be reported.

Beta-blockers can be categorized according to their relative cardioselectivity, lipid solubility, and intrinsic agonist activity (Table 30–1). *Cardioselectivity* refers to the degree of preferential affinity for $beta_1$-receptors, which predominate in the heart and are the principal target of anti-anginal therapy. At low to intermediate doses, cardioselectivity is demonstrated by atenolol, metoprolol, and acebutolol, but this effect fades as doses increase. Beta-blockers that lack cardioselectivity are more likely at low doses to cause side effects associated with $beta_2$-blockade (bronchospasm, peripheral vasoconstriction, and inhibition of glycogenolysis—see below).

Lipid solubility affects absorption, metabolism, serum half-life, and degree to which an agent crosses the blood–brain barrier. The more lipid-soluble an agent is, the more rapid its absorption, the shorter its half-life, and the more likely its entry into the central nervous system (CNS). Lipid-soluble preparations are, for the most part, hepatically metabolized. The most lipid-soluble beta-blocker is propranolol, followed by metoprolol, and then pindolol; the least lipid-soluble include atenolol and nadolol.

Agonist activity is an intrinsic characteristic of pindolol and acebutolol. At low doses, these drugs show some sympatholytic action and tend to cause less reduction in heart rate, contractility, and conduction than other beta-blockers. As doses increase, these effects are overpowered by their beta-blocking activity.

Adverse effects include the potential to induce *heart failure* in patients with preexisting left ventricular dysfunction. Preparations with some intrinsic beta-agonist activity may

Table 30-1. The Beta-blocking Agents

DRUG	HALF-LIFE (H)	LIPID SOLUBILITY	CARDIOSELECTIVITY	AGONIST ACTIVITY
Propranolol*	Up to 6	High	No	No
Metoprolol*	Up to 6	Moderate	Yes	No
Atenolol	Up to 24	Low	Yes	No
Nadolol	Up to 24	Low	No	No
Timolol	Up to 24	Low	No	No
Pindolol	Up to 12	Low	No	Yes
Acebutolol	Up to 12	Low	Yes	Yes
Labetalol	Up to 12	Low to moderate	No	No

*A sustained-release form of the drug is available.

be better tolerated. Not all patients worsen, but careful monitoring is essential. Use with other negatively inotropic drugs (eg, verapamil, disopyramide) should be avoided in patients with heart failure.

Other potentially adverse cardiac effects include slowing the SA node and AV conduction, leading to symptomatic *bradycardia* and *heart block*, especially in patients with underlying conduction system disease. Sinus arrest may ensue in such patients. A preparation with some intrinsic beta-agonist activity may be preferred if a beta-blocker is to be used in the setting of underlying conduction system disease. Close monitoring is critical to safe use.

By blocking beta$_2$-receptors, nonselective beta-blockers (and all preparations when used in full doses) may trigger bronchospasm, peripheral vasoconstriction, or inhibition of glycogenolysis. *Bronchospasm* is the most serious of these and may occur in any patient with a history of bronchospastic disease, even if asymptomatic at the time of initiating therapy. Many regard beta-blockers as relatively contraindicated in such persons. If used, a cardioselective preparation is preferred (eg, atenolol, metoprolol). There is a slight theoretical advantage to a selective preparation with some mild beta-agonist activity (eg, acebutolol) to help maintain bronchodilation.

Beta-blockers will blunt the *adrenergic response to hypoglycemia* and thus must be used with care in diabetics taking insulin. However, use of insulin is not an absolute contraindication to beta-blocker therapy (see Chapter 102).

Mild (5–10%) reductions in *HDL cholesterol* have been noted with use of some beta-blockers (eg, atenolol, nadolol, propranolol). The effect on HDL is variable. Those agents possessing intrinsic sympathomimetic activity have little or no influence on HDL. The effect on HDL has been invoked to explain the less-than-expected protection against fatal and non-fatal myocardial infarction observed when beta-blockers are used for treatment of hypertension. There are no data to support the HDL hypothesis, and beta-blockers remain a cornerstone of antihypertensive therapy in patients with coronary disease (see Chapter 26).

The CNS effects of beta-blockers are of considerable concern and often a cause for discontinuation of therapy. Anecdotal reports of *cognitive problems*, *depression*, *sexual dysfunction*, *altered sleep*, *nightmares*, and *fatigue* appeared soon after propranolol became widely available. Their frequency is particularly high in the elderly. Some suggest that the incidence of CNS side effects could be substantially reduced by use of lipid-insoluble preparations (eg, atenolol, nadolol, timolol), though the relative advantage of using lipid-insoluble beta-blockers remains a subject of contention.

The issue of an increased *risk of depression* with beta-blocker use also remains unresolved, pending data from prospective, randomized, placebo-controlled trials. In one of the few well-designed studies—comparing atenolol to nifedipine in elderly hypertensive patients—atenolol was found to impair neither cognition nor mood. Pending further data, it appears that depression or other forms of CNS dysfunction are not an absolute contraindication to beta-blocker therapy. Use of a lipid-insoluble preparation is probably preferable in such patients, provided there is careful monitoring of mood, sleep pattern, and sexual and cognitive functioning.

Although *coronary vasospasm* is a theoretical concern with use of beta-blocker therapy, it is rarely a problem clinically. Beta-blockers have proven useful in patients with variant angina but are usually used only in conjunction with agents that have coronary vasodilating capacity, such as the nitrates or calcium channel blockers. Their benefit is thought perhaps related to a decrease in platelet aggregation, oxygen demand, and other factors contributing to vasospasm or angina.

Peripheral vasoconstriction can occur with beta-blocker therapy, particularly in patients who suffer from vasospastic Raynaud's disease. However, as long as a low-dose, cardioselective program is used, the Raynaud's patient can usually tolerate beta-blocker treatment. Similarly, patients with peripheral atherosclerotic arterial disease rarely suffer a compromise in limb perfusion when taking a beta-blocker (see Chapter 34).

Abrupt withdrawal of beta-blockade can precipitate an exacerbation of angina, acute coronary insufficiency, or even infarction. Onset is characteristically within 2 to 6 days after abrupt cessation of therapy. Concern about withdrawal is particularly common in anginal patients who are about to undergo surgery and are likely to have most of their medications discontinued preoperatively. About 10 percent of stable anginal patients experience a serious rebound in symptoms when beta-blockade is suddenly terminated. Infarction and death may occur. Those at greatest risk are patients on large doses who have achieved much benefit from beta-blockade. It has been hypothesized that an "up-regulation" of beta-adrenergic receptors results from long-term blockade and makes these patients more sensitive to unopposed beta-adrenergic stimulation. Withholding beta-blockers for up to 48 hours can be done without risking any increase in angina. Patients who experience an exacerbation usually do so 2 to 6 days after abrupt discontinuation of therapy. Tapering therapy over the course of 1 to 2 weeks can minimize a precipitous reaction to withdrawal.

Individual Preparations. *Propranolol* is the prototype beta-blocker. Although usually well tolerated, its disadvantages include relatively little cardioselectivity, short serum half-life (4–6 h), and high lipid solubility that permits CNS penetration. A sustained-release preparation is now available, making for more convenient use. Available generically, it is among the least expensive of beta-blockers, especially in its basic generic form.

Metoprolol differs from propranolol in that it is relatively cardioselective at low to moderate doses and less likely to induce bronchospasm, making it useful in patients who also suffer from chronic obstructive pulmonary disease. *Atenolol* is also cardioselective, but it has the additional advantages of a longer half-life (up to 24 h), allowing once-daily administration, and low lipid solubility that limits CNS penetration. The cost has dropped considerably now that it is available generically. These features make it a particularly attractive choice.

Nadolol also has a long half-life and low lipid solubility; however, it is not cardioselective. *Timolol* is a more potent beta-blocker with a very narrow therapeutic range. It can be administered on a twice-daily basis and does not penetrate the CNS readily.

Pindolol and *acetebulol* possess some intrinsic sympathomimetic activity and, at low doses, produce less depression of contractility, conduction, and sinus node function than other beta-blockers. Acetebulol has the advantages over pindolol of being relatively cardioselective and less lipid-soluble. These agents are worth consideration in patients who might not otherwise tolerate beta-blockade due to marginal left ventricular function, bradycardia, or heart block. Their intrinsic beta-agonist activity makes them theoretically attractive for use in patients with coronary vasospasm. However, as noted earlier, variant angina does not appear to be a contraindication to use of beta-blockers, including those lacking beta-agonist activity.

Labetalol differs from other drugs in this class by having an additional alpha-blocking effect. This quality is sometimes useful in treatment of hypertension (see Chapter 26) but offers little advantage in the treatment of chronic stable angina. Adverse effects include greater degrees of postural hypotension and sexual dysfunction than seen with most other beta-blockers.

Selection. Proper choice requires consideration of the patient's overall clinical state, with special attention to any left ventricular dysfunction, conduction system disease, or bronchospasm. Those with *obstructive airway disease* should receive beta-blocker therapy cautiously, if at all, using a cardioselective preparation (eg, *atenolol* or *metoprolol*). Those with *left ventricular dysfunction*, conduction system disease, or sinus node problems might best tolerate a beta-blocker with some intrinsic adrenergic activity (eg, *pindolol* or *acebutolol*). If fatigue or mild depression is present, a beta-blocker with minimal CNS penetration (eg, atenolol or timolol) is worth consideration.

Compliance is facilitated by agents that can be administered on a once-daily or twice-daily basis (eg, atenolol, sustained-release preparations of propranolol and metoprolol, timolol). Sustained-release preparations appear as effective for control of angina as standard formulations that must be given several times a day.

Cost is an important consideration and can be critical to compliance. Generic formulations of propranolol and atenolol are available. Although propranolol lacks some theoretically advantageous properties, many patients take it without difficulty and need not be switched to one of the newer (and usually more expensive) agents. Generic atenolol represents an especially appealing value, since the agent has such an excellent drug profile and is now available at markedly reduced cost.

Initiation of beta-blocker therapy requires titration of dose against the *resting* and *exercise heart rates*. Lowering the resting heart rate to about 60 beats/min is usually considered evidence of sufficient beta-blockade, but may not be a relaible indicator in elderly patients. A subset of patients do not achieve adequate control of their angina at this level of beta-blockade. Further increases in dosage (and a slower resting heart rate) may be necessary to prevent chest pain. Such bradycardia is often well tolerated hemodynamically. Typical target heart rates are 50 to 60 beats per minute at rest, with an increase to 70 to 80 with moderate exercise and to no more than 100 with vigorous exercise. The true measures of adequate therapy remain the suppression of angina and improvement of exercise tolerance.

Calcium Channel Blockers

These agents inhibit calcium transport via the "slow" calcium channel of the cellular membrane in myocardial, vascular, and other smooth muscle tissues. The net effects range from coronary and systemic vasodilation to decreases in myocardial contractility and conductivity. Coronary vasodilation improves perfusion in those few patients prone to spasm. In the vast majority of stable anginal patients, benefit derives from a reduction in myocardial oxygen demand brought about by reductions in contractility and systemic blood pressure (afterload).

The first generation of calcium channel blockers include nifedipine, diltiazem, and verapamil. They represent a spectrum of activity (see below). Improvements in rates of infarction and cardiac death have yet to be demonstrated, though studies are pending in patients with stable angina. Patients with preserved LV function appear to do best (see below).

Nifedipine is the most active vasodilator of the calcium channel blockers. Its main effect is arterial. Both coronary and peripheral arterial dilatation are produced, making this agent useful for patients with coronary vasospasm and hypertension (see Chapter 26). Although nifedipine is negatively inotropic, its net effect on left ventricular function is minimal because the drug induces a strong beta-adrenergic reflex response to its arterial vasodilation. In some patients, a *reflex tachycardia* occurs. Its potent vasodilating effects produce a higher incidence of *flushing*, *hypotension*, *dizziness*, *leg edema*, and *headache* than occurs with other drugs in its class. Also, unlike the others, nifedipine has no clinically significant suppressant effect on the SA or AV nodes, making it safe for use in patients with underlying conduction system disease. Nifedipine has been shown to be effective in treatment of chronic stable angina, unstable angina, and variant angina.

Verapamil is the calcium channel blocker with the most pronounced net effects on myocardial contractility and conduction. Even though it effectively reduces afterload, it can precipitate *heart failure* in patients with underlying LV dysfunction and cause *heart block* in patients with conduction system disease. This potent effect on conduction tissue has made it extremely useful for treatment of supraventricular tachycardias (see Chapter 28). *Constipation* and *leg edema* are consequences of its dilating effect on gastrointestinal and venous smooth muscle.

Diltiazem is the best tolerated of the calcium channel blockers. Although it more closely resembles verapamil than nifedipine, its pharmacologic profile is unique. Compared to verapamil, it causes greater slowing of the SA node but has less influence on the AV junction, contractility, and vascular tone. In studies of its effects on mortality and reinfarction in post-myocardial infarction patients, there was no overall improvement in either mortality or reinfarction, but patients with normal LV function showed reductions in rates, while those with LV dysfunction showed rate increases, suggesting that benefit is limited to those with preserved LV function. Survival and infarction data in anginal patients who have never infarcted are awaited.

Second-Generation Dihydropyridines. These agents are marketed predominantly as antihypertensive agents and promoted for their "vascular selectivity." Some are already approved and others likely to be approved in the future for use in angina. Nifedipine was the first dihydropyridine, now followed by *nicardipine, isradipine*, and *felodipine*. Like nifedipine, they all induce arterial dilation and an initial reflex tachycardia but do not affect AV conduction or SA node activity. They are less negatively inotropic than earlier calcium channel blockers, but their safety for use in patients with LV dysfunction remains to be fully defined. These qualities appear to make them good candidates for combined use with a beta-blocker. Side effects are similar to those of nifedipine (flushing, peripheral edema, headache, light-headedness). Comparative studies of these agents and their roles in anginal therapy are awaited. Emerging data suggest felodipine may even be beneficial in patients with heart failure.

Choice of Calcium Channel Blocker for use in chronic stable angina depends to a large extent on the state of the patient's myocardium and conduction system (Table 30–2). Patients with sinus node dysfunction should not be started on diltiazem due to the risk of bradyarrhythmias; verapamil is relatively contraindicated in the presence of heart failure or conduction system disease. Nifedipine and the second generation drugs are the preferred calcium channel blockers in situations where cardiac side effects would not be well tolerated, although these agents are less effective against angina relative to the other calcium channel blockers. Moreover, their marked effects on noncardiac smooth muscle result in the highest incidence among calcium channel blockers of extracardiac side effects such as peripheral edema, flushing, and postural hypotension. All drugs in this class should be used with caution in patients with marked LV dysfunction (ejection fraction <40 percent), because many have a direct suppressant effect on the myocardium, an effect that might be enhanced by simultaneous use of beta-blocker therapy.

Designing the Medical Regimen

Pending more data on the morbidity and mortality associated with use of particular anti-anginal agents, design of the starting medical regimen remains an attempt to match drug action with the patient's underlying pathophysiology and clinical state. Subsequent adjustments and additions to the medical regimen are made empirically, based on symptomatic response to therapy (ie, frequency and severity of anginal episodes) and severity of side effects. As more long-term outcomes data become available, they can be incorporated into the decision making process. Studies to date (eg, those of beta-blockers) have concentrated on post-infarction patients. More data are needed on patients with stable angina and no history of infarction.

Single-Drug Regimens for Initial Therapy. Traditionally, *nitrates* are the agents of first choice, based on safety, modest cost, and efficacy in controlling symptoms. They are a reasonable choice for patients who have demonstrated a good response to nitroglycerin, whether for exertional or rest pain. A *beta-blocker* provides excellent control for patients with exertional chest pain and would be especially advantageous in patients who have a coexisting condition that would also benefit from beta-blockade (eg, hypertension or migraine). Moreover, they improve survival, at least in post-infarction patients. *Calcium channel blockers* can bring symptomatic relief to patients with stable angina, and especially to those with coronary vasospasm. For patients with spasm-induced variant angina, starting with nitrates or a calcium channel blocker is reasonable. In studies comparing isosorbide to nifedipine, control of variant angina was equivalent for both agents. The efficacy of the other calcium channel blockers relative to nitrates in patients with spasm remains to be determined. *Diltiazem* has a very low incidence of side effects and might be considered for single drug therapy if nitrates were poorly tolerated or failed to control symptoms.

Two-Drug Regimens. Patients with chronic stable angina who are not well controlled or who cannot tolerate full doses of single-agent therapy are candidates for consideration of a two-drug regimen. However, adding a second agent should not be done casually or before trying maximally tolerated doses of a single drug. Although drug actions can be complementary, adverse effects may also be additive and poorly tolerated, especially in the setting of poor LV function.

In patients inadequately controlled on *long-acting nitrates* alone, the addition of a *beta-blocker* is a reasonable next step. Their effects are complementary. The beta-blocker will slow any reflex tachycardia induced by nitrates, helping to reduce oxygen demand. Nitrates can help decrease preload and minimize any increase in left ventricular end-diastolic volume that may ensue from the negative inotropic effects of beta-blockade. In the treatment of angina, nitrates and beta-blockers are often used together.

Another two-drug strategy involves combining a *calcium channel blocker* with a *beta-blocker*. In theory, their effects

Table 30-2. Properties of Calcium-Channel Blockers

DRUG	CORONARY DILATION	PERIPHERAL ART. DIL.	AV NODE DEPRESSION	SA NODE DEPRESSION	NET EFFECT ON LV
nifedipine	+ +	+ + +	0	0	+/−
diltiazem	+	+ +	+	+ +	−
verapamil	+	+	+ +	+	− −
nicardipine	+ +	+ + +	0	0	0
felodipine	+ +	+ + +	0	0	0

on reducing myocardial oxygen demand should be additive. In clinical practice and in clinical studies, the results are more equivocal. Patients not adequately controlled by maximal doses of beta-blockers or calcium channel blockers alone usually show some improvement in exercise tolerance and frequency of angina with a two-drug strategy. Patients adequately controlled on monotherapy with either a beta-blocker or a calcium channel blocker typically do not achieve significant additional benefit from the addition of a second agent.

The problem with a beta-blocker/calcium channel blocker program is its additive and potent *suppression of LV function* and *AV conduction*. Not only are beta-blockers negatively inotropic, but so are the calcium channel blockers, including nifedipine (when sympathetic reflexes are blocked). Patients most in need of combined therapy for control of angina often have the most severe heart disease, with significant LV dysfunction (ejection fraction <0.40). In addition, poorly controlled patients may also have coexisting conduction system disease, which is apt to be made worse by a combination regimen, raising the risks of heart block, hypotension, and symptomatic bradyarrhythmias. Patients with conduction system disease who are free of LV dysfunction may tolerate the combination of a beta-blocker plus nifedipine (whose effects on conduction are minimal). LV function should still be closely monitored.

Patients who are poor candidates for the beta-blocker component of combination therapy (eg, bronchospastic disease, heart failure, severe conduction system disease) may benefit from a cautious trial of substituting a *calcium channel blocker*, especially one that slows the SA node and counters reflex tachycardia (eg, diltiazem). Such a program may be particularly effective in patients with stubborn vasospastic disease, but it must be undertaken with care because of the potential for hypotension and worsening angina.

Further studies are needed to better define optimal approaches to combination therapy and the role, if any, of the newer dihydropyridine-type calcium channel blockers. For now, careful individual tailoring of the two-drug anti-anginal regimen is essential.

Three-drug Regimens utilizing a *calcium channel blocker* in conjunction with a *beta-blocker* and *long-acting nitrates* are commonly prescribed for treatment of patients with severe chronic stable angina refractory to two-drug regimens. Adding a calcium channel blocker to long-acting nitrates and beta-blockade is the usual sequence and is typically justified on the grounds of suspected vasospasm or a need to decrease doses of the other agents due to bothersome side effects. Though these ideas are appealing and the practice common, there are no controlled data to support them.

Cautions. Combined use of a beta-blocker and a calcium channel blocker requires reduced doses of both agents due to the risks of adversely affecting contractility, chronotropy, conduction, and blood pressure. Concurrent use of potent arterial vasodilators (eg, captopril, prazosin, hydralazine) and agents with central alpha-adrenergic blocking effects (eg, clonidine, methyldopa) is also to be avoided due to the risk of serious hypotension. Care is also required when combination therapy is used in conjunction with digoxin therapy, because of potential for further suppression of conduction through the AV node.

Antiplatelet Therapy

With increasing appreciation for the roles of thrombosis and vascular reactivity in coronary artery disease, the question of inhibiting platelet function arises. Aspirin, dipyridamole, and sulfinpyrazone have been examined. Most studies have failed to demonstrate any statistically significant improvement in survival, with the exception of *aspirin* in patients with *unstable angina*. In patients with *stable angina*, the risk of infarction can be lowered by aspirin use. In a segment of The Physician's Health Study—a long-term, randomized, placebo-controlled primary prevention trial of low-dose aspirin (325 mg qod) in male physicians—participants with chronic stable angina demonstrated an 87 percent reduction in risk of myocardial infarction and a trend toward a reduction in risk of death from infarction; however, there was also a trend toward an increase in risk of stroke. Aspirin therapy did not prevent the onset of angina. More data on survival and stroke risk are needed before aspirin can be recommended for routine use in patients with chronic stable angina.

Invasive Therapy

The principal modalities of invasive therapy are *percutaneous transluminal angioplasty (PTCA)* and *coronary artery bypass graft (CABG)* surgery. Both procedures have become among the most commonly performed invasive therapies in the nation, with over 500,000 performed annually. Considerable debate has surrounded the indications for their use, because widespread performance prior to careful study has been the rule rather than the exception. The indications for CABG have become clearer with completion of major multicenter studies of survival, but some of the indications for PTCA are still contested, and the field remains in evolution. *Directional atherectomy* has enjoyed recent popularity, but randomized controlled studies find no evidence for benefit, but do note high rates of complications and increased costs.

Angioplasty. PTCA involves passing a balloon catheter into a stenosed vessel and inflating the balloon at the site of the narrowing to widen the lumen. It requires coronary angiography and surgical standby, given the risk of sudden vessel occlusion from manipulation. A *high-grade proximal stenosis* (>70%) that is smooth, concentric, less than 0.5 cm in length, and noncalcified is considered the lesion most amenable to PTCA treatment. The immediate success rate for PTCA in patients with favorable lesions is in excess of 85 percent. The risk of restenosis is 25 percent to 40 percent and greatest within the first 6 months of the procedure. After that, the reappearance of angina often represents progression of another lesion that was not dilated rather than late restenosis.

PTCA has been used predominantly as an *alternative to surgery* in symptomatic patients with *single-vessel disease* who *fail* to achieve relief with *medical therapy*. In addition, angioplasty has been studied as an *alternative to medical therapy* in stable anginal patients with single-vessel disease. In the multicenter, prospective, randomized Angioplasty Compared to Medicine (ACME) study, patients receiving PTCA demonstrated better symptomatic relief and exercise tolerance at 6 months of follow-up than those treated medically, but also greater risk of acute myocardial infarction. Selected patients with amenable two-vessel disease are also being studied, but preliminary data suggest no benefit over medical therapy.

There are a number of settings in which PTCA does not appear successful. As with bypass surgery, high rates of restenosis have occurred in patients with variant angina. Invasive therapy is not useful in patients with coronary vasospasm. In patients with left-main or three-vessel disease, the risk of PTCA is greater than that of CABG, which remains the treatment of choice in patients who can undergo surgery (see below).

For treatment of limited coronary disease, PTCA may eventually prove a reasonable alternative to other forms of medical and surgical therapy in properly selected patients, but more data are needed. As noted above, the high rates of restenosis make repeat PTCA procedures likely; this needs to be factored into the calculation of the relative costs and benefits of CABG versus PTCA. The long-term safety, efficacy, and cost-effectiveness of PTCA in comparison to medical therapy and bypass surgery remain to be defined.

PTCA is worth considering in patients with high-grade, proximal, single-vessel disease who remain disablingly symptomatic despite full medical therapy. For patients with preserved LV function who respond well to medical therapy and demonstrate good exercise tolerance, medical therapy is currently preferred, given the excellent prognosis. The literature should be followed closely, as there will be much data forthcoming. Sorely needed are prospective, randomized, controlled studies of cardiovascular morbidity and mortality comparing PTCA with CABG and medical therapy, similar to those done for bypass surgery. The hope that PTCA will prove a cost-effective alternative to surgery and superior to medical therapy for improving symptoms, preventing infarction, and lowering mortality remains to be demonstrated.

Bypass Surgery. Surgery clearly improves symptoms and functional status in patients who fail medical therapy. The pattern emerging from prospective, randomized, clinical trials of surgery versus medical therapy is that greatest benefit from surgery accrues to those with the worst prognosis.

The group at greatest risk are those with critical stenosis of the *left main coronary artery*. In the Veterans Administration (VA) study of bypass surgery in patients with stable angina, those with left-main disease randomized to surgery experienced a dramatic improvement in survival (average annual mortality fell to 3%). Also benefiting in the VA study were those with angiographic and clinical features of high risk (*three-vessel disease, LV dysfunction, resting ST depression, history of myocardial infarction or hypertension*). Only patients with combined high angiographic and clinical risks demonstrated improved survival from surgical therapy over the entire follow-up period, which now extends well over a decade. Patients in categories of lower risk did not benefit as much from surgery. Those having high risk in only one category (eg, three-vessel disease and impaired LV function but no clinical risk factors), experienced lesser benefit. Patients with normal LV function, low angiographic risk, and low clinical risk tended to do better throughout follow-up if treated medically, although their advantage was not statistically significant, except among patients with two-vessel disease.

The question of surgical efficacy in less seriously ill patients with chronic stable angina was addressed in the *Coronary Artery Surgery Study (CASS)*. It included patients with less serious illness (no left-main disease or severe angina); however, only high-risk patients—those with three-vessel disease and LV dysfunction—showed a statistically significant improvement in rates of infarction and cardiac death. Such findings also pertained to patients older than 65 years of age.

A third major bypass surgery study, the *European Coronary Artery Surgery Study*, confirmed improved survival with surgery in patients with left-main disease and also demonstrated survival benefit in those with three-vessel disease who had *preserved LV function* and in those with *two-vessel disease* who had a high-grade proximal stenosis of the left anterior descending coronary artery (*"left-main equivalent"* anatomy).

In sum, bypass surgery is superior to medical therapy for prevention of infarction and prolongation of survival in stable anginal patients at greatest risk, that is, those with left-main or three-vessel disease, especially if there is concurrent LV dysfunction. In patients at less risk, comparable results can be achieved with medical therapy. *Late graft occlusion* has reduced some of the apparent advantages of surgical therapy that were noted enthusiastically in earlier reports. Use of the left internal mammary artery for grafting reduces the rate of late graft occlusion to 15 percent at 10 years. Risk-factor modification remains important, even after bypass surgery.

Hundreds of thousands of patients currently undergo bypass surgery each year in hope of achieving prolonged survival. While surgery is clearly useful as a means of providing symptomatic relief to patients with incapacitating angina inadequately controlled by a full trial of medical therapy, there is little evidence it enhances survival, except in those with left-main or severe three-vessel coronary disease. Long-term follow-up reports from the VA, CASS, and European studies should continue to illuminate this issue.

Surgery for Patients with Coronary Spasm. Most studies of surgical therapy for patients with coronary spasm show disappointing results, with surgical groups experiencing significantly higher rates of mortality and nonfatal infarction. Surgical therapy should be considered only when medical therapy has failed and spasm has been documented in or about an area of fixed, critical stenosis and not in other vessels or distally.

Selecting Candidates for Surgery. Patients with *more than 50 percent stenosis* of the *left main coronary artery* and those with *severe three-vessel disease* (especially if accompanied by LV dysfunction) are the prime candidates for bypass surgery and need to be identified. They represent nearly 10 percent of patients with coronary artery disease. Although there is no simple pattern of symptoms, signs, or resting electrocardiographic changes that reliably identifies such patients, clusters of such clinical findings appear predictive and are the subject of ongoing study. Scoring systems and decision rules have been devised. Should they be validated, they could prove useful to identifying candidates for invasive testing. For now, *exercise stress testing* remains the best noninvasive means of identifying patients who should be considered for invasive evaluation by angiography (see Chapter 36).

Treatment of Risk Factors and Precipitants

Epidemiologic studies have documented a reduction of as much as 40 percent in age-adjusted deaths from cardiovascular disease over the past 3 decades. Data from the Framingham Study suggest that over half of the improvement is attributable to improved control of atherosclerotic risk factors and the remainder to improvements in treatment of coronary disease. Such data emphasize the importance of attending to cardiovascular risk factors in the design of a management program for the patient with angina.

Treatment of CHD Risk Factors. *Smoking* is not only a CHD risk factor but also a major aggravating factor for angina. The absorbed nicotine increases blood pressure and heart rate, thus increasing myocardial oxygen demand. Nicotine may also cause vasospasm, and the rise in carboxyhemoglobin from smoke inhalation cuts down on oxygen delivery. Even passive smoking (from being in a smoke-filled room) can reduce exercise tolerance in patients with stable angina. Cessation of smoking can be psychologically stressful and physically uncomfortable, but the immediate and long-term benefits greatly outweigh the short-term discomfort. The development of symptomatic coronary disease may provide a potent stimulus to smoking cessation; the effort often succeeds when the physician takes a strong interest in achieving it (see Chapter 54).

Treatment of *hypercholesterolemia* can reduce coronary risk. Adherence to a low–saturated fat, low-cholesterol diet should be an essential part of the medical program for all patients with coronary disease. A reduction in low-density lipoprotein (LDL) cholesterol is associated with a reduction in coronary risk (see Chapter 15). Aggressive treatment of hypercholesterolemia is indicated in patients at greatest CHD risk (which includes those with symptomatic CHD—see Chapter 27). Not only can there be a halt to disease progression, but modest degrees of plaque regression are achievable, and coronary morbidity and mortality may be reduced.

Hypertension is a potent CHD risk factor and must be controlled. It also contributes to myocardial oxygen demand by raising afterload. As noted above, a number of antihypertensive agents are effective for treatment of angina (eg, beta-blockers, calcium channel blockers—see Chapter 26).

Precipitants and Aggravating Factors of angina also require attention. As noted earlier, correction, where possible, of factors increasing myocardial oxygen demand is essential to a successful outcome. In addition to cigarette smoke and elevated blood pressure, severe *anemia* (see Chapter 82), *hyperthyroidism* (see Chapter 103), *heart failure* (see Chapter 32), and *hypoxemia* (see Chapters 46 and 47) are all capable of worsening both symptomatic and silent myocardial ischemia in the context of underlying coronary disease.

The contribution from *psychological stress* has become increasingly evident. Although the relation between acute stress and anginal episodes is widely recognized, only recently has it been appreciated how common stress-induced ischemia is in patients with coronary artery disease. Episodes of silent ischemia as well as symptomatic ischemia have been documented in stressful situations. Public speaking and difficult mental tasks can induce as much symptomatic and silent ischemia as exercise in patients with coronary artery disease. High levels of life stress and social isolation are independent predictors of death from coronary disease. The role of personality style, such as so-called Type A behavior, remains a subject of debate, though the evidence from studies of mental stress suggests that coronary patients who have a low tolerance for frustrating circumstances might be expected have an increased likelihood of ischemic stress responses.

Addressing the psychosocial stresses that the anginal patient encounters is critical. An adequate evaluation includes a thorough psychosocial history with emphasis on those factors contributing to stress and social isolation. Urging the hard-driving, impatient person to change his personality style is counterproductive, but counseling him on means of coping with frustration and introducing him to simple *relaxation techniques* (see Appendix of Chapter 226) may be better appreciated.

If acute anxiety or situational stress is known to predictably precipitate severe chest pain or significant silent ischemia, occasional prophylactic use of a *minor tranquilizer* may be warranted. However, frequent benzodiazepine use is strongly discouraged because it can lead to tolerance and even addiction (see Chapter 226); furthermore, tranquilizer use is no substitute for an adequate medical regimen. *Beta-blocker* therapy can be quite effective in limiting the adverse cardiac effects of anxiety by blocking the attendant adrenergic discharge.

Obesity increases myocardial work and lowers high-density lipoprotein (HDL) cholesterol, raising CHD risk. A weight reduction program is indicated in the patient who is more than 20 percent overweight. A low-saturated fat, low-cholesterol diet is a good starting place, supplemented by exercise (see Chapter 233).

Neither *coffee* nor *caffeine* consumption has been shown to increase the risk of coronary disease, though an oft-quoted epidemiologic study found a minor trend toward increased risk in patients consuming more than four cups of decaffeinated coffee per day. Modest *alcohol* consumption is of no harm. Consuming more than 2 oz/d is associated with an increase in blood pressure, which increases cardiovascular risk.

Exercise can significantly improve functional status, and exercise training may prolong survival, though the issue remains unresolved. Exercise can increase exercise capacity in patients with chronic stable angina by improving skeletal muscle efficiency, decreasing heart rate and blood pressure, and improving psychological well-being (see Chapters 18 and 31).

Patient Education

Patient education is pivotal, both to ensure proper compliance with what can be a rather complex medical regimen and to maximize functional status. An understanding of the rationale behind the medical regimen will facilitate its effective use. Counseling about prognosis and allowable activity can prevent unnecessary restriction of activity, relieve fear, and improve lifestyle. Of particular concern to many patients is the safety of engaging in *sexual intercourse*. The issue should be addressed openly and directly, even if the patient does not take the initiative to raise the subject. Failure to do so can lead to marital problems, depression, and a worsening of symptoms. Guidelines for engaging in sexual activity are similar to those for any other form of physical exertion. The oxygen demands of intercourse among married, middle-aged partners are about the same as those for climbing a flight of stairs. If intercourse takes place among unaccustomed partners, the physical and emotional stress may be considerably greater and the oxygen requirements increased substantially. If a patient has serious concerns as to how much activity he can safely tolerate, an exercise test may be of value for reassurance, especially if he is needlessly limiting himself.

Indications for Admission and Referral

Admission is required when the anginal pattern is increasing in frequency or severity or is becoming harder to control. Episodes that are starting to last more than 15 minutes and beginning to occur at rest as well as with exertion suggest progression to *unstable angina*, with its attendant increase in risk of acute infarction. Hospitalization may also be of benefit to judge the adequacy of a medical regimen and to check on compliance when a patient with stable angina reports insufficient relief of symptoms. Referral to a cardiologist for consideration of coronary angiography and angioplasty is indicated when maximum medical therapy has failed to control symptoms and when left-main or severe three-vessel disease is suspected. The same is true if tight aortic stenosis is a consideration (see Chapter 33).

Therapeutic Recommendations

- Help the patient to eliminate or reduce important risk factors such as smoking, hypertension, excess intake of cholesterol and saturated fat, life stress and social isolation, and marked obesity.
- Treat any concurrent aggravating factors such as hypertension, heart failure, severe anemia, hyperthyroidism, hypoxia, or critical aortic stenosis.
- Use nitroglycerin, 0.3 or 0.4 mg sublingually, for immediate symptomatic treatment of anginal episodes; instruct the patient to rest at the time of pain and to repeat the nitroglycerin if the pain does not resolve within 5 minutes. Advise patient to maintain a fresh supply of nitroglycerin and to discard any bottle that has been open for more than 6 months or any tablets that fail to burn sublingually or cause throbbing headache.
- Instruct the patient to use sublingual nitroglycerin prophylactically if anginal pattern is predictably related to events and short-term (<30 min) protection will suffice (eg, before carrying bundles, climbing a hill).
- If short term prophylaxis is insufficient or frequency and severity of episodes is too great for sublingual nitroglycerin alone, add a long-acting nitrate, a beta-blocking agent, or a calcium channel blocker to the program. Choice of agent is determined by the clinical situation:

1. Nitrates. For patients who respond well to nitroglycerin, begin an oral long-acting nitrate such as isosorbide dinitrate. Starting dose should be low to avoid severe headache (eg, 5 mg tid) and advanced slowly over 1 to 2 weeks in increments of 5 mg per dose. To minimize the high risk of developing nitrate tolerance, there should be at least one 10- to 12-hour interval per day between doses; the intervals between doses need not be equal. Increase dose until control is obtained, side effects become intolerable, systolic blood pressure falls to 100 mm Hg, resting heart rate increases more than 10 beats/min, or postural hypotension occurs. Nitroglycerin paste can be used as an adjunct to isosorbide therapy for nocturnal pain. Begin with 1 inch of the ointment applied to the precordium or any other part of the body before bed. Advance dose by ½ inch at a time until therapeutic end point of pain relief achieved. Use daytime for daily nitrate-free interval, if possible. Transdermal nitroglycerin patches can be used as a nocturnal substitute for nitroglycerin paste or as a convenient daytime substitute for isosorbide. Begin with a 5- or 10-mg patch; leave on for no more than 12 to 14 hours; allow for a daily 10- to 12-hour patch-free interval due to especially high risk of nitrate tolerance in patients using patches.
2. *Beta-blocking agents*. For patients with exertional angina as well as those who do not respond well to nitroglycerin or have another condition that would also benefit from beta-adrenergic blockade (eg, hypertension, migraine headache) and who have no serious contraindications to beta-blockade (eg, heart failure, heart block, asthma, tight aortic stenosis), begin a generically available, relatively cardioselective beta-blocking agent (eg, *atenolol* 50 mg qd). Dose can be increased every 3 to 4 days in 25- to 50-mg increments until control is achieved, heart rate falls below 40 to 50 beats/min, fatigue develops, or evidence of heart failure ensues.
   a. A beta-blocker agent can also be added to the regimen at the same time long-acting nitrates are begun; the effects of combined therapy are often synergistic, canceling out adverse cardiac side effects and achieving good control with smaller doses of each agent.
   b. If beta-blockade must be terminated, do so only in a tapering fashion over several days and have the patient reduce activity during this time.
3. *Calcium channel blockers*. Use as initial therapy if coronary vasospasm is strongly suspected; also use if nitrate and/or beta-blocker therapy does not adequately control symptoms or is poorly tolerated. *Sustained-release preparations* increase compliance and can reduce cost, but consider twice-daily administration to reduce risk of a trough in serum level and breakthrough of angina. Choose preparation based on the patient's cardiac status:
   a. For patients with angina complicated by LV dysfunction or conduction system disease, *nifedipine* and other dihydropyridine preparations (nicardipine, felodipine, isradipine) are the calcium channel blockers of

choice. They are also effective for patients who require blood pressure control. Start with a modest dose (eg, nifedipine 10 mg tid), and advance in 10-mg increments until control achieved or blood pressure falls below 100 mm Hg. Exert caution when using in combination with a beta-blocker, which can unmask nifedipine's negatively inotropic effects.

b. For patients with no LV dysfunction or disease of SA or AV nodes, consider *diltiazem* or *verapamil*, both of which are more effective for control of angina than nifedipine and less likely to cause such disturbing side effects as reflex tachycardia, headache, leg edema, and postural light-headedness. Diltiazem is usually started at 30 mg three times per day, verapamil at 80 mg three times per day. Monitor carefully for signs of heart failure, heart block, and bradycardia.

4. *Multi-drug regimens*. Consider a two-drug regimen (not counting use of sublingual TNG) *only if* full doses of a single-drug program fail to control symptoms or cannot be tolerated. Side effects can be additive.
   a. A *long-acting nitrates/beta-blocker* program is safe, effective, and low in cost. Therapeutic effects are additive; side effects are complementary. Use reduced doses of each.
   b. Consider a *calcium channel blocker/beta-blocker program* in patients with preserved LV function. Effects are complementary, and many side effects are cancelled out. However, *exert caution when prescribing in patients with LV dysfunction or conduction system disease—heart failure* and symptomatic *bradycardia* may be induced. Use reduced doses of each agent to minimize side effects and risk of *hypotension*. Avoid use of verapamil in such a program.
   c. A *calcium channel blocker/long-acting nitrates* program is uncommonly used. High risk of hypotension; side effects are additive. May be necessary in cases of stubborn coronary vasospasm.

- Routine use of aspirin for chronic stable angina cannot be recommended yet. Although low-dose therapy reduces the risk of myocardial infarction, there is a trend toward increased risk of stroke; a cardiovascular mortality benefit remains to be demonstrated.
- In patients well enough to undergo bypass surgery, consider exercise stress testing to screen noninvasively for evidence of poor prognosis and candidacy for angiographic study. Thallium imaging and measurement of ejection fraction with exercise may increase predictive value of test results (see Chapter 36).
- Begin a gentle exercise program for all patients (eg, walking 20 min three times per week) and a more intensive program for the highly motived one; obtain an exercise stress test first (see Chapter 31).
- Thoroughly review with patient and family the rationale and proper use of medications; encourage patient to help monitor efficacy of therapy. Counsel on allowable activity, encourage exercise as tolerated, and help avoid self-imposed unnecessary limits on activity.
- Consider angiography and invasive therapy for the patient who remains incapacitated by angina despite a full trial of medical therapy and for the patient who has noninvasive evidence suggestive of left-main or three-vessel disease +/- LV dysfunction. Also refer any anginal patient with evidence of critical aortic stenosis. Single-vessel disease with a proximal high-grade stenosis is an indication for consideration of angioplasty; more extensive disease is not. Bypass surgery is superior to medical therapy and improves survival only for patients with left-main and three-vessel disease, especially if there is LV dysfunction.
- Admit patients with unstable angina or worsening LV dysfunction promptly and obtain cardiac consultation.

A.H.G.

ANNOTATED BIBLIOGRAPHY

Baim DS. Angioplasty as a treatment for coronary artery disease. N Engl J Med 1992;326:56. *(A thoughtful editorial; argues that further improvements in short- and long-term outcomes will be necessary before PTCA can be considered a primary form of therapy.)*

Bonow RO, Kent KM, Rosing DR, et al. Exercise-induced ischemia in mildly symptomatic patients with coronary artery disease and preserved left ventricular function: Identification of subgroups at risk of death during medical therapy. N Engl J Med 1984;311:1339. *(Mildly symptomatic patients with three-vessel disease who had normal ejection fractions at rest but falls in ejection fraction with exercise had a poor prognosis.)*

Burris JF. β-Blockers, dyslipidemia, and coronary disease. Arch Intern Med 1993;153:2085. *(Addresses the question of adverse effect; finds no proof.)*

CASS Principal Investigators. Myocardial infarction and mortality in the coronary artery surgery study (CASS) randomized trial. N Engl J Med 1984;310,750. *(One of the landmark randomized studies on the efficacy and indications for bypass surgery. Neither prolongation of life nor prevention of infarction was demonstrated in mildly symptomatic patients.)*

Chesebro JH, Fuster V. Thrombosis in unstable angina. N Engl J Med 1992;327:192. *(Major role; discussion of the evidence and implications.)*

Cohn PF. Silent myocardial ischemia. Ann Intern Med 1988; 109:312. *(Excellent,terse review; includes discussion of mechanisms, detection, prognosis, and treatment; 61 refs.)*

Curfman GD. The health benefits of exercise: a critical reappraisal. N Engl J Med 1993;328:574. *(An editorial examining quality of data on the health benefits of exercise; notes most studies are observational.)*

DeCesare N, Bartorelli A, Fabbiocchi F, et al. Superior efficacy of propranolol versus nifedipine in double-component angina, as related to different influences on coronary vasomotility. Am J Med 1989;87:15. *(Interestingly, propranolol produced no important vasoconstriction, whereas nifedipine's effect was variable, ranging from vasodilation to vasoconstriction.)*

Dimsdale JE, Newton RP, Joist T. Neuropsychological side effects of beta-blockers. Arch Intern Med 1989;149:514. *(A review of 55 studies; concludes there is little evidence for a difference in CNS effects between the lipophilic and lipophobic preparations.)*

Elkayam U. Tolerance to organic nitrates: evidence, mechanisms, clinical relevance, and strategies for prevention. Ann Intern Med 1991;114:667. *(Best available review to date of nitrate tolerance; 134 refs.)*

Frishman WH, et al. Comparative effects of abrupt withdrawal of propranolol and verapamil in angina pectoris. Am J Cardiol 1982;50:1191. *(No rebound effect was noted in those on ver-*

apamil; 2 of 20 patients had severe exacerbation of symptoms when propranolol was withdrawn.)

Gersh BJ, Kronmal RA, Schaff HV, et al. Comparison of coronary artery bypass surgery and medical therapy in patients 65 years of age or older. N Engl J Med 1985;313:217. *(A non-randomized segment of the CASS study; benefit continued to be demonstrated in the elderly.)*

Grobbee DE, Rimm EB, Giovannucci E, et al. Coffee, caffeine, and cardiovascular disease in men. N Engl J Med 1990; 323:1026. *(An epidemiologic study of 45,000 men; no increase in risk of coronary disease.)*

Houston MC, Hodge R. Beta-adrenergic blocker withdrawal syndromes in hypertension and other cardiovascular diseases. Am Heart J 1988;116:515. *(Documents that withdrawal is usually mild, but of 338 patients developing withdrawal, 15 infarcted and 8 died.)*

Kotler TS, Diamond GA. Exercise thallium-201 scintigraphy in the diagnosis and prognosis of coronary artery disease. Ann Intern Med 1990;113:684. *(Authoritative review serving as the basis of a policy statement by the American College of Physicians in the same issue; 193 refs.)*

Luchi RJ, Chahine RA, Raizner AE. Coronary artery spasm. Ann Intern Med 1979;91:441. *(Excellent review of pathophysiology and its clinical implications; 118 refs.)*

Manson JE, Grobbee DE, Stampfer MJ, et al. Aspirin in the primary prevention of angina pectoris in a randomized trial of United States physicians. Am J Med 1990;89:772. *(A report from the Physician's Health Study indicating that alternate-day aspirin failed to reduce the incidence of symptomatic coronary disease.)*

Mark DB, Shaw L, Harrell FE Jr, et al. Prognostic value of a treadmill exercise score in outpatients with suspected coronary artery disease. N Engl J Med 1991;325:849. *(Demonstrates ability of the ECG stress test to distinguish high- from low-risk patients.)*

Morrow K, Morris CK, Froelicher VF, et al. Prediction of cardiovascular death in men undergoing noninvasive evaluation for coronary artery disease. Ann Intern Med 1993;118:689. *(Data on predictive value of noninvasive testing.)*

Muller JE, Tofler GH, Stone PH. Circadian variation and triggers of onset of acute cardiovascular disease. Circulation 1989; 79:733. *(The morning hours are the time of greatest risk.)*

The Multicenter Diltiazem Postinfarction Trial Research Group. The effect of diltiazem on mortality and reinfarction after myocardial infarction. N Engl J Med 1988;319:385. *(A major, randomized, multicenter study. Patients with normal LV function showed improved survival and lower rates of infarction; those with LV dysfunction showed reduced survival and increased rates of infarction; overall, the net effect was nil.)*

The Norwegian Multicenter Study Group. Timolol-induced reduction in mortality and reinfarction in patients surviving acute myocardial infarction. N Engl J Med 1981;304:801. *(This landmark trial demonstrated a 45 percent reduction in sudden death among post-MI patients attributable to beta-blockade with timolol.)*

Packer M. Combined beta-adrenergic and calcium-entry blockade in angina pectoris. N Engl J Med 1989;320:709. *(A critical review of studies on this approach to anginal treatment; finds the data supports its use only in patients with preserved LV function who fail full doses of single agent therapy; 128 refs.)*

Parisi AF, Folland ED, Hartigan P, et al. A comparison of angioplasty with medical therapy in the treatment of single-vessel coronary artery disease. N Engl J Med 1992;326:10. *(A randomized, multicenter study; PTCA was superior to medical therapy for relief of pain and exercise tolerance at 6 months, but there was an increased risk of acute infarction.)*

Parker JO, Farrell B, Lahey KA, et al. Effect of intervals between doses on the development of tolerance to isosorbide dinitrate. N Engl J Med 1987;316:1440. *(A placebo-controlled study in patients with chronic stable angina; onset of tolerance found with QID, but not tid or bid dosing.)*

Parker JO. Efficacy of nitroglycerin patches: Fact or fancy? Ann Intern Med 1985;102:548. *(An editorial reviewing the evidence for efficacy and raising the question of tolerance developing rapidly with patch use.)*

Parker JO, Van Koughnett KA, Farrell B. Nitroglycerin lingual spray: clinical efficacy and dose-response relation. Am J Cardiol 1986;57:1. *(Efficacy and dosing are nearly identical to sublingual TNG.)*

Popma JJ, Dehmer GJ. Care of the patient after coronary angioplasty. Ann Intern Med 1989;110:547. *(A very useful review for the primary physician, detailing not only the care of such patients but the risks and outcomes of the procedure; 153 refs.)*

Pryor DB, Shaw L, Harrell FE Jr, et al. Estimating the likelihood of severe coronary disease. Am J Med 1991;90:553. *(Describes a validated scoring system based on simple clinical findings that identifies high-risk patients; a potentially useful low-cost alternative.)*

Reichek N, Sutton, M. *Long-acting nitrates.* Ann Intern Med 1982;97:774. *(An editorial critically reviewing the efficacy of nitrate preparations.)*

Ridker PM, Manson JE, Gaziano JM, et al. Low-dose aspirin therapy for chronic stable angina: a randomized, placebo-controlled clinical trial. Ann Intern Med 1991;114:835. *(The Physicians' Health Study; risk of a first infarction reduced by 87 percent; survival did not improve significantly, and risk of stroke trended upward.)*

Rozanski A, Bairey CN, Krantz DS, et al. Mental stress and the induction of silent myocardial ischemia in patients with coronary artery disease. N Engl J Med 1988;318:1005. *(A controlled study; personally relevant stress was just as potent an inducer of ischemia as exercise.)*

Siegel D, Grady D, Browner WS, et al. Risk factor modification after myocardial infarction. Ann Intern Med 1988;109:213. *(Substantial reduction in CHD risk can be achieved with modest reduction in risk factors.)*

Silber S, Vogler AC, Krause KH, et al. Induction and circumvention of nitrate tolerance applying different dosage intervals. Am J Med 1987;83:860. *(An eccentric schedule that allowed 10–12 h of washout was most effective.)*

Skinner MH, Futterman A, Morrissette D, et al. Atenolol compared with nifedipine: effect on cognitive function and mood in elderly hypertensive patients. Ann Intern Med 1992;116:615. *(One of the few randomized, controlled, double-blinded, crossover studies on the CNS effects of a beta-blocker; no adverse effect on mood or cognitive function detected.)*

Strauss WE, Parisi AF. Combined use of calcium-channel and beta-adrenergic blockers for the treatment of chronic stable angina. Ann Intern Med 1988;109:570. *(A more favorable review of the data than that of Packer; suggests a role for adding a calcium-channel blocker when one desires to reduce the dose of beta-blocker; 77 refs.)*

Sytkowski PA, Kannel WB, D'Agostino RB. Changes in risk factors and the decline in mortality from cardiovascular disease: the Framingham Study. N Engl J Med 1990;322:1635. *(Documents a 40 percent decline in mortality, the majority of which is attributed to risk factor control.)*

Varnauskas E. Twelve-year follow-up of survival in the randomized European coronary surgery study. N Engl J Med 1988;319:332. *(A late follow-up report of one of the three major randomized studies of bypass surgery; confirms survival benefit for patients with left-main, three-vessel, and "left-main equivalent" disease.)*

Veterans Administration Coronary Artery Bypass Surgery Cooperative Study Group. Eleven-year survival in the Veterans Administration randomized trial of coronary bypass surgery for stable angina. N Engl J Med 1984;311:1333. *(Landmark study. Only those with a very high risk of dying (left-main disease, very severe three-vessel disease) demonstrated a benefit from surgery at 11 years of follow-up; earlier benefits found at seven years disappeared by year 11.)*

Viscoli CM, Horwitz RI, Singer BH. Beta-blockers after myocardial infarction: influence of first-year clinical course on long-term effectiveness. Ann Intern Med 1993;118:99. *(Benefit appears greatest in those whose clinical course is characterized by recurrent ischemic events, congestive heart failure, arrhythmias, or severe comorbidity.)*

Willard JE, Lange RA, Hillis LD. Use of aspirin in ischemic heart disease. N Engl J Med 1992;327:175. *(Comprehensive review; 86 refs.)*

Wong JB, Sonnenberg FA, Salem DN, et al. Myocardial revascularization for chronic stable angina: analysis of the role of percutaneous transluminal angioplasty based on data available in 1989. Ann Intern Med 1990;113:852. *(A decision analysis study done in an attempt to address the issues of PTCA vs bypass in the absence of randomized prospective study data.)*

31
Cardiovascular Rehabilitation and Secondary Prevention of Coronary Artery Disease

GREGORY D. CURFMAN, M.D.

Primary Care Medicine: Office Evaluation and Management of the Adult Patient, 3rd edition, edited by Allan H. Goroll, Lawrence A. May, and Albert G. Mulley, Jr. J.B. Lippincott Company, Philadelphia

The major goals of a program in cardiovascular rehabilitation are to improve functional capacity in patients with established heart disease and apply interventions aimed at halting the progression of the coronary atherosclerotic process and its clinical manifestations. The first goal can be accomplished in a majority of patients, and recent information indicates that the second goal may also be within reach. Because the interventions sometimes require major changes in the patient's lifestyle, the influence of the primary physician is critically important. One needs to know what interventions are effective and how to tailor a rehabilitation program to the needs and capabilities of the individual patient.

STRUCTURE OF A CARDIAC REHABILITATION PROGRAM

Cardiovascular rehabilitation programs have traditionally been divided arbitrarily into four phases, which describe the temporal sequence of rehabilitative measures followed in patients with coronary artery disease.

Phase I, Early Rehabilitation, occurs *during hospitalization* for an acute coronary event. The major goals of this phase include 1) prevention of physical deconditioning; 2) patient education regarding coronary risk factors; and 3) interventions aimed at preventing psychological disability resulting from the anxiety and depression that frequently follow an acute coronary event.

Physical deconditioning is avoided by initiating a program of low-level activity as soon as possible after clinical stability has been achieved. In practice, low-level activity can begin safely as soon as the third day after admission for an uncomplicated myocardial infarction (MI), as soon as symptoms have been controlled in patients admitted for medical therapy of angina, and as soon as the patient who has undergone coronary artery bypass surgery can walk.

Initial activity should consist of *slow walking* (60–80 steps/min); the heart rate should not exceed 15 to 20 beats/min above the resting level (or 10–15 beats/min above the resting value in patients receiving beta-adrenergic blocking agents). An alternative low-level activity program can be initiated during hospitalization with a *stationary bicycle ergometer* in the free-wheeling mode, where the systemic oxygen consumption is only 1.3 times resting oxygen consumption. This low level of activity is comparable in intensity to slow walking and is quite safe for most patients. Either mode effectively prevents skeletal muscle deconditioning and atrophy. Low-level activity also improves morale; patients feel that they are contributing positively to the recovery process.

Before hospital discharge, most patients should be observed by their physician while climbing a flight of stairs. This will provide confidence that such tasks can be performed safely and will often uncover specific questions about what should and should not be done during the first weeks at home. *Submaximal exercise testing* before hospital discharge has been recommended and is performed routinely in many centers. A treadmill exercise test to a 5-met level has been found to be safe even when performed within 10 days of an uncomplicated MI. Successful completion of an exercise test before discharge from the hospital helps to restore patient confidence and suggests that the recovery process is proceeding smoothly.

The information obtained from exercise testing has prognostic implications and may be useful in patient management. A negative submaximal test predicts an excellent prognosis during the subsequent year, whereas a test that is positive for ischemic electrocardiographic changes with or without anginal symptoms predicts a poorer outcome. In the latter instance, a more aggressive medical approach, coronary angioplasty, or coronary artery bypass surgery may be indicated (see Chapter 30).

Exercise testing can also be effective in exposing latent ventricular dysrhythmias and may help in selecting patients whose long-term prognosis may benefit from beta-adrenergic blocker therapy (see Chapters 29 and 30). In addition, the procedure helps in deciding which patients can safely undergo early discharge. Thallium scintigraphy in conjunction with submaximal exercise testing may sharpen risk stratification after myocardial infarction. Thallium scanning after administration of the coronary vasodilator dipyridamole is used by some physicians to stratify patients into risk categories.

Phase II, the Convalescence Phase, begins at the time of hospital discharge and continues for 3 to 6 weeks. The goal of Phase II rehabilitation is to return the patient to the level of physical conditioning that existed before the cardiac event. Since evidence from experimental animal models suggests that high-level physical activity soon after myocardial infarction may promote infarct expansion and possible ventricular aneurysm formation, the prescribed activity level remains relatively low during Phase II. Exercise intensity is regulated by monitoring peak heart rate, which should not exceed the level achieved during the predischarge submaximal exercise test. If the exercise test disclosed ischemic electrocardiographic changes, anginal symptoms, or ventricular dysrhythmias, then the heart rate during exercise training sessions should be maintained below the heart rate at which any of these pathologic events was observed. The exercise training modalities used during Phase II, as in Phase I, usually consist of *walking* and *stationary bicycling*. The process of educating the patient and the family about coronary risk factors is an important component of Phase II (see below).

Phase III, the Late Convalescence and Physical Training Phase, is designed to increase the patient's level of physical conditioning. Based on a *maximal exercise test* performed 3 to 6 weeks after discharge, the exercise prescription is rewritten to provide a greater *physiologic training* effect. This test allows the patient's heart rate and blood pressure responses to exercise to be quantified and provides another screening test for latent myocardial ischemia and ventricular dysrhythmias. The exercise training modalities used during Phase II can be broadened during Phase III to establish a balanced exercise program that will have long-term patient appeal. Upper extremity conditioning may be added, especially in patients for whom upper extremity work is important on the job. During Phase III, efforts to modify risk factors continue. These include *dietary interventions* to lower the total serum cholesterol and low-density lipoprotein (LDL) cholesterol concentrations, raise high-density lipoprotein (HDL) cholesterol concentration, and achieve ideal body weight (see Chapters 27 and 233). *Hypertension control* (see Chapter 26), and *smoking cessation* (see Chapter 54) are critically important. *Management of psychological stress* should also be addressed (see Chapter 226), particularly as the patient returns to work. A well-balanced cardiac rehabilitation program attends to all of these factors and should involve the patient's family as well as the patient.

Phase IV, the Maintenance or Follow-up Phase, completes the cardiac rehabilitation cycle. The goal is to encourage lifelong adherence to the health habits established during Phase III. Follow-up visits at 6- to 12-month intervals are important. Blood pressure and pulse measurement, serum lipid levels, and even repeat maximal exercise tolerance tests can provide useful feedback to the patient about his or her health practices and indicate areas that may require lifestyle change to minimize coronary risk. Further research is needed to improve our understanding about the most effective methods of achieving permanent lifestyle modification.

THE EFFECTS OF EXERCISE TRAINING ON CARDIAC REHABILITATION

Substantial information is now available to support the use of exercise training in conjunction with risk factor modification to reduce the morbidity and mortality of cardiovascular disease. Moreover, there is increasing evidence that physical activity is protective against the development of first manifestations of coronary artery disease (primary prevention—see Chapter 18).

Effects on Morbidity and Mortality. A number of studies indicate the important role that cardiac rehabilitation, broadly defined, plays in the secondary prevention of coronary disease. Two recent meta-analyses and one cumulative meta-analysis of controlled clinical trials of cardiac rehabilitation indicate that rehabilitation programs are effective in reducing morbidity and mortality after acute myocardial infarction. With respect to total mortality, cardiovascular mortality, and fatal reinfarction, cardiac rehabilitation reduced the relative risk of these end points by approximately 20 percent (relative risk 0.80). However, this beneficial effect was statistically significant only in programs that included smoking cessation, dietary modification, and stress reduction along with an exercise component. Rehabilitation programs based only on an exercise intervention had no significant effect on these three end points, although the relatively small number of patients in such programs reduces the statistical power to exclude a beneficial effect of exercise alone. Nonetheless, the data suggest that cardiac rehabilitation programs aimed at secondary prevention of coronary disease should incorporate measures to modify coronary risk factors (such as smoking cessation and dietary modification) along with an exercise intervention.

Mechanisms of Benefit. Regular physical exercise may benefit patients with coronary artery disease by a number of mechanisms. Among these is the *"physiologic training effect."* Because of the increase in peripheral oxygen extraction by working skeletal muscles and the increase in cardiac stroke volume that constitute the training effect, the cardiovascular system of the trained subject is able to deliver a given quantity of oxygenated blood to the peripheral tissues at a lower heart rate. Since systemic arterial pressure also tends to be somewhat lower during exercise in the trained state, the rate–pressure product (heart rate × systolic arterial pressure), which correlates closely with myocardial oxygen consumption under most physiologic conditions, is often substantially lower than in the untrained state. The benefit to the patient with ischemic heart disease is obvious; it becomes possible for the trained patient to exercise to a higher level before reaching the critical rate–pressure product at which myocardial ischemia develops.

Beta-adrenergic blockers benefit patients with angina pectoris in a similar fashion, by reducing heart rate and blood pressure during exertion. Unlike exercise training, however, beta-blocking agents also tend to *reduce the maximal cardiac output* that can be achieved during exertion, and thereby also decrease maximal oxygen consumption and exercise capacity.

Exercise training may benefit patients with cardiovascular disease by other physiologic mechanisms as well. Aerobic exercise training results in *dilatation of large coronary arteries*, and this effect may diminish the hemodynamic compromise from existing coronary artery lesions. Some evidence also suggests that exercise training may improve collateral blood flow to ischemic zones. Coronary blood flow under conditions of maximal coronary vasodilation may also be increased. Another important beneficial effect is an *increase in HDL cholesterol* concentration (see Chapter 15).

Other potentially important protective mechanisms of aerobic exercise include an *increase in fibrinolytic response* to occlusive stimuli in the trained state and an *increase in ventricular fibrillation threshold* (noted in animal studies). Exercise conditioning may alter the electrophysiologic properties of the myocardium, rendering it less vulnerable to ventricular dysrhythmia.

ESTIMATING THE AMOUNT OF EXERCISE NEEDED

How much exercise is needed to produce the beneficial physiologic effects discussed above remains unsettled. The generally accepted assumption is that one must achieve a physiologic training effect to obtain health benefits. Classic exercise physiology indicates that the training effect can usually be produced by any form of *aerobic (endurance) exercise* (running, jogging, fast walking, cycling, rowing, cross country skiing, swimming) that is performed at least four times a week for at least 30 minutes per exercise session, at an intensity resulting in a heart rate of 70 percent to 85 percent of a measured maximum. However, it is possible that less intense aerobic activity may also be effective in producing a training effect and the associated health benefits. Further investigation of this important question is clearly indicated and ongoing.

The traditional and simplest method of determining an effective exercise intensity for patients undergoing exercise training in a cardiac rehabilitation program is to *calculate 70 percent to 85 percent of a measured maximal heart rate*. The measured maximal heart rate is usually based on the results of an exercise stress test. The mode of exercise used for exercise testing should be specific to the type of exercise planned for the training program (eg, treadmill testing for a walking/jogging program, bicycle ergometer testing for a cycling program). Some authorities suggest other methods of calculating the target heart rate, but in practice, the traditional calculation is generally the most efficient. This exercise intensity translates to approximately 60 percent to 80 percent of maximal oxygen consumption.

The relationship between heart rate and oxygen consumption is not influenced by beta-adrenergic blockade. This point is important in cardiac rehabilitation, because many patients receive a beta-blocking agent as part of their post-myocardial infarction therapeutic regimen (see Chapter 30). Such patients require a formal graded exercise test under the influence of a beta-blocker if they are going to be taking a beta-blocker while engaged in an exercise training program.

OTHER INTERVENTIONS FOR SECONDARY PREVENTION OF MYOCARDIAL INFARCTION

Exercise training is but one means of rehabilitation and secondary prevention in the patient with coronary disease. As noted above, a balanced rehabilitation program should focus attention on other aspects of coronary risk, including hypertension (see Chapter 26), hypercholesterolemia (see Chapter 27), smoking (see Chapter 54), obesity (see Chapter 233), and psychological stress (see Chapter 226). In addition, the long-term use of pharmacologic agents has been applied in an attempt to achieve secondary prevention of coronary disease.

Beta-adrenergic Blockade. A number of randomized trials have indicated that beta-adrenergic blockade reduces the total mortality rate as well as the incidences of recurrent infarction and sudden death in patients following acute infarction. Two exemplary studies leading to this conclusion were the Norwegian timolol study (39% reduction in total mortality, 28% reduction in reinfarction rate) and the American Beta-blocker Heart Attack Trial (26% reduction in total mortality, 23% reduction in reinfarction).

Other agents for secondary prevention have been studied, including *antiplatelet agents* and *oral anticoagulants*. A number of trials have suggested a modest reduction in death or reinfarction with *long-term aspirin* therapy or anticoagulation with *warfarin*. Aspirin has also been found efficacious in preventing myocardial infarction among patients with unstable angina (see Chapter 30). Consequently, long-term prophylactic therapy with aspirin should be strongly considered for patients with acute myocardial infarction and unstable angina; therapy with warfarin should also be considered in post-infarction patients.

Angiotensin converting enzyme inhibitor therapy may also reduce mortality and reinfarction risks in post-infarction patients, as demonstrated in a controlled study with captopril among patients with an ejection fraction of less than .40 but no clinical signs of heart failure. The subsequent development of severe heart failure and the need for hospitalization for heart failure were also reduced. However, the beneficial effects were not evident until 1 year of therapy had been completed. Patients with left ventricular dysfunction following acute MI, who do not have active heart failure, should be considered candidates for long-term angiotensin converting enzyme therapy with captopril.

PATIENT EDUCATION

The patient who has suffered an acute coronary event is among those in greatest need of health education and individualized lifestyle counseling. Patient and family are apt to be depressed and frightened by the diagnosis of "coronary disease," believing the prognosis to be grim and fearing invalidism, especially if an infarction has occurred. They need to be informed that in the vast majority of uncomplicated cases, a return to job and regular activity is the rule rather than the exception.

Prognosis is a major concern of the patient and family. Long-term survival rates after infarction have been examined in prospective epidemiologic studies. Average annual mortality in the Framingham Study was 5 percent for men and 7 percent for women. Patients at greatest risk for late cardiac death were those with "malignant" ventricular irritability (see Chapter 29) beyond the acute phase of illness, azotemia, previous infarction, persistent congestive failure, angina, or advanced age. Once congestive heart failure ensued, 50 percent were dead within 5 years. Risk of postinfarction angina in the Framingham Study was 2.9 percent for men, 9.6 percent for women. Risk of heart failure was 2.3 percent.

Many of the complications of infarction are a function of the degree of myocardial damage. This is consistent with the observation that prognosis correlates with extensiveness of disease, a finding also supported by angiographic studies (see Chapter 30). As noted above, 1-year survival can be estimated from a limited treadmill exercise test done prior to discharge. Prognosis can be improved by use of beta-blockers and lowering of serum cholesterol.

Counseling needs to begin in the predischarge period. Realistic concerns as well as excessive fears of incapacitation may dramatically alter self-image and diminish self-respect. The most effective way of dealing with such fears is to specifically elicit and address the patient's and the family's concerns, discuss the plan for recovery and rehabilitation, and provide an activity prescription.

Specific statements concerning *exercise capacity* can be based on graded treadmill stress testing during the recovery period. Knowing what one should and should not do during various stages of the recovery process can help reduce some of the anxiety that accompanies having heart disease.

Activity guidelines should be given. Unsupervised activities during the first month following an MI should require no more than 3 mets (see Table 18–1). By the time 6 to 8 weeks have passed, tasks requiring up to 5 mets will be safe for most patients, provided a gradual increase in activity has not be interrupted by symptoms or complications. Specific guidelines, tailored to the patient's personal occupational and recreational interests, are essential.

Some concerns may not always be verbalized by the patient. One such concern is the safety of resuming *sexual activity*. Often, there is fear of sudden death during intercourse. The safety of sexual activity should be routinely discussed with the patient and spouse, even if the topic is not initially raised by them.

Sexual intercourse with a familiar partner requires about 3 to 5 mets. Thus, sexual activity can be safely resumed by most patients as early as 4 weeks post-MI. During the early return to full sexual activity, the patient should be advised to avoid coital positions that require sustained isometric exercise, such as upper torso weight bearing with the arms.

The period following an acute coronary event is also a time when patients are particularly receptive to counseling about changes in *lifestyle* that reduce coronary risk, such as smoking cessation (see Chapter 54) and dietary change (see Chapter 27). The primary physician is ideally suited to take advantage of this opportunity. A balanced cardiac rehabilitation program offers a very positive response to a very frightening event. In many instances, the results are extremely gratifying, with a patient who is healthier and more fit than before the acute coronary event.

ANNOTATED BIBLIOGRAPHY

Antiplatelet Trialists Collaboration. Secondary prevention of vascular disease by prolonged antiplatelet treatment. Br Med J 1988;296:320. *(A terse overview of clinical trials of antiplatelet agents.)*

Beta Blocker Heart Attack Trial Research Group. A randomized trial of propranolol in patients with acute myocardial infarction. JAMA 1982;247:1707. *(This large-scale randomized trial among men and women with one prior MI demonstrated a reduction in total mortality from 9.8 percent to 7.2 percent and in cardiovascular mortality from 8.5 percent to 6.2 percent.)*

Brown G, Alpers JJ, Fisher LD, et al. Regression of coronary artery disease as a result of intensive lipid-lowering therapy in men with high levels of apolipoprotein B. N Engl J Med 1990;323:1289. *(Intensive lipid-lowering therapy reduced the frequency of progression of coronary lesions, promoted regression, and reduced the frequency of cardiovascular events.)*

Curfman GD. Cardiac rehabilitation and secondary prevention of coronary artery disease. Transition, June 1984. *(Portions of the current chapter first appeared in this review; reproduced with permission.)*

Curfman GD. Shorter hospital stay for myocardial infarction. N Engl J Med 1988;318:1123. *(A summary of available data, indicating safety of shortened stay for patients with uncomplicated infarction.)*

Echt DS, Liebson PR, Mitchell LB, et al. Mortality and morbidity in patients receiving encainide, flecainide, or placebo. The Cardiac Arrhythmia Suppression Trial. N Engl J Med 1991; 324:781. *(In patients with asymptomatic ventricular arrhythmia following myocardial infarction, antiarrhythmic therapy resulted in poorer survival.)*

EPSIM Research Group. A controlled comparison of aspirin and oral anticoagulants in prevention of death of myocardial infarction. N Engl J Med 1982;307:701. *(No difference in mortality or reinfarction was noted.)*

Frishman WH, Furberg CD, Friedewald WT. Beta-adrenergic blockade for survivors of acute myocardial infarction. N Engl J Med 1984;310:837. *(A review of clinical studies, potential mechanisms, and clinical use.)*

Hennekens CH, Buring JE, Sandercock P, et al. Aspirin and other antiplatelet agents in the secondary and primary prevention of cardiovascular disease. Circulation 1989;80:749. *(A good summary of the role for antiplatelet therapy.)*

ISIS-2 (Second International Study of Infarct Survival) Collaborative Group. Randomized trial of intravenous streptokinase, oral aspirin, both, or neither among 17187 cases of suspected acute myocardial infarction: ISIS-2. Lancet 1988;2:349. *(All treatments were superior to placebo in the management of acute myocardial infarction.)*

Lau J, Altman EM, Jimenez-Silva J, et al. Cumulative meta-analysis of therapeutic trials for myocardial infarction. N Engl J

Med 1992;327:248. *(Summarizes data on the efficacy of cardiac rehabilitation in secondary prevention after myocardial infarction.)*

Lewis HD, Davis JW, Archibald DG, et al. Protective effects of aspirin against acute myocardial infarction and death in men with unstable angina. N Engl J Med 1983;309;396. *(Men treated for 12 weeks with buffered aspirin had a 51 percent lower incidence of death from acute infarction compared to placebo controls.)*

Norwegian Multi-Center Study Group. Timolol-induced reduction in mortality and reinfarction in patients surviving acute myocardial infarction. N Engl J Med 1981;304:801. *(The landmark trial demonstrating a 45 percent reduction in sudden death among post-MI patients.)*

O'Connor GT, Buring JE, Yusuf S, et al. An overview of randomized trials of rehabilitation with exercise after myocardial infarction. Circulation 1989;80:234. *(An important meta-analysis; efficacy of cardiac rehabilitation after MI when exercise rehabilitation was linked with modification of other coronary risk factors.)*

Pfeffer MA, Braunwald E, Moye LA, et al. Effect of captopril on mortality and morbidity in patients with left ventricular dysfunction after myocardial infarction. Results of the survival and ventricular enlargements trial. N Engl J Med 1992; 327:669. *(Compared to placebo, treatment with captopril improved long-term outcome.)*

Shaw LW. Effects of a prescribed supervised exercise program on mortality and cardiovascular morbidity in patients after myocardial infarction. Am J Cardiol 1981;48:39. *(Results of the National Exercise and Heart Disease Project, which examined the effects of a formal exercise program on prognosis.)*

Siegel D, Grady D, Browner WS, et al. Risk factor modification after myocardial infarction. Ann Intern Med 1988;109:213. *(Substantial reduction in CHD risk can be achieved with modest reduction in risk factors.)*

Smith P, Arnesen H, Holme I. The effect of warfarin on mortality and reinfarction after myocardial infarction. N Engl J Med 1990;323:147. *(Beneficial effects noted.)*

Theroux P, Waters DD, Halphen C, et al. Prognostic value of exercise testing soon after myocardial infarction. N Engl J Med 1979;301:341. *(Demonstrates both the safety and usefulness of such testing.)*

Van Camp SP, Peterson RA. Cardiovascular complications of outpatient cardiac rehabilitation programs. JAMA 1986;256:1160. *(Documents very low risk of cardiac events associated with supervised programs.)*

Viscoli CM, Horwitz RI, Singer BH. Beta-blockers after myocardial infarction: influence of first-year clinical course on long-term effectiveness. Ann Intern Med 1993;118:99. *(Benefit appears greatest in those whose clinical course is characterized by recurrent ischemic events, congestive heart failure, arrhythmias, or severe comorbidity.)*

32
Management of Chronic Congestive Heart Failure

Primary Care Medicine: Office Evaluation and Management of the Adult Patient, 3rd edition, edited by Allan H. Goroll, Lawrence A. May, and Albert G. Mulley, Jr. J.B. Lippincott Company, Philadelphia

Chronic congestive heart failure (CHF) ranks among the most serious of cardiac problems encountered in office practice. Of particular importance is the design of a treatment program properly tailored to the patient's underlying pathophysiology. The growing appreciation of both systolic and diastolic dysfunction and their respective roles in CHF has led to more precisely targeted therapy. Diuretics and digitalis remain basic components of pharmacologic therapy, complemented by angiotensin converting enzyme (ACE) inhibitors.

A carefully designed program helps to maximize outcomes and prevent such treatment complications as prerenal azotemia and dehydration. Successful management of CHF in the outpatient setting also requires identification and correction of treatable underlying causes and elimination of precipitating factors. Because multi-drug regimens are often necessary, thorough instruction is essential to limit complications and prevent unnecessary hospitalizations that result from poor compliance or drug toxicity.

PATHOPHYSIOLOGY, CLINICAL PRESENTATION, AND COURSE

Pathophysiology. The "congestive" manifestations of CHF—leg edema, orthopnea, paroxysmal nocturnal dyspnea (PND), rales, jugular venous distention—represent elevations in right or left ventricular filling pressures. Traditionally, filling pressure elevations have been viewed as a consequence of *systolic dysfunction* producing a backup of blood into the pulmonary and systemic venous systems. The hallmark of systolic dysfunction is a *reduced ejection fraction.*

However, as many as 40 percent of patients presenting with congestive failure appear to have reasonably well-preserved systolic function but suffer from *diastolic dysfunction*, manifested by increased resistance to diastolic ventricular filling. Such diastolic dysfunction has been demonstrated in patients with valvular, hypertrophic, ischemic, and cardiomyopathic diseases. Mechanisms include impairment of diastolic myocardial relaxation, valvular dysfunction, loss of myocardial distensibility, ventricular remodeling, and intracellular calcium overload. Diastolic dysfunction has also been noted in the setting of volume overload.

The emerging view of congestive heart failure is one of diastolic as well as systolic dysfunction. The role of *neurohumoral factors* has gained increasing recognition. Heart failure triggers a number of compensatory neurohumoral mechanisms, which ultimately become troublesome. For example, the initial fall in cardiac output activates *renin–angiotensin* production and *sympathetic* discharge, which temporarily help preserve cardiac output, but at the cost of an increase in preload and afterload. Eventually, the resultant venous hypertension and increased left ventricular work affect the failing heart, which cannot tolerate such increases in work, and cardiac output drops. Normal hearts respond to increased venous return via the Frank-Starling mechanism to increase cardiac output, but not the failing heart. The result is increased pulmonary and systemic hypertension and no improvement in cardiac output. The progressive decrease in cardiac output and rise in venous pressure trigger further neurohumoral activity, and a vicious cycle is established.

Clinical Presentation. Regardless of etiology, the clinical manifestations of CHF are quite stereotyped and reflect the magnitude of the fall in cardiac output and the rise in pulmonary and systemic venous pressures. Initially and in mild cases, the patient may complain of *fatigability*, *dyspnea on exertion*, or unexplained *weight gain*. There may be few overt physical signs of failure, but chest x-ray often shows *redistribution* of pulmonary venous flow to the upper lung fields and/or *cardiomegaly*. *Fatigue* becomes increasingly prominent as cardiac output falls. As pulmonary congestion increases, dyspnea worsens, *orthopnea* is noted, and *paroxysmal nocturnal dyspnea* may be reported. At this stage, *rales* become evident on auscultation of the lungs, but their absence does not rule out the presence of CHF. Sometimes failure-induced *bronchospasm* dominates the pulmonary examination. In severe cases, the chest film will show *interstitial pulmonary edema*. In chronic CHF, right-sided or bilateral *pleural effusions* are common. *Ankle edema*, *jugular venous distention*, and *hepatojugular reflux* are indicative of elevated systemic venous pressure; if CHF is predominantly left-sided, these findings may not be present. An *S_3 gallop* is among the most specific physical signs of failure, but it is often difficult to hear. If left ventricular (LV) dilation becomes very marked, a *mitral regurgitant murmur* may become evident. Pedal edema is one of the least specific signs of CHF; in the elderly, isolated pedal edema is more likely to be a result of venous insufficiency (see Chapter 22).

Partially treated CHF may present with atypical manifestations. For example, potent diuretic therapy may eliminate most congestive manifestations, while pump function remains depressed. Dyspnea, orthopnea, leg edema, rales, and even radiologic signs of CHF (see below) may be absent, and fatigue might dominate the clinical picture.

Clinical Course. Since congestive failure is not a single disease, it does not have a uniform natural history. Clinical course and response to therapy depend on the nature of the underlying etiology and the state of the myocardium at the time of presentation. For example, the appearance of CHF in a patient with aortic stenosis is an ominous prognostic sign associated with a mean survival of no more than a year or two. However, if the valve is replaced before irreversible myocardial decompensation has occurred, the prognosis is altered dramatically (see Chapter 33). Cases of CHF caused by alcohol abuse, thiamine deficiency, hypertensive heart disease, and hyperthyroidism also have favorable outcomes if detected and treated early. However, if uncorrected, they lead to cardiomyopathic changes and accelerated mortality.

The Framingham study has provided interesting epidemiologic data concerning CHF in the community setting prior to the advent of echocardiography and vasodilator therapy. The annual incidence rate for development of failure was 2.3 per 1000 for men and 1.4 per 1000 for women. The major causes were hypertension in one-third of the patients, hypertension in combination with coronary disease in another one-third, isolated coronary disease in about 10 percent, and valvular disease in another 10 percent. Sixty percent of patients had a serious noncardiac illness along with CHF. Five-year survival rates, regardless of cause, were only 50 percent. Later studies have shown significantly improved survival rates associated with the use of ACE inhibitors, even in patients with advanced disease (see below).

Several factors have been examined for their correlation with prognosis. In an important study, *plasma norepinephrine* levels were found by multivariate analysis to correlate strongly with mortality risk and were superior to such catheterization data as pulmonary wedge pressure, cardiac index, mean arterial pressure, and heart rate. The higher the plasma norepinephrine level, the poorer the prognosis. The high catecholamine level represents autonomic compensation for falling cardiac output, though such a compensatory mechanism is not without its own risks, especially for patients with underlying ischemic or hypertensive disease who cannot tolerate the increase in afterload.

DIAGNOSIS AND MONITORING OF HEART FAILURE

Heart failure is frequently a mistaken diagnosis. Since many of its manifestations are due to compensatory mechanisms, the typical clinical findings may be nonspecific and misleading. A common error is to attribute ankle edema or dyspnea to congestive heart failure. In a study of patients on digitalis for supposed CHF, 40 percent did not fulfill basic diagnostic criteria for the condition. *Right-sided heart failure* is easier to document than left-sided heart failure. It is defined as a right atrial pressure greater than 6 cm H_2O, manifested as a vertical distance from the level of the right atrium to the top of the jugular venous column that is greater than 6 cm. Ankle edema in the absence of jugular venous distention does not constitute a diagnosis of right heart failure. On the other hand and as noted earlier, the absence of ankle edema and jugular venous distention do not necessarily rule out heart failure, especially in the patient taking diuretics.

Left-sided heart failure is more difficult to diagnose solely on clinical grounds. By themselves, most findings on history and physical examination are neither very sensitive nor specific, but in conjunction with other evidence they can be quite helpful. A story of orthopnea and paroxysmal nocturnal dyspnea is suggestive, as are *basilar rales* on pulmonary examination. The finding of a *third heart sound (S_3)* is among the more specific of signs for systolic dysfunction, but it is often difficult to elicit and is sometimes present in elderly hypertensive patients with a normal ejection fraction. Other suggestive findings are found on *chest x-ray* and include upper zone flow redistribution, cardiomegaly, prominent interstitial markings, Kerley "B" lines, and perihilar haziness. Patients who develop CHF only during exertion may not show interstitial changes on a chest film done at rest, though cardiomegaly and upper zone redistribution may be present. Left atrial enlargement by electrocardiographic criteria in conjunction with cardiomegaly by chest film also have diagnostic value.

In the absence of definitive radiologic evidence of pulmonary edema, the diagnosis of CHF is best supported by the finding of upper zone redistribution and one of the other historical, physical, or laboratory findings just noted. In the absence of upper zone redistribution, the presence of any three other findings (eg, S_3, cardiomegaly, and basilar rales) constitutes reasonable evidence for the diagnosis.

More precise assessment of left ventricular function is afforded by use of *echocardiography*, which can help confirm the diagnosis of heart failure and identify its underlying pathophysiology. *Systolic dysfunction* is manifested by a *reduction in ejection fraction*. Wall motion abnormalities, chamber enlargement, and valvular disease can also be detected. *Diastolic dysfunction* can be detected by adding *Doppler* technology to the echocardiographic assessment. Doppler enables determination of blood flow across the mitral valve during diastolic filling of the left ventricle. In diastolic dysfunction, flow is reduced or delayed. The morphology of the Doppler wave helps identify the cause of abnormal flow and thus the mechanism of diastolic dysfunction.

Once the diagnosis of heart failure is made and its underlying pathophysiology determined, simple means can be used for *monitoring*, including patient weight, symptoms, physical examination, and chest x-ray. Repeated use of elaborate diagnostic technology for monitoring purposes is likely to raise costs considerably with little marginal benefit.

PRINCIPLES OF MANAGEMENT

The first task is to search for and treat a *reversible underlying etiology*. All too often, many cases are encountered at the time irreversible myocardial damage has occurred, but when a treatable cause is present and detected early, there is an opportunity for definitive measures to bring about a successful outcome. *Coronary artery disease* (see Chapter 30), *valvular disease* (see Chapter 33), *alcohol excess* (see Chapter 228), *hypertension* (see Chapter 26), *hyperthyroidism* (see Chapter 103), and *hypothyroidism* (see Chapter 104) are examples of conditions requiring etiologic therapy. A stereotypic approach with digitalis and diuretics that ignores etiology may be counterproductive or lead to loss of a unique therapeutic opportunity.

Attention must be directed to the presence of *precipitating factors*. Acute *ischemia* (see Chapter 30), severe *anemia* (see Chapter 82), *high fever* (see Chapter 11), *tachycardia* (see Chapters 28 and 29), *pneumonia* (see Chapter 52), *pulmonary embolization* (see Chapter 35), *excess salt intake*, marked *obesity* (see Chapter 233), and *excess exertion* or *emotional stress* may worsen or precipitate failure in patients with decreased myocardial reserve. Excessive doses of *beta-blockers* (see Chapter 30) or other negatively inotropic agents (eg, *verapamil*, *disopyramide*) may also bring on CHF. A careful search for these factors is essential.

Correct selection and application of drug treatment requires an understanding of the underlying pathophysiology. For example, digitalis can be helpful when there is a marked systolic dysfunction but is of little benefit when the ejection fraction is well preserved. Digitalis, diuretics, and vasodilators have specific roles determined by their different hemodynamic effects. Digitalis is used mainly for its positive inotropic action, diuretics for their ability to reduce volume, and vasodilators to lessen preload and afterload.

Digitalis

Indications for Therapy. Digitalis remains a cornerstone of treatment for congestive heart failure. Its ability to increase contractility makes it a potentially important agent for CHF patients with systolic dysfunction. It increases contractility by increasing intracellular calcium through inhibition of the myocyte sodium pump. Beneficial effects on neurohumoral mechanisms are also postulated. Symptomatic and physiologic benefits have been demonstrated in those with *severe systolic dysfunction* (ejection fraction <.40, audible third heart sound S_3, marked left ventricular dilation). In fact, the presence of an S_3 is a strong predictor of response to cardiac glycoside therapy. Patients with less compromised left ventricular function show little improvement. The overall response rate is about 12 percent among heterogeneous populations of CHF patients in sinus rhythm—mostly a reflection of the relatively small number of CHF patients with severe LV dysfunction. Despite the several centuries of digitalis use, its effect on survival remains unknown (though studies addressing this issue are in progress).

In patients with significant systolic dysfunction, digitalis enhances the results achieved by diuretics and ACE inhibitors (see below). Digoxin withdrawal leads to clinical deterioration in patients with a low ejection fraction. Their effects appear to be complementary. However, one should consider withdrawal of digitalis if it is being used in a patient who never had evidence of severe systolic dysfunction. An echocardiographic study might be useful for the determination. Use of digitalis prior to initiation of diuretic therapy seems unwise, in view of the relative safety of diuretic therapy, the narrow therapeutic range of digitalis (see below), and the seriousness of digitalis toxicity. Available data indicate no excess mortality when digoxin is used for systolic dysfunction in patients who have suffered recent myocardial infarction.

Digitalis remains the drug of choice for heart failure induced by *rapid atrial fibrillation* and some other supraventricular tachycardias (see Chapter 28). The drug is also of use acutely in patients with CHF resulting from *uncontrolled hypertension* or *severe aortic stenosis* but is no substitute for blood pressure reduction (see Chapter 26) or for valve surgery when the aortic stenosis is critical (see Chapter 28). Digitalis is of little use in heart failure resulting from hypertrophic cardiomyopathies, be they idiopathic or due to long-standing hypertension (a common etiology among outpatients, especially women). Patients with idiopathic hypertrophic subaortic stenosis may develop worsening outflow tract obstruction with use of digitalis.

Digitalis is also of no proven benefit in cases of mitral stenosis, as long as the patient is in sinus rhythm, and is of no use in patients with episodes of CHF due to recurrent, transient ischemia. The efficacy of digitalis in *cor pulmonale* is in question; the drug is occasionally beneficial, but the results are not impressive and the risks of toxicity are increased in the setting of hypoxia.

Initiation of Therapy. *Digoxin* is the preparation of choice in the vast majority of patients (see below). Those who are stable can be started on an oral *maintenance dose* without resorting to a loading dose. Using a daily maintenance dose of 0.25 mg, one can achieve therapeutic serum levels in 5 to

7 days. If the patient is less stable, but not so compromised as to require hospitalization, then an oral *loading dose* of 1.0 to 1.25 mg can be prescribed in divided doses over 24 hours.

The decision to initiate digitalis therapy should not be made casually. The incidence of digitalis toxicity was found to be 23 percent in a prospective study of 900 consecutive admissions to the Boston City Hospital general medical service prior to the advent of serum digoxin determinations. Mortality from digitalis intoxication has averaged 22 percent in published series. Use of serum concentration measurements seems to have helped limit the incidence of toxicity. However, one cannot depend on serum levels alone for the diagnosis of digitalis toxicity, because there is considerable overlap in serum concentrations among those with and without evidence of toxicity.

Digitalis Preparations. Numerous digitalis preparations are available; the physician should become familiar with one or two, learn their pharmacokinetics, and use them predominantly. *Digoxin* is the most widely used. In the past, some variations in bioavailability had been noted among different brands; this seems to have been corrected. Half-life of digoxin is 36 hours; onset of action is 1 to 2 hours when taken orally; absorption from the gastrointestinal (GI) tract ranges from 50 percent to 75 percent complete. Excretion is renal and decreases significantly with reduction in creatinine clearance. Higher doses are not needed in obese patients; their nonlipid extracellular fluid volume is normal.

If a patient presents taking a digitalis preparation other than digoxin, it is best to leave him on the drug he is used to. The exception to this generalization concerns patients taking *digitalis leaf*. Because of its variable and unpredictable composition of digoxin and digitoxin, digitalis leaf should be discontinued, and one of the preparations containing only a single active ingredient should be used instead. *Digitoxin* may be beneficial when digitalis must be given to a patient with renal failure, because elimination of digitoxin is not dependent on renal function. However, a major disadvantage with digitoxin is its long half-life of 4 to 6 days, making for serious problems if toxic levels occur. Digoxin can be used safely in renal failure as long as renal function and serum levels are frequently checked and necessary dosage adjustments made.

Monitoring Therapy. Digitalis therapy requires careful monitoring. *Serum levels* should be measured at least three or four times per year, more frequently if there are changes in the patient's renal or volume status. Monitoring should help reduce the incidence of digitalis toxicity. A sample should be drawn at least 6 hours after the last dose, since there is a 4- to 6-hour rise in serum level after an oral dose. In most instances, it is best to have the patient omit the day's dose when he comes to the office for a serum determination.

A number of factors can affect serum concentration, including renal function when digoxin is being used and hepatic function in digitoxin therapy.

Absorption of digitalis from the gut remains adequate in CHF but may fall in severe cases of malabsorption. Thyroid status can affect digitalis metabolism; hypothyroidism prolongs the half-life, and hyperthyroidism shortens it. Treatment of thyroid disease needs to be accompanied by an adjustment of dose.

The serum level of digitalis is not in itself diagnostic of *toxicity*, because there is considerable overlap in serum concentrations among those with and without evidence of toxicity; but if the *digoxin level* is *greater than 2.0 ng/mL*, the probability of encountering toxicity increases considerably. In one series, 80 percent of patients without evidence of toxicity had a digoxin level below 2.0 ng/mL; in 87 percent of those with toxicity, the level was above 2.0 ng/mL.

To avoid *digitalis toxicity*, even when the dose is closely followed, the physician needs to monitor factors that increase the "sensitivity" of the myocardium to the toxic effects of the drug. Such factors include *hypokalemia*, abnormalities in serum *calcium* and *magnesium*, organic heart disease, and pulmonary disease with acute *hypoxia*.

Digitalis Toxicity. Symptoms of digitalis toxicity can be divided into noncardiac and cardiac manifestations. Anorexia, nausea, vomiting, diarrhea, visual disturbances including yellow halos around lights, and in rare instances, delirium have been described since Withering's time. Arrhythmias are the predominant cardiac manifestation of toxicity. Digitalis can cause any type of rhythm and/or conduction disturbance because it affects automaticity of myocardial tissues as well as the conduction system. *Ventricular irritability* (especially bigeminy), *paroxysmal atrial tachycardia* with block, and *junctional tachycardia* are particularly characteristic of digitalis excess.

The unexplained onset of an arrhythmia in a patient on digitalis raises the possibility of drug-related toxicity. The drug should be withheld, a serum level obtained, potassium, calcium, and magnesium levels checked, and serious consideration given to immediate hospitalization for monitoring and parenteral antiarrhythmic therapy. The high incidence and mortality rate of this preventable and often treatable condition call for vigilance.

A few pitfalls in the use of digitalis are worth repeating. 1) Digitalis should not be used unless there is genuine evidence of severe chronic systolic dysfunction or atrial fibrillation. An all-too-common error is to assume that ankle edema in the elderly patient is a sign of CHF and an indication for starting digitalis. Most of the time the ankle edema is due to venous insufficiency; even if due to congestive heart failure, it may be a manifestation of diastolic dysfunction and respond better to diuretics or ACE inhibitors. 2) Digitalis should not be discontinued unless a reversible cause of pump failure has been fully corrected or there is no basis for using the drug in the first place. Patients who respond to digitalis need the drug chronically; they have been shown to deteriorate clinically and hemodynamically when the drug is withdrawn in experimental circumstances, even in the context of ACE inhibitor use. 3) Digitalis-induced ST-T wave changes on the electrocardiogram have no correlation with optimal or toxic dose levels and cannot be used for such determinations. Serum drug levels are necessary.

Diuretics

Diuretics are an important initial therapy when there is evidence of volume overload. Most patients with failure begin to retain sodium as cardiac output falls and renal perfusion diminishes. As noted earlier, the increase in volume initially helps to produce a rise in diastolic filling pressure and maintain cardiac output by the Frank-Starling mechanism. However, the degree of fluid retention is often excessive, resulting in pulmonary congestion and/or peripheral edema. Abnormalities in release of atrial natriuretic peptide, prostaglandin metabolism, and neurohumoral regulation are believed to be involved in the process of volume overload. The renin–angiotensin system also plays a central role.

Like digitalis, diuretics have been used empirically for decades in treatment of CHF without definitive study of their efficacy. In several recent controlled studies comparing the ACE inhibitor captopril to the potent diuretic furosemide in patients with mild to moderate CHF, patients did better acutely with diuretic therapy. However, diuretic therapy alone is usually insufficient for chronic treatment of CHF, in part because it stimulates the renin–angiotensin system and raises serum catecholamines, leading to increased afterload, reduced cardiac output, and further sodium retention. Although diuretics may be effective in controlling peripheral edema and pulmonary congestion, they do little to prevent the progression of heart failure or improve prognosis. Consequently, diuretics emerge as important treatment for relief of congestive symptoms, but they are insufficient for altering prognosis, especially in patients with a failing left ventricle. Overzealous use of diuretics may acutely worsen the situation by producing prerenal azotemia or a dangerous fall in filling pressure (as in critical aortic stenosis). Moreover, escalating diuretic therapy in mitral or aortic valve disease may inappropriately delay the timing of surgical therapy (see Chapter 33).

Selection of Agent and Initiation of Therapy. Diuretic therapy can be initiated with a *thiazide* (eg, 50 mg hydrochlorothiazide) when the symptoms of failure are mild or when the patient is asymptomatic but showing weight gain or x-ray findings indicative of early CHF. The degree of dyspnea on exertion and weight change are the simplest clinical parameters to follow for gauging response to therapy in mild cases. For patients with renal impairment and mild CHF, *metolazone* can be useful. It is similar in potency to the thiazides, but more effective in the setting of azotemia.

Patients with more severe CHF, manifested by dyspnea at rest, orthopnea, or paroxysmal nocturnal dyspnea, represent the other end of the spectrum. If it is judged reasonable to attempt outpatient management of such patients, a loop diuretic such as *furosemide* or *ethacrynic acid* is necessary. Small doses of loop diuretics may also benefit patients with mild to moderate failure that cannot be adequately controlled by thiazides. Caution is warranted when treating a patient for the first time with a loop diuretic, because a marked diuresis may be evoked, even from a small dose. If a thiazide had been used previously, it should be stopped rather than continued in conjunction with the loop diuretic, because the two agents are very potent when used together. The combination of a thiazide and loop diuretic is indicated in cases of failure refractory to large doses of the loop diuretic alone. The maximal effect of a loop diuretic can be achieved by using a large single daily dose, rather than smaller doses spread throughout the day.

In decompensated CHF, *absorption* of oral furosemide declines, which accounts for the oft-noted reduction in efficacy during an exacerbation of heart failure. Parenteral administration of the drug or high-dose oral therapy is required to achieve diuresis. At times, supplementing oral therapy with an occasional intravenous administration of a loop diuretic in the office will suffice to counter worsening failure refractory to oral therapy.

The *potassium-sparing diuretics* (amiloride, triamterene) are relatively weak agents used mainly in conjunction with thiazides and loop diuretics to prevent potassium depletion. Their onset of action is slow; full effect may take up to a week to become evident. The *mercurials* have dropped from use because of the need to administer them parenterally.

Monitoring Therapy. Monitoring *postural signs*, *blood urea nitrogen (BUN)*, and *creatinine* are essential to avoid excess volume depletion and severe prerenal azotemia. When a potassium-wasting diuretic is being used in conjunction with digitalis therapy, it is critical to carefully monitor the *serum potassium* (see Appendix). The incidence of digitalis toxicity rises appreciably in the setting of hypokalemia. *Magnesium depletion* may also be triggered by diuretic therapy and contribute to digitalis sensitivity and refractory hypokalemia. Use of a potassium-sparing drug necessitates watching for hyperkalemia and discontinuing chronic potassium supplementation once hypokalemia is corrected.

Diuretic Preparations. *Thiazides* are sulfonamide derivatives, believed to inhibit sodium reabsorption in the cortical tubule. Although the number of thiazide preparations is large, they differ only in cost and duration of action. *Hydrochlorothiazide* is the least expensive and is available generically. Thiazides cause modest potassium depletion, which can be clinically important if there is underlying heart disease, especially in the setting of ventricular irritability, ischemia, or use of digitalis. Under such circumstances, careful monitoring for hypokalemia and assiduous potassium supplementation are essential. Sometimes a potassium-sparing diuretic may be used instead of a potassium chloride supplement (see below). Hyperglycemia and hyperuricemia are commonly encountered when thiazides are used. They are usually of little clinical significance (see Chapter 21). During the first 7 to 10 days of therapy, the serum calcium may rise, but it will stay elevated indefinitely only in patients with underlying hyperparathyroidism. Absorption from the GI tract is rapid; onset of action is 1 hour, and half-life 12 to 24 hours.

Metolazone is another sulfonamide diuretic, an agent similar to the thiazides in site of action, but possessing a longer half-life and more effective for treatment of mild CHF in patients with impaired renal function. Metolazone has an effective half-life of 24 to 48 hours, compared to 12 to 24 hours for the thiazides. Being a sulfonamide, it shares many of the same side effects, such as hypokalemia, hyperglycemia, and hyperuricemia. The maximum daily dose is 10 to 20 mg. Metolazone can be combined with a loop diuretic for use in very refractory cases in which volume overload is a major problem.

Loop diuretics are potent agents that act at the loop of Henle. They include *furosemide*, *ethacrynic acid*, and *bumetanide*. Their absorption is rapid, and onset of diuretic action occurs within 30 to 60 minutes, lasting 4 to 8 hours. Caution must be exercised, since serious volume depletion may occur with their use. Prerenal azotemia (manifested by a BUN–creatinine ratio of more than 20:1), postural hypotension, light-headedness, and fatigue are clues to marked hypovolemia. Hypokalemia, hyperglycemia, and hyperuricemia may occur. Ethacrynic acid is potentially ototoxic, especially when used in combination with an aminoglycoside antibiotic such as kanamycin. Audiograms should be obtained if ethacrynic acid is to be given for a prolonged period.

Frequent urination is a common complaint in patients using these potent diuretics; evening doses should be avoided if possible. Starting dose of furosemide is 20 to 40 mg/d. If this amount does not produce the desired effect, the amount of the single dose should be increased rather than the frequency of doses. In many instances, one daily dose is sufficient, maximally effective, and well tolerated by the patient. Potassium loss can be countered by prescribing potassium supplements or adding a potassium-sparing diuretic (see further discussion).

Potassium-sparing diuretics (*spironolactone, triamterene,* and *amiloride*) are commonly used. The former is an antagonist of aldosterone, the latter two are not, but they clinically behave in a manner similar to spironolactone. All are weak diuretics when used alone and should never be used initially in CHF. Their role is to help preserve potassium and supplement diuresis. Serious hyperkalemia may occur, necessitating frequent serum potassium determinations and discontinuation of potassium supplements. These drugs should not be used in renal failure, since life-threatening hyperkalemia may ensue. Spironolactone has been known to cause gynecomastia; there is also a question of increased risk of carcinogenesis based on experiments in which high doses were given to rats.

Fixed combinations containing a potassium-sparing diuretic and a thiazide are heavily promoted and expensive (see Chapter 21), though they are convenient and facilitate compliance. Prior to prescribing such a preparation, the proper dose of each agent should be determined separately. The combination preparation is reasonable to use only if it can provide the exact dosages desired. Many combinations contain subtherapeutic thiazide doses.

ACE Inhibitors and other Vasodilators

Advances in understanding the effects of preload and afterload on cardiac output in the failing heart have added a new dimension to the treatment of congestive heart failure. Agents have been sought that would act safely both on the arterial bed (to reduce impedance to the ejection of blood from the left ventricle) and on the venous bed (to decrease preload and reduce pulmonary and systemic venous congestion). Initially, no single agent sufficed—prazosin, minoxidil, hydralazine, and the calcium channel blockers were all tried—though the *combined use* of *hydralazine* for arterial dilation and *isosorbide* for venodilation achieved significant afterload and preload reductions and symptomatic improvement. Isosorbide acts predominantly on capacitance vessels to reduce preload, though at the high doses required for use in CHF (up to 80 mg tid–qid), it also causes some arterial dilatation and modest decreases in systemic resistance. CHF patients with marked pulmonary and systemic venous congestion are especially good candidates. A landmark Veterans Administration study found a 20 percent to 30 percent reduction in mortality and marked improvement in hemodynamics with use of this combination in patients with mild to moderate heart failure.

With the advent of *ACE inhibitors* (captopril, enalapril, lisinopril, and others) came the opportunity to achieve both goals with a single agent, and in a more physiologically advantageous manner than previously achievable. These agents are very active on both the arterial and venous sides of the circulation, decreasing left ventricular filling pressure and increasing cardiac output. They bind to a receptor on the angiotensin converting enzyme, preventing the formation of angiotensin II—a potent vasoconstrictor and stimulant of renin and aldosterone secretion. Conventional vasodilator therapy triggers neurohumoral counterregulatory mechanisms that result in reflex vasoconstriction, adrenergic stimulation of the heart, and sodium retention; the ACE inhibitors do not set off such counterregulatory forces.

Unlike digitalis—whose efficacy is confined to patients with severe systolic dysfunction—ACE inhibitors have been found effective in most CHF patients, whether they are suffering from mild, moderate, or severe disease. Several landmark studies have documented this broad spectrum of efficacy. The CONSENSUS Study of enalapril in *severe* congestive heart failure (New York Heart Association class IV) demonstrated a 27 percent reduction in *overall mortality* and a 50 percent reduction in *mortality from progressive heart failure* compared with conventional therapy that included use of other vasodilators as well as diuretics and digoxin. Reductions in heart size, symptoms, and need for other medications were also found. The SOLVD Study examined the effects of enalapril on survival in patients with less severe heart failure (NYHA class II and III). There was a 22 percent reduction in deaths from progressive heart failure.

Selection of Vasodilator Agent. Most vasodilators have been found to improve circulatory dynamics when used acutely, but acute response does not predict efficacy of chronic therapy. An important double-blind, randomized comparison of enalapril versus hydralazine-isosorbide addressed this question in patients with mild to moderate heart failure (the Vasodilator-Heart Failure Trial). Two-year mortality was significantly lower in the enalapril group, especially in patients with less severe symptoms, but ejection fraction increased more in the hydralazine-isosorbide group. Both groups had similarly reduced death rates from progressive heart failure, but the hydralazine-isosorbide group had a higher rate of cardiac sudden death, perhaps due to the combination's greater stimulation of neurohumoral counterregulatory mechanisms. These data suggest that *ACE inhibitor therapy is superior* to nonspecific vasodilators (eg, hydralazine-isosorbide) in patients with chronic congestive heart failure, probably in part by not triggering potentially harmful neurohumoral counterregulatory mechanisms.

Debate continues on the *ACE inhibitor of choice*. In the few randomized, controlled studies directly comparing ACE inhibitors for treatment of chronic CHF, both long- and short-acting preparations proved hemodynamically effective, but the *long-acting agents* (eg, *enalapril, lisinopril*) demonstrate greater risk of prolonged hypotension and impairment of renal perfusion, especially when used in high doses, than do the *short-acting agents* such as *captopril*. The high affinity of the long-acting agents for the converting-enzyme receptor completely inhibits production of angiotensin II, whereas inhibition is less sustained with the short-acting drugs. Unfortunately, the number of comparative studies is small and their adverse findings perhaps exaggerated by their use of very high doses of ACE inhibitor (eg, 40 mg/d of enalapril) in conjunction with fixed doses of diuretic, which may have exacerbated hypotensive and renal perfusion risks. Subsequent placebo-controlled studies of long-acting agents used at much lower doses in conjunction with variable diuretic doses suggest less risk.

Duration of action is probably less important to selection of agent than is the need for careful titration of ACE inhibitor and diuretic doses. The advent of sustained-release captopril formulations may further blur the distinction between short- and long-acting preparations. Captopril is now available generically, lowering the cost of ACE inhibitor therapy. Quality-of-life study comparing captopril with enalapril in hypertensive patients suggests that captopril may be the better tolerated.

Initiating Therapy and Minimizing Adverse Effects. Vasodilator therapy with an ACE inhibitor should be considered if diuretics alone fail to control congestive symptoms, especially in patients with mild to moderate CHF and absence of a third heart sound—patients who are not candidates for digitalis. It is important to inquire into exercise tolerance. Patients may note improvement at rest with use of diuretics +/- digitalis, but if exercise tolerance remains limited, then a trial of ACE inhibitor therapy deserves consideration. Treatment need not be delayed until the end stages of CHF; vasodilator therapy has proven quite safe and well tolerated when used with care in CHF.

Since *hypotension* is common at the onset of therapy, it is recommended to start with *small doses* (eg, as little as 6.25 mg of captopril or 2.5 mg of enalapril) and *reduce concurrent diuretic therapy*. The dose is then increased gradually (eg, up to as much as 100 mg of captopril tid–qid or 10–20 mg of enalapril qd). Monitoring *blood pressure* is important not only to assure adequate renal perfusion, but also to minimize dizziness and falls. Most CHF patients are elderly and can be very susceptible to even mild degrees of cerebral hypoperfusion. Continuous blood pressure monitoring is needed, because onset of hypotension may be delayed a few weeks, yet persist.

Renal function should also be closely monitored (BUN, creatinine, and urinalysis). Any deterioration in renal function should result in dose reduction, which usually suffices. Patients with preexisting renal dysfunction and those receiving very large ACE inhibitor doses are at greatest risk for renal injury. Rarely is discontinuation of therapy necessary, though there have been case reports of proteinuria and membranous glomerulopathy linked to ACE inhibitor therapy that resolved only with cessation of therapy.

Since ACE inhibitors reduce aldosterone levels, the *serum potassium* may rise and should be monitored, particularly in patients receiving potassium supplementation or a potassium-sparing agent as part of their diuretic therapy. Such supplementation should be reduced or even discontinued. Other adverse effects are mostly idiosyncratic and include a dry, irritant *cough* (effecting as many as 10%), *neutropenia* (usually within the first 3 months and only with captopril, due to its sulfhydryl group), *loss of taste*, and *rash* (including necrotizing vasculitis).

The Newer Inotropic Agents

Despite the development of vasodilator therapy, the search continues for agents that will improve contractility better and more safely than digitalis. *Phosphodiesterase inhibitors* are potent enhancers of contractility, but experimental results have been marred by increased rates of cardiac death. Early reports noted impressive clinical improvement with such agents as *milrinone*, *flosequinan*, and *vesnarinone*, but follow-up revealed unacceptable rates of cardiac morbidity and mortality—flosequinan had to be recalled after receiving Food and Drug Administration approval. Vesnarinone improves survival and functional status when used in doses too small to affect phosphodiesterase, but in larger doses, cardiac mortality rises markedly.

These results underscore the importance of factors other than contractility in determining the outcome of CHF. Demonstrating improved contractility does necessarily predict improved outcome. Neurohumoral activation is believed to be a causative factor affecting CHF mortality. *Beta-blockers* have been used investigationally in an attempt to counter this potentially harmful sympathetic stimulation.

Oral Anticoagulation

Although the presence of CHF is not, per se, an indication for warfarin anticoagulant therapy, it does increase the risk of thromboembolic disease in a patient with an underlying predisposition for an embolic event. For example, the CHF patient who is put to bed rest is at increased risk of deep vein thrombophlebitis and deserves consideration for anticoagulation (see Chapter 35). The same holds true for the patient in atrial fibrillation who develops CHF (see Chapter 28). The initiation and monitoring of oral anticoagulant therapy require considerable attention to detail (see Chapter 83).

Concurrent Drug Use and Nonpharmacologic Measures

Use of medications that might depress left ventricular function or alter neurohumoral regulatory mechanisms should be undertaken with extreme care and only after the potential risk is weighed. For example, *beta-blocking agents, disopyramide,* and such calcium channel blockers as *verapamil* are myocardial suppressants; they are relatively contraindicated for use in CHF. In a study of the role of prostaglandins in CHF, it was discovered that use of prostaglandin inhibitors, such as the *nonsteroidal anti-inflammatory agent* indomethacin, caused a worsening of CHF in patients with advanced disease complicated by hyponatremia; patients without hyponatremia were unaffected.

Fortunately, some important medications are not contraindicated in CHF. For example, the *tricyclic antidepressants* do not cause a reduction in left ventricular performance; they are relatively well tolerated, though they occasionally cause postural hypotension in CHF patients. A study of the effects of *acute intake of alcohol* on patients with functional class III or IV CHF found no deleterious effect on cardiac function; in fact, a modest reduction in afterload was noted, though the authors hastened to add that they were not recommending alcohol as a vasodilator.

Salt Restriction has traditionally occupied an important place in supportive therapy. It is probably most helpful in preventing unnecessary exacerbations of failure. Patients are placed on a *no-added-salt diet*, which provides about *4 g of sodium per day*. The patient and family are instructed to prepare and serve meals without addition of salt and to avoid foods with large salt content, including canned ham (which is packed in salt water), bacon, catsup, canned soups, and other processed foods. Rarely is extreme salt restriction (eg, 1–2 g sodium diet) urged on the patient, since it is often unrealistic and unpalatable, leading to poor caloric intake and depression. Fluid restriction is reserved for severe cases that are complicated by hyponatremia.

The Activity Prescription has an important function in minimizing myocardial work demands while maintaining the patient's ability to live as fully as possible. The level of allowable activity needs to be tailored to the patient's medical status, lifestyle, and responsibilities. Patients with symptoms of failure on moderate exertion (NYHA class II disease) can continue to work as long as reasonable limits are placed on emotional and physical demands. It may be more stressful psychologically (and consequently physically) to have to quit one's job than to continue working in a somewhat more limited capacity. In most instances, the amount of allowable activity can be determined from an office visit by a careful history that elicits the degree of exertion that precipitates symptoms. At times, symptoms may be out of proportion to physical findings; taking a walk up a flight of stairs with the patient can provide helpful data regarding exercise tolerance. Treadmill testing is sometimes necessary to gauge exercise capacity, especially if the patient has coronary disease and it is unclear whether it is failure or ischemia that is limiting the patient. Regardless of etiology, a daily rest period and reduction of psychological stress are key means of lessening myocardial work in the patient with failure.

If weight is increasing, orthopnea worsening, and dyspnea on exertion more severe and brought on by less exertion, activity should be further restricted. A few days of bed rest are often beneficial and may obviate the need for hospitalization. The patient with failure who is put to bed should use a footboard or get out of bed periodically to avoid prolonged venous stasis and thrombus formation.

PATIENT EDUCATION

Because the medical program is often complex and the need for compliance is great, the physician must take the time to discuss with patient and family the rationale behind therapy and to set with them the guidelines for activity, diet, and use of medication. In this way they can become valuable partners in the treatment effort.

Patients should be instructed to weigh themselves each morning before breakfast and to keep a *weight record*. If their clinical status, weight, and medication program are stable, less frequent recordings are necessary. Patients are advised to call their physician if weight increases suddenly by more than 2 or 3 pounds, because this may be the earliest sign of increasing CHF and a forerunner of more severe symptoms. Reliable, intelligent patients may be instructed to adjust their diuretic doses according to weight. Debilitated or uncooperative individuals should have a family member or visiting nurse obtain weight recordings. Weight is among the most helpful parameters to follow in outpatient management of failure.

Patients and their families must know the identity of the medication being used. It is easy for the patient to become confused, because multiple-drug regimens are common and many of the pills are similar in appearance. Medication booklets are invaluable. Each tablet is taped to the page alongside its generic and brand names, dose schedule, indication for use, and warning signs of toxicity. For patients with poor eyesight, a family member or visiting nurse should put out and set aside the pills to be taken each day.

INDICATIONS FOR REFERRAL AND ADMISSION

Patients with markedly worsening or refractory failure should be considered for hospital admission. For the patient with stubbornly persistent disease, hospitalization provides the opportunity for valuable observation under controlled conditions that assure compliance with the medical regimen. Moreover, hospitalization provides opportunity to initiate additional therapy under close supervision and to search for a treatable underlying etiology that may have initially eluded detection. Cardiac consultation is indicated for the patient who appears refractory to standard therapy. Relatively young patients failing maximal medical therapy may be appropriate for consideration of transplantation, provided renal, pulmonary, hepatic, and central nervous system functions are preserved. Other indications for admission include evidence of digitalis toxicity, renal failure, hypotension, and inadequate support and supervision at home.

THERAPEUTIC RECOMMENDATIONS

- Identify the etiology of the CHF (eg, dysrhythmia, hypertension, valvular disease, ischemia, cardiomyopathy) and any precipitating factors (eg, fever, anemia, atrial fibrillation, infection, salt excess); treat these specifically if they are amenable to therapy, rather than relying solely on symptomatic measures to ameliorate the CHF.
- Initiate a no-added-salt diet (4 g sodium), but do not restrict water intake unless dilutional hyponatremia ensues.
- Begin diuretic therapy if there is evidence of volume overload or pulmonary venous congestion. If the CHF is *mild*, prescribe a thiazide (eg, *hydrochlorothiazide 50–100 mg/d*).
- If CHF is *more severe*, use a loop diuretic (eg, *furosemide 20–40 mg bid*). Be alert for a very brisk diuresis in patients who have never before received a loop diuretic. Exert particular caution with use of potent diuretics in situations

that require a high filling pressure (eg, critical aortic stenosis).

- In initial stages of loop diuretic use, divide daily dose to minimize the inconvenience of a large diuresis in the morning or evening that might interfere with activity. Avoid giving an evening dose if sleep is being interrupted by nocturia.
- If patient does not respond adequately to a loop diuretic dose that is being given in divided fashion, try combining the entire daily dose into one administration of the drug, before increasing total daily dose.
- If moderate doses of diuretic therapy do not suffice to relieve congestive symptoms, then *add* an *ACE inhibitor*, starting at a low dose to minimize the risks of hypotension and hypoperfusion (eg, *6.25 mg captopril tid or 2.5 mg enalapril qd*). Monitor blood pressure, potassium, BUN, and creatinine, and decrease diuretic dose if blood pressure falls or prerenal azotemia develops.
- Gradually advance ACE inhibitor therapy as needed to improve exercise tolerance and relieve congestive symptoms while continuing to monitor blood pressure, potassium, and renal function. Average captopril dose is 25 to 50 mg tid; for enalapril, the average dose is 10 to 20 mg qd.
- In patients with severe heart failure due to *marked systolic dysfunction* (manifested by a low ejection fraction, S_3, and marked LV dilation), consider starting *digitalis* therapy. Digitalis is also indicated when the cause of CHF is rapid atrial fibrillation, severe hypertension, or tight aortic stenosis. *Digoxin* is the digitalis preparation of choice, except in the setting of severe renal failure.
- If the candidate for digitalis is relatively stable, one can begin therapy with an oral maintenance dose program (eg, *digoxin .25 mg/d*), checking the serum level in 1 week and making any needed dose adjustments on the basis of clinical response and serum level.
- If the digitalis candidate has worsening heart failure but does not require immediate hospitalization, then one can start digitalis therapy with a loading dose of 1.0 to 1.25 mg of digoxin orally, given in 4 divided doses over 24 hours. Dose is then adjusted as above.
- Monitor patients on digitalis by following the heart rate, rhythm, and serum levels of *potassium*, *BUN*, *creatinine*, and *digoxin*. If prerenal azotemia develops, then obtain a serum digoxin level and reduce the dose until a serum digoxin level is available to guide further administration. One can estimate the required dose from available nomograms or use the serum level as a guide. Serum digoxin level should be drawn no sooner than 6 hours after the last dose, because there is a transient increase in serum level after an oral dose.
- If, on monitoring heart rate and rhythm, a cardiac dysrhythmia is noted, it should be investigated quickly. Dysrhythmias strongly suggestive of digitalis toxicity include paroxysmal atrial tachycardia with block, ventricular irritability (especially bigeminy), junctional tachycardia, and severe bradycardia.
- Monitor serum *potassium* in all CHF patients, but particularly closely in those taking digitalis. Hypokalemia, which results from diuretic therapy, should be avoided, because it enhances sensitivity to the toxic effects of digitalis, especially dysrhythmias.
- Prevent potassium depletion by dietary potassium supplementation or use of an oral potassium preparation (see Appendix). Alternatively, a potassium-sparing diuretic may be helpful. Oral potassium supplements and potassium-sparing diuretics should be used with extreme caution, if at all, in patients taking ACE inhibitors, since the latter increase serum potassium. If a potassium-sparing diuretic is used, chronic oral potassium supplementation should be stopped.
- If an oral potassium preparation is employed, begin with an agent that provides chloride as well as potassium in order to avoid diuretic-induced hypokalemic alkalosis; however, if possible avoid potassium chloride tablets, because they risk injury to the gastrointestinal mucosa.
- Monitor *serum magnesium* in patients taking digitalis and those with refractory hypokalemia. Diuretic-induced hypomagnesemia is common and may impair potassium repletion; it also enhances sensitivity to the toxic effects of digitalis.
- Consider oral anticoagulant therapy for CHF patients if prolonged bed rest, atrial fibrillation, or severe congestive cardiomyopathy ensue (see Chapter 83).
- Avoid, if possible, large doses and combinations of cardiac drugs with negative inotropic effects such as verapamil, disopyramide, and beta-blockers. If beneficial, use smallest dose possible.
- Provide patient and family with thorough instruction on the purpose and proper use of medications prescribed for CHF. Advise patient to check his or her weight regularly, measuring it before breakfast and calling if there is an unexplained weight gain of more than 2 to 3 pounds since the last reading.
- Advise bed rest for exacerbations of CHF, but discourage major reorganization of a patient's lifestyle unless symptoms are severe and refractory.
- Admit for refractory or markedly worsening CHF, suspected digitalis toxicity, or inadequate support and supervision at home.
- Obtain cardiac consultation for refractory or rapidly worsening cases, and consider transplantation for the relatively young patient with end-stage myocardial disease but preserved renal, hepatic, pulmonary, and neurologic function.

A.H.G.

ANNOTATED BIBLIOGRAPHY

Braunwald E. Ace inhibitors—a cornerstone of the treatment of heart failure. N Engl J Med 1991;325:351. *(An editorial summarizing the evidence for the central role of these drugs in treatment of CHF.)*

Chakko S, Woska D, Martinez H, et al. Clinical, radiographic, hemodynamic correlations in chronic congestive heart failure: conflicting results may lead to inappropriate care. Am J Med 1991;90:353. *(Critical look at methods for diagnosis of CHF.)*

Cohn JN, Johnson G, Ziesche S, et al. A comparison of enalapril with hydralazine-isosorbide dinitrate in the treatment of chronic congestive heart failure. N Engl J Med 1991;325:303. *(Enalapril proved superior to hydralazine-isosorbide, though mechanisms of action differed and suggested possible complementarity.)*

The CONSENSUS Trial Study Group. Effects of enalapril on mortality in severe congestive heart failure. N Engl J Med 1987;23:1429. *(Adding enalapril to conventional therapy reduced mortality and improved symptoms in this prospective, randomized, multicenter study of patients with severe heart failure.)*

Deedwania PC. Angiotensin-converting enzyme inhibitors in congestive heart failure. Arch Intern Med 1990;150:1798. *(A useful clinical review; 61 refs.)*

Feldman AM, Bristow MR, Parmley WM, et al. Effects of vesnarinone on morbidity and mortality in patients with heart failure. N Engl J Med 1993;329:149. *(Improved survival noted, but only when used in non-inotropic doses.)*

Fleg JL, Hinton PC, La Katta EG, et al. Physician utilization of laboratory procedures to monitor outpatients with congestive heart failure. Arch Intern Med 1989;149:393. *(High cost of monitoring documented among those using diagnostic studies for monitoring.)*

Grossman W. Diastolic dysfunction in congestive heart failure. N Engl J Med 1991;325:1557. *(Excellent basic science review of diastolic dysfunction that is clinically useful.)*

Jaeschke R, Oxman AD, Guyatt GH. To what extent do congestive heart failure patients in sinus rhythm benefit from digoxin therapy? A systematic overview and meta-analysis. Am J Med 1990;88:279. *(A meta-analytic study indicating that patients with severe systolic dysfunction do best.)*

Lee DC, Johnson RA, Bingham JB, et al. Heart failure in outpatients: a randomized trial of digoxin versus placebo. N Engl J Med 1982;306:699. *(Only CHF patients with an S3 and other signs of severe systolic dysfunction showed benefit from long-term digoxin therapy.)*

Packer M. The search for the ideal positive inotropic agent. N Engl J Med 1993;329:201. *(An editorial addressing the significance of the increase in mortality seen with use of many positively inotropic agents.)*

Packer M, Carver JR, Rodeheffer RJ, et al. Effect of oral milrinone on mortality in severe chronic heart failure. N Engl J Med 1991;325:1468. *(Hemodynamic effects were beneficial, but long-term cardiovascular morbidity and mortality were increased with the use of this potent inotropic agent.)*

Packer M, Gheorghiade M, Young JB, et al. Withdrawal of digoxin from patients with chronic heart failure treated with angiotensin-converting-enzyme inhibitors. N Engl J Med 1993; 329:1. *(Withdrawal of digoxin associated with an increased risk of worsening in patients with systolic dysfunction.)*

Packer M, Lee WH, Yushak M, et al. Comparison of captopril and enalapril in patients with severe chronic heart failure. N Engl J Med 1986;315:847. *(Both were effective, but enalapril use was more likely to cause hypotension and renal dysfunction; unfortunately, only very large doses were used.)*

Smith TW. Digoxin in heart failure. N Engl J Med 1993;329:51. *(An editorial summarizing evidence for efficacy.)*

The SOLVD Investigators. Effect of enalapril on survival in patients with reduced left ventricular ejection fractions and congestive heart failure. N Engl J Med 1991;325:293. *(Enalapril reduced mortality and hospitalization in this important randomized, prospective, multicenter trial of patients with mild to moderate heart failure.)*

Spirito P, Maron BJ. Doppler echocardiography for assessing left ventricular diastolic function. Ann Intern Med 1988;109:122. *(A review of the technique for diagnosis of diastolic dysfunction; 70 refs.)*

Testa MA, Anderson RB, Nackley JF, et al. Quality of life and antihypertensive therapy in men—a comparison of captopril with enalapril. N Engl J Med 1993;328:907. *(Captopril was the better tolerated.)*

Whang R. Magnesium deficiency: pathogenesis, prevalence, and clinical implications. Am J Med 1987;82(suppl 3A):24. *(A terse review of this important problem, especially in patients taking digitalis and diuretics.)*

Appendix: Potassium Supplementation

Patients with heart failure have considerable underlying heart disease, and many take digitalis and diuretics; as such, they are at greatly increased risk for hypokalemia-induced arrhythmias. Prompt correction and prevention of hypokalemia are essential. There is less consensus regarding the need for such assiduous treatment of hypokalemia in patients without underlying heart disease; a potassium as low as 3.0 mg/dL is usually rather well tolerated.

Individual responses to potassium-wasting diuretics and requirements for potassium replacement vary widely, necessitating regular monitoring of the serum potassium level, which is not an exact measure of total body potassium, but rather a rough guide.

Supplements may be taken in the form of dietary additions or potassium-containing preparations. The amount needed is usually determined empirically, ranging from 0 to 60 mEq/d over and above normal dietary potassium intake. For patients on thiazides, dietary replacement often suffices. When a loop diuretic is used, the potassium loss may be greater, necessitating a potassium preparation (unless a potassium-sparing agent is used.) *Dietary supplements* are the most palatable way to provide potassium. There are 15 mEq in a 10-oz glass of orange, pineapple, or grapefruit juice; a medium-sized banana; a baked potato; or two oranges. Tomato juice has almost twice the potassium content of orange juice, but most brands have added salt to enhance taste.

Salt Substitutes contain potassium chloride (KCl), but some are also 50 percent sodium chloride. Even those that are pure KCl do not provide sufficient potassium to serve effectively as a supplement.

Patients who need to maintain normokalemia but cannot do so by dietary means require a *potassium preparation.* There is a plethora of these on the market. Oral supplements combine potassium with any of a number of different anions. Only the chloride form is effective in correcting the hypokalemic alkalosis that results from diuretic use. However, any form will prevent potassium depletion unless there is concurrently severe sodium chloride depletion.

Potassium Chloride Elixir remains the safest and least expensive. The 10 percent solution contains 20 mEq of potassium per tablespoon (15 mL). It is most easily taken in orange juice; some find it unpalatable, even when mixed in fruit juice. However, when faced with the high cost of alternatives, many patients who complain of its taste are willing to reconsider using it. Its safety, chloride content, and ability to deliver more potassium per dose than most other preparations strongly recommend it. Citrus flavored *effervescent* tablets dissolved in water provide an alternative to the elixir preparation, but at greater cost and without much improvement in taste.

Potassium Chloride Tablets of many types have been produced. The earliest preparations caused a high incidence of mucosal injury, leading to gastrointestinal ulceration, bleeding, obstruction, and perforation. A second generation of tablet preparations was devised by encoating them in a *wax matrix* in order to slow release and reduce mucosal injury. Examples include Slow-K, Kaon-Cl, Klotrix, K-Tab, and others. Encoating did decrease the risk of gastrointestinal complications, but did not eliminate it. Complications continue to occur, often in unpredictable fashion.

Microencapsulation represents another release strategy. KCl is prepared in small crystals, each coated with a polymer permeable to water, theoretically helping to disperse the potassium while minimizing locally high concentrations. Endoscopic data suggest some improved safety over other tablet forms, but cost is almost 10 times that of the elixir for an equivalent dose. Moreover, since each tablet contains only 8 mEq of potassium, multiple tablets are needed each day to provide the 15 to 45 mEq usually required.

Potassium Gluconate and Bicarbonate preparations are available, some in the form of liquids, others as effervescent tablets. Although they tend to be more palatable, disadvantages include high cost and absence of chloride to counter alkalosis.

If all attempts at potassium supplementation fail, then a potassium-sparing diuretic is indicated. Combinations with a thiazide are now available in generic formulation and may provide a reasonable and inexpensive alternative to diuretic plus potassium supplementation in patients requiring both a thiazide and tight potassium control. Refractory hypokalemia requires checking for hypomagnesemia (see above).

A.H.G.

ANNOTATED BIBLIOGRAPHY

Micro-K potassium supplement. The Medical Letter 1982;24:71. *(This KCl preparation may be safer than previously available slow-release preparations, but at greatly increased cost.)*

Slow-release potassium. Medical Letter 1978;20:29. *(Small bowel ulceration continues to be reported in patients using these preparations.)*

33
Management of Acquired Valvular Heart Disease

RICHARD R. LIBERTHSON, M.D.

Primary Care Medicine: Office Evaluation and Management of the Adult Patient, 3rd edition, edited by Allan H. Goroll, Lawrence A. May, and Albert G. Mulley, Jr. J.B. Lippincott Company, Philadelphia

As a result of increased physician awareness and improvements in noninvasive diagnostic techniques, the diagnosis of acquired valvular heart disease is being made earlier in the course of illness. Outpatient management has become commonplace because symptoms are frequently absent or mild at the time the condition is discovered. Although consultation with a cardiologist is often obtained, the responsibility for long-term care usually falls on the primary physician.

To properly manage the patient with valvular heart disease, the primary physician must be familiar with the condition's natural history, early warning signs of hemodynamic deterioration, and indications for and types of medical and surgical therapies. Of major importance is the proper timing of referral for consideration of invasive therapy.

NATURAL HISOTRY

Mitral Stenosis (MS)

Most cases of MS are *rheumatic* in origin, even though as many as 50 percent of patients cannot give a history of rheumatic fever. The symptom-free interval averages about 10 years (range is 3–25 y). In most instances, symptoms develop gradually over a decade, roughly paralleling the progression of stenosis; however, some people remain relatively free of complaints until stenosis becomes severe. Left atrial and pulmonary venous pressures increase substantially as valve area falls below 1.5 cm^2, and at this point patients typically experience *dyspnea on exertion*. Any stimulus that rapidly increases blood flow or decreases the time available for diastolic filling can precipitate a sudden increase in pulmonary congestion and result in acute shortness of breath. Strenuous activity, fever, emotion, and onset of atrial fibrillation are often responsible for acute dyspnea.

Progressive narrowing of the valve orifice is accompanied by worsening exercise tolerance and increasing dyspnea. In patients with tight stenosis (valve area <1.0 cm^2), the period from onset of symptoms to incapacity averages 7 years, but the decline can be precipitous with the onset of atrial fibrillation or pneumonia. Chronic marked increase in pulmonary venous pressure often leads to fixed *pulmonary hypertension*. Cardiac output usually falls with onset of severe pulmonary hypertension, and fatigue may become a prominent symptom. The right ventricle hypertrophies in response to the rise in pulmonary artery pressure, and *right-sided heart failure* and death ensue unless intervention occurs; deterioration may be rapid at this stage.

Atrial fibrillation complicates 40 percent to 50 percent of cases of symptomatic mitral stenosis. The correlation between development of atrial fibrillation and the severity of stenosis is slight and not due solely to the degree of left atrial enlargement. The loss of atrial systole and the increase in heart rate that characterize atrial fibrillation markedly reduce flow across the mitral valve and boost left atrial pressure. Premature atrial contractions and paroxysmal atrial fibrillation often precede sustained atrial fibrillation due to mitral stenosis.

Systemic embolization occurs in 10 percent to 20 percent of patients with MS. Age and presence of atrial fibrillation are the major determinants of risk; severity of stenosis is not a determinant, and, in fact, embolization may be a presenting symptom of MS.

In sum, there is typically a symptom-free period of about 10 years. Patients then begin to note dyspnea on exertion over the next 10 years, which progresses in many instances in the following decade. Once symptoms are present on minimal exertion, survival becomes markedly reduced. Patients with New York Heart Association class IV disease (symptoms at rest) have been found to have a 5-year mortality rate of 85 percent. Some patients have disease that may remain stable for many years. In another subset of patients, symptoms do not develop until late in the illness.

Mitral Regurgitation (MR)

Rheumatic Mitral Regurgitation can remain asymptomatic for many years, because the left ventricle dilates and adjusts well to the increase in volume load. Onset of dyspnea and fatigue may not occur for decades. Symptoms take an average of 10 years to progress to the point of disability and need for surgery. It is not until very *late* in the course of the disease that myocardial reserve falters. Once the left ventricle fails, patients note *progressive dyspnea* and *fatigue*; symptoms become present at rest (functional class IV disease). If pulmonary hypertension develops, signs of right-sided heart failure will ensue. Prognosis is poor at this stage.

Atrial fibrillation is found in more than 75 percent of cases, but the abrupt episodes of pulmonary congestion that typify mitral stenosis complicated by atrial fibrillation are less frequent in MR, although rupture of one of the chordae tendineae can result in sudden deterioration.

Nonrheumatic Forms of Chronic MR are commonly encountered in the outpatient setting. Etiologies include mitral valve prolapse, papillary muscle dysfunction, and calcified mitral valve annulus.

Mitral Valve Prolapse (MVP) is one of the most common valvular disorders, with prevalence estimates of 4 percent to 7 percent. The condition usually does not produce hemodynamically significant regurgitation, and the amount of regurgitant flow tends not to increase with time, though a small subset—those with an initial left ventricular diastolic dimension in excess of 60 mm—may eventually require mitral valve replacement. Patients with redundant valves on echocardiogram are at increased risk for sudden death, infective endocarditis, and cerebral embolization. However, for the vast majority the prognosis is excellent, and most are entirely asymptomatic. There is a slight increase in risk of *bacterial endocarditis*, especially in those with clinically evident regurgitation or a redundant valve. The American Heart Association suggests endocarditis prophylaxis for those with MVP who have evidence of mitral insufficiency; other authorities suggest prophylaxis for all MVP patients (see Chapter 16).

Some have raised the question of a relation between *panic disorder* and MVP, because of panic-like symptoms occurring in a small percentage of patients with MVP. Indeed, a small percentage of MVP patients do suffer from *autonomic dysfunction* and complain of palpitations, atypical chest pain, orthostatic dizziness, near-syncope, cold extremities, throbbing headaches, and neurasthenia and manifest tachyarrhythmias, orthostatic hypotension, and peripheral vasoconstriction. However, careful studies have found no causal link between MVP and autonomic dysfunction or panic disorder. A very small group of MVP patients have *ventricular irritability*; in rare instances there is a history of ventricular fibrillation and a family history of sudden death.

Papillary Muscle Dysfunction is responsible for as many as 10 percent of MR cases found clinically. Causes include ischemic injury, left ventricular dilatation, and cardiomyopathy. Ischemic heart disease is the most frequent etiology, with 40 percent of posterior infarcts and 20 percent of anterior infarcts accompanied by the development of papillary muscle dysfunction. The amount of regurgitant flow is highly variable. Severe MR and marked pulmonary congestion can occur, even in the context of only a minimal reduction in left ventricular ejection fraction. However, prognosis does depend on left ventricular systolic performance.

Calcification of the Mitral Annulus occurs in older people, often in conjunction with calcification of the aortic valve. The mitral lesion is usually not of hemodynamic significance, but heart block can develop if calcification extends into the ventricular septum.

Mixed Mitral Disease

Mortality is increased when significant stenosis and regurgitation occur simultaneously. In one large series of patients managed medically, the 10-year survival rate from the time of diagnosis was 33 percent.

Aortic Stenosis (AS)

Because of the marked ability of the left ventricle to hypertrophy and compensate for the pressure load, patients with AS can remain symptom-free for many years, even with tight stenosis (valve area <0.7 cm^2). This is especially true in young patients. However, it must be remembered that sudden death can occur in previously asymptomatic individuals with critical AS. Onset of *angina* and *effort syncope* suggest a hemodynamically critical lesion that is limiting cardiac output, although in as many as 30 percent to 60 percent of AS patients with angina, there coexists significant occlusion of a coronary vessel. Survival averages 3 years from the onset of angina or effort syncope. The development of *congestive failure* is an ominous sign, for it signals the inability of the myocardium to continue tolerating the severe pressure load; survival averages 2 years from the time failure is first noted. More than half of patients with AS die of congestive failure. Sudden death accounts for another 20 percent. The mean age of death for patients dying suddenly is 60 years; the mechanism of death in these cases is believed to be a dysrhythmia triggered by myocardial ischemia, though debate continues. The rate of stenosis is unpredictable and can progress rapidly over a few years, especially as the patient enters his sixties. Figures for survival are only averages; the range is wide, and many patients die soon after the onset of symptoms.

Age at clinical onset of AS is dependent in part on the underlying etiology. Significant AS appearing in a patient younger than 30 years of age is congenital in origin, due most often to a *bicuspid* valve. In approximately 15 percent of such patients, obstruction is caused by a discrete *subaortic membrane*. Patients presenting between ages 30 and 70 have either a bicuspid valve or a valve damaged by *rheumatic fever.* Those who present with significant AS caused by rheumatic fever average 10 to 15 years older than patients who present with rheumatic mitral stenosis, due to the more gradual progression of the illness when it involves the aortic valve. Nevertheless, the course can be one of rapid deterioration.

AS developing in the *elderly* is usually due to *primary degenerative calcification* of a normal aortic valve. Unlike AS caused by rheumatic disease with its fusion of valve commissures, calcific aortic stenosis results from calcific thickening of the valve leaflets and their loss of mobility. Patients with calcification of a bicuspid valve may present as early as the sixth decade; those with senile calcification of a tricuspid aortic valve present with stenosis in the eighth and ninth decades. By 80 years of age, half of the population has a systolic ejection murmur; in a small percentage, hemodynamically significant stenosis ensues.

Calcific AS of the elderly now accounts for the majority of new AS cases. Unlike rheumatic AS with its fixed valve orifice, the degree of stenosis in calcific AS varies with the strength of the left ventricle (LV). The weaker its contraction, the less the valve will open and the greater the outflow obstruction. A failing LV may cause a rapid downhill course. Thus, the contractile state of the LV is a critical determinant of the clinical course of calcific AS. Also, the degree of calcification may progress.

Aortic Regurgitation (AR)

Rheumatic Fever accounts for the largest number of AR cases. Most patients live for decades with little incapacity, as the left ventricle dilates to accommodate the extra volume load. The latent period from occurrence of rheumatic fever to onset of clinical manifestations is about 10 years. During the next decade, symptoms appear and progress. The onset of symptoms is typically gradual, with *palpitations* being among the earliest changes noted by the patient, followed by *dyspnea on exertion* and *fatigability*. Appearance of *left ventricular hypertrophy* (LVH) with strain and progressive *left ventricular dilation* are associated with a markedly increased risk of heart failure and death within 5 years. If exertional dyspnea worsens, other manifestations of congestive failure are likely to follow and signal the beginning of a rapidly declining phase of the disease due to left ventricular decompensation. At this stage, deterioration is rapid, with death occurring within 1 to 2 years of the onset of congestive failure. *Angina* is common, reported by almost 30 percent of patients; unlike the angina of aortic stenosis, it typically takes place *at rest* rather than on exertion. Angina becomes more frequent when there is worsening heart failure. *Sudden death* may also occur in patients with severe aortic regurgitation.

Nonrheumatic Causes of chronic AR include syphilis, myxomatous degeneration, bacterial endocarditis, and connective tissue disease. Aortic regurgitation secondary to untreated *syphilis* appears about 15 to 25 years after the initial infection and often has a more rapidly downhill course than AR caused by rheumatic fever. *Myxomatous degeneration* has been found in 10 percent to 15 percent of cases of AR studied pathologically. The process is progressive and becomes clinically evident between the ages of 30 and 60. Although *bacterial endocarditis* can damage a tricuspid aortic valve, particularly one that is fibrotic or calcific, it is far more likely to occur with a biscuspid valve. *Ankylosing spondylitis* is complicated by AR in about 3 percent of cases. The severity of the lesion is highly variable, and conduction defects are frequent. AR may appear before the onset of other symptoms, but in most instances it follows the appearance of arthritic symptoms by 10 to 20 years. The presence of severe AR shortens the otherwise normal life expectancy of patients with ankylosing spondylitis. *Reiter's syndrome* is associated with the development of AR in 5 percent of cases, typically in those with florid manifestations of the disease such as iritis, mucocutaneous changes, and extensive sacroiliac inflammation. Onset of AR occurs an average of 15 years after the disease is first noted, often preceded by conduction disturbances. The severity and course of the AR are highly variable.

Mixed Aortic Valve Disease. Many patients with AS have some degree of AR, and vice versa. Whenever the gradient across the aortic valve is greater than 25 mm Hg in the context of significant regurgitation, there begins to develop a substantial pressure load as well as an increased volume load on the left ventricle. The clinical course is similar to that for isolated AS of the same degree, although some clinicians believe there is an earlier onset of symptoms.

Combined Aortic and Mitral Disease. The etiology is mostly rheumatic; in fact, most cases of rheumatic fever produce some degree of multiple valve damage, though disease of one valve often dominates the clinical picture. Mitral stenosis may be overlooked in the setting of concurrent heart failure, pneumonia, or aortic valvular disease. In a study of 152 patients with echocardiographically significant MS, 15 percent of MS cases were unrecognized prior to ultrasound examination, yet most had an audible murmur on reexamination. The most common combination is aortic regurgitation in conjunction with mitral disease. Atrial fibrillation and systemic embolization are more frequent than in isolated AR, as is the severity of pulmonary symptoms. Less common is the coexistence of AS and MS. Symptoms and signs of AS are blunted by significant MS, such that pulmonary symptoms, atrial fibrillation, and systemic embolization may dominate the presentation, but there may be more angina and syncope than expected from isolated MS. Course is dictated by the severity of the individual lesions, but MS can delay the appearance of some of the manifestations of advanced AS.

ESTIMATING SEVERITY OF DISEASE

Mitral Stenosis

Symptoms provide crude indications of the severity of stenosis. *Dyspnea* correlates with increase in left atrial pressure and development of *pulmonary venous congestion*, but the relationship between degree of stenosis and elevation of left atrial pressure is variable. *Fatigue* occurs most often in the context of *pulmonary hypertension*, but the nonspecific nature of the symptom lessens its utility in estimating severity. *Hemoptysis* is related to pulmonary *venous hypertension* but does not necessarily imply severe stenosis. Thus, history alone may fail to detect severe stenosis that is unaccompanied by marked pulmonary congestion; however, a worsening of dyspnea and a decline in exercise tolerance suggest hemodynamic deterioration and require further investigation.

On physical examination, the interval between the second heart sound and the opening snap, referred to as the *S_2-OS interval*, and the duration and timing of the diastolic murmur provide additional clues of severity. The S_2-OS interval is a function of the elevation in left atrial pressure. The greater the pressure, the shorter the interval. Unfortunately, the degree of MS is not the only determinant of left atrial pressure; the interval can be affected by factors other than valve area, such as heart rate and left ventricular pressure. Moreover, the valve must be mobile to snap; in advanced disease, the valve may calcify and the snap becomes inaudible. Nevertheless, the S_2-OS interval is useful because it can be determined at the bedside and does provide data that may help in judging severity when considered in the context of other findings. Perhaps the most precise use of the interval is in separating hemodynamically insignificant disease from moderate and severe MS. An interval of greater than 0.11 second at rest with a heart rate of 70 to 80 beats/min argues against a significant lesion (although there are exceptions). Patients with moderate to tight stenosis usually demonstrate intervals less than 0.08 second which shorten with exercise. Proper estimation of the S_2-OS interval takes considerable practice.

The intensity of the *diastolic murmur* does not correlate with severity of stenosis, but its duration through diastole does. However, development of pulmonary hypertension may decrease cardiac output from the right side of the heart, result in a diminution of flow across the mitral valve, and consequently shorten the duration of the murmur.

Chest x-ray provides important evidence of severity. The earliest radiologic sign of MS is dilation of the left atrium, which is best seen on a lateral view in conjunction with a barium swallow to outline the esophagus. The finding is not a very reliable manifestation of severity. A better sign is redistribution of pulmonary venous blood flow, producing dilation of the upper zone pulmonary veins. Upper zone redistribution becomes prominent at a left atrial pressure of 25 mm Hg and parallels severity of stenosis. This change in pulmonary venous flow is very sensitive to changes in left atrial pressure, but it is not unique to mitral stenosis. Radiologic evidence of pulmonary hypertension (dilation of the right pulmonary artery to 15–18 mm, rapid tapering of vessels, and right ventricular enlargement) strongly suggests advanced mitral stenosis, though again the findings are not specific for MS. Presence of Kerley B lines, perihilar haze, and other manifestations of interstitial edema are seen in patients with severe dyspnea due to MS; the absence of interstitial edema on chest film does not rule out tight MS, but a patient with dyspnea at rest should always show these changes on chest x-ray; otherwise, one must question the etiology of the shortness of breath. In sum, no single radiologic finding is specific for severe MS, but x-ray data can provide important supporting evidence.

The *electrocardiogram (ECG)* is of limited utility for estimation of severity. The best ECG sign appears to be the *QRS axis*; a rightward shift to greater than +60 is associated with a valve area of less than 1.3 cm^2 in more than 85 percent of cases. The absence of the rightward shift in axis means little. The greater the pulmonary artery pressure, the more likely right ventricular hypertrophy will appear on ECG.

Cardiac ultrasound (echocardiography) is the most sensitive noninvasive method for evaluating mitral stenosis. *One dimensional (M-mode)* echocardiography readily identifies mitral valve thickening, calcification (when present), and the degree of limitation of valvular movement or excursion. *Two-dimensional (B-mode)* echocardiography provides definitive assessment by allowing direct visualization of the entire valve and its supporting apparatus, measurement of the valve orifice, left atrial and left ventricular chamber dimensions, and assessment of abnormality of other cardiac valves. The addition of *Doppler ultrasound* techniques—including *continuous wave* Doppler and *color-flow* study—to the ultrasound examination provides detailed delineation of valve anatomy, blood flow, and magnitude of obstruction. A scoring system based on data from these noninvasive studies has evolved which identifies candidates for transcatheter balloon dilation of the stenotic valve.

Cardiac catheterization is indicated when symptoms are progressive and cardiac surgery or balloon valvuloplasty is being considered (see below).

Mitral Regurgitation

A reasonable estimate of the severity of mitral insufficiency can be obtained by history and physical examination. *Dyspnea on exertion* and *fatigability* are early symptoms of hemodynamically significant regurgitation, although the absence of such symptoms does not rule out severe disease. On physical examination, severe MR produces *left ventricular enlargement* with a hyperdynamic, slightly diffuse, apical impulse displaced to the left but of normal timing and duration. In addition, there is a pansystolic murmur (its loudness does not correlate directly with severity), a loud third heart sound (S_3), often a mid-diastolic rumble from increased flow across the mitral valve, and at times wide splitting of the second sound due to shortening of left ventricular systole and early aortic valve closure. In contrast to other forms of valvular disease, a third heart sound may sometimes be audible in an MR patient in the absence of other signs of severe MR and need not represent a failing left ventricle.

In patients with advanced disease, cardiomegaly and left atrial enlargement are pronounced on *chest film*. A normal heart on chest x-ray and absence of an apical pansystolic murmur rule out significant mitral regurgitation. The *ECG* reflects both left atrial and left ventricular enlargement, but is hardly specific for MR. *B-mode cardiac ultrasound* is useful for identifying the specific process causing the MR, be it rheumatic fever, prolapse, a ruptured chordae tendineae, or endocarditis. Also readily ascertained are such important items as left atrial and left ventricular size and ejection fraction. In addition, the severity of disease can be ascertained by *Doppler study* that includes color-flow mapping.

Cardiac catheterization is indicated in patients with progressive symptoms and rapidly increasing heart size who are being considered for surgery. One needs to estimate degree of regurgitation, assess ventricular function, and check for the presence and severity of associated valvular and coronary disease.

Aortic Stenosis

There are numerous pitfalls in the clinical estimation of severity of AS, especially in the elderly. Nevertheless, careful history and physical examination can provide important clues. Effort *syncope*, *angina*, and symptoms of congestive *heart failure* point to advanced disease with markedly reduced chances of 5-year survival. At times, it is impossible to tell clinically if these worrisome symptoms are due to AS, because of the high prevalence of coexisting coronary disease. The presence of angina must be interpreted cautiously; cardiac catheterization and coronary angiography are generally necessary.

Delay in carotid artery upstroke is one of the most helpful physical signs of significant AS, especially in the young. A normal upstroke in a patient younger than 60 years of age is strong evidence against important stenosis; however, upstroke may appear normal in the elderly patient with severe stenosis because of a stiff, noncompliant carotid artery. Particularly when there are prominent transmitted carotid thrills, the *brachial arteries* may better reflect the severity of aortic stenosis and should also be assessed by palpation. When coincidental aortic regurgitation is present, the upstroke may also appear normal in the presence of marked stenosis. A misleading delay in carotid upstroke can occur from the combination of systemic hypertension and congestive heart failure. Elevation of systolic blood pressure does not rule out hemodynamically significant AS, though a pressure greater than 200 mm Hg and a pulse pressure in excess of 80 mm Hg are unusual when stenosis is marked.

In young patients, the *intensity* of the *murmur* often correlates with severity; however, while it is generally true that critical aortic stenosis is unlikely in a young ambulating person who has less than a 3/6 systolic ejection murmur, rare exceptions do occur. In patients with far advanced disease and a failing left ventricle, the murmur may decrease in intensity and appear insignificant as flow across the valve diminishes. In general, the longer the murmur takes to reach peak intensity, the greater the stenosis. Unfortunately, the *timing of maximal intensity* may not be delayed in some cases of severe stenosis, but if the murmur does peak after midsystole, the stenosis is usually significant. Because the murmur of AS in the elderly may lose its characteristic qualities, it is best to judge severity on the basis of symptoms and other findings.

A delay in the aortic component of the *second heart sound* (S_2) is another sign of significant AS. S_2 may be single or paradoxically split. Calcification and increased rigidity of the valve will often diminish the intensity of the aortic closing sound; it may become inaudible. A forceful *left ventricular impulse* noted on palpation of the precordium is a reliable indication of secondary left ventricular hypertrophy due to significant outflow obstruction.

The *ECG* can contribute to the evaluation by showing signs of left ventricular *hypertrophy* (increased voltage and a strain pattern in the precordial leads V_5 and V_6). The likelihood of finding a strain pattern (ie, ST and T wave depression in the apical and lateral leads), increases with the increase in gradient across the aortic valve. These ECG changes also identify patients at increased risk of sudden death, as fewer than 10 percent of patients succumbing to sudden death demonstrate a normal ECG. In children, the ECG is less helpful; even severe AS may not produce left ventricular hypertrophy and a strain pattern.

Cardiac ultrasound has become essential for assessment of AS, capable of determining degree of calcification, valve anatomy, chamber size, and LV contractility. In the elderly, the *degree of valvular calcification* correlates with severity of stenosis. The absence of significant calcification in a patient older than 60 years of age greatly reduces the probability of important valvular stenosis. Poststenotic dilation of the aorta suggests aortic valvular stenosis but does not have quantitative meaning. The findings of thickening and decreased mobility of the aortic valve leaflets suggest advancing disease. Echocardiography can help distinguish valvular from subvalvular stenosis and, if subvalvular, whether the stenosis is secondary to a discrete membrane, a fibromuscular bar, or a hypertrophic myocardium as in *hypertrophic cardiomyopathy*. In the young patient with normal left ventricular function, the echocardiogram can provide an indirect estimate of the magnitude of the obstructive gradient. The echocardiogram also delineates the magnitude of left ventricular wall thickening and any associated valvular abnormality, particularly rheumatic valve disease. The addition of *Doppler* techniques to the echocardiographic evaluation provides an accurate determination of valve area and helps detect any accompanying AR.

Cardiac catheterization is indicated in the young, asymptomatic patient with evidence of severe stenosis, as well as in any patient with known aortic stenosis who begins to develop symptoms of angina, heart failure, or syncope. Elderly patients who are deemed healthy enough to be candidates for surgery should also have coronary angiography performed to identify significant occlusive disease that may be the source of symptoms or may limit chances of surviving surgery without correction at the time of valve replacement.

Aortic Regurgitation

Severity of AR can usually be well assessed clinically in cases of isolated valvular insufficiency. Marked regurgitation that is long-standing produces dyspnea, a loud diastolic murmur that extends beyond mid-diastole, an S_3, a bounding pulse, and a widened pulse pressure. The absence of a wide pulse pressure does not rule out hemodynamically significant AR, nor does the degree of widening necessarily correlate quantitatively with severity. Changes in peripheral resistance alone can cause large variations in pulse pressure. ECG and x-ray evidence of left ventricular hypertrophy and enlargement are indicative of long-standing significant regurgitation and suggest worsening left ventricular function if they progress.

The *echocardiogram* with *Doppler* enhancement can determine left ventricular size and contractility and delineate the specific disease process in AR—be it rheumatic, annular dilation, or advanced luetic destruction. Signs of LV dysfunction by ultrasound study often precede symptoms and help determine the optimal time for consideration of surgery (see below). Doppler has a sensitivity approaching 100 percent for diagnosis of AR, especially when *color-flow* techniques are used, far superior to physical examination or B-mode echocardiography. Color-flow techniques can provide an excellent noninvasive estimate of regurgitant severity that is within 10 percent of that found at cardiac catheterization.

When aortic regurgitation occurs in the presence of coexisting aortic stenosis, mitral stenosis, or heart failure, the estimation of severity can be very difficult to judge on clinical grounds alone. Consultation with a cardiologist and catheterization are often needed.

PRINCIPLES OF MANAGEMENT

The major therapeutic objectives are to preserve exercise capacity, lifestyle, and life expectancy and to minimize the chances of endocarditis and systemic embolization. Proper timing of intervention is essential to successful treatment. A common management error is to inappropriately delay surgery or valvuloplasty, allowing irreversible myocardial decompensation to develop; this increases the risk of operation and reduces the postoperative benefit. A physician can be lulled into a false sense of security by continuing to control symptoms through repetitive escalations of medical therapy. The need for progressive increases in medication suggests worsening ventricular function and the need for interventional therapy. By ignoring the significance of such developments, the physician may miss the optimal opportunity for the best possible surgical outcome, long-term improvement, and survival.

Early in the course of illness, symptoms of pulmonary congestion can be treated with a mild diuretic regimen, ACE inhibitor, or digitalis (see Chapter 32), but more advanced stages of disease require invasive intervention. Life expectancy and quality of life are clearly improved by properly timed intervention. Advances in valuloplasty technique, prosthetic valve design, and operative technique have produced substantial reductions in interventional mortality. At present, mortality rates for patients undergoing valve surgery in major centers average less than 1 percent for mitral valvulotomy and less than 5 percent for mitral or aortic valve replacement. Operative mortality increases sharply when patients with advanced disease (eg, functional class IV) undergo surgery. However, patients with severe disease should not be denied an operation if they have sufficient myocardial reserve and thus a chance for meaningful survival.

The 5-year life expectancy rate for patients with class IV disease who live through valve replacement is usually less than 50 percent, but this figure is much better than the less than 5 percent rate for similar patients managed medically. Thus, even when surgery is inordinately delayed, it may still offer the patient some opportunity for prolonging survival. Contraindications to valve surgery include serious coexisting noncardiac illness that would compromise survival and the existence of end-stage myocardial decompensation that would make surgery for naught.

Prior to surgery, medical therapy should be directed at control of heart failure (see Chapter 32), maintenance of a near normal lifestyle, and avoidance of potentially dangerous complications, such as arrhythmias (see Chapters 28 and 29), bacterial endocarditis (see Chapter 16), and embolization (see Chapter 83). Most people can be well managed on an outpatient basis for many years prior to the need for interventional therapy, but escalation of medical therapy beyond the time when surgery is indicated must be avoided.

It is important to emphasize that patients who undergo valve surgery still have a "cardiac problem" after surgical correction, be it a prosthetic valve with a variable and still unknown late course, a need for anticoagulation and endocarditis prophylaxis, or an associated cardiac abnormality such as coronary, myocardial, or conduction system disease. All too often this is forgotten after the patient undergoes valve repair. Such patients need continued close follow-up and will always remain "cardiac patients."

Percutaneous balloon angioplasty is being used effectively and safely for relief of severe mitral valvular stenosis in selected patients. For young patients with valvular aortic stenosis, it has also proved to be efficacious. In the elderly with severe AS, results have been disappointing, with a high rate of mortality (approximately 30%) during short-term follow-up. Overall, balloon angioplasty has proven particularly useful as a palliative measure for patients who are too ill to tolerate the risk of open heart surgery.

THERAPEUTIC RECOMMENDATIONS AND INDICATIONS FOR REFERRAL AND ADMISSION

- Monitor all patients by periodic assessment of exercise tolerance, cardiopulmonary examination, chest x-ray, and cardiac ultrasound examination (including Doppler study).
- All patients with any form of valvular heart disease should receive *prophylaxis for bacterial endocarditis* (see Chapter 16).
- Patients younger than 35 years of age with previous rheumatic fever should be considered for *rheumatic fever prophylaxis* (see Chapter 17) particularly if they have frequent beta-streptococcal infections or exposure to young children.
- Onset of *atrial fibrillation* with a rapid ventricular response rate accompanied by acute hemodynamic deterioration is an indication for immediate hospital admission and treatment. Patients with slower rates who tolerate the atrial fibrillation can be digitalized on an outpatient basis (see Chapter 28).
- Occurrence of *systemic embolization* is an indication for urgent admission and intravenous anticoagulant therapy followed by long-term oral anticoagulant treatment (see Chapter 83). Some clinicians argue that valve surgery should be considered if embolization occurs; most concur that surgery is indicated if embolization happens repeatedly.

Mitral Stenosis

- Asymptomatic patients with mild to moderate stenosis need no restriction of activity. Those with evidence of tight stenosis and relatively few symptoms should be advised of the risk of precipitating symptoms by extreme exertion or pregnancy.

- Patients with mild dyspnea that occurs only on exertion can be started on a *mild diuretic* program (eg, hydrochlorothiazide 50–100 mg/d) and advised to follow a no-added-salt diet. Digitalis is of no benefit in isolated mitral stenosis unless there is atrial fibrillation. Extremely vigorous exertion and emotional upset should be avoided to prevent precipitating symptoms.
- Chronic *warfarin* oral anticoagulation is indicated for the patient with MS, particularly when there is atrial fibrillation (see Chapter 28).
- The development of *tight MS* (as evidenced by a short S_2-OS interval, prolonged diastolic murmur, left atrial enlargement and upper zone redistribution on chest x-ray, and narrowed valve orifice and reduced flow on ultrasound) necessitates *referral* to a cardiologist for consideration of invasive intervention, be it surgery or balloon angioplasty, even if few symptoms are reported. Consultation is also needed for worsening dyspnea that is inadequately controlled by a mild diuretic program and salt restriction.
- *Young patients* with evidence of isolated, tight MS with a pliable, noncalcified valve should be considered for interventional therapy early in the course of their illness, even before symptoms are disabling, because transcatheter or surgical *valvulotomy* can be performed. Both procedures provide long-lasting hemodynamic improvement.
- *Early referral* for cardiologic assessment is advisable, since percutaneous balloon mitral valvulotomy is an increasingly attractive alternative to surgical mitral commissurotomy in appropriately selected patients.
- *Older patients* with fibrotic valves (absent opening snap, heavy valve calcification, and limited motion) must undergo *valve replacement* if surgery is needed. Since surgical mortality and complications are greater for valve replacement than for valvulotomy, surgery need not be advised until symptoms are more disabling. However, surgery should not be delayed until symptoms occur at rest or on minimal exertion, because operative risk and long-term mortality increase substantially. A walk with your patient down a corridor or up a flight of stairs may be of great help in convincing both you and the patient that the time for surgery has arrived.
- Cardiac consultation for consideration of catheterization is indicated in the patient being considered for surgery when there is a question of *mixed mitral disease* or involvement of *multiple valves*, or when symptoms are out of proportion to objective evidence of disease.

Mitral Regurgitation

- *Asymptomatic* young patients need *no restriction* of activity.
- Onset of *fatigue* and *dyspnea* can be treated with initiation of a gentle diuretic program (eg, 50–100 mg/d hydrochlorothiazide) in conjunction with a no-added-salt diet. A modest diuretic program that adequately controls symptoms may suffice for years in patients with mild to moderate MR and is not an indication for surgery.
- The development of any *increase in dyspnea* that requires escalation of diuretic therapy is an indication for *cardiac consultation* concerning valve replacement. Progressive deterioration in clinical status and increasing heart size suggest presence of myocardial decompensation; prompt referral is indicated; medical therapy is no substitute for valve surgery.
- *Refractory congestive failure* due to MR is *not* a *contraindication* to *surgery*, though risk is increased. Prior to surgery, symptoms may be lessened by vasodilator therapy, particularly ACE inhibitors (eg, captopril 25–50 mg tid—see Chapter 32), which can diminish the magnitude of regurgitant flow by decreasing afterload. Use of vasodilators can benefit the inoperable patient.
- Patients with incapacitating dyspnea and pulmonary congestion thought to be caused by *papillary muscle dysfunction* should be referred to the cardiologist for catheterization to determine if valve replacement will be of benefit. In one series, those with ejection fractions above 0.35 had the best surgical survival. If there is coexisting coronary disease, it should be treated (see Chapter 30).
- *Valve reconstruction* is becoming an increasingly frequent option in MR, obviating the need for an artificial valve and its attendant risks in many cases.
- Patients with a *prolapsed mitral valve* rarely require treatment other than *endocarditis prophylaxis* (see Chapter 16). Dyspnea is uncommon and digitalis, diuretics, and salt restriction are unnecessary, since the magnitude of the regurgitation is usually insignificant and rarely progressive in the absence of a ruptured chordae or endocarditis. Occurrence of chest pain demands careful evaluation so that other etiologies are not mistakenly attributed to the valve disease (see Chapter 20). Palpitations are rarely due to a significant cardiac arrhythmia and usually do not require treatment (see Chapter 25).
- Patients with *calcification of the mitral valve annulus* should be followed for development of heart block. Regurgitant flow is usually small; consequently, dyspnea and pulmonary congestion are not major problems.
- Chronic *anticoagulation* is indicated in MR patients with atrial fibrillation, especially when accompanied by marked left atrial and left ventricular enlargement.

Aortic Stenosis

- *Asymptomatic* patients with mild AS do not require restriction of activity.
- Young, *asymptomatic* patients with evidence of *tight stenosis* should be advised against heavy physical exertion (eg, competitive sports) and referred to a cardiologist for consideration of catheterization and valvuloplasty or valve replacement. Cardiac catheterization is needed.
- Many *young patients* with tight AS may benefit from *transcatheter aortic balloon valvuloplasty*. Results in appropriately selected young patients are comparable to those achieved with surgical valvuloplasty.
- In *elderly* patients, especially those with fibrotic, calcified valves and associated aortic incompetence, *balloon valvuloplasty* is appropriate only as a *palliative* measure in those unfit for surgery.
- Onset of *angina*, *effort syncope*, or *congestive heart failure* dictates *prompt referral* for consideration of valve surgery. These are signs of critical stenosis and predict a poor prognosis unless definitive therapy is undertaken. Such pa-

tients are at risk for sudden death. Medical therapy is *no* substitute.

- *Congestive failure* can be treated symptomatically on a *temporary* basis by prescribing *digitalis* and a moderate *diuretic* program (eg, cautious use of furosemide 20–40 mg/d—see Chapter 32). Such therapy may help reduce pulmonary congestion and sustain cardiac output temporarily, but the need for a high diastolic filling pressure must be kept in mind; overzealous diuretic therapy can cause a precipitous fall in cardiac output.
- *Angina* can be treated symptomatically with *nitrates* pending surgery (see Chapter 30). Beta-blockers are contraindicated due to their negative inotropic effects. *Coronary angiography* is required at the time of cardiac catheterization to determine if there is coexisting significant coronary artery disease and the need for a bypass procedure at the time of valve replacement.
- Advanced age is not an absolute contraindication to valve replacement. Survival from surgery is predominantly a function of the patient's myocardial reserve. Consequently, even patients in their eighties need not be denied surgery if they are otherwise reasonable surgical candidates and demonstrate an adequate ejection fraction, even in the setting of severe AS.
- Because calcification of the aortic valve can progress rapidly over a few years, patients with AS should have careful longitudinal care and regular follow-up, even when disease appears hemodynamically insignificant and the patient is asymptomatic.

Aortic Regurgitation

- No activity restrictions are necessary in young, asymptomatic patients with mild regurgitation.
- Assess severity with an initial cardiac ultrasound examination that includes Doppler study, and follow patients having evidence of severe regurgitation with serial ultrasound examinations in addition to regular office assessments.
- Patients with evidence of *worsening left ventricular function* (LVH) with a strain pattern on ECG, increasing cardiomegaly on chest film, falling ejection fraction and increasing left ventricular end-systolic dimension on ultrasound examination) should be *referred* to a cardiologist for consideration of surgery, even in the *absence* of symptoms. Patients with a declining LV have an increased risk of ventricular tachycardia and an increased 5-year mortality rate. Early identification of high-risk patients is suggested in the hope of correcting AR prior to the development of irreversible myocardial decompensation, which may have already started by the time symptoms occur.
- Onset of mild symptoms of pulmonary congestion (dyspnea on climbing more than one flight of stairs) in the absence of evidence of significant LV dysfunction can be treated medically with digitalization, a mild diuretic (50–100 mg hydrochlorothiazide), or afterload reduction, but close clinical follow-up and frequent serial ultrasound examinations are essential to prevent inappropriate delay of surgery. Progression of dyspnea to onset after climbing less than one flight of stairs or worsening of LV function on follow-up ultrasound examination indicates the need for prompt cardiac consultation and consideration of surgery.
- Patients with dyspnea prompted by minimal exertion, orthopnea, or paroxysmal nocturnal dyspnea require prompt referral for surgery, because life expectancy is less than 1 year without surgery. Medical therapy with digitalis and diuretics may provide some symptomatic relief temporarily but must not be used in place of valve surgery at this stage of illness.

PATIENT EDUCATION

By far, the most essential elements of patient education are teaching the importance of endocarditis prophylaxis (see Chapter 16) and self-monitoring for early symptoms of cardiac decompensation. The patient with rheumatic heart disease also requires instruction in prophylaxis against Group A beta-streptococcal infection (see Chapter 17). The chances of compliance are certain to improve if time is taken to explain the rationale for prophylaxis and self-monitoring. Patients and their families should also be fully briefed on allowable activity, to avoid both unnecessary restriction and the risk of sudden death in the high-risk patient (eg, the young person with critical AS). If the safety of unlimited activity is in doubt, then a cardiac consultation may be helpful.

The patient's functional status and the proper timing of interventional therapy can be optimized by close, regularly scheduled follow-up and instructions to promptly report early symptoms of cardiac decompensation (eg, onset of exertional dyspnea). Patient confidence and a sense of partnership care are fostered by such follow-up. It is helpful to inform the patient of the treatability of his condition and its excellent prognosis when therapy is properly selected and timed. This provides the rationale for careful self-monitoring. If the patient cannot be depended on to relate symptoms accurately, then a family member or friend needs to be recruited to watch for early manifestations of worsening disease and monitor therapy. Detailed review of the medical program with all concerned cannot be overemphasized, given the very serious consequences from misuse of diuretics, digitalis, and anticoagulants in valvular disease. Of particular importance is warning against unauthorized self-escalation of the medical program when symptoms worsen.

ANNOTATED BIBLIOGRAPHY

Biem HJ, Detsky AS, Armstrong PW. Management of asymptomatic chronic aortic regurgitation with left ventricular dysfunction: a decision analysis. J Gen Intern Med 1990;5:394. *(The analysis strongly favors surgical intervention at the first signs of significant LV dysfunction, even though the patient may remain asymptomatic.)*

Brady ST, Davis CA, Kussmal WG, et al. Percutaneous aortic balloon valvuloplasty in octogenarians: morbidity and mortality. Ann Intern Med 1989;110:761. *(Hemodynamics improved but overall short-term mortality was very high [32 percent]; recommended as a palliative measure only.)*

Brunnen PL, Finlayson JD, Short D. Serious mitral stenosis with slight symptoms. Br Med J 1964;1:1958. *(Symptoms may be slight, but young patients with tight stenosis are at risk for sudden deterioration; pregnancy was a major precipitant.)*

Chen JTT, Beliar VS, Morris JJ, et al. Correlation of roentgen findings with hemodynamic data in pure mitral stenosis. Am J Roentgenol 1968;102:280. *(Prominent upper zone redistribution and pulmonary artery dilation correlated closely with severe mitral stenosis.)*

Collins JJ Jr. The evolution of artificial heart valves. N Engl J Med 1991;324:624. *(An editorial and terse but useful review for the general reader.)*

Folland ED, Kriegel BJ, Henderson WG, et al. Implications of third heart sounds in patients with valvular heart disease. N Engl J Med 1992;327:458. *(Indicative of failure in aortic stenosis, but not in mitral regurgitation.)*

Fowler NO, Van Der Bel-Kahn JM. Indications for surgical replacement of the mitral valve. Am J Cardiol 1979;44:148. *(A review that emphasizes timing of surgical therapy; 41 refs.)*

Galloway AC, et al. Current concepts of mitral valve reconstruction for mitral insufficiency. Circulation 1988;78:1087. *(Details the approach of reconstructing rather than replacing the regurgitant mitral valve.)*

Goldschlager N, Pfeifer J, Cohn D, et al. Natural history of aortic regurgitation. Am J Med 1973;54:577. *(Long symptomatic period, but once symptoms occur, irreversible myocardial changes may have already taken place.)*

Graboys TB, Cohn PF. Prevalence of angina and abnormal coronary arteriograms in severe aortic stenosis. Am Heart J 1977;93:683. *(Twenty percent of patients had at least one significant luminal stenosis.)*

Grayburn PA, Smith MD, Handshoe R, et al. Detection of aortic insufficiency by standard echocardiography, pulsed Doppler echocardiography, and auscultation. Ann Intern Med 1986; 104:599. *(Doppler was the superior method, though auscultation was better than standard echocardiography.)*

Greenberg B, Massie B, Bristow JD, et al. Long-term vasodilator therapy of chronic aortic insufficiency: a randomized double-blind, placebo controlled clinical trial. Circulation 1988;78:92. *(Vasodilator therapy can reduce left-ventricular volume; effect on clinical course remains to be determined.)*

Hammermeister KE, et al. Comparison of outcomes in men 11 years after heart-valve replacement with a mechanical valve or bioprosthesis. N Engl J Med 1993;328:1289. *(Useful data for selection of prosthesis.)*

Hoagland PM, Cook EF, Wynne J, et al. Value of noninvasive testing in adults with suspected aortic stenosis. Am J Med 1986;80:1041. *(Enables identification of patients with critical stenosis.)*

Lee RT, Bhatia SJS, St John Sutton MG. Assessment of valvular heart disease with Doppler echocardiography. JAMA 1989; 262:2131. *(Excellent review of this very important technologic addition to the assessment of valvular disease; 30 refs.)*

Marks AR, Choong CY, Sanfilippo AJ, et al. Identification of high-risk and low-risk subgroups of patients with mitral-valve prolapse. N Engl J Med 1989;320:1031. *(Those with valve thickening and redundancy were at greatest risk of complications.)*

Morganroth J, Jones RH, Chem CC, et al. Two-dimensional echocardiography in mitral, aortic, and tricuspid valve disease. Am J Cardiol 1980;46:1164. *(An authoritative review of ultrasound for diagnosis of valvular heart disease.)*

Oh JK, Taliercio CP, Holmes DR, et al. Prediction of the severity of aortic stenosis by Doppler aortic valve area determination. J Am Coll Cardiol 1988;11:1227. *(A prospective study of 100 patients coming to catheterization; excellent correlation found between Doppler and catheterization results.)*

Palacios IF, Block PC, Wilkin GT, et al. Follow-up of patients undergoing percutaneous mitral balloon valvulotomy: analysis of factors determining restenosis. Circulation 1989;79:573. *(The technique proved safe and effective in appropriately selected patients; detail criteria for selection.)*

Perloff JK. Evolving concepts of mitral valve prolapse. N Engl J Med 1982;307:369. *(MVP is a heterogeneous disease; in most, it is a harmless condition.)*

Roth RB, Palacios IF, Block PC. Percutaneous aortic balloon valvuloplasty: its role in the management of patients with aortic stenosis requiring major noncardiac surgery. J Am Coll Cardiol 1989;13:1039. *(An example of the palliative use of valvuloplasty.)*

Selzer A. Changing aspects of the natural history of valvular aortic stenosis. N Engl J Med 1987;317:91. *(Most of the AS now being encountered is due to calcific degenerative disease of the elderly; excellent review of its presentation and clinical course and how it differs from rheumatic AS; 116 refs.)*

Sherman W, Hershman R, Lazzam C, et al. Balloon valvuloplasty in adult aortic stenosis. Ann Intern Med 1989;110:421. *(A longitudinal study showing a high mortality rate; also addresses determinants of clinical outcome.)*

Sherrid M, Goyal A, Delia E, et al. Unsuspected mitral stenosis. Am J Med 1991;90:189. *(Hemodynamically significant disease detected by ultrasound was missed clinically due to concurrent aortic stenosis, heart failure, pneumonia, or just a low index of suspicion; most cases had an audible MS murmur on reexamination.)*

Siemienczuk D, Greenberg B, Morris C, et al. Chronic aortic insufficiency: factors associated with progression to aortic valve replacement. Ann Intern Med 1989;110:587. *(Measurement of LV size and function were predictive of need for valve replacement.)*

Taylor AA, Davies AO, Mares A, et al. Spectrum of dysautonomia in mitral valvular prolapse. Am J Med 1989;86:287. *(Dysautonomic responses occurred irrespective of the presence of MVP; refutes the purported etiologic link between these responses and MVP.)*

Primary Care Medicine: Office Evaluation and Management of the Adult Patient, 3rd edition, edited by Allan H. Goroll, Lawrence A. May, and Albert G. Mulley, Jr. J.B. Lippincott Company, Philadelphia

34
Management of Peripheral Arterial Disease

DAVID C. BREWSTER, M.D.

Treatment of peripheral arterial insufficiency has undergone a quiet revolution. Plaque regression has now been demonstrated with aggressive lipid-lowering therapy (see Chapter 27), and, in properly selected patients, percutaneous transluminal angioplasty (PTA) produces results that approach those of bypass surgery. In addition, great progress has been made in arterial reconstructive surgery for severe cases, making possible the salvage of limbs that would otherwise require amputation. The wealth of available therapeutic options and a relatively favorable natural history provide the symptomatic patient with substantial opportunity for improvement. The primary physician needs to know 1) the natural history of arterial occlusive disease so as to optimize the timing and intensity of therapy; 2) the techniques, efficacies, and indications for conservative therapy, including risk factor modification; and 3) the indications for angioplasty and bypass surgery. With so many treatment modalities available, the primary physician has to be skilled in the timing, selection, implementation, and coordination of care.

NATURAL HISTORY OF PERIPHERAL ARTERIAL DISEASE

The *prognoses* for the *limb* and for *symptoms* in patients presenting with claudication are quite good. The worst clinical courses occur among patients manifesting ischemic ulcers or rest pain, especially if they suffer from long-standing diabetes mellitus or persist in smoking. In a series of 529 diabetic patients from the Mayo Clinic followed over 5 years prior to the advent of surgical reconstruction, only 3 percent came to amputation within 5 years if the sole manifestation of their disease was claudication. Of the smokers who ceased smoking, none required amputation, but 11.4 percent who continued to smoke lost a limb. A more recent study of 104 patients with claudication who underwent angiography also noted a relatively benign prognosis. Over a 6-month to 8-year follow-up (average 2.5 y), 79 percent remained stable or improved, and only 5.8 percent came to amputation. When patients were divided into mild, moderate, and severe disease groups on the basis of distance walked before onset of claudication, it was found that prognosis paralleled severity; the group with most severe disease accounted for five of the six amputations. Nevertheless, even in the most severe cases, 69.4 percent stayed the same or improved, and only 15.1 percent came to amputation, underscoring the fact that progression to loss of limb is hardly inevitable.

Pooled data show that after 5 years from onset of symptoms, about half of patients remain symptomatically stable or improved. In the Framingham Study, only a third of patients presenting with intermittent claudication still had persistent symptoms 4 years later. In essence, prognosis is rather good, especially if major atherosclerotic risk factors can be brought under control.

While prognosis for the limb is favorable, *mortality* rates—both overall and cardiovascular—are high. In a 10-year prospective study of mortality in 565 men and women examined for peripheral arterial disease, the risk of dying from a cardiovascular cause was sixfold greater in those with peripheral arterial disease than in those of similar age, sex, and lipid profile without it. All-cause mortality rose threefold, due almost entirely to the increase in cardiovascular risk. Similar mortality figures have been reported in other studies, with combined mortality rates in the range of 30 percent, 50 percent, and 70 percent at 5, 10, and 15 years after onset of symptoms, respectively—a relative risk about three times that for patients of similar age and gender. Concurrent disease of the coronary arteries, cerebrovasculature, or aorta accounts for most of the increased mortality, underscoring the systemic nature of atherosclerosis and its adverse effect on prognosis. The prevalence of systemic atherosclerosis in patients with peripheral arterial insufficiency should not be surprising, given that up to 80 percent give a history of smoking, 40 percent have hypertension, 30 percent have lipid abnormalities, and 20 percent have diabetes.

PRINCIPLES OF MANAGEMENT

Medical Management

The basic objectives of medical management are to control or limit disease progression, increase exercise tolerance, and minimize risk of complications.

Smoking Cessation. The most important methods for achieving these objectives are cessation of cigarette smoking, regular daily exercise, and meticulous foot care. Smoking hastens progression of atherosclerosis and may further impair blood flow by inducing vasoconstriction. *Smoking cessation* ranks as a major priority for the patient with peripheral arterial disease. Cessation can reduce rest pain, claudication, risk of amputation, and need for bypass surgery. The risk of repeat occlusion after angioplasty or bypass falls by over two-thirds in those who quit. Moreover, quitting decreases cardiovascular morbidity and mortality. The chances of successfully quitting are greatest when a smoker becomes symptomatic from a complication of smoking; the physician's influence is considerable in this context. Nicotine gum or transdermal patch serves as a useful cessation aid by minimizing nicotine withdrawal, though nicotine may induce vasospasm (see Chapter 54). Since vasospasm usually does not play a major role in claudication, nicotine therapy is probably not contraindicated in these patients, but care is advised if it is going to be used.

Exercise. Daily exercise remains a cornerstone of the treatment program, even though it now appears unlikely that it stimulates redistribution of blood flow or development of collaterals in the ischemic limb. Suggested mechanisms include improvements in muscle metabolism, hemorrheology, walking technique, and pain threshold. Whatever the reason, physical training significantly increases the claudication-free walking distance. The programs showing the best results are those that combine supervised *group walking sessions* with additional sessions performed daily at home. The best candidates are those with stable intermittent claudication who are free of rest pain, ulceration, unstable angina, congestive heart failure, and severe lung disease or arthritis. Although group results are excellent, predicting outcome in an individual patient is difficult. Most who achieve benefit report it within 3 months of initiating an exercise program. Regularity of exercise is more important than intensity or duration, though at least 30 min/d of continuous leg exercise appears necessary. Any form of dynamic leg exercise will suffice, including stationary bicycling and stair-climbing as well as walking. An exercise program can also reduce cardiovascular risk (see Chapter 29).

Foot Care. Careful attention to foot care is vital to prevention of limb loss. It has been estimated that up to 80 percent of amputations required in diabetics are attributable to poor foot care. Feet need to be inspected daily, especially in diabetics with peripheral neuropathy that limits protective sensation. As little as an hour of patient education has been shown to reduce the amputation and ulceration rate by two-thirds.

Atherosclerotic Risk Factors. Aggressive treatment of *hyperlipidemia* can reduce or halt atherosclerotic plaque progression in peripheral vessels; modest plaque regression has also been demonstrated. Some decrease in risk and severity of symptomatic peripheral ischemic disease can be expected, but the most important benefit stems from the marked reductions in cardiovascular morbidity and mortality. Since patients with peripheral arterial disease are at high risk for life-threatening cardiovascular complications, they stand to gain considerably from aggressive lipid-lowering therapy (see Chapter 27).

If *hypertension* is present, it too deserves attention (see Chapter 14). The effect of blood pressure reduction on progression of peripheral vascular disease remains unknown, but treatment clearly reduces morbidity and mortality from stroke and cardiovascular disease. Choosing an agent on the basis of its effect on peripheral vascular tone does not appear to be critical, though some patients complain of worsening symptoms on beta-blocker therapy. Controlled studies have failed to confirm an adverse effect with beta-blockers. Antihypertensive agents with vasodilating potential (eg, calcium channel blockers) do not materially improve claudication symptoms. Angiotensin converting enzyme inhibitors are contraindicated if there is coexisting renal artery stenosis.

Weight reduction can be helpful by lessening work load and reducing metabolic demands of the extremities. In addition, weight reduction may also help lower lipid levels, glucose intolerance, and cardiovascular risk (see Chapter 10).

To date, there is no evidence that "tight" *control of diabetes* improves the clinical course of peripheral arterial disease (see Chapter 102). Perhaps that is because diabetic peripheral vascular disease begins earlier and progresses more rapidly than that of other patients. Moreover, large vessels may remain relatively patent while small vessels become occluded. Neuropathy aggravates the situation by contributing limb injury. Whether improved glucose control lessens neuropathic disease is unresolved. Foot care is essential.

Patients with extensive premature peripheral arterial disease (occurring before age 50) may suffer from heterocyclics for *homocystinuria* and should be tested for impaired homocysteine metabolism. Patients with the condition may respond to vitamin B_6 or folate.

Vasodilators, Antiplatelet Agents, and Other Drugs. Pharmacologic treatment of arterial insufficiency remains disappointing. *Vasodilators* have failed to demonstrate a significant effect on symptoms or clinical course. This reinforces the view that vasoconstriction plays little role in claudication. *Pentoxifylline*, an agent that appears to increase erythrocyte deformability and blood viscosity and reduce platelet activity, has been promoted as a potentially useful drug for treatment of symptomatic peripheral arterial disease. A randomized, double-blind, multi-center study revealed a modest increase in patients' walking distance at some centers, but there were multiple interventions and the increase was only 18 percent of that reported for exercise programs. Other studies have produced equally equivocal and inconsistent findings. High cost, nausea, and dizziness further limit pentoxiphylline's appeal and relegate the drug to a minor role in patients who fail other forms of conservative therapy.

Antiplatelet agents hold some promise. *Aspirin* and aspirin plus *dipyridamole* were found to reduce progression of peripheral atherosclerotic disease compared to placebo in a 2-year angiographic study. There are no data on symptomatic effects. Compelling many clinicians to use aspirin in patients with claudication are the heightened risks of stroke and cardiovascular disease, which do seem to be reduced by aspirin use (see Chapters 30 and 171). Other agents that block specific inducers of atherosclerosis are under investigation, including *omega-3 fatty acids*, *calcium channel blockers*, and *prostaglandin* E analogues. *Oral anticoagulants* have no role in chronic management of peripheral arterial disease.

Certain drugs are powerful peripheral vasoconstrictors and should be used with *caution*, if at all, in patients with severe disease, especially in those with ulcers or rest pain. *Ergot derivatives* are a classic example; *alpha-agonists* also may aggravate ischemic symptoms and impede healing of skin lesions. As noted earlier, randomized controlled studies did not find that use of *beta-blockers* compromised perfusion or worsened symptoms, despite anecdotal reports.

Interventional Therapies

Patients who continue to have disabling symptoms despite implementation of a full medical regimen (smoking cessation, exercise program, control of cardiovascular risk factors) are potential candidates for interventional therapy. With the advent of angioplasty and improvements in surgical technique, the threshold for invasive therapy has been lowered, but the decision to consider such treatment should not be taken lightly or made prematurely. The relatively favorable natural history of peripheral vascular disease and the excellent responses to medical measures argue for resorting to interventional therapy only after other approaches have failed and the patient is incapacitated or a limb is at risk. Persisting inability to walk two blocks and carry out activities of daily living are typical functional criteria for consideration of interventional therapy. Rest pain and a nonhealing ulcer are even more compelling reasons.

Before referring the patient for interventional therapy, a full set of *noninvasive studies* (including duplex or triplex ultrasound scanning and segmental blood pressures) should be ordered to more precisely document the location and severity of disease (see Chapter 23). The best candidates for interventional measures are those with proximal disease and preserved distal runoff. Patients who prove to have predominantly small vessel disease (eg, diabetics) do not benefit much from interventional therapy unless there is concurrent proximal disease that can be alleviated. *Angiography* will be necessary to make the final determination, but detailed noninvasive study can help screen patients and minimize unnecessary angiography, with its attendant risks of intimal dissection, groin hematoma, and dye-induced renal failure.

Percutaneous Transluminal Angioplasty (PTA) has emerged as a cost-effective alternative to bypass surgery, especially for the patient with segmental stenosis of the aortoiliac or femoral artery. In a prospective randomized trial of PTA versus surgery in patients with lesions amenable to angioplasty, PTA produced short- and long-term results similar to those of surgery. The cost of PTA is one-fifth that of surgery; durability of result is moderately less, reducing but not eliminating the cost differential.

The procedure is typically performed at the time of angiography, using a balloon catheter inserted percutaneously at a remote site, usually the femoral artery, and manipulated fluoroscopically within the diseased segment of artery. With balloon inflation, the obstructing plaque is cracked and vessel lumen enhanced.

Results are best for short segmental stenoses in proximal vessels. Patency rates, both immediate and long-term, are a function of location. Aortoiliac procedures average a 90 percent immediate success rate, and 80 percent are patent at 5 years; for a femoral lesion, the rates average 75 percent and 50 percent, respectively. Risks include groin hematoma, dissection, renal ischemia, and distal embolization. The overall complication rate averages 10 percent, with about 2 percent to 5 percent being serious enough to warrant surgical intervention. Mortality is less than 0.5 percent. As expected, experienced teams in centers performing large numbers of PTAs have the best results and the fewest complications.

PTA is suitable for about 30 percent of patients being considered for interventional therapy. The remainder tend to have more widespread or distal occlusive disease. PTA has a lower morbidity and mortality than standard surgery, making it an especially attractive option in patients who are bad surgical risks because of severe underlying disease. In addition, it may be combined with surgery; for example, correcting a proximal iliac stenosis by balloon angioplasty and bypassing a more distal lesion with a femoropopliteal graft. Poor candidates for PTA include those with a complete occlusion, a stenotic lesion greater than 10 cm in length, multiple serial stenoses, calcified or eccentric plaque, or poor distal runoff.

Recanalization Techniques. Because angioplasty cannot be performed on a totally occluded vessel, there has been considerable interest in *recanalization techniques*. *Laser* methods and *mechanical arthrectomy* devices have been applied to allow percutaneous catheter-based opening of atherosclerotic arteries. The initial enthusiasm and commercial promotion of such devices have proven premature. With current technology, these techniques can sometimes serve as an *adjunct* to conventional balloon angioplasty, carving out a small channel in a limited area of total occlusion so that a standard PTA balloon catheter may traverse the lesion. This is likely to be an area of rapid development. The literature should be followed for well-designed studies of this emerging technology.

Surgical Therapy. In patients with *claudication alone*, surgery should be considered only in those who are so severely disabled that their ability to earn a living is compromised, their desired lifestyle is intolerably limited, and their vascular lesions are not amenable to PTA. The role of arterial reconstruction for claudication alone remains controversial. In general, the physician must attempt to determine the significance of ischemic symptoms in each patient. The patient's age, work requirements, social circumstances, and general state of health must all be considered. When doubt exists, referral for a surgical opinion is often useful.

Surgical referral is clearly indicated in patients with *advanced ischemia* resulting in *ischemic rest pain*, nonhealing *ischemic ulcerations*, or *gangrene*. Such limbs are clearly at risk, and arterial reconstruction is indicated, if feasible, to maximize chances of limb salvage. In such circumstances, patients should be referred for surgical investigation as soon as possible, before tissue necrosis or infection become too extensive. The morbidity and mortality of common revascularization procedures is in many instances less than that associated with major amputation. For poor-risk patients, various "extra-anatomic" reconstructions are also available, which may be done with even more safety.

Many patients with significant arterial insufficiency that requires surgery also have underlying coronary disease that is hemodynamically critical. The coronary disease may be clinically silent due to the exercise restrictions stemming from severe claudication. Such patients have high rates of perioperative morbidity and mortality. *Dipyridamole–thallium stress testing* before surgery helps to identify high-risk patients who would benefit from coronary revascularization prior to peripheral vascular surgery (see Chapter 36).

Great progress has been made in the surgical management of arterial insufficiency. With an experienced surgeon, careful preoperative cardiac evaluation, and good anesthetic and postoperative management, the patient may anticipate successful correction of aortoiliac occlusive disease, with a mortality risk of only 1 percent to 2 percent, and excellent long-term patency of approximately 85 percent to 90 percent at 5 years. Femoropopliteal or tibial artery bypass may be done with even greater safety, although long-term patency is somewhat less, with approximately 70 percent to 75 percent of saphenous vein grafts still patent at 5 years. If the saphenous vein is unavailable for use, a number of suitable alternative prosthetic grafts have been developed within recent years. With improvement of direct reconstructive methods, lumbar sympathectomy is rarely considered a primary mode of treatment.

PATIENT EDUCATION

Patient education is vital, because a favorable outcome requires strong patient participation in the treatment program (cessation of smoking, daily exercise, foot care, risk factor reduction). Compliance is facilitated by the patient's understanding the atherosclerotic basis of the problem, the factors that may aggravate the severity of symptoms, and the rationale behind the measures recommended. Many patients come to the physician with reluctance to walk and fear of limb loss. The benefits of exercise, the likelihood of improvement, and the low risk of limb loss are usually of great comfort and reassurance to the patient and family. The importance for foot care must be repeatedly emphasized, especially in the diabetic. A single hour of detailed foot care instruction can greatly reduce the risk of limb loss. Also important to stress is that even the most trivial foot injury or lesion requires prompt attention. Specific instructions for an appropriate exercise program are essential; recommending such a program can provide a considerable psychological boost.

The psychologic management of the patient is essential in preventing depression and invalidism. Emphasis should be on the generally favorable prognosis and the patient's ability to improve his own condition. Frequent follow-up in the early stages of the treatment program is reassuring and helps maximize compliance. The patient with new claudication should be seen at least every 2 to 3 months to assess exercise tolerance and inspect the feet for potential pressure points and ulcers.

INDICATIONS FOR REFERRAL AND ADMISSION

Patients with disabling claudication who fail to respond to conservative therapy and have noninvasive evidence of proximal disease should be referred for consideration of PTA. Patients needing direct referral for consideration of bypass surgery are those with such severe disease (rest pain, nonhealing ulcers, early gangrene) that they are at risk for losing the limb. Urgent hospitalization is indicated for the patient with early gangrenous changes or signs of infection in an ischemic extremity. Those with refractory claudication whose lifestyle or livelihood are *intolerably* compromised by the inability to walk distances and who appear by noninvasive testing to have disease too distal or too diffuse for PTA are also potential candidates for surgery. The final determination regarding candidacy for angioplasty or surgery requires angiography, but noninvasive screening can maximize the appropriateness of the referral.

THERAPEUTIC RECOMMENDATIONS

- *Cessation of smoking*. Total cessation is essential, both to limit disease progression and to prevent reocclusion after interventional therapy. The patient must be firmly told that he or she *must* stop smoking completely. Smoking as little as 5 cigarettes per day can compromise a limb. The physician must be unequivocal about this, as patients often interpret halfhearted advice as only a suggestion (see Chapter 54).
- *Daily exercise*. In the patient with claudication, the best exercise is daily walking. Patients are advised to walk to the point of discomfort, stop briefly, and then resume walking. At least 30 minutes of relatively continuous walking each day is recommended. A weekly group session can be extremely useful. An exercise bicycle can be used as an alternative mode of exercise. It is important to emphasize to the patient that pain does not indicate harm or damage to the leg, and that exercise can help rather than aggravate the condition. Any tendency to restrict activity, sometimes to the point of invalidism or confinement to the home, should be avoided, unless severe ischemia is present.

  Patients with more advanced ischemia and rest pain at night may benefit from raising the head of the bed on 6- to 8-inch blocks so that the feet and legs are made slightly dependent; gravity may aid blood flow enough to allow more comfortable sleep.
- *Foot care*. This aspect of preventive medicine is of extreme importance, particularly in the diabetic patient who often lacks protective sensation due to neuropathy and who may be more susceptible to infection. Because there is often a great deal of confusion about what is meant by "foot care," its components require elaboration:

  1. *Inspection*. The feet should be inspected daily for any scratches, cuts, fissures, blisters, or other lesions, particularly around the nail beds, between the toes, and on the heels.
  2. *Washing*. The feet should be washed daily with mild soap and lukewarm (never hot) water. Rinse thoroughly and dry gently but completely, particularly between the toes. Excessive soaking, leading to maceration, should be avoided.
  3. *Lanolin*. A moisturizing cream such as lanolin or Eucerin should be applied to the skin of the foot and heel but not between the toes. A light film, well rubbed in, will prevent drying and cracking of the skin, which is often the genesis of a lesion, particularly on the heel. The cream should not be applied thickly or allowed to "cake" on the foot.

4. *Lambswool.* A small amount of lambast or dry cotton or gauze may be placed between the toes to prevent lesions, which may occur if toes are allowed to rub together, particularly if orthopedic deformities of the toes are present.
5. *Powder.* An antifungal powder, such as nystatin, should be applied between the toes if excessive moisture or maceration is a problem.
6. *Proper footwear.* Properly fitting shoes with ample space in the forefoot are essential. Special shoes are rarely necessary.
7. *Podiatry.* Nails should be cut with extreme care, in good light, and only if vision is normal. They should be cut straight across and even with the end of the toe, never close to the skin or into the corner of the nailbed. Any abnormality of the nails as well as any corns or calluses should be treated by the physician or podiatrist.
8. *Avoidance of trauma.* Never use adhesive tape on the skin (paper tape is better), or any strong antiseptic solution. Avoid heating pads, hot packs, heat lamps, and scalding hot water. Never walk barefoot.

It is the physician's responsibility to educate his patients in these points, and to urge them to contact him at the first sign of difficulty.

- *Weight reduction* (see Chapter 233).
- *Control of other risk factors* (eg, hypertension [see Chapter 26], hyperlipidemia [see Chapter 27]). In patients with premature disease, test for homocystinuria and treat with vitamin B_6 and folic acid supplements if positive.
- Referral

1. *Patients with claudication alone.* PTA is worth considering if the pain is disabling and refractory to a full trial of medical therapy and noninvasive study suggests only focal proximal disease. Referral for consideration of surgery is indicated only in patients who have failed medical therapy, have disease that appears amenable to surgery but not PTA, and are so significantly disabled by claudication that their livelihood or lifestyle is intolerably compromised by their inability to walk distances. Final decision requires angiography, but noninvasive study to screen for appropriate candidates is essential.
2. *Patients with more severe disease.* People with rest pain, nonhealing ulcers, or early gangrene who have a limb which is in jeopardy should be considered for operation with some urgency.
3. Consider preoperative dipyridamole–thallium stress testing to identify patients with high cardiac risk who might need coronary bypass grafting prior to peripheral arterial surgery.

ANNOTATED BIBLIOGRAPHY

Brewster DC, Cambria RP, Darling RC, et al. Long-term results of combined iliac balloon angioplasty and distal surgical revascularization. Ann Surg 1989;210:324. *(Good long-term results for combined interventional therapy.)*

Coffman JD. Vasodilator drugs in peripheral vascular disease. N Engl J Med 1979;300:713. *(Best study on the issue; no evidence that they work.)*

Criqui MH, Langer RD, Fronek A, et al. Mortality over a period of 10 years in patients with peripheral arterial disease. N Engl J Med 1992;326:381. *(Relative risk of all-cause mortality was 3.0, due mostly to a sixfold increase in risk of cardiovascular death.)*

Duffield RGM, Lewis B, Miller NE, et al. Treatment of hyperlipidaemia retards progression of symptomatic femoral atherosclerosis. Lancet 1983;2:639. *(Aggressive therapy produced a two-thirds reduction in progression.)*

Ernst E, Fialke V. A review of the clinical effectiveness of exercise therapy for intermittent claudication. Arch Intern Med 1993;153:2357. *(A supervised, high-intensity program of at least 2 months works best.)*

Hallett JW Jr. Foot care. In: Hallett JW Jr, Brewster DC, Darling RC (eds): Manual of Patient Care in Vascular Surgery. Boston, Little, Brown, 1982:171. *(Good discussion of the key elements of proper foot care, with appropriate references.)*

Hess H, Miewtaschik A, Deischel G. Drug-induced inhibition of platelet function delays progression of peripheral occlusive arterial disease; a prospective double-blind arteriographically controlled trial. Lancet 1985;1:415. *(Best available angiographic data suggesting aspirin and dipyridamole may be beneficial, but no clinical outcomes data provided.)*

Jonason T, Bergstrom R. Cessation of smoking in patients with intermittent claudication. Acta Med Scand 1987;221:253. *(Cessation of smoking greatly improves prognosis.)*

Jonason T, Ringvist I. Diabetes mellitus and intermittent claudication: relation between peripheral vascular complications and location of the occlusive atherosclerosis in the legs. Acta Med Scand 1985;218:217. *(Increased risk of amputation in diabetics may be due to their increased prevalence of diffuse and distal disease.)*

Johnston W, Rae M, Jogg-Johnston SA, et al. Five-year results of a prospective study of percutaneous transluminal angioplasty Ann Surg;1987:206:403. *(Excellent prospective study of a large series of patients undergoing iliac and femoropopliteal PTA; results related to site, anatomic extent of disease, and severity of symptoms.)*

Krupski WC. The peripheral vascular consequences of smoking. Ann Vasc Surg 1991;3:291. *(A thorough review of the vascular effects and possible mechanisms by which tobacco usage causes or aggravates atherosclerotic disease.)*

Malone JM, Snyder M, Anderson G, et al. Prevention of amputation by diabetic education. Am J Surg 1989;158:520. *(A single 1-hour educational program on foot care resulted in a marked decrease in the amputation rate.)*

McAllister FF. The fate of patients with intermittent claudication managed nonoperatively. Am J Surg 1976;132:593. *(One hundred patients with intermittent claudication followed for an average of 6 years; 78 percent either improved or remained stable. The study argues for restraint in bypass grafting.)*

Perler BA, Osterman FA, White RA Jr, et al. Percutaneous laser probe femoropopliteal angioplasty: a preliminary experience. J Vasc Surg 1989;10:351. *(A sobering report of generally poor results and high recurrence rate when typical peripheral occlusive disease is treated by laser.)*

Radack K, Wyderski RJ. Conservative management of intermittent claudication. Ann Intern Med 1990;113:135. *(The best review of the evidence for efficacy of walking, smoking cessation, and pentoxiphylline; 99 refs.)*

Reiber GE, Pecoraro RE, Koepsell TD. Risk factors for amputation in patients with diabetes mellitus. Ann Intern Med 1992;117:97. *(Identifies important clinical features that were predictive.)*

Wilson SE, Wolf GL,Cross AP. Percutaneous transluminal angioplasty versus operation for peripheral arteriosclerosis. Report of a prospective randomized trial in a selected group of patients. J Vasc Surg 1989;9:1. *(In a group of patients with lesions amenable to PTA, short and long-term success rates were similar for both surgery and PTA.)*

Wong T, Detsky A. Preoperative cardiac risk assessment for patients having peripheral vascular surgery. Ann Intern Med 1992;116:743. *(High risk of infarction makes preoperative assessment essential; good review of the data.)*

35

Management of Peripheral Venous Disease

DAVID C. BREWSTER, M.D.

Primary Care Medicine: Office Evaluation and Management of the Adult Patient, 3rd edition, edited by Allan H. Goroll, Lawrence A. May, and Albert G. Mulley, Jr. J.B. Lippincott Company, Philadelphia

Problems of the peripheral venous system (varicose veins, venous insufficiency, and phlebitis) are extremely prevalent, especially among the elderly. Many physicians do little for the more mundane complaints referable to the venous system because of lack of knowledge and confusion about pathophysiology and proper management. Such attitudes are unfortunate, because neglected venous problems can cause considerable disability and place the patient at serious risk. The primary management of venous diseases is still largely nonoperative, and great benefit is possible with well-conceived office care.

PATHOPHYSIOLOGY AND CLINICAL PRESENTATION

The high frequency of venous disorders of the lower extremities is unique to humans and reflects the consequences of an upright posture and gravity. In order to return blood from the periphery to the right heart, the venous system in the legs must work against the force of gravity without the aid of organs specifically designed for this purpose. A number of factors work to lessen venous pressure in the leg and propel blood toward the heart. These include the "muscular pump" effect of the exercising calf musculature, the negative intrathoracic pressure created by the "bellows effect" of the chest wall with respiration, and the presence of multiple valves in both superficial and deep venous systems. The last prevents reflux of blood and serves to reduce pressure in the veins that would otherwise equal the weight of an uninterrupted column of blood from the heart to the foot (approximately 100 mm Hg).

A knowledge of basic anatomy of the venous system is vital to evaluation and management of lower extremity venous problems. The existence of two venous systems, superficial and deep, is well known. A third system linking the superficial and deep systems, the communicating or perforating veins, is less well recognized but of great importance. Valves also exist in the communicating veins, permitting flow from the superficial to the deep system but preventing retrograde flow.

When functioning properly, these three systems work in coordinated fashion. The deep system, composed of paired anterior and posterior tibial and peroneal veins, popliteal veins, and superficial and deep femoral veins, handles approximately 80 percent to 90 percent of venous return, while the superficial network of greater and lesser saphenous systems is much less important in this respect.

Clinical disorders of the venous system usually stem from obstruction to venous return due to thrombosis of the vein lumen or from incompetent venous valves that allow reflux of blood and persistent elevation of venous pressure in the leg and foot.

Varicose Veins

The superficial veins lie in the subcutaneous tissue and lack the support afforded by muscle and fascial compartments, making them most prone to difficulty. Varicose veins are extremely common and probably affect some 10 percent to 20 percent of the adult population to some degree. They are more common in women, who also seem more likely to consult a physician for advice.

A family history of varicosities is present in the majority of patients and lends support to the concept of a hereditary or congenital etiology. It is unclear whether the primary problem is a congenital incompetence of valves or a weakness of the venous wall itself, which causes dilation of the vein lumen and subsequent valve inadequacy. In any event, a self-perpetuating cycle ensues of venous reflux leading to further vein dilation and valve failure.

In time, the poorly supported superficial veins widen, elongate, and become tortuous. In a smaller percentage of patients the initial defect may be in the communicating veins, where poorly functioning valves allow abnormal flow toward the superficial system, causing eventual overdistention. In other patients, acquired factors such as old trauma or venous thrombosis may play a role. Factors that raise intraluminal vein pressure, such as repeated pregnancies, obesity, or wearing of tight garments that constrict the thigh, may be of importance. The final common pathway remains valvular incompetence.

Varicosities most commonly involve the veins of the greater saphenous system and its tributaries and therefore occur principally in the medial and anterior thigh, calf, and ankle regions. The lesser saphenous system may also be involved, producing varicosities of the posterior calf and lateral ankle region. The exact distribution of involved branches is of real importance only when considering surgical correction.

The presenting symptoms of varicose veins are extremely variable and often seem to bear little relationship to the apparent severity of the varicosities. Complaints are more frequent in women, particularly young women at the time of the menstrual period. Clearly, hormonal factors that favor fluid retention may aggravate venous distension, but in many such patients the main concern is over the cosmetic appearance of minor varicosities.

Typically, patients complain of local aching or burning pain in the area of the varicosities, particularly at the end of the day after having been on their feet at work. "Tiredness," "heaviness," or a "bursting" sensation are commonly reported. Itchiness due to a stasis dermatitis may occur in the region of a severe and chronic varix, especially in the region of an incompetent perforating vein. Mild swelling of the ankle region may occur; however, this is relatively unusual with uncomplicated varicose veins. Similarly, ulceration due solely to varicose veins is rare. Severe swelling or recurrent ulceration almost always implies problems with the deep venous system (see below).

Large varices may be subject to trauma and bleeding. Much more commonly, however, the distended vein with sluggish blood flow may thrombose, leading to superficial phlebitis.

Chronic Venous Insufficiency

Chronic venous insufficiency, also called the *postphlebitic syndrome,* is a common chronic disorder that is particularly disabling if stubborn venous ulcers develop. Although the superficial venous system may be secondarily involved with varicose veins, the principal defect lies in the deep venous system.

A documented history of deep venous thrombosis (DPT) can be obtained in fewer than one-half of patients with chronic venous insufficiency, but it is felt to be the underlying etiology in most instances. Deep venous thrombosis can often be clinically silent, as documented by prospective ^{125}I-fibrinogen scanning studies in postoperative patients. Despite subsequent recanalization of deep venous occlusions, the phlebitic inflammatory process deforms or destroys venous valves in the deep system, and their incompetency results in reflux and increased venous pressure. Communicating veins undergo similar changes through valvular damage or simply by exposure to chronically elevated pressure from the deep venous system. Some authorities feel a congenital valvular incompetence may also play a role, similar to varicose veins of the superficial system. Regardless of cause, high venous pressure generated by muscular contraction forces blood through damaged valves in communicating veins toward the superficial system, resulting in "ambulatory venous hypertension." Such venous hypertension results in edema, usually most prominent in the calf and ankle region. Indeed, swelling is one of the hallmarks of chronic venous insufficiency and usually differentiates the problem from simple varicose veins. Swelling of the thigh may occur, denoting valvular incompetence at the iliofemoral level as well. Generally, this is less severe and less troublesome than the edema of the lower leg.

Venous hypertension leads not only to interstitial fluid accumulation but also to extravasation of plasma proteins and red blood cells into subcutaneous tissues. In time, this results in brawny induration of the skin and pigmentation of the thickened but fragile tissue. The presence of edema and continual high venous pressure results in reduced local capillary flow and relative hypoxia, which further increase the likelihood of tissue breakdown and subsequent healing difficulties. Eventually these processes and accompanying infection lead to damage of the lymphatics, aggravating swelling and local tissue breakdown.

The presenting complaints of patients with chronic venous insufficiency usually center around swelling or ulceration of the lower leg. Chronic recurrent swelling causes a sensation of tightness or bursting, as well as heaviness or aching of the limb. Naturally, this is often worst at the end of the day, and may largely disappear overnight.

Thrombophlebitis

The cause of acute thrombus formation in the venous system is often unclear, but in most instances factors contributing to the three basic elements of Virchow's triad (intimal damage, stasis, and hypercoagulability) can be identified. *Superficial thrombophlebitis* almost always occurs in varicose veins and is clearly a result of static blood flow in these channels. Trauma may occasionally be implicated. In the upper extremity, the cause is most often iatrogenic following intravenous cannulation. On examination, there will be pain and tenderness along the course of the vein, which may also be palpated as a tender cord or knot. There is often an inflammatory erythema locally.

Superficial thrombophlebitis that occurs in several locations over a short time span is sometimes called *migratory superficial phlebitis.* It can be an important clue to a more serious underlying problem such as occult malignancy, especially carcinoma of the pancreas. A hypercoagulable state seems to occur because of the tumor.

Deep venous thrombophlebitis (DVT) is notoriously variable and often subtle in its clinical presentation. Classically, the patient complains of pain in the limb, worse with motion, walking, or dependency and better with rest or elevation of the extremity. Leg edema below the level of the clot, pain on compression of the knee, a *Homans' sign* (calf pain produced by dorsiflexion of the foot), and a palpable cord are cited as the classic physical findings. With extensive deep venous thrombosis, a dusky cyanosis may appear. Engorged or prominent superficial veins are also suggestive of deep venous obstruction. Unfortunately, most classic findings have proven to be disappointingly low in sensitivity and specificity. A patient reporting little or no pain and showing no calf tenderness may harbor extensive deep venous clots, while another with impressive pain, calf tenderness, and an apparently positive Homans' sign may be clot-free. *Unilateral leg edema* may be the only finding; it stands out as the most sensitive indicator of DVT.

EVALUATION

Varicose Veins

On physical examination one should note the extent and location of the varicosities and, more importantly, look for signs suggesting pathology in the deep venous system: thrombophlebitis, stasis changes, ulceration, or swelling. Complaints of leg pain should be carefully evaluated to rule out other possibilities, such as arterial insufficiency, orthopedic or joint disorders, or neurologic problems. Severe varicosities occurring at a young age suggest a congenital arteriovenous malformation, while varicosities appearing after trauma should always raise the question of an arteriovenous fistula, which also may produce a bruit.

Venous Insufficiency

Venous insufficiency needs to be distinguished from other causes of leg edema such as lymphatic obstruction, hypoalbuminemia, and deep vein thrombophlebitis (see Chapter 22). Any accompanying leg ulcers must be differentiated from those due to arterial insufficiency, which tend to be more "punched out" in appearance and localized to the dorsum or lateral aspect of the foot or ankle. A history of claudication, rest pain relieved by dependency, absent pulses, bruits, dependent rubor, and atrophic skin changes also helps distinguish arterial disease from venous insufficiency. Noninvasive studies can be helpful (see Chapter 23).

Superficial Thrombophlebitis

Physical examination should strive to exclude other diagnoses that may be confused with superficial thrombophlebitis, such as cellulitis or lymphangitis. In the latter two, one notes the absence of a palpable thrombosed vein, widespread distribution of erythema and swelling beyond the course of a vein, and identification of a possible focus of infection. Musculoskeletal and neurologic causes of pain and tenderness should be sought, such as a Baker's cyst in the popliteal fossa (see Chapter 152), or radicular pain (see Chapter 147). Swelling of the extremity should also be carefully noted, as isolated superficial phlebitis should not contribute to generalized edema.

Deep Vein Thrombophlebitis

Detection of deep vein thrombophlebitis is critical; undetected and untreated, it may lead to pulmonary embolization. The initial evaluation of the patient who complains of unilateral leg edema—with or without calf pain—must include consideration of DVT. Truly unilateral swelling, particularly extending above the knee, makes venous thrombosis more likely, but cellulitis and lymphedema must also be considered. Pain alone is an unreliable symptom. The findings of calf tenderness and a "positive" Homans' sign are by no means conclusive. Numerous studies have demonstrated the relative inaccuracy of diagnosis by history and physical examination, which is incorrect in up to 50 percent of cases.

The dilemma, then, is accurate diagnosis. *Contrast venography* is the most definitive technique for detecting deep venous thrombosis and is often referred to as the "gold standard" of diagnostic evaluation to which other methods are usually compared. Routine venography, however, has several disadvantages that make it impractical or even undesirable. For example, the test can be quite uncomfortable and is associated with a small risk (1%–3%) of inducing phlebitis. Moreover, it is costly, technically unsuccessful in up to 20 percent of candidates, and requires considerable expertise for both its performance and interpretation.

For these reasons, considerable effort has gone into developing noninvasive methods as an alternative to contrast venography and hospitalization for diagnosis and treatment of DVT. Ultrasound, plethysmography, and nuclear scanning have received the most attention. After a decade of experience with these techniques, *duplex scanning (two-dimensional ultrasound combined with Doppler ultrasound)* has emerged as the most sensitive and specific of available methods, especially when Doppler is enhanced by *color-flow* technology (*triplex scanning*). Sensitivity and specificity for DVT above the knee—where risk of embolization is greatest—exceed 95 percent. The test is much less sensitive for DVT below the knee, because 40 percent of studies below the knee are technically inadequate. However, the risk of embolization for clot below the knee is negligible, though there is a 20 percent to 30 percent chance of clot propagation. If propagation is suspected (eg, leg edema worsens and extends above the knee), then repeat scanning is indicated. Drawbacks of duplex and triplex scanning include high cost of equipment and required time and expertise.

A widely available noninvasive alternative to duplex scanning is *plethysmography*. Sensitivity for detection of DVT above the knee approaches 90 percent to 95 percent for impedance plethysmography, especially when serial studies are performed, but specificity can be disappointing, producing a high rate of false-positives. *^{125}I-fibrinogen scanning* had been a promising technology for prospective study of DVT; labeled fibrinogen is taken up by clot as it forms. However, the HIV risk associated with use of pooled fibrinogen and the time required for results (24–48 h) have greatly discouraged its use. (See Chapter 22 for more detailed discussion of these tests and the workup for DVT.)

Several conclusions can be drawn from information provided by noninvasive evaluation in detecting DVT. Patients with strongly positive studies can be considered to have DVT involving veins above the knee and anticoagulated without venography. Conversely, patients with normal studies can be confidently observed without anticoagulants, with minimal risk. Repeat noninvasive studies are indicated if the patient's symptoms worsen. When laboratory studies are equivocal, tests should be repeated in 48 to 72 hours. Finally, venography is needed for detection of iliac vein occlusion, for patients with a worrisome disparity between clinical and laboratory findings, and for postphlebitic patients, who are likely to have chronically abnormal and therefore unreliable noninvasive studies.

Noninvasive studies have made a great contribution to the evaluation of patients with possible DVT. The cost savings alone related to patients found to be free of DVT, in whom venography, anticoagulation, and hospitalization are avoided, is enormous. The necessity of firmly establishing the diagnosis by means other than history or physical examination cannot be overemphasized.

MANAGEMENT

Varicose Veins

Management of varicose veins can very often be satisfactorily accomplished by nonoperative means, based on appreciation of the principal problem of valve incompetence and poor soft tissue support. Untreated, most varicose veins will slowly worsen and may lead to increasing difficulty and disability. All patients will benefit from proper *elastic support* of medium weight, together with periodic *elevation* of the extremity at intervals during the day. Elastic support is best achieved by a properly fitted surgical stocking obtained from a hospital or commercial surgical company such as Jobst. The various stockings sold in department or drug stores are usually of too light weight and improper fit. Ace wraps are cumbersome and often applied improperly, creating a "tourniquet" effect at the knee level. A below-knee stocking is preferred, because proper compression is difficult to achieve in the thigh, above-the-knee stockings are difficult to keep up, and patient compliance is considerably less. Fortunately, varicosities in the thigh are much less often associated with symptoms or complications.

In addition, obese patients are urged to *lose weight,* and women are reminded to *avoid* the use of *tight garters* or panty girdles, which will constrict superficial venous return at the thigh level. *Prolonged standing* should be avoided as much as feasible.

Sclerotherapy has some enthusiasts but is not generally recommended. The technique involves injection of a sclerosing agent into the vein lumen followed by application of a pressure dressing maintained for several weeks. An inflammatory reaction causing eventual fibrosis and obliteration of the vein lumen is hoped for. Although occasionally used for a small isolated varix (eg, a residual vein following surgical therapy), sclerotherapy is not indicated for the primary treatment of varicose veins.

Indications for surgical referral include persistently symptomatic varicose veins (particularly if a conservative program has been tried), cosmetic dissatisfaction, or recurrent episodes of superficial thrombophlebitis. The option of surgical therapy should probably be discussed initially, because some patients, particularly young women, will prefer this to chronic use of elastic support. In most instances of primary varicose veins, an excellent result can be expected from surgery with extremely low morbidity and a hospitalization of only 2 to 3 days. In experienced hands, the "recurrence" rate of varicose veins should be less than 10 percent.

Venous Insufficiency

Treatment of venous insufficiency is best initiated before the occurrence of venous ulceration, which will follow in many untreated cases. An understanding of the pathophysiology again emphasizes the importance of elastic support and periodic elevation of the extremity. *Patient education* is essential, because compliance is poor otherwise. A *knee-length heavyweight elastic stocking* is prescribed and must be worn religiously from the moment the patient gets out of bed until retiring at night. The leg is best elevated on a pillow or by raising the entire foot of the bed at night. *Periodic elevation* during the day is essential in most patients; it must be emphasized to the patient that the leg should be above the level of the heart for this to be effective. This must be done as often as necessary to prevent formation of edema. *Mild diuretic therapy* (eg, hydrochlorothiazide 50 mg qd) may be of some help in stubborn edema. The chronic and incurable nature of the problem must be made clear to the patient, with reassurance given that symptoms and problems are controllable and preventable by strict adherence to the above program.

Progression to the point of *ulceration* creates a much more troublesome problem. The ulcers may occur with even minor and unrecalled trauma because of atrophic, vulnerable skin and subcutaneous tissues. They usually occur in the lower medial leg just above the medial malleolus, usually overlying an incompetent communicating vein. These lesions will be refractory to all methods of care as long as venous hypertension from the incompetent deep system continues to be transmitted to the superficial tissues. Secondary infection (bacterial or fungal) is common, further impairing any chance for local tissue repair.

Management at this stage is much more difficult, time-consuming, and often expensive. Preferred treatment is an extended period of *bed rest* with *elevation* of the involved extremity well above heart level at all times, combined with *wet to dry saline dressings* to the ulceration, applied three times daily (see also Chapter 197). Hopefully such a program can be carried out at home by the family, perhaps with the help of a visiting nurse. Healing may be anticipated over a 2- to 4-week period. Hospitalization is generally not necessary unless dictated by social circumstances. Any infection should be cultured and treated appropriately with oral antibiotics; staphylococci and gram-negative rods are common. The patient should be urged to exercise the calf muscles repeatedly while in bed, ideally against a footboard, to minimize the occurrence of acute deep venous thrombosis.

Alternatively, particularly for patients who cannot afford extensive time off their feet, an *Unna paste venous boot* may be employed. Properly applied, this medicated bandage can supply good compression, does not require much patient cooperation, and allows the patient to remain ambulatory. Such boot dressings are best changed every 7 to 10 days. With some experience, many venous ulcers may be successfully handled in this fashion. Once healed, chronic use of a heavyweight elastic stocking is resumed.

Surgical referral is advisable for recurrent or nonhealing ulcerations, because surgical interruption of incompetent communicating veins underlying these areas, together with stripping and ligation of associated superficial varicosities, may be indicated. In recent years, some surgeons have reported good results with direct repair of incompetent venous valves, or interposition of a competent valve from an arm vein into the deep venous system of the leg. Insufficient long-term experience exists, however, to ascertain the usefulness of such surgical therapy at this time.

Superficial Thrombophlebitis

Superficial thrombophlebitis in the lower leg is best managed by a combination of local heat and compression with a good elastic stocking. Anti-inflammatory agents such as aspirin or one of the other nonsteroidal drugs may be useful. Antibiotics have no role. Women taking birth control pills should probably discontinue their use. The patient should avoid sitting or standing, but remain ambulatory to minimize the chance of developing any associated clot in the deep venous system. Pain and inflammation usually resolve within 1 to 2 weeks.

If superficial phlebitis extends above the knee, consideration of anticoagulation or ligation of the saphenous vein at the level of the saphenofemoral junction in the groin may be indicated, and surgical consultation should be considered. This is particularly true if the process has ascended while under treatment and observation. The rationale for such a policy is the increased risk of extension of thrombus into the deep system.

Deep Vein Thrombophlebitis

Deep vein thrombophlebitis above the knee is associated with a high risk of thromboembolization and requires immediate *hospitalization* for *heparin* therapy and subsequent initiation of *oral anticoagulation* with *warfarin*. There are no definitive data on how long to continue oral anticoagulation, although it is customary to maintain therapy for 3 months after the first episode and for longer periods if there are recurrences. Data from randomized studies comparing chronic standard- and low-dose warfarin programs show that the low-dose regimen minimizes bleeding complications without sacrificing efficacy (see Chapter 83).

Thrombolytic agents (streptokinase, tissue plasminogen activator) have been studied in patients with DVT, with the hope that effective clot lysis will minimize the chances of developing postphlebitic syndrome. The risk of postphlebitic syndrome is greatest in patients with proximal DVT. The best results have been achieved in patients with proximal vein DVT treated within 3 days of onset of symptoms; most studies have used streptokinase. Clot lysis occurs in about 50 percent of instances, more readily in proximal veins. There is an increased risk of bleeding; overall, clinical outcomes have been mixed. Patients who do best over the long term are those who experienced rapid and complete clot lysis. Only patients with new onset of proximal DVT (in the iliac or femoral system) should be considered potential candidates for thrombolytic therapy.

Deep vein thrombophlebitis below the knee poses much less risk of embolization so long as the clot does not propagate up into the thigh. Risk of propagation ranges from 10 percent to 30 percent. Risk of embolization from a clot that stays below the knee is small. For example, in a study of outpatients with clinically suspected DVT, 289 had initial and follow-up impedance plethysmograms over 10 days that remained negative for DVT above the knee. Of these 289 patients, only one developed a pulmonary embolus during the 10 days of follow-up, and it was minor, for a short-term risk of 0.3 percent. Even if only one-third of patients clinically suspected of a DVT below the knee actually have one, then the risk would increase, but still only to 1 percent. None of the 289 patients with normal studies received anticoagulation, and none embolized during a 6-month follow-up period.

These data suggest that for outpatients suspected of having DVT but without evidence of extension above the knee, hospital admission and anticoagulation are not necessary. Exceptions might include those at greatly increased risk of propagation, such as patients who are bedridden or have an underlying carcinoma and a resultant hypercoagulable state. All patients with suspected DVT below the knee require careful and close follow-up during the acute phase of the illness. Repeat noninvasive study, using plethysmography or duplex scanning, is indicated if there is any clinical suspicion of propagation, such as edema extending up into the thigh.

ANNOTATED BIBLIOGRAPHY

Anderson DR, Lensing AW, Wells PS, et al. Limitations of impedance plethysmography in the diagnosis of clinically suspected deep-vein thrombosis. Ann Intern Med 1993;118:25. *(The sensitivity and specificity were less than in most reports, pointing out limitations of the technology.)*

Cranley JJ, Canos AJ, Sull WJ. The diagnosis of deep venous thrombosis: Fallibility of clinical symptoms and signs. Arch Surg 1976;111:34. *(Documentation of the inaccuracy of clinical diagnosis.)*

Davidson BL, Elliott CG, Lensing AWA, et al. Low accuracy of color Doppler ultrasound in the detection of proximal leg vein thrombosis in asymptomatic high-risk patients. Ann Intern Med 1992;117:735. *(Although the test has performed excellently in most settings, it has its shortcomings, as noted in this report from a study of arthroplasty patients.)*

Heijber H, Buller HR, Lensing AWA, et al. A comparison of real-time compression ultrasonography for the diagnosis of deep-vein thrombosis in symptomatic outpatients. N Engl J Med 1993;329:1365. *(Ultrasound proved superior, with a higher positive predictive value: 94% versus 83%.)*

Hobb JJ. Surgery and sclerotherapy in the treatment of varicose veins. Arch Surg 1974;109:793. *(Good review of treatment for this common problem, focusing on the advantages and proper indications for the use of each modality.)*

Huisman MV, Buller HR, Ten Cate JW, et al. Serial impedance plethysmography for suspected deep venous thrombosis in outpatients. N Engl J Med 1986;314:823. *(A study of 426 outpatients with clinically suspected DVT; risk of embolization was low in patients presenting with disease below the knee; serial impedance plethysmography was sensitive for detection.)*

Hull RD, Rascob GE, Hirsh J, et al. A cost-effectiveness analysis of alternative approaches for long term treatment of proximal venous thrombosis. JAMA 1984;252:239. *(An analysis and review of data from randomized trials of alternative anticoagulant therapies, indicating that low-dose oral therapy is the safest and most cost-effective.)*

Juergens JL, Lofgren KA. Chronic venous insufficiency (postphlebitic syndrome, chronic venous stasis). In: Juergens JL, Spittell JA Jr, Fairbairn JF II (eds): Peripheral Vascular Diseases. Philadelphia, WB Saunders, 1986:809. *(Excellent discussion of the pathophysiology and clinical management of chronic venous insufficiency.)*

Powers LA. Distal deep vein thrombosis: what's the best treatment? J Gen Intern Med 1988;3:288. *(Best critical review of available data, much of which is methodologically incomplete; 54 refs.)*

Rogers LQ, Lutcher CL. Streptokinase therapy for deep vein thrombosis: a comprehensive review of the English literature. Am J Med 1990;88:389. *(Concludes that streptokinase can be of value in properly selected patients, namely those with proximal DVT treated within 7 days of onset of symptoms; 76 refs.)*

Strandness DE, Langlois Y, Kramer M, et al. Long term sequelae of acute venous thrombosis. JAMA 1983;250:1289. *(Long-term sequelae including hyperpigmentation, pain, and swelling were not uncommon and were associated with occluded on incompetent distal deep veins.)*

White RH, McGahan JP, Daschbach, et al. Diagnosis of deep-vein thrombosis using duplex ultrasound. Ann Intern Med 1989; 111:297. *(A review of available studies; concludes that diagnostic accuracy for proximal DVT is very high; 51 refs.)*

Primary Care Medicine: Office Evaluation and Management of the Adult Patient, 3rd edition, edited by Allan H. Goroll, Lawrence A. May, and Albert G. Mulley, Jr. J.B. Lippincott Company, Philadelphia

36
Exercise Stress Testing

GREGORY D. CURFMAN, M.D.

The exercise stress test has become a widely employed method for the detection of coronary artery disease. Assessments of exercise capacity, ventricular dysrhythmias, severity of coronary disease, and efficacy of anti-ischemic therapy can also be accomplished by exercise testing. At present, the predominant method of exercise testing is continuous electrocardiogram (ECG) monitoring of the patient during exercise on a treadmill or stationary bicycle. Thallium imaging techniques improve diagnostic accuracy in the detection of coronary disease but also add substantially to the cost. The primary physician needs to know the sensitivity, specificity, and predictive value of the ECG exercise test and the factors that affect the study measurement in order to appropriately select the study and properly interpret its results.

PHYSIOLOGIC BASIS OF THE TEST

A complete assessment of the cardiovascular system often requires an evaluation of cardiovascular function under conditions of the enhanced metabolic demands of exercise. Evaluation of the heart in the resting state only reveals part of the story. The exercise stress test assesses the ability of the coronary circulation to supply sufficient blood to meet the increase in myocardial oxygen requirements generated by exercise. Since the rate of oxygen extraction by the heart is relatively fixed, increased oxygen supply is usually achieved by an increase in coronary blood flow. When coronary artery stenosis limits adequate blood supply, ischemia may result, often manifested by anginal chest pain, ECG changes, or perfusion defects on a thallium scan. The demand placed on the coronary circulation can be quantified; the product of heart rate times systolic blood pressure closely parallels the measured myocardial oxygen consumption during isotonic exercise. Heart rate alone is almost as good an indicator of oxygen consumption. Since known quantities of work are being performed, the exercise stress test can provide a measure of exercise capacity as well as aid in the detection of coronary disease.

APPROACHES TO EXERCISE TESTING

Exercise testing for the detection of coronary disease most often uses dynamic (isotonic) rather than sustained-contraction (isometric) exercise. Isotonic exercise permits smoother increases in the rate–pressure product to be accomplished, allowing the patient's ischemic threshold to be approached gradually. Nevertheless, isometric exercise testing (eg, by sustained handgrip) can be of use in special situations, such as in assessing the safety of isometric activities in patients with known coronary disease.

Protocols for isotonic exercise testing are divided into maximal and submaximal types, depending on the level of exercise achieved during the test. A *maximal test* is defined as one in which systemic oxygen consumption reaches a plateau before exercise is terminated. Only by making serial measurements of oxygen consumption can one be certain that maximal exertion has been achieved. Because it is often not convenient to measure oxygen consumption during routine exercise testing, maximal effort is usually approximated by exercising the individual to his or her age-adjusted predicted maximal heart rate. Values for maximal predicted heart rate can be obtained from standardized tables or regression formulas, but the value 220 minus age in years for men (or 210 minus age for women) provide reasonable approximations of the true maximal heart rate. If a patient is receiving a beta-adrenergic blocking agent, the maximal predicted heart rate is not useful in judging when maximal effort has been accomplished. In this situation maximal effort can be approximated by having the patient exercise to exhaustion. The level of effort expended during the test can be assessed semiquantitatively using the scale of perceived exertion developed by Borg (a 15-point scale, numbered between 6 and 20). If perceived effort is "very very hard" (19 or 20 on Borg's scale) at the termination of the test, it can be reasonably assumed that maximal exertion has been closely approximated.

A *submaximal exercise test* is by definition one in which maximal systemic oxygen consumption is not achieved. The test may be terminated prematurely by design (at a certain percentage of predicted maximal heart rate or at a given level of systemic oxygen consumption), or it may be terminated because of the appearance of angina, marked ischemic electrocardiographic changes, cardiac arrhythmias, severe hypertension, or hypotension. Tests terminated prematurely because a certain percentage of predicted maximal heart rate has been achieved are generally less useful than maximal exercise tests. Such submaximal tests provide little information about exercise capacity, and they often give less diagnostic information. In general, it is best to continue the test to the predicted maximum heart rate, to maximal perceived effort, or until a pathologic event (angina, ischemia, arrhythmia, hypotension) occurs. One clinical situation in which submaximal testing has proved useful is in patients early (within 2 wk) *after myocardial infarction*. In this setting submaximal exercise testing to a 5 met level (1 met = 3.5 mL O_2 consumed/kg/min) has been useful in identifying patients at higher risk for subsequent coronary events and death and has also been found to be safe. Many physicians prefer instead to perform a symptom-limited exercise test 1 month after myocardial infarction, in lieu of an earlier submaximal test.

Most maximal and submaximal tests are *multistage*, that is, graded amounts of work are performed, with a progressive increase in work load between stages. The objective of graded exercise is to obtain the greatest increase in heart rate before musculoskeletal fatigue limits the amount of exercise that the patient can perform. The previously used Master's exercise test was a single stage step test in which the intensity and amount of exercise were fixed; the test had a high rate of false-negative results because many patients did not sufficiently increase their heart rates during the performance of the test. Another disadvantage of Master's test was its inability to provide continuous ECG monitoring; ECGs were taken before and after exercise only, often reducing the amount of information available from the test.

Exercise Devices and Monitoring. Currently the *treadmill* and *bicycle ergometer* are the most popular devices used for exercise testing. Slightly higher values for maximal oxygen consumption can usually be obtained on the treadmill than on the bicycle ergometer, because a somewhat larger muscle mass is called on during treadmill exercise. Many different exercise testing protocols are available for the treadmill and bicycle. Although the treadmill protocol developed by Bruce is very popular, it has the disadvantages of unequal changes in work load between stages, and a very abrupt increase in work load at stage IV, which is too vigorous for many cardiac patients. The protocols developed by Balke are characterized by a constant increment in work load from one stage to the next and by a constant treadmill speed (walking pace), which is tolerated well by most patients.

Walking protocols are generally preferred over protocols that require running for diagnostic purposes in unfit populations. Bicycle ergometer protocols usually consist of 2- to 3-minute stages in which work load is increased by 10 to 30 watts per stage, depending on the level of physical conditioning of the subject. For both treadmill and bicycle tests, it is best to select a protocol that will allow the patient to reach maximal exertion within a 10- to 12-minute period. A longer test may be limited by the subject's endurance, and a shorter test usually increases the work load too rapidly.

Continuous *ECG monitoring* is employed during exercise testing. A modified V_5 lead (CM_5) is the one most commonly monitored. The sensitivity of the test can be increased by employing a three-lead system, since the CM_5 lead may not detect inferior ischemic changes. Further increases in sensitivity can be expected from recording 12-lead ECGs during exercise. In many laboratories, three leads are recorded each minute during exercise and 12 leads are recorded every 3 minutes. Because ischemic changes may not occur on the ECG until *after* exercise, monitoring is continued for at least 5 to 7 minutes into the recovery phase.

SENSITIVITY, SPECIFICITY, AND PREDICTIVE VALUE

ECG Testing

Myocardial ischemia may be manifested during the exercise stress test by ECG changes, by abnormal blood pressure and heart rate responses, by angina, or by anginal equivalents, such as severe dyspnea. ECG changes, particularly alterations in ST segments that occur during exercise in the context of ischemia, have received the most attention and study. The sensitivity and specificity of ST segment changes in the diagnosis of coronary disease have been determined by correlating ECG findings with the results of coronary angiography.

A number of factors affect the sensitivity and specificity of the exercise test, including *severity of the underlying coronary disease* and the ECG criteria used for diagnosis of ischemia. For example, test sensitivity using the criterion of ST segment depression increased in one study from 40 percent to 76 percent as the extent of disease went from one-vessel to three-vessel stenosis. The *magnitude of ST segment depression* required for diagnosis affects sensitivity and specificity. One can achieve an increase in sensitivity by reducing the amount of ST depression required for the designation of ischemia, but at the cost of lowering specificity and obtaining more false-positive results. An analysis of pooled data showed that when the criterion for diagnosis of ischemia was 1 to 1.5 mm of ST depression, sensitivity was 23.3 percent and specificity 89 percent. When the amount of ST depression required was raised to 1.5 to 2 mm range, sensitivity fell to 8.8 percent, but specificity rose to 97.8 percent. This trade-off between sensitivity and specificity is characteristic of all tests having a quantitative standard for diagnosis (see Chapter 2).

Other aspects of *ST segment* change have been examined to improve sensitivity and specificity. The configuration of the ST segment has been subjected to careful study. A downsloping ST segment (Fig. 36–1) was found to have a specificity of 99 percent. Horizontal or plane depression of the ST segment had a specificity of 85 percent, and a slowly upsloping ST segment (≥1.5 mm ST depression at 0.08 sec after the J point) had a specificity of 68 percent. Simple J-point depression without a slowly upsloping ST segment is a non-

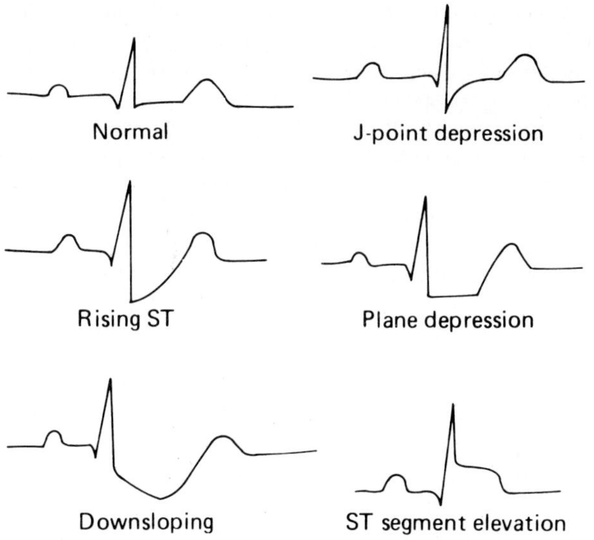

Figure 36-1. Exercise-induced ST segment changes.

specific finding and *not* diagnostic of ischemia. When the criterion for an ischemic response was at least 1 mm of downsloping or horizontal ST segment depression, the exercise test was found to have a sensitivity of 64 percent and a specificity of 93 percent. When a slowly upsloping ST was added to the list of acceptable criteria for ischemia, sensitivity increased to 76 percent, but at the expense of specificity, which fell to 82 percent.

A number of other factors alter the sensitivity and specificity of the ECG exercise test, including the *type of exercise protocol* used (submaximal tests appear to be less sensitive) and the *number of leads* used (a three-lead system improves sensitivity by about 10 percent over a single-lead system). The specificity of ST segment changes is limited by the fact that ST segment depression is not unique to coronary disease. Patients with valvular or hypertensive disease, nonischemic myocardial disease, and preexcitation syndromes may demonstrate ST segment depression during exercise in the absence of ischemia. In addition, left ventricular hypertrophy, recent glucose ingestion, hypokalemia, and sedatives may produce *false-positive results*. Digitalis glycosides are notorious for their ability to cause deviations in ST segments. If possible, it is best to discontinue digitalis for at least 48 hours prior to testing. If this is not feasible, then exercise-associated ischemia should not be diagnosed until at least 2 minutes of ST segment depression is observed. Studies have also suggested that false-positive responses may be more common in women than in men by a factor as high as 3. In all of these situations, the use of thallium scintigraphy in conjunction with exercise testing may improve the diagnostic value of the test.

Investigators have searched for *other changes* that occur during the exercise test that might help to better identify patients with coronary disease. The changes in ST segments that occur with exercise do not provide a definite answer but rather a probability statement of the likelihood of the patient having coronary disease. Among other variables studied have been the *timing and duration of ST segment changes*, the presence and severity of *ventricular dysrhythmias and heart rate and blood pressure changes*, and the coexistence of *exercise-induced angina*. In a series of 302 patients undergoing exercise testing and coronary angiography, the occurrence of *typical angina* during exercise had a sensitivity of 51 percent and specificity of 90 percent, compared with 76 percent sensitivity and 76 percent specificity for ST segment changes alone. In essence, exercise-induced angina had about the same diagnostic significance as did ST segment changes, especially when predictive values for these changes in the appropriate populations were compared.

Three exercise-induced variables have been used to predict *prognosis*: the duration of exercise, the maximal extent of ST segment deviation during or after exercise, and the presence and severity of angina. When used to compute a treadmill exercise score, these variables provide an accurate prediction of subsequent mortality in an outpatient population with suspected coronary disease. Those subjects with the best exercise scores had a 4-year survival rate of 99 percent, while those with the worst had a 4-year survival rate of only 79 percent.

Knowledge of test sensitivity and specificity and attempts to improve them still do not provide the clinician with an estimate of the probability that coronary disease is present when a positive test result is encountered (ie, the predictive accuracy or predictive value positive of the test). Figures for the predictive accuracy of the exercise stress test have varied greatly from series to series, and between men and women, presumably because of wide differences in the prevalence of underlying coronary disease in the populations studied. The predictive accuracy of any diagnostic test is directly related to the prevalence of the disease in the population examined (see Chapter 2). As a result, a test will have a low predictive accuracy when disease prevalence is low, regardless of how sensitive and specific the test is.

Asymptomatic patients with few or no risk factors for coronary disease who are subjected to exercise testing and demonstrate "ischemic" changes are less likely to have underlying coronary disease and more likely to have a false-positive test. Therefore, asymptomatic subjects with an abnormal stress test should be screened carefully for possible causes of a false-positive response. In asymptomatic populations, abnormal ST segment responses should be viewed as a "risk factor" for coronary disease rather than as definite evidence of the disease. In these individuals, the incidence of coronary disease is about 6 percent, rising to 12 percent by the sixth decade.

It is important to recognize another shortcoming of the use of exercise testing to screen asymptomatic populations. The majority of patients who die suddenly from coronary disease do not have flow-limiting coronary artery lesions; instead they have severe atherosclerotic lesions that cause sudden death when they suddenly rupture and occlude the coronary vessel. Exercise testing may not be effective in the detection of such non–flow-limiting lesions. Other studies have indicated that exercise testing is not a cost-effective way of screening otherwise healthy people for coronary disease.

Prevalence of coronary disease has been found to be 16 percent in patients with nonanginal chest pain, 50 percent in those with atypical pain, and 89 percent when typical angina is present. Consequently, the predictive value of a positive test is expected to be greatest in *patients with typical angina,* but in such instances the history of angina is almost as good as the test's predictive value (about 90%) in diagnosing coronary disease. The very high figures initially reported for the diagnostic utility and accuracy of the exercise test resulted from studies conducted on a referred population that had a high probability of coronary disease in the opinion of the referring physicians; these were the people in whom angiography was deemed most appropriate.

In essence, the exercise test adds little to the diagnosis of coronary disease in patients with typical angina, although exercise testing may be very useful in such patients to quantitate the amount of exertion required to induce ischemia, to obtain preliminary information about the extent of coronary disease (see Chapter 30), and to assess the efficacy of antianginal therapy. Also, exercise testing in asymptomatic persons may produce false-positive responses, and care must be taken to avoid factors that may lead to a false-positive result. Exercise testing in asymptomatic subjects may also fail to detect a considerable number of persons destined to die suddenly as the first manifestation of coronary disease. The test may be of diagnostic help in *patients with atypical anginal pain* as long as the criteria for atypical pain are rather rigid (eg, at least two or three characteristics of classic angina must be present). In such settings, the predictive accuracy has been on the order of 40 percent to 50 percent. In general, exercise testing has its greatest diagnostic usefulness in those whose pretest likelihood of having coronary disease is moderate. An example would be a man older than 50 years of age with an atypical chest pain syndrome and one or two coronary risk factors. In this situation a positive exercise test would substantially increase the posttest likelihood of underlying coronary disease, and a negative test would substantially reduce it.

Radionuclide Scanning

Further attempts to improve the sensitivity and specificity of the exercise test have led to the development of radionuclide imaging techniques, such as the use of *thallium 201,* which is taken up by myocardial cells via the sodium pump, similarly to potassium ions. Thallium is distributed to the myocardium according to the regional coronary blood flow, and underperfused areas will take up less of the isotope and will appear as "cold" spots on the perfusion scan. When thallium 201 is injected intravenously during exercise, myocardial uptake of the isotope is determined by regional differences in myocardial blood flow at the time of injection. Areas of myocardium that appear underperfused during exercise may "fill in" later during the 2 to 4 hours after exercise. Therefore, sequential scanning during and after exercise is required to diagnose hemodynamically significant coronary stenoses. Thallium scintigraphy has proved especially valuable in patients who have resting repolarization abnormalities on the ECG or left bundle branch block, both of which render interpretation of the standard exercise test difficult. Thallium scanning is also useful in patients whose standard exercise test results are suspected to be false-positive or false-negative.

Thallium scanning not only helps in detection of ischemia but it also facilitates the estimation of disease severity and prognosis. It can demonstrate the extent of underperfused myocardium (sometimes referred to as the "amount of myocardium at risk"). Diffuse ischemia suggests high-risk coronary disease (three-vessel or left-main stenosis) and the need to consider coronary angiography (see Chapter 30). Uptake of thallium by the lungs, a sign of left ventricular dysfunction, is another indicator of poor prognosis. However, thallium scanning adds substantially to the cost of exercise testing, often tripling it. The study should not be used as a routine screening procedure.

Dipyridamole–thallium imaging represents a technique for noninvasively assessing coronary perfusion in patients unable to undergo exercise testing. Dipyridamole induces maximal coronary vasodilation; when used in conjunction with thallium myocardial imaging, the test has a sensitivity and specificity for detection of significant coronary disease comparable to that of exercise thallium imaging.

Exercise Echocardiography

Echocardiographic assessment of cardiac wall motion during exercise is being conducted at some centers for the diagnosis of coronary artery disease. The methodology is technically demanding and requires considerable expertise to detect regional wall-motion abnormalities. Its role in evaluation of the patient with suspected coronary disease and its cost-effectiveness remain to be determined.

OTHER APPLICATIONS OF EXERCISE TESTING

The severity of known coronary disease can be assessed by electrocardiographic exercise stress testing. Factors correlating with the severity and extent of disease include the depth of ST segment depression, early onset of ST changes, persistence of ST segment depression past 8 minutes into the recovery period, downward sloping ST configuration, hypotensive response at low work loads, and impairment of heart rate response to exercise (see Chapter 30). In addition, the occurrence of both angina and ischemic changes during exercise has been reported to predict an increased likelihood of multivessel disease.

Assessment of prognosis of patients in the early postinfarction period may be aided by exercise testing. The greater the work load tolerated, the better the prognosis. Patients who developed angina on a limited exercise test conducted just before hospital discharge had twice the rate of postinfarction angina. Those with no ST segment changes had a 2.1 percent 1-year mortality, compared with a 27 percent mortality for those who did develop ST segment depression during exercise testing.

Determination of Exercise Capacity can be provided by the exercise stress test, since the patient is made to perform known quantities of work under direct observation and continuous ECG monitoring. This determination is essential for designing a safe cardiac rehabilitation program and may help to reassure the patient who is unnecessarily restricting activity out of fear of sudden death or infarction. The work level achieved during the test can be used to define the degree of incapacity (when it is in question) as well as provide guidelines for establishing safe levels of daily activity for the patient.

Detection of Ventricular Dysrhythmias can sometimes be facilitated by exercise testing, especially if the rhythm disturbance is believed to be exercise-induced. However, except in a few cases of ventricular tachycardia, ambulatory ECG (Holter) monitoring was found in a careful study to be superior for detecting most types of ventricular irritability. Ambulatory monitoring should be obtained in conjunction with an exercise test if the objective is optimal detection of dysrhythmias (see Chapters 25 and 29).

Safety and Contraindications

Reported mortality in a multi-center study involving 170,000 exercise tests was 0.01 percent. There was no relationship to the type of test or to exercise intensity. Morbidity requiring hospitalization was 0.2 percent. Safety is enhanced by a pre-examination history, a physical examination, and a resting ECG. Patients with unstable angina, uncompensated congestive failure, severe anemia, high-grade heart block, severe aortic stenosis, cor pulmonale, or severe hypertension should not undergo testing. A physician should be present throughout, and a defibrillator and other resuscitation equipment should be in the room. The test should be terminated if blood pressure or heart rate falls suddenly during exercise, or if exhaustion, angina, faintness, marked ST changes, severe hypertension, or serious arrhythmias (ventricular tachycardia, heart block, etc.) occur. When performed by experienced personnel, exercise testing is very safe and is one of the most useful noninvasive tests for evaluating cardiovascular function and disease.

ANNOTATED BIBLIOGRAPHY

Bartel AG, Behar US, Peter US, et al. Graded exercise stress tests in angiographically documented coronary artery disease. Circulation 1974;49:348. *(Classic paper demonstrating that the depth of ST segment depression correlated with severity and extent of coronary disease.)*

Bonow RO. Prognostic applications of exercise testing. N Engl J Med 1991;325:887. *(A brief editorial summarizing the current state of the art.)*

Bruce RA. Methods of exercise testing. Am J Cardiol 1974;33:715. *(A concise and thorough discussion of the differences in various methods of stress testing by one of the pioneers in the field.)*

Chaitman BR. The changing role of the exercise electrocardiogram as a diagnostic and prognostic test for chronic ischemic heart disease. J Am Coll Cardiol 1986;8:1195. *(An excellent, comprehensive review.)*

DeBusk RF. Specialized testing after recent myocardial infarction. Ann Intern Med 1989;110:470. *(Reviews exercise testing and other diagnostic tests for risk stratification after acute myocardial infarction.)*

Epstein SE, Quyyumi AA, Bonow RO. Sudden cardiac death without warning: possible mechanisms and implications for screening asymptomatic populations. N Engl J Med 1989; 321:320. *(An interesting discussion of the pitfalls of using exercise testing to screen asymptomatic persons for coronary disease.)*

Gill JB, Ruddy TD, Newell JB, et al. Prognostic importance of thallium uptake by the lungs during exercise in coronary artery disease. N Engl J Med 1987;317:1485. *(Evaluates uptake of thallium by the lungs during thallium scintigraphy in relation to other prognostic indicators in coronary artery disease.)*

Goldschlager N. Use of the treadmill test in the diagnosis of coronary artery disease in patients with chest pain. Ann Intern Med 1982;97:383. *(An analytic review of the exercise stress test including an algorithmic approach to atypical chest pain and a description of the role of thallium stress scintigraphy.)*

Leppo JA, Boucher CA, Okada RD, et al. Serial thallium-201 myocardial imaging following dipyridamole infusion. Circulation 1982;66:649. *(Diagnostic utility for detection of ischemic disease equalled that of exercise stress testing.)*

Mark DB, Shaw L, Harrell FE, Jr, et al. Prognostic value of a treadmill exercise score in outpatients with suspected coronary artery disease. N Engl J Med 1991;325:849. *(This exercise score incorporates exercise duration, ST segment change, and the occurrence of angina into a single predictive index.)*

Martin CM, McConahay DR. Maximum treadmill exercise electrocardiography. Circulation 1972;46:956. *(Provides data on the changes in sensitivity and specificity associated with different diagnostic criteria. When 0.5 mm ST depression is used, false-positive rate equals 43 percent; it falls to 11 percent with 1.0 mm criteria.)*

Morrow K, Morris CK, Froelicher VF, et al. Prediction of cardiovascular death in men undergoing noninvasive evaluation for coronary artery disease. Ann Intern Med 1993;118:689. *(Data on use of a predictive rule utilizing clinical findings and results from exercise stress testing.)*

Moss AJ, Benhorin J. Prognosis and management after a first myocardial infarction. N Engl J Med 1990;322:743. *(A useful review of risk stratification after a first myocardial infarction.)*

Pollack ML, Wilmore JH, Fox FM, et al. *Exercise in Health and Disease.* Philadelphia,: WB Saunders, 1984. *(A textbook containing valuable information about exercise testing and the role of exercise in health promotion.)*

Rifkin RD, Hood WB. Bayesian analysis of electrocardiographic exercise stress testing. N Engl J Med 1977;297:681. *(Argues that the results of the stress test should be viewed as a probability statement, rather than as "positive" or "negative"; emphasizes the predictive value of various test results and the dependence of the predictive value on the prevalence of the disease in the population being studied.)*

Sox HC Jr, Littenberg B, Garber AM. The role of exercise testing in screening for coronary artery disease. Ann Intern Med 1989;110:456. *(A cost-effectiveness analysis of exercise testing as a screening test for coronary disease.)*

Theroux PT, Waters DD, Halphen C, et al. Prognostic value of exercise testing soon after myocardial infarction. N Engl J Med 1979;301:341. *(Performance of a limited treadmill test just prior to hospital discharge provided useful prognostic information.)*

Weiner DA, McCabe C, Heuter DC, et al. The predictive value of anginal chest pain as an indicator of coronary disease during exercise testing. Am Heart J 1978;96:458. *(The occurrence of anginal pain during exercise was found to be as predictive of coronary disease as ischemic ECG changes alone.)*

Weiner DA, Ryan TJ, McCabe CH, et al. Exercise stress testing. N Engl J Med 1979;301:230. *(A detailed study of data from the Coronary Artery Surgery Study examining the influence of the prevalence of coronary artery disease on the diagnostic accuracy of stress testing.)*

Primary Care Medicine: Office Evaluation and Management of the Adult Patient, 3rd edition, edited by Allan H. Goroll, Lawrence A. May, and Albert G. Mulley, Jr. J.B. Lippincott Company, Philadelphia

4
Respiratory Problems

37
Screening for Lung Cancer

Lung cancer is the most common fatal malignancy among males and females in the United States. In recent years, it has claimed the lives of as many men as tumors of the colon and rectum, prostate, pancreas, and stomach combined. The incidence of lung tumors in males has been rising dramatically since 1930. More recently, there has been a dramatic increase among women. Approximately 10 percent of American men and 5 percent of American women alive today will develop lung cancer during their lifetime; of these, 85 percent will die of the disease.

Most people are aware of the epidemic proportions of the lung cancer problem. Many have lost friends or relatives and know the grim prognosis of the disease. However, screening of asymptomatic individuals, whether it is restricted to those at high risk, can offer little reassurance. Efforts to improve the prognosis by early detection have been thwarted by the insensitivity of available tests, poor compliance with screening programs among patients at high risk, and the aggressive natural history of most lung tumors. Without an understanding of these limitations, the primary care provider may expend resources that produce little more than exaggerated fear in some patients and inappropriate reassurance in others. Knowledge of the risk factors, the natural history, and the validity of available diagnostic tests provides a basis for the reasoned approach to many pulmonary symptoms (see Chapters 40 to 44).

EPIDEMIOLOGY AND RISK FACTORS

The epidemiology of lung cancer is dominated by its association with smoking. The dramatic increase in cancer death rates among men and the more recent increase among women can be attributed to increases in cigarette consumption. A dose-response relationship between duration and intensity of cigarette smoking and risk of lung cancer has been documented in men and women. When compared with nonsmokers, risks of lung cancer increase fivefold, 10-fold, and 20-fold for men who smoke less than ½ pack, ½ to one pack, and one to two packs per day, respectively. A decrease in risk has been demonstrated in smokers who are able to stop and in those who smoke filter-tipped cigarettes. A decrease in the prevalence of smoking among adults since 1965 should be followed by a declining incidence of lung cancer. Cigar and pipe smokers incur much less risk, but again a dose-response relationship has been documented (see Chapter 54).

The association between smoking and cancer is strongest for the epidermoid (squamous cell) and small cell undifferentiated (oat cell) tumors. The relationship is less certain for adenocarcinoma (alveolar cell) and large cell undifferentiated (anaplastic) histologic types.

The observation that lung cancer occurs in males far more often than in females can be explained for the most part by differences in smoking patterns. In fact, lung cancer without a smoking history is more common among women. A slight apparent excess of lung cancer cases also occurs in urban areas and among low-income groups. The presence of polycyclic organic matter in urban pollution and in some occupational environments (see Chapter 39) may provide a partial explanation. Exposure to asbestos, chromate, nickel, uranium, or radon gas has also been associated with significantly increased rates of lung cancer. The combined effect of such exposures and smoking is generally more than additive. For example, smokers exposed to asbestos have a 90-fold greater risk of lung cancer than nonexposed nonsmokers.

NATURAL HISTORY OF LUNG CANCER AND EFFECTIVENESS OF THERAPY

Lung cancer's rapidly progressive and usually inexorable course frustrates screening efforts. The 5-year survival rate is between 5 percent and 10 percent. At the time of symptomatic presentation, 75 percent of patients have lesions that are clearly unresectable. Of the remainder, 60 percent prove to be unresectable because of mediastinal involvement discovered by further evaluation or at thoracotomy. Five-year survival rates after resection in the relatively few remaining patients vary from about 10 percent for patients with oat cell tumors to 30 percent for patients with squamous cell tumors.

Reports of 5-year survival rates based on the symptoms present at the time of diagnosis are more relevant to the question of early detection. In a group of patients with overall 5-year survival of 7 percent, the 6 percent who were discovered while asymptomatic had an 18 percent survival rate, compared with 10 percent to 15 percent for patients with local symptoms and 6 percent for those with systemic symptoms. Nearly one-third of the patients had symptoms of metastatic disease; all died within 5 years.

There are reports of higher survival rates after resection of *in situ* lung cancer diagnosed by means of chest x-ray or sputum cytology followed by bronchoscopy, but this may represent little more than selection of slow-growing or otherwise benign lesions. Some highly speculative estimates of growth rate suggest that squamous cell carcinoma and adenocarcinoma take as long as 10 and 25 years respectively to reach a size likely to be detected by radiography. If such estimates are accurate and if there is wide variability in natural history, overestimation of benefits of early detection are likely due to the problems of lead time and time-linked bias sampling (see Chapter 3).

SCREENING AND DIAGNOSTIC TESTS

Chest Radiograph

A controlled British study of semiannual chest x-rays in more than 29,000 men detected 101 lung tumors over a 3-year period. Seventy-six were detected in a control population of 25,000. The overall 5-year survival rates among cancer patients from the screened and control groups were 15 percent and 6 percent, respectively. Of the 101 cancers in the screened group, only 65 were detected by routine chest x-ray; the remainder presented symptomatically during screening intervals.

The value of chest x-ray screening was also addressed by the Philadelphia Pulmonary Neoplasm Project, which attempted to screen more than 6000 male volunteers older than 45 years of age with semiannual x-ray examinations. Lung cancer developed in 121 patients during a 10-year period, with an ultimate mortality rate of 92 percent at 5 years. The poor results were attributed to poor patient compliance with screening, patient and physician delay, advanced age or concomitant illness contraindicating surgical therapy, and inadequate sensitivity of the screening method.

Three additional randomized trials of lung cancer screening were conducted by members of the Cooperative Early Lung Cancer Group. Separate studies at the Mayo Clinic, Memorial Sloan-Kettering Cancer Center, and Johns Hopkins Hospital each enrolled more than 10,000 male smokers. In the Mayo study, those randomized to the close surveillance group were screened with both sputum cytology and chest x-ray examinations every 4 months, while control patients were advised, but not reminded, to have such studies annually. At Memorial Sloan-Kettering and Johns Hopkins, patients were randomized to receive either annual chest x-ray and 4-monthly sputum cytologies or annual chest x-ray alone. The findings of these studies indicate that screening, particularly sputum cytology examinations, may advance the time of diagnosis, with more cancers detected in an earlier stage. However, there was no difference in survival between screening groups at Memorial Sloan-Kettering and Johns Hopkins, suggesting that there is no benefit from the addition of cytology to annual radiographic screening. Furthermore, in the Mayo study, there was no significant difference in lung cancer mortality rates in the screened and control groups despite the fact that more than twice as many post-surgical stage I lung cancers were found in the screened group than among controls.

It should be kept in mind that false-positive chest x-rays may engender considerable fear as well as the morbidity associated with confirmatory diagnostic tests. Although the specificity of radiographic screening has been shown to be in the range of 90 percent to 97 percent, it is still too low to give an acceptable predictive value. A Veterans Administration study of lung cancer screens found 438 false-positive x-rays compared with 97 true-positive readings for suspected neoplasm. In the Memorial Sloan-Kettering study described above, 10,040 persons were screened with both chest x-ray and cytology. Approximately 10 percent had abnormal chest x-rays leading to additional studies to rule out cancer. The predictive value of such a positive finding in this and other recent studies has been in the range of 1 percent to 5 percent.

Cytologic Screening

The sensitivity of cytologic screening varies with the cell type and location of the tumor and the methods of specimen collection. It used to be thought that a single cytologic specimen would detect about 70 percent of squamous cell lesions and that three specimens would increase sensitivity to 90 percent. However, data from the recent large randomized trials indicate that cytologic examination is much less sensitive. Only 10 percent of cancers in the Memorial Sloan-Kettering study and 13 percent of those in the Mayo study were detected initially by cytology alone. Presumably, these disappointing findings can be explained by the spectrum problem, that is, decreased sensitivity for early rather than late stage tumors (see Chapter 3). The low sensitivity can also be explained by the relatively low proportion of cancers that were squamous cell, which is the histologic type most likely to be detected by cytologic examination. The specificity of sputum cytologic examination is high, in the range of 98 percent to 99 percent. In the Memorial Sloan-Kettering Prevalence screen of 10,040 men, only seven had cytology classified as marked atypia or cancer before they were found not to have cancer. Though rare, such false-positive findings are highly problematic often requiring meticulous bronchoscopic examination to sixth- and seventh-generation bronchi.

It should be noted that, as *diagnostic* tests, chest x-ray and cytologic examination are complementary. In a Veterans Administration study, cytology alone had an overall screening sensitivity of 33 percent and a specificity of 98 percent; x-ray screening had a sensitivity of 42 percent and specificity of 98 percent; the sensitivity for combined radiographic and cytologic examination was 63 percent. X-ray examination is more sensitive for peripheral lesions, whereas cytologic examination is more sensitive for central squamous cell tumors.

SUMMARY AND CONCLUSIONS

- Lung cancer is a major cause of morbidity and mortality, especially among men. The incidence is increasing among women.

- Smoking is the overwhelming risk factor for lung cancer. Occupational exposures also are relevant.
- Little is known about the presymptomatic natural history of lung cancer. It is presumed to be very variable. The 5-year survival despite all forms of therapy is 5 percent to 10 percent. Survival is slightly better when an asymptomatic lesion is detected.
- Cytologic examination of the sputum and chest x-ray are complementary diagnostic tests. However, neither is sensitive nor specific enough to serve as a screening test.
- Large-scale early detection programs have demonstrated little benefit. Such efforts to improve prognosis have been thwarted by the usually rapid course of lung cancer, the characteristics of the patients at risk, and the relative insensitivity of available tests.

A.G.M.

ANNOTATED BIBLIOGRAPHY

(Additional references concerning the relationship of lung cancer to smoking follow Chapter 54.)

Berlin NI, Buncher CR, Fontana RS. Results of the initial screen (prevalence). Early lung cancer detection: introduction. Am Rev Respir Dis 1984;130:549. *(This introduction is followed by three papers describing prevalence screen results from Hopkins, Mayo and Sloan-Kettering studies.)*

Boucot KR, Weiss W. Is curable lung cancer detected by semiannual screening? JAMA 1973;224:1361. *(Reviews the data of the Philadelphia Pulmonary Neoplasm Project, in which 5-year survival in men offered semiannual x-ray screening was only 8 percent.)*

Eddy DM. Screening for lung cancer. Ann Intern Med 1989; 111:232. *(Well-reasoned analytic review that includes discussion of Hopkins, Mayo, and Sloan-Kettering studies.)*

Flehinger BJ, Kimmel M, Melamed MR. The effect of surgical treatment on survival from early lung cancer. Implications for screening. Chest 1992;101:1013. *(Post-study analysis of Hopkins, Mayo and Sloan Kettering data with focus on outcomes for patients with stage I cancer.)*

Fontana RS, Sanderson DR, Woolner LB, Taylor WF, et al. Screening for lung cancer. A critique of the Mayo Lung Project. Cancer 1991;67:1155. *(A review of the Mayo trial, including results of follow-up for five years beyond the six-year study period.)*

Hammond EC, Selikoff IJ, Seidman H. Asbestos exposure, cigarette smoking and death rates. Ann NY Acad Sci 1979;330: 473. *(Includes data from 18,000 insulation workers: relative risks of 90 and 50 for 2 pack and ½ pack smokers, respectively, compared to nonexposed nonsmokers.)*

Hubbell FA, Greenfield S, Tyler JL, et al. The impact of routine admission chest x-ray films on patient care. N Engl J Med 1985;312:209. *(The impact of routine admission chest x-rays on the care of 742 consecutive patients admitted to a VA hospital was negligible; in only one case was a new pulmonary malignancy detected, but outcome was unaffected.)*

Kabat GC, Wynder EL. Lung cancer in nonsmokers. Cancer 1984;53:1214. *(A case–control study focusing on risk factors other than smoking; includes review of passive smoking risk studies.)*

Roscoe RJ, Steenland K, Halperin WE. Lung cancer mortality among nonsmoking uranium miners exposed to radon daughters. JAMA 1989;262:629. *(Estimated 12-fold relative risk for exposed nonsmokers.)*

Wynder EL, Goodman MT. Smoking and lung cancer: some unresolved issues. Epidemiol Rev 1983;5:177. *(Comprehensive review with special attention to passive smoke inhalation and the low yield cigarette.)*

Primary Care Medicine: Office Evaluation and Management of the Adult Patient, 3rd edition, edited by Allan H. Goroll, Lawrence A. May, and Albert G. Mulley, Jr. J.B. Lippincott Company, Philadelphia

38

Screening for and Prophylaxis of Tuberculosis

HARVEY B. SIMON, M.D.

Active tuberculosis (TB) remains a relatively uncommon occurrence in ambulatory practice, though its prevalence is beginning to increase again in some populations, especially among patients infected with the human immunodeficiency virus (HIV) and the urban poor. Being a contagious yet potentially treatable condition, TB is always an important consideration in patients presenting with hemoptysis (see Chapter 42), chronic cough (see Chapter 41), or fever and weight loss (see Chapters 9 and 10). Tuberculin reactivity remains prevalent. On a daily basis, the primary physician faces the questions of whether to test for reactivity and how to respond when it is present. These issues have become particularly problematic in the care of HIV-positive individuals.

EPIDEMIOLOGY AND RISK FACTORS

Until the mid 1980s, the number of reported TB cases in the United States was declining at an annual rate of about 6 percent, with most new cases occurring among the institutionalized elderly who represented a remaining pool of latent endogenous infection (prevalence of tuberculin skin test positivity 20 percent; prevalence of active disease, 2.4 percent). Since 1985, there has been a marked reversal, with a 16 percent *increase* in the annual rate, accounted for by substantial outbreaks of new infection among HIV-positive persons, intravenous drug abusers, the urban poor (especially the homeless), and immigrants from countries in Asia and Latin America where TB is prevalent. Among HIV-infected individuals, the risk of acquiring TB increases by upwards of 200-fold and the chances of developing active disease from 10 percent per lifetime to 10 percent per year. Other population groups with a disproportionately high incidence of TB include alcoholics and patients with a history of gastrectomy, neoplasia, or other debilitating diseases.

NATURAL HISTORY OF TUBERCULOSIS AND EFFECTIVENESS OF THERAPY

Natural History

Mycobacterium tuberculosis is transmitted by way of fresh droplet nuclei expelled by an individual with cavitary disease. It cannot be spread by hands, utensils, or other fomites, although organisms can be cultivated from room dust. While inoculation can occur via the gastrointestinal tract, the vast majority of infections in the United States begin in the lung (see Chapter 49). Until the HIV epidemic, it was rare for primary infection to result in early progressive disease; young children were at greatest risk for this complication. However, among HIV-positive patients, the risk of rapid progression to active disease is substantial, with one study showing an attack rate of 10 percent and a mean incubation period of only 80 days. In immunocompetent hosts, exposure stimulates an immune response that develops over a period of several weeks, and the disease enters a latent stage.

Approximately 5 percent to 15 percent of new tuberculous infections eventually progress to serious disease. Risk is greatest during the years immediately following infection. Only 3 percent to 5 percent of patients without clinical disease 5 years after infection will suffer late reactivation.

Effectiveness of Therapy

Three strategies may be used in the prevention of clinical infection: 1) biologic prophylaxis of uninfected individuals with BCG vaccine; 2) chemoprophylaxis of newly or recently infected individuals with isoniazid (INH); and 3) INH chemoprophylaxis of selected individuals with latent infection.

Biologic prophylaxis utilizing *bacillus Calmette-Guérin (BCG) vaccine* is widely practiced in countries where TB is prevalent. The vaccine is used for prevention in uninfected individuals; it has no value in infected persons. BCG vaccine contains a live, attenuated strain of *Mycobacterium bovis*, which has little virulence in humans. It produces a positive tuberculin test in recipients; it should not be administered to individuals who react positively to the purified protein derivative (PPD) tuberculin skin test. The vaccine has been in clinical use since 1922, but its role remains controversial. Early trials demonstrated that BCG could prevent TB in up to 80 percent of recipients, but subsequent trials on the Indian subcontinent failed to demonstrate efficacy. Even though recent studies in Great Britain and Canada suggest that the vaccine may be up to 60 percent effective, BCG is not currently recommended for routine use in the United States. The relatively low incidence of new tuberculous infections in the U.S. still makes case-finding and INH prophylaxis a more effective approach (see below). Whether the new outbreaks of TB in the U.S. will require a reconsideration of biologic prophylaxis—especially among high-risk populations—remains to be seen.

Chemoprophylaxis of newly or recently infected individuals, as identified by recent conversion to tuberculin reactivity, is an important method of preventing clinical disease. Even in HIV-infected patients, chemoprophylaxis appears to significantly reduce the risk of progression from latent infection to active disease. In patients who have not received chemotherapy, a positive skin test implies the presence of a few dormant but viable tubercle bacilli, which have the potential for reactivation. In a sense then, patients with positive tuberculin skin tests serve as their own reservoir for future clinical disease. It has been demonstrated that the administration of *INH* daily for 6 to 12 months reduces the risk of reactivation by up to 80 percent. Since the risk of progressive disease is greatest soon after infection, recent converters to tuberculin reactivity are most likely to benefit from such therapy.

Current guidelines for INH chemoprophylaxis depend on the patient's *age*, the *strength of the tuberculin reaction*, and the presence of *other risk factors*:

- Patients with *HIV infection*, those with *close exposures* to active pulmonary TB, and those with radiologic evidence of *old TB on chest x-ray* (see Chapter 49) are at highest risk for developing TB. People in these categories who have *skin reactivity* of *5 mm* or more are candidates for INH prophylaxis, regardless of their age.
- Patients who are HIV-positive, anergic, and belong to a group with an high prevalence of TB (>10% [see Chapter 7]) are candidates for INH prophylaxis.
- Patients who have important but somewhat less potent risk factors include those who are *immunosuppressed*, *abuse drugs intravenously*, or have other disorders known to increase the risk of TB. They are candidates for INH prophylaxis if their PPD skin test shows *10 mm* or more of reactivity, regardless of their age.
- *Recent tuberculin converters* who are *younger than age 35* should be considered for INH prophylaxis if their skin test has *increased by 10 mm*. Recent converters *older than 35* should be considered for prophylaxis if their skin test reactivity increased by *15 mm*.
- Patients *younger than age 35* who have no risk factors but who belong to a *high-incidence population* (eg, immigrants, low-income and medically underserved, prison inmates, homeless) should be considered for prophylaxis if their skin test reactivity is *10 mm* or more.
- Patients who have *no risk factors* and who belong to a *low-incidence group* are candidates for INH prophylaxis only if they are *younger than age 35* and have a PPD skin test of more than *15 mm*.

When INH is used for prophylaxis, it should be administered *daily* for periods of *6 to 9 months*, except in the case of *HIV-positive* individuals and those with *old TB* by chest x-ray criteria; the latter require *12 months* of INH.

Enthusiasm for INH prophylaxis must be tempered by the significant side effects of the drug and the emergence of drug-resistant strains in patients (especially those who are

HIV-positive) who fail to complete a full course of therapy (estimated to be at least 20%). INH can be *hepatotoxic*. Liver injury is quite rare in patients younger than age 20 and occurs in no more than 0.2 percent of those between ages 20 and 34. On the other hand, among patients older than 50, more than 2 percent may develop INH-induced liver disease (see Chapter 49).

SCREENING AND DIAGNOSTIC TESTS

The tuberculin skin test, far more sensitive and specific than the chest x-ray, is the most useful test for the diagnosis of past or present tuberculous infection. The *Mantoux test* using the intradermal injection of Tween-80 stabilized *purified protein derivative (PPD)* is more reliable than multiple-puncture tests, such as the tine test. Three strengths of PPD are available: the *"first strength"* contains *1 tuberculin unit (TU)*; the *"intermediate strength," 5 TU* units; and the *"second strength," 250 TU*.

The intermediate-strength PPD is the standard test material. The tuberculin skin test should be interpreted 48 to 72 hours after injection; the diameter of *induration* (not erythema) determines the interpretation. Until recently, a single standard was used to interpret the tuberculin skin test in all people: 0 to 4 mm was "negative"; 5 to 9 mm was "doubtful"; and 10 mm or more was "positive." As noted above, authorities such as the Centers for Disease Control and Prevention (CDC) now recommend that different skin test criteria be applied to different population groups, to provide a more accurate assessment of risk.

The current CDC *criteria for skin test positivity* include:

- *5 mm* of induration for patients who are HIV-positive or have other major defects in cell-mediated immunity and for patients who are very likely to have TB, such as close contacts with documented cases and patients with chest x-ray films that strongly suggest TB (see Chapter 49);
- *10 mm* of induration for members of high-incidence populations;
- *15 mm* of induration for individuals with no identifiable risk factors.

First-strength PPD should be reserved for patients in whom a very strong reaction is anticipated. Second-strength PPD should be reserved for individuals with negative reactions to a lower strength. A positive second-strength test in the face of a negative or doubtful intermediate-strength test is suggestive of infection with atypical mycobacteria and resultant cross-sensitization to PPD. Obviously, a positive tuberculin test does not by itself prove active disease. Repeated tuberculin skin tests can produce a booster effect; among hospital employees or other populations in which repeated skin testing may be necessary, a booster effect may be mistaken for tuberculin conversion. Confusion can be avoided by repeating negative or doubtful skin tests 1 week later: any increase in the diameter of induration can be attributed to the booster effect. In contrast, increased reactivity that occurs at 1 year, but not at 1 week, should be attributed to newly-acquired infection.

False-negative reactions have been documented in up to 20 percent of patients with tuberculosis, particularly in those individuals who are immunocompromised from HIV infection, overwhelming or advanced disease, malnutrition, or debility. Many of these patients are anergic. Approximately 50 percent of patients with clinical acquired immunodeficiency syndrome (AIDS) may have falsely negative PPD tests in the setting of active TB. The development of anergy is a poor prognostic sign. The lowering of the criterion for a positive skin test in HIV-positive patients to 5 mm of induration is an attempt to improve test sensitivity. The CDC recommends that skin testing of such patients should include use of two other antigens (*Candida*, mumps, or tetanus toxoid) to test for anergy and facilitate interpretation of the tuberculin skin test result.

In addition to the immunologic incompetence of the host, false-negative skin tests may result from mishandling of the antigen or from faulty injection technique. Tuberculin should never be transferred from one container to another, and skin tests should be given as soon as possible after the syringe is filled. Subcutaneous rather than intradermal injection may result in false-negative reactions. Since tuberculin sensitivity develops 2 to 10 weeks after initial infection, early skin tests may be negative in newly-infected individuals.

Tuberculin skin testing is highly specific; however, cross-reactivity with atypical mycobacterial antigens may cause intermediate skin test reactions to occur in people who have not been exposed to *M. tuberculosis*. More often, individuals infected with atypical mycobacteria will have positive second-strength PPD reactions and weak or negative intermediate PPD results.

RECOMMENDATIONS AND CONCLUSIONS

- As long as the tuberculin skin test and INH remain useful for case-finding and prophylaxis respectively, biologic prophylaxis with BCG for PPD-negative patients is not recommended. Should prevalence rise considerably or skin-test anergy become more of a problem, then the need for immunization, especially among high-risk groups, may require reconsideration.
- The tuberculin skin test can be useful in apparently healthy individuals, especially children and young adults. Because of its prognostic value and the importance of recent conversion, the PPD status of such healthy individuals should be determined. Healthy individuals with a high risk of exposure to TB, such as those in the health professions, should have tuberculin testing on an annual basis so long as they remain PPD-negative.
- PPD testing should be performed in all HIV-infected patients. Other high-risk individuals should also be tested, including intravenous drug abusers, homeless persons, Hispanic and Asian immigrants, prisoners, residents of chronic care facilities, and those who are immunosuppressed or have other chronic illnesses known to increase the risk of TB. Anergy testing with two other antigens (*Candida*, mumps, or tetanus toxoid) should be part of skin testing in such patients.
- INH prophylaxis should be considered for tuberculin-positive individuals, based on the strength of the PPD reaction, the presence of risk factors, and age. Positive reactors require a minimum of 6 to 9 months of daily INH prophylaxis (300 mg/d); those at highest risk (HIV-positive, old TB on chest x-ray) require 12 months of daily pro-

phylactic treatment. Care must be taken to ensure compliance to prevent emergence of drug-resistant strains.

- Anergic, PPD-negative, HIV-positive patients from groups with a high prevalence of TB (>10%) should be considered for INH chemoprophylaxis.

ANNOTATED BIBLIOGRAPHY

American Thoracic Society/Centers for Disease Control. Diagnostic standards and classification of tuberculosis. Am Rev Respir Dis 1990;142:725. *(Standards for the administration and interpretation of the tuberculin skin test.)*

Boyd JC, Marr JJ. Decreasing reliability of acid-fast smear techniques for detection of tuberculosis. Ann Intern Med 1975; 82:849. *(Misleading title but very useful article pointing out high specificity [99 percent] of smears but low predictive value [45 percent] because of low prevalence; sensitivity 22 percent.)*

Centers for Disease Control. Guidelines for preventing the transmission of tuberculosis in health-care settings, with special focus on HIV-related issues. MMWR Morbid Mortal Wkly Rep 1990;39:RR-17. *(Important advice on preventing nosocomial infection; items germane to outpatient care included.)*

Centers for Disease Control. Purified protein derivative (PPD)—tuberculin anergy and HIV infection: guidelines for anergy testing and management of anergic persons at risk of tuberculosis. MMWR Morbid Mortal Wkly Rep 1991;40(suppl RR-5):27. *(Recommends use of two additional antigens for skin testing and treatment of anergic patients who are HIV-positive and come from groups with a prevalence of TB greater than 10 percent.)*

Centers for Disease Control. Update: tuberculosis elimination—United States. MMWR Morbid Mortal Wkly Rep 1990;39:153. *(A concise overview of the epidemiology of tuberculosis and approaches to its control.)*

Centers for Disease Control, Advisory Committee for the Elimination of Tuberculosis. Screening for Tuberculosis and tuberculous infection in high-risk populations, and the use of preventive therapy for tuberculous infection in the United States. MMWR Morbid Mortal Wkly Rep 1990;39:RR-8. *(Recommends aggressive testing and treatment.)*

Centers for Disease Control, Advisory Committee for the Elimination of Tuberculosis. Use of BCG vaccines in the control of tuberculosis. MMWR Morbid Mortal Wkly Rep 1989;37:663. *(CDC guidelines for BCG prophylaxis.)*

Dooley SW, Jarvis WR, Martone WJ, et al. Multi-drug resistant tuberculosis. Ann Intern Med 1992;117:257. *(A terse summary of this worrisome condition and means of prevention.)*

Frieden TR, Sterling T, Pablos-Mendez A, et al. Emergence of drug-resistent tuberculosis in New York City. N Engl J Med 1993;328:521. *(High prevalence among those who are HIV-positive, IV drug abusers, and those previously treated.)*

Gordin F. Tuberculosis control: back to the future? JAMA 1992;267:2649. *(An editorial reviewing current methods of control and their adequacy in the setting of HIV disease.)*

Graham MH, Nelson KE, Solomon L, et al. Prevalence of tuberculin positivity and skin test anergy in HIV-1-seropositive and -seronegative intravenous drug users. JAMA 1992;267:369. *(Finds both a high rate of anergy in HIV-positive patients, especially in those with low CD4 counts, and reductions in diameter of response; suggests that the criterion for positivity be reduced to 2 mm.)*

Huebner RE, Villarino ME, Snider DE. Tuberculin skin testing and the HIV epidemic. JAMA 1992;267:409. *(An editorial recommending careful anergy testing and addressing the optimal definition of a positive skin test.)*

International Union Against Tuberculosis Committee on Prophylaxis. Efficacy of various durations of isoniazid preventive therapy for tuberculosis: five year follow-up of the IUAT trial. Bull World Health Organ 1982;60:555. *(A cooperative European study of 27,830 tuberculin-positive adults with fibrotic pulmonary lesions. Fifty-two weeks of INH produced a 75 percent reduction in TB; 24 weeks of treatment provided a 65 percent reduction. Hepatitis occurred in 0.5 percent of the INH recipients, as compared with 0.1 percent in placebo recipients. For the 52-week regimen, the benefit/risk [tuberculosis averted/INH hepatitis] ratio was 2.1; for 24 weeks the ratio was 2.6.)*

Selwyn PA, Hartel D, Lewis VA. A prospective study of the risk of tuberculosis among intravenous drug abusers with HIV infection. N Engl J Med 1989;320:545. *(Documents a very high risk of infection, even in those who are PPD-negative.)*

Stead WW, Lofgren JP, Warren E, et al. Tuberculosis as an endemic and nosocomial infection among the elderly in nursing homes. N Engl J Med 1985;312:1483. *(A study of 25,000 elderly nursing home residents showing a high prevalence of tuberculin reactivity and active disease; risk of new infection was great.)*

Thompson NJ, Glassrath JL, Snider DE Jr, et al. The booster phenomenon in serial tuberculin testing. Am Rev Respir Dis 1979;119:387. *(A good discussion of the booster phenomenon with guidelines for serial skin testing in high-risk population groups.)*

Wadhawan D, Hira S, Mwansa N, et al. Isoniazid prophylaxis among patients with HIV-1 infection. In: Proceedings of the Seventh International Conference on AIDS. Florence, Italy, 1991:2. Abstract WB 2261. *(INH prophylaxis reduced the risk of progression from infection to active disease in these high-risk patients.)*

Primary Care Medicine: Office Evaluation and Management of the Adult Patient, 3rd edition, edited by Allan H. Goroll, Lawrence A. May, and Albert G. Mulley, Jr. J.B. Lippincott Company, Philadelphia
© 1995

39

Prevention and Evaluation of Occupational Respiratory Disease

L. CHRISTINE OLIVER, M.D.
JOHN D. STOECKLE, M.D.

Occupational lung disease, one of the 10 leading causes of work-related health problems in the United States, results from inhaled organic and inorganic dusts, irritant gases, and toxic fumes, which adversely affect both the upper and lower respiratory tracts. Although the true scope of occupational respiratory illness and disease is unknown, some estimates can be given. It has been estimated that approximately 65,000 males in the United States have clinically diagnosable asbestosis; moreover, it is predicted that 19,000 cases of mesothelioma and 55,000 cases of lung cancer will occur by the year 2009 in males with a history of occupational exposure to asbestos. Persons permanently disabled by respiratory disease due to previous exposure to cotton dust number about 30,000; active cotton mill workers partially disabled, about 85,000. Ten percent of active coal miners and 20 percent of retired miners have coal worker's pneumoconiosis (CWP). The U.S. Department of Labor has estimated that over one million workers are exposed to silica and that approximately 60,000 have silicosis.

Yet these figures underestimate the extent of occupational pulmonary disease. The reasons are several. First, since clinical findings of work-related respiratory disease resemble those of nonoccupational respiratory disease, diagnosis is often missed. Second, the latency period between exposure and the subsequent development of disease is often long, obscuring the causal relationship. Third, physicians often underdiagnose because they have inadequate training in occupational medicine. Fourth, occupational disease is underreported by health personnel. Moreover, the estimates do not include "paraoccupational" lung disease resulting from bystander exposure, from household contact with toxins carried home on work clothes, and from neighborhood exposures. Asbestos-related disease has been reported in family members of asbestos workers and in individuals living in close proximity to shipyards and asbestos-manufacturing plants. Chronic beryllium disease has resulted from residence in the neighborhood of beryllium plants, and asthma from residence near grain elevators.

It is critical that the primary physician be familiar with occupational lung diseases and their diagnosis if unnecessary morbidity is to be avoided. Since acute respiratory symptoms due to toxic exposure are nonspecific, recognition of their relationship to the toxic agent is essential. Continued exposure may result in needless, irreversible functional abnormalities. The diagnosis of established chronic occupational respiratory disease is also important. In such instances, the rate of functional deterioration or the risk of secondary disease such as neoplasia may be reduced by removal from the exposure, control of infection, and elimination of smoking.

PATHOPHYSIOLOGY AND CLINICAL PRESENTATION

Inhaled dusts, gases, and fumes exert their effect on the respiratory tract in several ways. The first and most obvious is that of *direct irritation*. Excessive mucous secretion, cough, airway hyperreactivity, chest tightness or pain, dyspnea, pneumonitis, or pulmonary edema may develop. With such irritant gases as nitrogen dioxide (NO_2) and phosgene, a delay of 12 to 24 hours may precede the onset of pulmonary edema.

Second, dusts may be retained in the lungs, provoking a *fibrotic or granulomatous response*. To reach the lung, substances must have a particle size of 5 μm or less. Related to level of exposure, latency periods preceding the onset of clinical disease can be 15 to 20 years.

Third, *hypersensitivity* and abnormal function of the immune system may play a role in the development of occupational lung disease. Hypersensitivity is important etiologically in hypersensitivity pneumonitis and in certain types of occupational asthma. Increased circulating levels of immunoglobulins, rheumatoid factor (RF), antinuclear antibody (ANA), and alpha$_1$-antitrypsin have been observed in individuals with asbestosis. Reported peripheral blood T-lymphocyte abnormalities appear to be related to duration of asbestos exposure and to radiographic outcome. Elevated titers of circulating ANA and RF are seen in association with silicosis. Individuals with chronic beryllium disease are reported to have alterations in circulating T-lymphocytes and a high rate of blast transformation of lymphocytes in peripheral blood and bronchoalveolar lavage compared to controls.

Fourth, *other host factors* are also important. Asbestos acts synergistically with cigarette smoke to increase the risk for lung cancer. The prevalence of bronchitis and airways obstruction is increased in smoking welders and coal miners compared to their nonsmoking coworkers. Finally, *social and economic factors* and work practices often determine the geographic proximity of home site to industrial sources of air pollution and affect the likelihood that family members will bring potentially toxic materials home on work clothes.

Occupational respiratory disease can be classified clinically, as shown in Table 39–1.

Industrial Bronchitis

Industrial bronchitis is characterized by cough and sputum. It may be associated with chronic airways obstruction. Acute bronchitis is self-limited. Chronic bronchitis is cough and sputum on most days, for 3 months or more per year, for 2 consecutive years or more. A nonspecific manifestation

Table 39-1. Classification of Occupational Respiratory Disease

Industrial Bronchitis
Causal agents: welding fumes, coal dust, sulfur dioxide, vanadium pentoxide
Pulmonary Fibrosis
Causal agents: asbestos, coal dust, silica, beryllium, talc, kaolin, and organic materials such as thermophilic actinomycetes, aspergillus, and animal proteins
Obstructive Airways Disease
Occupational asthma
Causal agents: toluene diisocyanate (TDI), phthalic anhydride, nickel, chromium, platinum salts, formaldehyde, *Bacillus subtilis* proteolytic enzyme, grains, animal products, epoxy resins, Western red cedar, mahogany, and oak
Byssinosis
Causal agents: cotton, flax, and hemp
Cancer
Causal agents: asbestos, arsenic trioxide, hexavalent chromium, nickel, bischloromethyl ether (BCME), chloromethylmethyl ether (CMME), vinyl chloride monomer, and radiation
Noncardiogenic Pulmonary Edema
Causal agents: nitrogen dioxide (NO_2), phosgene, chlorine, ammonia, and sulfuric acid

of airway irritation and inflammation, bronchitis may result from exposure to such agents as coal dust and silica, the irritant gases sulfur dioxide and chlorine dioxide, welding fumes, and vanadium pentoxide fumes.

Interstitial Lung Disease

Coal Worker's Pneumoconiosis (CWP) results from the deposition of coal dust in peribronchial tissues, with the formation of dust macules and the distention of terminal bronchioles. Occurrence and extent of disease depend both on the level of dust exposure and the rank of the coal, with anthracite being more fibrogenic than bituminous. CWP occurs in two forms: "simple pneumoconiosis," characterized by the presence of small dust nodules, usually less than 5 mm in diameter; and "complicated pneumoconiosis" or "progressive massive fibrosis" (PMF), characterized by large masses of dust and collagen tissue. The most prevalent respiratory symptom is chronic bronchitis, unrelated to radiographic appearance of the lungs and more common in smoking miners. Physiologic abnormalities on lung function testing are variable, and with the exception of single breath diffusing capacity for carbon monoxide ($DLCO_{SB}$), unrelated to radiographic appearance in simple CWP. Reduced $DLCO_{SB}$ is associated with category "p" opacities (<1.5 mm in diameter) of simple CWP and with advanced PMF. Airway obstruction may be seen in PMF and in association with chronic bronchitis.

Asbestosis is fibrosis of the lung parenchyma or pleura as a result of asbestos exposure. Pleural plaques may contain calcium. An early finding, usually occurring within 10 years of exposure, is the so-called "benign asbestos effusion." It may be unilateral or bilateral and often leaves behind residual pleural thickening at the costophrenic angle. Severity of asbestos-related pulmonary fibrosis is related both to total dose and to latency. In epidemiologic studies, parenchymal asbestosis is more closely associated with dose, while pleural asbestosis is more closely related to latency. Respiratory symptoms are nonspecific and depend on extent of disease. Physical examination may reveal characteristic dry end-inspiratory crackles at the lung bases and clubbing. Physiologic abnormalities include restrictive mechanics and impaired gas exchange. Small airways dysfunction, probably resulting from peribronchiolar fibrosis, may be an early finding. The posterior–anterior chest radiograph typically reveals irregular densities in the lower lung zones or the pleural plaques. Lateral views of the chest are useful in detecting *calcified hemidiaphragmatic plaques,* a hallmark of asbestos exposure. The value of oblique views in detecting pleural plaques is inversely related to risk for developing disease. Extensive pleural thickening has been associated with respiratory failure; the presence of pleural plaques has been associated with increased risk for subsequent development of lung cancer, mesothelioma, and parenchymal fibrosis. The full effect of exposure to asbestos from asbestos-containing materials in schools and other public buildings remains to be determined. Asbestosis has been reported in school custodians, and malignant mesothelioma in custodians and building occupants.

Silicosis results from exposure to silicon dioxide (SiO_2) or quartz, which is fibrogenic. Silica exposure occurs in a wide variety of occupational settings. Particularly important is bystander exposure. It is often the case that sandblasters are given respiratory protection, whereas workers around them are not. Like CWP, silicosis may occur in a simple nodular form or in a "complicated" form with PMF. Latency and severity of disease are directly related to level of dust exposure. Silicosis may occur after 1 to 2 years of high-level exposure. It may be complicated by mycobacterial or fungal infection. Radiographic abnormalities characteristically precede functional abnormalities and initially occur as small rounded opacities involving the upper lung zones. Hilar lymph nodes may become enlarged with "eggshell" calcifications. Physiologic abnormalities reflect the peribronchiolar location of the silicotic nodules and consist of small airways dysfunction and impaired gas exchange in the early stages. With PMF, obstruction, restriction, or a mixed pattern may develop.

Acute and Chronic Beryllium Disease results from the inhalation of beryllium. At risk are workers engaged in the manufacture of beryllium-containing products and in the electronics and aircraft industries. Acute disease follows inhalation of relatively high concentrations of beryllium. Its irritant effect on the respiratory tract may produce nasopharyngitis, tracheobronchitis, or clinical pneumonitis. Chronic beryllium disease is a systemic granulomatous disorder often confused with sarcoidosis. Chest radiograph typically reveals a diffuse reticulonodular infiltrate, with hilar lymphadenopathy in about 40 percent of patients. Lung function tests may reveal obstruction or restriction and/or impaired gas exchange. The angiotensin$_I$-converting enzyme (ACE) is elevated in about 50 percent of individuals with active sarcoidosis, a finding that may be useful in distinguishing this entity from chronic beryllium disease. Elevated levels of beryllium in urine or tissue suggest the diagnosis and provide definitive evidence of exposure. The blast transformation of pulmonary lymphocytes on in vitro exposure to beryllium confirms the diagnosis.

Hypersensitivity pneumonitis (extrinsic allergic alveolitis) occurs following exposure to organic material. Causal agents include thermophilic actinomycetes, aspergillus, and serum and urine protein from animals and fish. Clinical disorders include farmer's lung, bird fancier's lung, bagassosis, humidifier fever, and animal handler's lung. Both acute and chronic reactions may occur. Chest radiograph may reveal miliary or larger discrete opacities in the middle and lower lung zones. Repeated exposure may result in recurrence of symptoms and ultimately in the development of chronic disease, with interstitial fibrosis on chest radiograph and impaired lung function on physiologic testing. The acute phase may be mild and pass relatively unnoticed. Antigen-specific precipitins appear in about 90 percent of cases.

So-called "benign pneumoconioses" occur following exposure to certain inert dusts. Chest radiograph reveals interstitial opacities. Lung function generally remains intact. These pneumoconioses follow exposure to iron oxide (siderosis), tin oxide (stannosis), barium (baritosis), and zirconium.

Obstructive Airways Disease

Occupational Asthma is reversible airway hyperreactivity caused by inhalation of substances in the workplace. These substances can be divided into three groups: high molecular weight, low molecular weight (less than 1000 Daltons), and irritant gases or fumes. The condition occurs in both nonatopic and atopic individuals. Symptoms include chest tightness, wheezing, dyspnea, and cough. Lung function tests may reveal small airways dysfunction and an obstructive defect that is partially reversible following administration of bronchodilators. Lung function may be observed to decline over the work shift or gradually over the work week. A fixed level of obstruction may ultimately develop. The longer the duration of exposure after onset of symptoms, the more likely is the development of irreversible changes.

Byssinosis is characterized by respiratory symptoms and obstructive airways disease and follows exposure to cotton, flax, and hemp dust. It is seen most commonly in the United States among cotton textile workers. Symptoms of chest tightness and dyspnea, with reduction in air flow rates, initially appear on the first day of the work week after a 2-day absence from work. These abnormalities may become persistent, resulting in chronic and irreversible disease with continued exposure. Diagnosis depends to a large extent on occupational history. The bract of the cotton plants is thought to contain the as-yet unidentified causal agent.

Cancer

Occupational exposures causally associated with cancer of the respiratory tract involve arsenic, chromium (hexavalent), nickel, vinyl chloride monomer, radiation, and possibly fumes from the welding of stainless steel. The chemicals bischloromethyl ether (BCME) and chloromethylmethyl ether (CMME) have been shown to cause small cell carcinoma of the oat cell type. Asbestos causes bronchogenic carcinoma, as well as mesothelioma, a tumor of the pleura and peritoneum. Asbestos and cigarette smoke act synergistically to increase the risk for lung cancer by 50 to 70 times, while asbestos alone increases the risk by a factor of three to five. Smoking does not affect the risk for malignant mesothelioma. Asbestos also increases the risk for cancers of the larynx in smokers and in cancer of the gastrointestinal tract in selected, heavily exposed populations.

NATURAL HISTORY OF DISEASE AND EFFECTIVENESS OF CONTROL

Although much remains to be learned about the natural history of most occupational lung diseases, practical control steps can be taken. It is worthwhile to distinguish agents that commonly cause acute symptoms and, with repeated exposures, may produce irreversible disease from other agents that produce disease evident only after a long asymptomatic latent period.

Byssinosis and asthma due to diisocyanate exposure are examples of acute reversible diseases that can progress to chronic, irreversible diseases with repeated exposure. Both are characterized by acute symptoms of coughing and wheezing that occur when the worker is re-exposed after a brief absence from work. Chronic obstructive changes can develop in those whose exposure continues despite symptoms. Some workers exposed to enzyme detergents have similar acute symptoms; progressive loss of elastic recoil is possible if exposure continues. Disorders due to organic dusts (farmer's lung) and toxic metals (beryllium) also produce both acute and chronic syndromes that are related to level and duration of exposure.

In contrast, diseases due to mineral dusts, such as CWP and asbestosis, become clinically manifest only after a long asymptomatic latent period. The clinical findings of coal worker's pneumoconiosis usually follow 10 years of exposure. Similarly, 10 to 20 years of low-level exposure is usually required to produce detectable pulmonary asbestosis. In the case of pleural asbestosis, exposure usually precedes the development of disease by 20 to 30 years. Silicosis also has a long latent period unless exposure is intense. Despite improved dust control, termination of exposure has been advised for people with identifiable pulmonary disease. However, the extent to which progression of the disease can be influenced by cessation of exposure after the appearance of detectable abnormalities is not known.

DIAGNOSIS

Eliciting the *occupational history* is the most important step in the diagnosis of occupational respiratory disease. Although a chronologic lifetime work history is ideal, it is often unnecessary in the primary care setting. Three questions will usually suffice: 1) What is your current job? 2) What was your previous job? and 3) What is your usual job, that is, the one you have worked at the longest? It is important to obtain not only job title but also job description. Specific information about type, level, and duration of exposures is needed. It is important to characterize the temporal relationship of symptoms and disease to work, and to inquire about similar illness in coworkers and family members.

Lung function and other laboratory tests provide valuable diagnostic information. Reduction in the $DLCO_{SB}$ may be the only abnormality in developing pulmonary fibrosis. Small airways dysfunction may be an early sign of interstitial or obstructive lung disease. Pre- and post-shift *spirometry* is often useful in the diagnosis of occupational asthma or byssinosis. If history and clinical findings suggest the diagnosis of pneumoconiosis, *chest radiograph* should be interpreted according to the ILO System of Classification, developed by the International Labor Organization for standardization and more specific radiographic characterization and quantification of pneumoconiosis. *Bronchial provocation* by inhalation under carefully controlled conditions can be a useful tool in the diagnosis of occupational asthma.

Thorough documentation is essential not only for design of a treatment program, but also for disability and compensation determinations.

CONCLUSIONS AND RECOMMENDATIONS FOR PREVENTION

The role of the primary care physician in the prevention of occupational respiratory disease is as follows:

1. To appropriately recognize and diagnose work-related respiratory illness and disease.
2. To inform the patient of the diagnosis, making certain that he is aware of any occupational etiology. Ascertaining patient understanding is important because of statutes of limitation associated with legal remedies, such as worker compensation.
3. To inform the employee and/or a regulatory agency such as the Occupational Safety and Health Administration (OSHA) of any serious or potentially life-threatening hazards to the patient or coworkers to facilitate a workplace evaluation and eliminate the toxic exposure.
4. To encourage patients to abstain from habits such as smoking that are inherently toxic to the lungs and exacerbate the respiratory effects of occupational exposures.
5. To treat respiratory infections without delay. Unfortunately, there is often no specific treatment for occupational lung disease.
6. To institute appropriate medical surveillance for subsequent pulmonary disease.

Elimination of exposure through the use of rigorous engineering controls is the ultimate goal in prevention. Removal from the job should be a "court of last resort."

ANNOTATED BIBLIOGRAPHY

Becklake MR. Asbestos-related diseases of the lung and other organs: Their epidemiology and implications for clinical practice. Am Rev Respir Dis 1976;114:55. *(Comprehensive review.)*

Bouhuys A, Heapty LJ, Schilling RSF, et al. Byssinosis in U.S. N Engl J Med 1967;277:170. *(Chronic irreversible disease occurs mainly in reactors, those with acute reversible symptoms.)*

Centers for Disease Control. Release of the 1992 supplement to work-related lung disease surveillance report. JAMA 1993; 269:465. *(Source for epidemiologic data.)*

Chan-Yeung M, Malo JL. Occupational asthma update. Chest 1988;93:407. *(Very useful discussion for the general reader.)*

Frumkin H, Berlin J. Asbestos exposure and gastrointestinal malignancy: review and meta-analysis. Am J Ind Med 1988; 14:79. *(Evidence for an association.)*

Goodman LR. Radiology of asbestos disease. JAMA 1983;249: 644. *(Succinct, illustrated summary of characteristic findings.)*

Hammond EC, Selikoff IJ, Seidman H. Asbestos exposure, cigarette smoking and death rates. Ann NY Acad Sci 1979; 330:473. *(Study of independent and interactive contributions of asbestos exposure and cigarette smoking to death from lung cancer in 17,800 asbestos insulation workers.)*

Kriebel D, Sprince NL, Eisen EA, et al. Beryllium exposure and pulmonary function: a cross sectional study of beryllium workers. Br J Ind Med 1988;45:167. *(Detailed documentation of the changes that occur.)*

Kreiss K, Newman LS, Mroz MM, et al. Screening blood test identifies subclinical beryllium disease. J Occ Med 1989;31: 603. *(Utility of the lymphoblast transformation test for diagnosis of pulmonary beryllium disease.)*

Oliver LC, Sprince, Greene R. Asbestos-related disease in public school custodians. Am J Ind Med 1991;19:303. *(Reports increased risk associated with building exposures.)*

Oliver LC. Occupational and environmental asthma: legal and ethical aspects of patient management. Chest 1990;98:220S. *(Two very difficult issues in the care of these patients.)*

Parkes WR. Occupational Lung Disorders. Boston, Butterworths, 1982. *(Chapters 7,8,11,12 provide detailed discussion of silicosis, CWP, hypersensitivity pneumonitis, and occupational asthma with exceptional photography.)*

Sprince NL, Oliver LC, McLoud TC, et al. Asbestos exposure and asbestos-related pleural and parenchymal disease: associations with immune imbalance. Am Rev Respir Dis 1991; 143:822. *(Evidence for an immunologic component to asbestos-related injury.)*

Stoeckle JD, Hardy HL, Weber AL. Chronic beryllium disease, a report of 60 cases and selective review of the literature. Am J Med 1969;46:545. *(Exposures occurred primarily during the manufacture of fluorescent lamps. Cor pulmonale was the usual cause of death.)*

Ziskind M, Jones RN, Weill H. Silicosis. Am Rev Respir Dis 1976;113(5):643. *(Comprehensive review of silicosis, with discussion of history, sources and nature of exposures, pathogenesis, and clinical findings.)*

Primary Care Medicine: Office Evaluation and Management of the Adult Patient, 3rd edition, edited by Allan H. Goroll, Lawrence A. May, and Albert G. Mulley, Jr. J.B. Lippincott Company, Philadelphia

40
Evaluation of Chronic Dyspnea

Dyspnea is the subjective sensation of difficult or uncomfortable breathing. Patients commonly complain of "shortness of breath" to describe their respiratory difficulty. *Acute dyspnea* is most often a manifestation of sudden left ventricular dysfunction (see Chapter 32), bronchospasm (see Chapter 48), pneumonia (see Chapter 52), pulmonary embolization (see Chapter 20), or anxiety (see Chapter 226). The patient usually presents in the urgent care setting. Patients with chronic dyspnea, even when severe, are more likely to come to the office for care. Long-standing dyspnea can usually be evaluated safely in the outpatient setting, provided the patient's condition is not rapidly deteriorating.

Heart and lung diseases account for most cases of chronic dyspnea. At times the differentiation can be difficult; moreover, these etiologies often coexist. In such instances, diagnosis requires determining which cause is predominant. In evaluating the chronically dyspneic patient, one needs to check for precipitants and reversible components, in addition to ascertaining the cause. Also important are assessment of functional status, severity of deficits, and prognosis.

PATHOPHYSIOLOGY AND CLINICAL PRESENTATION

The pathophysiology of dyspnea is multifactorial and complex. In most instances, it results from cardiac or pulmonary decompensation and is provoked by stimulation of receptors responsive to metabolic changes, pulmonary interstitial stretch, respiratory muscle tension, and central respiratory command. Shortness of breath is experienced when ventilatory demand exceeds the actual or perceived capacity of the lungs to respond. The work of breathing may be increased by altered chest wall mechanics, decreased lung compliance, airway obstruction, increased ventilatory requirements, or exogenous factors such as obesity.

There are several important clinical settings in which dyspnea occurs. *Congestive heart failure* (CHF) can cause dyspnea as pulmonary capillary pressure rises and fluid accumulates in the interstitium, leading to a fall in pulmonary compliance and a sense of difficulty breathing. The earliest symptom is often dyspnea on exertion. More severe failure is manifested by orthopnea and finally paroxysmal nocturnal dyspnea. Basilar crackles (rales) and a third heart sound are important signs of left-sided heart failure and pulmonary venous hypertension; the third heart sound is one of the most specific signs of CHF. Peripheral edema and jugular venous distention are common manifestations of right-sided heart failure, but these findings are very nonspecific, particularly leg edema (see Chapter 22). Contributing and precipitating factors include fever, acute ischemia, excessive dietary sodium intake, dysrhythmias, concurrent use of agents that are negatively inotropic (eg, beta blockers, disopyramide, verapamil), and poor compliance with medical regimen (see Chapter 32).

Besides CHF, there are a number of other causes of pulmonary venous hypertension that result in increased pulmonary capillary pressure and dyspnea. *Mitral stenosis* is the most important etiology in this class of conditions.

Airway obstruction at any level of the respiratory tract can lead to difficulty breathing. *Tracheal stenosis* resulting from intrinsic disease or extrinsic compression is characterized by dyspnea in conjunction with stridor and inspiratory retraction of the supraclavicular space. *Chronic obstructive pulmonary disease* (COPD) (see Chapter 47) is the leading cause of airway obstruction. *Chronic bronchitis* is the subcategory of COPD that is defined as cough and sputum production that persists for 3 months or more in 2 consecutive years. Characteristically, these patients have a long-standing history of smoking, productive cough, and a slowly progressive decline in exercise capacity. In advanced stages, they may become plethoric, cyanotic, and cough incessantly; the term "blue bloater" has been applied to such patients. Tobacco-stained fingers, wheezes, coarse rales, rhonchi, and prolonged expiratory phase of respiration are often present on examination. Signs of cor pulmonale (right ventricular heave, jugular venous distention, leg edema) are late findings indicative of severe, advanced disease.

Another group of COPD patients are those with *emphysema*. Sputum production is minimal compared to that in patients with bronchitis, and there is less mismatching of ventilation and perfusion; consequently, hypoxia and cyanosis are less prominent. Gradual deterioration in exercise capacity takes place over many years. Patients with advanced emphysema appear thin and barrel-chested. They may purse their lips during expiration to keep their poorly supported airways from collapsing. The chest is hyperresonant, breath sounds are distant, and a few end-expiratory wheezes may be noted; expiration is prolonged.

COPD patients who suffer from *bronchiectasis* have a clinical presentation similar to those with chronic bronchitis, except their physical findings are more localized, their clinical course is punctuated by more frequent episodes of pneumonia, and their sputum tends to be more copious and sometimes bloody.

Asthma is another of the obstructive airway diseases. It usually produces attacks of acute dyspnea, but airway obstruction may persist for a prolonged period after an acute episode and result in more chronic respiratory complaints, including exercise intolerance, cough, and sputum production. At times, sputum production may be the predominant early symptom and may be mistaken for infection. Diffuse wheezes are commonly noted on examination; in severe cases there is use of accessory muscles, retraction, and pulsus paradoxus. Exercise-induced asthma is common in young people and may contribute to recurrent dyspneic episodes (see Chapter 48).

Diffuse *interstitial lung disease* alters pulmonary compliance and may lead to a disturbance in the balance between ventilation and perfusion. The process is usually very gradual, and often patients have few symptoms when pulmonary involvement is mild or even moderate; however, tachypnea and cyanosis ensue in severe cases. Diffuse, "dry," midexpiratory crackles are often heard on auscultation. As the interstitial process progresses, dyspnea and hypoxia worsen and exercise tolerance deteriorates (see Chapter 46).

Kyphoscoliosis is the major chest wall deformity capable of seriously impairing pulmonary musculoskeletal mechanics. Advanced cases can even terminate in cor pulmonale and respiratory failure. Among the extrapulmonary etiologies hindering lung mechanics are severe *obesity*, marked *ascites* (see Chapter 71) and large *pleural effusions* (see Chapter 43). Dyspnea is often the chief complaint in such patients.

Pulmonary hypertension represents a serious cause of chronic dyspnea and has a poor prognosis. It may be primary or secondary and is characterized by a fixed elevation in pulmonary artery pressure and resultant right heart strain. Common physical findings include an accentuated pulmonic component of the second heart sound, a right ventricular third heart sound, the murmur of tricuspid regurgitation, and peripheral edema.

Secondary pulmonary hypertension occurs with conditions that chronically elevate pulmonary artery pressure, such as *recurrent pulmonary embolization*, *chronic hypoxemia*, *pulmonary parenchymal disease*, and *left-sided heart failure*. Some forms of secondary disease have subtle presentations and can easily be mistaken for primary disease. For example, pulmonary hypertension due to recurrent pulmonary embolization typically occurs in patients with few symptoms of embolization. With the exception of recalling perhaps a single episode of pleuritic chest pain and acute dyspnea, the majority of patients report few symptoms before the onset of pulmonary hypertension. Those with symptomatic, recurrent embolization rarely develop significant pulmonary hypertension. The reason for this paradox remains unclear. The source of emboli is believed to be the proximal deep veins of the legs.

Primary pulmonary hypertension is a diagnosis of exclusion, found most commonly among women between ages 20 and 40. Mean age is about 35, with a ratio of women to men of 1.7:1. Dyspnea is the most frequently reported symptom, followed by fatigue, near syncope, and Raynaud's phenomenon. An immunologic basis for the condition is suspected in many of these patients, because of the high frequency of anti-nuclear antibody (ANA) seropositivity, especially in women. Immunologically mediated endothelial damage is postulated. Hyperventilation may result and be mistakenly attributed to anxiety.

Anxiety attacks are often confused with more serious etiologies, because the patient may appear to be in severe respiratory distress. The patient often reports chest tightness or claims that he cannot get in enough air. The florid, acute case is represented by the hyperventilation syndrome (see Chapter 226), but commonly there is a less dramatic, chronic feeling of dyspnea and fatigue that is affected little by exertion. Frequent sighing, multiple bodily complaints, nervousness, and a normal physical examination are typical of such patients.

Table 40-1. Common Causes of Chronic Dyspnea

Cardiac
1. Congestive heart failure
2. Other causes of pulmonary venous congestion (mitral stenosis, mitral regurgitation)

Pulmonary
1. Chronic obstructive pulmonary disease
2. Pulmonary parenchymal disease (including interstitial diseases)
3. Pulmonary hypertension
4. Severe kyphoscoliosis
5. Exogenous mechanical factors (ascites, massive obesity, large pleural effusion)
6. Chronic asthma

Psychologic
1. Anxiety

Hematologic
1. Severe chronic anemia

DIFFERENTIAL DIAGNOSIS

The causes of chronic dyspnea encountered in the office setting are listed in Table 40–1.

WORKUP

History. History remains the single most useful diagnostic modality. In studies of dyspnea, the diagnosis is established by history in about 75 percent of instances. However, differentiating dyspnea due to cardiac disease from that resulting from pulmonary pathology can be a challenge. Both etiologies share a number of clinical features. For example, exertional dyspnea is common to both. A frequent misconception is that paroxysmal nocturnal dyspnea is unique to heart failure. Excessive airway secretions from chronic obstructive lung disease often pool at night and lead to airway obstruction, causing dyspnea and forcing the patient to sit up to clear his airway. The occurrence of wheezing is a nonspecific manifestation of large airway bronchospasm, whether it is caused by heart failure or obstructive lung disease.

In general, a past history dominated by chronic cough, sputum production, recurrent respiratory infections, occupational exposure, or heavy smoking points more to lung disease than to a cardiac origin. However, unless there is a strong history of previous lung disease or substantial sputum production, it may be very hard to distinguish a cardiac from a pulmonary source on the basis of history alone. Moreover, both may coexist concurrently. Physical findings and laboratory studies are often necessary for a better differentiation (see below).

Dyspnea that is a manifestation of a chronic anxiety state may superficially mimic cardiopulmonary disease and cause some confusion. Onset at rest in conjunction with a sense of chest tightness, suffocation, or inability to take in air are characteristic features of the history. Also, there is little evidence of significant heart or lung disease, though there may be much fear of it. Multiple bodily complaints, history of emotional difficulties, absence of activity limitations, and lack of exacerbation on exercising argue for a psychogenic cause. Unfortunately, patients with pulmonary hypertension may have episodes that can resemble anxiety-induced bouts of dyspnea; sometimes a young patient with primary pulmonary hypertension is incorrectly labeled "neurotic."

It is helpful to define as precisely as possible the degree of activity that precipitates the sensation of dyspnea, to estimate the severity of disease, determine the extent of disability, and detect changes over time. One means of achieving these objectives is to relate symptoms to the patient's daily activities and interpret the degree of restriction in terms of the expected endurance of a patient of similar age.

Factors that may contribute to the occurrence or worsening of dyspnea should be documented, including cigarette smoking, occupational exposure, excessive salt intake, weight gain, and increasing sputum production. The occupational history is particularly important, as the relationships between exposures and lung disease are becoming increasingly evident (see Chapter 39).

The patient should be asked about hemoptysis; the symptom raises the possibilities of bronchiectasis, endobronchial malignancy, embolization with infarction, and pneumonia. Suspicion of embolization requires an inquiry into pleuritic chest pain, leg edema, and other symptoms of deep vein thrombophlebitis (see Chapter 22) as well as such risk factors as chronic venous insufficiency, inactivity, and—in young women—use of oral contraceptives and pregnancy. Careful inquiry for historical evidence of recurrent pulmonary embolization is particularly important in the context of encountering pulmonary hypertension.

Physical Examination should begin with a check for tachycardia, tachypnea, fever, and hypertension. Weight increase must not be forgotten, for it may be an early sign of worsening congestive failure (see Chapter 32). The patient's respiratory efforts need to be observed carefully to obtain an estimate of the amount of work expended in breathing; contractions of the accessory muscles of respiration suggest severe difficulty. Retraction of the supraclavicular fossa implies tracheal stenosis that has become critical. Pursed-lip breathing and a prolonged expiratory phase are signs of significant outflow obstruction. The best way to observe airflow obstruction is to have the patient take a deep breath and blow out as hard and as fast as he can. The chest is examined for increased A–P diameter (suggestive of COPD) and deformity resulting from kyphoscoliosis or ankylosing spondylitis. Retraction of the intercostal muscles on inspiration is characteristic of emphysema.

The chest should be percussed for dullness and hyperresonance and auscultated for wheezes, crackles, and quality of breath sounds. Unfortunately, the elicitation of wheezing on maximal forced exhalation has proven neither sensitive nor specific for the diagnosis of asthma and cannot be recommended as a technique for uncovering underlying airway hyperreactivity. Crackles suggest fluid in the airway, as occurs with bronchitis, pneumonitis, and CHF. A normal lung examination does not rule out pulmonary pathology, but it does lessens its probability and its likelihood of being severe. Cardiac examination should focus on signs of left-sided heart failure (see Chapter 32), on detection of left-sided heart murmurs (see Chapters 21 and 33), and on signs of pulmonary hypertension and its consequences (accentuated and delayed P_2, right ventricular heave, right ventricular S_3, right-sided systolic regurgitant murmur of tricuspid insufficiency, jugular venous distention, and peripheral edema). It is important to recognize that many of the signs of right-sided heart failure may be a consequence of long-standing pulmonary disease and therefore are not specific for a cardiac etiology. The abdomen is examined for ascites and hepatojugular reflux; the legs are checked for edema and other signs of phlebitis (see Chapters 16 and 30). Finally, the mental status is checked for manifestations of an anxiety disorder; particularly germane is excessive sighing.

Laboratory Studies. The *chest x-ray* is essential to evaluation and should be studied for pulmonary venous redistribution, effusions, interstitial changes, hyperinflation, infiltrates, enlargement of the pulmonary arteries (indicative of pulmonary hypertension), cardiac chamber enlargement, and valve calcification. Upper zone redistribution of pulmonary blood flow is among the earliest x-ray findings of CHF (see Chapter 32); however, redistribution may also occur in COPD from destruction of vessels in the lower lung fields. The x-ray diagnosis can be made with a high degree of accuracy if any two of the following criteria are met: depression and flattening of the diaphram with blunting of the costophrenic angles on PA film; irregular lucency of the lung fields; abnormally enlarged retrosternal space; diaphragmatic flattening or concavity on the lateral film. Chest radiography is sometimes useful for detection of interstitial lung disease, because physical findings may be minimal. However, x-ray findings may also be unimpressive, necessitating further study (see below). When an infiltrate is present, *Gram's stain* of the *sputum* and *culture* are often informative, especially when the patient is febrile, coughing more than usual, or reports a change in sputum.

Sputum cytology is indicated under similar circumstances, particularly if there is onset of hemoptysis. A *Zeil-Nielson stain* for acid-fast bacilli and sputum *culture for tuberculosis* are also important components of the workup when an infiltrate is detected (see Chapter 49).

Simple *pulmonary function tests* can be reliably performed in the office on an inexpensive spirometer. The *FEV_1* and *vital capacity* are the most informative of these measurements for detecting obstructive and restrictive defects, and for determining severity. The ratio of FEV_1 to vital capacity is markedly reduced in clinically important obstructive disease. In restrictive disease, the ratio is close to 1.0, but the vital capacity is significantly reduced. An FEV_1 can also provide prognostic information. A reading of less than 1.0 L/sec is associated with a poor 5-year survival rate among patients with COPD (see Chapter 47). Patients suspected of having tracheal stenosis may require *flow-volume studies* to identify the lesion and determine its severity; referral is indicated.

Arterial blood gases (ABGs) are not routinely available in most office settings, but they are worth obtaining when there is a question of deteriorating ventilation. Hospitalization should be considered when the PCO_2 is inappropriately elevated for the respiratory rate and repeat determinations reveal further PCO_2 increases. Drawing ABGs before and after exercise is helpful in assessing the severity of diffuse interstitial disease. A fall in PO_2 is evidence of a significant degree of interstitial disease. When use of accessory muscles is noted and the patient appears to be worsening, prompt hospital admission should be carried out, rather than taking time to obtain ABGs in the office.

A *single-breath carbon monoxide diffusing capacity* test may be the earliest sign of interstitial fibrosis. The test is particularly useful in evaluation of dyspnea associated with suspected occupational interstitial disease (see Chapters 39 and 46).

Sometimes the combination of history, physical examination, chest x-ray, and pulmonary function tests is not sufficient to determine the relative contributions of heart disease and lung disease to the patient's dyspnea. When findings are equivocal, it may be helpful to order a *cardiac ultrasound* examination, a readily available noninvasive means of determining chamber size, valvular anatomy, and left ventricular function. Ejection fraction will be reduced in the setting of LV dysfunction and relatively preserved in patients who suffer predominantly from lung disease. Cardiac ultrasound in conjunction with *Doppler* study is an excellent means of detecting important treatable causes of pulmonary hypertension, such as tight mitral stenosis (see Chapter 33) and sometimes pulmonary embolization. An old-fashioned but occasionally useful test, the *circulation time*, is prolonged by 4 or more seconds beyond the upper limit of normal (16 seconds) in patients with CHF.

The neurotic patient with anxiety-induced dyspnea often benefits from having a chest radiograph and simple pulmonary function tests; the confirmation of a well-functioning respiratory system may provide some reassurance and lessen concern over bodily symptoms. At times, a *walk with the patient* up and down a few flights of stairs is just as convincing for both physician and patient. Climbing stairs with the patient complaining of dyspnea is also useful in those with suspected cardiopulmonary disease, for exercise tolerance can be quantitated in terms of flights climbed and the heart and respiratory rates attained.

Evaluation of Pulmonary Hypertension. Finding evidence suggestive of pulmonary hypertension (dyspnea; signs of right-sided heart strain on physical examination and electrocardiogram; prominent main pulmonary artery and hilar vessels in conjunction with decreased peripheral vessels on chest x-ray) necessitates consideration of its treatable causes, such as recurrent pulmonary embolization, sleep apnea (see Chapter 8), and mitral stenosis (see Chapter 33). Although pulmonary hypertension is typically quite advanced by the time the diagnosis is made, efforts at earlier recognition and identification of treatable causes are imperative if prognosis is to be improved.

Echocardiogram has shown considerable promise in the noninvasive diagnoses of cor pulmonale, pulmonary hypertension, and their antecedent etiologies. The *perfusion lung scan* has proven to be a safe, noninvasive means of screening for recurrent pulmonary embolization and differentiating it from primary pulmonary hypertensive disease. In primary disease, the scan may be normal or show a subsegmental or diffuse patchy peripheral distribution of labeled albumin. In secondary disease due to recurrent pulmonary emboli, the scan shows multiple segmental or large subsegmental defects. Any segmental or large subsegmental perfusion defect in a patient with pulmonary hypertension is an indication for consideration of *pulmonary angiography*. Simultaneous ventilation scanning usually does not add enough specificity to the evaluation in this context to obviate the need for angiography.

SYMPTOMATIC MANAGEMENT AND PATIENT EDUCATION

Relief of dyspnea requires attention to *exacerbating factors* as well as to the underlying etiology. Symptomatic management begins with correcting reversible forms of airway obstruction (see Chapters 47 and 48) and precipitants of left ventricular dysfunction (see Chapter 32). Any concurrent respiratory tract infection needs treatment (see Chapter 52). If there is a large pleural effusion (see Chapter 43), a severe anemia (see Chapter 82), or an acute situational stress (see Chapter 226), it too should receive prompt attention. Environmental irritants ought to be eliminated (see Chapter 39). All patients with dyspnea should be advised to stop smoking; often the onset of even mild dyspnea is sufficient stimulus to quit, especially when combined with the physician's urging (see Chapter 54).

Attention to the underlying etiology cannot be overemphasized, whether it is heart disease (see Chapters 30, 32, 33), lung disease (see Chapters 47, 48, 52), a mechanical factor such as massive obesity (see Chapter 233), or an anxiety disorder (see Chapter 226). Dyspneic patients with such disorders greatly appreciate knowing the cause of their discomfort and its prognosis, especially when it differs from their perception.

Many patients with chronic dyspnea request *home oxygen therapy*. Such requests are reasonable if the patient suffers from a condition causing chronic hypoxemia, provided there is no evidence of carbon dioxide retention and the attendant risk of suppressing respiratory drive. Nocturnal oxygen therapy is particularly useful in preventing pulmonary hypertension in patients suffering from chronic hypoxemia, but it must be used with care (see Chapter 47). Patients without significant hypoxemia—even those with chronic emphysema—do not benefit from oxygen therapy.

Selected patients with lung or heart disease may benefit from an *exercise program*; exercise tolerance is often improved, although the effect on survival remains unproven (see Chapters 18, 30, 31, 47). It is important that patients be reminded to note the level of activity that they can tolerate and report any decrease. Precipitants of worsening exercise tolerance should also be watched for.

Use of *anxiolytics* is helpful only in patients whose dyspnea is a manifestation of a severe anxiety disorder. Even then, extreme caution must be exercised in chronic use of such medications (see Chapter 226). Prescribing tranquilizer use for a patient with heart or lung disease who is anxious because of trouble with breathing is more likely to exacerbate the respiratory problem than to help it.

INDICATIONS FOR REFERRAL AND ADMISSION

Patients with underlying heart or lung disease who experience a worsening of their chronic dyspnea deserve prompt consideration for hospital admission, especially when the change is rapid. It may represent acute left ventricular decompensation, ventilatory failure, or hypoxemia. Acute anxiety can superficially mimic cardiopulmonary decompensation and needs to be ruled out (see above) before hospitalization is authorized. Pulmonary consultation may be helpful in the patient with suspected pulmonary hypertension, both for design of the diagnostic assessment and for selection of the treatment plan if a secondary cause is identified. For the patient found to have pulmonary hypertension secondary to recurrent pulmonary embolization, a referral to a surgeon experienced in performing thromboendarterectomy deserves consideration.

A.H.G.

ANNOTATED BIBLIOGRAPHY

Baumstark A, Swensson RG, Hessel SJ, et al. Evaluating the radiographic assessment of pulmonary venous hypertension in chronic heart disease. Am J Radiol 1984;142:877. *(Suggests the assessment can be quite accurate; sensitivity 0.75 and specificity 0.88.)*

Come PC. Echocardiographic recognition of pulmonary arterial disease and determination of its cause. Am J Med 1988;84:384. *(Provides evidence for the utility of ultrasound in the identification and differential diagnosis of pulmonary hypertension.)*

D'Alonzo GE, Bower JS, Dantzker DR. Differentiation of patients with primary and thromboembolic pulmonary hypertension. Chest 1984;85:457. *(The pattern on perfusion lung scan is different.)*

Hull RD, Hirsch J, Carter CJ, et al. Pulmonary angiography, ventilation lung scanning, and venography for clinically suspected pulmonary embolism with abnormal perfusion lung scan. Ann Intern Med 1983;98:891. *(Details the indications for each; angiography remains the definitive test.)*

King DK, Thompson BT, Johnson DC. Wheezing on maximal forced exhalation in the diagnosis of atypical asthma. Ann Intern Med 1989;110;451. *(Wheezing proved neither sensitive nor specific.)*

Lee DC, Johnson RA, Bingham JB, et al. Heart failure in outpatients. N Engl J Med 1982;306:699. *(Includes a discussion of clinical findings indicative of the diagnosis and predictive of response to therapy.)*

Jones NL. Exercise testing in pulmonary evaluation: clinical application. N Engl J Med 1975;293:647.*(Describes the use of exercise pulmonary function tests in evaluating dyspnea; preceded by article, N Engl J Med 1975;293:341, detailing methods and physiology of exercise testing.)*

Liss HP, Grant BJB. The effect of nasal flow on breathlessness in patients with chronic obstructive lung disease. Am Rev Respir Dis 1988;137:1285. *(Nasal cannular delivery of room air provided as much improvement in dyspnea as cannular delivery of oxygen.)*

Man GCW, Hsu K, Sproule BJ. Effect of alprazolam on exercise and dyspnea in patients with chronic obstructive lung disease. Chest 1986;90:832. *(No benefit was found in patients who had normal PO_2 levels.)*

Mulrow CD, Lucey CR, Farnett LE. Discriminating causes of dyspnea through clinical examination. J Gen Intern Med 1993;8:383. *(Clinical assessment had a 70% accuracy.)*

Nicklaus TM, Stowell DW, Christiansen WR, et al. The accuracy of the roentgenologic diagnosis of chronic pulmonary emphysema. Am Rev Respir Dis 1966;93:889. *(In patients with severe disease, the sensitivity of the chest x-ray was 0.91 and specificity 0.96; these figures would be greatly reduced in patients with less severe disease.)*

Pratt PC. Role of conventional chest radiography in diagnosis and exclusion of emphysema. Am J Med 1987;82:998. *(A review arguing that a high degree of accuracy can be achieved if validated criteria are used; 40 refs.)*

Raffin TA. Indications for arterial blood gas analysis. Ann Intern Med 1986;105:390. *(A critical review of uses for blood gas; 76 refs.)*

Rich S, Levitsky S, Brundage BH. Pulmonary hypertension from chronic pulmonary embolism. Ann Intern Med 1988;108:425. *(A review exploring the often confusing relationship between these two conditions; 87 refs.)*

Rich S, Dantzker DR, Ayers SM, et al. Primary pulmonary hypertension: a national prospective study. Ann Intern Med 1987;107:216. *(Findings from a national registry; best available data on clinical and epidemiologic features.)*

Tobin MJ. Dyspnea: pathophysiologic basis, clinical presentation, and management. Arch Intern Med 1990;150:1604. *(Useful review with emphasis on pathophysiology; also good discussion of hyperventilation syndrome; 97 refs.)*

Primary Care Medicine: Office Evaluation and Management of the Adult Patient, 3rd edition, edited by Allan H. Goroll, Lawrence A. May, and Albert G. Mulley, Jr. J.B. Lippincott Company, Philadelphia

41
Evaluation of Chronic Cough

A chronic cough (one lasting longer than 3 weeks) poses a challenging evaluation problem because the list of etiologies ranges from the trivial to the life-threatening. Patients present because of fear that "something is wrong," with fear of acquired immunodeficiency syndrome (AIDS), cancer, tuberculosis (TB), and pneumonia leading the list of concerns. Relief from symptoms is another precipitant of coming for an evaluation. The primary physician must keep in mind more worrisome etiologies (eg, bronchogenic carcinoma and TB) and be aware that cough may be an important though atypical presentation of such common conditions as asthma and gastroesophageal reflux. The objective is to conduct a complete yet efficient evaluation that avoids both unnecessary testing and excessive delay. A difficult issue is when to refer for bronchoscopy.

PATHOPHYSIOLOGY AND CLINICAL PRESENTATION

The physiological function of cough is to remove foreign substances and mucus from the respiratory tract. It is a three-phase mechanical process that involves a deep inspiration, increasing lung volume, muscular contraction against a closed glottis, and sudden opening of the glottis. The maneuver produces and sustains a high linear air velocity to expel material from the respiratory tree.

Cough is a reflex response that is mediated by the medulla but is subject to voluntary control. The afferent limb may involve receptors in the larynx, respiratory tree, pleura, acoustic duct, nose, sinuses, pharynx, stomach, or diaphragm. The receptors respond to mechanical, inflammatory, or irritant stimuli. The trigeminal, glossopharyngeal, phrenic, and vagus nerves can carry the afferent signal. The efferent limb of the cough reflex involves the recurrent laryngeal, phrenic, and spinal motor nerves, which innervate the respiratory muscles.

The most common cause of chronic cough is *cigarette smoking*, which may trigger the cough reflex by direct bronchial irritation or may induce inflammatory changes and mucus production, stimulating a self-propagating productive cough. Chronic bronchitis may ensue. Chronic cough and decreased flow rates have been observed in teenagers after only 3 to 5 years of smoking. Pipe and cigar smoking cause lesser degrees of difficulty.

Environmental irritants play a major role in production of cough in patients living in industrialized urban areas. Pollutants that are frequently involved are heavy smog, sulphur dioxide, nitrous oxide, and industrial gases such as ammonia. In Britain, the relationship between air quality and production of cough has been documented. The dusts and particulate matter that are capable of producing pneumoconioses can contribute to the problem (see Chapter 39). The excessive drying of normal airway moisture that takes place in centrally heated homes—humidity may fall below 10 percent unless a humidifier is utilized—can result in a persistent dry cough during the winter months.

Carcinoma of the lung may present with cough in its early stages, particularly when an endobronchial lesion is present. Often the cigarette smoker notes a change in the pattern of his or her chronic "cigarette cough." *Hemoptysis* is noted in about 5 percent to 10 percent of early cases. Other clues are localized wheezing and purulent sputum suggestive of obstruction. In later stages, cough is present in conjunction with weight loss, anorexia, and dyspnea. In some instances, a systemic syndrome (eg, inappropriate ADH secretion, hypertrophic pulmonary osteoarthropathy, dermatomyositis, peripheral neuropathy) may precede appearance of tumor.

Cough may be the predominant manifestation of *asthma*. Studies of asthmatics have emphasized that cough can occur in the absence of wheezing or abnormalities on routine pulmonary function testing. The cough is characteristically worse at night and can be triggered or exacerbated by exposure to environmental irritants, allergens, or cold. Exercise is a common stimulant. In such cases the bronchorrheal component of asthma predominates, but methacholine or carbachol challenge will often unmask the obstructive manifestations (see Chapter 48).

Inflammation anywhere along the upper or lower respiratory tract is capable of producing cough, for receptors capable of transmitting impulses that stimulate cough are believed to be distributed throughout the respiratory system. The greater the inflammatory stimulus, the larger the white cell response and the more purulent the sputum. (The green coloration of very purulent sputum is due to the degeneration of white cells.) A number of patients experience a dry persistent cough after an upper respiratory infection; the cough may last more than 8 weeks and is unrelated to postnasal drip or airway hyperreactivity. The pathophysiology of this cough is believed to be related to airway epithelial damage.

Chronic bronchitis is among the most common causes of chronic cough and sputum production. The condition is defined clinically as the presence of a productive cough that persists for at least 3 months for 2 consecutive years. A morning cough is often prominent, and bronchospasm is a frequent accompaniment (see Chapter 47). *Bronchiectasis* is also characterized by cough and sputum production, but it differs clinically from bronchitis in that there are more likely to be repeated bouts of hemoptysis and pneumonia. Copious amounts of purulent sputum are often produced. Chronic cough and sputum production commonly persist between episodes of pneumonia. Focal destruction of supporting lung tissue leads to dilation of bronchi and focal findings of rhonchi and wheezes on physical examination. A history of suppurative pneumonia in childhood is sometimes elicited.

Nasal and *otic problems* are often overlooked as sources of chronic cough. *Chronic allergic rhinitis* (see Chapter 222) with resultant postnasal drip ranks as one of the leading causes of chronic cough productive of clear sputum. The nasal mucosa may be edematous and the pharyngeal mucosal "cobblestoned" in appearance. Similarly, *sinusitis* (see Chapter 219) may be associated with a persistent cough and sputum production due to excessive retropharnygeal mucus drainage. It accounts for up to a third of patients with postnasal drip. Sinus tenderness and purulent nasal drainage are typical manifestations, but they may be absent even in the presence of significant mucosal thickening on sinus films. Even impacted cerumen and external otitis have been implicated in stimulating the cough reflex (see Chapter 218).

Interstitial lung disease and *extraluminal compression* may stimulate mechanical receptors and result in a nonproductive cough. Fibrotic diseases of the interstitium and pulmonary edema are examples of intrapulmonary etiologies, and hilar adenopathy, aortic aneurysm, and neoplasm are important extraluminal mass lesions. *Chronic interstitial pulmonary edema* produces nocturnal cough due to increased venous return at night, which worsens heart failure (see Chapter 32). When failure is severe, frothy pink or blood-tinged sputum may be noted.

Psychogenic cough is more prevalent in children but may occur in adults; characteristically, it is nonproductive, occurs at times of emotional stress, and ceases during the night.

Gastroesophageal reflux sometimes leads to chronic cough. Mechanisms include 1) esophageal irritation with stimulation of an esophageal-tracheobronchial reflex and 2) nocturnal aspiration of gastric juices. Cough may be the only presenting symptom.

The advent of *angiotensin converting enzyme (ACE) inhibitors* has been associated with an unexpectedly high incidence of dry nocturnal cough, with reports of 10 percent to 15 percent of patients being affected. First reported with use of enalapril, the cough has been documented with the taking of most long-acting ACE inhibitor preparations. Patients complain of an irritant feeling. The cough usually does not respond to switching to another ACE inhibitor, though reduction in dose may help. In about 50 percent of instances, the cough is so annoying that ACE inhibitor therapy must be terminated.

DIFFERENTIAL DIAGNOSIS

The common causes of chronic cough are listed in Table 41–1. In a series of 139 consecutive cases of chronic cough encountered in the community setting, the cause was hyperactive airway disease in 21 percent, postnasal drip in 19 percent, postinfectious in 9 percent, chronic bronchitis in 4 percent, gastroesophageal reflux in 4 percent, and in a few cases, occupational lung disease and psychiatric illness. In a referral setting study, a postnasal drip syndrome accounted for 41 percent of cases, asthma for 24 percent, esophageal reflux for 21 percent, and chronic bronchitis for 5 percent. Cough was the sole presentation of asthma in 28 percent of asthmatics and of reflux in 43 percent of patients with reflux. In a quarter of cases, there was more than one cause identified. Sinusitis accounted for 38 percent of postnasal drip cases. Rarer etiologies of chronic cough include irritation of the pleura, diaphragm, or pericardium. Case reports of truly rare causes of cough include osteophytes of the cervical spine and pacemaker malfunction.

Table 41-1. Important Causes of Chronic or Persistent Cough

Environmental Irritants
1. Cigarette smoking (cigar and pipe smoking to a lesser degree)
2. Pollutants (sulfur dioxide, nitrous oxide, particulate matter)
3. Dusts (all agents capable of producing pneumoconioses)
4. Lack of humidity
Lower Respiratory Tract Problems
1. Lung cancer
2. Asthma (including variant asthma)
3. Chronic obstructive lung disease (especially bronchitis)
4. Interstitial lung disease
5. Congestive heart failure (chronic interstitial pulmonary edema)
6. Pneumonitis
7. Bronchiectasis
Upper Respiratory Tract Problems
1. Chronic rhinitis
2. Chronic sinusitis
3. Disease of the external auditory canal
4. Pharyngitis
5. ACE inhibitors
Extrinsic Compressive Lesions
1. Adenopathy
2. Malignancy
3. Aortic aneurysm
Psychogenic Factors
Gastrointestinal Problems
1. Reflux esophagitis

WORKUP

Although some causes of chronic cough are readily apparent, presentations of even the common etiologies may be subtle, necessitating careful investigation. The initial focus of the workup should be on screening for the serious etiologies (cancer, tuberculosis, heart failure) and checking for the common treatable conditions (asthma, bronchitis, esophageal reflux, postnasal drip). In the most detailed study of workup for chronic cough, history was the highest yielding with 70 percent of patients having a true positive finding, physical examination was second with 49 percent, and laboratory studies third with an average 22 percent true positive rate.

History. A careful history and description of the cough, combined with a review of aggravating and alleviating factors and any associated symptoms, can provide useful information, though there is much overlap in presentations. A cough that worsens when the patient lies down suggests postnasal drip, esophageal reflux, bronchiectasis, bronchitis, and heart failure. One accompanied by production of clear sputum is consistent with a hypersensitivity mechanism, whereas persistent purulence suggests chronic infection (eg, chronic sinusitis, bronchiectasis, or tuberculosis), and bloody sputum raises the spectre of cancer, tuberculosis, and bronchiectasis (see Chapter 42). Associated symptoms of orthopnea, dyspnea on exertion, and paroxysmal nocturnal dyspnea implicate heart failure; dyspnea may also reflect pneumonitis or asthma. By definition, chronic bronchitis is diagnosed by the history of a chronic productive cough 3 months of the year for two consecutive years. The diagnosis is reinforced by a reduction in the cough with cessation of smoking or avoidance of environmental irritants.

Although reports of postnasal drip, throat clearing, and nasal discharge are characteristic of conditions causing a postnasal-drip syndrome, some of these symptoms may also occur in patients with asthma or even esophageal reflux, though they are not typical of them. Chronic throat clearing is also consistent with a psychogenic etiology. While heartburn or a sour taste in the mouth are reported by the majority of patients whose cough is due to reflux, as many as 40 percent of those whose cough proves linked to reflux do not report these symptoms. Hoarseness is usually indicative of tracheobronchial disease with laryngeal involvement but may represent a tumor impinging on the recurrent laryngeal nerve.

The history should also detail smoking habits, environmental and occupational exposures, use of ACE inhibitors, and review for previous allergies, asthma, sinusitis, recent respiratory infection, and tuberculosis exposure.

Physical Examination should emphasize the upper respiratory tract, chest, and cardiovascular system. The physician needs to examine the skin for cyanosis and clubbing; the pharynx for postnasal discharge, mucosal edema, and tonsillar enlargement; the nose for polyps, discharge, and obstruction; the sinuses for tenderness; and the ears for impacted cerumen or otitis. The trachea is palpated for position and the neck for masses and adenopathy. Auscultation and percussion of the lungs (including the apices) are done to detect wheezing, crackles, and signs of consolidation or effusion. Generalized wheezing is associated with obstruction from asthma or bronchitis, but localized wheezing may be a sign of tumor. Wheezing only on maximal forced exhalation was found to be neither sensitive nor specific for the diagnosis of variant asthma. During cardiac examination, the physician should evaluate the jugular venous pulse for elevated systemic venous pressure, palpate for chamber enlargement, and listen for an S_3, all indicative of heart failure.

Laboratory Studies. Testing can very often be held to a minimum when careful history and physical examination are performed. For example, when history is suggestive of chronic rhinitis causing post-nasal drip, one can proceed directly to a diagnostic trial of antihistamines and decongestants without resorting to laboratory testing. Alternatively, a topically active corticosteroid nasal spray may be used for the trial. Similarly, the suspected asthmatic may be given a diagnostic trial of inhaled steroids (see Chapter 48). In most cases of chronic cough, only a few, well-chosen studies are usually necessary. The *chest radiograph* is essential when there is historical or physical evidence that raises the question of carcinoma, pneumonitis, tuberculosis, heart failure, or bronchiectasis. However, the test is overused and not necessary in the nonsmoker who presents with a persistent cough after a recent upper respiratory infection and a normal physical examination. The chest film may be used to provide reassurance, but a careful explanation and follow-up in 4 to 6 weeks should suffice. The search for pneumonitis should be reserved for patients with a history of disease related to infection by the human immunodeficiency virus (HIV) or findings suggestive of ongoing infection (persistent production of purulent sputum, night sweats, fever, a respiratory rate greater than 25/min, rales, asymmetric respirations, increased vocal fremitus).

Sinus films are usually unnecessary when the history is positive for postnasal drip. In fact, the correlation between films and symptoms considered typical of sinusitis may be poor. In rare instances, a patient who has eluded diagnosis may have an occult sinusitis identified by sinus films, with greater than 6 mm of mucosal thickening identified on x-ray study. However, routine sinus films are unnecessary.

When there is purulent sputum or an infiltrate identified on chest x-ray, every effort should be made to obtain *sputum for examination*. Patients who give a history of producing purulent sputum in conjunction with cough, but who cannot raise sputum at the time of examination, should be instructed to drink a few glasses of water and remain a while to see if sputum can be raised. Inducing sputum with use of a saline spray may also be helpful. A surprisingly common omission in evaluating a cough productive of purulent sputum is failure to obtain and examine the sputum.

An important component of the sputum examination is the *Gram's stain*. In those at high risk for tuberculosis (eg, recent immigrants, immunocompromised hosts), an *acid-fast stain* for tubercle bacilli is needed. *Culturing* the sputum is also important, especially when tuberculosis is a possibility, because the acid-fast examination is not a very sensitive test and the diagnosis cannot be ruled out with certainty until three early-morning sputum samples have failed to produce growth by 4 to 6 weeks (see Chapters 38 and 49).

Sputum cytology—obtaining three early-morning sputum samples—can be a useful screening test for pulmonary neoplasm (see Chapters 37, 42, and 53) when clinical findings raise suspicion (history of smoking, hemoptysis, nodule on chest x-ray). Pulmonary histiocytes must be demonstrated on each specimen to prove that the sample of pulmonary secretions is adequate. A "negative" test in the absence of histiocytes is the source of many false-negative results.

Because sputum cytology is not a particularly sensitive test, it cannot be used to rule out lung cancer. When tumor remains in differential diagnosis, *fiberoptic bronchoscopy* requires consideration. It is also helpful for evaluation of obstructing lesions and infiltrates that elude diagnosis, since biopsies, washings, and cultures can be taken. However, if the chest film is normal and there is no hemoptysis or history of smoking, then the yield from bronchoscopy is very low and further workup for cancer unlikely to be productive.

Cough of Obscure Etiology. When the etiology remains elusive despite the extensive workup described above, consideration of *variant asthma* and *gastroesophageal reflux* is indicated. These conditions account for a substantial proportion of hard-to-diagnose cases of chronic cough. As noted earlier, the history and physical exam may not reveal the characteristic symptoms and signs that are typically associated with these conditions. Effective testing and avoidance of a falsely positive diagnosis necessitates a knowledge of test performance for these conditions among patients with chronic cough. Traditional *spirometry* with *bronchodilator administration* was found in one study to have only a 50 percent positive predictive value in patients with chronic cough, due to a high false-positive rate (33%), though sensitivity was excellent (approaching 100%). *Methacholine challenge* to induce bronchospasm shows a similarly high degree of sensitivity, but a lower false-positive rate (22%), giving a slightly better positive predictive value (60%). Both tests rule out asthma if they are normal.

The diagnosis of esophageal reflux is harder to make in the absence of typical symptoms. Whereas a history of retrosternal burning traveling upwards has a predictive value of more than 90 percent for gastroesophageal reflux, its absence does not rule it out. Prolonged *esophageal pH monitoring* has proven the most effective test for esophageal reflux in patients with chronic cough. In the best study of its efficacy, the test had a positive predictive value of more than 95 percent, with few false-positives and false-negatives. Monitoring of pH was far superior to barium swallow, which had a high false-negative rate. An alternative to pH monitoring is a *diagnostic trial of H_2-blocker therapy* (see Chapter 61).

However, 1 to 2 months of therapy may be necessary to demonstrate a definitive reduction in cough. Thus, pH monitoring may be the most rapid means of diagnosis of reflux-induced cough. Patients with reflux symptoms do not need radiologic study or endoscopy unless cancer or obstruction is a concern (see Chapter 61).

SYMPTOMATIC THERAPY AND PATIENT EDUCATION

The most effective means of stopping the cough is to identify and treat the underlying cause (see Chapters 47–49, 61, and 222). An empiric trial of an etiologic therapy is sometimes worth a try for diagnostic purposes (see above), but certain etiologic therapies should not be used empirically—especially antibiotics in the absence of proven infection. Symptomatic management is distinguished from empiric etiologic therapy. It is directed at eliminating precipitants and suppressing the cough. The goal is to prevent complications that may result from prolonged forceful coughing, such as sleeplessness, musculoskeletal pain, rib fractures, pneumothorax, exhaustion, pneumomediastinum, post-tussive syncope (see Chapter 24), and rupture of subconjunctival or nasal veins. The occurrence of any of these complications may be a reason for occasionally suppressing a cough that has not been completely diagnosed.

The first priority and simplest manipulation is to remove or reduce irritants. Of paramount importance is *cessation of smoking* and passive exposure to cigarette smoke; this alone eliminated cough in 77 percent and reduced it in another 17 percent of patients within a month. Second, a proper *humidification* should be maintained. If a humidifier is used, it should be kept clean, because it can become colonized with bacteria or fungi and cause infection or hypersensitivity pneumonitis. Third, adequate internal *hydration* should be encouraged, with at least 1500 mL of fluid consumed daily. These simple measures alone may abolish cough in many patients.

The patient with a chronic cough secondary to established underlying lung disease requires careful education. The patient must be informed that sputum should be expectorated when possible. Patients with chronic bronchitis or bronchiectasis can be taught how to cough with quiet, forceful expirations and how to perform *postural drainage* to promote removal of mucus from the bronchioles. Postural drainage is best timed before meals and at bedtime. *Ipratropium* is sometimes helpful in reducing night-time cough in the COPD patient (see Chapter 47).

Patients with chronic cough often request and need *temporary cough suppression* to allow uninterrupted sleep or when complications of cough arise. A wide variety of agents have been used to treat cough. The most effective are the *narcotic antitussives*, which act centrally to suppress the medullary cough center. Other preparations are expectorants or mucolytic agents, which merely help to mobilize sputum. They can have a mild placebo effect as well, but it is not an impressive one. When cough significantly interferes with sleeping or eating, a narcotic cough suppressant should be used. *Codeine* is the drug of choice. It should be used in relatively small doses of 8 to 15 mg, at intervals of 3 to 4 hours, according to the patient's needs. In many instances a dose before bedtime will suffice. Liquid and tablet preparations are equally effective. If a small dose does not suppress the cough, doses of up to 60 mg every 3 to 4 hours may be tried. It is worth noting that many patients expect to use a syrup for cough suppression; prescribing the drug in syrup form may provide some psychologic benefit. Patients for whom a narcotic antitussive is prescribed should be given small quantities and followed closely to ensure that the cough resolves and excessive use does not result. The obvious exception to this precaution is the patient with incurable lung cancer, who should receive the doses necessary to provide relief from the discomfort of persistent cough.

Nonnarcotic antitussives lack addiction potential but are not as effective as codeine. The most popular and effective over-the-counter cough suppressant is *dextromethorphan*, which has a mild suppressant effect. Many over-the-counter preparations contain *alcohol, sympathomimetics,* and *antihistamines*. The mucolytic effects of alcohol are minimal. The sympathomimetics are of little use except in patients whose cough derives from chronic vasomotor rhinitis (see Chapter 222). The antihistamines are most useful for patients with allergic upper airway disease (see Chapter 222) and a helpful adjunct for sleep when used before bed. Some over-the-counter agents dull the peripheral sensory receptors; this is the rationale for putting mild topical anesthetics in sprays, syrups, and cough lozenges. They are of questionable utility.

Expectorants are heavily consumed. There are over 60 preparations containing guaifenesin; terpin hydrate is another popular expectorant. These agents are often combined with an effective cough suppressant and, as such, are associated with a beneficial effect, but by themselves they have no proven effect and represent an unnecessary expense. They are given when the patient insists on something for cough but lacks clear indications for cough suppression, or because the patient believes expectorants help.

Patients with cough due to asthma respond to inhaled topically active *corticosteroids* and *bronchodilators* (see Chapter 48). Topical steroid therapy may also help in allergic rhinitis (see Chapter 222). Patients with persistent cough after a recent respiratory tract infection and no signs of pneumonitis may benefit from a short course of inhaled steroid therapy, which presumably lessens residual inflammatory changes. Time is another effective therapy.

Patients with suspected reflux should respond to a course of anti-reflux therapy with *antacids* and *H_2-blockers* (see Chapter 61), though as noted above, the benefits may not be apparent for several weeks.

INDICATIONS FOR REFERRAL

Although endobronchial cancer is a feared etiology, it is not a common cause of chronic cough in the absence of other findings, especially in the patient with a normal chest x-ray. However, the undiagnosed patient with risk factors for cancer (smoking, occupational exposure) requires a consultation for consideration of bronchoscopy, particularly if the chest x-ray is abnormal. The patient with a normal chest x-ray and no risk factors can probably be followed expectantly without resorting to bronchoscopy, since the likelihood of a positive study is small.

A.H.G.

ANNOTATED BIBLIOGRAPHY

Bloustine S, et al. Ear cough (Arnold's reflex). Otol Rhinol Laryngol 1976;85:406. *(A clinical survey of 688 patients that revealed an incidence of the ear cough reflex of 1.74 percent, a reminder to examine the ear.)*

Corrao W, Braman SS, Irwin RS. Chronic cough as the sole presenting manifestation of bronchial asthma. N Engl J Med 1979;300:633. *(Six patients whose asthma presented as cough and had no prior history of wheezing.)*

Diehr P, Wood RW, Bushyhead J, et al. Prediction of pneumonia in outpatients with acute cough—a statistical approach. J Chron Dis 1984;37:215. *(A study of nearly 2000 patients presenting with cough with and without radiographic evidence of pneumonia. A discriminate analysis scoring system is presented.)*

Ing AJ, Ngu MC, Breslin ABX. Chronic persistent cough and clearance of esophageal acid. Chest 1992;102:1668. *(Acid reflux is an important etiology; impaired clearance of acid found.)*

Irwin RS, Corrao WM, Pratter MR. Chronic persistent cough in the adult: the spectrum and frequency of causes and successful outcome of specific therapy. Am Rev Respir Dis 1981; 123:413. *(A series of 49 intensively studied patients revealing 12 with asthma, 14 with postnasal drip, 9 with asthma plus postnasal drip [usually following upper respiratory infection], 6 with bronchitis, 5 with esophagitis, and one each of malignant, cardiac, or interstitial origin.)*

Irwin RS, Curley FJ, French CL. Chronic cough: the spectrum and frequency of causes, key components of the diagnostic evaluation, and outcome of specific therapy. Am Rev Respir Dis 1990;141:640. *(A prospective study of a systematic anatomic diagnostic evaluation protocol; asthma, postnasal drip, and esophageal reflux accounted for a large percentage of cases; detailed data on utility of various diagnostic modalities.)*

Irwin RS, Curley FJ. The treatment of cough. Chest 1991;99:1477. *(A comprehensive review of symptomatic therapies; 68 refs.)*

King DK, Thompson BT, Johnson DC. Wheezing on maximal forced exhalation in the diagnosis of atypical asthma. Ann Intern Med 1989;110:451. *(The maneuver proved neither sensitive nor specific for the diagnosis of asthma.)*

Israeli ZH, Hall WD. Cough and angioneurotic edema associated with antiotensin-converting-enzyme inhibitor therapy. Ann Intern Med 1992;117:234. *(A review of pathophysiology and clinical presentation.)*

Laudon RG. Smoking and cough frequency. Rev Respir Dis 1976;114:1033. *(A paper that confirms that smokers cough more frequently than nonsmokers.)*

McFadden FR, Jr. Exertional dyspnea and cough as preludes to acute attacks of asthma. N Engl J Med 1975;292:555. *(Wheezing may be absent as an early manifestation of an acute attack, and cough may dominate the clinical picture.)*

Poe RH, Harder RV, Israel RH, et al. Chronic persistent cough: Experience in diagnosis and outcome using an anatomic diagnostic protocol. Chest 1989;95:723. *(Irwin's protocol does not work as well in the community setting; about 14 percent remain undiagnosed.)*

Prater MR, Bartter T, Akers S, et al. An algorithmic approach to chronic cough. Ann Intern Med 1993;119:977. *(Describes a sequential workup with use of response to antihistamine-decongestant medication.)*

42
Evaluation of Hemoptysis

Primary Care Medicine: Office Evaluation and Management of the Adult Patient, 3rd edition, edited by Allan H. Goroll, Lawrence A. May, and Albert G. Mulley, Jr. J.B. Lippincott Company, Philadelphia

Because of its well-known associations with cancer and tuberculosis, hemoptysis is an alarming symptom for both patient and physician. Hemoptysis refers to coughing up of either blood-tinged or grossly bloody sputum. In the office, the primary physician is usually confronted with a patient who has noted sputum streaked with blood. Most patients prove to have inconsequential lesions, but a thorough evaluation is necessary because the seriousness of the etiology does not correlate with the amount of blood coughed up.

PATHOPHYSIOLOGY AND CLINICAL PRESENTATION

Inflammation of the tracheobronchial mucosa accounts for many cases of hemoptysis. Minor mucosal erosions can result from *upper respiratory infections* and *bronchitis;* blood-streaked sputum is often noted, especially if coughing has been vigorous and prolonged. Patients with *bronchiectasis* are more subject to recurrent episodes of grossly bloody sputum, because necrosis of the bronchial mucosa can be quite severe. Up to 50 percent of those with bronchiectasis experience hemoptysis. In the United States, hemoptysis occurring with *tuberculosis (TB)* is usually caused by mucosal ulceration, although potentially fatal bleeding can occur when a blood vessel adjacent to a cavitary lesion ruptures. About 10 percent to 15 percent of patients with TB report some form of hemoptysis; most of these episodes are minor, involving sputum tinged with small amounts of blood. Endobronchial inflammatory injury from granuloma formation is the mechanism of hemoptysis associated with *sarcoidosis;* small amounts of blood-streaked sputum are occasionally noted.

Mucosal injury can also be a consequence of *bronchogenic carcinoma.* Disruption of endobronchial tissue may be minimal and cause little more than a trace of hemoptysis from time to time; hemorrhage is rare. Between 35 percent and 55 percent of patients with proven bronchogenic carcinoma report at least one episode of hemoptysis during the course of their illness; it is the presenting symptom in about 10 percent of cases. The amount of bleeding can vary considerably and need not be impressive. For example, in one study, malignancy was the cause in 25 percent of patients with minimal amounts of hemoptysis. However, most patients have a positive smoking history and an abnormal chest x-ray.

Carcinoma metastatic to the lung rarely results in hemoptysis. *Bronchial adenomas* are quite vascular, and they are commonly central and endobronchial in location; as a consequence, they frequently bleed, and recurrent episodes of hemoptysis are reported in about half of cases.

Injury to the pulmonary vasculature is an important source of hemoptysis. *Lung abscess* may result in damage to adjacent vessels and frequently presents with bloody as well as purulent sputum. *Necrotizing pneumonias,* such as those produced by *Klebsiella,* can cause substantial vascular disruption; 25 percent to 50 percent of patients cough up tenacious, bloody sputum referred to as "currant jelly." *Aspergillomas* are also capable of vascular injury; hemoptysis is the most common symptom of the condition. The patient with an aspergilloma is typically a compromised host with prior cavitary disease from TB, bronchiectasis, or the like. *Pulmonary infarction* secondary to embolization is characterized by sudden onset of pleuritic pain in conjunction with hemoptysis; embolization without infarction does not cause hemoptysis. Pulmonary contusion from blunt *chest trauma* may present with hemoptysis following a nonpenetrating blow to the thorax.

Marked elevations in pulmonary capillary pressure can cause vascular injury and extravasation of red cells. The pink, frothy sputum of *pulmonary edema* is a manifestation of this process. More grossly bloody sputum sometimes occurs in severe *mitral stenosis* when a dilated pulmonary-bronchial venous connection ruptures. Vasculitic injury is responsible for the hemoptysis found in *Wegener's granulomatosis* and *Goodpasture's syndrome*. Hematuria often accompanies both conditions. Hereditary vascular malformations are subject to recurrent bleeding. *Arteriovenous malformations* may be accompanied by an audible bruit on auscultation of the lung. In *hereditary hemorrhagic telangiectasia,* there is often a family history of bleeding problems or prior episodes of bleeding from multiple sites; telangiectasias may be visible in the buccal cavity and on the skin. Bleeding into the interstitium characterizes *idiopathic pulmonary hemosiderosis*. This rare disease, uncommon in adults, is manifested by diffuse interstitial infiltrates, anemia, and hemoptysis.

Hemoptysis may be the first sign of a *bleeding disorder* or *excessive anticoagulant therapy;* however, there is usually an underlying bronchopulmonary lesion as well.

DIFFERENTIAL DIAGNOSIS

Acute and chronic bronchitis are the most common etiologies, followed by bronchogenic carcinoma, TB, pneumonia, and bronchiectasis. Most prevalence figures are obtained from chest clinics and inpatient units serving preselected populations of patients with either abnormal chest x-rays or unexplained hemoptysis; therefore, they cannot be readily extrapolated to the primary care setting. In everyday office practice, the nasal mucosa and oropharynx are more often the source of blood-tinged sputum than is the lower respiratory tract. The recent resurgence of TB (see Chapter 38), more widespread use of fiberoptic bronchoscopy, and increases in cigarette smoking and lung cancer in women also must be kept in mind when interpreting data from published clinical series, which are more than 10 years old. In a recent fiberoptic bronchoscopy study done in a general hospital setting that included both inpatients and outpatients, bronchitis accounted for 37 percent, bronchogenic carcinoma for 19 percent, tuberculosis for 7 percent, and bronchiectasis for only 1 percent. The briskness of bleeding did not correlate with etiology. The more common and important etiologies of hemoptysis are listed in Table 42–1.

Table 42-1. Important Causes of Hemoptysis

Gross Hemoptysis
1. Tuberculosis (with cavitary disease)
2. Bronchiectasis
3. Bronchial adenoma
4. Bronchogenic carcinoma (uncommon)
5. Aspergilloma
6. Necrotizing pneumonia
7. Lung abscess
8. Pulmonary contusion
9. AV malformation
10. Hereditary hemorrhagic telangiectasia
11. Bleeding disorder or excessive anticoagulant therapy
12. Mitral stenosis (with rupture of a bronchial vessel)
13. Immune alveolar disease

Blood-streaked Sputum
1. Any of the causes of gross hemoptysis
2. Upper respiratory tract infection
3. Chronic bronchitis
4. Sarcoidosis
5. Bronchogenic carcinoma
6. Tuberculosis
7. Pulmonary infarction
8. Pulmonary edema
9. Mitral stenosis
10. Idiopathic pulmonary hemosiderosis
11. Immune alveolar disease

WORKUP

As noted earlier, most cases of blood-tinged sputum encountered in the primary care setting, especially those seen during the winter, are upper respiratory in origin. Such cases do not require further investigation. To avoid unnecessary workup for a pulmonary etiology, the history and physical examination should first focus on the nasal and oropharyngeal mucosa. Only in the absence of an upper respiratory bleeding source need further workup proceed in the manner detailed in the following paragraphs.

History. Evaluation of the patient with a suspected lower respiratory source of hemoptysis should begin with consideration of the epidemiology of the serious underlying causes. Concern about pulmonary neoplasm should be highest in the older male with a long history of heavy smoking or asbestos exposure. The elderly patient with evidence of old disease on chest x-ray should be presumed to have reactivated tuberculosis infection. The adolescent with hemoptysis may have a new infection due to recent tuberculosis exposure. The compromised host with previous cavitary disease is at risk for an aspergilloma.

The patient's description of the sputum associated with hemoptysis can be of some diagnostic help. Pink sputum is suggestive of pulmonary edema fluid; putrid sputum is indicative of a lung abscess; currant-jellylike material points to a necrotizing pneumonia; copious amounts of purulent sputum mixed with blood are consistent with bronchiectasis. The commonly described blood-streaked sputum is nonspecific.

History should also be examined for previous bleeding episodes, family history of hemoptysis, hematuria, concurrent pleuritic chest pain, known heart murmur or history of rheumatic fever, lymph node enlargement, blunt chest trauma, symptoms of heart failure (see Chapter 32), and use of anticoagulant drugs. Determining the amount of blood produced is not particularly helpful for diagnostic purposes beyond establishing whether the hemoptysis was gross or scant. As noted above, it is important to be certain that there is no history of a coexisting nasopharyngeal problem or source of gastrointestinal bleeding that the patient may be mistaking for true hemoptysis.

Physical Examination is directed at detecting nonpulmonary sources of bleeding as well as evidence of chest pathology and systemic disease. The vital signs should be checked for fever and tachypnea, the skin for ecchymoses and telangiectasias, and the nails for clubbing. Clubbing is associated with neoplasm, bronchiectasis, lung abscess, and other severe pulmonary disorders (see Chapter 45). Nodes are examined for enlargement, suggestive of sarcoidosis, TB, and malignancy (see Chapters 12 and 51). The neck is noted for jugular venous distention, consistent with heart failure, and severe mitral disease. Examination of the chest should include a search for bruits, signs of consolidation, wheezes, crackles, and chest wall contusion.

The history and physical findings can be used to determine the pace at which workup should proceed, as well as the selection and sequence of laboratory tests. The patient with minimal hemoptysis may be evaluated on an outpatient basis, as long as the patient is given explicit advice to return immediately if severe bleeding ensues. The patient with a suspected bleeding diathesis should not be sent home.

Laboratory Studies. The *chest x-ray* is essential to assessment. As alluded to earlier, the vast majority of patients with hemoptysis due to bronchogenic carcinoma have an abnormal chest x-ray. In addition to uncovering a mass lesion, chest films may reveal an abscess, infiltrate, interstitial change (see Chapter 46), hilar adenopathy, signs of congestive failure (see Chapter 32), or evidence of significant mitral stenosis (see Chapter 33). Less common radiologic findings include peribronchial cuffing, indicative of bronchiectasis, and a crescentic radiolucency surrounding a coin lesion, characteristic of an aspergilloma. However, in the majority of instances, the chest film is normal and consideration of further study is warranted.

The *sputum Gram's stain* is essential if the sputum appears grossly purulent or the patient is febrile. An *acid-fast stain* for tubercle bacilli is also essential, not only for diagnosis but for a rough assessment of infectivity (see Chapter 49). The sensitivity of the acid-fast smear depends on the diligence with which the search for pathogenic organisms is made. In one series, only 20 percent of culture-positive samples were identified in advance by acid-fast smear. It should also be remembered that despite a very high specificity, the predictive value of a positive smear may be as low as 50 percent when the sputum specimens of low-risk patients are examined. A *tuberculin skin test* should be performed if the patient's PPD reactivity status is not known. It must be remembered, however, that approximately 7 percent of all adults (25% of adults over age 50) will have positive reactions. (See Chapters 38 and 49).

Sputum cytologies should be obtained in all patients in whom there is no clear diagnosis. The sensitivity of a single sputum cytology examination has been shown to be about 70 percent in the detection of squamous cell lesions, lower for other cell types. Three consecutive cytologic examinations increase sensitivity to 90 percent.

Fiberoptic bronchoscopy can be extremely helpful for diagnosis when used thoughtfully. Its most common indication is to exclude the possibility of tumor. However, the test should not be viewed as a routine part of the hemoptysis evaluation, because yield is extremely low in situations where the risk of malignancy is very low (eg, the nonsmoker under the age of 50 with a normal chest x-ray). Bronchoscopy enhances the sensitivities of cytologic and bacteriologic studies when washings for specimens are obtained during the procedure, and the test has proven capable of detecting otherwise occult endobronchial cancers in patients at increased risk for lung malignancy (eg, age >50, male gender, history of smoking), even if the chest x-ray is nonlocalizing. Patients with a high-risk profile, "positive" or "suspicious" cytology, or a radiologic abnormality are appropriate candidates for consideration of endoscopy. Subjecting low-risk patients to bronchoscopic examination is wasteful and unlikely to affect management or outcome. Moreover, the cost and morbidity associated with bronchoscopy are not trivial.

Serious complications are rare with fiberoptic bronchoscopy, but they do occur. In a review of 48,000 procedures, fewer than 100 life-threatening cardiovascular or respiratory complications were reported, most often in older individuals with COPD and coronary disease. Hypoxia occurs commonly following bronchoscopy.

Bronchoscopy is mandatory in all patients with massive hemoptysis who are being seriously considered for surgery, to localize the bleeding site. Rigid bronchoscopy is preferred in this situation.

Additional diagnostic tests may be indicated in specific clinical settings; for example, *chest computed tomography (CT) scan* may better define a suspicious lesion seen on chest x-ray. *Bleeding studies*, such as a prothrombin time (PT), partial thromboplastin time (PTT), platelet count, and bleeding time are needed if more than one site of bleeding is noted.

Cryptogenic Hemoptysis refers to patients with hemoptysis who have a normal or nonlocalizing chest x-ray and a nondiagnostic fiberoptic bronchoscopy. What to do in such a situation can be perplexing. Prognosis appears to be favorable, with over 90 percent of these patients experiencing resolution of their hemoptysis by 6 months and no cases of cancer, active TB, or other serious pathology emerging subsequent to the initial evaluation. The combination of a careful history and physical examination, in combination with a chest x-ray and proper use of bronchoscopy, appears to effectively exclude cancer, active tuberculosis, and other must-not-miss pathologies, making repeat bronchoscopy, pulmonary angiography, CT scanning, and bronchography of little use in these patients. In one study, bronchial inflammation (bronchitis) was the most common etiology, followed by the sequelae of old tuberculous disease.

INDICATIONS FOR REFERRAL AND ADMISSION

Hemoptysis patients who are believed to be at increased risk for an underlying malignancy (abnormal chest x-ray, male sex, age >50, smoking history) are candidates for referral and consideration of bronchoscopy. Patients with brisk bleeding need urgent hospitalization.

A.H.G.

ANNOTATED BIBLIOGRAPHY

Adelman M, Haponik EF, Bleecker ER, et al. Cryptogenic hemoptysis: clinical features, bronchoscopic findings, and natural history in 67 patients. Ann Intern Med 1985;102:829. *(Prognosis was excellent and no cases of cancer, TB, or other serious etiologies were missed by the combination of a careful history and physical examination combined with a chest x-ray and bronchoscopy.)*

Fontana RS, Sanderson DR, Taylor WF, et al. Early lung cancer detection. Am Rev Respir Dis 1984;130:561. *(Results of screening with sputum cytology and x-ray examination were not very impressive.)*

Leatherman J, Davies SF, Hoidal JR. Alveolar hemorrhage syndromes: diffuse microvascular lung hemorrhage in immune and idiopathic disorders. Medicine (Baltimore) 1984;63:343. *(Comprehensive review.)*

Johnston H, Reisz G. Changing spectrum of hemoptysis. Arch Intern Med 1989;149:1666. *(A bronchoscopic study of both inpatients and outpatients from the general hospital setting emphasizing that bronchiectasis is waning as a cause of hemoptysis; bronchitis was first, followed by cancer, and TB.)*

Poe RH, Israel RH, Marin MG, et al. Utility of fiberoptic bronchoscopy in patients with hemoptysis and a nonlocalizing roentgenogram. Chest 1988;93:70. *(Utility was greatest in patients who were male, were older than age 50, and had a history of smoking.)*

Santiago S, Tobias J, Williams AJ. A reappraisal of the causes of hemoptysis. Arch Intern Med 1991;151:2449. *(Bronchogenic carcinoma, bronchitis, and idiopathic disease were the leading causes.)*

Smiddy JF, Eliot RC. The evaluation of hemoptysis with fiberoptic bronchoscopy. Chest 1973;64:158. *(An early prospective study that established the utility of fiberoptic bronchoscopy in evaluating hemoptysis. The source of bleeding was located in 66 of 71 patients.)*

Surratt PM, Smiddy JF, Gruber B. Deaths and complications associated with fiberoptic bronchoscopy. Chest 1976;69:747. *(Fifty-two severe respiratory complications and 27 severe cardiovascular complications in nearly 50,000 procedures.)*

Weaver LJ, Solliday N, Cugell DW. Selection of patients with hemoptysis for fiberoptic bronchoscopy. Chest 1979;76:719. *(Critical look at who needs bronchoscopy.)*

Primary Care Medicine: Office Evaluation and Management of the Adult Patient, 3rd edition, edited by Allan H. Goroll, Lawrence A. May, and Albert G. Mulley, Jr. J.B. Lippincott Company, Philadelphia

43
Evaluation of Pleural Effusions

Most pleural effusions encountered in the office are discovered as incidental findings and often pose a diagnostic challenge because etiology is frequently unclear. Of major concern are the possibilities of tumor and infection. Outpatient evaluation of a pleural effusion requires skill in performance of a diagnostic thoracentesis in the office and the differentiation of a transudate from an exudate. The primary physician should be able to carry out the initial evaluation of a pleural effusion safely in the ambulatory setting, provided the patient's respiratory status is satisfactory and there is no evidence of serious acute illness.

PATHOPHYSIOLOGY AND CLINICAL PRESENTATION

The pleural cavity normally contains a small volume of serous fluid that serves as a lubricant. About 17 mL of such fluid are formed each day by transudation from the parietal pleural surface and reabsorbed predominantly by the visceral pleura through lymphatic stomata into the lymphatic system. When there is excessive transudation of fluid or an exudative process involving the pleural surfaces, an effusion forms. Once more than 200 mL are formed, the effusion becomes visible radiographically. Effusions are classified pathophysiologically as transudates or exudates. Clinically, the distinction is based on pleural fluid protein and lactate dehydrogenase (LDH) concentrations. An effusion is *transudative* if any two of the following three criteria are met: the ratio of *pleural fluid protein:serum protein is less than 0.5;* the ratio of *pleural fluid LDH:serum LDH is less than 0.6;* or the *pleural fluid LDH is less than two-thirds of the upper limit of normal for the serum LDH.* If these ratios or levels are exceeded, the effusion is exudative.

Transudates

Increased hydrostatic pressure in the pulmonary interstitium and decreased colloid oncotic pressure produce transudates. Increased hydrostatic pressure below the diaphragm, as occurs in ascites or peritoneal dialysis can also result in a transudative pleural effusion. Because transudates are rarely associated with pleural inflammation, they are not usually accompanied by pleuritic pain, but may lead to shortness of breath if they are large enough to interfere with respiratory mechanics. They may be unilateral but are often bilateral. Physical examination of the lung reveals dullness and diminished breath sounds. If the effusion has produced some atelectasis, there may be bronchial breath sounds and increased vocal fremitus above the effusion. Most transudates have a protein concentration of less than 3.0 g/100 mL, but chronic transudates may show higher concentrations and mimic an exudative process.

Congestive Heart Failure is among the most common causes of transudative effusions. Left heart failure increases pulmonary capillary pressure (see Chapter 32), which forces excess fluid into the interstitium. Right ventricular failure contributes by raising central venous pressure, which elevates the hydrostatic force in the capillaries of the parietal pleura and diminishes fluid reabsorption. Most effusions due to congestive failure are *bilateral,* but at times there can be an *isolated right-sided* effusion; isolated left-sided effusions due to congestive failure are rare. The reason for the right-sided preference is unknown. Symptoms and signs of congestive failure (see Chapter 32) are usually evident. Over 85 percent of effusions resulting from heart failure have protein concentrations less than 3.0 g/100 mL. The concentration may be greater if the effusion is chronic or the patient has recently been undergoing a brisk diuresis. The pleural fluid is usually clear, but it may be bloody and have red cell counts in excess of 5000/mL.

Pulmonary Embolization has been found to be accompanied by pleural effusion in up to 50 percent of cases. The effusions are usually small and not dependent on occurrence of pulmonary infarction. There is considerable variation in cell count, differential, and protein concentration. The transudative effusion associated with a pulmonary embolus may result from localized interstitial edema. The effusions that result from infarction are more likely to be bloody. Bilateral effusions can be seen when emboli affect both lungs. A small effusion on chest x-ray in a patient with pleuritic chest pain can be an important clue (see Chapter 20).

Other Causes of Transudation. In the *nephrotic syndrome,* a similar, but more generalized interstitial edema may ensue and lead to effusion. *Overexpanded extracellular volume* due to severe *hypoalbuminemia* or *salt retention* can produce a transudative effusion, but edema fluid first collects in parts of the body where hydrostatic pressures are greatest (eg, lower extremities) before fluid appears in the pleural space. Cardiomegaly may be in evidence, but overt signs of congestive failure are usually absent. Generalized edema is rare before the serum albumin falls below 2.0 to 2.5 g/100 mL.

Intraabdominal diseases are occasionally responsible for transudative effusions. Between 5 percent and 10 percent of patients with *ascites* due to *cirrhosis* develop a *right-sided* pleural effusion; the composition of the effusion resembles that of the ascitic fluid. In cases of *pancreatitis* or a *subphrenic abscess,* a *"sympathetic effusion"* with the characteristics of a transudate sometimes forms; it soon changes into an exudate.

Pleural effusions are common after *coronary bypass graft surgery* and do not imply serious pathology. The same holds for the *postpartum* patient. Transudates may form in the setting of *pericardial disease, myxedema,* and *sarcoidosis;* the mechanism(s) remain unknown.

Exudates

Exudates result from inflammatory or infiltrative disease of the pleura and its adjacent structures; damage occurs to capillary membranes, and protein-rich material accumulates in the pleural space. Obstruction to lymphatic flow can also produce an exudative effusion. Because most exudates form as a consequence of pleural injury, they are often accompanied by pleuritic chest pain, especially in the acute phase when a friction rub may be heard before much fluid accumulates. The fluid is initially free-flowing but may become walled-off and loculated when there is a marked inflammatory response. The protein content is usually greater than 3.0 g/100 mL. The fluid is typically deep yellow or cloudy in appearance. The leukocyte count is often greater than 1000 cells per milliliter; a count greater than 10,000 is suggestive of an empyema, particularly if most of the cells are neutrophils.

Neoplasms are often responsible for the development of effusions. The majority of pleural fluid accumulations due to malignancies have the characteristics of exudates, although at times the protein concentration is less than 3.0 g/100 mL. Mechanisms of exudate formation include pleural metastasis with increased permeability and obstruction of lymphatic outflow. The formation of a malignant effusion is often a poor prognostic sign, particularly if the pH of the fluid is less than 7.3 and the glucose is less than 60 mg/dL, indicating extensive pleural involvement with tumor.

Bronchogenic carcinoma is the tumor most frequently associated with a pleural effusion. Fluid collects in most instances as a direct result of pleural invasion; unilateral effusions are the rule. Patients report dyspnea when the effusion is large and occasionally complain of pleuritic chest pain. The pleural fluid is usually clear and straw-colored, but it may be bloody and its glucose level may be very low. The white cell count is typically around 2500/mL, with most cells being lymphocytes. Malignant cells are found in about 60 percent of instances. Unfortunately, the disease and its effusions are progressive; thoracentesis is followed by rapid reaccumulation.

Pleural effusions due to *metastatic carcinoma* are more likely to be bilateral than those due to bronchogenic carcinoma, because they occur as a consequence of lymphatic obstruction or diffuse seeding of the pleura. When effusions are due to seeding, cytologic examination of the pleural fluid is positive in up to 90 percent of cases. Carcinoma of the *breast* is the leading metastatic tumor producing pleural effusions, accounting for 25 percent of all malignant effusions. The characteristics of the pleural fluid are similar to those of effusions due to bronchogenic carcinoma. *Lymphoma* is another major cause of malignant bilateral pleural effusions, responsible for up to 20 percent of cases. The formation of a large effusion is a sign of advanced disease; there is often evidence of pleural, parenchymal, and lymph node involvement by the time a significant effusion appears. The pleural fluid may be a transudate or an exudate; most of the cells are lymphocytes. Cough and dyspnea accompany parenchymal involvement, but pleuritic pain is rare.

Mesotheliomas have become an increasingly important source of effusion as the incidence of *asbestos exposure* has increased. Only malignant mesotheliomas produce important pleural fluid accumulations. The latent period for mesothelioma formation ranges from 20 to 40 years after asbestos exposure; the degree of exposure may appear inconsequential (see Chapter 39). Chest pain, cough, and shortness of breath result from extensive pleural disease and large effusions. The fluid may be bloody and often contains malignant cells, but they are sometimes hard to identify cytologically, necessitating chromosomal analysis. The fluid may be high in *hyaluronic acid.* Because the tumor is only locally invasive, there are no signs of extrathoracic disease.

Impressive effusions can form as a consequence of *benign ovarian neoplasms (Meigs' syndrome).* The tumor produces ascites, and fluid tracks across the diaphragm and into the thorax. The effusion is typically on the right, but may be left-sided or even bilateral; it is exudative in quality, free of malignant cells, and similar in composition to the ascitic fluid from which it derives. Removal of the ovarian tumor results in prompt resolution of the effusion.

Infections are an important source of exudative pleural effusions, but among the *acute bacterial pneumonias* encountered in ambulatory patients effusions are uncommon. For example, only about 5 percent of patients with *pneumococcal pneumonia* develop an effusion, and it is usually small and transient. Such effusions are termed *parapneumonic* to imply that bacteria need not have entered the pleural space to cause the effusion. The term *empyema* is reserved for cases in which organisms are recovered from the pleural fluid, either by Gram's stain or culture. Empyema is a rare, but worrisome event, seen in less than 1 percent of pneumococcal pneumonias that present in the outpatient setting, with most cases occurring when proper antibiotic therapy is delayed. Cough, sputum production, fever, chills, and pleuritic pain may be prominent. Early on, the pleural fluid appears serous and may be sterile, but it quickly turns purulent and organism-positive with empyema formation. In some instances, the pleural fluid offers the only opportunity for recovery of the causative organism. Characteristics of the pleural empyema fluid include a white cell count in excess of 5000 to 10,000/mL, with neutrophils predominating. The concentration of glucose is typically less than 20 mg/100 mL. Pleural scarring may be substantial if the empyema fluid is allowed to remain.

Viral pneumonitis and *mycoplasmal pneumonia* are sometimes associated with pleural effusions in the course of illness, but the effusions are small, transient, and of little consequence (see Chapter 52).

The effusion due to *postprimary tuberculosis (TB)* represents a delayed hypersensitivity reaction to spillage of organisms into the pleural space during early bacteremia or subclinical parenchymal disease (see Chapter 49). The effusion is almost always *unilateral.* The patient may be relatively free of symptoms or complain of lethargy, fever, and weight loss; at times, the clinical picture is dominated by acute onset of pleuritic pain and fever. Cough and sputum are conspicuously absent. The chest x-ray may show little more than an isolated effusion, but the intermediate-strength tuberculin skin test is usually positive. The pleural fluid has the qualities of an exudate; the *glucose* concentration may be *low.* The white cell count averages 1000 to 2000 cells/mL; lymphocytes predominate; mesothelial cells are scarce (less than 2%). Neutrophils may be seen early in the course of the illness. Organisms are rarely found on acid-fast stain of the fluid and can be cultured from the fluid in only 25 percent of cases. Most of these effusions resolve spontaneously within a few months and leave little or no residual; however, symptomatic pulmonary parenchymal involvement eventually develops in over half of such patients (see Chapter 47).

Rheumatoid Disease, particularly *systemic lupus erythematosus,* can produce transient pleuropericardial inflammation during the course of the disease, usually after other signs and symptoms have appeared. There may be a brief period of pleuritic pain. On occasion, pleural involvement may be the disease's initial clinical presentation. In most instances, the pleural fluid has the characteristics of a exudate and may demonstrate low glucose and serum complement levels.

Rheumatoid arthritis is much less likely to produce a pleural effusion than is lupus, but the fluid often persists. Less than 5 percent of patients experience pleuropericardial involvement; these individuals usually have a history of extraarticular manifestations and joint symptoms. Occasionally, the effusion is the first manifestation of rheumatoid disease. The effusion is an exudate, with a predominance of lymphocytes and a very low (less than 20 mg/100 mL) glucose concentration. Although the fluid may contain rheumatoid factor, its presence is not unique to this disease.

Intraabdominal Pathology can lead to the production of an exudative pleural effusion, particularly when recent abdominal surgery, intestinal perforation, or hepatobiliary disease is complicated by development of a *subdiaphragmatic abscess.* In addition to gastrointestinal symptoms, these patients may complain of pleuritic pain, fever, weight loss, and malaise. Often symptoms are nonspecific, causing considerable delay in the decision to seek medical help. The diaphragm on the involved side (which is the right in two-thirds of cases) is elevated and moves poorly on fluoroscopy. A pathognomonic subdiaphragmatic air–fluid level may be present on chest film. The pleural fluid is usually sterile, although it may have a high leukocyte count. If the diaphragm has been perforated, an empyema can form. The pleural effusion associated with *pancreatitis* may begin as a transudate but usually becomes exudative. The effusions are most often on the left but may be bilateral or right-sided. The fluid characteristically has a *high amylase* concentration and is blood-tinged in one-third of cases.

DIFFERENTIAL DIAGNOSIS

Although the etiologies of pleural effusions can be conveniently divided into those conditions that produce transudates and those that result in exudates (see Table 43–1), it is important to keep in mind that a number of conditions can cause both. In such conditions, the initial effusion is transudative but turns exudative as the disease process continues. Chronic congestive heart failure is the etiology most frequently encountered in the ambulatory population. Neoplasms account for the majority of cases seen in referral populations. In a series reported from the Mayo Clinic, bronchogenic carcinoma was the leading cause of malignant pleural effusions, accounting for 30 percent, followed by breast carcinoma (25%) and lymphoma (20%). Infection is the third most common etiology of fluid in the pleural space, with TB still accounting for a substantial proportion of effusions subjected to full evaluation. Bloody effusions are most often due to neoplasms but are also seen with congestive heart failure, pulmonary embolization with infarction,

Table 43-1. Important Causes of Pleural Effusions

Transudates
Congestive heart failure
Hypoalbuminemia, severe
Salt-retention syndromes
Ascites due to cirrhosis
Early phases of a sympathetic effusion
Neoplasm (on occasion)
Peritoneal dialysis
Postpartum
Cardiac bypass graft surgery
Exudates
Neoplasms
Bronchogenic carcinoma
Breast cancer
Lymphoma
Mesothelioma
Meigs' syndrome
Infections
Tuberculosis (and atypical myobacteria in AIDS patients)
Bacterial pneumonia (including empyema)
Viral pneumonitis
Mycoplasmal pneumonia
Pneumocystis pneumonia
Pulmonary embolization
Connective tissue disease
Rheumatoid arthritis
Systemic lupus erythematosus
Intra-abdominal disease
Subphrenic abscess
Pancreatitis
Idiopathic

TB, and pancreatitis. About 15 percent of effusions remain unexplained; most idiopathic effusions are exudates.

Among acquired immunodeficiency syndrome (AIDS) patients, infectious etiologies account for over two-thirds of cases, with bacterial, mycobacterial, and pneumocystis pneumonias accounting for most. Hypoalbuminemia is the leading noninfectious cause of effusion among patients with advanced human immunodeficiency virus (HIV) disease.

WORKUP

The diagnosis of pleural effusion is usually suggested by the findings of dullness and diminished breath sounds upward from the lung base and confirmed by chest x-ray. The first task after identifying the effusion is to assess the degree, if any, of respiratory compromise associated with the effusion. The vital signs should be checked for tachypnea and tachycardia, the skin should be checked for cyanosis, and the chest should be checked for use of accessory muscles of respiration. Patients with objective evidence of substantial respiratory compromise should be admitted to the hospital for further workup. Those who are comfortable can proceed with an outpatient assessment. Although radiologic features may suggest a diagnosis, the history and physical examination complemented by examination of the pleural fluid are essential to an accurate assessment.

History

The patient should be asked about the presence of fever, cough, sputum production, chest pain, dyspnea, edema, abdominal pain, prior history of malignant, hepatic, renal, or HIV disease, exposure to TB or asbestos, and symptoms of rheumatoid disease (see Chapter 146). Cough, fever, and sputum production in conjunction with pleuritic chest pain suggest pneumonitis with pleural involvement. Pleuritic pain is also consistent with embolization, malignancy, and pleural inflammation with adjacent pericarditis due to connective tissue disease. Dyspnea may be induced by the effusion alone, but the symptom is indicative of congestive heart failure when accompanied by orthopnea and paroxysmal nocturnal dyspnea. A history of peripheral edema raises the possibilities of hypoalbuminemia, volume overload, and congestive failure. A history of alcohol abuse, recent abdominal surgery, or abdominal pain or distention points to a source below the diaphragm.

Physical Examination

In addition to the assessment for respiratory compromise, the vital signs are checked for fever and weight change. The integument is inspected for petechiae, purpura, spider angiomas, jaundice, clubbing (see Chapter 45), manifestations of rheumatoid disease (see Chapter 146), and rashes. The neck is noted for jugular venous distention and tracheal deviation; the lymph nodes are checked for enlargement; and the breasts are checked for masses. On lung examination, the level of the effusion and extent of involvement are determined. It is worth noting any compression of adjacent lung, suggested by egophony and bronchial breath sounds heard above the effusion. A pleural friction rub may be audible but is usually lacking when there is a considerable accumulation of fluid. The heart should be checked for an S_3 indicative of pump failure, and a three-component friction rub suggestive of pericarditis. The abdomen is examined for signs of ascites, organomegaly, focal tenderness, and peritonitis (see Chapter 58). The pelvic examination is done to rule out the presence of an ovarian mass, and the extremities are noted for edema, calf tenderness, and signs of joint inflammation.

Laboratory Evaluation

The centerpieces of the laboratory workup are the chest x-ray and pleural fluid analysis. The *chest x-ray* should be studied for pleural-based densities, infiltrates, signs of congestive heart failure (see Chapter 32), hilar adenopathy, coin lesions, and loculation of fluid (detection of which requires lateral decubitus views). Elevation of a hemidiaphragm and presence of a subdiaphragmatic air–fluid level are important radiologic signs of a subphrenic abscess. The location of the effusion may be helpful. Among transudative effusions due to cardiac failure, unilateral effusions tend to be right-sided, and bilateral effusions usually are asymmetric with more fluid on the right side. On the other hand, effusions associated with pericarditis, or with pancreatitis, tend to be left-sided.

When an etiology is not readily evident from the history, physical examination, and chest film, then a *diagnostic thoracentesis* is indicated. Of course, there are instances when thoracentesis need not be done on the first visit. Such instances include the afebrile patient with clinical evidence of congestive heart failure, the postpartum woman who is otherwise well, the patient who has had bypass graft surgery, and the young patient with a small effusion in conjunction with a viral or mycoplasmal pneumonia. These individuals can be followed expectantly with repeat chest films; failure of the effusion to clear with resolution of the presumptive etiology is an indication for thoracentesis.

A diagnostic thoracentesis can be done safely and comfortably in the office on patients who have free-flowing effusions confirmed by lateral decubitus films. Ultrasound has been increasingly used to help guide thoracentesis, but it has not been shown to enhance the safety or yield to the procedure except in situations of very small effusions. Thoracentesis for loculated effusions is more difficult and has a greater risk of pneumothorax; it is best not to tap such effusions in the office.

There are a few pitfalls in thoracentesis technique that must be avoided. A common error is to enter the chest too far below the meniscus of the effusion, risking penetration of the diaphragm or entering the diaphragmatic sulcus, which is likely to be sealed off from the effusion by lung tissue. To define the proper entry point, the lung fields should be percussed and auscultated to determine the upper border of the effusion. Because pleural fluid rises in a meniscus where it comes in contact with the parietal pleura, the needle should be passed into the chest one interspace *above* the upper border of the effusion as determined by examination. A few millimeters of penetration into the pleural space at the level of the meniscus allows full drainage without the complications of a low entry. Injury to the neurovascular bundle along the inferior surface of the rib is avoided by aiming the needle just above the rib's *superior* margin, accomplished by "walking the needle" over the anesthetized surface of the rib. Pneumothorax is minimized by withdrawing or changing needle position as soon as air bubbles begin to appear or one feels the visceral pleura contacting the needle tip; the onset of coughing is common at this stage. The patient should be advised to resist the impulse to cough because the act may impale the lung on the needle. Use of a large-bore Intracath (14 or 16 gauge) minimizes the risk of needle injury to the lung. A post-thoracentesis chest film should be obtained to be sure that a significant pneumothorax has not been produced.

The laboratory analysis of pleural fluid should begin with determination of *protein* and *LDH concentrations*. A simultaneous serum sample should also be sent for protein and LDH levels. As noted earlier, the three most useful findings to distinguish a pleural exudate from a transudate are *pleural LDH level (>200 units), pleural-to-serum LDH ratio (>0.6),* and *pleural-to-serum protein ratio (>0.5)*. The presence of any two of three has a sensitivity in excess of 90 percent and a specificity of 99 percent. If this first step indicates that the effusion is a transudate, no further laboratory analysis of the fluid is indicated. In fact, because of the poor specificity of white and red blood cell counts, glucose level, amylase level, and even bacterial cultures (due to contamination), such tests performed on transudates may be misleading.

If any of the criteria for an exudate are met, the laboratory analysis should include *differential cell count, bacterial culture* (including cultures for anaerobes and mycobacteria), and *cytologic examination*. Although, a high white blood cell count may indicate infection, it is a nonspecific finding. A lymphocyte predominance is suggestive of TB or malignancy but does not help in distinguishing between the two. The sensitivity of cytologic examination depends on the mechanism of the malignant effusion and extent of disease; it may be as high as 95 percent in advanced disease with extensive pleural involvement, but as low as 50 percent in early disease. However, a positive cytology is highly specific when reported by an experienced pathologist.

In certain circumstances, other tests may be useful. *A low pleural fluid glucose level* (<60 mg/dL) is associated with TB, other serious infections, and advanced pleural involvement with malignancy. A *low pleural fluid pH* (less than 7.30) has a similar meaning. Conversely, when the pleural fluid pH is low, the pleural fluid cytologic examination is likely to be positive if there is an underlying cancer. Very low glucose levels (<30 mg/dL) are most consistently associated with the effusion of rheumatoid arthritis. An elevated *amylase* level may point to pancreatitis as the cause of effusion, but it can also be seen in malignant effusion. Specific tumor markers have not proven useful, except in the case of *chromosomal analysis* for identifying malignant mesothelioma. Similarly, measurement of *complement levels* (CH50, C3, and C4) should be reserved for the rare instance when it is necessary to confirm that an exudative effusion in a patient with rheumatoid disease is due to underlying disorder and not another condition. Pleural fluid antinuclear antibody (ANA) measurement may be useful in further establishing the diagnosis of lupus pleuritis.

In about 15 percent of cases, the etiology of an exudative effusion is not evident after complete laboratory analysis of the pleural fluid from an initial thoracentesis. If the suspicion of malignancy persists, repeat thoracentesis is indicated. Sensitivity approaches 90 percent with submission of fluid specimens from three separate pleural taps in patients with underlying malignancy. Test sensitivity is particularly high if there is advanced pleural involvement by tumor, as suggested by a pleural fluid pH of less than 7.30 and a glucose less than 60 mg/dL. *Pleural biopsy* alone may be less sensitive than cytologic examination of pleural fluid in detecting malignancy, but the two tests are complementary, with a sensitivity in excess of 90 percent when used together. Pleural biopsy is most useful in detecting TB, having a sensitivity of 60 percent to 80 percent. Again, the biopsy information is complementary; fluid culture or pleural tissue (or both) will make the diagnosis of TB in up to 95 percent of those with the disease. Pleural tissue, as well as pleural fluid, should be submitted for mycobacterial culture.

When contemplating pleural biopsy, it should be anticipated that the majority of specimens will disclose only nonspecific inflammatory changes. Although as many as 20 percent of such patients will eventually have the diagnosis of malignant effusion made, the majority will have their effusion resolve spontaneously without serious sequelae. When there is a history of hemoptysis or a pulmonary abnormality on chest x-ray, *fiber optic bronchoscopy* may prove useful.

INDICATIONS FOR ADMISSION AND REFERRAL

The patient with respiratory discomfort is best evaluated on an inpatient basis, especially if the patient is HIV-positive or when embolization, severe congestive failure, acute empyema, or an intraabdominal crisis is likely. Few of these patients present to the physician in the office; however, the patient with a chronic, but enlarging collection of pleural fluid is apt to be encountered. The person who appears to be tolerating the effusion without much discomfort can be evaluated and managed on an outpatient basis as long as there is no evidence suggestive of an empyema or a subphrenic abscess, conditions that require surgical attention. Referral is appropriate when malignancy or TB is suspected and pleural biopsy or fiber optic bronchoscopy is deemed necessary.

SYMPTOMATIC MANAGEMENT

The patient can be made comfortable before establishing a diagnosis. Pleuritic pain often responds to indomethacin; the drug has the advantage over narcotics in that it does not have any suppressive effect on respiration. Removal of fluid is indicated when the effusion is compromising respiratory efforts. Usually no more than a liter should be removed at one time to avoid intravascular volume depletion on reequilibration. Malignant pleural effusions are notoriously difficult to treat in the setting of advanced disease with marked pleural involvement (pleural fluid pH less than 7.30 and glucose less than 60 mg/dl). Comfort measures are preferable to repeated attempts at sclerosing therapy under such circumstances (see Chapter 92).

A.H.G.

ANNOTATED BIBLIOGRAPHY

Chang S-C, Perng R-P. The role of fiber optic bronchoscopy in evaluating the causes of pleural effusions. Arch Intern Med 1989;149:855. *(Useful in patients with a pulmonary abnormality on chest x-ray or hemoptysis.)*

Fine NL, Smith LR, Sheedy PF. Frequency of pleural effusions in mycoplasma and viral pneumonias. N Engl J Med 1970; 283:790. *(Small transient effusions are common in these conditions, but large effusions are rare.)*

Frist B, Kahan AV, Koss LG. Comparison of the diagnostic value of biopsies of the pleura and cytologic evaluation of pleural fluids. Ann Intern Med 1972;77:507. *(Among 106 cases of malignant effusion, 97 percent had positive fluid cytology and 38 percent positive pleural biopsies; together, the tests had a sensitivity approaching 100 percent.)*

Hughson WG, Friedman PJ, Feigin DS, et al. Postpartum pleural effusion: A common radiologic finding. Ann Intern Med 1982;97:856. *(In a small prospective study, a majority of asymptomatic women had pleural effusions within 24 hours after delivery.)*

Hunder GG. Pleural fluid complement in systemic lupus erythematosus and rheumatoid arthritis. Ann Intern Med 1972;76: 356. *(Complement levels are low.)*

Joseph J, Strange C, Sahn SA. Pleural effusions in hospitalized patients with AIDS. Ann Intern Med 1993;118:856. *(Although not a study of outpatients, the findings provide etiologies to consider when encountering an HIV-positive patient, especially one with AIDS.)*

Light RW, Ball WC. Glucose and amylase in pleural effusion. JAMA 1973;225:259. *(TB and malignant effusions were not universally associated with low glucose values.)*

Light RW, et al. Cells and pleural fluid. Arch Intern Med 1973;132:854. *(Reviews the diagnostic significance of cell counts; concludes that the finding of many mesothelial cells is incompatible with TB; red cell counts greater than 100,000 suggested neoplasm, infarction, or trauma; predominant lymphocytes were consistent with TB and neoplasm.)*

Light RW, et al. Pleural effusions: The diagnostic separation of transudate and exudate. Ann Intern Med 1972;77:507. *(A classic article that details rigorous criteria for the separation of transudates from exudates.)*

Peterman TA, Speicher CE. Evaluating pleural effusions. JAMA 1984;252:1051. *(Advocates a two-stage procedure identifying exudates with rapid determination of protein and LDH values, thereby eliminating need to order additional tests for transudates.)*

Poe RE, Israel RH, Vtell MJ, et al. Sensitivity, specificity, and predictive values of closed pleural biopsy. Arch Intern Med 1984;144:325. *(Sensitivity was 68 percent for malignant disease.)*

Sahn SA. The pleura. Am Rev Respir Dis 1988;138:184. *(An exhaustive review of pleural pathophysiology and pleural effusion.)*

Sahn SA, Good JT, Jr. Pleural fluid pH in malignant effusions. Ann Intern Med 1988;108:349. *(A pH less than 7.30 correlated with advanced pleural involvement with tumor and a very poor prognosis.)*

Weiss JM, Spodick DH. Association of left pleural effusion with pericardial disease. N Engl J Med 1983;308:696. *(Patients with pericarditis tend to have unilateral pleural effusions that are left sided or bilateral effusions that are larger on the left; this is in contrast to the right-sided dominance in congestive heart failure.)*

44
Evaluation of the Solitary Pulmonary Nodule

Primary Care Medicine: Office Evaluation and Management of the Adult Patient, 3rd edition, edited by Allan H. Goroll, Lawrence A. May, and Albert G. Mulley, Jr. J.B. Lippincott Company, Philadelphia

Solitary nodules are found at a rate of one to two per 1000 routine chest x-rays. The discovery is a worrisome finding because it raises the possibilities of primary lung cancer and solitary metastasis from a nonpulmonary source. The patient is usually asymptomatic and undergoing chest x-ray for either an unrelated issue or screening. Granulomas and hamartomas account for the majority. About 30 percent prove to be malignant. Pulmonary malignancies with the greatest potential for cure present as solitary nodules. Consequently, thorough assessment is of utmost importance. On the other hand, the majority of these lesions are not cancers, and to subject all patients to invasive studies and excision can lead to much unnecessary morbidity. The primary physician needs to determine the likelihood of malignancy on the basis of clinical and radiologic findings to identify the patient who requires referral for consideration of bronchoscopy, percutaneous needle biopsy, or thoracotomy. Workup can be initiated on an outpatient basis.

PATHOPHYSIOLOGY AND CLINICAL PRESENTATION

Solitary pulmonary nodules characteristically appear in the middle or lateral lung fields, surrounded by normal lung and unaccompanied by satellite lesions. They have smooth contours and are usually round ("coin" lesions) or oval. Neoplastic, granulomatous, vascular, and cystic processes are the principal pathologic mechanisms responsible for nodule formation. The nodule displaces normal aerated lung parenchyma and does not cause symptoms unless there is airway obstruction, pleural invasion, interference with respiratory mechanics, or involvement of blood vessels or nerves. Inflammatory lesions double in volume in less than 5 weeks; malignancies take between 1 and 18 months to double; benign nodules take longer. A solitary nodule that does not change in size over 2 years is benign. The older the patient, the greater the chances that the nodule is malignant; the probability is less than 2 percent below age 30 and increases by 10 percent to 15 percent with each succeeding decade. A history of smoking greatly increases the probability that the nodule is malignant, as does concurrent weight loss, headache, or bone pain.

Benign and malignant solitary lung nodules may have similar appearances on chest x-ray. However, the distribution *patterns of calcification* are different and of diagnostic utility. Benign lesions tend to have calcium deposited in central, peripheral, concentric, "popcorn," or homogeneous patterns, whereas eccentric patterns of calcification are more characteristic of malignancies (see below and Figure 44–1).

Among lung cancers, adenocarcinomas tend to be located peripherally; squamous and small cell cancers are usually more central in location. However, squamous cell cancers that are located peripherally tend to cavitate.

DIFFERENTIAL DIAGNOSIS

Healed infectious granulomas account for the majority of solitary nodules. In most series, 20 percent to 40 percent prove to be cancers. Of these, more than 75 percent are *primary lung cancers*, the remainder are *metastatic lesions*. Tumors of the *breast, colon,* and *testicles* are particularly prone to metastasize to the lung. Of the 60 percent to 80 percent of solitary pulmonary nodules that prove to be benign, 85 percent to 90 percent are granulomas; most are *tuberculous,* but, in endemic areas, *histoplasmosis* and *coccidiomycosis* are important considerations. Benign pulmonary tumors such as *hamartomas* account for about 5 percent of benign nodules. The remainder are *bronchogenic cysts, hydatid cysts, pseudolymphomas, arteriovenous malformations,* and *bronchopulmonary sequestrations*. Extrapulmonary lesions, such as skin lesions, moles, nipples, chest wall and rib lesions, and pleural plaques, may be confused with solitary lesions of lung parenchyma.

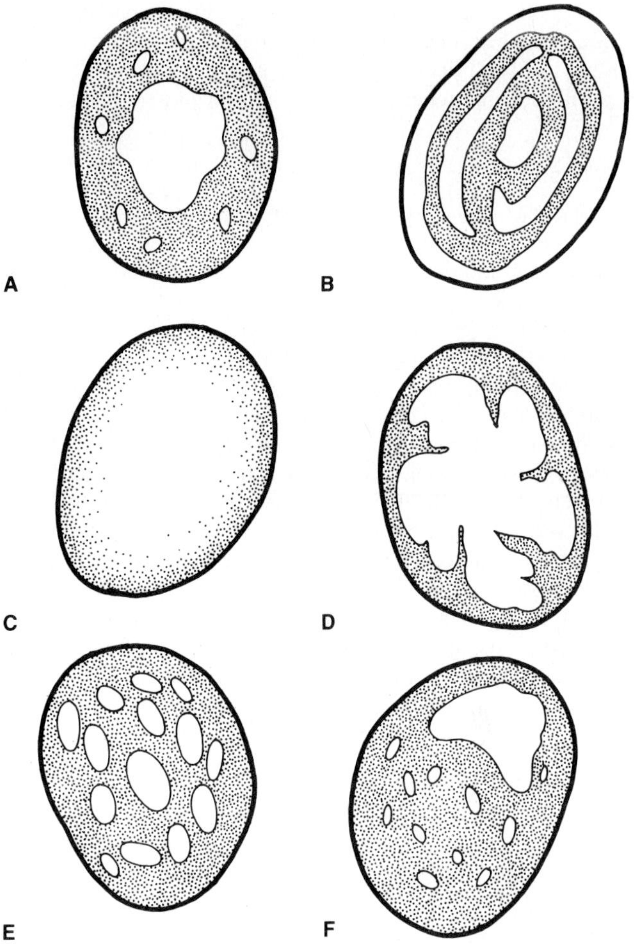

Figure 44-1. Patterns of calcification in solitary pulmonary nodules include (**A**) central, (**B**) laminated, (**C**) diffuse, (**D**) popcorn, (**E**) stippled, and (**F**) eccentric, **A** through **D** are virtually always benign; **E** and **F** may be benign or malignant.

WORKUP

The major issue posed by a solitary nodule is the chance of an early resectable lung cancer. Many surgeons argue that the risk of thoracotomy is small and potential benefit is considerable, because resection of a nodule that proves to be an early primary lung cancer may provide the patient with a chance for cure. They note that for resected bronchogenic carcinomas and solitary lung metastases presenting as solitary nodules, average 5-year survivals are 60 percent and 35 percent, respectively. On the other hand, pulmonologists have argued that lesions that possess many of the criteria of benignity can be managed conservatively, and that definitive tissue diagnosis can be approached by bronchoscopy or needle biopsy without resorting to early thoracotomy, which has a surgical mortality ranging from 1 percent to 10 percent. A review of the literature reveals passionate advocates on both sides. Conclusive data taking into account morbidity and mortality of both approaches are still lacking.

The task of the primary care physician is to make the best possible clinical estimate of cancer risk based on history, physical examination, and appearance of the nodule on chest x-ray and computed tomography (CT). Proper patient selection is the best means of maximizing the yield from invasive study and surgical intervention and minimizing the false alarm rate and unnecessary morbid procedures.

History

The age of the patient and history of smoking are important determinants of cancer risk. The likelihood ratio for malignancy in men increases markedly with age, estimated at 0.1 for those less than age 35 to 5.7 for those over 70. Likelihood ratios for smoking range from 0.15 for never having smoked to 3.9 for currently smoking over two packs per day. The probability of cancer is 50 percent for patients in their 60s but less than 2 percent for those under 30. Although symptoms are often absent, it is worth inquiring into bone pain, headache, weight loss, and other symptoms suggestive of malignancy. A history of hemoptysis (even if minimal; see Chapter 42), known previous breast, bowel, or testicular cancer also increases the likelihood of malignancy. History of exposure to tuberculosis (TB) or residence in an area in which histoplasmosis or coccidiomycosis is endemic raises the possibility of a granulomatous etiology but does not rule out malignancy. A family history of hemorrhagic telangiectasia can be a valuable clue.

Physical Examination

The physical examination is generally unrevealing, but a breast or testicular mass, occult blood in the stool, clubbing (see Chapter 45), cutaneous or mucosal telangiectasia, and an audible bruit over the chest wall (suggestive of a vascular etiology) should be excluded. Perhaps the most important part of the physical examination is careful palpation of lymph nodes, particularly those in the supraclavicular and axillary regions. If enlarged, such nodes can be biopsied, which may eliminate the need for thoracotomy or other invasive procedures.

Laboratory Studies

Chest X-ray *appearance* of the lesion and its *doubling time* are among the most useful data for determining the chances of malignancy. Assessment of doubling time—the period during which the tumor doubles in volume—can be especially helpful, but possible immediately only if there are *previous chest films* available. It is important to keep in mind that doubling refers to volume, not diameter. In doubling, the diameter of the lesion need increase by only 28 percent, not 100 percent. A doubling time of greater than 2 years or less than 30 days makes malignancy unlikely.

Every effort should be made to locate old chest x-rays before further studies are undertaken. If no old films are available and it is determined reasonable to follow the patient expectantly (see below), then serial films should be obtained, beginning with one 3 weeks from the time of initial evaluation and then at intervals of 3 to 6 months for the next year, decreasing to every 6 to 12 months thereafter.

If previous films are unavailable, careful evaluation of the *radiologic appearance* of the nodule is indicated. A most helpful sign is the presence of *calcification*. Laminated or concentric calcification is specific for granulomas. Central, diffuse, or homogeneous patterns of calcification are, with rare exceptions, also associated with benign lesions. However, radiographically visible calcium in stippled or eccentric patterns can occur in malignancies as well as in benign lesions. Moreover, a primary cancer may engulf a preexisting calcified granuloma or scar; eccentricity of the calcium in the nodule should raise this possibility (see Figure 44-1).

Location, size, and *shape* of the nodule as it appears on chest x-ray are less valuable distinguishing signs. Both cancers and tuberculous granulomas are more common in the upper and middle lobes than in the lower lobes. Small lesions are more likely to be benign but, if malignant, are still at a stage when detection and definitive diagnosis may have the greatest positive impact. Ill-defined borders suggest a primary malignancy, as does lobulation of the margin of the nodule. However, smooth borders are also seen with metastatic lesions. Cavitation occurs with nearly equal frequency in cancers and granulomas.

Computed Tomography (CT) has become the imaging technique of choice for evaluation of the solitary pulmonary nodule. It provides much better definition of the lesion and pattern of calcification than does chest x-ray, reducing the false-negative rate associated with reliance on chest x-ray appearance alone. What appears to be a single nodule on plain film may actually be one of several lesions on CT and indicative of metastatic disease. CT is useful for guiding needle biopsy and allows assessment of the mediastinum, which is useful in staging lesions that are suspected to be malignant (although its sensitivity and specificity for staging have been found wanting in patients with lesions less than 3 cm; see Chapter 53).

Taking thin sections (high-resolution CT) or using iodinated contrast can sometimes uncover calcification not visible by standard CT, can better confirm hamartomas and arteriovenous (AV) malformations, and can enhance appearance of malignant nodules.

Magnetic Resonance Imaging (MRI) is inferior to CT for imaging solitary pulmonary nodules. It does not detect calcification well but does reveal the mediastinum better than does CT, and is useful for imaging chest-wall invasion, aortopulmonic window adenopathy, and superior sulcus tremors.

Ancillary Studies. An intermediate strength *tuberculin skin test* should be implanted (see Chapter 38). If sputum is available, it should be stained for *acid-fast organisms* and *cultured for TB*. In endemic areas, *fungal cultures* and histoplasmin complement fixation titers may be of importance.

Sputum cytologic examination is the least invasive means of identifying a malignancy. Three first morning samples should be obtained on consecutive days. Yield is highest when the sample contains pulmonary histiocytes (a sign of a deep sample) and the lesion is in the upper lobes, centrally located, communicating with a bronchus, or greater than 2 cm in diameter (see Chapter 37). Although specificity is high in experienced hands, sensitivity has been found wanting in many studies, with figures ranging from 13 percent to 77 percent. Thus, a negative study does not rule out the diagnosis. Moreover, the importance of distinguishing a small cell carcinoma from other cell types (see Chapter 53) often necessitates obtaining tissue for diagnosis. Because of these shortcomings, some have argued that sputum cytology is not worth the effort, except in patients who are too ill to undergo invasive study.

Conservative Approach to further evaluation is reasonable in patients determined to have little chance of cancer after noninvasive evaluation. Withholding invasive study is a legitimate management option in patients with lesions that have not enlarged in 5 years, and in young nonsmoking patients with radiologic evidence that suggests benignity (central, laminated, diffuse, or "popcorn" pattern of calcification; sharp borders). Careful follow-up with serial chest films taken in the schedule noted above is essential, because some malignancies can be slow-growing.

Invasive Diagnostic Measures deserve consideration if the risk of malignancy persists after noninvasive evaluation. Thoracotomy with resection represents the most direct and definitive means of diagnosis (and treatment), but it is associated with a perioperative mortality risk of 1 percent to 10 percent and considerable morbidity (see Chapter 53). Less morbid options include bronchoscopy with transbronchial biopsy and needle aspiration biopsy under fluoroscopic or CT control.

Fiberoptic bronchoscopic examination with bronchial brushing and biopsy may make a diagnosis if a bronchus appears to enter the lesion on CT, but sensitivity is substantially lower (10%–30%) when nodules are small (<2 cm) and well circumscribed. *Transthoracic needle aspiration* is a far more valuable approach to diagnosis. Sensitivity for detection of malignancy approaches 95 percent when the nodule is accessible to the transthoracic approach. Accurate pathologic diagnosis is facilitated by using a large-bore needle rather than a "skinny" one and taking multiple samples. Specific histologic types of malignant lesions can often be identified.

Mediastinoscopy and thoracotomy are indicated when preprocedure probability of an early resectable primary lung cancer is high (see Chapter 53) and the patient is a good operative risk. Patients with severe obstructive or restrictive disease should first undergo formal pulmonary function testing.

Choice of Diagnostic Approach depends on the estimated probability of malignancy, location of the lesion, the ability and willingness of the patient to tolerate the event (or the uncertainty, if watchful waiting is a consideration), and the availability of the needed technical expertise. The decision to proceed must also take into account the patient's ultimate willingness and tolerance for treatment of cancer.

The high-probability patient who can tolerate surgery and is determined to have a resectable lesion (see Chapter 53) should undergo thoracotomy and resection. Patients at intermediate probability of malignancy might be best approached by transthoracic needle biopsy if it appears technically feasible. Very-low-risk patients are reasonable candidates for careful follow-up by serial x-ray study.

In sum, the optimal approach to evaluation of the patient with a solitary pulmonary nodule remains problematic, because outcome data are lacking. It appears that a conservative approach to evaluation is justified in patients judged to be at low risk for malignancy based on epidemiologic, historical, physical, and x-ray criteria. Patients at high risk for malignancy require a tissue diagnosis. A patient who falls between these two groups poses a dilemma, which should be shared with the patient so that a satisfactory plan can be devised.

PATIENT EDUCATION AND INDICATIONS FOR REFERRAL

Patients suspected on clinical and radiologic grounds of having a malignancy should be referred for tissue diagnosis. Decisions regarding need for and type of invasive procedure should be made in conjunction with surgical and radiologic consultants. In situations where the probability of malignancy is unclear, the patient needs to be informed about the lack of diagnostic confidence based on noninvasive study, as well as the nature of further testing that would be undertaken. Patients who cannot emotionally tolerate the uncertainty should be advised to undergo a definitive procedure to end the constant worry about the possibility of malignancy. The patient who can live with such uncertainty and is reluctant to have a thoracotomy or biopsy could be followed with serial chest films at 3- to 6-month intervals for 2 years.

A.H.G.

ANNOTATED BIBLIOGRAPHY

Becker GL, Whitlock WL, Schaefer PS, et al. The impact of thoracic computed tomography in clinically staged T1, N0, M0 chest lesions. Arch Intern Med 1990;150:557. *(Finds that CT was not helpful for staging the suspected lesion in patients with lung nodules less than 3 cm.)*

Cummings SR, Lillington GA, Richard RJ. Estimating the probability of malignancy in solitary pulmonary nodules. Am Rev Respir Dis 1986;134:449. *(Utilizes prevalence, diameter of nodule, age, smoking history, calcification pattern, and type of edge; very useful.)*

Fulkerson WJ. Fiberoptic bronchoscopy. N Engl J Med 1984;311:511. *(Reviews the indications, contraindications, and complications as well as diagnostic yield of fiberoptic bronchoscopy and endobronchial biopsy.)*

Godwin JD. The solitary pulmonary nodule. Radiol Clin North Am 1983;21:709. *(A valuable clinical review including extensive discussion of the role of CT examination.)*

Khouri NF, et al. Transthoracic needle aspiration biopsy of benign and malignant lung lesions. Am J Roentgenol 1985;144:281. *(Diagnostic yield well in excess of 80% and helped by use of wide aspiration needle, which facilitates diagnosis of benign lesions.)*

Lillington GA. The solitary pulmonary nodule. Chest 1976;70:322. *(An editorial that argues by example that early thoracotomy for every nodule, particularly in young people, would be uneconomic. It is suggested that needle biopsy or watchful waiting has a legitimate role in patients with low probability of malignancy.)*

Lillington GA. The solitary pulmonary nodule. Am Rev Respir Dis 1974;110:699. *(A classic review of the problem.)*

Lillington GA, Stevens GM. The solitary nodule: The other side of the coin. Chest 1976;70:322. *(An editorial arguing that early thoracotomy in persons of low risk is probably unnec-*

essary; suggests needle biopsy or watchful waiting as alternatives.)

MacDougall B, Weinerman B. The value of sputum cytology. J Gen Intern Med 1992;7:11. *(Sensitivity and specificity were found lacking, and the test was found to be of limited use in the work-up of suspected lung cancer.)*

Nathan MH. Management of solitary pulmonary nodules: An organized approach based on growth rates and statistics. JAMA 1974;227:1141. *(A very conservative approach is advocated: observation of the nodule with serial x-rays for calculation of doubling time.)*

Swenson SJ, et al. Solitary pulmonary nodule: CT evaluation of enhancement with iodinated contrast material. Radiology 1992; 182:343. *(Improved detection of malignancy suggested.)*

Swenson SJ, Jett JR, Payne WS, et al. An integrated approach to evaluation of the solitary pulmonary nodule. Mayo Clin Proc 1990;65:173. *(A critical review of diagnostic studies; 79 refs.)*

Toomes H, et al. The coin lesion of the lung: A review of 955 resected coin lesions. Cancer 1983;51:534. *(A useful series for statistics on types of lesions identified.)*

Webb WR. MR Imaging in the evaluation and staging of lung cancer. Semin Ultrasound, CT, MR 1988;9:53. *(Useful for chest wall, superior sulcus, and aortopulmonic window assessment.)*

45
Evaluation of Clubbing

Primary Care Medicine: Office Evaluation and Management of the Adult Patient, 3rd edition, edited by Allan H. Goroll, Lawrence A. May, and Albert G. Mulley, Jr. J.B. Lippincott Company, Philadelphia

The term *clubbing* refers to enlargement and sponginess of the nail beds of the fingers and toes and reduction in the angle created by the nail and the dorsum of the distal phalanx. Clubbing is sometimes accompanied by a chronic subperiosteal osteitis, *hypertrophic osteoarthropathy.* Patients rarely complain of clubbed fingers; it is the physician who detects this abnormality as an incidental finding on physical examination. Because clubbing or hypertrophic osteoarthropathy may be the first clinical sign of a serious underlying condition, such as a pulmonary neoplasm, it is important for the primary physician to recognize these findings and investigate their possible causes.

PATHOPHYSIOLOGY AND CLINICAL PRESENTATION

Hypotheses explaining the pathogenesis of clubbing and osteoarthropathy implicate autonomic influences, arteriovenous (AV) shunting, and bloodborne substances. The precise pathophysiology remains uncertain, but it is known that intrathoracic vagotomy can abolish clubbing and osteoarthropathy, as can correction of an AV shunt or removal of a pulmonary tumor.

Pathologic examination of clubbed fingers reveals increased vascularity. In hypertrophic osteoarthropathy, the periosteum is found to be edematous, hyperemic, and infiltrated by mononuclear cells. There is periosteal elevation, new bone formation, and endosteal resorption in the distal ends of long bones, metacarpals, and metatarsals. Soft tissue swelling in the distal ends of the fingers and toes may lead to clubbing.

Clubbing is usually asymptomatic. Patients with hypertrophic osteoarthropathy may complain of pain in the wrists, ankles, hands, and feet; erythema and effusions are sometimes noted. Hypertrophic osteoarthropathy may precede clubbing or occur without it, but most often the two appear together. Clubbing often takes place in the absence of osteoarthropathy. Either finding may develop before the clinical presentation of one of the conditions associated with it.

Idiopathic hypertrophic osteoarthropathy, sometimes referred to as pachydermoperiostosis, is a benign condition that must be distinguished from hypertrophic osteoarthropathy secondary to systemic disease. These patients show periosteal new bone formation, swelling of the joints, and thickened and furred skin as well as clubbing. The benign syndrome can be differentiated from secondary hypertrophic osteoarthropathy by its development in adolescence, slow growth, paucity of joint symptoms, and absence of concurrent hepatic or pulmonary disease.

DIFFERENTIAL DIAGNOSIS

Clubbing and hypertrophic osteoarthropathy occur in 2 percent to 12 percent of patients with *lung cancer,* developing with equal frequency in patients with large cell, squamous cell, or adenocarcinomas, but rarely in the setting of small cell cancer. Metastatic lung tumors are rarely responsible for such changes. With the decline in the incidence of *chronic pulmonary infectious* diseases (such as tuberculosis, lung abscess, and bronchiectasis), carcinoma of the lung has emerged as the leading cause of hypertrophic osteoarthropathy. Clubbing and osteoarthropathy are seen in patients with cyanotic congenital heart disease with *right-to-left shunts,* subacute bacterial *endocarditis, inflammatory bowel disease,* and *biliary cirrhosis.* Clubbing is a classic sign of chronic *hypoxemia* in patients with chronic obstructive lung disease. In addition, there are *hereditary* or idiopathic forms of clubbing and hypertrophic osteoarthropathy that have no clinical significance. Unilateral clubbing is associated with impairment of the vascular supply to the arm that occurs with aortic, subclavian, or innominate artery lesions. Jackhammer operators may develop clubbing.

Clubbing must be differentiated from a number of other phalangeal conditions that resemble it. Many normal people, particularly African-Americans, have increased curvature of the nails. Infections of the terminal phalanges such as felons and chronic paronychia may be confused with clubbing, as may thyroid acropachy.

WORKUP

The evaluation of clubbing should begin with confirmation of the characteristic physical findings: *loss of the angle* made by the nail and *increase* in the *ballotability* of the nail bed. Hypertrophic osteoarthropathy is identified by *x-ray of the long bones;* the typical changes are increase in periosteal thickness and new bone formation at distal ends. Once it is clear that clubbing or hypertrophic osteoarthropathy is present, evaluation for an underlying etiology can commence.

History. Before an elaborate search for a serious illness is undertaken, it should be established whether clubbing has been lifelong and is present in other family members, indicative of the harmless familial variety. Symptoms such as cough, sputum production, hemoptysis, and dyspnea point to a respiratory problem and may have already triggered an evaluation of the lungs (see Chapters 40 to 42). The patient should be questioned about history of a heart murmur and exercise intolerance, as well as prior liver disease, crampy lower abdominal pain, diarrhea, bloody stools, and joint complaints. Smoking and other risk factors related to development of lung cancer (see Chapter 37) should be assessed. Exposure to tuberculosis also needs to be ascertained (see Chapter 38).

Physical Examination requires a check for fever, tachypnea, tachycardia, cyanosis, tobacco stains, jugular venous distention, barrel chest, wheezes, rhonchi, rales (crackles), signs of consolidation or effusion, heart murmur, skin lesions of hepatocellular disease, and signs of cirrhosis. Lymph nodes should be palpated for enlargement, and joints should be checked for hypertrophic changes and signs of inflammation.

Laboratory Studies. The only mandatory laboratory study is a *chest x-ray,* because an early pleural, pulmonary, or mediastinal neoplasm may be asymptomatic. A complete blood count (CBC) and stool examination for occult blood may be of help. Further evaluation of the liver, thyroid, heart, or bowel should be undertaken only if symptoms or physical findings suggest pathology in these areas. Patients with new onset of clubbing and a long smoking history should be followed for the development of pulmonary neoplasm; periodic examinations including sputum cytology and chest x-ray are appropriate.

Differentiating Osteoarthropathy From Rheumatoid Disease can be difficult. An extensive review of patients with clubbing and lung cancer showed that the symptoms of osteoarthropathy were often mistaken for arthritis and predated the diagnosis of neoplasm by a mean of 4.9 months. Frequent complaints of bilateral joint discomfort in the small joints, such as the wrists and hands, and an adequate response to aspirin or nonsteroidals tended to persuade physicians that they were dealing with rheumatologic disease. It was also noteworthy that they found acute elevations in acute phase reactants and a positive rheumatoid factor in 1 of 14 as well as antinuclear antibody in 5 of 12. The symmetric involvement of small peripheral joints and the tendency to develop synovitis presents a significant diagnostic dilemma with some patients having a syndrome indistinguishable from that of an inflammatory arthritis.

SYMPTOMATIC MANAGEMENT AND PATIENT EDUCATION

There is no symptomatic therapy for clubbing. It is an innocuous cosmetic disturbance. Discomfort in the bones and joints secondary to hypertrophic osteoarthropathy can be treated with aspirin. Rarely, there are disabling joint symptoms; these may require extreme therapies such as corticosteroids or intrathoracic vagotomy. Resection of the underlying lung cancer may reduce joint pain and swelling of the fingers. Such therapeutic options should be undertaken in consultation with a consultant familiar with the problem.

Patient education is important in any condition where the physician discovers a potential sign of disease that is not obvious to the patient. It is likely that patients will be disturbed by the investigation and by the possibility of serious disease. The physician must take time to inform the patient that clubbing can be a harmless finding as well as a helpful guide to the early diagnosis of disease. The patient who smokes should be strongly advised to quit (see Chapter 54).

A.H.G.

ANNOTATED BIBLIOGRAPHY

Pineada CJ, Fonseca C, Martinez-Lavin M. The spectrum of soft tissue and skeletal abnormalities of hypertrophic osteoarthropathy. J Rheumatol 1990;17:626. *(Detailed description of characteristic findings.)*

Segal AN, Mackenzie AH. Hypertrophic osteoarthropathy: A ten-year retrospective analysis. Semin Arthritis Rheum 1985; 12:220. *(Authoritative review with extensive study of 16 patients with hypertrophic osteoarthropathy; the differentiation from rheumatoid disease can sometimes be difficult.)*

Stenseth JH, Clagett OT, Woolner LB. Hypertrophic pulmonary osteoarthropathy. Dis Chest 1967;52:62. *(Review of 888 pulmonary neoplasms, revealing a 9.2 percent incidence of hypertrophic osteoarthropathy.)*

Primary Care Medicine: Office Evaluation and Management of the Adult Patient, 3rd edition, edited by Allan H. Goroll, Lawrence A. May, and Albert G. Mulley, Jr. J.B. Lippincott Company, Philadelphia

46
Approach to the Patient with Sleep Apnea

Sleep apnea is an important condition that often gets overlooked because its symptoms (eg, daytime tiredness, snoring) may be mistaken by the patient for normal phenomena of everyday life. A growing appreciation of its potentially serious consequences has heightened physician and lay awareness of this seemingly harmless problem. The primary care physician needs to be cognizant of sleep apnea's early manifestations so a timely work-up can commence and treatment can be instituted before the onset of pulmonary hypertension and cor pulmonale.

PATHOPHYSIOLOGY AND CLINICAL PRESENTATION

Sleep apnea may result from central suppression of respiration (as occurs with congestive heart failure and diseases of the central nervous system [CNS]) or from airway obstruction. The latter is the more common problem in the office setting and is technically referred to as obstructive apnea. The obstruction occurs when the normal mechanisms that sustain the patency of the pharyngeal airway collapse during sleep. Much debated are the precise mechanisms for this collapse, but reduction in upper airway dilator muscle activity is believed to play a part. The reduction leads to obstruction in susceptible patients—those who have an anatomically narrow pharyngeal airway (eg, the very obese). When the obstruction is partial, loud snoring occurs. Full obstruction interrupts ventilation and, if sufficiently prolonged, results in hypercarbia and hypoxemia. Restoration of breathing usually requires arousal from sleep. The nightly occurrence of multiple apneic episodes and disturbed sleep pattern causes daytime tiredness and hypersomnolence. Chronic persistence of nighttime arterial desaturation can lead to pulmonary hypertension and even cor pulmonale, especially in patients with concomitant lung disease. In addition, systemic hypertension and cardiac arrhythmias may develop if arterial blood gases become markedly disturbed.

The patient with obstructive sleep apnea typically presents complaining of excessive daytime tiredness and hypersomnolence. The visit may have been triggered by the insistence of his bed partner, who reports excessive, loud snoring and disturbed sleep, perhaps even noting periods of irregular or halted breathing. Although the vast majority of patients are male and markedly obese, the condition is not limited to such individuals. It is estimated that as many as 2 percent to 5 percent of adult males suffer from obstructive sleep apnea.

DIFFERENTIAL DIAGNOSIS

Because obstructive sleep apnea may present as tiredness, it must be differentiated from other causes of chronic fatigue (see Chapter 8). In patients who present with interrupted sleep, other sleep disturbances deserve consideration (see Chapter 232). Those whose presentation is predominantly one of nocturnal difficulty breathing require consideration of heart failure (see Chapter 32) and chronic obstructive lung disease (see Chapter 47), and other causes of snoring (see Chapter 223).

Conditions contributing to obstructive sleep apnea include marked obesity (body mass index in excess of 25 kg/m^2), tonsillar hypertrophy, severe nasal obstruction, and a pharyngeal tumor.

WORKUP

The best way to recognize the condition is to have a high index of suspicion for its presence when an obese, hypertensive male presents complaining of excessive daytime tiredness and hypersomnolence. A check with a bed partner, if available, about loud snoring, interrupted sleep, and irregular respiratory activity will further suggest the diagnosis. A multivariate analysis found that male gender, age greater than 50, body mass index greater than 20 percent of normal, and loud snoring at night were predictive of a positive sleep study, but had a sensitivity no greater than overall clinical assessment. Unless the condition is far advanced and there are signs of pulmonary hypertension (eg, right ventricular heave, loud pulmonic component of the second heart sound, jugular venous distention), the physical examination is likely to be unremarkable, with the exception of blood pressure elevation. However, a check of the upper airway, looking for tonsillar hypertrophy and a narrowed nasopharyngeal airway, is occasionally rewarding. In addition, a review of symptoms and signs of hypothyroidism (see Chapter 104) is indicated, and a thyroid-stimulating hormone (TSH) should be ordered if there is sufficient suspicion for this readily reversible, albeit uncommon, cause of sleep apnea.

Few laboratory studies are of value. Most patients have a normal hematocrit, and arterial blood gases will be normal in the office. Home monitoring for arterial desaturation is undergoing evaluation and may prove useful in the future, but the technology remains to be validated. The definitive diagnostic procedure in symptomatic patients strongly suspected of sleep apnea is a formal *polysomnographic study* that includes continuous monitoring of *arterial oxygen saturation*. The best means of properly selecting patients for this expensive procedure is a careful history. Other screening tests are under consideration, but their cost-effectiveness has not been proven.

There are no definitive criteria for a positive study because the upper limit for apneic periods in normals is not well-defined. However, most authorities agree that 30 to 40 apneic periods per hour in a symptomatic patient with arterial desaturation during sleep is strong grounds for initiation of therapy. A lesser frequency of apneic episodes (10 to 30/h) is a more common finding and necessitates careful consideration of the overall clinical picture before recommending treatment. Decreased survival has been found in patients with 20 or more apneic periods per hour of sleep and in those with underlying lung disease.

PRINCIPLES OF MANAGEMENT

Treatment does improve survival of patients with obstructive sleep apnea, but a proper matching of disease severity with treatment intensity is critical to achieving the best possible outcome. Patients with preexisting lung disease plus sleep apnea have a worse prognosis than those with no underlying lung disease and should be treated more aggressively. Minimally symptomatic patients with no concurrent pulmonary disease can be followed expectantly, but those who are obese should be prescribed a *weight reduction program*. Weight reduction is also the centerpiece of the treatment program for those who are more symptomatic because it can greatly ameliorate or even cure sleep apnea. Design of a comprehensive, personalized program of weight reduction is essential to a successful weight loss effort (see Chapter 233).

Nighttime nasal administration of *continuous positive airway pressure (CPAP)* is becoming as an important component of the treatment program for obstructive sleep apnea. A sealed nasal mask is worn at night connected to a blower apparatus that pneumatically sustains sufficient airway pressure to maintain upper airway patency. Patient acceptance is steadily improving, and compliance now exceeds 80 percent, facilitated by rapidly advances in apparatus design.

Surgical approaches are worth consideration if symptoms are severe and an obstructing anatomic anomaly is found or if more conservative measures have failed. Surgical excision of obstructing tonsils, a nasal mass, or a pharyngeal tumor can be curative. Surgery has also been applied to patients with severe obstructive disease, even in the absence of a single, identifiable, obstructing lesion. The procedure used most for this purpose has been the *uvulopalatopharyngoplasty (UPPP)*. In performing the UPPP, the surgeon excises the uvula, part of the soft palate, and any redundant pharyngeal tissue. The problem with recommending such surgery is that only about half of patients obtain a satisfactory result. Moreover, it has not been possible to predict in advance who will benefit from the surgery. As a result and with the improvements in CPAP therapy, UPPP is becoming a less utilized treatment option.

Pharmacologic approaches have not proven effective. Progesterone and protriptyline have been studied but have failed to demonstrate benefit. Avoidance of agents that might suppress respiration deserves attention. Sleep apnea patients should cease evening use of alcohol and should avoid sedative use. *Dental appliances* have proven useful in a small number of patients, but their efficacy and acceptability for long-term use remain to be determined.

INDICATIONS FOR REFERRAL

Obese male patients with severe daytime tiredness and hypersomnolence should be considered candidates for referral and consideration of a formal sleep study, especially if there is a corroborating history by the patient's bed companion of loud, persistent snoring, disturbed sleep, and abnormal respirations. The presence of marked obesity and hypertension should further raise the level of suspicion about an obstructive sleep disorder and should prompt the consultation. Referral is best made to a pulmonary specialist experienced in the conduct and interpretation of polysonography, although it should be made clear that the purpose of the consultation is for assessment of candidacy for formal sleep testing, not for automatic performance of polysonographic study. Consultation with a pulmonary specialist experienced in treatment of sleep disorders can also be very useful in the patient who fails to improve with weight loss and needs consideration of CPAP and surgical approaches to therapy.

PATIENT EDUCATION

Patients brought in by a spouse who complains of their excessive snoring require detailed information on the potential seriousness of this seemingly harmless condition. Unless they suffer from disabling daytime tiredness and excessive sleepiness, they are unlikely to appreciate the significance of their condition. Patient education is also essential as regards treatment. The effectiveness of weight loss in alleviating upper airway soft tissue obstruction makes the teaching of a comprehensive approach to weight reduction (see Chapter 233) an essential component of the office encounter.

A.H.G.

ANNOTATED BIBLIOGRAPHY

Connaughton JJ, Catterall JR, Elton RA, et al. Do sleep studies contribute to the management of patients with severe chronic obstructive pulmonary disease? Am Rev Respir Dis 1988;138:341. *(Finds that nighttime hypoxemia is not an independent risk factor for mortality in patients with COPD and thus argues that sleep study is unnecessary.)*

Fletcher EC, Schaaf JW, Miller, et al. Long-term cardiopulmonary sequelae in patients with sleep apnea and chronic lung disease. Am Rev Respir Dis 1987;135:525. *(The combination of sleep apnea and chronic lung disease increases the risk of cor pulmonale and worsens the prognosis, but treatment of the apnea improves right ventricular function.)*

He J, Kryger MH, Zorick FJ, et al. Mortality and apnea index in obstructive sleep apnea. Chest 1988;94:9. *(Increased mortality in patients demonstrating 20 or more apneas per hour of sleep; CPAP improved survival.)*

Kuna ST, Sant'Ambrogio G. Pathophysiology of upper airway closures during sleep. JAMA 1991;266:1384. *(Excellent review of the mechanisms of upper airway obstruction in sleep apnea.)*

Pack AI. Simplifying the diagnosis of obstructive sleep apnea. Ann Intern Med 1993;119:528. *(Editorial summarizing available diagnostic methods and their limitations.)*

Roehrs T, Zorick F, Wittig R, et al. Predictors of objective daytime sleepiness in patients with sleep-related breathing disorders. Chest 1989;95:1202. *(Daytime hypersomnolence strongly related to apnea-induced sleep disruption.)*

Schmidt-Nowara WW, Meade, et al. Treatment of snoring and obstructive sleep apnea with a dental orthosis. Chest 1991;99:1378. *(A promising, but preliminary report of some improvement.)*

Strohl KP, Cherniack NS, Gothe B. Physiologic basis of therapy for sleep apnea. Am Rev Respir Dis 1986;134:791. *(Useful review of pathophysiology and the pathophysiologic basis of available treatment options.)*

Viner S, Szalai JP, Hoffstein V. Are history and physical examination a good screening test for sleep apnea? Ann Intern Med 1991;115:356. *(Age, body mass index, male sex, and snoring were predictive of sleep apnea in this logistic regression study, but sensitivity was not much better than subjective clinical assessment.)*

Young T, Palta M, Dempsey J, et al. The occurrence of sleep-disordered breathing among middle-aged adults. N Engl J Med 1993;328:1230. *(Prevalence was 24 percent among men and 9 percent among women, with sleep apnea among 4 percent of men and 2 percent of women—much higher than previously estimated.)*

47
Management of Chronic Obstructive Pulmonary Disease (COPD)

Primary Care Medicine: Office Evaluation and Management of the Adult Patient, 3rd edition, edited by Allan H. Goroll, Lawrence A. May, and Albert G. Mulley, Jr. J.B. Lippincott Company, Philadelphia © 1995

Chronic obstructive pulmonary disease (chronic bronchitis/emphysema) is a major cause of total disability, second only to coronary artery disease. Its prevalence approaches 30 per 1000. Because COPD is incurable and often irreversible, the prime goal of management is to preserve function and limit complications. In many instances, functional impairment can be minimized and exercise tolerance can be improved. Treatment objectives include cessation of smoking (see Chapter 54), immunization against influenza and pneumococcal infection, control of bronchospasm and inflammation, mobilization of secretions, improvement of exercise tolerance, and effective treatment of pneumonia and chronic hypoxemia, should they occur. The primary physician needs to know how and when to use bronchodilators, corticosteroids, oxygen, pneumococcal and influenza vaccines, physical therapy measures, exercise training, and antibiotics in the management of patients with COPD. Physician attitude is also an important determinant of successful outcome.

PATHOPHYSIOLOGY, CLINICAL PRESENTATION, AND COURSE

COPD is a subset of the obstructive pulmonary diseases (which also include asthma, bronchiectasis, and cystic fibrosis). This diverse set of conditions share a pathophysiologic common denominator: slowing of the expiratory flow rate. This slowing manifests itself as a *reduction in the ratio of the forced expiratory volume (FEV_1) to forced vital capacity (FVC or VC)*. The earliest manifestation of COPD appears to be an increase in small airway resistance.

The COPD patient may present clinically with any combination of cough, sputum production, wheezing, and shortness of breath. The presentation is a function of the severity of illness and the degrees of chronic bronchitis and emphysema to the clinical picture. Most patients have mixed disease, although one pathophysiology often predominates.

Emphysema is characterized as pathologic enlargement of the airspaces distal to the terminal bronchioles due to destruction of the alveolar walls and its constituent components. This destructive process remains incompletely understood but probably is due to an excess of alveolar protease activity. Alveolar tissue contains both proteases and antiproteases, with neutrophil-derived elastase being the most important protease and $alpha_1$-antitrypsin being the prime antiprotease. Alveolar wall destruction is believed to result when there is a reduction in antitrypsin activity or an increase in elastase levels. Cigarette smoking increases the risk of COPD by about 30 times, perhaps by causing an influx of elastase-rich neutrophils into the alveoli or by oxidative inactivation of antitrypsin. Patients with a hereditary deficiency of $alpha_1$-antitrypsin (less than 80 mg/L) are at greatly increased risk of developing emphysema, although they account for less than 3 percent of cases.

Whatever the mechanism, the net result pathologically is fragmentation of pulmonary elastic tissue, leading to destruction of alveolar architecture as well as of the capillary bed that lies within the alveolar wall. There results a fall in expiratory flow rates as the lung's normal elastic recoil and radial traction on airways are lost and the poorly supported noncartilaginous airways collapse during expiration. There is some evidence of a reversible cholinergic component of airway obstruction responsive to atropine. Inspiratory flow rates are normal because airway caliber is normal. *Pulmonary compliance* increases with the decline in elasticity. The size of the pulmonary capillary bed is reduced, causing *carbon monoxide diffusing capacity (DLCO)* to drop. The reduction in size of the vascular bed parallels the fall in alveolar surface area. Thus, ventilation still roughly matches perfusion, and significant hypoxemia does not ensue.

The *clinical picture* is dominated by *dyspnea*, particularly on exertion. Cough is only a minor complaint, and sputum production is scant. The patient with advanced disease is *thin* and *tachypneic*, often using accessory muscles of respiration and *pursed-lip breathing*. The latter helps keep noncartilaginous airways from collapsing during expiration. Cyanosis is uncommon, because PO_2 is only minimally reduced. The neck veins may seem distended, but only on expiration. The *anterior–posterior diameter* of the chest is *increased;* the percussion note is hyperresonant; and the *breath sounds* are *distant*. There are usually no signs of cor pulmonale, although the right ventricular impulse may be prominent due to displacement by hyperinflated lungs. As noted, hypoxemia is minimal and there is little, if any, carbon dioxide retention until the end stages of the disease. The chest x-ray demonstrates hyperinflation and hyperlucency, especially at the apices—except in those with antitrypsin deficiency, whose x-ray changes are greatest at the bases.

Chronic Bronchitis. Inflammation of the cells lining the bronchial wall in conjunction with hyperplasia of the mucous glands and narrowing of small airways are the predominant pathologic features of chronic bronchitis. Etiology of the condition is poorly understood, but chronic infection and airway hyperreactivity are believed to play important roles. Smoking is a major precipitant, along with prolonged exposure to air pollution and other bronchial irritants. However, even after withdrawal of such irritants the inflammatory process often continues unabated. Airway edema, excess mucus production, and loss of ciliary transport result. Obstruction to airflow occurs with inspiration as well as with expiration. Widespread bronchial narrowing and mucous plugging produce *hypoxemia* due to mismatching of ventilation and perfusion. *Hypercarbia* results from impeded ventilation. Chronic hypoxia and hypercarbia increase pulmonary arterial resistance and may lead to development of pulmonary hypertension and eventually cor pulmonale. Sudden worsening may precipitate acute right heart failure in severe chronic bronchitis. Compared to emphysema, chronic bronchitis causes much less parenchymal damage; diffusing capacity, lung volumes, and compliance are not greatly altered.

Chronic bronchitis patients are typically colonized with *Haemophilus influenzae* and *Streptococcus pneumoniae*. However, the role of infection in the genesis of acute exacerbations remains unsettled, but evidence from double-blind, randomized, placebo-controlled trials demonstrates little difference in outcome between patients given prophylactic tetracycline and those given a placebo.

The person with chronic bronchitis is often a smoker who presents with a history of chronic, productive cough. By definition, the cough must be present for at least 3 months each year, during 2 consecutive years. At first, the sputum production and cough occur just in the winter months, but soon the patient becomes symptomatic year round, with a history of frequent exacerbations. By the time dyspnea on exertion sets in, the disease is well advanced. Patients may report having to sit up at night to breathe; at times this may be a manifestation of congestive heart failure, which is not uncommon, but more careful questioning often reveals that the difficulty was precipitated by cough and relieved by raising sputum. As noted above, cor pulmonale and right heart failure may ensue if there is chronic hypoxemia and pulmonary hypertension.

The chronic bronchitic patient is typically male and in his fifties at the time of presentation. He appears *plethoric* and *cyanotic* at the stage of severe disease, a time when many first come for help. Tobacco stains on the fingers and teeth are common, and there may be signs of cor pulmonale (distended neck veins, a right ventricular heave, a right ventricular gallop, and peripheral edema). The lungs sound noisy; *crackles* and *wheezes* are readily evident. The expiratory phase of respiration is prolonged. Because of the mismatching of ventilation with perfusion, *hypoxemia* may be found on measurement of arterial blood gases. The PCO_2 rises as the patient's ability to move air effectively declines. *Secondary polycythemia* is common, and the chest x-ray shows increased bronchovascular markings.

Clinical Course. The clinical course of COPD is generally *progressive*, although some individuals seem to reach a plateau clinically—especially if they stop smoking. Before the onset of symptoms, one can often detect an increase in the *closing volume* and a decrease in the *maximum midexpiratory flow rate* (sensitive measures of small airway disease); measures of large airway resistance are usually within normal limits during this phase of illness. The presymptomatic, *small airway stage* of COPD may represent a period of reversible disease; however, early fibrotic changes have been found in airways of such patients. It is unresolved whether intervention at the time of early small airway abnormalities will alter the course of disease and improve prognosis.

Longitudinal studies of symptomatic patients have shown a steady deterioration in pulmonary function with time. Using the forced expiratory volume at 1 second (FEV_1) as the measure of obstruction, an annual average decrease in flow rate of 50 to 70 mL/sec has been noted. By the time the FEV_1 declines to 1 L/sec, the mean annual mortality approaches 10 percent. The rate of decline in FEV_1 can be halted if the patient stops smoking. The onset of resting tachycardia and signs of cor pulmonale are other indicators of a poor prognosis. Prognosis appears better for asthmatic bronchitis than for emphysema, perhaps because of better treatment modalities.

Several parameters are emerging as prognostically useful (Table 47–1). In one important study, significant reductions in 12-year survival were found among patients with marked reduction in the ratio of FEV_1 to forced vital capacity (FVC), a substantial drop in FEV_1 or FVC, hypoxemia, hypercarbia, cor pulmonale, or decreased diffusing capacity. The FEV_1 may be a more useful predictor of prognosis in advanced disease than the ratio of FEV_1 to FVC. In late disease, the FEV_1 often slows in its rate of decline and the FVC may fall more rapidly, thus preserving their ratio even in the setting of clinical deterioration. However, once the FEV_1 falls below 1 L/sec, it is less able to distinguish survivors from nonsurvivors. Other predictors of poor prognosis included heavy smoking and rate of decline of expiratory flow rates over time. Interestingly, the group with the lowest 12-year probability of survival still had a 40 percent chance of remaining alive.

Other investigators have found mixed venous oxygen concentration to be an important prognostic indicator; pulmonary hemodynamics were not predictive. Differences in patient populations make rigid extrapolation from studies of prognosis to individual patients unwise, but the parameters identified can be of qualitative use clinically. It remains difficult to predict survival in individual patients.

Although prognosis for patients with COPD is not good, recent British and American studies have shown that stable, chronically hypoxemic patients ($PO_2 < 60$) achieve prolonged survival when treated with continuous oxygen therapy. The exact mechanism of improved survival is not known, but pulmonary hypertension and secondary polycythemia decreased, and neuropsychiatric functioning improved. As noted above, cessation of smoking is critical to improving the chances of survival.

WORKUP

Although the selection of treatment modalities is partially empirical, it is still helpful to identify the predominant pathophysiologic defects, their severity, effect on the patient's functional status, and any aggravating or precipitating factors. Clarification of these issues can help focus therapy and serve as a baseline for monitoring efficacy of treatment.

Table 47-1. Predictors of Poor Prognosis in COPD

1. FEV_1 <40% of predicted; especially less than 1.0 L/min
2. FEV_1/FVC <0.40
3. Arterial PO_2 <55 mm Hg
4. Presence of cor pulmonale
5. CO_2 retention
6. FVC <80% of predicted
7. Decreased single-breath diffusing capacity
8. Decreased mixed venous oxygen concentration

History. One should obtain a careful description of symptoms and activity limitations experienced in daily life, both at rest and with exercise. A detailed smoking history and environmental or work exposures to pulmonary irritants should be sought and specified. Quasiquantitative estimates of exercise capacity (eg, flights of stairs that can be climbed or distance that can be walked on level ground) are helpful, as is some indication of progression of symptoms over time. Presence of leg edema and worsening exercise tolerance suggest onset of right heart failure in the patient with chronic bronchitis.

Physical Examination. It is important to note any tachypnea, tachycardia, degree of prolongation of expiratory phase, cyanosis, clubbing, use of accessory respiratory muscles, wheezes, signs of consolidation, and evidence of cor pulmonale (jugular venous distention, peripheral edema, right ventricular heave, loud pulmonic closure sound, and right ventricular S_3).

Laboratory Studies are first directed at quantifying the degree of obstructive defect *and* determining the response to bronchodilators. Small airway disease can be detected during the asymptomatic phase of illness by ordering *closing volume* and *maximal midexpiratory flow rate* determinations. The degree of obstruction in larger airways can be assessed by measuring expiratory flow rates on an office spirometer; the most helpful measurement is the *ratio of the forced expiratory volume at 1 second (FEV_1) to the vital capacity*. Crude estimates of obstruction can be provided by the FEV_1 alone. Results are compared to predicted values. Patients with a 50 percent reduction in FEV_1 are often dyspneic on exertion; by the time the FEV_1 falls to 25 percent of predicted, they may complain of shortness of breath at rest. Determination of expiratory flow rates before and after inhalation of a bronchodilator (eg, albuterol) can provide a quick estimate of the benefit a patient may derive from bronchodilator therapy. The failure to obtain an improvement in flow rate from a few inhalations of a bronchodilator does not rule out the possibility of benefit, but it suggests the likelihood is not great.

A *chest x-ray* is helpful both for diagnosis of COPD and detection of its complications, such as heart failure, pneumonia, or a pneumothorax. The diagnosis of emphysema can be made with a high degree of accuracy if two or more of the following criteria are present: flattening of the diaphragm and blunting of the costophrenic angle on PA view, irregularity of lung field lucency, enlargement of the retrosternal space, flattening or concavity of the diaphragmatic contour on lateral view. *Arterial blood gases* provide measures of oxygenation and ventilation. Hypoxemia and hypercarbia are manifestations of severe chronic bronchitis. Blood gases are particularly useful for documenting acute decompensation. In patients with severe chronic bronchitis, baseline studies of blood gases should be performed, so that gases obtained at times of marked subjective worsening can be compared to baseline determinations. *Hematocrit* and *hemoglobin* concentration provides a rough indication of the severity and chronicity of hypoxemia and the possible need for phlebotomy. The electrocardiographic abnormalities that appear in COPD generally reflect the severity of the lung disease and the presence of cor pulmonale. The *electrocardiogram (ECG)* should be studied for sinus tachycardia, multifocal atrial tachycardia, peaked P waves (P pulmonale), and signs of right ventricular hypertrophy (eg, tall R wave in V_1 and deep S in lead V_6. Examination of the *sputum* is mandatory when acute pneumonitis is suspected.

PRINCIPLES OF MANAGEMENT

The prime goal of treatment is to improve the patient's functional status so that he can better carry out his daily activities. Elimination of precipitants and risk factors, prevention and treatment of infection, control of bronchospasm, mobilization of secretions, and avoidance of chronic hypoxia are the principal objectives of management. With the exception of chronic oxygen therapy in hypoxemic patients, treatment does not prolong survival and therefore must be evaluated by the patient's subjective response. The success of treatment is strongly influenced by the physician's interest and the participation of patient and family in the program.

Avoidance of Precipitants and Risk Factors

Smoking Cessation. Regardless of severity of disease or the types of deficits present, all COPD patients must stop smoking and should be urged to do so in emphatic terms. A surprisingly large number of patients report little or no warning about smoking from their physicians; studies indicate that the physician's advice does lead some patients to cease smoking, especially those who are symptomatic (see Chapter 54).

Reduction in exposure to other pulmonary irritants should be advised. Readily avoidable pulmonary irritants include aerosol deodorants, hairsprays, paint sprays, and insecticides. An occupational history should be reviewed (see Chapter 39) for important worksite irritants. Change in job or residence (for patients living in areas of severe air pollution) may be necessary, but should be urged only when the relationship between exposure and disease is strong; otherwise, the advice might cause more harm than good.

Immunization Against Influenza is essential for all COPD patients. Trivalent influenza vaccine should be given each fall, at least 6 weeks before the onset of the influenza season. Serious reactions are rare unless the patient is allergic to egg protein. Mild fever and myalgias are sometimes noted. Due to ever-changing viral strains, vaccination must be done yearly (see Chapter 6). Should an outbreak of influenza occur, protection for patients who were not immunized can still be provided by prescribing oral *amantadine*. Amantadine is effective against known strains of influenza A. Recent studies demonstrated a protection rate of 78 percent against clinical disease. Its effects are additive to those of influenza vaccine, and it can be given to very sick vaccinated patients who require maximum protection (see Chapter 6). *Rimantidine,* a new alpha-methyl derivative of amantidine, is as effective but less likely to cause central nervous system side effects.

Pneumococcal Vaccine is equally important for COPD patients. Available preparations incorporate the capsular antigens of 23 species that are responsible for 90 percent of the pneumococcal pneumonia occurring in the United States. Mild erythema and pain at the injection site are the only common adverse reactions to the vaccine. The vaccine is administered as a single intramuscular injection of 0.5 mL. Repeat doses of the vaccine are not recommended as necessary at the present time; antibody titers are remaining high in those vaccinated as long as 5 years ago (see Chapter 6).

There is no blunting of antibody response or increased frequency of adverse reactions when both the pneumococcal and influenza vaccines are given simultaneously. The only disadvantage is difficulty in determining the cause of hypersensitivity should a reaction occur.

The Question of Prophylactic Antibiotics. There is conflicting evidence on the use of prophylactic antibiotics. The original studies done in England suggested benefit from prophylactic use of antibiotics during the winter months, reducing the number of exacerbations and days lost from work. Studies in the United States and Canada show a more modest benefit from antibiotic use and only in patients with acute, severe exacerbations of symptoms in the setting of purulent sputum. Thus, empirical treatment with antibiotics is reasonable when there is strong clinical evidence of infection (fever, change to purulent sputum loaded with white cells) and a deterioration in pulmonary status.

Because *pneumococci* and *H. influenzae* are the predominant organisms colonizing patients with COPD, *amoxicillin* is a reasonable first choice of antibiotic when there is evidence of infection. For patients allergic to penicillin, *tetracycline* or *trimethoprim–sulfamethoxazole* is a reasonable alternative, although they are not effective against pneumococci. *Cefaclor,* an orally administered cephalosporin, is active against both pneumococci and *H. influenzae;* its major disadvantage is high cost.

Augmentation Therapy for Alpha$_1$-Antitrypsin Deficiency. Patients with emphysema who have significant antitrypsin deficiency (less than 80 mg/dL) are candidates for augmentation therapy (weekly or monthly infusions of alpha$_1$-antitrypsin). Only symptomatic patients with clinical evidence of emphysema and sufficiently low antitrypsin levels are considered appropriate candidates for augmentation therapy, because not all patients with low concentrations develop emphysema. A history of smoking rules out candidacy.

Bronchodilation

In the absence of curative or disease-altering therapy, symptomatic relief through reduction of airway resistance becomes a priority. Bronchodilators remain a mainstay of treatment. Their mechanisms of action are diverse, complex, and less well understood than previously thought. In addition to bronchodilation, they may have other beneficial effects, such as ability to improve mucociliary clearance, diaphragmatic action, and cardiac contractility, and to inhibit mediator release.

Beta-agonists constitute an increasingly important class of bronchodilators. Isoproterenol was the prototype, now replaced by the more bronchially selective and longer-acting inhaled beta$_2$ agents (albuterol, metaproterenol, terbutaline, fenoterol, bitolterol). Although most are available in both oral and inhaled preparations, the *inhaled* one is *preferred* because it is more rapidly acting, associated with fewer cardiac side-effects, yet just as long-acting (up to 6 hours). At high doses, cardioselectivity is lost. Oral terbutaline produces severe tremulousness in some patients when used at full doses, although tremor may decrease with continued use. The convenience and rapid onset of action of inhaled beta-agonists sometimes lead to excessive use and the potential for *tachyphylaxis*. Reliance on inhalation therapy must be accompanied by thorough patient education regarding proper inhalation technique and frequency of administration (see below).

The role of administering beta-agonist therapy by means of *intermittent positive-pressure breathing* (IPPB) for treatment of COPD has been carefully studied and found to be lacking in demonstrable benefit. A long-term (33 month), multicenter controlled study conducted to settle the controversy surrounding the efficacy of this expensive, although popular treatment modality found no statistically significant differences in mortality, rate and duration of hospitalization, and change in lung function or quality of life among those taking bronchodilator by IPPB or compressor nebulizer. Moreover, there were no differences in response among any clinically relevant subgroups, such as those with more severe disease, copious sputum, or emphysema. Modern metered-dose aerosol inhalers have replaced IPPB in COPD.

Anticholinergic Agents with atropinelike activity have long been known to affect bronchodilation. With the advent of *ipratropium,* an inhaled, topically active, poorly absorbed anticholinergic preparation, comes the ability to deliver anticholinergic therapy conveniently and with minimal side-effects. Inhaled ipratropium has proven equal in bronchodilating capacity to maximal doses of beta-agonists. Its rather slow onset of effect, but sustained action make it best suited for maintenance use. Volume of sputum may be reduced without increasing its viscosity.

Anticholinergic side effects of blurred vision, urinary outflow obstruction, and rapid heart rate are rarely a problem when the drug is used in proper doses. Bedtime administration appears particularly effective in some patients.

Theophylline and Its Derivatives have been a standard component of COPD therapy for years, being inexpensive and symptomatically helpful. However, questions have arisen as to their ability to improve objective measures of airflow and their cardiovascular safety, especially in settings where hypoxemia or reduced clearance may be a problem (eg, congestive heart failure, hepatocellular insufficiency, use of cimetidine or erythromycin). In addition, evidence of effective bronchodilation is inconsistent.

Nonetheless, some patients report considerable subjective benefit, perhaps related to improved diaphragmatic function and myocardial contractility. A major randomized controlled trial demonstrated improvement in respiratory function and dyspnea in patients with severe COPD, with much of the benefit attributed to enhanced respiratory muscle performance. Intravenous aminophylline for acute exacerbations of COPD has not proven effective. Some patients with COPD experience a worsening of airway hyperreactivity at night. Use of a long-acting, controlled-release theophylline formulation before bed may help such patients.

These methylxanthine preparations are available in oral and rectal formulations. Absorption of an oral dose approaches 90 percent; rectal administration is associated with erratic absorption and the potential for suddenly high serum concentrations that can cause dangerous side-effects. The oral route is preferred. Sustained-release preparations can provide therapeutic serum levels (10 to 20 g/mL) for 12 to 24 hours. Wide variability in level for a given dose is due to individual differences in clearance, which is predominantly hepatic. As noted above, decreased clearance and increased serum levels occur with heart failure, hepatocellular disease, and drugs such as cimetidine and erythromycin; smoking and barbiturates increase clearance.

Serious side-effects include *ventricular dysrhythmias* and *seizures*. Such adverse effects usually occur only when serum levels rise precipitously, but can develop when serum levels are in the "normal" range if there is concurrent heart failure or hypoxemia.

A formerly popular, but irrational combination preparation of theophylline, a beta-agonist (in subtherapeutic dose), and a barbiturate is to be avoided. In the setting of hypoxemia, the sympathomimetic ingredients may potentiate toxicity; moreover, the barbiturate hastens clearance of theophylline and may reduce respiratory drive in patients with CO_2 retention.

Choice of Agent. The decision to employ bronchodilators and the choice of agent are somewhat empirical; trial and error are usually necessary to arrive at an optimal program. It is not always possible to predict who will respond to bronchodilators on the basis of response to a single exposure of an inhaled beta-agonist, but those who show considerable improvement in FEV_1 are good candidates for a trial of therapy. All COPD patients with evidence of a severe obstructive defect should be considered for a trial of bronchodilators. Even COPD patients with airflow obstruction that appears fixed and irreversible (less than a 15 percent improvement in FEV_1 after inhaling a bronchodilator) may experience a significant improvement in symptoms or ventilatory function after an empiric course of bronchodilator therapy. A limited empirical trial is probably reasonable but should not be continued unless there is clear-cut subjective or objective benefit. There is no evidence that bronchodilator therapy improves prognosis.

Corticosteroids

Recent research on the importance of inflammation in obstructive lung disease has refocused interest on corticosteroids. Their anti-inflammatory effects appear to reduce mucosal edema, inhibit prostaglandins that cause bronchoconstriction, and increase responsiveness to beta-adrenergic agents. By addressing the inflammatory components of COPD, they can control an acute bronchospastic exacerbation as well as mitigate the bronchospasm and airway inflammation characteristic of chronic stable COPD. Meta-analytic study finds a modest (10%) chance of a reasonable (20%) improvement in FEV_1 among patients with stable chronic COPD. But definitive evidence of greater benefit remains elusive. Oral prednisone has been shown in short- to medium-term studies to achieve 30 percent or greater improvement in FEV_1 over baseline measurements compared to all other bronchodilators. Steroid-related side-effects limit the benefit of long-term steroid therapy (see Chapter 105). Morbidity may be reduced by 1) tapering oral dosage as soon as control of bronchospasm is attained; and 2) switching to alternate-day therapy or use of an inhaled, nonabsorbable corticosteroid.

The availability of topically active, relatively nonabsorbable, metered-dose *inhaled corticosteroid* preparations (triamcinolone, beclomethasone, flunisolide) has created a resurgence of interest in long-term inhaled steroid therapy for COPD, but efficacy of inhaled steroids has not been thoroughly studied. Recent reports suggest some improvement in functional measures and prognosis, but more data are needed before inhaled steroids can be considered a mainstay of COPD therapy.

Oxygen Therapy

Survival is prolonged in COPD patients who are chronically hypoxemic (PO_2 less than 55 mm Hg) when they receive long-term *continuous oxygen therapy*. The more continuous the therapy, the better the effect; round-the-clock oxygen therapy is superior to nocturnal oxygen administration. Maximum benefit requires at least *18 hours/d* of continuous administration. Less than 12 hours/d is unlikely to be of any help. Nighttime oxygen therapy was thought to be worthwhile in those COPD patients with only nocturnal hypoxemia, but such therapy proved incapable of reducing pulmonary hypertension or improving survival. Most COPD patients with profound nocturnal hypoxemia also are hypoxic during the day and require continuous administration of oxygen. Concern about the potential of continuous oxygen therapy to worsen carbon dioxide retention has not been borne out. A study of the effect of supplemental oxygen on gas exchange in hypercarbic hypoxic patients with severe COPD found no clinically important increases in PCO_2 during sleep (when CO_2 retention is at its worst) and concluded that oxygen therapy can be used safely in such patients.

Indications for supplemental oxygen therapy are a resting *PO_2 less than 55 mm Hg* or a *PO_2 less than 60 mm Hg* if there is evidence of concurrent *right heart failure* or *secondary polycythemia* (see Chapter 80). Nasal prong administration usually suffices and should deliver enough oxygen to increase the PO_2 to 65 mm Hg. Some recommend adding an additional 1 L/min of flow during sleep and exertion.

The need for *short-term supplemental oxygen* comes up during consideration of *air travel*. Prediction of need for oxygen and tolerance of the cabin environment can be accomplished by preflight measurement of the arterial PO_2 and FEV_1. A formula has been derived using these parameters to predict arterial oxygen at cruising altitude. Alternatively, one can have the patient inhale a hypoxic gas mixture (17.2% O_2) that simulates the cabin environment of a jet aircraft at cruising altitude. Although there are no established guidelines for when oxygen supplementation is needed, a drop in PO_2 to below 50 mm Hg or the development of symptoms are reasonable indications for oxygen supplementation during flights longer than 2 hours. Airlines will provide an oxygen supply if notified at least 48 hours in advance of travel; their units provide flows of 2 to 4 L/min of 25 percent or 30 percent oxygen. Patients are usually not allowed to bring their own oxygen tanks into the cabin of domestic airlines.

Brief administrations of oxygen have been given to *improve exercise tolerance* in COPD patients. Studies on the effects of such oxygen use have been conflicting. When unblinded, exercise tolerance improves. When blinded and done in controlled fashion, little benefit can be demonstrated. Most hypoxemic COPD patients are chronically hypoxic and require continuous oxygen supplementation. The small subset of patients who are only hypoxemic and markedly dyspneic with exercise are the best candidates for a trial of short-term oxygen supplementation. A convenient means of identifying such patients is to measure their diffusing capacity during routine pulmonary function testing, rather than trying to obtain arterial blood gases just after or during exercise. A diffusing capacity above 55 percent has been shown to be 100 percent specific in excluding arterial hypoxemia during exercise; sensitivity was 68 percent. If oxygen is to be tried, it should be limited to those who have a reduced diffusing capacity and demonstrate consistently better performance on oxygen than on air when both are administered in single-blind fashion. Pulse oximetry during exercise is another means of identifying patients who might benefit from oxygen supplementation.

Control of Secretions and Exercise

Secretions. Patients bothered by heavy, tenacious sputum may obtain benefit by maintaining good *fluid intake*, ensuring adequate *humidification* of the indoor environment (particularly in centrally heated homes), and practicing *postural drainage* when clearance of secretions is difficult and cough is incapacitating. The simplest method of postural drainage is to have the patient lean over the side of the bed, rest the elbows on a pillow placed on the floor, and cough as a family member or visiting nurse gently pounds on the chest. For hydration, ultrasonic nebulizers are no better than the simple maintenance of good systemic hydration, although the moisture they deliver does reach deep into the tracheobronchial tree. Occasionally, bronchospasm can be triggered by a nebulizer, and its reservoir can become contaminated and serve as a source of airway infection. Nebulized detergents are of no proven use, but *mucolytic agents* such as acetylcysteine are capable of thinning secretions; they are usually reserved for patients on respirators and not commonly used in outpatient practice. Oral *expectorants* are very popular with some bronchitic patients, who report improved ability to raise sputum; however, they are without proven clinical efficacy. These preparations need not be denied to the patient who feels that they are of benefit but should not be the mainstay of the therapeutic program. Glyceryl guaiacolate and potassium iodide are the most frequently prescribed expectorants; many are available without a prescription.

Exercise Training. Among the simplest and most effective measures for improving exercise tolerance is an *exercise training* program. Walking has proven to be the best form of exercise for increasing the duration and intensity of activity in COPD patients. Exercises that involve the arms and upper body appear to compromise respiratory mechanics. Three or four sessions per day of walking are recommended, ranging from 5 to 15 minutes each. The pace and duration of activity are matched to the patient's capabilities; most begin the program walking at a half-maximal pace and build gradually over a period of several weeks. At the end of the training period, heart and respiratory rates for a given level of activity are decreased; oxygen consumption also falls. Tests of ventilatory function are not significantly changed, but increases of 25 percent are attained in maximum duration and intensity of exercise. Many patients enjoy marked improvement in ability to carry out their daily activities.

Breathing exercises may have some beneficial effect, particularly in those who readily panic and hyperventilate when dyspneic or show evidence of respiratory fatigue. Teaching the anxious individual to take slow, deep, relaxed breaths and exhale against pursed lips can lessen the work of moving air, provide a sense of control over breathing, and encourage a more relaxed respiratory pattern. Inspiratory muscle training is popular in some centers, with encouraging reports of improvement in exercise performance among patients who experience respiratory muscle fatigue. However, the importance of diaphragmatic dysfunction and the need for exercises continue to be debated.

Management of Cor Pulmonale

Patients with chronic cor pulmonale can often be made more comfortable by careful attention to their volume status, degree of hypoxemia, and hematocrit. Reduction of excess intravascular volume can reduce edema; *diuretic therapy* (see Chapter 32) is an effective means of volume control. As noted earlier, continuous *low-flow oxygen* therapy is indicated in cor pulmonale patients who are chronically hypoxic. Survival is improved, although the precise mechanism of improvement is unknown; pulmonary vascular resistance and secondary polycythemia are only modestly decreased. Whether oxygen therapy prevents development or worsening of cor pulmonale is unsettled.

Focus is shifting to examination of cardiac output as a determinant of survival in patients with cor pulmonale. Augmented cardiac output is a normal response to a fall in PO_2. Many patients with cor pulmonale maintain a high cardiac index. It is suspected that a fall in cardiac output may be a determinant of poor prognosis. If this proves to be the case, then increased efforts at improving cardiac output may be indicated.

Previous attempts at inotropic therapy have produced equivocal results. *Digitalis* seems to help some patients, but not uniformly or predictably. The incidence of digitalis toxicity is high, aggravated by hypoxemia; clinical response is often equivocal. The drug is worth a try in patients with reduced cardiac output, especially if there is concurrent left ventricular dysfunction (see Chapter 32), but should be continued only in those who show an objective as well as subjective response to therapy. Patients who do appear to improve with digitalis should be given a minimum maintenance dose and should be monitored closely for manifestations of digitalis toxicity (see Chapter 32).

Vasodilators (calcium-channel blockers and angiotensin-converting enzyme [ACE] inhibitors) have proved disappointing, with little improvement in cardiac output or pulmonary artery resistance noted with sustained use in most patients. In some instances, systemic hypotension and even hypoxemia may result.

Phlebotomy is indicated only for urgent treatment when secondary erythrocytosis is severe enough to markedly reduce blood viscosity, significantly impair oxygen delivery, and cause an exacerbation of cor pulmonale. The risk of such decompensation is greatest when the hematocrit rises above 55 percent.

Monitoring Therapy

Symptomatology remains one of the most important measures of efficacy. Semiquantitative reports from the patient on such parameters as number of stairs climbed or distance walked can be useful. Subjective assessment of bronchospasm has been found to correlate surprisingly well with FEV_1 measurement in asthmatics, and this probably is valid for COPD patients as well. Important aspects of the physical examination to be monitored include ratio of inspiration to expiration, respiratory rate, heart rate, jugular venous pressure, right ventricular impulse, and extremities (for edema). In patients with known CO_2 retention it is worth testing for asterixis, an indication of worsening ventilatory status with further carbon dioxide retention and encephalopathy. Serial determination of arterial blood gases, FEV_1, and FVC can help in objectively following the course of disease and detecting acute deteriorations.

PATIENT EDUCATION

The first priority is to stress the importance of cessation of smoking; this should be followed by design of specific program (see Chapter 54). Patients should be encouraged to maintain as much activity as possible and be provided with an exercise program if they can be motivated to comply. Patient, family, and physician should be involved in setting reasonable and realistic activity goals. Advice regarding adequate hydration and pulmonary toilet is basic to the care of chronic bronchitis patients. Patients likely to panic and hyperventilate when they become dyspneic often benefit from being taught slow, relaxed, deep breathing to institute in such circumstances.

Careful instructions regarding the indications and adverse effects of therapy can help the patient to carry out the prescribed program properly. Complex regimens should be written down and reviewed with both patient and family. It is essential to warn patients with CO_2 retention against unauthorized use of tranquilizers and sedatives, because of the risk of further suppressing their respiratory drive. Patients using inhalers should receive thorough instruction on their proper use (see Chapter 48); many treatment failures are due to poor technique. Such patients also require warning that excessive use of $beta_2$-agonists can lead to tachyphylaxis and cardiac side-effects; persistent overdoses of inhaled steroids (more than 20 puffs per day) can cause adrenal suppression.

Part of the patient education process should include instruction on self-monitoring and reporting of functional status. The involvement of the patient and the interest and concern of the physician have a considerable effect on the progress made by the COPD patient.

INDICATIONS FOR ADMISSION AND REFERRAL

The patient with acute respiratory decompensation, especially if accompanied by signs of encephalopathy (eg, asterixis, lethargy) should be urgently admitted to the hospital; no oxygen should be administered on the way to the hospital for fear of further suppressing the respiratory drive. Those with refractory bronchospasm, severe cor pulmonale, or acute pneumonitis also require inpatient management. Consultation with a specialist in pulmonary medicine is indicated when considering chronic use of systemic steroids for refractory bronchospasm, long-term continuous oxygen therapy for chronic hypoxemia, augmentation therapy, and inotropic agents for cor pulmonale.

THERAPUETIC RECOMMENDATIONS

- Insist on complete *cessation of smoking* and design for the smoker a comprehensive smoking cessation program (see Chapter 54).
- Advise the patient to reduce exposure to known environmental irritants (see Chapter 39) and allergens (see Chapters 48 and 222).
- Design, with patient participation, an *exercise program;* walking is probably the best exercise to use, although any aerobic exercise will suffice. Begin with an easily achieved level of activity (eg, half-maximal pace) and increase slowly in small increments. Frequency is three to four times daily, with duration ranging from 5 to 15 minutes.
- Administer trivalent *influenza vaccine* (0.5 mL IM) in the fall of each year to all COPD patients (except those having a known allergy to eggs) and at least 6 weeks before the usual winter onset of the flu season. Consider administering amantadine to unvaccinated COPD patients during an influenza epidemic (see Chapter 6).
- Administer *pneumococcal vaccine* to all COPD patients; dose is 0.5 mL IM and need be given only once; it can be given at the same time as the influenza vaccine.
- Consider for augmentation therapy with $alpha_1$-antitrypsin only those nonsmoking emphysematous patients who are symptomatic and who have an antitryspin level of less than 80 mg/dL.
- Advise patients bothered by heavy sputum production to keep well hydrated and to humidify the indoor environment (particularly those living in centrally heated homes). Nebulized detergents and oral expectorants are of no proven benefit. Teach postural drainage techniques to patients bothered by difficulty in raising sputum.
- Teach slow, relaxed, deep breathing to patients likely to hyperventilate when dyspneic; consider targeted inspiratory muscle training in patients with severe COPD; a respiratory therapist may be of help in the teaching effort.
- For patients who have obvious bronchospasm or dyspnea on exertion and a substantial reduction in expiratory flow rate (eg, FEV_1 <1.5 to 2 L/sec or FEV_1/FVC <0.50), begin a trial of bronchodilator therapy. Use an inhaled metered-

dose preparation of *either* the topically active, nonabsorbed anticholinergic *ipratropium* or a *beta$_2$-adrenergic agent* (eg, albuterol). Dosage for both is two puffs from a measured-dose inhaler q6h. Judge response on the basis of change in exercise tolerance and expiratory flow rates after about 1 week of therapy. Response to a single dose of inhaled bronchodilator does not predict response to continuous treatment. Be sure patient is instructed in and demonstrates proper inhaler technique (see Chapter 48).

- Consider combination inhaled bronchodilator therapy only if full doses of a single agent cannot be used. The sequencing and timing of combination inhaler therapy do not seem to matter.
- For patients using a beta-agonist, warn about dangers from overuse. Use with caution in patients with heart disease, because these agents are only relatively cardioselective and only at low doses.
- For patients using ipratropium, total daily dose should not exceed 12 inhalations per day. Prevent spray from getting into the eyes, especially in patients with narrow-angle glaucoma, although there is no danger of worsening glaucoma if used properly (negligible systemic absorption at prescribed doses).
- There is no evidence that delivery of inhaled bronchodilators by an IPPB apparatus provides any benefit. The use of such expensive therapy is not recommended.
- Patients failing to achieve adequate bronchodilation or unable to tolerate beta-agonist or anticholinergic therapy can be given a trial of a topically active, *inhaled corticosteroid* preparation such as beclomethasone, triamcinolone, or flunisolide. The medication is delivered by metered-dose hand-held nebulizer. Dose is two puffs qid. Reserve oral, *systemic corticosteroids* (eg, prednisone 20 to 40 mg/d) for severe flares or refractory bronchospasm. Taper and switch to alternate-day or high-dose inhaled therapy as soon as possible (see Chapters 48 and 105).
- If control of symptoms remains inadequate, especially at nighttime, consider adding a *long-acting, controlled-release theophylline* preparation before bed (eg, Uniphyl 400 mg qhs). Monitor symptoms closely for response after about 1 week of therapy before deciding to continue therapy. Check serum theophylline level (therapeutic range 10 to 20 g/mL) to be sure safe levels are not exceeded. Use with extreme caution in patients with cardiac arrhythmias.
- The use of empiric antibiotic therapy for acute exacerbations of chronic bronchitis remains controversial. An increase in sputum quantity only does not appear to warrant antibiotics. Initiate empiric antibiotic therapy for patients with new onset of grossly purulent sputum in conjunction with worsening respiratory status (dyspnea, increased wheezing). Initial drug of choice is *amoxicillin,* 500 mg tid. *Doxycycline,* 100 mg bid, and *trimethoprim–sulfa* double-strength, one tablet bid, are alternatives for penicillin-allergic patients. *Cefaclor,* 250 mg tid, is worth consideration if there is concern about resistant *H. influenzae* as the predominant organism.
- For patients with cor pulmonale, begin a diuretic program (eg, *furosemide* 20 to 40 mg/d) when peripheral edema begins to occur; increase program as needed to control fluid accumulation caused by systemic venous hypertension. Phlebotomize the patient with secondary erythrocytosis (hematocrit in excess of 55%) when there is acute decompensation (worsening of right heart failure or hypoxemia).
- Consider *continuous low-flow oxygen* therapy for patients with a PO_2 less than 55 mm Hg or less than 60 mm Hg in the setting of erythrocytosis or cor pulmonale. Such patients may require phlebotomy to keep their hematocrit below 55.
- Consider a short-term trial of digitalis therapy (eg, digoxin, 0.25 mg/d) in patients with severe right heart failure; treat for 2 weeks and check for objective signs of improvement (eg, decreased edema, lower jugular venous pressure, reduced heart size). Use with care in the setting of hypoxemia, and check serum levels regularly. Monitor closely for evidence of digitalis toxicity (see Chapter 32).
- Review entire treatment program thoroughly with patient and family; encourage patient participation in setting goals and monitoring functional status.

A.H.G.

ANNOTATED BIBLIOGRAPHY

American Thoracic Society. Standards for the diagnosis and care of patients with chronic obstructive pulmonary disease (COPD) and asthma. Am Rev Respir Dis 1987;136:225. *(Very useful position paper.)*

Anthonisen NR. Long-term oxygen therapy. Ann Intern Med 1983;99:519. *(Fine review of the recent evidence suggesting improvement in survival with chronic oxygen treatment; 60 refs.)*

Anthonisen NR, Manfreda J, Warren CPW, et al. Antibiotic therapy in exacerbations of chronic obstructive pulmonary disease. Ann Intern Med 1987;106:196. *(Prospective, placebo-controlled, randomized, double-blind, crossover trial; empiric antibiotic therapy had a 68 percent success rate compared to 55 percent for placebo.)*

Anthonisen NR, Wright EC. IPPB trial group: Bronchodilator response in chronic obstructive pulmonary disease. Am Rev Respir Dis 1986;133:814. *(Patients with COPD do manifest some bronchodilator responsiveness.)*

Aubier M, DeTroyer A, Sampson M, et al. Aminophylline improves diaphragmatic contractility. N Engl J Med 1981;305: 249. *(A finding that may justify a trial of aminophylline despite documented poor bronchodilator effect.)*

Bates JH. The role of infection during exacerbations of chronic bronchitis. Ann Intern Med 1982;97:130. *(Summary of the controversy and some thoughts about why the issue remains unresolved.)*

Burrows B, Blood JW, Traver GA, et al. The course and prognosis of different forms of chronic airways obstruction in a sample from the general population. N Engl J Med 1987;317:1309. *(Patients with emphysema had a 10-year mortality of 60 percent; those with asthmatic bronchitis had a lesser mortality.)*

Callahan CM, Dittus RS, Katz BP. Oral corticosteroid therapy for patients with stable chronic obstructive pulmonary disease. Ann Intern Med 1991;114:216. *(A meta-analysis showing a modest benefit.)*

Celli B, Rassulo J, Make BJ. Dyssynchronous breathing during arm but not leg exercise in patients with chronic airflow obstruction. N Engl J Med 1986;314:1485. *(Leg exercise did not interfere with lung mechanics, but arm exercise did.)*

Dillard TA, Berg BW, Rajagopal KR, et al. Hypoxemia during air travel in patients with chronic obstructive pulmonary disease. Ann Intern Med 1989;111:362. *(Arterial PO_2 declined to significantly low levels; oxygen supplement is urged for patients with severe COPD during air travel.)*

Dompeling E, van Chayck CP, van Grunsven PM, et al. Slowing the deterioration of asthma and chronic obstructive pulmonary disease observed during bronchodilator therapy by adding inhaled corticosteroids. Ann Intern Med 1993;118:770. *(Prospective, randomized clinical trial showing improvements in flow rate, symptoms, and number of exacerbations.)*

Easton PA, Jadue C, Dhingra S, et al. A comparison of the bronchodilating effects of a beta-2 adrenergic agent (albuterol) and an anticholinergic agent (ipratropium bromide), given by aerosol alone or in sequence. N Engl J Med 1986;315:735. *(Equal efficacy demonstrated; no benefit when a second agent was added to maximum doses of the first.)*

Ferguson GT, Cherniack RM. Management of chronic obstructive pulmonary disease. N Engl J Med 1993;328:1017. *(Useful, brief review; 50 refs.)*

Goldstein RS, Vivekanand R, Bowes G et al. Effect of supplemental nocturnal oxygen of gas exchange in patients with severe obstructive lung disease. New Engl J Med 1984;310:425. *(Nocturnal oxygen therapy did not induce clinically worrisome increases in PCO_2 during sleep in COPD patients with resting hypoxia and hypercarbia; argues for safety of continuous oxygen therapy in patients with CO_2 retention.)*

Gross NJ. Ipratropium bromide. N Engl J Med 1988;319:486. *(Superb review of inhaled anticholinergic therapy; 110 refs.)*

Harver A, Mahler DA, Daubenspeck JA. Targeted inspiratory muscle training improves respiratory muscle function and reduces dyspnea in patients with chronic obstructive pulmonary disease. Ann Intern Med 1989;111:117. *(One of the most careful studies of the respiratory muscle training approach to COPD treatment.)*

Himelman RB, Stsruve SN, Brown JK, et al. Improved recognition of cor pulmonale in patients with severe chronic obstructive pulmonary disease. Am J Med 1988;84:891. *(Echocardiogram proved the most sensitive diagnostic method and superior to clinical findings and chest film.)*

Intermittent Positive Pressure Breathing Trial Group. Intermittent positive pressure breathing therapy of COPD: A clinical trial. Ann Intern Med 1983;99:612. *(Multicenter controlled trial of 985 patients showing that IPPB was no better than nebulizer for administration of bronchodilator therapy.)*

Kanner RE, Renzetti AD, Stanish WM, et al. Predictors of survival in subjects with chronic airflow limitation. Am J Med 1983;74:249. *(A 12-year prospective study identifying important determinants of prognosis and confirming findings of earlier studies.)*

Kerstjens HAM, Brand PLD, Hughes MD, et al. A comparison of bronchodilator therapy with or without inhaled corticosteroid for obstructive airway disease. N Engl J Med 1992;327:1413. *(Inhaled steroids reduced morbidity and obstruction.)*

Lertzman MM, Cherniack RM. Rehabilitation of patients with chronic obstructive pulmonary disease. Am Rev Respir Dis 1976;114:1145. *(Still useful review of rehabilitative modalities in the management of chronic obstructive pulmonary disease.)*

Lipworth BJ, McDevitt DG, Struthers AD. Prior treatment with diuretic augments the hypokalemic and electrocardiographic effects of inhaled albuterol. Am J Med 1989;86:653. *(Identifies an important contributor to arrhythmias associated with beta agonist use.)*

Matthay RA, Niederman MS, Wiedemann HP. Cardiovascular pulmonary interaction in chronic obstructive pulmonary disease with special reference to pathogenesis and management of cor pulmonale. Med Clin North Am 1990;74:571. *(Detailed review of treatment modalities for cor pulmonale, including vasodilators, oxygen, and phlebotomy.)*

Murciano D, Auclair H-M, Pariente R. A randomized, controlled trial of theophylline in patients with severe chronic obstructive pulmonary disease. N Engl J Med 1989;320:1521. *(Documents improvements in respiratory function and symptoms; attributes them to enhanced respiratory muscle performance.)*

Nicotra MB, Rivera M, Awe RJ. Antibiotic therapy of acute exacerbations of chronic bronchitis: A controlled study using tetracycline. Ann Intern Med 1982;97:18. *(Double-blind, randomized, placebo-controlled trial in 40 moderately ill COPD patients; found no difference between patients on tetracycline and those taking placebo.)*

Owens GR, Rogers RM, Pennock BE, et al. The diffusing capacity as a predictor of arterial oxygen desaturation during exercise in patients with COPD. N Engl J Med 1984;310:1218. *(Diffusing capacity measured during routine pulmonary function testing at rest correlated well with degree of hypoxemia during exercise; a simple way to determine who would benefit from oxygen supplementation during exercise?)*

Petty TL. Circadian variations in chronic asthma and chronic obstructive pulmonary disease. Am J Med 1988;85(suppl 1B):21. *(Review of the phenomenon and its treatment; 21 refs.)*

Pratt PC. Role of conventional chest radiography in diagnosis and exclusion of emphysema. Am J Med 1987;82:998. *(Detailed discussion of using the chest film to make and exclude the diagnosis of emphysema; very high predictive value when validated criteria are used.)*

Rochester DF. The diaphragm in "COPD": better than expected, but not good enough. N Engl J Med 1991;325:961. *(Editorial arguing that the goals of respiratory therapy should be directed at preventing diaphragmatic weakness not fatigue.)*

Rodrigues J, Niederman MS, Fein AM, et al. Nonresolving pneumonia in steroid-treated patients with obstructive lung disease. Am J Med 1992;93:29. *(Fungal infection accounted for most and was usually missed.)*

Shim CS, Williams MH. Aerosol beclomethasone in patients with steroid-responsive COPD. Am J Med 1985;78:655. *(Double-blind, randomized crossover trial comparing oral prednisone with inhaled beclomethasone. Beclomethasone did not prove to be an adequate substitute for oral corticosteroid therapy.)*

Shim CS, Williams MH. Bronchodilator response to oral aminophylline and terbutaline versus aerosol albuterol in patients with COPD. Am J Med 1983;75:697. *(Randomized, double-blind crossover study indicating that the aerosol route is superior to the oral one for administration of bronchodilators in COPD.)*

Silverman EK, Pierce JA, Province MA, et al. Variability of pulmonary function in alpha-1-antitrypsin deficiency: clinical correlates. Ann Intern Med 1989;111:982. *(Finds that many patients with the deficiency do not necessarily have pulmonary impairment attributable to the deficiency.)*

Similowski T, Yan S, Gautherier AP, et al. Contractile properties of the human diaphragm during chronic hyperinflation. N Engl J Med 1991;325:917. *(Finds that diaphragmatic function is preserved in stable COPD and that treatment to improve diaphragmatic function is not indicated.)*

Stoller JK, Gerbarg ZB, Feinstein A. Corticosteroids in stable chronic obstructive lung disease. J Gen Intern Med 1987;2:29.

(*A meta-analysis suggesting a possible benefit, but finding many methodologic shortcomings in available studies.*)

Sunderrajan EV, Byron WA, McKenzie WN, et al. The effect of terbutaline on cardiac function in patients with stable chronic obstructive lung disease. JAMA 1983;250:2151. (*Even small doses of terbutaline significantly increased right and left ventricular ejection fraction in patients with severe COPD.*)

Timms RM, Khaja FU, Williams GW, et al. Hemodynamic response to oxygen therapy in chronic obstructive pulmonary disease. Ann Intern Med 1985;102:29. (*Detailed data showing a modest response; patients with the best response had the best prognosis; normalization was rarely observed.*)

Tougaard L, Krone T, Sorknaes A, et al. Economic benefits of teaching patients with chronic obstructive pulmonary disease about their illness. Lancet 1992;339:1517. (*Cost of care reduced.*)

Wewers MD, Casolaro A, Sellers SE, et al. Replacement therapy for alpha-1-antitrypsin deficiency associated with emphysema. N Engl J Med 1987;316:1055. (*Infusions did reverse biochemical abnormalities.*)

Wewers MD, Gadek JE. The protease theory of emphysema. Ann Intern Med 1987;107:761. (*Concise summary of this suspected pathophysiology.*)

Primary Care Medicine: Office Evaluation and Management of the Adult Patient, 3rd edition, edited by Allan H. Goroll, Lawrence A. May, and Albert G. Mulley, Jr. J.B. Lippincott Company, Philadelphia

48
Management of Asthma

Asthma is predominantly an outpatient condition, affecting about 2.5 percent of the population. It is characterized by airway hyperreactivity and bronchospasm leading to reversible airway obstruction. A renewed appreciation for the inflammatory nature of the condition has markedly altered the approach to therapy, with antiinflammatory agents superseding bronchodilators as the first line of treatment. Although there are no cures for asthma, effective means of control are available, with inhaled, topically active preparations providing excellent control with minimal systemic side effects. Bronchodilators such as the beta$_2$-adrenergic agents, theophylline, and ipratropium have been relegated to a secondary role. The primary physician needs to be skilled in the use of these agents and able to design a practical program that minimizes the frequency and severity of attacks. Many emergency room visits for treatment of asthma are avoidable.

PATHOPHYSIOLOGY, CLINICAL PRESENTATION, AND COURSE

Pathophysiology

The pathogenesis of asthma remains incompletely understood. Both *sensitization* and *inflammation* appear to play important roles. A positive correlation has been found between cumulative exposure to the *dust mite allergen* and risk of sensitization, but as many as one-fourth of all asthmatics have no evidence of atopy. Regardless of the precipitant, *inflammation* sustains bronchial hyperreactivity, accounting for the success of anti-inflammatory agents and the failure of purely bronchodilating drugs to prevent attacks (see below).

Many precipitants and mediators of the bronchoconstriction, edema, and mucous production that characterize asthma have been identified; however, precise roles and interrelationships remain to be elucidated. The list of mediators includes *prostaglandin* D_2, *leukotrienes* (slow-reacting substance of anaphylaxis), *eosinophilic chemotactic factor*, and *histamine*.

Asthma appears to have an early and a late phase. The *acute bronchconstrictive phase* involves the rapid development of reversible airway obstruction in response to stimuli that fail to affect normal persons. Stimuli include allergens such as molds, sulfites, animal danders, and pollens; aspirin; exercise; emotional stress; viral respiratory infections; and respiratory irritants such as perfumes and dusts.

Allergen-induced asthma involves immunologically triggered release of bronchoconstricting substances from sensitized pulmonary mast cells. Sensitization occurs when IgE attaches to these cells and combines with the allergen, setting in motion a complex set of intracellular biochemical events that ends with degranulation of mast cells and release of biochemical mediators.

In addition to the initial mediator-induced bronchospasm, asthmatic patients experience a second or *late-phase reaction* occurring 6 to 12 hours later. This late-phase reaction is believed to be a manifestation of the inflammatory response, being more refractory to bronchodilator treatment than the initial one. Neutrophil chemotactic factor is believed to play a role. Even some patients with exercise-induced asthma experience a late reaction.

Elements of a *neurogenic pathway* have also been elucidated. Bronchial smooth muscle is responsive to autonomic influences; it is unsettled whether the effect is direct or by way of biochemical mediators. Vagal stimulation and cholinergic drugs cause bronchial constriction; beta-adrenergic stimulation appears capable of countering the cholinergic influences. Bronchial irritants and emotional stress are thought to precipitate bronchospasm, in part, by way of triggering vagal reflexes. The nerve endings of asthmatics have been found devoid of the bronchodilatory neuropeptide vasoactive intestinal polypeptide.

Traditionally, asthma has been divided clinically into "extrinsic" and "intrinsic" categories, with extrinsic disease believed to be a manifestation of immunologic reactivity to environmental antigens, and intrinsic disease thought to be unrelated to allergen exposure. However, patients in both groups have demonstrated IgE-related reactivity, challenging the notion of separate allergen- and nonallergen-related categories of asthma. Nonetheless, the categories are still used clinically (see following discussion).

Clinical Presentation

Regardless of precipitant, the pathophysiologic final common pathway is airway inflammation, with bronchial edema, smooth muscle contraction, and excessive mucus production. Clinical manifestations include *wheezing, dyspnea, cough,* and *sputum.* Presentations range from pure bronchospasm with little cough and sputum, to a predominance of bronchorrhea and coughing that mimics bronchitis or an upper respiratory tract infection. In fact, cough and sputum production may be the initial symptoms of an asthmatic attack. *Nocturnal exacerbation* of symptoms is common, linked to the diurnal variation in blood catecholamines and vagal tone.

Extrinsic Asthma. Although classifying asthma according to allergen-responsiveness may be an oversimplification, the categories extrinsic and intrinsic do describe two relatively distinct clinical presentations. Patients with *extrinsic asthma* typically give a history of atopy, onset of symptoms during childhood or adolescence, predictable seasonal occurrence, and response to environmental stimuli. However, the condition can occur at any age, and attacks may take place seasonally or year-round, precipitated by such common household allergens as the house-dust mite, animal dander, or fungal spores. Anxiety, inhalation of airway irritants, and exposure to perfumes and strong household odors can also precipitate asthmatic episodes in these patients. The course of attacks is usually self-limited, although some patients have severe bouts requiring hospitalization. Prognosis is relatively good, with 70 percent found to be symptom-free 20 years after onset.

Intrinsic Asthma. Patients with *intrinsic asthma* usually begin having symptoms in the third or fourth decade. Although there is no identifiable extrinsic allergen associated with attacks in these patients, they do demonstrate elevations in serum IgE similar to patients with intrinsic disease. There can be much sputum production, sometimes making differentiation from chronic bronchitis difficult. Minor upper respiratory tract infections often precipitate attacks. Some patients present with exertional dyspnea or cough and no demonstrable wheezing, although expiratory flow rates are clearly reduced. Patients with intrinsic asthma are sometimes more refractory to treatment than those with extrinsic disease.

Other Important Clinical Presentations include postexertional asthma, asthma associated with nasal polyps and aspirin sensitivity, and occupational asthma. *Postexertional asthma* is a form of airway hyperreactivity most common in children and adolescents. The stimulus is believed to be a reduction in the temperature of inhaled air, leading to mediator release in susceptible patients. Both initial and late phase reactions have been identified. Vigorous exercise on a cold dry day is particularly apt to trigger an attack; airway temperature can get quite low in such circumstances. The association between *nasal polyps* and *aspirin sensitivity* is a curious but important familial one. The bronchospasm may be marked.

Occupational asthma has gained increasing recognition as an important cause of work-related disability. Exposure to irritant or toxic pollutants in the workplace and inhalation of allergens are the main sources of difficulty. Cold air, low concentrations of sulfur dioxide, fluorocarbons, and inert dusts are common irritants that stimulate reflex bronchospasm. Toxic gases such as high concentrations of sulfur dioxide, halogens, ammonia, acid fumes, and solvent vapors cause inflammatory bronchoconstriction. Important allergens include animal proteins, enzymes, grain and cereal dusts, seeds, vegetable gums, and legumes. Other substances have pharmacologic activity; there are histamine-releasing compounds in cotton dust, organic acids in wood dust, and numerous chemicals with anticholinesterase activity. Some agents provoke asthma through multiple mechanisms; toluene diisocyanate (TDI) has reflex, pharmacologic, beta-blocking, and IgE effects.

Patients with occupational asthma due to toxic or irritant substances characteristically report a direct relation between exposure and onset of symptoms. Those with allergen-induced disease note no symptoms at time of first exposure followed by occurrence of marked wheezing after even minor repeat contact with the allergen (anamnestic response). Typically, patients with occupational asthma are symptom-free during days off from work, only to have a flare-up on returning (see Chapter 39).

Clinical Course

Regardless of the type of asthma, subclinical but significant bronchospasm remains for days to weeks after the wheezing of an acute attack subsides. The continuing bronchial hyperresponsiveness is believed related to ongoing inflammation. Often, small airways may remain constricted even after large airways have relaxed. The clinical recurrences that commonly develop shortly after the apparent resolution of an acute attack are most often not new episodes but relapses. No single clinical or laboratory parameter reliably predicts relapse (see below).

The long-term consequences of asthma are few. There is no evidence that it leads to such permanent pulmonary parenchymal damage as development of chronic bronchitis or emphysema. Overall mortality for all forms of asthma is 0.1 percent per year; the rate increases markedly to 3.3 percent for patients with episodes of status asthmaticus. There was a 6.2 percent annual increase in asthma-related mortality during the 1980s. The cause for this increase is unclear, but some speculate that overdependence on beta-agonist therapy and delay or omission in use of an anti-inflammatory may be an important contributing factor.

PRINCIPLES OF MANAGEMENT

The goals of therapy are to prevent attacks and effectively reduce bronchial hyperresponsiveness in patients who suffer attacks. Before initiating therapy, it is important to verify that the patient's wheezing is not due to a nonasthmatic cause of bronchospasm, such as pulmonary edema, embolization, foreign body, or infection (see Chapters 32, 40 to 42).

Management of Acute Attacks and Chronic Active Disease

Most patients with acute asthmatic attacks can be managed on an outpatient basis, provided that proper therapy is promptly and fully instituted. The vast majority of patients seeking emergency room care do not need parenteral therapy. In a prospective study of 140 asthmatic patients who came for emergency room care, most presented because they had no available medication, underutilized or improperly administered their medication, relied on over-the-counter preparations, or used fixed combination tablets or suppository forms that did not permit proper dosing.

With the renewed appreciation for the central role of inflammation in asthma and the awareness of increased morbidity and mortality associated with overreliance on bronchodilators comes the need to institute a major change in asthmatic treatment. *Antiinflammatory therapy* (corticosteroids and cromolyn) now emerges as the *cornerstone* of treatment, with *bronchodilators* relegated to an *adjunctive* role.

The consensus view is that all patients with active disease should be started and maintained on continuous anti-inflammatory therapy and that bronchodilators should be used only for symptomatic relief of mild acute exacerbations and for prevention of postexertional flares. The previous reliance on chronic bronchodilator therapy as the first line of treatment is now discouraged because of its association with increased morbidity and mortality, probably due as much to delay in instituting anti-inflammatory therapy as to any intrinsically harmful effects from high doses of bronchodilators. The principal anti-inflammatory agents are the glucocortico steroids and cromolyn; a new anti-inflammatory drug, nedocromil, has shown considerable promise in initial trials.

Glucocorticosteroids are the anti-inflammatory agents of choice in most adults with asthma. Their precise mechanism of action in asthma is not known, but the 6- to 12-hour delay noted between time of administration and onset of effect suggests that protein synthesis is required. The topically active, inhaled preparations (beclomethasone, triamcinolone, flunisolide) are preferable to oral therapy because systemic absorption is minimal at usual doses, virtually eliminating the risk of steroid-related adverse effects. Although highly effective, oral and parenteral preparations of systemic glucocorticoids (eg, prednisone, methylprednisolone, hydrocortisone) should be reserved for refractory cases, and then only for as short a period as possible. The adverse consequences of prolonged daily use of systemic glucocorticoids (osteoporotic fractures, adrenal suppression, skin changes, aseptic necrosis of bone, aggravation of diabetes mellitus; see Chapter 105) make such therapy ill-advised except in the most refractory of cases.

Topically active, inhaled glucocorticoids were developed in an effort to achieve the advantages of chronic steroid therapy without the systemic side effects. Prospective, randomized, controlled studies have shown them capable of slowing the clinical course of disease and improving functional status. The principal metered-dose aerosol preparations include *beclomethasone dipropionate* (Vanceril; Beclovent), *flunisolide* (Aerobid), and *triamcinolone acetonide* (Azmacort). All are topically active, equally effective for treatment of asthma, poorly soluble in water, and with little systemic effect at therapeutic doses (up to 20 puffs/d from a metered dose inhaler). Cough and wheezing occur into about 20 percent of patients using beclomethasone, compromising compliance. The symptoms are believed related to a small amount of the dispersant oleic acid present in all brands of the inhaled steroid preparation. Switching to an alternative inhaled steroid resolves the problem. Oral *thrush* and *hoarseness* are sometimes problems with prolonged use, but can be prevented by rinsing and gargling with water after each dose or by using a spacer (see below). Twice-daily regimens are nearly as effective as a qid program and are helpful in maximizing compliance.

Although the inhaled preparations can spare chronic use of systemic steroids, care must be taken when switching from a course of prolonged oral steroids to inhaled therapy. Inhaled steroids are not sufficiently absorbed to prevent adrenal insufficiency in patients with adrenal–pituitary suppression secondary to long-term systemic glucocorticoid use. Patients previously maintained on long-term systemic corticosteroids have gone into shock and died when switched abruptly to topical therapy. Cortrasyn testing for adrenal–pituitary responsiveness should be considered before switching from oral therapy to an inhaled program if systemic therapy has been maintained for more than 4 weeks at suppressive doses (see Chapter 105). A period of slow tapering or extended alternate-day therapy may be necessary before assuming an inhaled steroid program. Even if oral therapy cannot be eliminated immediately, the dose may be reduced by adding an inhalation program.

Onset of action is within 2 to 8 hours, but, when therapy is begun, 24 to 48 hours may pass before symptomatic improvement is noted. Response is dose-related and lasts about 6 to 8 hours. During periods of stress and flare-ups of asthma, topical therapy should be supplemented with large doses of systemic steroids; adrenal responsiveness may still be submaximal; moreover, topical medication may not penetrate obstructed airways where it is needed most.

The most frequent complication is mild *oropharyngeal candidiasis;* it responds well to nystatin mouthwash or clotrimazole troches and can be prevented by rinsing the mouth and pharynx with water after each dose. Some patients complain of hoarseness or throat irritation after inhaling beclomethasone; slight reduction in dose usually suffices. Some patients find that inhalation of beclomethasone triggers bronchospasm; use of an adrenergic agent beforehand will prevent it. As with any inhaler, proper technique is essential to obtaining a good therapeutic response (see below).

High-dose inhaled steroid therapy (20 puffs or more per day) has been advocated for refractory cases as an alternative to systemic steroid therapy. It appears to be more effective than alternate-day prednisone but is associated with such "systemic" complications as cataracts, skin changes, and adrenal suppression. Slightly lower doses of inhaled steroids (<20 puffs per day) are associated with a much reduced risk of adverse effects.

Prednisone is the prototype oral glucocorticosteroid. Half-life is 12 to 24 hours. Administration of as little as 15 mg/d beyond 2 weeks may begin to suppress the adrenal–pituitary axis (see Chapter 105). A short-term course of prednisone is optimal for control of a severe acute attack that is refractory to all other measures. Such a course (eg, 7 to 10 days), beginning at high dose (40 to 60 mg/d) and administered on a rapidly tapering schedule is often effective and will not result in adrenal suppression. A placebo-controlled, double-blind, randomized study of such prednisone use demonstrated that the group treated with steroids had significantly fewer symptoms and a lower rate of relapse than those not receiving steroid therapy.

Only patients with chronic disabling bronchospasm refractory to all other forms of therapy should be considered for long-term, daily systemic steroid treatment. In most instances, regular use of a topically active steroid aerosol preparation supplemented by bronchodilator treatment for mild exacerbations will suffice, with short courses of high-dose systemic therapy reserved for severe exacerbations. As noted earlier, one might try an alternate-day steroid regimen, which causes less adrenal suppression and fewer steroid-related adverse effects than does daily therapy if it proves difficult to withdraw oral steroid therapy entirely.

Beta-Agonists. Catecholamines with beta-adrenergic activity are potent bronchodilators useful for *acute treatment* of flares of *bronchospasm* that are mild to moderate in severity, although they have no direct anti-inflammatory action and thus no effect on airway hyperresponsiveness. A wide variety of adrenergic agents are used for asthma, ranging from the very rapidly acting, short duration, nonselective isoproterenol to the long-acting, semiselective, $beta_2$-agonists such as albuterol and metaproterenol. The advent of the inhaled, semiselective $beta_2$-agonists provides bronchodilation that is rapid in onset, sustained, and relatively free of extrapulmonary side effects. As noted above, excessive dependence on these agents at high doses is associated with an increased risk of morbidity and mortality from asthma. The mechanism is unclear, although delay in instituting anti-inflammatory therapy is suspected as much as a direct toxic effect. In a study of prolonged use, greater than 6 months of continuous beta-agonist treatment led to a deterioration in control.

The inhaled selective $beta_2$-agonists have become the *bronchodilator of choice* for treatment of asthma, because of their relative selectivity for bronchial beta-receptors, rapid onset (2 to 5 minutes) when taken by the aerosol route, sustained duration of action (up to 6 hours), and paucity of systemic side effects. *Albuterol* (Proventil; Ventolin), *metaproterenol* (Alupent; Metaprel), *bitolterol* (Tornalate), *terbutaline* (Brethine; Bricanyl), and *pirbuterol* (Maxair) are the major drugs in this class for use in asthma. Most are available in both oral and inhaled forms; terbutaline is available for subcutaneous injection. The inhaled preparations are preferred, being more rapid in onset and less likely to cause systemic side effects.

A few of the older adrenergic agonists may be encountered. *Isoethrane* (Bronkosol; Bronkometer) is a bronchoselective catecholamine that has been widely used for years, particularly as part of intermittent positive-pressure breathing (IPPB) therapy. It also comes in hand-held nebulizer form. Because it has a short duration of action and a potential for tachyphylaxis, its role has been supplanted by the newer noncatecholamine $beta_2$-agonists. Moreover, the efficacy of IPPB therapy has been found no better than that available from a hand-held nebulizer (see Chapter 47). *Ephedrine* is an older drug that causes release of endogenous catecholamines, with nonselective beta-adrenergic effects. It too has been largely replaced by the newer $beta_2$-agonists but is still available in irrational fixed-combination preparations (eg, Tedral; Marax), which should be avoided.

All semiselective $beta_2$-agents cause some *cardiotonic effects* when used in high doses. Metaproterenol is somewhat less $beta_2$-selective than the others and may cause more cardiac stimulation. *Tremor* is common, particularly at the onset of oral therapy; it may be sufficiently disabling to cause termination of therapy, although it usually diminishes over time. Tremor has been particularly troublesome in patients taking terbutaline, although it has also been noted with metaproterenol use. Significant *tachyphylaxis,* manifested as failure to respond to parenteral epinephrine, has been a concern but not noted to a worrisome degree, except in the context of prolonged regular use.

Choice of agent in this class should be individualized, based on degree of selectivity needed and tolerance to such side effects as tremor. Albuterol is a reasonable choice for most patients requiring an inhaled semiselective beta-agonist.

Theophylline and Its Derivatives. The methylxanthines *theophylline* and *aminophylline* (a derivative salt of theophylline) were the first orally active bronchodilators. Their role has become more limited as faster, safer, more effective therapies have been developed. For acute outpatient exacerbations, they are slower in onset of action, less potent, and less well tolerated than the newer inhaled $beta_2$-agonists. For reducing the frequency and severity of bronchospastic flares, they are less well tolerated and less effective than inhaled corticosteroids. Nonetheless, they continue to help some patients, particularly those bothered by nocturnal exacerbations (see below), and they can reduce systemic steroid requirements in some patients with refractory disease. Their low cost, clearly defined and readily measured therapeutic range (10 to 20 g/mL), and availability of sustained-release preparations facilitate utilization.

The utility and safety of methylxanthine therapy have been challenged. The narrow therapeutic range, failure in emergency room studies to demonstrate additional bronchodilation beyond that achieved by beta-agonists alone, and association with increased risks of cardiopulmonary toxicity blunted enthusiasm for their use. Debate continues as to their role in *urgent care settings,* where some reduction in need for hospital admission has been noted, even in the absence of additional bronchodilation. Efficacy may be related to other modes of action, such as improvements in diaphragmatic function, myocardial contractility, mucociliary transport, as well as inhibition of anaphylactic mediator release and suppression of mast cell response.

Adverse effects are proportional to serum level, with levels in excess of 20 g/mL associated with a marked increase in risk of toxic side effects. When levels exceed 35 g/mL, life-threatening *ventricular arrhythmias* can occur. *Seizures* refractory to standard anticonvulsant therapy have occurred without warning when serum levels go above 40 g/mL. The minor gastrointestinal and neurologic side effects are largely dose-related but occur in some patients at normal or even subtherapeutic serum levels. *Nausea, vomiting, reflux, and diarrhea* are the common minor gastrointestinal effects. It was erroneously thought that the oral route of theophylline administration was responsible for the gastrointestinal upset; this theory lead to the use of subtherapeutic oral doses and manufacture of rectal suppository preparations. Suppositories should not be used; they have erratic rates of drug release and absorption; serum levels are unpredictable. Common minor neurologic side effects include *agitation, tremor, and insomnia*.

Pharmacokinetics include onset of action within 15 minutes with use of liquid hydroalcoholic preparations, longer for other preparations. Rapidly absorbed theophylline preparations produce wide swings in serum levels; slow-release formulations give more stable serum concentrations and need be administered only every 12 to 24 hours. Half-life of oral theophylline or aminophylline averages 6 hours but can range from 4 to 8 hours; there is much individual variation due to differences in clearance rates.

Clearance is predominantly by hepatic biotransformation. Impairment of hepatic microsomal activity (as occurs with advanced age, erythromycin, cimetidine, oral contraceptives, caffeine, and perhaps influenza vaccination) raises serum levels and prolongs duration of action. Clearance increases with smoking, eating of charcoal-broiled foods, phenytoin, and phenobarbital.

Preparations include *theophylline elixir,* which contains alcohol to speed absorption. Because it is more expensive, shorter in duration of action, and more likely to produce erratic serum levels than other oral theophylline preparations, it is rarely used. *Aminophylline* is much lower in cost and longer-acting. *Sustained-release formulations* are more cost-effective, providing 12 to 24 hours of therapeutic serum levels. Generic versions are available. They are well-suited for nighttime use in patients with nocturnal exacerbations. Because aminophylline *suppositories* produce erratic absorption and unpredictable serum levels, they are not recommended. *Combination preparations,* containing theophylline in fixed dose combination with ephedrine, barbiturates, and expectorants, are not recommended because they do not permit adjustment of theophylline dose without increasing the intake of the other components.

Dosage must be individualized because of wide variation in clearance. Serum levels can be used to guide dosing, although need to achieve a therapeutic serum level has declined as more effective agents have become available. Serum levels are useful for detection of toxic concentrations and best obtained from blood drawn 4 to 6 hours after the last dose. Initiation of outpatient theophylline therapy is best carried out gradually over the course of 1 week, which helps to minimize adverse effects. Obese patients need not be given extra high doses; area of drug distribution does not increase proportionally.

Anticholinergics. *Ipratropium,* a topically active muscarinic blocking agent similar to atropine, is available in a metered-dose inhalation preparation. It is particularly useful in COPD, where its bronchodilating effects rival those of beta-agonists (see Chapter 47). Its efficacy is considerably less in asthma, although it may add some marginal bronchodilation to beta-agonist therapy, being longer-acting although slower in onset. Unlike atropine, it is poorly absorbed, has little systemic effect, and can be used in patients with glaucoma and prostatism. Care should be taken to avoid spray contact with the eyes in patients with narrow-angle glaucoma.

Leukotriene Receptor Antagonists. Investigational uses of drugs that inhibit leukotriene activity (eg, zileuton) show benefit and suggest a possible role in future treatment programs. These agents achieve bronchodilation and symptomatic improvement.

Prophylaxis

Once an acute attack subsides, the goal of management shifts to prevention of future episodes. Identification of the responsible allergen is sometimes helpful, especially in industrial settings (see Chapter 39) and in patients with extrinsic asthma. Avoidance of exposure and desensitization are too often overlooked as important components of the management program. *Desensitization* therapy (using intradermal injections of offending allergens; see Chapter 222) has been shown in controlled study to reduce frequency and severity of asthmatic episodes and may obviate or reduce the need for systemic steroid therapy. Patients with refractory extrinsic asthma should be considered for allergen testing and desensitization, especially when a well-defined and unavoidable allergen (eg, a pet or dust-mites) is suspected. *Avoidance* of the offending agent is good therapy where practical (eg, in industrial situations or when air pollution is heavy); unfortunately, this is not always feasible, and other methods of prophylaxis have to be used.

The limitations of immunotherapy and avoidance are not critical in view of the availability of effective pharmacologic agents for prophylaxis. As noted earlier, the recognition of inflammation's pivotal role in sustaining airway hyperresponsiveness has led to a renewed *emphasis* on *anti-inflammatory therapy* and a *reduction* in dependence on chronic *bronchodilator treatment*. Cromolyn sodium, the inhaled steroids, and prednisone are the important anti-inflammatory agents for prophylaxis.

Cromolyn Sodium is a unique and important prophylactic agent that works by preventing degranulation of mast cells. It is especially effective for *prevention* of episodes in children, especially episodes that are *exercise- or allergen-induced*. Many adults also benefit, including up to 60 percent of those with intrinsic asthma. Cromolyn should be considered before a patient is committed to more toxic therapy, such as long-term systemic prednisone. A 4- to 8-week empiric trial is needed to assess efficacy, because there is no way to predict response and prophylactic effect may take weeks to emerge. Because the drug possesses no direct bronchodilating activity, it should not be used for treating bronchospastic attacks.

Cromolyn is taken by the *inhaled* route. Its availability in an aqueous solution has reduced the frequency of reactions to the often irritating powdered formulation. The dose schedule for patients with chronic asthma is one capsule qid.

For prophylaxis of exercise-induced asthma, the patient inhales 30 minutes before exercise or exposure to a known allergen. (Patients with exercise-induced asthma who cannot tolerate cromolyn can take a few inhalations of a *beta$_2$-adrenergic aerosol* before engaging in activity.) Cromolyn is expensive, but it is free of adverse side effects and should be considered a first-line drug in asthma prophylaxis.

Corticosteroids. Patients who do not respond to cromolyn or need more rapid prophlaxis are candidates for a trial of *inhaled steroid* therapy (beclomethasone, flunisolide, triamcinolone). Two inhalations qid usually suffices, although higher doses are advocated for stubborn cases and during flares. Up to 20 puffs/d can be taken without inducing significant adrenal suppression or other systemic side effects. *Systemic steroids* (eg, prednisone) can prevent attacks in patients with a history of life-threatening asthma or recurrent disabling attacks that cannot be controlled by any other means. Risk of systemic steroid side effects is high (see Chapter 105). Alternate-day regimens are less adrenally suppressive and better tolerated. Occasionally, very high-doses of inhaled steroids (16 to 32 inhalations/d) can be substituted for alternate-day prednisone, but some systemic effects do occur (eg, cataracts, skin changes, mild adrenal suppression). Patients with extrinsic asthma may also benefit from use of a topically active steroid applied as a nasal spray during the peak of ragweed season (see Chapter 222).

Other Agents. *Methylxanthines* may have some steroid-sparing capability, and use of a long-acting preparation may be worth considering, especially in patients with nocturnal exacerbations (see above). *Methotrexate* has been studied as a steroid-sparing therapy for patients dependent on systemic steroid therapy. Preliminary results are encouraging, but more study is needed before this immunosuppressive approach can be recommended.

Antibiotics have a limited role in prophylaxis. Although viral upper respiratory infections frequently precipitate attacks—making *influenza vaccine* a must—bacterial infections do not. The occurrence of heavy sputum production has often been mistakenly attributed to infection when it was actually a manifestation of the asthma. However, in cases where bacterial infection is strongly suggested by sputum Gram's stain and confirmed by sputum culture, prompt treatment with an appropriate antibiotic (see Chapter 43) is important.

Choice of Therapy

Mild Intermittent Disease. The inhaled beta$_2$-adrenergic agents are the drug class of choice for patients with mild intermittent asthmatic episodes, including *exercise-induced* asthma. Use of metered-dose therapy with a beta$_2$-agent (eg, albuterol) is convenient, rapid in onset, sustained in duration of action, and associated with a minimum of extrapulmonary side effects. *Cromolyn* is excellent for prevention of exercise-related episodes.

Mild Chronic Disease. *Inhaled topical steroid therapy* is the treatment of choice (eg, beclomethasone, two inhalations qid). Higher doses may be necessary. If so, the program may be prescribed as a twice-daily regimen to facilitate compliance. *Nocturnal attacks* can be prevented by use of a long-acting *controlled-release theophylline* preparation before bed; serum theophylline levels should be monitored.

Acute Disease. An *inhaled beta$_2$-agonist* (eg, albuterol, three puffs q6h) is the initial treatment of choice. Those with stubborn bronchospasm that lessens but does not fully resolve within 24 hours of initiating nonsteroidal bronchodilator therapy may achieve control from a short, rapidly tapering course of oral steroids. Prompt initiation of a 7- to 10-day course of *oral corticosteroid* therapy (eg, prednisone) beginning at full doses (eg, 40 to 60 mg/d) is indicated if symptoms persist and fail to respond within the first day of symptoms. Tapering should be followed by a course of inhaled steroids. Delay in initiating steroid therapy and over-reliance on beta-agonists can be dangerous.

Chronic Refractory Disease. Daily doses of *oral corticosteroids* may be required to provide adequate control, although regular use of inhaled steroids, sometimes at increased dose (eg, 20 inhalations/d) has dramatically reduced the number of patients requiring long-term systemic steroid therapy or at least reduced the dose necessary to maintain control. In a study of 371 patients with chronic refractory disease followed for 1 year, 78 percent were well controlled without oral steroids or with only short-term prednisone therapy when inhaled steroids were added to the program. High doses of inhaled steroids (16 to 32 inhalations/d) may even be superior to alternate-day prednisone, although cost and inconvenience are greater and, as noted earlier, some degree of adrenal suppression may ensue.

Monitoring Therapy

Assessments of symptoms, signs, and expiratory flow rates remain the basic means of monitoring asthmatic patients and judging severity of illness. In a carefully conducted study of 96 asthmatic patients, *self-estimates of severity* and daily change in airway obstruction correlated better with peak expiratory flow rate measurements than did the clinical assessment of their physicians.

Certain physical findings, such as the *ratio of inspiration to expiration,* help to semiquantitatively judge the degree of bronchospasm. However, wheezes and related physical findings are not sensitive indicators of airway obstruction. The absence of wheezes does not indicate resolution of bronchospasm (see below). *Pulsus paradoxus* and *sternocleidomastoid retraction* are signs of severe obstruction, suggesting an FEV_1 of less than 1 L/sec, but these findings are not inevitably present when expiratory flow rates are very low. Moreover, there is much variation between the degree of paradox and severity of bronchospasm.

Spirometry provides additional sensitivity. Careful studies correlating physical findings with spirometric readings have shown that the *forced expiratory volume* at 1 second (FEV_1) is still prolonged at the time wheezes disappear. Even after the FEV_1 has returned to normal, measures of small airway obstruction (eg, *maximum midexpiratory flow rate*) continue to indicate bronchospasm. Patient use at home of a *hand-held flow meter* can facilitate monitoring.

The clearing of wheezes signifies little more than partial resolution of large airway bronchospasm; small airway bronchoconstriction may still be prominent and slower to resolve. Failure to continue therapy beyond resolution of audible wheezes and the acute phase of bronchoconstriction is partially responsible for the high rate of relapse that accompanies acute episodes treated only while wheezes persist.

Sputum and blood eosinophil counts correlate with response to therapy in patients treated with steroids for an acute attack. Although blood eosinophilia is not an invariable feature of an acute exacerbation of asthma, it does decline with improvement of expiratory flow rate. The same holds true for sputum eosinophilia. The usefulness of the eosinophil count for predicting relapse and response to therapy is unsettled.

Arterial blood gases provide important information in severe cases, particularly adequacy of ventilation. A PCO_2 that is inappropriately high for the respiratory rate indicates ventilatory failure and urgent need for hospitalization. However, because arterial blood gases are not readily available in most office settings, decisions usually must be made without them. A *chest x-ray* rarely provides information of use in decision making.

Thus, some of the most easily obtained parameters (the patient's subjective assessment of severity, ratio of inspiration to expiration, pulsus paradoxus, sternocleidomastoid retraction, and FEV_1) are among the more meaningful guides to clinical status and severity of illness.

The Seemingly Refractory Patient

One of the most common reasons why outpatient treatment fails is *improper inhaler technique*. In a study of 30 asthmatic patients, 47 percent were found to be using improper technique and not getting an adequate dose of medication. Correct use of an inhaler is an essential skill for every asthmatic patient (see discussion of Patient Education).

Another important cause of treatment failure is *underutilization of anti-inflammatory medication* and *overdependence on bronchodilators,* often due to slow onset of steroid action, fear of steroid side effects, and ignorance of the inflammatory nature of the illness. Other common mistakes include reliance on *nonprescription agents,* such as inhalers with low doses of an adrenergic agent, and use of suboptimal prescription drugs, such as theophylline suppositories or fixed combination agents containing ephedrine. Over-the-counter epinephrine inhalers are too short-acting to provide adequate relief from an attack. *Use of theophylline suppositories* is also ill-advised due to erratic absorption. The *fixed-combination agents* containing subtherapeutic doses of theophylline (120 mg per tablet) in combination with ephedrine (25 mg per tablet) provide too little theophylline and excess adrenergic stimulation if more than four tablets are taken in a 24-hour period. The result is poor bronchodilation and marked adrenergic side effects. These preparations often contain barbiturates as well, which speed theophylline clearance and pose the added risks of ventilatory suppression and dependence.

Management of the Pregnant Patient

Fetal morbidity and mortality are increased if asthma goes uncontrolled during pregnancy. Most asthma drugs are safe to use both during pregnancy and when breast-feeding, although in some instances data are lacking due to the difficulty of performing controlled studies. Epinephrine increases the risk of fetal malformations, and the safety of the $beta_2$-agonists and cromolyn remains to be established; until safety is proven, they should be avoided if possible. Use of beclomethasone appears without serious consequence, and even systemic steroids can be prescribed if necessary. Theophylline is safe, as is penicillin. Erythromycin is a reasonable alternative in penicillin-allergic patients; tetracycline is contraindicated because it damages fetal liver, bone, and teeth. Some barbiturates have been linked to fetal malformations; many fixed-combination preparations contain barbiturates and should not be prescribed.

PATIENT EDUCATION

Patients need to be made partners in management of their asthma, because good compliance and proper use of medication can minimize the severity and frequency of attacks. Instruction in preventive measures is always appreciated. The bedroom environment deserves particular attention. Covering the mattress and pillows with impermeable materials limits exposure to dust mite allergen, a potential trigger of asthma and its exacerbations. Wall-to-wall carpets are another source of such allergens and should be avoided. Because asthma is a condition characterized by periodic exacerbations, every patient who is capable of understanding his or her medications should be given instructions for initial self-treatment of an attack along with strong advice to call the physician if relief does not come quickly. Patients need to know that excessive delay may lead to refractory bronchospasm. Home use of a *hand-held flow meter* has helped encourage patient participation in monitoring and adjusting treatment.

Addressing patient concerns and providing written information facilitates *compliance*. Many worry about becoming "dependent" on medication or "immune" to it. These fears need to be addressed openly. A medication booklet that lists prescribing information, side effects, and indications for use alongside a picture of the medication can be helpful to patient and family. Often, patients mistakenly stop the wrong medication or cease therapy altogether because they were fearful or unfamiliar with the side effects of their medications.

Patients who develop bronchospasm from air pollution, pollens, or exercise need an *activity prescription*. Staying indoors, avoiding physical exertion, and using air-conditioning on particularly bad days are helpful. Those with exercise-induced asthma need not restrict themselves as long as prophylactic measures suffice; however, very cold dry days may be difficult.

Those with asthma due to occupational exposure or household factors need careful *counseling* when considering such difficult alternatives as leaving a job, giving up a favorite pet, or moving to a new location. Often less extreme measures are adequate (see above). A number of patients with allergic asthma request advice about desensitization treatment. Allergen testing and consideration of trial of such therapy are reasonable if episodes are frequent and incapacitating, and a single allergen is identified (see Chapter 222).

Patients receiving steroids deserve an extra measure of instruction, particularly when switching over from systemic to aerosol therapy. Writing out the tapering schedule and emphasizing the importance of taking systemic steroids at the time of an exacerbation or major stress will help minimize the risk of adrenal insufficiency.

The pregnant patient with asthma will be reluctant to take medication. Detailed counseling about which medications can be used with safety and the importance of asthma control to the health of the fetus are needed to ensure compliance and alleviate concern.

Inhaler Technique. With the growing importance of inhaled metered-dose therapy, proper inhalation technique is essential. Delivery of drug to distal airways is facilitated by *increased duration of breath-holding* and *prolongation and moderation of inspiratory flow*. Rapid inspirations deposit drug in the upper airway; very deep ones are no better than moderate ones. During periods of respiratory distress, a greater number of inhalations is needed to deliver an adequate dose to distal airways due to increase in inspiratory flow rate. Thus patients need to be instructed to increase the number of inhalations during a period of respiratory distress if benefit does not appear forthcoming, although extreme care is warranted when increasing beta-agonist dose, because systemic absorption will occur from drug deposited in the proximal airway.

Correct inhaler use involves coordinating inspiration with actuation of the metered-dose inhaler, a skill that takes some practice to master. There are two recommended approaches: 1) placing the inhaler between the closed lips, actuating the inhaler, breathing in, and holding the breath; 2) holding the mouthpiece 3 to 4 cm from the lips of an open mouth, releasing the medication at the beginning of a full 5-second inspiration, and holding the breath for 10 seconds. The latter technique is a bit more difficult but capable of delivering twice the dose to the lower respiratory tract if the inspiration is moderate, prolonged, and accompanied by breath holding.

Many patients make the mistake of inhaling first, then actuating the canister, holding their breath for 2 or 3 seconds more, and exhaling before taking the first inhalation. Others inhale through the nose. Because many patients cannot perform aerosol inhalation correctly after a demonstration, they need to practice under observation. Moreover, about half forget how to do it when tested on follow-up. Repeat checks of technique are important.

Upwards of 40 percent of patients cannot master such techniques and require use of an *inhalation aid,* often referred to as a *"spacer."* Commercially available spacers are aerosol-holding chambers that not only eliminate the need for hand–breath coordination, but also cut down on oropharyngeal deposition of steroid.

INDICATIONS FOR ADMISSION

One of the most difficult determinations is predicting the need for hospitalization at the time of initial presentation. Ability to make such predictions is particularly important for the care of patients with severe attacks who visit the office or emergency room. Some have argued that response to maximum nonsteroidal therapy is a good predictor of immediate outcome and need for admission. Most studies provide little evidence that any one parameter is predictive, although one group noted that patients who sat bolt upright on admission to the emergency room had a strong likelihood of requiring admission. Another group developed an index of multiple clinical parameters selected by multivariate discriminant analysis to predict need for hospitalization. Pulse rate greater than 120/min, respiratory rate greater than 30/min, pulsus paradoxus greater than 18 mm Hg, peak expiratory flow rate less than 120 L/min, moderate to severe dyspnea, accessory muscle use, and wheezing made up the presenting clinical parameters used in the index. Although in the investigators' setting the index was capable of distinguishing between those who needed admission and those who did not (sensitivity, 95%; specificity, 97%), it did not function nearly as well when applied prospectively by other investigators in their emergency room settings.

Lacking more definitive means of prediction, clinical status and response to therapy remain the most helpful guidelines for decision making. Consideration of hospital care is indicated for patients with an acute attack who manifest any one of the following:

1. Subjective report of severe difficulty breathing
2. Failure to respond fully and promptly to inhaled beta-agonist therapy that is followed promptly by full doses of prednisone
3. Use of accessory muscles of respiration (sternocleidomastoid retraction)
4. More than 10 mm Hg of pulsus paradoxus
5. FEV_1 less than 1.0 L/sec
6. Arterial PCO_2 inappropriately high for respiratory rate
7. Underlying cardiac condition
8. Inadequate home situation or a history of poor compliance

THERAPEUTIC RECOMMENDATIONS

Prophylaxis

- Identify and advise avoidance of any known allergens or environmental irritants.
- Consider immunotherapy (desensitization) for those with a single known precipitating allergen.
- Begin a trial of cromolyn therapy in children, adolescents, and those with exercise-induced asthma; an adequate trial is 4 to 8 weeks. Dose for continuous prophylaxis is two puffs of the aqueous solution qid, or two puffs ½ hour before vigorous activity. Alternatively, prevention of exercise-induced asthma can be achieved with a few inhalations of a $beta_2$-adrenergic agent (eg, albuterol) 30 minutes before exertion.
- For adults with mild chronic asthma, consider either a trial of cromolyn or an inhaled corticosteroid (eg, beclomethasone) in a dose of two puffs qid.
- Consider adding a long-acting theophylline preparation at bedtime (eg, Uniphyl, 400 mg qhs) to prevent nocturnal

exacerbations not fully controlled by inhaled steroids or cromolyn; regularly monitor the serum theophylline level.

- If standard doses of inhaled steroids do not suffice (even when supplemented by long-acting theophylline), then advance to high-dose inhaled steroid therapy (16 to 24 inhalations/d, which can be prescribed in bid fashion to facilitate compliance).
- If maximal inhaled steroidal therapy fails to provide adequate prophylaxis, then add alternate-day oral corticosteroid therapy (eg, prednisone, 10 to 20 mg qod). If alternate-day prednisone plus inhaled steroids do not suffice, increase alternate-day prednisone dose (eg, to 20 to 40 mg qod) or switch to daily therapy (eg, 20 mg qd). Taper daily therapy to the smallest dose necessary to prevent attacks.
- Do not rely on bronchodilators for prophylaxis, except in the case of minor exercise-induced asthma.
- Administer trivalent influenza vaccine each fall at least 6 weeks before start of the flu season. Also administer pneumococcal vaccine (see Chapter 6).

Acute Asthmatic Attacks

- If attacks are mild and infrequent, prescribe an inhaled $beta_2$-agonist (eg, albuterol, two to three puffs qid) to be used at the first sign of an attack.
- If the beta-agonist alone does not promptly suffice, begin a short course of oral corticosteroid therapy with prednisone 40 to 60 mg/d, tapering rapidly over 7 to 10 days.
- To facilitate tapering and maintenance of control, add an inhaled corticosteroid (eg, beclomethasone, three puffs qid) to the oral steroid program. Continue it as the systemic steroid program is phased out.
- Advise the patient to keep well hydrated to prevent mucous plugging during an attack.
- Patients with a stubborn attack unaccompanied by worrisome prognostic signs or incapacity can be treated on an outpatient basis with a more prolonged course of prednisone therapy, provided the overall trend is toward improvement and the patient is reliable; if there is any doubt, consider hospitalization.
- Taper systemic steroids slowly if the patient has been taking prednisone long enough to cause hypothalamic–pituitary–adrenal suppression (see Chapter 105). At times of stress and flare-ups, increase inhaled steroid therapy to 16 to 20 puffs per day and consider resuming full doses of systemic steroid therapy (eg, 40 to 60 mg prednisone per day) until episode passes.
- Arrange prompt emergency room care for parenteral theophylline and systemic corticosteroids if there are signs of severe airway obstruction (pulsus paradoxus, $FEV_1 < 1$ L/sec, use of accessory muscles of respiration, and so forth).
- Avoid overreliance on bronchodilators and use of antianxiety agents, sedatives, fixed combination preparations, and rectal theophylline suppositories.
- Be sure patient is fully informed about medications, their side effects, and proper use. Demonstrate and check technique of inhaler use. Consider teaching use of the hand-held flow meter to encourage patient participation in monitoring and adjusting therapy. Directly elicit and address any patient concerns.

A.H.G.

ANNOTATED BIBLIOGRAPHY

Aelony Y. "Noninvasive" oral treatment of asthma in the emergency room. Am J Med 1985;78:929. *(Most patients were fully controlled by nonparenteral means, arguing that most emergency room visits are unnecessary.)*

Altman LC, Findlay SR, Lopez M, et al. Adrenal function in adult asthmatics during long-term daily treatment with 800, 1,200, and 1,600 mcg triamcinolone acetonide. Chest 1992;101:1250. *(Inhalation therapy produced no major suppression of adrenal function.)*

Baigelman W, Chodosh S, Pizzuato D, et al. Sputum and blood eosinophils during corticosteroid treatment of acute exacerbations of asthma. Am J Med 1983;75:929. *(Eosinophil counts correlated with objective measures of response.)*

Barnes PJ. New concepts in the pathogenesis of bronchial hyperresponsiveness and asthma. J Allergy Clin Immunol 1989; 83:1013. *(A discussion of the role of inflammation in the pathogenesis of asthma.)*

Burrows B, Lebowitz MD. The beta-agonist dilemma. N Engl J Med 1992;326:560. *(An editorial reassessing the role of beta-agonist therapy; argues for a secondary rather than primary role.)*

Burrows B, Martinez FD, Halonen M, et al. Association of asthma with serum IgE levels and skin-test reactivity to allergens. N Engl J Med 1989;320:271. *(Prevalence closely related to serum IgE levels; patients with both extrinsic and intrinsic asthma had evidence of immunologic hyperreactivity.)*

Busse WW. The precipitation of asthma by upper respiratory infections. Chest 1985;87:44S. *(A review of the mechanisms underlying viral-induced asthma.)*

Chan-Yeung M. Occupational asthma. Am Rev Respir Dis 1986; 133:686. *(Useful review of occupations and compounds associated with occupational asthma; guides elimination of environmental precipitants.)*

Dompeling E, van Chayck CP, van Grunsven PM, et al. Slowing the deterioration of asthma and chronic obstructive pulmonary disease observed during bronchodilator therapy by adding inhaled corticosteroids. Ann Intern Med 1993;118:770. *(A prospective, randomized clinical trial showing improvements in flow rate, symptoms, and number of exacerbations.)*

Ernst P, Spitzer WD, Suisse S, et al. Risk of fatal and near fatal asthma in relation to inhaled corticosteroid use. JAMA 1992; 268:3462. *(Risk markedly reduced by its use.)*

Fiel B, Swartz MA, Glanz K, et al. Efficacy of short-term corticosteroid therapy in outpatient treatment of acute bronchial asthma. Am J Med 1983;75:259. *(A double-blind, placebo-controlled study showing reductions in symptoms and rate of relapse.)*

Greenberger PA. Beclomethasone diproprionate for severe asthma during pregnancy. Ann Intern Med 1983;98:478. *(Prevalence of congenital malformations was within the normal range among patients using the drug during pregnancy.)*

Gross NJ. Ipratropium bromide. N Engl J Med 1988;319:486. *(Excellent review of anticholinergic therapy in asthma; 110 refs.)*

Israel E, Rubin P, Kemp JP, et al. The effect of inhibition of 5-lipoxygenase by zileuton in mild to moderate asthma. Ann Intern Med 1993;119:1059. *(A leukotriene pathway inhibitor with bronchodilating capability; a potentially useful new class of antiasthmatic agents.)*

Mathison DA, Stevenson DD, Simon RA. Asthma and the home environment. Ann Intern Med 1982;97:128. *(Editorial describing the allergens associated with house dust, household pets, ubiquitous fungi, and nonallergic irritants.)*

Mayo PH, Richman J, Harris HW. Results of a program to reduce admission for adult asthma. Ann Intern Med 1990;112:864. *(Educational program in conjunction with a vigorous medical regimen resulted in a two- to threefold reduction in admission rate.)*

McFadden ER. Methylxanthines in the treatment of asthma: the rise, the fall, and the possible rise again. Ann Intern Med 1991;115:323. *(Editorial reviewing the changing view of methylxanthine use and suggesting a retained role.)*

McFadden ER. Exertional dyspnea and cough as preludes to acute attacks of bronchial asthma. N Engl J Med 1975;292: 555. *(Intermittent episodes of cough and breathlessness represented variants of asthmatic attacks.)*

McFadden ER, Gilbert Ileen. Asthma. N Engl J Med 1992;327: 1928. *(Review that concentrates on pathophysiology and treatment based on advances in its understanding; 148 refs.)*

McFadden ER Jr. Dosages for corticosteroids in asthma. Ann Rev Respir Dis 1993;147:1306. *(Recommendations by a leading authority.)*

Mullarkey MF, Lammert JK, Blumenstein BA. Long-term methotrexate treatment in corticosteroid-dependent asthma. Ann Intern Med 1990;112:577. *(Encouraging report on use of immunosuppressive therapy in place of systemic steroids.)*

Newhouse MT, Dolovich P. Control of asthma by aerosols. N Engl J Med 1986;315;870. *(Best article on metered-dose inhaler use.)*

Petty TL. Circadian variations in chronic asthma and chronic obstructive pulmonary disease. Am J Med 1988;85:(suppl 1B): 21. *(Documents worsening pulmonary status during nighttime.)*

Pope AM. Indoor allergens—assessing and controlling adverse health effects. JAMA 1993;269:2721. *(Brief summary of this increasingly important issue.)*

Rubinstein I, Levison H, Slutsky AS, et al. Immediate and delayed bronchoconstriction after exercise in patients with asthma. N Engl J Med 1987;317:482. *(Eight of 53 patients were found to have a delayed response as well as an acute one; argues for more than a simple single mediator.)*

Selner JC. Helping asthmatic patients control their environment. J Respir Dis 1986;8:83. *(Useful practical advice.)*

Shim CS, Williams MH. Cough and wheezing from beclomethasone dipropionate aerosol are absent after triamcinolone acetonide. Ann Intern Med 1987;106:700. *(Twenty percent of patients could not tolerate the drug; the dispersant oleic acid is believed to be the cause of the problem.)*

Shim C, Williams MH. Evaluation of the severity of asthma: Patients versus physicians. Am J Med 1980;68:11. *(Patients better at estimating severity and change in expiratory flow rates than their physicians.)*

Shim C, Williams MH. The adequacy of inhalation of aerosol from canister nebulizers. Am J Med 1980;69:891. *(Almost half of patients studied were not using their inhalers properly, and, even after training, many still required further instruction and follow-up.)*

Shim C, Williams MH, Jr. Effects of odors in asthma. Am J Med 1986;80:18. *(Significant decline in FEV_1 and worsening of symptoms with exposure to one or more common odors.)*

Spitzer WO, Siussa S, Ernst P, et al. The use of beta-agonists and the risk of death and near death from asthma. N Engl J Med 1992;326:501. *(Important paper; documents increased risk of severe disease and death associated with prolonged use.)*

Stephenson BJ, Rowe BH, Haynes RB, et al. Is this patient taking the treatment as prescribed. JAMA 1993;269:2779. *(An excellent piece on compliance with asthma therapy.)*

Turner ES, Greenberger PA, Patterson R. Management of the pregnant asthmatic patient. Ann Intern Med 1980;93:905. *(Detailed review of this special aspect of asthma management; 126 refs.)*

Weinberger M, Hendeles L. Slow-release theophylline: Rationale and basis for product selection. N Engl J Med 1983;308:760. *(Detailed review of these preparations; 35 refs.)*

Weiss KB, Wagenner DK. Changing patterns of asthma mortality. JAMA 1990;264:1683. *(An annual increase of 6.2 percent found in the 1980s.)*

Welsh PW, Reed CE, Conrad E. Timing of once-a-day theophylline dose to match peak blood level with diurnal variation in severity of asthma. Am J Med 1986;80:1098. *(Nocturnal use especially effective.)*

Wrenn K, Slovis CM, Murphy F, et al. Aminophylline therapy for acute bronchospastic disease in the emergency room. Ann Intern Med 1991;115:241. *(Admission rate greatly reduced, even though no additional bronchodilation produced.)*

49
Management of Tuberculosis

HARVEY B. SIMON, M.D.

Primary Care Medicine: Office Evaluation and Management of the Adult Patient, 3rd edition, edited by Allan H. Goroll, Lawrence A. May, and Albert G. Mulley, Jr. J.B. Lippincott Company, Philadelphia

Tuberculosis (TB) may be encountered by the primary care physician as either a positive tuberculin skin test in the absence of active infection (an estimated 7% of the U.S. population may fall into this category) or as active TB, which is becoming increasingly common among human immunodeficiency virus (HIV)-positive persons and other high-risk populations (see Chapter 38). Over the years, diagnosis and treatment have shifted from the sanatorium and the specialist to the community and the primary physician.

Rapid diagnosis and treatment of TB are impaired by several factors, including inadequate sensitivity of skin testing and sputum smears, a wide variety of clinical presentations—many of which are subtle, nonspecific x-ray findings—several weeks required for confirmatory cultures and antibiotic sensitivities, long treatment regimens (with associated compliance problems), and emergence of drug-resistant strains. In addition, many clinicians have little experience with the disease and often do not suspect its presence. Even patients admitted to university hospitals may experience a delay in diagnosis, with some cases recognized only at autopsy. In addition, the management of TB has undergone such tremendous changes that studies have demonstrated suboptimal management by many general physicians in the United States. Clearly, diagnosis and treatment of TB pose major challenges for the primary physician.

PATHOPHYSIOLOGY AND EPIDEMIOLOGY

Virtually all cases are acquired through *person-to-person aerosol* transmission of a nonmotile, acid-fast, gram-positive rod. People with active pulmonary infection shed infected droplets, which are then airborne into the environment. Because most infectious patients discharge relatively few organisms, casual contacts have a low risk of infection, and most secondary cases occur in household members, schoolmates, or other close contacts of the index case. TB is more common in immigrants and population groups where there is crowding, poverty (especially homelessness), or a high risk of HIV infection (see Chapter 38). Among HIV-infected patients, risk increases 100- to 200-fold. Serious outbreaks (with attack rates of 10%) have been reported among patients in hospital wards with a large concentration of acquired immunodeficiency syndrome (AIDS) patients.

Most persons harboring the tubercle bacillus mount an immune response sufficient to prevent progression from *primary infection* to clinical illness; they manifest a positive skin test. About 5 percent of infected persons (rate higher for AIDS patients) fail to contain the primary infection and progress to *active primary disease* within 2 years of initial infection. In the past, primary infection occurred almost entirely in childhood, but, as the epidemiology of tuberculosis has changed (see Chapter 38), primary tuberculosis is now also seen in adults, particularly among elderly nursing home residents and patients on AIDS wards. This suggests that *nosocomial tuberculosis* may be developing into an important problem. A worrisome characteristic of some nosocomial outbreaks has been the emergence of organisms *resistant* to multiple antituberculous drugs.

Another 5 percent of infected patients (again, rate higher in AIDS patients) experience *reactivation of latent endogenous infection,* most often within 2 to 4 years of the initial infection or at times of lowered host resistance (eg, adolescence, postpartum, chronic debilitating illness). However, reactivation can occur many decades after initial infection, as reported among elderly nursing home residents. Upwards of one-fifth of patients with reactivated disease have histories of inadequately treated clinical TB. In many instances, a discrete insult to host defenses such as steroid therapy, alcoholism, malnutrition, neoplastic disease, HIV infection, or gastrectomy can be implicated, but at times it is impossible to identify the reason for reactivation.

The vast majority of "new" cases in the United States still represent reactivated disease. Only a small fraction of clinically active TB is due to direct progression of primary infection. Even in HIV-infected patients and residents of nursing homes, the bulk of active disease is due to reactivation. However, reports from AIDS wards and nursing homes raise the spectre of an increase in incidence of primary infection proceeding directly to active TB.

Atypical mycobacterial infections are probably acquired from inhalation or ingestion of organisms from sources in nature; there is no evidence for person-to-person transmission. Patients with AIDS are particularly susceptible, especially in the late phases of their illness.

CLINICAL PRESENTATION AND COURSE

Primary Infection. As noted above, more than 90 percent of patients are entirely asymptomatic at the time of primary infection and can be identified only through conversion of the tuberculin skin test from negative to positive. The majority of these patients have a normal chest x-ray. Among the 10 percent who progress directly to symptomatic disease, four broad syndromes can be identified: 1) *Atypical pneumonia* is the most common, characterized by fever and nonproductive cough. Chest x-rays may show unilateral lower lobe patchy parenchymal infiltrates or paratracheal or hilar adenopathy. Although such patients should receive full antituberculous chemotherapy when diagnosed (see below), the disease usually resolves, even without treatment. 2) *Tuberculous pleurisy* and effusion are accompanied by fever, cough, pleuritic chest pain, and occasionally dyspnea. Chest x-rays reveal unilateral pleural effusions, often without identifiable parenchymal lesions. The tuberculin test is almost always strongly positive. Diagnosis depends on examination and culture of the pleural fluid or on percutaneous needle biopsy of the pleura, because sputum cultures are positive in only 30 percent of such cases. 3) *Direct progression* from primary disease to upper lobe involvement is another presentation. 4) Early *systemic dissemination,* which used to be seen exclusively in children, now occurs in HIV-infected patients. In addition to these major manifestations, patients with primary TB may present with *hypersensitivity reactions* such as *erythema nodosum.*

Reactivation (Postprimary) Tuberculosis. As noted above, this is still the most common clinical form of TB. Symptoms usually begin insidiously and progress over a period of many weeks or months before diagnosis. Constitutional symptoms are often prominent, including *anorexia, weight loss,* and *night sweats.* Most patients have *low-grade fever,* but higher temperatures and even chills may be seen occasionally when the disease progresses more rapidly. In addition, most patients present with pulmonary symptoms, including *cough* and *sputum production.* Dyspnea is relatively uncommon in the absence of underlying chronic lung disease. A frequent complaint is *hemoptysis,* often in the form of bright red streaks of blood caused by bronchial irritation. Although physical examination is usually nondiagnostic, chest x-rays are highly suggestive of the diagnosis. Typical features include *infiltration* in the *posterior apical* pulmonary segments, which may be unilateral or bilateral, and which progresses to frank *cavitation.* Apical lordotic views and chest tomography may be helpful in documenting cavitary disease. Occasionally, postprimary TB may involve the lower lung fields, and in rare instances the chest x-ray may appear normal. The tuberculin skin test is positive in about 80 percent of patients with reactivation tuberculosis; patients with advanced disease are often malnourished and anergic.

Extrapulmonary Tuberculosis. Approximately 20 percent of all newly recognized cases of TB in the United States are extrapulmonary. Although the frequency of pulmonary TB is constant, the incidence of extrapulmonary disease is increasing, due largely to HIV-positive patients (see below). Although the clinical features of extrapulmonary TB vary widely, certain generalizations are possible. Past history is not a reliable guide to the diagnosis. Only 25 percent of patients have a past history of TB; of these, virtually all have been inadequately treated. There is typically a long latent period between the first episode of infection and the extrapulmonary presentation. Approximately 50 percent of patients with extrapulmonary disease have entirely normal chest x-rays; most of the others have stigmata of old inactive pulmonary disease, whereas a minority have coexisting active pulmonary infection. Although extrapulmonary disease can involve all organ systems, either singly or in various combinations, the most commonly affected areas are the genitourinary tract, the musculoskeletal system, and the lymph nodes.

The most common type of extrapulmonary TB is infection of an individual organ system. The patient is most often afebrile and can be entirely free of constitutional complaints. The illness typically pursues an indolent course characterized by local organ dysfunction and eventual destruction rather than by progressive general decline. In fact, the clinical presentation in these individuals more often suggests neoplastic disease than infection. The tuberculin skin test is almost always positive. Clinical syndromes in this category include genitourinary tuberculosis, tuberculous arthritis and osteomyelitis, tuberculous lymphadenitis, and many others.

HIV-positive patients with TB may experience extrapulmonary disease and dissemination early on. Intravenous drug abusers and nonwhite populations are at highest risk. When CD4+ counts are well preserved (see Chapter 13), tuberculous infection usually causes pulmonary disease that resembles TB in HIV-negative individuals. However, in more severely immunocompromised HIV patients, TB is often extrapulmonary and may be severe, widespread, and atypical in presentation. A high incidence of tuberculous *meningitis* has been reported among HIV-positive patients, often in conjunction with *diffuse lymphadenopathy* and representing the first manifestation of AIDS. The occurrence of extrapulmonary TB in patients with HIV infection fulfills the criteria for the diagnosis of AIDS.

In HIV-infected patients with disseminated disease, the purified protein derivative (PPD) skin test is often negative. Chest x-rays are normal in more than 10 percent of patients. When infiltrates do occur, they are often nonspecific and involve the lower lobes. Despite these atypical features, the diagnosis can usually be established, if suspected, without much difficulty by visualizing or culturing the causative organism from the sputum or extrapulmonary sites.

Atypical Mycobacterial Infection. Clinical infection with *atypical mycobacteria* is not seen often in primary care practice. Representative syndromes caused by these organisms include cervical adenitis in children (scrofula), pulmonary infection, and cutaneous disease (swimming pool granuloma). Disseminated disease occasionally takes place in immunosuppressed individuals. For example, *Mycobacterium avium-intracellulare* has been a major problem causing disseminated infection in patients with AIDS. Unlike tuberculous infection in HIV-positive patients, which can occur in the early stages of illness, *M. avium-intracellulare* infection does not cause disseminated disease until late.

DIAGNOSIS

The tuberculin *skin test* is the most sensitive test for diagnosis of infection with *M. tuberculosis* (see Chapter 38); it is far more sensitive than the chest x-ray. A positive tuberculin test does not by itself prove there is active disease but does indicate that infection has occurred. Negative tuberculin reactions have been documented in 20 percent of patients with TB, particularly those individuals with overwhelming or advanced disease, malnutrition, and debility. In HIV-positive patients, especially those with low CD4+ counts, false-negative skin-test rates have been as high as 50 percent. Many of these individuals are anergic, so that simultaneous skin testing with *Candida*, mumps, tetanus toxoid, or streptokinase-streptodornase antigens can be useful in demonstrating overall immunologic impairment. The Centers for Disease Control and Prevention (CDC) recommends anergy testing for interpretation of tuberculin testing in all HIV-infected persons, using two antigens in addition to PPD (see Chapter 38).

When there is active pulmonary disease, the diagnosis of pulmonary TB can usually be confirmed by examination of the *sputum*, taking precautions to *avoid spread of organisms during efforts to obtain sputum*. If patients are not able to produce sputum spontaneously, attempts should be made to *induce sputum* with the aid of hydration, pulmonary physiotherapy, intermittent positive-pressure breathing (IPPB), and mucolytic agents. *Bronchoscopy* or *bronchoalveolar lavage* may be necessary for obtaining appropriate specimens. Although *cultures* are necessary for a positive diagnosis and are more sensitive than smears, sputum specimens should be examined microscopically either by the traditional *Ziehl-Neelsen (acid-fast) stain*, or by the newer Truant *fluorescent stain*. Sputum or bronchoscopic washings should be examined both directly and after concentration by centrifugation and digestion. Carefully collected individual specimens are preferred to a 24-hour pool of sputum and saliva. Cultures of first morning fasting *gastric aspirates* are also helpful. Because gastric acid is toxic to mycobacteria, the collection bottles should contain a buffer such as sodium bicarbonate. Smears of gastric juice are misleading, because of the potential presence of saprophytic mycobacteria, and should not be performed.

Tissue biopsy is often required for diagnosis of tuberculous pleurisy or extrapulmonary disease, because sputum and gastric samples are usually negative for organisms in these situations.

PRINCIPLES OF TREATMENT

Prophylaxis in Uninfected Individuals. In many parts of the world where tuberculosis is common, bacille Calmette-Guérin (BCG) vaccine is used for the prevention of primary infection. It is intended only for prophylaxis and should not be given to patients with positive skin tests (see Chapter 38). Because the incidence of tuberculosis is relatively low in the United States, BCG is not routinely recommended in this country. Close contacts of patients with active pulmonary tuberculosis should be considered for *isoniazid (INH)* therapy, particularly if they are children, adolescents, nursing home residents, or immunocompromised individuals (see Chapter 38).

Prophylaxis in Tuberculin Converters and Those with Latent Disease. Prevention of active tuberculosis can be achieved with INH. An estimate of the risk of reactivation of tuberculosis needs to be weighed against the chances of drug-induced hepatitis (see Appendix) to select patients for INH prophylaxis (see Chapter 38 for detailed guidelines). Patients with a positive skin test should be evaluated to exclude active infection. One needs to check for cough, fever, sputum production, pleuritic chest pain, lymphadenopathy, meningeal irritation, pleural effusion, pulmonary consolidation, and enlargement of the liver or spleen. A chest x-ray is essential, and complete blood count, differential, urinalysis, and liver function tests (particularly the alkaline phosphatase) may provide clues of active disease (eg, "sterile" pyuria or isolated alkaline phosphatase elevation). If no active infection is identified, the patient should be reassured, and the potential risks and benefits of INH therapy should be explained so the patient can participate in therapeutic decisions.

Treatment of Patients with Active Tuberculosis. Antituberculous drugs are the cornerstone of therapy. Because the patient will be noncontagious shortly after starting therapy, most treatment can be administered on an outpatient basis after a brief period in the hospital. The chemotherapy of tuberculosis is different from other antimicrobial programs and proceeds according to a unique set of principles:

1. Multidrug regimens and completion of a full course of therapy are necessary to prevent the emergence of drug-resistant organisms.
2. Single daily dosages are preferred.
3. Prolonged chemotherapy is necessary. With combinations of newer agents, shorter regimens of 6 to 9 months have been found to be effective. However, HIV-infected persons require treatment for 1 year or longer. When INH and rifampin cannot be used simultaneously because of patient intolerance or drug resistance, older, more prolonged regimens of 18 to 24 months are necessary.
4. Supervised, twice-weekly regimens provide a reasonable treatment alternative for the noncompliant patient.
5. No matter what regimen is chosen, it is important to follow patients closely to ensure compliance and to monitor for drug efficacy and toxicity.
6. Because chemotherapy will control the organisms, surgery is reserved for the treatment of complications such as restrictive pericardial scarring.
7. Elaborate programs of rest and diet have no place in modern treatment of tuberculosis.
8. Prolonged surveillance beyond 1 year after completion of a full course of therapy is generally not necessary due to the efficacy of current chemotherapeutic regimens; however, immunosuppressed patients and those with drug-resistant organisms require more prolonged follow-up.

Most patients with clinically active pulmonary tuberculosis should be hospitalized for the initial phases of therapy. As little as 2 weeks of multidrug therapy will greatly decrease the infectiousness of these patients, although a few mycobacteria may still be present on sputum smears or cultures. Hence, short-term admission to a general hospital is preferred, with early home care for patients who are reliable and clinically stable. Patients with extrapulmonary tuberculosis are much less infectious and can sometimes be managed entirely as outpatients.

CASE REPORTING AND PATIENT EDUCATION

All cases of tuberculosis should be reported promptly to public health authorities, so that contacts can be investigated and appropriate control measures can be instituted. However, it must be remembered that, particularly in elderly patients, the diagnosis of tuberculosis still carries social stigma and dire prognostic implications. Reassurance and education are therefore of great importance. It should be stressed that tuberculosis occurs in all social and economic classes, that modern chemotherapy is truly curative, and that prolonged periods of hospitalization and isolation are no longer necessary.

Patients who are candidates for INH prophylaxis should understand the risks and benefits of INH therapy. If INH therapy is recommended and accepted, the patient should be instructed to discontinue the medication and report to the physician if adverse effects are noted, including skin rash, fever, fatigue, anorexia, abdominal distress, jaundice, or peripheral neuropathic symptoms. The importance of full compliance with the drug regimen, be it for prophylaxis or treatment of active disease, must be stressed.

THERAPEUTIC RECOMMENDATIONS

Prophylaxis

For more information, see Chapter 38.

- The decision to use INH for prophylaxis involves weighing the risk of drug-induced hepatotoxicity (see Appendix at the end of this chapter) against the benefit of preventing active disease. The older the patient, the greater the risk of hepatitis, although the benefit usually outweighs risk, especially in populations with a high incidence of infection and active disease. (See Chapter 38 for detailed guidelines.)
- Prompt diagnosis and institution of an effective, individualized treatment program are essential to preventing spread of disease and emergence of resistant organisms. Of particular importance is the early recognition of TB in HIV-infected patients. A high index of suspicion and an awareness of its potentially atypical presentations (eg, disseminated disease, meningitis) are essential.

Active Disease

- Patients with active disease require *combination chemotherapy*. Those with mild to moderate pulmonary or extrapulmonary disease can be treated with either of two regimens: 1) *INH plus rifampin* taken daily for 9 months; or 2) *INH, rifampin, and pyrazinamide* daily for 2 months followed by 4 months more of daily INH and rifampin. The relapse rates and toxicities are similar for both. The latter program produces more rapid sputum conversion and achieves greater patient compliance.

- For *immunosuppressed patients* (such as those who are HIV-positive) and for patients with advanced pulmonary or extrapulmonary disease, it is desirable to initiate chemotherapy with at least *three drugs. INH and rifampin plus pyrazinamide or ethambutol* may be used in these circumstances. If the clinical response is favorable, it is reasonable to simplify the program to INH and rifampin after 2 or 3 months; however, therapy should be continued for a total of 1 year, especially in HIV-infected patients.
- Patients who have failed previous chemotherapy and those who have immigrated from Latin America and Southeast Asia within the past 15 years are at high risk of harboring *drug-resistant organisms*. Such organisms are more likely to be resistant to INH and streptomycin than to rifampin or ethambutol. Consequently, such patients should be treated with *INH, rifampin, ethambutol, and possibly pyrazinamide* until the results of sensitivity testing are available.
- If INH and rifampin cannot be administered simultaneously because of patient intolerance or drug resistance, multiple drug therapy should be continued for 18 to 24 months. Treatment programs should be individualized on the basis of the patient's tolerance and the organism's sensitivities. Ideally, INH or rifampin should be administered with pyrazinamide or ethambutol. *Streptomycin* is also helpful for initial therapy, but the need for intramuscular administration and its vestibular toxicity limit patient acceptance of long-term use.
- *Noncompliant patients* may benefit from intermittent chemotherapy administered under *direct medical supervision*. Many regimens are available. One calls for daily INH, rifampin, and pyrazinamide for 2 months, followed by *high-dose INH* (900 mg) and *conventional-dose rifampin* (600 mg) administered under direct observation *twice weekly* for an additional 4 months.
- For use in *pregnancy,* INH, rifampin, and ethambutol all appear to be safe.
- After completion of therapy, all patients should be followed for 1 year, monitoring for evidence of recurrence. Longer follow-up is appropriate for those with drug-resistant organisms and HIV-positivity, and suspected poor compliance.
- *Hospitalization* should be considered in the *initial stages of active pulmonary disease* to minimize risk of spread. Two weeks of chemotherapy usually suffice to render the patient noninfectious.
- With the exception of *M. kansasii* and *M. marinum,* the majority of atypical mycobacteria are drug resistant, making therapy difficult. So-called second-line antituberculous agents are sometimes necessary (see Appendix). Consultation with a specialist in mycobacterial disease is indicated.

Appendix: Antituberculous Chemotherapeutic Agents

Isoniazid (INH). Introduced into clinical use in the early 1950s, INH remains the single most important antituberculous drug. Of importance is the excellent tissue penetration of this small, water-soluble molecule. The distribution of INH includes the central nervous system (CNS), tuberculous abscesses, and intracellular sites. The major metabolism of INH is by hepatic acetylation. Although metabolites are excreted by the kidneys, it is not necessary to modify INH doses except in advanced renal failure. INH is available both orally and parenterally; it is an inexpensive drug. The usual dose is 5 mg per kilogram of body weight, which averages 300 mg per day for the adult. For initial therapy of life-threatening disease, doses of 10 to 15 mg per kilogram per day may be used.

The major adverse effects of INH include:

- *Neurotoxicity,* ranging from peripheral neuropathy (which can be prevented by administration of 50 mg of pyridoxine daily) to much less common manifestations, including encephalopathy, seizures, optic neuritis, and personality changes.
- *Hypersensitivity* reactions including fever, rash, and rheumatic syndromes with or without positive antinuclear antibodies.
- *Hepatocellular injury,* including serious clinical hepatitis in less than 2 percent, but a transient, clinically insignificant rise in transaminase in 10 percent to 20 percent. Risk of clinically significant hepatitis increases with age.

The U.S. Public Health Service does not recommend routine *transaminase (SGOT/ALT)* determinations in individuals who are reliable and who are able to comply with directions for reporting symptoms of hepatitis. However, transaminase determinations can be helpful, particularly insofar as they give the physician an opportunity to reinforce instructions and also because the surveillance is reassuring to most patients. The problem with following the transaminase level is that between 10 percent and 20 percent of individuals receiving INH can be expected to show mild transient elevations, which will return to normal even during continued therapy and are of no clinical significance.

Although precise data are lacking, a reasonable approach is to routinely determine the transaminase at monthly intervals for the first 3 months of therapy, because most elevations develop during this period. In symptomatic patients with an elevated transaminase, INH should be discontinued and liver function tests should be monitored. In asymptomatic individuals with a mild elevation (up to 2.5 times normal), the drug can be continued, but the patient should be monitored weekly. If the transaminase fails to return to normal in 3 to 4 weeks, it seems prudent to discontinue the INH. On the other hand, even if a patient is asymptomatic, a single, more substantial transaminase elevation may be grounds to discontinue the agent. Again, it must be emphasized that these are "rules of thumb" rather than precise guidelines.

Rifampin is a major antituberculous drug and rivals INH in its efficacy. Rifampin is a large, fat-soluble molecule that achieves excellent tissue penetration, including into the CNS. The drug is excreted by the liver; modification of dosage is not required in renal failure but may be necessary in hepatic insufficiency. It is available in both oral and parenteral formulations. The average adult dose is 600 mg per day, taken once daily. Unlike INH and ethambutol, rifampin is actually a broad-spectrum antimicrobial, acting against some atypical mycobacteria, *M. leprae,* many bacteria (including staphylococci, meningococci, and various gram-negative bacilli), trachoma agent, and some viruses. Patients should be cautioned to expect *orange discoloration of urine, sweat,* tears, and saliva, which is of no clinical significance.

Toxicities include *hypersensitivity* reactions (fever, rash, or eosinophilia), *hematologic* toxicities (thrombocytopenia, leukopenia, and hemolytic anemia), and *hepatitis,* including elevated transaminases in up to 10 percent. Drug interactions occur; rifampin antagonizes the effect of warfarin, quinidine, oral contraceptives, and methadone. Rifampin should never be used in high-dose intermittent therapy because toxic reactions (including hemolytic anemia, thrombocytopenia, and hepatic failure) occur frequently. However, use of intermittent therapy (600 mg given twice weekly) appears to be well tolerated. Rifampin is expensive.

Pyrazinamide, a derivative of nicotinic acid, was introduced in 1952, but was not widely used until its incorporation into short-course regimens in the 1980s. Like INH and rifampin, it is bactericidal, a major asset in short-course therapy. The drug is well absorbed from the gastrointestinal (GI) tract and is widely distributed in body tissues and fluids, including the cerebrospinal fluid. It is excreted by mixed hepatic and renal mechanisms. Major toxicities are hepatic dysfunction, hyperuricemia, and hypersensitivity. The usual dose is 20 to 35 mg per kilogram per day (maximum: 3 g).

Ethambutol was introduced clinically in the United States in 1967 and represented a major advance in antituberculous chemotherapy. Although ethambutol penetrates tissues well—including the CNS when the meninges are inflamed—it is not bactericidal; it is only bacteriostatic. The drug is excreted by the kidneys. Dose modification in renal failure should be based on serum ethambutol levels (available through the manufacturer) and monitored in patients with renal failure who require the drug. The major toxicities of ethambutol include hypersensitivity reactions, such as fever and rash, and optic neuritis, which is dose related and usually manifested first by a loss of color vision. Less common side effects include neuritis, GI intolerance, headache, and hyperuricemia. The cost of ethambutol is moderate. The usual dose is 15 mg per kilogram per day; 25 mg per kilogram per day may be used for the first 2 months. Color vision and visual acuity should be monitored periodically because of a small risk of retinal injury; for this reason the drug is usually not administered to young children.

Streptomycin, the first effective antituberculous drug, remains useful. Like other aminoglycosides, streptomycin has only a fair tissue distribution, being inactive at an alkaline pH in an anaerobic milieu and penetrating the cerebrospinal fluid very poorly. It must be given parenterally. Streptomycin is excreted by the kidneys, and dosage should be reduced in patients with renal failure. Major toxicities include hypersensitivity reactions and *eighth nerve toxicity,* especially to the vestibular division, resulting in vertigo. The cost of streptomycin is moderate. The drug is active against a variety of organisms in addition to *M. tuberculosis,* although many gram-negative bacilli have become resistant due to widespread use over many years.

The "Second-Line" Antituberculous Drugs tend to be both less effective and more toxic than the standard agents, but occasionally are of critical importance in patients with drug-resistant tuberculosis or atypical mycobacterial infection, and in those who cannot tolerate the standard therapies. Three of these agents are administered orally, including *para-aminosalicylic acid (PAS), ethionamide,* and *cycloserine.* For many years, PAS was considered a first-line drug, but its relatively weak tuberculostatic action and very high incidence of GI intolerance has relegated it to a secondary role. Two other drugs available parenterally—kanamycin and capreomycin—are pharmacologically similar to streptomycin.

Newer Drugs. With the emergence of new multidrug-resistant strains comes an accelerated search for new antituberculous agents. Several fluoroquinolone antibiotics have shown activity against *M. tuberculosis,* including *ciprofloxacin.* The drug has also shown activity against strains of *M. intracellulare,* the cause of serious infection in patients with advanced AIDS.

ANNOTATED BIBLIOGRAPHY

American Thoracic Society. Diagnosis and treatment of disease caused by nontuberculous mycobacteria. Am Rev Respir Disease 1990;142:940. *(Excellent review and approach to atypical mycobacterial infections.)*

Berenguer J, Moreno S, Laguna F, et al. Tuberculous meningitis in patients infected with the human immunodeficiency virus. N Engl J Med 1992;326:668. *(HIV-infected patients are at an increased risk for TB meningitis.)*

Cohn DL, Catlin BJ, Peterson KL, et al. A 62-dose, 6-month therapy for pulmonary and extrapulmonary tuberculosis: a twice-weekly, directly observed, and cost-effective regimen. Ann Intern Med 1990;112:407. *(Demonstrates efficacy of a strategy for poorly compliant patients.)*

Combs DL, O'Brien RJ, Geiter LJ. USPHS tuberculosis short-course chemotherapy trial 21: Effectiveness, toxicity, and acceptability. Ann Intern Med 1990;112:397. *(A 6-month regimen of INH and rifampin plus pyrazinamide during the first 8 weeks was similar in outcome measures to a 9-month regimen of only INH and rifampin.)*

Davidson PT. Treating tuberculosis: What drugs, for how long? Ann Intern Med 1990;112:393. *(Editorial reviewing shorter-course regimens.)*

Dooley SW, Jarvis WR, Martone WJ, et al. Multidrug-resistant tuberculosis. Ann Intern Med 1992;117:3. *(Editorial summing up current knowledge of this serious condition and approaches to coping with it.)*

Edlin BR, Tokars JI, Grieco MH, et al. An outbreak of multidrug-resistant tuberculosis among hospitalized patients with the acquired immunodeficiency syndrome. N Engl J Med 1992;

326:1514. *(Documents nosocomial transmission of multidrug-resistant infection among AIDS patients.)*

Frieden TR, Sterling T, Pablos-Mendez A, et al. Emergence of drug-resistant tuberculosis in New York City. N Engl J Med 1993;328:521. *(High prevalence among those who are HIV-positive, IV drug abusers, or previously treated.)*

Goble M, Iseman MD, Madsen LA, et al. Treatment of 171 patients with pulmonary tuberculosis resistant to isoniazid and rifampin. N Engl J Med 1993;328:527. *(Overall response rate is only about 50 percent; risk proportional to number of drugs received before current therapy.)*

Horsburgh CR. *Mycobacterium avium* complex infection in the acquired immunodeficiency syndrome. N Engl J Med 1991; 324:1332. *(Review of this important opportunistic mycobacterial infection in AIDS patients.)*

Kramer F, Modilevsky T, Waliany AR, et al. Delayed diagnosis of tuberculosis in patients with human immunodeficiency virus infection. Am J Med 1990;89:451. *(Delay in therapy was common among patients with HIV infection; high index of suspicion needed.)*

Small PM, Schecter GF, Goodman PC, et al. Treatment of tuberculosis in patients with advanced human immunodeficiency virus infection. N Engl J Med 1991;324:289. *(Conventional therapy was effective in sterilizing the sputum, improving the chest x-ray, and preventing relapse.)*

Snider DE, Roper WL. The new tuberculosis. N Engl J Med 1992;326:703. *(Editorial addressing the emergence of drug-resistant strains and the rapid transmission of infection among HIV-infected patients.)*

Stead WW. Pathogenesis of the sporadic case of tuberculosis. N Engl J Med 1967;277:1008. *(Lucid and important overview of the "unitary concept" of the pathogenesis of TB. This excellent paper clarifies relationship among primary infection, inactive disease, and reactivation tuberculosis.)*

Stead WW, Kerby GR, Schlueter DP, et al. The clinical spectrum of primary tuberculosis in adults. Ann Intern Med 1968, 68:73. *(Classic clinical study of primary TB, which includes an excellent summary of the wide spectrum of events that may occur after initial infection by* M. tuberculosis.*)*

Stead WW, Lofgren JP, Warren E, et al. Tuberculosis as an endemic and nosocomial infection among the elderly in nursing homes. New Engl J Med 1985;312:1483. *(Exogenous infection can occur in the elderly and nosocomial TB may be an important problem in nursing homes.)*

Stead WW, To T, Harrison RW, et al. Benefit–risk considerations in preventive treatment for tuberculosis in elderly persons. Ann Intern Med 1987;107:843. *(INH treatment of nursing home patients who had definite skin test conversions was beneficial and outweighed the risk of hepatitis.)*

50
Management of the Common Cold

HARVEY B. SIMON, M.D.

Primary Care Medicine: Office Evaluation and Management of the Adult Patient, 3rd edition, edited by Allan H. Goroll, Lawrence A. May, and Albert G. Mulley, Jr. J.B. Lippincott Company, Philadelphia

Upper respiratory tract infections are among the most frequent reasons for office visits; nevertheless, physicians see only a small fraction of patients with such problems, because most treat their symptoms at home with over-the-counter remedies or simply wait for the illness to pass by itself. Upper respiratory infections (URIs) are the leading cause of absenteeism, accounting for an average of almost 7 days lost from work per person per year. Although a viral etiology accounts for the overwhelming proportion of cases, the physician must be alert for specifically treatable bacterial processes. In addition, familiarity with agents available for symptomatic relief is necessary because patients turn to their physicians when home remedies fail to help.

PATHOPHYSIOLOGY AND CLINICAL PRESENTATION

The upper respiratory tract is composed of two distinct types of epithelial surfaces. The oropharynx and nasopharynx are lined by a stratified squamous epithelium and are normally teeming with a varied microbial flora. In addition, many potentially pathogenic bacteria can temporarily reside on these epithelial surfaces as "colonizers" without causing true infection. With a few exceptions, such as herpes simplex and Epstein-Barr virus, viruses are not usually long-term members of the normal flora of the respiratory tract.

Numerous host defense mechanisms protect the upper airway from infection. Mechanical defenses tend to prevent penetration of organisms from the nasopharynx and oral cavity into more vulnerable areas. These defenses include the cough, gag, and sneeze reflexes, viscous mucous secretions entrap particulate material, and ciliary action propels such particles outward. In addition, local immunologic defenses attempt to deal with organisms that have breached the mechanical barriers. These defenses include lymphoid tissue, secretory IgA antibodies in respiratory secretions, and a rich vasculature capable of rapidly delivering phagocytic leukocytes.

The common cold is caused by viral agents (although about 30% of pharyngitis cases are chlamydial in origin and another 5% to 10% each are due to mycoplasma and group A streptococcus; see Chapter 220). *Rhinoviruses* are the most common viral agent associated with upper respiratory tract illness. Because there are over 110 antigenic serotypes, there is no cross-immunity and reinfection with another serotype right after a recent cold is common.

Mechanisms of transmission include *aerosolization* of virus-laden respiratory secretions, and direct *mucous membrane contact* with virus from contaminated hands, other skin surfaces, and even table tops. Touching one's eyes or nose effects the inoculation. The timeless motherly warning that "you'll catch cold if you get wet or damp" has not been borne out by experimental study; at least such conditions are not sufficient in themselves to cause illness. However, there is evidence from prospective controlled study suggesting that *psychological stress* can increase the risk of infection, although the effect is not great.

Numerous viral agents including rhinoviruses, respiratory syncytial virus, adenoviruses, influenza viruses, and parainfluenza viruses can cause an identical clinical picture. Incubation periods for viral URIs range from 1 to 5 days; virus shedding lasts up to 2 weeks. Typical symptoms include coryza, pharyngitis, laryngitis, headache, malaise, and fever, in various combinations. Ear and sinus discomfort are often present as well, but these symptoms are caused by mucosal edema, which impairs drainage, rather than by acute viral infection of these regions (see Chapters 218 and 219).

Whether known as the common cold, nasopharyngitis, or URI, these problems generally resolve spontaneously. Common viral URIs rarely progress to pneumonia; most colds resolve spontaneously within 1 week, although symptoms may linger for several weeks.

PRINCIPLES OF MANAGEMENT

Prevention. The best things one can do to avoid "catching" a cold are to avoid aerosol exposure, wash hands, and keep hands away from mucous membranes (conjunctivae, nasal and oral mucosae). Gargling with "antiseptic" mouthwash is of no benefit. Initial studies on use of inhaled alpha$_2$-interferon showed promising results for prevention of rhinovirus infection, but such approaches remain experimental. The enthusiasm that surrounded use of high-dose vitamin C (ascorbic acid) for prophylaxis waned as controlled studies failed to demonstrate efficacy. Similarly, zinc lozenges proved no better than placebo in controlled trials.

Symptomatic Relief. Therapeutic efforts are directed toward relieving nasal congestion, headache, and grippelike symptoms and preventing complications such as otitis, sinusitis, and lower respiratory tract infection. Millions of dollars are spent annually on over-the-counter cold remedies. Most contain a combination of ingredients, including antihistamines, sympathomimetic amines, and analgesics. Some even contain more than one antihistamine or sympathomimetic. Antitussives, caffeine, vitamin C, belladonna alkaloids, and expectorants are common additives as well. Antacids, laxatives, quinine, and papaverine are occasionally found.

Decongestants can be helpful not only for providing symptomatic relief, but also for preventing sinus and eustachian tube obstruction that could result in sinusitis and otitis media, respectively. *Alpha-adrenergic agents* are the most commonly used decongestants. They work by causing generalized vasoconstriction and thus reducing formation of secretions. Because they produce systemic vasoconstriction, sympathomimetics may raise blood pressure when used in doses sufficient to alleviate nasal congestion. There is no oral adrenergic agent that provides selective local vasoconstriction; *nasal sprays* are more effective for this purpose but may be associated with rebound congestion after the drug effect subsides, leading to abuse of the spray. According to most authorities, nasal sprays are good for short-term therapy, whereas oral preparations are better when use is to continue longer than 10 days, because chronic spray applications interfere with ciliary action and irritate and dry the nasal mucosa, producing swelling.

Analgesics are useful for relief of the headache, fever, and achiness that often accompany a cold. *Aspirin* and *acetaminophen* have similar analgesic and antipyretic effects and are key ingredients in the combination cold remedies. However, both have been found capable of delaying the immune response to experimental rhinovirus infection and causing a slight increase in nasal signs and symptoms, although neither prolongs viral shedding. Nonprescription doses of *ibuprofen* showed similar effects, though *naproxen* did not. All remain clinically useful for symptomatic relief of the headache, myalgias, and fever that may accompany a cold. Salicylate derivatives such as salicylamide are sometimes used, although they are much less effective than aspirin. Of all analgesics, plain aspirin is, by far, the least costly; the other agents can be expensive.

Expectorants are included in many preparations in the belief that they stimulate the flow of mucus. There is no evidence to support this view, although these agents are widely prescribed and requested by patients. More important is adequate *hydration*. Hydration helps loosen secretions and prevent upper airway obstruction and the complications that may ensue from it. *Warm fluids* (including tea and, yes, chicken soup) can increase the rate of mucous flow, providing some symptomatic relief, as can *inhaling steam* (another of grandmother's remedies), or using a dilute saline nasal spray.

Research suggesting that increasing nasal mucosa temperature to 37°C could limit viral replication and decrease nasal congestion led to renewed interest in inhalation of warm humidified air. Double-blinded study of inhaling steam through use of an active device showed no significant benefit over placebo therapy, although both were associated with considerable subjective improvement. An expensive heated nebulizer device (the Viralizer) has been heavily promoted as a means of promptly and completely relieving cold symptoms, especially if supplemented by hexylresorcinol or phenylephrine sprays introduced into the nebulizer. Controlled study has failed to confirm such excessive claims.

Cough suppressants, including narcotics such as *codeine* and non-narcotic agents such as *dextromethorphan,* are effective and useful symptomatically, especially in allowing the patient to sleep uninterrupted by cough. In many patients, a decongestant is even more effective in suppressing cough, because postnasal drip accounts for much of the cough stimulus. These agents are commonly available in combination with expectorants, although they may be prescribed alone, thereby saving the patient money.

Antihistamines exert an atropine-like drying effect, which might actually exacerbate symptoms of congestion and cause upper airway obstruction by impairing flow of mucus. Use of these agents for a cold is *irrational,* because cold symptoms have no allergic mechanism. Nonetheless, nonprescription antihistamines are widely consumed, especially as combination cold remedies. Sedation is a major side effect of most nonprescription over-the-counter antihistamines and probably their only benefit to patients suffering from a cold. Prescription antihistamines have no place in the treatment of colds.

Atropine, laxatives, caffeine, and antacids are present in subtherapeutic doses in combination preparations; they have little impact on symptoms and only increase costs. As noted above, the vitamin C included has not been shown to have any effect, even when given in gram doses.

PATIENT EDUCATION

Among the most frustrating experiences in primary care practice is the request by patients suffering from a cold for *antibiotics*. Explaining that antibiotics have no role in an uncomplicated viral URI can be time-consuming at best and has the potential to develop into a power struggle. A proactive approach is to send educational materials to patients at the beginning of the URI season. Pamphlets and other informational materials are much appreciated by patients and can help cut down on unnecessary visits and telephone calls. They should include helpful hints at self-care and the indications for seeking medical attention (eg, high fever, marked pain or tenderness in an ear or sinus, increasingly purulent sputum, dyspnea, pleuritic chest pain). In addition, the role of antibiotics in treatment of viral URI should be reviewed (ie, only for complications such as otitis and sinusitis) as well as the risks of unnecessary antibiotic therapy (eg, allergic reactions, alteration of bacterial flora, emergence of resistant strains). Unnecessary office visits and telephone calls have been reduced by as much as 30 percent to 40 percent through well-designed educational efforts.

If all else fails, one can call the pharmacist and prescribe an antibiotic appropriate for treatment of a URI complication such as sinusitis or otitis media (eg, amoxicillin), but with instructions to dispense only if the patient develops clear-cut symptoms of such a complication (eg, marked sinus tenderness or ear pain accompanied by fever; see Chapters 218 and 219).

THERAPEUTIC RECOMMENDATIONS

Prevention is difficult, but hand washing, keeping fingers away from mucous membranes, and avoidance of droplet exposure might help. Relief from cold symptoms and avoidance of complications are facilitated by rest, fluids, aspirin, and perhaps inhalation of steam. A cough suppressant before bed (eg, 15 mg codeine sulfate) and a nasal decongestant spray (eg, phenylephrine; see Chapter 219) may aid in symptomatic management and are superior to expensive combination agents, which often contain irrational mixtures or subtherapeutic doses of active ingredients. Proactive patient education just before the beginning of the cold season may help reduce unnecessary office visits, telephone calls, and requests for antibiotics. Vitamin C has no proven role in prevention or alleviation of symptoms. Antihistamines and antibiotics are of no use in an uncomplicated viral URI.

ANNOTATED BIBLIOGRAPHY

Cohen S, Tyrrell DAJ, Smith AP. Psychological stress and susceptibility to the common cold. N Engl J Med 1991;325:606. *(Careful, controlled, prospective study showing a significant, although not particularly strong relation between stress and risk of getting a cold.)*

Coulehan JL, Eberhard S, Kapner L, et al. Vitamin C and acute illness in Navajo schoolchildren. N Engl J Med 1976;295:973. *(Double-blind placebo-controlled trial in 868 schoolchildren, failing to show prophylactic or therapeutic benefit.)*

Douglas RG, Lindgren KM, Couch RB. Exposure to cold environment and rhinovirus common cold. N Engl J Med 1968; 279:742. *(Your mother is wrong! Exposure to moisture and cold does not increase susceptibility to URIs, at least not in this study of volunteers experimentally infected with rhinovirus.)*

Douglass RM, Moore BW, Miles HB, et al. Prophylactic efficacy of intranasal alpha$_2$-interferon against rhinovirus infections in the family setting. *(Report on this experimental use of interferon for prevention of colds; worked only for rhinovirus disease.)*

Gaffey MJ, Kaiser DL, Hayden FG. Ineffectiveness of oral terfenadine in natural colds. Pediatr Inf Dis J 1988;7:223. *(No benefit in controlled study; histamine is not a mediator of cold symptoms.)*

Garibaldi RA. Epidemiology of community-acquired respiratory tract infections in adults. Am J Med 1985;78(6B):32. *(Good review of epidemiology and pathophysiology of URIs.)*

Graham NMH, Burrell CJ, Douglas RM, et al. Adverse effects of aspirin, acetaminophen, and ibuprofen on immune function, viral shedding, and clinical status in rhinovirus-infected volunteers. J Infect Dis 1990;162:1277. *(Documents modest reductions in immune function and slight increases in symptoms; no effect on virus shedding.)*

Lanc RS, Barsky AJ, Goodson JD. Discomfort and disability in upper respiratory tract infection. J Gen Intern Med 1988;3: 540. *(Severity of symptoms was linked in part to the patient's emotional state.)*

Macknin ML, Mathew S, Medendorp SVB. Effect of inhaling heated vapor on symptoms of the common cold. JAMA 1990; 264:989. *(No benefit over control group, although both showed improvement.)*

Oral cold remedies. Medical Letter 1975;17:89. *(Critiques over-the-counter oral cold remedies and warns against their high cost, irrational combination of agents, and frequent use of subtherapeutic doses of active ingredients.)*

Simon HB. The immunology of exercise: A brief review. JAMA 1984;252:2735. *(Your mother is wrong again! There is no evidence that exercise lowers "resistance" to respiratory or other infection; nor is it protective.)*

Sperber SJ, Hendley JO, Hayden FG, et al. Effects of naproxen on experimental rhinovirus colds. Ann Intern Med 1992; 117:37. *(Beneficial effect on headache, malaise, myalgia, and cough; no effect on virus shedding or antibody response.)*

Stergachis A, Newmann WE, Williams KJ, et al. The effect of self-care minimal intervention for colds and flu on the use of medical services. J Gen Intern Med 1990;5:23. *(Simple self-care pamphlet did not affect medical utilization, but includes an excellent discussion of other such interventions that did.)*

Tyrrell D, Barrow I, Arthur J. Local hyperthermia benefits natural and experimental common colds. BMJ 1989;298:1280. *(Raising nasal temperature decreased symptoms and viral replication.)*

Primary Care Medicine: Office Evaluation and Management of the Adult Patient, 3rd edition, edited by Allan H. Goroll, Lawrence A. May, and Albert G. Mulley, Jr. J.B. Lippincott Company, Philadelphia

51
Management of Sarcoidosis

HARVEY B. SIMON, M.D.

Sarcoidosis is a disease characterized by formation of noncaseating granulomas, particularly in the lung but also occurring throughout the body. The precise etiology remains unknown, but activation of T-cell lymphocytes in the lung plays an important role in the pathogenesis of granuloma formation. In the United States, sarcoidosis is ten times more prevalent in African Americans than whites; people of Scandinavian descent also have a high incidence of the disease. Females outnumber males. Onset is most often between ages 20 and 45.

Although a large percentage of patients with sarcoidosis are asymptomatic, diverse and clinically important syndromes do result. Granuloma formation in the lung can be especially damaging, as can involvement in a number of other organ systems (eg, eye, gastrointestinal tract). Once diagnosis is established, the prime management decision regards need for corticosteroid therapy. Improved methods of monitoring disease activity have enhanced the clinician's ability to treat sarcoidosis effectively, while minimizing the risk of adverse effects from long-term steroids. The primary physician needs to know the most efficacious means of establishing the diagnosis, determining disease activity, and deciding on the need for and duration of therapy with systemic steroids.

PATHOPHYSIOLOGY, CLINICAL PRESENTATION, AND COURSE

Pathophysiology. The cause of sarcoidosis is unknown. A variety of infectious and exogenous agents have been suggested as inciting factors, but whether one or several agents are involved remains conjectural. It is suspected that the granulomas and inflammatory reactions of sarcoidosis are due to an abnormal immunologic response to a provocative agent in susceptible hosts.

Although the etiology of sarcoidosis is unknown, the pathogenesis of its granulomatous inflammation is being clarified. Bronchoalveolar lavage studies reveal that the early stage of pulmonary sarcoid consists of an alveolitis, with an increased number of T-lymphocytes. Helper T-cells predominate, and there are an increased number of "activated" lymphocytes capable of secreting various soluble mediators or lymphokines, which may recruit monocytes and transform them into the macrophages of granulomas. The alveolitis of early disease and subsequent granulomatous inflammation are reversible, either spontaneously or with corticosteroid therapy, but the fibrosis that characterizes advanced chronic sarcoidosis is irreversible once it forms.

In contrast to the increased numbers and activity of helper T-cells in the lungs, the peripheral blood of patients with sarcoidosis may show a decreased number of T-lymphocytes; this may account for the depressed cell-mediated immunity and cutaneous anergy observed in many such patients. However, the blood of patients with sarcoid often reflects increased activity of B-lymphocytes, accounting for the hypergammaglobulinemia and elevated antibody levels and circulating immune complexes that are often observed.

The granulomas of pulmonary sarcoidosis often resolve spontaneously, leaving the lung morphologically unscathed. However, in about 20 percent of patients, the process is more destructive and is characterized by interstitial fibrosis, obliteration of capillaries, and destruction of pulmonary architecture. The end stage is formation of cystic spaces interspersed with bands of connective tissue.

Clinical manifestations of sarcoidosis reflect the sites of granulomatous inflammation. The most common presentation, especially in young adults, is *bilateral hilar adenopathy,* which occurs in 50 percent of patients and is often detected on routine chest x-ray. About 25 percent present with bilateral hilar adenopathy and *pulmonary infiltrates,* and 15 percent present with infiltrates alone. Disease in the hilum is not associated with invasion or compression of bronchi or nodal calcification. *Erythema nodosum* or *uveitis* (manifested by red, watery eyes) may accompany hilar adenopathy. Some patients complain of *cough, shortness of breath, wheezing,* or chest discomfort, as well as constitutional symptoms of *fever, malaise,* and *fatigue.*

Although pulmonary symptoms are the most frequent, sarcoidosis may present with extrathoracic disease, including *hepatomegaly, splenomegaly,* or uveitis. Other presenting manifestations include *fever of unknown origin,* granulomatous *hepatitis,* salivary and lacrimal gland enlargement, *arthritis,* peripheral *adenopathy,* and skin lesions. *Hypercalcemia* due to increased sensitivity to vitamin D is reported in 10 percent to 30 percent, but it is sustained in only 2 percent to 3 percent. Cardiac conduction abnormalities, such as heart block, and neurologic abnormalities (including facial palsies) are each seen in about 5 percent of cases. In addition, there are many case reports of unusual presentations.

DIAGNOSIS

The diagnosis of sarcoidosis is sometimes a clinical challenge, because the condition may be hard to distinguish from other interstitial lung diseases (see Appendix to this chapter). However, *asymptomatic, bilateral hilar adenopathy* with or without uveitis or erythema nodosum is likely to be due to sarcoidosis. In a retrospective series of 100 patients with bilateral hilar adenopathy, conducted before the advent of acquired immunodeficiency syndrome (AIDS), all 30 who were asymptomatic had biopsy-proven sarcoidosis. Moreover, 50 of 52 with bilateral hilar adenopathy and negative physical examinations also had the disease. All 11 patients with neoplasms were symptomatic, and 9 had easily identifiable extrathoracic tumor on physical examination. Among symptomatic patients, all with erythema nodosum or uveitis had sarcoid. Thus, the patient with bilateral hilar adenopathy who is asymptomatic, is human immunodeficiency virus (HIV)–negative, and has a negative physical examination or has erythema nodosum or uveitis does not necessarily require a biopsy to confirm the diagnosis of sarcoidosis. Nevertheless, some clinicians prefer to obtain a tissue diagnosis in all cases of sarcoidosis, including those with asymptomatic bilateral hilar adenopathy.

A decision to *biopsy* must be made by viewing the potential for discovering treatable conditions and balancing this probability against the risks associated with the procedure. For the tissue diagnosis of hilar adenopathy, *mediastinoscopy* is the most direct approach and is usually well tolerated. For the documentation of pulmonary sarcoid, *fiberoptic bronchoscopy* with *transbronchial biopsy* is favored. This procedure has a reported sensitivity of 60 percent to 80 percent. In addition, bronchoscopy allows direct visualization of the bronchial tree so that it can be helpful in ruling out tumor and obtaining samples of secretions by *bronchoalveolar* lavage for laboratory study. The major complication of transbronchial lung biopsy is pneumothorax; this is infrequent in experienced hands.

In patients with extrathoracic sarcoidosis, accessible sites for biopsy include skin lesions and enlarged peripheral lymph nodes. Biopsy of conjunctivae, salivary glands, and liver may reveal noncaseating granulomas, even when there is no clinical evidence of sarcoid in these tissues. Because of the low morbidity of salivary gland and conjunctival biopsies, these may be particularly useful. It must be remembered that the histologic appearance of sarcoid granulomas is not etiologically specific. Therefore, the other known causes of noncaseating granulomas must be ruled out, including tuberculosis, syphilis, berylliosis, brucellosis, Q fever, biliary cirrhosis, Wegener's granulomatosis, drug reactions, and local sarcoidal reactions in nodes draining solid tumors. Hodgkin's disease is particularly difficult to exclude with mediastinoscopy in patients presenting with unilateral or asymmetric hilar adenopathy.

The *Kveim test* has also been used in the diagnosis of sarcoidosis. The test requires the intracutaneous injection of heat-sterilized human sarcoid tissue, usually spleen. A positive reaction consists of the development of epithelioid granulomas detected on skin biopsy of the injection site at 4 to 6 weeks. The delay period, variability of the material available for injection, and the high incidence of false-positive and false-negative results (due to impure batches of antigen) have limited the usefulness of the Kveim reaction. Furthermore, Kveim antigen is not readily available.

Other abnormalities that may be present in patients with sarcoidosis include cutaneous anergy, hyperglobulinemia, abnormal liver function tests, and elevated levels of lysozyme; none of these findings is specific, but together they are supportive of the diagnosis. Similarly, bone films of the hands may reveal changes suggestive of sarcoid.

Serum levels of *angiotensin-converting enzyme (ACE)* are elevated in about 70 percent of patients with active sarcoidosis, but ACE determinations lack both sensitivity and specificity for establishing a diagnosis of sarcoidosis. ACE levels have been studied as markers of disease activity and therapeutic responsiveness, but results have proved disappointing in clinical practice (see below). The same is true of *gallium-67 (^{67}Ga) scanning,* although it can help identify extrathoracic disease.

STAGING, NATURAL HISTORY, AND CLINICAL COURSE

Staging. Intrathoracic sarcoidosis can be divided into *four stages*. In *stage 0,* the chest x-ray is normal. In *stage I,* only bilateral hilar adenopathy is present; most patients are asymptomatic, the lung parenchyma appear normal on chest film, and pulmonary function tests show normal mechanics (although carbon monoxide diffusion capacity may be impaired). In *stage II,* both hilar adenopathy and pulmonary infiltrates are present; pulmonary function tests show predominantly restrictive defects. In *stage III* disease, pulmonary infiltrates are present, accompanied by obstructive and restrictive defects; however, hilar adenopathy has resolved. In *stage IV,* there is advanced fibrosis, bullae, and cysts.

Natural History. Patients with clear lungs and asymptomatic hilar adenopathy have an excellent prognosis. In one large series of untreated cases, complete remission occurred in over 75 percent within 5 years. In 50 percent with untreated pulmonary parenchymal involvement, complete resolution was seen within 2 years. In one-third of those in whom clearing did not occur, severe fibrosis developed. Overall, at 5 years, 87 percent were clinically well, 10 percent had died of respiratory failure, and 3 percent were disabled by pulmonary disease.

Most natural history data derive from referral centers. In a report from a nonreferral setting, 86 patients were followed for 10 years in a primary care practice; only 12 developed pulmonary fibrosis, and none experienced respiratory failure or cor pulmonale. This latter study suggests that the course of sarcoid may be more benign than has been reported from referral centers, which are more likely to attract complicated cases.

In general, patients with stage I disease have an 80 percent chance of spontaneous remission, those with stage II disease have about a 50 percent remission rate, and those with stage III have about a 20 percent to 40 percent chance of spontaneous remission. Stage IV represents irreversible, advanced disease.

Extrathoracic complications are infrequent. Hepatic granulomas are present often, but development of clinically symptomatic *granulomatous hepatitis* is much less common; hepatic failure and portal hypertension are rare. Cranial and peripheral *neuropathies* tend to occur early in the disease and are usually transient; however, in some patients, significant neurologic damage is seen. *Uveitis* affects about 15 percent, comes on acutely, and often resolves spontaneously. More worrisome is chronic iridocyclitis; it presents as pain and blurring of vision and may go on to produce cataracts, secondary glaucoma, and blindness. As noted above, *hypercalcemia* persists in about 2 percent to 3 percent, although it may be found transiently in up to 30 percent. Cardiac granulomata are found in 20 percent of sarcoidosis cases that come to autopsy, but less than 5 percent of patients experience difficulties with conduction or impulse formation. Rarely, infiltration of the myocardium produces pump failure.

The course of patients with sarcoid may occasionally be complicated by *infections* such as tuberculosis, aspergillar fungus balls, candidiasis, and cryptococcosis, attributable in part to the disease and in part to the use of long-term steroid therapy.

PRINCIPLES OF MANAGEMENT, THERAPEUTIC RECOMMENDATIONS, AND MONITORING

The *goals* in the treatment of sarcoid include *relief of symptoms* and *prevention* of significant impairment of organ function. As noted earlier, the natural history of sarcoid is variable, but often favorable. Hence, the indications for therapy are frequently unclear. Patients who present with stage I disease (asymptomatic bilateral hilar adenopathy or erythema nodosum) usually have a benign course, so that no treatment is indicated unless symptoms develop. Even patients with stage II or stage III disease may undergo spontaneous remission, and there is no way to identify who will progress and who will remit. There is no evidence that treatment in the early phases of pulmonary sarcoid prevents progression to pulmonary fibrosis.

The view that emerges from available studies is that treatment should be reserved for patients who are symptomatic and have evidence of active pulmonary disease (dyspnea on exertion, abnormal pulmonary function studies, infiltrate on chest x-ray). The use of gallium scanning and ACE determinations have also been used to provide evidence of disease activity, but in clinical practice have not proven to be particularly accurate. Additional indications for treatment include important extrathoracic disease, such as uveitis, conduction abnormalities, hypercalcemia, neuropathy, and severe skin involvement (see below).

The principal treatment for sarcoidosis is *systemic corticosteroid therapy*. The great variability in the disease's clinical course and the previous lack of sensitive indicators of disease activity have made it difficult to document rigorously the efficacy of steroid therapy. Older studies relied on such crude measures as symptoms, x-ray findings, and pulmonary function tests. Recent evaluations have examined the effect of corticosteroids on more direct indicators of the disease process (see below) and have found marked suppression of the alveolitis, but little influence on anatomic abnormalities present before initiation of steroid therapy.

Most authorities recommend commencing with large doses of steroids (eg, 40 to 60 mg prednisone) given on a daily basis for anywhere from 6 weeks to 6 months, followed by tapering or switching to alternate-day therapy if measures of disease activity indicate response. Improvement is usually evident by 2 to 3 weeks. Steroid therapy is most effective if instituted before development of pulmonary fibrosis. However, there is no evidence that prophylactic treatment is worth the adverse effects of chronic steroid use (see Chapter 105).

Steroids consistently produce subjective improvement in dyspneic patients with early sarcoidosis and may even reduce pulmonary infiltrates when they are due to alveolitis or granulomatous changes. Lung volumes usually improve, but not necessarily the diffusing capacity, which may be permanently altered by destructive changes. Relapses after cessation of therapy are frequent, necessitating close monitoring for at least 12 months after discontinuation of treatment. *Alternate-day steroid therapy* (eg, 15 to 25 mg qod) has proved successful as a maintenance program in some patients, controlling disease when given after an initial course of daily steroids; this approach minimizes the adverse effects of long-term steroid therapy (see Chapter 105).

Adrenal corticosteroids are also indicated for active ocular disease. Every sarcoid patient should have an ophthalmologic examination, especially if visual symptoms develop. Topical steroids may be used, but systemic therapy is usually added. Treatment is also indicated in the presence of significant or progressive involvement of any organ. Onset of hepatitis, facial nerve palsies, meningitis, myocardial conduction defects, hypercalcemia, or persistent constitutional symptoms (fever, fatigue) are other indications for treatment.

Monitoring. Whenever steroid therapy is carried out, objective documentation of response to treatment is essential. Because the predominant pathologic process in sarcoidosis is an alveolitis leading to granuloma formation and because corticosteroids work by suppressing the alveolitis, the optimal means of monitoring disease activity and response to therapy would be to follow measures of the alveolitis. *Chest x-ray, lung volumes,* and *diffusing capacity* (DLCO) have been unable to distinguish between extent of alveolitis and anatomic derangement. Although these parameters are certainly useful for determining severity of disease, they are relatively insensitive measures of disease activity and suboptimal for judging adequacy of therapy or the need for continued treatment. Even the sensitivity of the diffusing capacity for measuring disease extent has come under question. In one study, the DLCO was well preserved whereas lung volumes and measures of oxygenation (eg, alveolar–arterial oxygen gradient and O_2 saturation) showed declines.

Attempts to improve on such crude measures of disease activity have been discouraging. Tests generally reflective of inflammation, such as the erythrocyte sedimentation rate and serum globulins, proved inadequate. Initial studies of *ACE levels, gallium scanning,* and serial *bronchoalveolar lymphocyte counts* were encouraging, but later controlled study found them no more sensitive for monitoring and managing steroid therapy than the combination of serial chest x-ray, diffusing capacity, and lung volumes. Some authorities still argue that following ACE (which is believed to be produced by epithelioid cells within the sarcoid granuloma) can be useful in those patients with very high levels before therapy, a situation most common in stage II disease.

Until better tests are devised (an ongoing effort), the best available approach to monitoring appears to be either serial examination of the combination DLCO, chest x-ray, and lung volumes or serial ACE determinations if the initial serum ACE level is markedly elevated.

PATIENT EDUCATION

The diagnosis of sarcoidosis is far more common than are serious consequences of the disease. The nature of the disease should be carefully explained, with emphasis on its relatively benign, self-limited nature in the asymptomatic patient. Patients who are treated with steroids should be counseled about the side effects and risks inherent in such treatment (see Chapter 105). The need for careful follow-up must be emphasized in both the asymptomatic patient (to detect the development of functional abnormalities) and the patient with symptoms (to document objective benefits of treatment). Patients should be instructed about early signs of important complications, such as red eyes, blurred vision, eye pain, and dyspnea on exertion, so that therapy is not unnecessarily delayed.

ANNOTATED BIBLIOGRAPHY

Crystal RG, Roberts WC, Hunningham GW, et al. Pulmonary sarcoidosis: A disease characterized and perpetuated by activated lung T-lymphocytes. Ann Intern Med 1981;94:73. (*Comprehensive review of exciting new insights into the pathogenesis and immunology of sarcoidosis; 280 references.*)

Dunn TL, Watters LC, Cherniack, et al. Gas exchange at a given degree of volume restriction is different in sarcoidosis and idiopathic pulmonary fibrosis. Am J Med 1988;85:221. (*Study comparing measures of disease severity; diffusing capacity less sensitive measure of disease than volume change and degree of oxygenation.*)

Harkleroad LE, Young RL, Savage PJ, et al. Pulmonary sarcoidosis: Long-term follow-up of the effects of steroid therapy. Chest 1982;82:84. (*Although only 25 patients were entered into this alternate-case steroid trial, a 15-year follow-up was available; no discernible benefit from early steroid therapy.*)

Israel HL, Fouts DU, Begys RA. A controlled trial of prednisone treatment of sarcoidosis. Am Rev Respir Dis 1973;107:609. (*Prospective study of 90 patients; at 3 months, those on prednisone showed improvement in all parameters measured, but over the long term, no significant differences.*)

James DG. Kveim revisited, reassessed. N Engl J Med 1975;292:859. (*Reviews the test, its sensitivity, and specificity.*)

Johns CJ, Macgregor MI, Zachary JB, et al. Extended experience in the long-term corticosteroid treatment of pulmonary sarcoidosis. Ann NY Acad Sci 1976;278:722. (*192 cases of severe disease treated with prednisone; clinical improvement resulted from treatment; relapses frequent when therapy was terminated, necessitating long-term therapy with 10 to 15 mg of prednisone, often for years.*)

Koontz CH, Joyner LR, Nelson RA. Transbronchial lung biopsy via the fiber optic bronchoscope in sarcoidosis. Ann Intern Med 1976;85:64. (*Test sensitivity was 63 percent, with a higher probability of a positive biopsy in symptomatic patients.*)

Lawrence EC, Teague RB, Gottlieb MS, et al. Serial changes in markers of disease activity with corticosteroid treatment in sarcoidosis. Am J Med 1983; 74:747. (*Initially encouraging data on value of the gallium scan and ACE levels for monitoring response to steroid therapy; see Turner-Warwick reference below for a more sanguine view.*)

Lieberman J, Schleissner LA, Nosal A, et al. Clinical correlations of serum angiotensin-converting enzyme (ACE) in sarcoidosis. A longitudinal study of serum ACE, 67 gallium scans, chest roentgenograms and pulmonary function. Chest 1983;84:522. (*Another early, enthusiastic report.*)

Reich JM, Johnson RE. Course and prognosis of sarcoidosis in a nonreferral setting. Analyses of 86 patients observed for 10 years. Am J Med 1985;78:61. (*Course may be more benign than that reported for referral center populations.*)

Siltzbach LE, James DG, Neville E, et al. Course and prognosis of sarcoidosis around the world. Am J Med 1974;57:847. (*Terse summary of clinical findings showing no differences of significance among different races and ethnic groups.*)

Turner-Warwick M, McAllister W, Lawrence R, et al. Corticosteroid treatment and pulmonary sarcoidosis: Do serial lavage lymphocyte counts, serum converting enzyme measurements, and gallium-67 scans help management? Thorax 1986;41:903. (*These studies proved no more sensitive than chest film and pulmonary function tests.*)

Winterbauer RH, Belic N, Moores KD. Clinical interpretation of bilateral hilar adenopathy. Ann Intern Med 1973;78:65. (*Classic paper from the pre-HIV era, providing evidence that asymptomatic patients with bilateral adenopathy only need not undergo biopsy for definitive diagnosis.*)

Appendix: Evaluation of Interstitial Lung Disease

When a chest x-ray shows a diffuse infiltrative pattern that is labelled "interstitial" in appearance, a wide variety of diagnostic possibilities emerge, ranging from sarcoidosis and rheumatoid disease to pneumoconiosis and idiopathic pulmonary fibrosis. With such a large number of diagnostic possibilities at hand, an efficient approach to workup is essential. The primary physician's role is to narrow the differential by careful attention to important elements of the history and physical examination, supplemented by a few well-chosen initial laboratory studies.

Pathophysiology and Clinical Presentation

Most conditions that cause this diffuse parenchymal x-ray pattern are not truly "interstitial," because in addition to involving the area between the alveolar epithelium and the capillary endothelial basement membrane, they may also affect the gas-exchanging portion of the lung (including the alveolar epithelium, the alveolar space, and the pulmonary microvasculature.

Most of the interstitial lung diseases begin with parenchymal injury followed by an inflammatory response and collagen deposition. It is the widespread nature of the injury and inflammatory response—often compromising the alveolar walls—that accounts for the pathophysiology and clinical presentation. In a few instances, the process is invasive or infiltrative rather than inflammatory; in others, there is a filling of the alveolar space with an outpouring of material.

The physiologic consequences of such alveolar compromise are development of a *restrictive defect* manifested by a reduction in forced vital capacity and a *ventilation–perfusion mismatch* due to inflammation and fibrosis of the gas-exchanging surfaces causing reductions in carbon monoxide diffusing capacity and PO_2. Symptoms may be minimal, although progressive dyspnea is the rule, at times accompanied by a dry cough. The lungs may be clear to auscultation, or basilar crackles may predominate.

Differential Diagnosis

The conditions responsible for interstitial lung disease can be grouped according to their underlying pathophysiology: drug-induced inflammatory response, connective tissue disease, pneumoconiosis, alveolar filling disease, primary lung disease, and idiopathic disease (Table 51–1).

The most common causes are sarcoidosis and idiopathic pulmonary fibrosis, although in industrial settings the pneumoconioses may predominate.

Workup

History should focus on the duration of symptoms, speed of progression, and presence of fever, hemoptysis, pleuritic chest pain, and symptoms of extrathoracic disease (eg, joint pain, lymphadenopathy, skin changes). Most conditions have a chronic, progressive course, but acute onset with *fever* and a rapidly progressive course suggest a hypersensitivity pneumonitis, usually due to organic antigen exposure (ranging from cocaine to bird droppings). Fever, bothersome dry cough, plus a subacute course (2 to 10 weeks) accompanied by a patchy, bilateral air-space process characterizes bronchiolitis obliterans organizing pneumonia, where a lymphocytic infiltrate and granulation tissue occupy the distal airways and alveoli. *Productive cough* is rare in interstitial lung disease, but its occurrence indicates fluid-filled alveoli, as can happen in diffuse alveolar cell carcinoma. *Hemoptysis* suggests conditions that cause diffuse alveolar bleeding (eg, Goodpasture's syndrome, lupus, severe mitral stenosis, idiopathic pulmonary hemosiderosis). Bleeding that originates from or occurs in the context of the upper airway disease is a hallmark of Wegener's granulomatosis. *Pleuritic pain* indicates that the inflammatory process has spread to involve the pleura, which is characteristic of the connective tissue diseases and some drug-induced etiologies. Sudden severe pleuritic pain and acute dyspnea raise the question of a spontaneous pneumothorax, which occurs with many of the primary lung diseases such as histiocytosis X and lymphangiomyomatosis.

Table 51-1. Differential Diagnosis of Interstitial Lung Disease

Pneumoconiosis
Silicosis
Asbestosis
Coal worker's pneumoconiosis
Berylliosis
Organic dusts (pigeons, turkey, duck, chicken, humidifer)
Drugs
Chemotherapeutic agents (busulfan, bleomycin, methotrexate)
Antibiotics (nitrofurantoin, sulfonamides, INH)
Gold
Amiodarone
Penicillamine
Lupus-like reactions (hydralazine, procainamide)
Radiation
Connective Tissue Disease
Systemic lupus erythematosis
Rheumatoid arthritis
Scleroderma
Polymyositis
Primary Lung Diseases
Sarcoidosis
Histiocytosis X
Lymphangiomyomatosis
Lymphangetic carcinomatosis
Lipoidosis
Alveolar Filling Disease
Diffuse alveolar bleeding (Goodpasture's syndrome, lupus, mitral stenosis, idiopathic pulmonary hemosiderosis)
Alveolar proteinosis
Alveolar cell carcinoma
Eosinophilic pneumonia
Lipoid pneumonia
Other
Idiopathic pulmonary fibrosis
Bronchiolitis obliterans organizing pneumonia
Lymphocytic interstitial pneumonia

Adapted from Schwarz MI. In Kelley WN. Textbook of Internal Medicine. JB Lippincott, Philadelphia, 1989;2060.

The presence of extrapulmonary symptoms—especially if they predate the development of lung findings—can be diagnostic. Polyarticular *joint complaints* and *skin changes* characterize the connective tissue/rheumatoid diseases and sarcoidosis, with the latter often associated with reports of *lymph gland enlargement*. Patients with idiopathic pulmonary fibrosis may complain of arthralgias, but symptoms of joint inflammation are absent. A history of renal disease, especially *nephritis* can be a tip-off for Goodpasture's syndrome and lupus, although in the former, pulmonary disease usually predates renal involvement.

Drug and occupational histories are among the most important parts of the clinical assessment. Chronic use of such chemotherapeutic agents as methotrexate, busulfan, bleomycin, and cyclophosphamide may result in interstitial lung changes, as might prolonged use of nitrofurantoin, gold, amiodarone, or penicillamine. High-dose procainamide can lead to a lupus-like serositis syndrome. Radiation therapy may trigger a diffuse pneumonitis 6 to 12 weeks after treatment, followed by fibrosis. Occupational exposures, including distant ones, to inorganic dusts such as silicone, asbestos, talc, beryllium, and coal deserve careful review. Patients with a hypersensitivity pneumonitis should be queried about exposure to organic dusts on the job; typically, symptoms are worse at work. Nasal inhalation of cocaine has been reported as a cause of hypersensitivity pneumonitis and needs to be checked for. A *smoking* history is always pertinent. It is uncommon for nonsmoking patients with Goodpasture's syndrome to develop lung disease.

Physical examination is particularly useful for signs of extrathoracic disease; the lung findings are usually nonspecific. The skin is checked for signs of connective tissue disease (rheumatoid nodules, malar flush, sclerodermal changes) and sarcoidosis (see above) and the lymph nodes are checked for sarcoid-related enlargement. Patients with complaints of hemoptysis should have a careful upper airway examination looking for signs of necrotizing changes in the nasal passages and sinuses that typify Wegener's granulomatosis. The joints are examined for evidence of inflammation (swelling, warmth, redness, effusion) which is indicative of rheumatoid disease but also occurs with sarcoidosis and Wegener's granulomatosis. Enlargement of the liver and spleen are oft-noted features of sarcoidosis and occasional findings in advanced connective tissue disease and histiocytosis X.

As noted earlier, the lung examination is typically nonspecific and may even be grossly normal. Bibasilar rales are common in many forms of interstitial lung disease, especially the drug-related, pneumoconiotic, idiopathic, and connective tissue varieties. In those conditions that result in alveolar filling, the rales are likely to be "wet" in quality, whereas those without fluid in the alveoli produce "dry" crackles (sometimes referred to as "Velcro" rales) on end-inspiration. Cardiac examination is checked for mitral stenosis if there is a history of hemoptysis and for signs of cor pulmonale and right heart failure (right ventricular heave or S_3, increased intensity of the second heart sound, jugular venous distention, peripheral edema) resulting from chronic hypoxemia-induced pulmonary hypertension.

Chest x-ray findings are usually nonspecific but can be helpful. Radiologic adjectives for the diffuse changes associated with interstitial disease include such terms as "ground glass," "reticular (linear)," "reticulonodular," and "nodular." The lower lobes tend to be more involved than the upper ones and there is a "honey-combing" or cystic appearance to the lung fields as fibrous tissue replaces normal alveoli. Exceptions to these generalizations are the upper lobe predilection and nodular infiltrates of silicosis, berylliosis, chronic hypersensitivity pneumonitis, and histiocytosis X.

Unfortunately, no particular x-ray pattern is diagnostic, although a few emerge as useful. The alveolar filling diseases tend to produce alveolar densities in an ill-defined or "fluffy" nodular pattern; an air-bronchogram might ensue as involved alveoli become silhouetted by uninvolved airway. The blossoming of such a pattern in a patient with previously known interstitial disease suggests a superimposed process such as alveolar cell carcinoma or active inflammation. Frankly nodular infiltrates are seen with sarcoidosis and Wegener's granulomatosis due to granuloma formation; nodular infiltrates may even occur with the pneumoconioses and hypersensitivity pneumonitis.

X-ray findings outside the lung parenchyma are important and worth noting. Concurrent appearance of pleural involvement suggests connective tissue disease, asbestosis, and occasionally sarcoidosis. Bilateral hilar adenopathy can be pathognomonic of sarcoidosis (see above). Diffuse infiltrates, hilar adenopathy, and pneumothorax point to histiocytosis X. A thin rim of calcium in the hilar nodes is characteristic of silicosis.

Pulmonary function tests help confirm the interstitial nature of the disease (particularly when x-ray findings are minimal) and provide a baseline to judge disease course, although they correlate poorly with degree of pathologic change. As noted earlier, the ratio of *forced expiratory volume* (FEV_1) to *forced vital capacity* (FVC) increases and demonstrates a restrictive pattern due to a steady reduction in FVC. Some interstitial conditions (eg, lymphangiomyomatosis, histiocytosis X) can also cause airway obstruction and may reduce the FEV_1. The DLCO is typically reduced, although it may be preserved until rather late in the course of illness when mismatching of ventilation and perfusion become prominent. *Arterial blood gases* are initially normal, but with disease progression, hypoxemia, hypocarbia, and a respiratory alkalosis ensue. The hypocarbia is a manifestation of tachypnea, triggered predominantly by the increased work of breathing due to stiffening of the lung from progression of the fibrotic process.

Laboratory Studies. There are few routine noninvasive laboratory studies of diagnostic value. A simple, yet often overlooked one is *urinalysis,* which can provide important evidence of glomerular injury (red cells, casts, albuminuria) suggesting connective tissue disease, Wegener's granulomatosis, and Goodpasture's syndrome. Most other tests should be ordered only when findings from the history, physical, and chest film provide a reasonable pretest probability of the condition in question. Unselective testing is associated with a high rate of false-positive results (see Chapter 2). If connective tissue disease is suspected, then *rheumatoid factor, ANA,* and *deoxyribonucleic acid (DNA) binding* studies (see Chapter 146) and a *urinalysis* should be considered. Hypersensitivity pneumonitis, especially if drug-induced, may produce 10 percent to 20 percent eosinophils on the *peripheral smear* examination, but test sensitivity is low (20%). The *ACE* level is useful for gauging disease activity but lacks sensitivity for the diagnosis of sarcoidosis. *Precipitating antibodies* are frequently ordered when inhalation of a potentially sensitizing organic dust is suspected, but the test does not distinguish between an etiologic role and exposure. Patients suspected of having Goodpasture's syndrome are usually positive for *antiglomerular basement membrane antibody.* In Wegener's granulomatosis, the *antineutrophil cytoplasmic autoantibodies* are positive in only 60 percent of cases, but specificity is high (95+%).

Fiberoptic bronchoscopy with *bronchoalveolar lavage* provides an opportunity to sample the cellular and fluid contents of the distal airways (counts of total white cells, macrophages, lymphocytes and lymphocyte subsets, neutrophils, and eosinophils; malignant cells; antibodies). Alterations in the normal cellular profile may aid diagnosis as can the discovery of malignant cells. However, because of considerable overlap among etiologies, the findings are usually nonspecific. Lavage data sometimes help stage illness and predict response to therapy.

With the exception of patients with connective tissue disease, pneumoconiosis, or drug- or radiation-induced disease, most patients with interstitial lung disease usually require a tissue diagnosis. *Transbronchial biopsy* allows a low-morbidity means of obtaining tissue during bronchoscopy. Unfortunately, it rarely establishes a definitive tissue diagnosis. Most forms of interstitial disease that necessitate a tissue diagnosis require more tissue than is availed by the transbronchial approach. However, when sarcoidosis, lymphangitic carcinomatosis, or an alveolar filling disease is suspected, a transbronchial biopsy may suffice. In most other instances, an *open-lung biopsy* is required.

Indications for Referral and Admission

Referral to a pulmonary medical specialist is indicated when the diagnosis remains elusive after completion of the noninvasive segment of the evaluation and the need for lavage or a tissue diagnosis is being considered. A thoughtful consultation may save the patient an unnecessary procedure and help select those patients most likely to warrant an invasive evaluation. Hospitalization is indicated when there is severe ventilation–perfusion mismatching leading to clinically significant hypoxemia ($PO_2 < 55$ mmHg).

A.H.G.

ANNOTATED BIBLIOGRAPHY

Cooper JAD, White DA, Matthay RA. Drug-induced pulmonary disease: Part I: cytotoxic drugs; Part II: noncytotoxic drugs. Am Rev Respir Dis 1986;133:321,488. *(Comprehensive, authoritative review.)*

Crystal RG, Bitterman PB, Rennard SI, et al. Interstitial lung disease of unknown cause. Disorders characterized by chronic inflammation of the lower respiratory tract: Parts 1 and 2. N Engl J Med 1984;310:154,235. *(Definitive review and description of these important and difficult diseases, usually referred to as idiopathic pulmonary fibrosis.)*

Ettinger NA, Albin RJ. A review of the respiratory effects of smoking cocaine. Am J Med 1989;87:664. *(Includes description of an acute hypersensitivity interstitial pneumonitis.)*

Gibson PG, Bryant DH, Morgan GW, et al. Radiation-induced lung injury: A hypersensitivity pneumonitis. Ann Intern Med 1988;109:288. *(Interesting data on mechanism and review of clinical presentation.)*

Haupt M, Moore GW, Hutchins GM. The lung in systemic lupus erythematosis. Am J Med 1981;71:791. *(Analysis of pathologic changes in 121 patients.)*

Hunninghake GW, Fauci AS. Pulmonary involvement in the collagen vascular diseases. Am Rev Respir Dis 1979;119:471. *(Classic and comprehensive review.)*

Leatherman JW, Davies SF, Hoidal JR. Alveolar hemorrhage syndromes: Diffuse microvascular lung hemorrhage in immune and idiopathic disorders. Medicine 1984;63:343. *(Comprehensive review, including discussion of conditions that also cause renal injury.)*

Nolle B, Specks U, Ludemann J, et al. Anticytoplasmic antibodies: Their immunodiagnostic value in Wegener granulomatosis. Ann Intern Med 1989;111:28. *(Sensitivity averaged 63 percent during active disease; specificity 95 percent.)*

Reynolds HY. Bronchoalveolar lavage. Am Rev Respir Dis 1987;135:250. *(Excellent review of the procedure, its findings, and diagnostic utility.)*

Primary Care Medicine: Office Evaluation and Management of the Adult Patient, 3rd edition, edited by Allan H. Goroll, Lawrence A. May, and Albert G. Mulley, Jr. J.B. Lippincott Company, Philadelphia

52
Approach to the Patient With Acute Bronchitis or Pneumonia in the Ambulatory Setting

HARVEY B. SIMON, M.D.

Respiratory tract infections are among the most common acute problems seen in office practice; the majority are limited to the upper airway (see Chapters 50, 218, 219, and 220). The cough, fever, chest discomfort, and dyspnea that may accompany lower respiratory infections provoke great concern in the patient, and the physician should respond with a careful evaluation designed to elucidate three basic issues: 1) Is the process limited to the trachea and bronchi, or is a frank pneumonia present? In general, patients with bronchitis respond well to ambulatory care, whereas some patients with pneumonia may need hospital admission. 2) Is the patient at increased risk for cardiopulmonary complications? The elderly patient with underlying cardiac or chronic lung disease may decompensate acutely from bronchitis alone, whereas otherwise healthy young individuals have a much greater tolerance for these infections. 3) What is the causative organism—is it bacterial or nonbacterial? Bacterial processes are usually more severe and require antibiotics, whereas viral infections are managed symptomatically.

The assessment and decision-making process become considerably more complicated if the patient is human immunodeficiency virus (HIV)–positive. Not only does the range of organisms increase to include *Pneumocystis carinii* and other opportunistics but also the chances of serious clinical deterioration rise if treatment is not prompt and etiologic. (See Chapter 13 for a detailed discussion of the prevention and management of lower respiratory tract infection in the HIV-positive patient.)

PATHOPHYSIOLOGY AND CLINICAL PRESENTATION

The distinction between bronchitis and pneumonia is anatomic rather than etiologic; the same organisms can cause both syndromes, and patients may present with similar complaints, including fever, malaise, cough, and sputum production. Muscular-type chest wall discomfort produced from coughing occurs in both conditions, but individuals with pneumonia are more likely to have pleurisy or dyspnea as well as higher temperatures, chills, hypoxia, and a more "toxic" appearance. Similarly, although either type of infection can lead to sputum production, patients with bacterial pneumonia generally produce more sputum and are more likely to have hemoptysis.

The clinical distinction between bronchitis and pneumonia is based predominantly on physical examination and chest x-ray findings. Patients with bronchitis can have clear lungs or diffuse rhonchi or wheezes due to large airway secretions and bronchospasm, whereas individuals with pneumonia classically have rales, rhonchi, bronchial breath sounds, and dullness to percussion over the involved areas of lung. Pleural effusions may accompany pneumonia. The chest x-ray in acute bronchitis usually reveals no infiltrate or signs of consolidation in contradistinction to the x-ray of the patient with pneumonia. But even this most clear-cut distinction between bronchitis and pneumonia can be misleading because changes of chronic lung disease can simulate new infiltrates in some patients with bronchitis, whereas dehydration can minimize x-ray abnormalities in patients with pneumonia.

Patients with pneumonia are far more likely to experience complications such as hypoxia, cardiopulmonary failure, local suppuration (lung abscess or empyema), and spread of infection to other organs by way of the bloodstream. Clinical presentations are, in part, a function of the causative organism.

Gram-Positive Organisms. *Streptococcus pneumoniae* is still the most common cause of bacterial bronchitis and pneumonia, accounting for up to 30 percent to 50 percent of all bacterial pneumonias. It is especially likely to be the agent infecting healthy young ambulatory patients, but it may affect all age groups. Classic clinical features include abrupt onset of fever with a single rigor, cough with rusty sputum, and pleuritic chest pain. Radiologic evidence of lobar consolidation is typical, but infiltrates can be patchy, especially in patients with chronic lung disease. The sputum Gram's stain reveals abundant polymorphonuclear leukocytes and gram-positive diplococci (classically lancet shaped) in pairs or short chains.

The most common complication of pneumococcal pneumonia is bacteremia, which occurs in about one-third of patients. Blood-borne distant sepsis (septic arthritis, peritonitis, meningitis, and so forth) is much less common. Sterile pleural effusions are common, whereas empyema is less frequent, and lung abscess is a rare complication. Delayed resolution of radiographic abnormalities is a relatively common occurrence and may take up to 6 to 8 weeks.

Staphylococcus aureus is the etiologic agent in up to 10 percent of bacterial pneumonias. Except in infancy, when it can be a primary infection, staphylococcal pneumonia most commonly follows a viral respiratory tract infection, particularly *influenza*. It may also occur as a nosocomial infection or as a result of bacteremic seeding of the lungs, especially in patients with staphylococcal endocarditis or intravenous (IV) drug abuse. Patients with staphylococcal pneumonia of respiratory or bloodstream origin are usually extremely ill. *Staphylococcus aureus* produces tissue necrosis, and the distinctive feature of staphylococcal pneumonia is the tendency to produce multiple small lung abscesses. Healing usually leaves some degree of residual fibrosis. Abundant polymorphonuclear leukocytes and gram-positive cocci in pairs, clumps, and clusters are found on the sputum Gram's stain. Local suppurative complications, including lung abscess, empyema, and pneumothorax, are relatively common. Bacteremia with metastatic seeding of distant sites such as endocardium, bone, joints, liver, and meninges may occur.

Pneumonia caused by *group A streptococci* is a rather uncommon infection, but has occurred in epidemics, especially in closed groups such as military units. Occasionally, streptococcal pneumonia can occur after primary influenza pneumonia. Streptococcal pneumonia usually begins abruptly with fever, cough, and severe debility. Chest pain is prominent in most patients. The distinctive clinical and radiologic feature is rapid spread in the lung, with resultant early empyema formation. Initially, the empyema fluid may be thin, possibly due to the many enzymes elaborated by group A streptococci, but later frank purulence occurs. Other complications such as lung abscess, bacteremia, metastatic infection, and poststreptococcal glomerulonephritis are uncommon. In patients with streptococcal pneumonia, the sputum Gram's stain reveals numerous polymorphonuclear leukocytes and gram-positive cocci in pairs and short to long chains.

Gram-Negative Organisms. Although *Haemophilus influenzae* has long been recognized as a common cause of bronchitis in adults with chronic lung disease, there has recently been a greater recognition of frank pneumonias caused by this organism, sometimes with bacteremia. Most cases of bronchitis are caused by untypeable strains of *H. influenzae*, but pneumonias are often caused by the more invasive encapsulated strains, especially type b. Radiographically, a bronchopneumonia pattern is typical. Abundant polymorphonuclear leukocytes and small pleomorphic gram-negative coccobacillary organisms are the characteristic findings in the sputum of patients with pneumonia or bronchitis due to *H. influenzae*. Complications of *H. influenzae* pneumonia in adults are uncommon, but in patients with underlying chronic lung disease or HIV-infection, the illness may be particularly severe with hypoxia and respiratory failure developing.

Klebsiella pneumoniae typically produces pulmonary infection in debilitated patients, especially *alcoholics*, and is one of the only gram-negative bacillary pneumonias to occur with any frequency in ambulatory patients. It usually presents as an acute illness; rarely it may cause chronic pneumonitis. The organism has a high propensity to produce tissue necrosis, which accounts for the hemoptysis, dense lobar consolidation, and high incidence of abscess formation seen in this illness. Abundant polymorphonuclear leukocytes and large gram-negative bacilli, occasionally with thick capsules, are characteristically seen on sputum Gram's stain. Lung abscess is a common complication and is really part of the natural evolution of the disease. Empyema may occur.

Other gram-negative bacillary pneumonias were once rare, but have increased over the past 15 years and now account for up to 20 percent of bacterial pneumonias. They are principally hospital-acquired infections and remain rare in the ambulatory population. Patients with gram-negative bacillary pneumonia are typically debilitated from other illnesses and frequently have received antibiotic therapy, which alters their respiratory flora, thus accounting for the presence of these otherwise unusual pathogens. These pneumonias may result either from aspiration of gram-negative organisms present in the upper airway (often related to inhalation therapy), or from seeding of the lungs in the course of gram-negative bacteremia. *Bacteremic pneumonias* are characterized by multiple small areas of infection in both lungs. Abundant polymorphonuclear leukocytes and gram-negative bacilli are seen on sputum Gram's stain. Complications including lung abscess, empyema, and bacteremia with metastatic spread of infection may occur.

Moraxella (Branhamella) catarrhalis is a gram-negative coccus that morphologically resembles the Neisseria family, but differs in biochemical and deoxyribonucleic acid (DNA) characteristics. It is found in the oropharynx of normal hosts and had not been considered pathogenic until the 1980s when it was established as the cause of lower respiratory tract infection in some patients with chronic obstructive pulmonary disease (COPD). In up to 60 percent of COPD patients, it is the only organism isolated from the lower respiratory tract; overall, it is the second most common COPD isolate after *Streptococcus pneumoniae*. In over 80 percent of *Moraxella catarrhalis* infections, there is *underlying pulmonary disease*. Diabetes, alcoholism, malignancy, and steroid use are other known risk factors. The principal means of spread is believed to be endogenous from upper to lower airway, although hand-to-hand infection has been documented. The organism is also a common isolate in *children* with acute *otitis media*.

There appears to be a concentration of cases in the *winter* months, perhaps indicating a relation to preceding viral infection. The typical lower respiratory tract infection that ensues is mild and sometimes even self-limited. The organism is readily identified by Gram's stain, and almost all sputum cultures are positive. Chest x-ray shows an interstitial or interstitial-airspace infiltrate. Bacteremia is rare, and full recovery with prompt response to antibiotics is the rule, although about two-thirds of isolates are positive for beta-lactamase.

Legionnaires' Disease. First identified in 182 patients in the 1976 Philadelphia outbreak, Legionnaires' disease is now recognized as an important cause of pneumonia around the world. The causative organism, *Legionella pneumophila,* is a filamentous, fastidious bacillus that survives in water and, to a lesser extent, soil. Human infection is acquired by inhalation of contaminated aerosols; person-to-person transmission is unknown. Legionnaires' disease may occur in sporadic cases or epidemics; hospital water supplies can be contaminated, and nosocomial infections can occur. Middle-aged and elderly patients are most often affected, and immunosuppressed patients are particularly vulnerable. Nine serogroups of *L. pneumophila* have been recognized, and at least seven other *Legionella* species can cause human disease. The most important of these, *L. micdadei,* causes "Pittsburgh-agent" pneumonia in immunosuppressed patients.

The spectrum of clinical illness due to *Legionella* infection ranges from mild upper respiratory disease (Pontiac fever) and self-limited atypical pneumonia to potentially fatal Legionnaires' disease and opportunistic infections in immunocompromised hosts. After a short prodrome, the full-blown form of Legionnaires' disease begins acutely with high fever, nonproductive cough, and dyspnea. *Pleuritic chest pain* occurs in about one-third of cases. Extrapulmonary manifestations such as *diarrhea, confusion,* and *renal dysfunction* are common and can be clues to diagnosis. Although the typical patient is severely ill, milder cases have been recognized.

A pretibial rash and relative bradycardia occur in a few patients, but in most the physical examination is nonspecific. A modest leukocytosis and interstitial infiltrates or areas of patchy consolidation are characteristic laboratory abnormalities. The urinalysis may show *red cells,* and renal and liver function tests may be abnormal; hypoxia can occur. Sputum is typically absent or scant. The sputum Gram's stain fails to reveal pathogens, but *L. pneumophila* can sometimes be visualized in sputum or other specimens by direct immunofluorescent staining. The organisms can be cultured on charcoal yeast extract agar, and *Legionella* antigens can be detected in the urine of some patients. In most instances, the diagnosis is made serologically (see later discussion).

Mixed Flora. *Aspiration pneumonias* are usually mixed infections caused by the aerobic and anaerobic streptococci, bacteroides, and fusobacteria, which are harmless normal flora of the upper airway, that cause pneumonia if they attain a foothold in lung parenchyma. Predisposing factors include alteration of consciousness (drugs, anesthesia, alcohol, head trauma) and diminution of gag reflex, permitting aspiration to occur. Patients usually are mildly to moderately ill but can be toxic, especially if lung abscess or empyema occurs. It must be stressed that hospitalized patients and ambulatory patients receiving antibiotics may have altered respiratory flora. Aspiration of mouth organisms in such individuals may result in staphylococcal or gram-negative bacillary pneumonia, as discussed previously, rather than the pulmonary infection due to normal upper respiratory flora, as considered here. The sputum from patients with aspiration pneumonia may be malodorous and characteristically shows abundant polymorphonuclear leukocytes and mixed flora, including gram-positive cocci in pairs and chains and pleomorphic gram-negative rods on Gram's stain. Lung abscess and empyema are fairly common complications of aspiration pneumonia, especially if therapy is delayed.

Nonbacterial Organisms. *Mycoplasma pneumoniae* is one of the most common causes of nonbacterial pneumonia and accounts for up to 20 percent of all pneumonias in some urban populations. It is the leading cause of the *atypical pneumonia syndrome* (fever, dry cough, nonspecific infiltrate on chest film) in otherwise healthy adults. The organism spreads by way of respiratory droplets and appears to have a long incubation period, so that slow spread among family members or other closed groups over a period of many weeks is characteristic. Although all ages can be affected, the greatest incidence of mycoplasmal pneumonia is in *older children* and *young adults*. The disease usually begins gradually. In addition to a *nonproductive cough* with fever and malaise, *headache* is a rather constant symptom. Physical examination discloses fine rales, which are typically less extensive than the *patchy alveolar densities* (usually confined to one of the lower lobes) seen on chest x-ray. Occasionally, examination of the tympanic membrane will also show a bullous myringitis. Laboratory studies reveal a normal white blood cell count and differential in most cases. The sputum is scant, with a predominance of *mononuclear cells*. *Mycoplasma* organisms are very small and lack cell walls; hence, they cannot be visualized with conventional microscopy. Mycoplasma pneumonia is usually a mild, self-limited illness, but it can produce severe pneumonia in children with sickle cell anemia, in immunosuppressed hosts, and in the elderly. Uncommon complications include hemolytic anemia, encephalitis, Guillain-Barré syndrome, myopericarditis, and Stevens-Johnson syndrome.

Chlamydia. The *Taiwan Acute Respiratory Disease (TWAR)* strain of *Chlamydia pneumoniae* causes pneumonia in *young adults*. Unlike psittacosis, which is a true zoonoses that spreads only from animal to man, *C. pneumoniae* appears to spread from person-to-person by respiratory droplets and to cause "atypical pneumonia"—mild pneumonia without sputum production. In populations of young adults, TWAR accounts for about 10 percent to 20 percent of atypical pneumonias; mycoplasma accounts for 30 percent, and viruses account for 20 percent. The clinical features of TWAR pneumonia resemble those of mycoplasma: after a prodrome of pharyngitis lasting up to 2 weeks, a nonproductive cough and fever occur. Pulmonary infiltrates are mild. The infection is usually self-limited; rare fatalities have been reported in debilitated patients. Prolonged bouts of bronchitis (sometimes with sinusitis) have been recognized in adults with COPD.

Viruses. Many viruses are capable of producing upper and lower respiratory tract infections, including adenoviruses, respiratory syncytial virus, and parainfluenza virus. These infections are clinically indistinguishable except when part of a distinctive systemic viral illness such as rubeola in children or varicella in adults. Cytomegalovirus is a common cause of viral pneumonia in the immunocompromised host. The most important cause of viral pneumonia is influenza, which can be recognized by its epidemic spread and marked systemic symptoms such as fever and myalgias. Influenza pneumonia may be a mild or fulminant illness capable of causing lethal respiratory failure. Bacterial pneumonia, especially of the pneumococcal, staphylococcal, or streptococcal variety, is a frequent complication.

Psittacosis is caused by a member of the *Chlamydia* group of obligate intracellular parasites, which are also responsible for lymphogranuloma venereum and trachoma. The disease is transmitted from parrots or other birds (including pigeons and turkeys) to humans. The clinical features of psittacosis are indistinguishable from those of other nonbacterial pneumonias, with prominent headache, nonproductive cough, and fever. Occasionally, a faint macular rash or splenomegamy develops.

Q Fever. Caused by *Coxiella burnetii,* Q fever is unique among rickettsial infections in that pneumonia is prominent, there is no rash, and spread is through inhalation of infected dust particles rather than by way of the bite of an insect vector. The organisms reside principally in animals; human contact with cattle, sheep, goats, or with infected animal hides or hide products is the most important epidemiologic factor, and is often the only clue to diagnosis. The clinical features of Q fever are similar to those of the other nonbacterial pneumonias, except that hepatitis occurs in up to one-third of patients.

Fungi and Other Opportunistic Organisms. Immunosuppressed patients (eg, those taking corticosteroids, HIV-positive patients) are at heightened risk for a community-acquired opportunistic infection (eg, *Aspergillus, Candida, cytomegalovirus,* or *Pneumocystis;* see Chapter 13). HIV-positive patients are also at enhanced risk of *primary tuberculosis* (see Chapter 49). Some fungal infections may occur in immunocompetent hosts. For example, in the Midwest and West, exposure to spore-containing dusts may lead to *histoplasmosis* or *coccidiodomycosis* respectively, characterized in its initial phases by a nonproductive cough, flulike illness, liver or splenic enlargement, alveolar infiltrates, and sometimes hilar adenopathy; however, most often the chest film is normal.

DIFFERENTIAL DIAGNOSIS

The differential diagnosis of community-acquired pneumonia is listed in Table 52–1. In a study from England, pneumococcal infection was the most common cause, followed by *H. influenzae* and influenza A and B.

In addition to the conditions listed in Table 52–1 and detailed above, noninfectious diseases can occasionally mimic infectious processes. Bronchial asthma (see Chapter 48) and hypersensitivity pneumonitis (see Chapter 51) are common examples. The radiologic findings associated with chronic pulmonary diseases, especially chronic bronchitis (see Chapter 47), and bronchiectasis (see Chapter 41), may be misleading if previous x-rays are not available. Atelectasis, pulmonary infarction, pulmonary edema (see Chapter 32), and lung tumors may also be confused with pneumonia.

WORKUP

The first task is to differentiate lower respiratory tract infection from the other causes of cough and fever cited above (see Chapters 32, 41, 42, and 51). Once this has been accomplished, the focus quickly shifts to a search for etiology, especially for treatable conditions such as those due to bacterial infection.

Table 52-1. Differential Diagnosis of Pneumonia

- I. Bacterial pneumonias
  - A. Gram-positive
    1. *Pneumococcus*
    2. *Streptococcus*
    3. *Staphylococcus aureus*
  - B. Gram-negative
    1. *H. influenzae*
    2. *Klebsiella*
    3. *Proteus, Escherichia coli, Pseudomonas* and others (usually in hospitalized patients)
    4. Legionnaire's disease
    5. *Moraxella*
  - C. Mixed
    1. Aspiration pneumonia
  - D. Mycobacterial
    1. Tuberculosis
- II. Nonbacterial pneumonias
    1. *Mycoplasma*
    2. Viral
    3. Psittacosis
    4. *Chlamydia pneumoniae*
    5. Q fever
    6. *Pneumocystis carinii*
    7. Fungi

History. A careful description of symptoms, their onset, and their clinical course can be helpful in distinguishing between bacterial and nonbacterial etiologies. Although this distinction may be difficult in individual patients, certain broad generalizations can be offered. Patients with bacterial pneumonias are more likely to have abrupt onset of illness and to be clinically sicker with higher temperatures, a higher incidence of chills, more copious sputum production, and a greater likelihood of developing significant pleural effusions. Although both types of pneumonia can affect all ages, nonbacterial pneumonias are more common in older children and young adults. Such patients characteristically report a more gradual onset of symptoms with only moderate fever. Patients with viral and mycoplasmal pneumonias will often complain of a severe hacking cough, but substantial sputum production is unusual.

The clinical context of the illness at hand has important etiologic implications. A recent viral upper respiratory infection is a common precipitant of gram-positive and *Moraxella* infections. An exposure history is particularly important as regards tuberculosis (see Chapter 49), mycoplasmal, and chlamydial pneumonias. A history of smoking or chronic lung disease (see Chapters 47, 48, and 51) increases the risks of pneumococcal, *H. influenzae,* and *Moraxella* infections. A history of HIV-positivity greatly raises the likelihood of opportunistic infection from *Pneumocystis,* cytomegalovirus, *Mycobacterium tuberculosis,* and fungi, although common organisms are also common in HIV-positive patients (see Chapter 13). Aspiration is suggested when pneumonia occurs in the setting of impaired cough and gag reflexes due to sedative use, recent head trauma, intoxication, or neurologic disorders.

A history of recent travel raises the question of unusual bacterial or fungal processes; and occupational exposures or animal (Q fever) and bird (psittacosis) contacts further broaden the differential diagnosis (see Chapter 51). The occurrence of such extrapulmonary symptoms as diarrhea and confusion in conjunction with the pneumonia suggests Legionnaires' disease.

Physical Examination. The patient with bacterial pneumonia generally looks sicker, and the chest examination usually reveals signs of consolidation or at least localized rales and rhonchi. In contrast, the chest examination of patients with nonbacterial pneumonias typically shows only fine rales, and often the physical findings are less extensive than the radiologic abnormalities.

Physical examination also helps to assess the overall status of the patient. High fever, marked tachycardia, hypotension, cyanosis, signs of hypercapnia (asterixis, confusion, papilledema), and alterations of mentation are indications for emergency hospitalization (see below).

Physical findings can have etiologic significance. A relative bradycardia in the setting of fever, tachypnea, and pneumonia is suggestive of Legionnaires' disease. The skin should be checked for a viral exanthem, the pretibial rash of Legionnaires' disease, and manifestations of acquired immunodeficiency syndrome (AIDS; eg, Kaposi's sarcoma; see Chapter 13). The fundi of an immunocompromised host are examined for retinitis indicative of cytomegalovirus infection, and the tympanic membranes are examined for bullous myringitis that may accompany mycoplasmal disease. The heart should be auscultated for the presence of a new murmur, especially if the patient has a history of IV drug abuse. Neurologic examination should include testing for meningeal signs, level of mentation, and ability to protect the airway.

Laboratory Studies. When the patient is only mildly ill and has clear lungs, laboratory studies can be limited to a *sputum Gram's stain, sputum culture,* and a *white blood cell count* with *differential.* When pneumonia is suspected by history or physical examination, PA and lateral *chest x-rays* are useful for confirmation. If the patient appears quite ill, *blood cultures* should be obtained. *Thoracentesis* should be considered if pleural fluid is present. The fluid is sent for Gram's stain, culture, and protein, glucose, and lactate dehydrogenase (LDH) determinations (see Chapter 43).

Laboratory studies help distinguish between viral and bacterial causes. Patients with bacterial pneumonias are more likely to have a polymorphonuclear leukocytosis. If the chest x-ray reveals lobar or segmental consolidation, abscess formation, or significant pleural effusions, then bacterial pneumonia is more likely; a patchy infiltrate can occur in either type of process, but a true interstitial infiltrate suggests a nonbacterial etiology (see Appendix of Chapter 51).

Examination of sputum is the key to diagnosis. The sputum of the patient with bacterial pneumonia is typically thick and green to brownish in color. It may be blood tinged. A good sputum specimen for microscopic examination and culture is crucial. If the patient cannot expectorate spontaneously, methods of inducing sputum production should be tried, especially if the patient is immunocompromised and at risk for such infections as *Pneumocystis* pneumonia and tuberculosis. Caution should be exercised in obtaining sputum so as to minimize the risk of aerosol spread (this is especially important in patients suspected of tuberculosis; see Chapter 49). If these methods fail, transtracheal aspiration can be considered, but some argue that the yield from such invasive methods is low and does not warrant their morbidity risk.

Gram's stain of sputum from patients with bacterial pneumonia usually reveals abundant polymorphonuclear leukocytes and will often disclose the primary pathogen; finding intracellular organisms is especially diagnostic. Common mistakes in the interpretation of the sputum Gram's stain include examination of samples contaminated with mouth flora and inadequate decolorization. The finding of a wide variety of organisms, few polymorphonuclear leukocytes, and many epithelial cells is diagnostic of an inadequate specimen. However, the finding of mixed flora is not per se a sign of an inadequate specimen, because aspiration will also produce a sputum filled with mixed flora, but there will also be many polymorphonuclear leukocytes and few epithelial cells. Another error is inadequate alcohol decolorization of the specimen (the polymorphonuclear leukocytes should be pink), leading the examiner to mistaking a gram-negative organism for a gram-positive one. Proper staining is important when the responsible organisms are cocci. Finding gram-negative cocci suggests *Moraxella,* and gram-negative coccobacillary forms are indicative of *H. influenzae.*

Patients with nonbacterial pneumonias generally produce only scant quantities of thin sputum, although in the case of influenzal pneumonia, it can be bloody; the Gram's stain is noteworthy for an absence of bacteria and a scant cellular response. In patients with mycoplasmal pneumonia, *mononuclear cells* may predominate.

The value of the *sputum culture* depends on obtaining a deep specimen. Often, sputum production is scant, as in cases of atypical pneumonia. Culturing an inadequate specimen is a waste of time. All cultures should be obtained and sent before antibiotics are started. Some organisms are too fastidious to grow from sputum samples; other means of definitive diagnosis may be necessary. For example, pneumococci may fail to grow out from sputum samples but can be isolated from *blood cultures* drawn during the early bacteremic phase of the illness.

Legionnaires' disease can be diagnosed by culture of the organism, antibody staining, or serologic study. In most instances, serologic study confirms the diagnosis. A single *antibody titer* of 1:256 is presumptive evidence, but confirmation requires demonstration of a fourfold rise in titer between acute and convalescent specimens, and a convalescent titer of at least 1:128. The organism can be isolated and cultured from sputum, lung, or pleural fluid, using charcoal yeast extract agar. Identification is sometimes made by *fluorescent antibody staining* of sputum.

Most *viral pneumonias* can be diagnosed on clinical grounds and epidemiologic evidence. Specific diagnosis depends on either serologic studies (which are retrospective) or viral cultures (which are not widely available). Recognition of influenza is important because contacts can be protected by prophylactic use of amantadine; diagnostic confirmation is worth seeking when influenza is suspected.

Mycoplasma can be grown in the laboratory only on specialized media. An important clue to diagnosis is the presence of cold agglutinins in the serum. Low titers (< 1:64) can occur in other disorders such as adenovirus and influenza infections, but high or rising titers are strongly suggestive of *Mycoplasma pneumoniae* infection. Cold agglutinins may be absent, particularly in patients with mild disease, and specific serologic tests are then required. A DNA probe can be used to identify organisms rapidly in sputum specimens.

A new interstitial infiltrate in a patient who is HIV-positive raises the question of infection with *Pneumocystis* or another opportunistic organism. Coexisting oral candidiasis, a marked elevation in serum LDH, and an elevated sedimentation rate suggest *Pneumocystis*. Criteria for initiation of therapy range from dyspnea and hypoxia to visualization of the organism in sputum or bronchoalveolar lavage samples (see Chapter 13).

For *psittacosis,* a history of bird exposure is the key to diagnosis, and specific serologies are required for confirmation. The diagnosis of Q fever depends on specific serologies.

PRINCIPLES OF MANAGEMENT

Many patients with community-acquired lower respiratory tract infections, especially those with acute bronchitis or mild pneumonia due to virus, *H. influenzae,* pneumococci, *Mycoplasma, Chlamydia,* and *Moraxella* can be managed on an outpatient basis, provided that they are alert, reliable, have help available to them, and have no signs of serious compromise (see Indications for Admission below). Oral antibiotic regimens can achieve therapeutic serum antibiotic levels. In a study of community-acquired pneumonia in England, about three-quarters of patients were able to be managed at home; overall mortality was 3 percent.

Certain general principles of management apply, regardless of etiology. Adequate *hydration* is essential to help clear secretions; this can be achieved by fluid intake and local airway humidification. *Expectorants* such as guaifenesin may be helpful to some patients in loosening the sputum, although there is no objective evidence that they make a significant difference in outcome. *Pulmonary physical therapy* may help with mobilization of secretions, but prospective trials have failed to demonstrate that this time-honored intervention improves outcome (see Chapters 41 and 47).

In general, the cough reflex should not be suppressed in patients with bacterial infections, because coughing is an important mechanism for clearing secretions. However, if severe paroxysms of coughing produce respiratory fatigue or severe pain, temporary relief may be obtained with small doses of *codeine,* especially before bed (see Chapter 41). Chest pain should be treated with analgesics that do not suppress cough. *Aspirin* should be tried first, but in children with influenza used only with caution due to risk of Reyes' syndrome. For more severe pain, *nonsteroidal antiinflammatory agents* or codeine may be needed. If narcotics are used, the patient must be carefully monitored for respiratory depression and excessive cough suppression. Fever can be controlled with aspirin or acetaminophen (see Chapter 11). If *oxygen* is administered before hospitalization, only very low FIO_2s (24% to 28%) should be used. Individuals with chronic lung disease who retain CO_2 depend on their hypoxic drive; excessive oxygen therapy may precipitate respiratory depression (see Chapter 47).

More specific therapy depends on the etiologic agent involved. Although culture and sensitivity testing require at least 24 to 48 hours to provide definitive information, the clinical setting, chest x-ray, and sputum Gram's stain usually enable the physician to make a reasonable presumptive diagnosis and to initiate therapy promptly. Treatment can be modified as necessary on the basis of culture results. For example, young, otherwise healthy patients with *atypical pneumonia* can be started on *erythromycin,* which will cover *Mycoplasma,* pneumococcal disease, and *Chlamydia.*

THERAPEUTIC RECOMMENDATIONS

Tables 52–2 and 52–3 summarize therapeutic recommendations for lower respiratory tract infections (acute bronchitis and pneumonia). Treatment is similar for both, although with pneumonia, the risk of complications is greater and may necessitate more intensive therapy.

Pneumococcal Disease. *Penicillin* is the drug of choice. Therapy should be continued until the patient has been afebrile for 3 to 5 days or for a total course of 10 to 14 days. A healthy young patient with disease confined to one lobe and a supportive home environment can be given an initial dose

Table 52-2. Antibiotics of Choice for Outpatient Treatment of Lower Respiratory Tract Infections

ORGANISM*	DRUG OF CHOICE	ALTERNATE DRUGS
S. pneumoniae (pneumococcus)	Penicillin	Cephalosporins Erythromycin Lincomycin Clindamycin
Haemophilus influenzae	Ampicillin or amoxicillin	Tetracycline Trimethoprim-sulfamethoxazole
Mycoplasma pneumoniae	Erythromycin or tetracycline	
Q fever	Tetracycline	Chloramphenicol
Psittacosis	Tetracycline	

*Lower respiratory infections due to group A streptococcus, *Staphylococcus aureus,* Legionnaire's disease bacillus (*Legionella pneumophilae*), *Klebsiella pneumoniae, Pseudomonas aeruginosa, E. coli, Proteus mirabilis,* and other gram-negative bacilli require hospitalization for parenteral antibiotic therapy; the same is true for aspiration pneumonia due to mixed "normal" mouth flora.

of intramuscular procaine penicillin and continued on oral penicillin (eg, phenoxymethyl penicillin, 500 mg qid) at home with close follow-up. The elderly and the immunocompromised may need consideration of hospitalization for initial treatment with IV penicillin until substantial improvement occurs (see below). Table 52–2 lists alternatives for penicillin-allergic patients; tetracyclines should *not* be used because many pneumococci are resistant to them. *Prophylaxis* against future pneumococcal infection is available with use of *polyvalent pneumococcal vaccine* (see Chapters 6 and 47). Although there are 83 capsular types of pneumococci, each with its own type-specific immunity, a relatively small number of serotypes account for most human infections. The vaccine incorporates 23 capsular types, which together account for about 90 percent of pneumococcal pneumonias in the United States, and field trials suggest that it may be up to 80 percent effective in preventing pneumonia due to these 23 types. All patients who have undergone splenectomy or who have sickle cell disease should be vaccinated because of their unique susceptibility to fulminating pneumococcal sepsis. In addition, immunosuppressed patients, the elderly, and people with chronic heart or lung disease are prime candidates for vaccination (see Chapters 6 and 47). Mild local pain and erythema are the only common adverse reactions to the vaccine, which is administered in a single 0.5-mL intramuscular or subcutaneous dose. Repeat doses of vaccine are not recommended, although it appears that antibody responses decline with advancing age. The response rate in the elderly is aided by vaccination before age 55. The vaccine can be given at the same time as influenza vaccine. Many patients received the original pneumococcal vaccine, which had 14 capsular antigens. It is uncertain whether patients who received the old vaccine should be revaccinated, but very high-risk patients probably should be.

Staphylococcus Aureus. A parentally administered semisynthetic penicillin (or penicillin if the organism is not a penicillinase producer) is the drug of choice, requiring hospitalization. Therapy should be continued until clinical and x-ray healing is apparent; this usually requires at least 2 to 4 weeks.

Table 52-3. Antibiotic Dosage Regimens for Ambulatory Therapy of Acute Bronchitis and Mild Cases of Pneumonia in Adults

DRUG	DOSE*	MAJOR TOXICITY†
Penicillin‡	250–500 mg every 6 h	Hypersensitivity
Ampicillin‡	250–500 mg every 6 h	Hypersensitivity GI intolerance
Amoxicillin‡	250–500 mg every 8 h	Hypersensitivity GI intolerance
Erythromycin	250–500 mg every 6 h	GI intolerance Hypersensitivity
Trimethoprim-sulfamethoxazole	2 tablets every 12 h or 1 double-strength tablet every 12 h	Hypersensitivity
Tetracycline	250–500 mg every 6 h	GI intolerance Hypersensitivity
Clindamycin	150–300 mg every 6 h	Enterocolitis Hypersensitivity
Cephalexin‡§	250–500 mg every 6–8 h	Hypersensitivity

*All doses are for average-sized adults with normal renal and hepatic function. Consult manufacturer's recommendations for details.

†Only major toxicity is listed; see manufacturer's literature for additional adverse reactions. In addition, all antibiotics predispose individuals to superinfection with resistant organisms and should be used with caution.

‡Cross-sensitivity is shared among all of the penicillins. In addition, patients who are allergic to penicillins may be allergic to cephalosporins.

§Other cephalosporins used orally include cephradine (similar to cephalexin), cefaclor (somewhat more active than cephalexin against *H. influenzae*), cefadoxril (can be given q12h).

Streptococcus Pyogenes. Parenteral penicillin is the treatment of choice, requiring hospitalization. Therapy should be continued until clinical resolution, usually at least 2 weeks.

H. Influenzae Infection. For initial therapy of uncomplicated *H. influenzae* bronchitis in an immunocompetent patient, *amoxicillin* should suffice. However, an increasing number of ampicillin/amoxicillin-resistant strains have been recognized, although such strains still constitute a minority. For patients with suspected *H. influenzae* pneumonia who can be managed on an outpatient basis (see below), it is advisable to begin treatment with an alternative to amoxicillin, pending results of sensitivity testing. Appropriate choices for oral therapy include *trimethoprim-sulfamethoxazole, amoxicillin-clavulanic acid,* a *tetracycline,* or a second-generation oral cephalosporin such as *cefaclor* or *cefuroxime axetil.* If susceptibility testing reveals no drug resistance, then switching to ampicillin or amoxicillin is warranted (generic amoxicillin can be one-tenth the cost of cephalosporins). Immunocompromised and frail patients require admission for parenteral therapy with cefuroxime, ampicillin-sulbactam, or a third-generation cephalosporin. Chloramphenicol remains an effective parenteral alternative. In general, patients with bronchitis should be treated for 7 to 10 days, and patients with pneumonia should be treated for 10 to 14 days. The new macrolide antibiotic *clarithromycin* is also effective against *H. influenzae.*

***Klebsiella* and Other Enterobacteriaceae.** Hospital admission for parenteral antibiotic therapy is required. A wide range of antibiotics are reasonable for initial therapy, including gentamicin, the third-generation cephalosporins, aztreonam, ciprofloxacin, and imipenem-cilastatin. Final choice is based on results of susceptibility testing.

Legionnaires' Disease. Therapy during outbreaks is often initiated on clinical and epidemiologic grounds before the diagnosis is confirmed. *Erythromycin* remains the drug of choice. For seriously ill patients, 1 g IV four times daily is required; treatment failures have been reported when seriously ill patients are given oral erythromycin. Mild cases may be managed on an outpatient basis with 500 mg erythromycin four times daily for 7 to 10 days. Close follow-up is mandatory.

Aspiration Pneumonia. A patient who aspirates cannot protect his or her airway and must be admitted to the hospital. Penicillin is the traditional drug of choice, but clindamycin has proven superior in prospective randomized trials.

***Mycoplasma* and *Chlamydia*.** Oral *erythromycin* or *tetracycline* is effective. The penicillins are ineffective. Treatment should be continued for 1 to 2 weeks.

Moraxella. Outpatients with *Moraxella* infection can be started on *erythromycin, trimethoprim-sulfamethoxazole, cefaclor,* or *amoxicillin-clavulanic acid.* Oral antibiotic therapy usually suffices. A high prevalence of beta-lactamase makes amoxicillin an inadequate first choice but may be reasonable after sensitivity testing. Ciprofloxacin and third-generation cephalosporins are excellent for severely ill patients.

Viruses. Although there is no treatment for viral pneumonia, *prophylaxis* against influenza is extremely important. All elderly patients and those with underlying cardiopulmonary and chronic disease should be vaccinated annually with *polyvalent influenza vaccine* in the fall of each year. The vaccine is 70 percent to 80 percent protective, and it is prepared annually to correspond with the wild strains in circulation. The vaccine is made of purified, killed virus. There have been no reports of an increased incidence of Guillain-Barré syndrome with use of routine influenza vaccine; swine flu vaccine used only in 1976 was associated with an increased risk of neurologic complications. Serious reactions are rare, unless the patient is allergic to egg protein. Minor febrile responses and myalgias are sometimes noted.

Patients not immunized and at high risk of contracting influenza can be given oral *amantadine.* At a dose of 100 mg twice per day, it can prevent or at least blunt clinical illness in 70 percent to 90 percent of patients exposed to influenza A (it has no activity against influenza B). Unfortunately, it must be taken daily during the period of risk to provide protection, and it causes neurologic side effects (insomnia, dizziness, and confusion), particularly in the elderly. As such, it is best used during an epidemic to protect the frail unvaccinated population until an emergency vaccination program can be completed. Rimantadine, the new alpha-methyl derivative of amantidine, has the advantage of fewer neurologic side effects.

Atypical Pneumonia Syndrome. Most otherwise healthy young ambulatory patients with fever, nonproductive cough, and nonspecific infiltrate have a self-limited disease that will resolve without treatment. However, because *Mycoplasma* and *Chlamydia*—and possibly *Moraxella*—are the most likely etiologies in this patient population, an empirical course of *erythromycin* can be used to shorten duration of illness. Erythromycin is also likely to help in cases of *Legionella* infection presenting as mild atypical pneumonia; diagnosis and treatment may be based on epidemiologic grounds (eg, epidemic outbreak, common water source suspected).

Often, epidemiologic data determine initial treatment decisions in patients with atypical pneumonia. When there has been travel to an area endemic for histoplasmosis or coccidiomycosis, then *ketoconazole* requires consideration. Possible exposure to *Chlamydia psittaci* from handling of birds necessitates beginning with a *tetracycline.* Patients with AIDS who come down with an atypical pneumonia require prompt consideration for *Pneumocystis carinii* infection. *Trimethoprim-sulfamethoxazole* is usually the drug first administered and has proven effective when given parenterally. However, there is a high incidence of allergic reactions to the agent among AIDS patients, necessitating a switch to pentamidine (see Chapter 13).

Tuberculosis. For more information, see Chapter 49.

MONITORING THERAPY

Temperature, respiratory rate, chest examination, and white cell count provide a reasonable estimate of recovery. Repeating chest x-rays at frequent intervals is wasteful if the patient is progressing well clinically. It is important to recognize that clearing of radiologic findings often lags far behind clinical resolution; continued presence of a slowly resolving infiltrate is neither a sign of poor response to therapy nor indicative of serious prognosis. This is particularly true for pneumococcal disease, in which the patient feels much better although x-rays may still show an infiltrate up to 6 weeks later. However, x-ray examination is important for detection of complications such as lung abscess and empyema, and films should be obtained when the patient's condition is worsening or fever is not resolving.

INDICATIONS FOR ADMISSION

As alluded to repeatedly, one of the most important decisions in the care of the patient with a community-acquired lower respiratory infection is the proper setting for care. There is little question as regards the immunocompetent, otherwise healthy young patient with an acute bronchitis or the seriously ill patient with overt respiratory compromise. In between are the many patients who are elderly or have underlying cardiopulmonary disease and present in the ambulatory setting with a lower tract infection; they are the source of concern.

One validated set of criteria for high risk and need for admission derive from the Appropriateness Evaluation Protocol, a triage instrument used by quality assurance and review organizations. It specifies six criteria, any one of which is grounds for admission: 1) *marked vital sign abnormality* (pulse greater than 140 per minute, systolic blood pressure < 90 mmHg, or respiratory rate > 30); 2) *altered mental status;* 3) arterial *PO_2 less than 60 mmHg* on room air; 4) a *suppurative pneumonia-related infection* (eg, empyema, endocarditis; 5) *severe acute electrolyte, hematologic, or metabolic abnormality* (eg, BUN > 50 mg per deciliter; hematocrit < 30; serum, WBC < 1000; Na < 130 mg per deciliter); 6) an *acute coexistent medical condition* (eg, myocardial infarction.)

Prospective testing of these criteria found them relatively insensitive for predicting a complicated outpatient course. Multiple regression analysis identified *age over 65, comorbid illness* (especially cardiopulmonary disease), *temperature over 101°F* (38.3°C), *immunosuppression* (including HIV disease), and *high-risk organism* (*Staphylococcus* or gram-negative rods) as more sensitive criteria. The complication rate ranged from 40 percent for the presence of one risk factor to 100 percent for all four. The presence of more than one of these risk factors was deemed a basis for admission, whereas the presence of just one was considered grounds for a cautious, closely watched trial of outpatient therapy. Much research continues on refinement of decision rules for hospitalization of patients with community-acquired pneumonia.

Irrespective of these criteria, need for admission is often based on the *quality of the home environment* and presence of an organism necessitating *parenteral therapy*. With home IV therapy becoming increasingly practical and cost-effective, the ability to treat at home should increase, shortening the course of inpatient therapy or even obviating the need for admission in carefully selected instances.

PATIENT EDUCATION

Patients treated on an ambulatory basis need to be instructed to maintain a good fluid intake (approximately 2000 mL of liquid daily) to avoid inspissation of secretions and poor pulmonary toilet. Temperature should be taken and recorded each evening. Caution against overuse of any cough suppressant is important; emphasis should be on nighttime use only, allowing for sleep but permitting cough and mobilization of sputum during the day. Many patients think all coughing is bad; they need to understand its role in clearing the airways so they do not abuse their medication. If the patient is a smoker, he or she should be strongly urged to cease smoking, if he or she has not already done so. In fact, this is an excellent opportunity to encourage the patient to quit, because many do at this time (see Chapter 53). The patient and his or her family should be instructed to watch for evidence of worsening (such as unremitting fever, drowsiness, dyspnea) and to call at first sign of difficulty.

ANNOTATED BIBLIOGRAPHY

Austrian R, Gold J. Pneumococcal bacteremia with special reference to bacteremic pneumococcal pneumonia. Ann Intern Med 1964;60:759. *(Classic study of clinical features and prognostic indicators in bacteremic pneumococcal pneumonia.)*

Douglas RG, Jr. Amantadine as an antiviral agent in influenza. N Engl J Med 1982;307:617. *(Summarizes studies on amantadine and argues for its use during epidemics of influenza A.)*

Fang G-D, Fine M, Orloff J, et al. New and emerging etiologies for community-acquired pneumonia with implications for therapy. Medicine (Baltimore) 1990;69:307. *(Excellent data on community-acquired etiologies.)*

Fine MJ, Smith DJ, Singer DE. Hospitalization decision in patients with community-acquired pneumonia: A prospective cohort study. Am J Med 1990;89:713. *(Provides a decision rule and criteria for admission based on a multivariate analysis.)*

Health and Public Policy Committee, American College of Physicians. Pneumococcal vaccine. Ann Intern Med 1986;104: 118. *(Strongly recommends use of the vaccine; guidelines provided.)*

Jay SJ, Johannson WG, Pierce AK. The radiographic resolution of *Streptococcus pneumoniae* pneumonia. N Engl Med 293: 798, 1975 *(Classic study showing that delayed resolution of radiographic abnormalities is typical.)*

Katz MH, et al. Risk stratification of ambulatory patients suspected of pneumocystis pneumonia. Arch Intern Med 1991; 51:105. *(LDH elevation > 220, ESR > 50, diffuse or perihilar infiltrate on chest x-ray, and oral candidiasis predicted* Pneumocystis *infection in a population of homosexual young men.)*

Kirilloff LH, Owens GR, Rogers RM, et al. Does chest physical therapy work? Chest 1985;88:436. *(One of several prospective studies that fail to demonstrate efficacy.)*

Kleemola SRM, Karjalainen JE, Raty RKH. Rapid diagnosis of *Mycoplasma pneumoniae* infection: clinical evaluation of a commercial probe test. J Infect Dis 1990;162:70. *(Sensitivity 95 percent; specificity 85 percent testing sputum samples with this DNA probe.)*

La Force MA. Community-acquired lower respiratory tract infections: Prevention and cost-control strategies. Am J Med 1985;78(6B):52. *(Provocative paper examining the utility of diagnostic, preventive, and treatment modalities.)*

Levy M, Dromer F, Brioin N, et al. Community-acquired pneumonia: Importance of initial noninvasive bacteriologic and radiographic investigations. Chest 1988;93:43. *(Argues against invasive diagnostic techniques even if initial sputum examinations are nondiagnostic.)*

Mansel JK, Rosenow EC, Smith TE, et al. *Mycoplasma pneumoniae* pneumonia. Chest 1989;95:639. *(Excellent review of this important cause of atypical pneumonia.)*

Marrie TJ, Grayston JT, Wang S-P, et al. Pneumonia associated with the TWAR strain of *Chlamydia*. Ann Intern Med 1987; 106:507. *(Documents that TWAR can cause serious pneumonia in older patients as well as mild acute respiratory disease in younger ones.)*

Mayer RD. Legionella infections: A review of five years of research. Rev Infect Dis 1983;5:258. *(Excellent overview of the epidemiology, pathogenesis, diagnosis, and management of this important infection.)*

Musher DM, McKenzie SO. Infections due to *Staphylococcus aureus*. Medicine 1977;56:383. *(Review of staphylococcal infections, including aerogenous and bacteremic pneumonias.)*

Neu HC. New macrolide antibiotics: Azithromycin and clarithromycin. Ann Intern Med 1992;116:517. *(More useful for their expanded spectrum [eg, against Lyme disease and atypical mycobacteria] than for treating those conditions already well covered by erythromycin; although more effective against* H. influenzae.*)*

Nolan PE, Bass JB. New drugs for treating lung infection. Chest 1988;94:1076. *(Useful review that includes both oral and parenteral agents.)*

Rodrigues J, Niederman MS, Fein AM, et al. Nonresolving pneumonia in steroid-treated patients with obstructive lung disease. Am J Med 1992;93:29. *(COPD patients on steroids had a high risk of opportunistic infection when pneumonia did not clear with antibiotic therapy.)*

Ruf B, Schurmann D, Horbach SI, et al. Prevalence and diagnosis of *Legionella* pneumonia: A 3-year prospective study with emphasis on application of urinary antigen detection. J Infect Dis 1990;162:1341. *(The infection accounted for more than 3 percent of ambulatory pneumonias.)*

Sarubbi FA, Myers JW, Williams JJ, et al. Respiratory infections caused by *Branhamella catarrhalis:* Selected epidemiologic features. Am J Med 1990;88(suppl 5A):9S. *(Finds a seasonal pattern; occurring in both pediatric and adult populations; many isolates are beta-lactamase positive.)*

Schlamm HT, Yancovitz SR. *Haemophilus influenzae* pneumonia in young adults with AIDS, ARC, or risk of AIDS. Am J Med 1989;86:11. *(Finds high risk of potentially serious pneumonia from* H. influenzae *infection in this group.)*

Sims RV, Steinmann WC, McConville JH, et al. The clinical effectiveness of pneumococcal vaccine in the elderly. Ann Intern Med 1988;108:653. *(Documents 70 percent efficacy in the elderly.)*

Woodhead MA, MacFarlane JT, McCraqcken JS, et al. Prospective study of the aetiology and outcome of pneumonia in the community. Lancet 1987;1:671. *(A British study;* Pneumococcus *was the most frequent pathogen [36 percent of cases];* H. influenzae *accounted for 10 percent; in 45 percent no etiology was identified; mortality 3 percent.)*

Wright PW, Wallace RJ, Shepherd JR. A descriptive study of 42 cases of *Branhamella catarrhalis* pneumonia. Am J Med 1990;88(suppl 5A):2S. *(Describes a mild clinical illness occurring in many patients with underlying pulmonary disease.)*

53
Approach to the Patient with Lung Cancer

Primary Care Medicine: Office Evaluation and Management of the Adult Patient, 3rd edition, edited by Allan H. Goroll, Lawrence A. May, and Albert G. Mulley, Jr. J.B. Lippincott Company, Philadelphia

Lung cancer continues to be the leading cause of cancer deaths in the United States and is the second most common cause of cancer among men and women, trailing prostate and breast cancers, respectively. Cigarette smoking accounts for 95 percent of lung cancers in men and 85 percent of those in women (see Chapter 54). Once established, most forms of lung cancer are minimally responsive to therapy, although there are important exceptions. The primary physician needs to be skilled in prevention (see Chapter 54); alert to early signs of lung cancer (see Chapters 41, 42, and 44); capable of conducting the workup, staging, and monitoring of the disease; and knowledgeable about treatment options and their effects on survival and quality of life.

PATHOLOGY, CLINICAL PRESENTATION, AND COURSE

The common types of bronchogenic carcinoma are designated as squamous cell, adenocarcinoma, large cell, and small cell. Each has its own epidemiologic and clinical characteristics, although, with the exception of small-cell disease, they share a similar natural history and response to therapy. Consequently, lung cancers are often classified as small cell (SCLC) and non-small cell (NSCLC).

Small-Cell Lung Cancer (SCLC). Small-cell carcinoma (formerly known as oat-cell carcinoma) is typically central in location and accounts for 25 percent of cases. Growth is rapid, with 50 percent to 75 percent manifesting evidence of metastatic disease beyond the chest at the time of clinical presentation and initial staging. These tumors derive from endocrine cells of the bronchial mucosa and can produce a variety of paraneoplastic syndromes (see Chapter 92). Untreated, the course of illness is rapid with median survival of only a few months. However, these tumors are very responsive to chemotherapy (see below).

Non-Small-Cell Lung Cancers (NSCLC). A quarter to a third of NSCLC patients present with localized disease (stages I and II). Another quarter to a third have locally or regionally advanced disease (stages IIIa and b), and a third to half present with advanced disease with distant metastases (stage IV). Survival is a function of stage at time of presentation, with nearly 40 percent of the first group surviving 5 years, 7 percent of the second group, and less than 1 percent of the last.

Squamous-cell (epidermoid) carcinoma is the most common lung cancer. It is predominantly a disease of men and accounts for more than 40 percent of all cases. Like most other bronchogenic carcinomas, there is a strong association with smoking. Most of these tumors occur centrally and can produce bronchial obstruction. They tend to ulcerate and may cause bleeding.

Adenocarcinomas are responsible for about 25 percent of lung cancers and many of those that present peripherally. They sometimes arise in areas of fibrosis secondary to prior pulmonary parenchymal damage. This cell type is less closely associated with smoking than others.

Undifferentiated large-cell carcinomas are, in most instances, probably a form of adenocarcinoma. Unlike well-differentiated adenocarcinomas, they are often centrally located and bronchoscopically visible as an endobronchial mass lesion. These cancers tend to metastasize hematogenously relatively early, leading to disease in the bones, liver, and brain.

Clinical presentation is partially a function of the tumor's location; *central endobronchial* lesions may produce symptoms *early* in the course of illness. *Hemoptysis, cough, sputum* production, and a *localized wheeze* are among complaints reported in early phases; however, the frequency with which these symptoms are noted in early disease is low. Hemoptysis occurs as a presenting symptom in only 7 percent to 10 percent of patients with lung cancer, although up to 40 percent will report hemoptysis at some time in their illness. On occasion, a systemic syndrome, such as hypertrophic osteoarthropathy (see Chapter 45), peripheral neuropathy, or inappropriate antidiuretic hormone (ADH) secretion, may precede other evidence of disease (see Chapter 92). Symptoms of *advanced disease* include *anorexia, weight loss, nausea* and vomiting, *hoarseness* (recurrent laryngeal nerve involvement), *pleuritic chest pain, bone pain,* and *neurologic deficits.*

Of the patients presenting with metastasis or destined to develop metastasis, the most frequent sites include extension to local or regional *lymph nodes* within the chest (25% to 45%), *liver* (30% to 45%), *bone* and *bone marrow* (20% to 40%), and *central nervous system* (CNS; 20% to 35%).

Clinical Course and Prognosis. Overall 5-year survival remains at a dismal 13 percent, essentially unchanged in the past two decades. The poor prognosis is related in part to the advanced stage of disease at the time of diagnosis. Unfortunately, local and regional disease are most often asymptomatic. Because the median survival for patients with lung cancer is less than 12 months, late metastasis is rare. There are important exceptions to these dim statistics, in particular the improvement in survival for SCLC and those with NSCLC who have surgically resectable tumors.

As noted above, clinical course is different for SCLC and NSCLC. For *NSCLC,* clinical course and survival are a function of surgical–pathologic stage. The staging scheme for NSCLC has been revised according to the tumor–node–metastasis system (TMN; see Table 53–1 and Chapter 86). Survival improves markedly with surgical resectability. For example, those patients fortunate enough to have their disease confined to the lung (stage I) have a 5-year survival approaching 50 percent. With involvement of hilar and mediastinal lymph nodes, survival rates decrease significantly, but less so than was previously thought if complete tumor resection is achieved. Unfortunately, only a small minority of patients presents with surgically curable disease. Screening efforts have failed to provide satisfactory early detection (see Chapter 37). Preliminary data suggest that monoclonal antibodies directed against some tumor antigens may correlate inversely with prognosis.

SCLC differs substantially from NSCLC in that prognosis is more independent of anatomic distribution at the time of diagnosis. Before the advent of contemporary chemotherapy, median survival was 1 to 3 months; it has increased severalfold to 7 to 16 months, depending on extent of disease. Five-year survival remains poor (5% to 10%), due

Table 53-1. Staging and Survival in Non-Small-Cell Lung Cancer

STAGE	TUMOR	NODES	METASTASES	5-YEAR SURVIVAL
I	T1 or T2	N0	M0	50%
II	T1 or T2	N1	M0	30%
IIIa	T1-2 or T3	N1 or N0	M0	15%
IIIb	any T	any N	M0	<5%
IV	any T	any N	M1	0%

T1 = lesions up to 3 cm in diameter
T2 = lesions > 3 cm
T3 = invasion of mediastinum, diaphragm, or chest wall
T4 = invasion of heart, great vessels, or malignant pleural effusion
N0 = no nodal involvement
N1 = tracheobronchial or hilar node involvement
N2 = ipsilateral mediastinal nodes
N3 = contralateral or supraclavicular nodes
M0 = no metastasis
M1 = systemic metastasis

*Staging for small cell lung cancer is designated as either "limited disease" (confined to the thorax) or "extensive disease" (metastasis outside the thorax).

Adapted from Mountain CF. A new international staging system for lung cancer. Chest 1986;89(suppl 4):225S.

to the high probability of metastasis, even among those who present with limited disease.

WORKUP AND STAGING

The basic approach to diagnosis and staging is to begin with noninvasive studies and proceed to increasingly invasive ones only as necessary. Staging is done to determine prognosis and treatment and, in particular, to assess resectability of the tumor. The advent of computed tomography (CT) scanning has greatly facilitated noninvasive assessment of hilar and mediastinal node involvement. Invasive studies should only be considered if the results will have a marked effect on treatment plans. Many patients with lung cancer have concurrent chronic lung disease and may be seriously compromised by a complication of an invasive study. The histopathologic diagnosis of lung cancer may be obtained with a variety of procedures ranging from sputum cytology to thoracotomy (see Chapters 37 and 44).

Diagnosis

Chest x-ray is the primary diagnostic modality, with the appearance of the lesion and its doubling time helpful in distinguishing benign from malignant disease. Although there are reports of lesions as small as 3 mm being detected, most are not visible until they are at least 5 mm or more in diameter. The finding of a calcified nodule can be helpful, especially if the pattern of calcification is eccentric (see Chapter 44).

Computed tomography (CT) of the chest aids diagnosis by confirming the presence of a suspected lung mass and, if calcium is present, by clarifying its calcification pattern. CT has become critical to staging by determining the presence and extent of hilar and mediastinal node involvement (see below).

Sputum cytology may provide evidence of lung cancer and even cell type. Test sensitivity ranges from 25 percent to 75 percent, depending on the site of the tumor. Optimal collection requires obtaining three deep, first-morning samples. The presence of pulmonary histiocytes indicates an adequate specimen. A negative cytologic examination does not rule out cancer, especially in patients with peripheral lesions.

The yield of cytologic testing can be greatly enhanced by use of *fiberoptic bronchoscopy* complemented by *washings, brushings,* or *forceps biopsy.* For centrally located visualized lesions, washings provide a diagnosis in nearly 80 percent of instances; for brushings, yield is 92 percent; and for forceps biopsy, 93 percent. Yield falls for peripheral lesions: it is 20 percent to 30 percent for peripheral lesions less than 3 cm in diameter, and about 40 percent to 70 percent for those larger than 3 cm. The complication rate is low in experienced hands, with hypoxemia, hemorrhage, pneumothorax, or laryngospasm occurring in 0.1 percent to 0.3 percent of cases. On occasion, *transbronchial biopsy* is deemed the best means of establishing the diagnosis (eg, in suspected alveolar cell carcinoma; see Chapter 51). Risk of pneumothorax rises to 5 percent.

For peripheral lesions, the *percutaneous transthoracic fine-needle biopsy*—usually guided by CT or chest fluoroscopy—has proven accurate for diagnosis of lung cancers. Reports on the diagnostic accuracy of these radiologically guided procedures quote sensitivity in excess of 90 percent and specificity over 95 percent when performed by skilled radiologists using "fine-needle" techniques that allow not only aspiration, but removal of a tiny core of material as well. However, sensitivity and specificity may be compromised by the inadequacy of the specimen sometimes obtained, which occasionally is an aspirate of cytologic material rather than a solid core of tissue; in such instances, the architectural relationships may be obscured or unavailable in cytologic specimens. Pneumothorax ensues in close to 30 percent, but it is usually small, of little clinical consequence, and resolves spontaneously without need for a chest tube. Hemorrhage is rare, unless a vascular lesion is biopsied. For patients with limited pulmonary reserve who may be unable to tolerate any degree of pneumothorax, a controlled *thoracotomy* may also be preferable to needle aspiration.

Scalene node biopsy is indicated when these peripheral nodes are noted to be enlarged; it can save the patient extensive testing for both diagnosis and staging.

Staging

Staging is performed to determine prognosis and select therapy. The principal challenge is to assess surgical candidacy, which requires accurate evaluation of hilar and mediastinal lymph nodes. Contralateral involvement of these regional nodes by tumor places the patient in stage IIIb and out of consideration for curative surgical therapy, but ipsilateral disease is no longer de facto grounds for rejection of surgical candidacy. The challenge is to accurately evaluate these regional nodes.

Chest x-ray contributes to staging by providing data on tumor size and may show evidence of spread to chest wall or regional nodes if there is a marked degree of involvement, although sensitivity is low.

Chest CT with contrast has been used extensively in hopes of improving the sensitivity of radiologic staging. Although sensitivity and specificity of CT for diagnosis of mediastinal disease appear to be reasonable for patients with clinical stage I disease who have a lung lesion greater than 3 cm (T2N0M0), results for those with earlier stage I disease (T1N0M0—lung nodule < 3 cm) have been disappointing. False-positive and false-negative rates of 5 percent to 10 percent have been reported for diagnosis of contralateral mediastinal node involvement in such patients. This has led some authorities to warn against reflexively ordering a CT scan in patients with early stage I disease or depending too heavily on its findings for decision making (eg, ruling in or out surgical candidacy solely on the basis of a CT result). For patients with a pulmonary lesion greater than 3 cm, CT with contrast continues to be a useful noninvasive step for assessment of the hilum and mediastinum, but a negative CT scan does not rule out microscopic spread from central or late peripheral lesions.

CT is sensitive for detection of metastasis below the diaphragm (to liver and adrenals); upper abdominal views should be obtained at the time of chest CT examination. If positive and confirmed by needle biopsy, CT would indicate stage IV disease and inappropriateness of surgery.

For judging tumor involvement of the chest wall, *magnetic resonance imaging (MRI)* is superior to CT. MRI is also better for assessment of disease in the superior sulcus and for definition of subcarinal nodal involvement.

Although symptomatic metastasis to head and bone are relatively common, routine use of *head CT* and *bone scanning* is wasteful, unless there is clinical evidence of disease referable to these sites (see Chapter 86).

More invasive staging techniques are indicated when the patient's surgical candidacy remains in question after CT scanning. Many thoracic surgeons believe that all patients should undergo *mediastinoscopy* for evaluation of the mediastinum and hilum before thoracotomy, because the presence of microscopic tumor in the contralateral mediastinum is a contraindication to resection. Under general anesthesia, a cervical incision is made and mediastinal node biopsy is carried out under direct visualization. They argue that sensitivity of CT is insufficient, even in the setting of more advanced or central disease, in which the likelihood of microscopic nodal involvement is high. The debate and efforts to improve mediastinal staging continue.

Advances in needle biopsy and fiberoptic endoscopy techniques have enhanced the roles of *transthoracic* and *transbronchial needle-aspiration biopsy* in staging of lung cancer. These techniques offer a less morbid alternative to mediastinoscopy for tissue-based assessment of mediastinal spread. They do not require general anesthesia or a formal surgical procedure and can be performed under CT guidance. Mediastinoscopy can be reserved for those in whom these procedures are inconclusive.

The remainder of staging is determined by the tumor's cell type. For patients with *inoperable non-small-cell carcinoma,* further staging is of little value, because the information would have minimal impact on decision making or estimation of prognosis. Staging is considerably different for patients with *small-cell carcinoma*. Because the disease usually presents with evidence of bilateral nodal involvement, the issue is extent of disease rather than resectability. The goal is to distinguish between limited and extensive disease (the latter implies spread beyond the hemithorax of origin and regional nodes). Almost 25 percent of patients have marrow invasion, and marrow biopsy is done routinely. CT scanning of common sites of metastatic disease (eg, brain) may also be useful if the result will affect plans for therapy (see below).

PRINCIPLES OF MANAGEMENT

Small-Cell Disease

Small-cell disease is biologically unique among bronchogenic cancers in that its cells are extremely sensitive to chemotherapy and radiation, probably due in part to their rapid rate of proliferation. Surgical treatment is usually not possible, because 85 percent of patients have extensive disease at time of presentation. Irrespective of whether disease is limited to the chest or disseminated, the treatment of choice is *combination chemotherapy*. For patients with limited disease, *radiation* is given as adjunctive therapy. As noted above, survival irrespective of stage has been prolonged four- to fivefold by chemotherapy. However, cure rates are very low. Only about 10 percent of limited-stage patients survive 5 years, although those who survive 2 years have a greater than two-thirds chance of relapse. Essentially all patients with extensive disease die within 2 years.

Chemotherapy. Since introduction of combination chemotherapy in the 1970s, there have been a modest additional improvement in survival rates and considerable progress in reducing treatment morbidity, complexity, and duration. The use of a reduced-dose regimen of *etoposide* plus *cisplatin* after a course of three-drug therapy (cyclophosphamide, doxorubicin, vincristine) has improved survival and reduced marrow suppression. Shorter courses of therapy (no more than 4 to 6 months) are standard; longer courses are without additional benefit. In the elderly, single-dose etoposide appears to provide up to 80 percent of the response without significant compromise of survival.

Radiation. Patients with limited disease experience a 90-percent response rate to irradiation. Survival appears to improve when radiation is used as an adjunct to chemotherapy, although toxicity increases. The optimal means of combining both modalities is under active study, with preliminary data on a synergistic effect noted for concurrent use of cisplatin and radiation.

Surgery has almost no role in SCLC, because of the nearly universal occurrence of occult disease beyond the initial lesion.

Non-Small-Cell Disease

Surgery offers the only hope for cure. The procedure of choice is a *thoracotomy with resection*. About 35 to 45 percent of patients presenting with NSCLC will have potentially resectable disease, but only 60 percent have successful resections. For the latter group, the 5-year survival or cure rate ranges from 25 percent to 40 percent. Thus, at best, less than 10 percent of patients who present with NSCLC can expect a cure. Two concurrent trends dominate the surgical approach to NSCLC: expanding candidacy to patients with stage IIIa disease and reducing the extend of resection in patients with stage I disease. Patients with a single ipsilateral mediastinal disease are now being considered surgical candidates. Previously, mediastinal nodal involvement was considered an incurable lesion, but those with ipsilateral disease that can be grossly removed have shown a 5-year survival ranging from 15 percent to 30 percent.

Patients with localized disease are being treated with less radical, more conservative surgery. The goal is to preserve as much functional lung tissue as possible, especially in patients with underlying lung disease. Previously, pneumonectomy was performed in more than 70 percent of patients, incorporating the hilar as well as mediastinal lymph nodes. A regional excision that employs wedge or segmental resection for stage I peripheral lobe lesions is now preferred. The general surgical dictum is to employ the minimal degree of surgery necessary to remove all macroscopic evidence of tumor.

Surgical excision is particularly indicated for nodules with long doubling times or long disease-free intervals, especially if the nodules are solitary and unassociated with extrathoracic disease. The subsequent use of radiation therapy may augment local control, allowing for lesser surgery.

Radiation therapy is used both for curative intent and for palliation. Preoperative radiation therapy may promote the resectability of tumors and possibly extend survival rates. The superior sulcus tumor is one instance in which preoperative radiation therapy has improved the likelihood of cure despite contiguous extension of the tumor to bone or the chest wall. In general, when surgery is used in combination with prior radiation, the resection almost always needs to be a pneumonectomy; in principle, surgery must incorporate all sites that were diseased before the radiation therapy.

When used as sole therapy with *curative intent,* results have been disappointing. Patients with NSCLC respond poorly to irradiation as a curative therapy, but achieve good intrathoracic control of tumor, even eradication. In a major randomized trial of definitive radiation therapy for patients with unresectable stage III cancer, higher rates of regression and better disease control in the chest were observed with use of the high-dose therapy (60 Gy); however, there was no improvement over baseline 5-year survival, which remained at 5 percent. Although radiation may achieve local control, it does little to prevent relapse, which most often is the result of distant metastases. This has led to attempts to combine chemotherapy with irradiation (see below).

Chemotherapy for NSCLC has a far more limited role than in SCLC. It has been used as adjuvant therapy before surgery in patients with extensive, but surgically resectable disease (eg, stage III), after surgery, and in those with inoperable disease undergoing radiation therapy. The goals are to improve local control and decrease risk of distant metastasis. Results have been modest at best, but some improvements in survival are being noted. *Cisplatin,* in particular, has shown promise, although its side effects can be disabling (see Chapter 88). For example, a large prospective randomized study of concurrent cisplatin plus radiation in patients with inoperable but nonmetastatic NSCLC demonstrated marked improvement over radiation alone (16% versus 2% 3-year survival). However, the benefit was attributable only to improvement in local control. Cisplatin has produced some improvement in survival for patients with stage IV disease, although the improvement in survival has to be weighed against drug-induced morbidity. Further refinement of chemotherapy and its use in combination modality programs offers promise, but much work remains to be done.

Management of Stage III Disease deserves special comment because more than 60 percent of patients with NSCLC present with inoperable disease. The majority of patients with stage III bronchogenic carcinoma develop distant metastases regardless of control of the primary tumor. Survival is a function of the rate and extent of systemic dissemination. Substantial advances in therapy are required before genuine hope can be offered to the patient with this stage of disease. Encouraging developments include the improved survival associated with surgical treatment of patients with stage IIIa disease, and with concurrent administration of cisplatin and radiotherapy for stage IIIb disease.

MONITORING

Monitoring patients with surgically resectable and potentially curable lung cancer is conditioned by the fact that there is little one can do for metastatic disease. Thus, monitoring is more specifically directed at searching for a new primary tumor in this high-risk population. Chest films are indicated at regular intervals, ranging from every 3 months during the first 2 years to every 4 to 12 months in later years. Routine monitoring for recurrent disease outside the chest is unnecessary in the absence of specific symptoms suggesting bone, liver, or brain metastasis.

Monitoring patients with extensive disease is directed at assessing the efficacy of therapy. One needs to select one or more objective measures of tumor burden (see Chapter 86) that can be followed conveniently to gauge response to treatment. Chest x-ray, CT scan, and bronchoscopy are commonly used.

MANAGEMENT OF COMPLICATIONS

Superior Vena Cava Syndrome. Obstruction of the superior vena cava by lung tumor produces the classic clinical syndrome of facial edema, proptosis, suffusion of the conjunctivae, and dilation of the veins of the upper thorax and neck. Asymptomatic neck vein distention is an early manifestation. In late stages, the patient may complain of relentless headache. In patients with lung cancer, the syndrome is invariably caused by tumor extending into the right side of the mediastinum and compressing the venous system adjacent to the mediastinal lymph nodes. The secondary effects of compression are thrombosis and tumor invasion; if untreated, neurologic function may be compromised. The histopathologic types of lung cancer that lead to the syndrome are variable, but most commonly the culprit is undifferentiated small-cell carcinoma. (See Chapter 92).

The approach to evaluation and therapy has undergone some revision in recent years. Previously, it was believed that emergency radiation therapy was indicated regardless of whether a tissue diagnosis was available; the view was that the risk of an invasive procedure to obtain tissue outweighed its potential contribution to design of a treatment plan. More recent data indicate that the risk of evaluation in patients lacking a tissue diagnosis is low and that chemotherapy may be superior to radiation in some instances (eg, small-cell cancer). Because superior vena cava syndrome may be the initial presentation of lung cancer, the issue of need for tissue diagnosis is frequently encountered in this setting. When the result will change the mode of therapy, tissue diagnosis should be attempted, taking care to minimize risk to the patient.

Even when a tissue diagnosis is not obtained, response to radiotherapy is rather good; in unselected series, more than 70 percent of patients demonstrate a response. Although patients with superior vena cava syndrome secondary to lung cancer have an inoperable tumor, the prognosis is no worse than for other patients with stage III lung cancer.

Malignant pleural effusion is another important complication. It occurs in 10 percent to 15 percent of patients with carcinoma of the lung and may be secondary to direct pleural implantation or a consequence of mediastinal obstruction to lymphatic drainage of the pleural surface. Only 20 percent to 30 percent of pleural effusions that develop as a consequence of bronchogenic carcinoma are cytologically confirmed, and many are transudates. Pleural biopsy is often required for definitive diagnosis.

The median survival for patients who develop a malignant pleural effusion is less than 3 months; therefore, the effusion should be monitored and treated only when it causes significant respiratory discomfort. The use of intrapleural chemotherapeutic agents (eg, bleomycin, fluorouracil) or chemical irritants, such as tetracycline, talcum powder, or quinacrine, may be effective in 50 percent to 60 percent of patients. The specific choice of agent for sealing the pleura is determined by the morbidity of the treatment. The chemotherapeutic agents such as bleomycin and fluorouracil are relatively innocuous. On the other hand, nitrogen mustard and the "inert" irritants may result in a major secondary inflammatory response with reactive effusion and fever. Quinacrine (Atabrine) must be instilled repeatedly over a 5- to 7-day period to be maximally effective. Radiation therapy to the mediastinum or to the pleura has been of limited effectiveness. Surgical drainage with an intrathoracic tube for 2 to 3 days may result in a secondary inflammatory response adequate to seal the pleural space.

Tumor–humoral syndromes are associated with small-cell carcinomas. Because the tumor is derived from endocrine cells of the bronchial mucosa, it is capable of producing adrenocorticotropic hormone (ACTH), ADH, and even on occasion, serotonin. The clinical pictures that may result are Cushing's syndrome, inappropriate ADH secretion, and carcinoid syndrome, respectively. In an autopsy series of 85 patients with small-cell carcinoma, it was found that patients who manifested a paraneoplastic syndrome tended to have a more benign clinical course and longer survival; in addition, there was a significantly lower incidence of metastases to the CNS.

Complications of surgical therapy include prolonged air leakage due to a bronchopleural fistula, and postoperative intrapleural infection with empyema formation. Both are potentially serious and require prompt surgical attention. Pulmonary insufficiency is uncommon as a result of careful preoperative pulmonary evaluation of candidates for resection; however, pneumonia in the remaining lung can lead to respiratory compromise.

Complications of chemotherapy are those related to the use of such agents as cisplatin, cyclophosphamide, adriamycin, methotrexate, and nitrosoureas (see Chapter 88). Use of certain chemotherapeutic agents (eg, nitrosoureas, methotrexate) during the induction phase of radiation therapy in patients with small-cell cancer is suspected of accounting for some late complications seen in long-term survivors, such as risk of other malignancies.

Complications of radiation therapy include radiation pneumonitis, esophageal stricture, pericardial and myocardial fibrosis, rib fractures secondary to radiation-induced osteonecrosis, and radiation fibrosis.

PATIENT EDUCATION

Most laymen believe that lung cancer is fatal. Although prognosis and efficacy of treatment are indeed poor in most types of lung cancer, the patient with a newly discovered, suspicious pulmonary nodule needs to know that there are major differences in prognosis based on tissue type and stage of disease at time of presentation. Before completion of workup and staging, this background information can help sustain the patient and family through a worrisome period of uncertainty and provide a rationale for the procedures that need to be done.

Once the diagnosis and extent of disease are known, prognosis and treatment options should be shared with the patient and family. When surgical cure is a genuine possibility and the patient can tolerate the surgery, it should be urged. However, in lung cancer, in which prognosis is often so poor, treatment plans should be formulated jointly, eliciting and respecting the patient's preferences and willingness to undergo treatment. A realistic assessment for the patient and family of prognosis and the pros and cons of treatment are essential for effective decision making. All too often, inappropriately aggressive forms of therapy are rushed into, mostly for the sake of "doing something." Studies have found that socioeconomically advantaged patients tend to undergo more aggressive forms of therapy, although when controlling for disease stage, there is no evidence of improved survival.

Patients with incurable disease need to know their prognosis, which is best given in amounts of detail consistent with their desire to know. The news of lung cancer in a loved one is very upsetting to family members, who will try to shield the patient from the information. Facilitating communication between family and patient is essential to preserving the patient's quality of life and helping the family to cope (see Chapter 87).

A.H.G.

ANNOTATED BIBLIOGRAPHY

Ahmann FR. A reassessment of the clinical implications of the superior vena cava syndrome. J Clin Oncol 1984;2:961. *(Argues that diagnostic workup is safe and useful for proper selection of treatment modality. Based on review of over 1800 cases.)*

Becker GL, Whitlock WL, Schaefer PS, et al. The impact of thoracic computed tomography in clinically staged T1, N0, M0 chest lesions. Arch Intern Med 1990;150:557. *(CT did not prove useful due to an unacceptable number of false-positive and false-negative results; argues that routine CT scanning is not indicated in such patients.)*

Bunn PA, Licheter AS, Makuch RW, et al. Chemotherapy alone or with chest radiation therapy in limited stage small-cell lung cancer: A prospective randomized trial. Ann Intern Med 1987;106:655. *(Modest enhancement of benefit from addition of radiation therapy.)*

Dillman RO, Seagren SL, Propert KJ, et al. A randomized trial of induction chemotherapy plus high-dose radiation versus radiation alone in stage III non-small cell lung cancer. N Engl J Med 1990;323:940. *(Encouraging results with use of combined modality therapy.)*

Einhorn LH, Crawford J, Birch R, et al. Cisplatin plus etoposide consolidation following cyclophosphamide, doxorubicin, and vincristine in limited small-cell lung cancer. J Clin Oncol 1988;6:451. *(A reduced, simplified regimen for chemotherapy of small-cell disease.)*

Errett LE, Wison J, Chiu RCJ, et al. Wedge resection as an alternative procedure for peripheral bronchogenic carcinoma in poor-risk patients. J Thorac Cardiovasc Surg 1985;90:656. *(Example of the trend toward less radical surgery in selected patients.)*

Greenberg ER, Chute CG, Stukel T, et al. Social and economic factors in the choice of lung cancer treatment. N Engl J Med 1988;318:612. *(Controlling for stage of illness, patients of higher socioeconomic status tended to undergo more aggressive therapy without evidence of improved survival.)*

Ihde DC. Chemotherapy of lung cancer. N Engl J Med 1992; 327:1434. *(Excellent review; 107 references.)*

Johnson BE, Grayson J, Makuch RW, et al. Ten-year survival of patients with small-cell lung cancer treated with combination chemotherapy with or without irradiation. J Clin Oncol 1990; 8:396. *(National Cancer Institute's long-term experience in the treatment of small-cell cancer with chemotherapy.)*

Lee JS, Hong WK. Prognostic factors in lung cancer. N Engl J Med 1992;327:47. *(Editorial summarizing progress in use of monoclonal antibodies for prediction of prognosis in lung cancer.)*

Lin AY, Ihde DC. Recent developments in the treatment of lung cancer. JAMA 1992;267:1661. *(Excellent, authoritative, yet terse review for the general reader; good guide to the plethora of data from clinical trials; 33 references.)*

de la Monte SM, Hutchins GM, Moore GW. Paraneoplastic syndromes and constitutional symptoms in prediction of metastatic behavior of small cell carcinoma of the lung. Am J Med 1984;77:851. *(Autopsy series of 85 patients indicating that patients with paraneoplastic syndromes had a more benign clinical course and less CNS metastasis.)*

Mountain CF. A new international staging system for lung cancer. Chest 1986;89(suppl 4):225S. *(Newly adopted and widely used staging system.)*

Perez CA, Pajak TF, Rubin P, et al. Long-term observations of the pattern of failure in patients with unresectable non-oat-cell cancer of the lung treated with definitive radiotherapy: Report by the Radiation Oncology Group. Cancer 1987;59:1874. *(Major study showing that disease control was good, but survival was unaffected due to metastatic disease.)*

Pignon J-P, Arriagada R, Ihde DC, et al. A meta-analysis of thoracic radiotherapy for small-cell lung cancer. N Engl J Med 1992;327:1618. *(Modest improvement in survival in patients with limited disease treated with chemotherapy.)*

Ries LAG, Hankey BF, Miller BA, et al. Cancer Statistics Review 1973–1988. Bethesda, MD: National Cancer Institute; 1991. NIH publication 91-2789. *(Little progress in overall 5-year cancer survival: went from 12 percent to 13 percent.)*

Schaake-Konig C, Bogaert WVD, Dalesio Otilla, et al. Effects of concomitant cisplatin and radiotherapy on inoperable non-small-cell lung cancer. N Engl J Med 1992;326;524. *(Significant increase in 3-year survival achieved by combining cisplatin with radiotherapy; local radiation-enhancing effect noted, but 3-year survival still inadequate at 16 percent.)*

Silverberg E, Boring CC, Squires TS. Cancer Statistics 1990;40:9. *(Authoritative overview of survival data.)*

Spiro SG, Souhami RL, Geddes DM, et al. Duration of chemotherapy in small-cell lung cancer. Br J Cancer 1989;59:578. *(Efficacy of reduced duration demonstrated.)*

Woodring JH. Lung cancer. Radiol Clin North Am 1990;28:489. *(Monograph on lung cancer diagnosis and staging from the radiologist's perspective.)*

54
Smoking Cessation

NANCY A. RIGOTTI, M.D.

Primary Care Medicine: Office Evaluation and Management of the Adult Patient, 3rd edition, edited by Allan H. Goroll, Lawrence A. May, and Albert G. Mulley, Jr. J.B. Lippincott Company, Philadelphia

Cigarette smoking is the major preventable cause of death in the United States. Strong evidence documents benefit from cessation of smoking, even for the elderly and patients who have already developed chronic tobacco-related disease. Although the health risks of smoking are widely recognized and the prevalence of smoking has fallen dramatically in the past two decades (from 40% to about 25%), millions of Americans continue to smoke, a substantial fraction more heavily than ever, and adolescents continue to take up the habit in large numbers. Nevertheless, many people are eager to quit and often come to the primary physician for advice. Numerous studies have shown that physicians can change a patient's smoking habits. The primary care physician needs to be expert in motivating patients to quit and in advising them on the best means to accomplish their goal. This requires knowledge about available smoking cessation techniques and an appreciation of how and when to use them.

EPIDEMIOLOGY OF SMOKING AND QUITTING

Since 1964, when the Surgeon General's Report first publicized the health risks of smoking, there has been a decline in cigarette smoking by adults in the United States. This decline in the percentage of the population that smokes is averaging about 1.1 percentage points per year, with the percentage of smokers falling to about 25 percent. This decrease is largely attributable to the increasing number of smokers who have quit, rather than to a fall in the number of smokers taking up the habit. About 30 percent of smokers report attempting to quit each year. As less addicted smokers quit, the proportion of heavy smokers (> 25 cigarettes per day) has increased from about one in four to one in three. Smoking in adolescence—the time when smoking usually begins—has fallen little since its peak in the 1970s. Adolescent girls are smoking in numbers comparable to boys; the historical gender difference continues to narrow. This is worrisome because women who smoke during the reproductive years incur special risks with pregnancy and oral contraceptive use. Smoking is increasingly prevalent among populations that are nonwhite, poor, or of low educational status.

Most smokers claim they are aware of the health hazards of smoking and say they would like to quit, but most have difficulty doing so. Although the success rate for any single quitting attempt is low, smokers who repeatedly try to quit increase their likelihood of success. Lighter smokers are more successful than heavier smokers. Smokers most likely to quit are those who expect their attempt to succeed, who have a strong belief in their personal control over events, feel competent and personally secure, and have a good social support system. The smoking habits of the spouse and, in some studies, friends, are important; those with nonsmoking spouses are more likely to succeed. Patients with *depression* or a history of depression have a hard time initiating smoking cessation and a poor success rate (40% that of nondepressed patients) when they try.

More than 90 percent of former smokers quit on their own without assistance from physicians, groups, patches, gum, hypnosis, acupuncture, or psychological counseling. Those who benefit most from an assisted method are heavy, more addicted smokers. Their chances of successfully quitting are about half that of smokers who quit on their own. Receiving advice from a physician about smoking cessation doubles the chances of a patient making an attempt to quit. Smokers who quit using the "cold turkey" approach are more likely to remain abstinent than those who taper. Some reduction in cigarette consumption and switching to a different brand can be part of a smoker's preparation for quitting—being especially helpful in building a sense of confidence and control—but is no substitute for setting a definite date for abrupt and total cessation.

Health concerns are the most common reasons given by former smokers for quitting. However, the risks of lung cancer and heart disease are less often cited than are minor smoking-related ailments such as cough, dyspnea, and sore throat. Minor symptoms may successfully motivate a smoker to quit by making personally salient the more serious health risks of smoking. Illness in one smoker can influence other smokers to quit (eg, the friend or family member in the intensive care unit), as can personally sustaining a serious smoking-related illness, such as a heart attack. The likelihood that a smoker will quit increases with the severity of the illness. Although fewer than 5 percent of smokers in the general population quit each year, cessation rates are higher among individuals with newly diagnosed coronary heart disease. Many studies report that approximately one-third of smokers surviving a myocardial infarction stop smoking permanently. Increased rates of cessation are also reported in smokers with chronic obstructive pulmonary disease. During pregnancy, 20 percent of women smokers stop smoking, but the majority resume smoking after delivery. Many smokers quit temporarily when they have an acute respiratory illness.

Other reasons for quitting cited by former smokers include a desire to exert self-control over one's life, aesthetic objections to the smoking habit, and fear of setting a bad example for others. The cost of cigarettes exerts little influence among adults.

WHY PEOPLE SMOKE

Smoking is a complex behavior initiated and maintained for different reasons. The influence of peers and parents appears to be most important in the initiation of smoking. Adolescents whose parents and friends smoke are more likely to begin smoking. Once the smoking habit is established, it is sustained by many factors.

Both pharmacologic and psychological models have been proposed to explain what maintains smoking behavior. The *psychological model* regards smoking as a learned behavior that continues because it is rewarding to the smoker. Certain situations, such as finishing a meal, become strongly associated with smoking and trigger the urge to smoke. Smokers also use cigarettes to handle environmental stress and regulate emotions, especially strong negative emotions like anger.

A strong association between *depression* and smoking has been documented. Depressed patients are more likely to be smokers and, as noted above, less likely to attempt quitting or succeed at quitting. It is hypothesized that smoking may represent a form of self-medication for the depressed patient, with nicotine alleviating a dysphoric mood through activation of central neuroreceptors. Such a response would strongly reinforce smoking and might trigger a craving for cigarettes during times of depressed mood. Moreover, withdrawal of nicotine during an attempt at smoking cessation might trigger symptoms of depression, which has been reported in studies of patients with a history of depression who attempt to quit.

The *pharmacologic model* emphasizes physical addiction to nicotine. The evidence for smoking as an addiction is strong, and nicotine has been established as the addicting substance in tobacco smoke. According to this model the smoker smokes to maintain a constant blood level of nicotine and thereby avert the *withdrawal syndrome,* characterized by falls in heart rate, blood pressure, basal metabolic rate, and changes in electroencephalogram (EEG) rhythms and rapid eye movement (REM) sleep patterns. Craving for nicotine is the most common subjective complaint of withdrawal, but other symptoms include restlessness, irritability, inability to concentrate, daytime drowsiness and fatigue, sleep disturbances, headache, nausea, alteration in bowel habits, and increased appetite. Symptoms begin within hours after cessation of smoking, but their duration and severity are highly variable, representing different degrees of nicotine addiction among smokers. There is no simple test to measure nicotine addiction, but heavily addicted smokers tend to have their first cigarette shortly after arising (ie, within 30 minutes), smoke more and stronger cigarettes, and have difficulty not smoking for even a few hours.

The pharmacologic model can explain initial difficulties with cessation but cannot explain why smokers have difficulty remaining abstinent after the first few days or weeks. In fact, the majority of smokers who stop temporarily resume smoking within a few months.

Table 54-1. Smoking Cessation Strategy for Office Practice

1. Assess smoking habits
   A. Smoking and quitting history
   B. Interest in cessation
   C. Identify potential motivating factors
2. Advise every smoker to stop smoking
3. Motivate the smoker to attempt to quit
   A. Emphasize benefits of cessation
   B. Focus on short-term changes
   C. Tailor to the clinical situation
      1. Asymptomatic smoker
      2. Acute respiratory illness
      3. Chronic cardiopulmonary illness
      4. Pregnancy
   D. Address common fears
4. Ask for a commitment to quit
5. Help the smoker to quit
   A. Physician counseling/nurse counseling
   B. Self-help materials
   C. Nicotine patch or gum
   D. Referrals to formal smoking withdrawal programs
   E. Anticipate problems
      1. Withdrawal symptoms
      2. Weight gain
6. Follow-up
   A. Put smoking on the problem list
   B. Follow-up visits with nurse or physician
   C. Continued monitoring at each visit

TECHNIQUES FOR SMOKING CESSATION

The methods of smoking cessation range from unassisted "cold turkey" to formal treatment programs administered in a group setting, with a host of interventions in between. As noted, the vast majority of smokers quit in unassisted fashion. As might be expected from the multidimensional nature of the smoking problem, no single method suffices. The most effective approaches address both principal components of the smoking problem: 1) nicotine addiction; and 2) behavioral dependency on cigarettes. Combining a number of approaches into a personalized, comprehensive program appears to be the most successful strategy.

Strategies that combine pharmacologic and behavioral techniques appear to be the most effective. Pharmacologic methods are used to relieve symptoms of nicotine withdrawal, freeing the patient to focus on behavioral efforts (Tables 54–1 and 54–2).

Maintaining long-term tobacco abstinence remains the challenge in smoking cessation treatment. Short-term cessation rates of 70 percent to 80 percent are common among programs. However, a predictable and rapid return to smoking follows initial cessation. A 1-year cessation rate of 30 percent to 35 percent is considered the standard for an effective smoking cessation program.

Pharmacologic Methods

The principal pharmacologic approach is to relieve symptoms of withdrawal by continuing some nicotine exposure, although at reduced and tapering doses. The nicotine must be given by a route independent of inhalation, so as not to continue reinforcing the behavior of smoking. Nicotine is available in a chewing gum and transdermal patch for this purpose. Other pharmacologic approaches to minimizing withdrawal symptoms have included use of clonidine, minor tranquilizers, and drugs that mimic the autonomic effects of nicotine.

Transdermal nicotine—"the patch"— represents a second-generation form of nicotine reduction therapy, following introduction of nicotine gum over a decade ago (see below). It provides a convenient means of maintaining nicotine ex-

Table 54-2. A Behavioral Program for Smoking Cessation

RATIONALE	SUGGESTIONS FOR THE SMOKER
Preparing to Quit	
1. Increase motivation	Write out a list of reasons to quit.
2. Make a commitment	Set a quit date. Sign a contract with family, friends.
3. Develop social supports	Enlist the support of nonsmoking friends, relatives, coworkers.
4. Self-monitoring to identify smoking cues	Keep a record of each cigarette smoked, noting circumstances, time, and how highly desired. Wrap this around cigarette pack with rubber band.
5. Progressive restriction	Eliminate least desired cigarettes; delay smoking first morning cigarette; smoke only at certain times or places.
6. Aversive conditioning	Fill a glass bottle with all your cigarette butts ("butt bottle").
7. Satiation	Oversmoke on the day before quitting.
Initial Cessation	
1. Avoid smoking cues	Eliminate all cigarettes, ashtrays, lighters from home and car. Spend the quitting day in places where smoking is not permitted.
2. Positive reinforcement	Reward self with a treat on quitting day.
3. Aversive conditioning	Look at "butt bottle" frequently. Wear rubber band on wrist and snap it when urge to smoke occurs.
4. Substitute oral stimuli	Chew on straws, toothpicks, carrot sticks, sugarless candy or gum.
5. Substitute activities for hands	Rubber bands, paper clips.
Relapse Prevention—Maintaining Nonsmoking	
1. Avoid smoking cues	Spend time in places where smoking is not permitted. Substitute situations associated with smoking (coffee, alcohol, end of meal) with other behaviors (tea, soft drink, brushing teeth, or taking a walk at end of meal).
2. Positive reinforcement	Treat self with money saved by not smoking.
3. Aversive conditioning	Wear rubber band on wrist and snap it when urge to smoke occurs.
4. Strategies to cope with urges to smoke	Take slow deep breaths. Relaxation training Incompatible activity (take a shower) Contact a nonsmoking friend.

posure and preventing nicotine withdrawal symptoms while the smoker addresses the behavioral component of the smoking problem. Once the habit is broken, nicotine supplementation is stopped. A smoker on nicotine reduction therapy is already weaning off nicotine because the patch's pharmacokinetic properties differ from those of inhaled smoke. Nicotine delivered transdermally provides more constant nicotine levels than the peaks and troughs characteristic of smoking.

The *effectiveness* of the patch is related to its ease of administration. In randomized clinical trials of at least 6 months' duration, nicotine patches have been shown to be superior to placebo in helping smokers to stop smoking; the cessation rates of smokers using the nicotine patch were approximately double the rates of smokers receiving placebo patches. Data comparing the patch to gum are pending, but the patch is likely to prove superior because it is easier to use, facilitating compliance.

Patches are neither a panacea nor appropriate for everyone. They should be prescribed only to smokers who: 1) want to quit and are willing to set a quitting date; 2) have a significant amount of nicotine addiction (ie, smoke more than one pack per day, smoke first cigarette within 30 minutes of arising, report withdrawal symptoms on prior attempts at quitting); 3) will not smoke while using the patch; and 4) will follow a behavioral program (individual or group) in conjunction with patch use.

Four different nicotine patches are available in the United States. Three products are for use 24 hours per day; one is used 16 hours per day and removed at bedtime. No studies have directly compared the safety or efficacy of the four patches to determine whether any is superior. All four have been demonstrated to be more effective than placebo.

Proper use involves beginning patch application on the day of quitting. The patch is applied to any nonhairy skin site and worn for 16 or 24 hours. Because of possible skin irritation, the patch site should be rotated. Once applied, the patch is impervious to external water (shower, swimming), but it can come loose with perspiration. As such, it should put on after exercise. Most patches come in multiple strengths. Most smokers should use the patch for 2 to 3 months starting with the strongest dose (21 mg per day), and gradually tapering to lower-dose patches (14 mg per day and 7 mg per day). Those who weigh less than 100 lb are advised to begin with the 14 mg per day strength. A typical program might use the 21 mg per day patch for 4 to 6 weeks, switching to the 14 mg per day strength for 2 to 4 weeks, and then to the 7 mg per day patch for 2 to 4 weeks. Some argue that patients who smoke less than one pack per day can begin with a 14 mg per day patch, but such patients may not be sufficiently addicted to nicotine to need the patch in the first place.

Side effects are relatively few. The most common is skin irritation, which is usually minor. It is reduced by frequent change in patch location. Insomnia is also reported, probably due to the stimulant effect of a constant level of nicotine. The 16-hour patch might be useful for patients bothered by insomnia, or a 24-hour patch can be removed at bedtime. Rash, headache, nausea, vertigo, myalgias, and dyspepsia have been reported, but not dependence or abuse, although experience is still too limited to rule out the possibility. There have been isolated case reports of myocardial infarction in patients who continue to smoke while using the patch. In clinical trials, only 5 percent of patients stopped therapy because of side effects. Because of the vasoconstrictive action of nicotine, patients with recent myocardial infarction, unstable angina, peripheral vascular disease, serious arrhythmias, and women who are pregnant or breast-feeding should avoid patch use.

Patient education is critical. Many patients view the patch as a simple, passive means of quitting, one that requires little effort on their part. Some even continue to smoke while using the patch, under the mistaken belief that it should be used for tapering. Proper patient selection and education are essential to the safe and effective use of the patch. The patch is effective only when combined with behavioral smoking cessation therapy.

Nicotine chewing gum was the original form of nicotine reduction therapy. It also provides an oral substitute for cigarettes. Nicotine, released from the gum by chewing, is absorbed through the oral mucosa, resulting in blood levels lower but more constant than those achieved by smoking. Exposure to the other harmful constituents of cigarette smoke is avoided. In some studies patients using the gum also gained less weight after cessation of smoking than smokers not using the gum. The preparation initially available contained 2 mg of nicotine. A 4 mg gum was approved for use in 1993 and is probably more effective.

Nicotine gum is more effective than placebo when used in conjunction with a behavioral program for self-selected, motivated smokers attending a smoking withdrawal clinic; 1-year cessation rates of 30 percent to 50 percent have been reported, representing an advance over behavioral treatments alone. The gum, like the patch, may be especially useful in smokers heavily addicted to nicotine. When the gum is prescribed by physicians for less motivated patients, cessation rates are lower, and its effectiveness is less certain. Like the patch, the gum is effective only for helping the patient to quit; it is not a substitute for behavioral therapy. Studies of long-term abstinence show little benefit from gum use if there is no behavioral program.

To use the gum, smokers are instructed to pick a target date when they will stop smoking. After that, they chew the gum whenever they have an urge to smoke, usually consuming a dozen pieces daily at the onset. Gum use should continue for 2 to 3 months. Five percent to 10 percent of users develop dependence and have difficulty stopping. It is important to emphasize to the patient that best results are obtained when gum use is accompanied by a program that teaches behavioral skills.

Side effects are mostly a consequence of overly vigorous chewing and release of excess nicotine—sore jaw, mouth irritation or ulcers, nervousness, dizziness, nausea, vomiting, hiccups, intestinal distress, headache, and excess salivation. To reduce these symptoms, smokers should chew the gum very slowly, just enough to detect a slight tingling taste in the mouth. Contraindications to use are the same as those for the transdermal patch (see above).

In addition to side effects, factors limiting effectiveness include poor compliance (as many as 50% fail to fill their prescription and 35% use the gum for too short a period), improper chewing technique, and adherence to dental appliances and bridgework. Smokers starting the gum need detailed instruction in its proper use. Nicotine absorption may be compromised by use of acidic beverages (eg, coffee, carbonated drinks). By lowering the pH of saliva, they have been found to block nicotine absorption when taken during or immediately before gum use. Advice to refrain from them around the time of gum use clears the problem.

Other Agents. *Clonidine,* the centrally acting adrenergic blocking agent, has been shown to lessen the symptoms of opiate and alcohol withdrawal and has been tried for smoking cessation. Initial studies were encouraging, but randomized controlled studies with sufficient follow-up duration found clonidine to be no better than placebo.

Lobeline (Nikoban), a non-nicotine substitute whose autonomic effects mimic those of nicotine, is no more effective than placebo. *Minor tranquilizers* have been prescribed as a means of blunting the anxiety and irritability of nicotine withdrawal, but they are no better than placebo. Furthermore, because their daily use for more than a few days is associated with significant risks of tolerance and dependency (see Chapter 226), they are not appropriate for use in smoking cessation, where several weeks of daily use would be required.

Antidepressant therapy may prove an important pharmacologic adjunct to smoking cessation, given the high prevalence of depression among smokers and the difficulty that depressed patients have in successfully quitting. Controlled trials of antidepressant therapy are in progress.

Behavioral Methods

The behavioral model of smoking has inspired a host of techniques to manipulate environmental cues that trigger or reward smoking. These techniques form the core of most smoking cessation programs (see Table 54–2).

Stimulus-control strategies require the individual to identify and control environmental stimuli that trigger smoking. Cues are first identified by *self-monitoring*. For example, the smoker might be asked to carry a sheet of paper wrapped around the cigarette pack on which he records the circumstances in which each cigarette is smoked. Environmental cues, identified from this daily log, are then progressively avoided or modified so that they no longer trigger smoking. The behavior is separated from its triggers by *progressive restriction* of the situations in which smoking is permitted. At a point in the relearning process, smoking stops altogether.

Controlled studies have not demonstrated impressive long-term cessation with this approach alone. Smokers may decrease their cigarette consumption but are less successful at total cessation, and those who stop have a high relapse rate. By itself, the technique is more effective in preparing the smoker to quit than in achieving long-term cessation.

Aversive conditioning techniques pair an unwanted act like smoking with an unpleasant stimulus to make the act less likely to occur. The most effective aversive stimulus is cigarette smoke, which is unpleasant even to a heavy smoker. In the best-known technique, *rapid smoking,* the smoker is required to inhale every 6 seconds until unable to tolerate further smoking because of nausea, headache, or lightheadedness. *Smoke holding* is a variation on rapid smoking, believed to have similar aversive effects with less health risk. A related technique is *satiation;* smokers purposely double or triple their base smoking rate for up to a day before cessation. The safety of rapid smoking and satiation has been a concern because of the smoker's intense exposure to nicotine and carbon monoxide. However, no serious medical complications have been reported with supervised use of rapid smoking among healthy people and even those with mild cardiopulmonary disease, although the technique is not advised for those with more symptomatic heart or lung disease.

Rapid smoking and other aversive techniques are effective for initial abstinence, producing high rates of short-term cessation, but relapse occurs rapidly unless other techniques are employed.

Hypnosis. There is much interest in hypnosis among patients, many of whom hope it offers an effortless way to stop smoking. Most studies evaluating hypnosis have been uncontrolled, with small samples and brief follow-up; they report abstinence rates of 20 percent to 25 percent at 1 year, comparable to the standard achieved by behavioral programs. The elements identified as most predictive of success include multiple sessions, supportive therapists, motivated clients, and individualized hypnotic suggestions based on specific motivations for smoking.

Acupuncture, like hypnosis, is widely requested by smokers. Needles are inserted at acupuncture points, often around the ear. Advocates claim the procedure can reduce the urge to smoke and even lead to long-term cessation. Success appears related to belief in its efficacy. Randomized, control trials are few; those that are available found no long-term benefit when used alone. Acupuncture might prove useful for temporary relief of withdrawal symptoms in addicted patients.

Organized Group Programs. Both nonprofit and commercial organizations offer group programs for smoking cessation. Most programs have a high dropout rate and have not been adequately evaluated. The oldest and best known is the Five-Day Plan developed in 1963 with sponsorship of the Seventh Day Adventist Church. It consists of meetings on five consecutive nights and is low in cost. Techniques used are health education, encouragement to quit, and nonspecific support.

Adding behavior modification techniques to group programs has improved their effectiveness. SmokEnders is a commercial program consisting of weekly meetings run by exsmokers. In one long-term study, 70 percent of smokers were not smoking at the end of the program and 39 percent remained abstinent 4 years later. However, on reanalysis, the long-term cessation rate was 24 percent, equivalent to the standard rates achieved by other behavioral programs. The American Cancer Society and the American Lung Association offer similar group programs at lower cost. More intensive group programs with extended follow-up offered in the medical setting have achieved better results. Patients who appear to benefit most from such programs are women, middle-aged persons, those who are heavy smokers and have made multiple attempts to quit, and persons who are more educated. Overall, however, fewer than 5 percent of smokers who successfully quit use a group program.

Individual Aids. Booklets, audiovisual aids, telephone services, and nonprescription filters are available to help the smoker who wishes to quit on his own. Few have been evaluated. *Self-help manuals* range from booklets with practical tips on how to quit to longer books containing comprehensive programs of behavior modification. Many are available at minimal cost through nonprofit organizations like the American Cancer Society, the American Lung Association, and the National Cancer Institute.

These groups also sponsor *telephone services* that provide education, encouragement, advice, and referrals. Use of the American Lung Association manuals has produced cessation rates of 12 percent at 1 month and 5 percent at 1 year.

A series of progressively stronger *filters,* which gradually restrict the tar and nicotine delivery from the smoker's own cigarettes, has not proved to be effective.

THE PHYSICIAN'S ROLE

Counseling Smoking Cessation

Because health is the most common reason given by former smokers for quitting, the physician is in a unique position to encourage smoking cessation. The potential importance of the physician's role is heightened by the increased likelihood of cessation occurring in smokers who develop the symptoms of cardiopulmonary disease or who become pregnant. Such patients are particularly motivated to quit and are more responsive to intervention efforts. The chances of making an attempt to quit are doubled by a physician's urging and advice. Providing no more than brief advice to stop smoking to all patients has been shown to be more effective than doing nothing for promoting cessation, and it is a cost-effective medical practice. Doing more—ie, brief, structured smoking cessation counseling—has, in randomized controlled trials, increased patients' efforts to stop smoking and, in some trials, their rates of long-term smoking cessation as well. Surveys indicate that physicians are not taking advantage of their opportunity to alter their patients' smoking habits. Fewer than one-half of current smokers recall being told to quit by a physician. In fact, physician's advice can make a difference. Physicians who devote more time to counseling smokers can expect to be even more effective. In one study, a regularly scheduled follow-up visit for smoking counseling was more effective than one-time advice. The physician can be most effective by advising all smokers to quit and providing more counseling to susceptible smokers—those with respiratory symptoms or the recent diagnosis of a serious smoking-related disease. Physician components identified by the National Cancer Institute as particularly helpful to the cessation effort include making the office a smoke-free site, identifying all smokers in the practice, asking them at each visit about smoking and advising cessation at every appropriate opportunity, helping them set a quit date, providing them with educational and self-help materials, prescribing nicotine reduction therapy when indicated, and arranging follow-up to sustain cessation. A team approach using the nurse to provide more in-depth counseling and follow-up after physician introduction to cessation can enhance outcomes and reduce expenditure of physician time (see Table 54–1).

Preventing Relapse

Follow-up is critical. Studies of physician intervention show that scheduling follow-up visits to discuss smoking increases patients' cessation rates. The importance of continuing to work with the former smoker throughout the first year of cessation cannot be overemphasized, particularly the person with evidence of nicotine addiction. Such patients need to be prepared by the physician to recognize and manage nicotine withdrawal symptoms, prescribed a nicotine reduction program, and followed-up within 2 weeks of quitting. Only after a full year of cessation can the patient be considered an exsmoker. In the interim, repeat visits for reinforcement and support are essential to a successful outcome.

Weight gain must be addressed. Failure to do so risks ignoring a major cause of late relapse. Weight gain may be particularly upsetting to the person who quits out of a desire to improve appearance and personal hygiene. Nicotine increases energy expenditure. With cessation, such excess expenditure is lost, leading to weight gain unless the patient decreases caloric intake or increases physical activity. Most smokers gain some weight after stopping smoking, with men averaging 2.8 kg and women 3.8 kg. The risk of large weight gain (>13 kg) is low, occurring in about 10 percent of men and 13.5 percent of women. African Americans and heavy smokers (more than 15 cigarettes per day) are also at increased risk. However, weight gain does not cancel the health benefits of smoking cessation. The physician needs to prepare the patient who plans to quit for the risk of weight gain. Prescribing a program of *exercise* (see Chapter 18) can be one of the best complements to the smoking cessation effort, facilitating weight control and providing an enhanced sense of well-being.

Depression also requires attention. Before quitting, the physician should evaluate the patient for an underlying depression (see Chapter 227), because it can be a major cause of smoking and a barrier to successful cessation (see above). If major depression is present, it must be treated before smoking cessation is attempted. Although routine use of antidepressant therapy is not recommended as an aid in smoking cessation, a trial of such therapy is indicated in the smoker who has evidence of major depression. Patients with a history of depression, but not depressed before quitting are at increased risk for a relapse during the withdrawal period. Depression needs to be watched for and responded to (see Chapter 227).

RECOMMENDATIONS

Smoking cessation strategy for office practice is summarized in Table 54-1.

1. *Assess smoking habits.* Smoking habits should be assessed as a part of every encounter in ambulatory practice. A smoking history should be taken from all smokers to assess the patient's current interest in quitting and to anticipate difficulties with cessation, such as a high level of nicotine addiction or lack of social support. The smoker's prior cessation efforts and current medical and social situation can help guide treatment recommendations.
2. *Advise every smoker to stop smoking.* A firm statement to stop smoking should be made to all smokers at every visit. Total cessation is the goal.
3. *Motivate the smoker to attempt to quit.* This is the physician's primary role. The strategy should focus on health concerns, tailored to the individual's clinical situation. The approach should be positive, emphasizing the benefits of cessation and including short-term benefits, such as increased exercise tolerance or improved taste and smell. The contribution of smoking to any of the patient's current symptoms should be emphasized.

   The asymptomatic smoker may be the most difficult one to motivate. Most smokers do have minor smoking-related symptoms that would improve with cessation, such as morning cough or limited exercise tolerance. Smokers unable to quit for their own sake may do so for their children's health or to insure a safe pregnancy.

   Smokers with an *acute respiratory illness* commonly stop smoking for a few days on their own. The physician can suggest that the smoker take advantage of the period of reduced desire to stop smoking permanently. For the smoker with a *chronic disease* associated with smoking, the physician should point out the potential for reduced symptoms, improved function, and slowed progression of disease. Radiologic or pulmonary function tests are not recommended for asymptomatic smokers because they do not detect early disease, and a normal result may give inadvertent reassurance to a smoker that his or her health is not being jeopardized.

   Smokers reluctant to attempt cessation often harbor a specific concern, such as a fear of failure, weight gain, withdrawal symptoms, or loss of a pleasurable habit or a way to handle life stresses. Helping the smoker to clarify this concern and to develop counterarguments can be helpful. If the smoker remains unwilling to consider cessation, the physician should stop with a strong antismoking recommendation, but should make a renewed effort at subsequent visits.
4. *Ask for a commitment to quit.* Encourage the smoker to set a date on which he or she will stop smoking, preferably within 4 weeks. Ideal quitting dates are landmarks like a birthday, anniversary, New Year's Day, or times when life stresses are minimized, such as the first day of a vacation. The physician should record the date in the medical record, as a reminder to follow the patient's progress.
5. *Help the smoker quit.* The physician should be prepared to offer a personalized and detailed cessation program that will maximize the patient's chances of success and build confidence. Specific behavioral suggestions should be offered (see Table 54-2). Smokers concerned about weight gain should be advised to begin a concurrent exercise program and keep low-calorie snacks readily at hand. The addicted, heavy smoker should be educated about withdrawal symptoms and considered a candidate for nicotine reduction therapy (transdermal nicotine patch or gum), especially if there is a history of severe withdrawal or marked weight gain on prior attempts. The patch or gum should be prescribed only in conjunction with a behavioral program; it is not sufficient by itself. Total abstinence is a precondition to prescribing reduction therapy, and the patient should be warned of the potential risks of smoking while using the patch. Smokers who develop increased cough and sputum immediately after cessation should be reassured that this is temporary, common, and results from a return of ciliary clearance activities in the respiratory tract.

   The majority of smokers will initially elect to stop on their own, and an individual attempt should be the physician's initial recommendation. These smokers will benefit from self-help material. For heavy smokers who have failed unassisted quitting attempts, consideration of an assisted program is indicated. Providing information about and referral to such community smoking cessation programs is important.

   If there is an underlying depression, it should be treated specifically before attempting cessation. If depression develops subsequently, it too should be treated directly (see Chapter 227).
6. *Follow-up.* Continued monitoring of the smoking habit is essential. Listing the problem on the patient's medical problem list will remind the physician to make its management part of the patient's continuing care. One or more return visits for follow-up will increase patients' success rates. The first follow-up should be scheduled shortly after the quit date. At follow-up, smokers who quit should be congratulated but cautioned of the need to maintain vigilance against relapse. Exsmokers should be monitored carefully during the first year after cessation, when most relapses occur. For smokers whose attempts to quit were unsuccessful, the physician should focus on positive aspects, such as the duration of time the smoker was abstinent, and encourage another attempt. By careful questioning, the physician should determine what circumstances led the effort to fail so that the physician should encourage the patient to learn from the experience in order to increase the chance of success in the next attempt to quit.

ANNOTATED BIBLIOGRAPHY

Agee LL. Treatment procedures using hypnosis in smoking cessation programs: A review of the literature. J Am Soc Psychosom Dent Med 1983;30:111. *(Identifies those components predictive of success with hypnosis.)*

Anda RF, Williamson DF, Escobedo LG, et al. Depression and the dynamics of smoking. JAMA 1990;264:1541. *(Epidemiologic data showing that depressed smokers were 40 percent less likely to quit than nondepressed ones.)*

Benowitz NL. Pharmacologic aspects of cigarette smoking and nicotine addiction. N Engl J Med 1988;319:1318. *(Comprehensive review of the pharmacokinetics of nicotine, its effects on the cardiovascular, nervous, and endocrine systems, and smoker's regulation of nicotine intake. Makes the case for smoking as an addiction to nicotine.)*

Benowitz NL, Jacob P, Kozlowski LT, et al. Influence of smoking fewer cigarettes on exposure to tar, nicotine, and carbon monoxide. N Engl J Med 1986;315:1310. *(Patients tended to oversmoke their cigarettes to maintain intake of nicotine, greatly reducing the health benefit of smoking fewer cigarettes.)*

Burt A, et al. Stopping smoking after myocardial infarction. Lancet 1974;1:305. *(Controlled prospective study of infarction survivors demonstrating effectiveness of brief physician advice in-hospital, supplemented by nurse follow-up after discharge.)*

Centers for Disease Control. Cigarette smoking among adults—United States. JAMA 1992;267:3133. *(Prevalence declining by about 1.1 percent per year since 1987.)*

Cohen SJ, Stookey GK, Katz BP, et al. Encouraging primary care physicians to help smokers quit. Ann Intern Med 1989;110:648. *(Randomized controlled trial of two practical interventions: use of nicotine gum and labeling of charts; achieved a two- to fivefold increase in quitting rate at 12 months.)*

Cummings SR, Coates TJ, Richard RJ, et al. Training physicians in counseling about smoking. Ann Intern Med 1989;110:640. *(Randomized trial; changed the way physicians counseled, but percentage of smokers who achieved long-term cessation increased by only 1 percent to 2 percent; useful discussion of reasons for the poor results and implications.)*

Cummings SR, Rubin SM, Oster G. The cost-effectiveness of counseling smokers to quit. JAMA 1989;261:75–79. *(A careful analysis demonstrating that brief advice during routine office visits is at least as cost-effective as other accepted preventive medical practices.)*

Department of Health and Human Services. The health benefits of smoking cessation: A report of the Surgeon General. Washington, DC: Government Printing Office, 1990, DHHS Publication No. (CDC) 90-8416. *(Authoritative and comprehensive update on smoking cessation.)*

Duncan CL, Cummings SR, Hudes ES, et al. Quitting smoking: Reasons for quitting and predictors of cessation among medical patients. J Gen Intern Med 1992;7:398. *(Health concerns were the most common reason for quitting, and addiction was the greatest barrier; education, social pressure, provider advice, and formal programs increased chances of quitting.)*

Fielding JE, Phenow KJ. Health effects of involuntary smoking. N Engl J Med 1988;319:1452. *(Comprehensive review of knowledge, demonstrating increased risk of lung cancer among nonsmokers exposed to passive smoke.)*

Fiore MC, Novotny TE, Pierce JP, et al. Methods used to quit smoking in the United States: Do cessation programs help? JAMA 1990;263:2760. *(Important epidemiologic study of smoking cessation methods; among the best available data.)*

Franks P, Harp J, Bell B. Randomized controlled trial of clonidine for smoking cessation in a primary care setting. JAMA 1989;262:3011. *(Clonidine had no effect on withdrawal symptoms or short-term rate of smoking cessation.)*

Fuller JA,. Smoking withdrawal and acupuncture. Med J Aust 1982;1:28. *(Finds that it helped reduce withdrawal symptoms only.)*

Glantz SA, Parmley WW. Passive smoking and heart disease. Circulation 1992;83:1. *(Reviews evidence supporting increased risk of cardiovascular mortality among individuals exposed to passive smoke.)*

Glassman AH, Helzer JE, Covey LS, et al. Smoking, smoking cessation, and major depression. JAMA 1990;264:1546. *(Finds that when patients with a history of depression stop smoking, depressive symptoms and even major depression may follow.)*

Glynn T, Manley M. How to help your patients stop smoking: a National Cancer Institute manual for physicians. Bethesda, MD: National Institutes of Health, 1989. *(A practical, step-by-step model for physicians and their office staffs to use in counseling smokers. Available free by calling (800) 4-CANCER.)*

Greene HL, Goldberg RJ, Ockene JK. Cigarette smoking: The physician's role in cessation and maintenance. J Gen Intern Med 1988;3:75. *(Detailed review of what physicians can do to affect the smoking behavior of their patients; 122 references.)*

Henningfield JE, Radzius A, Cooper TM, et al. Drinking coffee and carbonated beverages blocks absorption of nicotine from nicotine polacrilex gum. JAMA 1990;264:1560. *(Possible reason why some patients fail to benefit from nicotine gum.)*

Hollis JF, Lichtenstein E, Vogt TM, et al. Nurse-assisted counseling for smokers in primary care. Ann Intern Med 1993;118:521. *(Physician burden reduced, quitting rate enhanced.)*

Kawachi I, Colditz GA, Stampfer MJ, et al. Smoking cessation in relation to total mortality rates in women: a prospective cohort study. Ann Intern Med 1993;119:992. *(As in men, the risk of total mortality among female former smokers declines to approach that of never smokers 10–14 years after cessation.)*

Kottke TE, Battista RN, DeFriese GH, et al. Attributes of successful smoking cessation interventions in medical practice: A meta-analysis of 39 controlled trials. JAMA 1988;259:2883. *(Good analysis of available data, although many studies of suboptimal design.)*

LaCroix AZ, Lang J, Scherr P, et al. Smoking and mortality among older men and women in three communities. N Engl J Med 1991;324:1619. *(Finds that mortality risk continues into later life, making cessation efforts worthwhile and capable of improving life expectancy in elderly persons.)*

Lam W, Sacks HS, Sze P, et al. Meta-analysis of randomized controlled trials of nicotine chewing gum. Lancet 1987;2:27. *(Meta-analysis demonstrating effectiveness of gum in smoking cessation clinics but not in physician office.)*

Manley MW, Epps RP, Glynn TJ. The clinician's role in promoting smoking cessation among clinic patients. Med Clin North Am 1992;76:477. *(Presents the rationale, validation, and actual steps of the National Cancer Institute's model for counseling smokers in primary care office practice.)*

Perkins KA, Epstein LH, Marks BL, et al. The effect of nicotine on energy expenditure during light physical activity. N Engl J Med 1989;320:898. *(Nicotine increases energy expenditure markedly during light exercise; a possible mechanism for weight gain during cessation of smoking.)*

Rigotti NA, Singer DE, Mulley AG, Thibault GE. Smoking cessation following admission to a coronary care unit. J Gen Intern Med 1991;6:305. *(25% of smokers admitted to a coronary care unit were not smoking one year later. Lighter smokers and those with the new diagnosis of coronary artery disease were most likely to stop smoking.)*

Russell MAH, Wilson C, Taylor C, et al. Effect of general practitioners' advice against smoking. Br Med J 1979;2:231. *(Careful randomized controlled study in which routine advice to stop smoking resulted in a significant increase in cessation that was sustained over 1 year.)*

Tonnesen P, Norregaard J, Simonsen K, et al. A double-blind trial of a 16-hour transdermal nicotine patch in smoking cessation. N Engl J Med 1991;325:311. *(Study of patch therapy without a behavioral component; excellent short-term efficacy, but at 1 year only 17 percent continued off cigarettes; emphasizes need for combination approach.)*

Transdermal Nicotine Study Group. Transdermal nicotine for smoking cessation. Six-month results from two multicenter controlled clinical trials. JAMA 1991;266:3133. *(Documents efficacy, especially at 6 weeks, but with substantial relapse after 6 months.)*

Williamson DF, Madans J, Anda RF, et al. Smoking cessation and severity of weight gain in a national cohort. N Engl J Med 1991;324:739. *(Average weight gain was 3.8 kg in women and 2.8 kg in men; major weight gain of more than 13 kg occurred in 9.8 percent of men and 13.4 percent of women.)*

Wilson D, Wood G, Johnston N, et al. Randomized clinical trial of supportive follow-up for cigarette smokers in a family practice. Can Med Assoc J 1982;126:127. *(Patients scheduled for regular return visits to their family physician for continued smoking counseling were more likely to quit than those receiving one-time advice from their physician.)*

Primary Care Medicine: Office Evaluation and Management of the Adult Patient, 3rd edition, edited by Allan H. Goroll, Lawrence A. May, and Albert G. Mulley, Jr. J.B. Lippincott Company, Philadelphia

5
Gastrointestinal Problems

55
Screening for Gastric Cancer

For unknown reasons, the incidence of gastric cancer in the United States has been decreasing at a rate of 2 percent to 4 percent per year for the past several decades. During the 1930s, the death rate for gastric cancer was greater than 30 per 100,000; during the 1970s, the rate was approximately 10 per 100,000. At present, an American has an approximately 1-percent chance of developing gastric malignancy over his or her lifetime. Nevertheless, mortality remains high; approximately 75 percent of the 25,000 Americans who develop gastric cancer each year eventually die from the disease.

The usual insidious onset of the disease and the lack of suitable screening tests have thwarted preventive measures. Advances in endoscopic instrumentation, allowing more complete visualization of the stomach, have raised questions about unmet potential in prevention of gastric cancer deaths among high-risk populations. Some recommendations for routine endoscopic evaluation have sparked controversy. The primary care physician must understand the natural history of gastric cancer and the limitations of diagnostic tools in the detection of early disease.

EPIDEMIOLOGY AND RISK FACTORS

There is a marked international variation in the incidence of gastric cancer. Among the countries with the highest incidences are Japan, Chile, Finland, and Iceland. Incidence also varies, predictably, with age and sex. Men are twice as likely to develop gastric cancer in most countries. More than 60 percent of cases occur in people over age 65. Fewer than 10 percent of cases occur in people younger than age 30. The incidence among nonwhites and people in low socioeconomic groups in the United States is twice that among whites and the more well-to-do.

Genetic factors do not play a major role in determining risk for gastric cancer. It has been documented that migrants from areas of high risk (eg, Japan) eventually acquire the lower rates of their new home (eg, the United States). A genetically determined minor risk factor for gastric cancer is blood group; people with type A blood have a 10-percent increase in risk of developing gastric cancer.

A number of environmental factors have been suggested as explanations for the geographic variability of gastric cancer incidence. Phenol, present in all smoked foods, and the high salt concentration in salted fish and meat products have been linked to the high incidence of gastric cancer in Finland, Iceland, and Japan. Talc-treated rice has been implicated in Japan and Northern China. Provinces in Chile with high gastric cancer rates are agricultural, with high concentrations of nitrate present in the soil and drinking water. Nitrosamines, derived from nitrates and secondary amines, are suspected causes of gastric cancer in Chile and, to a lesser extent, in the United States, where nitrates and nitrites are used as food additives in meat and fish.

A number of pathologic conditions, including gastric polyps and adenomas, have been associated with increased risk of stomach cancer. Gastric polyps are relatively infrequent; a prevalence of less than 0.5 percent has been documented in one autopsy series. The vast majority of polyps are hyperplastic and not associated with increased cancer risk. People with adenomas, particularly villous adenomas, have the same risk of cancer when the adenomas are found in the stomach as when they are in the colon. Some authorities have argued that peptic ulcer disease predisposes patients to gastric cancer. Carcinoma is found in approximately 3 percent of surgically resected gastric ulcers. It is likely, however, that ulceration follows carcinoma rather than vice versa. This association is the basis for the clinical practice of biopsying or resecting suspicious-appearing or persistent gastric ulcers.

A number of studies have demonstrated a statistical association between atrophic gastritis and gastric cancer. Achlorhydria and atrophic gastritis are common. Prevalence increases with age. An incidence of 1 percent per year of gastric cancer among patients with atrophic gastritis has been demonstrated in one study with yearly radiographic examination. The atrophic gastritis associated with pernicious anemia is also a risk factor for gastric cancer. Evidence indicates that patients with pernicious anemia have at least a fourfold increase in risk. Some studies have found even higher rates.

Prior gastric surgery for benign ulcer disease has long been considered a risk factor for subsequent gastric cancer. Increased risk was not evident early after surgery, but several Scandinavian studies suggested that those who lived more than 10 to 15 years after surgery faced a two- to threefold increase in gastric cancer risk. Recommendations for annual endoscopic examination followed. More recently, a large population-based study conducted in Olmstead County, Minnesota, found gastric cancer to be no more common among patients with prior gastric surgery than among the population at large.

NATURAL HISTORY OF GASTRIC CANCER AND EFFECTIVENESS OF THERAPY

Gastric cancer typically has an insidious presentation. The most common initial symptom is epigastric discomfort. Later symptoms include early satiety, indigestion, weight loss, and other systemic symptoms. The percentage of patients who survive 5 years has not improved significantly in recent years; it remains at 20 percent of unselected cases. The patients who are operated on early in the course of their disease have a 60 percent to 90 percent 5-year survival rate. Recent population-based studies from Japan confirm that 5-year survival rates of 70 percent can be achieved among patients with gastric cancer detected by screening. Furthermore, follow-up for 15 years suggests that the cancer death hazard rate decreases rapidly for 7 years after detection and treatment of cancer, and then remains very low.

Among highly selected patients with "early gastric cancer," defined as gastric cancer confined to the mucosa or submucosa but not extending to the muscularis propria, resection may be curative for as many as 95 percent. Intensive screening efforts in Japan have increased the proportion of gastric cancers detected in this early stage from approximately 5 percent to 30 percent. Efforts have not been as successful elsewhere, where fewer than 10 percent of cases meet criteria for early gastric cancer. The duration of the asymptomatic detectable period is unknown, but early gastric cancer has been found as long as 3 years after biopsies were originally misread as benign. The natural history of early gastric cancer appears to include protracted cycles of healing and ulceration.

SCREENING AND DIAGNOSTIC TESTS

None of the tests generally used in the United States for the *diagnosis* of gastric carcinoma are suitable for wide-scale screening efforts.

Gastric Cytology. Unlike cervical cytopathology, the collection and examination of specimens for gastric cytopathologic analysis is a laborious process. Samples must be obtained either by endoscopic scraping or by gastric lavage. Examination of the resulting slides usually takes 2 to 3 hours rather than the several minutes sufficient for the screening examination of cervical Pap smears. Many studies have demonstrated the sensitivity of gastric cytopathology studies to be approximately 90 percent. It is not known how much this figure is influenced by the spectrum of disease, that is, how sensitive cytology can be for the early, curable cancer. Specificity in a laboratory with experienced personnel should be approximately 97 percent to 98 percent. False-positive results are often found in association with healing gastric ulcer and other gastric pathology. Although cytopathology is useful for further diagnosis in documented cases of abnormality of gastric mucosa, it cannot be recommended for indiscriminate screening.

Endoscopy. Similarly, endoscopy must be considered a diagnostic rather than a screening procedure. Sensitivity in making the diagnosis of gastric cancer is 90 percent. However, recent evidence suggests that endoscopic visualization is much less sensitive for early cancers, with a visual diagnosis being made in fewer than 50 percent of cases in some series. Multiple biopsies of any and all suspicious lesions can increase the sensitivity to 90 percent.

Diagnostic Radiology. The sensitivity of contrast studies in the diagnosis of gastric cancer has been reported to be as high as 95 percent. Obviously, however, it is least sensitive in cases of early disease and is too expensive and time consuming to be considered a screening test in asymptomatic patients. In Japan, where gastric cancer is the leading cause of cancer death, radiographic techniques have been adapted to mass screening. These modifications in the standard contrast studies have been shown to have a sensitivity and specificity of 90 percent.

Stool analysis for occult blood (described in detail in Chapter 56) is an appropriate screening procedure for all gastrointestinal malignancies. Yearly guaiac testing has been recommended as part of the general screening for all adult patients. This is especially important for patients with identified increased risk of gastric cancer, such as those with a history of pernicious anemia or documented atrophic gastritis.

CONCLUSIONS AND RECOMMENDATIONS

- Despite a significant downward trend in incidence, gastric cancer remains a disease of high morbidity and mortality.
- The yearly analysis of stool for occult blood is indicated in all adult patients. This is especially important for those with a history of pernicious anemia, atrophic gastritis, or other gastric pathology.
- The value of gastric cytology, endoscopy, and contrast studies as routine procedures in high-risk patients is unproven. They are diagnostic procedures and should generally be reserved for symptomatic patients or patients with occult blood demonstrated by stool analysis.

A.G.M.

ANNOTATED BIBLIOGRAPHY

Ackerman NB. An evaluation of gastric cytology: Results of a nation-wide survey. J Chron Dis 1967;20:621. *(Survey of practices in U.S. hospitals indicating wide variation in validity of techniques. Not generally used for screening purposes but rather in response to symptoms or radiographic abnormalities.)*

Bedikian AY, Chen TT, Khankhanian N, et al. The natural history of gastric cancer and prognostic factors influencing survival. J Clin Oncol 1984;2:305. *(Useful review of natural history with an emphasis on clinical determinants of survival.)*

Farley DR, Donohue JH. Early gastric cancer. Surg Clin North Am 1992;72:401. *(Review of early gastric cancer and surgical issues.)*

Green PHR, O'Toole K. Early gastric cancer. Ann Intern Med 1982;97:272. *(Editorial reviewing endoscopic screening programs, which concludes that benefit remains unproven.)*

Hitchcock CR, MacLean LD, Sullivan WA. Secretory and clinical aspects of achlorhydria and gastric atrophy as precursors of gastric cancer. J Natl Cancer Inst 1957;18:795. *(Review of data indicating increase of 4.5 and 21.9 times in risk among patients with achlorhydria and pernicious anemia. Recommends frequent radiographic studies.)*

Hoerr SO. Prognosis for carcinoma of the stomach. Surg Gynecol Obstet 1973;137:205. *(Five-year survival rates ranging from 83 to 11 percent depending on stage; overall 5-year survival rate of 18 percent.)*

Kurihara M, Shirakabe H, Yarita T, et al. Diagnosis of small early gastric cancer by x-ray, endoscopy, and biopsy. Cancer Detect Prev 1981;4:377. *(Sensitivity of double-contrast x-ray 75%; endoscopy plus biopsy >95%.)*

Logan RFA, Langman MJS. Screening for gastric cancer after gastric surgery. Lancet 1983;2:667. *(Accepts evidence for increased risk but, nevertheless, does not favor endoscopic screening.)*

Muramaki R, Tsukuma H, Ubukata T, et al. Estimation of validity of mass screening program for gastric cancer in Japan. Cancer 1990;65:1255. *(Radiographic techniques adapted for mass screening for gastric cancer in Japan achieve sensitivity and specificity of 90 percent.)*

Schafer LW, Larson DE, Melton LJ, et al. The risk of gastric carcinoma after surgical treatment for benign ulcer disease. N Engl J Med 1983;309:1210. *(No evident increase in the risk of gastric cancer after surgical treatment for benign peptic ulcer disease led the authors to conclude that there is no indication for endoscopic surveillance in this population.)*

Yamazaki H, Oshima A, Muramaki R, et al. A long-term follow-up study of patients with gastric cancer detected by mass screening. Cancer 1989;63:613. *(Includes survival curves and hazard rates for more than 1000 patients with gastric cancer detected by mass screening in Japan.)*

Primary Care Medicine: Office Evaluation and Management of the Adult Patient, 3rd edition, edited by Allan H. Goroll, Lawrence A. May, and Albert G. Mulley, Jr. J.B. Lippincott Company, Philadelphia

56
Screening for Colorectal Cancer

MICHAEL J. BARRY, M.D.

Colorectal cancer (CRC) is the second most common malignancy found in both men and women, accounting for about 12 percent of cancer deaths. Americans face a lifetime probability of developing a carcinoma of the colon or rectum of approximately 5 percent to 6 percent. The majority of colorectal cancers that present clinically have already spread beyond the intestinal wall, resulting in a poor 5-year survival rate. However, cancers detected and removed while disease is still localized are associated with a 5-year survival in excess of 80 percent. CRC's long asymptomatic period, the availability of screening tests that can find localized disease, and the effectiveness of early therapy suggest that screening for large bowel tumors should be a primary care priority. Evidence from prospective, randomized, controlled study that screening for CRC actually reduces mortality is now emerging for the first time.

EPIDEMIOLOGY AND RISK FACTORS

The incidence of colorectal cancer is greater in economically developed societies. The high-fat, low-fiber *diet* prevalent in Western societies has been implicated in the etiology of these cancers by increasing secretion of bile acids. Such acids, along with their intestinal microflora-derived metabolites, are believed to have carcinogenic or cocarcinogenic potential.

Advancing *age* is an important risk factor, with the incidence of CRC rising from about 75 per 100,000 in the sixth decade to 300 per 100,000 in the eighth decade.

Family history is also a risk factor. Having a first-degree relative with CRC raises personal risk two- to threefold, with risk greatest when cancer diagnosed at an early age (<45 years old) and when other first-degree relatives also develop colorectal cancer. Autosomal dominant familial adenomatosis confers a risk of colorectal cancer of about 50 percent by age 40, and a number of other familial polyposis and familial cancer syndromes also increase risk greatly.

Ulcerative colitis, particularly pancolitis of more than 10 years' duration, increases a patient's risk of CRC five- to tenfold, although isolated ulcerative proctitis probably does not confer any additional risk. There is controversy as to whether Crohn's disease is associated with a clinically significant increase in risk of CRC.

Most CRCs are believed to arise from *adenomatous polyps*. The prevalence of adenomatous polyps increases with age, occurring in 30 percent of 50-year-olds (3% > 1 cm), 40 percent of 60-year-olds (4% > 1 cm), and 50 percent of 70-year-olds (5% > 1 cm). Once a person has had an adenomatous polyp removed, it has been suggested that there is a higher future risk for CRC. However, the magnitude of future risk, if any, is uncertain, especially if the index polyp is small (< 1 cm).

Patients with *resected colorectal cancers* have a threefold increase in risk of metachronous cancer in other locations of the colon. Recurrences of index cancers are usually extramural and not amenable to detection by screening.

The prevalence of *synchronous colonic neoplasia* is high and important to consider in the evaluation of the patient with a positive screening test. Synchronous adenomas occur in 40 percent to 50 percent of patients with an index polyp; 3 percent to 5 percent with a carcinoma will harbor a second one.

NATURAL HISTORY OF COLORECTAL CANCER AND EFFECTIVENESS OF THERAPY

Sporadic polyps are common lesions, with the most common being small hyperplastic outcroppings of the colonic

Table 56-1. Polypoid Lesions of the Colon and Rectum. Relation of Size to Cancer (1116 polypoid lesions, Massachusetts General Hospital, 1954–1963)

DIAMETER (CM)	PERCENTAGE CANCEROUS
Less than 0.5	0.5
0.5–0.9	1
1.0–1.4	1.8
1.5–1.9	6
2–2.4	10
2.5–3.4	23
3.5 or larger	29

Behringer GE. Changing concepts in the histopathologic diagnosis of polypoid lesions of the colon. Dis Colon Rectum 1970;13:116–118.

mucosa; these lesions do not have malignant potential. Adenomas are truly neoplastic and may contain malignancy. The risk of malignancy depends on histology and size of the adenoma, with size being the more important determinant. In one study, invasive cancer was found in only 0.5 percent of colonoscopically removed polyps from 0.5 to 0.9 cm in diameter, but in almost 15 percent of polyps greater than 3 cm in diameter. Villous adenomas are the polyps with the highest malignant potential, tending to be larger and more sessile than other adenomatous polyps. Mixed tubovillous adenomas and those with pure tubular histology are associated with less risk (Table 56–1). About 10 percent of polyps have villous histology, tubular adenomas account for 70 percent, and the remainder have mixed histology. The probability and time frame for a nonmalignant polyp to develop into an invasive cancer are not well defined, although these are important variables in estimating the effectiveness of screening strategies. Interestingly, although the prevalence of polyps increases with age (see above), average polyp size does not, suggesting that most polyps do not progressively enlarge.

Symptoms occur late in the course of CRC growth. Duration of the asymptomatic detectable period is estimated to be several years. When cancers are found after symptomatic presentation, 60 percent have already disseminated to regional nodes or distant organs. Five-year survival rates vary dramatically with the stage of disease at the time of diagnosis. Tumors confined locally to the bowel wall (Duke's stage A) or pericolic fat (Duke's B) have an 80-percent 5-year survival, whereas tumors with regional lymph node metastases (Duke's C) have a 46-percent 5-year survival, which drops to 5 percent with distant metastases.

SCREENING TESTS

Digital Examination

In older series, up to 40 percent of CRCs were within reach of the examining finger; however, recent series based on colonoscopic data suggest this figure is now only about 10 percent. Although many experts recommend performing this time-honored examination on an annual basis starting at age 40, the U.S. Preventive Services Task Force has recently concluded that there is insufficient evidence to recommend for or against this screening maneuver in office practice.

Fecal Occult Blood Testing (FOBT)

Intermittent occult bleeding occurs with some asymptomatic CRCs and large polyps. Serial sampling of stools for occult blood can be performed to identify this bleeding. Guaiac-impregnated filter paper slides (Hemoccult II and others) are capable of detecting very small amounts of fecal blood, which will be present in some patients with CRC. The fact that colonic tumors selectively enrich the stool surface with blood enhances the sensitivity of guaiac testing of stool samples. Stool sampling is best performed serially because of the intermittent nature of the bleeding (eg, two samples from a stool on each of 3 days).

A six-test guaiac stool test sequence has a sensitivity of 30 percent to 70 percent for CRC. The lower figure is probably more accurate for early cancers in asymptomatic patients. Sensitivity falls when prepared slides are stored for more than 4 days before developing. Rehydration of the sample before application of developer can increase sensitivity, but at the cost of a loss in specificity. False-positive tests may occur from nonmalignant lesions, iron use, aspirin, nonsteroidal antiinflammatory drugs, rare red meat, or foods with high peroxidase activity. A specificity of 97 percent to 98 percent can be attained by omitting rare red meat, horseradish, cantaloupe, or uncooked fresh vegetables (especially broccoli, turnip, radish, cauliflower) 2 days before the first sample is collected. High doses of vitamin C increase the false-negative rate.

In large population studies of persons over age 50, about 3 percent to 4 percent of screened persons will have a positive FOBT, with a positive predictive value of 10 percent for CRC and 40 percent for cancers and polyps. Most of these polyps are too small to cause detectable bleeding but are found serendipitously when follow-up studies are performed after a positive occult blood test. Using rehydration, the positivity rate increases to over 9 percent, but the positive predictive value falls to 2.2 percent for cancers and to 30 percent for cancers plus adenomas.

HemoQuant is a newer test for fecal occult blood, based on a direct measurement of stool hemoglobin content. It is not affected by high-peroxidase foods. However, sensitivity and specificity for detection of colorectal neoplasia appear no better than that achieved with use of Hemoccult II. Moreover, HemoQuant can be more cumbersome and more expensive than guaiac-based tests.

Individuals with a positive fecal occult blood test require a thorough evaluation for colorectal neoplasia. Smaller polyps produce guaiac positivity only on occasion, but their high prevalence makes them the most common lesions found during the evaluation of patients with occult bleeding. *Colonoscopy* or the combination of *sigmoidoscopy* and *air-contrast barium enema* are acceptable alternatives for follow-up evaluation of the patient with a test positive for occult blood. Colonoscopy offers the advantage of allowing a biopsy or polypectomy during the same examination and is probably the more sensitive for detecting smaller polyps. However, given the uncertain natural history of these lesions and the cost of polypectomy (both initially and for any necessary future colonoscopic surveillance), it is not clear if this higher sensitivity is an advantage or disadvantage.

The best outcome measure of screening efficacy is *reduced CRC mortality,* as judged by prospective, randomized, controlled clinical trials with a long period of follow-up. One such study, The Minnesota Colon Cancer Study, demonstrated a 33-percent reduction in cumulative colorectal cancer mortality (from 8.3 to 5.9 per 1000 over 13 years) as a result of annual occult blood screening. This trial used a six-sample annual testing protocol, followed by colonoscopy for persons testing positive. The guaiac cards were rehydrated, which increased the true positive rate of testing from 81 percent to 92 percent, but increased the false-positive rate from 2 percent to 10 percent. As a result of this decrease in specificity, 38 percent of screenees underwent colonoscopy during the study. The cumulative incidence of colorectal cancer was almost identical in both the screened and control groups, suggesting most of the benefit came from early detection of established cancers, rather than from preventing future cancers by resecting polyps. Compared with the control group, screened patients demonstrated a shift to detection of earlier cancers.

As seen from the Minnesota study, rehydration of the guaiac card increases its sensitivity, but it increases also the number of colonoscopies needed, the cost of screening, and the false-positive rate. Whether this approach is the most cost-effective one remains to be determined.

Proctosigmoidoscopy

About 25 percent of cancers are within the range of the rigid sigmoidoscope. An intermediate length flexible sigmoidoscope (35 cm) may be more preferable to patients in terms of comfort than either the rigid instrument or the longer (65 cm) flexible endoscope. The risk of a bowel perforation—the major complication of proctosigmoidoscopy—is low (about 1 to 2 per 10,000 rigid exams). The risk with flexible scopes has been less well studied. The number of cancers found per 1000 examinations ranges from 1.5 for the rigid scope to 4 for the long flexible scope. Adenomatous polyps are found in up to 20 percent of persons screened. When adenomatous polyps are detected and removed at sigmoidoscopy, the patient is usually followed-up by colonoscopy to examine the rest of the colon. The cost-effectiveness of colonoscopic follow-up study remains uncertain.

Sigmoidoscopy can clearly find localized cancers and polyps for removal, but the key question is the procedure's effect on CRC mortality rates when used for periodic screening. Data from prospective studies are pending, but a retrospective, case-control study of periodic rigid sigmoidoscopy for CRC screening suggested a 60 percent to 70 percent reduction in CRC mortality risk. As expected, the protective association appeared specific for cancers within reach of the sigmoidoscope; the exposure odds were not reduced for more proximal cancers.

The American Cancer Society recommends proctosigmoidoscopy every 3 to 5 years after two negative examinations 1 year apart, beginning at age 50 for patients at average risk. Lacking data from prospective randomized trials, the U.S. Preventive Services Task Force believes there is insufficient evidence to recommend for or against this test in asymptomatic persons of average risk.

An Overall Screening Strategy

The most commonly recommended approach to screening for CRC is a combination of *annual fecal occult blood testing* and *proctosigmoidoscopy every 3 to 5 years,* starting at age 50 for average-risk persons. Screening might start at age 40 for those at higher risk (eg, positive family history). Some experts have suggested as an alternative less frequent total-colon examinations. In one cost-effectiveness analysis, the combination of annual occult blood tests and an air-contrast barium enema every 5 years was particularly attractive. The high cost of colonoscopy weighs strongly against its periodic use as a screening test.

When adenomatous polyps greater than 0.5 cm are found at proctosigmoidoscopy, referral for colonoscopy to search for synchronous disease as well as to remove the index polyp for histology is recommended.

CONCLUSIONS AND RECOMMENDATIONS

- The relatively high prevalence of colorectal cancer, its slow evolution from adenomatous polyp to cancer, and the accumulating evidence that available screening tests reduce mortality from this disease suggest that an aggressive approach to colorectal cancer screening is appropriate.
- However, uncertainty about the optimal strategy for screening and its cost-effectiveness, as well as the small absolute benefits seen, mean that screening cannot be considered mandatory for patients of average risk, although high-risk persons should be screened.
- Identify degree of risk by checking for a history of familial polyposis, colon cancer in a first-degree relative, ulcerative colitis with pancolonic involvement, and prior history of CRC.
- *High-risk* individuals (ie, those with ulcerative pancolitis longer than 10 years or familial polyposis) should be referred to a gastroenterologist for periodic colonoscopy. Most authorities would include patients with a history of colorectal cancer in this group as well.
- *Intermediate-risk* individuals (ie, those who have had a large (> 1 cm) adenomatous polyp or a family history of CRC in a first-degree relative) should have annual fecal occult blood testing, supplemented by periodic proctosigmoidoscopy approximately every 3 to 5 years. Some authorities recommend periodic total colon examination (air-contrast barium enema or colonoscopy) for such patients, although data regarding efficacy are inconclusive.
- *Average-risk* patients (ie, those with no risk factors other than age) are reasonable candidates for a personalized approach to CRC screening, beginning at age 50. The physician should review with the patient the benefits and risks of available screening strategies and plan an individualized approach to future CRC screening.
- *Fecal testing* for occult blood, if selected, should be done annually, with two samples obtained on each of 3 days,

during which dietary peroxidases and rare red meat are restricted. Any positive test should be followed by colonoscopy or the combination of sigmoidoscopy plus air-contrast barium enema. (This is preferable to repeating any positive test obtained on an undefined diet.)

- Performing a single guaiac test on stool obtained at the time of office digital rectal examination is of inadequate sensitivity and of uncertain specificity.
- Rehydration of stool guaiac cards increases sensitivity, but also results in a fivefold increase in the number of screenees who need a subsequent total-colon examination. The cost-effectiveness of this approach to guaiac testing remains to be determined.
- *Proctosigmoidoscopy* can be added to the fecal occult blood test every 3 to 5 years for persons willing to accept some short-term discomfort in exchange for some possible reduction in cancer risk (see Appendix).
- Neither fecal occult blood testing nor proctosigmoidoscopy is sensitive enough to preclude further evaluation in patients with symptoms or signs suggestive of colorectal cancer.
- The literature should be watched closely for the several additional large CRC screening trials that are in progress. They should provide additional evidence for the efficacy of CRC screening and needed data on cost-effectiveness of different screening strategies.

ANNOTATED BIBLIOGRAPHY

Ahlquist DA, et al. Pattern of occult bleeding in asymptomatic colorectal cancer. Cancer 1989;63:1826. *(Documents the relatively low sensitivity of guaiac tests for asymptomatic cancers.)*

Allison JE, Feldman R, Tekawa IS. Hemoccult screening in detecting colorectal neoplasm: Long-term follow-up in a large group practice setting. Ann Intern Med 1990;112:328. *(Practice-based analysis of the operating characteristics of a fecal occult blood test.)*

Cannon-Albright LA, Skolnick MH, Bishop DT, et al. Common inheritance of susceptibility to colonic adenomatous polyps and associated colorectal cancers. N Engl J Med 1988;319: 533. *(First-degree relatives have an increased risk of colorectal cancer.)*

Eddy DM. Screening for colorectal cancer. Ann Intern Med 1990;113:373. *(Sophisticated mathematical models examine the cost-effectiveness of colorectal cancer screening with a variety of test strategies.)*

Friedman GD, Selby JV. Colorectal cancer: Have we identified an effective screening strategy? J Gen Intern Med 1990;5:S23. *(General review, also describes a case-control study designed to test the efficacy of colorectal cancer screening.)*

Hardcastle JD, et al. Randomized controlled trial of faecal occult blood screening for colorectal cancer: Results for first 107,349 subjects. Lancet 1989;1:1160. *(Describes the predictive value of occult blood testing.)*

Knight KK, Fielding JE, Battista RN. Occult blood screening for colorectal cancer. JAMA 1989;261:587. *(General review of the procedure.)*

Lindsay DC, et al. Should colonoscopy be the first investigation for colonic disease? Br Med J 1988;296:167. *(Randomized trial of colonoscopy versus rigid sigmoidoscopy and air-contrast barium enema in the workup of colonic disease.)*

Mandel JS, Bond JH, Church TR, et al. Reducing mortality from colorectal cancer by screening for fecal occult blood. N Engl J Med 1993;328:1365. *(Randomized prospective study; demonstrates a large relative reduction in mortality risk, although the absolute reduction in risk is small.)*

Neugut AI, Pita S. Role of sigmoidoscopic screening for colorectal cancer. Gastroenterology 1988;95:492. *(Thorough review.)*

Ransohoff DF, Lang CA. Screening for colorectal cancer. N Engl J Med 1991;325:37. *(General review, including implications of detecting adenomatous polyps.)*

Ransohoff DF, Lang CA. Small adenomas detected during fecal occult blood test screening for colorectal cancer: The impact of serendipity. JAMA 1990;264:76. *(High predictive value of occult blood tests for polyps is the result of their high prevalence, rather than the fact that they bleed.)*

Rex DK, et al. Screening colonoscopy in asymptomatic average-risk persons with negative fecal occult blood tests. Gastroenterology 1991;64:100. *(The negative predictive value of fecal occult blood testing.)*

St John DJB, McDermott FT, Hopper JL, et al. Cancer risk in relatives of patients with common colorectal cancer. Ann Intern Med 1993;118:785. *(Risk increased if cancer present in first-degree relative, especially if diagnosed at early age and if other first-degree relatives affected.)*

St John DJB, Young GP, McHutchison JG, et al. Comparison of the specificity and sensitivity of Hemoccult and HemoQuant in screening for colorectal neoplasia. Ann Intern Med 1992; 117:376. *(Cross-sectional study, in which Hemoccult performed better than HemoQuant.)*

Selby JV, Friedman GD. Sigmoidoscopy in the periodic health examination of asymptomatic adults. JAMA 1989;261:595. *(Reviews the evidence used in the deliberations of the U.S. Preventive Services Task Force regarding proctosigmoidoscopic screening.)*

Selby JV, Friedman GD, Collen MF. Sigmoidoscopy and mortality from colorectal cancer: The Kaiser Permanante Multiphasic Evaluation Study. J Clin Epidemiol 1988;41:427. *(Critical reexamination of the reduction in mortality from colorectal cancer noted from recommending sigmoidoscopy to patients in a health promotion program.)*

Selby JV, Friedman GD, Quesenberry CP Jr, et al. Effect of fecal occult blood testing on mortality from colorectal cancer. Ann Intern Med 1993;118:1. *(Retrospective, case-control study suggesting that mortality risk might be lowered, but confidence intervals wide; more data needed.)*

Selby JV, Friedman GD, Quesenberry CP, et al. A case-control study of screening sigmoidoscopy and mortality from colorectal cancer. N Engl J Med 1992;326:653. *(Retrospective study indicating a survival benefit with screening by proctosigmoidoscopy.)*

Simon JB. Colonic polyps, cancer, and fecal occult blood. Ann Intern Med 1993;118:71. *(Editorial examining the quality of available data on the natural history of polyps and the utility of fecal occult blood testing.)*

Vasen HF, Hartog Jager FCA, Menko FH. Screening for hereditary nonpolyposis colorectal cancer. Am J Med 1989;86:278. *(Screening found worthwhile.)*

Wagner JL, Herdman RC, Wadhwa S. Cost effectiveness of colorectal screening in the elderly. Ann Intern Med 1991;115: 807. *(Presents data supporting cost-effectiveness of screening the elderly.)*

Willett WC, Stampfer MJ, Colditz GA, et al. Relation of meat, fat, and fiber intake to the risk of colon cancer in a prospective study among women. N Engl J Med 1990;323:1664. *(Epide-*

miologic study showing that high intake of animal fat [or red meat] increases risk of colon cancer.)

Winawer SJ. Colorectal cancer screening comes of age. N Engl J Med 1993;328:1416. *(Editorial summarizing available data on utility of screening.)*

Winawer SJ, et al. Randomized comparison of surveillance intervals after colonoscopic removal of newly diagnosed adenomatous polyps. N Engl J Med 1993;328:901. *(Longer interval just as effective as the shorter one.)*

Winawer SJ, Andrews M, Flehinger B, et al. Progress report on controlled trial of fecal occult blood testing for the detection of colorectal neoplasia. Cancer 1980;45:2959. *(Examines additional value of occult blood testing when added to sigmoidoscopy alone.)*

Appendix: Proctosigmoidoscopy and Other Anorectal Examinations

Lawrence S. Friedman, M.D.

Proctosigmoidoscopy is a basic technique for evaluating patients with gastrointestinal complaints and a useful screening method for colorectal cancer screening (see above). *Rigid sigmoidoscopy* can be performed during an office visit. The necessary equipment is inexpensive to purchase, easy to master, and simple to maintain; the scope section is disposable, facilitating cleanup. The development of the flexible *fiberoptic sigmoidoscope* makes possible visualization of bowel previously beyond reach. However, fiberoptic instruments are much more expensive to purchase and maintain, and harder to master and clean. The ultimate role for fiberoptic sigmoidoscopy in primary care practice remains unsettled. The primary care physician should at least be capable of performing a competent rigid sigmoidoscopic examination.

ANORECTAL EXAMINATION

An anorectal examination is indicated in all patients who are to undergo sigmoidoscopy and should be incorporated into all complete physical examinations in adults. No bowel preparation is necessary, but the physician must establish rapport with the patient by taking a history and performing other parts of the physical examination first. Apprehension and embarrassment may be minimized by explaining each step, describing the anticipated sensations, and draping the patient to expose only the perineum.

Inspection. The patient may be examined in either the knee–chest or left lateral decubitus (Sims') position. After retraction of the buttocks, the perianal skin and anal orifice are inspected for fecal material (reflecting poor hygiene, painful lesions that make cleansing difficult, or incontinence), drainage, dermatoses, scars, prolapsed hemorrhoids, fistulas, fissures, abscesses, hematomas, condylomata, and carcinomas. Lesions are described anatomically (eg, anterior, right-sided), not with reference to the face of a clock. Perineal and sacrococcygeal tissues should be palpated with the gloved but unlubricated index finger for tenderness, induration, fluctuance, or masses.

Palpation. Digital examination of the rectum is then performed by placing the gloved, lubricated index finger at the anal orifice and gently inserting as the patient bears down. The small finger may be used in patients with painful or stenotic anal lesions. Anesthetic ointment may be helpful if a tender lesion is present. The anal sphincter tone and strength of contraction are noted, and the finger is swept circumferentially as it is advanced into the rectum. Abnormalities sought include fissures, fistulous tracts, abscesses, villous and pedunculated polyps, and cancers. Rarely, foreign bodies may be encountered. Internal hemorrhoids are not palpable unless they are thrombosed. In inflammatory bowel disease the mucosa may feel gritty. Stool in the rectum is deformable, distinguishing it from other rectal masses. The rectal ampulla should be checked carefully (Fig. 56–1); it is often overlooked and may harbor a neoplasm.

The average effective depth of insertion of the index finger is 7.5 cm. In women, care must be taken not to mistake the cervix for a rectal "tumor" along the anterior rectal wall; the cervix is smooth and symmetric. In men, the prostate and, if possible, the seminal vesicles should be examined. Finally, on withdrawal, the examining finger should be inspected for the character of feces and the presence of blood, pus, or mucus. A test for occult blood should be performed, unless gross blood is evident.

Anoscopy

Anoscopy may be a useful adjunct to the anorectal examination, particularly in the evaluation of bright red rectal bleeding, perianal pain, or suspected hemorrhoids. Anoscopes are metal or disposable plastic tubes with a diameter of 2 cm at the tip and a length of 7 cm. A built-in light source may be present or an external light source may be required, depending on the make of anoscope. With the patient in the same position as for the anorectal examination, the lubricated anoscope is held in the right hand with the thumb pressing on the obturator as the instrument is introduced with slow gentle pressure. The instrument is first directed along the longitudinal axis of the anal canal toward the um-

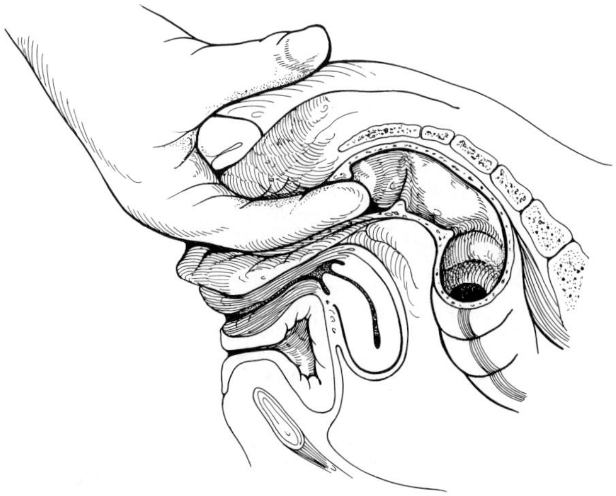

Figure 56-1. Digital examination.

bilicus and then pointed more posteriorly at the anorectal angle. It is inserted the full length and held in the left hand so that the flange rests against the anus. The obturator is removed, and the anoscope is slowly withdrawn as the mucosa is examined.

The normal anal mucosa is pink with a visible delicate network of submucosal vessels. In patients with proctitis the vascular pattern is typically obliterated and the mucosa may be friable (ie, it may bleed easily on gentle swabbing). Anoscopy is particularly helpful in identifying hemorrhoids, which may appear as purple bulges into the lumen; occasionally blood may be seen to issue from a hemorrhoid. Fissures may be identified at the anal verge.

SIGMOIDOSCOPY

In asymptomatic individuals, sigmoidoscopy can be an important screening procedure for early detection of colorectal cancer (see above). About one-third of colorectal cancers are within reach of the rigid sigmoidoscope, and over 50 percent are within reach of the flexible sigmoidoscope. It appears that asymptomatic rectal cancers discovered by sigmoidoscopy are less advanced and survival rates are better than in patients with symptomatic cancers. Screening by flexible sigmoidoscopy has been shown capable of improving survival in patients with colorectal cancer, although cost-effectiveness is still a subject of debate. Also unresolved is the optimal frequency of surveillance (see above).

Sigmoidoscopy provides for direct visualization of the colonic mucosa. As such, it is an essential part of the evaluation of patients presenting with a host of complaints or problems referable to the large bowel (Table 56–2). Also, sigmoidoscopy can supplement barium studies by providing additional observations of abnormalities detected on barium enema, such as polyps and other suspected mass lesions. In patients with known inflammatory bowel disease, sigmoidoscopy is useful for monitoring disease activity and response to therapy.

Table 56-2. Indications for Sigmoidoscopy

Symptoms
Rectal pain
Rectal discharge
Bright red bleeding per rectum
Hematochezia
Persistent or recurrent diarrhea
Change in bowel habits
Chronic constipation
Unexplained weight loss
Signs
Abdominal or rectal mass
Enlarged sentinel lymph node
Guaiac-positive stool
Unexplained hepatic nodule or enlargement or other signs of metastatic cancer
Laboratory Abnormalities
Unexplained iron deficiency anemia
Mass or polyp on barium enema
Other laboratory manifestation of metastatic disease from unknown primary lesion
Screening
Patients at high risk for colorectal malignancy (ulcerative colitis, familial polyposis)
Patients at average risk of malignancy (controversial)

Rigid Sigmoidoscopy

Preparation. Satisfactory cleansing of the bowel can be achieved in most patients with a single tap water or phosphasoda (Fleet) enema administered 45 minutes before sigmoidoscopic examination. If the examination has been scheduled in advance, the patient can be instructed to self-administer one or two enemas at home on the morning of examination. Adequate preparation is particularly advisable in older individuals, who often have large amounts of retained stool in the rectal vault.

In patients with diarrhea or suspected inflammatory bowel disease, it is preferable to forego enema cleansing before sigmoidoscopy. These patients can usually achieve adequate preparation by having a bowel movement just before the examination. Moreover, because enemas may induce edema and erythema of the mucosa, prior enema administration may make it impossible for the observer to distinguish subtle mucosal changes caused by proctitis from those induced by the enema.

Because of the low risk of endocarditis associated with sigmoidoscopy in patients with valvular heart disease, antibiotic prophylaxis is not recommended except for patients with prosthetic valves (see Chapter 16). Sedation and analgesia are seldom necessary but may be used in patients with painful anal lesions.

Technique. The patient is examined in the same position as for the rectal and anoscopic examinations. The left lateral decubitus (Sims') position is better tolerated than the knee–chest position by older and debilitated patients and may be less embarrassing to patients in general. However, knee–chest permits greater range of scope motion. If available, a tilt-table designed for sigmoidoscopy minimizes the discomfort for the patient and eliminates the rather awkward position required of the examiner when Sims's position is used.

The sigmoidoscope is a rigid metal or disposable plastic tube, 25 cm long and approximately 1.5 cm in diameter. Newer rigid sigmoidoscopes have distal fiberoptic lighting, a proximal magnifying lens, and a connection for air insufflation. Additional standard equipment includes long cotton swabs, suctioning apparatus, and biopsy and grasping forceps.

The lubricated instrument is inserted with the right hand holding the obturator firmly in place and with gentle pressure against the anal sphincter as the patient bears down. Alternatively, if the rectal examination is performed with the left index finger, the sigmoidoscope may be guided over the withdrawing examining finger to avoid having to dilate the anal sphincter a second time. The sigmoidoscope is initially directed toward the umbilicus and then posteriorly at the anorectal junction (Fig. 56–2).

Once past the anorectal ring, the obturator is withdrawn, and the sigmoidoscope is advanced with the lumen in view at all times. Unless stool is present, insertion is easy until the rectosigmoid junction is reached at about 12 to 15 cm from the anus. At this point the lumen bends forward sharply and to the left. The patient may experience painful spasm

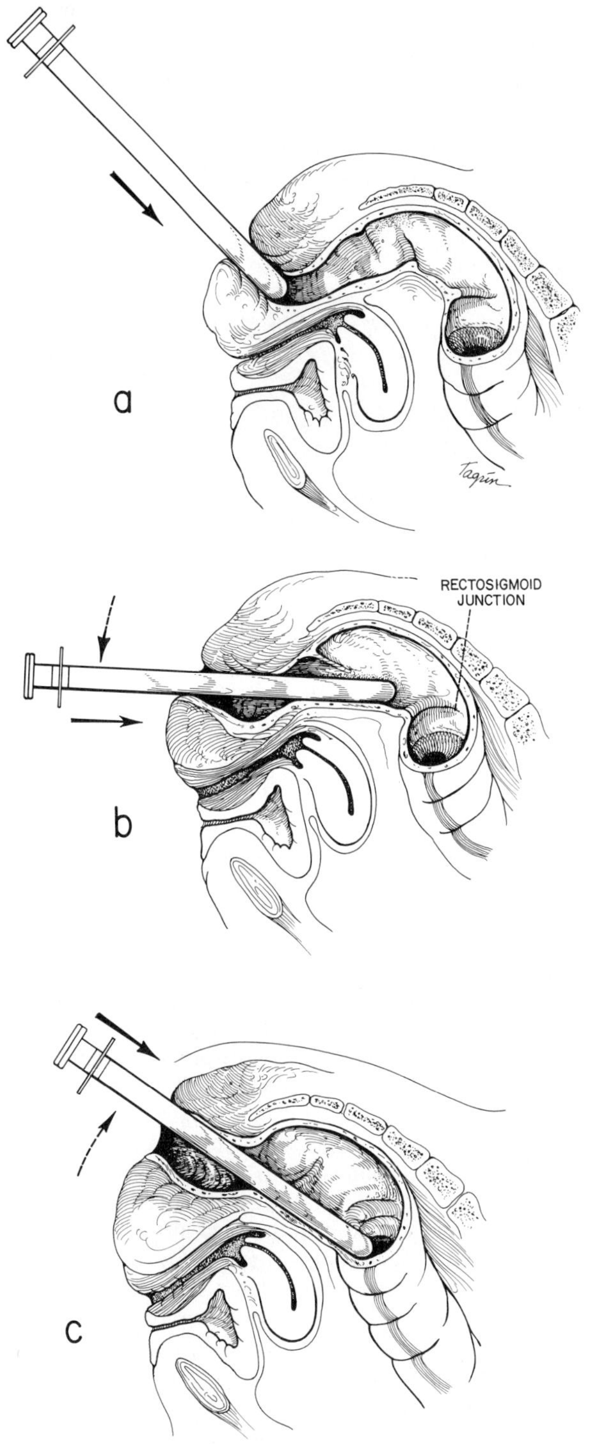

Figure 56-2. Overview of rigid sigmoidoscopic examination: **(A)** Tip of sigmoidoscope is inserted into anal canal in direction of umbilicus; **(B)** At anorectal junction (about 3 cm from anus) tip is deflected toward sacrum; **(C)** At rectosigmoid junction (about 12 to 15 cm from anus) tip is deflected anteriorly and to left.

and should be reassured and instructed to breathe slowly and deeply to ensure relaxation of abdominal muscles as the instrument is slowly advanced. Air insufflation should be kept to a minimum to avoid painful colonic distention. When a tight bend in the lumen is encountered and the direction of the lumen is not obvious, it is best to withdraw the sigmoidoscope slightly until a smooth crescentic band of mucosa appears in the field of view. This band always represents the anterior aspect of the mucosa as it bends behind the band, and the sigmoidoscope can be advanced again just beyond the band and deflected in the same direction, where the lumen should be expected to appear (Fig. 56–3). It is important not to push the sigmoidoscope blindly and to desist when the mucosa blanches or the patient experiences severe pain.

Although it is desirable to pass the sigmoidoscope the entire 25 cm, complete insertion is often not possible. In fact, even in the hands of an experienced sigmoidoscopist, the average depth of insertion is 16 to 20 cm. Furthermore, it is important to note whether the sigmoidoscope is advancing up the lumen or merely distending the rectal mucosa.

Examination of the mucosa is conducted on slow withdrawal of the instrument. The tip is swept circumferentially to visualize all areas of the wall, and air is injected in small amounts to flatten out folds and allow adequate inspection. As noted earlier, the normal mucosa is pale pink with a visible network of submucosal blood vessels. Occasionally some blood produced from enema tip trauma may be present. The mucosa should be examined and described; any lesions should be noted, and the distance from the anal verge should be recorded. Occasionally blood may be found to come from a point above the reach of the instrument; this should be noted.

Biopsies of suspicious lesions and abnormal mucosa may be obtained with angled forceps. Mucosal biopsies should be shallow and taken from the posterior rectal wall, where the risk of perforation is small. Bleeding from biopsy sites usually stops with pressure from a swab or by application of silver nitrate sticks. Because of the risk of perforation, barium enema examination should be avoided for at least 5 days after a sigmoidoscopic biopsy.

The entire sigmoidoscopic examination should take from 2 to 5 minutes. However, the goal should never be speed, but rather thoroughness and assurance of patient comfort.

Complications. Perforations are rare, occurring in no more than one in 10,000 sigmoidoscopies, and are more likely if the examiner persists in pushing the sigmoidoscope forward in a bowel that is fixed at any point, as by tumor. Bleeding from biopsy sites is infrequent. Arrhythmias have been reported rarely.

Flexible Fiberoptic Sigmoidoscopy

The most widely used flexible fiberoptic sigmoidoscopes are 60 to 65 cm long with large-caliber suction and biopsy channels, full control of tip deflection by two hand dials, and controls for air insufflation and water instillation. The diameter of the shaft is 11 mm, making the instrument narrower and longer than the rigid sigmoidoscope. The control dials and buttons are managed with the left hand as the examiner views the colon through the eyepiece; advancement of the instrument up the colon is accomplished with the right hand. Acute angulations of the colon are traversed by various combinations of tip deflection, shaft twisting, and repetitive back-and-forth motions; however, even accomplished sigmoidoscopists may encounter difficulty in advancing the

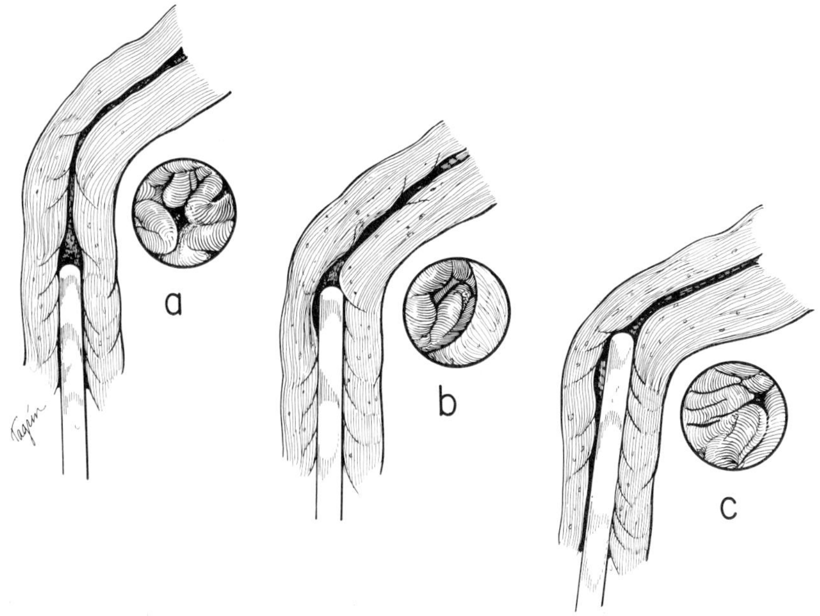

Figure 56-3. Maneuvering a rigid sigmoidoscope past an angulation in the sigmoid colon: **(A)** Advancement of sigmoidoscope through straight portion of colon; view through scope shows concentric lumen with radiating mucosal folds. **(B)** As bend in colon is reached, a crescentic band of mucosa is seen in front of the lumen as it bends. To maneuver past this angulation the scope is first withdrawn 1–2 cm as the tip is deflected *away* from the lumen. The scope is then readvanced slowly as the tip is deflected back toward the lumen *behind* the crescentic mucosal band. **(C)** Lumen reappears as the bend is tranversed.

instrument through very sharp angles. The procedure can be done in the office or clinic, usually with no sedation or anesthesia, and with a preparation of only one or two phospha-soda enemas. However, competency in 60 cm fiber optic flexible sigmoidoscopy generally requires about 25 procedures performed under supervision.

Flexible Versus Rigid Sigmoidoscopy. The advantage of the flexible sigmoidoscope over the rigid sigmoidoscope is its ability to examine a longer segment of colon. Whereas the average depth of insertion of the rigid instrument is no more than 20 cm, the average depth of insertion for the flexible instrument in the hands of experienced endoscopists is about 50 cm. Consequently, the diagnostic yield of flexible sigmoidoscopy is greater than that of rigid sigmoidoscopy. For example, in comparative studies, the flexible instrument identified two to six times more neoplasms and detected some abnormalities, such as diverticula, not generally within reach of the rigid sigmoidoscope. In addition, the flexible instrument is tolerated by the patient as well or better than the rigid instrument.

The apparent advantages of flexible sigmoidoscopy must be weighed against the observation that, as a screening test, it detects no more than two-thirds of colorectal polyps and cancers. Moreover, patients undergoing either rigid or flexible sigmoidoscopy for gastrointestinal symptoms may still require additional tests, such as a barium enema or colonoscopy, to complete the evaluation. Thus, the decision to perform flexible rather than rigid sigmoidoscopy in a given instance may be more a matter of physician preference, cost, and convenience than of an apparent improvement in diagnostic yield. The most clear-cut advantage of flexible over rigid sigmoidoscopy would appear to be in the screening of asymptomatic patients for colorectal cancer, in which case a barium enema or colonoscopy would not be performed unless indicated (see above).

Other factors to consider in deciding whether to use flexible instead of rigid sigmoidoscopes in a clinical practice are expense and convenience. Flexible fiberoptic instruments are much more expensive than disposable plastic rigid sigmoidoscopes and are more likely to be damaged and require occasional costly repairs. In addition, the flexible instrument must be cleaned thoroughly between patients, and the average duration of examination is at least 10 minutes, so that the time involved in using the instrument per patient is much greater for the flexible than the rigid instrument. Moreover, cleaning and proper care of the flexible sigmoidoscope include U.S. government-mandated disinfection procedures between each case. In a busy clinical practice, use of the flexible sigmoidoscope may be less practical and efficient than use of the rigid instrument.

Consensus is that rigid sigmoidoscopy is preferred when a careful examination for rectal pathology is desired, when one is monitoring activity of ulcerative colitis or evaluating the cause of an infectious colitis, and when one wants to avoid contaminating a flexible scope. Flexible sigmoidoscopy is the more sensitive test for colorectal cancer screening, although whether it is more cost-effective than rigid sigmoidoscopy remains to be determined. It is preferred when determining the source of recurrent rectal bleeding, evaluating a radiologically detected lesion in the sigmoid colon, searching for colitis in a patient with normal rectal mucosa, and evaluating a patient with suspected diverticulitis (see Chapter 75).

The flexible sigmoidoscope has not been widely evaluated in a primary care setting staffed by physicians with no prior experience with fiberoptic instruments. Preliminary data suggest that nearly any physician can learn to use the flexible instrument, but only with supervised instruction. The diagnostic yield of the flexible sigmoidoscope in the hands of primary care physicians has not been evaluated, either in comparison with the rigid instrument or in comparison with experienced endoscopists. Recently, a shorter 30-cm flexible sigmoidoscope has been introduced and in preliminary studies appears to be easy to learn to use with minimal instruction. Whether the shorter instrument has sufficient advantage over the longer one to justify its commercial distribution has not been determined. Until experience with flexible sigmoidoscopy has been more thoroughly evaluated in the primary care setting, it would seem wise for primary physicians to master the technique of rigid sigmoidoscopy and to consider learning the technique of flexible sigmoidoscopy only if they are willing to commit sufficient time to develop true proficiency. Unless expertise has been achieved, the primary care physician should refer patients in need of flexible sigmoidoscopy to a gastroenterologist or a surgeon skilled in performing the examination.

ANNOTATED BIBLIOGRAPHY

American Society for Gastrointestinal Endoscopy. Flexible Sigmoidoscopy: Guideline for Clinical Application, 1986. *(A booklet that summarizes the training requirements for primary care physicians to use a flexible scope. Most experts suggest 7 to 10 procedures to use the 35-cm scope and 15 to 30 procedures to master the 60-cm scope.)*

Bohlman TW, Katon RM, Lipshutz GR, et al. Fiberoptic pansigmoidoscopy: An evaluation and comparison with rigid sigmoidoscopy. Gastroenterology 1977;72:644. *(In 120 patients, the flexible instrument was inserted nearly three times as far [55 cm versus 20 cm] and identified pathologic lesions three times as often [39 percent versus 13 percent] as the rigid instrument.)*

Coller JA. Technique of flexible fiberoptic sigmoidoscopy. Surg Clin North Am 1980;60:465. *(Detailed and well-illustrated description of the technique.)*

Lehman GA, Buchner DM, Lappas JC. Anatomical extent of fiberoptic sigmoidoscopy. Gastroenterology 1983;84:803. *(A 60-cm examination, achieved in 50 percent of those examined, viewed the entire sigmoid colon 80 percent of the time.)*

Levin B. Screening sigmoidscopy for colorectal cancer screening. N Engl J Med 1992;326:700. *(Editorial arguing for its use in colorectal cancer screening, but also pointing out its limitations.)*

Madigan MR, Halls JM. The extent of sigmoidoscopy on radiographs with special reference to the rectosigmoid junction. Gut 1968;9:355. *(Failure to insert the rigid sigmoidoscope to 25 cm in a majority of patients was usually due to the acute angulation of the rectosigmoid junction.)*

McCarthy BD, Moskowitz MA. Screening flexible-sigmoidoscopy: Patient attitudes and compliance. J Gen Intern Med 1993;8:120. *(Seventy-five percent agreed to the procedure; only 14% said they would not do it again.)*

Nivatvongs S, Fryd DS. How far does the proctosigmoidoscope reach? A prospective study of 1000 patients. N Engl J Med 1980;303:380. *(Average depth of insertion of rigid sigmoidoscope was 19.5 cm to 20.3 cm in males and 18.6 cm in females.)*

Schrock TR. Examination of the anorectum, rigid sigmoidoscopy, and flexible fiberoptic sigmoidoscopy. In Sleisenger MH, Fordtran JS (eds). Gastrointestinal Disease, 4th ed., pp 1570–1576. Philadelphia, WB Saunders, 1989. *(Comprehensive discussion of indications for and techniques of both rigid and flexible sigmoidoscopy.)*

Selby JV, Friedman GD, Quesenberry CP, et al. A case-control study of screening sigmoidoscopy and mortality from colorectal cancer. N Engl J Med 1992;326:653. *(Retrospective study indicating a survival benefit with screening by proctosigmoidoscopy.)*

Weissman GS, Winawer SJ, Baldwin MP, et al. Multicenter evaluation of training of non-endoscopists in 30-cm flexible sigmoidoscopy. CA 1987;37;26. *(Results suggest that nonendoscopists should initially use the 30-cm scope.)*

Primary Care Medicine: Office Evaluation and Management of the Adult Patient, 3rd edition, edited by Allan H. Goroll, Lawrence A. May, and Albert G. Mulley, Jr. J.B. Lippincott Company, Philadelphia

57
Prevention of Viral Hepatitis

JULES L. DIENSTAG, M.D.

Viral hepatitis is a contagious disease estimated to afflict more than 500,000 people in the United States each year. Although the majority of those infected are either asymptomatic or minimally symptomatic, a small proportion may develop fulminant disease. Several thousand deaths per year are related to the disease. Five distinct types of viral hepatitis are recognized: A, B, C (formerly labeled non-A, non-B), D, and E (formerly labeled the enteric form of non-A, non-B).

In general, outbreaks of hepatitis are often traced to a source of hepatitis A virus (HAV) or, in developing countries, to hepatitis E virus (HEV). Occasionally, clusters of hepatitis B follow exposure of several persons to contaminated needles or blood products. Among urban adults presenting to a primary care physician with sporadic cases of hepatitis, hepatitis B accounts for approximately 50 percent of cases, hepatitis C for 15 percent to 30 percent, and hepatitis A for the remainder. More than 95 percent of transfusion-associated cases are attributable to hepatitis C; however, the frequency of transfusion-related cases has been dramatically reduced by the recent introduction of sensitive screening tests for hepatitis C (see below). Hepatitis D is due to a defective virus that infects only in the presence of infection with hepatitis B virus.

Prevention of infection and prophylaxis against clinical disease are prime objectives in the management of viral hepatitis. The primary physician has major responsibility for these tasks, because patients and their contacts often present at a time when infectivity is high. Prevention of viral hepatitis requires a knowledge of the common modes of viral transmission, the periods of maximal communicability, and the efficacy of globulin preparations and vaccines.

EPIDEMIOLOGY AND RISK FACTORS

Hepatitis A virus is shed in the feces, and transmission occurs predominantly by the *fecal–oral* route. Prior exposure to hepatitis A is manifested by the presence of antibody to hepatitis A virus (anti-HAV), which confers life-long immunity. More than 80 percent of patients over age 60 are positive for anti-HAV; acute infection is rare in this age group. Because children and adolescents are least likely to have had previous exposure to the virus, they are the most susceptible to infection. Spread of infection is greatest when poor sanitary conditions and crowding exist. In a New York City study, 75 percent of low-income people had evidence of prior infection, compared with 20 percent to 30 percent of residents in middle- to upper-income neighborhoods. In developed countries, the prevalence of anti-HAV and of immunity to the virus has fallen successively since the end of World War II. There is no carrier state.

Hepatitis B used to be considered a disease that resulted from *parenteral exposure,* but *nonpercutaneous transmission* is a common mode of spread. Perinatal transmission from mother to offspring is common in developing nations. Patients with hepatitis B infection have been found to harbor hepatitis B surface antigen (HBsAg) in saliva, semen, vaginal secretions, and breast milk, as well as in the serum. Spouses of patients with acute hepatitis B and people with a large number of sexual partners (eg, male homosexuals) are maximally subjected to sources of nonpercutaneous transmission and have a markedly increased risk of contracting infection. About 0.1 percent of healthy blood donors are positive for HBsAg; the percentages increase markedly for intravenous (IV) drug abusers and patients in some dialysis units. Surgeons, laboratory technicians, oral surgeons, and other medical personnel exposed to blood and body fluids are at increased risk of contracting hepatitis B. Spread of infection from health personnel who are HBsAg carriers is a rare event, usually resulting from inadvertent patient exposure to their blood from cuts or abrasions.

The development and application of sensitive screening methods for detection of HBsAg have essentially eliminated posttransfusion hepatitis type B. Reliance on blood obtained from volunteer donors, which is less likely to contain the virus, as well as blood-donor exclusion practices and screening tests to prevent transfusion-transmittted acquired immunodeficiency syndrome (AIDS) and hepatitis C have also contributed to reducing the frequency of hepatitis B after transfusion.

Hepatitis C, initially labeled "non-A, non-B hepatitis," was first recognized in *transfusion* recipients and found to be the predominant type of hepatitis after transfusion. In the 1970s, it occurred in up to 10 percent of transfusion recipients, usually within 1 to 3 months of receiving volunteer-donated blood. The frequency of infection fell with exclusion of blood donors at risk for human immunodeficiency virus (HIV) infection and was further reduced by use of screening tests for HIV (see Chapter 13), surrogate tests for hepatitis C (eg, alanine aminotransferase [ALT], antibodies to hepatitis B core antigen), and finally direct testing for anti-hepatitis C virus (HCV). Currently, the risk of hepatitis C after transfusion is barely measurable. Hepatitis C can be spread by *any percutaneous route,* such as needlestick inoculation (3% to 10% risk of infection) or self-injection among IV drug users. Risk is felt to be extraordinarily low from sexual transmission or perinatal transmission. About 40 percent of cases occur in persons with no identifiable risk factors.

Hepatitis D or delta hepatitis is caused by a defective ribonucleic acid (RNA) virus that requires *coinfection with hepatitis B* (a deoxyribonucleic acid [DNA] virus) to support its replication. Infection with this agent occurs either simultaneously with acute hepatitis B infection or is superimposed on chronic hepatitis B. Like hepatitis B, hepatitis D is transmitted by percutaneous inoculation and intimate contact. In nonendemic areas, such as the United States and western Europe, hepatitis D has been confined primarily to populations with frequent *percutaneous exposures,* such as drug addicts and hemophiliacs. In endemic areas, such as the Mediterranean countries, hepatitis D is transmitted primarily through *intimate contact.*

Hepatitis E is a disease prevalent in India, Asia, and underdeveloped countries, transmitted by the *fecal–oral* route, with virus shed in the stool.

NATURAL HISTORY

Both hepatitis A and E are self-limited and do not lead to chronic liver disease; however, hepatitis B, C, and D can lead to chronic hepatitis.

Hepatitis A has an average incubation period of 30 days (range, 15 to 45 days) from the time of exposure to the onset of symptoms. An early manifestation of disease is elevation of the serum aminotransferase level, which occurs about a week before onset of flulike symptoms. However, fecal shedding of HAV has been found to occur even before the rise in aminotransferases and up to 2 weeks before the development of symptoms. HAV disappears from stool within 2 to 3 weeks, usually coinciding with the onset of jaundice and resolution of prodromal symptoms. A fall in viral titer parallels a rise in antibody titer, which persists indefinitely. Initially, the *anti-HAV* is of the *IgM* class; during convalescence anti-HAV of the *IgG* class becomes predominant. Therefore, a diagnosis of acute hepatitis A can be made by demonstrating IgM anti-HAV in a single serum sample. No episodes of chronic hepatitis or a carrier state have been found to result from hepatitis A infection. Fatalities are rare; fewer than 5 percent of cases of fulminant hepatitis are due to type A virus infection.

Hepatitis B infection is a much more variable disease. The incubation period averages 12 weeks, with a range of 4 weeks to 6 months. About 2 to 4 weeks before the onset of symptoms, *HBsAg* appears in the serum, followed by a rise in aminotransferase levels and symptoms. Antigen usually is cleared from the serum by 4 to 6 months; persistence of antigenemia beyond 6 months is considered chronic infection.

Symptoms of acute hepatitis B typically last 4 to 6 weeks, but there is much variation, ranging from clinically inapparent disease to fulminant hepatocellular failure and death. Age, immunologic competence, undefined host factors, and virulence of the virus are postulated to be among the determinants of disease severity.

Approximately 1 percent to 2 percent of patients with clinically apparent disease acquire *chronic infection* and continue to have circulating HBsAg. A much larger number of cases of chronic hepatitis B do not originate as clinically apparent acute illness, making the number of chronic cases much larger than would otherwise be anticipated. Among patients with chronic hepatitis B, some remain *asymptomatic carriers,* whereas a proportion progress to *chronic active hepatitis,* the progressive form of chronic hepatitis B. The fatality rate for acute hepatitis B is about 0.1 percent; however, among those requiring hospitalization, the mortality rate is 1 percent.

Antibody to surface antigen (anti-HBs) is produced early during infection but becomes detectable with commercially available serologic assays only as HBsAg disappears. Over 95 percent of patients acquire detectable levels of anti-HBs; they persist indefinitely.

Antibody to the nucleocapsid core of hepatitis B virus (HBV; anti-HBc) appears in the circulation within a week or so after HBsAg becomes detectable and persists indefinitely. Occasionally, during late acute infection, an interval occurs in which HBsAg has already disappeared, and anti-HBs has not yet become detectable. This so-called window period can be identified by the presence of anti-HBc; however, this window period is rarely encountered. Most instances in which anti-HBc occurs in the absence of HBsAg and anti-HBs represent HBV infection in the remote past. In rare instances, isolated anti-HBc represents a false-positive test, while in patients at high risk for blood-borne infections (eg, intravenous drug users), isolated anti-HBc may represent low-level HBV infection in which the level of HBsAg does not exceed the detection threshold.

A test for anti-HBc of the IgM class (IgM anti-HBc) can distinguish between acute or relatively recent acute hepatitis B (IgM positive) and remote infection or chronic carriage (IgM negative, anti-HBc of the IgG class). In a small proportion of cases of acute hepatitis B, HBsAg does not reach the threshold for detection; in such cases, a diagnosis of acute hepatitis B can be established by detecting IgM anti-HBc.

Hepatitis B e antigen (*HBeAg*) is a product of the gene that codes for the nucleocapsid core; its presence signifies the presence of a state of high virus replication. As such, patients with HBeAg have a high level of circulating virions, high infectivity, and substantial liver injury. HBeAg becomes detectable in *all* patients early during acute hepatitis B, and, therefore, there is no clinical utility to the test during early acute hepatitis B; however, if circulating HBeAg persists beyond the first 3 months of acute hepatitis, the likelihood of chronic infection is increased. Testing for HBeAg is more important during chronic infection, for the presence of HBeAg denotes a more highly *replicative* chronic infection, associated with increased infectivity (eg, 20–25% infectivity of a needlestick) and liver injury (eg, chronic active hepatitis). When anti-HBe can be detected in the absence of HBeAg during chronic infection, the patient can be classified as having a less replicative infection, with limited infectivity (eg, 0.1% infectivity of a needlestick) and liver injury (chronic carrier).

Hepatitis B virus DNA (HBV DNA) is a more quantitative marker of HBV replication, and is helpful in following patients with chronic disease and in monitoring the success of antiviral therapy (see Chapter 70).

Hepatitis C has a mean incubation period of 7 weeks (range, 2 to 15 weeks), with most cases occurring after 5 to 10 weeks of incubation. Improved assays for *antibodies to hepatitis C virus (anti-HCV)* turn positive during acute infection and remain so indefinitely in most patients. They can be used for routine diagnostic purposes during acute hepatitis C. Because of occasional nonspecificity of immunoassays for anti-HCV, a supplemental confirmatory test is needed when a positive result is encountered in a patient at very low risk for blood-borne infection (eg, the asymptomatic blood donor with no risk factors). In such instances, a *recombinant immunoblot assay (RIBA)* can be performed to identify the viral or nonviral proteins responsible for the positive test. The most sensitive test for hepatitis C infection is one that measures *HCV RNA*.

Only a quarter of patients with acute, transfusion-associated hepatitis C become icteric, compared with two-thirds of those with transfusion-induced hepatitis B. However, up to 50 percent of patients with acute hepatitis C progress to *chronic infection* and liver injury, regardless of the mode of acquisition. Among those with chronic hepatitis following acute hepatitis C, 20 percent may progress to cirrhosis over the first decade of illness, even in patients with mild liver disease. On the other hand, morbidity over the first 20 years after acute hepatitis C is limited.

Hepatitis D (delta hepatitis) is being recognized with increasing frequency in the United States. Its incubation period is similar to that for hepatitis B, and, when both hepatitis B and hepatitis D infections are acquired simultaneously, a single clinically apparent episode of hepatitis may ensue. There is a slight increase in the risk of *fulminant hepatitis* when the two infections occur simultaneously, but, in general, the outcome of simultaneous acute hepatitis B and D is no different from the outcome of hepatitis B alone. In contrast, among patients with chronic hepatitis B infection, superimposed hepatitis D may lead to severe, fulminant hepatitis, convert a mild or asymptomatic chronic hepatitis B infection into a severe form of chronic hepatitis (*chronic active hepatitis*), or accelerate the course of chronic active hepatitis. A diagnosis of delta hepatitis is made by demonstrating the appearance of *antibody to hepatitis D (anti-HDV)*.

Hepatitis E has a mean incubation period of about 40 days, slightly longer than that for hepatitis A. Its clinical course is similar to that of hepatitis A, except that more patients experience a *cholestatic illness* and the likelihood of fulminant disease is higher (1% to 2%, 10% to 20% in pregnant women). The disease is *self-limited* and does not progress to chronic infection. The virus is excreted in stool early, and antibodies to HEV become detectable during acute illness. Serologic tests are under development.

PRINCIPLES OF PROPHYLAXIS

The principal means of prophylaxis are minimizing exposure to hepatitis viruses and use of globulin preparations and vaccines. In many instances, globulin prophylaxis does not prevent infection, but it may reduce the chances of developing clinical hepatitis. Precautions against contact with the hepatitis patient are most appropriate during the prodromal stage of illness, when the patient sheds virus most heavily or when there is often little clinical evidence of hepatitis, making avoidance of contact with the virus difficult. Consequently, immunotherapy emerges as the mainstay of prophylaxis.

Hepatitis A. Prophylaxis for hepatitis A can be accomplished by use of standard *immune globulin* (IG). This globulin preparation contains high titers of anti-HAV and is about 80 percent effective in preventing clinical disease. The mechanism by which IG protects the exposed patient was believed to be passive–active immunization, in which passively administered antibody acts to minimize clinical illness but does not prevent infection. Newer analyses suggest that IG more often prevents infection entirely. IG must be administered within 1 to 2 weeks of exposure to be most effective. Patients with a prior history of serologically documented hepatitis A need not receive IG because they are already protected by their own anti-HAV.

Household contacts and small groups experiencing a common source outbreak (eg, an athletic team) should be given IG prophylaxis, if the outbreak is identified early enough. During the early phase of clinical hepatitis, when jaundice first appears, there may still be some shedding of virus; precautions such as avoiding intimate contact and careful washing of hands after contact are probably reasonable for a week or two longer. The patient should not serve food to others and may minimize transmission of virus by using disposable dishes and utensils.

Routine immunoprophylaxis is not necessary for casual contacts at work or school. Preexposure prophylaxis is recommended for those who travel to areas of the world where hepatitis A is endemic. Formalin-inactivated hepatitis A vaccines have been developed and have been shown to be safe, immunogenic, and effective in preventing hepatitis A. When they become commercially available, they are likely to replace immune globulin for preexposure prophylaxis.

Hepatitis B. Prophylaxis of hepatitis B is achieved by providing the susceptible person with protective antibody, anti-HBs. This can be accomplished by passive immunization with immune globulins containing anti-HBs. *Hepatitis B immune globulin (HBIG)* is prepared from the plasma of persons with high-titer anti-HBs and contains anti-HBs at titers in the range of 1:100,000 or higher. HBIG appears to attenuate clinical illness, rather than prevent infection. It is recommended in conjunction with vaccine for postexposure prophylaxis (see below).

Active immunization has become possible with the advent of *hepatitis B vaccine*. The original vaccine was prepared from the plasma of hepatitis B carriers. Although this vaccine underwent multistep inactivation that destroyed the infectivity of all known viruses (including HIV), concerns over the origin of the vaccine from high-risk persons limited its acceptance. In 1987, a recombinant vaccine became available, derived from recombinant yeast into which the gene for surface antigen had been inserted. Such vaccines have replaced plasma-derived vaccines in the United States.

Hepatitis B vaccine has been recommended as *preexposure prophylaxis,* primarily for population subgroups considered to be at high risk of exposure to HBV (eg, health and laboratory workers exposed to blood, hemodialysis staff and patients, residents and staff of custodial institutions, promiscuous persons, IV drug users, patients requiring repeated administration of blood products or clotting factors, and household and sexual contacts of chronic HBsAg carriers). Although these groups remain targets for vaccination, the attempt to vaccinate them has not been successful in limiting the spread of HBV within the general population of developed countries. Frequency has actually increased. Attempts to vaccinate population subgroups targeted for vaccination have not been successful—fewer than 10 percent have actually been vaccinated, and 30 percent to 40 percent with acute hepatitis B do not belong to any of these recognized risk groups. Therefore the U.S. Public Health Service has recommended that universal vaccination in childhood should be adopted. Whether for high-risk groups or for universal childhood vaccination, three deltoid injections of the vaccine are recommended, the first two are given 1 month apart and the third is given at 6 months. Doses vary according to age group and vaccine manufacturer.

For *postexposure prophylaxis* in susceptible persons who sustain an exposure to hepatitis B, a combination of *HBIG* and hepatitis B vaccine is recommended. Babies born to mothers with chronic hepatitis B (or acute hepatitis B during the third trimester of pregnancy), heterosexual contacts of patients with acute hepatitis B, and those who sustain HBsAg-positive needlesticks should receive HBIG plus hepatitis B vaccine. The HBIG provides immediate, high-level, passively acquired anti-HBs, and the vaccine adds long-lasting immunity and probably attenuation of clinical illness in the postexposure setting. HBIG should be administered as soon as possible after exposure (eg, no later than 48 hours after a needlestick, in the delivery room for babies). The first dose of vaccine can be given simultaneously or within a few hours in newborns, within a week in those sustaining needlestick exposures, or within 2 weeks in those with sexual exposure. Because early prophylaxis is paramount after an HBsAg needlestick, HBIG should be administered immediately and without delay to wait for the results of antibody testing. There is no interference between hepatitis B vaccine and HBIG, even when administered simultaneously.

Hepatitis B vaccine consists entirely of HBsAg protein (no core proteins are included), allowing one to distinguish between immunization and infection by assaying for presence of antibody to core protein (anti-HBc).

Although determination of the HBeAg status of the contact case or inoculum source may provide information about relative infectivity, HBeAg status should not be a criterion for providing prophylaxis to contacts. The delay necessitated by waiting for HBeAg testing may invalidate efforts at prophylaxis, and infectivity can occur in the absence of HBeAg, although the likelihood is reduced. Nonintimate household contacts do not require prophylaxis, nor do casual contacts at work.

The *duration of protection* after hepatitis B vaccine is not definitively known but appears to be at least 5 to 7 years. Even after anti-HBs levels fall below detectable levels, new exposures in nature are likely to be accompanied by an anamnestic immune response, and adequate immunity against clinically apparent infection and chronic infection appear to be maintained. Based on these observations, authorities have not recommended routine booster vaccination in immunocompetent persons. Booster doses are recommended for hemodialysis patients who lose protective levels of anti-HBs after vaccination, and a booster in the early teens (before sexual exposure) is worth considering for those vaccinated in childhood.

Reducing the spread of hepatitis B has been aided by screening *blood donors* for HBsAg. The person discovered to be an *asymptomatic carrier* requires attention. If the person is a health care worker who is free of symptoms and has normal liver function tests, he or she need not be removed from work unless proven to be a source of infection. However, health care workers and professionals with HBeAg who perform "exposure-prone" invasive procedures are advised to have their privileges evaluated by an expert review panel. Liver function and HBsAg status should be evaluated every 4 to 6 months to monitor for active disease. *Food handlers* have not been implicated in the transmission of hepatitis B and, when HBsAg-positive, they need not be restricted. However, during acute hepatitis with symptoms, for their own comfort, they should be advised to refrain from work like anyone else with acute hepatitis B.

Risk of exposure to HBsAg ceases when antigen disappears from the bloodstream; this is usually within 6 to 8 weeks of infection. Repeat serum determinations of HBsAg can help define when precautions may be relaxed.

Hepatitis D (Delta Hepatitis). Prevention of delta hepatitis in persons susceptible to HBV infection can be achieved by administering hepatitis B vaccine. Once immune to HBV, a person is immune to hepatitis D as well. For HBsAg carriers, there is no effective immunoprophylaxis against infection with the delta agent. For them, prevention of delta hepatitis requires limitation of percutaneous and intimate contacts with patients known to be infected with hepatitis D.

Hepatitis C. The incidence of posttransfusion hepatitis C has been dramatically reduced by excluding commercially donated blood and persons at high risk of transmitting blood-borne disease as well as by screening prospective donors for evidence of HCV infection (eg, presence of anti-HCV, elevated aminotransferase). Immune globulin and HBIG are of no proven benefit in preventing transfusion-associated hepatitis C. However, some authorities recommend a single IG injection for needlestick, sexual, or perinatal exposure to hepatitis C, although efficacy has never been demonstrated and the anti-HCV in IG is not neutralizing. There is no vaccine for hepatitis C, and the acquisition of neutralizing antibody after naturally acquired hepatitis C is considered rare. Still, efforts to develop a protective vaccine based on immunization with envelope proteins is being pursued.

Hepatitis E. Immunoprophylaxis for hepatitis E is not available. Whether globulins prepared in developed countries where hepatitis E is rare protect against HEV infection in Asia and other parts of the world where hepatitis E is common is not known.

RECOMMENDATIONS AND PATIENT EDUCATION

Hepatitis A Precautions (To Be Continued Until a Week After the Onset of Jaundice)

- Advise the patient to wash hands thoroughly after use of the toilet.
- The patient need not be confined to home, but intimate contact should be avoided.
- Prohibit the patient from handling and serving food to others.
- Advise others to avoid contact with the patient's fecal material and to wash hands thoroughly if contact is made.

Hepatitis A Prophylaxis

- Administer IG to household contacts within 2 weeks of exposure: the dosage is 0.02 mL per kilogram; average adult dosage is 2 mL intramuscularly.
- Administer IG for contacts in an epidemic and for travelers to areas in which hepatitis A is endemic; the dose is the same as for household contacts, unless travel is prolonged; then the dose should be 0.06 mL per kilogram every 4 to 6 months.

Hepatitis B Precautions (To Be Continued Until HBsAg Clears from the Serum)

- All blood donors should be screened for HBsAg.
- Use volunteer blood, rather than blood from commercial donors.
- Preferentially use disposable syringes and needles.
- Have patient use separate razor, toothbrush, and other personal items.
- Have any materials containing HBsAg handled carefully, particularly blood samples and other bodily fluids; use of gloves is required. Following universal precautions when handling clinical materials makes additional precautions unnecessary.
- Recommend avoidance of intimate contact, but confinement to home is unnecessary.
- Hands should be washed thoroughly after direct contact with the patient or with the patient's blood or body fluids.

Hepatitis B Prophylaxis

Preexposure.

- Administer three 1-mL (0.5-mL for those under age 10) intramuscular injections of hepatitis B vaccine at 0, 1, and 6 months to persons in high-risk groups. (Doses may vary according to manufacturer.) High-risk groups include health workers exposed to blood, residents and staff of custodial institutions, household and sexual contacts of chronic HBsAg carriers, promiscuous male homosexuals and promiscuous heterosexuals, patients with hereditary hemoglobinopathies and clotting disorders who require long-term therapy with blood products, and hemodialysis patients.

Postexposure.

- Administer HBIG intramuscularly, 0.06 mL per kilogram of body weight (approximately 5 mL), to those who sustain an accidental percutaneous or transmucosal exposure with HBsAg-positive blood or body secretions or needles/instruments contaminated with HBsAg-positive material. This globulin injection should be administered as soon after exposure as possible; although globulin injections are recommended up to 7 days after inoculation, their efficacy is nil beyond 2 days. Passive immunoprophylaxis with HBIG should be followed by a complete three-injection course of hepatitis B vaccine; these injections can be started at the same time as HBIG or within the first few days to a week after exposure.
- Administer HBIG, at the dose cited above, to sexual contacts of patients with *acute* hepatitis B as soon after exposure as is practical. Because recognition of hepatitis in a sexual contact is often delayed, early prophylaxis is usually impossible. In one study, prophylaxis within 30 days of recognized exposure was effective, but current recommendations call for prophylaxis within 14 days of exposure. HBIG should be followed by a complete three-injection course of hepatitis B vaccine in all sexual contacts of patients with acute hepatitis B.
- Administer 0.5 mL of HBIG intramuscularly to newborns of HBsAg-positive mothers immediately after birth, preferably in the delivery room. This should be followed by a complete three-injection course of hepatitis B vaccine, 0.5 mL per dose, preferably to be started within 7 days of birth (Dose may vary according to manufacturer).
- No prophylaxis is necessary for casual contacts or nonintimate household contacts.
- Universal vaccination of all children shortly after birth is now recommended.

Hepatitis D Prophylaxis

- Vaccination against hepatitis B prevents hepatitis D in those susceptible to hepatitis B.
- For those already infected with hepatitis B, prevention of hepatitis D relies on limiting percutaneous and intimate contact with persons known to harbor hepatitis D virus (HDV) infection.

Hepatitis C Precautions and Prophylaxis

- Precautions are the same as those for hepatitis B (ie, limitation of exposure to infected patients' blood and body fluids).
- The best means of limiting transfusion-associated hepatitis C is to rely exclusively on volunteer rather than commercial blood donors and to screen donors for anti-HCV.
- Although immune globulin has not been shown to be effective in preventing transfusion-related hepatitis C, some authorities recommend that IG be administered for exposures in which the inoculum size is much smaller than in transfusion settings (ie, to those who sustain a needlestick, to sexual contacts of acute cases of hepatitis C, and to babies born to mothers with hepatitis C). A single 0.06 mL/kg (0.5-mL for newborns) has been suggested.

ANNOTATED BIBLIOGRAPHY

Aach RD, Stevens CE, Hollinger FB, et al. Hepatitis C virus infection in post-transfusion hepatitis: An analysis with first- and second-generation assays. N Engl J Med 1991;325:1325. *(When second-generation assays are used, the frequency of hepatitis C in blood recipients can be reduced to levels indistinguishable from those observed in nontransfused controls.)*

Alter MJ, Hadler SC, Margolies HS, et al. The changing epidemiology of hepatitis B in the United States: Need for alternative vaccination strategies. JAMA 1990;263:1218. *(Argument for a policy of universal hepatitis B vaccination in childhood.)*

Alter MJ, Margolies HS, Krawczynski K, et al. The natural history of community-acquired hepatitis C in the United States. N Engl J Med 1992;327:1899. *(Confirms the high frequency of hepatitis C, even in persons acquiring their acute infections sporadically; persistent asymptomatic viremia was universal, even in those who recovered clinically.)*

Bloom BS, Hillman AL, Fendrick AM, et al. A reappraisal of hepatitis B virus vaccination strategies using cost-effectiveness analysis. Ann Intern Med 1993;118:298. *(Most cost-effective is screening newborns and routine administration to 10-year-olds.)*

Centers for Disease Control. Protection against viral hepatitis: Recommendations of the Immunization Practices Advisory Committee (ACIP). MMWR 1990;39:1. *(Official recommendations of the U.S. Public Health Service for use of hepatitis B vaccine and HBIG for pre- and postexposure prophylaxis.)*

Dienstag JL. Non-A, non-B hepatitis. I. Recognition, epidemiology, and clinical features; II. Experimental transmission, putative virus agents and markers, and prevention. Gastroenterology 1983;85:439,743. *(Two-part review compiled before discovery of hepatitis C; many of the concepts noted in the review were confirmed with isolation of the hepatitis C virus.)*

Donahue JG, Munoz A, Ness PM, et al. The declining risk of post-transfusion hepatitis C virus infection. N Engl J Med 1992; 327:369. *(Frequency reduced to 0.57 percent per patient and 0.03 percent per unit of blood with testing for hepatitis C.)*

Genesca L, Esteban JI, Alter HJ, et al. Blood-borne non-A, non-B hepatitis: Hepatitis C. Semin Liver Dis 1991;11:147. *(Detailed review of new information since discovery of the virus in 1988.)*

Hadler SC, Francis DP, Maynard JE, et al. Long-term immunogenicity and efficacy of hepatitis B vaccine in homosexual men. N Engl J Med 1986;315:209. *(Detectable anti-HBs per-*

sisted for 5 years in 85 percent of patients, with levels considered protective persisting in 63 percent of patients; clinically apparent and chronic infection rarely, if ever, occurred.)

Hoofnagle JH. Type D (delta) hepatitis. JAMA 1989;261:1321. *(Brief, but authoritative review.)*

Hoofnagle JH, Di Bisceglie AM. Serologic diagnosis of acute and chronic viral hepatitis. Semin Liver Dis 1991;11:73. *(Reviews serologic and virologic events useful for diagnosis of viral hepatitis types A, B, C, and D.)*

Houghton M, Weiner A, Han J, et al. Molecular biology of the hepatitis C viruses: Implications for diagnosis, development, and control of viral disease. Hepatology 1991;14:381. *(Review by the discoverer of the virus.)*

Katkov WN, Dienstag JL. Prevention and therapy of viral hepatitis. Semin Liver Disease 1991;11:165. *(Review addressing key issues related to hepatitis B vaccine, with brief consideration of hepatitis A vaccine.)*

Koretz RL, Abbey H, Coleman E, et al. Non-A, non-B posttransfusion hepatitis: Looking back in the second decade. Ann Intern Med 1993;119:110. *(A long-term follow-up study.)*

Krawczynski K. Hepatitis E. Hepatology 1993;17:932. *(Authoritative review.)*

Krugman S, Giles J. Viral hepatitis: New light on an old disease. JAMA 1970;212:1019. *(Classic paper on natural history of hepatitis A and B and efficacy of gamma-globulin for prevention of hepatitis A.)*

Lemon SM. Type A viral hepatitis: New developments in an old disease. N Engl J Med 1985;313:1059. *(Excellent review.)*

McMahon BJ, Helminiak C, Wainwright RB, et al. Frequency of adverse reactions to hepatitis B vaccine in 43,618 persons. Am J Med 1992;92:254. *(This survey adds to the overwhelming evidence of the vaccine's safety.)*

Mulley AG, Silverstein MD, Dienstag JL. Indications for use of hepatitis B vaccine, based on cost-effectiveness analysis. N Engl J Med 1982;307:644. *(Hepatitis B vaccine, despite its high cost, actually saves medical care costs if administered to population groups with a sufficiently high risk of infection.)*

Seeff L, Buskell-Bales Z, Wright EC, et al. Long-term mortality after transfusion-associated non-A, non-B hepatitis. N Engl J Med 1992;327:1906. *(Mortality did not exceed that in control groups of transfused patients who did not develop hepatitis.)*

Szmuness W, Stevens CE, Harley EJ, et al. Hepatitis B vaccine: Demonstration of efficacy in a controlled clinical trial in a high-risk population in the United States. N Engl J Med 1980;303:833. *(Classic paper describing the landmark controlled trial of hepatitis B vaccine in homosexual men, establishing the safety and efficacy of the vaccine in preventing clinical and subclinical cases of hepatitis B.)*

Werzberger A, Mensch B, Kuter B, et al. A controlled trial of formalin-inactivated hepatitis vaccine in healthy children. N Engl J Med 1992;327:453. *(The vaccine was 100 percent effective in preventing clinically apparent disease.)*

Primary Care Medicine: Office Evaluation and Management of the Adult Patient, 3rd edition, edited by Allan H. Goroll, Lawrence A. May, and Albert G. Mulley, Jr. J.B. Lippincott Company, Philadelphia

58
Evaluation of Abdominal Pain

JAMES M. RICHTER, M.D.

One of the most challenging problems faced by the primary physician is the outpatient assessment of the patient with abdominal pain. When the pain is acute in onset, triage decisions have to be made regarding the need for hospital admission and surgical intervention. If the pain is chronic or recurrent, the physician must design a safe, cost-effective plan for workup that will efficiently distinguish among a myriad of possible etiologies. In many instances, the exact cause of pain is not immediately evident, necessitating a few basic studies to better define the underlying pathophysiology, narrow the differential diagnosis, and effectively guide further assessment and treatment. Also important is the need to decide on the proper speed and extent of evaluation.

PATHOPHYSIOLOGY AND CLINICAL PRESENTATION

The major mechanisms of abdominal pain include obstruction of a hollow viscus, peritoneal irritation, vascular insufficiency, mucosal ulceration, altered bowel motility, capsular distention, metabolic imbalance, nerve injury, abdominal wall injury, and referral from an extraabdominal site.

Clinical presentations of abdominal pain are determined, in part, by the site of involvement. Although generalizations concerning the location of pain are crude, a few are clinically useful. Lower esophageal pain is usually subxyphoid or substernal but may be referred to the back. Gastric and duodenal disease produces epigastric discomfort, which sometimes radiates into the back. Pain from the small bowel is usually periumbilical but likely to occur in the right lower quadrant when the terminal ileum is involved. Most colonic pain is felt in the lower abdomen, particularly the left lower quadrant; with rectosigmoid problems, referral may be to the sacrum. Disease of the transverse colon may give upper abdominal or even periumbilical discomfort. Gallbladder and common bile duct obstruction result in epigastric or right upper quadrant complaints, with characteristic radiation to the scapular region. Pancreatic pain is usually epigastric or midline, with radiation into the back. Diffuse pain is seen with generalized peritonitis, metabolic disturbances, and psychogenic illness, although all may produce focal complaints.

Obstruction. Pain receptors in the bowel, biliary tree, and ureters respond to distention and increased wall tension. The severity of the pain is a function of the speed of onset as well as the degree of distention. Obstruction that develops slowly over weeks to months may be relatively subtle in presentation, compared with the more dramatic picture produced by acute obstruction. In acute obstruction, the pain is severe and "colicky" or wavelike in nature; it makes the patient restless. The pain of acute *small bowel* obstruction is greatest when the obstruction is jejunal. The patient is often comfortable between bouts of pain. Severity decreases with time as bowel motility diminishes. Complete strangulation of small bowel is associated with steady pain from secondary vascular insufficiency or peritoneal irritation. Vomiting is common, particularly in proximal obstruction; when the problem is distal, vomiting is less frequent. Flatus and passage of small amounts of stool may occur at the outset, but they soon cease if the obstruction is complete. Diarrhea is noted in some cases of partial obstruction. On examination, the patient appears restless during bouts of pain. The temperature is typically normal or only mildly elevated. The abdomen may be distended, especially when the obstruction is distal. High-pitched, hyperactive bowel sounds are characteristic, but not always present. Tenderness to palpation is not impressive, unless ischemia or leakage of bowel contents has occurred and caused peritoneal soilage. The stool is usually negative for occult blood.

Large bowel obstruction is, in most instances, less painful and associated with less vomiting than is obstruction of the small intestine. Constipation or change in bowel habits often precedes complete obstruction. Diarrhea may occur with partial obstruction. Distention is greater than that seen in small bowel obstruction. Stools are frequently positive for occult blood, because malignancy and diverticular disease are common etiologies.

In cases of bowel obstruction, the white blood cell count may be normal, even in association with a strangulating obstruction (ie, with compromise of the intestinal blood supply in addition to blockage of the lumen). A plain radiograph of the abdomen (supine and upright) in patients with small bowel obstruction often shows distention of loops of small bowel with high air–fluid levels. This, together with an absence of gas in the large bowel (distal to the obstruction) is characteristic of small bowel obstruction. The radiographic appearance of colonic obstruction varies with the competency (or incompetency) of the ileocecal valve. If the valve is competent, less small bowel dilatation ensues.

Sudden *obstruction* of the *cystic duct* by a stone produces acute pain, sometimes referred to as biliary "colic." Obstruction and dilatation that occur gradually are often painless. Unlike the cramping pain of acute intestinal obstruction, the pain of acute cystic duct obstruction is mostly steady, lasting over an hour after sudden onset. In *acute cholecystitis,* the typical pain is maximal in the right upper quadrant or epigastrium, radiating to the scapular region, accompanied by nausea, vomiting, and fever without jaundice; at times there is only mild epigastric discomfort (see Chapter 69). *Murphy's sign* (inspiratory arrest in response to right upper quadrant palpation) may be seen, and right upper quadrant tenderness to percussion or pressure over the gallbladder is also a suggestive finding. Laboratory investigation usually reveals a leukocytosis and sometimes a modest alkaline phosphatase elevation. In an occasional case, slight hyperbilirubinemia may occur, usually after the initial onset of symptoms.

In *common duct obstruction,* the pain is more likely to be epigastric and less severe. Jaundice is noted soon after onset. Emesis may be prominent. Physical examination reveals a tender right upper quadrant, but, compared with acute cholecystitis, tenderness is less focal and deeper. A palpable gallbladder suggests gradual progressive development of ductal obstruction, typical of that due to malignancy. Alkaline phosphatase is markedly elevated as is the serum bilirubin.

Obstruction within the *urinary tract* can present as abdominal pain. Acute ureteral blockade by a stone is extremely uncomfortable. Onset is sudden and the pain is cramping, beginning in the back and flank and radiating into the lower abdomen and groin. If acute pyelonephritis develops, upper abdominal pain, fever, and chills may ensue. Acute bladder outflow obstruction presents as lower abdominal distention and suprapubic pain. Symptoms of prostatism (see Chapter 134) may precede the episode.

Peritoneal irritation may cause severe pain, because of the rich innervation of the parietal peritoneum. Focal injury results in well-localized discomfort that is described as sharp, aching, or burning. Spread of the irritant process leads to more generalized abdominal pain. Severity is related to the nature of the irritant and the speed at which the noxious exposure occurs. There can be reflex spasm of the overlying abdominal wall musculature, producing involuntary guarding. Rebound tenderness is prominent on physical examination. Most important, the pain is accentuated by pressure changes in the peritoneum, thus, palpation, coughing, or movement may increase the pain, leading the patient to lie still, in contrast to the restlessness of patients with "colicky" pain. Focal peritonitis of the retroperitoneum, which is characteristic of *early appendicitis,* may be tested by having the patient lie on the left side and extend the right hip (*psoas sign*). Bowel sounds are often reduced or absent, especially when the irritation is generalized. The origin of the peritoneal irritant need not be intraabdominal.

Familial Mediterranean fever (FMF) is an autosomal recessive disorder that causes recurrent, severe attacks of peritoneal irritation. The condition occurs among Armenians and Sephardic Jews and presents in childhood or early adulthood. It is characterized by brief, but severe attacks of fever, peritoneal irritation, pleuritis, and synovitis. Patients complain of abdominal swelling and severe pain. Marked elevations in the sedimentation rate and acute phase reactants accompany attacks. Amyloidosis is a serious consequence, sometimes resulting in renal impairment. Colchicine provides dramatic relief from the pain of an acute attack and also prevents amyloid deposition and renal impairment.

Vascular disorders such as acute *arterial insufficiency* (due to atherosclerosis or embolus) may present with severe abdominal pain, although mild, constant pain may be the only symptom for several days. The pain of mesenteric arterial insufficiency may occur in the absence of tenderness and rigidity, and the diagnosis is not necessarily considered until signs of peritonitis and shock from peritoneal soilage ensue. *Dissection* or rupture of an abdominal aortic aneurysm produces severe acute abdominal pain that often radiates to the back or genitalia. *Mesenteric venous thrombosis* is a less common cause of intestinal ischemia than arterial occlusion. It may present similarly, although it often has a more slowly progressive course. Both aortic dissection and mesenteric thrombosis typically result in pain complaints that are in excess of those elicited by physical examination.

Chronic arterial insufficiency may precede an acute episode of infarction, especially in cases of progressive atherosclerotic narrowing. The patient complains of episodes of cramping or dull midabdominal pain that come on 15 to 30 minutes after a meal and can last up to 2 or 3 hours. This so-called *abdominal angina* is greatest at times of maximal demand for blood supply to the bowel (eg, after a large meal). Some patients lose considerable amounts of weight because of the fear that eating will induce pain. Ischemic, abdominal pain also results from vascular occlusive crises of sickle cell anemia.

Mucosal ulceration or inflammation of the gastrointestinal (GI) tract is often accompanied by pain. Although the exact mechanism of pain in *peptic ulcer disease* remains incompletely understood, it is believed that acid plays a major role. This hypothesis is supported by the observation that neutralization of acid often provides immediate relief. Pain pattern of duodenal ulcer disease usually parallels the acid-peptic cycle (see Chapter 68). Unless there is perforation or penetration into the pancreas, the pain is mostly confined to the epigastrium. Patients use such terms as "gnawing," "aching," and "burning" to describe their discomfort. Radiation of pain into the back in patients with duodenal ulcer suggests perforation into the pancreas.

Inflammation of the mid or lower intestine, as seen with acute *gastroenteritis* and acute flares of *inflammatory bowel disease* (see Chapter 73), can disturb motility and absorption. In most instances, the pain is diffuse, but occasionally it is focal and can simulate appendicitis or other surgical conditions. Fever, nausea, and vomiting are often prominent in the early stages of gastroenteritis; bowel sounds are usually hyperactive.

Altered Bowel Motility. This mechanism predominates in functional bowel disturbances, of which *irritable bowel syndrome* is the best example. Spasmodic, nonpropulsive segmental contractions of large bowel result in high intraluminal pressures manifested by cramping lower abdominal pain. Constipation alternating with diarrhea and mucous stools are typical findings, as are pain relieved by defecation, more frequent and loose stools with the onset of pain, and a feeling of incomplete evacuation (see Chapter 73). Psychiatric disturbances, especially *anxiety* and *mood disorders,* are common in persons with irritable bowel syndrome who seek medical attention. Symptoms may arise from any area of the intestinal tract—esophagus, stomach, small intestine, and biliary tree, as well as the colon. The result is a broad spectrum of presentations that includes nausea, vomiting, dyspepsia, and flatulence, as well as cramping abdominal pain. Altered motility and chronically increased intraluminal pressures may lead to *diverticular disease* (see Chapter 75).

Intestinal pseudoobstruction refers to a syndrome in which the clinical features of intestinal obstruction are found in the absence of a lesion, causing mechanical obstruction of the lumen. It may be chronic, with recurrence or persistence of symptoms, or it may occur acutely (so-called acute ileus). Symptoms can include vomiting and abdominal distention; diarrhea or constipation may also be seen. Plain films of the abdomen demonstrate intestinal dilatation, suggesting partial obstruction. It is noteworthy that the syndrome of chronic pseudoobstruction may precede the recognition of associated systemic diseases by many years (see below).

The causes of *acute ileus* include peritonitis (resulting from a variety of causes), systemic infections, ischemic bowel injury, abdominal operations (a common etiology), abdominal trauma, pharmacologic agents (especially anticholinergics and narcotics), and metabolic disturbances (particularly hypokalemia).

Chronic intestinal pseudoobstruction is often idiopathic, although it may occur in the setting of scleroderma, Parkinson's disease, drug use (opiates, phenothiazines, tricyclic antidepressants, or antiparkinsonian medications), hypercalcemia, diabetes, myxedema, amyloidosis, radiation enteritis, and chronic laxative abuse.

Capsular Distention. Distention of the well-innervated capsule surrounding an organ can be another source of constant, *aching* abdominal pain. *Hepatic* capsular distention may result from hepatic swelling secondary to hepatitis, congestive heart failure, fatty infiltration, or subcapsular hematoma and may result in right upper quadrant pain. The pain of *splenic* capsular distention, as may occur secondary to blunt trauma, from an auto accident, is located in the left upper quadrant. With subdiaphragmatic peritoneal irritation, the patient may experience pain radiating to the ipsilateral shoulder. With splenic trauma, there can be a deceptive period of many hours before peritoneal signs develop if a subcapsular hematoma temporarily retards the spilling of blood into the peritoneum.

Metabolic disturbances may mimic intraabdominal etiologies. *Porphyria* and *lead poisoning* sometimes simulate bowel obstruction, because they can cause cramping abdominal pain and hyperperistalsis. *Acute intermittent porphyria (AIP)* presents with moderate to severe colicky abdominal pain, which may be localized or generalized. Abdominal symptoms may be the result of intestinal dysmotility; vomiting and diarrhea are also common complaints. Fever and leukocytosis may be present but on examination the abdomen is found to be soft. Proximal muscle pain and a range of neuropsychiatric symptoms accompany the abdominal pain. The clinical features of *hereditary coproporphyria* and *variegate porphyria* are similar to those described for AIP; skin lesions may be prominent. A Watson-Schwartz test for urinary porphobilinogen may suggest the diagnosis of an acute attack in all three of these entities.

Lead poisoning may also present with abdominal pain. Such pain is typically wandering, poorly localized, colicky, and accompanied by a rigid abdomen. Encephalopathy, peripheral neuropathy, and anemia are associated features. The *urine coproporphyrin* test is a more reliable indicator of this entity than is a serum lead level, which can be normal.

Ketoacidosis has been found to present with severe abdominal pain in 8 percent of instances and may be accompanied by emesis and an elevated white cell count. These symptoms are due, at least in part, to gastroparesis, which may occur in ketoacidosis. However, it should be remembered that acute intraabdominal events such as cholecystitis may be the precipitants of ketoacidosis.

C'1 esterase inhibitor deficiency may result in episodic *angioneurotic edema* and severe abdominal pain. If this diagnosis is suspected, it is useful to check the serum level of C4, which is low in C'1 esterase inhibitor deficiency.

Nerve injury from encroachment or irritation is an important mechanism of abdominal pain. The source of pain may be intraabdominal, as occurs when a pancreatic cancer invades adjacent splanchnic nerves, or it may be extraabdominal, as in herpes zoster irritating a nerve root that supplies an abdominal wall dermatome. Abdominal pain occurs in about 75 percent of patients with *cancer of the pancreas;* it is usually epigastric and most common in patients with tumor involving the body or tail of the pancreas. Sometimes the pain radiates to the back or is confined to it. Pancreatic malignancy also causes pain by other mechanisms, including obstruction of the common or pancreatic duct. Nerve root irritation from *herpes zoster* may be mistaken for an intraabdominal process, especially before the rash appears. Often, the patient complains of a severe lancinating pain resembling an intraabdominal source. There may be associated rectus muscle spasm simulating peritonitis, but, unlike peritoneal irritation, there is no effect on bowel function and palpation may actually alleviate the rectus muscle spasm. The pain of herpes infection often precedes the rash by several days and may persist after the skin clears, particularly in the elderly (see Chapter 192).

Abdominal wall pathology can also be mistaken for disease inside the abdominal cavity. Traumatic injury to the musculature of the wall produces pain that is constant, aching, and exacerbated by movement or pressure on the abdomen. The muscles may be in spasm, simulating the involuntary guarding of peritonitis. When a generalized myositis is responsible for the muscle pain, discomfort occurs in the limbs as well as in the abdomen. Occasionally, a tender mass in the wall, such as a rectus sheath hematoma, is found to be the source of difficulty.

Referred pain from a process originating in the chest is sometimes an etiology of abdominal complaints. Pulmonary infarction and pneumonia of the lower lobes are among the chest problems that may present as pain in the upper abdomen; at times reflex muscle spasm even accompanies the pain. Upper abdominal pain, nausea, and vomiting may be the principal manifestations of an acute inferior myocardial infarction. Fortunately, most intrathoracic sources of abdominal pain are accompanied by symptoms and signs of cardiac or pulmonary disease.

DIFFERENTIAL DIAGNOSIS

Because the number of possible causes of abdominal pain is large, it is helpful to consider the differential diagnosis in terms of pathophysiologic mechanisms (Table 58–1). Etiologies causing obstruction, peritoneal irritation, and vascular insufficiency are among the most dangerous. About 70 percent of mechanical small bowel obstruction is due to adhesions or external hernias; 90 percent of large bowel obstruction is attributable to diverticular disease and carcinoma. Acute arterial insufficiency results most often from systemic embolization due to atrial fibrillation, severe atherosclerotic occlusive disease, and hypoperfusional states. Pelvic pathology is a common extraabdominal source of peritoneal irritation.

Table 58-1. Principle Mechanisms of Abdominal Pain

Obstruction	**Altered Motility**
1. Gastric outlet	1. Gastroenteritis
2. Small bowel	2. Inflammatory bowel disease
3. Large bowel	3. Irritable bowel syndrome
4. Biliary tract	4. Diverticular disease
5. Urinary tract	
Peritoneal Irritation	**Metabolic Disturbance**
1. Infection	1. Diabetic ketoacidosis
2. Chemical irritation (blood, bile, gastric acid)	2. Porphyria
3. Systemic inflammatory process	3. Lead poisoning
4. Spread from a local inflammatory process	**Nerve Injury**
	1. Herpes zoster
	2. Root compression
	3. Nerve invasion
Vascular Insufficiency	**Muscle Wall Disease**
1. Embolization	1. Trauma
2. Atherosclerotic narrowing	2. Myositis
3. Hypotension	3. Hematoma
4. Aortic aneurysm dissection	
Mucosal Ulceration	**Referred Pain**
1. Peptic ulcer disease	1. Pneumonia (lower lobes)
2. Gastric cancer	2. Inferior myocardial infarction
	3. Pulmonary infarction
	Psychopathology
	1. Depression
	2. Anxiety
	3. Neuroses

Other pathophysiologic mechanisms, such as nerve injury, metabolic imbalance, abdominal wall disease, and disordered motility may produce symptoms that superficially mimic a more worrisome etiology; but usually conditions associated with these mechanisms are more annoying than dangerous (an important exception is diabetic ketoacidosis). Pain referred from an extraabdominal site is more of a problem; significant cardiac disease (eg, inferior myocardial infarction) or pulmonary pathology (eg, lower lobe pneumonia) may present as abdominal pain.

WORKUP

The first priority in the office evaluation of the patient with abdominal pain is to determine the likelihood of serious pathophysiology and the pace and extent of workup. Patients with acute pain need to be examined promptly for evidence of obstruction, peritoneal irritation, vascular compromise, and cardiopulmonary disease. The evaluation of chronic pain can be assessed at a more gradual pace, allowing time to get to know the patient and his or her problem before rushing into extensive testing.

History should include a complete description of the pain including localization, characterization, area of referral, time course of onset and resolution, and precipitating and alleviating factors. The chronologic sequence of symptom occurrence should be clearly outlined.

In addition to carefully obtaining a complete description of the patient's pain, checking for specific items is needed: prior abdominal surgery, previous episodes of obstruction, known gallbladder or kidney stones, presence and nature of vomitus, passage of flatus, time of last bowel movement, occurrence of diarrhea, constipation or change in bowel habits, effect of movement on pain, presence of fever and rigors, development of distention, difficulties in urination, and presence of any cardiac or pulmonary symptoms. Inquiry into pregnancy and symptoms of pelvic pathology, such as dyspareunia, abnormal vaginal discharge, and irregular menstrual bleeding, should be included in the assessment of every woman with abdominal pain.

Frequently confounding variables in the assessment are the patient's perception of and response to the pain. Substantial variation in pain perception, as well as communication, may be due to factors other than the pain itself. Patients display widely varying tolerances to pain, yet the physician must learn to interpret accurately the "true" quality and quantity of the patient's experience. Psychological and ethnic factors alter expression and response to pain and must be taken into consideration, especially in cases of chronic abdominal pain. A thorough psychosocial history is essential in the context of eliciting the pain complaint and determining its effect on daily living. Exploring patient fears, concerns, and expectations is critical to understanding the patient, designing an effective treatment plan, and communicating a sense of caring and understanding.

Physical Examination. Particular attention ought to be paid to the patient's *general appearance*. The patient who appears reluctant to change position and keeps still is likely to have peritoneal irritation, whereas the patient with obstruction is often restless. It is important to check the *vital signs* for postural changes in blood pressure or heart rate, because obstruction, peritonitis, and bowel infarction can produce large losses of intravascular volume. Any hypotension, atrial fibrillation, or fever should be noted; however, absence of fever does not rule out serious pathology, especially in the elderly or chronically ill patient. The *skin* is examined for jaundice, other stigmata of chronic liver disease, clubbing or spooning of the fingernails, signs of trauma, excoriations, prior surgical scars, evidence of dehydration, edema, or dermatomal rash. In addition, the sclerae are noted for icterus. The *chest* is checked for splinting, a pleural friction rub, and signs of consolidation (particularly in the lower lobes), and the *heart* is checked for murmurs, chamber enlargement, and signs of heart failure (see Chapter 32).

The *abdominal examination* should be performed with care to avoid unnecessary discomfort. A sharp increase in pain with coughing demonstrates rebound tenderness without the need for palpation and release. Examination of the abdomen includes checking for the presence of distention, altered bowel sounds (increase or absence), a hepatic rub or a vascular bruit, tenderness, guarding, rebound, hepatosplenomegaly, and masses (including a dilated aorta, loops of bowel, stool, or a distended bladder or uterus). An increased abdominal venous pattern suggests portal hypertension; periumbilical adenopathy suggests pancreatic cancer.

Pelvic and rectal examinations are essential parts of the evaluation, checking for masses and tenderness. These examinations are certainly more revealing if done gently. The fecal occult blood test is also mandatory.

If psychogenic pain or a major degree of psychocultural overlay is suspected, deep palpation ought to be done while the patient is distracted. Distracting an anxious patient while gently performing deep palpation may be the best way to demonstrate a lack of tenderness. One method used is to push deeply while auscultating with a stethoscope in a patient who is anxious about palpation.

In an *elderly person* with no history of somatizing, the presence of significant abdominal pain out of proportion to tenderness subsequently elicited by physical examination suggests vascular compromise. The elderly person with an acute intraabdominal process may at first show few signs of serious illness. Peritoneal signs may be absent or minimal. The only early clues may be unexplained mild fever, tachycardia, and vague abdominal discomfort. A high index of suspicion is needed.

Examining for nerve and muscle wall injury is often overlooked in the urgency of searching for more worrisome pathology. Two important signs of nerve involvement are pain in a dermatomal distribution and hyperesthesia. Both occur with nerve injury due to herpes zoster or nerve root impingement; however, hyperesthesia is also seen with focal peritoneal irritation. Testing is performed by gentle stroking of the skin overlying the area of pain. The rash of herpes may not appear until the time of the follow-up assessment. Abdominal wall pathology may be discovered by careful palpation of the wall for masses and muscle tenderness and by exacerbation of pain on contracting the muscles, as occurs with sitting up. Any pain on sitting up should not be confused with that due to involuntary muscle spasm from peritoneal irritation. The limbs should also be checked for muscle tenderness, which is suggestive of a generalized muscle disorder.

Laboratory Tests. Relatively few laboratory tests are needed at the time of initial assessment. Studies are aimed at determining the likelihood of obstruction, peritonitis, acute vascular insufficiency, metabolic abnormality, and cardiac or pulmonary disease.

The Complete Blood Count (CBC) and Differential. These tests are often helpful in confirming the presence of an acute inflammatory process. Although very nonspecific, the CBC and differential are reasonably sensitive in patients able to mount a normal acute inflammatory response. Unfortunately, the CBC may show little change in the elderly or chronically ill patient, even in an acute intraabdominal emergency. The differential ought to be ordered even if the white cell count is "normal," because a shift to immature forms sometimes occurs without a significant elevation in the white count. At times a relatively benign condition such as viral gastroenteritis may produce an impressive elevation in the white cell count (as high as 20,000 cells per cubic centimeter) accompanied by a marked shift to immature forms, simulating the peripheral blood picture of a patient with more worrisome disease. The CBC and differential must be carefully interpreted in the context of the entire clinical picture and not used alone to decide whether to admit the patient.

Pregnancy Testing. Because of the seriousness of an ectopic pregnancy, every woman of reproductive age who presents with lower abdominal pain should be considered a candidate for pregnancy testing. A *serum HCG beta subunit* is the preferred test.

Plain films of the abdomen, supine and upright, are essential if one suspects bowel obstruction or perforation. Multiple (ie, three) air–fluid levels, distention of the small bowel, and absence of gas in the large bowel are characteristic of complete small bowel obstruction; unfortunately, such findings are present in fewer than 50 percent of cases of bowel strangulation, especially in the early stages of obstruction. Partial mechanical obstruction may produce some loops of bowel with air–fluid levels, but there is also gas in the colon; the same findings are found in patients with adynamic ileus. In colonic obstruction with a competent ileocecal valve, only the large bowel appears distended, but if the valve is not competent, both the large and small bowel demonstrate distention and gas, mimicking the findings of adynamic ileus. Distinguishing partial small bowel obstruction from ileus requires repeat films or a barium study. Suspected obstruction of the large bowel is an indication for a barium enema and is usually a contraindication to performing an upper GI series.

On the plain film, free air under the diaphragm indicates perforation of a viscus; absent psoas shadows suggest retroperitoneal bleeding, abscess, or mass; and displaced stomach or bowel (determined by gas patterns) may be caused by compression from a tumor. Plain films are also helpful in finding a biliary or renal stone, abdominal aortic calcification suggesting an aneurysm, or pancreatic calcification due to pancreatitis. Calcification has been found on plain film of the abdomen in over 60 percent of abdominal aneurysms. A cross-table lateral view best demonstrates the lesion.

Although useful, plain films of the abdomen are commonly overused in evaluating abdominal pain. Limiting this study to patients with moderate to severe tenderness or high clinical suspicion of bowel obstruction, urinary tract calculi, trauma, ischemia, or gallbladder disease (regardless of degree of tenderness) was found in a retrospective study to be capable of reducing utilization by more than 50 percent without any significant reduction in the rate of detecting clinically important pathology. Plain films were not useful for detecting unsuspected pathology, especially in patients with mild tenderness on examination.

Using plain films to "rule out" serious pathology is possible only for bowel obstruction and perforation, in which the sensitivity of the plain film approaches 100 percent. Sensitivity for detection of other conditions is much lower.

Other initial tests can aid the evaluation. A *urinalysis* should be checked for pyuria, hematuria, bacteria, sugar, and ketones. Mild to moderate ketonuria is common when the patient has not eaten and is unrelated to diabetes; the diagnosis of ketoacidosis requires urine ketones in large concentrations (see Chapter 102). Red cells in the urine of a patient with flank pain suggest a stone in the ureter (see Chapter 135).

The *BUN, glucose electrolytes,* and *amylase* levels should be measured. Elevation of the serum amylase occurs not only in pancreatitis, but also in intestinal obstruction, perforated ulcer, and biliary tract disease; additional information is needed to identify the source of the elevation (see Chapter 72). Although not especially specific, the serum amylase is sensitive.

Serum electrolytes can be helpful in cases of vomiting, diarrhea, or adynamic ileus; tests of renal and liver function, and blood sugar should also be determined when clinical findings are suggestive.

The initial investigation of acute upper abdominal pain should also include a *chest film* and *electrocardiogram,* looking for pleuropulmonary disease in the lower lobes and acute ischemic changes in the inferior myocardium. In patients with diarrhea, a microscopic *examination of the stool* for polymorphonuclear leukocytes is indicated (see Chapter 64).

In patients with ascites or those who have sustained abdominal trauma, an abdominal *paracentesis* with a small needle can add valuable information (see Chapter 71). This procedure should be performed in the lower abdomen where there is less chance of perforating a viscus or a large blood vessel. Nontympanitic areas of the right lower quadrant, left lower quadrant, or the linea alba (midline) are the usual sites.

The patient with acute colicky pain but no signs of obstruction or inflammation may have lead poisoning and should have urine samples checked for *coproporphyrin.* Serum lead levels are unreliable. The person with acute intermittent porphyria may also present with colicky pain. Often such individuals are thought to be psychiatrically disturbed because of abnormal behavior during an attack. The diagnosis is suggested by periodic attacks of cramping pain, constipation, nausea and vomiting, and neuromuscular symptoms in conjunction with the altered psychological state. The *Watson-Schwartz test* for *urinary porphobilinogen* is a reliable screening test for acute intermittent porphyria in patients who are symptomatic.

Once it is determined that acute obstruction, peritonitis, bowel ischemia, and worrisome metabolic and cardiopulmonary diseases are unlikely, further evaluation can be carried out on an outpatient basis, at a more gradual pace. Among the most productive diagnostic measures is repetition of the history and physical examination. Many serious etiologies may lead to a worsening of the clinical picture in a few days; this is particularly true for bowel ischemia, which initially may have an indolent presentation. Any patient sent home with undiagnosed acute pain requires careful follow-up and reexamination.

Radiologic Contrast Studies, Imaging, and Endoscopy. Selection ought to be judicious and based on the need to confirm or rule out specific diagnoses. Blind searches that involve "running the bowel" in the absence of suggestive clinical evidence are wasteful, potentially misleading, and uncomfortable for the patient. Recurrent epigastric or right upper quadrant pain in conjunction with an elevated alkaline phosphatase level is an indication for *ultrasonography* of the gallbladder and biliary tree (see Chapters 62 and 69).

Epigastric pain that parallels the acid-peptic cycle or responds to food or antacids suggests acid-peptic disease. There is little need for an *upper GI series* or *endoscopy* if the patient is under the age of 40 and the risk of gastric or esophageal malignancy is judged to be very low. Such patients can be safely treated for presumed ulcer disease without documenting the lesion. However, failure to respond to therapy or the presence of worrisome symptoms (melena, hematemesis, weight loss) necessitates a full evaluation, as does the occurrence of ulcer symptoms in older patients, who are at increased risk of gastric cancer (see Chapter 55).

Suspicion of small bowel pathology (suggested by periumbilical pain) is an indication for upper GI series with small-bowel follow-through. A lymphoma or carcinoid tumor may cause an intermittent partial obstruction.

All patients with lower abdominal pain and evidence of bleeding (be it gross or occult) should be evaluated by *colonoscopy* or the combination of *barium enema* and *sigmoidoscopy* to identify the source (see Chapter 63). However, the very young patient with constipation and obvious hemorrhoidal bleeding need undergo only a sigmoidoscopy to rule out associated rectosigmoid pathology. Sufferers of lower abdominal pain who have no bleeding, weight loss, or change in bowel habits are less likely to benefit from radiologic or endoscopic evaluation unless their symptoms are particularly severe or chronic.

At times, there is little clinical indication for a contrast study, but the patient insists on having an upper GI series or barium enema done to rule out a particular concern. The contribution of a normal test result to the peace of mind of the patient has to be taken into account when deciding which tests to obtain.

Sigmoidoscopy is a simple procedure with which much information about rectosigmoid masses or mucosal abnormalities can be obtained; it complements the barium enema. *Colonoscopy* may be useful, especially when hematochezia is prominent and cancer or colitis is a consideration. This study allows for biopsy of suspicious lesions, polypectomy, and assessment of the extent of disease in patients with inflammatory bowel disease.

The patient with flank pain, hematuria, or pyuria may have a renal source for their abdominal pain. An *intravenous pyelogram* may help in looking for disease in the kidneys or ureters or for displacement of a ureter by an abdominal or retroperitoneal mass. *Renal ultrasonography* can reveal a stone or ureteral dilatation. *Pelvic ultrasonography* is indicated when a uterine or ovarian mass is noted on bimanual examination.

Abdominal ultrasonography and computerized body tomography have come to play important roles in the evaluation of abdominal pain, making major contributions toward the noninvasive detection of pancreatic malignancy and other abdominal tumors. *Ultrasonography* has become the test of choice for diagnosis of gallstones (see Chapter 69) and useful for detection of biliary and ureteral obstructions (see Chapters 62 and 135, respectively). It can help identify ascites and sometimes localize intraabdominal abscesses. Ultrasonography has been instrumental in the detection of pancreatic tumors. The test's sensitivity for diagnosis of *pancreatic carcinoma* is reported to range from 65 percent to 85 percent. Specificity is a bit lower, but can be greatly enhanced by using ultrasound to guide *needle biopsy* of a suspicious lesion. Large amounts of bowel gas and fat limit the sensitivity of the ultrasonogram and result in a fraction of studies that are technically inadequate or indeterminate; however, its relatively low cost, its noninvasive nature, and the absence of radiation exposure make it an excellent screening test for detecting pancreatic disease.

Computed tomography (CT) has shown sensitivity and specificity similar to those of ultrasonography for detection of pancreatic cancer, but it has also shown a much lower rate of indeterminate readings (in one study, 4% versus 23%). CT is less dependent on the skill of the operator to yield a high-quality image than is ultrasonography, but it is more expensive and involves radiation exposure. In addition to imaging the pancreas, it provides excellent views of the liver, retroperitoneum, and spine. Both ultrasonography and CT visualize the common bile duct, portal vein, and hepatic artery and detect any displacement, encroachment, or encasement of the major intraabdominal vessels and organs.

Endoscopic retrograde cholangiopancreatography (ERCP) is more sensitive and more specific for detecting pancreatic cancer than ultrasonography, but success is very dependent on the skill of the endoscopist. Patients suspected of harboring a pancreatic malignancy should be screened with an ultrasound study. If the study is not technically adequate, then CT or ERCP should be ordered. If a mass is found, needle aspiration biopsy is usually needed to confirm a diagnosis of malignancy. Although much progress has been made in identifying a pancreatic mass in symptomatic patients, early detection in the asymptomatic period remains an elusive goal.

Evaluation of Undiagnosed Abdominal Pain. A most vexing problem arises when the cause of abdominal pain remains undetermined despite a careful medical evaluation. There may be pressure from patient and family to look still harder for a serious cause and a tendency, out of frustration, to order progressively more invasive studies in search of such an etiology. Certainly, further anatomic study is indicated in patients with a strongly positive family history of bowel malignancy (see Chapter 56), significant weight loss, presence of a mass, unexplained iron-deficiency anemia, or a stool test that is positive for occult blood. However, more often the cause of undiagnosed abdominal pain is an underlying *psychological disturbance* that leads to a chronic functional disturbance of bowel function.

Abnormal illness behaviors characterize patients with psychosocial problems that present as bodily complaints like abdominal pain (see Chapter 230). Such behaviors include an exaggerated presentation with disability out of proportion to the degree of detectable disease, chronic complaints that defy precise diagnosis, persistent attempts to validate suffering, excessive dependence on the physician and others for care, avoidance of health-promoting behaviors, and attempts to maintain the sick role. Other clinical features suggesting a psychologically dysfunctional state include a history of multiple bodily complaints, a nonprogressive clinical course that may span many years, lack of relation between symptoms and physiologic stimuli, inconsistent or distractible physical findings, and presence of somatic symptoms suggestive of depression (early morning awakening, fatigue, decreased libido, altered appetite).

Such behaviors and clinical features are likely to divert attention from the patient's psychosocial suffering and root causes unless recognized, understood, and responded to appropriately (see Chapters 226, 227, and 230). In the absence of worrisome objective findings, one should avoid relentless testing of these patients and concentrate more on their underlying psychosocial problems. This can be facilitated by soliciting the patient's perspective during the initial description of symptoms. Of particular importance is eliciting the patient's concerns, beliefs, and expectations. Also pertinent are data on the patient's daily functioning at work and at home, social supports, and psychological state. The abdominal pain may be only a symptom of psychosocial suffering. Although the patient, family, or friends may be pressing for a medical diagnosis, the real need is for care rather than a diagnostic label. The risk of a missed anatomic diagnosis is less than 3 percent when the initial evaluation is normal and evidence of abnormal illness behavior and clinical features of psychological disturbance are present.

While attending to the psychosocial nature of the problem, care must be taken to neither deny the reality of the patient's pain and suffering nor to emphasize the psychosocial nature of the problem any more than the patient is willing to accept. A careful and detailed history (with attention to the patient's perspective) plus a pertinent physical examination that addresses patient concerns along with simple screening laboratory tests should suffice. Patients with a clinical picture suggestive of functional disease may benefit from inquiry into psychosocial issues, such as concurrent stresses and losses and the effect of the pain on the patient's life and daily activities. However, to suggest at the outset that the problem is probably psychogenic before completing a careful evaluation that addresses patient concerns is to invite resistance and hostility. Requests for aggressive testing can be denied on the basis of available data as long as one responds in caring fashion with a plan for careful longitudinal follow-up and an attitude of open-mindedness. In this manner, a working partnership can be established rather than an adversarial relationship.

Sometimes a diagnostic trial of increased fiber is worth considering. A positive response can be informative. A tablespoon of psyllium in 8 oz of water or a bowl of bran cereal per day is a simple means of enhancing dietary fiber intake and may help ease symptoms. One should be aware that increasing milk intake through use of cereal increases lactose intake and may trigger symptoms of lactose intolerance in susceptible patients (see Chapter 64).

Psychiatric consultation is indicated when there is evidence of serious depression (see Chapter 227) or excessive somatization (see Chapter 230). In patients with neurotic complaints presenting with irritable bowel syndrome, thorough reassurance (which includes addressing patient concerns) delivered in sympathetic fashion can be most effective, especially when combined with a trial of increased dietary fiber. If low-grade depression is suspected, a course of *antidepressant therapy* may be warranted (if constipation is a problem, one should select an antidepressant with minimal anticholinergic effects; see Chapter 227). Such empirical approaches to patients with psychogenic abdominal pain may effect symptomatic relief without the need to resort immediately to formal psychotherapy.

The patient with chronic or recurrent abdominal pain that defies explanation poses one of the most difficult problems in clinical medicine. In a study of 30 such patients presenting to a general internist, most had epigastric pain, distention, belching, and nausea without vomiting or weight loss. Symptoms often began at the time of a personal loss or other emotional stress. Depression was commonly found. When treatment was directed at depression, the pain disappeared in many instances. In a study of 64 patients with abdominal pain of unknown etiology, two-thirds of the patients were women. The younger the age and shorter the duration of the symptoms, the better the chances were for improvement. Older women with pain for more than 3 months were least likely to improve or to be diagnosed. Of those subjected to laparotomy, a diagnosis was obtained in only 10 percent; the rate of improvement was the same as for those who did not undergo exploration. In 15 percent of the total study population, a cause for the patient's abdominal pain was found, but in only 6 percent did the condition require surgery. Thus, very few patients with abdominal pain of unknown etiology are endangered by continued observation, as long as signs of serious pathophysiology are absent. The morbidity of exploratory laparotomy in such patients greatly exceeds the benefit. Unexplained pain that is present for less than 2 weeks is likely to resolve spontaneously, but such improvement is unlikely when pain has persisted for more than 3 months.

INDICATIONS FOR ADMISSION AND REFERRAL

Any evidence suggestive of peritoneal irritation, obstruction, or acute vascular compromise is an indication for immediate hospitalization and surgical consultation. Sometimes further observations made in the hospital can save the patient a surgical procedure, but no patient with the possibility of a condition that might require urgent surgery should be sent home from the office. Elderly patients are especially prone to subtle presentations.

Where the diagnosis is unclear but urgent admission does not seem warranted, assiduous, close follow-up is mandatory. Repeated histories and examinations may yield the diagnosis and hence allow proper treatment. Such factors as the degree of distress manifested by the patient, the degree of temperature elevation, white blood count elevation or other laboratory abnormalities, and the ability of the patient to eat and drink all need to be assessed. Judgment also must be made as to whether a patient with undiagnosed abdominal pain should undergo more invasive testing. In general, patients with unexplained abdominal pain in conjunction with recurrent nausea and vomiting, jaundice, fever, weight loss of greater than 10 percent of body weight, or the presence of blood in the stool will require more extensive evaluation; consultations with the gastroenterologist, surgeon, and radiologist may provide valuable assistance. Further evaluation in these cases may include endoscopy, ERCP, abdominal CT, small bowel studies, or laparoscopy. Conversely, the internist can feel comfortable following the patient who appears well and has an otherwise normal history, physical examination, and screening laboratory results. For the worried patient, a session with the gastroenterologist to talk over concerns can be useful and may obviate need for further testing.

The patient with unexplained pain that has defied outpatient diagnostic attempts may benefit from further assessment in the hospital, especially if a need for large amounts of pain medication has developed. Admission provides an opportunity for 24-hour observation, specialty consultation, and assessment of the need for further study.

SYMPTOMATIC THERAPY

Although treatment is most effective when the etiology has been determined and based on a thorough evaluation, pain relief may be a high priority for the patient even before a definitive diagnosis is arrived at. However, patients with acute abdominal pain of unknown etiology should not be given analgesics, because these may obscure important findings. Although the patient with undiagnosed chronic pain often requests pain medication, regular use of narcotics ought to be avoided, because the risk of addiction is extremely high; many such patients have underlying psychopathology and a strong potential for narcotic abuse. However, the patient with terminal cancer must not be denied the relief afforded by narcotics, even if the cause of pain is not fully defined (see Chapter 91).

As noted above, *therapeutic trials* are sometimes informative and may bring relief from troublesome symptoms. Patients suspected of having peptic ulcer disease can be given an empiric course of *antacids* or *histamine$_2$-blocker* therapy, provided there is no suspicion of a malignancy (see Chapter 68). As detailed earlier, those with probable irritable bowel syndrome might be tried on a *high-fiber diet;* sometimes adding an *anticholinergic* preparation may provide added benefit (see Chapter 74). *Antidepressant* therapy may prove beneficial to the patient with abdominal pain of unclear etiology who manifests symptoms of major depression (see Chapter 227), although drug-induced constipation may ensue and worsen the problem, if it is not due to depression.

Patients with refractory functional disease linked to underlying psychosocial distress are among the hardest to help, especially when illness behavior is greatly distorted. Although formal psychiatric care may be necessary, the primary physician can help to modify illness behavior by a series of simple actions. One is to provide the patient with techniques to increase control over the illness. Useful approaches include participation in treatment decisions, learning relaxation techniques, and beginning an exercise program. Even the keeping of a symptom diary can help provide a sense of control.

Equally important for such patients is reinforcement of positive behaviors and removal of rewards for symptoms. Follow-up should be scheduled at regular intervals rather than as needed for symptoms. However, setting limits to time and availability is appropriate, with no more than 20 minutes necessary for a visit and unscheduled visits discouraged. During the visit, the focus should be on accomplishments rather than symptoms ("what have you been able to do" rather than "how do you feel"). Reports of accomplishments are best received with positive reinforcement and requests for elaboration, whereas complaints of suffering and symptoms should be responded to by a neutral stance and no request for elaboration, unless worrisome new symptoms are reported. Finally, setting realistic treatment goals is critical. Emphasis needs to be on improving quality of life and not on removal of symptoms, which may not be possible.

ANNOTATED BIBLIOGRAPHY

Anuras S, Shirazi S. Chronic pseudoobstruction. Am J Gastroenterol 1984;79:525. *(The syndromes of acute and chronic colonic pseudoobstruction are differentiated; 99 references.)*

Baron TH, Ramirez B, Richter JE. Gastrointestinal motility disorders in pregnancy. Ann Intern Med 1993;118:366. *(Constipation is common; mechanisms reviewed.)*

Council on Scientific Affairs, American Medical Association. Ultrasonic imaging of the abdomen. JAMA 1991;265:1726. *(Expert panel report on its utility; 56 refs.)*

Donaldson RM, Joyce CM, Feinstein AR. Effect of restraints on diagnostic approaches to abdominal pain and weight loss. Am J Med 1986;81:641. *(Provocative study examining test utilization when quests for economy and "team" approaches to test ordering are initiated.)*

Drossman DA, McKee DC, Sandler RS. Psychosocial factors in the irritable bowel syndrome: A multivariate study of patients and non-patients with irritable bowel syndrome. Gastroenterology 1988;95:701. *(Patients had a higher rate and degree of psychological disturbance than both nonpatients and normals.)*

Drossman DA, Thompson WG, Talley NJ, et al. Identification of subgroups of functional gastrointestinal disorders. Gastroenterol Int 1990;3:159. *(Consensus panel report on diagnostic guidelines for identification of functional disease and a recommendation that use of diagnostic studies be limited.)*

Eisenberg RL, Heineken P, Hedgcock MW, et al. Evaluation of plain abdominal radiographs in the diagnosis of abdominal pain. Ann Intern Med 1982;97:257. *(Effort to develop criteria for the ordering of abdominal films in patients with abdominal pain.)*

Friedman G. American College of Gastroenterology Committee on FDA-Related Matters. Irritable bowel syndrome I: A practical approach. Am J Gastroenterol 1989;84:803. *(Emphasizes use of fiber and other simple measures.)*

Greenlee HB. Acute large bowel obstruction: An update. Surg Annu 1982;14:253. *(Comprehensive review.)*

Hill OW, Blendis L. Physical and psychological evaluation of "non-organic" abdominal pain. Gut 1967;8:221. *(High frequency of epigastric discomfort, distention, nausea, and belching without vomiting or weight loss; bereavement or emotional upheaval often initiated symptoms.)*

Mitchell CM, Drossman DA. The irritable bowel syndrome: Understanding and treating a biopsychosocial illness disorder. Ann Behav Med 1987;9:13. *(Comprehensive and multidimensional review of the disorder, with helpful recommendations for management.)*

Moosa AR. Diagnostic tests and procedures in acute pancreatitis. N Engl J Med 1984;311:639. *(Reviews critically the host of tests available.)*

Ottinger LW. Mesenteric ischemia. N Engl J Med 1982;307:535. *(Terse review of clinical presentations, diagnosis, and treatment.)*

Richter JM, Christensen MR, Simeone JH, et al. Chronic cholecystitis: An analysis of diagnostic strategies. Invest Radiol

1987;22:111. *(Analysis of clinical utility of ultrasonography and other studies in the evaluation of abdominal pain.)*

Sarfeh IJ. Abdominal pain of unknown etiology. Am J Surg 1976;132:22. *(Over two-thirds of cases were in women; improvement most likely in younger patients with symptoms less than 2 weeks' duration; laparotomy did not influence the rate of improvement; it established diagnosis in only 1 of 23 patients explored.)*

Scott PJ, et al. Benefits and hazards of laparotomy for medical patients. Lancet 1970;2:941. *(Exploration established a diagnosis in 69 of 81 patients with extensive medical workups and no firm diagnosis. A remediable cause was found in 40 percent, but the incidence of morbidity was 45 percent, and perioperative mortality was 15 percent.)*

Shatila AH, et al. Current status of diagnosis and management of strangulation obstruction of the small bowel. Am J Surg 1976;132:299. *(Compares presentations of simple obstruction and strangulation; clinical differentiation often not reliable.)*

Silen W. Cope's Early Diagnosis of the Acute Abdomen, 18th ed. London, Oxford University Press, 1991. *(Concise, systematic approach to diagnosis of acute abdominal problems. Emphasis is on history and physical findings; required reading for the primary physician; a classic work.)*

59
Evaluation of Nausea and Vomiting

Primary Care Medicine: Office Evaluation and Management of the Adult Patient, 3rd edition, edited by Allan H. Goroll, Lawrence A. May, and Albert G. Mulley, Jr. J.B. Lippincott Company, Philadelphia

Nausea and vomiting are extremely common presenting complaints, ranking in one study of primary care practice second only to symptoms of upper respiratory tract infection. Although in most instances the symptoms are due to self-limited disease, they may be a manifestation of a more serious underlying illness. The primary care physician needs to recognize the more worrisome causes of nausea and vomiting, provide relief from these debilitating symptoms, and correct any important fluid and electrolyte disturbances.

PATHOPHYSIOLOGY AND CLINICAL PRESENTATION

Two major central nervous system centers are involved in the vomiting reflex—the vomiting center and the chemoreceptor trigger zone. Irritation of vagal and sympathetic afferents in the pharynx, heart, peritoneum, mesentery, bile ducts, stomach, and bowel triggers impulses to the vomiting center in the medullary reticular formation. Gastric irritation, distention of a hollow viscus, myocardial ischemia, increased intracranial pressure, metabolic disturbances, drugs, pharyngeal stimulation, and emotional upset are important noxious stimuli that act through this pathway. Vestibular disturbances, centrally acting drugs, and metabolic derangements stimulate the chemoreceptor trigger zone in the floor of the fourth ventricle, which, in turn, activates the vomiting center. A cortical pathway to the vomiting center has been postulated to account for some forms of psychogenic vomiting.

The act of vomiting is a stereotyped response that varies little regardless of cause. Even so-called projectile vomiting (which is characterized by forceful emesis without prior nausea or retching), supposedly limited to cases of increased intracranial pressure, occurs in other conditions. Moreover, nausea, retching, and nonprojectile vomiting are seen with increased intracranial pressure.

Nausea and vomiting may be only one part of a symptom complex or may dominate the clinical picture (as in psychogenic vomiting, early pregnancy, digitalis toxicity, and metabolic disturbances). Although there is considerable overlap among clinical presentations, some causes of nausea and vomiting are more likely to occur independent of meals, whereas others are characteristically associated with food intake. For example, early morning nausea and vomiting is typical of *metabolic etiologies*. Up to 75 percent of cases of diabetic ketoacidosis are accompanied by nausea and vomiting. Emesis and nausea are found among as many as 90 percent of patients in addisonian crisis. Uremia may be heralded by similar symptoms; nausea often improves with correction of any associated hyponatremia, but can be refractory. *Binge drinkers* experience early morning nausea and dry heaves from excessive alcohol intake.

Early pregnancy is associated with mild early morning nausea and vomiting in over 50 percent of instances. The problem is severe in fewer than 1 percent of cases, leading to electrolyte abnormalities, dehydration, and weight loss. Most cases are mild; symptoms begin after the first missed period and terminate by the fourth month. Women with severe cases often have a history of vomiting in response to psychosocial stress. Disturbed motility is also noted in many cases. The diagnosis of pregnancy is sometimes overlooked.

In contrast to the causes of early morning vomiting, symptoms can be triggered shortly after eating by psychoneurotic illness, bile reflux, peptic ulcer disease, and gastritis. *Psychogenic vomiting* is characterized by years of recurrent emesis. It can often be traced back to childhood and is more common when there is a family history of vomiting. Patients report that symptoms appear just after eating and can be sufficiently controlled voluntarily to avoid vomiting in public. Some patients admit to inducing emesis; most are surprisingly untroubled by the problem. Nausea accompanies almost all episodes. A study of 20 patients with psychogenic vomiting revealed a marked predominance of women who were engaged in hostile relationships; abdominal pain and depression were uncommon.

Bulimia is a form of psychogenic emesis in which self-induced vomiting occurs, often after a period of binge eating. Preoccupation with being thin and preponderance among young women with poor self-image are characteristic. Laxative abuse frequently complicates the clinical picture (see Chapter 234).

A *pyloric channel ulcer* or *acute gastritis* may be associated with marked postprandial emesis. The vomiting in ulcer disease is believed due in part to irritation, edema, and spasm of the pyloric sphincter mechanism. Concurrent bleeding can lead to vomiting of coffee-ground material. Patients who undergo surgery for peptic ulcer may be troubled by recurrent *bilious vomiting,* which is believed due to reflux of bile into the stomach or gastric remnant. Patients vomit bile within 15 minutes of eating; little food is present. Nausea and a bad taste in the mouth are present on awakening in the morning.

Gastric retention results in vomiting of food eaten more than 6 hours previously. A succussion splash is detectable on examination, and food is seen in the stomach on upper GI series. In chronic cases there may be gastric outflow obstruction or atony secondary to diabetic neuropathy, anticholinergic use, or gastric malignancy. Transient gastric dilatation is a frequent concomitant of pancreatitis, peritonitis, gallbladder disease, and hypokalemia. A *cyclic idiopathic* form of nausea and vomiting has been described with gastric hypomotility demonstrated.

Acute episodes of vomiting accompany a host of conditions, ranging from the self-limited to the life-threatening. The most common is *viral gastroenteritis.* After many years of attributing this illness to viral infection, investigators have finally isolated and identified the responsible viruses. Explosive bouts of nausea and vomiting in conjunction with watery diarrhea, cramping abdominal pain, myalgias, headache, and fever are typical. Recovery is rapid in most instances, but symptoms may linger for 7 to 10 days. Similarly, anorexia, nausea, and vomiting often dominate the prodromal stage of *acute viral hepatitis* (see Chapter 70).

Acute gastroenteritis that results from *food poisoning* due to *Salmonella* or *Shigella* infection has a similar clinical presentation and course; onset is 24 to 48 hours after exposure to the contaminated food. Domestic fowl and their eggs represent the largest single reservoir of *Salmonella* infection. Inadequate cooking is often responsible for human infection. Intake of pastries and similar items containing *staphylococcal enterotoxin* causes symptoms indistinguishable from viral gastroenteritis, except that onset is within 1 to 6 hours after eating the spoiled food, fever is rare, and complete clearing takes place by 24 to 48 hours. *Clostridial food poisoning* rarely produces prominent nausea and vomiting.

Persons with travel to an epidemic area are at risk for contracting *cholera,* especially if they have eaten raw or undercooked seafood or had drinks chilled with contaminated ice. South America is the latest area to experience an epidemic. High U.S. sanitary standards for the handling of sewage, water, and food have so far prevented outbreaks from spreading to this country. The causative organism is a toxigenic strain of *Vibrio cholerae,* elaborating an enterotoxin that induces secretion of water and electrolytes from the intestinal mucosa. Mild infection is characterized by a nonspecific diarrheal illness. In 3 percent to 5 percent of cases, the disease is much more severe (*cholera gravis*) and presents as profuse watery diarrhea with flecks of whitish mucus ("rice-water stools"), vomiting, and dehydration. Vomiting is exacerbated by the acidosis that results from bowel bicarbonate loss. Circulatory collapse, altered consciousness, renal failure, and death are possible outcomes.

Peritoneal irritation and acute obstruction may precipitate acute emesis, usually in the context of severe abdominal pain (see Chapter 58). *Intestinal obstruction,* especially of the proximal small bowel, produces marked nausea and vomiting of bilious material. Distention may be lacking, but intermittent cramping abdominal pain is characteristic. Feculent emesis is found in distal small bowel obstruction. In *acute pancreatitis,* emesis is seen in 85 percent of patients; however, upper abdominal pain radiating into the back is the cardinal symptom, occurring in 95 percent of patients (see Chapter 72). Anorexia, nausea, and vomiting are early symptoms in more than 90 percent of patients with *acute appendicitis;* usually emesis clears early. As with pancreatitis, pain typically precedes other symptoms. *Acute pyelonephritis* may mimic a gastrointestinal etiology, by causing nausea, vomiting, and abdominal pain. *Acute cholecystitis* sometimes triggers acute emesis, but less regularly than does *acute cholangitis* due to sudden obstruction of the common duct.

Myocardial infarction may activate vagal afferents and produce nausea, vomiting, and epigastric discomfort simulating intraabdominal disease. A prospective series of 62 patients with acute infarction revealed nausea and vomiting at the outset in 69 percent of those with inferior infarctions and 27 percent of those with anterior infarctions.

Neurologic emergencies can provoke severe bouts of acute emesis. In *midline cerebellar hemorrhage,* nausea and vomiting are profuse, in association with severe gait ataxia; meningeal signs and headache are seen as well. Within a few hours the patient may become comatose and die unless promptly diagnosed and treated (see Chapter 165). One-third of patients with *increased intracranial pressure* experience vomiting. When it is sudden, forceful, and not preceded by nausea it is termed "projectile," but this presentation is not specific. Concurrent bifrontal or bioccipital headache is the rule. *Migraine headaches* and *vestibular disease* are less worrisome neurologic causes of acute emesis (see Chapters 165 and 166). The former is suggested by photophobia and throbbing unilateral headache, the latter by vertigo.

Of the many *drugs* that induce vomiting, *digitalis* intoxication is among the most serious. Anorexia is an early sign, followed by nausea and vomiting due to stimulation of the chemoreceptor trigger zone. Visual disturbances such as colored haloes are suggestive of the diagnosis (see Chapter 32). Hypokalemia and dehydration induced by vomiting may precipitate or worsen digitalis toxicity.

Most *cancer chemotherapeutic agents* and *radiation therapy* produce substantial nausea and vomiting, with cisplatin being among the most problematic of chemotherapic agents. The mechanism of nausea and vomiting is believed to involve drug-induced release of serotonin from enterochromaffin cells, leading to activation of serotonin receptors on visceral afferent fibers and stimulation of the vomiting center and chemoreceptor trigger zone. Drugs that block such serotonin receptors have proven uniquely effective (see below and Chapter 91).

Drug withdrawal as well as drug excess may trigger emesis. Nausea, dry heaves, and retching beginning at about 36 hours are characteristic features of opiate withdrawal syndrome. Sweats, chills, and restlessness precede other symptoms; the vomiting peaks by 72 hours and subsides (see Chapter 235).

DIFFERENTIAL DIAGNOSIS

Table 59–1 lists some of the more common and important conditions associated with prominent nausea and vomiting. Causes of simple regurgitation are omitted from the list because they are usually manifestations of esophageal difficulties (see Chapter 61) and unaccompanied by emesis. The etiologies are listed for convenience according to clinical presentation; however, it is important to keep in mind that there can be considerable overlap and variation in the clinical picture. For example, some causes listed as being accompanied by abdominal pain may present with just isolated emesis.

WORKUP

History and physical examination supplemented by a few well-chosen laboratory studies are sufficient for diagnosis in most cases.

Table 59-1. Some Important Causes of Nausea and Vomiting

NAUSEA/VOMITING AS PREDOMINANT OR INITIAL SYMPTOMS
Acute
1. Digitalis toxicity
2. Ketoacidosis*
3. Opiate use
4. Cancer chemotherapeutic agents
5. Early pregnancy
6. Inferior myocardial infarction*
7. Drug withdrawal
8. Binge drinking
9. Hepatitis
Recurrent or Chronic
1. Psychogenic vomiting
2. Metabolic disturbances (uremia, adrenal insufficiency)
3. Gastric retention (gastroparesis, outlet obstruction)
4. Bile reflux postgastric surgery
5. Pregnancy
NAUSEA/VOMITING IN ASSOCIATION WITH ABDOMINAL PAIN†
1. Viral gastroenteritis
2. Acute gastritis
3. Food poisoning
4. Peptic ulcer disease
5. Acute pancreatitis
6. Small bowel obstruction and pseudoobstruction
7. Acute appendicitis
8. Acute cholecystitis
9. Acute cholangitis
10. Acute pyelonephritis
11. Inferior myocardial infarction
NAUSEA/VOMITING IN ASSOCIATION WITH NEUROLOGIC SYMPTOMS
1. Increased intracranial pressure
2. Midline cerebellar hemorrhage
3. Vestibular disturbances
4. Migraine headaches
5. Autonomic dysfunction

*Abdominal pain is sometimes present.
†Abdominal pain is sometimes absent.

History should focus on such details as timing of symptoms, their relation to meals, characteristics of the vomitus, and associated complaints. Early-morning onset points to metabolic disturbances, alcoholic binge, and early pregnancy. Emesis precipitated by meals suggests psychogenic vomiting, pyloric channel ulcer, and gastritis. Onset a few hours after eating raises the possibility of gastric-outflow tract obstruction, gastric atony, or bowel obstruction. Emesis of food that was ingested more than 12 hours earlier strongly suggests gastric stasis and an organic etiology, as does vomiting of large volumes (> 1500 mL per day). However, absence of such features hardly rules out organic disease.

Vomiting blood or coffee-ground material is indicative of gastritis and ulcer disease. Bilious vomitus means that the pyloric channel is open. When the material vomited is pure gastric juice, peptic ulcer disease and Zollinger-Ellison syndrome are suggested. Lack of acid suggests gastric cancer. Feculent material is a sign of distal small-bowel obstruction and blind-loop syndrome.

The history needs to include inquiry into abdominal pain, fever, jaundice, weight loss, abdominal surgery, external hernias, family history of emesis, symptoms of diabetes, prior renal disease, ischemic heart disease, drug use (eg, digitalis, narcotics), visual disturbances, headache, ataxia, vertigo, last menstrual period, and concurrent emotional stresses and conflicts. Gentle questioning about self-image, binge eating, and self-induced emesis is indicated when the patient is a young woman suspected of bulimia.

Epidemiologic data need to be obtained, particularly any exposure to commonly contaminated foods (eg, raw shellfish, pastries, poultry) or hepatitis, and travel to an area where there is poor sanitation and outbreaks of cholera. Vomiting in conjunction with diarrhea sufficient enough to cause severe dehydration in an adult suggests cholera, especially if there are supportive epidemiologic data.

Physical examination requires a check for postural hypotension (indicative of marked volume depletion or circulatory collapse), malignant hypertension, irregularities of rate and rhythm, Kussmaul breathing, pallor, hyperpigmentation, jaundice, papilledema, retinopathy, nystagmus, stiff neck, abdominal distention, visible peristalsis, abnormal bowel sounds, succussion splash, peritoneal signs, focal tenderness, organomegaly, masses, flank tenderness, muscle weakness, ataxia of gait, and asterixis. If there is a history of vertigo in conjunction with nausea, then Bárnáy's maneuver (see Chapter 166) might reproduce symptoms and confirm the diagnosis of a vestibular etiology.

Patients suspected of having a "functional" disorder should be checked carefully for signs of autonomic insufficiency. Finding postural hypotension, lack of sweat, or blunted pulse and blood pressure responses to Valsalva's maneuver suggests autonomic dysfunction and a bowel motility problem as the underlying etiology of the nausea and vomiting.

Laboratory Studies. In patients with emesis accompanied by acute abdominal pain, the first priority is to rule out an acute surgical etiology such as bowel obstruction, peritonitis, or blockage of a hollow viscus. *Plane and upright films of the abdomen* are indicated when such etiologies are suspected (see Chapter 58). Acute nausea and vomiting without associated abdominal pain may also be a clue to serious illness. If the patient is a known diabetic, ketoacidosis should be suspected and *serum ketones* should be checked. In a patient with strong risk factors for coronary artery disease, an *electrocardiogram* should be obtained; inferior ischemia may present as gastrointestinal upset (see Chapter 20). Hepatitis might present like acute gastroenteritis, with anorexia, nausea, and vomiting; a *transaminase* determination can be diagnostic. The onset of pancreatitis may be dominated by emesis; a serum *amylase* is indicated. Acute onset of nausea and vomiting in conjunction with ataxia of gait and a stiff neck is very suggestive of a midline cerebellar hemorrhage; an emergency *head CT scan* of the posterior fossa is needed.

Acute vomiting of unclear etiology without focal signs should also be pursued by carefully checking medications and *serum levels*. If a digitalis preparation is being taken, the drug should be withheld, an electrocardiogram obtained, a serum level ordered, and a potassium supplement prescribed if the potassium level is below 4.0 mg per 100 mL (see Chapter 32).

Recurrent vomiting of unknown etiology raises the question of a psychogenic cause. The patient with psychogenic vomiting may be recognized by the characteristic history of chronic emesis, with vomiting around mealtime, partial suppressibility, and a conflict-ridden social situation. The need for additional studies in such cases is best individualized, because some patients may insist on further testing whereas others may be comforted by knowing that extensive studies are not necessary. Any woman of childbearing age whose vomiting is suspected to have a psychogenic cause should always have a *pregnancy test* (the serum human chorionic gonadotropin [HCG] beta-subunit is the most sensitive; see Chapter 112) before concluding that emesis is emotional in origin.

Elimination of pregnancy and psychogenic causes leaves metabolic disorders and gastric pathology among possible antecedents of recurrent emesis. Metabolic disease is suggested by vomiting that occurs in the early morning. A *urinalysis* and determinations of the serum *BUN, creatinine, electrolytes,* and *glucose* should be obtained. An *upper GI series* can confirm gastric outlet obstruction or retention. Sometimes *endoscopy* is necessary for assessment of the stomach (see Chapter 68). The suspicion of hepatitis can be confirmed by obtaining a transaminase level (see Chapter 70).

Therapeutic Trials. A therapeutic trial may have diagnostic utility and provide symptomatic relief. When there is suspicion of a motility disorder, a short course of a prokinetic agent such as *metoclopramide* or *cisapride* can be useful. A therapeutic response is very suggestive of a motility disturbance. Patients suspected of having an underlying affective disorder sometimes respond to a 4- to 8-week trial of *antidepressant medication;* an agent with minimal anticholinergic activity (eg, trazodone, desipramine, or fluoxetine) is preferred to minimize chances of gastrointestinal side effects.

INDICATIONS FOR REFERRAL AND ADMISSION

Hospital admission for parenteral fluid and electrolyte replacement is indicated if there is postural hypotension, especially if the patient is elderly. Prompt hospitalization also is needed if there is evidence of bowel obstruction, increased intracranial pressure, or other gastrointestinal, neurologic, or metabolic emergency.

Patients who remain undiagnosed after extensive evaluation, unresponsive to therapeutic trials, and without evidence or suspicion of an underlying psychiatric disturbance deserve consideration for gastric emptying and motility studies. These studies are done at only a few specialty centers; referral should be made in consultation with a gastroenterologist. Patients suspected of psychogenic vomiting need psychiatric consultation, because they may be seriously disturbed. Suicidal attempts are not uncommon among bulimics and others with psychogenic emesis. Referral to a mental health professional skilled and experienced in the treatment of patients with eating disorders is optimal for those suffering from bulimia (see Chapter 234).

SYMPTOMATIC RELIEF

When a cause is identified, but treatment of the underlying condition does not adequately control the symptoms, antiemetic drug therapy may help provide symptomatic relief. The available agents work by suppressing the vomiting center, the chemoreceptor trigger zone, or peripheral receptors. Symptomatic therapy must not be used in lieu of making a diagnosis.

The phenothiazines are indicated for initial symptomatic treatment of vomiting caused by drugs, metabolic disorders, and gastroenteritis. They suppress the chemoreceptor trigger zone and probably the vomiting center and peripheral receptors as well. *Prochlorperazine* (*Compazine*) and *promethazine* (*Phenergan*) are the phenothiazines used most often for vomiting. Prochlorperazine can be given in doses of 5 to 10 mg orally, every 6 hours, or 25 mg rectally, tid. The oral dose of promethazine is 12.5 to 25.0 mg every 6–8 hours; the rectal dose is 25 mg tid. This class of drugs is not effective for motion sickness or vestibular disease. Trimethobenzamide (Tigan) is a centrally acting nonphenothiazine antiemetic useful for emesis due to central causes. Oral dose is 250 mg tid. Rectal suppositories are given tid. Like all centrally acting agents, it can cause drowsiness, especially in the elderly.

For symptomatic relief of *vestibular disturbances,* the antihistamine *meclizine* (*Antivert*) has proven useful, acting on the vestibular system and the chemoreceptor trigger zone and to help control the nausea and vomiting associated with vestibular dysfunction. Because meclizine can suppress or blunt important clues of vestibular disease, it should not be used unless a diagnosis has been established. Other antihistamines enjoy considerable popularity for treatment or prevention of *motion sickness* because, compared to meclizine, they provide either more rapid onset of action (eg, *dimenhydrinate* [Dramamine]) or more prolonged effect (eg, *transdermal scopolamine*). The average dosage of meclizine is 25 mg qid for vestibular disease. A single transdermal scopolamine patch applied behind the ear several hours before a trip will provide prophylaxis for up to 3 days. Anticholinergic side effects (constipation, dry mouth, giddiness) are common. Meclizine is teratogenic in animals and is not indicated for vomiting due to pregnancy. All antihistamines can cause drowsiness and should not be used before driving or use of machinery.

For patients with emesis due to gastroparesis, the prokinetic agents *metoclopramide* (10 mg pc and qhs) and *cisapride* (10 mg pc and qhs) can help. The latter does not act centrally and thus causes few central nervous system side effects, making it more tolerable for chronic use, particularly in the elderly.

A few specific problems require elaboration:

The nausea and vomiting associated with *cancer chemotherapy* can be especially uncomfortable and demoralizing. A wide variety of agents have been tried empirically, ranging from phenothiazines to tetrahydrocannabinol (as found in marijuana). Few provide truly satisfactory control, particularly when cisplatin is required. The selective serotonin S3 receptor antagonist *ondansetron* has proven remarkably effective and safe, probably by virtue of its ability to block the effects of cisplatin-induced serotonin release from enterochromaffin cells. Anticholinergic therapy with high-dose *metoclopramide* has also been used, but cisplatin was superior and better tolerated in double-blinded crossover study (see Chapter 91).

Morning sickness is best treated with small morning feedings and support; the goal is to try to avoid use of antiemetics. No antiemetic is approved for use in pregnancy. The more prolonged, severe form of nausea and vomiting due to pregnancy (hypemesis gravidarum) may remit with hypnosis or supportive psychotherapy, but drug therapy is sometimes necessary. *Vitamin* B_6 (25 mg/d) has proven useful in controlled trials and appears safe. *Metoclopramide* has also been used for years in severe cases without reports of fetal injury. Approval for *Bendectin* has been withdrawn because of concern for teratogenic effects.

Psychogenic vomiting is best approached by attention to the conflicts troubling the patient. No controlled studies have been done on the effectiveness of antiemetics; fortunately, patients often do not request medication for symptomatic relief.

In *hepatitis*, nausea and vomiting may respond to very cautious use of phenothiazines. However, because they are metabolized by the liver and in rare instances can cause cholestasis, they should be used only in limited doses for short periods of time (see Chapter 70).

A.H.G.

ANNOTATED BIBLIOGRAPHY

Abell TL, Kim CH, Malagelda J-R. Idiopathic cyclic nausea and vomiting—A disorder of gastrointestinal motility? Mayo Clin Proc 1988;63:1169. *(Gastrointestinal motor disturbances found.)*

Ahmed S, Gupta R, Brancato R. Significance of nausea and vomiting during acute myocardial infarction. Am Heart J 1977; 95:671. *(Nausea and vomiting occurred in 69 percent of patients with inferior infarctions, compared with 27 percent of those with anterior infarctions.)*

Baron TH, Ramirez R, Richter JE. Gastrointestinal motility disorders during pregnancy. Ann Intern Med 1993;118:366. *(Pathophysiology of vomiting in pregnancy.)*

Biggs J. Vomiting and pregnancy. Drugs 1975;9:299. *(Terse review of clinical presentation and therapy.)*

Bothe F, Beardwood J. Evaluation of abdominal symptoms in the diabetic. Ann Surg 1937;105:516. *(Classic study; 75 percent of patients in ketoacidosis had nausea and vomiting; 8 percent had severe abdominal pain and elevated white counts simulating an acute abdomen; intraabdominal disease can precipitate ketoacidosis.)*

Cubeddu LX, Hoffman IS, Fuenmayor NT, et al. Efficacy of ondansetron (GR 38032F) and the role of serotonin in cisplatin-induced nausea and vomiting. N Engl J Med 1990;322:810. *(Randomized, placebo-controlled study demonstrating that ondansetron is effective and safe.)*

Hill OW. Psychogenic vomiting. Gut 1968;9:348. *(High frequency of hostile living situations and symptoms coming on at mealtime.)*

Malagelda JR, Camillieri M. Unexplained vomiting: A diagnostic challenge. Ann Intern Med 1984;101:211. *(Useful review of approaches to this difficult situation. Details neuromuscular disorders that may present as unexplained emesis; 61 references.)*

Richards RD, Valenzuela GA, Davenport KG, et al. Objective and subjective results of a randomized, double-blind, placebo-controlled trial using cisapride to treat gastroparesis. Dig Dis Sci 1993;38:811. *(Found effective.)*

Rimer D. Gastric retention without mechanical obstruction. Arch Intern Med 1966;117:287. *(Good review of the problem, detailing the causes of this condition; 73 references.)*

Sahakian V, Rouse D, Sipes S, et al. Vitamin B_6 is effective for nausea and vomiting of pregnancy. Obstet Gynecol 1991; 78:33. *(A randomized, placebo-controlled, double-blind trial.)*

Swerdlow DL, Ries AA. Cholera in the Americas. JAMA 1992;267:1495. *(Terse and excellent review of epidemiology, clinical presentation, diagnosis, and treatment; 42 references.)*

Primary Care Medicine: Office Evaluation and Management of the Adult Patient, 3rd edition, edited by Allan H. Goroll, Lawrence A. May, and Albert G. Mulley, Jr. J.B. Lippincott Company, Philadelphia

60
Evaluation of Dysphagia and Suspected Esophageal Chest Pain

Dysphagia is the unpleasant sensation of difficulty swallowing due to neuromuscular or anatomic pathology involving the esophagus (and sometimes the oropharynx). Such pathology may also trigger substernal chest pain and simulate angina (see Chapter 20). Odynophagia refers to painful swallowing, which usually results from serious mucosal inflammation. Because esophageal dysfunction and pain may be a manifestation or mimicker of important pathology, it deserves to be fully assessed and not dismissed as a trivial problem or glibly invoked to account for symptoms.

PATHOPHYSIOLOGY AND CLINICAL PRESENTATION

Dysphagia implies an abnormality in swallowing and arises from either a loss of coordinated motor activity or from mechanical obstruction, be it intrinsic narrowing or extrinsic compression of the esophagus.

Transfer dysphagia (also referred to as *oropharyngeal dysphagia*) usually occurs as a consequence of neurologic or neuromuscular disease and presents as choking or difficulty initiating swallowing. In many instances, other neurologic symptoms dominate the clinical picture, but at times, difficulty swallowing is the major complaint, with aspiration and regurgitation of fluid into the nose. The problem is particularly common among the very elderly. Cortical and brainstem lesions due to stroke, tumor, and degenerative disease are important causes. In addition, medications with central effects (eg, benzodiazepines, L-dopa, phenothiazines) may blunt the swallowing mechanism. Unlike esophageal disease, oropharyngeal dysphagia is accurately localized to the suprasternal area. Those with neuromuscular etiologies report liquids more difficult to swallow than solids, nasal regurgitation, coughing, and aspiration. Patients with anatomic narrowing and mechanical obstruction of the pharynx or upper esophagus have more difficulty with solids than liquids.

Achalasia, the most common cause of motor dysphagia, is a slowly progressive motility disorder with a chronic course. The pathologic hallmark is a loss of cells in the myenteric ganglia. Lesions in the dorsal vagal nucleus and vagal trunks have also been described. There is speculation that these changes represent damage caused by a neurotropic virus. As a consequence of losing smooth muscle ganglion cells, the esophagus functions poorly, has episodes of aperistalsis, and demonstrates exquisite sensitivity to gastrin and cholinergic agents. The gastroesophageal sphincter fails to relax properly, leading to functional obstruction at the gastroesophageal junction. In addition, there is a *loss of peristaltic activity* in the distal esophagus. Dysphagia and substernal chest pain ensue. The resting pressure at the lower esophageal sphincter (LES) rises, and barium study shows absence of peristalsis and delay in esophageal emptying. Paradoxically, vigorous nonpropulsive (tertiary) esophageal contractions resulting in chest pain may be observed early in the disease in young patients. Swallowing liquids and solids are equally difficult, yet by eating slowly and drinking small amounts, the patient may be able to consume a full meal. Pain is reported by 70 percent to 80 percent of patients, especially if they eat or drink rapidly, but pain is not an invariable accompaniment and only 2 percent of patients with chest pain due to esophageal disease have achalasia. Very cold liquids or emotion may provoke symptoms. Patients find that repeated swallowing or performing a rapid Valsalva maneuver can help pass material into the stomach. Regurgitation is common and can be provoked by changes in position or by physical exercise; pulmonary aspiration sometimes results. Patients may demonstrate foul breath because of retained esophageal material. Squamous cell carcinoma of the esophagus is sometimes a complication of achalasia; it occurs in 5 percent to 10 percent of patients.

Carcinoma-induced achalasia is seen with tumors at the gastroesophageal junction. Adenocarcinoma of the stomach is the most common of these neoplasms. The mechanism by which tumor induces achalasia is unclear, but manometric findings are identical to those of primary achalasia. Patients are typically over age 50 and complain of marked weight loss and symptoms of dysphagia that are less than a year in duration.

Scleroderma can impair neuromuscular function and result in a decrease in LES tone as well as a lack of propulsive motor activity. *Reflux* is more of a problem than is dysphagia (helping to distinguish scleroderma from other motility disorders), but as many as 20 percent of patients may suffer some difficulty in swallowing. About 75 percent of patients with scleroderma have esophageal involvement, as part of the CREST syndrome (*c*alcinosis, *R*aynaud's, *s*clerodactyly, and *t*elangiectasia).

Diffuse esophageal spasm is characterized clinically by nonprogressive dysphagia and substernal chest pain that may mimic angina (see below and Chapter 20). Radiologically and manometrically, patients manifest nonpropulsive *simultaneous contractions* (tertiary contractions) throughout the entire esophagus (especially the distal portion) in more than 10 percent of wet swallows. Such contractions are also observed in normal persons under conditions of emotional stress and dry swallows, leading some to view this condition as little more than a transient abnormality in motor function induced by stress. However, as noted above, the condition may also be an early manifestation of neuromuscular disease that progresses to achalasia. Unlike achalasia, diffuse esophageal spasm is intermixed with periods of normal peristaltic activity. Dysphagia is noted with both liquids and solids. Diffuse esophageal spasm accounts for about 10 percent of cases of noncardiac chest pain due to abnormal esophageal motility. Some asymptomatic patients manifest the radiologic and manometric criteria for esophageal spasm but rarely experience discomfort.

Nutcracker esophagus is a picturesque radiologic description applied to patients experiencing *very high amplitude contractions* in the distal esophagus. The resultant pressures exceed the mean by more than two standard deviations. These peristaltic contractions are not only of exceptionally high amplitude, but also of long duration. Unlike diffuse esophageal spasm, there are no simultaneous contractions and only occasionally is there impairment of esophageal function leading to dysphagia. The principal symptom is *chest pain* (see below), with nutcracker esophagus accounting for about half of all cases of noncardiac chest pain due to an esophageal motility disturbance. Occasionally reflux precipitates the contractile abnormalities. About 3 percent to 5 percent of patients develop achalasia, and degenerative changes are noted in ganglia and nerves, suggesting to some a possible link to achalasia. Supersensitivity to gastrin and cholinergic agents can be demonstrated.

Hypertensive lower esophageal sphincter is characterized by increased resting LES pressure, but normal relaxation and peristalsis, with no impediment to bolus passage. About half of the patients have high-amplitude contractions consistent with nutcracker esophagus.

Mechanical obstruction differs clinically from motor dysfunction in that the patient has more difficulty with solids than with liquids. The duration of symptoms is shorter (less than 1 year) for patients with malignancy than it is for those with benign causes of obstruction; progression is often rapid. Most patients with tumor are over age 50 and report marked weight loss. The location of discomfort does not necessarily correlate with the site of obstruction, because the pain may be referred. Spontaneous pain is not a common feature of neoplasm involving the esophagus. Patients with stricture due to severe esophagitis usually have a long-standing history of reflux.

Inflammatory lesions of the pharynx or esophagus may cause *odynophagia* (pain on swallowing). There is no disturbance of esophageal motility, but swallowing is made difficult by the pain. Even saliva may be irritating. *Radiation therapy, tablet ingestion,* and *infection* are important causes of this severe esophageal irritation. Tetracycline, quinidine, potassium tablets, nonsteroidal antiinflammatory agents, and iron preparations have been implicated. The elderly are at greatest risk because they are likely to consume more tablets, use less water, and have age-related decreased saliva production. The discomfort will often be associated with the tablets and will generally decrease over a period of a few days.

Infectious esophagitis caused by *Candida, herpes simplex,* or *cytomegalovirus* is being increasingly recognized in immunocompromised patients and those on long-term broad-spectrum antibiotics, and in the growing number of patients immunocompromised with acquired immunodeficiency syndrome (AIDS). Onset may be rapid and accompanied by fever, chills, nausea, vomiting, and epigastric pain. Viral or fungal esophagitis rarely occurs in immunologically intact individuals; when it does, it is usually short-lived and self-limited.

Esophageal chest pain is most often associated with prolonged or severe contractile waves, although distention of stretch receptors and stimulation of chemoreceptors may also contribute. Certain investigators have suggested that some patients subject to attacks of esophageal chest pain may have an esophageal version of irritable bowel syndrome, with motor dysfunction and increased sensitivity to distention and chemical stimuli. They wonder whether there might be an "irritable gut syndrome," with a common pathophysiology extending from the esophagus to the rectosigmoid. They note that many patients with esophageal chest pain also report symptoms of irritable bowel syndrome.

Chest pain is particularly prevalent in patients with nutcracker esophagus; the condition accounts for about half of patients presenting with noncardiac chest pain and abnormal esophageal motility. The chest pain associated with esophageal motor disorders can mimic angina in terms of pain location (substernal), quality (tightness), radiation (into the arm or back), and response to nitroglycerin (prompt relief). Adding to the confusion with coronary pain is the fact that esophageal chest pain need not be accompanied by dysphagia, although sometimes heartburn is reported as a preceding symptom. The pain is frequently nocturnal, awakening the patient from sleep. Chest discomfort need not occur in relation to swallowing, but sometimes is triggered by drinking very hot or very cold liquids.

Conditions confused with dysphagia. Sometimes *globus hystericus,* a condition seen in anxiety disorders, is confused with dysphagia. The patient complains of a constant "lump in the throat," although there is no actual difficulty swallowing food, but there is a perception of obstruction. An involuntary tightening of the cricopharyngeal muscle has been observed in some patients with this condition and may account for symptoms. Symptoms are unrelated to swallowing, and esophageal function is normal.

DIFFERENTIAL DIAGNOSIS

The causes of dysphagia can be divided into motor and obstructive categories and are often subdivided according to whether they affect the upper or lower esophagus (Table 60–1). Most esophageal cancers are of the squamous cell variety, although half of those in the distal half of the esophagus are adenocarcinomas, suggesting that they arise in the cardia of the stomach. True dysphagia must be distinguished from conditions that may produce esophageal pain without interfering with the mechanics of swallowing, as occurs with most forms of esophagitis and motor disorders with propulsive, but high-amplitude contractions (eg, nutcracker esophagus). The patient with globus hystericus reports a constant sensation of something in the throat, but swallows normally.

Table 60-1. Differential Diagnosis of Dysphagia

Motor Disease
Pharyngeal (transfer dysphagia)
- Pseudobulbar palsy
- Myasthenia gravis
- Multiple sclerosis
- Amyotrophic lateral sclerosis
- Parkinson's disease

Transesophageal
- Achalasia
- Scleroderma
- Diffuse esophageal spasm

Distal
- Nutcracker esophagus
- Hypertensive lower esophageal sphincter

Obstructing Lesions
Upper esophageal
- Tumor
- Zenker's diverticulum
- Sideropenic webs (Plummer-Vinson syndrome)
- Goiter
- Enlarged lymph nodes
- Cervical spine osteophytes

Lower esophageal
- Carcinoma
- Stricture (chronic reflux, corrosive agents, intubation)
- Webs and rings
- Foreign bodies
- Food impaction
- Mediastinal tumors
- Aortic aneurysm

Odynophagia
Opportunistic esophageal infection (cytomegalovirus, herpes, *Candida*)
- Tablet-induced irritation
- Severe reflux esophagitis

No detailed population studies have been done on the prevalence of dysphagia and the relative frequencies of its etiologies. However, in a study of 910 patients with noncardiac chest pain, 28 percent were found to have abnormal esophageal motility. Of these 28 percent, 48 percent had a nutcracker disease, 36 percent had nonspecific esophageal motility dysfunction, 10 percent had diffuse esophageal spasm, and 2 percent had achalasia.

WORKUP

History

A tentative diagnosis can often be made by history. A British study found that history alone could provide an accurate diagnosis in about 80 percent of cases. The most important historical features include the duration and progression of symptoms, relation of symptoms to solids and liquids, effect of cold on swallowing, and response to swallowing a bolus. Inquiry into these aspects of the problem help in the important task of differentiating a motor disorder from mechanical obstruction. Motor disease is suggested by gradual onset, slow progression, chronic course, equal difficulty with liquids and solids, aggravation of symptoms on swallowing cold substances, and passage of a bolus by repeated swallowing, forceful drinking, Valsalva maneuver, or throwing back the head and shoulders. Mechanical obstruction is characterized by more rapid onset and progressive course, more difficulty with solids than with liquids, no aggravation with cold foods, and regurgitation on trying to swallow a bolus. As noted above, the location of discomfort helps to locate the lesion only if it is very high or very low in the esophagus; a distal lesion may cause pain referred to the neck. Hiccups point to difficulty in the terminal portion of the esophagus. Intermittent dysphagia that occurs only with solid food is indicative of a lower esophageal (Schatzki's) ring.

Other historical features also have some discriminative value, including presence of pain, reflux, and neurologic defects. Pain in conjunction with dysphagia suggests spasm or achalasia, although pain may occur in these conditions without concurrent difficulty in swallowing. Pain on swallowing saliva alone is characteristic of mucosal inflammation. A history of heartburn in conjunction with difficulty swallowing solids argues strongly for a stricture secondary to chronic reflux esophagitis, especially if the problem is chronic. Scleroderma also is suggested when symptoms of reflux occur with dysphagia (as well as by complaints of skin changes and cold extremities). Dysphagia that comes on only after activity, in association with motor aphasia, diplopia, or dysphonia, is indicative of myasthenia. Tremor or difficulty in initiating movement suggests Parkinson's disease (see Chapter 174). Other historical facts to note are recent use of topical upper respiratory or inhaled steroid aerosols, broad-spectrum antibiotics, and concurrent immunodeficiency (eg, AIDS).

The pace of illness is important to note. Very acute dysphagia suggests infection, irritation, or food impaction. Rapid progression is due to tumor until proven otherwise, whereas slow progression is most consistent with a motor disorder. Weight loss may occur with any etiology, but in a Mayo Clinic study it was more predictive of an obstructive one.

Physical Examination

The skin is noted for pallor, signs of scleroderma (sclerodactyly, telangiectasias, calcinosis), and hyperkeratotic palms and soles (a rare finding suggestive of esophageal carcinoma). The mouth should be examined carefully for inflammatory lesions, ill-fitting dentures, and pharyngeal masses. The human immunodeficiency virus (HIV)-positive patient with oral candidiasis has an increased risk of esophageal involvement. Lymph nodes are palpated in the neck and elsewhere for enlargement suggestive of neoplasm and infection (see Chapter 12), and the thyroid is palpated for a goiter that might extrinsically compress the esophagus. The abdomen is checked for masses, tenderness, organomegaly, and occult blood in the stool (suggestive of neoplasm and esophagitis). Neurologic examination should be thorough and should include testing for motor dysfunction, looking for tremor, rigidity, and fatigability as well as cranial nerve deficits, abnormal Babinski's response, and abnormal gag reflex.

Laboratory Studies

The history and physical examination usually provide sufficient evidence to distinguish oropharyngeal from esophageal dysphagia, and a mechanical form of esophageal dysphagia from a neuromuscular one. Making such a determination before laboratory testing helps focus the laboratory workup, interpret the results, and avoid unnecessary studies.

Barium swallow is usually the first step in the diagnostic evaluation of the dysphagic patient and is especially important if a structural impediment to swallowing is suspected. Its sensitivity is excellent for determining the location and severity of an obstructing mass lesion or stenosis, but it often lacks precision in identifying the nature of the lesion, particularly in distinguishing cancer from postinflammatory scarring and stenosis. For example, some gastric carcinomas may show little more than intrinsic narrowing. Endoscopic biopsy (see below) may be necessary, especially when the history is suspicious of malignancy (eg, rapid progression, marked weight loss).

By providing fluoroscopic evidence of esophageal function, the barium swallow can sometimes help in documenting motor disorders, although test sensitivity is not high. Early achalasia and esophageal spasm may produce few findings on a routine barium swallow, especially when symptoms are infrequent. The characteristic radiologic features of achalasia include dilatation of the distal two-thirds of the esophagus, segmental contractions, and termination of the distal esophagus into a narrowed segment (often referred to as a "break") caused by the tonically contracted LES. When the patient is upright, an air–fluid level may be present on the barium esophagram. If diffuse esophageal spasm occurs during barium examination, it produces multiple tertiary contractions and differs from achalasia in that there is no break. Functional assessment of dysphagia is facilitated by performing all barium studies with the patient in the supine position to cancel the effect of gravity, and by dipping a piece of bread into barium to better trace the movement of solid food. *Video studies of the oropharyngeal phase* of swallowing are essential in the evaluation of suspected oropharyngeal dysphagia, not only for diagnosis, but also to determine the risk of aspiration. Radiologic expertise is required for the interpretation of such films.

Upper GI endoscopy and biopsy are needed when an intrinsically obstructing lesion is discovered and there is concern about it being malignant. As noted above, even stenoses may represent early cancer and should be considered for endoscopy and biopsy if the clinical context is suggestive (eg, age greater than 50, progressive clinical course). On occasion, even the patient with achalasia may require endoscopy, particularly when contraction of the LES is so persistent that stenosis cannot be ruled out by barium study alone. Stretching of the sphincter can be accomplished at the same time. However, endoscopy for truly x-ray–negative dysphagia is generally of low yield.

Acute onset of odynophagia suggests severe esophageal inflammation and, in an immunocompromised host, raises the possibility of an infectious etiology. Endoscopic examination is needed to examine for plaques, vesicles, and pseudomembranes. Brushings and biopsies are obtained as needed and prepared appropriately for fungi, giant cells, and intranuclear inclusion bodies. All patients with new onset odynophagia require endoscopic evaluation.

Manometry. Strong clinical suspicion of motor dysfunction or failure of the barium swallow to reveal a probable etiology raises the question of proceeding to manometry. Although potentially diagnostic, manometry often gives indeterminate data. Many patients suspected of achalasia or esophageal spasm fail to show typical manometric findings at the time of testing. Furthermore, others who are symptom-free may demonstrate abnormalities when tested. Still others end up being placed in a category of nonspecific motility disease. Nevertheless, many authorities insist on manometric data before concluding a patient has esophageal spasm or a related motor disorder. The diagnosis of nutcracker esophagus is especially dependent on manometric data.

Provocative testing is most useful and worth serious consideration when the physician is confronted with a patient who complains of *atypical chest pain*. Once cardiac disease is ruled out (see Chapter 20), an esophageal etiology is high on the list of possible explanations. Provocative testing provides a ready means in the office of identifying an esophageal origin for an atypical pain, although it does not specify a mechanism and it is of less use in the evaluation of dysphagia. The objective of provocative testing is to reproduce the patient's exact symptoms. Two tests have proven most useful: the Bernstein or acid perfusion test and edrophonium (Tensilon) infusion.

The Bernstein test was initially used to confirm symptoms due to reflux, but a positive test has also proven specific for esophageal chest pain even in the absence of documented reflux. Seven to 27 percent of cases of noncardiac chest pain have been associated with a positive Bernstein test and deemed to be of definite esophageal cause, although evidence of acid reflux may not be found on 24-hour pH monitoring. The test consists of instilling a small amount of acid through a nasogastric tube placed in the esophagus.

Edrophonium testing grew out of a desire to find a safe and well-tolerated means of stimulating esophageal contractions. Ergonovine was originally tried, and although it was successful in reproducing symptoms, its risks of serious cardiac side effects negated its usefulness. Edrophonium (a relatively gentle muscarinic agonist) has proven superior to acid perfusion, bethanecol, and pentagastrin in reproducing atypical chest pain complaints, with 24 percent to 34 percent of patients having a positive test (reproduction of pain during wet swallows). As with the Bernstein test, edrophonium only identifies an esophageal origin for the pain, it does not specify the mechanism (correlation between response to edrophonium and manometric findings is poor). Side effects from a rapid bolus of intravenous edrophonium (80 μg/kg body weight) included mild degrees of lightheadedness, nausea, and abdominal cramps, but not the tachycardia, hypertension, or coronary vasoconstriction seen with ergonovine.

Twenty-four-hour ambulatory monitoring of both *intraesophageal* pH and *pressures* is becoming increasingly available and may prove useful, especially in cases that defy explanation despite comprehensive testing. Esophageal pH monitoring over 24 hours has emerged as a useful tool in the evaluation of noncardiac chest pain, providing an opportunity to correlate acid reflux with occurrence of symptoms.

In a study comparing traditional esophageal tests (manometry, Bernstein test, and edrophonium) with 24-hour PH monitoring, the latter led the field in providing an explanatory correlation in 46 percent of instances of chest pain versus 19 percent for both edrophonium and the Bernstein test, the next best studies. A single manometric study was of little use. Because no gold standard is available, determinations of sensitivity and specificity are not possible.

As just noted, abnormal motor activity may be difficult to detect at the time of a particular study or may be induced by the study and have little to do with the patient's problem. Round-the-clock pressure monitoring opens up new avenues of evaluation. The precise indications for such testing remain to be defined; studies are ongoing.

SYMPTOMATIC RELIEF AND PATIENT EDUCATION

Motility Disorders. A conservative approach sometimes suffices in patients with mild motor disease. The dysphagic person with achalasia is often able to manage reasonably well by *eating slowly, drinking small quantities* at a time, and *avoiding cold foods*. A trial of *sublingual nitrates* or *calcium-channel blockers* before eating may sufficiently relax spastic smooth muscle in patients with mild to moderate dysfunction to provide relief.

Patients with *atypical chest pain* due to esophageal disease benefit greatly from knowing definitively that their pain is not indicative of heart disease. Thorough explanation after a careful evaluation can greatly reduce morbidity and even the frequency of symptoms. Given the presumed relation of atypical chest pain to esophageal spasm, nitrates and calcium-channel blockers have been used. The results have been variable, which is not surprising, given the variable relation of spasm to pain; however, benefit does accrue for some patients, making a trial of these agents worthwhile. *Antireflux therapy* (see Chapter 61) can be an important component of the treatment program when the workup suggests acid reflux as a trigger of symptoms. *Antidepressants* with little anticholinergic activity, such as trazodone, have proven effective in patients suspected of having a psychiatric precipitant to esophageal motor dysfunction. *Relaxation techniques* and other *behavioral methods* are worth a try in those with stress-induced esophageal motor dysfunction (see Chapter 226). *Anticholinergic therapy* has been disappointing. When there is *odynophagia* and an inflammatory lesion is suspected as the precipitant, especially when opportunistic infection might be the cause (as in patients with HIV disease), then antifungal or antiviral therapy may be needed (see Chapter 13).

Patients with severe achalasia get little relief from dietary or drug manipulations; *esophageal dilatation* or *myotomy* is needed. Myotomy is more effective but requires major surgery and often produces severe reflux that does not respond to antireflux surgery. Consequently, pneumatic esophageal dilation is usually the most effective invasive procedure for treatment of severe motor disease. Dysphagia is relieved immediately, while there remains sufficient LES pressure to prevent bothersome reflux.

Obstructing Lesions. Regardless of etiology and pending definitive diagnosis, all patients suspected of having obstruction should be advised to take predominantly liquids or soft solids. The goal is to provide an adequate caloric intake that can be swallowed with a minimum of discomfort. Patients with mechanical obstruction often require dilatation or surgery, but there are many exceptions. The person with a lower esophageal ring is best treated by advising slow intake of small amounts; dilatation does not work very well. Restoration of adequate iron intake will reverse the pathologic changes of sideropenic dysphagia, unless a carcinoma has ensued in the pharynx. Carcinoma of the upper or middle third of the esophagus is often unresectable and best treated by radiation therapy; considerable palliation is sometimes achieved. Treatment of oropharyngeal dysphagia due to obstruction is approached surgically (eg, removal of a Zenker's diverticulum or large goiter), whereas attention to the underlying neurologic deficit is necessary in cases due to motor dysfunction, although myotomy may help as well. The patient with globus hystericus can be given thorough reassurance, although symptoms are not likely to resolve easily.

INDICATIONS FOR REFERRAL

Patients with oropharyngeal dysphagia who aspirate more than 10 percent of a barium test bolus and show barium residue in the oropharynx with subsequent swallows are at great risk of aspiration and need referral for consideration of a nonoral means of nutrition. In addition, those with evidence of sufficient neuromuscular disease to cause oropharyngeal dysphagia might benefit from a neurologic consultation. The patient with an obstructing lesion requires endoscopic evaluation and referral to a gastroenterologist or surgeon for consideration of endoscopic biopsy. The patient who is referred for further evaluation and therapy should still be followed closely by the primary physician, especially to monitor nutritional status.

A.H.G.

ANNOTATED BIBLIOGRAPHY

Achem SR, Kotts BE, Wears R, et al. Chest pain associated with nutcracker esophagus: A preliminary study of the role of gastroesophageal reflux. Am J Gastroenterol 1993;88:187. *(Reflux may play a role in up to a third of patients.)*

Bernstein LM, Baker LA. A clinical test for esophagitis. Gastroenterology 1958;34:760. *(Original description of the acid perfusion test.)*

Browning TH. Diagnosis of chest pain of esophageal origin: A guideline of the patient care committee of the American Gastroenterological Association. Dig Dis Sci 1990;35:289. *(Consensus statement offering evaluation guidelines.)*

Clouse RE, Lustman PJ. Psychiatric illness and contraction abnormalities of the esophagus. N Engl J Med 1983;309:1337. *(Documents the association between psychiatric conditions, including depression and anxiety states, and symptomatic esophageal motility disorders, many presenting as chest pain.)*

Cohen S. Esophageal motility disorders and their response to calcium channel antagonists: The sphinx revisited. Gastroenterology 1987;93:201. *(Poor response to these muscle relaxants challenges the view of a simple etiologic association.)*

Dalton CB, Castell DO, Richter JE. The changing face of the nutcracker esophagus. Am J Gastroenterology 1988;83:358. *(Detailed characterization of the condition in view of accumulating data.)*

Dipalma JA, Prechter GC, Bradie CE. X-ray negative dysphagia: Is endoscopy necessary? J Clin Gastroenterol 1984;6:409. *(Endoscopy in x-ray–negative dysphagia is generally of low yield.)*

Edwards DAW. Discriminative information in the diagnosis of dysphagia. J R Coll Physicians Lond 1975;9:257. *(Critical discussion of important historical data; diagnostic accuracy by history alone is close to 80 percent.)*

Goff JS. Infectious causes of esophagitis. Annu Rev Med 1988; 39:163. *(Excellent review of these important causes of odynophagia.)*

Hewson EG, Sinclair JW, Dalton CB, et al. Twenty-four-hour esophageal monitoring: The most useful test for evaluating noncardiac chest pain. Am J Med 1991;90:576. *(Test identified an esophageal etiology in 46 percent of instances.)*

Hurwitz AL, Duranceau A. Upper esophageal sphincter dysfunction: Pathogenesis and treatment. Am J Dig Dis 1978;23:275. *(Review of the causes of oropharyngeal dysphagia and a presentation of the results of cricopharyngeal myotomy as a method of relieving symptoms; 48 references.)*

Janssens J, Vantrappen G, Ghillebert G. 24-hour recording of esophageal pressure and pH in patients with noncardiac chest pain. Gastroenterology 1986;90:1978. *(Correlations between pressure, pH, and chest pain were often variable.)*

Katz PO, Dalton CB, Richter JE, et al. Esophageal testing of patients with noncardiac chest pain or dysphagia. Ann Intern Med 1987;106:593. *(Provocative testing proved best in those with chest pain; manometric studies were superior in those with dysphagia.)*

Kilman WJ, Goyal RK. Disorders of pharyngeal and upper esophageal sphincter motor function. Arch Intern Med 1976;136: 592. *(Thorough discussion of oropharyngeal motor diseases.)*

Kim CH, Weaver AL, Hsu JJ, et al. Discriminant value of esophageal symptoms. Mayo Clin Proc 1993;68:948. *(Further evidence of the value of a careful history; authors develop a discriminant model, but not one based on a primary care population.)*

Mukhopadhyay AK, Graham DY. Esophageal motor dysfunction in systemic diseases. Arch Intern Med 1976;36:583. *(Connective tissue disease, metabolic problems, and neuromuscular disorders are reviewed.)*

Richter JE, Bradley LA, Castell DO. Esophageal chest pain: Current controversies in pathogenesis, diagnosis, and therapy. Ann Intern Med 1989;110:66. *(Best review to date, with interesting discussion of the "irritable gut" hypothesis; 119 references.)*

Richter JE, Castell DO. Diffuse esophageal spasm: A reappraisal. Ann Intern Med 1984;100:242. *(Argues for a manometric diagnosis of spasm; critical review of diagnostic criteria.)*

Richter JE, Dalton CB, Bradley LA, et al. Oral nifedipine in the treatment of non-cardiac chest pain in patients with the nutcracker esophagus. Gastroenterology 1987;93:21. *(Disappointing results, although these agents show ability to decrease pressure.)*

Richter JE, Wu WC, Johns DN, et al. Esophageal manometry in 95 healthy adult volunteers: Variability of pressures with age and frequency of "abnormal" contractions. Dig Dis Sci 1987; 32:83. *(Documents the nonspecificity of many manometric findings and the overlap with asymptomatic patients.)*

Tavitian A, Raufman JP, Rosenthal L. Oral candidiasis as a marker for esophageal candidiasis in the acquired immunodeficiency syndrome. Ann Intern Med 1986;104:54. *(A useful clinical marker.)*

Ward BW, Wu WC, Richter JE, et al. Long-term follow-up of symptomatic status of patients with noncardiac chest pain: Is diagnosis of esophageal etiology helpful? Am J Gastroenterology 1987;82:215. *(The reassurance provided reduced morbidity and even frequency of episodes.)*

Wilcox CM. Esophageal disease in the acquired immunodeficiency syndrome: Etiology, diagnosis, and management. Am J Med 1992;92:412. *(Thorough review.)*

Young LD, Richter JE, Anderson KO, et al. Effects of psychological and environmental stressors on peristaltic esophageal contractions in healthy volunteers. Psychology 1987;24:132. *(Data suggesting that stress can induce esophageal motor dysfunction.)*

61

Approach to the Patient With Heartburn and Reflux

JAMES M. RICHTER, M.D.

Primary Care Medicine: Office Evaluation and Management of the Adult Patient, 3rd edition, edited by Allan H. Goroll, Lawrence A. May, and Albert G. Mulley, Jr. J.B. Lippincott Company, Philadelphia

Heartburn is a common gastrointestinal complaint. In one survey of presumably normal hospital staff, 7 percent reported suffering from daily heartburn and 36 percent experienced heartburn at least once a month. The term *heartburn* typically refers to retrosternal burning that radiates upward, due to reflux of gastric acid up into the esophagus. It is characteristically exacerbated by large meals, supine posture, or bending over, and alleviated, at least temporarily, by antacids. Heartburn ranges in severity from an occasional episode of postprandial discomfort without sequelae to a syndrome of severe esophageal inflammation, stricture, bleeding, and even esophageal carcinoma. Evaluation and management are best carried out in stepwise fashion.

PATHOPHYSIOLOGY AND CLINICAL PRESENTATION

The modern concept of reflux esophagitis emerged in 1935 with the proposal that esophagitis was caused by "the irritant action on the mucosa of free hydrochloric acid and pepsin." Through the 1940s and 1950s gastroesophageal reflux was believed to be related primarily to anatomic factors, specifically to the presence of a *hiatus hernia*. Many patients still refer to a "hiatus hernia" when suggesting a cause for their heartburn. Although there may be some modest predisposition to reflux disease among patients with hiatus hernia, careful studies refute a close association between hiatus hernia and gastroesophageal reflux. However, recent studies indicate that a certain amount of intraabdominal esophagus is necessary for optimal esophageal function and sphincter competence, and peristalic clearing of acid is impaired in patients with a hiatus hernia.

Esophageal manometry studies in the 1960s showed that the physiologic action of the *lower esophageal sphincter (LES)* is critical to maintaining a pressure barrier between the stomach and the esophagus. Subsequent studies suggested that the pathogenesis of reflux disease is multifactorial, depending on more than just a decrease in the resting tone of the LES. Transient inappropriate relaxations of the LES, decreased secondary peristalsis, and defective mucosal resistance have all been implicated. Inability to clear acid from the esophagus and delayed gastric emptying are other potentially important etiologic factors.

The LES is a complicated region of smooth muscle modulated by the interaction of hormonal, neural, and dietary factors. The hormone gastrin increases its resting tone, whereas estrogens, progesterone, glucagon, secretin, and cholecystokinin all decrease sphincter pressure. Vagus nerve input helps maintain resting tone, as does alpha-adrenergic stimulation. Pharmacologic agents that increase sphincter tone include bethanechol, metoclopramide, pentobarbital, histamine, edrophonium, and antacids. Anticholinergics, theophylline, meperidine, and the calcium-channel blockers all decrease the resting tone. Tobacco, ethanol, chocolate, and foods with high concentrations of fat or carbohydrate all decrease LES pressure and increase heartburn. Citrus fruits and fruit juices often exacerbate symptoms; the mechanism by which they cause heartburn is not clear. Although pregnancy may cause reflux because of increased intraabdominal pressure, the primary reason for heartburn in pregnancy is reduced sphincter pressure due to increased circulating levels of progesterone and estrogen. Reflux can be precipitated in normal persons by exercise, with jogging after meals the most common cause.

Much emphasis has been placed on measurement of *lower esophageal sphincter pressures,* but there is enormous variation and overlap between patients with symptomatic gastroesophageal reflux and normal subjects. Normal pressure ranges from 12 to 30 mm Hg. Although single pressure determinations are fraught with inaccuracies, it is reasonable to assume that LES pressures of less than 6 mm Hg are apt to allow reflux, and that pressures greater than 20 mm Hg should prohibit it. Pressures between 6 and 20 mm Hg are found in both patients and controls. Recent studies using 24-hour intraesophageal pH monitoring suggest that in many patients reflux occurs as a result of transiently inappropriate sphincter relaxations rather than low basal tone.

Other factors involved in reflux disease include alterations in esophageal mucosal resistance to caustic liquids, impaired esophageal clearance (secondary peristalsis), and prolonged rates of gastric emptying. Saliva may be an important protective mechanism, inducing peristalsis as well as aiding in washout, dilution, and neutralization of acid refluxed into the esophagus.

Heartburn predictably accompanies gastroesophageal reflux. The patient characteristically complains of retrosternal ache or burning within 30 to 60 minutes of eating, especially after large meals. Symptoms are made worse by lying down or bending over; many patients learn to avoid lying down after meals. Reflux may trigger *chest pain* than can mimic cardiac angina, with some patients describing chest heaviness or pressure that, like angina, may radiate to the neck, jaw, or shoulders (see Chapters 20 and 60).

In some cases, *regurgitation* of fluid or food particles may occur, particularly at night. The patient may describe soiling of the pillow with gastric contents or may awake because of coughing or a strangling sensation. *Nocturnal aspiration* is occasionally associated with gastroesophageal reflux and can cause recurrent pneumonias, bronchospasm, and chronic cough. A *reflex salivary hypersecretion* or *"water brash"* is sometimes described by patients with reflux. Water brash is especially common in children, but direct questioning is often required to determine its occurrence. Hoarseness, sore throat, and the feeling of a lump in the throat are other common otolaryngologic manifestations of reflux.

Pain or difficulty swallowing usually suggests long-standing reflux disease with *either* active inflammation, stricture, or both. Solid food may stick in the distal esophagus (with or without stricture formation), although food usually passes into the stomach after repeated swallows or drinking liquids, unless there is a fairly tight obstruction (see Chapter 60). Chronic gastroesophageal reflux may result in alteration of the distal esophageal mucosa, from the usual stratified squamous epithelium to a columnar epithelium. This mucosal change is called *Barrett's esophagus* and is associated with esophageal ulcers, strictures, hemorrhage, and increased risk of adenocarcinoma. Classic radiologic presentation is a midesophageal ulcer or stricture. *Bleeding* may accompany reflux esophagitis, and be either slow and chronic, resulting in iron-deficiency anemia, or brisk, resulting in hematemesis.

DIFFERENTIAL DIAGNOSIS

The diagnosis of gastroesophageal reflux disease is secure when the patient describes heartburn and experiences regurgitation of stomach contents. However, many patients report only a dull substernal discomfort or ache, and in such circumstances the physician must consider myocardial ischemia, esophageal spasm, high-amplitude esophageal peristalsis, cholelithiasis, and mediastinal inflammation. Gastroesophageal reflux may accompany peptic ulcer disease (particularly in gastric hypersecretory conditions) and cancer of the gastroesophageal junction. Esophageal infections with opportunistic organisms such as cytomegalovirus, herpes virus, and *Candida albicans* can cause heartburn in the immunocompromised host. Reflux esophagitis may also accompany intestinal dysmotility syndromes, including idiopathic intestinal pseudoobstruction, or secondary pseudoobstruction due to scleroderma. Diabetic gastroparesis may predispose a patient to reflux and heartburn, because of retarded emptying of gastric contents.

WORKUP

History. The characteristic history of a retrosternal burning sensation radiating upward, associated with large meals and supine posture, is virtually diagnostic of reflux disease. An attempt should be made to identify any aggravating factors such as intake of fatty foods, concentrated sweets, alcohol, peppermint, coffee, tea, anticholinergics, calcium-channel blockers, and theophylline compounds. Drugs capable of causing esophageal injury (nonsteroidal antiinflammatory drugs, quinidine, wax matrix potassium chloride tablets, tetracycline) should also be checked for. Inquiry should be made regarding response to antacids. Surgery near the gastroesophageal junction, for example, prior antireflux surgery or vagotomy, may predispose the patient to reflux disease. A history of Raynaud's phenomenon raises the possibility of scleroderma. Consideration of achalasia, malignancy, esophagitis, and stricture is indicated if dysphagia is part of the clinical presentation (see Chapter 60).

Physical Examination. The physical examination is generally unrevealing, but several points are worth special attention. Sclerodactyly, calcinosis, and telangiectasia suggest underlying scleroderma (see Chapter 146). The epigastrium should be carefully examined for the presence of a mass lesion, and the stool should be examined for presence of occult blood.

Laboratory Studies. No single test is accepted as the standard for the diagnosis of reflux disease. Fortunately, a careful history is sufficient for the diagnosis in the majority of patients, and laboratory tests are needed only in atypical or severe cases. When a classic reflux story is elicited, initial therapy can be instituted on the basis of history alone for simple heartburn in a young patient.

The most sensitive and specific test is *24-hour esophageal* pH *monitoring*, but it is very expensive, not universally available, and usually unnecessary. However, it does allow correlation of activity to symptoms and reflux of acid and can be of help in confusing situations, such as atypical chest pain (see Chapter 60). Nevertheless, history still remains the mainstay of diagnosis.

If there is dysphagia, painful swallowing, significant weight loss, or occult blood loss, the patient should undergo a *barium swallow* and *upper gastrointestinal (GI) series* or *endoscopy* to rule out a neoplasm or a complication of acid-peptic disease. Suspected damage to esophageal mucosa due to reflux disease can be assessed by endoscopy in conjunction with *biopsy*. The barium swallow may show inflammation, ulceration, or stricture, but it is normal in most cases. It remains widely used for reflux, but its sensitivity may be as low as 25 percent and it is far less accurate than a careful history. Its main utility is in searching for stricture and tumor.

In atypical cases, the *Bernstein acid perfusion test* is often employed to see if symptoms are due to reflux; however, the Bernstein test is rarely needed when the patient gives a classic description of heartburn, and the test requires careful interpretation because false-positives are common. It is of more use determining if chest pain is due to acid reflux (see Chapter 60).

SYMPTOMATIC MANAGEMENT

Otherwise healthy patients with classic history of uncomplicated reflux can be treated empirically, employing step 1 and step 2 measures (Table 61–1). In many instances, these measures will suffice. If the patient fails to respond or if heartburn is complicated by dysphagia, weight loss, anemia, or stool test positive for occult bleeding, then, as noted earlier, a more comprehensive diagnostic investigation is indicated. A detailed evaluation is especially important in older patients, in whom the risk of malignancy is increased.

Dietary Measures and Suppression of Gastric Acid Production. Therapy for reflux disease is best approached in a stepwise fashion, beginning with simple nonpharmacologic measures and *adding* pharmacologic intervention as needed. The first and most important steps are *dietary intervention, lifestyle modification,* and *antacids* (see Table 61-1, step 1). Attention to these measures is essential to a good outcome; they will often suffice. Even if additional therapy is needed, these conservative measures constitute the foundation of all treatment programs and must not be omitted. They represent the most cost-effective approach to therapy for the majority of patients.

An H_2*-blocker* can be added if necessary (step 2). In many instances, H_2-blockers are used in place of high-dose

Table 61-1. Treatment of Esophageal Reflux

Step 1.
a. Dietary manipulations—avoidance of foods high in fat or carbohydrate (chocolate can be particularly problematic, being high in both)
b. Weight reduction if obese
c. Avoidance of large evening meals near bedtime or before exercise
d. Elevation of the head of the bed with 6-inch blocks under the bedposts (pillows are not adequate)
e. Avoidance, if possible, of medications that decrease sphincter tone, including theophylline compounds, calcium-channel blockers, meperidine, and anticholinergics
f. Avoidance, if possible, of drugs that may injure the esophageal mucosa (tetracycline, quinidine, wax matrix KCl tablets, NSAIDs)
g. Avoidance of cigarettes, alcohol, coffee
h. Antacids after meals and at bedtime

Step 2. Add:
a. Oral H_2-blocker (bid regimen best, eg, ranitidine 150 mg, cimetidine 800 mg, famotidine 20 mg)

Step 3. Add:
a. Omeprazole (20–40 mg/day); limit to no more than 3–6 months; drug of choice for erosive esophagitis

Step 4. Add:
a. Metoclopramide (a dopamine antagonist); 10–15 mg qid *or*
b. Cisapride (a dopimine antagonist); 10–20 mg qid *or*
c. Bethanechol (a cholinergic agent) 25 mg qid), *or*

Step 5. Consider:
a. Antireflux surgery for incapacitating refractory disease

antacid therapy, providing better and more convenient round-the-clock symptom relief and esophageal healing. A twice-daily, full-dose regimen achieves best results (eg, cimetidine 800 mg bid, ranitidine 150 mg bid, or famotidine 20 mg bid), although in milder cases of reflux, a once-daily dose at the time of maximal symptoms will suffice, especially if combined with antacids.

Patients with symptoms refractory to full implementation of dietary and lifestyle modifications in conjunction with high doses of H_2-blockers and those with erosive esophagitis are candidates for *omeprazole* therapy (step 3). A single daily dose of this gastric proton pump inhibitor achieves nearly complete suppression of gastric acid production. It has demonstrated efficacy in the healing of erosive lesions and controlling refractory symptoms. However, relapses after completion of therapy are common, and the safety of chronic therapy is not yet established. Rats given large omeprazole doses for prolonged periods develop gastric carcinoid tumors, perhaps in response to the high gastrin levels that ensue. Omeprazole is approved for no more than 3 months of continuous use at a time, although sometimes repeated courses or more chronic use is necessary in severe cases. A common approach to prevention of relapse is to follow a course of omeprazole with a maintenance program of chronic H_2-blocker therapy. Use of omeprazole for step-2 care has been suggested, but not prospectively tested in controlled trials.

Prokinetic Therapy. A few patients will report persistent symptoms despite the above measures. In such situations prokinetic drugs have been used in an attempt to increase LES pressure and halt reflux (step 4). The leading choice is the dopamine receptor antagonist *metoclopramide*. The drug augments gastric emptying and raises LES tone. It is most useful for patients with reflux without heartburn and those with gastroparesis. However, up to a third of patients may not tolerate the drug because of its central nervous system side effects. *Cisapride,* a dopamine antagonist that does not cross the blood–brain barrier, represents an advance in prokinetic therapy; side effects are minimal.

The alternative prokinetic agent is the potent anticholinergic *bethanechol,* which raises LES pressure, increases salivary flow, and improves acid clearance by the esophagus. The drug is contraindicated in those with asthma and other conditions in which anticholinergic therapy may aggravate symptoms.

Antireflux surgery (fundoplication, crural tightening, and return of the esophagogastric junction to below the diaphragm) represents a more aggressive approach to treatment (step 5). It is best reserved for patients who experience disabling refractory symptoms or such complications as stricture, bleeding, Barrett's esophagus, or pulmonary aspiration. Results are best in younger patients and those with preserved function of the esophageal body. A major complication of surgery is difficulty with gastric emptying, which can lead to chronic bloating. Normal gastric emptying should be demonstrated before subjecting a patient to surgery. It appears that a substantial percentage of surgical repairs break down after 5 years, although symptoms do not necessarily return. Reoperation may be necessary.

Chronic Care. Management of gastroesophageal reflux disease can be a challenge. Relapse rates are high, often necessitating indefinite continuation of dietary, postural, behavioral, and even pharmacologic measures. H_2-blocker therapy may be required chronically (sometimes, reduced doses will suffice). Although effective, omeprazole cannot be recommended for indefinite use until its long-term safety is established; follow-up H_2-blocker therapy is the best means of preventing relapse. Antireflux surgery represents a final option for patients with a serious complication or refractory disease, but durability of the repair is a concern.

Patients with long-standing severe reflux may develop columnar epithelialization of the distal esophagus (*Barrett's esophagus*) as a response to chronic acid injury. Such patients are at increased risk of developing esophageal adenocarcinoma (annual incidence 0.6% per year). Some specialists advocate annual endoscopic surveillance screening of such patients, but biopsy is often necessary to detect dysplasia or early malignancy. The cost-effectiveness of such monitoring remains unsettled, although some authorities recommend endoscopic biopsy every 2 to 3 years. The condition is not reversible.

In some patients, chronic reflux has resulted in respiratory problems, particularly *chronic cough,* believed due to nocturnal reflux and subsequent aspiration (see Chapter 41). Pharyngitis, nocturnal coughing and choking spells, and wheezing have also been described. A trial of antireflux therapy is indicated when a patient with chronic pulmonary complaints reports symptoms of reflux. Several weeks of treatment may be needed to allow for airway healing before symptom resolution is noted. Any use of theophylline for pulmonary complaints in patients with reflux should be stopped, because it might aggravate the problem by reducing LES pressure (see Chapter 48).

PATIENT EDUCATION

Successful management depends on the patient's compliance with medications, diet, and postural measures. A thorough explanation of the mechanisms of reflux and its aggravating factors helps provide a rational basis for the patient's action. Patients need to realize that no single measure will alleviate the discomfort of reflux, but when all are performed together, relief is extremely likely. The lack of direct connection between hiatus hernia and reflux also deserves mention because it is a common misunderstanding and often leads to a belief that surgery is required for treatment.

ANNOTATED BIBLIOGRAPHY

Achkar E, Carey W. The cost of surveillance for adenocarcinoma complicating Barrett's esophagus. Am J Gastroenterol 1988; 83:291. *(Annual incidence 0.6 percent; yearly surveillance cost $62,000 and 78 lost days of work to find one cancer.)*

Altorki NK, Skinner DB. Pathophysiology of gastroesophageal reflux. Am J Med 1989;86:685. *(Useful review; emphasizes LES physiology and role of the intraabdominal esophagus; 61 references.)*

Castell DO. Medical therapy for reflux esophagitis. Ann Intern Med 1986;104:112. *(Useful editorial on treatment modalities and a phased approach to therapy.)*

Cohen S. Pathogenesis of gastrointestinal reflux disease. Ann Intern Med 1992;117:1051. *(Editorial reviewing mechanisms.)*

Cohen S. Pathogenesis of coffee-induced gastrointestinal symptoms. N Engl J Med 1980;303:122. *(Suggests that LES dysfunction and gastroesophageal reflux are the cause of coffee-induced heartburn in susceptible individuals.)*

Fink SM, McCallum RW. The role of prolonged esophageal pH monitoring in the diagnosis of esophageal reflux. JAMA 1984;252:1160. *(Indications for use.)*

Gaynor EB. Otolaryngologic manifestations of gastroesophageal reflux. Am J Gastroenterol 1991;86:801. *(Voice change, chronic cough, and lump in throat are among the ENT symptoms reported.)*

Harvey RF, Hadley N, Gill TR. Effects of sleeping with the bedhead raised and of ranitidine in patients with severe peptic oesophagitis. Lancet 1987;2:1200. *(Both were better than either alone; each was equally effective alone.)*

Helm JF, Dodds WJ, Pelc LR, et al. Effect of esophageal emptying and saliva on clearance of acid from the esophagus. N Engl J Med 1984;310:284. *(Documents the importance of proper emptying and saliva on mucosal integrity.)*

Hetzel DJ, Dent J, Reed WD, et al. Healing and relapse of severe peptic esophagitis after treatment with omeprazole. Gastroenterology 1988;95:903. *(Rate of healing excellent, but high incidence of relapse.)*

Hillman AL, Bloom BS, Fendrick AM, et al. Cost and quality effects of alternative treatments for persistent gastroesophageal reflux disease. Arch Intern Med 1992;152:1467. *(A decision–analysis study suggests omeprazole may be best for patients who fail step-1 therapy.)*

Holt S, Howden CW. Omeprazole: Overview and opinion. Dig Dis Sci 1991;36:385. *(Pharmacology and use in clinical practice; 93 references.)*

Jonsell G, DeMeester P. Comparison of diagnostic methods for selection of patients for antireflux operations. Surgery 1984; 95:2. *(Review of what should be done before subjecting patients to surgery.)*

Kitchin LI, Castell DO. Rationale and efficacy of conservative therapy for gastroesophageal reflux disease. Arch Intern Med 1991;151:448. *(Review stressing the importance of dietary, lifestyle, and antacid regimens.)*

Kraus BB, Sinclair JW, Castell DO. Gastroesophageal reflux in runners. Ann Intern Med 1990;112:429. *(Finds that it does occur during running and responds to prophylactic ranitidine.)*

Lieberman DA, Keefe EB. Treatment of severe reflux esophagitis with cimetidine and metoclopramide. Ann Intern Med 1986; 104:21. *(Demonstrates symptomatic and endoscopic improvement, but frequency of side effects was high.)*

Richter JE. A critical review of current medical therapy for gastrointestinal reflux. J Clin Gastroenterol 1986;8(suppl I):72. *(Superb review of studies on efficacy of therapy; 69 references.)*

Richter JE, Castell DO. Drugs, foods, and other substances in the cause and treatment of reflux esophagitis. Med Clin North Am 1981;65:1223. *(Review of precipitants and importance of attending to them in treatment.)*

Sabesin SM, Berlin RG, Humphries TJ, et al. Famotidine relieves symptoms of gastroesophageal reflux disease and heals erosions and ulcerations. Results of a multi-center, placebo-controlled, dose-ranging study. Arch Intern Med 1991;151:2394. *(A 20-mg bid regimen was superior to a single 40-mg dose.)*

Sloan S, Rademaker AW, Kahrilas PJ. Determinants of gastroesophageal junction incompetence: Hiatal hernia, lower esophageal sphincter, or both. Ann Intern Med 1992;117:977. *(Fresh look at pathophysiologic mechanisms; evidence for both.)*

Spechler SJ. Barrett's esophagus: What's new and what to do. Am J Gastroenterol 1989;84:220. *(Cancer risks, diagnosis and management.)*

Spechler SJ, et al. Comparison of medical and surgical therapy for complicated gastroesophageal reflux disease in veterans. N Engl J Med 1992;326:786. *(In men with complicated disease, surgery was better than intensive medical therapy [although omeprazole was not used].)*

Thamik KD, Chey WY, Shah AN, Gutierrez JG. Reflux esophagitis: Effect of bethanechol on symptoms and endoscopic findings. Ann Intern Med 1980;93:805. *(Shows efficacy of cholinergic therapy for reflux disease.)*

Winnan GR, Meyer CT, McCallum RW. Interpretation of the Bernstein test. A reappraisal of criteria. Ann Intern Med 1982;96:320. *(Reviews technique and sources of confusion in interpretation of results.)*

62
Evaluation of Jaundice

JAMES M. RICHTER, M.D.

Primary Care Medicine: Office Evaluation and Management of the Adult Patient, 3rd edition, edited by Allan H. Goroll, Lawrence A. May, and Albert G. Mulley, Jr. J.B. Lippincott Company, Philadelphia

The onset of jaundice usually prompts the patient or the patient's family to seek medical attention. When associated symptoms are minimal, the patient is likely to present on an ambulatory basis, concerned about hepatitis or cancer. The primary physician needs to distinguish jaundice due to hepatocellular dysfunction (which can be managed medically) from that due to biliary tract obstruction (which usually requires an anatomic intervention). More specific determination of etiology is a secondary task that is less important to initial decision making. Effective clinical assessment necessitates familiarity with the mechanisms and clinical presentations of jaundice as well as the indications for and limitations of the noninvasive diagnostic studies available in the outpatient setting.

PATHOPHYSIOLOGY AND CLINICAL PRESENTATION

The mechanisms responsible for jaundice include excess bilirubin production, decreased hepatic uptake, impaired conjugation, intrahepatic cholestasis, extrahepatic obstruction, and hepatocellular injury. Clinically, jaundice becomes noticeable when the serum bilirubin reaches 2.0 to 2.5 mg per 100 mL The yellow hue may be mimicked by carotenemia, but in the latter there is no scleral icterus. Deeply jaundiced patients often demonstrate a greenish tinge resulting from the oxidation of bilirubin to biliverdin.

Excess bilirubin production results from accelerated red cell destruction. Occasionally, markedly ineffective erythropoiesis may be responsible. The excessive amounts of hemoglobin and resultant bilirubin released into the bloodstream overwhelm the normal liver's capacity for uptake, and an unconjugated hyperbilirubinemia ensues. Total bilirubin rises as a result of the increased indirect fraction. All tests of hepatocellular function are normal (as are urine and stool appearances). Symptoms, signs, and laboratory tests point to hemolysis or ineffective erythropoiesis (see Chapter 78).

Decreased uptake and conjugation are other mechanisms of unconjugated hyperbilirubinemia. The only evidence of hepatocellular dysfunction is an increase in unconjugated bilirubin. Frequently there is a concurrent, acquired illness such as an infection, cardiac disease, or cancer. Hereditary conditions, such as Gilbert's and Crigler-Najjar syndromes are often responsible. *Gilbert's syndrome* is the most common cause. It is a benign disorder that produces recurrent self-limited episodes of mild jaundice. Typically, the unconjugated fraction rises to no more than 1.5 to 3.0 mg per 100 mL In Gilbert's syndrome, fasting and minor illness can precipitate jaundice.

Intrahepatic cholestasis may occur at a number of levels: intracellularly (eg, hepatitis), at the canalicular level (when estrogen-induced), at the ductule (phenothiazine exposure), at the septal ducts (primary biliary cirrhosis), and at the intralobular ducts (cholangiocarcinoma). Regardless of site, there are similarities in presentation. Jaundice begins gradually; pruritus is common. The liver is large, smooth, and nontender; it may be firm but not rock hard. Splenomegaly is unlikely except in primary biliary cirrhosis. Stools are pale, and steatorrhea is present in severe cases. There is a hyperbilirubinemia, predominantly of the conjugated fraction, with marked alkaline phosphatase elevation, mild transaminase rise, and normal serum albumin. Urine is dark and positive for bilirubin. Prothrombin time may be prolonged due to malabsorption but is reversible by vitamin K injection.

Extrahepatic obstruction occurs when stone, stricture, or tumor block the flow of bile within the extrahepatic biliary tree. A history of gallstones, biliary tract surgery, or prior malignancy may be elicited. The gallbladder is sometimes palpable, especially when there is gradual development of obstruction, allowing time for painless dilatation of the biliary tree. Sudden onset with pain results from passage of a stone that becomes wedged into the common duct; fever and sepsis may follow shortly thereafter, indicating cholangitis. Weight loss is a nonspecific finding, but when it is marked and accompanied by jaundice, it suggests carcinoma of the head of the pancreas or metastatic disease obstructing the common duct. Extrahepatic obstruction and intrahepatic cholestasis may be identical in presentation. The liver is usually enlarged; tenderness is minimal unless cholangitis or rapid distention occurs. A rock-hard mass strongly points to malignancy. As in intrahepatic cholestasis, conjugated bilirubin exhibits the greatest rise in association with a high serum alkaline phosphatase and a mild to moderate increase in the transaminase level. Any prolongation of prothrombin time is at least partially reversible with parenteral vitamin K. Urine is dark because of the conjugated bilirubinuria. Stools are pale from absence of bile.

Hepatocellular disease is typified by hepatitis, with prodromal symptoms of anorexia, nausea, abdominal pain, and malaise preceding jaundice (see Chapters 52 and 70). Hepatic tenderness and some hepatomegaly are common. There may be ecchymoses. Transaminases may reach dramatic levels, except in cases of hepatitis C and alcoholic hepatitis, in which the rise is no more than five times normal. The alkaline phosphatase rises modestly to two to four times above the baseline. Urine is dark, and stools are pale. There may be evidence of decreased protein synthesis. The prothrombin time is the first measure of synthetic function to become abnormal, because the half-lives of the clotting factors made in the liver are less than 7 days. If synthetic function remains depressed beyond 2 weeks, the serum albumin begins to fall. Chronic hepatocellular disease may lead to fibrosis and cirrhosis with portal hypertension, peripheral edema, ascites, gynecomastia, testicular atrophy, bleeding, and encephalopathy (see Chapter 71).

DIFFERENTIAL DIAGNOSIS

The causes of jaundice are extensive but can be grouped according to major pathophysiologic mechanisms and type of hyperbilirubinemia (conjugated or unconjugated; Table 62–1). It is important to recognize that more than one mechanism can be operating in a given case. The vast majority of cases are due to obstruction, intrahepatic cholestasis, or hepatocellular injury. In young patients, hepatitis predominates. In the elderly, stones and tumor are often responsible. Drugs account for many cases of intrahepatic cholestasis and often mimic extrahepatic etiologies.

WORKUP

History and physical examination often provide a diagnosis or at least indicate whether the underlying pathophysiology is hepatocellular injury or biliary obstruction. In a study of 61 cases of jaundice documented by liver biopsy, history and physical examination alone correctly identified 70 percent of viral hepatitis cases, 80 percent of cirrhosis cases, and 77 percent of those with obstructive jaundice.

History. Key historical items found useful for discriminating among etiologies included presence of abdominal pain (indicative of obstruction) and history of alcoholism, exposure to hepatitis, and flulike onset (all suggestive of a hepa-

Table 62-1. Differential Diagnosis of Jaundice by Pathophysiologic Mechanisms

A. Unconjugated hyperbilirubinemias (urine negative for bilirubin)
   1. Increased bilirubin production
   2. Decreased hepatic uptake of bilirubin
   3. Decreased conjugation
B. Conjugated hyperbilirubinemias (urine positive for bilirubin)
   1. Hepatocellular disease
   2. Intrahepatic cholestasis
   3. Extrahepatic obstruction

tocellular etiology). Of little discriminant value were history of weight loss, pruritus, nausea, vomiting, and distaste for tobacco. Dark urine and pale stools confirm a conjugated hyperbilirubinemia but do not distinguish between hepatic and obstructive disease. Absence of abdominal pain does not rule out obstruction, especially that which develops slowly from tumor growth or primary biliary cirrhosis. History should also be checked for other hepatocellular disease risk factors (eg, previous blood transfusion, travel to an area endemic for hepatitis, raw shellfish consumption, intravenous drug abuse, high-risk sexual practices, use of potentially hepatotoxic drugs). History of gallstones, previous biliary tract surgery, and high fever point toward an obstructive cause. Family history of episodic jaundice in the setting of an intercurrent illness is consistent with Gilbert's disease. Intrahepatic cholestasis is a consideration if the patient reports use of estrogens, phenothiazines, and other drugs that can cause cholestasis.

Physical Examination. Findings that favor a diagnosis of advanced hepatocellular disease include a small liver, signs of portal hypertension (ascites, splenomegaly, prominent abdominal venous pattern), asterixis, peripheral edema (from hypoalbuminemia), spider angiomata, gynecomastia, and palmar erythema. Mild to moderate hepatic enlargement and mild tenderness to punch are also consistent with early or mild hepatocellular disease, especially that due to acute viral hepatitis. A palpable gallbladder (Courvoisier's sign) suggests malignant obstruction of the common bile duct. Marked hepatic enlargement (6 cm or more below the inferior costal margin) occurs in some instances of extrahepatic obstruction as well as with advanced hepatic infiltration, severe passive hepatic congestion, and metastatic cancer to the liver. If obstruction is acute in onset, there may be some associated guarding, rebound tenderness, and fever. The finding of ecchymoses is consistent with both obstructive and hepatocellular mechanisms. The same is true for detection of pale stools and dark urine.

Laboratory investigation can be used to identify the predominant pathophysiology and to assess severity, especially when history and physical findings are nondiagnostic. Testing begins with a check of the *urine for bilirubin,* a simple, inexpensive, yet often overlooked test, which can be performed quickly in the office. Because only conjugated bilirubin appears in the urine, its presence indicates a conjugated hyperbilirubinemia and the possibility of cholestasis, obstruction, or hepatocellular injury; its absence argues for excess bilirubin production, decreased uptake, and impaired conjugation. Determinations of *direct* and *indirect serum bilirubin* levels quantitatively confirm urinary findings and indicate disease severity.

An elevation predominantly of the unconjugated bilirubin fraction and a negative urinary bilirubin should initiate a search for hemolysis (see Chapter 79), ineffective erythropoiesis, hereditary causes of jaundice, and concurrent systemic illness. Standard "liver function tests" add little to the assessment of unconjugated hyperbilirubinemia; they are normal or very mildly and nonspecifically elevated.

Conjugated hyperbilirubinemia and a positive urine necessitate a check of *transaminases* (SGOT, SGPT)—newer nomenclature refers to them as the *aminotransferases* (AST, ALT)—*alkaline phosphatase, prothrombin time,* and *serum albumin.* Mechanical obstruction and intrahepatic cholestasis are characterized by marked rises in *alkaline phosphatase* (greater than four to five times normal) and modest elevations in *transaminases* (two to three times normal). Hepatocellular disease characteristically causes a proportionately far greater rise in serum transaminase levels than in alkaline phosphatase concentrations. As noted earlier, two exceptions are hepatitis C and alcoholic hepatitis, where transaminases may be only mildly elevated (no more than two to three times the upper limits of normal). SGPT (ALT) elevations are more specific for liver disease; SGOT also rises with myocardial or skeletal muscle injury.

Unfortunately, not all conditions in which the alkaline phosphatase is markedly elevated have an obstructive pathophysiology. An intrahepatic cholestatic picture occasionally occurs in some cases of hepatocellular injury, such as with viral, alcoholic, and drug-induced forms of hepatitis. However, a low alkaline phosphatase (under 50 IU per 100 mL) is rarely seen in the presence of extrahepatic obstruction. Elevations in alkaline phosphatase also occur in settings of increased bone metabolism. Bony etiologies can be distinguished from hepatobiliary ones by measuring the *heat stable fraction* of the enzyme or the *5′ nucleotidase* (which are of hepatobiliary tract origin).

Further separation of hepatocellular disease from cholestatic and obstructive conditions can be attempted by studying measures of liver synthetic function. A prolonged *prothrombin time* unresponsive to parenteral vitamin K is strongly suggestive of hepatocellular failure. Cholestasis and obstruction may also produce prolongation of the prothrombin, but it can be reversed by vitamin K. *Serum albumin* levels fall when substantial hepatocellular injury has occurred and synthetic capacity has been suppressed for a few weeks. Interpretation of the albumin level requires consideration of dietary intake and sources of possible protein loss.

In most instances, hepatocellular disease can be distinguished from cholestasis and extrahepatic obstruction on the basis of clinical data, liver function tests, and response to vitamin K.* On the other hand, cholestasis and obstruction may be indistinguishable without further testing. The dis-

*Instances of anaphylaxis have been reported with intravenous use of vitamin K. Intramuscular or subcutaneous administration is preferable.

tinction is critical to management, because mechanical obstruction requires direct surgical, endoscopic, or radiologic intervention to restore bile flow.

Clinical evaluation and liver function tests have a sensitivity of 90 percent for detection of obstruction, but they have a predictive value of only 75 percent; 25 percent of patients suspected on clinical grounds of having obstruction turn out to have hepatocellular disease with a cholestatic picture. Thus, the clinical impression of obstruction must be confirmed by imaging techniques. When the clinical likelihood of obstruction is low, imaging studies are generally unnecessary.

Liver biopsy is sometimes important for determining the cause of hepatocellular injury (see also Chapters 70 and 71) but is unwise in the setting of possible obstructive jaundice because it can lead to bile peritonitis if there is obstruction. Once obstruction is ruled out or relieved, biopsy is an important consideration if more precise identification of the underlying hepatocellular illness is required.

Study of the biliary tree is necessary to differentiate intrahepatic cholestasis from extrahepatic obstruction and can be achieved by ultrasonography, computed tomography (CT), percutaneous transhepatic cholangiography, and endoscopic retrograde cannulation.

Ultrasonography has emerged as the noninvasive study of choice in the evaluation of jaundice. Specificity is better than 90 percent. Sensitivity ranges from 47 percent to 90 percent, depending on the duration and degree of bile duct obstruction. Cases of early, acute, or intermittent obstruction may be missed unless ultrasound study is repeated after the ducts have had a few days to dilate. False-positive results may occur from ductal dilatation that persists after cholecystectomy or relief of obstruction. In about half of cases, ultrasonography cannot indicate the level of obstruction, nor is it particularly good at detecting the cause of the obstruction, unless it is due to a mass in the head of the pancreas. Stones in the common duct are frequently missed. Ultrasound studies done in patients with overlying bowel gas or marked obesity are often of inadequate technical quality, necessitating a repeat study or CT.

CT is similar to ultrasonography in sensitivity, specificity, and predictive value for diagnosis of obstructive jaundice. It has many of the same shortcomings plus greater expense and radiation exposure. As such, it is a second-choice test after ultrasonography. However, results are not obscured by overlying bowel gas or fat and there is better ability to detect the level of obstruction than with ultrasound. Moreover, if surgical intervention is being considered, the test is helpful in providing more definitive anatomic information. Nonetheless, cholangiography is usually still necessary.

If obstruction is strongly suspected on clinical grounds (even if the ultrasonography or CT is negative) or if additional anatomic detail is required for planning treatment, *percutaneous transhepatic cholangiography* or *retrograde cannulation* of the common bile duct is indicated. Both procedures are relatively safe, have similar complication rates, have similar rates of visualization, and provide equally diagnostic information. The predictive value of a positive test is very high, but occasionally stones are missed in dilated ductal systems. Some authorities suggest that proceeding directly to one of these procedures and skipping noninvasive study is indicated when there is very strong clinical suspicion of obstruction.

Transhepatic cholangiography is technically simple in patients with dilated intrahepatic ducts; however, 3 percent to 10 percent of patients experience cholangitis, hemorrhage, or bile leakage. Retrograde cholangiography is more difficult but allows examination of the ampulla and pancreas and has a slightly lower incidence of serious complications. For patients who may have a retained common duct stone after cholecystectomy, the opportunity to perform an endoscopic papillotomy makes the retrograde cholangiogram advantageous. Techniques have been developed for draining an obstructed biliary tract either endoscopically or transhepatically. Overall, both procedures are valuable diagnostically and have therapeutic uses as well; final selection is based on the clinical circumstance as well as on local availability and expertise. Selection should be made in consultation with a surgeon, radiologist, or gastroenterologist experienced in evaluating obstructive jaundice.

Other studies deserve comment, more for their limited usefulness than because they are indicated in evaluation of jaundice. *Plain films* of the abdomen and *upper gastrointestinal (GI) series* rarely provide diagnostic information. Hepatobiliary scintigraphy is better suited for diagnosis of cholecystitis; it provides poor anatomic resolution and often cannot aid in distinguishing between intrahepatic cholestasis and extrahepatic obstruction. *Cholescintigraphy* is useful for diagnosis of acute cholecystitis and cystic duct obstruction (see Chapter 69), but it has no value in the evaluation of jaundice and can be misleading.

INDICATIONS FOR ADMISSION, CONSULTATION, AND REFERRAL

Most patients with jaundice turn out to have acute viral hepatitis and can be managed on an ambulatory basis, unless they are unable to maintain their hydration or begin to show evidence of severe hepatocellular failure (see Chapter 71). Admission is mandatory when jaundice is complicated by fever and peritoneal signs indicative of cholangitis. Intravenous antibiotics and prompt surgical consultation are required.

As noted earlier, when there is clinical suspicion of extrahepatic obstruction, consultation with a gastroenterologist, surgeon, or radiologist experienced in the evaluation of jaundice can be very useful, especially when there is difficulty differentiating between intrahepatic cholestasis and extrahepatic obstruction.

When hepatocellular disease is suspect, and there is evidence of hepatic failure, portal hypertension or encephalopathy, or when jaundice persists longer than 3 months, liver biopsy may be indicated for definitive diagnosis. Consultation should be sought with a gastroenterologist familiar with liver disease and needle biopsy techniques.

SYMPTOMATIC RELIEF

Mild jaundice in itself is innocuous, but more marked elevations in bilirubin may produce considerable pruritus. Presumably the mechanism involves bile salt deposition in the skin, although recent evidence refutes this view. Cholestyramine has been used successfully to treat pruritus and is worth a try in patients who are uncomfortable. One 9-g packet of the powder containing 4 g of cholestyramine resin is mixed in orange juice or apple sauce and taken three times a day. Absorption of fat-soluble vitamins may be impaired by cholestyramine, and oral or parenteral supplements of vitamins A, D, and K can be prescribed. Absorption of drugs may also be interfered with; drugs should be taken at least 1 hour before cholestyramine. Constipation or diarrhea is a minor common side effect.

ANNOTATED BIBLIOGRAPHY

Datta D, Sherlock S. Cholestyramine for long term relief of the pruritus complicating intrahepatic cholestasis. Gastroenterology 1966;50:323. *(Cholestyramine is effective; 4 to 7 days of therapy are required before relief is obtained.)*

Felsher B, Rickard D, Redeker A. The reciprocal relation between caloric intake and the degree of hyperbilirubinemia in Gilbert's syndrome. N Engl J Med 1970;283:170. *(Increase in unconjugated bilirubin occurred with fasting or low-caloric intake—approximately 400 calories.)*

Frank BB, Members of the Patient Care Committee of the American Gastroenterological Association. Clinical evaluation of jaundice. JAMA 1989;262:3031. *(Comprehensive, but terse overview of the approach to the jaundiced patient.)*

Levine R, Klatskin G. Unconjugated hyperbilirubinemia in the absence of overt hemolysis. Am J Med 1964;36:541. *(High proportion traceable to a concurrent illness rather than a hereditary condition.)*

Matzen P, Malchow-Moller A, Brun B. Ultrasound, computed tomography, and cholescintigraphy in suspected obstructive jaundice. Gastroenterology 1983;84:1492. *(Presents data on test sensitivity and specificity.)*

Mueller PR, van Sonnenberg E, Simenone JF. Fine needle transhepatic cholangiography. Ann Intern Med 1982;97:567. *(Radiologist's view of this technique and its central role in the evaluation of biliary obstruction.)*

O'Connor KW, Snodgrass PJ, Swonder JE, et al. A blinded prospective study comparing four current noninvasive approaches in the differential diagnosis of medical versus surgical jaundice. Gastroenterology 1983;84:1498. *(Demonstrates the importance and accuracy of clinical evaluation.)*

Richter JM, Silverstein MD, Schapiro RH. Suspected obstructive jaundice: A decision analysis of diagnostic strategies. Ann Intern Med 1983;99:46. *(Comparison of comprehensive diagnostic strategies for the investigation of suspected obstructive jaundice.)*

Scharschmidt BF, Goldberg HI, Schmid R. Approach to the patient with cholestatic jaundice. N Engl J Med 1983;308:1515. *(Good review of tests available for workup of obstructive jaundice.)*

Schenker S, Balint J, Schiff L. Differential diagnosis of jaundice: Report of a prospective study of 61 proved cases. Am J Dig Dis 1962;7:449. *(Classic study of the merits of clinical features and laboratory tests in the differential diagnosis of jaundice.)*

Sherman KE. Alanine aminotransferase in clinical practice. Arch Intern Med 1991;151:260. *(Review of this increasingly used aminotransferase for detection of hepatocellular injury; 26 references.)*

63
Evaluation of Gastrointestinal Bleeding

DEBRA F. WEINSTEIN, M.D.
JAMES M. RICHTER, M.D.

Primary Care Medicine: Office Evaluation and Management of the Adult Patient, 3rd edition, edited by Allan H. Goroll, Lawrence A. May, and Albert G. Mulley, Jr. J.B. Lippincott Company, Philadelphia

Ambulatory patients frequently report gastrointestinal (GI) bleeding to the primary physician. They may complain of *melena* (tarry-black stools), *hematochezia* (bright red or maroon blood per rectum), or *hematemesis* (vomiting fresh or changed blood). Sometimes, GI bleeding may be evident only as a *positive screening test for fecal occult blood*. Decisions regarding the nature and pace of the evaluation of GI bleeding depend on the characteristics, severity, and acuity of the problem. Proper decision making requires a knowledge of the probability of a serious underlying lesion and of the sensitivity and specificity of contrast studies, endoscopy, and stool guaiac testing.

PATHOPHYSIOLOGY AND CLINICAL PRESENTATION

Hematemesis usually represents bleeding proximal to the ligament of Treitz, although the site of blood loss may, on rare occasions, be in the jejunum. The absence of hematemesis does not, however, exclude the possibility of active upper GI bleeding. *Melena* is usually seen with blood loss proximal to the ileocecal valve, where hemoglobin is converted into hematin, which gives the stool its tarry appearance. Right colonic bleeding may also cause melena when transit is slow. *Hematochezia* most often originates in the left colon or anorectal region, although very brisk movement of blood from the right colon, small bowel, or even stomach can lead to a similar presentation. *Occult GI bleeding* may be indicated by a positive test for fecal occult blood or may be suggested by the presence of iron deficiency anemia without apparent cause. The source may be anywhere in the GI tract.

Manifestations of blood loss are a function of the rate and chronicity of bleeding. *Postural hypotension* (orthostatic fall of > 10 mm Hg of blood pressure and/or an increase of > 10 beats per minute in heart rate on moving from supine to standing) in the setting of known bleeding suggests serious acute hemorrhage and intravascular volume depletion. *Fatigue* and *exertional dyspnea* are typical presenting symptoms of someone with slow, but chronic blood loss. Patient descriptions of the volume of bleeding are frequently unreliable.

DIFFERENTIAL DIAGNOSIS

The chief causes of GI bleeding can be conveniently grouped by clinical presentation (Table 63–1). Hematemesis prompts consideration of important upper GI etiologies. Melena requires consideration of upper GI causes as well as small intestinal and right colonic sources. Hematochezia raises the question of anorectal or colonic disease and, if brisk, a small bowel or even upper GI lesion. The prevalence of specific disorders varies with the population studied, diagnostic methods employed, and time of investigation in relation to bleeding.

Melena or Hematemesis. A British series of 277 patients with melena or hematemesis provides representative prevalence figures in a population composed of both outpatients and patients seen in emergency rooms. More than 85 percent of the patients in this study underwent endoscopy; diagnosis was also made by upper GI series or at surgery: 20 percent had duodenal ulcers, 15 percent had gastric ulcers, 12 percent had Mallory-Weiss tears, 11 percent had esophageal varices, 5 percent had gastritis, and 1 percent had gastric cancer. In 21 percent, no cause was found (half of these patients did not undergo endoscopy), and in 5 percent-multiple lesions were detected. Patients with chronic renal failure are at increased risk of bleeding, with angiodysplasia and esophagitis being the most common sources.

Hematochezia. In the setting of severe *hematochezia,* age has a major influence on the differential diagnosis. In young adults, Meckel's diverticulum, inflammatory bowel disease, and polyps lead the list of causes. In adults to age 60, diverticulosis, inflammatory bowel disease, and polyps are the predominant etiologies, followed by malignancy and a-v malformations. In those over age 60, the vascular ectasias, diverticulosis, malignancy, and polyps are responsble for most cases.

In a study of 311 patients who complained of *mild–moderate anorectal bleeding* and were evaluated by careful physical examination, sigmoidoscopy, and barium enema, 79 percent had lesions of the anal canal, 15 percent had rectal and colonic disease, and 7 percent had perianal skin problems. Leading causes were hemorrhoids in 54 percent, fissure in ano in 18 percent, neoplasm in 6.5 percent, and inflammatory bowel diseases in 5 percent. In 8 percent no cause was found at the time of the examination. The majority of neoplasms were more than 10 cm above the anus, beyond the reach of digital examination.

In a series of 239 patients with *undiagnosed rectal bleeding* subjected to colonoscopy, 40 percent had significant lesions; 16 percent were found to have polyps; 10 percent had inflammatory bowel disease; 9 percent had carcinomas missed by barium enema; and 3 percent had diverticular disease, hemangiomas, or other causes. In a large percentage of these patients, no cause was found. In a study of anemic competitive runners, an increase in fecal hemoglobin was detected.

Patients with GI bleeding while on *anticoagulant therapy* are likely to have an underlying lesion, and warrant thorough evaluation. In a study examining 3800 courses of anticoagulant therapy, GI bleeding occurred in 45 patients. In 32 patients, a source was determined: 13 had hemorrhoids, 9 had peptic ulcers, 7 had neoplasms, and 3 had other lesions.

Nosebleeds and respiratory-tract bleeding must be considered in the differential diagnosis of melena and guaiac-positive stools. A false-positive stool guaiac test result can be produced by use of glycerol guaiacolate, the popular expectorant, or a meal of rare red meat. Black stools may result from bismuth (Pepto-Bismol), iron, charcoal, or spinach intake; red stools can occur from eating large quantities of beets.

Table 63-1. Differential Diagnosis of GI Bleeding

Hematemesis
Esophageal varices
Esophagitis
Esophageal ulceration
Mallory-Weiss tear
Esophageal cancer
Gastritis or duodenitis
Gastric or duodenal ulcer
Gastric neoplasm (carcinoma, lymphoma, or rarely leiomyoma/sarcoma)
Telangiectasia
Angiodysplasia, especially in patients with renal failure
Melena
All causes of hematemesis plus:
Meckel's diverticulum
Crohn's disease
Small bowel neoplasms (rare)
Hematochezia
Hemorrhoid
Anal fissure
Colonic polyp
Colorectal carcinoma
Angiodysplasia
Diverticular disease
Inflammatory bowel disease
Any upper GI or small bowel lesion if bleeding is brisk

WORKUP

History and physical examination may provide information regarding the location and severity of bleeding, but additional investigations are usually necessary to determine the exact cause. In the previously mentioned series of 311 cases of anorectal bleeding, history and physical examination alone yielded a definite diagnosis in 28 percent. Nevertheless, history and physical examination have important roles that may obviate the need for more invasive testing or help in selecting an optimal procedure.

History. Before proceeding with an extensive workup, the physician ought to be certain that the report of blood loss is accurate. Dark stools must not be mistaken for genuine melena, and one should check for intake of substances that may turn stool black. Factors that may produce a false-positive stool Hemoccult test should be considered, but a positive test ought not be dismissed lightly.

An approximate bleeding site can be determined by the nature of the blood loss, that is, whether it is melena, hematemesis, or hematochezia. A crude estimate of rate and severity can be obtained by asking about postural lightheadedness. The actual volume lost is not reliably obtained from the history, although reports of very large amounts should be taken seriously.

When the patient complains of voluminous blood loss or lightheadedness, a careful check for postural change in vital signs is indicated before proceeding with a complete ambulatory assessment. Immediate hospital admission should be arranged if blood pressure falls more than 10 mm Hg to 15 mm Hg, or the heart rate increases by more than 10 to 15 beats per minute when the patient stands up from a supine position. Measurement of the hematocrit in the acute phase of blood loss may show deceptively little decline if there has not been sufficient time for reequilibration of intravascular volume.

Once it is clear that the degree of blood loss does not pose an immediate hazard, office evaluation can proceed. When hematemesis is reported, sources of esophageal, gastric, and duodenal bleeding must be sought. A history of cirrhosis, chronic liver disease, or alcoholism raises suspicion of esophageal varices. Use of aspirin, alcohol, and antiinflammatory agents suggests bleeding due to ulceration or gastritis. A history of peptic ulcer or the presence of epigastric pain responsive to antacids or related to food intake raises the possibility of bleeding from a gastric or duodenal ulcer. It is worth noting, however, that another explanation for bleeding may be present in patients with a history typical of ulcer disease and that more than one potential bleeding site may be discovered (eg, esophageal varices).

When no hematemesis is noted, the source may still be from above the ligament of Treitz; however, small bowel and colonic lesions must be considered as well. Diarrhea, urgency, tenesmus, and lower abdominal cramping suggest inflammatory bowel disease (see Chapter 73). With ulcerative colitis, diverticulosis, and other forms of rectosigmoid disease, there is often some frank rectal bleeding. Brisk rectal bleeding is particularly common with diverticular disease. Weight loss or change in bowel habits raises suspicion of colonic cancer. A history of diverticular disease may be a clue to the cause of blood loss, but a coincident carcinoma must be ruled out. Many patients with rectal bleeding admit to past or present hemorrhoidal problems, but in almost half of the cases another lesion is found to be the cause of blood loss. Although note should be taken of oral anticoagulant use, most patients who experience GI bleeding while taking warfarin have an underlying pathology.

Physical Examination. As noted above, when there is evidence of acute bleeding, the evaluation should begin with postural signs and a cardiopulmonary examination to assess severity of volume loss and presence of any hemodynamic compromise. Next, the skin is inspected for pallor, ecchymoses, petechiae, telangiectasias, and stigmata of chronic liver disease (eg, jaundice, palmar erythema, spider angiomata). The nose and pharynx are examined for sources of bleeding. Lymph nodes are palpated for enlargement (eg, left supraclavicular adenopathy suggests an intraabdominal malignancy) and the abdomen is palpated for organomegaly, ascites, and masses. Anorectal lesions are sought on inspection and digital examination; the stool is checked for color and occult blood (see Chapter 56). Anoscopy is an essential part of the examination for patients who complain of anorectal symptoms.

If the patient describes convincing hematemesis, one may assume that the bleeding is from the upper GI tract, but if there is evidence of recent significant bleeding of uncertain origin, a nasogastric tube should be passed to aspirate gastric contents and test for the presence of blood. The guaiac test may be insensitive for heme unless the acidic aspirate is neutralized with a few drops of sodium hydroxide (NaOH).

Laboratory studies should be obtained to determine the chronicity and magnitude of blood loss as well as the presence of coincident disease. Hemoglobin concentration should be measured in all patients; however, if blood loss is acute, the hemoglobin concentration may not yet accurately reflect the severity of blood loss. A low mean corpuscular volume (MCV) suggests the possibility of iron deficiency due to chronic GI blood loss. Studies of coagulation (platelet count, prothrombin time [PT], and partial thromboplastin time [PTT]) and tests of liver and renal function are useful in checking for factors that may exacerbate bleeding.

Hematochezia. In stable patients, the main concern is the possibility of colon cancer; risk increases with age. Less than 5 percent of such cancers occur in patients under age 40 and less than 1 percent in those under age 30. Thus, if the physical examination or anoscopy reveals a bleeding hemorrhoid or other cause of local anal pathology in a young patient, it may be unnecessary to proceed with further tests. The finding on sigmoidoscopy of guaiac-negative stool from above the bleeding point also provides reassurance. On the other hand, 80 percent of colorectal malignancies are found in patients over 50. When a person over 50 presents with rectal bleeding, a thorough search for tumor is required even if a local lesion such as a hemorrhoid is discovered. Twenty-seven percent of patients with carcinoma of the rectum and 10 percent of those with carcinoma of the sigmoid have been noted to have coincidental hemorrhoids.

There are increasing data describing yields of diagnostic procedures. In the series of 311 patients with bright red rectal bleeding subjected to history, physical examination, sigmoidoscopy, and barium enema, the history diagnosed 5 percent, the physical examination raised the figure to 28 percent, and the addition of *sigmoidoscopy* provided an explanation in 90 percent. *Barium enema* raised the yield in this series only another 3 percent, probably because of the unusually large number of lesions in this study that were within reach of the sigmoidoscope. However, cumulative data suggest that only 30 percent of colonic malignancies can be viewed by sigmoidoscopy. Consequently, persons with rectal bleeding in the age group at high risk for large bowel malignancy should undergo additional study. Barium enema has a sensitivity of 70 percent to 90 percent for detecting carcinoma and 70 percent for polyps larger than 5 mm in diameter. Cancers most often missed are in the cecum or rectosigmoid or are obscured by concurrent diverticulosis or ulcerative colitis. Air-contrast techniques improve the results.

The advent of *colonoscopy* has improved the identification of bleeding sources. About 40 percent of patients with frank rectal bleeding or occult blood loss in conjunction with a normal sigmoidoscopy and barium enema are found to have previously undetected lesions when studied by colonoscopy. About 10 percent have cancers, another 10 percent have polyps, 10 percent have inflammatory bowel disease, and 5 percent have telangiectasia. Furthermore, carcinomas and polyps were detected in 20 percent of patients in whom only diverticula were seen with barium enema. Although the precise role for colonoscopy is not yet entirely settled, most patients over the age of 50 with bleeding are candidates for colonoscopy, either primarily or if barium enema and sigmoidoscopy are normal or show only diverticula.

Hematemesis. Endoscopy has proven superior to barium studies. The sensitivity of the upper GI series is around 60 percent, compared with 95 percent for endoscopy. Esophagitis, Mallory-Weiss tears, and gastritis are readily seen by endoscopy, although they are often undetectable radiologically. Moreover, barium obscures mucosal detail and interferes with endoscopy for 24 to 48 hours. Thus, for suspected acute brisk upper GI bleeding, endoscopy is the procedure of first choice, with barium study reserved as a supplementary procedure for patients with inactive bleeding, unexplained chronic blood loss, or suspected small bowel disease.

The question of whether early endoscopy results in improved outcome for hematemesis (and should therefore be applied broadly) remains unresolved. Several studies have failed to demonstrate a significant difference in outcome among patients who have undergone diagnostic endoscopy as compared with those who have had an upper GI series. However, *therapeutic* endoscopy was not routinely applied in such trials. Until further data become available, a reasonable approach is to pursue endoscopy in patients considered at high risk for recurrent bleeding (such as those with evidence of chronic liver disease or a transfusion-requiring initial bleed) and those with persistent bleeding despite medical therapy. In addition, it may be useful to perform upper GI endoscopy to exclude esophageal and gastric mucosal features indicative of high risk for rebleeding (eg, a "visible vessel" in an ulcer crater).

Melena. Because melena may occur from an upper or lower GI source, one needs to decide which part of the GI tract to evaluate first. The decision needs to be individualized to the patient at hand, although in general, an upper GI site is a more likely source of bleeding.

Occult Bleeding. The evaluation of occult GI bleeding is generally aimed at detecting asymptomatic neoplasms at a curable stage. Because colonic adenomas and carcinomas are the most common GI neoplasms, evaluation of the colon has greatest utility in this setting. A cost-effectiveness analysis comparing different strategies for evaluating a positive test for fecal occult blood has suggested that colonoscopy would save more lives at lower cost than the combined use of barium enema and flexible sigmoidoscopy. Of seven strategies evaluated, barium enema (without sigmoidoscopy) had the lowest cost-effectiveness ratio but would save fewer lives than colonoscopy. The use of colonoscopy plus barium enema was the only strategy predicted to save more lives than colonoscopy alone but does so at significantly higher cost (see Chapter 56).

If no etiology for occult bleeding is identified within the colon, evaluation of the upper GI tract and small bowel may be considered, although the yield for detection of cancer is likely to be low. In a study of 26 patients followed for 2 to 8 years after a negative colonoscopy or barium enema/sigmoidoscopy, only one patient was later found to have a gastric cancer. In five others, a nonmalignant upper GI source emerged as the cause of the occult bleeding. A prospective study of patients with iron deficiency anemia found that site-specific symptoms were predictive of the location of the bleeding source. Upper GI sources were common. Synchronous sources of blood loss were rare, making further evaluation unnecessary when an obvious source was found.

PROPHYLACTIC AND SYMPTOMATIC MANAGEMENT

Patients at high risk for upper GI bleeding (such as those with varices or a prior history of upper GI bleeding, especially if exposed to anticoagulants or high doses of nonsteroidal antiinflammatory drugs [NSAIDs]) are candidates for prophylactic measures. Propranolol has been successful for prevention of a first bleed in patients with known varices (see Chapter 71). *Sclerotherapy* is not indicated for primary prophylaxis because it may actually increase mortality in patients with varices. As noted, *endoscopic ligation* is reasonable in those at high risk of recurrent variceal bleeding. *H_2-blockers* and *omeprazole* may be helpful in selected patients with a history of bleeding from an ulcer or gastritis (see Chapter 68). Patients taking steroids do not appear to require such prophylaxis unless there is an additional risk factor for bleeding.

Modest falls in hematocrit that accompany chronic low-grade GI blood loss can be treated with oral iron ($FeSO_4$, 300 mg tid) to make up for the resulting iron deficiency (see Chapter 84). Marked, but gradual, decreases in hematocrit are usually well tolerated unless the patient has cardiopulmonary disease. Most patients do not need transfusion unless they are symptomatic. Oral iron usually produces a prompt reticulocytosis and at least partial correction of the anemia (see Chapter 82). Patients with presumed anal bleeding can be given fiber supplements or stool softeners to decrease mechanical trauma to the lesion (see Chapter 65).

INDICATIONS FOR ADMISSION AND REFERRAL

The patient with a story of recent or ongoing brisk bleeding, especially if it is accompanied by orthostatic hypotension or other symptoms or signs of hemodynamic compromise, requires emergency ward evaluation. Prompt hospitalization is indicated for the person with a profound anemia, even in the absence of evidence for dramatic blood loss. Some patients with less severe, even possibly chronic GI blood loss also deserve consideration for hospitalization if they have a comorbid condition that might be aggravated by anemia (eg, ischemic heart disease). For most others, evaluation can proceed safely on an ambulatory basis if the patient does not have serious cardiopulmonary disease and is responsible enough to recognize and promptly report signs of worsening blood loss or volume depletion. Referral to a gastroenterologist should be considered for patients who are potential candidates for endoscopy, as well as for patients in whom the source of bleeding remains elusive after initial evaluation.

ANNOTATED BIBLIOGRAPHY

Barry MJ, Mulley AG, Richter JM. Effect of workup strategy on the cost-effectiveness of fecal occult blood screening for colorectal cancer. Gastroenterology 1987;93:301. *(Comparative analysis of seven potential strategies for evaluating the colon in asymptomatic patients with guaiac-positive stool.)*

Boley SJ, Brandt LJ, Frank MS. Severe lower intestinal bleeding. Clin Gastroenterol 1981;10:65. *(Useful enumeration of etiologies by age of patient.)*

Carson, JL, Strom BL, Schinnar R, et al. The low risk of upper gastrointestinal bleeding in patients dispensed corticosteroids. Am J Med 1991;91:223. *(Risk was 2.8 cases per 10,000 person months; argues against prophylactic therapy unless other risk factors present.)*

Conn HO. To scope or not to scope. N Engl J Med 1981;304:967. *(Thoughtful editorial addressing this difficult question. Good summary of available data.)*

Coon U, Willis P. Hemorrhagic complications of anticoagulant therapy. Ann Intern Med 1974;133:386. *(More than half of patients who bled on anticoagulant therapy had an identifiable underlying GI lesion.)*

Dooley CP, Larson AW, Stacen H, et al. Double-contrast barium meal and upper gastrointestinal endoscopy. Ann Intern Med 1984;101:538. *(Literature review; endoscopy was substantially more sensitive—92 percent vs. 5 percent—and more specific—100 percent vs. 91 percent—than double-contrast barium swallow, but no "gold standard.")*

Foster DN, Miloszewski K, Losowsky M. Stigmata of recent hemorrhage in diagnosis and prognosis of upper gastrointestinal bleeding. Br Med J 1976;1:1173. *(Duodenal ulcer, gastric ulcer, Mallory-Weiss lesions, and esophageal varices led the list of causes.)*

Goulston KJ, et al. Evaluation of rectal bleeding. Lancet 1986; 2:261. *(Colorectal malignancies would have been missed on clinical basis alone.)*

Graham DY. Aspirin and the stomach. Ann Intern Med 1986; 104:390. *(Comprehensive review. Notes that degree of mucosal injury seen by endoscopy does not predict risk or degree of bleeding.)*

Griffiths WJ, Neumann DA, Welsh JD. The visible vessel as an indicator of uncontrolled or recurrent gastrointestinal hemorrhage. N Engl J Med 1979;300:1411. *(Important sign of high risk for a repeat upper GI bleed.)*

Knight KK, Fielding JE, Battista RN. Occult blood screening for colorectal cancer. JAMA 1989;261:587. *(General review of the procedure.)*

Laine L, El-Newihi HM, Migikovsky B, et al. Endoscopic ligation compared with sclerotherapy for the treatment of bleeding esophageal varices. Ann Intern Med 1993;119:1. *(Endoscopic ligation caused fewer local complications and eradicated varices more rapidly.)*

Layne EA, Mellow MH, Lipman TO. Insensitivity of guaiac slide for detection of blood in gastric juice. Ann Intern Med 1981;94:774. *(Sensitivity of the guaiac test was low, but it was greatly enhanced by neutralizing the acid with a few drops of NaOH.)*

Lindsay DC, et al. Should colonoscopy be the first investigation for colonic disease? Br Med J 1988;296:167. *(Randomized trial of colonoscopy versus rigid sigmoidoscopy and air-contrast barium enema in the workup of colonic disease.)*

Peterson WL, Barnett CC, Smith HJ, et al. Routine early endoscopy in upper gastrointestinal tract bleeding. N Engl J Med 1981;304:925. *(Randomized controlled trial; no advantage found for early endoscopy, except in those with alcoholic liver disease or continued bleeding.)*

Rockey DC, Cello JP. Evaluation of the gastrointestinal tract in patients with iron-deficiency anemia. N Engl J Med 1993; 329:1691. *(Lesions are frequently found; site-specific symptoms help predict location and direct workup.)*

Shapiro RH. The visible vessel: curse or blessing. N Engl J Med 1979;300:1438. *(Editorial reviewing the utility of endoscopy, with emphasis on defining a high-risk group of patients with upper GI bleeding.)*

Steer ML, Silen W. Diagnostic procedures in gastrointestinal hemorrhage. N Engl J Med 1983;309:646. *(Concise but very useful review of the operating characteristics of endoscopy, radionuclide imaging, angiography, barium contrast studies, and exploratory surgery.)*

Stewart JG, Ahlquist DA, McGill DB, et al. Gastrointestinal blood loss and anemia in runners. Ann Intern Med 1984; 100:843. *(Documents an increase in fecal hemoglobin level associated with competitive running, which may explain anemia and iron deficiency among long-distance runners.)*

Sutton FM. Upper gastrointestinal bleeding in patients with esophageal varices: what is the most common source of bleeding? Am J Med 1987;83:273. *(Varices account for the vast majority of bleeding episodes, although coexisting sources are not uncommon.)*

Wilcox CM, Truss CD. Gastrointestinal bleeding in patients receiving long-term anticoagulant therapy. Am J Med 1988;84: 683. *(Half of episodes were upper GI in origin; a lower GI origin was noted in 33 percent. Undiagnosed cases were associated with a very low risk of encountering a malignancy later.)*

Zuckerman GR. Upper gastrointestinal bleeding in patients with chronic renal failure. Ann Intern Med 1985;102:588. *(Upper GI angiodysplasia was the most common source; esophagitis was also prevalent.)*

Primary Care Medicine: Office Evaluation and Management of the Adult Patient, 3rd edition, edited by Allan H. Goroll, Lawrence A. May, and Albert G. Mulley, Jr. J.B. Lippincott Company, Philadelphia

64
Evaluation and Management of Diarrhea

JAMES M. RICHTER, M.D.

Diarrhea is an affliction familiar to everyone. It is clinically characterized as the frequent passage of unformed stools. Most episodes are brief, self-limited, and well-tolerated without need for medical attention. However, when diarrhea becomes severe or chronic, a thoughtful evaluation is needed to ensure proper management. As the physician of first contact, the primary physician needs to be skilled in the care of patients suffering from diarrhea. Major tasks include making an expeditious clinical diagnosis of acute diarrheas, deciding when to use antibiotic therapy, preventing and treating traveler's diarrhea, efficiently evaluating patients with chronic diarrhea, and providing symptomatic relief while evaluation is in progress. Diarrhea in the HIV-infected patient requires special attention (see Chapter 13).

PATHOPHYSIOLOGY AND CLINICAL PRESENTATIONS

Diarrhea is a change in a patient's bowel habits, manifested by increased stool volume, looseness, and frequency. The pathophysiologic common denominator is an increased water content of stools, which may be due to increased fluid secretion, decreased water absorption, or altered bowel motility. At times several mechanisms are operative. *Increased fluid secretion* can be triggered by inflammation, hormones, or enterotoxins. The resulting secretory diarrhea has the characteristics of a stool volume that remains in excess of 500 mL per 24 hours despite fasting, a low stool osmolality, and a normal stool electrolyte concentration. *Decreased reabsorption of fluid* occurs with abnormalities of the bowel mucosa, loss of reabsorptive surface, or the presence of unabsorbable osmotically active materials in the bowel lumen, such as lactose in patients with lactase deficiency. Patients with diarrhea due to decreased reabsorption typically respond to fasting with a decrease in stool volume to less than 500 mL per 24 hours; stool osmolality is increased, and its sodium and potassium concentrations are low. *Altered bowel motility* decreases the contact time with the bowel mucosa, limiting fluid reabsorption; it can ensue after vagotomy or may be hormonally triggered, as in hypergastrinemia.

Clinical presentation depends, in part, on the site of involvement. *Small bowel diarrheas* tend to result in passage of large, loose stools in conjunction with periumbilical or right lower quadrant pain. There may be diarrhea after meals or after eating certain foods, but this is also seen with patients suffering from malabsorption, osmotic diarrhea, a fistula, or the dumping syndrome. *Large bowel diarrheas*, especially those due to disease of the left colon and rectosigmoid, are manifested by passage of frequent, small, loose stools in conjunction with crampy, left lower quadrant pain or tenesmus.

Acute Diarrheas

A diarrhea is categorized as "acute" if its duration is less than 2 weeks. Infectious etiologies dominate and include viral, bacterial, and parasitic agents. Bacteria may cause diarrhea by producing a toxin in contaminated food or after ingestion, or by invading the bowel mucosa. Some parasites invade the bowel wall, whereas others cling to it and coat the absorptive surface.

Viral gastroenteritis has long been the most common cause of acute diarrhea in the United States, although it was not until the late 1970s that the responsible organisms were finally isolated and identified. Epidemics of viral gastroenteritis are particularly common. More than 40 percent of outbreaks of nonbacterial gastroenteritis investigated by the Centers for Disease Control during a 5-year period were linked to the Norwalk virus. In children, rotavirus infection is a common cause. Outbreaks have been found to occur during all seasons and include waterborne, foodborne, and person-to-person modes of transmission. They last about a week. Vomiting is the prominent symptom in children, diarrhea in adults. After an incubation period of 48 to 72 hours, symptoms usually begin abruptly with diarrhea, nausea, vomiting, headache, low-grade fever, abdominal cramps, and malaise; they resolve spontaneously within 24 to 96 hours. The diarrhea tends to be predominantly of the small bowel variety and secretory in quality. Abdominal examination reveals diffuse tenderness (without guarding) and hyperactive bowel sounds. The white count is usually normal but may be elevated. Stools are usually free of leukocytes, but occasionally white cells are found, mimicking an invasive etiology.

Staphylococcus aureus is a common contaminant of custard-filled pastries and processed meats. The organism produces an enterotoxin that causes nausea, vomiting, abdominal cramps, and diarrhea within 2 to 8 hours of eating the contaminated food. Symptoms usually last less than 12 hours. A common-source pattern and lack of fever are typical.

Clostridium perfringens is another common food contaminant, especially of foods that have been warmed on steam tables. The organism releases an enterotoxin after sporulation in the intestine. Consequently, the incubation period of 8 to 24 hours is a bit longer than that for staphylococcal food poisoning. Symptoms include diarrhea, abdominal cramps, and occasionally, some vomiting. It, too, has a common-source epidemiology, and there is no fever.

Bacillus cereus is a toxin-producing bacterial contaminant of rice and bean sprouts. One form of toxin-induced illness leads to vomiting but no diarrhea; in another, there is severe abdominal cramping and diarrhea. The incubation period is 8 to 16 hours after ingestion of contaminated food. The symptoms are self-limited.

Salmonella species cause diarrhea by invading the bowel wall. Achlorhydric patients who lack the antibacterial action of normal gastric acidity are at increased risk. The most common form of *Salmonella* infection is a self-limited diarrheal illness resulting from ingestion of contaminated food (eggs and poultry are the major sources). Children are at greatest risk; late summer and fall are the times of peak incidence. Although most episodes of salmonellosis are mild, debilitated patients are at risk for serious bacteremia. In the typical outpatient case, symptoms begin 12 to 36 hours after ingestion and resolve within 5 days, although diarrhea may persist for up to 2 weeks. The initial presentation is rather nonspecific although indicative of a small bowel process: watery diarrhea, cramps, nausea, vomiting, and fever. In addition to colonization, an enterotoxin is released that stimulates the secretory diarrhea. In later stages, invasion spreads to the large bowel and leukocytes may be noted in the stool. A distinguishing feature of salmonellosis is that the leukocytes are often mononuclear cells. In severe cases, dysentery can develop.

Typhoid fever, a rare but "must-not-miss" form of *Salmonella* disease, is caused by infection with *Salmonella typhi.* About 500 cases occur in the United States each year, mostly among young people. Infections are both waterborne and foodborne. Although only a small percentage of patients with typhoid fever develop diarrhea, it does occur. The classic and most severe form is a "pea-soup" diarrhea developing in the third week of illness. Early symptoms suggestive of the condition are progressive fever, relative bradycardia, evanescent rash on the trunk ("rose spots"), splenomegaly, cough, headache, and right lower quadrant abdominal pain.

Shigella infection produces an invasive diarrheal illness. Transmission is by the fecal–oral route, and stubborn reservoirs include day care centers, Indian reservations, urban ghettos, and rural villages in developing countries. Young children are at greatest risk and often the source of infection within a family. The illness proceeds in two stages. First, there is colonization in the small bowel, resulting in a watery diarrhea and periumbilical pain, followed in a few days by invasion of the large bowel producing small frequent stools, tenesmus, and polymorphonuclear leukocytes on smear. In florid cases, the patient has fever, toxicity, bloody diarrhea, nausea, vomiting, and cramps. Most often the disease is more subtle and may be difficult to distinguish from other diarrheal illnesses accompanied by fever.

Campylobacter jejuni infection is responsible for more cases of diarrhea in the United States than either *Salmonella* or *Shigella*. Infection derives most often from animal sources such as poultry and household pets; fecal transmission between people also occurs. The incubation period is 2 to 7 days. Clinically, the illness resembles that caused by *Salmonella* or *Shigella;* however, symptoms may persist longer. The relapse rate is as high as 20 percent, although the illness is usually self-limited and resolves within a week. In half of all cases, a Gram's stain of the stool shows characteristic curved gram-negative rods arranged in "seagull wing" fashion. The organism grows best on a special medium incubated at 42°C; it will not grow on plates customarily used for isolation of *Salmonella* and *Shigella*.

Yersinia enterocolitica also causes an illness that resembles salmonellosis. Patients become infected by eating contaminated meat or dairy products. The incubation period is 12 hours to 3 days. An intense regional lymphoid reaction may arise in the terminal ileum (the portal of entry for the organism) and result in a clinical picture of fever, right lower quadrant abdominal pain, and diarrhea that can simulate the onset of Crohn's disease. From 10 percent to 40 percent of patients develop fever, arthralgias, polyarthritis, or erythema nodosum. The illness is usually self-limited.

Vibrio parahemolyticus and *non-toxin–producing V. cholerae* are pathogenic *Vibrio* species that have caused outbreaks of diarrheal disease among people eating raw seafood, particularly oysters and sushi-style red snapper and salmon. The incubation period is measured in hours to several days. The illness that ensues is usually mild and self-limited, although an occasional patient may present with fever, nausea, vomiting, and crampy diarrhea.

Cryptosporidiosis is a protozoan infection being recognized with increasing frequency, especially among *immunocompromised patients,* such as those with acquired immunodeficiency syndrome *(AIDS).* In these patients, the infection can produce a profuse watery diarrhea with stool volumes that may exceed 3 L per day. Although the illness is usually self-limited, it may persist in immunocompromised hosts. Otherwise healthy, immunocompetent patients develop a mild illness; they become infected from occupational contact with animal dung; symptoms resolve spontaneously within 5 to 21 days.

Diarrhea in homosexual men may additionally ensue from infection with *Neisseria, Giardia, Entamoeba histolytica, Campylobacter, Chlamydia, Shigella,* or *Salmonella.* In a study of 194 homosexual men, a polymicrobial origin was identified in a major proportion of those presenting with diarrhea, tenesmus, and rectal pain.

Drug-induced diarrheas may occur as a result of excessive fluid secretion (alcohol, phenolphthalein, and castor oil), reduction of fluid absorption (magnesium-containing antacids), or stimulation of bowel motility (caffeine-containing beverages and herbal teas). Almost any drug can cause gastrointestinal (GI) upset and diarrhea (Table 64–1). In addition, broad-spectrum antibiotics can also cause diarrhea by allowing overgrowth of potentially pathogenic, toxin-producing species such as *Clostridium difficile* and by disrupting the ability of normal colonic flora to salvage unabsorbed carbohydrate. Normally, unabsorbed carbohydrate is metabolized by colonic bacteria, supplying the large bowel with short-chain fatty acids. Obliteration of colonic flora deprives the bowel of such fatty acids for its metabolism and leaves an unabsorbed carbohydrate load. The result is a crampy, osmotic diarrhea. Symptoms may begin acutely or develop as late as 2 months after cessation of the antibiotic.

Traveler's Diarrheas

Patients traveling from industrialized to developing nations are at considerable risk for developing diarrhea. Etio-

Table 64-1. A Differential Diagnosis of Diarrhea

ACUTE DIARRHEA	CHRONIC OR RECURRENT DIARRHEA
Viruses	**Protozoa**
Bacterial Toxins	*Giardia lamblia*
Staphylococcus	*Entamoeba histolytica*
Clostridium	*Cryptosporidia*
Bacteria	**Inflammation**
Salmonella	Ulcerative colitis
Shigella	Crohn's disease
Escherichia coli	Ischemic colitis
Campylobacter	Pseudomembranous colitis
Yersinia	**Drugs**
Bacillus cereus	Laxatives
Vibrio parahaemolyticus	Antibiotics
Vibrio cholerae	Quinidine
Protozoa	Guanethidine; other antihypertensive agents
Giardia lamblia	Caffeine
Entamoeba histolytica	Digitalis
Drugs	**Functional**
Laxatives	Irritable bowel syndrome
Antibiotics	Diverticulosis
Caffeine	**Tumors**
Alcohol	Bowel carcinoma
Functional	Villous adenoma
Anxiety	Islet-cell tumors
Acute Presentations of Chronic or Recurrent Diarrhea	Carcinoid syndrome
(See next column)	Medullary carcinoma of thyroid
	Malabsorption
	Sprue
	Intestinal lymphoma
	Bile-salt malabsorption
	Whipple's disease
	Pancreatic insufficiency
	Lactase deficiency
	Other disaccharidase deficiencies
	Alpha-beta lipoproteinemia
	Postsurgical
	Postgastrectomy dumping syndrome
	Enteroenteric fistulas
	Blind loops
	Parasympathetic denervation
	Short bowel syndrome
	Other
	Cirrhosis
	Diabetes mellitus
	Heavy-metal intoxication
	Other neurogenic diarrheas
	Hyperthyroidism
	Addison's disease
	Pellagra
	Scleroderma
	Amyloidosis

logic agents include *Escherichia coli, Salmonella, Shigella, Entamoeba histolytica, Giardia lamblia, Salmonella typhi,* and *Vibrio cholerae.*

Toxigenic Escherichia coli are responsible for a large proportion of cases labeled as "traveler's diarrhea" or "turista." The agent is transmitted by poor food-handling practices and contaminated water. With enterotoxin production, a watery diarrhea ensues because of the toxin's promotion of fluid secretion in the small bowel. Invasive *E. coli* strains can also cause a dysentery syndrome.

Entamoeba histolytica usually exists in a commensual relationship with the host, and most patients harboring the protozoan are asymptomatic carriers. Occasionally, this relationship breaks down and the ameba invades the colonic wall, resulting in an acute bloody diarrhea. The clinical presentation ranges from mild to fulminant illness. Occasionally the illness is mistaken for inflammatory bowel disease (see Chapter 65) and may have a protracted course with exacerbations and remissions. Asymptomatic carriers such as returning tourists and immigrants are often the source of infection in developed countries. Because amebiasis does not have a soil phase, it is not restricted to warmer climates. Well-documented outbreaks have occurred in the United States and Europe, in addition to those that originate in developing countries. Amebiasis can be spread by sexual contact and is prevalent among promiscuous homosexuals.

Giardia lamblia ranks as a leading parasitic cause of diarrhea, especially overseas, but also in the United States. Infection with the flagellated protozoan is particularly common where water supplies are contaminated by human sewage, but the organism is also endemic to such areas as the Rocky Mountains and Leningrad. The exact means by which *Giardia* causes diarrhea remains unsettled, although heavy infestations can lead to malabsorption by coating large areas of the small bowel, particularly the lower duodenum and upper jejunum. The majority of patients with giardiasis are asymptomatic, but the organism is being recognized more frequently as an important cause of acute, intermittent, and chronic diarrheas in the United States. The ensuing loose stools may be watery or greasy; mucus is often present, but blood is rare. The patient may complain of epigastric or periumbilical discomfort. Mild steatorrhea and malabsorption occur with heavy parasite burdens.

Cholera is the prototypical secretory diarrheal disease. It results from drinking water contaminated with *Vibrio cholerae.* Most outbreaks are pandemic in the Indian subcontinent, Southeast Asia, Africa, and the Middle East. Isolated outbreaks have been reported in Mediterranean countries. In the United States, rare outbreaks sometimes occur along the Gulf Coast. The disease ranges in severity from a mild illness to fulminant, life-threatening diarrhea with copious production of gray, watery, mucoid ("rice water") stool. In severe cases, fluid losses may reach over 1 L per hour, accompanied by vomiting, muscle cramps, and severe thirst. Being a noninvasive diarrhea involving the small bowel, cholera causes no tenesmus and the stool contains no leukocytes. Dehydration, serious volume depletion, and a metabolic acidosis may ensue. In mild cases, the patient reports painless, nonbloody diarrhea of abrupt onset.

Chronic and Recurrent Diarrheas

Although the number of etiologies is vast, consideration of a few exemplary conditions provides a good sense of the range and types of presentations.

Irritable bowel syndrome (see Chapter 74) is the most common of the motility disorders responsible for chronic diarrhea. It can present as diarrhea alternating with constipation, or as chronic, recurrent diarrhea. Some studies report a high frequency of associated psychiatric disease. In addition to diarrhea and constipation, patients may complain of distention, cramping, and mucus-laden stools. The condition waxes and wanes over many years. Neither fever nor fecal leukocytes are present. Any rectal bleeding that may occur is secondary to anal trauma from straining and passage of hard stool.

The *inflammatory bowel diseases* (see Chapter 73) are typical of the diarrheas that result from inflammatory destruction of the bowel wall. Abdominal pain, bloody stools, purulent discharge, and fever are seen in patients with active disease affecting the large bowel. Extraintestinal manifestations occur and may involve the skin, joints, liver, and heart. Microscopic examination of the stool reveals red cells and leukocytes.

Pseudomembranous colitis develops when normal bowel flora are suppressed by use of broad-spectrum antibiotics, allowing *Clostridium difficile* (a cytotoxin-producing gram-negative rod found in 6 percent of normal adults) to proliferate. The antibiotics most often responsible are *ampicillin* and *clindamycin,* but other broad-spectrum agents have also been implicated. Immunocompromised patients, the elderly, and those with underlying bowel disease are most susceptible. Fever, abdominal pain, profuse watery stools, and fecal leukocytes are typical clinical features; the illness may range from mild to severe. Symptoms usually start after the initiation of a course of antibiotics, but onset can be delayed for as much as 4 to 8 weeks after cessation of therapy. Symptoms sometimes persist for months, mimicking inflammatory bowel disease. The sigmoidoscopic finding of nodular, inflammatory ulcers or yellow-white mucosal plaques is characteristic.

Diabetic enteropathy results from diabetes-induced autonomic neuropathy (see Chapter 102). When the small bowel is involved, the ensuing stasis allows bacterial overgrowth. The bacteria deconjugate bile acids, leading to fat malabsorption. With involvement of the large bowel, the patient experiences distressing nocturnal diarrhea. Postural hypotension, impotence, and other symptoms and signs of autonomic insufficiency may accompany the diarrhea and suggest the diagnosis.

The *dumping syndrome* is another motility disorder, seen most commonly in patients who have undergone vagotomy and gastroenterostomy. Patients complain of sweating, postural lightheadedness, tachycardia, and diarrhea following meals. Concentrated carbohydrates are most likely to trigger symptoms. Lying down minimizes symptoms, as does avoidance of concentrated sweets. Symptoms begin shortly after surgery and often subside within 12 months; they sometimes persist. Besides altered motility, other mechanisms, such as osmotic factors, are believed to be operative in this syndrome, although their precise contributions remain to be elucidated.

Villous adenoma of the rectosigmoid causes a secretory, noninflammatory chronic diarrhea. Watery diarrhea, independent of food and fluid intake, is typical; severe potassium depletion can result. In some patients with this tumor, excessive secretion of mucus occurs, with loss of sufficient protein to produce hypoalbuminemia and a protein-losing enteropathy syndrome.

Malabsorption of fat or carbohydrate can lead to an osmotic diarrhea. Some of the osmotically active substances may also stimulate increased bowel secretion of fluids and electrolytes. Malabsorption of *fat* characteristically presents as foul, bulky, greasy stools. Patients may note that the stools seem to be "sticky" and difficult to flush down the toilet. Steatorrheic stools "float" not because of their fat content but because of an increase in trapped gas. Associated symptoms are a function of the severity of the caloric and vitamin deficiencies that ensue and may include weight loss, ecchymoses, bone pain, glossitis, muscle tenderness, and peripheral neuropathy. Cramping lower abdominal pain typically precedes bowel movements.

Malabsorption of lactose due to *lactase deficiency* is the prototype of carbohydrate malabsorption diseases leading to an osmotic diarrhea. It is particularly common among African Americans, Indians, Asians, and Jews; onset is typically in adulthood. A secondary form of the disease may develop in patients suffering from extensive disease of the small bowel. Patients report nausea, bloating, cramps, and diarrhea after ingesting more than their customary intake of milk products. Weight loss and steatorrhea are absent or mild; appetite remains good. Avoidance of milk products (except for yogurts containing live cultures, which provide lactase) terminates symptoms. Diagnosis is confirmed by an abnormal lactose tolerance test or a hydrogen breath test (detects excessive hydrogen production from bacterial metabolism of undigested lactose).

Chronic laxative abuse is an important and often occult etiology of chronic diarrhea. Patients suffering from bulimia (see Chapter 234) tend to use laxatives chronically and surreptitiously in a relentless attempt to lose weight. Depending on the type of agent used, either a secretory or osmotic diarrhea may develop. Agents associated with secretory diarrheas include castor oil and phenolphthalein preparations. Osmotic diarrheas occur when the patient takes a preparation that contains magnesium (eg, milk of magnesia) or another poorly absorbable substance. These substances appear in the stool and can be tested for if laxative abuse is suspected. Patients who abuse laxatives may present with unexplained dehydration, electrolyte depletion, or preoccupation with weight loss.

Incontinence

A number of patients who complain of "diarrhea" actually suffer from incontinence. Typically, their stool volumes are normal (less than 250 mL per day), although their stools may be soft. Poor sphincter tone and evidence of stool incontinence are found on physical examination.

DIFFERENTIAL DIAGNOSIS

Acute Diarrhea. The differential diagnosis for acute diarrhea is dominated by infectious agents (see Table 64–1). Viruses are the single most important, frequent cause. Staphylococcal toxin, clostridial toxin, and ingestion of *Campylobacter, Salmonella, Shigella,* and enteropathogenic *Escherichia coli* are common bacterial etiologies. *Giardia* and amebae are less frequent sources of acute diarrhea in the United States. Drugs are important and common causes of diarrhea, especially antibiotics, laxatives, magnesium-containing antacids, and other agents such as quinidine. Alcohol and caffeine-containing beverages should be considered. Most causes of chronic diarrhea are also capable of acute presentations.

Chronic Diarrhea. The differential diagnosis is even more extensive for chronic diarrhea. The infectious agents and drugs discussed under acute diarrheal disease may be responsible, but the likelihood of parasites such as amebae or *Giardia* increases. Inflammatory bowel diseases must also be considered. Absorption defects resulting from sprue, bile-salt deficiency, lactase deficiency, intestinal lymphoma, Whipple's disease, and pancreatic insufficiency may cause chronic diarrhea. The patient who has had GI surgery may develop diarrhea on the basis of postgastrectomy dumping syndrome, fistulas, blind loops, loss of parasympathetic innervation, or extensive bowel resection. Diarrhea may be caused directly by neoplasms, particularly villous adenoma. Diarrhea alternating with constipation raises the possibility of colonic carcinoma, irritable bowel syndrome, or diverticular disease of the bowel. A variety of extraintestinal conditions may be responsible, including cirrhosis, alcoholism, pellagra, and heavy-metal intoxications from lead, mercury, or arsenic. Occasionally, chronic diarrhea may develop with endocrinopathies such as Addison's disease, hyperthyroidism, and diabetes mellitus.

WORKUP

The first task is to confirm that the problem is indeed diarrhea and not simply an occasional loose stool or frequent defecation of formed stools. The term *diarrhea* specifically denotes the frequent passage of unformed stools. Once diarrhea is confirmed, one should seek an etiologic diagnosis to guide therapy, especially in severe or persistent cases.

Acute and Traveler's Diarrheas

History. The *nature of the bowel movements* should be determined, including their frequency, consistency, volume, and the presence of gross blood, pus, or mucus (Tables 64–2 and 64–3). *Associated symptoms* such as fever, abdominal pain, and rash also deserve attention. Fever, blood, or pus suggests an invasive process, although blood may also result from anal pathology or irritation unrelated to the etiology of the diarrhea. Mucus that is free of leukocytes is a hallmark of irritable bowel syndrome. The macular "rose spot" rash on the trunk is an important clue for typhoid, a rare, but "must-not-miss" diagnosis. Patients with periumbilical or right lower quadrant pain and copious volumes of watery stool are likely to have a small bowel etiology. Those with left lower quadrant discomfort or tenesmus and frequent, small volumes of stool are probably suffering from an etiology that involves the large bowel.

Epidemiologic information is critical to making an etiologic diagnosis of acute diarrhea, because the clinical presentation is often nonspecific. Travel, food intake, and personal contacts require careful review. In more than 50 percent of cases, *"traveler's diarrhea"* results from exposure to enterotoxigenic *Escherichia coli; Salmonella, Shigella, Giardia,* and *Campylobacter* account for the remainder. Although most cases occur with travel to developing nations, this is not always true (eg, risk of giardiasis with travel to Leningrad or the Rocky Mountains).

Onset of diarrhea within hours of ingesting a potentially contaminated food is suggestive of *food poisoning;* this is confirmed by checking if others were similarly affected. Foodborne illness with a short incubation period and no fever indicates ingestion of a preformed enterotoxin. Presence of fever and a slightly longer incubation period are characteristics of an infectious etiology (see Table 64-3). Custard-filled pastries, processed meats, foods warmed on steam tables, eggs, poultry, raw seafood, raw milk, rice, and bean sprouts are among the foods often implicated in food poisoning.

Person-to-person spread is an important source of infection that needs to be explored. Among *male homosexuals,* diarrhea often has a polymicrobial etiology; *Neisseria, Chlamydia, Entamoeba histolytica, Lymphogranuloma venereum, Giardia,* and *Campylobacter* are additional pathogens to consider. *Children* who attend day care centers may contract rotavirus, *Giardia, Shigella,* cryptosporidiosis, or *Campylobacter.*

A good *drug history* is essential; any drug may cause diarrhea. It is particularly important to question for use of laxatives, magnesium-containing antacids, excess alcohol, caffeine-containing beverages, herbal teas, antibiotics, digitalis, quinidine, loop diuretics (furosemide, ethacrynic acid), antihypertensive agents, and excessive intake of sorbitol-containing "sugar-free" gums and mints.

Physical Examination. Vital signs must be checked for postural changes, a reflection of significant volume depletion. Any elevation in temperature or loss of weight needs to be noted. The skin is examined for rashes, the lymph nodes for enlargement, and the abdomen for tenderness, guarding, rebound, abnormal bowel sounds, organomegaly, and masses. A rectal examination and fecal occult blood test complete the physical evaluation.

Laboratory Studies. The laboratory workup should be individualized. The patient who feels well except for frequent loose stools requires no immediate laboratory testing. On the other hand, the patient who is ill with fever, nausea, abdominal cramps, or other systemic symptoms requires more extensive evaluation, beginning with a *methylene blue stain* of *stool or mucus.* A drop of the sample is placed on a microscope slide and mixed thoroughly with two drops of methylene blue solution. After a cover slip is placed over the mixture, it is ready for viewing under the microscope. If methylene blue is not available, a *Wright's stain* or Gram's stain will suffice to demonstrate the presence of leukocytes. Finding large numbers of white cells suggests an inflammatory or invasive diarrhea, such as occurs with *Shigella, Salmonella, Campylobacter,* invasive *Escherichia coli,* and *Entamoeba.* The presence of mononuclear cells is characteristic

Table 64-2. Important Features of Some Acute Diarrheas

ETIOLOGY	NATURE OF THE DIARRHEA W/S	OB	GB	ASSOCIATED SYMPTOMS AND SIGNS	EPIDEMIOLOGIC DATA	LABORATORY RESULTS
Viral	+/+	−	−	n, v, fever, myalgias abdominal cramps, headache	Occurs in short-lived epidemics	WBC: nl or elevated Stool: usually no WBC
Staphylococcus aureus	−/+	−	−	n, v, no fever	Custards; incubation: 2–8 h	WBC: nl Stool: no WBC
Clostridium perfringens	+/+	−	−	n, v, no fever	Steam tables incubation: 8–24 h	WBC nl Stool: no WBC
Bacillus cereus	+/+	−	−	n, v, no fever	Rice, sprouts	WBC: nl Stool: no WBC
Salmonella	+/−	+	+	n, v, fever, in some cases dysentery	Eggs, turtles, poultry	Stool: WBC + Culture +
Salmonella typhi	+/+ "Pea soup"	+	−	Rose spots, HA, splenomegaly, bradycardia, fever, toxic	Water, food	Stool: monos, culture +
Shigella	+/− Dysentery	+	−	n, v, fever, toxic in severe cases	Ghettos; day care centers; Indian reservations	Stool: WBC + Stool: WBC + Culture +
Campylobacter	+/− Dysentery	+	+	n, v, fever	Poultry, pets	Stool: WBC + Culture +
Yersinia	+/+	+	−	Simulates Crohn's disease and appendicitis; joint complaints	Dairy products, meat	Stool: WBC + Culture +
Vibrio sp.	+/+	−	−	n, v, cramps, occasionally fever	Raw seafood; 2-day course	Stool culture +
Cryptosporidia	+/−	−	−	occasionally n, v, cramps, dehydration	AIDS patients, immuno-suppressed	Stool for o & p +
Giardia	See Table 64-3					
Entamoeba histolytica	See Table 64-3					

W/S = watery/soft
OB = occult blood
GB = gross blood
n = nausea
v = vomiting
HA = headache
o & p = ova and parasites
\+ = present
− = absent
nl = normal
WBC = white blood cells

Table 64-3. Important Features of Traveler's Diarrheas

ETIOLOGY	NATURE OF THE DIARRHEA W/S	OB	GB	ASSOCIATED SYMPTOMS AND SIGNS	EPIDEMIOLOGIC DATA	LABORATORY RESULTS
Escherichia coli	+/−	−	−	Usually no fever; although occasionally toxicity	Contamination of water, food	Stool: WBC −; can also be +
Entamoeba histolytica	+/+ dysentery	+/−	+/−	Can simulate inflammatory bowel disease, asymptomatic carriers	Returning tourists; immigrants	Stool + for o & p; + serology
Giardia	−/+	−	−	Upper abdominal pain	Contamination of water supply	Stool + for o & p
Vibrio cholerae	+/− "rice water"	−	−	Marked dehydration, cramps, vomiting	Contamination of water supply	Stool: WBC −
Shigella	See Table 64-2					
Salmonella	See Table 64-2					

of salmonellosis. An occasional white cell is of no pathologic significance. Leukocytes may be absent from the stool in the early phases of shigellosis and pseudomembranous colitis.

In selected instances, a *Gram's stain* of the stool will give etiologic information. For example, in about half the cases due to *Campylobacter,* the Gram's stain will demonstrate gram-negative rods arranged in characteristic gull-wing configuration. If either occult blood or leukocytes are present in the stool, appropriate *bacterial cultures* should be obtained. Detection of *Campylobacter* or *Yersinia* requires plating on specific medium at 42°C; the usual medium for *Salmonella* and *Shigella* will not suffice.

Patients with gross blood or large numbers of leukocytes in the stool and severe illness should undergo *sigmoidoscopy* to examine the appearance of the colonic mucosa; samples of the mucus and cultures can also be obtained (see evaluation of chronic diarrhea for details). Preparatory enemas and cathartics should be avoided so as not to distort the appearance of the bowel wall (see Chapter 56).

If the diarrhea persists for 2 weeks or more, a secondary evaluation is indicated. Stools should once again be examined for blood and leukocytes. A second stool should be sent for bacterial culture, and a fresh specimen should be examined for *ova and parasites*. Ova and parasite examinations are fraught with limitations that must be kept in mind. If *giardiasis* is a consideration, at least three stool samples are necessary, because excretion of the organism is intermittent. Aspiration of jejunal contents or passage of a string into the upper jejunum may be necessary to demonstrate trophozoites; such efforts usually produce positive results in infected patients. Identifying *Entamoeba histolytica* trophozoites by stool examination can be difficult; their visualization is easily impaired by the presence of barium, bismuth, and kaolin compounds. False-negative stool examinations also result from preparatory enemas (which lyse the organism) and antibiotics (tetracycline and sulfonamides reduce shedding of trophozoites into the stool).

If symptoms persist and the diagnosis remains uncertain, the patient requires further assessment for a chronic or recurrent diarrheal syndrome (see below). The patient who becomes markedly dehydrated or toxic is a candidate for hospital admission, or at least several hours of intravenous fluid replacement in an emergency room.

Chronic or Recurrent Diarrhea

History. If an acute episode of diarrhea has not resolved within 2 weeks or a pattern of recurrent diarrhea develops, several additional etiologies must be considered (see Table 64–1). The history is reviewed for new findings as well as for a *characterization of the diarrhea* and any *associated symptoms* (Table 64–4). Rectosigmoid pathology is suggested by frequent passage of small, loose stools in association with crampy, left lower quadrant abdominal pain or tenesmus.

Table 64-4. Features of Representative Chronic Diarrheas

ETIOLOGY	NATURE OF THE DIARRHEA W/S	OB	GB	ASSOCIATED SYMPTOMS AND SIGNS	LABORATORY RESULTS
Irritable bowel syndrome	−/+ Mucus prominent	−	−	Bloating, intermittent alternating constipation	Stools: − for WBC/RBC
Ulcerative colitis	+/+	+	+	Fever, abdominal pain, extraintestinal disease, bowel ulcers/inflammation	Stools: + for WBC/RBC Endoscopy: +
Crohn's disease	−/+	+/−	+/−	Abdominal pain, obstruction, skip areas	Proctoscopy +/− WBC +; O & P −
Pseudomembranous colitis	+/+	+/−	+/−	Simulates inflammatory bowel disease clinically; bowel ulcers/plaques	Stools: + for *Clostridium difficile* toxin/WBC/RBC
Diabetic enteropathy	+/+	−	−	Signs of autonomic insufficiency; occasionally malabsorption	Stools: + for fat (in small bowel type)
Dumping syndrome	+/+	−	−	Gastric surgery; occurs with meals; sweats, tachycardia	Normal
Malabsorption of fat	−/+ Steatorrhea	−	−	Weight loss, vitamin deficiency, sprue, pancreatic disease	Stools: + for fat
Lactase deficiency	+/+	−	−	Associated with milk products, cramping, bloating	Abnormal lactose tolerance test
Laxative abuse	+/+	−	−	Wasting, bulimia, dehydration	Stool + for laxatives
Villous adenoma	+/− Secretory, mucus	+	−	Protein wasting, no relation to meals	Hypokalemia, low albumin
Colon cancer	+/+	+	+	Change in bowel habits	Iron deficiency

CHO = carbohydrate
O & P = ova and parasites
+ = positive
− = negative
w/s = watery/soft
OB = occult blood
GB = gross blood

Small bowel disease is a consideration when there are large, loose bowel movements in conjunction with periumbilical or right lower quadrant pain, or when diarrhea occurs shortly after a meal or ingestion of certain foods. *Diarrhea following meals* should lead to a search for malabsorption, an osmotic etiology, the dumping syndrome, or a fistula. The presence of foul, bulky, *greasy stools* further supports the diagnosis of fat malabsorption. *Bloody stools* require investigation for neoplasm, invasive infection, and inflammatory bowel disease. The presence of *fever* has similar diagnostic implications. *Frothy stools* and *excessive flatus* are signs of fermentation of unabsorbed carbohydrates. *Alternating diarrhea and constipation* point to irritable bowel syndrome, as does *mucus* in the stool. The absence of intermittent constipation in a patient complaining of chronic diarrhea does not rule out the diagnosis.

Recent *travel* in conjunction with diarrhea that persists for more than 2 weeks raises the possibilities of giardiasis and amebiasis; pseudomembranous colitis is a consideration if the traveler has a recent intake of antibiotics. The slow resolution of traveler's diarrhea suggests postdysentery lactase deficiency and postdysentery irritable bowel syndrome.

A thorough review of drug intake is mandatory. A history of surreptitious *laxative abuse* may be hard to elicit, but inquiring gently and nonjudgmentally into feelings of low self-esteem and body image may provide suggestive information when a young, intense woman presents with chronic diarrhea and wasting. Previous abdominal surgery should be specified, looking for procedures that may have produced blind loops and allowed for bacterial overgrowth. *Sexual history* is relevant; promiscuous male homosexuals have an increased risk of polymicrobial enteritis (see above). A *psychosocial history* is needed to check for factors that may contribute to an irritable bowel syndrome.

Physical Examination. A complete physical examination is mandatory and may confirm suspected causes as well as establish the severity of the disease. Any fever, dehydration, postural hypotension, or cachexia should be noted. The skin should be inspected for jaundice, pallor, and rash. The abdomen is examined for distention, ascites, hepatomegaly, tenderness, rebound, and masses. Rectal examination may reveal fecal impaction, perirectal fistula, or a patulous anal sphincter. Stool is tested for occult blood.

Laboratory. Blood tests are helpful but rarely diagnostic. They should include a *complete blood count* for evidence of anemia and leukocytosis, *serum electrolytes* for detection of serious losses and imbalances, *amylase* for pancreatic disease, *liver function tests* and *prothrombin time* for hepatobiliary disease, and *serum calcium* and *glucose* for metabolic conditions that can lead to diarrhea. Eosinophil counts are normal in most parasitic infections that cause diarrhea; worms, not protozoan, stimulate peripheral eosinophilia. Previously ordered, but not very sensitive or specific markers of malabsorption, are the serum carotene and serum B_{12} levels.

Sigmoidoscopy performed without cleansing enemas is a potentially definitive procedure (see Appendix to Chapter 56). It should always be done when there is blood or pus in the stool or other evidence of rectosigmoid pathology. The presence of mucosal ulceration, plaques, friability, and bleeding should be noted. The finding of mucus in the absence of evidence for inflammation helps confirm the diagnosis of irritable bowel syndrome, whereas the presence of pus directs the evaluation toward infection and inflammation. Nodular inflammatory ulcers and yellow-white mucosal plaques are characteristic of pseudomembranous colitis. Ulceration is also noted with inflammatory bowel disease and amebic colitis.

Amebic disease and pseudomembranous colitis are often mistaken for inflammatory bowel disease. Patients with recent antibiotic exposure and an inflammatory exudate require evaluation for pseudomembranous colitis. Their *stool* should be assayed for *Clostridium difficile* toxin, although it must be understood that some patients without disease harbor the organism and might show detectable amounts of toxin in the stool.

If there is ulceration of the rectosigmoid mucosa and suspicion of *amebic disease* on the basis of epidemiologic data, *fresh mucosal smears* should be made. Proper technique for identification of trophozoites involves sampling the periphery of the ulcers with a glass rod or metal spatula; cotton swabs are inadequate, because the organisms adhere too firmly and do not readily transfer to a slide. Multiple *stool examinations for ova and parasites* can also be ordered. False-negative examinations for trophozoites are common and result from use of preparatory enemas, recent exposure to antibiotics, and concurrent use of barium, bismuth, or kaolin.

When there is serious clinical and epidemiologic suspicion of amebic disease and yet ova and parasite examinations are negative, *serologic testing* is indicated. The standard test is an indirect hemagglutination (IHA) assay. A positive titer is in excess of 1:128. It takes 2 to 4 weeks for seroconversion to occur. By the time most patients with amebic disease present with diarrhea, they are seropositive. Serologic testing is 85 percent sensitive in the setting of intestinal disease and 95 percent sensitive with extraintestinal, spread. Serologic testing is useful in nonendemic areas, where most people are seronegative, but less meaningful among patients from endemic areas, where there may be a high frequency of seropositivity from carrier states and chronic exposure.

Other patients who ought to have *stools* searched for *ova and parasites* include those who have traveled to areas endemic for *Giardia*, homosexuals (who have an increased incidence of giardiasis), and immunocompromised hosts, including those with AIDS (who are at risk for a host of pathogens including *cryptosporidiosis;* see below). Fresh loose stools are needed for identification of trophozoites; less fresh specimens can be used for detection of ova. Several stool examinations may be necessary. Sometimes small bowel aspiration or even biopsy is necessary to establish the diagnosis of giardiasis or cryptosporidiosis.

Three other stool tests deserve note. A simple and quick test in patients suspected of laxative abuse is to *alkalinize the stool;* if it contains phenolphthalein (a common ingredient of many over-the-counter laxatives), it will turn pink. Patients suspected of fat malabsorption should have a stool sample subjected to *Sudan stain* for qualitative detection of fat. Those with a positive qualitative study are candidates for a *72-hour quantititative stool fat determination*. Normally, stool fat should not exceed 6 percent of daily fat intake. Stool fat in excess of 6 g per day while the patient is on a test diet of 100 g of fat per 24 hours indicates fat malabsorption. Other studies of help in defining the location and nature of a suspected malabsorption problem include a D-xylose test for detection of small bowel disease or a *Chymex* test (an indirect measure of chymotrypsin) for pancreatic insufficiency. For suspected lactase deficiency, a *lactose-tolerance test* can be obtained, although a diagnostic trial of restricting milk products for several days is more practical.

Barium enema and *upper GI series* best demonstrate anatomic abnormalities (blind loops, fistulas, and tumors). A barium enema is useful when inflammatory bowel disease and malignancy are being considered. However, the radiologic appearance of the bowel is not always definitive (eg, amebiasis can simulate the picture of inflammatory bowel disease). It is important to remember that barium obscures identification of ova and parasites, necessitating completion of stool collections before obtaining a barium study. *Sigmoidoscopy* or *endoscopy* is indicated for elusive cases and suspected inflammatory bowel disease; the procedure allows for direct visualization, mucosal smears, and biopsy (see Appendix).

Therapeutic Trials sometimes obviate the need for more elaborate studies. As noted above, cessation of diarrhea in response to *restriction of milk products* strongly supports the diagnosis of lactose intolerance. Other recognized empiric trials include a course of *antibiotic therapy* in patients suspected of blind-loop syndrome, a trial of *metronidazole* for patients with a travel history and clinical picture consistent with giardiasis, and use of *pancreatic enzymes* in patients believed to be suffering from pancreatic insufficiency.

Diarrhea in the AIDS Patient

Often, patients with AIDS experience acute or chronic diarrhea. They are especially susceptible to the common infectious etiologies as well as such uncommon ones as *Cryptosporidia, Mycobacterium avium intracellulare, herpes simplex, cytomegalovirus, Neisseria gonorrhoeae,* and *Chlamydia trachomatis*. Evaluation should focus on finding the pathogen and may require sigmoidoscopic biopsy to obtain tissue for viral or mycobacterial culture (see Chapter 13).

Chronic Diarrhea of Unknown Etiology

Patients who remain undiagnosed after an extensive evaluation often turn out to have irritable bowel syndrome or surreptitious laxative abuse. The latter is most prevalent among young, professional women who are preoccupied with their weight and have low self-esteem and a poor body image (see Chapter 234). An otherwise unexplained hypokalemia is also suggestive of laxative abuse.

If a diagnosis has not been made, it may be worthwhile to characterize the type of diarrhea further by determining *stool volume, osmolality,* and *electrolyte content*. A stool volume of less than 200 mL per day is strongly suggestive of irritable bowel syndrome. Osmotic diarrheas show increased stool osmolality and low sodium and potassium concentrations. The differential diagnosis of osmotic diarrhea includes ingestion of nonabsorbable solutes (magnesium, bran), maldigestion of food, and malabsorption of osmotically active substances (eg, carbohydrates). Stool volumes in excess of 1 L per day indicate a secretory diarrhea. Occult etiologies include surreptitious laxative abuse, villous adenoma, carcinoid syndrome, pancreatic cholera (from secretion of vasoactive intestinal peptide), and other similarly rare conditions.

Recently, two new conditions associated with refractory chronic diarrhea have been recognized, labeled as *collagenous colitis* and *lymphocytic colitis*. These illnesses occur predominantly in women and cause chronic, watery diarrhea, often complicated by steatorrhea and malabsorption. Colonic appearance is grossly normal, but biopsy reveals collagenous or lymphocytic infiltrates. The small bowel usually is normal, but may show spruelike changes in those with lymphocytic disease. The latter may present as patients with spruelike malabsorption unresponsive to a gluten-free diet. Diagnosis requires biopsy at the time of sigmoidoscopy, even if the colonic mucosa appears grossly normal.

PRINCIPLES OF MANAGEMENT

Acute Diarrheas

The vast majority of acute diarrheal illness should be managed by *maintaining hydration* and waiting for the spontaneous resolution of symptoms. Often, hydration can be maintained by use of oral fluids, even in cases of profuse diarrhea. Solutions rich in electrolytes and sugar facilitate absorption of water. An 8-oz glass of fruit juice to which is added a pinch of table salt and a half teaspoon of honey or a teaspoon of table sugar makes a well-tolerated replacement solution. Nondiet cola drinks that have been allowed to stand and lose their carbonation are a reasonable substitute. Either can be taken along with a similar-size glass of water containing one-quarter teaspoon of baking soda to replenish losses in stool electrolytes, which in acute infectious diarrhea are sodium (Na):125 mEq per liter, potassium (K):20 mEq per liter, bicarbonate (HCO_3):45 mEq per liter, and chlorine (Cl):90 mEq per liter.

Absorbent preparations are commonly used for symptomatic therapy of simple acute diarrhea. Solutions of *kaolin* and *pectin* have no proven benefit but seem to be harmless; however, they should not be relied on in the treatment of severe diarrhea. Doses of *bismuth subsalicylate (Pepto-Bismol)* in excess of those recommended on the bottle (eg, 2 to 3 tablespoons every 3 hours) are sometimes effective (see below). *Opiates* such as *diphenoxylate* (dispensed as a combination with small amounts of atropine [Lomotil] to discourage abuse) and *loperamide* are effective in the symptomatic treatment of diarrhea by directly inhibiting the motility of the intestinal smooth muscle. Diphenoxylate and loperamide are derived from meperidine but have less effect on the central nervous system. They should be used cautiously, if at all, in conditions in which toxic megacolon is possible (eg, inflammatory bowel disease). Their use should also be restricted in certain bacterial diarrheas, such as shigellosis, to avoid prolonging the clinical course. The usual dose of diphenoxylate is 2.5 to 5 mg, every 4 hours, up to 20 mg per day. Loperamide is given as 2 or 4 mg, every 4 hours, up to 16 mg daily. Lower maintenance dosages will often be sufficient after initial control is achieved. Other opiates are potent antidiarrheal agents but carry a higher risk of addiction; they are useful when their coincident analgesic activity is needed. Deodorized tincture of opium (0.5 to 1 mL), paregoric (4 mL), or codeine (30 to 60 mg) can be given orally every 4 hours. *Anticholinergics* are useful only for irritable bowel syndrome (see Chapter 74).

Antibiotics have not been used routinely for acute bacterial diarrheas, because most infections are self-limited. Antibiotics have minimal effect on the course of illness and may prolong the asymptomatic bacterial carrier state. Moreover, one risks triggering an antibiotic-induced diarrhea. Exceptions include typhoid fever and severe cases of shigellosis, pseudomembranous colitis, *Campylobacter,* and *Yersinia*. In addition, elderly debilitated patients and others who would be endangered by a *Salmonella* bacteremia (persons with prosthetic heart valves or sickle cell anemia) should receive a course of antibiotics to limit distant complications. *Salmonella bacteremia* and *typhoid fever* can be treated with parenteral *ampicillin* or oral *chloramphenicol;* in milder cases, oral *trimethoprim-sulfamethoxazole* (one double-strength tablet bid for 2 weeks) suffices.

New data suggest that empiric use of a broad-spectrum fluoroquinolone antibiotic (eg, *ciprofloxacin* or *norfloxacin* 500 mg bid) in patients suspected of having acute bacterial diarrhea can reduce the intensity of the diarrhea and may shorten the duration of symptoms, without triggering serious adverse effects. Confirmation of initial studies is required, but the benefits seem particularly impressive in the setting of traveler's diarrhea (see below) and in those with culture-positive disease or severe illness. However, usefulness is limited by delay in elimination of *Salmonella* and induction of resistance in *Campylobacter.*

Patients suffering severe dysentery caused by *shigellosis* can be treated with oral *amoxicillin* (500 mg tid for 3 to 5 days), but antibiotic sensitivity testing is needed because amoxicillin-resistant strains are common. *Trimethoprim-sulfamethoxazole* (one double-strength tablet bid for 3 to 5 days) is an excellent alternative. Pending stool culture results, a few days of empiric therapy for shigellosis is reasonable if the epidemiologic history is suggestive and the patient is experiencing severe bloody diarrhea. Antiperistaltic drugs are contraindicated. *Campylobacter* is sensitive to oral *erythromycin* (500 mg qid for 7 days). Most patients with *Yersinia* infection have a self-limited illness, but toxic patients are candidates for oral *chloramphenicol* (50 mg per kilogram per day in four divided doses for 7 to 10 days) or parenteral therapy.

Pseudomembranous colitis usually resolves without antibiotic treatment, but oral *vancomycin* liquid suspension (as little as 125 mg qid for 7 to 10 days) and *metronidazole* (250 mg tid for 5 to 10 days) have both proven equally capable of controlling the disease, although relapses occur in 10 percent to 20 percent necessitating retreatment. Metronidazole is preferred for initial use because it is less expensive. *Cholestyramine* (one packet in water tid) is used in conjunction with antibiotics to help bind the enterotoxin; it has proven useful in difficult cases, as has *rifampicin* and *bacitracin*.

Symptomatic patients suffering from diarrhea due to parasitic infection also benefit from definitive antimicrobial therapy. *Entamoeba histolytica* responds to *metronidazole* (750 mg tid for 5 to 10 days) for treatment of trophozoites and *diiodohydroxyquin* (650 mg tid for 21 days) for elimination of cysts. *Giardiasis* is treated with quinacrine (100 mg tid for 7 days) or metronidazole (250 mg tid for 7 to 10 days). Retreatment is often necessary.

Traveler's Diarrhea

The objectives of treatment of traveler's diarrhea include prevention of illness and provision of symptomatic relief. Although much attention has been given to pharmacologic agents for prophylaxis, care in what one eats and drinks remains the single most important means of preventing traveler's diarrhea. Avoid use of local water supplies when they are in question. This includes foregoing fresh vegetables, which may have been washed in such water, and even the use of ice cubes. Drinking bottled water is preferable.

Because the majority of "turista" cases are caused by enterotoxigenic *Escherichia coli, chemoprophylaxis* has been aimed at combating this organism. *Trimethoprim sulfa (TMS)* (one double-strength tablet/d) and *ciprofloxacin* (500 mg/d) can reduce the risk of diarrhea, which ranges from 20 to 30 percent. For symptomatic relief of acute diarrhea, ciprofloxacin (500 mg bid) for 3 days is effective, as is TMS (one double-strength tablet bid). Some resistance to TMS is emerging, making ciprofloxacin the preferred agent. *Doxycycline,* a tetracycline derivative, taken on the day of travel (200 mg) and daily (100 mg) while away has also proven useful, although as many as 40 percent of the toxigenic *E. coli* strains are resistant to the drug, and the drug often causes GI upset and photosensitivity. Prophylaxic use of antibiotics had been in vogue, but the growing awareness of antibiotic-induced diarrhea, the high frequency of bacterial resistance to some agents, and the efficacy of bacterial resistance to some agents, and the efficacy of bismuth-containing agents is leading to less reliance on antimicrobials.

Bismuth subsalicylate (Pepto-Bismol) has proven effective in both prophylaxis for and treatment of traveler's diarrhea when used in large doses (60 mL qid). Unlike antibiotics, it has the advantage of not altering the normal bowel flora. Its mechanism of action is believed to involve inhibiting bacterial colonization by toxigenic bacterial strains. Bismuth turns the stools black; it is useful to alert patients of this side effect so its occurrence does not cause alarm.

Many find taking *diphenoxylate* or *loperamide* more convenient for symptomatic relief of traveler's diarrhea; in most instances, it can be used for brief periods with safety, except when *Shigella* or *Salmonella* infection is a serious consideration (ie, when there is fever or rectal bleeding). Loperamide has also been a useful adjunct to antibiotic treatment of symptomatic disease.

Antibiotic treatment is indicated in acute, severe cases. Ciprofloxacin (500 mg bid) and TMS (one double-strength tablet bid) are both effective, especially when used with loperamide (2 mg after each loose stool, up to 16 mg/d). A 3-day course of antibiotics usually suffices. Giving travelers a 3-day antibiotic supply plus loperamide to carry with them is reasonable and appreciated. Ciprofloxacin is probably preferred due to emergence of TMS-resistant strains of *E. coli*.

Chronic Diarrhea

To be effective, therapy for chronic diarrhea needs to be etiologic. For example, steroids and sulfasalazine are needed to control diarrhea caused by exacerbations of inflammatory bowel disease (see Chapter 73). Malabsorption due to pancreatic insufficiency necessitates use of enzyme supplements (see Chapter 72). Steatorrhea due to sprue responds to a gluten-free diet. Patients with "refractory sprue" may have lymphocytic or collagenous colitis, which may respond to sulfasalazine or prednisone. Lactase deficiency requires limitation of milk products or use of exogenous lactase. The dumping syndrome necessitates small feedings. Persistent pseudomembranous colitis is an indication for antibiotic therapy (see above). Cessation of surreptitious laxative use cures the diarrhea that accompanies it (see Chapter 234). In the setting of irritable bowel syndrome, a high-fiber diet is indicated if the clinical picture is predominantly one of constipation interspersed with brief episodes of diarrhea, but, if diarrhea predominates, loperamide can be useful for symptomatic relief (see Chapter 74).

Unlike treatment of acute diarrhea where many causes are self-limited and nonspecific measures aimed at symptomatic relief are appropriate, effective management of chronic diarrhea requires an etiologic diagnosis and specific therapy. Simply suppressing symptoms without identifying a cause may delay identification of a serious underlying condition (eg, colon cancer).

Chronic Diarrhea of Unknown Etiology. For patients who remain undiagnosed after an extensive workup, yet appear otherwise well, a trial of therapy for irritable bowel syndrome (see Chapter 74) is reasonable. Many such patients with unexplained diarrhea turn out to have a bowel motility disorder and associated psychosocial stresses. Clues to the diagnosis include absence of weight loss, normal laboratory studies, and a suggestive psychosocial history. Failure to respond after 4 weeks of therapy should lead to gastroenterologic consultation. One should not resort to nonspecific antidiarrheal agents for treatment of undiagnosed patients.

INDICATIONS FOR ADMISSION AND REFERRAL

Most patients with diarrhea can be managed on an outpatient basis. However, those who are unable to maintain their hydration orally and become significantly volume depleted (posturally hypotensive) require serious consideration for hospital admission and parenteral fluid replacement. Sometimes, several hours of intravenous fluids given in the emergency room will suffice and obviate an admission. Infants, elderly persons, and those with chronic or debilitating illnesses are particularly vulnerable to the complications of volume depletion and deserve closest watching. Patients with inflammatory diarrheas manifested by bloody, purulent diarrhea, and fever are also candidates for possible admission.

Referral to a gastroenterologist is indicated for patients with complicated inflammatory bowel disease, undiagnosed chronic diarrhea, or a requirement for colonoscopy or intestinal biopsy. One particularly difficult issue worthy of consultation is the need for small bowel sampling in patients with suspected parasitic disease who have repeatedly negative stool examinations for ova and parasites.

PATIENT EDUCATION

Because most acute diarrheas are self-limited, the patient with no evidence of serious underlying pathology can be reassured and advised to concentrate on maintaining hydration. The sugar and electrolyte preparations described in this chapter are easy to take and should be encouraged. Many people think that taking fluids will seriously worsen their diarrhea, and they request opiates or antibiotics; the proper role for such agents needs to be reviewed and their unrestricted use should be limited. Many ask if kaolin-pectin preparations are helpful; there is no evidence that they alter symptoms or the course of the illness, but neither are they harmful. Although antibiotics have been in vogue for prophylaxis of traveler's diarrhea, patients should be informed of the emergence of resistant strains, the potential complications of antibiotic use, and the efficacy of bismuth preparations. A few bottles of a bismuth preparation (eg, Pepto-Bismol), a few tablets of diphenoxylate for "emergencies," and advice to use bottled water and avoid foods likely to be contaminated (eg, raw vegetables washed with local water) represent reasonable alternatives to antibiotic prophylaxis. Patients with chronic undiagnosed diarrhea need to be prepared for a potentially extensive evaluation. In the meantime, advice on perianal care is much appreciated and ought not to be overlooked while investigation proceeds.

Perianal Hygiene. Much can be done to relieve the perianal discomfort that accompanies severe unrelenting diarrhea. *Sitz baths* for about 10 minutes two or three times a day can be soothing, followed by gentle drying with absorbent cotton (not toilet paper or towels). Washing with warm water on *absorbent cotton* after each bowel movement is also helpful in lieu of using toilet paper, which can be irritating. Also important is avoidance of soap. A short course of *hydrocortisone cream* may be useful when there is considerable anal inflammation. Some patients report that cleaning gently with cotton pads soaked with *witch hazel* (Tucks) provides considerable relief. Ointments containing topical anesthetics should be avoided; they can be irritating in themselves.

Recovery Phase. After resolution of diarrhea, it is best to avoid milk and dairy products for approximately another 7 to 10 days, because mild lactose intolerance commonly accompanies many cases. The best foods to begin eating are easily digested, high-carbohydrate substances such as bananas, rice, baked potato, and applesauce. Continued repletion of fluid is important.

ANNOTATED BIBLIOGRAPHY

Afzalpurkar RG, et al. Self-limited nature of chronic idiopathic diarrhea. N Engl J Med 1992;327:1849. *(Clinically useful data on this difficult problem.)*

Bartlett JG. Antibiotic-associated diarrhea. Clin Infect Dis 1992; 15:573. *(Authoritative review of pseudomembranous colitis and other forms of diarrhea related to antibiotics.)*

Bayless TM, et al. Lactose and milk intolerance: Clinical implications. N Engl J Med 1975;292:1156. *(Study of the prevalence, characteristics, and diagnosis of lactose intolerance in adults.)*

Blaser MJ, et al. Campylobacter enteritis in the United States: A multicenter study. Ann Intern Med 1983;98:360. *(*Campylobacter *was more frequently isolated than both* Salmonella *and* Shigella *combined.)*

Cann PA, Read NW, Holdsworth CD, et al. Role of loperamide and placebo in the management of irritable bowel syndrome. Dig Dis Sci 1984;29:239. *(Placebo-controlled trial showing reduction in urgency and frequency of bowel movements.)*

Cover TL, Aber RC. *Yersinia enterocolitica*. N Engl J Med 1989;321:16. *(Comprehensive review of this pathogen; 201 references.)*

DuBois R, Lazenby AJ, Yardley JH, et al. Lymphocytic enterocolitis in patients with "refractory sprue." JAMA 1989;262: 935. *(Description of this now recognized cause of chronic, watery diarrhea and steatorrhea.)*

DuPont HL, Ericsson CD. Prevention and treatment of traveler's diarrhea. N Engl J Med 1993;328:1821. *(Excellent review.)*

DuPont HL, Hornick RB. Adverse effect of Lomotil therapy in shigellosis. JAMA 1973;260:1525. *(Lomotil therapy may cause fever and toxicity may be prolonged in patients with shigellosis.)*

Eastham EJ, Douglas AP, Watson AJ. Diagnosis of *Giardia lamblia* infection as a cause of diarrhea. Lancet 1976;2:950. *(Retrospective review of 31 patients found that* Giardia *is not considered often or early enough.)*

Ericsson CD, DuPont HL, Mathewson JJ, et al. Treatment of traveler's diarrhea with sulfamethoxazole and trimethoprim and loperamide. JAMA 1990;263;257. *(Randomized, double-blind study finding that combination therapy was the most effective.)*

Gebhard RL, Gerding DN, Olson MM, et al. Clinical and endoscopic findings in patients early in the course of *Clostridium difficile*–associated pseudomembranous colitis. Am J Med 1985;78:45. *(Useful description of early clinical and sigmoidoscopic appearance of the bowel mucosa.)*

Goodman LJ, Trenholme GM, Kaplan RL, et al. Empiric antimicrobial therapy of domestically acquired acute diarrhea in urban adults. Arch Intern Med 1990;150:541. *(Randomized controlled trial; empiric ciprofloxacin effective for suspected acute bacterial diarrhea; TMS was not.)*

Gorbach SL, et al. Traveler's diarrhea and toxigenic *Escherichia coli*. N Engl J Med 1975;292:933. *(Classic report documenting that traveler's diarrhea is often due to enterotoxigenic* Escherichia coli.*)*

Graham DY, Estes NK, Gentry LO. Double-blind comparison of bismuth subsalicylate and placebo in the prevention and treatment of enterotoxigenic *E. coli*–induced diarrhea in volunteers. Gastroenterology 1983;85:1017. *(Study of 32 volunteers confirming the effectiveness of bismuth subsalicylate in preventing diarrhea.)*

Guerrant RL, Shields DS, Thorson SM, et al. Evaluation and diagnosis of acute infectious diarrhea. Am J Med 1985;78:91. *(Presents a generalizable approach.)*

Harris JC, DuPont HL, Hornick RB: Fecal leukocytes in diarrheal illness. Ann Intern Med 1972;76:697. *(Classic article that established that fecal leukocytes indicate inflammatory causes of diarrhea, such as shigellosis, salmonellosis, typhoid fever, invasive* E. coli, *and inflammatory bowel disease.)*

Kapikian AZ. Viral gastroenteritis. JAMA 1993;269:627. *(A terse discussion of virology, epidemiology, prophylaxis, and treatment.)*

Kolars JC, Levitt MD, Aouji M, et al. Yogurt, an autodigesting source of lactose. N Engl J Med 1984;310:1. *(Yogurt is well tolerated by lactase-deficient patients; yogurts containing live cultures release lactase and permit digestion of lactose.)*

Murphy GS, Bodhidatta L, Echeverria P, et al. Ciprofloxacin and loperamide in the treatment of bacillary dysentery. Ann Intern Med 1993;118:582. *(Found effective.)*

Palmer DL, et al. Comparison of sucrose and glucose in the oral electrolyte therapy of cholera and other severe diarrhea. N Engl J Med 1977;292:1107. *(Discussion of the uses and limitations of oral fluid and electrolyte therapy in severe diarrhea.)*

Palmer KR, Corbett CL, Holdsworth CD. Double-blind, crossover study comparing loperamide, codeine and diphenoxylate in the treatment of chronic diarrhea. Gastroenterology 1980; 79:1272. *(Loperamide was more effective than diphenoxylate, as effective as codeine, and had fewer side effects than either agent.)*

Quinn TC, Goodell SE, Fennell C, et al. The polymicrobial origin of intestinal infections in homosexual men. N Engl J Med 1983;309:576. *(An important finding.)*

Read NW, et al. Chronic diarrhea of unknown etiology. Gastroenterology 1980;78:264. *(Clinical features, evaluation, and follow-up of 27 such patients; checklist for evaluation is presented.)*

Silva J, et al. Treatment of *Clostridium difficile* colitis and diarrhea with vancomycin. Am J Med 1981;71:815. *(Oral vancomycin proved extremely effective and terminated symptoms within 7 days in all patients tested.)*

Simon D, Brandt LJ. Diarrhea in patients with acquired immunodeficiency syndrome. Gastroenterol 1993;105:1238. *(Comprehensive update, especially of pathogens that establish the diagnosis of AIDS.)*

Taylor DN, Sanchez JL, Candler W, et al. Treatment of traveler's diarrhea: Ciprofloxacin plus loperamide compared with ciprofloxacin alone. Ann Intern Med 1991;114:731. *(The addition of loperamide was helpful, especially during the first 24 hours.)*

Valdovinos MA, Camilleri M, Zimmerman BR. Chronic diarrhea in diabetes mellitus: Mechanisms and approach to diagnosis and treatment. Mayo Clin Proc 1993;68:691. *(Detailed consideration of the consequences of autonomic neuropathy.)*

Wistrom J, Jertborn M, Ekwall E, et al. Empiric treatment of acute diarrheal disease with norfloxacin: A randomized, placebo-controlled study. Ann Intern Med 1992;117:202. *(Efficacy demonstrated, especially in the very ill and those with positive cultures.)*

Primary Care Medicine: Office Evaluation and Management of the Adult Patient, 3rd edition, edited by Allan H. Goroll, Lawrence A. May, and Albert G. Mulley, Jr. J.B. Lippincott Company, Philadelphia

65
Approach to the Patient With Constipation

Constipation is a universal affliction of Western civilization. In the United States, this malady accounts for over 2.5 million physician visits a year. It is among the most frequent reasons for self-medication and is particularly troublesome in the elderly. More than $500 million are spent annually in the United States on laxatives; a survey of Londoners revealed 30 percent admitting to recent laxative use.

There is no uniform definition of constipation. To some, it means movements that are too infrequent or stools that are too hard. Others complain of incomplete or difficult evacuation. Among normal people, bowel habits vary widely, and there are diverse perceptions of what constitutes normal function. Population studies show that most normal people have more than three bowel movements per week, with men likely to have at least five. Stools less than 35 g per day are well below the lower limit of normal.

The primary physician must be able to uncover any underlying pathology as well as to provide symptomatic relief to those without a structural lesion. The prevalence of excessive laxative use and inadequate dietary fiber make it imperative that the physician be knowledgeable about the actions and adverse effects of available laxative preparations as well as dietary alternatives to their use.

PATHOPHYSIOLOGY AND CLINICAL PRESENTATION

The process of elimination of fecal waste requires two processes: filling of the rectum by colonic transport and reflex defecation of stool. Constipation may arise secondary to interference with either of these processes. The time it takes food to reach the anus is partially a function of the amount of fiber in the diet. Normal people placed on a diet containing 15 g of bran fiber per day have twice the number of movements per week of those on an uncontrolled diet. Patients with constipation solely on the basis of low dietary fiber usually have intermittent complaints that fully resolve with alteration of diet alone.

Exercise has an important effect on propulsion of bowel contents. Colonic transit has been observed to be significantly greater in physically active people than in those who get little exercise. Previously active persons often become constipated when put to bed on account of illness. Less dramatic, but probably no less important, is the leading of a *sedentary lifestyle;* constipation is common in inactive people.

Metabolic and endocrine disturbances can slow colonic transport. Hypokalemia, hypercalcemia, hypothyroidism, and diabetes are the most important of these in terms of frequency or potential reversibility. *Hypokalemia* can produce a generalized ileus and is most often seen in patients who take diuretics. Chronic laxative abuse may also produce hypokalemia; characteristically, there is surreptitious use of laxatives and diuretics, self-induced vomiting, pathologic desire to lose weight, and a personality disorder. Such patients present with fatigue and electrolyte disturbances. When constipation is caused by *hypothyroidism,* other manifestations of the disease are usually present, although sluggish bowel movements may be the presenting complaint. Constipation is a bothersome problem in some patients with *diabetes:* 20 percent of those with neuropathy report severe difficulty. Significant *hypercalcemia* (serum calcium greater than 12 mg per 100 mL) can slow bowel motility.

Mechanical obstruction from tumor, stricture, or volvulus may be responsible for the new onset of constipation. Cramping abdominal pain and distention in conjunction with a marked change in bowel habits are characteristic. Constipation occurs in more than 50 percent of patients with *colorectal cancers;* it is usually a symptom of advanced disease but may be the presenting complaint. Constipation is a more common presentation of *Crohn's disease* than is diarrhea, because transmural involvement predisposes to scarring and obstruction (see Chapter 74).

Drug use may precipitate constipation. *Opiates* and agents with anticholinergic activity such as *antidepressants* are frequently implicated. *Calcium-channel blockers* may slow down bowel motility, and *cholestyramine* may induce constipation by binding bile salts. *Aluminum hydroxide* and *calcium carbonate* antacids are constipating. Habitual use of *laxatives* is associated with impaired motor activity. The typical clinical picture is a long history of chronic constipation or a desire to feel "well cleaned out," followed by increasing laxative dependence, decreasing response, and ultimately a sluggish, poorly contracting bowel. Whether there is a prior underlying motor disorder or actual damage from laxative use is unsettled.

Psychiatric disease and psychosocial distress have important roles. An underlying *depression* is often contributory, and bowel complaints may be one of many somatic symptoms (see Chapter 227). In *irritable colon syndrome,* there is an increased prevalence of somatization, anxiety, and phobias, which have been linked to triggering disturbances of bowel function. Situational stress appears to play a similar role. Patients complain of chronic abdominal discomfort related to alterations in bowel habits and relieved by defecation and of irregular bowel movements, typically diarrhea alternating with constipation (although one may predominate). Passage of mucus, sense of incomplete evacuation, and bloating or distention add to the clinical picture. The exact mechanisms by which emotional difficulties lead to constipation remain unclear, but their contribution is widely recognized. Disturbances in bowel motility and visceral perception have been documented. Constipation ensues when there is an excessive degree of nonpropulsive contractions and segmentation of bowel contents. At other times, excessive propulsive activity is noted, typically after meals, resulting in diarrhea.

Neurologic impairment may present as constipation. *Spinal cord injury* that leads to compression of the cauda equina can halt bowel motility and also cause urinary retention as well as incontinence. *Multiple sclerosis* may compromise bowel function, as can ganglionic abnormalities. In most instances, other neurologic deficits are present. Disease limited to loss of neurons in the bowel wall typically presents as chronic, refractory constipation; it may date from childhood or, as noted above, be associated with long-standing laxative use. A permanently damaged neuromotor apparatus may also occur as a consequence of *scleroderma*.

Inhibition of the rectal defecation reflex has been documented in cases of painful local anal pathology, neurogenic disease, chronic use of laxatives, and voluntary suppression. Patients with this problem are found to have stool packed into the rectal ampulla. *Voluntary suppression* of the urge to defecate is usually a concomitant of a hectic daily pace or travelling. The resulting intermittent constipation may lead to excessive use of laxatives and enemas and damage to the reflex emptying mechanism.

Some authorities believe that *inadequate fluid intake* may play a role, although this is not well established. Water is known to be an effective means of distending the stomach and stimulating intestinal activity. The consistency of stool is a function of how much water it contains, which is a result, in part, of how much is taken into it.

DIFFERENTIAL DIAGNOSIS

The causes of constipation can be grouped according to pathophysiology: impaired motility, neurologic disorders, obstruction, local anorectal pathology (Table 65–1).

Table 65-1. Important Causes of Constipation

MECHANISM	ETIOLOGY
Impaired motility	Inadequate dietary fiber Inactivity Laxative abuse Irritable colon syndrome Diverticulitis Hypothyroidism Hypokalemia Diabetes Hypercalcemia Pregnancy Scleroderma Drugs (opiates, anticholinergics, tricyclic antidepressants, ganglionic blockers, calcium- and aluminum-containing antacids, sucralfate, disopyramide, calcium-channel blockers, antihistamines)
Neurologic dysfunction	Multiple sclerosis Spinal cord injury Neurogangliomatosis
Psychosocial dysfunction	Depression Situational stress Anxiety Somatization Phobias

WORKUP

History. Evaluation begins with definition of the size, character, and frequency of bowel movements, followed by a determination of the problem's chronicity. Acute constipation is more often associated with organic disease than is a long-standing problem. Chronic complaints that wax and wane over months and years point to a functional disturbance, often compounded by habitual laxative use. Inquiry is needed into symptoms that suggest an underlying gastrointestinal problem, such as abdominal pain, nausea, cramping, vomiting, weight loss, melena, rectal bleeding, rectal pain, and fever. Anorexia, bloating, belching, flatus, mucus in the stool, headache, depression, and anxiety should also be recorded; these symptoms may be associated with constipation of any etiology but often accompany functional disorders.

It is helpful at the first visit to take a history of working, eating, and bowel habits. Inquiry into dietary fiber intake and physical activity is essential. Use of medications, including nonprescription agents (especially laxatives and antacids,) need to be detailed. The patient's perspective and concerns should be elicited, and a careful psychosocial history obtained, with attention to situational stresses, anxieties, and methods of coping.

Physical Examination. One begins by recording the patient's weight and noting overall nutritional status. Skin is checked for pallor and signs of hypothyroidism (see Chapter 104). The abdomen is examined for masses, distention, tenderness, and high-pitched or absent bowel sounds. Rectal examination includes careful inspection and palpation for masses, fissures, inflammation, and hard stool in the ampulla. The last finding rules out significant obstruction and poor colonic motility and suggests that the problem is inadequate rectal emptying. The stool is noted for color and consistency and tested for occult blood. Anal sensitivity and reflexes are noted. Disordered innervation of the anus is indicated by finding that the anal canal opens wide when the puborectalis muscle is pulled posteriorly. Anoscopy is needed to identify internal hemorrhoids, fissures, tumors, and other local pathology. Neurologic examination should be performed to search for focal deficits and delayed relaxation phase of the ankle jerks, suggestive of hypothyroidism. Mental status examination includes checking for signs of depression (see Chapter 227), anxiety (see Chapter 226), and somatization (see Chapter 230).

Laboratory Studies. Radiologic investigation is of limited use unless evidence from history and physical examination suggests a specific etiology, such as obstruction. Acute onset of constipation requires ruling out obstruction and ileus, especially when accompanied by abdominal discomfort; plain supine and upright films of the abdomen, plus measurements of serum potassium and calcium levels are indicated. Suspicion of colonic obstruction requires colonoscopy or sigmoidoscopy plus barium enema. Finding pigmented colonic mucosa is common in patients who abuse anthraquinone laxatives such as castor oil or senna. Any hint of diabetes can be verified by urinalysis or serum glucose (see Chapter 93) and of hypothyroidism by thyroid-stimulating hormone determination (see Chapter 104).

An important diagnostic concern in the elderly is the possibility of constipation being due to a colonic neoplasm. Blood in the stool, weight loss, or iron-deficiency anemia mandates colonoscopy or sigmoidoscopy followed by barium enema (see Chapter 56). More than 25 percent of patients with colorectal carcinomas present with constipation. However, the elderly person with no evidence of obstruction, anemia, or occult blood loss can probably be followed expectantly for a few weeks on a conservative program that includes more dietary fiber, increased exercise, and monitoring of stool guaiacs before it is decided whether to subject the patient to colonoscopy or barium enema. If symptoms resolve and stools are negative for occult blood, the probability of malignancy or obstruction is low, and the patient need not undergo further testing at that time. A return visit for repeat assessment ought to be scheduled within 4 to 8 weeks.

When the cause of constipation is obscure, it is helpful to stop all nonessential medications. The codeine in a cough suppressant, the calcium in an over-the-counter antacid, or the iron in a multiple vitamin may be responsible for an otherwise puzzling diagnostic problem.

SYMPTOMATIC MANAGEMENT AND PATIENT EDUCATION

Symptomatic management is appropriate for the patient with a functional etiology, but only after obstruction and other forms of serious organic pathology have been ruled out. The first intervention after a careful work-up is to *reassure* the patient that there is no evidence for a serious underlying illness. Cancer is a common fear, especially in elderly patients with new onset of constipation. Careful *patient education* about diet and use of laxatives is the next priority. Explanation is needed to reassure the patient that a daily bowel movement is not essential to good health and that comfortable patterns of elimination depend on good living and eating habits. *Daily exercise* should be prescribed and based on the patient's physical capacity (see Chapter 18). The patient should *stop taking laxatives,* enemas, and nonessential drugs that may suppress colonic motility. The *fiber* content of the diet should be increased by adding bran, fruits, green vegetables, and whole-grain cereals and breads. Most studies show that 15 g of fiber per day is needed for the best effects, but the amount can be individualized. A large breakfast including bran cereal, juice, milk or coffee, and whole-grain bread is helpful. It is important to inform the patient with chronic constipation that normal function may take many weeks to return. Often, immediate results are expected; when they do not appear, the patient becomes despondent, stops the program, and returns to laxative and enema use.

Some patients refuse to eat bran because it makes them feel bloated and gassy. The patient can be reassured that these side effects usually resolve within a month of continued use. If dietary and exercise efforts fail or the patient insists on medication, a nondigestible fiber residue such as ground *psyllium* seed (Metamucil) can be beneficial. It acts to increase bulk by means of its hydrophilic properties, but it must be taken with plenty of fluids to prevent formation of an obstructing bolus; the usual dose is one teaspoon in 8 oz of liquid, three times a day. Controlled study of psyllium's efficacy showed significant improvement in symptoms with its use. However, the placebo group showed an equally large improvement, suggesting that explanation, reassurance, and increased attention are also important to improved bowel function.

Some elderly patients will remain refractory to the above measures and press for prescription of a laxative. As noted earlier, most laxatives are inappropriate for long-term use. However, the nonabsorbable saccharide laxatives *lactulose* and *sorbitol* have been shown to be safe and effective when used chronically in the elderly. These agents induce a potent osmotic effect, retaining fluid in the bowel lumen and softening the stool. Sorbitol is about a tenth of the cost of lactulose and has been shown in double-blind cross-over study to be equal in effect and slightly better tolerated. Side effects include excessive flatulence, bloating, and cramping.

When fecal impaction is present, a *hypertonic enema* (eg, Fleet's) will often relieve the situation. In addition, the patient can be instructed to squat over the toilet by standing on a chair in front of the bowl, providing a more favorable position for evacuating the rectum. Only rarely does one need to resort to disimpaction.

Trying to establish a convenient, uninterrupted *time for defecation* each day may be useful; 15 to 20 minutes after breakfast provides a good opportunity, because spontaneous colonic motility is greatest during that period. Continuing this routine each day regardless of travel or situational stress ought to be encouraged. Although there are no controlled studies proving the efficacy of this approach, it seems to help some people, although days or weeks can pass before success is noted.

Prevention of constipation during an illness that requires bedrest can be achieved by use of a high-fiber diet, bulk agents, and a commode, in preference to a bedpan. Correction of any coincident hypokalemia is important (see Chapter 32). There is no evidence that prophylactic use of laxatives or stool softeners is effective. A randomized controlled study of dioctyl sodium sulfosuccinate (Colace), a popular and expensive stool softener, failed to demonstrate any effect on the quality or frequency of stools. Use of minor tranquilizers in overly anxious patients has little direct effect on constipation. When severe depression requires use of antidepressants, the least constipating agent should be selected (ie, one with minimal anticholinergic activity). All tricyclic antidepressants have at least some anticholinergic activity, but desipramine, nortriptyline, and trazodone seem to have the least. Alternatively, a nontricyclic antidepressant such as fluoxetine might be a reasonable choice (see Chapter 227).

The importance of establishing a trusting, therapeutic patient–doctor relationship cannot be overemphasized, especially in patients with irritable colon syndrome, where the probability of underlying psychosocial distress is high. One facilitates the establishment of trust by eliciting concerns and perspective and taking time to explain and answer questions. A patient who has used a particular agent for decades needs to be told why it is being removed from the program; otherwise, chances of compliance are small. Chronic laxative users should be warned that it may take 4 to 6 weeks before spontaneous bowel movements return. Patience and sympathetic support can be rewarding, but expectations of quick results must not be raised (see also Chapter 74).

A.H.G.

ANNOTATED BIBLIOGRAPHY

Almy TP. Management of the irritable bowel syndrome. Ann Intern Med 1992;116:1027. *(Editorial perspective on this difficult problem.)*

Baron TH, Ramirez B, Richter JE. Gastrointestinal motility disorders in pregnancy. Ann Intern Med 1993;118:366. *(Constipation is common; mechanisms reviewed.)*

Burkitt D, Walker A, Paintner N. Effect of dietary fibre on stools and transit times and its role in causation of disease. Lancet 1972;2:1408. *(Classic paper on fiber and its link to constipation and other bowel problems.)*

Camilleri M, Prather CM. The irritable bowel syndrome: Mechanisms and a practical approach to management. Ann Intern Med 1992;116:1001. *(Excellent review [78 references] and a balanced, pathophysiologic approach to therapy.)*

Cann PA, Read NW, Holdsworth CD. What is the benefit of coarse wheat bran in patients with irritable bowel syndrome? Gut 1984;25:168. *(Double-blind, placebo-controlled study demonstrating efficacy.)*

Connell A, Hilton C, Irvine R, et al. Variation of bowel habits in two population samples. Br Med J 1965;2:1095. *(Population study helping to define the range of normal for bowel activity and the prevalence of constipation.)*

Darlington RC. Over-the-counter laxatives. J Am Pharm Assoc 1966;6:470. *(Data on spending for over-the-counter preparations; dated but enlightening and still valid.)*

Drossman DA, Thompson WG. The irritable bowel syndrome: Review and a graduated multicomponent treatment approach. Ann Intern Med 1992;116:1009. *(Emphasizes the biopsychosocial model and the importance of the patient–doctor relationship to a successful outcome.)*

Goodman J, Pang J, Bessman A. Dioctyl sodium sulfosuccinate: An ineffective prophylactic laxative. J Chronic Dis 1976; 29:59. *(Randomized prospective study of patients admitted to the hospital. The drug made no difference in quality or frequency of stools.)*

Graham DY, Moser SE, Estes MK. The effect of bran on bowel function and constipation. Am J Gastroenterol 1982;77:599. *(Twenty grams of wheat or corn bran reduced transit time by 50 percent and improved constipation clinically in 6 of 10 constipated women.)*

Holdstock D, et al. Propulsion in the human colon and its relationship to meals and somatic activity. Gut 1970;11:91. *(Physical activity was found to stimulate mass movements, and inactivity reduced them.)*

Hull C, Greco RS, Brooks DL. Alleviation of constipation in the elderly by dietary fiber supplementation. J Am Geriatr Soc 1980;28:410. *(In an institutional geriatric population, adding bran prevented constipation and reduced laxative use.)*

Katz L, Spiro H. Gastrointestinal manifestations of diabetes. N Engl J Med 1966;275:1350. *(A classic review; constipation is a frequent gastrointestinal complaint of diabetics.)*

Kirwn WO, Smith AN. Colonic propulsion in diverticular disease, idiopathic constipation and the irritable bowel syndrome. Scand J Gastroenterol 1974;12:331. *(Transit time is prolonged in all three diseases and can be significantly reduced by bran.)*

Lederle FA, Busch DL, Mattox BS, et al. Cost-effective treatment of constipation in the elderly: A randomized double-blind comparison of sorbitol and lactulose. Am J Med 1990;89:597. *(Demonstrates efficacy and comparability; useful in elderly patients with refractory functional disease.)*

Longstreth GF, Fox DD, Youkeles MS, et al. Psyllium in irritable bowel syndrome: A double-blind study. Ann Intern Med 1981;95:53. *(Both treatment and control groups showed equally impressive degrees of improvement, suggesting that other factors are also operative.)*

Matthews. Making "connxtions": Enhancing the therapeutic potential of patient–clinician relationships. Ann Intern Med 1993;118:973. *(Useful piece with important insights into the treatment of patients with functional bowel disease.)*

Oster JR, Materson BJ, Rogers AI. Laxative abuse syndrome. Am J Gastroenterol 1980;74:451. *(Review article outlining this important cause of chronic constipation.)*

Roth HP, Fein SB, Shurman JF. The mechanisms responsible for the urge to defecate. Gastroenterology 1957;32:717. *(Describes normal process of defecation and provides physiologic basis for understanding disease states.)*

Sonnenberg A, Koch TR. Epidemiology of constipation in the United States. Dis Colon Rectum 1989;32:1. *(Accounts for over 2.5 million physician visits per year.)*

66
Approach to the Patient With Anorectal Complaints

Primary Care Medicine: Office Evaluation and Management of the Adult Patient, 3rd edition, edited by Allan H. Goroll, Lawrence A. May, and Albert G. Mulley, Jr. J.B. Lippincott Company, Philadelphia

Anorectal complaints often go incompletely evaluated. Although they are usually a result of minor conditions such as hemorrhoids or fissures, etiologies range beyond the trivial to inflammatory bowel disease, cancer, and infection. In addition, anorectal problems generate a substantial amount of worry and discomfort. As a result, they deserve careful consideration by the primary care physician. An increasingly frequent diagnostic challenge is the evaluation of anorectal problems in male homosexuals.

PATHOPHYSIOLOGY AND CLINICAL PRESENTATION

Anorectal complaints result from traumatic, vascular, infectious, inflammatory, neurologic, and malignant etiologies. Symptoms include pain, discharge, itching, mass, and fecal incontinence. *Pain* is most often a manifestation of anal pathology; anal and perianal skin are richly innervated with pain-sensitive nerve fibers; rectal tissue is relatively insensitive to pain. A fissure, distention by abscess or hemorrhoid, invasion by tumor, or marked inflammation can lead to considerable discomfort. Secondary anal sphincter spasm may ensue, prolonging and intensifying the pain. *Discharge* ensues from inflammation of the rectal mucosa or drainage of an abscess. Cancer, abscess, and thrombosed hemorrhoids can produce an anorectal *mass;* condylomata acuminata may also cause anal skin nodularity. *Itching* represents a minor form of skin irritation seen with a variety of mechanical and inflammatory lesions; it is intensified by moisture in the perianal area. Chronic itching leads to excoriation, edema, thickening, fissuring, and lichenification of the perianal skin. *Bleeding* is a common and important manifestation of anorectal pathology; its causes range from hemorrhoids and fissures to carcinoma and inflammatory bowel disease (see Chapter 63).

Hemorrhoids are the most common anorectal problem, affecting about half of patients over the age of 50. They represent dilatations of the anorectal vascular network. Epidemiologically, they are associated with diets high in fat and low in fiber. Theories explaining the etiology of hemorrhoids invoke a number of mechanisms, including increased venous pressure secondary to upright posture and straining at stool, arteriovenous communications in rectal tissue, and prolapsed cushions of tissue secondary to loss of support. Clinically, hemorrhoids are associated with pregnancy, portal hypertension, and constipation. The relative absence of hemorrhoids in African populations that have high-residue diets has led to the suggestion that an increase in dietary fiber might prevent the development of hemorrhoids.

Although the traditional view is that hemorrhoids are venous varicosities resulting from straining at stool, they do not always present in a fashion consistent with this postulate. For example, hemorrhoids develop in early pregnancy in many young women, long before there is significant intraabdominal pressure from a large fetus. Moreover, hemorrhoidal bleeding is characteristically arterial in quality (bright red) rather than the dark variety that would be expected from a strictly venous source. Nonetheless, many patients with hemorrhoids have been found to have increased resting anal sphincter pressures, which supports the hypothesis that increased anal pressure causes straining at stool. The straining stresses and compromises the rectal mucosa's supporting fibrous tissue, allowing the now poorly supported mucosa to slide down and become entrapped by the sphincter. Venous engorgement ensues as a consequence of the entrapment.

Hemorrhoids may be classified by presentation as *first degree* when they merely bleed, *second degree* if they prolapse on high pressure but return spontaneously, and *third degree* when the anal suspensory ligament is stretched to the point of permanent prolapse. Hemorrhoids are considered to be *internal* when derived from the superior hemorrhoidal plexus above the dentate line, and *external* when located below the dentate line and covered by squamous epithelium. External hemorrhoids are covered by pain-sensitive anal skin and arise from the inferior hemorrhoidal plexus. Internal hemorrhoids are covered by the much less pain-sensitive rectal mucosa and represent dilations of the superior hemorrhoidal plexus.

Pain, incomplete defecation, constipation, excessive moisture, rectal itching, bleeding, or detection of a prolapsed mass are the common presentations. Clinical presentation depends in part on the location of the hemorrhoid and the presence of complications. External hemorrhoids that have thrombosed present as tender bluish swellings. Internal hemorrhoids often bleed, but only when they prolapse do they present as a mass; when irreducible, they are subject to thrombosis. Recurrent bleeding may be seen with either type; sudden rupture may cause rather dramatic, although relatively harmless, bright red bleeding. Hemorrhoids are regularly encountered as incidental findings on physical examination. Skin tags are evidence of previous hemorrhoids that have thrombosed, leaving connective tissue. The most bothersome complications of hemorrhoids include bleeding, prolapse, and thrombosis.

Fistula-in-ano is a communication between the anal canal and the perianal skin. It is usually nontender. The external opening may be single or multiple, with a granulation tissue bud and chronic seropurulent drainage. Occasionally, an indurated cord of tissue may be palpable, extending from the external fistulous opening toward the anal canal. The fistula may result from rupture or surgical drainage of a perirectal abscess; other etiologies include Crohn's disease, carcinoma, tuberculosis, radiation therapy, lymphogranuloma venereum, and anal fissures. Patients complain of persistent and irritating drainage of blood, pus, or mucus.

Perirectal abscess and fistula-in-ano are two stages of the same disease process, beginning as an infection in the anal glands that empty into the anal crypts at the mucocutaneous junction, and subsequently spreading into the adjacent tissue. The abscess thus formed often drains through the perianal skin. Symptoms and signs are a function of the size and location of the abscess. The first manifestation is rectal pain, which may occur before any mass becomes palpable. Patients characteristically complain of constant, throbbing pain in the perianal region or in the rectum. A mass may be identified externally on examining the anus or internally on palpating the rectum. Perirectal abscess formation is a particularly important problem in patients with Crohn's disease, immunodeficiency states, and hematologic disorders.

An *infected pilonidal cyst or sinus* is most common in males between ages 16 and 30. These are midline, in the area of the natal cleft. Multiple sinuses may be present. Recurrent secondary infections are frequent.

Carcinoma of the perianal skin or anorectal tract typically does not cause pain until relatively late in its clinical course, often in the setting of a large ulcerated bleeding lesion. Earlier lesions present as painless nodules or plaques. Pruritus, mucoid drainage, and change in bowel habits are more subtle manifestations that sometimes occur.

Proctalgia fugax, as the term implies, is fleeting but severe rectal pain believed to be related to spasm of the levator ani and coccygeal muscles. Although usually brief, symptoms can last for more than 30 minutes. Suspected precipitants include chronic trauma from poor posture; psychogenic factors may also be operative. There are no associated physical findings, except for muscle tenderness on digital examination.

Proctitis, inflammatory disease of the rectum, has a wide variety of etiologies ranging from infection and trauma to radiation and inflammatory bowel disease. Regardless of the cause, the presentation is usually one of mucopurulent discharge, rectal bleeding, and, in severe cases, rectal pain and tenesmus. Patients with *ulcerative proctitis* demonstrate on sigmoidoscopy an inflamed rectal mucosa and a clearly demarcated upper border, above which the mucosa is normal. Systemic symptoms and extraintestinal manifestations are rare when the disease is limited to the rectum. The risk of carcinoma is small, and fewer than 10 percent to 15 percent of patients develop diffuse colitis.

Infectious proctitis occurs mostly among promiscuous *male homosexuals* who engage in frequent rectal intercourse with multiple partners. Gonorrhea, amebic disease, chlamydia, and herpes simplex infections are prominent in this population (see below). *Gonococcal proctitis* is especially common. The rate of asymptomatic carriage of gonorrhea among promiscuous male homosexuals is reportedly as high as 60 percent to 70 percent. Symptomatic gonococcal proctitis presents with discharge and rectal discomfort (see below). Diarrhea is the hallmark of symptomatic *amebic infection, shigellosis,* and *Campylobacter* infection (see Chapter 64). *Herpes simplex* proctitis can be a very painful condition, accompanied by tenesmus, constipation, rectal ulceration, and discharge. Involvement of the sacral nerve roots can lead to bladder and erectile difficulties, paresthesias, and pain in the thighs and buttocks.

Solitary rectal ulcer is a rare condition of unknown etiology associated with rectal discharge, bleeding, and occasionally, dull pain. The characteristic finding on sigmoidoscopy is a single shallow ulcer 7 to 10 cm from the anus; its borders may be heaped or nodular. Chronicity is the rule; complications are rare. These must be distinguished from cancer and lymphogranuloma venereum by biopsy.

Pruritus ani (chronic perianal itching) is not a diagnosis but rather a syndrome that results from a variety of mechanical and inflammatory lesions. Anatomic lesions that produce chronic discharge (such as *fistulas, fissures,* and *hemorrhoids* with intermittent mucosal eversion) can result in pruritus ani. There are a variety of infectious etiologies. *Anogenital warts (condylomata acuminata)* are viral in origin and generally transmitted by sexual contact. They may be confined to the perianal region or also involve the penis, vulva, and anal canal. Multiple, soft, filiform excrescences characterize these lesions, which may enlarge, become confluent, and even bleed. *Gonococcal proctitis* can lead to anal soreness, burning, and purulent discharge. Infestations with *pinworm (Enterobius vermicularis)* typically cause nocturnal anal itchiness, especially among children but sometimes spread to involve adult family members. Nocturnal symptoms are due to the daily evening migration of the female pinworm downward to deposit eggs on the perianal skin. Anal involvement is characteristic of some systemic dermatologic diseases, such as *psoriasis* and scabies. *Contact dermatitis* or *eczema* resulting from use of a topical agent is common and can complicate the diagnosis of the original cause of pruritus. Applied initially as a remedy for itching, the agent may only aggravate the problem by causing skin sensitization. Itching is intensified by moisture in the perianal area and often aggravated by use of topical agents applied in an attempt to quell symptoms. Passage of *alkaline stools* (as occurs in severe diarrhea) can have an irritant effect on the anal skin. Persistent anal itching may be a form of *neurodermatitis;* such patients characteristically present with multiple excoriations. *Candidal infection* is found among diabetics, homosexuals, and those recently taking broad-spectrum antibiotics; perianal erythema and itching are presenting manifestations.

Fecal impaction ranks as one of the major sources of anorectal discomfort among the elderly and bedridden. Chronic, incomplete evacuation leads to formation of an obstructing bolus of desiccated hard stool in the rectum. Symptoms of anal discomfort and constipation are typical, but anorexia, malaise, or nonspecific lower abdominal fullness may be all that is reported. Paradoxically, diarrhea rather than constipation is sometimes the only complaint, because of the collection of liquid stool distending the proximal colon and passing around the obstructing bolus. Unless this is corrected by disimpaction, complications such as intestinal obstruction, rectal prolapse, and even bowel perforation may ensue.

Fecal incontinence follows damage to the normal anal sphincter mechanism. Perianal disease, anal surgery, and neurologic disease can have devastating psychosocial consequences when they compromise the anal sphincter. Some patients lose the ability to sense rectal distention as well as to constrict the external sphincter. In others with only a weakened sphincter, the prognosis is less grim; biofeedback methods can be employed to help them regain continence.

Anorectal problems in homosexuals and others engaging in receptive anal intercourse can be complex in etiology and presentation. In a major study, more than 80 percent of homosexual men presenting to a venereal disease clinic with anorectal or intestinal symptoms were infected with one or more sexually transmissible anorectal or enteric pathogens. Three principal syndromes were noted: a *proctitis* characterized by anorectal pain, lesions, and discharge, but no evidence of disease above the rectum; a *proctocolitis* that, in addition to proctitic manifestations, included diarrhea, tenesmus, and inflammation extending into the sigmoid mucosa; and an *enteritis* (see Chapter 64) that consisted of diarrhea and abdominal pain, but no anorectal symptoms or signs.

As noted above, gonococcal, herpetic, chlamydial, and syphilitic forms of proctitis occur with increased frequency among these patients. In the carefully documented venereal disease clinic study of 119 symptomatic patients and 75 randomly selected asymptomatic homosexual men mentioned earlier, the prevalence of anorectal *gonorrhea* was reported to be 31 percent among those with symptoms. In the same series, *herpes simplex* virus was cultured from 19 percent of symptomatic men; all isolates were type 2. Rectal mucosal ulcerations were present in the majority and yielded herpes virus. *Syphilis* was also common in this series; 3 percent of symptomatic individuals were found to have anal chancres, another 3 percent had evidence of secondary anorectal syphilitic disease (erythematous nodular or indurated rectal mucosal lesions that were biopsy positive).

A clinical and sigmoidoscopic picture of *proctocolitis* occurred in about 15 percent of cases. Such patients complained of anorectal discomfort, tenesmus, diarrhea, constipation, and abdominal cramps. On sigmoidoscopy, inflammatory changes started at the rectum and extended beyond 15 cm into the sigmoid colon. *Campylobacter, Entamoeba histolytica, Chlamydia,* and *Clostridium difficile* were significantly correlated with the enterocolitis; often more than one organism was recovered. Polymicrobial infection is commonplace among symptomatic male homosexuals with many sexual partners.

Although much of the proctitis in this population is infectious in origin, *culture-negative proctitis* occurs with some frequency and has been linked to exposure to the *coloring agents* and scents found in some of the lubricants used for anal intercourse. Several etiologies may present simultaneously. The patient complaining of hemorrhoidal pain may actually have concurrent gonorrhea, allergic proctitis, and chlamydial infection. Traumatic complications of rectal intercourse include prolapsed hemorrhoids, anal fistulas and fissures, perirectal abscesses, rectal ulcers, and anal tears. Foreign bodies are sometimes recovered.

DIFFERENTIAL DIAGNOSIS

The differential diagnosis of anorectal problems can best be considered in anatomical terms, depending on whether symptoms and signs are predominantly anal, anorectal, or rectocolitic (Table 66–1). This is particularly true when considering the causes of anorectal disease in male homosexuals (Table 66–2).

Table 66-1. Differential Diagnosis of Anorectal Problems

PROBLEM	DIFFERENTIAL DIAGNOSIS
Anal discomfort	Hemorrhoids Fissure-in-ano (hard bowel movement, cancer, venereal disease) Fistula-in-ano (perirectal abscess, Crohn's disease, carcinoma, radiation, TB, lymphogranuloma venereum) Perirectal abscess (Crohn's disease, immunodeficiency, hematologic disorders) Infected pilonidal cyst Carcinoma of the anal epidermis Infections (syphilis, candidiasis, condylomata accuminata)
Rectal discomfort	Proctitis (ulcerative, gonococcal, amebic, herpetic) often accompanied by discharge and bleeding Perirectal abscess Impaction Proctalgia fugax Solitary rectal ulcer
Pruritus ani	Excess moisutre (poor hygiene), pinworms, eczema, scabies, diabetes, liver failure, irritants (topical agents, alkaline stools), fissure, early cancer, neurodermatitis, anal infections (see above)
Incontinence	Rectal surgery, neurologic disease, perianal disease

Table 66-2. Differential Diagnosis of Anorectal Problems in Male Homosexuals

SYNDROME	ETIOLOGY
Proctitis	*Neisseria gonorrhea* Herpes simplex *Chlamydia* (nonlymphogranuloma strains) Syphylis Condylomata acuminata Trauma Chemical irritants
Proctocolitis	*Campylobacter* *Shigella* *Entamoeba histolytica* *Chlamydia* (lymphogranuloma strains)
Enteritis	*Giardia lamblia*

WORKUP

History. Although a careful physical examination is the single most important part of the evaluation, history can provide important epidemiologic and etiologic information. Determining whether the condition is predominantly anal (local pain only), anorectal (local anal pain plus rectal discomfort, tenesmus, rectal discharge, constipation), or rectocolonic (rectal discomfort, tenesmus, rectal discharge, plus diarrhea, abdominal pain, bloating, nausea) helps to focus the evaluation.

Patients with anal complaints ought to be questioned about masses, nodules, focal tenderness, history of hemorrhoids, psoriasis, passage of hard stool, bleeding, discharge, generalized itching, nocturnal pattern, and recent trauma. Detailed inquiry into the use of topical medications (many of which are sensitizing), involvement of other household members or sexual partners, and hygienic practices should also be made.

For those with anorectal involvement, check into symptoms of inflammatory bowel disease (see Chapter 73), obtain a careful and detailed sexual history focusing on numbers of partners and practice of receptive rectal intercourse, and note any reports of inguinal adenopathy (seen with herpes and lymphogranuloma), sacral root paresthesias, and difficulty with micturition (other telltale symptoms of herpes simplex infection). Those with rectocolonic symptoms are likely to have either inflammatory bowel disease or a polymicrobial infection from rectal intercourse; consideration of associated symptoms and risk factors is indicated.

Physical Examination. Thorough and gentle inspection of the anus and perianal region is the *sine qua non* of successful diagnosis of anorectal problems. One examines the anal skin for erythema, eczema, psoriatic patches, ulcerations, vesicles, fistulas, fissures, condylomata, nodules, hemorrhoids, and inflammatory changes. The presence of perianal or rectal ulcers in association with proctitis in a male homosexual is indicative of syphilis or herpes simplex. If the lesions appear as scaling plaques, a look at the skin of the extensor surfaces of the extremities might provide additional evidence for a diagnosis of psoriasis. In a very anxious patient with multiple excoriations over other parts of the body, suspect neurodermatitis as the cause of pruritus ani. If an inflamed anorectal mucosa is encountered, gonorrhea needs to be considered and inquiry into rectal intercourse needs to be pursued.

Stretching the perianal skin will reveal fissures, which come into view at the anal verge, most often in the posterior midline but occasionally in the anterior midline. With chronic fissures, there is scarring and induration as well as an associated hypertrophied anal papilla at the pectinate line; a skin tag marks the external limit. Crohn's disease is likely in those with multiple fissures, recurrent fistulas, or perirectal abscesses. A painless hard nodule or plaque in the anal region may represent carcinoma. When the lesion is ulcerated, the diagnosis is more obvious and the disease is more advanced.

Digital rectal examination is almost always an essential component of the examination. However, in the presence of a painful fissure, it can be an extremely painful procedure that is likely to alienate the patient and cause such pain as to make adequate examination impossible. The same applies to use of anoscopy in such patients. On the other hand, rectal examination should never be deferred in patients who are not acutely and severely uncomfortable.

One needs to check for masses (both fluctuant and firm), discharges, ulcerations, and other mucosal changes as well as test the stool for occult blood. Ascribing anorectal symptoms to hemorrhoids without performing as complete an examination as possible is a common reason for delay in diagnosis of carcinoma.

Palpation for enlarged lymph nodes should not be overlooked. Prominent inguinal adenopathy is characteristic of herpetic and chlamydial infections (lymphogranuloma venereum species).

Diagnostic Studies. Unless the patient has a very painful lesion, *anoscopy* needs to be performed (see Appendix, Chapter 56) to visualize the canal and mucosa adequately and obtain samples of any discharge. One inspects for mucosal inflammation, fissure, fistula, mass, plaque, ulcer, and discharge. Patients with rectal inflammation, fistula formation, nonhealing fissures, bleeding, or diarrhea are candidates for *sigmoidoscopy*. Involvement of the sigmoid mucosa suggests inflammatory bowel disease (see Chapter 74) and infectious forms of colitis (see Chapter 64). Patients with atypical fissures, especially those that fail to heal, painless hard anorectal nodules, and mucosal ulcerations are candidates for *biopsy* to rule out malignancy, inflammatory bowel disease, and chronic infection (syphilis, tuberculosis). Children complaining of nocturnal pruritus ani can be evaluated for pinworm infestation by taking a cellophane tape impression of the anus and microscopically examining it under low power for the characteristic eggs.

Male homosexuals engaging in receptive anal intercourse with many sexual partners should undergo *anoscopy* to determine the nature of rectal involvement and to obtain samples of mucus for *Gram's stain* and *culture on Thayer-Martin plates*. A positive Gram's stain is excellent presumptive evidence of gonorrhea, although a negative smear does not rule out the diagnosis. Any chancrelike lesions should be subjected to *dark-field* examination for spirochetes. A *serologic test for syphilis* is also obtained.

Homosexual patients with evidence of rectal pathology on anoscopy require *sigmoidoscopy;* establishing the extent of mucosal involvement helps narrow the list of possible etiologies. Those with a *proctocolitis* picture of mucosal involvement extending above 15 cm or symptoms of colitis (diarrhea, nausea, abdominal cramping) should be *cultured for Campylobacter, Chlamydia* (lymphogranuloma strains), and *Shigella* and have their stools examined for the *ova and trophozoites* of *Entamoeba histolytica*. Those with *proctitis* only (no mucosal disease above 15 cm) are more likely to have gonorrhea, herpes simplex, or chlamydial infection (nonlymphogranuloma strains) and can be cultured accordingly. Viral cultures are not necessary, because the diagnosis of herpes simplex proctitis can usually be made on the basis of its characteristic clinical presentation (severe anorectal pain, multiple perianal ulcers, rectal ulceration, inguinal adenopathy, difficult micturition, impotence, and paresthesias in the S_4 and S_5 distributions).

SYMPTOMATIC MANAGEMENT AND INDICATIONS FOR REFERRAL

Fissure. Patients with anal pain due to *fissure* should initially be treated symptomatically. Lubricants, such as mineral oil, and agents providing a soft, bulky stool, such as methylcellulose, will decrease trauma and counteract the attendant sphincter spasm. Frequent warm sitz baths provide intermittent relief of pain and spasm. Topical analgesics are of limited use and may result in skin sensitization. Systemic analgesics are sometimes necessary, but if narcotics are used, increased constipation may occur. If the pain has not improved by conservative measures in several days to weeks, the patient should be referred for surgical treatment, which has a high success rate. In general, chronic or recurrent fissures will require surgery more often than acute or superficial fissures. In patients in whom the pain of fissure precludes digital or instrumental examination at the first visit, these may be done at the time of surgical treatment under adequate anesthesia.

Perirectal abscess will not resolve on antibiotics alone; the proper treatment is surgical drainage. Antibiotic therapy should be reserved for patients with extensive cellulitis, signs of systemic infection, immunosuppression, valvular heart disease, or intravascular prostheses. Incision and drainage of a perirectal abscess usually requires anesthesia and is not often an office procedure. Similarly, the treatment for an infected pilonidal sinus is surgical drainage, which is accomplished satisfactorily under local anesthesia.

Fistula-in-ano. The only successful treatment is surgical. However, patients with inflammatory bowel disease should not undergo surgery for fistula because this will usually fail as long as there is any active proximal disease. Surgery is reserved for palliation of complications of fistula (ie, drainage of recurrent perirectal abscess).

Suspicion of carcinoma and need for biopsy require surgical consultation, as does the patient with severe recurrent discomfort from *hemorrhoids* (see Appendix).

Pruritus ani. Specific therapy is related to identification of a specific etiology (eg, diabetes in the patient with candidiasis). Identification of the cause may be a challenging exercise to the primary physician. Pruritus resulting from anatomic lesions will generally remit with correction of the underlying cause. *Anogenital warts* are effectively treated with topical application of 25 percent podophyllin in tincture of benzoin repeated every 1 to 2 weeks. The patient is instructed to bathe between 6 and 12 hours after the application. Care should be taken to avoid applying the compound to intact skin. If anoscopy reveals intraanal warts at the initial examination, curettage and electrocoagulation under anesthesia will be necessary.

Pinworms. All family members should be treated simultaneously. Pyrantel pamoate (Antiminth) is the drug of choice; a one-time oral dose of 11 mg per kilogram of body weight usually suffices. Preventive measures are difficult to enforce, except for handwashing before meals and after bowel movements. The best prevention is simultaneous treatment of all members of the household.

Idiopathic. No specific cause is found. Pruritus appears to be a form of neurodermatitis affecting the perianal skin. However, the symptoms are often relieved by careful attention to *perianal hygiene* after bowel movements, keeping the perianal skin dry with application of witch hazel, and using topical steroid ointments (0.25% hydrocortisone ointment) for several weeks to break the cycle of itching and skin changes caused by scratching. When contact dermatitis is thought to be caused by topical agents, the offending medication should be discontinued.

Gonorrheal proctitis. See Chapter 116.

Homosexuals. While awaiting cultures, those with a nonspecific *proctitis* (inflammation limited to the lower 15 cm of the bowel and no ulcers) should be treated empirically by covering for gonorrhea and *Chlamydia* (see Chapters 137 and 141). Both infections may be present simultaneously. The presence of ulceration suggests syphilis and herpes simplex, but does not rule out concurrent gonorrhea and chlamydial infection; polymicrobial infection is found in about 25 percent of patients.

Fecal incontinence. Patients have achieved some benefit from *biofeedback* technique. However, only those who retain some degree of rectal sensation are candidates for biofeedback. The technique requires responding to the feeling of rectal fullness. Manometry is sometimes helpful to retrain the anal sphincter response to rectal distention.

PATIENT EDUCATION

When poor or excessive personal hygiene, application of irritating agents, or neurotic behavior is responsible for symptoms, the relationship between rectal discomfort and precipitants should be explained so the patient can take appropriate corrective action. Patients who obtain temporary relief of symptoms by applying a topical sensitizing agent may be reluctant to halt their medication if no other therapy is advised. Daily sitz baths can be prescribed in its place. Prevention through counseling is an important component of therapy in male homosexuals. Patients need to know that receptive anal sex with multiple partners carries a very high risk of intestinal infection and that they should certainly refrain from sexual activity if they become symptomatic.

A.H.G.

ANNOTATED BIBLIOGRAPHY

Alexander-Williams J. Causes and managements of anal irritation. Br Med J 1983;287:1528. *(Good review with the British clinical approach.)*

Goodell SE, Quinn TC, Mkrtichian PA, et al. Herpes simplex virus proctitis in homosexual men. N Engl J Med 1983;308:868. *(Documents the high frequency and distinctive clinical presentation of this infection.)*

Jensen SL, et al. Management of acute anal fissure. Br Med J 1986;292:1167. *(Sitz baths and bran worked best.)*

Lebedeff DA, Hochman EB. Rectal gonorrhea in men: Diagnosis and treatment. Ann Intern Med 1980;92:463. *(Prospective study of 1200 men detailing the clinical presentation, utility of Gram's stain and culture, and response to therapy.)*

Lieberman DA. Common anorectal disorders. Ann Intern Med 1984;101:837. *(Superb review with 107 references.)*

Owen WF. Sexually transmitted disease and traumatic problems in homosexual men. Ann Intern Med 1980;92:805. *(Good review of the multitude of problems faced by homosexual men practicing receptive anal intercourse; 60 references.)*

Quinn TC, Goodell SE, Fennell C, et al. Infections with *Campylobacter jejuni* and *Campylobacter*-like organisms in homosexual men. Ann Intern Med 1984;101:187. *(Describes the clinical presentation of infection with this class of organisms; about 25 percent of symptomatic patients were infected with the organism.)*

Quinn TC, Goodell SE, Mkrtichian E. *Chlamydia trachomatis* proctitis. N Engl J Med 1981;305:195. *(*Chlamydia trachomatis *of LGV immunotypes is associated with severe acute proctitis that mimics Crohn's disease.)*

Quinn TC, Stamm WE, Goodell SE, et al. The polymicrobial origin of intestinal infections in homosexual men. N Engl J Med 1983;309:576. *(Important paper documenting the polymicrobial nature of intestinal infection in this population.)*

Ramanujmps PRA, Sad ML, Abcarian H, et al. Perianal abscesses and fistulas: A study of 10,023 patients. Dis Colon Rectum 1984;27:595. *(Largest available series.)*

Smith LE, Henrich SD, McCullah RD. Etiology and treatment of pruritus ani. Dis Colon Rectum 1982;25:358. *(Practical article on mundane but important issue.)*

Wald A. Biofeedback therapy for fecal incontinence. Ann Intern Med 1981;95:146. *(Technique proved helpful in those who retain some degree of rectal sensation.)*

Appendix: Management of Hemorrhoids

Hemorrhoids are a source of much misery, although they are of no consequence unless they thrombose, prolapse, or bleed. Therapy is directed toward relief of symptoms and should be accomplished with a minimum of discomfort, cost, and time lost from work. Simple approaches to pain relief and sensible modification in bowel habits to prevent progression constitute the essentials of medical therapy. The primary physician must be certain that symptoms are attributable to hemorrhoids, alleviate any anxiety about neoplasm, provide conservative medical therapy, and decide on the need and timing of surgery.

PRINCIPLES OF MANAGEMENT

In most cases it is not necessary to remove hemorrhoids to treat them effectively. Symptomatic relief and a halt to progression can usually be achieved by use of simple local measures and minor changes in diet. For a painful attack, a *cold pack* applied for the first few hours offers considerable relief. Hot *sitz baths* (with a little salt added to the water to make it a more isotonic solution) are soothing and effective when used at least once or twice daily for about 20 to 30 minutes. Softening the stool helps minimize straining and can be accomplished by increasing *dietary fiber* and making short-term use of *stool softeners* (eg, dioctyl sodium sulfosuccinate). Irritant laxatives should be avoided. Patients should set aside a regular time each day to have an unhurried bowel movement and avoid vigorous wiping. Stubborn itching and inflammation respond well to *topical corticosteroids; hydrocortisone cream* and suppositories are adequate and relatively inexpensive. Topical hydrocortisone cream (1%), which can be purchased without a prescription, provides good relief from itching due to mild inflammation of anal tissue. It has been added to many of the popular over-the-counter (OTC) preparations, although generic hydrocortisone is the least expensive formulation.

A host of *over-the-counter preparations* are heavily promoted. Many contain a topical anesthetic, such as benzocaine or pramoxine. *Benzocaine* may produce some temporary pain relief, but it is quite sensitizing; the resultant allergic response may actually worsen symptoms. *Pramoxine* is another topical anesthetic found in popular OTC preparations (Anusol, Tronolane Cream, and so forth). It is similar in efficacy to benzocaine, acting within 3 to 5 minutes of application and lasting several hours, but is less sensitizing. However, the cream formulation can still be irritating because of the presence of paraben preservatives. *Preparation H* is among the best-selling and most widely advertised of OTC hemorrhoidal therapies. It contains shark liver oil, live yeast cell derivatives, and phenyl mercuric nitrate; none of these agents, singly or in combination, has been shown to have any beneficial effect on hemorrhoids, although they are promoted as being able to shrink hemorrhoids and reduce inflammation.

Hemorrhoids that bleed repeatedly, prolapse, produce intractable pain, or thrombose deserve surgical evaluation. Internal hemorrhoids that have been bleeding persistently or prolapsed can be removed in the surgeon's office by using *rubber-band ligation*. A rubber band is placed at the base of the hemorrhoid; within a week the lesion sloughs. Sometimes multiple attempts are necessary. *Injection of sclerosing agents* (eg, 5% phenol in oil) into the upper pole of an internal hemorrhoid is another means of dealing with internal hemorrhoids; the procedure has fallen out of favor because of its association with scarring of the anal canal. *Cryosurgery* is relatively painless and does not require anesthesia, but it produces a foul-smelling discharge for about a week and, occasionally, stricture is a late occurrence. Excruciatingly painful external hemorrhoids that have thrombosed can be excised under local anesthesia, and the *clot can be removed*. Excellent nonsurgical results have been reported using heat delivered through an infrared *photocoagulating probe* for treatment of first- and second-degree hemorrhoids. The heat is directed to the root of the hemorrhoid to interrupt its vascular supply, causing it to contract.

Definitive *hemorrhoidectomy* is the treatment of last resort. In contrast with the other surgical therapies mentioned, it requires hospitalization, and the recovery period can extend over several weeks. Moreover, there is a risk of compromising the competence of the anal sphincter. Nevertheless, it does represent a serious treatment option for patients with disabling, refractory disease.

THERAPEUTIC RECOMMENDATIONS

- Advise frequent hot sitz baths for relief of pain. At the initial recognition of pain, the patient can apply a cold pack for the first few hours, then take hot baths three or four times a day.
- If inflammation and itching are present, prescribe a suppository preparation containing a steroid (eg, hydrocortisone). If symptoms are predominantly external, prescribe 1 percent or 2.5 percent hydrocortisone cream.
- Topical anesthetics may be useful for the acute relief of severe pain. If this form of therapy is to be used, an agent that is minimally sensitizing (eg, pramoxine) should be chosen.
- Treat constipation by having the patient increase dietary fiber and use a stool softener, such as dioctyl sodium sulfosuccinate, 100 mg tid. After resolution of acute symptoms, the high-fiber diet should be continued.
- For thrombosed hemorrhoids:

  1. Instruct the patient to lie prone with ice applied to the thrombosed hemorrhoid.
  2. Prescribe oral analgesics; codeine may be required.
  3. Prescribe stool softeners.
  4. Conservative therapy should be successful in 3 to 5 days; otherwise refer the patient for surgical removal of the clot, which will relieve the pain promptly.

- Intractable symptoms require surgical therapy. The specific method chosen depends on the surgical expertise available in the community.

PATIENT EDUCATION AND PREVENTION

Instruction in proper diet and bowel habits is extremely helpful.

- Advise the patient to increase the intake of dietary fiber; suggest bran, carrots, green vegetables, and fruits with skin. Consider use of a psyllium preparation. Some people find foods such as chili, onions, and alcohol irritating. If this applies to your patient, suggest avoidance of them.
- Emphasize the importance of providing a regular time to have bowel movements. After bowel movements, the patient should avoid vigorous wiping; patting ought to suffice, and it minimizes irritation.
- Instruct the patient not to linger on the toilet or strain at stool. Long periods of standing should be avoided.
- Caution the patient against use of irritant laxatives.
- At the first sign of recurrent symptoms, institute frequent hot sitz baths.
- Instruct the patient to pat dry rather than wipe or rub.

A.H.G.

ANNOTATED BIBLIOGRAPHY

FDA Advisory Review Panel on OTC Hemorrhoidal Drug Products. Fed Register 1980;45:35576. *(Concludes it is unclear whether topical anesthetics are effective for treatment of hemorrhoids.)*

Johnson JF, et al. The prevalence of hemorrhoids and chronic constipation. Gastroenterol 1990;98:380. *(Best data, with divergent patterns noted.)*

Lieberman DA. Common anorectal disorders. Ann Intern Med 1984;101:837. *(Extensive review of the anatomy and physiology of the anus and rectum with special attention to hemorrhoids, fissure-in-ano, pruritus ani, and fecal incontinence; required reading for all primary physicians.)*

Murie JA, Sim AJ, MacKenzie I. Rubber band ligation versus haemorrhoidectomy for prolapsing haemorrhoids. Br J Surg 1982;69:536. *(Long-term prospective clinical trial showing that ligation is effective, except for permanently prolapsed painful lesions.)*

Prasad GC, et al. Studies on etiopathogenesis of hemorrhoids. Am J Proctol 1976;27(3):33. *(Excellent review of the pathogenesis of hemorrhoids.)*

Stern H, McLeod R, Cohen Z, et al. Ambulatory Procedures in anorectal surgery. Adv Surg 1987;20:217. *(Includes discussion of hemorrhoid treatments offered by the surgeon in the office setting.)*

To tie; to stab; to stretch, perchance to freeze (editorial). Lancet 1975;2:645. *(Concludes that hemorrhoidectomy should be reserved for failure of other methods.)*

Primary Care Medicine: Office Evaluation and Management of the Adult Patient, 3rd edition, edited by Allan H. Goroll, Lawrence A. May, and Albert G. Mulley, Jr. J.B. Lippincott Company, Philadelphia

67
Approach to the Patient With an External Hernia

MICHAEL N. MARGOLIES, M.D.

Abdominal hernias are exceedingly common, often causing occupational disabilities and posing the risk of incarceration and strangulation of bowel. Fortunately, adequate evaluation can usually be performed in the office by means of history and physical examination. The primary physician must distinguish between patients who require surgical referral and those who may be managed expectantly.

PATHOPHYSIOLOGY AND CLINICAL PRESENTATION

Pathophysiology. A hernia is a defect in the normal musculofascial continuity of the abdominal wall that permits the egress of structures not normally passing through the parietes. In general, the significant feature of hernia is not the size of the protrusion or the sac, but the size and rigidity of the defect in the abdominal wall. Fixation and rigidity of the hernial ring are the features that lead to incarceration and strangulation. The distinction between congenital and acquired hernia is not often clear, because many hernias that appear after trauma or straining represent a congenital predisposition, such as indirect inguinal hernia in the adult. This distinction has little bearing on management, although it may make considerable difference to the patient who may be compensated if the hernia can be attributed to trauma at work. Some of these hernias are incidental to, and antedate, the perceived injury.

Disorders resulting in increased intraabdominal pressure may contribute to the appearance of a hernia and affect the postoperative management as well. For example, chronic cough due to cigarette smoking or bronchitis can precipitate or worsen herniation; the same is true of symptomatic prostatism.

Clinical Presentation. The symptoms of an *uncomplicated* or *reducible external hernia* are related not to its size but to the degree of pressure on its contents. Patients with large scrotal hernias containing much intestine may have few symptoms other than a dragging sensation. A mass appears on standing, which reduces when the patient is supine. Pain may be intermittent, disappearing when the hernia is reduced. Patients with small hernias containing an entrapped knuckle of bowel may have rather severe pain and nausea. Many patients with femoral, umbilical, or epigastric hernias may be entirely unaware of their existence.

An *irreducible* or *incarcerated hernia* is one in which the contents cannot be replaced into the abdomen. Here the mass remains palpable with the patient relaxed and in the supine position. A *strangulated hernia* is an irreducible one in which the blood supply to the entrapped bowel loop has been compromised, resulting in small bowel obstruction and infarction. These patients complain of colicky abdominal pain, nausea, and vomiting and show signs of small bowel obstruction with distention, tympany, and hyperperistalsis. In addition, careful examination demonstrates a tender, irreducible groin or ventral hernia.

Indirect inguinal hernias, which account for one-half of all hernias in adults, pass through the internal abdominal inguinal ring along the spermatic cord through the inguinal canal, and exit through the external inguinal ring. In the male, these can descend into the scrotum. *Direct inguinal hernias* pass through the posterior inguinal wall medial to the inferior epigastric vessels, through Hesselbach's triangle. *Femoral hernias* pass through the femoral canal inferior to the inguinal ligament and become subcutaneous in the fossa ovalis. It is often difficult to distinguish between these three forms, especially when there is incarceration and the sac is large.

Indirect inguinal hernias are eight to ten times more common in men than in women, whereas femoral hernias are three to five times more common in women than in men. Nevertheless, the most common hernia in women is the indirect inguinal type. The diagnosis is less often made in women because physical examination of the external inguinal ring is more difficult. Direct hernias increase in incidence with advancing age and are the least likely of the external hernias to incarcerate or strangulate. Strangulation is common in femoral hernias.

The majority of patients with strangulated inguinal hernias are aware of the hernia before strangulation. In contrast, nearly half of those with strangulated femoral hernias are unaware of the hernia before strangulation. In addition, groin pain and tenderness are absent in a significant percentage of cases of strangulated femoral hernia.

The commonly encountered *ventral hernias* include umbilical, epigastric, and incisional varieties. Ventral hernias are often more obvious with the patient standing. *Umbilical hernias* pass through the umbilical ring and represent failure of the ring to obliterate after birth. In the infant, these often close spontaneously within the first 2 years of life. In the adult, they are more common in women and are associated with obesity, multiparity, and cirrhosis with ascites. Umbilical hernias are often missed because they are obscured by subcutaneous fat. There is a high risk of incarceration and strangulation and a greater mortality than with inguinal hernia because large bowel is frequently entrapped.

Incisional hernias are those that develop in the scar of a previous laparotomy or in a drain site. They are associated with a previous postoperative wound infection, dehiscence, malnutrition, obesity, and smoking. They are more common in vertical than in transverse scars. Incisional hernias often have multiple defects and several rings. They are frequently irreducible or only partially reducible because of adhesions within the sac. Patients with very large incisional hernias may be remarkably free from symptoms of intestinal obstruction, although incarceration is common; strangulation is relatively uncommon because of the usually large size of the defects.

Epigastric hernias occur through the linea alba between the xiphoid process and the umbilicus. They may be difficult to detect in the obese patient and must be looked for in patients with epigastric pain. Incarcerated epigastric hernia may produce symptoms that mimic peptic ulcer disease or biliary colic.

DIFFERENTIAL DIAGNOSIS

Recognizing a hernia usually presents little difficulty, although distinguishing one type of inguinal hernia from another can sometimes be complicated. Differential diagnosis of an entrapped femoral hernia includes not only inguinal hernia but femoral lymphadenopathy, saphenous varix, psoas abscess, and hydrocele. On occasion it is impossible to differentiate an incarcerated femoral hernia from a single enlarged femoral lymph node (the lymph node of Cloquet). Other causes of groin pain or swelling include muscle strain, hip arthritis, inguinal adenopathy, and undescended testicle.

WORKUP

Diagnosis and evaluation of external hernias require no more than a brief history and careful physical examination; laboratory and radiologic studies are unnecessary unless major complications have resulted.

History. The patient is questioned about groin pain, swelling, ability to reduce the hernia, circumstances of onset, and aggravating and alleviating factors, such as exacerbation on standing, straining, or coughing. Acute onset of colicky abdominal pain, nausea, and vomiting suggest entrapment and strangulation in a patient with a known hernia.

Physical examination is directed toward differentiating herniation from other causes of inguinal swelling or pain and distinguishing among 1) hernias that are uncomplicated and require no therapy; 2) those that can be repaired electively; and 3) those in which emergency surgery is the safest course. The physical examination is also important in distinguishing the anatomic type of hernia, because prognosis and likelihood of incarceration and strangulation differ among the various types.

The patient should be examined in both the supine and standing positions. Inspection is often as important as palpation for detection. Examination should include a Valsalva maneuver to increase intraabdominal pressure. In the male, small inguinal hernias are looked for by invaginating the scrotal skin while the patient is standing. To detect ventral hernias, the patient should be supine and then asked to lift the head from the examining table and to bear down to tense the abdominal wall.

Palpation follows and is best done with the patient standing. In the male, one inserts the index finger into the inguinal canal by following the spermatic cord. Distinguishing a direct from indirect hernia can be difficult. An indirect hernia projects more inferiorly, and protrusion into the scrotum is almost always a sign of it. To detect a femoral hernia, one palpates the fossa ovalis, inferior to the inguinal canal. If a groin hernia is detected, one should gently attempt to reduce it while the patient relaxes the abdominal muscles.

If a hernia is irreducible, the physician should look for local tenderness, discoloration, edema, fever, and signs of small bowel obstruction. It is often difficult to distinguish a simple incarceration from early strangulation; for this reason these two lesions are managed identically by immediate referral to a surgeon. Surgical exploration is the only way to be certain that no compromised bowel is trapped in the hernia sac. Conversely, when signs of small bowel obstruction are present, it is essential to examine thoroughly for a strangulated femoral hernia because groin pain and tenderness may be absent.

The groin area also is checked for lymphadenopathy and other masses that do not change with position or Valsalva. If there is groin pain but no mass, then a musculoskeletal etiology is suggested and a careful examination of hip movement is indicated.

A few conditions are believed to have more than a chance association with hernias, and some argue that they should be screened for. Whether the adult patient with a recent hernia is more likely to have an occult carcinoma of the colon remains a source of controversy. It had been suggested that patients undergo routine sigmoidoscopic examination and barium enema. However, if the patient reports no change in bowel habits and the stools are repeatedly guaiac negative, it is unnecessary to submit the patient to more extensive investigation for occult malignancy. Symptoms and signs of prostatism are frequently present in the elderly male with hernia and may require relief before herniorrhaphy. The entire abdomen ought to be examined for masses, hepatomegaly, and ascites, which are sometimes associated with hernia formation.

PRINCIPLES OF MANAGEMENT AND INDICATIONS FOR REFERRAL

Patients with an *asymptomatic,* easily *reducible inguinal hernia* can be managed expectantly without resorting to surgery. Surgery is elective, but should probably be carried out if the patient is young. Should pain ensue or signs of incarceration develop, then surgery may be indicated. Patients with a *symptomatic reducible inguinal hernia* should undergo elective repair for relief of symptoms and prevention of strangulation. Reduction by means of a truss may be unsatisfactory even in patients with relative medical contraindications to surgery. Moreover, surgical repair can be done under local anesthesia in the high-risk patient, and newer techniques make for less perioperative morbidity.

In patients with a *nontender incarcerated inguinal hernia* of recent onset, but without signs of inflammation or bowel obstruction, it may be safe to attempt gentle reduction ("taxis"). This is best accomplished with the patient supine and the hips and knees flexed. If gentle pressure over the hernial sac fails to reduce the mass further, efforts should be abandoned and the patient should be referred for surgery forthwith. Often the patient has more experience in reducing his own hernia than the physician. Patients with evidence of strangulated groin hernias should be subjected to immediate operation regardless of medical contraindications; if untreated, death will result from bowel necrosis.

Patients with *reducible femoral hernias* should undergo prompt elective repair because of the high incidence of strangulation. Whenever there is a question of an incarcerated femoral hernia, it is safest to proceed immediately with surgical exploration.

In *umbilical hernias,* surgery is unnecessary if on physical examination there is a small asymptomatic fascial defect without protrusion. When herniation is detected, however, umbilical defects should be repaired, because there is a high risk of incarceration and strangulation. The danger of strangulation is compounded by the greater likelihood of colonic entrapment with a resultant higher mortality rate than in hernias in which small intestine is strangulated. Therefore, all incarcerated umbilical hernias should be managed as if they were strangulated. Elective umbilical herniorrhaphy should be avoided in patients with ascites; instead, efforts should be directed toward reducing the ascites (see Chapter 71). The problem in patients with cirrhosis and ascites is made more difficult when the skin overlying the sac thins out and poses the risk of rupture.

Patients with small neck *incisional hernias* or tender incarceration should undergo repair on an urgent basis. Patients who have trophic changes or ulceration in the skin overlying incisional hernias are also candidates for urgent surgery. In some instances, cellulitis of the skin overlying the hernia sac occurs and is difficult to distinguish from strangulation of the contents of the sac. Management of large incarcerated incisional hernias that occur in the abdomen in very obese patients is a particular problem. Major efforts should be directed toward weight reduction before repair if it is possible to procrastinate. If there is doubt, however, as to the presence of intestinal obstruction or viability of the contents of the sac, the advice of a surgeon should be sought promptly.

Factors contributing to hernia formation should be corrected if possible. Prostatectomy is occasionally required after repair of hernia, and the patient with symptoms of prostatic obstruction should be advised of this possibility. Patients with chronic bronchitis and emphysema, or with chronic cough due to cigarette smoking, should be urged to stop smoking promptly to diminish symptoms caused by the hernia and to decrease the possibility of postoperative complications.

PATIENT EDUCATION

Patients who are to be managed conservatively must be taught to watch for signs of complications. It is the responsibility of the physician to instruct the patient in the symptoms of incarceration and strangulation and in the urgency of seeking help should they occur. If the patient is deemed incompetent to make such observations and to obtain help promptly, a strong case can be made for proceeding with surgery. Patients scheduled for elective surgery also require instruction, because incarceration occasionally occurs before the planned operation.

Many patients with asymptomatic or mildly symptomatic reducible hernias will be reluctant to undergo surgery because their symptoms are minimal. If they fall into the high-risk group (eg, femoral or small neck incisional hernias), they should be informed of the strong likelihood of strangulation and the minuscule morbidity and mortality associated with surgery.

Patients who are advised to have surgery appreciate estimates of time to walking (same day for local anesthesia); time to resumption of full activity (6 weeks); risk of recurrence (1–10%); and effect on sexual function (none).

ANNOTATED BIBLIOGRAPHY

Flanagan L Jr, Bascom JV. Repair of the groin hernia: Outpatient approach with local anesthesia. Surg Clin North Am 1984; 64:257. *(An increasingly common approach that reduces cost considerably.)*

Gilbert AI. An anatomic and functional classification for the diagnosis and treatment of inguinal hernia. Am J Surg 1989; 157:331. *(Useful, terse summary.)*

68
Management of Peptic Ulcer Disease

Primary Care Medicine: Office Evaluation and Management of the Adult Patient, 3rd edition, edited by Allan H. Goroll, Lawrence A. May, and Albert G. Mulley, Jr. J.B. Lippincott Company, Philadelphia

Peptic ulcer disease continues to be a major source of morbidity and a health problem of substantial importance. Prevalence estimates for active disease range from 1.5 percent to 2.0 percent. About 350,000 new cases are diagnosed annually. Five percent to 10 percent of the population will experience peptic ulcer disease in their lifetime. Males outnumber females by two to one. Duodenal ulcers account for 80 percent of cases. In men, peak prevalence of duodenal ulcer occurs between ages 45 and 54; for gastric ulcer, peak occurs between ages 55 and 64.

New advances in understanding peptic ulcer pathogenesis (the roles of *Helicobacter* infection and prostaglandin inhibition, the action of the proton pump) have led to marked improvements in pharmacologic therapy and enhanced outcomes.

The goals of management are to alleviate pain, promote healing, limit complications, and prevent recurrences while minimizing the costs and side effects of treatment. The primary care physician must be well-versed in the medical management of peptic ulcer disease, capable of designing and implementing an effective ulcer regimen and identifying in timely fashion patients who require referral for endoscopy or surgery.

PATHOPHYSIOLOGY AND CLINICAL PRESENTATION

Most peptic ulcers arise in the stomach and duodenum, areas exposed to gastric acid and pepsin. Although the precise mechanisms of ulcer formation remain incompletely understood, the process appears to involve the interplay of acid production, pepsin secretion, and mucosal defense mechanisms.

Gastric Acid Production and Mucosal Defenses. *Excess acid* production is the hallmark of duodenal ulcer disease, with significant increases noted in basal and peak acid outputs, parietal and chief cell masses, and responses to food and hormonal stimulation. Zollinger-Ellison syndrome (with its associated hypergastrinemia and parietal cell overproduction) is the prototypical acid hypersecretory condition resulting in ulcer formation. Some patients with duodenal ulcer demonstrate *rapid gastric emptying,* which raises the acid exposure of the proximal duodenum. *Pepsin* secretion is also elevated in duodenal ulcer disease. Gastric acid production is relatively normal in patients with gastric ulcers.

An appreciation for the importance of *mucosal defense mechanisms* is emerging. Major determinants of mucosal integrity include mucus secretion, bicarbonate production, mucosal blood flow, and cellular repair mechanisms. *Compromise of the mucous barrier* may result from increased mucus degradation, decreased secretion, or production of defective mucus. Bile acids, pepsin, pancreatic enzymes, and mechanical forces contribute to mucus degradation. *Gastric prostaglandin* production appears important to sustaining mucus production, bicarbonate secretion, and mucosal repair. By helping to maintain a neutral pH and aqueous environment at the surface of the gastric epithelium, mucus and bicarbonate protect the mucosa from acid, pepsin, and other potentially injurious agents.

The Role of Aspirin and Nonsteroidal Antiinflammatory Drugs (NSAIDs). The relation of *aspirin* and nonaspirin *nonsteroidal antiinflammatory drugs (NSAIDs)* to ulcer disease is due largely to their potent inhibition of gastric mucosal prostaglandin synthesis. With chronic use, all NSAIDs (including enteric-coated and nonaspirin salicylates and NSAID prodrugs) are capable of producing solitary deep gastric ulcers. The risk of clinically important ulceration is estimated by the U.S. Food and Drug Administration (FDA) to be 2 percent to 4 percent per patient-year of NSAID use, based on study of 11,000 patients and eight different NSAIDs. There are no major differences among NSAID preparations in ulcer risk (despite highly advertised claims to the contrary). About 15 percent of chronic NSAID users demonstrate gastric ulceration at endoscopy. Risk generally increases with dose and duration of therapy, but up to a fourth of complications have been observed within the first month of therapy. The elderly are at greatest risk (reported relative risk about 4.0).

NSAID use is not associated with new duodenal ulceration, but preexisting duodenal ulceration may be exacerbated and complicated by NSAID use. It is estimated that over half of ulcer complications associated with NSAID use occur in patients with preexisting duodenal ulcers. Much of the ulcer morbidity associated with NSAID use may be related to preexisting, subclinical disease.

In addition to prostaglandin inhibition, many NSAID preparations produce acute diffuse mucosal injury by means of a direct erosive effect. Endoscopic study has shown significant mucosal injury from both plain and tablet forms of buffered aspirin, although not with enteric-coated aspirin preparations, unless there is delayed gastric emptying. Similar acute erosions occur with uncoated NSAIDs, but not with enteric-coated preparations or prodrug formulations. Such diffuse acute injury is rarely associated with symptoms or clinically significant ulceration, although minor occult bleeding may ensue. Smoking, alcohol use, alcohol-related disease, and preexisting peptic ulcer disease greatly increase risk of ulcer and ulcer complications in NSAID-treated patients. There is suspicion that concurrent *Helicobacter pylori* infection also may predispose the patient to NSAID-related injury.

The role of *Helicobacter pylori* infection is increasingly appreciated as a major, if not the major precipitant of peptic ulcer disease. The organism has been found in over 95 percent of cases of duodenal ulcer and ulcer recurrence and has also been isolated from patients with gastritis, gastric ulcer, and even gastric carcinoma. Its eradication can speed ulcer healing and greatly reduce rates of recurrence. Cures of recurrent peptic ulcer disease have been associated with eradication of *H. pylori* infection. The organism does not appear to cause ulcers per se, but rather seems to make the mucosa more susceptible to the injurious actions of acid and pepsin. Acid hypersecretors may be particularly vulnerable to ulcer formation in the context of *Helicobacter* infection and subject to slow healing and a high rate of recurrence. The prevalence of *H. pylori* infection increases with age, approaching 90 percent in ulcer patients over age 65. Mode of transmission is unclear, although person-to-person, fecal–oral spread is suspected because there are clusters in families.

Other Precipitants. A host of psychological, dietary, pharmacologic, and hereditary factors have been implicated in causation or aggravation of ulcer disease. *Stress* has long been considered a key precipitant, a view supported by a higher incidence of chronic stress in ulcer patients than in controls, increased acid production in response to stress, and a more prolonged course and poorer prognosis in those with chronic severe anxiety. In addition, psychological studies have found that patients who develop ulcers view life stresses more negatively than do controls. Acid hypersecretion and ulcer formation have been observed in small-scale studies of patients undergoing severe emotional stress; with subsidence of stress, acid secretion falls and ulcers heal. Confirmation of these small-scale observations will strengthen the association between stress and ulcer disease.

Smoking is an important risk factor, identified by epidemiologic studies. For example, cigarette smokers are twice as likely to develop ulcers as nonsmokers. Risk of gastric ulcer correlates with the number of cigarettes smoked, and those with ulcers show increased rates of smoking. Rates of recurrence are dramatically increased in those who smoke; healing is markedly slowed. Impaired prostaglandin production has been demonstrated in the gastric mucosa of smokers.

Alcohol and *coffee* have also been implicated. Coffee, including decaffeinated forms, stimulates acid secretion, as do other caffeine-containing beverages, but evidence proving ulcer causation is lacking. *Ethanol* can compromise the mucosal barrier and cause gastritis, and beer is almost as potent a stimulant of acid secretion as gastrin. Nonetheless, data on the link between alcohol use and ulcer disease are conflicting. However, patients with alcohol-related cirrhosis are at increased risk of ulcer formation and complications.

The contribution of *glucocorticosteroids* to ulcer formation has been debated ever since these agents first became available. Multiple randomized controlled trials have produced conflicting results, as have two major meta-analyses examining pooled data from such trials. The first analysis concluded that steroids did not cause ulcers unless they were administered for more than 30 days or in a total dose exceeding the equivalent of 1000 mg of prednisone. The second analysis, which was done 7 years later, included additional studies but excluded others; it found that the incidence of ulcers varied directly with steroid dosage and was significantly increased, even in patients treated for less than a month or receiving less than 1000 mg. Although the increase in risk was double that of patients not taking steroids, it remained low at about 2 percent. Data from a recent case-control study of prescription data in Tennessee may help to explain the discrepancies. It found that risk is nil if one controls for concurrent NSAID use. However, there were few subjects taking more than 30 mg per day of prednisone; thus, the data do not rule out an ulcerogenic effect at higher steroid doses. In sum, even if steroids do increase the chances of ulcer formation, the risk is small as long as NSAIDs are not being taken concurrently.

Heredity plays some role. Parents, siblings, and children of ulcer patients have increased incidences of ulcer, and studies of twins show greater concordance (eg, both twins affected) among identical than among fraternal twins. Increased meal-stimulated gastrin release and pepsin secretion have been found to be hereditary traits among ulcer patients and their families.

Clinical Presentation. Peptic ulcers usually occur at or near mucosal transition zones, areas thought to be particularly vulnerable to the effects of acid, pepsin, bile, and pancreatic enzymes. Gastric ulcers are found in the atrium at the lesser curvature, near the junction of the acid-secreting parietal cells, and the antral mucosa. Duodenal ulcers arise mostly at the junction of the antrum and duodenum.

The clinical presentations of gastric and duodenal peptic ulcers are somewhat similar but rather nonspecific. Patients may present with pain, bleeding, or obstruction, or they may be symptom free. Epigastric pain, relieved by antacids and occurring in clusters of daily symptoms for a few weeks separated by pain-free periods of months, is characteristic of peptic disease. Duodenal ulcer pain is classically relieved by food, absent before breakfast, and responsible for awakening the patient at night; it starts 2 to 3 hours after a meal. However, careful studies of patients with documented duodenal ulcers have shown that in some individuals pain is often worsened by meals, present before breakfast, and continuous rather than periodic. Gastric ulcer pain is more likely to be precipitated by food and often radiates from the epigastrium to the back or substernal region. It, too, can awaken the patient and be relieved by food. In both conditions, the pain may be dull, aching, gnawing, or burning in quality, consistent with its visceral quality.

Symptoms may be absent and dissociated from mucosal changes. Silent disease is particularly common among the elderly and those using NSAIDs. A complication is the first clinical manifestation of ulcer disease in about 25 percent of those with ulcer disease unrelated to NSAID use; the figure is considerably higher in the setting of NSAID use.

Natural History and Clinical Course. Because most patients receive some form of treatment, available data reflect clinical course more than true natural history. Studies done before the advent of aggressive use of antacids or H_2-receptor antagonists showed that a large majority of ulcers heal completely by 4 weeks, although large ones in the stomach can take up to 12 weeks. The majority of patients in such studies became pain-free within the first 4 weeks; however, there was little correlation between cessation of pain and healing of the ulcer. Recurrences were frequent. The 5-year recurrence rates ranged from 30 percent to 90 percent. Although it was rare for a patient to have more than two or three repeat gastric ulcers, multiple recurrences were not unusual for those with duodenal ulcers. There was no correlation between recurrence rate and ulcer size, duration of symptoms, or location. Recurrent ulcers healed just as rapidly and completely as original lesions. The rate of developing a major complication, such as hemorrhage, perforation, or obstruction was less than 1 percent per year. Bleeding was slightly more common from duodenal than from gastric ulcers and two to three times more common than perforation.

With advances in medical therapy, the clinical course of peptic ulcer disease has improved markedly. Ninety to 95 percent of ulcers heal if therapy is continued for 12 weeks. Proton pump blockers (eg, omeprazole) produce even more dramatic results, particularly in patients with otherwise refractory disease. Although prevention of ulcer recurrence has been demonstrated with chronic use of H_2-receptor antagonists and proton pump inhibitors, risk returns to its previous level once drug therapy is discontinued. Even with continuation of adequate maintenance therapy, some silent breakthrough ulceration can be demonstrated by repeat endoscopy, but it is usually of no clinical consequence. Eradication of *H. pylori* infection greatly reduces the risk of recurrence and increases the probability of cure (see below).

Medical therapy can also lower the risks of hemorrhage, perforation, and obstruction, but shows little advantage over placebo for pain relief, in part because of a very strong placebo effect. Surgical therapy has also affected the clinical course. Antrectomy lowers recurrence rates for duodenal ulcer to 5 percent per year; selective proximal gastric vagotomy also substantially lowers recurrences, although to a lesser extent (see below).

WORKUP

A presumptive diagnosis of acid-peptic disease can often be made on clinical grounds alone (see Chapter 58). As long as the risk of underlying gastric cancer is inconsequential (age $<$ 40 years, no early satiety, weight loss, or stool test positive for occult blood) and there are no associated complications (eg, bleeding, perforation, or obstruction), a clinical suspicion of ulcer disease need not be confirmed by barium study or endoscopy to initiate therapy. Patients over the age of 40 are at greater risk of gastric cancer and should undergo either upper gastrointestinal (GI) series or endoscopy to document the nature and location of the lesion when there is strong clinical suspicion of ulcer disease.

The *choice of diagnostic procedure* remains a subject of debate. Endoscopists correctly argue that *gastroscopy* is superior to *barium study* for detection of gastric ulcer, malignancy, and *H. pylori,* because brushings, biopsy, and cultures can be performed at the same time. Radiologists counter that by using air-contrast techniques, they can approach the sensitivity of endoscopy with a procedure that is one-third the cost, safer, and more comfortable for the patient. The debate continues; test selection should be individualized. The patient with recurrent disease should undergo endoscopy to check for *H. pylori* infection, as should the elderly person who may have a gastric carcinoma presenting as an ulcer.

A related diagnostic dilemma is what to do when barium study reveals a benign-appearing gastric ulcer. About 4 percent of all gastric ulcers prove to be malignant, with many manifesting radiologic signs of cancer. Radiologic criteria for malignancy include irregular shape, nodular base, absence of radiating gastric folds, folds that are blunted or stop before the ulcer, and rigidity of adjacent stomach. Ulcers in the fundus are at increased risk of being malignant; those within 1 cm of the pylorus are almost always benign. Using these criteria, sensitivity of barium study for detection of gastric malignancy is reported to be in the range of 80 percent to 85 percent, compared with 95 percent for endoscopy with biopsy and brushing. However, if all gastric ulcer patients are routinely subjected to endoscopy, it would cost tens of thousands of dollars to find a single case of cancer. Because the prognosis is not particularly good for patients with a malignant gastric ulcer (the 5-year survival is 25% to 35%), the potential for benefit by adding endoscopy to every gastric ulcer patient's work-up does not appear very great. A less costly alternative is to refer for endoscopy and biopsy only those patients with a radiologically suspicious gastric ulcer and those with ulcers that fail to heal fully (see below). The literature should be followed for further cost–benefit studies.

Detection of H. pylori infection can be achieved by *endoscopic biopsy* with identification of the organisms on routine or specially stained specimens, by *culture of biopsy specimen* or aspiration contents, by *breath testing* for urease activity, and by *serologic testing* (which indicates exposure only).

PRINCIPLES OF THERAPY

Treatment Objectives and Therapeutic Options

The major objectives of therapy are to speed healing, reduce pain, and prevent complications and recurrences while minimizing the costs and side effects of therapy. Although peptic ulcer disease represents a heterogeneous set of disorders, the overall approach to medical therapy is similar and centers on reducing gastric acidity and protecting the mucosal barrier. Antacids are used to neutralize acid; histamine H_2-receptor antagonists and proton pump inhibitors block acid secretion. Sucralfate serves to form a cytoprotective coating over the injured mucosa, perhaps also absorbing pepsin and inactivating bile acids. Eradication of *Helicobacter* infection removes an important source of mucosal compromise. Avoidance of substances potentially injurious to the gastric mucosa (aspirin, NSAIDs), cessation of smoking, and reduction in stress complement the therapeutic effort. Use of prostaglandin analogues such as misoprostol helps prevent recurrence of NSAID-induced gastric ulceration and bleeding. Surgery remains an option for treatment of refractory disease and complications.

Choice of Approach

With a host of effective therapies at hand and a relatively favorable natural history of disease, selection of therapy is a matter of individualizing treatment to the needs and preferences of the patient. Regardless of pharmacologic approach selected, smoking cessation, avoidance of aspirin and NSAIDs, and stress reduction are among the nonpharmacologic measures that should be part of every program. Antacids, H_2-blockers, sucralfate, and omeprazole all speed ulcer healing. Antacids have the advantages of low cost and safety (little is absorbed); however, compliance becomes a problem because of the need for frequent doses. Cost is far greater for H_2-blocker therapy, but these agents are well-tolerated, convenient to use, and, with a few exceptions (see below), free of major adverse effects. Like antacids, sucralfate acts locally but must be taken frequently. It too is costly and may cause some GI upset. Omeprazole is reserved for refractory or complicated disease; cost is very high, and there is a concern about risk of inducing carcinoid tumors (see below). Eradication of *Helicobacter* infection should be considered when the organism is found, and is especially important in patients with refractory or recurrent disease. Misoprostol helps to counter the prostaglandin inhibition associated with NSAID use and reduces the risk of ulcer formation. Combination programs are common, although data on efficacy are inconclusive.

Nonpharmacologic Therapies

Diet. Contrary to common belief, there is no evidence that any particular dietary manipulation promotes healing or reduces acidity. The one exception is that avoidance of eating before bedtime probably reduces nocturnal acid levels by removing the postprandial stimulus to acid secretion. Otherwise, bland diets, frequent feedings, small feedings, and avoidance of spices, fruit juices, and acidic foods have never been shown to affect the course of ulcer disease. Milk is also without specific benefit; in fact, its high content of protein and calcium stimulates gastric acid secretion. Some patients claim that certain foods "disagree" with them; these can be avoided, but not for the sake of altering acid production. Intake of *coffee* (including decaffeinated forms) and other caffeinated beverages ought to be limited, but need not be eliminated entirely; their link with ulcer disease is not especially strong.

Avoidance of Agents Injurious to the Mucosal Barrier. A program to speed healing, limit recurrences, and prevent complications should address acute and chronic use of agents injurious to the mucosal barrier. *Aspirin* and most *NSAIDs* should be avoided, if possible, because they greatly increase risk and refractoriness to therapy. Using *enteric-coated* and *prodrug* NSAID formulations and taking them with meals might mitigate the superficial erosive injury but do little to prevent the deep ulcers that ensue from chronic use of these potent prostaglandin inhibitors. Consequently, if NSAID therapy must be continued, other means must be used to ensure their safe use (see below).

Although not an independent risk factor, *alcohol* should be probably restricted because it may impair healing and cause complications. Although *glucocorticosteroids* may exacerbate the chance of developing an ulcer in the context of NSAID therapy, they pose little direct risk, and concurrent use of a prophylactic regimen is not required unless other risk factors are present or large doses (eg, > 30 mg per day of prednisone) are going to be used for prolonged periods.

Alleviating Emotional Stress. Those with difficult home or work situations may benefit from counseling by the primary physician. Treatment begins with a careful history eliciting pertinent psychosocial information. The very act of discussing these issues and the opportunity to ventilate one's feelings to a supportive listener may lessen tension and help point the way to solutions. A short course of minor tranquilizer therapy is sometimes helpful to augment supportive psychotherapy and help the patient cope with the combination of stress and illness (see Chapter 226). Before the days of cost-containment, very stressed patients were hospitalized to facilitate ulcer healing; however, only stays in excess of 4 weeks were shown to be effective.

Smoking impedes the healing of peptic ulcers and might interfere with the action of H_2-receptor antagonists. For example, gastric ulcer patients who continue to smoke have blunted responses to cimetidine therapy. Cessation should be urged during recovery from an ulcer. Although the role of smoking as a causative factor in ulcer disease is less well-established, there is ample medical justification to advise its discontinuation (see Chapter 54).

Pharmacologic Therapies

Antacids remain a mainstay of therapy because they are effective, inexpensive, and safe. The preferred preparations are those containing magnesium hydroxide, aluminum hydroxide, or a combination of the two. Those containing calcium carbonate (eg, Tums, Rolaids) have considerable acid-neutralizing capacity, but result in calcium-stimulated rebound hypersecretion of acid and can cause hypercalcemia and systemic alkalosis. When taken in qid regimens, they have been shown endoscopically to be more effective than placebo and comparable to H_2 blockers and sucralfate in promoting healing of duodenal ulcers. Effectiveness in gastric ulcer disease and in preventing recurrences of gastric and duodenal ulcers are less well-established. These agents are no more effective than placebo for relief of pain due to duodenal ulcer, although they are better than placebo for symptoms attributable to gastric ulcer. This effect on gastric ulcer pain and the recently demonstrated efficacy of frequent but nonneutralizing antacid doses has stimulated speculation, especially for aluminum-containing antacids, as to mechanisms of action beyond simple acid neutralization (eg, protective coating, inactivation of irritant bile acids, and stimulation of prostaglandin synthesis).

The *buffering capacities* of liquid antacid preparations vary considerably, ranging from 6 to 128 mEq per 15 mL. Liquids are superior to tablets in buffering capacity (Tables 68–1 and 68–2). Calcium carbonate preparations are among the most potent in neutralizing capacity, but, as just noted, their usefulness is limited by the fact that they stimulate rebound acid secretion. The most effective liquid antacids contain magnesium and aluminum hydroxides. When the aluminum hydroxide mixes with acid, nonabsorbable aluminum salts are formed, which are constipating. The magnesium salts formed are also poorly absorbed but frequently cause diarrhea, an effect that may not be completely canceled by the constipating action of the aluminum. If diarrhea becomes a problem, one can alternately use an antacid containing only aluminum hydroxide. Many of the liquid antacids contain considerable amounts of sodium. A low-sodium preparation is sometimes needed to avoid sodium excess in patients who must restrict salt intake. Tables 68–1 and 68–2 list

Table 68-1. Characteristics of Major Liquid Antacids

PREPARATION	NEUTRALIZING CAPACITY (mEq/mL)	VOLUME FOR 140 mEq (mL)	SODIUM CONTENT (mg/5 mL)	RELATIVE COST*	BUFFERS
Maalox TC	4.2	33	<1.0	1.0	Al/$MgOH_2$
Titralac	4.2	33	11.0	0.7	$CaCO_3$
Delcid	4.1	34	1.5	1.0	Al/$MgOH_2$
Mylanta II	3.6	39	1.0	1.5	Al/$MgOH_2$
Camalox	3.2	44	2.5	1.2	Al/$MgOH_2$ $CaCO_3$
Gelusil II	3.0	47	1.3	1.7	Al/$MgOH_2$
Basaljel ES	2.9	48	23.0	2.4	$AlCO_3$
Riopan	2.7	50	<1.0	1.5	Magaldrate
Mylanta	2.5	55	<1.0	1.7	Al/$MgOH_2$
Alternagel	2.4	60	2.0	1.9	$AlOH_2$
Maalox Plus	2.3	61	1.0	1.7	Al/$MgOH_2$
Maalox	2.3	61	1.0	1.5	Al/$MgOH_2$
Gelusil	2.2	64	<1.0	1.9	Al/$MgOH_2$
Riopan Plus	1.8	78	0.7	1.5	Al/$MgOH_2$
Di-Gel	1.8	80	15.0	2.2	Al/$MgOH_2$
Amphogel	4	100	7.0	2.9	$AlOH_2$

*Reference cost is that of a 140-mEq dose of Maalox TC liquid. (Source: Green Book, 1986)

relative strengths of common liquid and tablet antacids and their sodium content.

Studies correlating healing with acid-neutralizing capacities indicate that substantial doses of antacids are needed in the treatment of duodenal ulcer; however, as little as 120 mEq per day has proved effective in healing gastric ulcers. Previous failures to demonstrate the effectiveness of antacids may have been due to inadequate doses. About 140 mEq at a time is necessary to bring the gastric pH into the 3.5 to 5.0 range. Typical 30-mL doses of many popular antacids provide only 60 mEq. Although contents listed on labels of weak and strong antacid preparations are similar, the relative amounts and solubilities of ingredients do vary, accounting for differences in potency.

The *timing* of the antacid dose affects the degree of acid neutralization. If given with a meal, the antacid is wasted because food is a perfectly adequate buffer. When antacid is given 1 hour after eating, gastric acidity is minimized for another 1 to 2 hours, countering the food-induced stimulation of acid secretion. A second dose 3 hours after a meal provides another hour of acid neutralization and tides the patient over to the next meal.

Table 68-2. Characteristics of Major Antacid Tablets

PREPARATION	NEUTRALIZING CAPACITY (mEq/tablet)	DOSE FOR 140 mEq (tablets)	SODIUM CONTENT (mg/tablet)	RELATIVE COST*	BUFFERS
Camalox	16.7	8	1.5	1.2	Al/$MgOH_2$
Basaljel	15.4	9	2.0	1.5	$AlCO_3$
Mylanta II	11.0	13	1.3	2.0	Al/$MgOH_2$
Tums	10.5	13	2.7	1.2	$CaCO_3$
Alka II	10.5	13	2.0	1.2	$CaCO_3$
Riopan Plus	10.0	14	0.3	1.7	Al/$MgOH_2$
Titralac	9.5	15	0.3	1.2	$CaCO_3$
Gelusil II	8.2	17	2.1	2.5	Al/$MgOH_2$
Rolaids	6.9	20	53.0	2.0	$AlCO_3$
Maalox Plus	5.7	25	1.4	2.5	Al/$MgOH_2$
Digel	4.7	30	10.6	2.5	Al/$MgOH_2$ $MgCO_3$
Amphogel	2.0	70	7.0	8.5	$AlOH_2$

*Reference cost is that of a 140-mEq dose of Maalox TC liquid. (Source: Green Book, 1986)

Side effects are relatively few, but important to recognize. *Diarrhea* is common as a result of the cathartic effect of insoluble magnesium salts. Alternating with an antacid containing only aluminum hydroxide can help. Antacids enhance the absorption of dicumarol and L-dopa and decrease absorption of H_2 blockers, phenothiazines, sulfonamides, INH, and penicillin. Potent antacids can cause premature release of aspirin from enteric-coated tablets when both are taken simultaneously. *Phosphate depletion* is possible in patients using an aluminum-containing antacid; insoluble aluminum phosphate forms. In renal failure, excess aluminum may accumulate and cause central nervous system (CNS) toxicity. There is also concern although no proof about the relation of dementia to serum aluminum excess in the elderly (see Chapter 169). Excess sodium absorption has already been mentioned. Magnesium-containing antacids should be avoided in renal failure due to risk of *hypermagnesemis;* the small amounts of magnesium absorbed cannot be eliminated. Calcium can be absorbed and precipitate *hypercalcemia* if renal function is depressed. Calcium also triggers rebound acid secretion, making such antacids irrational choices.

A *cost-effective* antacid regimen for duodenal ulceration employs an agent with a high degree of neutralizing capacity and low cost per therapeutic dose. Several liquid preparations have such qualities and stand out as the best buys; moreover, they are also among the lowest in sodium (see Tables 68–1 and 68–2). Compared to tablets, they are less expensive but not as convenient to use; tablets are particularly well-suited for use at work. Although antacids are safe and effective, their cost and inconvenience can mount when they must be taken seven times a day. Trying to achieve adequate acid neutralization with antacid tablets alone can become difficult; at least eight tablets must be taken just to obtain 140 mEq of acid-neutralizing capacity. For treatment of gastric ulcer, acid neutralization is less of an issue and much smaller doses may suffice (eg, two to three extra-strength tablets of an aluminum-containing antacid [Mylanta Double Strength or Extra-Strength Maalox Plus taken qid]). Compared to H_2-blocker therapy or sucralfate, antacid regimens are about one-fourth the cost.

Histamine H_2-Receptor Antagonists. The development of agents capable of inhibiting parietal cell acid production represented a major advance in the medical therapy of peptic ulcer disease. These drugs block the parietal cell's histamine H_2 receptor, resulting in a 50 percent to 80 percent reduction in basal, postprandial, and vagally stimulated acid production. The available preparations include cimetidine, ranitidine, famotidine, and nizatidine. Despite advertising claims of major differences among these agents, they are remarkably similar in efficacy. There are no clinically significant differences in rates of ulcer healing or prevention of relapse. About 75 percent of duodenal ulcers are healed by 4 weeks, and 84 percent to 97 percent by 8 weeks; 55 percent to 65 percent of gastric ulcers are healed by 4 weeks, and 80 percent to 90 percent by 8 weeks. Recurrence rates after completion of therapy range from 45 percent to 70 percent at 3 months to 75 percent to 90 percent at 1 year and are no different from those noted with other treatments. However, recurrence rates can be markedly reduced by treatment of underlying *Helicobacter* infection. Rarely is chronic H_2-blocker therapy necessary if *Helicobacter* infection is eradicated.

Cimetidine was the first H_2 blocker and is now available in generic formulation. It is rapidly and completely absorbed after oral administration. Peak blood levels occur 45 to 90 minutes after a 300-mg dose. Originally, tid or qid dosing was recommended, but equivalent results have been achieved with a single 800-mg dose at bedtime or 400 mg bid. A low-dose maintenance program (400 mg qhs) has been shown to reduce substantially the recurrence rate to 15 percent to 25 percent per year. Absorption is reduced 10 percent to 20 percent by concurrent intake of magnesium- or aluminum-containing antacids; a 2-hour staggering of doses helps maximize benefit, although it is not essential. Absorption is not affected by meals. Most of the drug is excreted unchanged in the urine; 15 percent is metabolized by the liver. Patients in renal failure require reduction in frequency of administration (eg, q12h when the serum creatinine rises above 3.0 mg per deciliter). The drug crosses the placental barrier.

Its *side effects* and *adverse reactions* are relatively minor and occur infrequently (in fewer than 5% of patients). In controlled studies, the frequency of side effects was indistinguishable from that for placebo; however, in long-term studies, the frequency of adverse reactions exceeds that for placebo. The most commonly experienced adverse reactions include diarrhea, nausea, vomiting, rash, dizziness, and headache. The incidence of each is less than 1 percent. The *CNS effects* are most prominent in the elderly, the very young, those with renal or liver disease, and those receiving high doses. Lethargy, confusion, slurred speech, agitation, and visual hallucinations have been reported, particularly in the elderly. The drug crosses the blood–brain barrier in humans. *Gynecomastia* and *sexual dysfunction* rank among the most troubling of side effects and are especially prevalent among patients taking the drug at high dosages for treatment of Zollinger-Ellison syndrome (>2400 mg per day). The causes are believed to involve the drug's ability to impair estradiol metabolism and bind to androgenic receptors, which also results in a small reduction in sperm count. Cimetidine slows hepatic drug metabolism by *inhibiting microsomal enzymes*. These effects are dose-related but occur with as little as 800 mg per day. Clearance is reduced by 20 percent to 30 percent, raising serum half-lives. Although such impairment is usually not clinically significant, it can be important when hepatically metabolized drugs with a narrow therapeutic range are in use (eg, *warfarin, benzodiazepines, phenytoin, procainamide,* and *theophylline compounds*). Cimetidine also reduces hepatic metabolism of *propranolol* and *carbamazepine* by about 20 percent. The net effect is a potentiation of drug effect. Dose reductions are essential, as is monitoring of serum levels. The effect of cimetidine on hepatic microsomal enzymes lasts for about 2 weeks after the drug is stopped. *Ketoconazole* absorption is reduced by up to 65 percent when the drug is taken within 2 hours after a cimetidine dose, necessitating administration at least 2 hours before intake of an H_2 blocker.

Isolated cases of *bone marrow suppression* have been reported in the setting of severe underlying illness and multiple drug use. Small, clinically insignificant decreases in *creatinine clearance* are sometimes noted. The effect is dose-related and more common when daily doses exceed 2000 mg per day. On occasion, the creatine clearance might fall by as much as 25%, but no permanent renal injury results. Frank *hepatotoxicity* is rare, but transient two- to threefold increases in aminotransferase (transaminase) levels do sometimes ensue, although usually disappearing even with continuation of therapy.

Ranitidine, famotidine, and nizatidine followed development of cimetidine and are more potent on a weight basis. Their single-dose ability to inhibit acid secretion is equal or superior to that of cimetidine, and the effect of a single dose lasts 12 to 24 hours. They can promote healing in a proportion of patients with refractory gastric ulcer, duodenal ulcer, or Zollinger-Ellison syndrome who did not respond to cimetidine. A single dose at night has been found to be as effective as cimetidine in preventing recurrence of duodenal ulcer, reducing recurrence rates to less than 25 percent.

Absorption after oral administration ranges from 45 percent for famotidine to 100 percent for nizatidine, a difference that is not clinically important. Concurrent intake of food does not reduce absorption, but use of aluminum or magnesium antacids does by 10 percent to 20 percent. About 30 percent of each of these agents is metabolized by the liver. Metabolites plus unmetabolized drug are excreted by the kidneys. Drug half-life is prolonged in renal failure. Like cimetidine, ranitidine is excreted in breast milk.

Their *side effect profiles* are similar and only slightly different from cimetidine (due at least in part to less clinical experience with the newer agents). *Headache* occurs in about 5 percent of famotidine patients and in 3 percent of those taking ranitidine; migraine may be exacerbated. *Confusion* is slightly less common with these agents than with cimetidine but still may occur, especially in elderly patients taking large doses. There are no reports of gynecomastia, but *impotence* has been encountered among a few patients taking extremely high doses. The only reported cases of bone marrow suppression are a few isolated instances of thrombocytopenia in patients taking famotidine. Renal function is unimpaired, but hepatoxicity has been noted in a few instances. There is less interference with *microsomal enzyme* function than with cimetidine, but it may occur with ranitidine, although usually only at high doses. Clearances of warfarin, theophylline, benzodiazepines, phenytoin, and procainamide appear normal, but metabolism of propranolol may be slowed as might absorption of ketoconazole.

Choice of H_2 Blocker. When prescribed in therapeutic doses, these agents are similar in efficacy and side effects. Drug–drug interactions are slightly more common with cimetidine, because inhibition of hepatic microsomal enzymes occurs at lower doses. Most other adverse effects are typically minor and usually of concern only when these drugs are used in the elderly or when very large doses are prescribed (as in treatment of hypersecretory states). The predominant difference among H_2 blockers is cost, with generic cimetidine being the least expensive (about half the cost per day). In the past when recommended schedules for cimetidine dosing were tid or qid, the once- or twice-daily dosing of the newer H_2 blockers offered a considerable compliance advantage. But now that bid cimetidine dosing has been shown to be effective, this advantage is less important, although the newer H_2 blockers may have a slight advantage in efficacy. With ranitidine becoming available generically, it too may offer a reduced-cost option. Billions of dollars per year are spent on H_2-blocker therapy, necessitating a cost-conscious approach to their use.

Sucralfate is a complex of aluminum hydroxide and sulfated sucrose, which is believed to act by forming a barrier on the ulcer base, inhibiting pepsin activity and binding bile salts. It has no acid-neutralizing activity, and little is absorbed, although aluminum salts are released and some aluminum is absorbed. In properly controlled trials, the drug is comparable to cimetidine and ranitidine for healing of duodenal ulcers. Prevention of recurrences with maintenance therapy (1 g bid) appears slightly less effective than for H_2 blockers. Fewer randomized, placebo-controlled studies are available on sucralfate and the healing of gastric ulcers. Available data suggest some benefit, but more data are needed, and the drug is not yet FDA-approved for this condition. Although some clinicians add sucralfate to H_2-receptor antagonist therapy to promote healing of gastric ulcers, evidence to support this approach is lacking. The claim that sucralfate preferentially heals ulcers in smokers has not been substantiated.

Sucralfate is most effective when taken 1 hour before meals and at bedtime, although twice-daily administration of double-strength doses has proven adequate for treatment of duodenal ulcer. The main side effect is constipation. The drug binds phosphate and has been reported to cause hypophosphatemia and aluminum toxicity in patients with chronic renal failure. Sucralfate may interfere with the GI absorption of tetracycline, fluoroquinolone antibiotics (eg, ciprofloxacin, norfloxacin), digoxin, phenytoin, and, to a clinically insignificant degree, H_2 blockers. There are no data on safety in pregnancy, nursing, or advanced age. The cost of daily sucralfate therapy is intermediate between that of cimetidine and other H_2 blockers.

Prostaglandin Analogues (Misoprostol). Recognition of the important role that gastric prostaglandins play in maintaining the integrity of the gastric mucosa stimulated interest in prostaglandin analogues for treatment of peptic ulcer disease. Although more effective than placebo, misoprostol proved less effective than H_2 blockers for treatment of peptic ulcers. However, peptic ulcers due to use of *NSAIDs* (which inhibit prostaglandin synthesis) appear to respond well to misoprostol. Although full acid-neutralizing doses of antacids, H_2 blockers, and use of omeprazole can help heal and maintain healing of both gastric and duodenal ulcers accompanying continued NSAID use, they have not been able to prevent NSAID-induced gastric ulcers. Misoprostol is the only agent FDA-approved for prevention of gastric ulcers in patients requiring chronic NSAID therapy. (There are no comparable data on its efficacy in preventing aspirin-induced ulcers.)

Because GI side effects are common with misoprostol intake (see below), its use for prophylaxis of NSAID-induced peptic ulcer disease should be reserved for those with high risk for and little tolerance to the GI hazards of NSAID use (eg, patients with previous peptic ulcer disease, the elderly, the debilitated). The best prophylaxis for such patients is to avoid NSAID use altogether, but if NSAIDs are essential, then the side effects of misoprostol are probably worth suffering for the NSAID benefit and protection from ulceration.

Dose-related *diarrhea* is common (20% with 100-μg qid doses, 40% with 200-μg qid doses). Reduction in dose is often necessary, but lowering dose from 200 to 100 μg qid reduces the protective effect of the drug. Use with meals helps to reduce the severity of diarrhea. The drug is an *abortifacient,* contraindicated in pregnancy or suspected pregnancy. Use in sexually active women of childbearing age should be done with proper warning and detailed patient education.

Misoprostol is very expensive. Cost-effectiveness has not been demonstrated. Although the drug has been shown to reduce significantly the risk of endoscopically measured ulcer disease, its ability to prevent clinically significant disease is still under study. In studies of primary prevention of NSAID-induced upper GI bleeding (an important complication of ulcer disease), misoprostol prophylaxis did not prove cost-effective. However, its use for secondary prevention was found cost-effective in patients with previous NSAID-related upper GI bleeding who had to continue NSAID therapy for a disabling condition. NSAID-induced primary duodenal ulceration is infrequent, but complications are common, and misoprostol might also help reduce their frequency (as might full doses of H_2 blockers). Studies are ongoing to better define the prophylactic, healing, and maintenance uses of misoprostol.

Omeprazole is the first of the gastric H^+/K^+-ATPase ("proton pump") inhibitors. It is the most potent of acid-inhibiting drugs, reducing 24-hour acid production by more than 90 percent with a single daily dose of 20 to 30 mg. This compares to 50 percent to 80 percent acid reduction with standard doses of H_2 blockers. Higher omeprazole doses achieve almost complete cessation of acid production. Speed of ulcer healing and pain reduction (40% to 80% at 2 weeks and 80% to 95% at 4 weeks) are greater with omeprazole than with standard doses of H_2 blockers. *Ulcers refractory to high doses of H_2 blockers* can be healed by 20 to 40 mg per day of omeprazole, and this situation appears to be one of its principal indications for use. However, rates of relapse are similar. It is also the drug of choice for *Zollinger-Ellison syndrome*.

Omeprazole is well tolerated. Important adverse effects include *drug–drug interactions* and an *increase in serum gastrin*. Drug–drug interactions include an increase in serum levels of some drugs metabolized by *hepatic microsomal enzymes* (benzodiazepines, phenytoin, warfarin, but not theophylline or propranolol), increased absorption of digoxin, and decrease in prednisone efficacy. Because of its potent inhibition of gastric acid production, omeprazole stimulates an increase in gastrin production. Short-term therapy produces increases two to four times above baseline; chronic administration is associated with larger elevations. Prolonged, very high gastrin levels have been associated with hyperplasia of enterochromaffin cells and development of carcinoid tumors in rats, but no increase in incidence of such tumors has been associated with omeprazole use in humans. Nonetheless, the drug is not yet FDA-approved for chronic administration. The raising of gastric pH increases the risk of bacterial infection. The safety and efficacy of long-term, alternate-day therapy for severe duodenal ulcer disease are being explored.

Treatment of *Helicobacter pylori* infection is emerging as an important consideration in many instances of recurrent or refractory peptic ulcer disease, be it gastric or duodenal. Ulcer recurrence after treatment is much more common in patients with persistence of *H. pylori* infection. Once infection is eradicated, the rate of recurrence falls significantly and often permanently. Patients with chronic symptomatic ulcer disease or an ulcer complication necessitating persistent maintenance therapy or consideration of surgery (see below) should first be tested for presence of *H. pylori* infection and treated for it. Patients who develop a recurrence while taking prophylactic therapy and those with two or more relapses should also be considered for diagnosis and treatment.

Triple therapy with *metronidazole, tetracycline* (or amoxicillin if patient is allergic to tetracycline), and *bismuth subsalicylate* appears necessary, because of rapid emergence of resistance to single-drug therapy. This regimen is usually given for 2 weeks. Compliance and antibiotic-induced diarrhea are common problems with the triple-therapy regimen. The reader is urged to watch the literature for refinements in indications and treatment modalities for *Helicobacter* infection.

Anticholinergic agents can suppress the parasympathetic muscarinic activity that triggers gastric acid secretion, especially the nocturnal surge. These agents are not nearly as potent as H_2-receptor antagonists in suppressing acid production. The frequency and severity of anticholinergic side effects make therapy intolerable for many patients. Because more effective, better tolerated agents are available, anticholinergics are rarely prescribed anymore.

Follow-up

Monitoring Response. If a *gastric* lesion was detected initially by x-ray film, has all the hallmarks of a benign lesion (see above), and symptoms resolve fully, then follow-up barium study or endoscopy can probably be forgone. Although some authorities advocate routine endoscopic or radiologic *documentation of healing,* there are no studies showing this to be cost effective in uncomplicated cases in which symptoms resolve within 4 to 6 weeks and do not recur. However, if there is suspicion of a refractory gastric ulcer (eg, persistent pain after 8 weeks despite a full medical regimen), then *endoscopic examination* and *biopsy* are needed, especially in patients over age 40, who are at increased risk of gastric cancer. Barium study is not sufficient, because even malignant ulcers may shrink in size in response to therapy. Earlier evaluation is indicated if there is evidence of bleeding or obstruction or other reason to be concerned about gastric carcinoma (see earlier).

In the case of a *duodenal* ulcer (where cancer risk is nil), follow-up radiologic or endoscopic evaluation should be restricted to instances where the results will influence clinical decision making. Persistence or recurrence of pain, symptoms of gastric outlet obstruction, and evidence of bleeding are among the indications for study. Periodic repetition of studies is unnecessary and expensive, even when typical symptoms recur, unless a different course of therapy such as surgery is contemplated. Following stool guaiacs and blood counts can help detect bleeding, as can careful questioning of the patient.

Duration of Therapy. Medical therapy should be continued for at least a full 4 weeks, the time needed for complete healing of duodenal ulcers in about 90 percent of patients. Resolution of pain cannot be used as a therapeutic endpoint; cessation of pain correlates poorly with completion of healing. Premature termination of therapy commonly occurs and increases the risk of symptomatic relapse. Patients who remain symptomatic after 4 weeks of therapy are likely to still have an unhealed ulcer; their treatment program should be extended for another 2 to 4 weeks. There is no need to change the program. Large gastric ulcers may take up to 12 weeks to heal.

Maintenance therapy is indicated for those with documented recurrences within 1 year, bleeding, concurrent need for NSAID therapy, or a condition necessitating use of anticoagulants (see Chapter 83). Maintenance programs with documented prophylactic efficacy include a nightly half-dose of H_2-blocker therapy. The efficacy of antacids for maintenance is unknown. Most authorities recommend continuing maintenance treatment for 1 year; the optimal duration of therapy remains unknown, as do the consequences of prolonged suppression of gastric acid production (see below). Although the relapse rate for medical maintenance therapy is ten times that of surgical therapy, most patients can be spared an operation. An alternative to daily maintenance therapy is empirical treatment of pain recurrences. The efficacy of this approach is yet to be determined, but it is used widely by patients.

Debate continues about the safety of chronically suppressing gastric acid production. There is concern that absence of acid will permit bacterial overgrowth, which in turn may lead to formation of the carcinogen nitrosamine. A once-daily ranitidine regimen allows sufficient acid secretion during a part of the day to suppress bacterial overgrowth.

Approach to Persistent Symptoms and Refractory Disease

Refractory cases ought to be evaluated for *Zollinger-Ellison syndrome,* especially when there are multiple ulcers, occurrences in unusual places, marked abdominal pain, or a secretory diarrhea (due to hypergastrinemia). Such patients often manifest evidence of multiple endocrine adenomatosis (concurrent hyperparathyroidism, pituitary tumors, and so forth). A fasting serum gastrin level in excess of 500 pg per milliliter in the presence of acid hypersecretion is diagnostic.

In addition to checking for worrisome etiologies, it is crucial to *check on compliance* and aggravating factors such as *smoking* and *stress*. Many instances of refractory disease and recurrence are closely linked to continued smoking, severe stress, and failure to follow a prescribed medical regimen. Concurrent *NSAID use* may also contribute to refractoriness. If an NSAID must be continued (eg, because of disabling rheumatoid disease), then prophylactic treatment may be required (see above). Sometimes, *increasing the dosage* of an agent may help. If the patient has been on low-dose maintenance therapy when a recurrence develops, full-dose therapy should be initiated. Those already on a standard dose of H_2-blocker therapy may benefit from doubling it. There is no convincing evidence that adding a second agent (eg, H_2 blocker plus sucralfate) achieves better results in treatment of refractory disease than do full doses of a single agent.

Switching to another agent is worth consideration when an ulcer fails to heal. Patients genuinely failing H_2-blocker treatment may respond to *omeprazole* or *triple therapy* for *Helicobacter infection* (see above). *Surgery* is a consideration in the setting of refractory disease, but its use has greatly decreased with advent of such effective medical therapies for refractory or recurrent disease as potent H_2 blockers, omeprazole, and triple therapy for *Helicobacter* infection).

Surgery

The *proximal gastric vagotomy* effectively limits recurrences without producing the disabling side effects associated with earlier forms of surgery for duodenal ulcer disease. The operation involves selective severing of the nerve supply to the acid-secreting fundus; the nerves to the antrum are left intact, preserving control of gastric emptying. The incidence of ulcer recurrences is slightly higher (10%) than with vagotomy and antrectomy (5%) but similar to vagotomy and pyloroplasty (12%). Surgical mortality is lower, and such potentially disabling postsurgical side effects as the dumping syndrome and diarrhea are much less common. The operation is technically demanding and should be considered only by surgeons specifically trained to perform it. The procedure should not be done in patients with delayed gastric emptying. Distal gastrectomy with excision of the ulcer remains the procedure of choice for gastric ulcer.

The most serious *indications for surgery* include brisk bleeding of 6 units to 8 units of blood in 24 hours (see Chapter 63), recurrent bleeding episodes, perforation, gastric outlet obstruction refractory to medical therapy, and failure of a benign gastric ulcer to heal after 15 weeks. Operations are most often done in patients who fail to respond to medical therapy and have disabling symptoms that interfere with their lives.

PATIENT EDUCATION

Enlisting the patient's active involvement and overcoming much of the mythology surrounding ulcer disease are prime objectives of the patient education effort. Before they go to the physician, many patients put themselves on bland diets, increase their intake of milk products, and purchase calcium carbonate antacid tablets in efforts at self-treatment. Some even take aspirin or over-the-counter NSAIDs for pain relief. Even when a medical program has been designed, common errors made by patients are stopping medication as soon as the pain disappears, taking antacids with meals (which wastes the antacid), taking cimetidine at the same time as antacids (which impairs cimetidine absorption), and stopping antacids when diarrhea develops. Patients taking misoprostol need to watch for diarrhea and reduce their dose by half should diarrhea become disabling. Women of childbearing age should be warned to use birth control if taking misoprostol and to avoid the drug outright if pregnant or not using birth control. Careful explanation and attention to detail are central to a successful medical program.

Use of coffee, alcohol, and tobacco need to be reviewed. Many physicians insist that coffee drinking be stopped, although this may cause more difficulty than is warranted by its role in pathogenesis. Cessation of smoking is essential and detailed cessation counseling is critical (see Chapter 54), because continuation of the habit greatly impedes healing. Alcohol intake should also be discouraged.

Counseling the patient with situational stress is often beneficial, but any suggestion to change jobs or family situations because an ulcer has developed is probably unwarranted and potentially counterproductive. There is no evidence that such extreme solutions contribute to healing, and they may actually heighten stress. One useful supplement to counseling is teaching simple relaxation techniques; these are especially useful for patients bothered by multiple somatic manifestations of stress (see Chapter 226).

The patient needs to be taught to watch for complications of ulcer disease. In particular, the manifestations of GI bleeding (see Chapter 63) should be well understood so that there is no delay in seeking help. If the question of elective surgery arises, the patient should be made a full partner in the decision, because there are few definite guidelines for operation. A value judgment is necessary, and the costs and benefits of surgery versus continued medical therapy need to be discussed.

INDICATIONS FOR REFERRAL AND ADMISSION

Refractoriness to therapy is an indication for referral to the gastroenterologist for review of the program and consideration of endoscopy. Admission is mandatory when symptoms of *hemorrhage, penetration, perforation,* or gastric *outlet obstruction* are present; both surgeon and gastroenterologist need to be consulted.

A most difficult issue is when and whom to select for *elective surgery*. Much has to do with the patient's preferences; gross generalizations are meaningless. Clearly those with recurrent major bleeds, gastric outlet obstruction, or evidence of malignancy need to be seen by the surgeon. Seventy-five percent of patients with intractable pain obtain relief when treated surgically, but subgroups with alcohol abuse, character disorders, or severe neuroses do poorly when operated on. The decision to resort to elective surgery for recurrent disease should be made in conjunction with the patient, weighing the small risk of operative mortality and the morbidity of postgastrectomy syndrome against the morbidity and cost of recurrent pain, time lost from work, and need for chronic drug therapy.

THERAPEUTIC RECOMMENDATIONS

- Avoid, or at least limit to the extent medically possible, the use of agents potentially injurious to the mucosa, including aspirin, NSAIDs, and perhaps chronic use of high-dose steroids.
- Insist on total *cessation of smoking* (see Chapter 54).
- Suggest a decrease in use of coffee (including decaffeinated forms) and other caffeine-containing beverages; however, complete cessation of intake is unnecessary.
- Do not restrict any foods or insist on a bland or milk-laden diet. Frequent small feedings are unnecessary, and a bedtime snack may stimulate nocturnal acid secretion. The patient should avoid only foods that cause discomfort.
- Begin an antacid program, H_2-receptor antagonist, or sucralfate, basing selection on patient preference, capacity for compliance, affordability, and potential for interaction with other medications the patient may be taking.
- If the patient is reliable, and one wants to minimize cost, systemic effects, and drug–drug interactions, *begin antacid therapy,* using a magnesium–aluminum hydroxide liquid antacid with high acid-neutralizing capacity and low sodium content (eg, Maalox TC or Mylanta Double Strength). Prescribe sufficient amounts to provide 140 mEq per dose for treatment of duodenal ulcer and 70 mEq per dose for gastric ulcer (see Table 68-1). Give doses 2 hours after meals and before bed. If diarrhea develops, alternate this with an aluminum hydroxide antacid (see Table 68-1). Recent data suggest that even lower doses, such as 50 to 75 mEq (two to three Mylanta Double Strength Tablets) qid will suffice.
- Begin *cimetidine* 400 mg per bid if one desires low-cost H_2-blocker therapy. Exert caution if patient is taking propranolol, warfarin, benzodiazepines, phenytoin, theophylline compounds, or other drugs metabolized by hepatic microsomes; cimetidine potentiates their effect. Avoid taking this drug at the same time as antacids, because absorption is reduced by 10 percent to 20 percent; separate them by at least 1 to 2 hours. Daily cost is about half that of other H_2 blockers, but two to three times that of antacids.
- Use one of the other H_2 blockers (eg, *ranitidine* 150 mg bid, *famotidine* 20 mg bid, or *nizatidine* 150 mg bid) under circumstances where cimetidine might be suboptimal (sexual or CNS dysfunction, taking drugs that are metabolized by hepatic microsomal enzymes,) or fails to achieve control of symptoms. Generic availability will lower the cost of their use.
- Begin *sucralfate* if the patient has been unable to tolerate antacids or H_2-receptor antagonists, but avoid it if compliance or constipation is a problem. The dosage is 1 g qid, taken 1 hour before meals and before bed. Avoid taking simultaneously with digoxin, tetracycline, phenytoin, or cimetidine; sucralfate inhibits their absorption.
- Thoroughly instruct the patient on how to carry out the therapeutic program and review common misconceptions.
- Attend to stress-related issues, but avoid recommending a major job or geographic change.
- For *duodenal ulcer,* continue full-dose therapy for 4 weeks; if symptoms have resolved by then, switch to maintenance therapy (one-half previous dose) for another 4 to 8 weeks to avoid relapse. If symptoms persist, continue until symptoms resolve. For *gastric ulcer,* continue full-dose treatment for 6 to 8 weeks or until symptoms resolve, whichever is longer, then switch to maintenance therapy for another 4 to 8 weeks.
- For patients refractory to initial therapy after 4 weeks, double the dose or switch to a more potent acid-suppressing agent (eg, *omeprazole* 20 mg qd).
- Until long-term use is proven safe, limit omeprazole therapy to no more than 8 to 12 weeks, if possible. Long-term therapy is appropriate and safe for treatment of Zollinger-Ellison syndrome.
- For patients with recurrences or refractory disease, check

for *Helicobacter pylori* infection by endoscopy or breath test. If present, eradicate with a 2-week course of triple therapy (*tetracycline* 500 mg q6h, *metronidazole* 250 mg qid, and *bismuth subsalicylate* two tablets qid); substitute amoxicillin for tetracycline if the latter is poorly tolerated.

- For refractory disease unresponsive to treatment for *Helicobacter,* examine endoscopically to rule out malignancy if not ruled out at time of initial presentation. Obtain brushings and biopsy of gastric ulcers that appear suspicious.
- Reemphasize importance of compliance, smoking cessation, and avoidance of NSAIDs.
- Treat recurrences in a fashion similar to the initial episode, but with emphasis on detection and eradication of *Helicobacter* infection, if present, and cessation of NSAID therapy.
- For patients with a history of peptic ulceration or upper GI bleeding who absolutely require chronic NSAID therapy for maintenance of function, consider *misoprostol* prophylaxis (200 μg with meals and before bed). Reduce dose if diarrhea is a problem. The drug appears no better than H_2 blockers for treatment of NSAID-induced peptic ulcers.
- Refer the patient with refractory pain, multiple ulcers, frequent recurrences, associated secretory diarrhea, or elevated serum gastrin level to the gastroenterologist for consideration of Zollinger-Ellison syndrome, as well as for review of the medical program and need for endoscopy. No follow-up examinations are needed for uncomplicated duodenal ulcers.
- Admit patients with evidence of bleeding, gastric outlet obstruction, or perforation and obtain surgical consultation.

A.H.G.

ANNOTATED BIBLIOGRAPHY

Anda RF, Williamson DF, Escobedo LG, et al. Smoking and the risk of peptic ulcer disease among women in the U.S. Arch Intern Med 1990;150:1437. *(First National Health and Nutrition Examination Survey; relative risk 1.8 overall, and increased with amount smoked; estimates 20 percent of all ulcers in women due to smoking.)*

Buchman E, Kaung DT, Dolank D, et al. Unrestricted diet in treatment of duodenal ulcer. Gastroenterology 1969;56:1016. *(Dietary restrictions made little or no difference.)*

Cantu TG, Korek JS. Central nervous system reactions to histamine-2 receptor blockers. Ann Intern Med 1991;114:1027. *(All H_2 blockers are capable of causing CNS effects, not just cimetidine.)*

Conn Ho, Blitzer BL. Nonassociation of adrenocorticosteroid therapy and peptic ulcer. N Engl J Med 1976;294:473. *(The first of two studies examining pooled data; concludes there is little association between steroids and risk of ulcer.)*

Cryer B, Feldman M. Effects of nonsteroidal anti-inflammatory drugs on endogenous gastrointestinal prostaglandins and therapeutic strategies for prevention and treatment of nonsteroidal anti-inflammatory drug-induced damage. Arch Intern Med 1992;152:1145. *(Comprehensive review; 193 references.)*

Curatolo PW, Robertson D. The health consequences of caffeine. Ann Intern Med 1983;98:641. *(Thorough review; examines the evidence linking caffeine with ulcer disease and acid secretion; 281 references.)*

Danilewitz M, Tim LO, Hirschowitz B. Ranitidine suppression of gastric hypersecretion resistant to cimetidine. N Engl J Med 1982;306:20. *(One of many reports showing the efficacy of switching to ranitidine when cimetidine does not work.)*

Dooley CP, Larson AW, Stace NH, et al. Double-contrast barium meal and upper gastrointestinal endoscopy. Ann Intern Med 1984;101:538. *(A randomized study that indicates superior sensitivity and specificity for endoscopy but admits that cost-benefit is not established.)*

Drake D, Hollander D. Neutralizing capacity and cost effectiveness of antacids. Ann Intern Med 1981;94:215. *(Excellent reference data on comparative characteristics of available antacids.)*

Edelson JT, Testeson AN, Sax P. Cost-effectiveness of misoprostol for prophylaxis against nonsteroidal anti-inflammatory drug-induced gastrointestinal tract bleeding. JAMA 1990; 264:41. *(Only secondary prophylaxis proved cost-effective.)*

Feldman M. Can gastroduodenal ulcers in NSAID users be prevented? Ann Intern Med 1993;119:337. *(The answer is yes, but this editorial provides a critical look at the clinical significance of the answer.)*

Friedman DG, Siegelaub AB, Seltzer C. Cigarettes, alcohol, coffee and peptic ulcer. N Engl J Med 1974;290:469. *(Increased prevalence of ulcer disease in smokers. Coffee consumption and alcohol were not independent predictors of ulcer disease.)*

Gabriel SE, Jaakkimainen L, Bombardier C. Risk for serious gastrointestinal complications related to use of nonsteroidal anti-inflammatory drugs. Ann Intern Med 1991;115:787. *(Relative risk increased by about three times; other risk factors include age greater than 60, concomitant NSAID use, and prior ulcer disease.)*

Galbraith RA, Michnovicz JJ. The effects of cimetidine on the oxidative metabolism of estradiol. N Engl J Med 1989;321: 269. *(Finds decreased metabolism of estradiol, which may account for some of the sexual dysfunction and gynecomastia associated with cimetidine use.)*

Graham DY. Treatment of peptic ulcers caused by *Helicobacter pylori*. N Engl J Med 1993;328:349. *(Editorial urging treatment of the organism when found in symptomatic patients with peptic ulcer disease.)*

Graham DY, Lew GM, Klein PD, et al. Effect of treatment of *Helicobacter pylori* infection on the long-term recurrence of gastric and duodenal ulcer. Ann Intern Med 1992;116:705. *(Randomized, controlled trial showing that eradication of the organism can lead to cure.)*

Graham DY, Smith JL. Aspirin and the stomach. Ann Intern Med 1986;104:390. *(Excellent review, emphasizing the differences between acute and chronic effects; 98 references.)*

Graham DY, White RH, Moreland LW, et al. Duodenal and gastric ulcer prevention with misoprostol in arthritis patients taking NSAIDs. Ann Intern Med 1993;119:257. *(Randomized, controlled, clinical trial showing reduction by misoprostol of rate of ulcer development.)*

Greenblatt DJ, Abernethy DR, Morse DS, et al. Clinical importance of the interaction of diazepam and cimetidine. N Engl J Med 1984;310:1639. *(Interaction not clinically important when diazepam used in modest doses; warns against extrapolating to large doses or use in the elderly.)*

Griffin MR, Piper JM, Daugherty JR, et al. Nonsteroidal anti-inflammatory drug use and increased risk for peptic ulcer disease in elderly persons. Ann Intern Med 1991;114:257. *(Risk substantial and increases with dose and recency of use.)*

Hentschel E, Brandstatter G, Dragosics B, et al. Effect of ranitidine and amoxicillin plus metronidazole on the eradication of *Helicobacter pylori* and the recurrence of duodenal ulcer. N Engl J Med 1993;328:308. *(Randomized controlled study showing that eradication of* Helicobacter pylori *infection significantly speeds healing and prevents recurrences.)*

Ippolitto A, Elashoff J, Valenzuela J, et al. Recurrent ulcer after successful treatment with cimetidine or antacid. Gastroenterology 1983;85:875. *(Recurrence rates after antacid therapy were 29 percent at 3 months and 56 percent at 6 months, compared with 36 percent and 55 percent after cimetidine.)*

Isenberg JI, Peterson WL, Elashoff JD, et al. Healing of benign gastric ulcer with low-dose antacid or cimetidine. N Engl J Med 1983;308:1319. *(Demonstrates efficacy for both cimetidine and low-dose antacids, although cimetidine was superior.)*

Jensen RT, Gardner JD, Raufman JP, et al. Zollinger-Ellison syndrome: Current concepts and management. Ann Intern Med 1983;98:59. *(Good review; 94 references.)*

Levant JA, Walsh JH, Isenberg J. Stimulation of gastric secretion and gastrin release by single oral doses of calcium carbonate. N Engl J Med 1973;289:555. *(Calcium carbonate causes rebound acid hypersecretion, although it is a good neutralizing agent.)*

Lipsy RJ, Fennerty B, Fagan TC. Clinical review of histamine$_2$ receptor antagonists. Arch Intern Med 1990;150:745. *(Compares cimetidine, ranitidine, famotidine, and nizatidine; differences are more subtle than previously thought; 99 references.)*

Mahl GF. Anxiety, HCl secretion and peptic ulcer etiology. Psychosom Med 1950;12:158. *(Classic study showing that acute anxiety raises acid secretion.)*

Maton PN. Omeprazole. N Engl J Med 1991;324;965. *(Comprehensive review; 181 references.)*

Maton PN, Vinayek R, Frucht H, et al. Long-term efficacy and safety of omeprazole in patients with Zollinger-Ellison syndrome: Prospective study. Gastroenterology 1989;97:827. *(Safety and efficacy demonstrated.)*

McCarthy DM. Sucralfate. N Engl J Med 1991;325:1017. *(Best recent review; 159 references.)*

Messer J, Reitman D, Sacks HS, et al. Association of adrenocorticosteroid therapy and peptic ulcer disease. N Engl J Med 1983;309:21. *(Second analysis of pooled data; finds that there is an increase in risk of ulcer disease, although the absolute risk is small.)*

Peterson WL. *Helicobacter pylori* and peptic ulcer disease. N Engl J Med 1991;324:1043. *(Excellent, terse review of the data; 97 references.)*

Peterson WL, Sturdevant RA, Frankl HD, et al. Healing of duodenal ulcer with an antacid regimen. N Engl J Med 1977; 297:341. *(Classic placebo-controlled study; documents the efficacy of high-dose [1000 mEq per day] therapy, surprisingly high rate of pain relief by placebo, and delayed healing in cigarette smokers.)*

Piper JM, Ray WA, Daugherty MS, et al. Corticosteroid use and peptic ulcer disease: Role of nonsteroidal anti-inflammatory drugs. Ann Intern Med 1991;114:735. *(Corticosteroid use was associated with increased risk of ulcer only in the context of concurrent NSAID use.)*

Pounder R. Silent peptic ulceration: Deadly silence or golden silence? Gastroenterology 1988;96:Suppl:626. *(Symptoms and ulceration are frequently dissociated.)*

Rutter M. Psychological factors in short-term prognosis of physical disease. 1. Peptic ulcer. J Psychosom Res 1963;7:45. *(Another classic; severe anxiety prolonged recovery and makes relapse more likely.)*

Sogtag S, Graham DY, Belisto A, et al. Cimetidine, cigarette smoking, and recurrence of duodenal ulcer. N Engl J Med 1984;311:689. *(Finds that smoking is a major factor in recurrence of duodenal ulcer.)*

Soll AH. Pathogenesis of peptic ulcer disease and implications for therapy. N Engl J Med 1990;322:909. *(Extremely useful review of new developments; 66 references.)*

Soll AH, Weinsten WM, Kurata J, et al. Nonsteroidal anti-inflammatory drugs and peptic ulcer disease. Ann Intern Med 1991;114:307. *(UCLA conference summarizing available data and showing a relationship; 80 references.)*

Spiro HM. Is the steroid a myth? N Engl J Med 1983;309:45. *(Editorial that examines the contradictory data on this topic.)*

Steinberg WM, Lewis JH, Katz DM. Antacids inhibit absorption of cimetidine. N Engl J Med 307:400, 1982. *(Original U.S. report of this important interaction; inhibition 10 percent to 20 percent.)*

Thompson JC. The role of surgery in peptic ulcer disease. N Engl J Med 1982;307:550. *(Editorial that nicely summarizes the indications for surgery and the procedures currently available.)*

Van Deventer GM, Elashoff JD, Reedy TJ, et al. A randomized study of maintenance therapy with ranitidine to prevent the recurrence of duodenal ulcer. N Engl J Med 1989;320:1113. *(Secondary prophylaxis was effective.)*

Walan A, Bader JP, Classen, et al. Effect of omeprazole and ranitidine on ulcer healing and relapse rates in patients with benign gastric ulcer. N Engl J Med 1989;320:69. *(Major European study showing omeprazole superior to H_2-blocker therapy.)*

Walsh JH. *Helicobacter pylori:* selection of patients for treatment. Ann Intern Med 1992;116:770. *(Recommended for patients with two or more recurrences of symptomatic peptic ulcer disease and for those with refractory disease.)*

Walt RP. Misoprostol for the treatment of peptic ulcer and antiinflammatory-drug-induced gastroduodenal ulceration. N Engl J Med 1992;327:1575. *(Very useful review of available data; only modest benefit proven; 69 references.)*

Wolfe MM. Diagnosis of gastrinoma: Much ado about nothing? Ann Intern Med 1989;111:697. *(Editorial suggesting that a screening serum gastrin level might be warranted in patients with duodenal ulcer.)*

69
Management of Asymptomatic and Symptomatic Gallstones

Primary Care Medicine: Office Evaluation and Management of the Adult Patient, 3rd edition, edited by Allan H. Goroll, Lawrence A. May, and Albert G. Mulley, Jr. J.B. Lippincott Company, Philadelphia

Gallbladder disease afflicts over 20 million Americans, with more than 500,000 undergoing cholecystectomy each year. Prevalence is particularly high among middle-aged, obese women (in part, due to the lithogenic effects of estrogen and the increased risk associated with even moderate degrees of weight gain and caloric excess—relative risk is 2 to 3). Most patients with gallstones are asymptomatic, whereas a few suffer from recurrent bouts of abdominal discomfort. Occasionally a complication such as acute cholecystitis, pancreatitis, or choledocholithiasis may ensue. The primary physician needs to help the patient choose between elective surgery, medical therapy, and expectant management.

CLINICAL PRESENTATION AND COURSE

Gallbladder disease may be asymptomatic or manifested by recurrent pain. Characteristically, *biliary colic* is rather sudden in onset, builds to a maximum within 1 hour, is steady, localized to the right upper quadrant or epigastrium, lasts 2 to 4 hours, and occasionally radiates to the left or right scapula. There is often nausea and vomiting. *Dyspeptic symptoms,* fatty food intolerance, belching, and bloating have also been attributed to chronic gallbladder disease, but the association has never been proven. Prospective studies have shown that such symptoms are just as common in middle-aged women without gallstones as in those with them. When patients with these symptoms are operated on, the dyspepsia often persists after cholecystectomy. Reflux of bile into the stomach has been noted in such individuals.

The rare patient with biliary colic, who has a normal gallbladder study on routine oral cholecystogram and ultrasound, may have acalculous gallbladder disease (an uncommon condition), or multiple small stones undetectable by conventional methods. These subtle forms of gallbladder disease may be discovered by observing delayed gallbladder emptying in response to a fatty meal or cholecystokinin.

The *clinical course* of untreated gallbladder disease is not known precisely. Two prospective studies, totaling 1300 patients who had at least one bout of pain, showed that over a follow-up period of 5 to 20 years, 30 percent had *recurrent pain,* and 20 percent experienced *complications* such as jaundice, cholangitis, or pancreatitis; half remained asymptomatic. Because all patients in these studies had pain requiring a hospital admission, this patient population probably represented a group with a greater likelihood of complications than one with a predominance of *asymptomatic* stones. In a more representative retrospective cohort study of 123 people with silent gallstones, there was no mortality from the condition and a 15-year accumulative probability of biliary pain of only 18 percent.

Although there is no certainty that the onset of complications will be preceded by episodes of biliary pain, a study of 600 patients found that more than 90 percent of patients who suffered a complication of gallbladder disease had prior warning symptoms of biliary colic, although these were often mild and ignored. Most patients with pain on presentation had similar patterns of pain on follow-up. When 112 patients with asymptomatic stones were followed without surgery for 10 to 20 years, 27 percent eventually complained of dyspepsia, 19 percent had biliary colic, and 4.5 percent experienced transient jaundice. No deaths resulted from delay of surgery.

In sum, the asymptomatic patient seems to have a relatively favorable prognosis. Individuals with recurrent pain have twice the rate of complications. Increased risk is also associated with stones larger than 2.5 cm, age over 60, and diabetes.

Some authorities believe there is a cause-and-effect relationship between gallstones and *carcinoma of the gallbladder.* The cancer occurs mostly in older women. The initial association with stone formation was based on circumstantial autopsy data. Community-based study has shown a much weaker association, pertaining only to men.

DIAGNOSIS

Asymptomatic Gallstones. Asymptomatic disease is usually detected as an incidental finding during radiologic or ultrasound investigation that encompasses the upper abdomen for a reason other than suspected gallbladder disease. With the advent and widespread application of ultrasound and computed tomography (CT) imaging techniques, the frequency of detection of asymptomatic disease has been on the increase.

Acute Cholecystitis. The occurrence of classic biliary colic provides strong presumptive evidence for the diagnosis of cholecystitis; dyspepsia and fatty food intolerance do not. Real-time *ultrasound* of the gallbladder is the test of choice for evaluation of patients with biliary coliclike pain and suspected acute cholecystitis. The only preparation necessary is 6 hours or more of fasting. The test takes about 15 minutes. Adequate images are obtained in about 98 percent of instances, although obesity can reduce visualization. Ultrasound can be performed rapidly, provides anatomic information, is low in cost, and allows examination of other potentially causative abdominal structures. Major criteria for a positive study are presence of stones or nonvisualization of the gallbladder (no fluid-filled lumen). Minor criteria include tenderness of the gallbladder during ultrasound examination, thickening of the gallbladder wall, and a rounded shape. Sensitivity and specificity are in excess of 90 percent.

Patients with a nondiagnostic ultrasound, but still strongly suspected of having acute cholecystitis (eg, presence of biliary colic), are candidates for *scintigraphy* with the radionuclide HIDA. The isotope is taken up by the liver and excreted into the bile. Images are obtained after 1 hour. The patient needs to be fasting (but no longer than 2 to 4 hours) and free of underlying hepatocellular disease and alcoholism (which cause false-positive tests). The gallbladder, common bile duct, and duodenum are visualized by 60 minutes in the normal person. Nonvisualization of the gallbladder after 1 hour is characteristic of acute cholecystitis (the common bile duct and duodenum remain visualized). Sensitivity and specificity approach that of ultrasound, but cost is greater, the test takes more time, and little anatomical information is provided. Sensitivity and specificity exceed 90 percent.

Ultrasound and scintigraphy have replaced the *oral cholecystogram* (OCG) for the diagnosis of acute cholecystitis, because they are just as sensitive and specific, yet provide results much faster and cause none of the gastrointestinal (GI) upset and diarrhea that are common with oral cholecystography.

Chronic Cholecystitis. *Ultrasound* is the diagnostic test of choice in patients with recurrent episodes of biliary colic. The *oral cholecystogram* has come back into use in patients who are being considered for lithotripsy or gallstone dissolution, because the test can provide information on gallbladder function and stone composition (see below).

PRINCIPLES OF MANAGEMENT

Available therapies include surgery, both traditional and laparoscopic, and gallstone dissolution, both chemical and physical. Given the rather benign natural history of asymptomatic stone disease, the primary physician faces the tasks of properly selecting the patient who requires treatment, as well as understanding the relative advantages and disadvantages of the treatment options. There have yet to be randomized controlled clinical trials comparing treatment options, necessitating extrapolation from available data on natural history of disease and on the risks and outcomes of interventions.

Asymptomatic Gallstones

There is no evidence that the vast numbers of patients with asymptomatic gallstones would benefit from surgery or stone dissolution. Although surgical mortality is only 0.5 percent, only 20 percent of asymptomatic patients will ever develop biliary colic and acute cholecystitis, and only a small fraction of these people will experience a complication such as pancreatitis. In most patients, the risks of conservative management are not much different from those of surgery, and involve far less expense, morbidity, and time lost from work. A substantial fraction of the 500,000 cholecystectomies done each year for asymptomatic gallstones and stones accompanied by dyspeptic symptoms (but not true biliary colic) could probably be avoided. Similarly, there is no evidence that stone dissolution therapy improves outcome in such patients, although data on this issue are sparse. Patients at high risk for gallbladder cancer might be reasonable candidates for prophylactic cholecystectomy, but few risk factors have been identified (other than calcified gallbladder and stones >3 cm).

Acute Cholecystitis

Patients presenting with symptoms of acute cholecystitis require hospitalization for prompt diagnosis, intravenous fluids, and surgical consultation. The elderly, diabetics, and other debilitated persons are at particularly increased risk. Although immediate surgery may not be necessary, inpatient care for assessment and initial supportive care are warranted. There is considerable debate among surgeons as to whether urgent surgery is indicated. Available analyses suggest there is little risk to delaying surgery until the acute inflammatory phase of the illness has receded, provided there are no acute complications such as choledocholithiasis or pancreatitis.

Symptomatic Gallstones

Symptomatic patients with recurrent attacks of biliary colic and confirmed gallstones should be advised to undergo *elective cholecystectomy,* provided they are reasonable surgical candidates. Before the advent of laparoscopic surgery, it was unclear which form of therapy was best for such patients, and several analytic studies found little difference between medical versus traditional surgical approaches. However, with development of minimally invasive surgical techniques, the decision has shifted in favor of gallbladder removal by laparoscopic cholecystectomy (see below). Here, the risk of complications from gallbladder disease (although relatively low) exceeds the risk of surgery. Patients unwilling or too frail to undergo general anesthesia and surgery are candidates for medical therapy, which aims at stone dissolution by use of bile acids, lithotripsy, ether instillation, or a combination of modalities.

Some patients will refuse all forms of treatment, preferring to "see how it goes." Such patients subject themselves to a small increase in mortality risk, but recent studies suggest the risk is actually modest and that the real issue is the patient's willingness to risk future attacks of pain and possible morbid complications (eg, pancreatitis). Patients with only a single episode of biliary colic are probably the best symptomatic candidates for an expectant approach to treatment, having a reasonable chance of remaining symptom-free into the future.

Surgery is the most definitive means of effecting a long-term cure. *Conventional open cholecystectomy* remains one of the most commonly performed of all surgical procedures, although laparoscopic cholecystectomy has become very popular and has replaced the traditional cholecystectomy in many settings. Mortality rates for conventional open cholecystectomy range from 0.3 percent to 0.5 percent in patients under the age of 50 and rise to 1.4 percent to 2.7 percent in those over age 70. Performing nonelective open cholecystectomy raises the risk fourfold (ie, up to 10% in the elderly). The complication rate from traditional elective surgery is 5 percent and doubles for nonelective surgery. Conventional surgery is successful; only about 4 percent experience chronic postoperative pain, with a retained stone often the cause. Surgery is sometimes undertaken to relieve dyspeptic symptoms, although results are inconsistent and usually disappointing. This is not surprising given the poor correlation between stones and dyspepsia.

Laparoscopic cholecystectomy provides the opportunity for a much less invasive procedure, with length of hospital stay reduced from 5 to 7 days to an average of 1.2 days. Over three-fourths of patients return to work within 10 days, compared to a month for conventional gallbladder surgery. The procedure takes about 30 minutes longer to perform than an open cholecystectomy. The reported complication rate among surgeons experienced in the technique is 5 percent, similar to that for open surgery in such patients, but the proportion of serious complications is reduced. The overall rate of bile duct injury is slightly higher (0.5% versus 0.2%), but in a major study fell to 0.1 percent after a 2.2 percent rate for the initial 13 cases. Only one case of trocar-induced bowel perforation occurred in over 1500 procedures, and there were no deaths attributable to surgery or a postoperative complication. The most common problem was superficial infection at the site of the insertion of the umbilical trocar. About 5 percent of cases had to be converted to open procedures, mostly due to poor visualization of the gallbladder. The procedure represents an excellent option in patients with uncomplicated, symptomatic gallstone disease. Suspicion of common duct stone necessitates consideration of an open procedure; however, common duct exploration is possible with laparoscopic surgery. If a common duct stone is found, the procedure needs to be converted to an open cholecystectomy or followed postoperatively by endoscopic retrograde cholangiopancreatography to achieve its removal. With increasing availability and surgical skill, this procedure is likely to become the treatment of choice for uncomplicated, symptomatic gallbladder disease.

Medical therapy has become an attractive option for patients who are poor surgical candidates or reluctant to undergo elective cholecystectomy. The objective is *stone dissolution* by biochemical means. Up to 80 percent of gallstones have cholesterol as the major constituent, making them potentially dissolvable in the presence of increased bile acid. A number of *bile acids* have been tried since the mid 1970s, but only the naturally occurring bile acid *ursodeoxycholic acid (ursodiol)* has proven both effective in dissolving stones and free of the serious GI side effects that accompanied trials of other bile acids, particularly *chenodiol* (which caused liver injury, diarrhea, and low-density lipoprotein [LDL] cholesterol elevations). Ursodiol is safe for long-term use. The agent not only dissolves stones directly, but also desaturates the cholesterol content of the bile by suppressing hepatic cholesterol synthesis and biliary cholesterol secretion. It is the only bile acid approved by the FDA for stone dissolution and has replaced chenodiol.

Gallstone dissolution is achievable in patients with small (2 cm) *cholesterol stones,* especially if there is a *functioning gallbladder* (as determined by OCG). The overall stone dissolution rate is just under 50 percent and higher for those with pure cholesterol stones (as determined by the OCG findings of floating radiolucent stones in a functioning gallbladder). Results are best in those with a few small stones. Many patients become pain-free even before full stone dissolution is achieved, and 40 percent become stone-free after 2 years of continuous bile acid therapy. Patients with larger or calcified stones fail to achieve complete stone dissolution.

The effects of therapy can be well documented by periodic oral cholecystogram or gallbladder ultrasound. Therapy is contraindicated in patients with inflammatory bowel disease or peptic ulcer, because the drug increases bile acids, which may be harmful to colonic and gastric mucosa. Stones recur at the rate of 15 percent per year. This high recurrence rate suggests a role for chronic suppressive therapy. Continued symptoms despite dissolution occur in about 4 percent.

Ursodiol is expensive, costing upwards of $2 to $3 per day. However, a major cost–benefit analysis showed that ursodiol treatment is a reasonable if not superior alternative to traditional surgery in elderly patients and in patients of all ages deemed poor surgical risks (although comparisons with laparoscopic surgery have not been performed). Some authorities have even advocated using ursodiol initially in all symptomatic patients and operating only on those who fail medical therapy. However, the excellent results reported with laparoscopic surgery, particularly the marked reductions in recovery time and perioperative morbidity, have probably tilted the equation back in favor of surgery for most patients who can tolerate general anesthesia.

Bile salt treatment has an adjuvant role in patients treated with lithotripsy or methyl-*tert*-butyl ether (see below). Stone fragments that remain after initial therapy are subjected to a course of ursodiol in an attempt to dissolve them. Bile salt treatment is also prescribed to prevent new stone formation.

Extracorporeal shock-wave lithotripsy is worth considering in the 10 percent of gallstone patients who have a small number of *calcium-containing stones* (with the calcium deposited in the core or along the rim) and a *functioning gallbladder.* Lithotripsy will effectively shatter such stones in over 95 percent of instances. Results are not as good if there are more than three stones or if they are greater than 3 cm in diameter. After the stone is shattered, follow-up therapy with ursodiol is required to achieve full dissolution or at least painless stone passage. The procedure is contraindicated in patients with acute cholecystitis or a coagulation deficit and can cause such adverse effects as cardiac arrhythmias, pain, bacteremia, hematuria, cutaneous abdominal wall petechiae, and transient liver injury. About 10 percent suffer stone-related symptoms after the procedure due to passage of stone fragments. Although transiently popular as a nonsurgical means of gallstone removal, lithotripsy has been supplanted lately by laparoscopic surgery. However, for patients with calcium-containing stones who are not surgical candidates, it remains a treatment option. The availability of lithotripsy has been limited by very high equipment costs and concerns about cost-effectiveness.

*Methyl-*tert*-butyl ether* dissolves cholesterol stones and has been used in a few centers to treat highly selected populations of patients with multiple or large cholesterol stones. Instilled directly into the gallbladder by way of a percutaneous catheter, the ether can dissolve stones in less than 3 days of continuous application. However, catheter placement and ether installation are difficult and potentially dangerous, necessitating an experienced team to perform the procedure. Stones reform in about 15 percent, and another 20 percent report biliary colic after treatment, probably due to a retained small, insoluble nidus. Ursodiol is often used as an adjunct.

In summary, medical therapy represents an alternative for symptomatic patients with cholesterol gallstones who are too sick or unwilling to undergo elective cholecystectomy. Definition of stone composition, size, and number is required, as is willingness to take bile acid medication for a prolonged period of time.

Dietary Measures and Avoidance of Lithogenic Drugs. *Obesity and Fat.* Although obesity and caloric excess are major risk factors for gallstone formation in women, there is no evidence that a low-fat, low-cholesterol diet per se alters the course of gallbladder disease. Some gallstone patients with dyspeptic symptoms feel better if they avoid fatty foods; however, the relationship between stones and fatty food intolerance is tenuous at best (see Chapter 74). Multivariate analysis shows that it is the number of calories consumed rather than the proportion of calories coming from saturated fat or cholesterol intake that seems to correlate best with risk. One case-control epidemiologic study did find a reduction in risk associated with increased consumption of vegetable protein and vegetable fat, but this finding needs confirmation. Although obesity and caloric excess can lead to stone formation, fasting and starvation diets are contraindicated because they cause bile to become very lithogenic. Perhaps modest weight reduction achieved in gradual fashion might be of some prophylactic value in high-risk patients such as obese women. Prospective study of dietary factors is sorely needed.

Alcohol and Tobacco. Daily consumption of small amounts of alcohol (about 1 oz per day) has been found in retrospective studies of women to correlate with a 20 percent reduction in risk of symptomatic gallstone disease. This closely parallels the 20 percent lower bile cholesterol saturation found among modest drinkers compared to controls. Smoking also appears to reduce risk in women, probably by its adverse effects on estrogen production and degradation. Risk of gallstone formation rises markedly with use of estrogen and clofibrate. Patients with known gallstones should not take them, and those taking such drugs should be monitored for gallstone formation. *Thiazide* use is associated with a modest increase in relative risk of gallstones (relative risk 2.0 to 2.9).

THERAPEUTIC RECOMMENDATIONS

- Patients with asymptomatic cholelithiasis can be managed expectantly, because the risk of developing symptomatic disease or a complication is only 1 percent per year.
- Patients with a single episode of biliary colic are also reasonable candidates for expectant management, as long as they continue free of recurrent pain.
- Patients with documented gallstones and recurrent biliary colic or a history of a complication of gallstone disease (cholecystitis, pancreatitis) should be advised to undergo elective cholecystectomy, provided they can tolerate general anesthesia and surgery. *Laparoscopic cholecystectomy* has become the surgical procedure of choice, reducing perioperative morbidity and shortening the recovery period when performed by a surgeon skilled in the procedure.
- Patients who are too frail or unwilling to undergo elective surgery should have an oral cholecystogram to determine stone composition, which helps guide selection of nonsurgical therapy.
- Symptomatic nonsurgical patients with a functioning gallbladder and radiolucent (ie, cholesterol) gallstones can be given a trial of bile acid therapy with *ursodiol* (10 to 15 mg per kilogram per day). Therapy is continued for at least 12 months and often for 24. Results are best in those with stones that are less than 2 cm in diameter and three in number. Presence of calcification rules out bile acid therapy. The effects of therapy should be monitored with a gallbladder ultrasound every 6 months.
- *Lithotripsy* is worth consideration in nonsurgical patients with calcium-containing stones. Results are best in those whose stones are less than 3 cm in diameter and less than four in number.
- Estrogen preparations, clofibrate, and other drugs that may trigger stone formation should be stopped, or dosages should be decreased.
- Restricting *fat* and *cholesterol* is of little or no benefit in altering the clinical course of gallstone disease. However, obesity and caloric excess are major risk factors, and gradual weight reduction through modest caloric restriction might be helpful. Fasting and starvation diets are to be avoided because they make the bile even more lithogenic. Modest *alcohol* consumption (less than 1 oz per day) is not harmful.
- Dyspeptic symptoms should not be considered grounds for medical or surgical treatment because their relation to gallstone disease is tenuous at best. Dyspeptic symptoms are likely to respond better to other measures (see Chapter 74).

PATIENT EDUCATION

The truly asymptomatic gallstone patient can be reassured of the low probability of becoming symptomatic or suffering a complication. Such patients can be followed expectantly and should not be pushed into surgery, medical therapy, or unnecessary dietary restriction. Previously, asymptomatic patients with large stones, diabetes, or advanced age were considered candidates for prophylactic stone removal, because they had an increased mortality risk from a complication. However, improvements in medical and surgical therapy have greatly reduced risk for such patients, making prophylactic surgical or stone-dissolution therapy unnecessary.

Because symptomatic patients have a slightly increased mortality risk and a modest chance of a complication, they need to be informed of the available therapeutic options so that patient preferences and treatment modality can be matched. The principal therapeutic benefit is a reduction in frequency of symptoms and in risk of complications; mortality benefit is small and almost clinically insignificant. The wish to refuse therapy can be respected, so long as the patient understands the risks of choosing expectant therapy. However, the short hospital stay, low morbidity, and speedy recovery afforded by laparoscopic cholecystectomy may be particularly appealing to previously reluctant symptomatic patients. Ursodiol is also well tolerated and may be an attractive option for qualifying patients fearful of any surgery.

Any dyspepsia should be clearly differentiated from biliary colic. Patients need to know that the link between dyspepsia and gallstones is not well founded and that the presence of dyspeptic symptoms is not an indication for surgery, lithotripsy, or medical therapy, although other measures might help (see Chapter 74).

INDICATIONS FOR REFERRAL AND ADMISSION

Patients with evidence of acute cholecystitis should be admitted to the hospital for evaluation, surgical consultation, and supportive measures. Consultation with a surgeon regarding elective cholecystectomy is also indicated for patients with recurrent biliary colic. Referral for consideration of laparoscopic cholecystectomy should be made exclusively to a surgeon skilled and experienced in performing the procedure. High levels of morbidity (eg, bile duct injury, perforation) and mortality have resulted from inadequately trained personnel performing the procedure. A gastroenterologic referral may be useful in patients who are deemed too frail to undergo elective surgery. Obtaining an oral cholecystogram before the referral helps to determine stone composition, which is essential to proper selection of medical treatment modality.

A.H.G.

ANNOTATED BIBLIOGRAPHY

American College of Physicians. Guidelines for the treatment of gallstones. Ann Intern Med 1993;119:620. *(Concensus recommendations.)*

Barkun AG, Ponchon T. Extracorporeal biliary lithotripsy. Ann Intern Med 1990;112:126. *(Review of experimental studies and clinical results; 71 references.)*

Broomfield PH, Chopra R, Sheinbaum RC, et al. Effects of ursodeoxycholic acid and aspirin on the formation of lithogenic bile and gallstones during loss of weight. N Engl J Med 1988;319:1567. *(Ursodiol prevented lithogenic changes in bile.)*

Carveth SW, Priestley JT, Gage R. Size and number of gallstones in acute and chronic cholecystitis. Mayo Clin Proc 1959; 34:371. *(Stones larger than 2.5 cm are more likely to precipitate attacks of cholecystitis than are smaller stones.)*

Cooperberg PL, Burhenne HJ. Real time ultrasonography in calculus gallbladder disease. N Engl J Med 302:1277, 1980. *(Sensitivity of 98 percent and a specificity of approximately 95 percent were reported. Comparison with oral cholecystography in a subsample showed greater sensitivity and the same specificity for ultrasound.)*

Dolgin SM, Schwartz JS, Kressel HY, et al. Identification of patients with cholesterol or pigment gallstones by discriminant analysis of radiographic features. N Engl J Med 1981;304:808. *(Describes oral cholecystogram findings that help identify patients with cholesterol stones; buoyancy was highly predictive of cholesterol composition; a discriminant function was used to facilitate categorization.)*

Gracie WA, Ransohoff R. The natural history of silent gallstones. N Engl J Med 1982;307:798. *(Retrospective cohort study of 123 people identified no mortality associated with asymptomatic gallstones and a 15-year accumulative probability of biliary pain of only 18 percent.)*

Health and Policy Committee, American College of Physicians. How to study the gallbladder. Ann Intern Med 1988;109:752. *(Consensus statement on recommended approaches to imaging the gallbladder.)*

Johnston DE, Kaplan MM. Pathogenesis and treatment of gallstones. N Engl J Med 1993;32:412. *(Comprehensive review.)*

Maclure KM, Hayes KC, Colditz GA, et al. Weight, diet, and the risk of symptomatic gallstones in middle-aged women. N Engl J Med 1989;321:563. *(Prospective data confirming the strong association between obesity and symptomatic gallstones; moderate overweight increases risk; alcohol decreases it.)*

Maringhini A, Moreau JA, Melton J, et al. Gallstones, gallbladder cancer, and other gastrointestinal malignancies. Ann Intern Med 1987;107:30. *(Community study showing only a minor increase in risk and much less risk than previously reported from autopsy studies.)*

Marton KI, Doubilet P. How to image the gallbladder in suspected cholecystitis. Ann Intern Med 1988;109:722. *(Best review of available methods; 103 references.)*

McSherry CK, Ferstenberg H, Calhoun WF, et al. The natural history of diagnosed gallstone disease in symptomatic and asymptomatic patients. Ann Surg 1985;202:59. *(Documents very favorable prognosis in 691 patients followed for an average of 5 years.)*

Mulley AG. Shock-wave lithotripsy. N Engl J Med 1986;314:845. *(Editorial suggesting caution regarding applicability of lithotripsy to therapy of gallstones.)*

NIH Consensus Development Panel on Gallstones and Laparoscopic Cholecystectomy. Gallstones and laparoscopic cholecystectomy. JAMA 1993;269:1018. *(Recent consensus view on the indications for laparoscopic gallbladder surgery.)*

Pastides H, Tzonou A, Trichopoulos D, et al. A case-control study of the relationship between smoking, diet, and gallbladder disease. Arch Intern Med 1990;150:1409. *(One of the few studies examining the relationship of these factors to symptomatic gallbladder disease.)*

Pickleman J, Gonzalez RP. The improving results with cholecystectomy. Arch Surg 1986;121:930. *(Review of outcomes in 389 consecutive cases; finds rates of mortality lower than previously reported and lower complication rates for the elderly and diabetics.)*

Price WH. Gallbladder dyspepsia. Br Med J 1963;3:138. *(Frequency and severity of dyspeptic complaints are unrelated to presence or absence of gallstones.)*

Ransohoff DF, Gracie WA. Treatment of gallstones. Ann Intern Med 1993;119:606. *(Authoritative review of risks and benefits of available treatment strategies, 92 refs.)*

Ransohoff DF, Gracie WM. Management of patients with symptomatic gallstones: A quantitative analysis. Am J Med 1990; 88:154. *(Decision analysis study indicating that survival benefit from surgery or medical therapy is modest, at best, and that management decisions should be based on considerations other than mortality.)*

Ransohoff DF, Gracie WA, Wolfenson LB, et al. Prophylactic cholecystectomy or expectant management for silent gallstones. Ann Intern Med 1983;99:199. *(Decision analysis suggesting a very small survival benefit for prophylactic cholecystectomy that may well be offset by monetary costs, morbidity, and time preferences.)*

Rosenberg L, Shapiro S, Slone D. Thiazides in acute cholecystitis. N Engl J Med 1980;303:546. *(Relative risk of acute cholecystitis among patients who used thiazide during the month before hospital admission was 2; for those who used thiazides for 5 or more years, the relative risk was 2.9.)*

Sackmann M, Delius M, Sauerbruch T, et al. Shock-wave lithotripsy of gallbladder stones. N Engl J Med 1988;318:393. *(Report of the first 175 cases, finding that results were best when combined with bile acid therapy.)*

Salen G, Tint GS. Nonsurgical treatment of gallstones. N Engl J Med 1989;320:665. *(Excellent editorial tersely reviewing the methods, indications, and results from nonsurgical therapies for gallstones.)*

Sauerbruch T. Gallstone lithotripsy by extracorporeal shock waves. Am J Surg 1989;158;188. *(Authoritative review by one of the pioneers of this form of therapy.)*

Schein CJ. Acute cholecystitis in the diabetic. Am J Gastroenterol 1969;51:511. *(Cholecystitis can be a lethal disease in the diabetic; documents increased risk in this subpopulation, although later studies have shown the risk to be lower than the one reported here.)*

Thistle JL, Cleary PA, Lachin JM, et al. The natural history of cholelithiasis: The National Cooperative Gallstone Study. Ann Intern Med 1984;101:171. *(Among 305 patients receiving placebo therapy, the most important predictor of biliary tract pain was a history of pain; only 4 percent required elective cholecystectomy in 2 years of follow-up.)*

Thistle JL, May RR, Bender CD, et al. Dissolution of cholesterol gallbladder stones by methyl-*tert*-butyl ether administered by percutaneous transhepatic catheter. N Engl J Med 1989;320:633. *(Report of successful application of this treatment modality.)*

Tint GS, Salen G, Colallilo A, et al. Ursodeoxycholic acid: A safe and effective agent for dissolving cholesterol gallstones. Ann Intern Med 1982;97:351. *(Ursodiol found to be an improved method of stone dissolution.)*

Weinstein MC, Coley CM, Richter JM. Medical management of gallstones: A cost-effectiveness analysis. J Gen Intern Med 1990;5:277. *(Finds medical therapy with ursodiol to be a cost-effective alternative to conventional surgery, especially in the elderly.)*

Primary Care Medicine: Office Evaluation and Management of the Adult Patient, 3rd edition, edited by Allan H. Goroll, Lawrence A. May, and Albert G. Mulley, Jr. J.B. Lippincott Company, Philadelphia

70

Management of Hepatitis

JULES L. DIENSTAG, M.D.

Viral and nonviral forms of hepatitis are more common than generally thought. More than 50,000 cases of viral hepatitis in the United States are reported to the Centers for Disease Control each year, although the actual number is estimated to be ten times as high. Before availability of tests for hepatitis C, hepatitis B accounted for 30 percent to 40 percent of cases of viral hepatitis, hepatitis A for 50 percent to 60 percent, and "non-A, non-B" hepatitis for 5 percent. Hepatitis C is now believed to be responsible for 20 percent to 40 percent of viral cases. Mortality from hepatitis types A, B, and C is well below 1 percent. Mortality from hepatitis E, rare in the United States but common in Asia and Central America, is about 1 percent to 2 percent (10% to 20% among pregnant women). The mortality rate of acute hepatitis D may reach 5 percent. In addition, a proportion of patients with acute types B, C, and D progress to chronic infection. Some become asymptomatic carriers; others develop chronic hepatitis, which is associated with an increased risk of cirrhosis and death. A subgroup of patients with chronic hepatitis have nonviral disease of an autoimmune etiology and a natural history and response to therapy different from that of viral hepatitis.

The primary physician needs to be skilled in the management of both viral and nonviral forms of hepatitis, because these are illnesses usually encountered in the outpatient setting. Effective outpatient management requires knowledge of diagnosis (see also Chapters 57 and 62), natural history, and treatment options. Immunosuppressive therapy for nonviral disease, interferon for viral disease, and transplantation for end-stage forms have widened the therapeutic options greatly. Although many treatment decisions require subspecialty consultation, the primary physician maintains responsibility for long-term management and should know the indications and contraindications for the various treatment options, as well as the best means of monitoring therapy and its side effects.

CLINICAL PRESENTATION AND NATURAL HISTORY

Acute Viral Hepatitis

In most instances, acute viral hepatitis is a self-limited illness; on the order of 85 percent of hospitalized patients and over 95 percent of outpatients recover completely and uneventfully within 3 months (except in hepatitis C, see below). A majority of persons with acute viral hepatitis never become jaundiced; their illness is mistakenly labeled as a nonspecific viral syndrome unless liver biochemical tests, such as aminotransferase levels, are ordered. A large proportion of patients remain asymptomatic, especially children. In elderly or immunologically compromised patients, the prognosis is more guarded, with increased risk of severe and protracted disease.

Prodromal symptoms occur after an *incubation period* of 2 to 4 (rarely 6) weeks for hepatitis A, 4 to 24 weeks for hepatitis B (with or without simultaneous acute delta hepatitis infection), and 3 to 15 weeks (80% within 5 to 10 weeks) for hepatitis C (shorter incubation periods of 1 to 4 weeks are common in factor-VIII-infusion-associated hepatitis C among hemophiliacs). Characteristically, *prodromal symptoms* consist of 1 to 2 weeks of malaise, anorexia, nausea, vomiting, change in senses of taste and smell, low-grade fever, right upper quadrant or midepigastric abdominal discomfort, and fatigue. Aminotransferase elevations may precede or coincide with the onset of prodromal symptoms.

If jaundice develops, it usually does so as prodromal complaints begin to subside, although persistence of prodromal symptoms is observed in more severe cases. By the time

6 to 8 weeks have elapsed, most patients are well on their way to full recovery. Occasionally, an isolated, mild aminotransferase elevation persists after clinical recovery. If it resolves within 3 to 6 months, the mild elevation has no prognostic significance.

Fulminant Acute Disease. This is the most ominous form of acute disease, characterized by overwhelming liver cell necrosis and signs of liver failure—encephalopathy, ascites, and coagulopathy. This complication is seen more often in cases of hepatitis B (especially when there is simultaneous delta hepatitis infection) than in those of hepatitis A or C, although, as noted earlier, the incidence is particularly high among pregnant women with hepatitis E. Before the availability of liver transplantation, the mortality of fulminant hepatitis approached 80 percent, despite the best intensive medical care.

Other Variants of Acute Hepatitis. In 5 percent to 10 percent of cases of acute type B hepatitis, the prodromal phase of illness may be characterized as a *serum-sickness-like syndrome,* with urticaria, arthralgias, fever, and polyarticular arthritis. Some patients with acute viral hepatitis, especially those with hepatitis A or E, have a *cholestatic* illness, with marked jaundice, elevation of serum alkaline phosphatase activity, and pruritus lasting 1 month to several months.

Approximately 5 percent to 10 percent of patients with viral hepatitis appear to suffer mild *relapses* during convalescence. Some of these apparent relapses actually represent instances of *second infections* with another hepatitis virus. Still, clinical and biochemical relapses have been documented in cases of hepatitis A and B. (Some relapses of hepatitis B may represent the clinical expression of simultaneous delta hepatitis infection.) Episodic swings in aminotransferase are common during acute and chronic hepatitis C. In some instances, these recurrent elevations are accompanied by a clinical "relapse."

Progression to Chronic Hepatitis. The risk of progression varies among the several types of viral hepatitis. Although an occasional case of hepatitis A may be slow to resolve and last more than 6 months, chronic hepatitis associated with hepatitis A has not been documented. Similarly, hepatitis E does not progress to chronic infection, but acute hepatitis B can, although at a very low rate (1% to 2%). When accompanied by high levels of hepatitis B virus (HBV) replication, patients with chronic hepatitis B tend to have chronic liver injury (chronic active or chronic persistent hepatitis; see below). Those with negligible virus replication become *asymptomatic carriers of surface antigen (HBsAg).*

The likelihood of chronic HBV infection is higher when acute infection occurs at birth or in *early childhood* or when acute infection occurs in an *immunocompromised host.* Most patients with chronic hepatitis B never experienced an acute hepatitis-like clinical illness, acquiring their infection subclinically. The likelihood of chronic hepatitis is not increased in patients with simultaneous acute hepatitis B and D (delta hepatitis).

Although most surface antigen carriers are asymptomatic and have a nonprogressive course, a small proportion may actually have subtle and insidious progression to chronic liver disease. Rarely, acute hepatitis-like exacerbations can occur. Such events may represent superimposed infection with another hepatitis virus (A, C, D) or reactivation of hepatitis B. Occasionally, an acute hepatitis-like elevation of aminotransferase activity represents a successful spontaneous seroconversion from highly replicative e-antigen-positive, HBV-deoxyribonucleic acid (DNA)-positive infection to relatively nonreplicative anti-HBe-positive, HBV-DNA-negative infection.

In *hepatitis C,* as many as 50 percent of patients experience elevations in aminotransferase that persist for more than a year after acute infection.

Histologic evidence of chronic hepatitis can be detected in liver-biopsy tissue. Among patients with transfusion-associated chronic hepatitis C, cirrhosis develops in 20 percent of cases within 10 years after onset of acute infection.

Clinical manifestations of progression to chronic hepatitis may be subtle, with little more than persistence of *mild symptoms and biochemical abnormalities* for 6 or more months. Many patients remain anicteric. There are no reliable early predictors of chronicity. In patients with hepatitis B, persistence of *surface antigenemia* or *e-antigenemia* increases the risk of chronic hepatitis, although early presence of either has no predictive value. Similarly, no reliable predictors of chronicity have been identified in patients with acute hepatitis C.

Toxic and Drug-Induced Hepatitis

Drugs can trigger hepatocellular injury through a direct toxic effect or by means of an idiosyncratic reaction. Some agents are associated with a cholestatic reaction, either as part of an idiosyncratic process or independent of it.

Direct Toxins. Directly toxic reactions are dose related and predictable. The latency period is short and there are no manifestations suggestive of a hypersensitivity reaction. *Acetominophen* is the most commonly used drug that is directly hepatotoxic, though only when taken in massive doses.

Idiosyncratic Reactions. These were once thought to be immunologically mediated, but are actually due to the hepatotoxic effects of drug metabolites. They are less predictable than direct toxins. Latency is variable, and there is little relationship to dose. In about 25 percent of patients, there are extrahepatic manifestations suggestive of a hypersensitivity reaction (eg, fever, rash, arthralgias, eosinophilia). Hepatitis due to *halothane, isoniazide, methyl dopa, valproic acid,* and *trimethoprim-sulfamethoxazole* has a strong idiosyncratic component.

Cholestatic Reactions. There are two cholestatic reactions: those in which there is little evidence of hepatitis, and those which result from an idiosyncratic reaction. Oral contraceptives cause the former, a reaction that is dose-related, though variable in onset. *Erythromycin* (especially the estolate preparation, but also other forms) and *chlorpromazine* are capable of causing a cholestatic idiosyncratic reaction. Like other idiosyncratic reactions, predictability and relationship to dose are minimal. *Anabolic steroids* also can cause cholestasis, often accompanied by a mild degree of hepatocellular injury.

Clinical Course. Severity of drug-induced hepatitis can range from an asymptomatic increase in liver enzymes to life-threatening illness. Prompt cessation of the drug is essential to limiting further hepatic injury; rechallenge may lead to an exaggerated reaction. Most cases are self-limited, provided that severe injury has not already occurred.

Chronic Hepatitis

Chronic Active Versus Chronic Persistent Disease. There are two general histologic categories of chronic hepatitis: chronic persistent and chronic active. The former tends to be more indolent, the latter more progressive. However, clinical differences between these two categories may be subtle, necessitating liver biopsy. *Chronic active hepatitis* is identified by the presence of a mononuclear-cell portal infiltrate that not only expands portal zones but also extends beyond the portal tract into the adjacent periportal lobular area with erosion of the limiting plate of periportal hepatocytes (*"piecemeal necrosis"*). Fibrous septae extending into the lobule are also characteristic, and a proportion of patients with chronic active hepatitis, up to 50 percent in some reported series, have cirrhosis on their initial liver biopsies. A more severe form of this lesion includes *"bridging necrosis,"* in which confluent necrosis and cell dropout span lobules (portal–portal and portal–central bridges).

In contrast, *chronic persistent hepatitis* represents mononuclear-cell inflammation confined to the portal tract; the limiting plate of periportal hepatocytes is not eroded, and hepatocellular necrosis and inflammation do not extend into the lobule. Some authorities distinguish yet another category of chronic hepatitis, *"chronic lobular hepatitis,"* in which the inflammatory process and hepatocellular necrosis involve the lobule but in which other features of chronic active hepatitis are absent. This morphologic pattern can be considered intermediate between chronic active and persistent hepatitis and resembles slowly resolving acute hepatitis.

The histologic differentiation of chronic active hepatitis from chronic persistent and lobular hepatitis is especially important for prognostic purposes. However, this distinction is probably more predictive in patients with autoimmune chronic liver disease (see below) than in the setting of chronic viral hepatitis. Nonetheless, chronic persistent hepatitis is generally a nonprogressive liver disorder with an excellent prognosis and only a modest risk of progression to cirrhosis. The same is true for chronic lobular hepatitis. In contrast, chronic active hepatitis tends to be a progressive disease, associated with an increased risk of cirrhosis and death.

Much of what is known about the natural history of chronic active and persistent hepatitis derives from observations in patients with autoimmune or idiopathic, but not viral chronic hepatitis. Extrapolations to viral hepatitis require some degree of caution. In viral chronic hepatitis, the level of virus replication is a more important determinant of progression than the histologic pattern.

Nonviral (Autoimmune, Idiopathic) Chronic Hepatitis. An autoimmune mechanism is believed to account for many cases of nonviral chronic hepatitis. Like other autoimmune diseases, the condition predominates in women between ages 20 and 40. An acute form with severe fatigue, jaundice, fever, amenorrhea, and anorexia sometimes occurs, but some present asymptomatically. There is a high incidence of extrahepatic manifestations, including arthritis, rash, thyroiditis, glomerulonephritis, and pleuropericarditis. Asymptomatic patients are typically discovered when an incidental modest elevation in aminotransferase is noted on routine testing. Marked elevation in *gamma globulin* (more than two times normal) is characteristic as are high titers of *antinuclear antibody* and antibody to *smooth muscle*. First-generation assays for antibody to hepatitis C may report false-positive readings in such patients. The bilirubin may be higher than in viral hepatitis. Histology and disease activity are particularly important determinants of prognosis for nonviral disease.

The *chronic active* variety may progress to cirrhosis and eventual death in patients with *severe* untreated disease (disabling symptoms, sustained aminotransferase elevations more than ten times normal, gamma globulin levels twice normal, bridging or multilobular collapse on biopsy). The 6-month fatality rate is 40 percent in patients with these findings. Bridging or multilobular necrosis on biopsy specimen is associated with cirrhosis in 40 percent and death in 20 percent after 5 years. In contrast, patients with *less severe disease* (piecemeal necrosis alone, minimal symptoms) are usually not at risk for death, and progression to cirrhosis is rare (3% to 10%).

Chronic persistent disease has a good prognosis in most cases but is not uniformly benign. This lesion has been documented to deteriorate to chronic active hepatitis and to progress to cirrhosis in certain patients, such as those with an initial histologic diagnosis of chronic active hepatitis whose liver biopsies improve with therapy and in immunosuppressed patients with a histologic diagnosis of chronic persistent hepatitis.

Viral Chronic Hepatitis. Histologic appearance also appears to serve as a determinant of prognosis for viral hepatitis. *Chronic persistent* disease is less likely to lead to cirrhosis than *chronic active* disease, but a quarter of patients with chronic persistent hepatitis B can still become cirrhotic. Similarly, a small number of those with *hepatitis C infection* and chronic persistent histology go on to end-stage liver disease. Superinfection with *hepatitis D* can cause progression to more severe liver disease among persons with chronic persistent hepatitis B.

Hepatitis B. The 5-year survival of chronic persistent hepatitis B is in excess of 95 percent, that of chronic active hepatitis B is about 85 percent, and that of chronic active hepatitis *with* cirrhosis associated with hepatitis B is about 50 percent. Progression to cirrhosis has been noted in 13 percent of those with chronic persistent hepatitis, in 16 percent of patients with "moderate" chronic active hepatitis (without bridging necrosis), and in 88 percent of those with severe chronic active disease (with bridging).

Other determinants of prognosis besides histology have been identified. *Level of virus replication* (as measured by serum concentration of HBV DNA and presence of e-antigen) is a key determinant of progression to cirrhosis in patients with chronic hepatitis B. Cirrhosis developed in 53 percent of those with persistent *HBV DNA,* but in none of those able to clear HBV DNA. In patients with chronic hepatitis B, *conversion from HBeAg to anti-HBe* may signal an improvement in liver histology, whereas superinfection with the *delta agent* is usually associated with a deterioration in histology (from chronic persistent to chronic active) in up to a third of patients and an acceleration of the disease process.

In sum, although histologic appearance is important, liver biopsy provides only a measure of disease at one point in time. Degree of virus replication activity may be the best predictor of prognosis. *Life-long infection* with HBV, such as occurs primarily among those infected at or shortly after birth, is associated with an increased risk of *hepatocellular carcinoma,* whether cirrhosis is present or not.

Hepatitis C. Episodic bursts of inflammatory activity often punctuate the clinical course of patients whose liver biopsies showed chronic persistent histology. Like hepatitis B, histologic features can change, with patients manifesting chronic persistent histology experiencing progressive disease. Even patients with clinically and histologically mild chronic hepatitis C can progress insidiously and slowly to cirrhosis. Chronic hepatitis C is predominantly a disease of chronic active histology. Generally, however, these patients rarely fulfill clinical or histologic criteria for severe chronic active hepatitis, and often, spontaneous improvement over time can be demonstrated. Still, despite this apparent relative benignity, chronic hepatitis C may progress insidiously, even in the absence of symptoms or marked elevations in aminotransferase activity, and may lead to cirrhosis in 20 percent within 10 years.

PRINCIPLES OF MANAGEMENT

Acute Viral Hepatitis

Being a generally benign and self-limited illness, acute viral hepatitis can be managed in most cases on an outpatient basis. Hospitalization should be reserved for high-risk patients (the elderly, immunocompromised persons, patients with difficult-to-manage underlying chronic diseases, and so forth) and those with marked prothrombin time prolongation, encephalopathy, ascites and edema, inability to maintain oral intake, hypoglycemia, or hypoalbuminemia. There is *no specific therapy* for acute viral hepatitis that will accelerate convalescence or prevent sequelae. The goals of care are to maintain *adequate nutrition* and *patient comfort,* to *avoid* additional *hepatocellular insults* from hepatotoxic medications and alcohol, and to *prevent the spread* of infection to others.

Neither specific dietary manipulations, corticosteroid therapy, nor strict bedrest has any beneficial effect on the course or prognosis of acute, uncomplicated or acute, severe viral hepatitis. *Oral contraceptives* need not necessarily be stopped, but *alcohol* intake should be omitted, and use of other drugs known to cause liver injury should be discontinued or monitored carefully. *Exercise* does not interfere with recovery; patients should be encouraged to engage in as much physical activity as they can tolerate without discomfort or undue fatigue.

The symptoms may be incapacitating. Nausea and vomiting can be controlled by cautious use of antiemetics; however, because phenothiazines cause cholestatic hepatitis in approximately 1 percent of patients, *nonphenothiazine antiemetics,* such as *trimethobenzamine,* should be used. Small, *frequent feedings,* especially in the morning when nausea is at a low ebb, can ensure adequate calorie intake. No specific foods need be restricted. In patients with cholestasis and pruritus, *cholestyramine* usually provides relief. Certainly, the identification of a patient with acute viral hepatitis should prompt consideration of prophylactic measures to limit the spread of infection to contacts (see Chapter 57).

Fulminant Acute Hepatitis. Neither corticosteroids nor any other specific medical therapy has proven effective. The best approach involves meticulous attention to details of the multisystem dysfunction that accompanies acute liver failure. Such patients should be admitted to an intensive care unit and considered for early referral to a transplantation center. *Liver transplantation* is the only intervention that has truly life-saving potential. With timely transplantation, survival rates of 50 percent to 60 percent are possible. Recurrent viral hepatitis may occur in the new liver, but not invariably.

Drug-Induced Hepatitis

Treatment is largely supportive. All possible offending agents should be stopped. Immunosuppressive and anti-inflammatory drugs are of no benefit.

Chronic Hepatitis

Treatment of chronic hepatitis depends on the type and severity of the disease. Histology is an important determinant of response to therapy, especially in patients with nonviral chronic hepatitis (see below). The goals of therapy are to relieve symptoms, prevent cirrhosis, and reduce the chances of mortality. Approaches to therapy of nonviral and viral types of chronic hepatitis are distinctly different.

Nonviral (Autoimmune or Idiopathic) Chronic Hepatitis. Because the *chronic persistent* form has an excellent prognosis, *no treatment,* beyond simple symptomatic relief, is indicated. The same is true for *chronic lobular* disease.

The *chronic active* form of nonviral hepatitis tends to be a more serious and progressive disease, but *severe cases* respond to *immunosuppressive-antiinflammatory therapy.* Randomized prospective trials have demonstrated clinical, biochemical, and histologic resolution in 80 percent of severe cases treated with *prednisone* or a *combination* of prednisone and *azathioprine*. Histologic features remitted to those of chronic persistent hepatitis or to normal within 6 to 36 months. Such intervention in severe cases significantly reduces mortality.

However, only 15 percent to 20 percent of patients with chronic active hepatitis fulfill criteria for severe disease. The need for and efficacy of immunosuppressive therapy in symptomatic patients with less severe disease remains unknown. In those with *mild* or *asymptomatic* illness, immunosuppressive therapy is not indicated, because the high probability of adverse effects from long-term high-dose glucocorticosteroid therapy (see Chapter 104) are likely to outweigh any potential benefit. More randomized controlled trials are needed to better define the efficacy of immunosuppressive therapy in such patients.

The Immunosuppressive Program. The immunosuppressive program consists of *high-dose prednisone* or *reduced-dose prednisone* in combination with *azathioprine*. In the prednisone-only program, treatment begins at 60 mg per day, and the dose is reduced over the course of a month to a maintenance level of 20 mg per day. The combination regimen is initiated with 30 mg per day of prednisone combined with 50 mg per day of azathioprine. The azathioprine dose remains constant, whereas the prednisone dose is reduced over the course of the first month to a maintenance level of 10 mg. About two-thirds of patients treated with the high-dose steroid-alone program experience severe steroid complications compared to <20 percent of those treated with the combination program. Azathioprine-induced *bone marrow suppression* or *hepatotoxicity* may occur in patients receiving the combination-therapy regimen, necessitating close monitoring. Occasionally unacceptable drug toxicity, intolerable gastrointestinal upset, compression fractures, or failure to respond necessitates premature cessation of therapy. Neither azathioprine alone nor alternate-day prednisone therapy has been found to be an effective alternative regimen. Lower dose corticosteroid-only regimens, without an initiating high-dose phase, have also been found effective.

Therapy is continued until there is objective evidence of remission (ie, a fall in *aminotransferase activity* to a level under twice normal and resolution of *morphologic features* of chronic active hepatitis). In responsive cases, symptoms improve within 6 months, aminotransferase levels within 12 months, and histology within 24 months. Rarely, more than 36 months are necessary to achieve remission. After 4 years, the likelihood of drug-induced complications becomes greater than the likelihood of beneficial drug effect. Nevertheless, some patients cannot be weaned from maintenance treatment and require indefinite continuation of therapy.

Once remission is achieved, therapy is discontinued by gradual tapering of prednisone over 6 weeks. Patients are monitored closely for signs of relapse, which occur in 50 percent of patients. Relapse is especially common in patients with cirrhosis, often necessitating prolonged therapy for many years or multiple courses of treatment. Approximately 20 percent of patients fail to respond to conventional doses but may respond to higher doses. Relapses usually occur early. If remission lasts more than 6 months after cessation of therapy, relapse is less likely. Most cases of relapse are accompanied by symptoms and biochemical abnormalities, but in 10 percent of cases, the only sign of relapse is a change in histology. After relapse, 80 percent of patients respond again to reinitiation of therapy. After cessation of therapy, again, the relapse rate is 50 percent.

Transplantation. For patients with end-stage disease who have sustained a life-threatening complication, referral to a liver transplantation program is an appropriate consideration. Spontaneous or recurrent hepatic encephalopathy, wasting, refractory ascites, variceal bleeding, and spontaneous bacterial peritonitis are among the indications for transplantation in patients with chronic liver disease.

Viral Chronic Hepatitis. The therapeutic approach differs substantially from that in patients with autoimmune disease. Immunosuppressive therapy is not effective and may even be detrimental, as in patients with chronic active hepatitis B, who experience an increase in viral replication.

Hepatitis B. Prospective randomized trials have demonstrated that hepatitis B patients with *compensated replicative chronic disease* (ie, with circulating HBV DNA and HBeAg) benefit from *interferon alfa*. About 40 percent experience seroconversion to nonreplicative infection. Treatment consists of a 16-week course of either daily subcutaneous injections of 5 million units or thrice weekly injections of 10 million units. About one-fourth of responders also lose detectable HBsAg. Improvements in serum aminotransferase and liver histology also occur. Successful interferon therapy is usually accompanied by a transient, acute hepatitis-like elevation in aminotransferase activity, believed to represent an enhancement of cell-mediated immune cytolysis of HBV-infected hepatocytes. The major *adverse effects* of interferon include flulike symptoms, marrow suppression, irritability (sometimes depression), and autoimmune thyroiditis (more rarely, other autoimmune disorders).

An alternative regimen relies on a short course of *steroid pretreatment* before interferon administration. The steroid pretreatment appears to improve the likelihood of response in patients with *minimally elevated* pretreatment aminotransferase activity. The steroids actually increase HBV replication; however a short course followed by abrupt withdrawal and administration of interferon appears to achieve an ultimate lowering of HBV DNA. The fall in viral replication is accompanied by an increase in aminotransferase, believed to result from a combination of the removal of the steroid stimulus to HBV replication and the destruction of virus-infected hepatocytes by cell-mediated cytolytic mechanisms unleashed by corticosteroid withdrawal. The pretreatment steroid program consists of 60 mg per day of prednisone for 2 weeks, 40 mg per day for 2 weeks, 20 mg per day for 2 weeks, and then abrupt cessation followed by administration of interferon.

These regimens are effective in patients with modest levels of HBV replication but are ineffective in those with very high levels of replication (HBV DNA > 200 pg per milliliter). Once seroconversion is achieved, relapse is rare. Among those who lose HBV DNA and HBeAg during therapy, loss of HBsAg has been observed over the course of the next 5 years in 60 percent to 70 percent. Subgroups not responding well to interferon include immunosuppressed patients and those who acquired infection in early childhood.

In *decompensated patients,* the acute hepatitislike exacerbation that accompanies successful interferon therapy may precipitate liver failure, making them poor candidates for routine interferon treatment. They may be candidates for *liver transplantation* or investigative protocols. The success of liver transplantation for chronic hepatitis B is 50 percent to 60 percent, reflecting failures in 20 to 30 percent due to aggressive HBV-induced injury to the allograft.

Hepatitis D. Corticosteroid therapy is ineffective, and the benefit of antiviral therapy remains to be demonstrated. Interferon achieves reductions in HDV RNA and a fall in aminotransferase, but cessation of therapy is followed almost invariably by a return of these parameters to pretreatment levels. Long-term, high-dose interferon therapy continued for a full year may produce more durable results. Liver transplantation has been successful in patients with end-stage disease, with an outcome better than that for hepatitis B alone.

Hepatitis C. Corticosteroids have never proven useful, but *interferon alfa* has and is now FDA-approved for treatment of chronic hepatitis C. After receiving a dose of 3 million units three times a week for 24 weeks, 50 percent of patients with chronic hepatitis C experience a normalization or near normalization of aminotransferase levels. Histologic improvement and reduction or loss of detectable HCV RNA also occur. The relapse rate after cessation of therapy is 50 percent and not reduced by increasing the dose or prolonging the duration of therapy. Sustained response occurs in fewer than 25 percent of patients. Those who relapse are candidates for resumption of therapy and almost invariably re-respond. Predictors of response and relapse are not known, although patients with established cirrhosis or high HCV RNA levels are less likely to respond. Pending development of better therapy, some authorities resort to treating relapses indefinitely with the lowest dose of interferon that maintains normal aminotransferase activity.

Candidates for antiviral therapy include those with compensated chronic hepatitis C. No consensus exists on treatment of patients with asymptomatic or mild disease. Decompensated patients are unlikely to respond. Liver transplantation is indicated for those with end-stage, decompensated chronic hepatitis C. Although reinfection of the allograft is universal, its clinical impact on the new liver is negligible in most cases.

A difficult problem is the asymptomatic patient incidentally found to have an elevated aminotransferase and, on further testing, antibody to hepatitis C. If the aminotransferase is less than twice normal, the patient can probably be followed expectantly. If it is greater than twice normal, consideration of liver biopsy is indicated if the results will help determine candidacy for interferon therapy. Alternatively, one could treat empirically with interferon. Consultation is indicated.

MONITORING COURSE AND RESPONSE TO THERAPY AND INDICATIONS FOR REFERRAL AND ADMISSION

Referral for consultation is indicated in most patients with fulminant and chronic forms of hepatitis, whether viral or nonviral, because treatment decisions are difficult and increasingly effective antiviral and immunosuppressive therapies are becoming available. However, responsibility for follow-up, monitoring, and long-term care remains with the primary physician, who must be knowledgeable about the major treatment modalities and proper methods of monitoring.

Acute Viral Hepatitis. The patient can be followed by observing symptoms and monitoring hepatocellular function. An *aminotransferase* level once weekly at the outset but then monthly is useful to judge the presence of ongoing disease, although the absolute level is not a particularly sensitive determinant of disease severity in the acute phase of illness. *Prothrombin time* is a good measure of hepatocellular synthetic function and should be checked when the patient first presents and when there is suspicion of worsening. *Serum bilirubin* also correlates with severity. A fall in *serum albumin* indicates reduced hepatocellular synthetic function, but because its half-life is 28 days, this change does not become apparent until late in the acute illness.

An office visit 1 to 2 weeks after the first presentation is often helpful to be sure there is no worsening and that the patient is managing satisfactorily. Thereafter, follow-up depends on how well the patient feels. At 3 months, a repeat aminotransferase, bilirubin, albumin, prothrombin time, and, in cases of hepatitis B, an *HBsAg* determination should be performed to ascertain disease activity, severity, and antigen status.

If symptoms and laboratory evidence of activity persist after 3 months, repeat evaluations at monthly intervals are indicated. *Liver biopsy* is not indicated in patients with acute viral hepatitis unless clinical suspicion of chronic hepatitis is present. Referral for biopsy is indicated for patients with suspected chronic active hepatitis (eg, hyperglobulinemia, autoantibodies). In patients with acute viral hepatitis who do not recover within 6 months, liver biopsy should be considered. A delay may be appropriate in patients who are continuing to improve at the 6-month mark.

Biopsy should be reserved for progressive or severe cases, either for prognostic information or as confirmation of disease severity before antiviral therapy is initiated. It is particularly important to obtain help from a hepatologist, gastroenterologist, or pathologist experienced in interpreting biopsy material obtained from patients with chronic hepatitis; diagnosis depends on histologic appearance and can be difficult.

Chronic Hepatitis. In *nonviral disease,* patients with mild *chronic persistent* hepatitis may be followed casually, but those who are symptomatic deserve careful monitoring and periodic reassessment to be sure there are no signs of progression. When *chronic active* disease has been identified, very close follow-up is vital. If prednisone and azathioprine are used, weekly and later monthly *platelet* and *white blood cell (WBC) counts* are required. *Aminotransferase, bilirubin,* and *gamma globulin levels* ought to be obtained at 2 weeks, then every 1 to 3 months to monitor response and to identify treatment failure. Patients with mild chronic active disease who do not receive therapy should be monitored in similar fashion and biopsied again if symptoms or biochemical parameters worsen.

In *viral chronic hepatitis,* therapeutic decisions may be made independently of histologic severity, but *liver biopsy* is indicated to establish the presence of necroinflammatory liver disease and to exclude other causes for abnormal liver chemistry tests (eg, infiltration with fat or iron). In patients considered for interferon therapy, a brief period of observation before instituting treatment is helpful to ensure that the patient is not in the process of spontaneous improvement. Once interferon therapy is started, monitoring of *WBC* and *platelet* counts is indicated at weeks 1, 2, and 4, and then monthly to detect any marrow suppression. Aminotransferases, bilirubin, and albumin are monitored monthly. For hepatitis B, similar monitoring of *HBV DNA* is indicated; HBeAg is checked at the end of therapy. Periodic monitoring of thyroid function (*thyroid-stimulating hormone* [*TSH*]) at 1- to 2-month intervals helps identify patients with thyroiditis who are candidates for reduction or cessation of interferon.

The need for and value of *repeat liver biopsies* at regular follow-up intervals are controversial. After the initial biopsy, which is necessary to initiate therapy, many authorities make subsequent decisions about duration and direction of therapy based on clinical and biochemical responses, without reliance on liver histology. Admission to the hospital is indicated for worsening mental status, bleeding, refractory ascites, or poor home environment. When decompensation does not respond readily to medical therapy, then referral to a *liver transplantation program* is indicated.

PATIENT EDUCATION

Hepatitis often affects previously vigorous people accustomed to full activity. The prolonged course and magnitude of malaise commonly precipitate a reactive depression. Thorough explanation of the disease's course, design of a sensible treatment program that actively involves the patient and family, and close follow-up can maximize compliance and minimize depression.

Instruction concerning diet and activity is central to a comprehensive treatment program. In particular, it is important to prevent unnecessary restriction of activity and to ensure adequate nutrition. Patients can be told to do as much as they feel like doing, as long as they avoid overtiring themselves. Small, frequent meals, especially in the morning, are tolerated best. No foods need be restricted, but carbohydrates seem to be the best-tolerated food when nausea is pronounced. Alcohol should be proscribed.

Patients and household members have many questions regarding transmissibility of the infection. Explicit instructions regarding preventive measures are greatly appreciated (see Chapter 57). Of particular concern is sexual activity, especially for young persons who might want to have children. In hepatitis B, risk of transmission by sexual intercourse is high. In hepatitis C, it is much lower, making it possible to allow unprotected intercourse for purposes of conception.

THERAPEUTIC RECOMMENDATIONS*

Acute Viral Hepatitis

- Maintain adequate caloric intake and a balanced diet. Small feedings are tolerated best, especially in the morning. No foods need be restricted.
- Ensure adequate rest, but activity need not be unduly restricted if the patient feels capable of it.
- Omit potentially hepatotoxic agents, especially alcohol.
- Treat severe pruritus with cholestyramine.
- Treat severe nausea and vomiting with a nonphenothiazine antiemetic, such as trimethobenzamide (Tigan) suppositories.
- Admit the patient to the hospital if signs of marked worsening of hepatocellular function occur (eg, encephalopathy, bleeding, prolongation of prothrombin time). Also consider admission for maintaining adequate caloric and fluid intake when symptoms are severe.
- Refer patients with fulminant hepatitis for consideration of liver transplantation.
- Check aminotransferase, prothrombin time, bilirubin, albumin/globulin, and HBsAg at onset and at 12 weeks; aminotransferase levels should be monitored at 1 to 4 week intervals during acute illness. Retest any patient with evidence of persistent symptoms or laboratory abnormalities every 4 weeks. Refer for liver biopsy those with a combination of failure to resolve infection and inflammation by 6 to 12 months and persistence of disabling symptoms.

*See Chapter 57 for prophylactic measures.

Drug-Induced Hepatitis

- Stop all drugs that might be responsible and institute supportive measures.
- Avoid re-challenging the patient with the same agent.

Nonviral Chronic Hepatitis

- Follow patients with chronic persistent hepatitis at regular intervals and rebiopsy if there are signs of marked worsening. Otherwise treat symptomatically. Steroids are not indicated.
- For patients with *severe chronic active disease* (multilobular or bridging necrosis, disabling symptoms, and marked aminotransferase and globulin elevations), begin high-dose *prednisone* (60 mg per day) or combination prednisone (30 mg per day) plus *azathioprine* (50 mg per day). Combination therapy is preferred for the elderly, diabetics, and others who cannot tolerate long-term high-dose steroids.
- Taper prednisone by 5 to 10 mg at a time over the course of a month until a maintenance dose of 10 mg per day (with 50 mg per day of azathioprine) or 20 mg per day is established.
- Monitor aminotransferase, bilirubin, and globulins at 2 weeks, then every 1 to 3 months. If the patient is taking azathioprine, obtain platelet and white cell counts at week 1 and 2 then monthly thereafter.
- Continue maintenance therapy for at least 24 to 36 months; then consider attempting discontinuation of therapy with a 6-week period of tapering medication.
- Obtain a consultation if there is failure to achieve clinical improvement within 2 to 8 months of initiating therapy; high-dose treatment may be indicated.
- Treat relapses in the same manner as new cases.

Viral Chronic Hepatitis

- Avoid immunosuppressive therapy in patients with viral chronic active hepatitis.
- Consider *interferon alfa* in patients with compensated chronic *hepatitis B* who demonstrate sustained presence of HBV DNA and HBeAg. If deemed appropriate by a consultant, begin a 16-week course of 5 million units administered subcutaneously daily or 10 million units every other day.
- Consider a short *pretreatment course* of *prednisone* if aminotransferase levels are near-normal. The steroid program

(60 mg per day, 40 mg per day, 20 mg per day for 2 weeks each) is withdrawn before starting interferon.

- Treat patients with compensated chronic *hepatitis C* who manifest sustained elevations of aminotransferase with *interferon* at a dose of 3 million units three times a week for 24 weeks. If relapse occurs when interferon is stopped, consider retreating for at least another 6 months. If a second relapse occurs, consider continuing therapy indefinitely at the lowest dose that will maintain normal aminotransferase levels.
- Consider *interferon alfa* for patients with *hepatitis D*. Long-term, high-dose therapy (a million units, 3 times/ week for up to 1 year) is required.
- Monitor patients receiving interferon by checking leukocyte, granulocyte, and platelet counts at weeks 1, 2, and 4 and monthly thereafter. Check aminotransferase levels monthly and TSH every 1 to 2 months. In patients with hepatitis B, monitor HBV DNA monthly and HBeAg at the end of therapy.
- Admit the patient to the hospital when there is evidence of marked worsening of hepatocellular function. Consider liver transplantation for patients with advanced hepatocellular failure.

ANNOTATED BIBLIOGRAPHY

Berk PD, et al. Corticosteroid therapy for chronic active hepatitis. Ann Intern Med 1975;85:523. *(Editorial arguing that steroid therapy should be applied very selectively.)*

Bisceglia AM. Interferon therapy for chronic viral hepatitis. N Engl J Med 1994;330:137. *(An editorial reviewing its efficacy.)*

Boyer JL. Chronic hepatitis—A perspective on classification and determinants of prognosis. Gastroenterology 1976;70:1161. *(Correlates histology with prognosis; a critical review; 66 references.)*

Czaja AJ. Chronic active hepatitis: The challenge for a new nomenclature. Ann Intern Med 1993;119:510. *(A review of etiologic agents, pathophysiology, and nomenclature, which can be confusing.)*

Czaja AJ, Wolf AM, Baggenstoss A. Laboratory assessment of severe chronic active liver disease during and after corticosteroid therapy: Correlation of serum transaminase and gamma globulin levels with histologic features. Gastroenterology 1981;80:687. *(These blood tests proved reliable indicators, making follow-up biopsy unnecessary in most instances.)*

Davis GL, Balart LA, Schiff ER, et al. Treatment of chronic hepatitis C with recombinant interferon alfa: A multicenter randomized controlled trial. N Engl J Med 1989;321:1501. *(The study that established its efficacy.)*

Di Bisceglie AM, Goodman ZD, Ishak KG, et al. Long-term clinical and histologic follow-up of chronic posttransfusion hepatitis. Hepatology 1991;14:969. *(A 20 percent progression to cirrhosis over a 10-year observation period in patients with hepatitis C, although most remained asymptomatic.)*

Dienstag JL. Non-A, non-B hepatitis. I. Recognition, epidemiology, and clinical features. II. Experimental transmission, putative virus agents and markers, and prevention. Gastroenterology 1983;85:439. *(Although written before identification of hepatitis C virus, its discussion of clinical features and outcome remains very useful; over 400 references.)*

Farci P, Mandas A, Coriana A, et al. Treatment of hepatitis D with interferon alfa-2a. N Engl J Med 1994;330:88. *(Response found in half of patients, but relapse common after treatment stopped; a randomized controlled trial.)*

Fattovich G, Brollo L, Alberti A, et al. Chronic persistent hepatitis type B can be a progressive disease when associated with sustained virus replication. J Hepatol 1990;11:29. *(Important natural history study; progression to chronic active disease hepatitis in one-third positive for HBV DNA.)*

Fattovich G, Brollo L, Giustina G, et al. Natural history and prognostic factors for chronic hepatitis type B. Gut 1991;32:294. *(Progression to cirrhosis in 13 percent of those with chronic persistent disease, in 16 percent with chronic active hepatitis without bridging necrosis, and in 88 percent with bridging necrosis; persistence of HBV DNA important to progression.)*

Gregory PB, Knauer CM, Kempson RL, et al. Steroid therapy in severe viral hepatitis: A double-blind, randomized trial of methylprednisolone versus placebo. N Engl J Med 1976;294:681. *(Steroid therapy not only failed to help, but was sometimes deleterious in patients with viral hepatitis.)*

Katkov WN, Dienstag JL. Prevention and therapy of viral hepatitis. Semin Liver Dis 1991;11:165. *(Summary of antiviral therapy for chronic hepatitis B, C, D.)*

Korenman J, Baker B, Waggoner J, et al. Long-term remission of chronic hepatitis B after alpha-interferon therapy. Ann Intern Med 1991;114:629. *(Loss of detectable HBV DNA associated with a 60 percent to 70 percent chance of losing HBsAg over 5 years.)*

Martin P, Munoz SJ, Friedman LJ, et al. Liver transplantation for viral hepatitis: Current status. Am J Gastroenterol 1992;87:409. *(Review of outcome in patients with fulminant and chronic viral hepatitis.)*

Perrillo RP, Schiff ER, Davis GL, et al. A randomized, controlled trial of interferon alfa-2b alone and after prednisone withdrawal for the treatment of chronic hepatitis B. N Engl J Med 1990;323:295. *(The study establishing efficacy of interferon for chronic hepatitis B.)*

Rizzetto M, et al. Chronic hepatitis in carriers of hepatitis B surface antigen, with intrahepatic expression of delta antigen: An active and progressive disease unresponsive to immunosuppressive treatment. Ann Intern Med 1983;98:437. *(Poor prognosis demonstrated.)*

Sagnelli E, et al. Serum levels of hepatitis B surface and core antigens during immunosuppressive treatment of HBsAg-positive chronic active hepatitis. Lancet 1980;2:395. *(Immunosuppressive therapy actually increased the level of hepatitis B virus replication.)*

Seeff LB, Beebe GW, Hoofnagle JH, et al. A serologic follow-up of the 1942 epidemic of post-vaccination hepatitis in the United States Army. N Engl J Med 1987;316:965. *(Documents that risk of progression from clinically apparent acute to chronic hepatitis B is very low—only 0.26 percent in this study.)*

Shindo M, Di Bisceglie AM, Hoofnagle JH. Long-term follow-up of patients with chronic hepatitis C treated with alfa-interferon. Hepatology 1992;15:1013. *(Those who experience a sustained response are often cured.)*

Sorrell MF, Shaw BWJ. A primer of liver transplantation for the referring physician. Semin Liver Dis 1989;9:159. *(Excellent reading for the nontransplantation physician.)*

Starzl TE, Demetris AJ, Van Thiel D. Liver transplantation. N Engl J Med 1989;321:1014,1092. *(Two-part review by the pioneers in the field.)*

Summerskill WHJ, Korman MG, Ammon HV, et al. Prednisone for chronic active liver disease: Dose titration, standard dose, and combination with azathioprine compared. Gut 1975;16:

876. *(Important double-blind randomized trial showing that prednisone or prednisone plus azathioprine was superior to placebo and azathioprine alone in treating severe chronic active hepatitis.)*

Tassopoulos NC, Papaevangelou GJ, Sjogren MH, et al. Natural history of acute hepatitis B surface antigen-positive hepatitis in Greek adults. Gastroenterology 1987;92:1844. *(Chronic infection developed in only 0.2 percent.)*

Weissberg JI, et al. Survival in chronic hepatitis B: An analysis of 379 patients. Ann Intern Med 1984;101:613. *(Five-year survival rates were 97 percent for patients with chronic persistent hepatitis, 86 percent for those with chronic active hepatitis, and 55 percent for those with chronic active hepatitis and cirrhosis. Age over 40, bilirubin elevation, ascites, and spider nevi associated with poor prognosis and high risk of death.)*

Wright EC, et al. Treatment of chronic active hepatitis: An analysis of 3 controlled trials. Gastroenterology 1977;73:1422. *(Critical review of major studies; concludes that a reduction in cirrhosis and mortality is achieved by steroids in patients with severe nonviral disease.)*

Primary Care Medicine: Office Evaluation and Management of the Adult Patient, 3rd edition, edited by Allan H. Goroll, Lawrence A. May, and Albert G. Mulley, Jr. J.B. Lippincott Company, Philadelphia

71
Management of Cirrhosis and Chronic Liver Failure

The best treatment is *prevention,* with emphasis on reducing alcohol consumption (see Chapter 228), limiting occupational hepatotoxin exposure, and preventing parenteral transmission of hepatitis B and C (see Chapters 57 and 58). The overall goal is to minimize hepatocellular injury and the risk of progressing to chronic liver failure and cirrhosis.

Cirrhosis represents an irreversible state of chronic liver injury. However, the cirrhotic patient may be kept comfortable, active, and independent if precipitants of hepatocellular injury can be eliminated and complications can be prevented. The responsibility for long-term management of patients with cirrhosis and chronic liver failure often rests with the primary care physician, who needs to be capable of dealing with such potential difficulties as ascites, peripheral edema, encephalopathy, infection, bleeding, renal dysfunction, and electrolyte imbalances.

CLINICAL PRESENTATION AND COURSE

Clinical presentation may be rather dramatic when ascites, encephalopathy, or brisk variceal bleeding brings the patient to medical attention. More subtle manifestations include splenomegaly, a firm liver edge, or such signs of hepatocellular failure as jaundice, palmar erythema, Dupuytren's contractures, spider angiomata, parotid and lacrimal gland hypertrophy, gynecomastia, testicular atrophy, loss of axillary and pubic hair, and clubbing. Hypogonadism and feminization are particularly prominent in male patients with cirrhosis due to alcoholism or hemochromatosis. Most findings are nonspecific and do not reflect the underlying etiology. More specific is the bronze appearance of the skin in patients with hemochromatosis or the appearance of antimitochondrial antibodies (anti-M2) in those with primary biliary cirrhosis. Nonspecific abnormalities in routine liver function tests are common, but the best measures of hepatocellular function are the serum albumin concentration and prothrombin time (PT). The PT is the first to become abnormal because of the short serum half-life (as little as 7 days) of the clotting factors that determine it.

Clinical Sequelae and Prognosis. *Portal hypertension, fluid retention,* and *encephalopathy* are the major sequelae of cirrhosis; they lead to *varices, ascites, hypersplenism, peripheral edema,* and *altered mental status.* Variceal bleeding occurs in 20 percent to 30 percent of all cirrhotic patients, one-third of whom die during the initial hospitalization, one-third rebleed within 6 weeks, and one-third survive 1 year or more. The principal causes of death in patients with cirrhosis are variceal bleeding, encephalopathy, and infection. In addition, patients with cirrhosis, especially those with chronic hepatitis B infection, are at increased risk for hepatocellular carcinoma.

Prognosis is determined by the nature, severity, and activity of the underlying illness. For example, continued alcohol consumption in the context of alcoholic hepatitis is associated with an 80 percent chance of developing cirrhosis, whereas absinthe lowers the risk to 15 percent. Even after *alcoholic cirrhosis* has developed, survival continues to be affected by alcohol ingestion. Five-year survival is 60 percent to 85 percent in those who abstain, compared with 40 percent to 60 percent for those who continue to drink. Onset of jaundice or ascites further decreases 5-year survival (to 30% in drinkers). A discriminant function (DF) using the serum bilirubin and prothrombin time (DF = 4.6[PT − control] + bilirubin [mg per 100 mL]) has been developed to predict survival. A DF greater than 32 indicates a short-term mortality risk of 35 percent. In a recent study of patients with symptomatic *primary biliary cirrhosis,* the average length of survival from the onset of symptoms was about 12 years, whereas the survival of asymptomatic patients did not differ from that of a control population matched for age and sex. The prognosis of patients with *postnecrotic cirrhosis* is difficult to assess because it is hard to date its onset; the cirrhosis develops insidiously over years from subclinical chronic active hepatitis.

Irrespective of etiology, development of ascites, encephalopathy, hyperbilirubinemia, hypergammaglobulinemia (from bypass of the hepatic reticuloendothelial system), and hypoalbuminemia are poor prognostic signs, as is decreased liver size. Worsening renal function is associated with a 33 percent 2-year mortality.

PRINCIPLES OF MANAGEMENT

Cirrhosis and Its Underlying Etiologies

Alcoholic cirrhosis requires complete *abstinence* from further alcohol intake, because prognosis is markedly worsened by continued drinking (see above). Attention to good nutrition, daily multiple vitamin supplements (including 1 mg of folic acid), and correction of any iron deficiency or electrolyte deficits are important supportive measures. The search continues for agents that might halt hepatic fibrosis and promote hepatocyte regeneration. Glucocorticosteroids and portacaval shunting have failed to demonstrate an improvement in survival, although corticosteroids do improve short-term survival in patients with acute alcoholic hepatitis. A randomized, placebo-controlled, long-term study of *colchicine* revealed a doubling of 5- and 10-year survival. The drug is an inhibitor of collagen deposition. However, confirmatory data are needed before it or other drugs found experimentally to improve survival (*e.g., propylthiouracil*) can be recommended. *Liver transplantation* is sometimes considered in patients who have become totally and permanently abstinent.

Primary biliary cirrhosis can cause severe pruritus, which may be relieved by *cholestyramine* in a dose of 4 g orally with meals. Because of decreased fat absorption from low intestinal bile-salt concentrations, these patients are particularly prone to develop deficiencies of the *fat-soluble vitamins*. They may require supplemental vitamin K (10 mg subcutaneously [SC] every 4 weeks), vitamin D (50,000 U orally two to three times a week or 100,000 U intramuscularly every 4 weeks) with oral calcium (1 g daily), and vitamin A (25,000 U orally per day). Night blindness unresponsive to vitamin A may be due to zinc deficiency, which is treated with oral *zinc sulfate* (220 mg per day). For patients with steatorrhea, *medium-chain triglyceride* preparations often help. *Azathioprine* and *colchicine* may have a beneficial effect on survival and are well tolerated. Corticosteroids and penicillamine do not improve survival and cause serious adverse side effects. *Liver transplantation* has proven to be a viable option.

Secondary biliary cirrhosis can be halted by relieving or bypassing the obstruction to bile flow.

Hemochromatosis is treated with weekly *phlebotomies* of 500 mL until the serum iron and ferritin levels fall to normal; then they are performed as needed.

Wilson's disease responds to *D-penicillamine* therapy, which should be administered in conjunction with a hepatologist experienced in using the drug, because of its potential for serious side effects.

Chronic active hepatitis may benefit from *corticosteroid* therapy or *interferon alfa,* depending on the etiology (see Chapter 70).

Complications

Ascites and edema result from increased portal pressure, hypoalbuminemia, secondary hyperaldosteronism, and impaired free water clearance. Its presence is strongly suggested by the clinical findings of a *fluid wave, shifting dullness,* and *peripheral edema.* Abdominal *ultrasound* can be used for confirmation and to rule out venoocclusive disease involving the hepatic veins or the hepatic region of the inferior vena cava (Budd-Chiari syndrome). Although ascites is not a hazard, gross ascites can cause abdominal discomfort and respiratory compromise; under such circumstances, it ought to be treated.

Diagnostic paracentesis is indicated before treatment is initiated in patients with new onset of ascites, worsening hepatic function, fever, or increasing encephalopathy to exclude infection and malignancy. Although it used to be felt that differentiating exudative from transudative ascitic fluid could aid in identifying infection and malignancy, such a differentiation has proven insufficiently sensitive and specific to be reliable. Fluid protein concentrations in excess of 2.5 g per deciliter are seen not only in conditions causing exudates, but also in patients with transudative processes subjected to diuresis. Moreover, the ascitic fluid protein concentration of patients with spontaneous bacterial peritonitis (SBP) is typically less than 1 g per deciliter. However, the *serum-to-ascites albumin gradient* (serum albumin concentration minus the ascites albumin concentration) can help differentiate portal hypertension from other causes of ascites, especially when the ascitic protein concentration is high. A gradient of greater than 1.1 mg per deciliter is indicative of portal hypertension; ascites in the presence of a gradient less than 1.1 suggests a mechanism other than portal hypertension. Ascitic fluid should also be sent for cytologic examination, cell count, and culture. A leukocyte count in excess of 2500 per milliliter is strongly suggestive of SBP in the patient with abdominal pain and fever. Culture is positive in over 80 percent of cases when 10 mL aliquots are injected into three blood culture bottles; Gram's stain is usually negative.

Management of ascites due to portal hypertension begins with *reduction in sodium intake.* Prescribing a 2 g sodium diet is a reasonable compromise between maximizing sodium restriction and dietary palatability. Adequate nutrition is critical. In the absence of encephalopathy, a daily protein intake of at least 50 g is recommended. Excessive *water* intake should be prohibited, and free water should be restricted to 1500 mL per day if hyponatremia ensues. An effective program of salt and water restriction requires a cooperative patient and a conscientious family. A dietitian can provide invaluable assistance. The patient should be instructed to check his or her weight daily. Measuring abdominal girth is an unreliable index of fluid loss because of variations due to gaseous distention of the gastrointestinal (GI) tract. About 15 percent of patients will respond to sodium and fluid restrictions alone. Bedrest is of no added benefit.

Diuretic therapy is indicated if a diuresis has not occurred spontaneously after a full week of salt restriction. *Spironolactone* is the agent of first choice, because it inhibits the hyperaldosteronism of portal hypertension. Being a specific aldosterone antagonist, it counters the hypokalemic alkalosis commonly seen in cirrhotic patients with ascites. Its diuretic action is mild and unlikely to cause rapid intravascular volume depletion. The initial dosage of spironolactone is 100 mg a day orally in divided doses. If diuresis does not follow within 1 week, the daily dosage may be increased by 100 mg every 4 or 5 days to a maximum of 400 mg daily (higher doses may cause hyperkalemic acidosis). It is useful to monitor urinary electrolyte concentrations, because diuresis should follow a significant rise in urinary sodium and a fall in urinary potassium. If natriuresis and diuresis do not occur on a maximal dosage of spironolactone, a loop diuretic such as *furosemide* (starting at 20 to 40 mg per day) may be added. *Bumetanide* or *metolazone* may be added to the diuretic program, but such potent diuretics must be used with extreme care to avoid precipitating renal failure, hypokalemia, and encephalopathy.

Monitoring BUN, creatinine, and electrolytes is critical during treatment of ascites. However, some cirrhotic patients with renal impairment do not manifest an elevated serum creatinine (believed related to reduced creatine synthesis by the liver). This reduces the sensitivity of the serum creatinine in some cirrhotic patients and can complicate monitoring of their renal status. Other measures of renal function may be required.

The maximum amount of ascitic fluid that can be mobilized in 24 hours is about 700 to 900 mL, although peripheral edema can be mobilized at a faster rate. This translates to a daily weight loss of 0.5 kg in patients with ascites alone and of 1 kg in those with both ascites and peripheral edema. Daily weight loss in excess of these amounts suggests overdiuresis, with its attendant risk of intravascular volume depletion leading to hepatorenal syndrome and encephalopathy. A falling urine output accompanied by orthostatic signs (rise in pulse and fall in blood pressure on change from supine to standing) suggest inadequate intravascular volume. An oral fluid challenge of several hundred milliliters of isotonic fluid can confirm the presence of hypovolemia by inducing a temporary increase in urine output.

Some patients with incapacitating ascites are *truly refractory* to sodium restriction and diuretics. For them, *large-volume paracentesis* and *peritoneovenous (LeVeen) shunting* become therapeutic considerations. Removal of more than 1 to 2 L of ascitic fluid at a time by paracentesis used to be considered unwise, because of the risk of precipitating serious intravascular volume depletion from the shift of intravascular fluid into the emptied peritoneal cavity. Moreover, protein depletion and increase in renin activity and aldosterone secretion might ensue. By infusing intravenous albumin (6 to 8 g per liter of ascitic fluid removed) at the time of paracentesis, large volumes (5 to 6 L) of ascitic fluid can be removed without precipitating adverse reactions. Results are comparable to those achieved by shunting procedures, although admissions for reaccumulation of fluid are more frequent (every 10 to 30 days). The best candidates are those with peripheral edema and relatively well-preserved renal function.

Before the development of large-volume paracentesis, peritoneovenous (LeVeen) shunting was the principal means of dealing with refractory ascites. Although effective in treating ascites, shunt placement does not improve survival. Moreover, insertion can precipitate disseminated intravascular coagulation. Infection and shunt obstruction are common complications. Compared to large-volume paracentesis, LeVeen shunting requires fewer readmissions for treatment of ascites, but an overall similar number of hospitalizations due to shunt occlusions. Its potentially serious complications and the advent of large-volume paracentesis has led to a decline in use of LeVeen shunts.

Hepatic encephalopathy is thought to be produced by one or more intestinally derived toxic substances that escape hepatic detoxification as a result of portasystemic shunting and hepatocellular dysfunction. Candidates include ammonia, benzodiazepine-like substances, mercaptans, phenol, neuroinhibitors, phenol, and short-chain fatty acids. Elevations of arterial and venous *ammonia levels* usually, but not always, correlate with the presence of hepatic encephalopathy. Venous levels may be falsely elevated when a tourniquet is left on too long at the time of blood drawing. Ammonia levels are useful in following the clinical state of individual patients. Important precipitating factors include GI bleeding, excessive dietary protein intake, hypokalemic alkalosis, infection, constipation, use of sedative or hypnotic drugs, surgical procedures, and volume depletion resulting from diuresis or paracentesis. Precipitants are identified in about 50 percent of patients; the prognosis is usually better in those with an identifiable contributory factor than in those in whom the onset of encephalopathy is associated only with worsening hepatic function.

Mild encephalopathy may be managed on an ambulatory basis. Aside from excluding GI bleeding, avoiding and correcting fluid and electrolyte disturbances, and discontinuing tranquilizers and sedatives, the mainstay of therapy is *restriction of dietary protein* intake to 30 to 40 g per day, while maintaining a daily caloric intake of 1500 kcal. Vegetable sources of protein are preferred over animal proteins because their metabolism produces less ammonia. Sometimes, oral *amino acid supplements* (high in branched-chain varieties and low in aromatic amines) are added to prevent negative nitrogen balance. Their efficacy in treatment of encephalopathy appears to be transient.

Simple gut cleansing with enemas or cathartics is effective when bleeding, constipation, or a large dietary protein intake has led to encephalopathy. Patients should be monitored with routine mental status examinations that include five-point star and signature testing and examination for asterixis.

Specific therapy for encephalopathy begins with *lactulose,* a synthetic, nonabsorbable disaccharide, which is metabolized to organic acids by enteric bacteria, causing an osmotic catharsis. In addition, lactulose suppresses the growth of ammonia-forming bacteria in favor of lactose-fermenting organisms. The initial dosage for patients with mild encephalopathy is 15 to 30 mL orally every 4 to 6 hours, with adjustments thereafter to produce two to three loose stools a day. Side effects of oral lactulose include diarrhea and abdominal distress, which usually resolve after a reduction in dosage.

Lactulose is as effective as *neomycin,* a poorly absorbed, broad-spectrum aminoglycoside antibiotic, which predated lactulose and is more toxic. It acts by decreasing the intestinal concentration of ammonia-forming bacteria. Prolonged use of doses of 4 g per day or more, especially in patients with renal insufficiency, may lead to ototoxicity and nephrotoxicity. The recommended maximum oral dose is 1 g twice daily. The drug also causes malabsorption. In patients who fail to respond to either lactulose or neomycin, the two may be given together; in some patients, the effect appears to be additive. *Metronidazole* may be used instead of neomycin; it is less toxic.

Variceal Bleeding. Primary and secondary prophylaxis against bleeding are the principal concerns of the primary care physician. In patients with known varices, risk of bleeding is high. Independent risk factors include marked hepatocellular dysfunction, ascites, encephalopathy, large varices, and presence of dilated venules on the varices. Risk of a first bleed is as high as 65 percent in the first year. Because clinical and endoscopic risk factors are independent and therefore not predictive of one another, some authorities recommend endoscopic assessment of all cirrhotic patients to determine risk and candidacy for treatment.

Patients judged to be at high risk are reasonable candidates for *beta-blocker therapy*. When prescribed in dosages that produce beta-blockade (a reduction in heart rate of about 25%), these agents can lower portal venous pressure and decrease the risk of variceal bleeding by about 50 percent. The rate of death from hemorrhage is also reduced. Although disappointing for secondary prophylaxis, beta-blockers have demonstrated efficacy for prevention of a first variceal bleed and should be considered for use in high-risk patients. Other agents are being investigated for their ability to further reduce portal pressure. Initial results with clonidine have been promising.

Injection sclerotherapy (involving endoscopic injection of sclerosing agents) is used to control acute variceal bleeding and, when repeated several times over 2 to 3 months, to prevent recurrences. Controlled trials have shown it to be superior to placebo in preventing repeat variceal hemorrhage, but having little impact on the risk of all-cause upper GI bleeding, which remains at close to 40 percent. Unresolved is its ability to prevent first bleeding. Like portasystemic shunt surgery (see below), sclerotherapy may only substitute one form of morbidity and mortality for another. Sclerotherapy has largely replaced portasystemic shunt surgery, which is now reserved for those who bleed despite repeated sclerotherapies.

Portasystemic shunt surgery remains the final treatment option for patients with recurrent variceal hemorrhage due to portal hypertension. While reducing the risk hemorrhage, shunt surgery increases the risk of encephalopathy. The likelihood of recurrent variceal bleeding is significantly reduced after portasystemic shunting, but long-term survival is not. Reasons for lack of improvement in survival include high operative mortality rates and no benefit to hepatic function, the principal determinant of survival. Consequently, portasystemic shunt surgery is not indicated in patients with varices who have never bled. Selective shunt procedures were developed to reduce the risk of encephalopathy, a common consequence of shunt surgery. For example, the selective *distal splenorenal shunt* attempts to preserve portal blood flow in patients with demonstrable preoperative portal perfusion. Its incidence of postoperative encephalopathy is lower than with conventional portacaval shunting, but long-term benefit is reduced as collateral channels develop. *Side-to-side portacaval* or *proximal splenorenal shunts* are the most effective operations for decompressing hepatic sinusoids and reducing ascites, but they still risk precipitating encephalopathy. For patients awaiting liver transplantation, the *transjugular intrahepatic portasystemic shunt* has proven safe and effective.

Coagulopathy results from reductions in vitamin K-dependent clotting factors (II, VII, IX, and X) secondary to decreased hepatic protein synthesis and increased plasma proteolytic activity. In addition, bile-salt deficiency, neomycin therapy, and malnutrition may contribute to malabsorption of vitamin K, and hypersplenism may account for thrombocytopenia. If a patient with cirrhosis is discovered to have a prolonged prothrombin time, a trial of *vitamin K* 10 mg subcutaneously daily for 3 days will correct hypoprothrombinemia caused by bile-salt deficiency, neomycin, or malnutrition but not hypoprothrombinemia related only to hepatocellular disease. In the absence of bleeding, measures to correct abnormal coagulation parameters are generally not indicated.

Role of Liver Transplantation. In the face of terminal hepatocellular failure, liver transplantation becomes a consideration. In properly selected patients, 5-year survival may be as high as 85 percent. The best candidates are those who are highly motivated, emotionally stable, and willing to comply with a medical program. Postnecrotic cirrhosis, primary biliary cirrhosis, and primary sclerosing cholangitis are among the primary indications. Alcohol-induced liver disease is a relative contraindication, as is hepatitis B liver disease, hepatocellular carcinoma, and renal failure. Absolute contraindications are acquired immunodeficiency syndrome (AIDS), extrahepatic sepsis, metastatic cancer, and severe cardiopulmonary disease.

THERAPEUTIC RECOMMENDATIONS AND MONITORING

General Measures

- The patient should maintain a caloric intake of at least 2000 to 3000 kcal per day.
- Use of alcohol or other hepatotoxic agents must be prohibited.
- The patient should avoid tranquilizers and sedatives.
- Monitor prothrombin time, serum albumin, and bilirubin to assess the severity and progression of hepatocellular dysfunction.
- Check stools at each visit for evidence of occult bleeding.
- Check for asterixis and other signs of encephalopathy at each visit.
- Check the abdomen for evidence of ascites (shifting dullness, fluid wave, bulging flanks). Ultrasound examination is useful to confirm the presence of ascites and rule out venoocclusive disease.

Management of Ascites

- Perform a diagnostic paracentesis in patients with the new onset of ascites or clinical deterioration in the setting of preexisting ascites. The fluid should be sent for cell count and differential, total protein and albumin concentrations, culture, and cytologic examination.
- Instruct patients with ascites to restrict daily sodium intake to no more than 2 g and to consume at least 50 g of protein per day. Consult with a dietitian and provide patient and family with specific menus and food lists.
- Restrict fluid intake to 1500 mL when there is marked hyponatremia (serum sodium concentration less than 125 mEq per liter).

- If salt restriction does not result in diuresis, begin spironolactone 100 mg daily in divided doses. If natriuresis and diuresis do not occur after 1 week, increase the daily dose of spironolactone by 100 mg every 4 to 5 days to a maximum of 400 mg per day.
- If spironolactone alone is ineffective in causing diuresis, add furosemide 20 to 40 mg per day to the regimen and cautiously increase dosage as necessary.
- Adjust diuretic dose so that no more than 0.5 kg of fluid (approximately 1 lb) is lost per day in patients with ascites alone, and no more than 1 kg per day (2 lb) in those with both ascites and peripheral edema. Halt diuretics at the first sign of intravascular volume depletion.
- Consider daily potassium supplementation (20 to 40 mEq KCl elixir) in patients receiving furosemide; administer cautiously, if at all, to patients concurrently taking a potassium-sparing diuretic such as spironolactone.
- Monitor serum potassium, BUN, creatinine, daily weight, and postural signs to avoid inducing intravascular volume depletion, renal failure, hypokalemia, and encephalopathy. Be aware that, in some patients, the serum creatinine may be falsely normal and remain within normal limits despite worsening renal function.
- Consider large volume paracentesis (5 to 6 L) with concurrent intravenous albumin infusion (6 to 8 g per liter of fluid removed) for patients with refractory ascites that is disabling. Admit for the procedure.

Encephalopathy

- At the first sign of encephalopathy, restrict dietary protein intake to 20 to 30 g per day. Obtain dietary consultation to construct a diet emphasizing plant protein over animal protein. Consider use of an oral supplement rich in branched-chain amino acids if protein intake is insufficient.
- Monitor mental status and check for asterixis; use five-point star or signature testing. Monitor venous ammonia levels; in drawing blood for a determination, avoid prolonged tourniquet application.
- When protein restriction fails to control encephalopathy, begin oral lactulose, 15 to 30 mL every 4 to 6 hours, with subsequent adjustments in the dosage to allow two to three soft stools a day. Add oral neomycin 1 g bid or metronidazole 250 mg tid if lactulose alone does not suffice.

Prevention of Variceal Bleeding and Bleeding due to Clotting Factor Deficiency

- Begin a beta-blocker (eg, propranolol 80 mg per day) for primary prevention in patients with risk factors for variceal bleeding (marked hepatocellular dysfunction, ascites, encephalopathy, large varices, and presence of dilated venules on the varices).
- Consider sclerotherapy and shunt procedures for prevention of recurrent variceal bleeding.
- Monitor prothrombin time and platelet count. Administer vitamin K (10 mg SC daily for 3 days) if there is prolongation of prothrombin time due to drug-induced bile-salt malabsorption, neomycin, or malnutrition. Platelet transfusions are unwarranted unless there is active bleeding in the context of a very low platelet count (see Chapter 81).

INDICATIONS FOR REFERRAL AND ADMISSION

Prompt hospitalization is required for patients with GI bleeding, worsening encephalopathy, increasing azotemia, signs of peritoneal irritation, or unexplained fever. Intractable ascites may respond to elective admission for large-volume paracentesis. Decisions about the management of refractory ascites, encephalopathy, variceal bleeding, and uncommon etiologies of cirrhosis (eg, primary biliary cirrhosis, Wilson's disease, hemochromatosis) are best made in consultation with a gastroenterologist skilled in treating liver disease. The same pertains to candidacy for liver transplantation. When urine output falls in the absence of a clear-cut explanation, a nephrologic consultation may be of considerable help, especially because creatinine level may not adequately reflect renal function.

PATIENT EDUCATION AND SUPPORT

It should be emphasized to the patient and family that prognosis can often be greatly improved and symptoms lessened by careful adherence to the prescribed medical program. In particular, dietary discipline and omission of alcohol are central to a successful outcome and should be stressed. Many of these patients are chronic alcoholics with low self-esteem. A nonjudgmental, sympathetic physician can be instrumental in providing support, raising self-esteem, and improving the chances of compliance (see Chapter 228). Depression is a frequent accompaniment of the later stages of chronic liver disease and is manifested by failure to comply with the medical regimen and outright expressions of wanting to die. Treatment is very difficult. Antidepressant drugs may cause oversedation and thus are risky. There are no simple measures, but the physician's concern and support can help enormously (see Chapter 227).

A.H.G.

ANNOTATED BIBLIOGRAPHY

Black M, Friedman AC. Ultrasound examination in the patient with ascites. Ann Intern Med 1989;110:253. *(Editorial urging its routine use in patients with new onset of ascites, both for its confirmation and to rule out a venoocclusive etiology.)*

Borowsky SA, Strome S, Lott E. Continued heavy drinking and survival in alcoholic cirrhotics. Gastroenterology 1981;80:1405. *(80 percent of those who continued to drink heavily died an average of 7.2 months after discharge; 95 percent of abstainers were still alive at 14 months.)*

Boyer JL, Ransohoff DF. Is colchicine effective therapy for cirrhosis? N Engl J Med 1988;318:1751. *(Urges caution in interpreting the very encouraging data that are emerging; see Kershenobich below.)*

Campra JL, Reynolds TB. Effectiveness of high-dose spironolactone therapy in patients with chronic liver disease and relatively refractory ascites. Dig Dis Sci 1978;23:1025. *(Doses as high as 600 mg per day found effective in patients with ascites presumed to be "refractory.")*

Christensen E, Neuberger J, Crowe J, et al. Beneficial effect of azathioprine and prediction of prognosis in primary biliary cirrhosis final results of an international trial. Gastroenterology 1985;89:1084. *(Improved survival demonstrated.)*

Conn HO, Leevy CM, Vlahcevic ZR, et al. Comparison of lactulose and neomycin in the treatment of chronic portal-systemic encephalopathy; a double-blind controlled trial. Gastroenterology 1977;72:573. *(Found to be equally effective and free of significant toxicity at the doses used.)*

Epstein M. Treatment of refractory ascites. N Engl J Med 1989;321:1675. *(Editorial summarizing data on LeVeen shunting and large volume paracentesis; argues that paracentesis may be preferable.)*

Fraser CL, Arieff AI. Hepatic encephalopathy. N Engl J Med 1985;313:865. *(Comprehensive review; 147 references.)*

Gines P, Arroyo V, Vargas V, et al. Paracentesis with intravenous infusion of albumin as compared with peritoneovenous shunting in cirrhosis with refractory ascites. N Engl J Med 1991;325:829. *(Randomized comparison showing equal effectiveness and similar total hospital days.)*

Graham DY, Smith JL. The course of patients after variceal hemorrhage. Gastroenterology 1981;80:800. *(One-third died in the initial hospitalization, one-third rebled within 6 weeks, and one-third survived at least 1 year. Long-term survival after the initial 2 weeks no different from that of unselected cirrhotics without bleeding.)*

Kaplan MM. Primary biliary cirrhosis. N Engl J Med 1987;316:521. *(Authoritative and very useful review for the generalist reader; 124 references.)*

Kershenobich D, Vargas F, Garcia-Tsao G, et al. Colchicine in the treatment of cirrhosis of the liver. N Engl J Med 1988;318:1709. *(Randomized, placebo-controlled study; 14 years of follow-up; survival doubled.)*

North Italian Endoscopic Club. Prediction of the first variceal hemorrhage in patients with cirrhosis of the liver and esophageal varices. N Engl J Med 1988;319:983. *(Multivariate analysis identifying risk factors predictive of bleeding.)*

Orrego H, Blake JE, Blendis LM, et al. Long-term treatment of alcoholic liver disease with propylthiouracil. N Engl J Med 1987;317:1421. *(Long-term, double-blind, randomized trial demonstrating reduction in mortality; about 50 percent of patients had cirrhosis.)*

Pagliaro L, D'Amico G, Sorensen TIA, et al. Prevention of first bleeding in cirrhosis: A meta-analysis of randomized trials of nonsurgical treatment. Ann Intern Med 1992;117:59. *(Beta-blockers prevent first bleeding in high-risk patients; sclerotherapy is of unproven efficacy for primary prophylaxis.)*

Papadakis MA, Arieff AI. Unpredictability of clinical evaluation of renal function in cirrhosis. Am J Med 1987;82:945. *(Some cirrhotics with reduced glomerular filtration have normal serum creatinine levels, which may remain within normal limits despite worsening of renal function.)*

Powell WJ Jr, Klatskin G. Duration of survival in patients with Laennec's cirrhosis. Am J Med 1968;44:406. *(Classic paper showing improved survival in cirrhotic patients who abstained from alcohol compared with those who continued to drink heavily.)*

Poynard T, Cales P, Pasta L, et al. Beta-adrenergic antagonist drugs in the prevention of gastrointestinal bleeding in patients with cirrhosis and esophageal varices. N Engl J Med 1991;324:1532. *(Analysis of pooled data showing reduction in risk of first bleeding and mortality from hemorrhage.)*

Rector WG, Jr, Reynolds TB. Superiority of serum-ascites albumin differences in "exudative" ascites. Am J Med 1984;77:83. *(Better than total protein for differential diagnosis.)*

Rikkers LF. Operations for management of esophageal variceal hemorrhage. West J Med 1982;136:107. *(Critical review of the various types of portasystemic shunt procedures and the indications for their use.)*

Ring EJ, Lake JR, Roberts JP, et al. Using transjugular intrahepatic portosystemic shunts to control variceal bleeding before liver transplantation. Ann Intern Med 1992;116:304. *(Prospective, uncontrolled trial; found safe and effective.)*

Shear L, Ching S, Gabuzda GJ. Compartmentalization of ascites and edema in patients with hepatic cirrhosis. N Engl J Med 1970;282:1391. *(Classic, elegant study; maximum rate at which ascites can be absorbed was 930 mL per 24 hours; concludes that the therapeutic aim in patients with ascites should be weight loss of no more than 0.5 kg daily.)*

Stanley MM, Ochi S, Lee KK, et al. Peritoneovenous shunting as compared with medical treatment in patients with alcoholic cirrhosis and massive ascites. N Engl J Med 1989;321:1632. *(Ascites alleviated, but survival unchanged.)*

Starzl TE, Demetris AJ, Van Thiel D. Liver transplantation. N Engl J Med 1989;321:1014,1092. *(Comprehensive review.)*

Williams JW, Simel DL. Does this patient have ascites? How to divine fluid in the abdomen. JAMA 1992;267:2645. *(Best review of the diagnostic utility of history and physical examination methods.)*

72
Management of Pancreatitis

JAMES M. RICHTER, M.D.

Primary Care Medicine: Office Evaluation and Management of the Adult Patient, 3rd edition, edited by Allan H. Goroll, Lawrence A. May, and Albert G. Mulley, Jr. J.B. Lippincott Company, Philadelphia

The primary physician encounters pancreatitis in three forms that lend themselves to ambulatory management: 1) recovery phase of acute pancreatitis; 2) chronic, mild relapsing pancreatitis presenting as recurrent abdominal pain; and 3) pancreatic insufficiency, with steatorrhea and weight loss.

In the United States, most cases of pancreatitis are a result of excess ethanol ingestion or biliary tract disease, chiefly among middle-aged alcoholic men and elderly women with gallstones, respectively. A penetrating duodenal ulcer, trauma, hypercalcemia, hypertriglyceridemia, vascular insufficiency, tumor, heredity, ampullary stenosis, and drugs such as thiazide diuretics, glucocorticosteroids, azathioprine, and sulfasalazine are also associated with pancreatitis. Frequently, no etiology is found. The course, response to therapy, and prognosis are largely functions of the etiology.

The primary physician must be able to distinguish acute pancreatitis from other causes of acute upper abdominal pain (see Chapter 58), pancreatic insufficiency from other causes of steatorrhea (see Chapter 64), and chronic abdominal pain due to pancreatitis from that due to pancreatic carcinoma and other important etiologies (see Chapters 58 and 76). Objectives of management include relief of pain, removal of precipitants, and assurance of adequate nutrition.

DIAGNOSIS, CLINICAL PRESENTATION, AND COURSE

Acute Pancreatitis. The manifestations of acute pancreatic disease are produced by inflammatory breakdown of pancreatic architecture, with release of digestive enzymes into the interstitium of the gland, leading to autolysis. Typically, acute pancreatitis produces constant epigastric, periumbilical, or left or right upper abdominal pain radiating to the back, often increased by food and decreased by upright posture. Vomiting can be persistent. Examination reveals abdominal tenderness and may include decreased bowel sounds, distention, and fever.

The diagnosis of acute pancreatitis is supported by increases in the serum amylase and serum lipase. The *serum amylase* is elevated principally in pancreatic disease, but may also be high in renal insufficiency, salivary gland disease, biliary tract obstruction, and such other intraabdominal conditions as perforated peptic ulcer, mesenteric infarction, and small bowel obstruction without detectable pancreatitis. The *serum lipase* is more specific but less sensitive; it is a good confirmatory test.

An *amylase–creatinine clearance ratio* of greater than 5 was thought to convey added specificity, but further study found it to be merely a nonspecific consequence of decreased renal amylase clearance that can occur in the setting of any severe, acute stress, including diabetic ketoacidosis and cutaneous burns. Assays for *trypsinogen* and *amylase isoenzymes* have been developed; they are useful confirmatory tests, but the serum amylase remains the best initial diagnostic study. At times *ultrasonography* can be used for diagnostic purposes; it shows edema of the gland, as well as any biliary tract pathology. Radiologic *contrast study* of the stomach and duodenum helps to rule out peptic ulcer disease when the etiology of the pain is unclear.

The *course* of acute pancreatitis depends on the severity of the disease and the underlying etiology. In a patient recovering from acute pancreatitis, symptoms are reliable indicators of disease activity. Elevated enzymes in an otherwise asymptomatic patient are usually of no significance. The serum amylase routinely falls to normal within several days but may remain elevated for weeks after an uncomplicated illness. In other instances, persistently elevated enzymes in an asymptomatic person may be a clue to the presence of a silent pseudocyst. If a mass is palpable or pain recurs, a pseudocyst should be ruled out by ultrasonography of the upper abdomen. *Pseudocysts* arise in about half of patients with severe pancreatitis, mostly in those with alcohol-induced disease. Spontaneous resolution occurs over 3 months in about 50 percent of patients; those with persistent lesions over 5 cm usually require surgical drainage.

Chronic pancreatitis characteristically presents and proceeds as bouts of mild to severe recurrent epigastric pain, often occurring in *alcoholic patients* after years of excessive drinking. Sometimes chronic pancreatitis is heralded by a severe attack of acute pancreatitis. At other times, there may be mild pain or simply the painless insidious onset of exocrine insufficiency and diabetes. The pain of chronic pancreatitis is not entirely constant and often varies in intensity over days to weeks. There may be exacerbations of pain, nausea, and vomiting after eating or drinking alcohol. Elevated serum *amylase* and *lipase* levels are helpful, but the sensitivity of these tests is lower than in acute pancreatitis.

Individuals who present with chronic recurrent abdominal pain and a history of relapsing pancreatitis usually do not present difficult diagnostic problems, but the patient without such a history requires more extensive assessment. A *plain film of the abdomen* may reveal *pancreatic calcification,* a late finding in alcoholic pancreatitis. *Ultrasonography* may demonstrate a diffusely enlarged gland, local mass, or pseudocyst. If ultrasound evaluation is normal and pancreatic disease is strongly suspected on clinical grounds, *computed tomographic (CT) scanning* of the upper abdomen should be performed. If a solitary mass is found, *needle biopsy* should be performed to help diagnose cancer. If uncertainty about cancer or chronic pancreatitis persists, *endoscopic retrograde pancreatography* may prove diagnostically useful. *Abdominal angiography* can be substituted for retrograde pancreatography, if the latter is unavailable or fails.

The *clinical course* of chronic pancreatitis is variable and depends on elimination of precipitating factors. Gallstones, particularly common bile duct stones, should be promptly removed, either surgically or endoscopically. Successful and early removal greatly reduces the risk of recurrent or chronic pancreatitis.

With recurrent disease, *pancreatic insufficiency* may gradually develop over years, manifested by weight loss and steatorrhea. Although mild glucose intolerance may occur early in the disease process, the onset of clinical *diabetes* is a late complication and a sign of advanced disease. There appears to be an increased risk of pancreatic cancer.

Pancreatic Insufficiency. Patients with pancreatic exocrine insufficiency complain of *weight loss* and frequent, greasy bowel movements (ie, steatorrhea). Weight loss is often striking but nonspecific in this population, which tends to substitute alcohol for other forms of nourishment. Steatorrhea is a late development, not seen until more than 80 percent of pancreatic exocrine function has been lost. Objective evidence of maldigestion may be obtained by a *qualitative examination for stool fat* with Sudan stain. Where this is not available, a 72-hour *quantitative stool fat* analysis can also be used to establish the presence of steatorrhea and a D-*xylose test* to exclude small bowel mucosal disease. The *bentiromide test* is a simple outpatient study for detecting pancreatic exocrine insufficiency. When bentiromide (500 mg) is given orally, it normally is acted on by pancreatic chymotrypsin to produce para-aminobenzoic acid, which is absorbed by the small bowel and excreted in the urine. In normal persons, greater than 50 percent is excreted in 6 hours. This test appears to have a sensitivity of 80 percent and a specificity of 90 percent for exocrine insufficiency. A trial of pancreatic enzyme replacement may be valuable diagnostically.

When significant uncertainty persists, direct pancreatic function tests, such as secretin stimulation, may be needed to demonstrate exocrine insufficiency objectively. A small group of patients with pancreatic insufficiency who do not give a history of alcoholism or recurrent abdominal pain should be evaluated for hemochromatosis and cystic fibrosis.

PRINCIPLES OF MANAGEMENT

Acute Pancreatitis. About 50 percent of patients have mild, self-limited disease and will recover spontaneously. Such patients with mild pain and no vomiting may be treated on an ambulatory basis with restriction of fat and protein and careful monitoring. Patients with more severe disease who require hospitalization generally tolerate a full diet before discharge from the hospital, although a *diet moderately restricted in fat* is often recommended to lessen the degree of pancreatic stimulation. *H_2-receptor antagonists, antacids,* and *anticholinergics* are frequently given with the hope of reducing the stimulus to pancreatic secretion, but are of no proven benefit. A patient who returns with severe pain and vomiting should be readmitted.

Identification and treatment or removal of precipitants, such as alcohol abuse, hypercalcemia, gallstones, and hypertriglyceridemia are essential to successful therapy. Of the conditions associated with pancreatitis, alcoholism is the most difficult to deal with. Even the pain of pancreatitis often does not dissuade the dedicated drinker from abusing alcohol. Nevertheless, the *treatment of alcoholism* should be undertaken with considerable effort (see Chapter 228), because there is much to gain by the cessation of drinking. A check for drugs associated with pancreatitis is indicated (thiazides, corticosteroids, estrogens, azathioprine).

All patients should undergo evaluation of the biliary tract by *ultrasonography* to rule out gallstone disease, a treatable cause of pancreatitis. The oral cholecystogram is less useful, because it may not visualize until 4 to 6 weeks after a bout of acute pancreatitis. After an acute episode, a *serum calcium* should be repeated, because *hypercalcemia* can be masked by the decrease in calcium that may result from an attack. Repeatedly marked elevations in *fasting triglyceride* concentration suggest the diagnosis of hypertriglyceridemia, which responds to gemfibrozil (see Chapter 27).

Chronic Pancreatitis. Patients with chronic pancreatitis may develop recurrent bouts of pain and vomiting indistinguishable from acute pancreatitis. Those with severe pain and inability to maintain hydration orally should be admitted. Others with less severe exacerbations may be managed on an outpatient basis. Many are bothered by chronic pain.

Initial treatment consists of eliminating causative factors (see above) and attempting to control the often disabling *pain.* Pancreatic enzymes and low-fat diets may decrease pancreatic secretion but do not reliably lessen the pain. Nonnarcotic analgesics (aspirin, ibuprofen, acetaminophen) should be tried but are usually inadequate, necessitating use of more potent agents. *Methadone* and *sustained-release morphine* are the narcotics best suited for long-term outpatient use. Sometimes, *tricyclic antidepressants* are useful adjuncts for pain control (see Chapter 227). The establishment of a *supportive doctor–patient relationship* complements pharmacologic pain control efforts.

Numerous *surgical procedures* have been designed to alleviate the pain of chronic pancreatitis; none is totally effective. Patients with persistent pain in the absence of gallbladder disease or alcoholism should have an endoscopic *retrograde pancreatogram* to search for a surgically treatable anatomic abnormality, such as pancreas divisum. If a markedly dilated duct is found, a modified *Puestow sphincteroplasty procedure* can be performed to improve drainage of pancreatic juices into the small bowel. The operation may provide reasonable pain relief without removal of pancreatic tissue. Large, persistent pseudocysts should be drained internally; however, reduction in pain is not consistently achieved. Sometimes partial or even subtotal pancreatectomies are attempted for control of pain; at best, results are equivocal.

In patients with severe active disease, the pancreas is progressively destroyed, and eventually the pain subsides as the disease "burns" itself out. Then the management priority shifts to treatment of pancreatic insufficiency.

Pancreatic Insufficiency. Management of pancreatic insufficiency begins with a therapeutic trial of oral pancreatic enzymes to judge efficacy of therapy. The patient who benefits from use of exogenous enzymes will tolerate the unpleasant taste and mild discomfort they cause. *Pancreatin* contains trypsin, amylase, and some lipase, whereas *pancrealipase* contains trypsin, amylase, and extra amounts of lipase. The usual dose is 0.5 g to 2.5 g with each meal. Because enzyme preparations are partially inactivated by gastric acid or require increased alkalinity in the duodenum, they may work better when given with antacids, bicarbonate, or H_2-receptor antagonists. *Medium-chain triglycerides* are often helpful, because they can be absorbed in the absence of lipase. Therapy can be assessed by monitoring symptoms, weight, and qualitative stool fat determinations. Clinically significant fat-soluble vitamin deficiencies are uncommon, perhaps because intact bile secretion prevents complete fat malabsorption.

Most patients with chronic pancreatitis have abnormal glucose tolerance tests. Mild glucose intolerance can be watched, but insulin dependence may occur. Hypoglycemia may be a problem, because loss of glucagon secretion leads to a "brittle" diabetic state, but ketoacidosis is rare. The vascular complications of diabetes are infrequent, but eventually occur if severe pancreatic insufficiency persists.

PATIENT EDUCATION

Most patients know little about the pancreas and its role in digestion. Moreover, few are aware of the connection between alcohol abuse and pancreatitis. Patient cooperation regarding diet, alcohol intake, and use of enzyme extracts may be facilitated by a better understanding of the function of the pancreas and the nature of pancreatitis. Also, patients with acute pancreatitis who are making good recoveries can be comforted by the fact that recurrence is not common when the underlying cause is treated.

The patient with intractable pain and narcotic dependence poses one of the most difficult problems encountered in clinical medicine. A major pitfall is the development of an adversarial relationship between patient and physician concerning the need for narcotics. Although there are no simple solutions, it is essential to elicit, understand, and respond to patient concerns, fears, and needs at the outset. A well-informed patient who has confidence in the physician and in him- or herself requires less pain medication than one who is scared, feels abandoned, and is in conflict with the physician.

INDICATIONS FOR ADMISSION AND REFERRAL

Some patients present with rather mild symptoms, but later develop a fulminant illness. Patients over age 55 are at risk for a serious progression, as are those who manifest fever, tachycardia, hyperglycemia, serum calcium below 8.0 mg per deciliter, or amylase over 1000 mg per deciliter at the time of initial presentation. Such individuals deserve admission for careful monitoring, even if they do not appear seriously ill at the outset. Patients who cannot maintain oral hydration also require admission. Patients with refractory pain might benefit from evaluation by a gastroenterologist skilled in endoscopic retrograde pancreatography. Surgical consultation is indicated if an anatomic abnormality, pseudocyst, or obstructive lesion is detected on work-up of the pancreas and biliary tract. Patients with chronic refractory pain may benefit from a psychiatric or pain management assessment, supplemented by tricyclic antidepressant therapy.

MANAGEMENT RECOMMENDATIONS

Recovery Phase of Acute Pancreatitis

- Begin feedings with foods rich in carbohydrates and low in protein and fat. Gradually increase the amount of protein in the diet as tolerated, followed by slow resumption of fat intake.
- Check for and treat any underlying alcohol abuse (see Chapter 228), hypertriglyceridemia (see Chapter 27), or hypercalcemia (see Chapter 96).
- Eliminate, if possible, use of drugs associated with pancreatitis (azathioprine, estrogens, thiazides, corticosteroids).
- Obtain ultrasound examination of the gallbladder and biliary tract; refer the patient for surgery if stones are found.

Chronic Pancreatitis

- Check for and treat any inciting cause, such as alcoholism, biliary tract disease, hypercalcemia, hyperlipidemia (see above).
- Readmit the patient if severe recurrent acute pancreatitis develops.
- Temporarily limit fat intake during flare-ups.
- Begin with mild analgesics for pain control, such as aspirin or acetaminophen 600 mg every 4 hours.
- Pain unrelieved by mild analgesia is an indication for a course of narcotic analgesics, such as methadone 5 or 10 mg every 6 or 8 hours.
- Further evaluation is needed to rule out carcinoma, pseudocyst, and biliary tract disease. Begin with ultrasonography and proceed to CT scan if ultrasonography is technically unsatisfactory.
- Refer the patient for surgery if a treatable lesion is found.
- Aggressive surgical procedures other than sphincteroplasty aimed at relieving ductal obstruction do not reliably relieve pain.
- Consider a trial of tricyclic antidepressant therapy (see Chapter 227) for patients with refractory pain. Psychiatric or pain management consultation may also help.

Pancreatic Insufficiency

- Give oral pancreatic extract with each feeding in doses of 0.5 to 2.5 g (two to eight tablets) with full meals and 0.5 g with snacks. Lack of effect may require addition of an antacid (eg, 60 mL of Mylanta with each meal) or H_2-receptor antagonist (eg, ranitidine, 150 mg bid) to neutralize gastric acid and prevent enzymes from becoming inactivated.
- Provide a high-calorie diet, rich in carbohydrate and protein.
- Supplement the diet with a medium-chain triglyceride preparation. Restrict fat in symptomatic steatorrhea.
- Monitor glucose tolerance and treat clinical diabetes, if present, with insulin, cautiously; these patients often exhibit "brittle" disease.

ANNOTATED BIBLIOGRAPHY

Agarwal N, Pitchumoni CS, Sivaprasad AV. Evaluating tests for acute pancreatitis. Am J Gastroenterol 1990;85:356. *(Current analysis of serologic and imaging studies.)*

Ammann RW, Akobintz A, Largiader F, et al. Course and outcome of chronic pancreatitis: A longitudinal study of a mixed medical–surgical series of 245 patients. Gastroenterology 1984;86:820. *(Excellent clinical course/natural history study.)*

Arvanitakis C, Cooke AR. Diagnostic tests of exocrine pancreatic function. Gastroenterology 1978;74:932. *(Excellent review of the major methods used to test exocrine function.)*

Bank S, Marks IN, Vinik AI. Clinical and hormonal aspects of pancreatic diabetes. Am J Gastroenterol 1975;64:13. *(Classic clinical description of pancreatic diabetes, its therapy, and its distinctive properties.)*

Karasawa E, Goldberg HI, Moss AA, et al. CT pancreatogram in carcinoma of the pancreas and chronic pancreatitis. Radiology 1983;148:489. *(Irregular calcified ducts are characteristic of chronic pancreatitis, whereas in pancreatic cancer, smooth or beaded dilatation is the most frequent finding.)*

Lowenfels AB, et al. Pancreatitis and the risk of pancreatic cancer. N Engl J Med 1993;328:1433. *(An association found.)*

Mallory A, Kern F, Jr. Drug-induced pancreatitis: A critical review. Gastroenterology 1980;78:813. *(Useful paper that includes how to separate the presumptive from the definite.)*

Marshall JB. Acute pancreatitis. Arch Intern Med 1993;153:1185. *(Comprehensive review of pathophysiology, diagnosis, and treatment; 156 refs.)*

Moosa AR. Surgical treatment of chronic pancreatitis: An overview. Br J Surg 1987;74:661. *(Excellent review of the data on surgical approaches to the problem.)*

Niederau C, Grendell JH. Diagnosis of chronic pancreatitis. Gastroenterology 1985;88:1973. *(Superb, absolutely comprehensive review of biochemical and imaging approaches to the diagnosis of chronic pancreatitis; 247 references.)*

Pitchumoni CS, Agarwal N, Jain NK. Systemic complications of acute pancreatitis. Am J Gastroenterol 1988;83:597. *(Best available review.)*

Richter JM, Schapiro RH, Mulley AG, et al. Association of pancreatitis and its treatment by sphincteroplasty of the accessory ampulla. Gastroenterology 1981;81:1104. *(Patients with pancreas divisum develop recurrent acute pancreatitis more frequently than people with normal anatomy.)*

Saunders JHB, Wormsley KG. Pancreatic extracts and the treatment of pancreatic exocrine insufficiency. Gut 1975;16:157. *(Provides a detailed review of pancreatic extracts, pancreatic replacement therapy, and the assessment of the efficacy of pancreatic replacement.)*

Steinberg WM, Goldstein SS, Davis SS, et al. Diagnostic assays in acute pancreatitis. Ann Intern Med 1985;102:576. *(Compares sensitivity and specificity of amylase, lipase, trypsinogen, and amylase isoenzymes; recommends use of amylase as the initial study.)*

Toskes P. Bentiromide as a test of exocrine function in adults with pancreatic exocrine insufficiency. Determination of appropriate dose of urinary collection interval. Gastroenterology 1983;85:565. *(Standardization of the bentiromide test as a simple outpatient test for pancreatic insufficiency.)*

Twersky Y, Bank S. Nutritional deficiencies in chronic pancreatitis. Gastroenterol Clin North Am 1989;18:543. *(Thorough and useful discussion of the problem and its management.)*

Van Dyke JA, Stanley RJ, Berland LL. Pancreatic imaging. Ann Intern Med 1985;102:212. *(Critical review of CT, ultrasound, and other imaging techniques; considers CT the best initial study, because ultrasonography often compromised by overlying bowel gas; 50 references.)*

73
Management of Inflammatory Bowel Disease

FREDRICK W. RUYMANN, M.D.
JAMES M. RICHTER, M.D.

Primary Care Medicine: Office Evaluation and Management of the Adult Patient, 3rd edition, edited by Allan H. Goroll, Lawrence A. May, and Albert G. Mulley, Jr. J.B. Lippincott Company, Philadelphia

Ulcerative colitis and Crohn's disease account for most of the inflammatory bowel disease seen in primary care practice. Abdominal pain, diarrhea, and bleeding are among the presenting manifestations. The first priority is to distinguish inflammatory bowel disease from other causes of diarrhea (see Chapter 64). The chronicity, potentially disabling symptoms, risk of malignancy (in the case of ulcerative colitis), and occasional refractoriness to medical therapy make management a major challenge. The primary care physician needs to know how to treat exacerbations, maintain remissions, and psychologically sustain these patients through difficult times. Competent care is based on a thorough understanding of the roles for medical and surgical therapy and skill in providing psychological support. Although patients with severe or refractory disease may need to be referred to the gastroenterologist, most others can be well-managed by the primary care physician.

PATHOPHYSIOLOGY, CLINICAL PRESENTATION, AND COURSE

Ulcerative colitis is an idiopathic, diffuse inflammatory disease of the *bowel mucosa.* Although pathogenesis remains poorly understood, there is growing evidence of a primary immune mechanism (eg, high prevalence of antibodies to intestinal epithelial antigens in asymptomatic relatives of patients as well as in patients themselves). The disease typically begins in adolescence or young adulthood, but may occur at almost any age. Whites are affected more often than African Americans. Prevalence is highest among Jews, and there is a tenfold increase in risk for having the disease among first-degree relatives of patients. The cardinal symptoms are bloody diarrhea and abdominal pain; in severe cases, fever, anorexia, and weight loss are present as well. The variability of presentations is remarkable, ranging from malaise and no symptoms referable to the colon, to fever, prostration, abdominal distention, and passage of large volumes of liquid stool.

The disease need not be confined to the bowel; extracolonic manifestations include arthritis, uveitis, jaundice, and skin lesions. The course is characteristically chronic, recurrent, and unpredictable. An insidious presentation does not predict a benign course, and a fulminant onset may be followed by long, relatively asymptomatic periods.

Ulcerative colitis almost always involves the *distal colon and rectum,* making diagnosis possible by sigmoidoscopy. The mucosa becomes edematous, obscuring the fine network of submucosal vessels. The moist, glistening mucosal surface is lost, and a granular appearance develops. The bowel wall is friable, bleeding spontaneously or when touched with a swab. In advanced cases, *pseudopolyps* and discrete *ulcers* may be seen. Smears of mucus from the bowel wall show polymorphonuclear leukocytes. Barium enema documents the extent of disease. Radiologic findings range from mucosal denudation to frank ulceration, with loss of haustral markings and a tubular appearance. There are *no skip areas. Liver* involvement occurs in the form of *pericholangitis and fatty infiltration;* these are common histologic findings in ulcerative colitis but are seldom symptomatic. Much less frequently, chronic active hepatitis, cirrhosis, or sclerosing cholangitis is seen. A migratory, *monoarticular arthritis* affecting the large joints develops in 10 percent of patients. This arthritis often coincides with an exacerbation of colitis and resolves with control of the underlying disease. *Ankylosing spondylitis* also occurs, but runs a course independent of the colitis. *Uveitis* or episcleritis may be seen at any time during the course of the disease. *Erythema nodosum, pyoderma gangrenosum,* or *oral aphthous ulcerations* are found in about 5 percent of patients, usually during active colitis.

The *prognosis* for patients with ulcerative colitis seen in the primary care setting is far better than that for patients studied in referral centers, who are likely to have more severe disease. A community-based study done over 10 years found that 87 percent went into complete remission after the first attack and only 8 percent developed chronic persistent disease. In 30 percent no further attacks occurred over 5 years, and in 74 percent disease was limited to the distal bowel (rectum or rectosigmoid). Overall mortality was no different from that of the general population, although it was increased in patients with severe first attacks or extensive disease.

The *risk of cancer* is enhanced and is a function of the extent and duration of disease and age at diagnosis. Risk begins to increase substantially after 8 years of illness. An important population study reported an absolute risk of colon cancer in patients with pancolitis to be 30 percent after 35 years from time of diagnosis. Those with pancolitis diagnosed before the age of 15 had an absolute risk of 40 percent. These figures are slightly lower than traditional risk estimates of 1 percent to 2 percent per year derived from referral center cohorts.

Ulcerative Proctitis. Typically, the patient with ulcerative proctitis is a young adult who presents with rectal bleeding and tenesmus. The bleeding is usually not severe; it is sometimes mistakenly attributed to hemorrhoids. Diarrhea or constipation may accompany the bleeding, but often there are only small frequent bowel movements associated with a small amount of mucus. On sigmoidoscopy, an edematous, friable rectal mucosa is observed; the bowel above the rectosigmoid is uninvolved. On barium enema or colonoscopy, the remainder of the large bowel is normal. The clinical presentation of ulcerative proctitis is not pathognomonic; the condition must be distinguished from infectious forms of proctocolitis, including acquired immunodeficiency syndrome (AIDS)-related etiologies (see Chapters 13 and 66).

Ulcerative proctitis is a variant of ulcerative colitis, distinguished by the limited extent of inflammation, its good prognosis, and paucity of serious complications. However, relapses are common. Fewer than 15 percent progress to generalized ulcerative colitis. The distant complications of ulcerative colitis are rare, and carcinoma of the rectum develops no more often than in unaffected individuals.

Crohn's disease is a chronic, relapsing inflammatory disorder of the alimentary tract, with a peak incidence in the second and third decades. The inflammation is characteristically *discontinuous,* with diseased segments of bowel separated by normal areas. Crohn's disease has a tendency to cause strictures, fistulas, and abscesses, because the granulomatous inflammatory process may extend through *all layers* of the bowel wall. The condition often affects the distal ileum and right colon, but frequently it involves only the small bowel or colon. It may occur in any portion of the alimentary tract, from the buccal mucosa to the anus.

Extraintestinal involvement occurs in 15 percent to 20 percent of cases, with *arthritis, ankylosing spondylitis, uveitis, erythema nodosum, aphthous oral ulcers,* and *pyoderma gangrenosum* being the predominant manifestations of disease outside the bowel. In addition, *cholelithiasis* and *nephrolithiasis* have a higher incidence in these patients than in the general population.

Symptoms vary, depending on the location and extent of disease. Diarrhea and abdominal pain (particularly in the right lower quadrant) are cardinal symptoms, occurring in almost 80 percent of patients. Weight loss, vomiting, fever, perianal discomfort, and bleeding are also common complaints. Constipation may be an early manifestation of obstruction. Symptoms can develop subtly or can present in fulminant fashion with the patient systemically toxic.

Physical examination may reveal a discrete abdominal mass, especially in the right lower quadrant, but usually a normal abdomen or doughy loops of bowel are found. Abdominal or perianal fistulous tracts are noted on examination in up to 10 percent of patients. Extraintestinal findings include inflamed joints, spinal deformities, erythema nodosum, pyoderma, uveitis, and aphthous ulcers.

Sigmoidoscopy is abnormal in fewer than 20 percent of cases; fistulous tracts and discrete inflammatory ulcers are sometimes encountered in the rectosigmoid. *Barium enema and upper gastrointestinal (GI) series* often show segmental involvement of large and small bowel, often with strictures, fistulas, and ulcers. The primary abnormality in Crohn's disease is submucosal, causing radiologic studies to sometimes appear normal. In such cases, *colonoscopy* aids diagnosis by demonstrating segmental disease and ulceration that may be missed on barium enema.

Prognosis. Although it is difficult to extrapolate from referral center data to patients seen in primary care settings, a pattern emerges of disease activity that waxes and wanes over many years. Disease-free intervals may last as long as several years or even decades, but recurrences are the rule. Several years of relief from symptoms may be afforded by surgical resection, but there is no evidence that any medical and surgical therapy alters the ultimate course of the illness. In referral center series, as many as 70 percent of patients ultimately require surgical resection.

WORKUP

Proper management requires confirming the diagnosis and determining the extent of disease. One proviso should be kept in mind: because these illnesses often occur in women of childbearing age, attempts should be made to minimize their x-ray exposure and carefully select only the most necessary radiologic studies.

Ulcerative Colitis

The diagnosis is usually based on the clinical presentation, sigmoidoscopic demonstration of inflammation, and the exclusion of bacterial and parasitic infections by culture and examination for ova and parasites (see Chapter 64). Because the disease almost invariably affects the distal colon and rectum, *sigmoidoscopy* is an essential component of the workup. The procedure is best performed without cleansing preparations, so as not to distort the appearance of the bowel mucosa (see Appendix in Chapter 56). In acute phases of the illness, the mucosa appears *friable* and inflamed; there is loss of the normal vascular pattern. As the disease progresses, a *purulent exudate* and discrete small *ulcers* may form. With severe colitis, there may be pus and spontaneous bleeding as well as large ulcers. Chronic phases of the disease are characterized by a *granular mucosa* and inflammatory *pseudopolyps* (tags of damaged mucosa and granulation tissue).

When the sigmoidoscopic picture is nonspecific, one should *culture and examine the stool* for *Clostridium difficile, Entamoeba histolytica, Campylobacter, Shigella, Salmonella,* and *Neisseria gonorrhea* (see Chapters 64 and 66). *Rectal biopsy* is indicated when one needs to confirm the diagnosis and exclude conditions such as Crohn's disease of the rectosigmoid, amebic colitis, pseudomembranous colitis, cytomegalovirus infection, and herpetic pancolitis. *Barium enema* or *colonoscopy* can be used to provide supportive evidence when the diagnosis is in doubt and helps document the extent of disease. However, they should not be performed during a flare-up because there is a small risk of perforation when the procedure is performed on an acutely inflamed bowel.

Assessing disease activity is critical to management, but can be difficult. Scoring systems based on clinical parameters are sometimes used in research settings but have little utility in clinical practice. A host of radionuclide imaging methods have been tried, but they lack specificity. Colonoscopy remains the mainstay of assessment.

Crohn's Disease

Crohn's disease of the colon may mimic ulcerative colitis clinically. Differentiating features include *"skip areas"* in the colon, significant *small bowel* involvement, *fistulas,* and *granulomas* on biopsy. The diagnosis is suggested by a history of recurrent postprandial lower abdominal pain and altered bowel habits in a young person; it is reinforced by finding on physical examination a mass or tenderness in the right lower quadrant. Radiologic contrast studies are needed for a more definitive assessment. The small bowel phase of an upper GI series shows *segmental narrowing,* areas with loss of the normal mucosal pattern interspersed with areas of normal mucosa, fistula formation, and the *"string sign"* (a narrow band of barium flowing through an inflamed or scarred area) in the terminal ileum.

Colonic disease may be documented by *air contrast barium enema,* with asymmetric segmental changes distinguishing Crohn's disease of the large bowel from ulcerative colitis. Disease of the terminal ileum can often be detected on barium enema; however, radiologic involvement of the terminal ileum is not unique to Crohn's disease. Some ulcerative colitis patients also demonstrate inflammatory changes in the terminal ileum ("backwash ileitis"), but they lack the skip pattern characteristic of Crohn's disease.

Sigmoidoscopy demonstrates rectosigmoid inflammation in the 20 percent to 50 percent of patients with disease in this area; however, the findings are often nonspecific (mild erythema). *Colonoscopy* is needed in difficult cases and helps in judging the extent and severity of disease. *Biopsy* can be diagnostic but is usually unnecessary unless the diagnosis remains unsubstantiated; it should be avoided when acute inflammation is present. *Disease activity* in the colon is best assessed by colonoscopy and in the small bowel by barium contrast study.

PRINCIPLES OF MANAGEMENT

Comprehensive management requires attending to the patient's medical, psychological, and nutritional needs. For the most part, treatment is empirical and directed at providing symptomatic relief. However, surgery does offer the possibility of cure for patients with ulcerative colitis, and studies have shown prophylactic benefit from sulfasalazine. The inflammatory bowel diseases are chronic illnesses that require long-term management and support for the patient and the family.

Ulcerative Colitis

Because the disease typically follows a relapsing course with acute exacerbations and intervals of remission, the approach to treatment depends on the patient's current clinical status. During remission, treatment is prophylactic; during flare-ups, the goal is control of the inflammatory process. For refractory and widespread disease, surgery requires consideration.

Dietary and Nutritional Measures. No specific diet improves or exacerbates ulcerative colitis. However, reduction in dietary *fiber* may be of some benefit during periods of active disease. In patients with inactive disease, 1 or 2 teaspoons of *psyllium* hydrophilic colloid (Metamucil) in water daily often helps to bind the stool. There is an increased incidence of lactase deficiency in these patients; an empirical trial of a *milk-free diet* is reasonable when diarrhea persists despite other evidence of clinical remission. Those who are anemic from blood loss need oral or parenteral *iron* supplementation (see Chapter 82). Oral iron may be poorly tolerated, necessitating parenteral administration. Anemia may also be due to folic acid deficiency. *Folic acid* supplementation is indicated when intake of leafy vegetables and fresh fruits is poor or when sulfasalazine is being taken (see below). Anemia may also be due to chronic disease and may not respond to dietary and nutritional measures.

Sulfasalazine. The drug is recommended as initial treatment for mild to moderate disease and for prevention of relapses. After oral administration, about 70 percent reaches the colon, where it is metabolized by intestinal bacteria, resulting in the local release of sulfapyridine and the salicylate analogue 5-aminosalicylate (5-ASA), which is felt to be the active moiety. Sulfasalazine's precise mechanism of action remains speculative. Hypotheses include effects on prostaglandin synthesis (particularly arachidonic acid metabolism) and inhibition of migration of polymorphonuclear leukocytes.

Randomized controlled studies have shown the drug to be effective as *initial treatment* for patients with mild to moderate symptoms when given in doses of 4 g per day for 2 to 4 weeks. About 80 percent of patients respond. Because sulfasalazine is less effective than corticosteroid therapy, it is reserved for relatively mild cases; however, combined use with steroids has been suggested for early treatment of severe disease.

Controlled studies have also documented the drug's efficacy for *prophylaxis* and maintaining remissions. In one major study, more than 65 percent of patients given maintenance doses of 2 g per day remained symptom-free for at least 1 year compared with 25 percent of patients given placebo. The prophylactic effect of maintenance therapy persists when the drug is continued beyond 1 year. The optimum dose is 2 g per day (4 g per day provides even better protection, but the frequency of side effects is markedly increased).

Sulfasalazine is usually well-tolerated, although minor *side effects* occur in about one-third of patients. *Rash and fever* are common hypersensitivity reactions to the sulfa moiety, whereas *nausea, vomiting, headache, and hemolysis* are common dose-related side effects. Patients unable to tolerate full doses of sulfasalazine because of gastrointestinal upset often do better when reintroduced to the drug more gradually. Taking it with meals also helps. Potential *hematopoetic effects* include anemia (from folic acid deficiency, hemolysis, or marrow suppression), granulocytopenia, and thrombocytopenia. *Low sperm counts* and qualitative sperm abnormalities have been noted in men taking the drug, usually after about 2 months of therapy; these conditions reverse when the medication is stopped. *Hepatitis* and *nephritis* have also been reported.

Drug interactions associated with sulfasalazine use include inhibition of folic acid absorption and a 25 percent reduction in *digoxin* bioavailability. Sulfasalazine's metabolism is slowed when *cholestyramine* or *broad-spectrum antibiotics* are used concurrently, an effect of uncertain clinical significance. *Ferrous sulfate* appears to have a similar effect on sulfasalazine, although iron absorption is not appreciably hindered; these drugs should not be taken at the same time.

Desensitization has been successful in patients with minor allergic reactions (rash, fever). Such patients are started on doses of a fraction of a tablet (1 to 30 mg per day were used in studies) and slowly advanced over 2 to 4 weeks until therapeutic doses are achieved. The drug has been used with safety in pregnant and nursing patients.

Newer 5-Aminosalicylate Agents. Although sulfasalazine is an excellent drug, a substantial number of patients cannot use it due to sulfa allergy. Consequently, much effort went into finding an sulfa-free means of delivering 5-ASA to the colon. Both oral and topical formulations have been developed. *Olsalazine* is the first oral drug of this group to be marketed commercially. It contains two 5-ASA molecules bound by an azo bond that is cleaved by bacteria in the colon, releasing the active moiety. In several controlled trials, oral 5-ASA agents performed as well as sulfasalazine in the treatment of active ulcerative colitis and in maintaining remissions. Patients who do not tolerate sulfasalazine deserve a trial of olsalazine, which has a lower incidence of side effects, probably from being sulfa-free. Other 5-ASA drugs under development (eg, *mesalamine*) are likely to offer differences in site of 5-ASA release. Preliminary data suggest capacity to reduce frequency of relapses.

Topical 5-ASA enemas were also developed as an alternative to sulfasalazine and represent a reasonable option in patients with distal colitis. Their safety profile is excellent, but cost is considerably higher than is the cost of a hydrocortisone enema. However, unlike steroid enemas, there is no concern about systemic steroid absorption.

Glucocorticosteroids. Steroids suppress the inflammatory process of ulcerative colitis. *Systemic preparations* are used in markedly symptomatic patients with *extensive disease*. Those without systemic toxicity can be well cared for at home by starting with the equivalent of 60 mg prednisone per day. Patients too ill for oral therapy (those with vomiting, high fever, or signs of bowel distention) should be admitted to the hospital. Once symptoms lessen, the dosage is gradually tapered over 4 to 8 weeks to the lowest dosage that maintains control. Whenever possible, every effort should be made to taper and terminate steroid therapy. The adverse effects of chronic steroid therapy can be disabling (see Chapter 105). In addition, only a small minority of ulcerative colitis patients benefit from chronic steroid use. In these patients, alternate-day steroid administration often suffices after a flare-up has been brought under control and poses much less risk of steroid side effects (see Chapter 105). Patients who require chronic, high-dose steroid therapy might benefit from a trial of steroid-sparing immunosuppressive therapy with *6-mercaptopurine (6-MP)* or *azathioprine* (see discussion of immunosuppressive therapy under treatment of Crohn's disease).

Patients with mild to moderate acute colitis limited to the distal colon can be treated with *rectally administered steroids*. Topical forms include hydrocortisone suppositories given one to three times daily or a retention enema given at night. These programs are capable of inducing remissions in patients with distal disease. The hydrocortisone will always reach the sigmoid; more proximal spread is variable. About one-third is absorbed systemically, but adrenal suppression is usually not a major problem unless very high doses of steroids are used. Steroid suppositories and foams in conjunction with sulfasalazine work well to control disease limited to the rectum (ulcerative proctitis).

Newer topical corticosteroids that possess potent anti-inflammatory properties without interfering with adrenal function are being studied. The topically active steroid beclomethasone has been found equally efficacious to hydrocortisone, but with less systemic absorption and no effect on serum cortisol levels.

When uveitis and colitis flare simultaneously, oral steroids are often effective for both. In the absence of active colitis, the uveitis may be treated with topical steroids and mydriatics. The best means of treating other systemic manifestations (erythema nodosum, pyoderma gangrenosum, and oral aphthous ulcerations) is to control the underlying disease. Patients with severe disease requiring daily steroids should receive calcium and vitamin D supplementation, because absorption may be impaired.

Opiates are useful for providing symptomatic relief of diarrhea during acute phases of illness and chronic active colitis. They must be used with *caution* in acutely ill patients because of the risk of precipitating *toxic dilatation*. Diphenoxylate, codeine, tincture of opium, paregoric, and loperamide all limit the number of bowel movements. They are given before meals and at bedtime. *Loperamide* is among the most effective and least addicting, but is considerably more expensive. *Codeine* is excellent for short-term use and superior to diphenoxylate in efficacy. *Tincture of belladonna* and other anticholinergics help to control cramps.

Psychological Support. Although psychological disturbances are more prevalent in patients with inflammatory bowel disease than in controls, there is little evidence that psychiatric disease is etiologically linked to the development of ulcerative colitis. However, recent data suggest a correlation between stress, immunologic dysfunction, and onset of symptoms. Formal psychotherapy directed at uncovering intrapsychic conflict has not proven useful, but a close, supportive, and empathetic patient–doctor relationship is invaluable to psychologically sustaining the patient through this illness (see below). Fears and worries about debility, surgery, colostomy, and body image contribute markedly to the psychosocial impairment and disability associated with this illness.

Surgery. An important and sometimes difficult issue is determining the necessity and timing of surgery. Indications for *elective surgery* include *high-grade dysplasia, suspected cancer,* and *unresponsiveness* of bowel or systemic symptoms to maximal medical management. For patients whose disease proves refractory to medical therapy, *total colectomy* offers complete cure of bowel disease and remission of most peripheral manifestations. Patients with severe, persistent disease requiring continuous, high-dose corticosteroids that cannot be tapered after 6 to 12 months also warrant serious consideration for surgery, as do those with frequent severe relapses or complications from prolonged exposure to systemic steroids.

Several surgical alternatives are available, although until recently little choice existed. The traditional procedure is *proctocolectomy with Brooke ileostomy.* It has the advantage of being the fastest and safest procedure. The disadvantages of an ileostomy include incontinence, need to frequently empty an external ileostomy appliance, skin excoriations, and potential need for stomal revision (in about 10% to 20%). One of the first alternatives developed was the *total proctocolectomy with continent ileostomy (Koch pouch).* This procedure creates a continent ileostomy that does not require wearing an appliance. It is best suited for proctocolectomy patients who desire control of stomal output.

Park's procedure (total colectomy, rectal mucosectomy, ileal reservoir, and ileoanal anastomosis) represents another surgical option available in centers with the necessary surgical expertise. It is particularly attractive to younger patients with preexisting fecal continence, because it provides the opportunity to retain such continence and avoid a stoma. Although there is likely to be some incontinence initially, this usually passes. About four to eight bowel movements per day are common, helped by chronic use of low-dose antidiarrheal therapy (eg, loperamide). Potential complications include pelvic infection, strictures, small bowel obstruction, and "pouchitis." Although complications occur in up to 30 percent, most patients are pleased with the procedure and its outcomes.

Regardless of the surgical procedure chosen, the morbidity of active disease and the threat of cancer must be weighed against the risks of major surgery. The mortality of elective colectomy is 1 percent to 3 percent, with the majority of patients having no postoperative complications. Stoma revision is necessary in 10 percent to 20 percent of cases.

Screening for Cancer. All patients with clinical or radiologic evidence of *pancolitis* of *7 or more years* should be considered for colon cancer screening. At this point, cancer risk begins to rise substantially. Because the bowel cancer is often multicentric, the best method of screening is *colonoscopy* with multiple biopsies. However, there is some debate about the cost-effectiveness of cancer screening and no agreement on its optimal frequency. Recommendations range from yearly to once every 3 years. Worrisome findings include *stricture* and *dysplasia.* Mild dysplasia is an indication for repeat study in 3 months. Severe dysplasia and stricture formation require consideration of colectomy; the risk of cancer is very high in the presence of such findings.

Crohn's Disease

Most patients can be treated on an outpatient basis by judicious use of medications and careful follow-up. A strong working alliance between the patient and primary physician is essential, because the disease is chronic, relapsing, and incurable.

Diet. Adequate nutrition is critical to the promotion of healing. Sufficient protein and calories must be provided, but in a manner that limits the stress put on an inflamed and often strictured bowel. Patients with cramps and diarrhea should have the *fiber* content of their diet *reduced;* those with steatorrhea will benefit from a *decrease* in *fat* intake to less than 80 g per day. An empiric trial of *restricting milk products* may terminate diarrhea due to lactase deficiency, which often accompanies the illness. More severely ill patients require partial *bowel rest,* which removes the stimulus that food has on bowel motility and secretion. *Elemental diet preparations* (eg, Magnacal, Ensure, Sustacal, Isocal) have been found to induce remission, improve symptoms, and decrease disease activity in patients with acute disease. They are convenient and usually well-tolerated sources of the extra nutrition needed during exacerbations. *Total parenteral nutrition* should be used in patients whose oral intake is not adequate or in whom surgery is indicated.

Vitamin and mineral deficiencies are common and must be corrected for proper healing and avoidance of such complications as anemia and bone disease. *Folic acid* supplementation is particularly important in patients taking sulfasalazine, which impairs its absorption. Patients who have had ileal surgery may need extra *vitamin* B_{12}. *Vitamin D* levels are likely to be low when intake is poor or steatorrhea is a problem. An oral supplement of 4000 IU or more usually suffices. Most vitamin and mineral deficiencies can be overcome by taking a multiple vitamin containing about five times the normal daily vitamin requirements and such minerals as iron, calcium, magnesium, and zinc.

Antidiarrheal Agents. The use of these agents in Crohn's disease is similar to that in ulcerative colitis (see above). The risks include addiction and exacerbation of obstructive symptoms.

Sulfasalazine and other 5-ASA Preparations. The National Cooperative Crohn's Disease Study demonstrated modest efficacy of sulfasalazine in patients with disease of the colon and no benefit in those with disease limited to the small bowel. Doses of 2 to 4 g per day are used to treat acute exacerbations of abdominal pain and diarrhea in patients with colonic involvement. Improvement typically occurs within 4 to 8 weeks. Chronic use of sulfasalazine does not maintain remissions. The drug in combination with corticosteroids is not better than steroids alone and has not been shown to have a steroid-sparing effect or allow more rapid tapering of steroids once a remission has been induced. The new oral 5-ASA preparations (see earlier) are best reserved for patients who do not tolerate sulfasalazine.

Metronidazole, in doses of approximately 10 to 20 mg per kilogram per day (eg, 250 to 500 mg tid) is effective in the treatment of patients with Crohn's ileocolitis or colitis and is a reasonable next step in patients who fail to respond adequately to sulfasalazine or a 5-ASA agent. In addition, uncontrolled studies have demonstrated healing of rectovaginal fistulas, abscesses, and proctocolectomy wounds. It appears that maintenance therapy at a lower dose can minimize recurrence of perineal disease. Patient acceptability is sometimes limited by gastrointestinal upset, metallic taste, and paresthesias.

Glucocorticosteroids. When a patient is acutely ill or has not responded to sulfasalazine, systemic steroids are indicated. Patients with small bowel involvement are especially responsive. *High doses* (eg, the equivalent of 60 mg prednisone per day) should be used initially. Steroids plus sulfasalazine are more effective than sulfasalazine alone in bringing an acute flare-up under control, but, like sulfasalazine, they are ineffective in preventing a relapse. Sulfasalazine has no steroid-sparing effect.

As acute disease activity subsides, the steroid dose is empirically tapered to the minimum necessary to control symptoms. Sometimes, *alternate-day regimens* will suffice to control disease activity; they have the advantage of minimizing the steroid side effects (see Chapter 105). As much as 4 months of steroid therapy may be necessary to treat an exacerbation.

Although steroids occupy a central place in the treatment of Crohn's disease, they are *ineffective for maintaining remissions* or preventing exacerbations. Prophylactic steroids are not indicated in Crohn's disease. Moreover, some extraintestinal manifestations and perianal disease do not respond well to glucocorticoids.

Immunosuppressive Agents. Although the precise pathogenesis of Crohn's disease remains to be defined, there does appear to be a component of immunologic hyperactivity manifested by high levels of selected T-cell populations and high prevalence of antibodies to intestinal epithelial antigens in patients with inflammatory bowel disease and in their asymptomatic relatives. This has led to interest in immunosuppressive treatment. Such therapy is recommended for consideration in all patients requiring chronic steroid therapy. In a major double-blind controlled study, *6-MP* proved effective, achieving or maintaining control and allowing a reduction or discontinuation of steroids in 75 percent of patients. In the same study, 65 percent of patients with fistulas had healing or potential healing while taking 6-MP. Other studies have demonstrated a role for 6-MP and also for *azathioprine* in maintaining remission achieved with other forms of therapy. Treatment is initiated at low doses (50 mg per day), increasing to as much as 1.5 to 2.0 mg per kilogram per day if no response is noted. Treatment is typically continued for about 12 months and then cessation is attempted. Unlike other forms of medical treatment for Crohn's disease, chronic immunosuppressive therapy has been shown to be capable of maintaining remission, especially in patients with fistulas or frequent relapses.

Limitations to immunosuppressive therapy include slow onset of action and potentially serious side effects. Onset of action may take as long as 3 to 6 months in some patients, necessitating a 6-month trial that includes a doubling of the starting dose. In addition, immunosuppressive therapy may induce infection, pancreatitis, bone marrow suppression, or drug-induced hepatitis. Monitoring of blood counts in essential. Despite the potential for such adverse effects, 6-MP and azathioprine have a good safety profile, especially if the dose is 50 mg per day or less. A total dose of 1.5 to 2.0 mg per kilogram per day should not be exceeded. Initiation of immunosuppressive therapy should not done without first consulting a gastroenterologist familiar with use of these agents.

Surgery. Unlike ulcerative colitis, surgery in Crohn's disease does not cure the patient. It is therefore best reserved for patients who have intractable disease, perforation, obstruction, or severe bleeding. It has been estimated that the probability of surgery is 78 percent at 20 years and 90 percent at 30 years from the onset of Crohn's disease symptoms. The objective of surgery is to remove grossly involved bowel and spare as much normal-appearing bowel as possible. Postoperative recurrence rates have been estimated to be 30 percent to 50 percent per decade and are inversely related to preoperative disease duration. The most common operation is removal of a diseased portion of the terminal ileum with an end-to-end ileocolonic anastomosis. For patients with colonic involvement, colectomy with an internal anastomosis connecting the ileum to the sigmoid or total proctocolectomy with Brooke ileostomy is the procedure of choice. Ileostomy is necessary in patients with marked rectosigmoid disease. Twenty percent to 40 percent of ileostomies need revision within 5 years because of disease in the stomal area.

Surgical treatment is undertaken with reluctance and only in the setting of severely disabling disease or serious complications. The patient presenting with obstruction may respond sufficiently to bowel rest, nasogastric suction, steroids, and other conservative measures, avoiding the need for immediate surgery, unless the obstruction persists or recurs quickly. In patients with multiple surgeries and much bowel already resected, stricturoplasty might be considered in lieu of yet another resection of bowel. All attempts should be made to use a conservative surgical approach to preserve functional bowel. Loss of bowel, especially right colon, can lead to disabling postsurgical diarrhea.

Management of the Pregnant or Nursing Patient with Inflammatory Bowel Disease

For patients with a flare-up of inflammatory bowel disease during nursing or pregnancy, both sulfasalazine and steroids are safe and effective. To maintain remission throughout pregnancy in ulcerative colitis, sulfasalazine should be continued in conjunction with folic acid supplementation. Metronidazole and immunosuppressive agents may be injurious to the fetus or nursing child and should be avoided. Women with ulcerative colitis are prone to suffer new attacks or exacerbations during the first trimester of pregnancy and have a spontaneous abortion rate of about 10 percent. Pregnancy seems to inhibit relapses during later trimesters. Women with active ulcerative colitis should be counseled to postpone getting pregnant until they have been in remission for about a year.

PATIENT EDUCATION

The education and support of the patient and the family are essential. Fears abound when patients are told they have ulcerative colitis or Crohn's disease. These diagnoses conjure up images of colostomy, recurrent hospitalizations, invalidism, and social isolation. It is important to emphasize that the vast majority of patients lead fully functional lives and many obtain satisfactory control of their disease through medical therapy.

Because these are chronic diseases that affect young adults, the questions of *conception, pregnancy, and childbearing* will arise. Although there is some familial pattern to the occurrences of the inflammatory bowel diseases, transmission is not purely genetic and there is ample evidence that while the disease is in remission, fertility is essentially normal and healthy full-term infants can be delivered. However, conception might be a problem when the male patient is taking sulfasalazine (see above).

The issue of *cancer risk* in patients with long-standing and extensive ulcerative colitis can be addressed directly and clearly, reassuring those with minimal disease that their risk is no greater than that of the general population. Even those with extensive disease appreciate knowing the magnitude of the risk.

The primary physician can do much to prepare the patient who requires *colectomy* and subsequent *ileostomy*. Thorough patient education combined with a caring approach that includes a willingness to listen to concerns and fears is invaluable and greatly appreciated. Many patients have fears and anxieties that they will not discuss unless they are broached by the physician. Also helpful in preparation for ileostomy is to have an ileostomy patient of the same age and sex discuss the procedure and its consequences with the surgical candidate. Seeing that one can go on to lead a fully active life is comforting. Where available, a local association of ostomates is a valuable resource. Finally, the more widespread use of ileoanal anastomosis in carefully selected patients may increase the acceptability of surgery.

Many patients can be taught to *adjust their medication* within a prearranged set of guidelines and limits. Dosages of sulfasalazine to be used for mild exacerbations can be specified and extra supplies of medication can be provided, allowing the patient to play an active role in his or her care and ensuring prompt treatment of a flare-up. Antidiarrheal agents can also be provided for as-needed use, but only to reliable patients who are not likely to abuse them. Patients should be *instructed to call* if fever develops, diarrhea worsens, bleeding occurs, or abdominal pain becomes marked.

The need for a steady exchange of information with the patient, including careful explanation of procedures and therapies, and the importance of close follow-up and availability cannot be overemphasized. Attentiveness and responsiveness help alleviate much of the fear and worry that accompany inflammatory bowel disease and support the development of an effective therapeutic alliance. Additional information and support is available to the patient from the local chapter of the National Ileitis and Colitis Foundation.

INDICATIONS FOR REFERRAL AND ADMISSION

Referral for gastroenterologic consultation is indicated when full dosages of sulfasalazine in combination with oral corticosteroids (± metronidazole in patients with Crohn's disease) fail to control symptoms. In addition, Crohn's disease patients who require high doses of chronic daily steroid therapy should be referred for consideration of immunosuppressive therapy. Ulcerative colitis patients with disabling, chronic, refractory disease ought to have a surgical consultation. The pancolitis patient with long-standing disease who is at increased risk for cancer needs referral for periodic colonoscopy and biopsy. Patients with extraintestinal disease should undergo an ophthalmologic consultation that includes a slit lamp examination to check for uveitis.

Prompt hospitalization for parenteral management is indicated for patients who are toxic, bleeding heavily, in severe pain, or too sick to obtain adequate nutrition orally. Bowel rest, nasogastric feeding of elemental diets, and parenteral steroids are prescribed, and surgical consultation is obtained, especially if there is severe bleeding, toxicity, distention, or evidence of peritoneal irritation. Home nasoenteric feeding has been demonstrated for carefully selected patients with malabsorption and weight loss refractory to conventional outpatient therapy. Nocturnal tube feedings of a low-fat elemental diet can correct such nutritional problems, but the program requires patients who can insert their own feeding tubes at night.

MANAGEMENT RECOMMENDATIONS

Ulcerative Colitis

General Measures

- Document mucosal inflammation with sigmoidoscopy.
- Reduce dietary fiber during an exacerbation.
- Advise adequate rest and sleep.
- Prescribe a *folic acid* supplement (1 mg per day) when leafy vegetables are restricted or sulfasalazine is being used.
- Add oral *iron* supplementation (300 mg ferrous sulfate tid) when there is considerable rectal bleeding and documented iron-deficiency anemia.
- Schedule visits frequently in the early phases of the illness to provide psychological support and close monitoring. Phone checks are helpful.
- Prescribe a short course of opiate therapy (eg, *loperamide* 2 to 4 mg or codeine 15 mg before meals and at bedtime) for temporary symptomatic control of troublesome diarrhea in patients with mild to moderate disease; avoid prolonged use and use in patients with severe disease (high risk of toxic dilatation).
- If mild diarrhea persists during remissions, initiate a trial of psyllium hydrophilic colloid (1 teaspoon in 8 oz of water once or twice daily); if this is still unsuccessful, try restricting milk products.
- Refer for consideration of periodic colonoscopy and biopsy those patients who have pancolitis lasting more than 8 years.

Mild to Moderate Disease

- Begin *sulfasalazine,* 500 mg qid with meals, and increase the dosage as tolerated over several days to 4 g per day. Continue this dosage for 2 to 4 weeks until symptoms abate, then decrease it to the smallest dosage that maintains control of symptoms (usually 2 g per day, although sometimes 4 g per day are required).
- Substitute a nonsulfa 5-ASA preparation (eg, *olsalazine*, 500 mg bid) in patients who are sulfa-allergic and cannot tolerate sulfasalazine.
- If sulfasalazine or olsalazine fails to achieve control within 3 weeks, add oral *prednisone;* begin with a dose of 40 mg per day. Initially give in divided doses for patients who are having symptoms round-the-clock, but change to a qAM program as soon as possible to limit the degree of adrenal suppression. Continue this dosage for 7 to 10 days.
- If control is achieved, begin tapering prednisone by 5 to 10 mg every 2 weeks to the lowest dosage necessary to suppress disease activity. An alternate-day program (using the same total weekly dose that maintains control) may be tried to minimize chronic steroid therapy side effects (see Chapter 105).
- Once steroids are tapered off and disease activity ceases, decrease sulfasalazine to a maintenance dose of 2 g per day and continue for at least 1 year to maintain remission. If olsalazine is being used, prescribe 1 g per day for maintenance.

Moderate to Severe Disease

- Start with *prednisone,* 60 mg per day in divided doses, and *sulfasalazine* at 4 g per day. Once the symptoms come under control, give the entire prednisone dose in the morning and begin tapering empirically by 5 mg per week. Continue the sulfasalazine at 1 g qid indefinitely.
- If food intake is inadequate over time because of nausea or abdominal pain, consider supplementing the diet with a nutritionally balanced, *low-residue liquid dietary preparation* (eg, Magnacal, Ensure, Sustacal, Isocal).
- Monitor carefully for marked blood loss, volume depletion, severe abdominal pain, distention, and peritoneal signs; any of these is an indication for prompt hospital admission, parenteral therapy, and urgent surgical consultation.
- Refer for consideration of steroid-sparing immunosuppressive therapy (6-MP or azathioprine) patients requiring persistently high doses of steroids.
- Refer for consideration of elective surgery, patients refractory to maximal medical therapy, those requiring daily steroids for prolonged periods (> 6 months), and those found on cancer screening to have a stricture or dysplasia.

Ulcerative Proctocolitis

- If disease is limited to the rectosigmoid, begin treatment with oral sulfasalazine (as noted above) or a topical agent. Enemas of *hydrocortisone* or *5-ASA* are both effective topically. Hydrocortisone can be administered rectally using a 100-mg *retention enema* taken once nightly, a 25-mg *suppository* once or twice daily, or a 90-mg *foam* preparation once or twice daily. Selection of preparation can be based on patient preference and empirical results. Use a 5-ASA enema if there is concern about steroid absorption and systemic side effects. Dose is 2 to 4 g per day for acute symptoms and 1 g per day for maintenance. Continue therapy until symptoms clear; continue sulfasalazine or isoleucine for prophylaxis.

Crohn's Disease

General Measures

- Document the extent of disease by barium studies or colonoscopy. Postpone barium enema and colonoscopy until disease activity subsides.
- Limit the fiber content of the diet in patients with cramps and diarrhea.
- Decrease the fat intake to less than 80 mg per day when there is steatorrhea.
- Conduct a trial of restricting milk products from the diet of patients with diarrhea; if the diarrhea promptly improves, continue with a lactose-restricted diet.
- Supplement the diet with a multivitamin preparation that contains five times the normal daily vitamin requirements plus iron, calcium, magnesium, and zinc.
- Consider short-course opiate therapy (eg, *loperamide* 2–4 g or codeine 15 mg with meals and before bed) for symptomatic relief of diarrhea; use caution, obstruction may be aggravated, and prolonged use can lead to narcotic dependence.
- Advise partial bowel rest and use of elemental, low-residue dietary preparations when cramps and diarrhea are severe.
- Admit for refractory disease, severe bleeding, toxicity, abdominal pain, abscess formation, or evidence of obstruction. Such patients need surgical consultation.

Colonic Disease

- Begin *sulfasalazine* (500 mg qid) and quickly increase the dosage to 1 g qid over several days; continue for 4 to 8 weeks. Use *olsalazine* (500 mg bid) for the sulfa-allergic patient. If there is a response, continue for 4 to 6 months and then stop if symptoms have ceased. Maintenance therapy does not prevent recurrences.
- If there is no response to sulfasalazine or olsalazine, *switch to metronidazole* in doses of 10 to 20 mg per kilogram per day (eg, 250 to 500 mg tid) and continue for a 4-week trial. If there is a satisfactory response, continue for 4 to 6 months, then stop if symptoms have ceased.
- If there is inadequate response to metronidazole, switch to *prednisone* 60 mg per day; qid dosages may be required at the outset for round-the-clock control.
- As disease activity subsides, give the entire dosage in the morning and begin tapering it to the lowest dosage that controls the symptoms (often as little as 5 mg per day). Continue this dosage until all evidence of disease activity ceases (as long as 4 months); an alternate-day schedule may suffice.
- For refractory disease or patients requiring chronic steroid therapy, refer for consideration of immunosuppressive therapy with 6-MP or *azathioprine* (both 50 mg per day).

Perianal Disease

- Prescribe *metronidazole* (750 to 2000 mg per day) for refractory perianal disease; a prolonged course of treatment may be necessary.

Ileal Disease

- The effectiveness of sulfasalazine for ileal disease is not well-established, although some patients with mild disease may benefit. Olsalazine (500 mg bid) may provide better results and is worth a 4- to 6-week trial. (There are no data on metronidazole in ileal disease.)
- If there is no response to olsalazine or if ileal symptoms are severe, then prescribe *prednisone* (60 mg per day) and use in the same fashion as for colonic involvement (see above).
- Consider use of *6-MP* or *azathioprine* (50 mg per day) for patients with fistulas, refractory symptoms, or persistent requirements for very high steroid dosages. A 6-month trial is often necessary. Treatment is continued for 12 months, and then cessation is attempted, although long-term therapy is sometimes necessary and successful in maintaining remission. Because immunosuppressive therapy can cause marrow suppression and carcinogenesis, gastroenterologic consultation is essential if it is to be used.

ANNOTATED BIBLIOGRAPHY

Bernstein LH, Frank MS, Brandt LJ, et al. Healing of perineal Crohn's disease with metronidazole. Gastroenterology 1980; 79:375. *(Documents the drug's usefulness in therapy of chronic perianal abscesses and fistulas.)*

Block GE. Surgical management of Crohn's colitis. N Engl J Med 1980;302:1068. *(Terse and useful review of available surgical approaches, including discussion of criteria for patient selection.)*

Camilleri M, Proano M. Advances in the assessment of disease activity in inflammatory bowel disease. Mayo Clin Proc 1989;64:800. *(Good review of a difficult issue.)*

Collins RH, Jr, Feldman M, Fordtran JS. Colon cancer, dysplasia, and surveillance in patients with ulcerative colitis. N Engl J Med 1987;316:1654. *(Provocative paper critical of routine surveillance in patients with ulcerative colitis.)*

Disanayake AS, Truelove SC. A controlled therapeutic trial of long-term maintenance treatment of ulcerative colitis with sulfasalazine. Gut 1973;14:923. *(Documents efficacy of sulfasalazine for prophylaxis; recurrence rate one-fourth that of the control group.)*

Donaldson RM. Management of medical problems in pregnancy: Inflammatory bowel disease. N Engl J Med 1985;312:1616. *(Practical approach to this important management issue.)*

Drossman DA. Psychosocial aspects of inflammatory bowel disease. Stress Med 1986;2:119. *(Good review of psychological and psychosocial dimensions.)*

Dworken HJ. Ulcerative colitis. A clearer picture. Ann Intern Med 1983;99:717. *(Reviews data on prognosis derived from community-based studies and argues for a more optimistic view of the illness.)*

Ekbom A, Helmick C, Zack H, et al. Ulcerative colitis and colorectal cancer: A population-based study. N Engl J Med 1990;323;1228. *(Best available data for estimation of risk for colorectal cancer.)*

Farmer RG, Whelan G, Fazio VW. Long-term follow up of patients with Crohn's disease. Gastroenterology 1985;88:818. *(Relationship between clinical pattern and prognosis.)*

Fiocchi C, Roche JK, Michener WM. High prevalence of antibodies to intestinal epithelial antigen in patients with inflammatory bowel disease and their relatives. Ann Intern Med 1989;110:786. *(Evidence suggesting that immune sensitization is a primary phenomenon.)*

Garrett, JW, Drossman DA. Health status in inflammatory bowel disease; review of biologic and behavioral considerations. Gastroenterology 1990;99:90. *(Outcomes appear to be a function of both disease and quality of life factors.)*

Gendry JP, Mary JY, Florent C, et al. Oral mesolamine (Pentasa) as maintenance treatment in Crohn's disease. A multi-center placebo-controlled study. Gastroenterology 1993;104:435. *(Relapse rate significantly reduced.)*

Glotzer DJ, et al. Comparative features and course of ulcerative and granulomatous colitis. N Engl J Med 1970;282:582. *(Classic review comparing and contrasting the two conditions.)*

Heymsfield SB, Smith-Andrews JL, Hersh T. Home nasoenteric feeding for malabsorption and weight loss refractory to conventional therapy. Ann Intern Med 1983;98:168. *(Interesting approach that allows properly selected patients with severe disease to remain at home.)*

Klotz UK, Maier K, Fischer C, et al. Therapeutic efficacy of sulfasalazine and its metabolites in patients with ulcerative colitis and Crohn's disease. N Engl J Med 1980;303:1499. *(Establishes that 5-aminosalicylate is the active moiety of sulfasalazine.)*

National Cooperative Crohn's Disease Study. Gastroenterology 1979;77:825. *(Multicenter prospective controlled trial demonstrating efficacy of sulfasalazine in acute disease of the colon. No improvement observed in patients with disease confined to the small bowel.)*

Orlein BA, Telander RL, et al. The surgical management of children with ulcerative colitis: The old vs new. Dis Colon and Rectum 1990;33:947. *(Reports the Mayo Clinic experience, including use of the newer approaches.)*

Peppercorn MA. Advances in drug therapy for inflammatory bowel disease. Ann Intern Med 1990;112;50. *(Especially useful is the discussion of the 5-ASA drugs, but also covers other aspects of medical therapy.)*

Peppercorn MA. Sulfasalazine: Pharmacology, clinical use, toxicity and related new drug development. Ann Intern Med 1984;101:377. *(All you ever wanted to know; 140 references.)*

Present DH, Korelitz BI, Wisch N, et al. Treatment of Crohn's disease with 6-mercaptopurine. N Engl J Med 1980;302:981. *(Long-term randomized double-blind study showing that 6-MP is effective in the management of refractory Crohn's disease. The accompanying editorial by Sleisenger puts the study's results into context.)*

Present DH, Meltzer SJ, et al. 6-mercaptopurine in the management of inflammatory bowel disease: short- and long-term toxicity. Ann Intern Med 1989;111:641. *(Reports an 18-year experience.)*

Rijk MC, van Hogezand RA, van Lier HJ, et al. Sulfasalazine and prednisone compared with sulfasalazine for treating active Crohn disease. Ann Intern Med 1991;114:445. *(Double-blind, randomized, multicenter trial showing that prednisone helped only in speeding initial improvement.)*

Robertson DAF, Ray J, Diamond I, et al. Personality profile and affective states of patients with inflammatory bowel disease. Gut 1989;30:623. *(Personality disturbances were frequent and correlated with duration of disease; many reported stress preceding onset of symptoms.)*

Singleton JW. Corticosteroids for Crohn's disease. Ann Intern Med 1979;90:983. *(Excellent editorial; argues for selective use.)*

Ursing B, Almy T, et al. A comparative study of metronidazole and sulfasalazine for active Crohn's disease. A Cooperative Crohn's Disease Study in Sweden. II. Results. Gastroenterology 1982;83:550. *(Metronidazole produced results comparable to those of sulfasalazine; moreover, the drug worked in some patients who failed to respond to sulfasalazine.)*

Whelan G, Farmer RG, Fazio VW. Recurrence after surgery in Crohn's disease, relationship to location and disease. Clinical pattern and surgical indication. Gastroenterology 1985;88: 1826. *(Six hundred and fifteen patients followed by the Cleveland Clinic from 1966 to the present show a high index of recurrence after operation.)*

Primary Care Medicine: Office Evaluation and Management of the Adult Patient, 3rd edition, edited by Allan H. Goroll, Lawrence A. May, and Albert G. Mulley, Jr. J.B. Lippincott Company, Philadelphia

74
Approach to the Patient With Functional Gastrointestinal Disease

Functional gastrointestinal (GI) disease accounts for a large proportion of the GI complaints seen in office practice, not only in the primary care setting but also in the referral practices of gastroenterologists. The international working group consensus definition of functional GI disease is "a variable combination of chronic or recurrent GI symptoms not explained by structural or biochemical abnormalities. They include symptoms attributed to the pharynx, esophagus, stomach, biliary tree, small and large intestine or anorectum." Included under the rubric of functional GI disease are two common, often troubling syndromes: *irritable bowel syndrome (IBS)* and *nonulcer dyspepsia*. The former is associated with large bowel discomfort or pain, disturbed defecation, and distention, often predominated by constipation, diarrhea, or gaseousness. The latter is characterized by upper abdominal discomfort, bloating, and nausea, which may or may not be related to meals. Another increasingly appreciated functional malady is *irritable esophagus* (sometimes referred to as esophageal spasm (see Chapter 61). In many cases of functional disease, there is a strong interplay between biopsychosocial factors and gut physiology.

The primary care physician needs to become expert in the recognition and management of these conditions, not only because they can mimic more serious disease (triggering unnecessary testing and worry), but also because they are the source of much functional impairment and substantial health care expenditures.

IRRITABLE BOWEL SYNDROME

Irritable bowel syndrome (IBS) is a functional disturbance of intestinal motility and visceral perception, strongly influenced by emotional factors. It accounts for about half of GI complaints seen by physicians. Epidemiologic studies suggest that nearly 20 percent of adults suffer from some form of the condition, although only a fraction actually seek medical attention. "Spastic bowel," "mucous colitis," and "spastic colitis" are less accurate terms sometimes used to connote the syndrome. When mistaken for organic disease, it can result in unnecessary testing or frustrating attempts at therapy. Careful diagnosis and a comprehensive approach to management (including a strong patient–doctor relationship) are essential to optimizing patient outcomes.

Pathophysiology and Clinical Presentation

The emerging pathophysiologic view of IBS is one of functional disturbances in motor activity and visceral perception, triggered or exacerbated by psychological distress and luminal irritants. *Abnormal motor function* is one of the hallmarks of this syndrome, capable of producing both *diarrhea* and *constipation*. Both may occur in alternating fashion or one may predominate. Nonpropulsive colonic contractions and slow-wave myoelectric patterns at two to three cycles per minute constitute about 40 percent of electrical and contractile activity at rest in patients with IBS, compared with 10 percent in normals. When excessive, these contractions may impede propulsion of stool, prolong transit time, and cause constipation. Diarrhea occurs when the increase in contractility is localized to the small bowel and proximal colon. A pressure gradient develops, causing accelerated movement of intestinal contents. Meals normally cause an increase in colonic contractions, but controlled study has shown that patients with irritable colon syndrome have a significantly exaggerated increase in motor response to food. Patients with diarrhea-predominant disease have more jejunal, fast, and high-amplitude contractions postprandially than do normal individuals, resulting in reduced colonic transit time.

Abnormalities in motor function may help explain the constipation and diarrhea, but do not adequately account for the *abdominal pain* and *anorectal discomfort* experienced. Recent balloon manometry studies of IBS patients demonstrate *excessive sensitivity* to balloon distention in the ileum, rectosigmoid, and anorectum. In patients with a predominance of diarrhea, there are reduced thresholds for initiation of reflex motor activity and discomfort; urgency is precipitated at abnormally small volumes of balloon distention. In patients with constipation, the threshold for reflex motor activity is abnormally high, and emptying is delayed. Fecal material collects and hardens, and the bowel becomes distended. Pain ensues.

The combination of abnormal motor and sensory functioning has the potential to cause the patient much discomfort. For example, increased sensitivity can trigger excessive reflex motor activity, leading to a cycle of anorectal discomfort or pain before a bowel movement, a sense of incomplete evacuation after one, and increased frequency of movements. There are also data suggesting that IBS patients experience alterations in flow of visceral sensory afferent data and abnormalities in its central processing, perhaps as a result of learned behavior or underlying psychopathology.

Situational stress has long been considered an important contributing factor. Hypermotility in response to stress has been documented in both normal persons and patients with IBS, but the latter show a significantly higher frequency of life stress.

In addition, a high prevalence of *psychopathology* has been uncovered in IBS patients presenting for care. Somatization, personality disturbances, anxiety, and depression are among the conditions frequently identified. Although it is well-recognized that psychological stress may alter bowel function, careful study of IBS reveals psychopathology to be more a *predictor of illness behavior* than a direct cause of the bowel disease. Psychiatric symptoms and poor coping skills usually predate bowel complaints. Disturbances in bowel function can be especially troubling to patients with preexisting psychopathology and more likely to precipitate medical encounters than might similar symptoms in otherwise well-adjusted persons. This finding has been invoked to explain why only a fraction of patients with IBS ever present for medical care. Patients with IBS who do not consult physicians have been found to be psychologically similar to controls.

What seems to characterize the patient persistently bothered by symptoms is the greater prevalence of serious situational stresses, psychopathology, and perhaps learned visceral responses to bowel discomfort and threatening situations. Such factors may modify the underlying pathophysiology and illness behavior, determining severity of symptoms, frequency of episodes, and thresholds for seeking and continuing with medical care.

Recently, a greater appreciation has emerged for *intraluminal factors* that might alter bowel motor function and cause it to behave in "irritable" fashion. These include selective *malabsorption* of certain sugars, such as *lactose* (the common dairy product sugar), fructose (the common citrus fruit sugar), and *sorbitol* (often found in "sugar-free" candy). Sorbitol is a common sweetener in candies and chewing gum and is capable of causing bloating and diarrhea if taken in large amounts, as are milk products in patients with lactose-intolerance. One study suggests that *food allergies* may play a role in some patients. *Bile acid* malabsorption has been detected in up to 10 percent of patients with diarrhea-predominant IBS. The resulting large quantities of fatty acids descending on the colon can trigger painful, rapid contractions leading to marked discomfort and diarrhea.

Clinical presentation is illustrated by a series of 50 patients treated in an outpatient unit. Most of the patients (62%) experienced onset of symptoms before age 40; 50 percent were under 30 at time of onset; and one quarter were under 20. *Chronicity* was the rule, with little change in symptoms over time, except for waxing and waning. Duration was in years. *Abdominal pain* was present in 90 percent, *mucous* stools in 36 percent, *pellet-like stools* in 38 percent, *diarrhea* alone in 10 percent, *excessive flatus* in 36 percent. Fifty percent considered their symptoms related to stress; 34 percent denied this; 66 percent manifested symptoms of anxiety or depression. The abdominal pain was most often in the left lower quadrant or lower abdomen (62%), but in 28 percent there were multiple sites of pain. Upper abdominal involvement occurred in 38 percent. The pain was typically achy rather than crampy, often relieved by a bowel movement or passage of flatus. It was unusual for the pain to awaken the patient. Radiation was variable, and even extended into the left chest and arm when gas was trapped in the splenic flexure.

Small, hard, infrequent stools and an empty rectal ampulla characterize the constipation. Prolonged retention of stool allows for full absorption of intestinal water content. The diarrhea is typically small in volume, associated with visible amounts of mucus, and may follow a hard movement by a few hours. There may be urgency. Dyspepsia and excessive gaseousness are also reported (see earlier). Weight loss is rare; symptoms usually parallel situational stresses. Rectal bleeding is absent unless there is coincident hemorrhoidal disease.

Clinical Course

IBS is a chronic, relapsing condition with no evidence of significant morbidity or mortality. A prospective British study providing follow-up at 2-month intervals over 3 years found that severity waxed and waned, but the constellation of symptoms remained remarkably constant. At 1 year, 50 percent were unchanged, 36 percent improved, 12 percent were symptom-free, and 20 percent were worse. The symptom-free period was usually less than a few months. One-third of employed patients lost time from work. There was no correlation between time lost and number of visits to the doctor; 40 percent made five or fewer visits, and 46 percent made none at all. At 2 years, a similar pattern was found. Only one patient remained symptom-free from the first year.

Studies on clinical course identified groups of patients with different prognoses. The group with symptoms triggered by a major life stress enjoyed long symptom-free periods after the acute problem abated, whereas those with continuous intestinal complaints in response to daily living rarely became asymptomatic.

Diagnosis and Initial Evaluation

Clinical criteria for diagnosis of IBS were specified by Manning and colleagues in the late 1970s. Although not derived quantitatively (eg, by multiple regression analysis), these symptom-based criteria have been largely validated and are widely used for suggesting the diagnosis of IBS. They include:

- Continuous or recurrent symptoms over several months of abdominal pain or discomfort relieved with defecation or associated with a change in frequency or consistency of stool and/or
- An irregular or varying pattern of disturbed defecation at least 25 percent of the time, consisting of two or more of the following: altered frequency; altered consistency; straining, urgency, or feeling of incomplete evacuation; passage with mucus; bloating or feeling of distention.

Although the sensitivity and specificity of the Manning criteria have, for the most part, been confirmed, there are some questions regarding the discriminant value of individual items. Moreover, some clinical situations require ruling out organic pathology that might resemble and be mistaken for IBS (see below). A combination of detailed history taking and careful physical examination, combined with selective, parsimonious testing and a few diagnostic trials of therapeutic measures will usually provide the best combination of completeness and cost-efficacy.

Because many IBS patients harbor fears of serious underlying disease, they commonly pressure physicians into ordering a plethora of diagnostic studies. Such cost-ineffective testing can be minimized by 1) conducting a detailed history and careful physical examination that specifically elicits and addresses patient concerns; 2) concluding the initial visit with a thorough review of key findings and their meaning (see below); and 3) using the clinical presentation to determine the need for any further diagnostic testing. Usually, the diagnosis of IBS can be made exclusively on clinical grounds. Prospective studies with up to 6 years of follow-up have shown only a 0 percent to 3 percent rate of missed diagnoses of organic disease in patients clinically labeled as having IBS.

When constipation predominates, it may be necessary to rule out a malignancy, particularly in patients over the age of 40 who have weight loss or a family history of colon cancer. In such patients, one needs to consider *flexible sigmoidoscopy with or without barium enema* or *colonoscopy* (see Chapter 65). In most others, a *stool test for occult blood* and a complete *blood count* (for microcytic anemia) should suffice. The absence of evidence for GI blood loss helps exclude organic disease. A clinical trial of *increased dietary fiber, stool softeners* (dioctyl sodium sulfosuccinate), or an *osmotic laxative* (psyllium) complements the diagnostic assessment. Patients taking diuretics should have a serum *potassium* checked, because hypokalemia may reduce bowel contractility and produce an ileus.

When diarrhea predominates, *dietary review* is essential for clues of intolerance to lactose or sorbitol. A check of the *blood sugar* is needed to rule out diabetes mellitus (which may present as diarrhea due to diabetic gastroenteropathy; see Chapter 102), as is a check of the *stool for ova and parasites*. A diagnostic trial of eliminating sorbitol-containing candies and restricting lactose-containing milk products (yogurts containing live cultures are relatively lactose-free) helps rule out contributions from intraluminal factors. A *lactose-hydrogen breath test* is an alternative means of testing for lactose intolerance. A trial of the bile acid-binding resin *cholestyramine* serves as a simple test for bile acid malabsorption. Should diarrhea persist undiagnosed, a *sigmoidoscopy with or without mucosal biopsy* might be reasonable to exclude inflammatory bowel disease and collagenous and lymphocytic forms of colitis (see Chapter 64).

Abdominal pain and bloating necessitate ruling out obstruction. During an episode of pain, a timely *plain film of the abdomen* should suffice. Such bloating and discomfort may also occur with lactose, fructose, or sorbitol intolerance, which can be tested for as detailed above.

Psychological Assessment. Because the prevalence of underlying psychopathology is very high in patients with IBS, definitive therapy often requires identifying and addressing the patient's psychological difficulties. In the context of conducting a thorough work-up, the clinician needs to sensitively elicit details of the patient's life situation, aspirations, accomplishments, frustrations, and losses. Concerns, fears, expectations, and responses to previous life stresses can also be very informative, as can the mental status of the patient on examination. *Anxiety* disorders are commonly identified (see Chapter 226), but *depression* (see Chapter 227) and *somatization* (see Chapter 230) often go unrecognized.

Principles of Management

Establishing a strong patient–doctor relationship, treating important underlying psychopathology, modifying diet, and supplementing these efforts with judicious use of medication constitute the basic approach to management of the patient with IBS. No single modality has proven successful in randomized, placebo-controlled studies. However, a strong patient–doctor relationship helps to minimize requests for repeated diagnostic evaluations and dependence on drugs for provision of symptomatic relief.

Establishing a Strong Patient–Doctor Relationship. The first rule in the care of IBS patients is to *take their symptoms seriously* and not dismiss them as inconsequential. Such an approach communicates a sense of caring and is essential to the formation of an effective patient–physician relationship, the *sine qua non* of IBS management. As noted earlier, it begins with a careful history and physical examination that addresses potentially serious etiologies, especially those of concern to the patient (eg, cancer, inflammatory bowel disease). One cannot overemphasize the therapeutic importance of such an initial evaluation.

Once IBS has been identified (usually by the end of the initial or second office visit), the physician needs to *review the diagnosis* with the patient. Anxious, emotionally troubled patients, such as those who present with IBS, often believe there is something seriously awry and will not accept a simplistic "there's nothing wrong with your bowels." They appreciate knowing the basis for their diagnosis and how more worrisome conditions were ruled out. In this way, the patient does not leave frustrated, feeling the "doctor cannot find what is wrong."

The establishment of a supportive *doctor–patient relationship* in conjunction with providing reassurance, explanation, and advice can have an important impact on outcome. When such care was given to patients in the prospective British study cited earlier, most reported feeling better, less concerned about their bowels, and more able to cope with their symptoms and the stresses of daily life. Although there were frequent relapses, these seemed to be less important when they occurred in the context of close medical support. The failure of many physicians to provide adequate support is suggested by the 20 percent rate of self-referral to alternative medicine practitioners noted in patients with IBS.

Management of Underlying Psychopathology. A distinguishing characteristic of patients who present to physicians with IBS is their high probability of underlying psychopathology. Often this is manifested by an exaggerated emotional response to bowel symptoms. Sometimes, the best intervention is withdrawing all previously prescribed medications and simply listening empathically to the patient's problems, helping him cope with his life situation.

When specific underlying psychopathology is identified, treatment should be directed toward it. Success rates are high in such circumstances. In a study of 67 patients with IBS, 56 were felt to suffer from *depression* and received a *tricyclic* agent. More than 50 percent become symptom-free, 33 percent improved, and 20 percent showed no benefit. Both *amitriptyline* and *desipramine* in low doses (50 to 100 mg qhs) have been found to be particularly effective in depressed IBS patients with diarrhea, due in part to their anticholinergic activity reducing bowel hyperactivity (see below). In patients with constipation, a tricyclic with strong anticholinergic effects may actually worsen symptoms. An antidepressant with minimal anticholinergic activity might be a better choice (eg, *fluoxetine*).

Many IBS patients suffer from *chronic anxiety,* but one must be careful not to prescribe anxiolytics chronically, because of their strong potential for inducing addiction and causing withdrawal syndromes (see Chapter 226). An *antidepressant with anxiolytic properties* may be a reasonable substitute (eg, *doxepin, nortriptyline,* or *trazodone;* see Chapter 227).

Treatment of patients with *somatization disorders* first requires withdrawing the vast array of medications prescribed by the multitude of physicians they have visited over the years, and then setting up regularly scheduled visits for them to talk about their symptoms and personal problems. Such supportive therapy by the primary physician often suffices to alleviate much of their complaining and need for medication (see Chapter 230).

When bowel symptoms are not due to a well-defined psychiatric illness, use of psychotropic agents is less effective and not recommended. Casual use of benzodiazepine/antispasmodic combinations should be avoided. A double-blind controlled study of 52 patients manifesting nonspecific anxiety showed that *diazepam* had no effect on bowel complaints compared with placebo.

Behavioral methods are worth considering in highly motivated patients. The emphasis is on changing behavior, rather than on gaining insight. They provide a sense of control and enhance health-promoting behaviors. *Relaxation techniques* help those with exaggerated sympathetic responses to stress. Patients are taught how to blunt such responses and relax skeletal muscles. *Biofeedback* is used predominantly for treatment of fecal incontinence, aiming for improved control over internal sphincter activity. The method is expensive, but promising. *Hypnosis* has been used successfully to reduce pain perception.

Psychotherapy represents an important treatment option for patients who seek to deal with their illness through better understanding. To be successful, the therapy has to be viewed as personally relevant. The goal is learning to understand and cope with psychosocial stresses. Controlled study has found psychotherapy plus medication to be superior to medication alone in reducing bowel symptoms. Methods range from traditional insight-focused therapy to cognitive-behavioral approaches, where the emphasis is on identifying stressors and thoughts that precipitate symptoms.

A *multifaceted approach* appears to be the best strategy. In a study of combined therapy that included medication, psychotherapy, and relaxation techniques, results were best when the treatment program used a combination of approaches. Predictors of a good response included presence of overt anxiety or depression, short duration of bowel symptoms, and absence of constant or diffuse pain.

Dietary Measures. Although a major part of the therapeutic effort in IBS involves redirecting the patient's attention away from his or her bowels, it is often necessary to provide patients with symptomatic relief before they are willing to turn their attention to the factors precipitating their symptoms. Dietary manipulations are sometimes helpful in this regard.

Foods that might exacerbate IBS should be avoided, including caffeinated beverages, alcohol, sorbitol-containing candies and gums, citrus fruits in those with fructose intolerance, and milk products in those who prove lactose intolerant. Reducing intake of such poorly digestible carbohydrates as beans and cabbage may help patients suffering from bloating, gas, and abdominal pain.

Many IBS patients insist they have *"food allergies"* as the cause of their symptoms. Although recent study suggests an increased incidence of food allergies in IBS, true food allergies are rare and typically cause acute hypersensitivity reactions, not chronic GI complaints. No changes in colonic motor activity have been found to occur in such patients on intake of the offending food. However, food intolerances (as noted above) are often noted in patients with IBS, and it may be worthwhile trying to avoid foods that seem poorly tolerated. Some food intolerances are mislabeled as IBS. For example, patients with gluten intolerance (adult celiac disease, nontropical sprue) may present with abdominal discomfort and diarrhea. Persistent diarrhea, bloating, cramping, and excessive flatus may be manifestations of underlying lactose intolerance. A 1- to 2-week trial of restricting a suspected offending food or substance is reasonable when clinical suspicion is high. On the other hand, patients who present having already restricted an unnecessarily large number of foods can have them added back. Rechallenging them with the purported offending agent rebuilds their confidence and avoids nutritional deficiency.

Increasing dietary fiber can help restore propulsive colonic motor activity. However, clinical studies examining bran and high-fiber diets have produced variable results, often no better than control diets due, in part, to a large placebo effect. In a double-blind trial of 50 patients eating a standardized bran biscuit or placebo, both groups reported subjective improvement in more than 50 percent of the subjects. A more recent controlled, but unblinded British study of 26 patients showed significant improvement in symptoms and colonic motor activity in the bran-fed group compared with controls. Certainly there is no harm in prescribing a high-fiber diet, and it may have other health benefits such as reducing the risk of colon cancer (see Chapter 76). However, some patients report worsening of bloating and gaseousness with initiation of a high-fiber diet due to bacterial metabolism of nondigestible fiber, although this subsides with time. It is best to start with the equivalent of about 1 tablespoon of bran daily and build up to 3 tablespoons per day as tolerated.

An alternative is to use *bulking agents,* such as the hydrophilic colloid *psyllium* (Metamucil). A total daily dose of 15 to 25 g per day is necessary to achieve benefit and most helpful in IBS patients bothered predominantly by constipation. *Low-residue diets* have been tried. There is no evidence that they are of any use.

Drug Therapy should proceed only in the context of a balanced program that includes patient education and support. Precipitously or prematurely resorting to pharmacologic measures in a hasty attempt to suppress symptoms completely can lead to frustration and excessive, even dangerous, escalations of drug intake. In fact, at the outset of therapy, it is often useful to *stop all nonessential medicines* that may affect bowel function, especially irritant laxatives. Nevertheless, there is a role for carefully selected, short-term applications of medication when some symptomatic relief is deemed necessary.

Diarrhea. Patients suffering from disabling diarrhea may benefit from use of an opiate derivative. Transit time is prolonged, water and ion absorption is enhanced, and anal sphincter tone is strengthened. These effects result in less diarrhea, rectal urgency, and fecal soiling. *Loperamide* (in doses of 2 to 4 mg qid) is the preferred opiate derivative, being less habit-forming and less likely to exert CNS effects than other derivatives, such as *tincture of opium* or *diphenoxylate.* Patients with diarrhea due to bile acid malabsorption experience improvement with *cholestyramine.* As noted earlier, those with an underlying depression may benefit from use of a tricyclic antidepressant with anticholinergic activity (eg, *amitriptyline* 50 to 100 mg per day).

Constipation. No drugs have been proven safe and effective for use in IBS patients suffering from constipation. The prokinetic agent *cisapride* is under investigation and may soon be available. It facilitates acetylcholine release from the myenteric plexus. Although transiently helpful in patients with constipation, the drug appears best for dyspeptic symptoms. *Metoclopramide* does not act on the lower bowel and is not recommended for use in IBS. Drugs with anticholinergic activity should be avoided, because they are likely to worsen constipation. As noted above, if antidepressants are needed, it is best to select a preparation without anticholinergic activity (eg, trazodone, fluoxetine).

Abdominal Pain and Distention. Patients suffering from postprandial pain and distention often request symptomatic relief. *Anticholinergic agents* have been used in such circumstances. The rationale is to reduce the cholinergic stimulation of colonic activity that occurs in response to a meal. The anticholinergic *dicyclomine* (10 to 20 mg before a meal) is the preparation most often recommended in this context. Although such agents have been shown to inhibit the postprandial increase in nonpropulsive colonic contractions, their clinical effectiveness is unproven. However, the consensus is that they are worth a try in cases in which nonpharmacologic measures have failed. They are best prescribed for short-term use. Chronic use should be avoided, because of the risk of worsening constipation and pain. *Combination preparations* containing a tranquilizer (eg, a benzodiazepine or a barbiturate) and an anticholinergic are promoted as *"bowel relaxants"* or *"antispasmodics."* They are heavily advertised, yet of no proven benefit and best avoided because of their habituation potential and poor efficacy. Whether the newer anxiolytics, which are nonsedating and free of habituation potential (eg, *buspirone* 15 to 30 mg per day), will prove beneficial remains to be proven. Studies are ongoing on the use of opioids, enkephalins, and other agents that have potential for blocking or modulating gut pain receptors.

Patient Education

Because IBS is a condition characterized by an exaggerated response to symptoms, patient education is central to effective management. As noted earlier, the basic elements of the patient education effort include addressing patient fears, providing a specific diagnosis, and explaining the pathophysiologic basis of symptoms. In patients with symptoms triggered by psychosocial stress, an explanation (perhaps aided by diagrams) of how such stress can lead to functional alterations in bowel motility helps patients to better understand their condition and cope with it.

When important situational stress or psychopathology is uncovered, it needs to be discussed openly so that the patient can begin to focus on the underlying issues rather than on bowel symptoms. Sometimes, having the patient keep a diary of symptoms, stresses, and feelings can help reveal connections that have otherwise eluded the patient. The major lesson to be mastered by patients with IBS is the relationship between their psychological state and symptoms, a message that often takes patience, sensitivity, and skill to communicate effectively. It is important not to push discussion and treatment of psychological issues beyond what the patient is prepared to accept. Patients initially unwilling to consider such issues should be respected, but once a supportive relationship is established, they often begin to cope better and spend less time obsessing about their bowels and more on the underlying issues triggering their "dis-ease."

Patients not psychologically minded can still be helped greatly by changing the focus of their care from cure of symptoms to improvement in functional status. At each office visit, instead of asking for an in-depth recitation of bowel complaints, the physician spends more time inquiring into how the patient is dealing with the demands of daily life and helping the patient to cope with them. The visit agenda shifts from eliminating symptoms to solving problems. Such a shift is often remarkably refreshing and revealing; it helps improve functional capacity and reduces the intensity of bodily complaints.

Indications for Referral and Admission

This is a condition in which a continuous relationship is essential, and any perceived need for referral should be acted on only after thorough discussion with the patient. In general, referral is helpful when there are refractory disabling symptoms, such as uncontrollable diarrhea, or when serious psychopathology is encountered. Less disturbed patients may also benefit from psychiatric referral, but only if the patient is accepting of a psychological dimension to the illness and is motivated to delve into it. A hospital admission may, in rare circumstances, be appropriate and very beneficial in helping the patient to learn new means of coping with stress and providing a respite from an intolerable living situation.

Management Recommendations

- Take the patient's bowel complaints seriously; do not minimize their importance or deny their "reality."
- Elicit a full psychosocial database as well as a complete history of the patient's bodily symptoms.
- Conduct a thorough work-up that includes a detailed investigation of all possible etiologies, both organic and psychological.
- Provide a thorough explanation of the diagnosis and directly address the patient's concerns and fears.
- Establish a supportive relationship and begin supportive psychotherapy for patients with underlying situational or psychosocial stresses.
- Identify, discuss, and treat specifically any underlying depression (see Chapter 227), anxiety disorder (see Chapter 226), somatization (see Chapter 230), or other psychiatric condition.
- When treating a depressed patient with antidepressant medication, consider its degree of anticholinergic activity and match it appropriately to bowel symptoms (eg, amitriptyline 50 to 100 mg qhs is helpful for the patient with diarrhea; fluoxetine 20 mg per day is a better choice in the IBS patient bothered by constipation; see Chapter 227).
- Stop all nonessential medicines that may affect bowel function, especially irritant laxatives.
- For the patient bothered predominantly by constipation, increase dietary fiber and recommend regular exercise. Add a bulking agent such as psyllium (Metamucil), 1 rounded teaspoon in 8 oz of water, tid, if constipation is still troublesome. A stool softener (eg, dioctyl sodium sulfosuccinate is sometimes helpful.
- If the patient finds abdominal pain and distention intolerable, resort to a trial of anticholinergic therapy (eg, dicyclomine 20 mg qid), but only if other measures have failed. It may also be useful for diarrhea. Use only for a short period of time. Tricyclic antidepressants with anticholinergic activity may also be worth a trial (eg, amitriptyline 50 to 100 mg qhs), but avoid these if constipation is bothersome.
- For the patient with diarrhea, evaluate first for underlying bowel pathology (parasitic disease, colitis, and so forth; see Chapter 64), then limit intake of potentially contributing substances such as caffeine, sorbitol-containing candies and chewing gums, alcohol, and dairy products (except for yogurt preparations). When short-term symptomatic relief is essential, prescribe a 2- to 5-day supply of loperamide, 1 tablet bid prn. Exercise caution with opiate use because of its addiction potential in this chronic condition.
- For patients with refractory diarrhea, consider a diagnostic trial of cholestyramine (4 g tid or qid), which will counter any concurrent bile acid malabsorption.
- Major dietary restrictions are usually unnecessary. However, if there is a strongly suggestive history of intolerance to a food or substance, consider a 1- or 2-week trial of omitting its intake. Sorbitol and lactose are the most common offenders.
- Despite the presence of chronic anxiety, avoid use of sedatives, tranquilizers, and combination preparations containing benzodiazepines or barbiturates. The risks of habituation and withdrawal outweigh any benefit. Antidepressants with anxiolytic activity (eg, amitriptyline, trazodone, doxepin) are reasonable alternatives, as might be the nonaddicting azapirone anxiolytics (eg, buspirone).
- Help redirect the patient's attention away from bowel symptoms and endless searches for cure and toward better coping with daily stresses; focus on accomplishments rather than symptoms, on taking control through exercise, good eating habits, and behavioral changes rather than on repeated recitation of symptoms.
- For motivated patients with well identified psychosocial stressors, consider referral for a combination of behavioral techniques and psychotherapy.
- See patient at regular intervals and be available for help at times of increased stress.

NONULCER DYSPEPSIA

Nonulcer dyspepsia is a poorly defined condition characterized by intermittent upper abdominal pain or nausea, which frequently, but not exclusively occurs with meals. The term *dyspepsia* literally means "bad digestion," although it is not meant to be synonymous with or inclusive of other symptoms of "indigestion" (such as heartburn, eructation, or regurgitation). Rather, the emphasis is on the abdominal pain, which resembles the discomfort of peptic ulcer disease; thus the phrase "nonulcer." Older terms for this condition also alluded to its ulcer-negative status, including "x-ray-negative dyspepsia" and "functional dyspepsia."

Nonulcer dyspepsia is twice as prevalent as ulcer-related dyspeptic disease and one of several GI conditions that can cause upper abdominal pain in the absence of an ulcer (see Chapter 58). Billions of dollars are spent annually on its evaluation and treatment, yet remarkably little is known about its pathogenesis. However, new data are emerging, and the primary care physician needs to understand the relative importance of diet, smoking, acid secretion, gastric motility, stress, and *Helicobacter* infection to fashion a rational and cost-effective treatment plan.

Pathophysiology, Clinical Presentation, and Course

The pathophysiology of nonulcer dyspepsia remains largely unknown. The most consistent abnormality is *disordered upper GI motility.* Gastric emptying is delayed, and gas transit is slowed. Distention and bloating are common and thought to be manifestations of this slowing. The efficacy of metoclopramide in relieving dyspeptic symptoms probably derives from its blocking of dopaminergic receptors, which inhibit upper GI motility and gastric emptying.

Although excess acid production may play some role in nonulcer dyspepsia (eg, in patients with duodenitis), it does not appear to be the predominant pathogenic factor. Patients and controls show little difference in *gastric acid secretion*. H_2-blocker therapy and antacids are little better than placebo in providing relief, although all three modalities achieve improvement in about 50 percent of cases.

Considerable interest has arisen in the importance of *Helicobacter* infection, because gastric inflammation is present in about half of cases and *H. pylori* has been implicated as a cause of gastritis and some forms of peptic ulcer disease (see Chapter 68). However, its contribution to dyspepsia remains controversial. For example, a recent British study of gastritis patients with and without dyspepsia revealed very high prevalences of *H. pylori* infection in both subgroups, but no consistently significant increase among those with dyspepsia. On the other hand, a careful American investigation found *H. pylori* to be more common in dyspeptic patients than in controls. More data are needed, especially on the long-term effects of eradicating *H. pylori* infection.

A number of other potential precipitants have been examined. *Stress responses* appear slightly altered, but no particular psychosocial factors have been identified. *Smoking, alcohol, coffee,* and *tea* were not found to have any relation to nonulcer dyspepsia. Although *fatty food intolerance* is a common complaint in dyspeptic patients, controlled studies using disguised meals fail to confirm fatty foods as precipitants. *Nonsteroidal antiinflammatory drugs (NSAIDs)* and *aspirin* are well-recognized gastric irritants, but in case-controlled studies no relation was found between their use and nonulcer dyspepsia.

Clinical presentation includes recurrent upper abdominal pain and nausea. In about half of instances, symptoms are associated with meals. Bloating and gaseous distention may accompany the pain. Reflux, biliary colic, painful or altered defecation, and chronic pain are not considered part of its presentation, but rather features of other forms of nonulcer upper abdominal pain.

Clinical course is benign, with little evidence that the condition ultimately leads to peptic ulceration or other forms of upper GI pathology. Previously, nonulcer dyspepsia was seen as part of a continuum that progressed to duodenitis and frank peptic ulceration, but this suspicion has not been confirmed (although there may be a small subset of patients for whom it might be true). Typically, the condition is chronic. Although it may wax and wane, it usually does not worsen substantially.

Workup

The diagnosis of nonulcer dyspepsia can usually be made on clinical grounds, but it may be necessary to rule out other important forms of upper abdominal pain. The differential diagnosis includes peptic ulcer disease, gastric cancer, esophageal reflux, biliary tract disease, chronic pancreatitis, and IBS. Upper GI endoscopy can readily identify and distinguish among many of these conditions—particularly peptic ulcer and gastric cancer—but the high frequency and harmlessness of nonulcer dyspepsia and the high cost of endoscopy make it wasteful to investigate everyone.

Endoscopy. Selectivity is necessary for cost-effective workup. If everyone were studied endoscopically at the time of initial presentation, the yield would be extremely low and the testing would be wasteful, because most will have nonulcer dyspepsia and a normal study. The major concerns are missing a gastric cancer or a bleeding peptic ulcer. Most authorities recommend a workup strategy based on risk stratification. Patients judged to be at low risk for gastric cancer or complicated ulcer disease are assigned to a 6- to 8-week course of *empiric antiulcer therapy* (H_2-blockers, antacids, or sucralfate plus cessation of NSAIDs, aspirin, smoking, alcohol, and caffeine). Patients deemed at higher risk are designated as reasonable candidates for immediate endoscopic study. Criteria suggested for designation of increased risk include age over 50, unexplained weight loss, protracted symptoms, persistent nausea and vomiting, dysphagia, jaundice, abdominal mass, and evidence of GI blood loss. Low-risk criteria include age under 40, recent onset of dyspeptic symptoms, and absence of weight loss, persistent vomiting, anemia, and stool blood test positivity. Subsequent endoscopic investigation of low-risk patients is reserved for those who fail to show some improvement after 7 to 10 days of full antiulcer therapy, those who do not clear after 6 to 8 weeks of empiric treatment, and those who quickly relapse when treatment is stopped.

Controversy persists as to whether H_2-blockers or antacids are the preferred initial empiric therapy. Some argue against use of H_2-blockers because of their ability to heal malignant gastric ulcers and mask symptoms; the same objections pertain as regards peptic ulceration, although the consequences are much less serious. Needed are prospective, controlled studies addressing the issue, although empiric antacid therapy has been shown in prospective study to be both safe and effective as a diagnostic strategy in low-risk patients. Its drawback is poor compliance, which may compromise results.

Other Studies. The clinical presentation can also determine the need for other investigations. Patients with heartburn are likely to have gastroesophageal reflux and may require *barium swallow* or *esophagoscopy* if the presentation is worrisome, although in most instances empiric therapy suffices (see Chapter 61). Patients reporting paroxysmal attacks of constant epigastric or right upper quadrant pain lasting a few hours and radiating into the back require consideration of biliary tract disease and the need for *abdominal ultrasound* and *liver function testing* (see Chapter 69). Unrelenting upper abdominal pain radiating into the back, especially if alcohol-related, suggests chronic pancreatitis. Serum *amylase* and abdominal ultrasound are indicated (see Chapter 72). Altered bowel habits in conjunction with upper abdominal pain argue for IBS involving the transverse colon; colitis and bowel cancer may need to be ruled out by *colonoscopy* or *barium enema* (see above).

Principles of Management

Given the poor understanding of the pathophysiology of nonulcer dyspepsia, it should not be surprising that there is little consensus on how best to treat the condition. Antacids, H_2-blockers, sucralfate, metoclopramide, dietary manipulations, and eradication of *H. pylori* infection have all been suggested, although the number of well-designed studies remains small.

Antiulcer Therapies. H_2-blockers, antacids, omeprazole, and sucralfate have all been tried. Contrary to common belief, there is little evidence that acid-inhibiting or acid-neutralizing treatment significantly improves symptoms in patients with nonulcer dyspepsia. Much of the confusion about the efficacy of such antiulcer therapy seems to result from a substantial placebo effect, the heterogeneous nature of patients with dyspepsia, and poor characterization of patients in many studies. Randomized, controlled trials have failed to demonstrate consistent benefit from use of antiulcer therapy in patients with carefully documented nonulcer dyspepsia. This correlates with data showing little excess acid production in most of these patients.

Nonetheless, antiulcer treatments are still widely prescribed for nonulcer dyspepsia, and many clinicians can cite anecdotal reports of improvement. Of interest, a recent set of randomized single-subject studies of dyspeptic patients showed that a brief 3-day course of cimetidine brought prompt relief, even to those with nonulcer dyspepsia. More and better data should be forthcoming. In the meantime, physicians are likely to continue prescribing antiulcer therapy empirically because there is little else to offer patients. If such therapy is to be offered, it should be given for a limited time and not continued if symptoms fail to resolve.

Enhancing Gastric Motility. If indeed nonulcer dyspepsia is a disease of altered upper GI motility, then drugs that facilitate such motility would be expected to be beneficial. *Metoclopramide* is the first of the dopaminergic blocking agents available for stimulating gastric motility. Short-term use has been helpful. Unfortunately, long-term administration of the drug is associated with risk of tardive dyskinesia, making it inappropriate for prolonged use. *Cisapride* is the first of another class of prokinetic agents that release acetylcholine at the myenteric plexus and stimulate upper GI motility. It appears better tolerated than metoclopramide, but data on its efficacy and long-term safety are still pending.

Eradication of *Helicobacter* infection has been advocated, based on the strong association between the organism and the occurrence of gastritis. However, at this time, the connection to nonulcer dyspepsia remains more tenuous, and eradication of the organism cannot yet be recommended until more data are available proving its efficacy.

Diet, Alcohol, Smoking, and Stress. There are no data indicating that a low-fat diet, restriction of alcohol, cessation of smoking, or reduction of stress have any effect on nonulcer dyspepsia. To be sure, these factors play important roles in other causes of upper abdominal pain and discomfort, but their elimination in nonulcer dyspepsia appears to be of little consequence.

Patient Education and Indications for Referral

Patients who present with recurrent upper abdominal pain are fearful of cancer and other serious forms of GI pathology. For many, the first priority is knowing that they do not have a life-threatening illness. As with any disorder that can mimic more worrisome illness, the patient's concerns should be taken seriously and addressed directly (see the Reassurance section on IBS above; the same principles and approach apply here).

Referral to a gastroenterologist is indicated when endoscopy is being considered. The most appropriate candidates are those at increased risk of gastric malignancy (see above). At times, a consultation with the gastroenterologist will help reassure the low-risk but overly concerned patient, although the need for such referrals can be kept to a minimum by thorough patient education and support.

A.H.G.

ANNOTATED BIBLIOGRAPHY

Irritable Bowel Syndrome

Almy T. Experimental studies on the irritable colon. Am J Med 1951;10:60. *(Classic paper on relation of stress to bowel activity.)*

Camilleri M, Prather CM. The irritable bowel syndrome: Mechanisms and a practical approach to management. Ann Intern Med 1992;116:1001. *(Best review of pathophysiology and a very useful mechanistic approach to treatment; 78 references.)*

Cann PA, Read NW, Holdsworth CD. What is the benefit of coarse wheat bran in patients with irritable bowel syndrome. Gut 1984;25:168. *(Bran did help pain, constipation, diarrhea, and urgency, as did placebo, except for constipation, which responded better with bran.)*

Cann PA, Read NW, Holdsworth CD, et al. Role of loperamide and placebo in management of irritable bowel syndrome. Dig Dis Sci 1984;29:239. *(Proved superior to placebo in patients with diarrhea, urgency, and incontinence.)*

Deutsch E. Relief of anxiety and related emotions in patients with gastrointestinal disorders. Am J Dig Dis 1971;16:1091. *(Diazepam relieved anxiety but did not improve bowel symptoms any better than did placebo.)*

Drossman DA, McKee DC, Sandler RS, et al. Psychosocial factors in the irritable bowel syndrome. A multivariate study of patients and nonpatients with irritable bowel syndrome. Gastroenterology 1988;95:701. *(Underlying psychopathology is a major predictor of becoming a patient.)*

Drossman DA, Thompson WG. The irritable bowel syndrome: Review and a graduated multicomponent treatment approach. Ann Intern Med 1992;116:1009. *(An outstanding review and the best on psychosocial factors and their management; 117 references.)*

Esler M, Goulston K. Levels of anxiety in colonic disorders. N Engl J Med 1973;288:16. *(Patients with predominant diarrhea were significantly more anxious and more neurotic by psychometric testing than normal persons or those with constipation and pain.)*

Greenbaum, Mayle JE, Vanegeren LE, et al. Effects of desipramine on irritable bowel syndrome compared with atropine and placebo. Dig Dis Sci 1987;32:257. *(The antidepressant was best in patients with diarrhea.)*

Guthrie E, Creed F, Dawson D, et al. A controlled trial of psychological treatment for the irritable bowel syndrome. Gastroenterology 1991;100:450. *(Best data on efficacy and patient selection.)*

Hislop I. Psychological significance of the irritable colon syndrome. Gut 1971;12:452. *(Fifty-six of 67 patients with irritable colon syndrome were treated with tricyclic antidepressants. More than 80 percent reported significant improvement.)*

Jones AV, McLaughlan P, Shorthouse M, et al. Food intolerance: A major factor in the pathogenesis of the irritable bowel syndrome. Lancet 1982;2:115. *(Evidence for intolerances to wheat, corn, dairy products, coffee, tea, and citrus fruits.)*

Klein KB. Controlled treatment trials in the irritable bowel syndrome: A critique. Gastroenterology 1988;95:232. *(Important paper on methodologic shortcomings of most studies; essential reading before reviewing the literature.)*

Kruis W, Thieme C, Weinzierl M, et al. A diagnostic score for the irritable bowel syndrome, its value in the exclusion of organic disease. Gastroenterology 1984;87:1. *(Elaborate regression study providing a weighted score with high specificity and sensitivity; blood in the stool rules out the diagnosis.)*

Longstreth GF, Fox DD, Youkeles MS, et al. Psyllium therapy in the irritable bowel syndrome. Ann Intern Med 1981;95:53. *(Randomized double-blind, controlled study; both treatment and controlled groups improved significantly, suggesting strong psychological overlay of symptoms and efficacy of supportive measures.)*

Manning AP, Thompson WG, Heaton KW, et al. Towards positive diagnosis of the irritable bowel syndrome. Br Med J 1978; 2:653. *(Most widely accepted criteria for diagnosis.)*

Merrick MV, Eastwood MA, Ford MJ. Is bile acid malabsorption underdiagnosed? An evaluation of accuracy of diagnosis by measurement of SeHCAT retention. Br Med J 1985;290:665. *(Diagnosis and the role for bile acid malabsorption.)*

Nanda R, James R, Smith H, et al. Food intolerance and the irritable bowel syndrome. Gut 1989;30:1099. *(Best available evidence for the role of food intolerances.)*

Newcomer AD, McGill DB. Clinical importance of lactose deficiency. N Engl J Med 1984;310:42. *(Editorial summarizing the data on lactose deficiency in clinical syndromes, including its role in IBS.)*

Prior A, Colgan SM, Whorwell PJ. Changes in rectal sensitivity after hypnotherapy in patients with irritable bowel syndrome. Gut 1990;31:896. *(Pain threshold raised, suggesting a mechanism and role for hypnotherapy in IBS.)*

Rumessen JJ, Gudmand-Hoyer E. Functional bowel disease: Malabsorption and abdominal distress after ingestion of fructose, sorbitol, and fructose-sorbitol mixtures. Gastroenterology 1988;95:694. *(Evidence for their role in some cases of IBS.)*

Schwarz SP, Taylor AE, Scharff L, et al. Behaviorally treated irritable bowel syndrome patients: A four-year follow-up. Behav Res Ther 1990;28:331. *(Lasting response demonstrated.)*

Smart HL, Mayberry JF, Atkinson M. Alternative medicine consultations and remedies in patients with irritable bowel syndrome. Gut 1986;27:826. *(Up to 20 percent make use of alternative treatment; suggests needs are not being met by their physicians.)*

Smith RC, Greenbaum DS, Vancouver JB, et al. Psychosocial factors are associated with health care seeking rather than diagnosis in irritable bowel syndrome. Gastroenterology 1990;98: 293. *(The title says it all.)*

Sullivan M, Cohen S, Snape W. Colonic myoelectric activity in irritable bowel syndrome. N Engl J Med 1978;298:878. *(Patients with IBS and abnormally prolonged increase in postprandial motor activity, which was reduced by an anticholinergic agent.)*

Svendsen JH, Munck LK, Andersen JR. Irritable bowel syndrome—prognosis and diagnostic safety. Scand J Gastroenterol 1985;20:415. *(Disease waxes and wanes; only rarely [0 to 3 percent of cases] is there a missed diagnosis of organic disease, even after 5 years of follow-up.)*

Talley NJ, Thieme C, Weinzierl M, et al. Diagnostic value of the Manning criteria in irritable bowel syndrome. Gut 1990;31:77. *(Best critique of these diagnostic criteria.)*

Treacher DF, et al. Irritable bowel syndrome: Is barium enema necessary? Clin Radiol 1986;37:87. *(Retrospective analysis of 114 patients; barium enema rarely revealed useful information in patients who had normal hematologic and biochemical screening, especially in those under age 50.)*

Van Outryve M, Milo R, Toussant J, et al. Prokinetic treatment of constipation-predominant irritable bowel syndrome: A placebo controlled study of cisapride. J Clin Gastroenterol 1991;13:49. *(Benefit demonstrated.)*

Waller S, Misiewicz J. Prognosis in the irritable bowel syndrome. Lancet 2:754, 1969 *(Symptoms wax and wane with little permanent resolution, but supportive therapy helps patients to cope.)*

Whitehead WE, Holtkotter B, Enck P, et al. Tolerance for rectosigmoid distention in irritable bowel syndrome. Gastroenterology 1990;98:1187. *(Sensation thresholds are altered.)*

Young S, Alper D, Norland C, et al. Psychiatric illness and the irritable bowel syndrome. Gastroenterology 1970;70:162. *(Seventy-two percent of patients with IBS in a general group practice have an underlying psychiatric illness; only 28 percent were properly recognized and diagnosed.)*

Zwetchkenbaum JF, Burakoff R. Food allergy and the irritable bowel syndrome. Am J Gastroenterol 1988;83:901. *(Disputes the role of food allergy; see also Nanda, above.)*

Nonulcer Dyspepsia

Bernersen B, Johnsen R, Bostad L, et al. Is *Helicobacter pylori* the cause of dyspepsia? Br Med J 1992;304:1276. *(Only small differences in* H. pylori *prevalences were found among those with and without dyspepsia.)*

Goodson JD, Lehman JW, Richter JM, et al. Is upper gastrointestinal radiography necessary in the initial management of uncomplicated dyspepsia? J Gen Intern Med 1989;4:367. *(Randomized controlled trial showing that low-risk patients randomized to an empiric course of antacids did just as well as those assigned to traditional radiologic study.)*

Health and Public Policy Committee, American College of Physicians. Endoscopy in the evaluation of dyspepsia. Ann Intern Med 1986;102:266. *(Recommends a 6- to 8-week course of empiric antiulcer therapy in low-risk patients before considering endoscopic evaluation.)*

Johannessen T, Petersen H, Kristensen P, et al. Cimetidine for symptomatic relief of dyspepsia. Scand J Gastroenterol 1992; 27:189. *(Evidence for benefit with H_2-blocker therapy.)*

Johnson AF. Controlled trial of metoclopramide in the treatment of flatulent dyspepsia. Br Med J 1971;2:25. *(Nausea and pain were relieved.)*

Nyren O, Adami HO, Bates S, et al. Absence of therapeutic benefit from antacids or cimetidine in non-ulcer dyspepsia. N Engl J Med 1986;314:339. *(Evidence against benefit from antiulcer therapy.)*

Rosch W. Cisapride in non-ulcer dyspepsia. Results of a placebo-controlled trial. Scand J Gastroenterol 1987;22:161. *(Promising results with this prokinetic agent.)*

Strauss RM, Wang TC, Kelsey PB. Association of *Helicobacter pylori* infection with dyspeptic symptoms in patients undergoing gastroduodenoscopy. Am J Med 1990;89:464. *(Prevalence of infection was greater in those with dyspepsia.)*

Talley NJ, McNeil D, Piper DW. Environmental factors and chronic unexplained dyspepsia: Association with acetaminophen but not other analgesics, alcohol, coffee, tea, or smoking. Dig Dis Sci 1989;33. *(Surprising, but well-documented findings.)*

Talley NJ, Phillips SF. Non-ulcer dyspepsia: Potential causes and pathophysiology. Ann Intern Med 1988;108:865. *(Exhaustive, but useful review with excellent discussions of disease mechanisms, possible precipitants, and workup, all with practical implications; 268 references.)*

Zell SC, Budhraja M. An approach to dyspepsia in the ambulatory care setting: Evaluation based on risk stratification. J Gen Intern Med 1989;4:144. *(Argues for a diagnostic approach that assigns low-risk patients to empiric antiulcer treatment rather than endoscopic study.)*

75
Management of Diverticular Disease

Primary Care Medicine: Office Evaluation and Management of the Adult Patient, 3rd edition, edited by Allan H. Goroll, Lawrence A. May, and Albert G. Mulley, Jr. J.B. Lippincott Company, Philadelphia

Diverticula, abnormal herniations of colonic mucosa through the muscularis, are extremely common and increase with age. Autopsy studies estimate their presence in 20 percent of people over 40 and in 70 percent of those over 70. About 15 percent of people with the condition develop attacks of *diverticulitis*, in which the diverticula become plugged and inflamed. It is possible that the recent emphasis on increasing the fiber content of the diet will reduce the incidences of diverticula and their complications in Western countries. The primary physician encounters many elderly patients with gastrointestinal (GI) complaints referable to diverticular disease. The physician must effectively and economically recognize and treat mild manifestations of disease, reduce the chances of complications, and decide when admission and surgical intervention are necessary.

PATHOPHYSIOLOGY, CLINICAL PRESENTATION, AND COMPLICATIONS

Pathophysiology. Increased intracolonic pressure causes herniation of colonic mucosa. Consequently, diverticula occur most frequently in the sigmoid where the colon is narrowest and pressure is highest. Diverticula show a predilection for points of relative weakness in the muscularis, especially where branches of the marginal artery penetrate the colonic wall. Current research indicates that the *low fiber content* of modern diets has a causal role, producing less bulky stool and increased intracolonic pressure. Conditions associated with abnormal colonic activity and segmentation, such as irritable colon syndrome, may contribute to the pathogenesis of diverticula; this remains speculative. The possibility of muscular degeneration has been suggested but remains unproven.

The diverticular sac can become inflamed when undigested food residues and bacteria get trapped in the thin-walled sac; blood supply is mechanically compromised and bacterial invasion ensues. Microperforations can occur, producing peridiverticular and pericolonic inflammation.

Clinical Presentation and Course. *Diverticulosis* is usually asymptomatic and often discovered incidentally on barium enema. However, colonic motor activity is sometimes disturbed, and intermittent left lower quadrant pain may result. Constipation is common, as is constipation alternating with diarrhea, and occasionally there is tenderness.

Diverticulitis is characterized by left lower quadrant pain, tenderness, fever, and leukocytosis in a patient with known diverticulosis. Frequently a tender mass is noted. The diagnosis is made clinically during an acute attack and confirmed later by barium enema, once the risk of perforation subsides. At times, the radiologic findings resemble those of cancer or Crohn's disease, and colonoscopy is needed for more definitive evaluation. In rare instances, there are extraintestinal manifestations (arthritis, pyoderma gangrenosum), which may simulate those of Crohn's disease and lead to misdiagnosis.

The major *complications* of diverticular disease are perforation, obstruction, and bleeding. *Perforations* may lead to abscess formation. The abscesses may spontaneously drain into the bowel or erode into an adjacent organ, such as the ureter, bladder, or vagina, forming fistulas. Perforations that fail to become walled off may cause peritonitis. Those that enter the vagina result in vaginal gas or feces; those that erode into the urinary tract lead to dysuria or pneumaturia. Chronic inflammation can thicken the bowel wall and cause *obstruction*. Erosion into a blood vessel may result in brisk rectal *hemorrhage*. Diverticular disease is one of the most common causes of lower GI hemorrhage and a leading consideration in patients who present with brisk rectal bleeding (see Chapter 63). In a 15-year study from the Lahey Clinic, the incidence of hemorrhage, obstruction, or perforation from diverticular disease was 15 percent.

DIAGNOSIS

As noted earlier, diverticulosis is usually an incidental finding in a patient undergoing a barium enema or colonoscopy for another reason. However, the diagnosis should also be considered in a patient presenting with relatively painless but brisk rectal bleeding. If the bleeding is not too severe, proctosigmoidoscopy can be performed to confirm the diagnosis and site of blood loss.

The diagnosis of acute diverticulitis should be suspected in an older patient who presents with new onset of left lower quadrant abdominal pain, low-grade fever, focal tenderness with or without guarding, and an elevated white blood cell count. In rare instances, the pain may be suprapubic or localized to the right lower quadrant if there is a redundant sigmoid or a right-sided diverticulum. Nausea, vomiting, and diarrhea or constipation may accompany the bowel complaints and simulate gastroenteritis. Absence of bowel sounds suggests peritoneal inflammation.

In situations of diagnostic uncertainty, confirmatory testing can be obtained. *Proctosigmoidoscopy* performed with a flexible sigmoidoscope can be done comfortably, safely, and with a minimum of bowel preparation when it is essential to rule out other causes of serious colonic pathology, such as inflammatory bowel disease and cancer. Inability to pass the flexible sigmoidoscope beyond the rectosigmoid junction due to acute bowel inflammation is strongly suggestive of acute diverticulitis. *Barium enema* will identify diverticulitis; contrast outside the bowel lumen is an important diagnostic feature. Some clinicians are reluctant to order a barium enema during the acute phase of illness, because of concern that performance of the enema might increase intraluminal pressure and cause bowel perforation. Although this concern is disputed, many postpone barium study until inflammation quiets down. The diagnostic accuracy of barium study has been questioned by some investigators, especially its ability to differentiate between diverticular disease and malignancy. They prefer endoscopic study. *CT scan* is an excellent, but expensive alternative to barium enema. It is especially useful for patients too sick to undergo invasive study, and also helpful for identifying abscesses and fistulas.

PRINCIPLES OF MANAGEMENT

Diverticulosis. The goals of therapy are prevention of symptoms, relief of pain, and avoidance of complications. Because diverticular disease is felt to be, in part, a manifestation of a low-fiber diet, *bran* has been tried in therapy. Prospective British studies of bran use have shown reversal of abnormal bowel physiology and reduction in symptoms in over 90 percent of cases. The average amount of bran needed to achieve an effect is 15 g per day. Some individuals are bothered by flatulence and bloating during the first 2 to 3 weeks of bran use, but this usually resolves as bran with continued bran intake.

Patients unable to tolerate bran may be treated with bulk agents such as *psyllium* (Metamucil). Irritant laxatives should be avoided. The efficacy of *anticholinergics* is controversial; painful spasm may be lessened, but the risk of constipation is increased, raising the likelihood of inspissation of fecal material. Indigestible materials (eg, seeds) that may block the mouth of a diverticulum should be omitted from the diet.

Diverticulitis can be treated at home when symptoms are mild and there is no evidence of peritonitis. The aim of therapy is to markedly reduce bowel activity to lessen the chance of perforation. *Rest* and clear *liquids* usually suffice. Strong analgesics and antipyretics should not be prescribed because they may mask signs of worsening inflammation. Broad-spectrum oral *antibiotics* such as amoxicillin or cephalexin are customarily used, especially when fever exceeds 101°F, although their efficacy is unproven.

An important decision in the therapy of diverticulitis is whether to treat the patient medically or opt for elective *surgical resection* of the involved bowel after initial resolution of symptoms. Proponents of surgical therapy argue that the frequency of complications warrants prophylactic operation once a patient experiences an attack of diverticulitis. The courses of 132 patients at Yale–New Haven Hospital with documented uncomplicated diverticulitis were analyzed. Of the 99 treated medically and 33 treated surgically, the rates of recurrence were almost identical. Moreover, three-quarters of the patients never had more than one attack. The increased length of hospitalization and postoperative morbidity were not balanced by a marked reduction in rate of recurrence or complications. However, the presence of abscess, perforation, or obstruction is an indication for surgery. Although controlled data are lacking, most authorities recommend treatment with a high-fiber diet after acute symptoms have ceased.

INDICATIONS FOR ADMISSION AND REFERRAL

The development of a temperature greater than 101°F, persistence of pain for more than 3 days, and increasing pain indicate need for admission. A markedly elevated white blood cell count may be the only clue to a deteriorating situation; many patients with diverticulitis are elderly and may not demonstrate much fever, abdominal pain, or peritoneal signs. The management of a patient with bleeding, abscess, or perforation requires surgical consultation; operative intervention may be urgent.

THERAPEUTIC RECOMMENDATIONS AND PATIENT EDUCATION

Diverticulosis. For the patient with known diverticula and occasional pain or constipation, the following recommendations should be observed:

- Increase the fiber content of the diet. The best sources are bran, root vegetables (particularly raw carrots), and fruits with skin. Bulk laxatives such as psyllium hydrophilic mucilloid (Metamucil) can be used in patients who cannot tolerate bran, but these are relatively expensive.
- Inform patients that any bloating or flatulence due to bran intake usually resolves with continued use.
- Advise patients to avoid foods with seeds or indigestible material that may block the neck of a diverticulum, such as nuts, corn, popcorn, cucumbers, tomatoes, figs, strawberries, and caraway seeds.
- Have patients avoid laxatives, enemas, and opiates because they are potent constipating agents.
- Anticholinergics are worth considering in patients with recurrent cramping pain, but they may increase constipation and the risk of inspissation of fecal material.
- Instruct patients to report fever, tenderness, or bleeding without delay.

Diverticulitis. For patients with mild diverticulitis (temperature less than 101°F, white cell count below 13,000 to 15,000), the following recommendations should be observed:

- Prescribe bedrest and a clear liquid diet.
- Use mild nonopiate analgesics for pain.
- Monitor temperature, pain, abdominal examination for

signs of peritonitis, and white blood cell count for elevation.

- Consider a broad-spectrum antibiotic (eg, amoxicillin 500 mg tid) if the patient is slow to improve.
- Arrange for prompt hospitalization if temperature goes above 101°F, pain worsens markedly, peritoneal signs develop, or white cell count continues to rise.

A.H.G.

ANNOTATED BIBLIOGRAPHY

Almy T, Howell DA. Diverticular disease of the colon. N Engl J Med 1980;302:324. *(Authoritative review; 119 references.)*

Boles R, Jordan S. Clinical significance of diverticulosis. Gastroenterology 1958;35:579. *(Classic natural history study; mean duration of follow-up 15 years. Frequency of hemorrhage, obstruction, or perforation was 15 percent.)*

Boulos PB, Karamanolis DG, Salmon PR, et al. Is colonoscopy necessary in diverticular disease? Lancet 1984;1:95. *(Authors argue that air-contrast barium enemas yield inaccurate results in one-third of cases; colonoscopy detected neoplasms in 31 percent of patients with diverticulosis.)*

Horner JL. Natural history of diverticulosis of the colon. Am J Dig Dis 1958;3:343. *(Study of 503 patients followed in the ambulatory setting for a mean of 8 years; incidence of diverticulitis was 15 percent.)*

Klein S, Mayer L, Present DH, et al. Extraintestinal manifestations in patients with diverticulitis. Ann Intern Med 1988;108: 700. *(Report of three cases of pyoderma gangrenosum and arthritis in patients with carefully documented diverticulitis.)*

Larson D, Masters S, Spiro H. Medical and surgical therapy in diverticular disease. Gastroenterology 1976;71:734. *(Patients followed for a mean of 9.8 years; no difference in outcome, and in about 75 percent of instances, no further problems occurred among those in either group.)*

Morris J, Stellato TA, Haaga JR, et al. The utility of computer tomography in colonic diverticulitis. Ann Surg 1986;204:128. *(Especially useful for patients too ill to undergo invasive study.)*

Nicholas GG, Miller WT, Fitts WT, et al. Diagnosis of diverticulitis of the colon: Role of barium enema in defining pericolic inflammation. Ann Surg 1972;176:205. *(Argues that the risk of the study is small, even in the setting of acute inflammation.)*

Painter N, Almeida A, Colebourne K. Unprocessed bran in treatment of diverticular disease of the colon. Br Med J 1972;2:137. *(Seventy patients treated with bran in a prospective but uncontrolled study. More than 90 percent showed marked improvement in symptoms.)*

Taylor I, Duthie H. Bran tablets and diverticular disease. Br Med J 1976;2:988. *(Cross-over trial of bran tablets, high roughage diet, and a bulk agent plus an antispasmodic; each improved bowel function, but bran was the most effective in relieving symptoms and normalizing colonic motor activity.)*

76
Management of Gastrointestinal Cancers

Primary Care Medicine: Office Evaluation and Management of the Adult Patient, 3rd edition, edited by Allan H. Goroll, Lawrence A. May, and Albert G. Mulley, Jr. J.B. Lippincott Company, Philadelphia

Recent developments in combining chemotherapy and radiation therapy with surgery for treatment of gastrointestinal cancer have added substantially to palliation and potential for cure, although mortality is still high (50% to 80%). Moreover, improvements in management of the gastrointestinal complications of cancer, such as obstruction, ascites, and cachexia, have improved the quality of life for these patients (see Chapter 91).

Gastrointestinal malignancies are among the most common tumors found in adults. The treatment of local disease is the province of the surgeon, but management of advanced disease is a responsibility coordinated by the primary physician in close conjunction with one's oncologic colleagues. It is important for the primary physician to know the indications, limitations, efficacy, and side effects of available treatment modalities to help counsel the cancer patient and make best use of therapies offered by the surgeon, radiation therapist, and oncologist.

ESOPHAGEAL CANCER

Carcinoma of the esophagus is difficult to diagnose and treat because symptoms usually do not occur until late in the course of illness. Although the tumor begins as a superficial mucosal lesion, it tends to spread silently under the mucosa and extend readily into the mediastinum, because the esophagus has no serosal surface barrier. As a result, by the time diagnosis is made, palliation is typically the only therapeutic option. Of the 9000 new cases of esophageal cancer diagnosed annually, less than 5 percent survive 5 years. Risk factors include *smoking* and *alcohol consumption,* and the malignancy may occur in conjunction with other tumors commonly associated with smoking, such as those of the lung, bladder, head, and neck.

Clinical Presentation and Diagnosis. Most tumors of the upper two thirds of the esophagus are of the squamous cell variety. Those of the lower third tend to be adenocarcinoma. Adenocarcinoma may appear in a *Barrett's esophagus,* a consequence of prolonged severe acid reflux disease (see Chapter 61). Typically, symptoms at time of presentation include *dysphagia* and progressive *inanition,* manifestations of late disease. Dysphagia indicates a markedly narrowed esophageal lumen and a substantial tumor burden. Tumor may extend regionally into the trachea as well as vertically up and down the esophageal mucosa and submucosa. Distant metastases occur in the liver and intraabdominal node-bearing areas. At the time of diagnosis, less than one-third of patients have cancer confined to the esophageal wall, the stage in which cure is possible with surgical resection.

Early symptoms may go unnoticed because they can be nonspecific (eg, a mild burning discomfort associated with swallowing, sometimes referred to as *odynophagia*). Barrett's esophagus is an important premalignant condition, with a significant potential for malignant degeneration. Reported prevalence of adenocarcinoma in a Barrett's esophagus ranges from 10 percent to 60 percent at time of initial evaluation, but incidence is less than 0.6 percent per year in follow-up.

Early diagnosis is among the best means of improving outcome and requires a high index of suspicion. New onset of odynophagia in a heavy smoker or drinker should trigger consideration of *endoscopy*, as should a chronic history of severe reflux disease, with its increased chances of a Barrett's esophagus and associated cancer risk. Although the presence of small nodules, minor erosions, thickened folds, or mucosal depressions is suggestive of early cancer, *mucosal biopsy* is required for definitive diagnosis. There is debate about the best means of managing the patient with a Barrett's esophagus. Some recommend annual endoscopic surveillance without biopsy. Others urge less frequent endoscopy (no more than every 2 to 3 years) but in conjunction with mucosal biopsy. The cost-effectiveness of these alternative approaches remains to be defined. Patients found to have dysplasia require more frequent tissue sampling. The development of persistent high-grade dysplasia is a worrisome finding. One promising low-cost alternative to endoscopic evaluation is *cytologic screening* performed by passing and retrieving a mesh-covered balloon. Initial results are encouraging.

Principles of Management. *Nutrition* is one of the first priorities. The morbidity of esophageal carcinoma is due largely to the severe dysphagia, odynophagia, and inanition that characterizes advanced disease. Many patients are unable to swallow their own saliva. Even partial obstruction leads to weight loss and cachexia. Good nutrition helps sustain immunologic competence and ability to tolerate the stresses of treatment. Blenderized diets and liquid diet supplements are helpful, and hyperalimentation is employed as a temporary means in patients with the potential for meaningful survival.

Once nutritional support has been provided, *staging* can be carried out. It is essential to determining candidacy for curative versus palliative therapy. Patients with tumor affixed to neighboring structures or with metastasis to the tracheobronchial tree, pleura, carinal area, or distantly to the abdomen are not candidates for curative therapy. The combination of *computed tomography (CT)* plus *endoscopic ultrasonography* has proven excellent for staging. CT (or magnetic resonance imaging [MRI]) can readily detect metastasis to the chest or abdomen but, by itself, is inadequate for delineating the extent of local disease. Ultrasound techniques are superb for the latter task.

There are few controlled studies available to help define the optimal approach to therapy. Most therapy is palliative, because few patients have curable lesions at the time of detection. The exception is the patient with early disease confined to the mucosa. *Total esophagectomy* in such patients is associated with 5-year survival rates of 50 percent to 80 percent. For most others, the issue is selecting the best form of palliative therapy, especially one that preserves or restores the ability to swallow.

Most authorities consider surgery the palliative treatment of choice, although perioperative complication rates and overall surgical mortality can be high. *Palliative surgical resection* is most successful in patients with disease confined to the distal esophagus. However, even partial esophagectomy is a major procedure. Overall mortality associated with surgery is close to 10 percent. The best results reported for palliative surgery include an 85 percent rate of symptomatic improvement, 17-month mean survival, and 20 percent 5-year survival.

For dysphagic patients too ill for surgery, palliation can be provided by endoscopic placement of a polyvinyl *stent*. Esophageal *dilatation* is useful for temporary relief. Gastrostomy may be of help for nutrition but provides no symptomatic relief from disabling dysphagia.

Radiation therapy has theoretical appeal because squamous cell cancers are radiosensitive, but the central intrathoracic location of these tumors adjacent to the heart, lungs, and spinal cord makes delivery of curative doses difficult. Attempts at radical curative radiation therapy are reserved for patients with cancer confined to the cervical esophagus, which is difficult to treat surgically and often requires laryngectomy. Preoperative radiation with lower doses (3000 to 4000 rad) can be safely delivered to help reduce tumor mass, but improved outcome has been hard to demonstrate in randomized studies. Moderate doses have also been used as a palliative measure to relieve dysphagia in patients who are not candidates for a surgical procedure; results are not satisfactory. The complication rate is high due to the tendency of a heavily irradiated esophagus to perforate and surrounding structures (mediastinum, trachea, spinal column) to experience radiation damage.

Use of lower radiation doses in *combination with chemotherapy* and surgery has produced encouraging results. Multidrug regimens (using cisplatin) in conjunction with radiation have produced major reductions in tumor size in up to 75 percent of patients, making some tumors amenable to surgical resection. Some patients treated preoperatively in this fashion showed no evidence of residual tumor at time of surgery. This finding has led to trials of chemotherapy plus radiation without surgery. Three-year survival rates of 10 percent to 40 percent have been reported, making such therapy a possible alternative for patients not deemed candidates for surgery. These encouraging reports still need confirmation in prospective, randomized, controlled trials of adequate size.

Laser therapy is available for palliation in patients too ill to undergo surgery or radiation. Results are encouraging, adverse effects are few, and therapy can be performed on an outpatient basis after an initial 2- to 3-day hospitalization. Relief is achieved, but there is no change in survival rate.

Prevention remains the most effective means of dealing with this devastating cancer. Efforts to encourage cessation of smoking (see Chapter 54) and alcohol abuse (see Chapter 228) can lower risk and are essential.

GASTRIC CANCER

There are approximately 20,000 new cases of gastric cancer in the United States each year and 14,000 deaths attributable to it annually. The incidence has been decreasing slightly over the past decade, but mortality remains relatively unchanged. Overall 5-year survival is about 10 percent. Improvement in outcome has been linked to advances in early diagnosis. Patients with early gastric carcinoma (disease confined to the mucosa and submucosa) have a 5-year survival in excess of 90 percent. Unfortunately, extension occurs rather early. Predisposing factors include *previous gastric surgery* (usually Billroth II anastomosis) and *atrophic gastritis* with achlorhydria and pernicious anemia. *Dietary nitrates* have been implicated as a risk factor. Increased prevalences occur among Native Americans, Asians, Hispanics, and Scandinavians.

About 95 percent of gastric malignancies are *adenocarcinomas,* with those that are well differentiated and circumscribed having a much better prognosis than those that are poorly differentiated and infiltrative. Lymphomas account for the majority of the remaining 10 percent.

Clinical Presentation, Course, and Diagnosis. Clinical presentation can be subtle, making early diagnosis difficult. Nonspecific abdominal pain, gastric ulceration with or without bleeding, weight loss, and obstruction are the major patterns of clinical presentation, but most are manifestations of advanced disease. About 75 percent of patients with early disease have *epigastric pain* as the initial complaint. Most are free of the nausea, vomiting, anorexia, and weight loss that characterize more advanced disease. *Gastric ulcer* is an important presentation, characterized by a suspicious appearance on barium study or a more benign-appearing radiologic defect that fails to heal completely or quickly recurs after 6 weeks of ulcer therapy (see Chapter 68).

Endoscopy with *brushings* and *biopsy* is the preferred method for definitive diagnosis and is indicated in patients over the age of 50 who present with epigastric pain unresponsive to 7 to 10 days of antacid therapy (see Chapter 74). In the absence of an ulcer, all atypical areas of mucosa should be biopsied. Endoscopy has largely replaced upper GI series for diagnosis, in part because it permits the obtaining of biopsy specimens.

The disease often progresses silently until signs of metastatic disease, such as enlargement of the *left supraclavicular lymph nodes* or *ascites,* become evident and cause the patient to seek medical attention. Spread occurs by direct extension as well as by seeding of the lymphatics, blood vessels, and peritoneal surface. Metastases develop locally as well as at distant sites, most frequently the *liver* (40%), *lung* (15%), and *bone* (15%). Among patients who come to surgery, approximately 80 percent are found to have *lymph node* metastases, whereas 40 percent have *peritoneal involvement* and 35 percent show spread to the liver or lung.

Principles of Management. *Surgery* is the primary mode of treatment, both for cure and palliation. Median survival for patients managed by complete surgical resection is in excess of 3 years. The 5-year survival rate varies according to location of the tumor: it is 25 percent in patients with distal lesions and 10 percent for those with proximal ones. When lymph node involvement is found, survival falls by 50 percent. The surgical loss of the stomach's food reservoir function necessitates small frequent feedings. Without careful patient education and use of high-calorie supplements, total gastrectomy can lead to malnutrition. Subtotal or total gastrectomy is optimal for management of bleeding or obstruction related to tumors at the gastroesophageal junction. *Linitis plastica* or total wall involvement of the stomach is incurable and not manageable by surgery.

Chemotherapy (using such agents as 5-fluorouracil [5-FU]) as the sole mode of treatment in patients with metastatic disease produces responses in almost 40 percent of patients. The average duration of response is 9 months, but there is no improvement in survival. Complete responses are rare. The efficacy of *adjuvant chemotherapy* after surgical resection remains controversial. The Gastrointestinal Tumor Study Group found in a randomized controlled trial that fluorouracil in conjunction with a nitrosourea after surgery improved survival and achieved a 20 percent cure rate. However, others have not been able to confirm these results, and the question remains unsettled. Unlike adenocarcinoma, gastric lymphomas are responsive to chemotherapy after gastrectomy (see Chapter 84), with 5-year survival approaching 40 percent. Combination chemotherapy is being considered for patients with primary gastric lymphoma that is unresectable.

Adenocarcinomas of the stomach are *not radiosensitive* at tolerable doses. Neither radiation used alone nor as part of an adjuvant program with chemotherapy has improved survival. Likewise, postoperative radiation does not seem to be of much benefit in patients with gastric lymphoma.

Patient monitoring should be guided by symptoms and not by routine testing for potential metastatic sites, because only palliative therapeutic options exist for patients with advanced disease.

PANCREATIC CANCER

Carcinoma of the pancreas is the fourth leading cause of cancer death in the United States. Mortality is high (close to 99% at 5 years); fewer than 20 percent survive 1 year. High death rates are due partially to difficulties in early detection, which stem from the tumor's retroperitoneal location. For decades, pancreatic cancer had been increasing in frequency, but incidence has plateaued since 1973. There are about 25,000 new cases annually. The disease is rare before age 45, but incidence rises rapidly thereafter. There is a slight male predominance.

Hypotheses regarding pathogenesis include concentration and excretion of carcinogens by acinar cells inducing neoplastic transformation among ductal cells. Established risk factors include heavy *alcohol consumption* and heavy *smoking*. Diabetes mellitus, chronic pancreatitis, and exposures to dry-cleaning chemicals and gasoline are also suspected contributing factors. The validity of a statistical association with coffee consumption has been disproved.

Clinical Presentation, Course, and Diagnosis. In most instances, the tumor remains silent until late in the course of disease, with presentation determined largely by the tumor's location. In about two-thirds of cases, the cancer begins in the head of the pancreas; in the remainder, it occurs in the body or tail. Disease that originates in the pancreatic head near the pancreaticobiliary junction may extend locally to obstruct bile flow and cause *painless jaundice*—one of the few potentially early symptomatic presentations of pancreatic cancer. Jaundice, with or without pain, is an eventual manifestation in about 50 percent of patients, although in many it is due to metastasis or late extension.

More often than not, symptoms are late in onset and nonspecific. Disease of the body or tail may present with vague upper abdominal or back *pain* or *discomfort,* unexplained *weight loss,* unexplained *depression,* or even migratory *thrombophlebitis*. Carcinomas of the tail may not cause symptoms until they metastasize. Pancreatic cancer is also an important cause of ectopic hormone production (insulin, glucagon, ACTH) and unexplained onset of *diabetes* or *pancreatitis*. Persistent *nausea* and *vomiting* suggest invasion and obstruction of the upper GI tract.

The *clinical course* of pancreatic carcinoma is dominated by regional extension into the retroperitoneum and liver. The tumor tends to spread perineurally and lymphatically. Median survival for patients with extrapancreatic tumor is 12 weeks from time of presentation, and 19 to 42 weeks for those with tumor confined to the pancreas.

Diagnosis no longer requires laparotomy, but tissue may still be needed because symptoms and signs may be nonspecific and there are no definitive blood tests. The workup begins with abdominal *ultrasonography* or *CT.* Both have the capacity to detect lesions as small as 2 cm and to image the biliary tree and pancreatic ducts. In many cases, both are ordered. Ultrasound is usually the initial study in patients with jaundice, because the test is readily available and provides a quick and inexpensive means of diagnosing common bile duct obstruction. It also can detect tumor before it distorts the pancreatic contour, an advantage it has over CT. CT provides better definition of the tumor and adjacent structures, helping to determine anatomy and detect metastasis to the liver and draining lymph nodes.

MRI techniques offer no advantages over CT, although advances in MRI may eventually prove useful. Pancreatic radionuclide scanning is not used due to poor diagnostic accuracy.

When a distinct pancreatic mass is identified, *fine-needle aspiration biopsy* can be performed percutaneously, guided by direct ultrasound or CT visualization. Limiting the yield from needle biopsy is the large zone of fibrosis and inflammation that typically surrounds the tumor. The procedure is the confirmatory test of choice in patients with disease felt to be metastatic or unresectable. Drawbacks include a substantial false-negative rate and the risk of seeding along the needle tract.

Patients with a mass at the pancreaticobiliary junction are excellent candidates for *endoscopic retrograde cholangiopancreatography (ERCP).* Early ampullary lesions causing jaundice can be visualized and biopsied directly, leading to prompt diagnosis, definitive treatment, and improved 5-year survival (as high as 50%). A pancreatogram is taken during ERCP, with ductal narrowing, obstruction, and extravasation of dye additional signs of malignancy (although they also can occur in chronic pancreatitis). An irregular stricture longer than 10 mm is characteristic of cancer. Cytologic sampling, especially that obtained by brushing, has a reported sensitivity approaching 85 percent, although results vary.

Serum tumor markers have always been appealing, although of limited use in diagnosis. *CA 19-9,* a tumor marker developed with monoclonal antibody technology, has been tested for its utility in detecting and monitoring pancreatic cancer. Although sensitive in the setting of advanced disease, the test is often normal in early stages. In addition, specificity has been disappointing; high levels have been reported in other GI cancers (bile duct, colon). It is not recommended for screening but can be useful in differentiating chronic pancreatitis from pancreatic cancer and in follow-up surveillance (provided levels were high before surgery and fall immediately after). Other serum tumor markers examined include carcinoembryonic antigen (CEA) and the ratio of testosterone to dihydrotestosterone. None has proven sufficiently sensitive or specific to warrant use in routine diagnosis.

Principles of Management. The chance for cure is limited because it depends on surgically removing the entire tumor, which is usually well advanced by the time it is detected. Careful *staging* is critical. One needs to distinguish between tumors that are localized and resectable, localized and not resectable, and metastatic. In addition, patients with duodenal obstruction need to be identified because they require operation.

CT with contrast is the staging procedure of choice for visualizing the tumor and detecting liver and large lymph node metastases. Such metastases rule out resectability. Microscopic nodal disease is not visible by CT, but neither is it considered a contraindication to surgery (although palliation rather than cure may be the objective). Many surgeons view data from *angiography* as useful—major vascular involvement indicates inoperability. The utility of a staging *laparoscopy* for patients being considered for surgery has become evident. Upwards of 40 percent of such patients are found at laparoscopy to have previously undetected peritoneal or omental metastases, which rule out resectability. These three tests are complementary and greatly increase the determination of surgical candidacy. They can save many patients from undergoing unnecessary laparotomy. If any one test is positive, only 5 percent will have a resectable tumor at laparotomy; but, if all 3 are negative, the rate increases to 78 percent.

Surgery. Only patients with relatively small lesions confined to the head of the pancreas are candidates for *curative surgery.* This accounts for no more than 5 percent to 22 percent of patients who present with the disease. The risks of surgery are great, the operations formidable, and postoperative complications serious. Operative mortality frequently approaches or even exceeds the 5-year survival rate. The decision to subject a patient with pancreatic cancer to a major operation with a high degree of operative mortality and only modest chances for substantially improved survival must be made individually.

The operation of choice is the *Whipple procedure* (pancreatoduodenectomy), which requires a surgical tour de force and should be attempted only by surgeons able to perform it with less than 5 percent mortality. Five-year survival rates are best in patients with a small (2 cm or less) tumor, approaching 30 percent at centers with surgical expertise in performing the operation. Survival increases to 57 percent if lymph nodes prove to be negative (unfortunately, an uncommon occurrence). Overall 5-year survival had been 5 percent, but reports of 15 percent to 25 percent are now appearing in conjunction with advances in staging, case selection, and operative technique. Regional pancreatectomy or total pancreatectomy provides no survival benefit.

Surgery is also recommended for *palliation*. Patients with biliary obstruction are candidates for biliary bypass or endoscopic stent placement, which can relieve jaundice and lower the risk of cholangitis. Surgical or percutaneous ablation of the celiac ganglion can provide relief from intractable pain.

Radiation therapy is applied to patients with localized, but unresectable disease. However, only when used in conjunction with 5-FU therapy does it prolong survival. Intraoperative radiation is also being promoted, but survival benefit remains to be defined. Preoperative courses of radiation and chemotherapy are being studied. Radiation therapy has also been used for control of intractable retroperitoneal pain; 4 to 6 months of relief have been reported.

Chemotherapy as a primary modality has a very limited role in this disease due to the debilitated, advanced state of most patients who present with inoperable disease. 5-FU has a response rate of about 20 percent, but there is no evidence of prolongation of survival compared to supportive therapy.

Supportive measures are essential, not only to patients who are dying of their disease (see Chapters 87), but also to those who have undergone pancreatectomy. In the latter group, insulin therapy and pancreatic enzyme preparations are needed. Insulin requirements are in the range of 20 to 30 units per day.

COLORECTAL CANCER

Colorectal cancer is one of the most common malignancies and, although one of the more potentially curable cancers, results in 50,000 deaths annually. Over 150,000 new cases develop each year. Among the suspected etiologic factors is an increased exposure to chemical carcinogens present within the bowel lumen. High-risk patients are those with a first-degree relative with colorectal cancer, long-standing pancolitis (see Chapter 73), familial polyposis, or Gardner's syndrome (polyps, osteomas, epidermoid cysts, soft tissue tumors). Loss of the tumor suppressor gene p_{53} has been found in colorectal cancer patients. High-fiber diets appear to lessen risk, perhaps because they speed transit time in the bowel. Intriguing epidemiologic data suggest that regular use of aspirin may reduce the risk of fatal colon cancer. Other preliminary data indicate that calcium supplementation can reduce epithelial proliferation in high-risk patients. Early diagnosis through screening has been a high priority in the approach to this condition, with screening sigmoidoscopy capable of reducing mortality (see Chapter 56).

Clinical Presentation, Course, and Diagnosis. The *clinical presentation* of colorectal cancer is related to the site of the tumor. Tumors of the ascending colon may be asymptomatic until late stages, producing little more than mild *iron deficiency* anemia or intermittently *guaiac-positive stools*. Tumors of the descending colon and rectosigmoid can cause symptoms earlier in the course of illness, presenting as *rectal bleeding* or *change in bowel habits* (diarrhea as well as constipation). At the time of surgery, 50 percent to 75 percent of patients demonstrate tumor that has penetrated the bowel wall; 60 percent of these show regional metastases.

Rectal cancers commonly present with occult or frank rectal bleeding, with or without an alteration in bowel habits. *Tenesmus* is usually a late symptom representing extension of the tumor beyond the bowel wall. Rectal or perianal pain is a consequence of the invasion of the pararectal structures in the sacral plexus. Tumor often arises on the posterior wall, making it particularly important to examine the rectal ampulla on routine rectal examination.

Prognosis depends on extent of penetration and local spread. A modification of the standard *Dukes' classification* serves as a useful system for staging (Table 76–1). Stage A patients have tumor limited to the submucosa and a 5-year survival in excess of 90 percent. Those with stage B disease have a 5-year survival ranging from 70 percent to 85 percent. Once the serosal surface and lymph nodes are involved, stage C, survival falls to 30 percent to 65 percent. Prognosis is also adversely effected by presence of polyploidy and mucin production in the tumor, and by preoperative elevation of serum CEA level (> 5 ng per ml).

The most common sites of metastasis are the *liver* (60% overall and 30% of solitary metastases) due to portal blood flow draining the intestines, the *peritoneal surface* (30%), and the *lung* (20%). Brain, skin, and local recurrences occur in less than 5 percent. Rectal cancers tend to invade locally and to recur in the pelvis alone or in association with distant metastases to the liver or lung, bypassing the intraabdominal cavity.

Diagnosis in a patient suspected of colorectal cancer is best accomplished by *colonoscopy* that extends to the cecum. The combination of flexible *sigmoidoscopy* plus *barium enema* is a second choice where colonoscopy is not available, but barium study does not allow for biopsy and the false-negative rate can be as high as 40 percent for single-contrast studies. Sensitivity is improved with use of air-contrast techniques, but elderly patients find such barium studies uncomfortable.

For patients in whom a cancer is detected in the rectosigmoid, a preoperative examination of the entire colon all the way to the cecum is required, either by colonoscopy or air-contrast barium enema, because about 3 percent of patients have synchronous tumors. Similarly, colonoscopy is needed when a benign adenomatous polyp is found on examination of the rectosigmoid.

Staging for colon cancer is based predominantly on findings at surgery and pathologic examination (see Table 76–1). Liver and CT scanning are not usually performed preoperatively because the results do not affect the decision to remove the tumor. However, *CT scan* or *MRI* of the pelvis can help determine extent of a rectal cancer and candidacy for surgery. A preoperative *CEA* level provides a baseline for postoperative monitoring of colorectal cancer and helps assess prognosis.

Treatment. *Surgery* is the primary modality of therapy, both for cure and for palliative purposes to prevent or relieve bowel obstruction. For colon cancer, *colectomy* is the procedure of choice. Because the tumor spreads lymphatically, adequate amounts of bowel on both sides of the lesion must be removed to avoid cutting into intramural lymphatics that may contain cancerous cells. Patients presenting with obstruction may benefit from a temporary diverting colostomy followed at a later date by reanastomosis. Resection of an

Table 76-1. Staging for Colorectal Cancer

STAGE	DESCRIPTION	5-YEAR SURVIVAL
A	Lesion confined to submucosa; nodes negative	>90%
B1*	Muscularis involved, but not serosa; nodes negative	80–85%
B2*	Lesion extends through serosa; nodes negative	70–75%
C1*	Lesion extends into muscularis only; nodes positive	70–75%
C1*	Lesion extends through serosa; 1–4 nodes positive	60–65%
C2*	Lesion extends through serosa; >4 nodes positive	30–40%

*Gastrointestinal Tumor Study Group Modification of Dukes' staging system.

Adapted from Steel G, et al. *Cancer Manual,* 8th ed. Massachusetts Division, Boston, American Cancer Society, 1990; 244.

isolated hepatic metastasis also provides opportunity for cure, although 5-year survival is only 25 percent.

Surgical management of rectal cancer consists of *abdominoperineal resection,* aided by adjuvant radiation therapy. When possible, an effort is made to preserve the anal sphincter. Tumors of the upper two-thirds of the rectum can usually be resected in conjunction with construction of an anastomosis; those of the lower third require an abdominoperineal resection with a permanent sigmoid colostomy. Sometimes unwise attempts are made to limit the resection to preserve the sphincter; inadequate surgical margins are taken, leading to local recurrence and death. Alternatives to abdominoperineal resection include local excision, fulguration, and intrarectal radiation therapy. Only patients with small exophytic tumors in the lower third of the rectum should be considered for such alternative therapy.

The recognition that adenomatous polyps, villoglandular polyps, and villous adenomas may harbor cancers or be premalignant has led to the recommendation of *polypectomy* when detected, aided greatly by fiberoptic colonoscopy. Cancer confined to the polyp is considered carcinoma *in situ;* detectable invasion of the stalk or muscularis necessitates *colectomy.*

Radiation therapy has no established role in colon cancer, in contrast to its important place in the treatment of rectal cancer. The tendency of rectal cancers that have penetrated the bowel wall to recur locally is high (30% to 50%). Adjunctive use of radiation therapy in such patients significantly reduces the risk of local recurrence. Patients with extensive local disease are irradiated preoperatively. This reduces tumor size and allows for subsequent resection. Postoperative radiotherapy is reserved for those whose findings at surgery suggest high risk of recurrence (ie, those with stage B2 or C). In addition, the application of adjuvant radiation therapy postoperatively has permitted an anterior resection with primary anastomosis in many patients who would otherwise require a colostomy.

Chemotherapy, consisting of postoperative application of *levamisole* and *5-FU,* can significantly reduce the risk of recurrence in patients with resected stage C colon cancers. Typically, treatment is begun as soon as possible after surgery. This therapy represents a major advance in the treatment of advanced disease. Before this development, 5-FU was used for advanced disease, with a 20 percent response rate but little chance of a meaningful prolongation of survival. The addition of leukovorin to 5-FU increases the response rate to 30 to 35 percent. At one point, claims were made for high-dose vitamin C. Randomized, double-blind control study has shown that such therapy is no better than placebo.

Monitoring. Attentive follow-up is essential because of the risk of a second bowel cancer (occurring in up to 5% of patients) and appearance of new polyps. Regularly scheduled *colonoscopy* should begin 6 months after surgery and take place every 24 to 36 months if no polyps are found and every 6 months if they are. Any encountered polyps are removed. If colonoscopy is unavailable or cannot reach the cecum, air-contrast *barium enema* is an adequate substitute. Early detection of recurrent or metastatic disease has been aided by sequential monitoring of the plasma *CEA*. The recommended interval for CEA determinations is every 6 months for the first 2 years, provided that the CEA was elevated before surgery and fell to low levels within 2 to 4 weeks after it. If the CEA rises by 30 percent or more per month from its postoperative level, then a search for curable recurrent disease should be undertaken. However, evidence that CEA surveillance is cost-effective and saves a significant number of lives is wanting. Careful patient selection is warranted.

A new primary in the bowel or a single metastasis to the lung or liver is amenable to curative resection. Besides the CEA, one should monitor symptoms (weight loss, fatigue, change in bowel habits), the physical examination (especially chest and abdomen), alkaline phosphatase, and the chest x-ray to help detect recurrent, but curable disease.

Supportive Therapy. Patients who have undergone abdominoperineal resection with permanent or temporary colostomy need careful counseling pre- and postoperatively to help them adapt to their situation. Becoming comfortable with the details of ostomy care as well as having an opportunity to discuss their fears and concerns (sexual function, odor, appearance, bag changes, recurrence of cancer) are essential components of the rehabilitation effort. Ostomy groups and stoma nurses are important resources for the patient, but there is no substitute for a supportive, understanding patient–physician relationship.

Management of Colorectal Polyps

As noted earlier, the patient found to have an adenomatous polyp should undergo colonoscopy to be sure all synchronous lesions are detected and removed. Patients found to have a villous, tubulovillus, or large (> 1 cm) adenomatous polyp of the rectosigmoid are at increased risk for subsequent colorectal cancer (incidence as high as 7%). The incidence of new cancer can be reduced by 70 to 90 percent by polypectomy. The optimal frequency for repeat colonoscopy is controversial. The best determinant of frequency is individual risk. Current concensus guidelines recommend performing the first follow-up study in 3 years, followed by one every 5 years if the first study is normal. Emerging data suggest that the first study after polyp removal need not occur for several years. About half of patients with adenomatous polyps have small tubular adenomas that are not associated with an increased cancer risk, even if there are multiple lesions. Such patients do not require follow-up colonoscopy. Patients with familial adenomatous polyposis are at very high risk of developing colorectal cancer (approximately 50% by age 40). Prophylactic colectomy is often recommended for such persons.

Encouraging epidemiologic data suggest that use of nonsteroidal antiinflammatory drugs (NSAIDs; eg, sulindac) may reduce risk, as may low–saturated fat diets high in fish, chicken, fiber, and vitamin A.

Synchronous Hepatic Metastases

Not uncommonly, hepatic metastases are discovered at the same time or even before discovery of the primary tumor, as is often the case with cancer of the colon. Synchronous metastases may represent up to 15 percent of new cases of colon cancer. In the presence of symptoms that are specifically derived from the primary tumor, such as bleeding or obstruction, a primary surgical resection is often undertaken if the patient has a life expectancy (on the basis of the hepatic metastases) that exceeds 2 months. In the presence of an asymptomatic primary tumor in the bowel, however, therapeutic efforts are directed first at the metastatic disease; if successful, a surgical approach to the primary tumor may be undertaken. This approach assumes that the median survival for patients with hepatic metastases does not exceed 6 months; therefore, in patients not responding to chemotherapy, the likelihood of dying of distant disease far exceeds the likelihood of significant complications from the primary tumor site.

A.H.G.

ANNOTATED BIBLIOGRAPHY

Esophageal Cancer

Achkar E, Carey W. The cost of surveillance for adenocarcinoma complicating Barrett's esophagus. Am J Gastroenterol 1988; 83:291. (*Cost of annual endoscopic surveillance was $62,000 per case found and approximately 1.2 days of work lost per person screened.*)

Cello JP, Gerstenberger PD, Wright T, et al. Endoscopic neodymium-YAG laser palliation of nonresectable esophageal malignancy. Ann Intern Med 1985;102: 610. (*Laser use to alleviate luminal obstruction; a promising therapy for patients with inoperable disease.*)

Coia LR, Engstrom PF, Paul A. Nonsurgical management of esophageal cancer. Report of a study of combined radiotherapy and chemotherapy. J Clin Oncol 1987;5:1783. (*Encouraging improvements in survival achieved.*)

Iizuka T, Ide H, Kakegawa T, et al. Preoperative radioactive therapy for esophageal carcinoma. Randomized evaluation trial in eight institutions. Chest 1988;93:1054. (*Therapy was well tolerated, but results were not impressive.*)

Lehr L, Rupp N, Siewert JR. Assessment of resectability of esophageal cancer by computed tomography and magnetic resonance imaging. Surgery 1988;103:344. (*Documents low sensitivity and specificity for disease extension into the mediastinum.*)

Leichman L, Steiger Z, Seydel HG, et al. Preoperative chemotherapy and radiation therapy for patients with cancer of the esophagus: A potentially curative approach. J Clin Oncol 1984;2:75. (*Discussion of a combined-modality approach to esophageal cancer in which 50 percent of patients coming to resection had no detectable tumor.*)

Mendenhall WM, Parson JT, Vogel SB, et al. Carcinoma of the cervical esophagus treated with radiation therapy. Laryngoscope 1988;98:769. (*One instance where radiation therapy may have great benefit and the potential to effect cure.*)

Schattenkerk ME, Obertop H, Mud HJ, et al. Survival after resection for carcinoma of the oesophagus. Br J Surg 1987; 74:165. (*Useful outcome statistics for surgical therapy.*)

Tio TL, Coene LO, Luiken HM, et al. Endosonography in the clinical staging of esophagogastric cancer. Gastrointest Endosc 1990;35:S2. (*Overall accuracy [89 percent] much better than that available from CT; overstaging 6 percent, understaging 5 percent.*)

Tsang TK, Hidvegi D, Horth K, et al. Reliability of balloon-mesh cytology in detecting esophageal carcinoma in a population of US veterans. Cancer 1987;59:556. (*Inexpensive method that may have promise; sensitivity 91 percent; specificity 94 percent.*)

Gastric Cancer

Eckardt VF, Giebler W, Kanzler G, et al. Clinical and morphological characteristics of early gastric cancer. Gastroenterology 1990;98:708. (*Very useful data on the presentation, diagnosis, clinical course, and outcome of early gastric cancer in the community setting.*)

Gastrointestinal Tumor Study Group. Controlled trials of adjuvant chemotherapy following curative resection for gastric cancer. Cancer 1982;49:1116. (*Prospective controlled trial in which adjuvant chemotherapy improved the cure rate for gastric cancer; unfortunately, results not confirmed by others.*)

Haber DA, Mayer RJ. Primary gastrointestinal lymphoma. Semin Oncol 1988;15:154. (*Useful review of this important gastric malignancy.*)

Health and Public Policy Committee, American College of Physicians. Endoscopy in the evaluation of dyspepsia. Ann Intern Med 1985;102:266. (*Recommends endoscopy in patients with dyspepsia who fail to clear after 6 to 8 weeks of full antiulcer therapy.*)

O'Brien MJ, Burakoff R, Robbins EA, et al. Early gastric cancer. Clinicopathological study. Am J Med 1985;78:195. (*Early gastric cancer now comprises a greatly increased portion of lesions leading to gastric resection, presumably due to use of endoscopic biopsy for benign-appearing gastric ulcers that fail to heal.*)

Pancreatic Cancer

Balthazar EJ, Chako AC. Computed tomography of pancreatic masses. Am J Gastroenterol 1990;85:343. (*Well-documented discussion of its utility in pancreatic cancer.*)

Cameron JL, Crist DW, Sitzmann JV, et al. Factors influencing survival after pancreaticoduodenectomy for pancreatic cancer. Am J Surg 1991;161:120. *(Small tumor size, negative nodes, and lack of vessel involvement predict good results.)*

Gordis L. Consumption of methylxanthine-containing beverages and risk of pancreatic cancer. Cancer Lett 1990;52:1. *(Critical and detailed review of all published data; concludes there is no increased risk.)*

Kalser MH, Barkin J, MacIntyre JM. Pancreatic cancer: Assessment of prognosis by clinical presentation. Cancer 1985;56: 397. *(Onset of symptoms is usually a sign of advanced disease, although jaundice may be an early manifestation in some.)*

Lowenfels AB, et al. Pancreatitis and the risk of pancreatic cancer. N Engl J Med 1993; 328:1433. *(Association found.)*

MacMahon B, Trichopoulos D, Warren K, et al. Coffee and cancer of the pancreas. N Engl J Med 1981;304:630. *(Study that started the controversy.)*

Parsons L, Palmer CH. How accurate is fine-needle biopsy in malignant neoplasia of the pancreas? Arch Surg 1989;124:681. *(Sensitivity 57 percent to 94 percent, few false-positives, but many false-negatives due to sampling errors and fibrosis and inflammation surrounding the tumor.)*

Steinberg W. The clinical utility of the CA 19-9 tumor-associated antigen. Am J Gastroenterol 1990;85:350. *(Useful for monitoring, but not for screening or early diagnosis.)*

Steiner E, Stark DD, Hahn PF, et al. Imaging of pancreatic neoplasms: Comparison of MR and CT. Am J Roentgenol 1989;152:487. *(MR was no better than CT.)*

Van Dyke JA, Stanley RJ, Berland LL. Pancreatic imaging. Ann Intern Med 1985;102:212. *(Critical review; argues that CT is the best initial study because ultrasound is often compromised by bowel gas.)*

Venu RP, Geenen JE, Kini M, et al. Endoscopic retrograde brush cytology: A new technique. Gastroenterology 1990;99:1475. *(Greatly enhances the diagnostic yield from ERCP.)*

Warshaw AL, Fernandez-del Castillo C. Pancreatic carcinoma. N Engl J Med 1992;326:455. *(Definitive review, including excellent discussion of surgical therapy; 186 references.)*

Wils JA. Current status of chemotherapy in metastatic pancreatic cancer. Anticancer Res 1989;9:1027. *(Useful review; no major breakthroughs.)*

Colorectal Cancer and Polyps

Atkin WS, Morson BC, Cuzick J. Long-term risk of colorectal cancer after excision of rectosigmoid adenomas. N Engl J Med 1992;326:658. *(Risk increased only in patients with villous, tubulovillous, or large adenomas.)*

Bond JH, for the Practice Parameters Committee of the American College of Gastroenterology. Polyp guideline: Diagnosis, treatment, and surveillance for patients with nonfamilial colorectal polyps. Ann Intern Med 1993;119:836. *(Recommends first surveillance after polypectomy at 3 years, then every 5 years.)*

Bresalier RS, Kim YS. Diet and colon cancer. N Engl J Med 1985;313:1413. *(Summarizes the data linking dietary factors and colon cancer.)*

Burt RW, Bishop T, Cannon LA, et al. Dominant inheritance of adenomatous polyps and colorectal cancer. N Engl J Med 1985;312:1540. *(Documents an autosomal dominant inheritance.)*

Creagan ET, Moertel CG, O'Fallon JR, et al. Failure of high-dose vitamin C therapy to benefit patients with advanced cancer. N Engl J Med 1979;301:1189. *(Despite anecdotal claims to the contrary, this careful study conclusively demonstrates that high-dose vitamin C is no more effective than placebo.)*

Fleischer DE, Goldberg SB, Browning TH, et al. Detection and surveillance of colorectal cancer. JAMA 1989;161:580. *(Review of consensus recommendations.)*

Fletcher RH. Carcinoembryonic antigen. Ann Intern Med 1986; 104:66. *(Thoughtful review indicating that surveillance by CEA can detect recurrences, but few lives are actually saved; 49 references.)*

Gastrointestinal Tumor Study Group. Prolongation of disease-free survival in surgically treated rectal carcinoma. N Engl J Med 1985;312:1465. *(Prospective randomized trial demonstrating benefit from adjuvant radiation plus chemotherapy for rectal cancer.)*

Giardiello FM. Treatment of colonic and rectal adenomas with sulindac in familial adenomatous polyposis. N Engl J Med 1993;328:1313. *(Some benefit suggested.)*

Gunderson LL, Sosin H. Areas of failure found at reoperation (second or symptomatic look) following "curative surgery" for adenocarcinoma of the rectum: Clinicopathologic correlation and implications for adjuvant therapy. Cancer 1974;34: 1278. *(High risk of local recurrence; rationale for use of adjuvant local radiation therapy.)*

Lipkin M, Newmark H. Effect of added dietary calcium on colonic epithelial-cell proliferation in subjects at high risk for familial colonic cancer. N Engl J Med 1985;313:1381. *(Shows a normalization of proliferation and raises the possibility of a role for added calcium in selected patients—very preliminary data, but interesting.)*

Mayer RJ. Does adjuvant therapy work in colon cancer? N Engl J Med 1990;322:399. *(Editorial succinctly reviewing the issue in view of new findings.)*

Moertel CG, Fleming TR, MacDonald JS, et al. Levamisole and fluorouracil for adjuvant therapy of resected colon carcinoma. N Engl J Med 1990;322:353. *(Major improvement in survival achieved for patients with advanced disease.)*

Ransohoff DF, Lang CA, Kuo HS. Colonoscopic surveillance after polypectomy: Consideration of cost effectiveness. Ann Intern Med 1991;114:177. *(Cost effectiveness is very sensitive to the risk of death from cancer after polypectomy.)*

Sandler RS, Freund DA, Herbst CA, et al. Cost effectiveness of preoperative carcinoembryonic antigen monitoring in colorectal cancer. Cancer 1984;53:193. *(Although the cost of identifying a resectable tumor with CEA monitoring ranged from $10,000 to $20,000, the actual cost might be less if more effective therapies were available.)*

Selby JV, Friedman GD, Quesenberry CP, et al. A case-control study of screening sigmoidoscopy and mortality from colorectal cancer. N Engl J Med 1992;326:653. *(Mortality from cancer of the distal colon and rectum reduced.)*

Thun MJ, Namboodiri MH, Heath CW. Aspirin use and reduced risk of fatal colon cancer. N Engl J Med 1991;325:1593. *(Intriguing epidemiologic data suggesting a protective effect.)*

Winawer SJ. Randomized comparison of surveillance intervals after colonoscopic removal of newly diagnosed adenomatous polyps. N Engl J Med 1993;328:901. *(Suggests that the interval need not be as short as previously thought.)*

Winawer SJ, Zauber AG, Ho MN, et al. Prevention of colorectal cancer by colonoscopic polypectomy. N Engl J Med 1993; 321:1977. *(Risk of cancer reduced by 70 to 90 percent; best prospective study.)*

6

Hematologic and Oncologic Problems

A

Hematology

Primary Care Medicine: Office Evaluation and Management of the Adult Patient, 3rd edition, edited by Allan H. Goroll, Lawrence A. May, and Albert G. Mulley, Jr. J.B. Lippincott Company, Philadelphia

77

Screening for Anemia

Anemia is a sign of illness rather than a diagnosis in itself. The incidental finding of a low hematocrit or hemoglobin level suggests a host of underlying conditions that range from the trivial to the life-threatening. Patients with fatigue or other subjective symptoms often ask about their "blood count." The absence of anemia in such instances is reassuring. But is the otherwise well patient likely to benefit from either the identification or treatment of asymptomatic anemia? The answer to this question depends on the prevalence and nature of conditions most likely to cause asymptomatic anemia and the relationship between hemoglobin level and those symptoms attributed to its reduction.

EPIDEMIOLOGY AND RISK FACTORS

By far the most common cause for asymptomatic anemia is *iron deficiency* due to inadequate dietary replacement of iron lost from the body. Daily iron requirements for males and postmenopausal females are between 0.5 and 1 mg. Because additional iron is needed by menstruating and pregnant women, their daily requirements are 2 mg and 2.5 mg, respectively. Because only 5 percent to 10 percent of the 10 to 20 mg of the iron contained in the average adult diet is absorbed, it is not surprising that iron deficiency is common in women of childbearing age. Population studies have found 10 percent to 20 percent of menstruating women to have abnormally low concentrations of hemoglobin (usually less than 12 g per 100 mL). Between 20 percent and 60 percent of pregnant women have hemoglobin levels below 11 g per 100 mL. Anemia is less likely to occur in women taking birth control pills and more likely to occur in women with intrauterine devices. Iron deficiency is rare in adult males; if present, it is a clear indication for diligent investigation of the gastrointestinal (GI) tract. Absorption of iron may be decreased after gastrectomy or in the presence of achlorhydria.

Sideroblastic and megaloblastic anemias are much less common. *Pernicious anemia,* the most common form of vitamin B_{12} deficiency, has a prevalence of 0.1 percent in individuals of Northern European extraction. It is much less common among other ethnic and racial groups. *Folate deficiency* is common during pregnancy and in patients with alcoholic liver disease, when it is often accompanied by sideroblastic anemia. Anticonvulsant drugs including phenytoin, primidone, and phenobarbital may interfere with folate absorption with resulting megaloblastic anemia. *Thalassemia minor* is a common cause of mild anemia in patients of Mediterranean or Far Eastern extraction. *Sickle cell disease* and trait, by far the most common hemoglobinopathy, is discussed separately (see Chapter 78).

NATURAL HISTORY OF ANEMIA AND EFFECTIVENESS OF THERAPY

Obviously, the natural history of anemia depends on the underlying cause. What symptoms can mild or moderate anemia be expected to cause? The hyperkinetic symptoms that follow compensatory increases in cardiac stroke volume and heart rate are rarely present before hemoglobin levels have fallen to 7.5 g per 100 mL. Other highly subjective symptoms including irritability, fatigue, and headache have been attributed to milder degrees of anemia. A British survey, however, found no relationship between the frequency of such symptoms and the level of hemoglobin (ranging from 8 to 12 g per 100 mL) among women found to have iron deficiency anemia during a screening program. There was indirect evidence that levels under 8 g per 100 mL were associated with symptoms severe enough to prompt presentation to a physician. Among the asymptomatic women identified by screening, no benefits from treatment were detected. It has been noted by some investigators that symptoms associated with vitamin B_{12} deficiency may predate onset of the anemia (see Chapters 79 and 82).

Most studies of screening for anemia have been conducted in the preoperative or inpatient setting. The few that have been done on outpatients have shown little benefit. In a Swiss study of the utility of the complete blood count in 595 outpatients attending a university-based clinic, 34 (5.8%) had a low hemoglobin level, and in only 3 (0.5%) was a new diagnosis made (iron deficiency without serious underlying pathology). Another report from Britain demonstrated a 10 percent prevalence of anemia among screened women. There was a noteworthy absence of treatable underlying conditions other than iron deficiency and, again, no demonstrable benefits from treatment.

SCREENING AND DIAGNOSTIC TESTS

The laboratory measurements of *hematocrit* and *hemoglobin concentration* are straightforward. Automated methods are reliable and reproducible when specimens are properly handled. Mean hematocrit for adult men at sea level is 46 percent, with a range of 41 percent to 51 percent; for women the mean is 42 percent and the range 37 percent to 47 percent. Slight differences may be noted when automated techniques are used to measure the hematocrit. Normal mean hemoglobin concentration is approximately 16 g per 100 mL for men, with a range of 14 to 18 g per 100 mL; for women the mean is 14 g per 100 mL and the range is 12 to 16 g per 100 mL. In men over 65, the mean falls to 13.5 g per 100 mL; in women over 65, 13.1 g per 100 mL. It must be remembered, as with all continuous laboratory variables, that the choice of a reference value for defining normality is arbitrary. This is particularly true in light of the unclear relationship between significant symptoms and mild "anemia."

CONCLUSIONS AND RECOMMENDATIONS

- Anemia is a common condition. It may be secondary to serious underlying disease or simple dietary deficiency. Determination of hemoglobin concentration or hematocrit is recommended as an important part of the evaluation of a variety of presenting complaints, including fatigue, weight loss, abdominal pain, and GI bleeding (see Chapters 8, 9, 58, and 63).
- Although determination of a complete blood count may provide clues in asymptomatic patients to the presence of early treatable disease, such as GI malignancy, more sensitive and more specific screening methods are available and preferred (eg, stool guaiac testing and sigmoidoscopy for early detection of colorectal cancer; see Chapter 56).
- There is no clear relationship between degrees of mild to moderate anemia and significant symptoms. No clearly measurable benefits after the treatment of mild anemia have been identified in screening studies.
- Thus, routine screening for anemia in nonpregnant, asymptomatic patients is not recommended.
- Iron deficiency anemia is common and important among pregnant patients and responsive to replacement therapy; screening for anemia is reasonable in this population.

A.G.M./A.H.G.

ANNOTATED BIBLIOGRAPHY

Committee on Iron Deficiency. Iron deficiency in the United States. JAMA 1968;203:407. *(Reviews prevalence studies of iron deficiency anemia.)*

Eddy DM. Screening for colorectal cancer. Ann Intern Med 1990;113:373. *(Sophisticated mathematical models examine the cost-effectiveness of colorectal cancer screening with a variety of test strategies.)*

Elwood PC, Shinton NK, Wilson IL, et al. Haemoglobin, Vitamin B_{12} and folate levels in the elderly. Br J Haematol 1971;21:557. *(Ten percent of males with hemoglobin less than 13 g per 100 mL; 10 percent of females less than 12.5 g per 100 mL. No megaloblastic anemia found.)*

Elwood PC, Waters WE, Greene WJW, et al. Symptoms and circulating haemoglobin level. J Chron Dis 1969;21:615. *(Symptoms not correlated with hemoglobin level in those found anemic on screening.)*

Elwood PC, Waters WE, Greene WJ, et al. Evaluation of a screening survey for anemia in adult nonpregnant women. Br Med J 1967;4:714. *(Not very extensive follow-up but no serious underlying disease detected among anemic women.)*

Ruttman S, Clemencon D, Dubach UC. Usefulness of complete blood counts as a case-finding tool in medical outpatients. Ann Intern Med 1992;116:44. *(One of the few studies done in the outpatient setting; yield 5.8 percent, but no significant pathology found in this middle-aged population.)*

U.S. Preventive Services Task Force. Guide to clinical preventive services: An assessment of the effectiveness of 169 interventions. Baltimore: Williams and Wilkins, 1989. *(Screening for anemia was not recommended for any age group.)*

Primary Care Medicine: Office Evaluation and Management of the Adult Patient, 3rd edition, edited by Allan H. Goroll, Lawrence A. May, and Albert G. Mulley, Jr. J.B. Lippincott Company, Philadelphia

78
Screening for Sickle Cell Disease and Sickle Cell Trait

Sickle cell disease is the most common of the clinically significant hemoglobinopathies. In the United States, the disease and trait occur almost exclusively among African Americans. During the late 1960s and early 1970s, sickle cell disease received a great deal of attention in the medical and lay press. The importance of screening for individuals with disease and trait was stressed. Some states legislated mandatory screening programs.

Sickle cell disease (the SS hemoglobin homozygous state) is usually identified during childhood. Patients whose anemia is not identified by screening are often diagnosed after presentation with impaired growth, increased susceptibility to infection, or painful crisis. Screening of adults is aimed at the identification of asymptomatic carriers of sickle trait (the AS hemoglobin heterozygous state). The principal objective is to reduce the prevalence of the homozygous condition by means of genetic counseling. Whether or not screening benefits the people screened has been debated. Screening performed without subsequent education and counseling can be harmful. An understanding of the natural history of sickle cell trait and disease, sensitivity to the concerns of affected patients, and selective use of available screening tests are all necessary if such harmful effects are to be avoided.

EPIDEMIOLOGY AND RISK FACTORS

Sickle cell disease has a prevalence of about 0.15 percent among African-American children in the United States. Double heterozygotes, including those with hemoglobin SC or S-beta-thal, are even less common. Prevalence of sickling disease is lower among adults, because the life span of SS homozygotes and double heterozygotes is decreased.

Screening surveys have documented a prevalence of sickle trait of 7.4 percent among African-American veterans and 8.7 percent in the African-American community of San Francisco. Some studies have shown regional differences in prevalence. Prevalence does not decrease with age. Sickle cell trait is present in low frequency in Southern Italy and higher frequency in parts of Greece. It remains a rare finding in Americans of Mediterranean extraction.

NATURAL HISTORY OF SICKLE CELL DISEASE AND EFFECTIVENESS OF THERAPY

The natural history of *sickle cell disease* is variable. Most children exhibit failure to thrive and suffer frequent infections. Anemia is usually moderate but can become severe, often as a result of infection or folate deficiency. The course is punctuated by painful crises precipitated by infection, dehydration, or hypoxia. Organ infarction, congestive heart failure, cholelithiasis, and skin ulcers are some of the complications of chronic disease. Because supportive care has been improved, life expectancy for patients with sickle cell disease has increased. However, it remains significantly shortened.

In contrast, life expectancy is not affected by *sickle cell trait*. AS red blood cells sickle at much lower oxygen tension than SS cells. The only clinical abnormality that occurs with any frequency among patients with sickle cell trait is painless hematuria, presumably the result of small infarcts of the renal medulla where red cells are particularly susceptible to sickling.

Concern about risk of sudden death during extreme physical exertion in patients with sickle trait has been raised by case reports and population studies of military recruits. Indeed, the presence of sickle trait was associated with an increased risk of otherwise unexplained sudden death among military recruits who were engaged in extreme exertion during basic training. This led to some concern and even suggestions that African-American recruits and athletes should be screened for sickle trait. Although the relative risk of sudden death might be elevated, the absolute risk still appears to be very small (about 1 in 3000 in the Army recruit study) and practically nil for exercise conducted by physically well-conditioned persons (no episodes of sudden death attributable to sickle trait among Olympic or professional athletes, even when performing at high elevations).

Thus, for untrained persons with sickle trait, there might indeed be a small increase in risk, especially at extremes of exertion and altitude, but under most other circumstances, sickle trait appears to be a benign condition. Some data even suggest that the reason for an occasional sudden death in patients with what appears to be ordinary sickle trait is the undiagnosed presence of an electrophoretically silent hemoglobin variant migrating like hemoglobin A but causing significant sickling in patients heterozygous for hemoglobin S.

If sickle trait is a generally benign condition, then the principal reason for screening adults is to provide genetic counseling. It is important to consider the effectiveness of such counseling. Evidence suggests that identification and counseling of heterozygotes do not alter marriage and parenthood decisions. The individual who does not wish to make such decisions on the basis of carrier status is not likely to benefit from screening. Some families have been traumatized by questions of paternity raised by indiscriminate screening. Because of the confusion among patients and physicians about differences between sickle cell disease and trait, unnecessary anxiety may be the most common result. Surveys have demonstrated that many internists and general practitioners do not sufficiently understand the implications of screening test results to properly counsel patients.

SCREENING AND DIAGNOSTIC TESTS

Screening tests for sickle cell trait are inexpensive and reproducible. Tests for sickling, including the use of 2 percent metabisulfite solution and the more expensive commercial methods, are positive in the presence of hemoglobin S but do not distinguish between homozygotes, heterozygotes, and double heterozygotes (hemoglobin S combined with thalassemia or hemoglobin C). Hemoglobin electrophoresis can also be performed inexpensively, although it is not a substitute for a test of sickling, because some nonsickling hemoglobin variants travel in the same electrophoretic band as hemoglobin S (eg, hemoglobin Lepore). Examining a peripheral blood smear and checking a reticulocyte count provide supportive data for diagnosis of sickle cell disease (see Chapter 79).

A number of techniques have been developed to diagnose sickle cell disease during early gestation of fetuses at risk. Chorionic biopsy has been used successfully to identify sickle cell disease during the first 6 to 8 weeks of pregnancy. The availability of prenatal diagnosis should be explained before screening. Careful counseling must also precede the responsible application of any prenatal diagnostic method. Risks of the procedure to mother and fetus, risks of false-positive and false-negative test results, and acceptability of therapeutic abortion should be discussed.

CONCLUSIONS AND RECOMMENDATIONS

- Sickle cell disease is a serious health hazard that usually presents during early childhood.
- Sickle cell trait is generally a benign condition. Although there is some question of increased relative risk of sudden death in untrained persons required to exert extreme physical effort at very high altitude, absolute risk is extremely low and nil in trained persons.
- Thus, the principal reason for screening adults for the presence of sickle trait is to facilitate genetic counseling.
- Indiscriminate screening followed by inadequate counseling may be harmful and is not likely to provide benefits to the individuals who will not revise marriage and parenthood decisions on the basis of test results.
- Screening for sickle trait should be offered to African-American adults in reproductive age groups. Implications of test results should be fully explained before testing is performed.

A.G.M./A.H.G.

ANNOTATED BIBLIOGRAPHY

Charache S. Sudden death in sickle trait. Am J Med 1988;84:459. *(Editorial summarizing the evidence; concludes risk is very small and clinically unimportant under most circumstances.)*

Farfel MR, Holtzman NA. Education, consent, and counseling in sickle cell screening programs: Report of a survey. Am J Public Health 1984;74:373. *(Of 52,000 persons screened in Maryland during a 1-year period, 25 percent were screened without informed consent.)*

Goossens M, Dumez Y, Kaplan L, et al. Prenatal diagnosis of sickle-cell anemia in the first trimester of pregnancy. N Engl J Med 1983;309:831. *(Earlier diagnosis of sickle cell disease is possible through chorionic biopsy techniques.)*

Kark JA, Posey DM, Schumacher HR, et al. Sickle-cell trait as a risk factor for sudden death in physical training. N Engl J Med 1987;317:781. *(Increased risk of sudden death found among sickle-trait recruits.)*

Kellon DB, Beutler E. Physician attitudes about sickle cell disease and sickle cell trait. JAMA 1974;227:71. *(Finds many primary care practitioners misunderstand the implications of sickle-cell screening.)*

Martin TW, Weisman IM, Zeballos RJ, et al. Exercise and hypoxia increase sickling in venous blood from an exercising limb in individuals with sickle cell trait. Am J Med 1989;87:48. *(At 4000 m, sickling increased significantly in venous blood, but not in arterial blood; oxygen consumption and exercise performance same as for controls.)*

Motulsky AG. Frequency of sickling disorders in U.S. blacks. N Engl J Med 1973;288:31. *(Estimates prevalence of double heterozygotes as well as SS disease at birth [1 in 625 with SS; 1 in 833 with SC; and 1 in 1667 with S-beta-thal] and in the population.)*

Murphy JR. Sickle cell hemoglobin in black football players. JAMA 1973; 225:981. *(Rate of Hb AS among African-American football players in the NFL was 6.7 percent.)*

Petrakis NL, Wiesenfeld SL, Sams BJ, et al. Prevalence of sickle-cell trait and glucose-6-PD-deficiency. N Engl J Med 1970; 282:767. *(An 8.7 percent prevalence of sickle trait among over 4000 San Francisco African Americans.)*

Sears DA. The morbidity of sickle cell trait. Am J Med 1978; 64:1021. *(Extensive review; although certain abnormalities do occur with increased frequency in sickle cell trait, survival is not impaired; 296 references.)*

Weisman IM, Zeballos RG, Johnson BD. Cardiopulmonary and gas exchange responses to acute strenuous exercise at 1270 meters in sickle cell trait. Am J Med 1988;84:377. *(Patients demonstrated normal responses.)*

Whitten CF. Sickle-cell programming—An imperiled promise. N Engl J Med 1973;288:319. *(Lists the arguments against indiscriminate screening.)*

Primary Care Medicine: Office Evaluation and Management of the Adult Patient, 3rd edition, edited by Allan H. Goroll, Lawrence A. May, and Albert G. Mulley, Jr. J.B. Lippincott Company, Philadelphia

79
Evaluation of Anemia

Anemia is a common problem in primary care practice, usually discovered in the context of routine testing or the evaluation of a specific complaint. It is not a diagnosis but rather a sign of underlying disease, particularly in men and nonmenstruating, nonpregnant women, in whom readily detectable pathology is found in over 50 percent of cases.

Because anemia is defined as a reduction in hematocrit or hemoglobin concentration, its definition is necessarily quantitative and arbitrary. Mean hematocrit or hemoglobin concentrations vary widely, depending on age distribution, gender, and altitude of residence of the populations tested. However, World Health Organization criteria for anemia based on hemoglobin concentration have become widely accepted in recent years: adult males below 13 g per deciliter; menstruating women, below 12 g per deciliter; pregnant women, below 11 g per deciliter. Such arbitrary cut-off values are essential for population-based studies, but the physician should recognize that they may have little meaning for the individual patient. The physician must also keep in mind that anemia is defined in terms of concentration. If plasma volume is expanded, a spurious diagnosis of anemia may be made when the total red cell mass and hemoglobin are normal. If plasma volume is contracted, a true anemia may be masked.

PATHOPHYSIOLOGY AND CLINICAL PRESENTATION

The pathogenesis of anemia is conceptually straightforward. There may be *blood loss, inadequate production,* or *excessive destruction;* often two or more mechanisms are operating simultaneously. Decreased production occurs when there are defects in stem cell proliferation or differentiation, deoxyribonucleic acid (DNA) synthesis, hemoglobin synthesis, or a combination of these deficiencies. Excessive destruction can result from membrane disorders, abnormal hemoglobins, enzyme deficiencies, and a host of extrinsic problems such as mechanical disruption or antibody-mediated injury.

Clinical presentation of the patient with anemia depends on abruptness of onset, severity, age, and ability of the cardiopulmonary system to compensate for the decrease in blood volume and oxygen-carrying capacity. When onset is gradual, symptoms may be minimal due to adequate time for compensatory adjustments to decreased hemoglobin. Important responses to anemia include an increase in 2,3-DPG (facilitating oxygen delivery to tissues) and expansion of the plasma volume.

There are few symptoms when the hematocrit is above 30, the anemia is gradual in onset, and the patient is otherwise healthy. However, if the hematocrit falls further, dyspnea and mild fatigue may begin to appear after strenuous exertion. Greater reductions in hematocrit result in cardiopulmonary symptoms that come with less activity. Age and cardiopulmonary reserve are also important determinants of symptoms. A potpourri of nonspecific complaints frequently accompanies anemia, including headache, tinnitus, poor concentration, palpitations, vague abdominal discomfort, anorexia, nausea, and diarrhea or constipation. Tachycardia and diminished peripheral resistance occur as the hemoglobin falls below 7.5 g per 100 mL; a systolic flow murmur due to high output is common. Pallor is an obvious finding best seen in the conjunctivae, but it is of little help in judging severity.

More specific clinical findings depend on the etiology, which can best be classified on the basis of red cell morphology (as determined by appearance on a Wright-stained peripheral smear or by autoanalyzer determinations of mean corpuscular volume (MCV) and degree of anisocytosis).

Microcytic Anemias

Iron deficiency results from inadequate dietary intake, inadequate absorption, or excessive blood loss. In mild cases the relation between the anemia and symptoms is tenuous. Fatigue, headache, and irritability are frequently noted by women with iron deficiency, but a community study of 295 anemic patients showed no correlation between symptoms and hemoglobin concentration. The headache, paresthesias, and burning tongue sometimes occurring in this condition have been thought to be caused by low tissue levels of cellular iron. Double-blind studies examining the effect of iron versus placebo in relieving symptoms are conflicting. Menorrhagia is another complaint attributed by some investigators to instances of iron deficiency, but this is disputed by others. Pica and dysphagia (due to an esophageal web) are classic, although rare, features today.

The physical findings that occur in iron deficiency are a bit more specific than are symptoms. Atrophic glossitis is commonly found, as is cheilitis. Koilonychia, with spooning, ridging, and thinning, is rare. Other physical findings and symptoms are manifestations of the underlying cause.

The earliest laboratory changes are depletion of marrow iron stores and a corresponding fall in serum ferritin. These are followed by a decrease in serum iron and an increase in transferrin, producing in many cases a reduction in the percent transferrin saturation to below 16 percent. The first change in the peripheral blood is a drop in the hematocrit and hemoglobin. An anisocytosis develops (manifested by an elevation in the red cell distribution width [RDW]). Later, with increasing severity of anemia (hemoglobin below 9 g per 100 mL), red cells become microcytic and eventually hypochromic.

Chronic blood loss is the most frequent cause of iron deficiency in adults. Malabsorption of iron and inadequate dietary intake are seldom major factors, although heavy antacid use and gastrectomy can inhibit iron uptake. Most menstruating women show depletion of iron stores, because the equivalent of 20 mg of iron is lost each month, and 500 mg iron is lost with each pregnancy, whereas daily normal iron intake provides only 1 mg. Long-distance runners have been shown to lose enough blood in their gastrointestinal (GI) tracts to produce iron deficiency anemia.

Anemia of chronic disease is a common accompaniment of chronic inflammatory disease and malignancy. In many instances, there is trapping of iron by activated macrophages, rendering the iron unavailable for erythropoesis. In addition, there is often some suppression of erythropoesis by humoral substances (interleukins, tumor necrosis factor, prostaglandins) elaborated in the course of the underlying chronic disease process. Interestingly, erythropoetin is inappropriately low in almost all cases. The anemia is usually moderate, with hemoglobin levels in the 7 to 11 g per deciliter range. Both serum iron and iron-binding capacity are reduced. The smear is most often normocytic but can be hypochromic and even microcytic, mimicking iron deficiency. The serum iron falls before anemia sets in; percent transferrin saturation may be less than 16 percent, again simulating iron deficiency. However, marrow iron stores and ferritin are normal or increased.

Another important anemia of chronic disease is that associated with *human immunodeficiency virus (HIV) infection,* which affects the bone marrow. Myelofibrosis occurs. Anemia is seen in about 15 percent of asymptomatic HIV-positive persons, in 45 percent with acquired immunodeficiency syndrome (AIDS)-related complex, and in 75 percent of those with untreated AIDS. For unknown reasons, erythropoetin is inappropriately low. The smear in most is normochromic-normocytic. Rouleaux formation due to circulating immune complexes sometimes develops, but hemolysis is uncommon. The anemia can be exacerbated by medications used in the treatment of HIV infection (zidovudine, pentamidine, trimethoprim, sulfonamides). Zidovudine is especially marrow toxic, causing anemia in about 30 percent of instances. Neutropenia and thrombocytopenia occur to a lesser extent. Patients most susceptible to the adverse hematologic effects of zidovudine are those with a low CD4 count, preexisting anemia, concurrent vitamin B_{12} deficiency, or neutropenia.

Thalassemia minor (thalassemia trait) is typically detected in asymptomatic patients undergoing an evaluation for a microcytic hypochromic anemia that does not respond to iron. A gene defect leads to impaired red cell maturation by causing an excess of either alpha or beta chains of hemoglobin to accumulate. The most prevalent form is beta-thalassemia trait, common among persons of Mediterranean ancestry. It associated with an increase in hemoglobin A_2. There are no characteristic physical findings. The red cell count is elevated, and the smear may reveal target cells, basophilic stippling, polychromatophilia, poikilocytosis, and anisocytosis in addition to microcytosis. Alpha thalassemia trait is seen among African Americans. The hemoglobin A_2 level is normal, but there is a mild anemia, hypochromia, and microcytosis.

Sideroblastic anemias are a heterogeneous set of disorders, including a primary type, which may be a preleukemic state; a congenital pyridoxine-responsive variant; and other variants associated with rheumatoid arthritis, polyarteritis, malabsorption, chronic alcoholism, cancer, porphyria, lead poisoning, and true pyridoxine deficiency. These, too, are conditions of abnormal red cell maturation. They can lead to significant anemia requiring repeated transfusion of red cells. Their hallmark is accumulation of nonheme iron within the mitochondria of the red cell. When stained for iron, immature red cells demonstrate a ring of stain around the nucleus (ringed sideroblasts). In the primary type, patients are typically over age 60 and may be on the way toward developing a myelodysplastic condition; liver or spleen are palpable in over 50 percent. The smear may be macrocytic, microcytic, or dimorphic. Cells can be hypochromic, leading to confusion with iron deficiency. Anisocytosis and poikilocytosis are pronounced. Serum iron is elevated, as is percent transferrin saturation. Marrow iron stains show many abnormal ringed sideroblasts.

Macrocytic Anemias

Vitamin B_{12} deficiency results most frequently from reduced gastric production of intrinsic factor, as occurs in pernicious anemia. The more than chance association with Hashimoto's thyroiditis and vitiligo has suggested an autoimmune mechanism. Blind loop syndrome, total gastrectomy, and terminal ileal disease are other causes. Dietary lack is rare, because vitamin B_{12} is available in everyday foods and body stores can hold up to a 3-year reserve. Onset is gradual. In pernicious anemia, symptoms usually become evident in the sixth decade. Sore tongue and numbness and tingling in the extremities are classic presentations, but anorexia, diarrhea, and other GI complaints may predominate. The neurologic manifestations are due to defects in maintenance of myelin integrity. They also include disturbances of position and vibratory sense (due to lesions in the posterior columns of the spinal cord), and incoordination, spasticity, and up-going toes (indicative of damage to the corticospinal tract). This neurologic syndrome of subacute combined degeneration is uncommon but may present in the absence of anemia as may memory loss, depression, and irritability.

By the time the anemia is discovered, it may be severe. Hypersegmented polymorphonuclear leukocytes are an early finding specific for the megaloblastic anemias. Oval macrocytes are also characteristic, although poikilocytosis is considerable. Classically, the MCV rises above 100, and the serum B_{12} falls below 100 pg per milliliter, but in up to a third of cases macrocytosis may be absent or the vitamin B_{12} level may be greater than 100. Macrocytosis may be absent if there is concurrent iron deficiency, but the hypersegmented polymorphonuclear leukocytes persist. In pernicious anemia, achlorhydria is found on stimulation testing.

Folate deficiency is more likely to follow inadequate dietary intake than is vitamin B_{12} deficiency, because body stores are limited to a 3-month reserve. Poor intake due to chronic alcohol abuse is the classic case. Increased demand sometimes occurs, as in pregnancy, hemolysis, malignancy, or severe psoriasis. Decreased uptake due to malabsorption or drugs (eg, phenytoin, other anticonvulsants) also can trigger the anemia. The same is true for folate antagonists such as methotrexate, trimethoprim, and triamterene. Hematologic features resemble those of vitamin B_{12} deficiency; there are no neurologic deficits.

Liver disease is responsible for a host of anemias, especially when accompanied by alcoholism and poor diet. It accounts for many macrocytic cases. Folate deficiency, marrow suppression, hypersplenism, bleeding, and bile salt alteration of the red cell membrane all contribute. The smear shows considerable poikilocytosis with spiculated red cells and some macrocytes; if folate deficiency occurs, a megaloblastic picture is superimposed.

Sideroblastic Anemia. (See above.)

Normochromic-Normocytic Anemias

Hemolytic anemias are a diverse group. Inherited forms are due to intrinsic red cell defects; acquired types depend primarily on extra-erythrocytic mechanisms such as immunologic or mechanical injury. Clinical presentations vary according to rate of destruction, compensatory adaptations, and underlying etiology. Jaundice sets in when the liver's capacity to conjugate the excess bilirubin from hemoglobin breakdown is exceeded; the serum level of unconjugated bilirubin climbs. Splenomegaly evolves as trapping of damaged red cells progresses. Sudden fever, chills, headache, back and abdominal pain, and hemoglobinuria characterize severe acute hemolysis.

The reticulocyte count is elevated unless there is an accompanying marrow defect. The peripheral smear usually appears normochromic-normocytic, but may be macrocytic due to release of immature forms during rapid red cell destruction and regeneration. Polychromatophilia is common, and nucleated red cells, stippling, schistocytes, and Howell-Jolly bodies may be noted. Spherocytes occur in *hereditary spherocytosis,* a condition of reduced cell membrane area resulting from a defect in synthesis of the membrane protein spectrin.

Sickle cell disease is the most prevalent hemolytic condition in the African-American population. *Sickle cell trait* is asymptomatic and anemia is absent, although mild hematuria due to sickling in the hypertonic renal medulla sometimes occurs. The peripheral smear is normal except for an occasional target cell. Hemoglobin electrophoresis reveals less than 50 percent of total hemoglobin to be of the S variety.

Patients homozygous for the sickle cell gene suffer *sickle cell anemia,* a much more serious condition characterized by painful crises precipitated by stress (especially infection).

Intravascular sickling ensues, the red cells become rigid, and vasoocclusion may result leading to arterial desaturation, hemolysis, and organ damage. Leg ulcers, hepatomegaly, hematuria, renal concentrating defects, and mild jaundice commonly occur. Patients report acute, severe pain in the lower extremities, back, or abdomen. Fever and leukocytosis may be present as well. Attacks typically last from a few hours to a few days, then resolve spontaneously. Aplastic crises develop when there is a concurrent illness that suppresses erythropoiesis. The smear is normochromic; sickled cells may be noted as well as target forms. Hemoglobin electrophoresis reveals a predominance of hemoglobin S. Addition of a reducing agent, such as metabisulfite, to a drop of blood causes the cells to sickle within a few minutes and confirms the diagnosis.

The red cell enzyme defect *glucose-6-phosphate dehydrogenase (G6PD) deficiency* is a sex-linked condition compromising the enzyme that maintains hemoglobin in an unoxidized state. In its episodic form seen in African Americans, hemolysis develops after exposure to oxidant compounds (sulfonamides, antimalarials) or infection. A chronic variety occurs in persons of Mediterranean ancestry.

Most *drug-induced hemolytic anemias* manifest an immune mechanism: adsorption to the red cell of drug–antibody complexes (quinidine); drug adsorption to the red cell forming a hapten, followed by binding of antidrug antibody (high-dose penicillin); or induction of a red cell "autoantibody" (long-term methyldopa). The hallmark of most drug-related hemolytic episodes is a positive direct Coombs' test. Withdrawal of the offending agent ends the process.

Autoimmune hemolytic anemias result from patients producing antibodies against their own red cells and are classified according to the type of antibody produced (IgG or IgM). Those of the *IgG class* are directed against the Rh antigen. Many are idiopathic; others occur in the context of lymphoma, lupus, or chronic lymphocytic leukemia. The diagnosis is made by detecting IgG and C3b proteins on the red cell surface. Macrophages that can detect these proteins bind the involved red cells. Hemolysis is mostly extravascular. The red cells are cleared by the spleen. The *IgM* form of autoimmune hemolytic anemia is a cold hemagglutinin condition. These antibodies are seen with mycoplasmal, Epstein-Barr virus (EBV) or cytomegalovirus (CMV) infection and with lymphoproliferative conditions. Cold agglutinin titers are markedly elevated in the setting of hemolysis (> 1:1000).

Aplastic anemias are usually idiopathic but may be linked to a marrow toxin (cytotoxic drugs, radiation), an idiosyncratic drug reaction (chloramphenicol, gold, sulfur compounds, carbamazepine) or a viral infection (hepatitis B, hepatitis C, CMV, HIV, parvovirus). Onset is gradual, with fatigue and bleeding noted first; infection is a later problem. There is no organomegaly. The smear appears normochromic-normocytic, but the number of platelets is diminished. There are no signs of increased red cell production. The reticulocyte count is zero, and a pancytopenia is present.

Renal Failure. The anemia of chronic renal failure is due to reduction in both production and survival or red cells. Lack of erythropoietin and metabolic injury to erythrocytes are postulated mechanisms. The severity of the anemia parallels the degree of azotemia. The smear is normochromic-normocytic; burr cells are sometimes prominent.

Hypothyroidism is associated with a number of anemic states. The most common is a mild normochromic-normocytic anemia. Iron deficiency may occur secondary to heavy menstrual bleeding. Also, a macrocytic picture that clears after administration of exogenous thyroid hormone is sometimes encountered. A true megaloblastic anemia due to vitamin B_{12} deficiency occurs in about 10 percent of hypothyroid patients with a macrocytic smear; the relation between hypothyroidism and pernicious anemia is unresolved, but an autoimmune mechanism is postulated.

Anemia of Chronic Disease. (See above.)

DIFFERENTIAL DIAGNOSIS

A practical method for organizing the many causes of anemia is to group them according to 1) the appearance of the Wright-stained smear of the peripheral blood; and 2) the electronically determined red cell indices. This method allows for classification of etiologies into normochromic-normocytic, hypochromic-microcytic, and macrocytic categories (Table 79–1) and facilitates workup.

The majority of patients who present with anemia have iron deficiency. In a London general practice, 95 percent of women and 50 percent of men with anemia had iron deficiency. In males and the elderly, this is likely to be due to occult bleeding from an underlying lesion. In the London

Table 79-1. Differential Diagnosis of Anemia (Representative Etiologies)

Microcytic (MCV < 80)
1. Iron deficiency
2. Anemia of chronic disease
3. Thalassemia trait
4. Sideroblastic anemia

Normocytic (MCV 80–100)
1. Hemolysis
   a. Drug-induced
   b. Autoimmune (idiopathic, collagen disease, lymphoma)
   c. Cold agglutinin-induced (viral infection, lymphoma)
   d. Hemoglobinopathy (sickle cell disease; G6PD deficiency)
   e. Hereditary spherocytosis
   f. Microangiopathy (heart valve, jogging, vasculitis, DIC).
2. Chronic disease, including HIV infection
3. Renal failure
4. Hypothyroidism
5. Myelofibrosis
6. Early stage of iron deficiency
7. Sideroblastic anemia
8. Mixed anemia (eg, iron and vitamin B_{12} deficiencies)

Macrocytic (MCV > 100)
1. Vitamin B_{12} deficiency
2. Folate deficiency
3. Aplastic anemia
4. Acute hemolysis or hemorrhage with brisk reticulocytosis
5. Chronic liver disease
6. Myelodysplastic syndromes
7. Hypothyroidism, severe

study, 95 percent of men with iron deficiency had blood loss from a GI source. In a British study of anemia in the elderly, 110 patients over age 65 who presented with anemia were evaluated; 70 percent had iron deficiency and about half had evidence of GI blood loss. In 40 percent of these cases, the etiology was listed as "undetermined," but many patients did not undergo full work-up because of advanced age. Prevalence of iron deficiency anemia among premenopausal women is conservatively estimated to be 15 percent, rising to well over 30 percent during pregnancy.

In the London survey, anemia was attributed to chronic disease in 4 percent (probably an underestimate) and to vitamin B_{12} deficiency in 8 percent. The British study of elderly patients reported 14 percent had folate deficiency and 9 percent had a low vitamin B_{12} level.

WORKUP

Diagnosis and Morphologic Categorization of Anemia

The diagnosis of anemia is based on measurement of the *hematocrit* or *hemoglobin concentration* of venous blood. Any abnormal test result needs to be repeated for confirmation before further evaluation is undertaken. Proper interpretation requires consideration of the patient's *intravascular volume status*. An overly expanded plasma volume will dilute the red cell mass and lead to a false-positive diagnosis. Conversely, dehydration can mask an underlying anemia.

Morphologic categorization helps focus the subsequent evaluation, which proceeds according to whether the anemia is micro-, macro-, or normocytic. Examination of the Wright-stained *peripheral blood smear* and autoanalyzer-determined *red cell indices* (MCV, mean corpuscular hemoglobin concentration [MCHC]) are the time-tested means of classifying anemias morphologically. Recent advances in flow cytometry have made possible an automated means of determining how much variability there is in the size of the patient's red cells. This measure of anisocytosis is referred to as the *red cell distribution width (RDW)*. Technically, the RDW is the coefficient of variation of cell volume; it serves as a means of detecting red cell heterogeneity, previously available only by examination of the peripheral smear. Although examination of the Wright-stained smear still provides morphologic information unattainable from other sources, the combined use of the MCV and RDW for initial classification of anemias markedly enhances interpretation based red cell indices (Table 79–2).

The peripheral smear and red cell indices should be examined in conjunction with one another; they provide complementary information. Overdependence on machine-generated indices can lead to errors in diagnosis. For example, anemia due to both iron and vitamin B_{12} deficiencies often produces a dimorphic population of microcytic and macrocytic red cells readily observed on peripheral smear, yet the electronically determined mean corpuscular red cell volume will calculate the average size and erroneously suggest a normocytic type of anemia. Moreover, some vitamin B_{12}-deficient patients with normal ferritin have normocytic indices.

The Wright-stained smear can also mislead when used alone, and it often lacks sensitivity. Cells that easily flatten

Table 79-2. Classification of Anemias by Use of Data from Automated Cytometry

MCV < 80 MICROCYTOSIS	MCV 80–100 NORMOCYTOSIS	MCV > 100 MACROCYTOSIS
Low RDW		
Anemia of chronic disease	Hypoproliferation (*eg*, renal failure)	Aplastic anemias
Most thalassemias	Hereditary spherocytosis	Myelodysplastic syndromes
	Anemia of chronic disease	
High RDW		
Iron deficiency	Sickle cell disease	Megaloblastic anemias
Sideroblastic anemia	Early iron deficiency	Acute hemolysis or hemorrhage
Hemoglobin H	Marrow infiltration Chronic hemolysis	Liver disease

out (as in liver disease) may appear larger on smear than they actually are; the MCV will give a more correct determination of size. The sensitivity of the smear in detection of iron deficiency has been found to be as low as 49 percent.

Determination of red cell size on the peripheral smear is facilitated by using the nucleus of the mature small lymphocyte as a good reference standard for normal red cell diameter. One can also make a control smear of known blood to help judge abnormalities. Use of the MCV and appearance on peripheral smear serves to classify the anemia morphologically and to facilitate evaluation.

Not all automatically determined cell indices have proven valuable. Careful studies suggest that the MCHC and the mean corpuscular hemoglobin (MCH) add little to the evaluation of anemia, although the MCHC still is used as a means of quantifying degree of hypochromia.

Workup by Morphologic Category—Microcytic Anemia

The basis for classification of microcytosis is the presence of small red blood cells on smear and an MCV below 82. A prime consideration should be iron deficiency and the important underlying conditions that might precipitate it, but thalassemia, anemia of chronic disease are also important to consider, and sometimes sideroblastic anemias.

History should focus on any abnormal blood loss, change in bowel habits, melena, heavy aspirin or nonsteroidal antiinflammatory drug (NSAID) use, family history of anemia (especially in those of Mediterranean descent), concurrent malignancy, HIV infection, symptoms of other chronic infections or chronic inflammatory disorders, number of pregnancies, pica, dysphagia, history of lead exposure, dietary iron intake, quantity of menstrual blood loss, gastric resection, changes in nails, and soreness of the tongue. *Physical examination* includes checking for glossitis, cheilitis, koilonychia, lymphadenopathy, hepatosplenomegaly, rectal mass, guaiac positivity, pelvic mass, and other signs of chronic infectious, inflammatory, and neoplastic disorders.

Laboratory results usually allow one to differentiate iron deficiency, thalassemia, sideroblastic anemia, and anemia of chronic disease, although some overlap does occur and may cause confusion and wasteful expenditures if tests are not thoughtfully selected.

Testing for Iron Deficiency. Recent studies confirm that the test of choice for screening and diagnosis of iron deficiency is the *serum ferritin*. It is the storage protein for iron and correlates best with marrow iron stores. Levels are somewhat higher in men than women and increase gradually with advancing age. The test is highly sensitive and specific for the diagnosis of iron deficiency. For example, a serum concentration of less than 15 g per liter has a predictive value for iron deficiency of greater than 90 percent when pretest probability is only 50 percent. A level greater than 100 g per liter virtually rules out the diagnosis.

Ferritin is also an acute-phase reactant that rises in response to inflammatory disease or hepatocellular dysfunction, potentially limiting its diagnostic utility in these settings. However, a serum ferritin below 50 g per liter in the setting of inflammatory or liver disease retains much of the test's predictive value for iron deficiency. Levels between 50 and 100 constitute a diagnostic "gray zone," necessitating careful attention to other clinical data for an accurate diagnosis. One can resort to determinations of serum iron and iron-binding capacity, bone marrow aspiration, or a diagnostic trial.

Measurements of *serum iron* and *total iron-binding capacity (TIBC)* have been traditional components of the workup for iron deficiency, but, under most circumstances, they add little information beyond that obtained from the ferritin determination and they lack its sensitivity or specificity. These tests need not be ordered routinely in patients with microcytic anemia. Nonetheless, *percent transferrin saturation* [(Fe/TIBC) × 100] of less than 16 has been used as a criterion for iron deficiency. However, the specificity of the test is limited by the finding that some patients with the anemia of chronic disease also have percent saturations that fall below 16 percent. The more typical pattern in anemia of chronic disease is a low iron and low TIBC in contrast to the low iron and increased TIBC characteristic of iron deficiency.

Bone marrow aspiration and examination of a sample stained for iron is the "gold standard" for diagnosis of iron deficiency, but up to 20 percent of aspirates are unsatisfactory, yielding insufficient marrow stroma. Ferritin testing has all but eliminated the need for marrow aspiration in the diagnosis of iron deficiency, but the test is sometimes necessary in confusing cases.

A *therapeutic trial* of oral iron therapy can also be used in the uncomplicated case as a simple alternative to ferritin level or marrow examination. The reticulocyte count is monitored over a 7- to 10-day period. A significant rise in the reticulocyte count is strong evidence for the diagnosis of iron deficiency.

Once iron deficiency is confirmed, the question of an occult gastrointestinal (GI) lesion arises, especially if the source of blood loss is not readily evident. Such idiopathic iron deficiency anemia is associated with a GI tract lesion in about two-thirds of cases. The most common upper GI lesion is peptic ulcer; colon cancer is the leading colonic lesion in this setting. Site-specific symptoms are predictive of the lesion's location. Concomitant lesions are present in less than 1 percent of cases, making it unnecessary to study both upper and lower GI tracts if a likely source is found on the first examination. Endoscopy is the test methodology of choice. Barium studies are considerably less sensitive, and their yield is nil in the setting of a negative endoscopic evaluation.

The vast majority of patients with no detectible lesion by upper and lower GI endoscopy have a favorable prognosis. Most respond to iron therapy. Those who do not are likely to have an underlying medical illness.

Testing for Thalassemia. If iron deficiency has been ruled out, the focus shifts to differentiating among anemia of chronic disease, thalassemia, and sideroblastic anemia. History is very important in this regard. A person of Mediterranean extraction without underlying chronic illness is likely to have thalassemia trait, necessitating a look at the *peripheral smear* for abnormalities of red cell morphology (eg, target cells, poikilocytosis) and a check of the *red cell count* for erythrocytosis. A *hemoglobin* A_2 level is ordered in such patients to confirm the diagnosis, but it may not be elevated if there is concurrent iron deficiency. A *hemoglobin electrophoresis* may be needed for the African-American patient suspected of thalassemia trait, because hemoglobin A_2 is not increased in alpha disease.

Differentiating Anemia of Chronic Disease from Sideroblastic Anemia. Once iron deficiency and thalassemia trait are deemed to be of low probability, then the task shifts to differentiating anemia of chronic disease from sideroblastic anemia. Here, the serum iron and TIBC may be of help. In the anemia of chronic disease, the serum iron and percent transferrin saturation are likely to be below normal or reduced; in sideroblastic anemia, both are often increased, as is the serum ferritin. Such an increase in the absence of another reason for iron overload suggests a sideroblastic state and the need for a bone marrow aspirate to search for ringed sideroblasts. To summarize:

1. The serum ferritin is the test of choice for iron deficiency; determinations of the serum iron, TIBC, and percent saturation are less diagnostic and need not be ordered routinely for the evaluation of suspected iron deficiency.
2. Examination of a peripheral smear (target cells, teardrops), and determinations of red cell count (for erythrocytosis) and hemoglobin A_2 level are indicated for the person suspected of thalassemia.
3. If iron deficiency and thalassemia have been ruled out, a transferrin saturation can help differentiate anemia of chronic disease from sideroblastic anemia. If both are elevated, a bone marrow aspirate should be considered for identification of ringed sideroblasts.

Macrocytic Anemia

The criteria for inclusion in this group are a MCV greater than 95, a normal MCHC, and macrocytes on smear. (Often the latter are hard to detect in mild cases.) Marked macrocytosis identified electronically is clinically significant. For example, in a study of 100 patients with MCV greater than 115, over half had folate or vitamin B_{12} deficiency; another 25 percent had liver disease or alcoholism accompanied by liver disease.

Megaloblastic versus Nonmegaloblastic. The first objective is to distinguish megaloblastic from nonmegaloblastic causes. The *peripheral smear* is the single most helpful test. Hypersegmented polymorphonuclear leukocytes (having nuclei with five or more lobes) are among the earliest and most specific signs of a megaloblastic anemia, seen in over 65 percent of cases. Oval macrocytes are also an early and characteristic finding but may be absent in the setting of concurrent iron deficiency. An increase in hypersegmented polymorphonuclear leukocytes can be screened for by counting the number of neutrophils with five or more lobes in a routine 100-cell differential. Finding three neutrophils with five lobes or even one with six is strong presumptive evidence for megaloblastic anemia.

Bone marrow aspiration may be needed in confusing situations (such as differentiating a sideroblastic anemia from a truly megaloblastic type or searching for megaloblastic changes in a patient with a low normal B_{12}), but in most instances a peripheral smear suffices. It must be remembered that megaloblastic marrow changes can revert to normal within 12 to 24 hours of therapy, and thus treatment should be delayed if marrow examination is anticipated. However, neutrophil hypersegmentation may persist for up to 2 weeks after initiation of vitamin replacement.

Folate versus Vitamin B_{12} Deficiency. Having identified a megaloblastic anemia, the focus shifts to folate versus vitamin B_{12} deficiency. History and physical examination can give important clues. A history of gastric surgery, inflammatory bowel disease, hypothyroidism, or raw fish intake (fish tapeworm) may provide the substrate for vitamin B_{12} deficiency. Neuropsychiatric symptoms and signs as well as those of subacute combined system disease further suggest vitamin B_{12} deficiency, as do the findings of vitiligo and glossitis. Alcoholism, poor nutrition, pregnancy, blood dyscrasias, sprue, severe psoriasis, and anticonvulsant intake suggest folate lack. Antimetabolite therapy with folate antagonists such as methotrexate can cause a megaloblastic picture with normal serum folate levels.

Obviously, *serum folate* and *vitamin B_{12}* determinations are helpful, but there are a number of pitfalls in interpreting the results. The bioassay for vitamin B_{12} is affected by recent antibiotic intake. Assays using radioactive cobalt or immunologic techniques are free of such interference. However, up to a third of patients with documented pernicious anemia will have vitamin B_{12} levels above 100 ng per liter (the oft-cited cut-off for diagnosis). Persistence in pursuing the diagnosis is necessary when clinical suspicion is high. Finally, vitamin B_{12} levels may be artificially low in patients with folate deficiency alone; folate and vitamin B_{12} levels must always be measured together. Recent green vegetable intake can cause a false rise in the serum folate level. Concomitant measurement of serum and red cell folate is needed to establish the diagnosis of a true folate deficiency. Serum measurements of *methylmalonic acid* and *total homocysteine* are becoming available and helpful in cases where the serum vitamin B_{12} or folate result is confusing: an increase in methylmalonate alone occurs in both vitamin B_{12} and folate deficiencies; both methylmalonate and total homocysteine are increased in vitamin B_{12} deficiency.

An empirical means of determining vitamin B_{12} or folate deficiency is to conduct a *therapeutic trial* of replacement therapy. Such a trial is appropriate when serum assays are unavailable or the results are equivocal. The hematocrit and reticulocyte counts are measured twice before administration, then followed every few days up to 10 days after a small but effective dose of vitamin B_{12} (eg, 100 μg IM) or folate (1 mg IM) is given. The trial is positive if a significant rise in reticulocyte count occurs within 10 days. It is important to use only small folate doses in such trials. Large folate doses can transiently and nonspecifically improve the hematologic picture in a patient with vitamin B_{12} deficiency and lead to its worsening by obscuring the diagnosis.

To distinguish vitamin B_{12} deficiency due to malabsorption from that due to lack of intrinsic factor, an *oral Schilling test* with and without intrinsic factor is used. An unlabeled intramuscular dose of 1000 μg of vitamin B_{12} is given to saturate binding sites. Then an oral dose of radioactive vitamin B_{12} without intrinsic factor is given, and both urine and plasma samples are taken to determine the amount of vitamin B_{12} absorbed. The test is repeated with the addition of intrinsic factor. In malabsorptive states, there will be no improvement with intrinsic factor, whereas there will be in pernicious anemia. One difficulty with the test is that vitamin B_{12} deficiency can cause malabsorption, confusing test interpretation. Thus, the test should be postponed until the deficiency is corrected. In addition, sensitivity is not very high; false-negative results occur in up to 30 percent to 40 percent of cases. The ability to assay the serum for *antiintrinsic factor antibody* presents an opportunity to test more directly for pernicious anemia; specificity is high so long as no vitamin B_{12} is injected within 48 hours of testing. There is no reliable test widely available for determining folate malabsorption.

Nonmegaloblastic macrocytic anemias can be divided into subgroups according to whether marrow activity is increased, normal, or decreased. To make this determination, a *reticulocyte count* is obtained. The normal range is 0.8 percent to 2.5 percent in males and 0.8 percent to 4.1 percent in females. To correct for the degree of anemia, the reticulocyte count is multiplied by the hematocrit and divided by 0.45. Increased reticulocytes are due to hemorrhage or hemolysis. Low normal or decreased counts occur in myxedema and liver disease. Marked reductions may occur in myelophthisic states and sideroblastic anemia. The patient should be questioned and examined carefully for symptoms of any of these conditions, and the smear should be studied again. In myelophthisic processes, there may be a particularly large number of teardrops on peripheral smear. A *bone marrow biopsy* is indicated when the reticulocyte count is low and there is concern about a sideroblastic anemia or a myelophthisic process.

To summarize:

1. Peripheral smear is examined for hypersegmented polymorphonuclear leukocytes and oval macrocytes.

2. If they are present, serum B_{12} and folate levels are ordered.
3. Alternatively, a diagnostic trial of a small dose of vitamin B_{12} or folate can be performed, monitoring reticulocyte count.
4. When vitamin B_{12} deficiency is detected, a Schilling test is helpful to differentiate between lack of intrinsic factor and malabsorption.
5. The reticulocyte count and peripheral smear examination are important to evaluation of nonmegaloblastic macrocytic cases; bone marrow biopsy is indicated if a sideroblastic or myelophthisic process is suspected.

Normochromic-Normocytic Anemia

This category encompasses a diverse group of conditions that can be classified according to marrow response as manifested by the *reticulocyte count.*

Elevated reticulocyte count suggests hemolysis or recent hemorrhage. If there is no evidence of recent brisk bleeding, then evidence of hemolysis and its precipitants should be sought. The history is reviewed thoroughly for medications (penicillins, cephalosporins, sulfa drugs, quinidine, methyl dopa), symptoms of sickle cell disease, family history of anemia, and symptoms of a viral infection (mononucleosis, CMV, viral hepatitis), lymphoproliferative disease, or systemic lupus. During physical examination the patient is checked for splenomegaly and signs of an underlying viral, lymphoproliferative, or connective tissue disease (see Chapters 12, 84, and 156). The laboratory assessment includes a check of hemolytic indices: *bilirubin, haptoglobin,* and *lactic dehydrogenase* (LDH). Haptoglobin is the most sensitive, but least specific due to its being an acute phase reactant. LDH and unconjugated bilirubin are less sensitive, but more specific for significant hemolysis. In a patient taking a potentially offending drug, a *direct Coombs' test* should be undertaken to assess the possibility of drug-related hemolysis. A drug-related or infection-related episode in an African-American patient should also raise the question of G6PD deficiency, especially when the drug is a sulfonamide or an antimalarial. An African-American patient presenting with painful episodes of hemolysis should have a smear examined, a *hemoglobin electrophoresis* obtained, and a *metabisulfite test* for sickling of red cells. If an underlying lymphoproliferative disorder or connective tissue disease is detected, then consideration of an immune hemolytic anemia is appropriate and a sampling of the blood for *IgG autoantibodies* is indicated. Concurrent viral infection or lymphoproliferative disease raises the question of an IgM-based hemolytic process and the need to check *cold hemagglutinin* levels. Bone marrow examination in cases of suspected hemolysis is unnecessary.

Reticulocyte count not appropriately elevated is grounds to search for a metabolic cause of marrow suppression, such as renal failure, myxedema, Addison's disease, and alcoholic liver disease. Even early forms of vitamin B_{12} deficiency and iron deficiency may present with relatively normal red cell indices, as can the anemia of chronic disease, necessitating a check for them (see above). If the *peripheral smear* shows considerable numbers of teardrop forms and fragmented cells, suggesting a myelophthisic process, a *bone marrow biopsy* is indicated (an aspiration of the marrow may only yield a dry tap).

A very low or absent reticulocyte count is suggestive of an aplastic anemia, especially if accompanied by evidence of pancytopenia on peripheral smear and cell counts. History of drug use (eg, chloramphenicol, phenylbutazone, antimetabolites, gold, zidovudine, pentamidine), toxin exposure (benzene, insecticides), or recent viral illness may provide a clue to etiology. In the majority of instances, the history is unrevealing. Bone marrow biopsy is indicated if the condition persists after all drugs are halted.

To summarize:

1. The reticulocyte count is checked.
2. If the count is elevated, evidence for recent hemorrhage or hemolysis is sought. Complementary tests for hemolysis include haptoglobin, bilirubin, and LDH. Confirmation of hemolysis leads to a search for a drug-induced etiology (direct Coombs' test), an autoimmune type (IgG or cold agglutinins), or a hemoglobinopathy (sickle-cell disease, G6PD deficiency).
3. If the reticulocyte count is not elevated, a search for underlying renal, endocrine, or liver disease should be undertaken, as well as an evaluation for early iron deficiency anemia, and anemia of chronic disease.
4. If the reticulocyte count is nil and the peripheral blood count and smear show a pancytopenia, or if the peripheral smear shows many teardrop forms and fragmented cells, then a marrow biopsy is necessary, especially if halting potentially offending medications does not result in prompt restoration of marrow function.

SYMPTOMATIC THERAPY

Few patients who present with an anemia of gradual onset require immediate correction of the anemia. The one exception is the patient with significant cardiopulmonary disease who may be compromised by a decrease in oxygen-carrying capacity (ie, hematocrit < 30). In almost all other instances, evaluation should proceed in an orderly manner and therapy should be withheld until a specific diagnosis can be made and a specific therapy can be implemented (see Chapter 82). The exception to this rule is the use of a therapy as a diagnostic trial (eg, vitamin B_{12} replacement). All too common is the practice of simultaneously prescribing multiple hematinics, which obscure important findings and the detection of serious underlying disease. The elderly and others with limited cardiopulmonary reserve should be admitted for inpatient evaluation and consideration of transfusion therapy when they are experiencing dyspnea, angina, or marked fatigue from their anemia.

PATIENT EDUCATION

Many patients think anemia is due to a vitamin or iron deficiency and consequently try self-treatment before seeing a physician. Others request vitamin therapy. A common error among both patients and physicians is to attribute symptoms of depression, such as fatigue and listlessness, to an underlying anemia. Unless the hematocrit is well below 30, or the patient has very little cardiopulmonary reserve, this attribution is unjustified (see Chapter 8). Finally, the patient needs to be told to what extent the anemia accounts for symptoms, what the possible causes are, and what the appropriate workup will be.

A.H.G.

ANNOTATED BIBLIOGRAPHY

Bessman JD, Gilmer PR Jr, Gardner FH. Improved classification of anemias by MCV and RDW. Am J Clin Pathol 1983;80:322. *(Description of the utility of automated cytometry in evaluation of anemia.)*

Beutler E. Glucose-6-phosphate dehydrogenase deficiency. N Engl Med 1991;324:169. *(Authoritative review; 85 references.)*

Beutler E. The common anemias. JAMA 1988;259:2433. *(Good summary of pathophysiology for the generalist reader.)*

Camitta BM, Storb R, Thomas ED. Aplastic anemia: Pathogenesis, diagnosis, treatment and prognosis. N Engl J Med 1982;306:645. *(Comprehensive review.)*

Carmel R. Pernicious anemia. The expected findings of very low serum cobalamin levels, anemia, and macrocytosis are often lacking. Arch Intern Med 1988;148:1712. *(The title says it all.)*

Cash JM, Sears DA. The anemia of chronic disease: Spectrum of associated diseases in a series of unselected hospitalized patients. Am J Med 1989;87:638. *(Although based on an inpatient sample, the spectrum may be wider than previously suspected.)*

Committee on Iron Deficiency. Iron deficiency in the United States. JAMA 1968;203:407. *(Still useful paper on natural history and epidemiology.)*

Crosby WH. Reticulocyte count. Arch Intern Med 1981;141:1747. *(Detailed discussion of this important test and its clinical significance.)*

Edwin E. The segmentation of polymorphonuclear neutrophils in hypovitaminosis B_{12}. Acta Med Scand 1967;182:401. *(Sixty-four percent of patients with vitamin B_{12} deficiency exhibited hypersegmentation on smear. Good discussion of errors in counting lobes.)*

Fry J. Clinical patterns and course of anemias in general practice. Br Med J 1961;2:1732. *(Clinical epidemiology from London general practice.)*

Guyatt GH, Oxman AD, Ali M, et al. Laboratory diagnosis of iron-deficiency anemia. J Gen Intern Med 1992;7:145. *(Detailed literature review; concludes ferritin is the test of choice; 73 references.)*

Huebers HA, Finch CA. Transferrin: Physiologic behavior and clinical implications. Blood 1984;64:763. *(Basic science of transferrin.)*

Rocker DC, Cello JP. Evaluation of the gastrointestinal tract in patients with iron-deficiency anemia. N Engl J Med 1993; 320:1691. *(High prevalence of GI lesions; site-specific symptoms predictive of site; concomitant lesions rare; prospective study.)*

Scadden DT, Zon LI, Groopman JE, et al. Pathophysiology and management of HIV-associated hematologic disorders. Blood 1989;74:1455. *(Excellent review of this increasingly important cause of anemia.)*

Stabler SP, Marcell PD, Podell ER, et al. Elevation of total homocysteine in the serum of patients with cobalamin or folate deficiency detected by chromatography-mass spectrometry. J Clin Invest 1988;81:466. *(New diagnostic approach.)*

Stewart JG, Ahlquist DA, McGill DB, et al. Gastrointestinal blood loss and anemia in runners. Ann Intern Med 1984; 100:843. *(Documents occult blood loss in runners.)*

Taymor M, Sturgis S, Yahia C. The etiological role of chronic iron deficiency in production of menorrhagia. JAMA 1974;187:323. *(Such bleeding may actually be the consequence as well as the cause of iron deficiency.)*

Thompson WG, Babitz L, Cassino C, et al. Evaluation of current criteria used to measure vitamin B_{12} levels. Am J Med 1987;82:291. *(Using an MCV < 95 or a vitamin B_{12} level < 100 may lead to missed diagnoses of true vitamin B_{12} deficiency.)*

Tudhope G, Wilson G. Anemia in hypothyroidism. Q J Med 1960;29:513. *(Classic study of 116 cases of hypothyroidism, revealing anemia in over 30 percent; pernicious anemia occurred in 7 percent.)*

Van der Weyden M, Rother M, Firkin B. Metabolic significance of reduced B_{12} in folate deficiency. Blood 1972;40:23. *(Low vitamin B_{12} levels found in folate deficiency; reduction is moderate and improves with folic acid replacement.)*

Wood M, Elwood P. Symptoms of iron deficiency anemia: A community survey. Br J Prev Soc Med 1966;20:117. *(In 295 patients studied, there was little correlation between symptoms and serum hemoglobin concentration.)*

Zauber NP, Zauber AG. Hematologic data on healthy very old people. JAMA 1987;257:2181. *(Increasing age alone does not cause anemia.)*

Primary Care Medicine: Office Evaluation and Management of the Adult Patient, 3rd edition, edited by Allan H. Goroll, Lawrence A. May, and Albert G. Mulley, Jr. J.B. Lippincott Company, Philadelphia

80
Evaluation of Erythrocytosis (Polycythemia)

An elevated red cell count, hemoglobin concentration, or hematocrit often occurs as an unexpected finding, noted coincidentally on obtaining an automated complete blood count. An absolute increase in circulating red cell mass is termed *erythrocytosis* or *polycythemia* (some use the term *erythrocytosis* for all conditions but those with an autonomous etiology). The upper limit of normal for a hematocrit is 52 percent for males, 47 percent for females. In the context of marked dehydration or severe chronic lung disease, the elevation comes as no surprise. In the absence of obvious concurrent disease, a search for an important underlying illness (eg, polycythemia vera, occult malignancy, right-to-left shunt, hemoglobinopathy) is warranted. The finding may even be spurious. In most instances, the primary physician should be able to distinguish among the variety of etiologies on clinical grounds, aided by a few simple laboratory studies.

PATHOPHYSIOLOGY AND CLINICAL PRESENTATION

Erythrocytosis, as opposed to a relative or spurious increase in hematocrit, is defined as an absolute increase in red cell mass. It may represent a stem cell defect, as in polycythemia vera, a response to hypoxia as in the reactive secondary polycythemias, or a manifestation of renal disease or extrarenal malignancy.

Polycythemia vera is a *myeloproliferative* disorder affecting all marrow elements, although erythrocytosis may be the presenting manifestation. The disease appears to occur secondary to an intrinsic cellular defect and is not dependent on erythropoietin. In fact, as might be expected, erythropoietin is lower in this condition than in any other. Polycythemia vera is characterized by abnormal proliferation of all blood elements in the bone marrow and a similar situation in *extramedullary sites,* producing absolute erythrocytosis, leukocytosis, thrombocytosis, splenomegaly, hyperuricemia, a hypercellular bone marrow and, often, myeloid metaplasia and myelofibrosis. The condition is uncommon, with an incidence in the United States of four to five cases per million per year, or about 1000 new cases per year. However, the prevalence is higher because survival is prolonged in the majority of patients. The peak age of onset is 50 to 60 years.

A small percentage of patients have a relatively benign course, with red-cell volume controlled by occasional phlebotomy, and pruritus and hyperuricemia controlled by medication. However, the disease can evolve into a malignant, disordered condition with the development of myeloid metaplasia, myelofibrosis, and acute leukemia.

It is not surprising that the presence of true polycythemia is often unsuspected, because symptoms develop gradually and are frequently vague and rather nonspecific. In early stages, the patient may be entirely asymptomatic, with an elevated hematocrit being the only manifestation. As the disease progresses, the white blood cell (WBC) and platelet counts also rise, and symptoms ensue as the red cell volume expands. Most symptoms are attributable to *hyperviscosity, hypervolemia,* and consequent sluggish blood flow, which take place when the hematocrit rises above 55. Headache, dizziness, vertigo, tinnitus, fullness of the head, and blurred vision are among the common neurologic symptoms. Patients may complain of angina pectoris or claudication when there is coexisting atherosclerotic disease. Generalized weakness, fatigue, sweating, and lassitude are frequently reported. Gastrointestinal complaints may predominate (eg, fullness, belching, epigastric discomfort). In polycythemia vera, a classic symptom is *pruritus* after bathing, believed due to abnormal histamine release. Also, gouty joint complaints occur in the context of marked secondary hyperuricemia caused by increased cell turnover. Left upper quadrant discomfort is a manifestation of the significant *splenomegaly* usually seen in polycythemia vera.

Bleeding may occur due to disturbed hemostasis that is a consequence of hyperviscosity and defects in platelet function. Patients may present with bleeding in uncommon sites, such as hepatic, mesenteric, or retinal veins, or with bleeding in the form of epistaxis, menorrhagia, easy bruisability, or oozing from the gums.

On examination, the patient has a deep red appearance; peripheral cyanosis and ecchymoses may be noted. Blood pressure is usually normal. Hepatomegaly is present in 40 percent and splenomegaly in 70 percent.

In about 60 percent to 70 percent of cases, the WBC rises above 12,000. Over half of patients experience increases in platelet count. The red cells appear normochromic and normocytic, unless iron deficiency develops. The erythrocyte sedimentation rate is frequently very low. Erythropoietin levels are never elevated (as opposed to other causes of polycythemia) and often low. Leukocyte alkaline phosphatase concentrations are increased in 80 percent, as are vitamin B_{12} levels due to an increase in vitamin B_{12}-binding proteins.

Reactive or secondary erythrocytosis represents the majority of cases of increased red cell mass. The increase is usually an appropriate physiologic response to tissue hypoxia and occurs when the Pao_2 falls chronically below 55 mm Hg or, more precisely, when the arterial oxygen saturation (Sao_2) drops below 92 percent. Obvious mechanisms of hypoxia include residence at high altitude and severe pulmonary disease, but cyanotic heart disease, increased carboxyhemoglobin from heavy cigarette smoking, and abnormal hemoglobins with high affinities for oxygen (resulting in poor tissue delivery) can have a similar deleterious effect on tissue oxygenation and trigger a reactive polycythemia.

Decreased tissue oxygenation is thought to be detected in the kidneys, causing release of erythrogenin, which acts enzymatically on a plasma protein substrate to form erythropoietin. There also seems to be a less sensitive nonrenal system for detecting tissue hypoxia and producing erythropoietin. Erythropoietin is a glycoprotein hormone that stimulates ribonucleic acid (RNA) synthesis, causing hematopoietic precursor cells to proliferate and differentiate into early erythroblasts. These cells mature at a faster than normal rate; early release of reticulocytes from the marrow and increased heme synthesis result. The increase in red cell mass improves tissue oxygenation, to the extent that hyperviscosity does not compromise it.

Pathologic secondary erythrocytosis results from inappropriate erythropoietin production, occurring autonomously in the absence of generalized tissue hypoxia. Renal disease and a host of extrarenal malignancies have been implicated. Inappropriate erythropoietin levels due to renal disorders and malignancies are unusual occurrences, but it is important to be aware of them, because polycythemia may be an early clue to their existence. About 1 percent to 3 percent of renal cell carcinomas have erythrocytosis as a manifestation, occurring at a time when cure is possible. Focal glomerulonephritis, hydronephrosis, renal artery stenosis, and polycystic kidney diseases are occasionally associated with elevations in erythropoietin and erythrocytosis. The mechanism is thought to involve a reduction in blood flow to renal tissue involved in erythropoietin production. Huge uterine myomas, cerebellar hemangiomas, and hepatomas are also causes, although the mechanisms are unclear; up to 10 percent of hepatoma patients in one series had erythrocytosis. In rare instances, an increase in circulating androgens is associated with polycythemia.

Relative (spurious) erythrocytosis (also referred to as Gaisböck's syndrome or stress erythrocytosis) denotes a heterogeneous set of conditions, characterized by an increase in hematocrit without an increase in red cell mass. One subset of patients has a high-to-normal erythrocyte mass and a low-to-normal plasma volume. The other has a normal erythrocyte mass and a low plasma volume. Most patients with relative erythrocytosis are obese, middle-aged, hypertensive men. About one-third of such patients experience thromboembolic complications. Those with a low plasma volume have the highest incidence of thromboembolization. The cause of relative polycythemia is unclear, but smoking appears to play a role. Loss of weight, cessation of smoking, control of hypertension, and implementation of exercise help alleviate the condition.

DIFFERENTIAL DIAGNOSIS

Patients with erythrocytosis can be separated on the basis of their underlying pathophysiology into three diagnostic categories: 1) polycythemia vera; 2) secondary erythrocytosis; and 3) relative (spurious) erythrocytosis. Secondary erythrocytosis can be subdivided into physiologic and pathologic varieties (Table 80–1).

WORKUP

The first task is to differentiate increased red-cell mass from decreased plasma volume and then, if the red-cell mass is increased, to determine whether it is due to a physiologic response or a pathologic one.

History. History of diuretic use, vomiting, diarrhea, hypertension, and stress suggest relative or spurious erythrocytosis. Important historical points suggesting a secondary, physiologic type include high-altitude residence, known congenital heart disease, history of heart murmur and cyanosis, smoking more than two packs per day, symptoms of chronic lung disease, familial occurrence, and history of renal disease. Patients with polycythemia vera give no such history but may volunteer vague or confusing symptoms related to hyperviscosity or bleeding, such as lassitude, headache, pruritus, sweating, easy bruising, abdominal pain, menorrhagia, or epistaxis. Pruritus worsened by bathing is especially characteristic.

Physical examination includes checking for hypertension, plethora, cyanosis, clubbing, ecchymoses, signs of chronic lung disease, heart murmurs associated with a right-to-left shunt, hepatic enlargement, splenomegaly, and abdominal and pelvic masses. Splenomegaly is very suggestive of polycythemia vera, but its absence does not rule out the diagnosis, particularly in the early phases of the disease.

Laboratory evaluation should begin with a *complete blood count, platelet count,* and *peripheral blood smear examination.* Two-thirds of patients with polycythemia vera have an elevated WBC, usually to 12,000 to 25,000 per cubic millimeter, and occasionally as high as 50,000 to 100,000 per cubic millimeter, with increased immature forms and basophils. Half of polycythemia vera patients have thrombocytosis, with platelet counts in the 450,000 to 1,000,000 per cubic millimeter range. Large, bizarre platelets and megakaryocytic fragments may be seen on the blood smear. In secondary and spurious forms of erythrocytosis, the WBC, platelet count, and blood smear are normal. In polycythemia vera, red cell morphology becomes abnormal with progression of disease. With the development of myeloid metaplasia, anisocytosis and poikilocytosis with tear-drop forms, ovalocytes, elliptocytes, and nucleated red blood cells are seen.

An *arterial blood gas* with *oxygen saturation* ($Sa{O_2}$) determination is important in the assessment of less obvious cases. A $Pa{O_2}$ less than 55 mm Hg and a $Sa{O_2}$ less than 92 percent indicate significant hypoxemia. In two-pack-per-day cigarette smokers, the $Sa{O_2}$ determination that is calculated from the measured $Pa{O_2}$ and a standard blood oxygen dissociation curve may be misleading. This method gives an erroneously high $Sa{O_2}$ if carboxyhemoglobin levels are elevated; polycythemia due to increased carboxyhemoglobin will be missed. This problem can be avoided by ordering an $Sa{O_2}$ determination that is measured directly rather than calculated from $Pa{O_2}$.

The diagnostic criteria for polycythemia vera are an elevated total red cell volume, normal $Sa{O_2}$, and splenomegaly. In the absence of splenomegaly, at least two of the following should be present: an elevation in *platelet count* (over 400,000 per cubic millimeter), *WBC* (over 12,000 per cubic millimeter), *leukocyte alkaline phosphatase, serum* B_{12} *level,* or unbound vitamin B_{12}-binding capacity.

If polycythemia vera and hypoxia-induced secondary polycythemia are ruled out, one should look for signs and symptoms of renal lesions and tumors, especially renal cell carcinoma. A *renal ultrasound* or *intravenous pyelogram (IVP)* with nephrotomograms is a reasonable screening test for such lesions; a positive study is followed by a contrast-enhanced *CT scan* of the abdomen. When there is a strong family history of polycythemia, one should obtain a *hemoglobin electrophoresis* in search of a mutant hemoglobin with

Table 80-1. Differential Diagnosis of Polycythemia

A. Polycythemia vera
B. Secondary polycythemia
   1. Physiologic (due to systemic hypoxia)
      a. High altitude
      b. Right-to-left shunt
      c. Heavy smoking
      d. Severe pulmonary disease
      e. Abnormal hemoglobin with high O_2 affinity
   2. Pathologic (no systemic hypoxia)
      a. Renal cell carcinoma
      b. Uterine myoma
      c. Cerebellar hemangioma
      d. Hepatoma
      e. Hydronephrosis
      f. Cystic kidney disease
      g. Renal artery stenosis
C. Relative polycythemia
   1. Marked volume depletion
      a. Protracted vomiting
      b. Persistent diarrhea
      c. Excessive diuretic use
   2. High-to-normal erythrocyte mass, low-to-normal volume
      a. Hypertensive, obese, middle-aged, male smoker

an abnormally high oxygen affinity. *Radioimmunoassay for erythropoietin* is best reserved for investigation of suspected pathologic secondary erythrocytosis, where the finding of inappropriate erythropoietin production would be important. Routine use of this expensive test in all patients with erythrocytosis is wasteful, unnecessary, and, in many instances, not particularly helpful.

Relative erythrocytosis should be suspected if the patient has signs of significant volume depletion or is an obese, middle-aged, hypertensive male smoker with a stressful lifestyle. Only when clinical evidence is insufficient to distinguish relative erythrocytosis from other forms should a *determination of red cell mass* be ordered. The calculation of red cell mass is rather elaborate and requires a laboratory experienced in its measurement. A radioisotope label (chromium-51) is administered to tag the red cells and perform the calculation. Body habitus needs to be taken into account when interpreting the result. Tall muscular individuals will have a greater red cell mass than short fat ones, because blood volume is greater in muscle than in fat. A normal red cell mass is diagnostic of relative erythrocytosis.

SYMPTOMATIC THERAPY

When possible, treatment should be etiologic (eg, correction of a right-to-left shunt, removal of a erythropoietin-secreting tumor). *Cessation of cigarette smoking* (see Chapter 54) is an important goal; in patients with relative erythrocytosis or reactive polycythemia due to heavy smoking and high carboxyhemoglobin levels, the hematocrit will begin to fall within a week and return to normal 3 to 4 months after smoking is terminated. For selected patients with severe chronic obstructive pulmonary disease (COPD), *chronic oxygen therapy* may help normalize arterial oxygen saturation (see Chapter 47).

The risks from erythrocytosis (hyperviscocity, thrombosis, impaired hemostasis) begin to rise substantially as the hematocrit moves into the 55 to 60 range. When the condition cannot be treated etiologically in prompt fashion, *phlebotomy* should be used. Phlebotomy improves oxygen delivery, relieves hyperviscosity symptoms, and prevents the thromboembolic and hemorrhagic complications associated with polycythemia. The target hematocrit is in the low to mid 40s, the level at which tissue oxygenation is optimal in normovolemic patients.

Phlebotomy is especially useful in patients with polycythemia vera and pathologic secondary erythrocytosis. Even in cases where the rise in red cell mass represents a physiologic accommodation to chronic hypoxemia, phlebotomy may be indicated if the erythrocytosis becomes excessive (hematocrit > 60) and threatens oxygen delivery. Reducing the hematocrit below 55 improves exercise tolerance in patients with severe COPD.

Phlebotomy is conducted by removing up to 500 mL of blood as often as every 2 to 3 days to achieve a hematocrit below 55. For patients who do not tolerate such large losses of volume (eg, the elderly), phlebotomy is limited to no more than 250 mL once or twice a week. Iron deficiency may ensue but should not be corrected in cases of polycythemia vera or pathologic secondary erythrocytosis, because it may stimulate a fulminant recurrence of red cell production. In patients with cardiopulmonary disease, enough modest iron replacement to correct microcytosis is probably beneficial, because microcytic erythrocytes increase blood viscosity and decrease oxygen delivery. The severely erythrocytic patient who is to undergo surgery requires phlebotomy to prevent compromised hemostasis. Preoperative phlebotomy should be followed by administration of a volume expander to correct volume depletion.

Treatment of Polycythemia Vera. Control of polycythemia vera with phlebotomy alone is usually possible in cases where platelet count and WBC remain relatively normal. Phlebotomy has been shown to increase median survival from 2 to 12 years. Frequency of treatments is a function of the hematocrit and symptoms. Most symptoms can be alleviated by reducing the hematocrit to around 50; however, continued frequent phlebotomy is recommended until a normal hematocrit is achieved (mid 40s in men, low 40s in women). A maintenance schedule can then be set up based on monthly monitoring.

Bothersome *pruritus* can be controlled by use of histamine blockers. The combination of an H_1 blocker (eg, *astemizole* 10 mg per day) and an H_2 blocker (eg, *cimetidine* 400 mg tid) will often suffice. Secondary *hyperuricemia* occurs in this disease and can lead to acute gout; *allopurinol* (300 mg per day) administered once daily prevents gouty attacks and should be considered when the uric acid rises above 9 to 10 mg per deciliter.

Myelosuppressive therapy deserves consideration when phlebotomy proves inadequate, thrombocytosis develops, or extramedullary hematopoiesis ensues. The optimal treatment is yet to be identified; a longitudinal investigation by the Polycythemia Vera Study Group has compared P_{32}, alkylating agents, and hydroxyurea. Although P_{32} and *alkylating agents* (eg, chlorambucil) are effective, they are also leukemogenic; as such, they are reserved for elderly patients. *Hydroxyurea* appears to be preferred, free of leukemogenic effects, yet capable of suppressing the disease. Its disadvantages include frequency of administration, large number of pills that must be taken, and far less sustained remissions than P_{32}. Patients who fail hydroxyurea therapy can be given a treatment of P_{32}, especially if they are elderly; it will induce a 6- to 24-month remission and is less leukemogenic than alkylating agents.

Thrombosis and bleeding are important complications of polycythemia vera. Prophylactic therapy with aspirin and Persantine has failed to halt thrombosis, but phlebotomy with volume expansion is helpful. Patients with persistent thrombocytosis have responded to *anagrelide,* a new agent with potent antiaggregating qualities that also reduces platelet counts. Recent studies of the agent are encouraging in terms of safety and efficacy.

In the later stages of the illness, painful splenic infarction or congestive splenomegaly may necessitate splenectomy. Transition to leukemia is associated with a lack of responsiveness to chemotherapy and a very poor prognosis.

PATIENT EDUCATION AND INDICATIONS FOR REFERRAL

Patient education is essential to encourage smokers to give up cigarettes (see Chapter 54) and COPD patients to follow a maximal program for improving oxygenation (see Chapter 47). The patient's understanding of the basis of the disease and its prognosis should help in achieving compliance (see Chapter 1). When polycythemia vera is diagnosed, patients should be referred to a hematologist for design of a treatment program. Referral is also appropriate when diagnosis is difficult and measurement of red cell mass or bone marrow biopsy is being considered.

A.H.G.

ANNOTATED BIBLIOGRAPHY

Anagrelide Study Group. Anagrelide, a therapy for thrombocythemic states. Am J Med 1992;92:69. *(Report of experience in 577 patients with this new anti-aggregating agent.)*

Balcerzak SP, Bromberg PA. Secondary polycythemia. Semin Hematol 12:353, 1975. *(Excellent review of pulmonary physiology related to tissue hypoxia-induced polycythemia and other classes of secondary polycythemia.)*

Berk PD, Goldberg JD, Donovan PD, et al. Therapeutic recommendations in polycythemia vera based on Polycythemia Vera Study Group Protocols. Semin Hematol 1986;23:132. *(Based on best available data.)*

Berk PD, Goldberg JD, Silverstein MN, et al. Increased incidence of acute leukemia in polycythemia vera associated with chlorambucil therapy. N Engl J Med 1981;304:441. *(Incidence of acute leukemia was 13 times that of patients treated with phlebotomy and 2.3 times that of those given P_{32}.)*

Brown SM. Spurious (relative) polycythemia: A nonexistent disease. Am J Med 1971;50:200. *(Patients with this condition were men with high normal red cell masses and low normal plasma volumes.)*

Chetty KG, Brown SE, Light RW. Improved exercise tolerance of the polycythemic lung patient following phlebotomy. Am J Med 1983;74:415. *(Patients with COPD show improved exercise tolerance when the hematocrit is lowered by phlebotomy to less than 55.)*

Cotes PM, Dore CJ, Yin JA, et al. Determination of serum immunoreactive erythropoietin in the investigation of erythrocytosis. N Engl J Med 1986;315:283. *(Not found to be of much value, except in identification of patients with pathologic secondary erythrocytosis.)*

Editorial. Polycythemia due to hypoxemia: Advantage or disadvantage? Lancet 1989;2:20. *(Fresh look at the pathophysiology.)*

Golde DW, Hocking WG, Koeffler HP, et al. Polycythemia: Mechanisms and management. Ann Intern Med 1981;95:71. *(Comprehensive review of pathophysiology, evaluation, and therapy.)*

Kaplan ME, Mack K, Goldberg JD, et al. Long-term management of polycythemia vera with hydroxyurea. Semin Hematol 1986;23:167. *(Found moderately effective and quite safe.)*

Lederle FA. Relative erythrocytosis: An approach to the patient. J Gen Intern Med 1987;2:128. *(Useful review; 31 references.)*

Milligan DW, MacNamee R, Roberts BE, et al. The influence of iron-deficient indices on whole blood viscosity in polycythemia. Br J Haematol 1982;50:467. *(Iron deficiency increases viscosity; replacement may be necessary in selected patients.)*

Perloff JK, Rosove MH, Child JS. Adults with cyanotic congenital heart disease: Hematologic management. Ann Intern Med 1988;109:406. *(Very useful paper on an often overlooked issue.)*

Smith JR, Landaw SA. Smokers' polycythemia. N Engl J Med 1978;298:6. *(Occurs in heavy smokers and resolves when smoking is stopped.)*

Thomas DJ, et al. Cerebral blood-flow in polycythemia. Lancet 1977;2:161. *(Documents marked reduction in blood flow that returns to normal after repeated phlebotomies.)*

Primary Care Medicine: Office Evaluation and Management of the Adult Patient, 3rd edition, edited by Allan H. Goroll, Lawrence A. May, and Albert G. Mulley, Jr. J.B. Lippincott Company, Philadelphia

81
Evaluation of Bleeding Problems and Abnormal Bleeding Studies

The bleeding problems encountered in the office setting range from abnormal screening studies to complaints of easy bruising, petechial rashes, or recurrent episodes of unexplained frank blood loss. Sometimes, the only manifestation is a low platelet count, prolonged prothrombin time (PT), or a delay in the bleeding time. When the volume of blood loss is small, rate of bleeding is slow, and risk of serious hemorrhage is low, evaluation may take place in the outpatient setting. The work-up involves examination of the intrinsic and extrinsic clotting systems as well as checking blood vessels, platelet function, and platelet quantity to identify which part of the hemostatic apparatus is at fault. Often a careful history and physical examination, supplemented by a few simple laboratory studies, can yield a clinically meaningful answer and guide therapy. An important objective is to determine if the problem is inherited or acquired. At times, an anatomic lesion coexists with a bleeding diathesis; the clinician always needs to address this possibility, especially when the bleeding originates from the lung (see Chapter 42), gastrointestinal (GI) tract (see Chapter 63), urinary tract (see Chapter 129), or vagina (see Chapter 111).

PATHOPHYSIOLOGY AND CLINICAL PRESENTATION

Hemostasis is achieved by the interplay of the coagulation cascade, platelets, and vessel wall. The platelets provide the initial primary hemostatic plug in response to vascular injury, followed secondarily by generation of fibrin at the site of damage. Blood coagulation is a carefully controlled process, limited by endogenous anticoagulants. Normal hemostasis represents a delicate balance between coagulant and anticoagulant factors. Any upset in this system of checks and balances may result in bleeding or thrombosis.

Disorders of primary hemostasis involve the platelets or vessel wall and present as spontaneous bleeding or bleeding into superficial tissues (skin, mucous membranes—including the lining of the bowel and genitourinary tract). Typical are the appearance of petechiae and slow oozing after trauma, rather than brisk bleeding. Menorrhagia or epistaxis may be a presenting complaint.

Disorders of secondary hemostasis involve the clotting factors or the fibrinolytic system and lead to bleeding that is characteristically deep and visceral, causing such problems as hemarthrosis, retroperitoneal hemorrhage, and deep hematomas.

Qualitative Platelet Disorders

Platelet function defects can be classified according to the step in platelet activity that is affected: adhesion, aggregation, activation, secretion, or acceleration of coagulation. Patients with isolated qualitative platelet defects have a prolonged bleeding time in conjunction with normal-appearing platelets that are adequate in number.

Defective Adhesion. The most important source of impaired adhesion is *von Willebrand's disease,* an autosomal dominant condition, causing decreased secretion or abnormal synthesis of a glycoprotein polymer (von Willebrand factor) needed for platelet adherence to a site of vascular endothelial injury. The release of von Willebrand factor in the classic form of the disease can be stimulated by desmopressin (DDAVP). Rarer forms of the disease are not corrected by DDAVP. Cryoprecipitate can also correct the problem. In addition, there is a deficiency of factor VIII procoagulant, giving rise to a prolongation in the partial thromboplastin time (PTT). Platelet agglutination fails to occur in the presence of the antibiotic ristocetin, a laboratory characteristic of this disease that is useful for its detection. Mucous membrane bleeding is a frequent manifestation. The severity of bleeding is variable and most severe among homozygous individuals, who may bleed from the GI tract; hemarthrosis is rare. There are also acquired forms of the disease, which occur in the context of lymphoma, other malignancies, and connective tissue disease.

An acquired adhesion defect occurs when high doses of *semisynthetic penicillins* or *cephalosporins* are taken; these agents can coat the platelet surface and reduce binding to glycoprotein.

Defective Activation and Secretion. Patients with activation problems have impaired production or impaired response to prostaglandin-dependent activators such as thromboxane A_2, which attracts platelets and constricts vessels. *Nonsteroidal antiinflammatory drugs* (NSAIDs) affect platelet activation and secretion by inhibiting cyclooxygenase, which helps convert arachidonic acid to thromboxane. In addition, they inhibit release of adenosine diphosphate (ADP) needed for platelet aggregation. Irreversible inhibition of cyclooxygenase occurs with even small single doses of aspirin and persists for the life span of the platelet (7 days). Reversible inhibition is seen with use of other NSAIDs and omega-3 fatty acids (found in oily fish). Severe bleeding does not result, but an underlying bleeding diathesis may be aggravated. In patients with *storage pool disease,* the ADP and serotonin contents of platelet granules are reduced or released prematurely, as occurs in patients who have undergone *cardiopulmonary bypass.* Bleeding is typically mild, and the bleeding time is only mildly prolonged.

Defective Aggregation. Patients with the rare hereditary defect in platelet aggregation, *Glanzmann's thrombasthenia,* are missing a bridging protein called glycoprotein IIb/IIIa. Their platelets cannot bind to fibrinogen and thus fail to aggregate by way of fibrinogen cross-links. *Clot retraction is abnormal;* the bleeding time is markedly prolonged. Serious bleeding can occur. Patients taking high doses of *semisynthetic penicillins* or *cephalosporins* also demonstrate reduced binding to fibrinogen.

Defective Acceleration of Coagulation. When platelets bind factors V and X on their surface, the rate of prothrombin conversion is greatly accelerated. Patients whose platelets cannot bind these clotting factors have a mildly prolonged PT, normal bleeding time, and normal tests of platelet aggregation.

Mixed or Unknown Defects in Function. A number of conditions are associated with poorly defined, but potentially important qualitative defects in platelet function. *Uremia* is the most important and is believed related to a dialyzable toxin. In addition to dialysis, correction of anemia, DDAVP, conjugated estrogens, and cryoprecipitate can reduce the prolongation in bleeding time. *Dysproteinemias* and *myeloproliferative diseases* also produce complex defects in platelet function, as can high parenteral doses of beta lactam *antibiotics.*

Quantitative Platelet Defects

A normal platelet count ranges from 150,000 to 300,000 platelets per cubic centimeter. *Thrombocytosis* (by definition, counts in excess of 400,000) may lead to impairment of platelet function, occasionally causing mucous membrane bleeding or hemorrhage following trauma or surgery. Bleeding from thrombocytosis most often occurs in the setting of myeloproliferative disease.

Thrombocytopenia, defined as a platelet count below 100,000, is associated with a prolongation in bleeding time. The diagnosis requires confirmation by viewing the peripheral smear, because spurious forms occur due to *in vitro* clumping of platelets in response to citrate or small amounts of circulating cold-agglutinin.

The risk of serious bleeding from true thrombocytopenia does not occur until the platelet count falls well below 50,000. Spontaneous bleeding arises as the count drops below 20,000. A petechial rash of the lower legs may be an initial manifestation. The lesions differ from those due to vasculitis in that they are painless, flat, nonpruritic, and without an erythematous blush. Hemorrhagic bullae in the buccal mucosa are another characteristic finding. Bleeding may initiate from the GI or urinary tract. Thrombocytopenia develops when there is increased platelet destruction (trauma, immune injury, disseminated intravascular coagulation [DIC], thrombotic thrombocytopenic purpura [TTP]), decreased production (marrow failure), or abnormal pooling (hypersplenism).

Increased destruction is the most common cause of thrombocytopenia. The primary mechanism is immunologic, occurring in association with drugs, viruses, lymphoproliferative disorders, and connective tissue diseases as well as idiopathically.

Idiopathic thrombocytopenic purpura (ITP) ranks among the major causes of platelet destruction. Although a platelet-bound IgG antibody has been detected in 80 percent of cases and found useful for diagnostic purposes, its pathophysiologic significance remains to be determined. Free antibody in the serum is less common and highly variable. The condition is most common in young adults, children, and women. In adults, the condition is more chronic, characterized by a waxing and waning course, few spontaneous remissions. It may present as bleeding in the context of aspirin or NSAID use, as an incidental finding on routine blood count, or as menorrhagia, epistaxis, or purpuric rash following a viral infection. The physical examination is otherwise normal, and the spleen usually is not palpable, although it might be slightly enlarged. There is no lymphadenopathy, hepatomegaly, or sternal tenderness, helping to distinguish it from other causes of immune thrombocytopenia (human immunodeficiency virus [HIV], connective tissue disease, lymphoproliferative disease). Mild fever is sometimes noted.

The immune thrombocytopenias associated with *chronic lymphocytic leukemia* (CLL) and *systemic lupus erythematosus* (SLE) follow clinical patterns similar to ITP. In addition, lymphadenopathy and splenomegaly are found in the majority of patients with CLL, and 25 percent have hepatomegaly as well. In SLE, arthritis and arthralgias are reported in 90 percent, skin rash in 70 percent, lymphadenopathy in 60 percent, and renal disease in 50 percent. Platelet counts below 100,000 are not frequent, being reported in about 15 percent of cases. *HIV infection* is also associated with an immune thrombocytopenia, affecting 10 percent of asymptomatic carriers and 30 percent of acquired immunodeficiency syndrome (AIDS) patients.

Drug-induced thrombocytopenia that results in increased destruction is idiosyncratic and immune-mediated. Heparin, H_2-blockers, quinidine, sulfonamides, and penicillins are common precipitants, although *any* drug may be responsible. Rapid fall in platelet count to levels below 10,000 can occur, and acute hemorrhage may ensue. Prompt return of the count to safe levels is typical as soon as the responsible drug is withheld.

Thrombotic thrombocytopenic purpura causes platelet consumption, rather than outright destruction, due to hyaline–platelet complexes forming in small vessels and trapping platelets. Unlike disseminated intravascular coagulation, there is no consumption of clotting factors or fibrin deposition. Cause is unknown, although an immune mechanism is postulated. A microangiopathic hemolytic anemia ensues. Fever develops and microvascular damage to the renal and central nervous systems (CNS) may become manifest. The lactic dehydrogenase can rise markedly. The combination of a peripheral smear showing schistocytes and thrombocytopenia in conjunction with fever, neurologic symptoms, and renal dysfunction comprise the clinical syndrome. Patients with the acute fulminant form of the disease are unlikely to present in the outpatient setting, but those with the chronic relapsing form may.

Decreased production implies bone marrow failure. The bone marrow may be suppressed by drugs, depressed after a viral infection, or replaced by tumor. Thrombocytopenias due to conditions causing *marrow failure* or a *myelophthisic process* usually occur in the context of a generalized pancytopenia (see Chapter 80). On occasion, individual *drugs* cause selective *inhibition of platelet production*. Chlorothiazide, tolbutamide, and ethanol are among the best documented. Megakaryocyte production suffers in *megaloblastic anemia* and quickly improves with replacement therapy. Transient thrombocytopenia may follow influenza, hepatitis, rubella, and other viral diseases. The thrombocytopenia of HIV disease involves viral invasion of megakaryocytes as well as increased peripheral destruction.

Increased pooling can be seen in disorders associated with an abnormally enlarged spleen. Splenomegaly results in excessive trapping and a fall in number of circulating platelets.

Defects of the Intrinsic Pathway

These conditions prolong the *PTT* (PT remains normal) by impairing the synthesis or functioning of intrinsic pathway clotting factors. Detection may be difficult because the PTT will not become prolonged until there is a greater than 75 percent reduction in concentration of a functioning intrinsic clotting factor. Fortunately, many clotting factor deficiencies do not cause serious bleeding, but the most common ones, the hemophilias, do.

Factor VIII and IX Deficiencies. *Hemophilias A* and *B* represent deficiencies of factors VIII and IX, respectively. They account for over 80 percent of patients with inherited bleeding diatheses and, being *X*-linked, affect only males. The risk of bleeding depends on the degree of factor deficiency. Patients with as little as 5 percent of normal concentrations experience little bleeding, except after surgery or major trauma; those with 1 percent to 5 percent may bleed after minor trauma; those with less than 1 percent undergo spontaneous hemorrhage, typically into muscle and weight-bearing joints. Bleeding can also occur into the CNS, genitourinary tract, and retroperitoneum. As noted, detection may be difficult if factor levels are in excess of 25 percent, because the PTT will be normal. Chromosomal mapping is being developed to help detect female carriers. Relatively early prenatal detection is available by deoxyribonucleic acid (DNA) analysis of chorionic villi tissue, provided tissue is also available from other affected family members. Fetal blood sampling for determination of antihemophilic factor levels may be done later in pregnancy by ultrasound-guided aspiration.

Factor XI deficiency occurs mostly among Ashkenazi Jews, inherited as an autosomal recessive disorder. A severe insult such as major trauma or surgery is needed to precipitate bleeding.

Other deficiencies of intrinsic pathway factors may cause a prolongation of the PTT but do not lead to clinical bleeding problems, even in the setting of major surgery or serious trauma.

Inhibitors. The *lupus anticoagulant* is an IgG antibody elicited in the setting of connective tissue disease and phenothiazine use. Bleeding complications are rare, but a hypercoagulable state is sometimes seen in patients with this anticoagulant, particularly pregnant women (leading to spontaneous abortion). Both the PTT and PT are prolonged because the antibody is directed against phospholipids used in both assays. Hemophiliacs who have had multiple antihemophiliac factor transfusions have close to a 15 percent risk of developing antihemophilic factor inhibitors, IgG antibodies against the replaced factors. Such antibodies are also noted in patients with connective tissue or lymphoproliferative disease, pregnancy, or advanced age.

Defects of the Extrinsic Pathway

The major clotting factors of the extrinsic pathway (II, VII, X) depend for their synthesis and modification on a healthy liver and an adequate dietary intake of vitamin K. Some vitamin K also derives from bacterial production by gut flora. Hereditary deficiencies of extrinsic pathway factors are rare. Most bleeding traced to the extrinsic pathway is due to impaired vitamin K production or liver disease. Causes include *hepatocellular insufficiency, cholestasis* (impairing absorption of lipid-soluble vitamin K), *poor dietary intake,* and use of *broad-spectrum antibiotics* that kill normal gut flora. The characteristic laboratory finding is a prolongation of the *PT.* Prolongation of the PT also occurs with warfarin anticoagulant therapy. *Warfarin* inhibits vitamin K-dependent, postsynthetic modification of factors II, VII, IX, and X; this prevents them from being able to bind calcium and achieve biologic activity (see Chapter 83).

Vascular Defects

Vascular defects are characterized by *purpuric bleeding* into the skin and mucous membranes in the absence of a detectable clotting factor or platelet abnormality. Ecchymoses and petechiae are the predominant manifestations. The most common form occurs as a result of aging, so-called *senile purpura.* Atrophy of connective and fatty tissues makes the vessels fragile and subject to ecchymotic bleeding, especially in areas of chronic sun exposure (face, neck, dorsum of hands, forearms). The skin fragility and easy bruising seen with *Cushing's syndrome* are believed to have a similar basis, due to the catabolic effects of prolonged corticosteroid excess. *Scurvy* causes defective collagen synthesis; affected patients may present with gingival bleeding or hemorrhage into subcutaneous tissue and muscle. Perifollicular bleeding is characteristic. *Purpura simplex* is a mild condition seen in otherwise healthy women; they experience ecchymoses mostly in the lower extremities (sometimes colorfully referred to as "devil's pinches"), especially during menstrual periods. Most cases are believed to be acquired, and some have been linked to use of NSAIDs.

Hereditary disorders of connective tissue (eg, *Marfan's syndrome, Ehlers-Danlos syndrome*) produce structural defects in supporting connective tissue and in major vessels. Bleeding ranges from easy bruising to serious hemorrhage. In *Rendu-Weber-Osler disease,* the developmental anomaly is *telangiectasia* formation due to lack of vessel support and contractility. Bleeding from these thin, convoluted networks of venules and capillaries might result from minor trauma or occur spontaneously. The telangiectatic lesions are violaceous, flat, usually no larger than a few millimeters, and range in shape from pinpoint to spidery. They occur on mucous membranes, face, trunk, palmar, and plantar surfaces. Lesions also arise in major viscera, leading to risk of serious hemorrhage. The clinical course is often one of repeated hemorrhagic episodes.

A host of pharmacologic agents can induce purpuric bleeding in the absence of demonstrable platelet or clotting factor abnormalities. *Drug-induced vascular purpura* is thought to have an autoimmune mechanism, with antibodies directed at the endothelial surface, although the responsible antibodies have yet to be identified. Drugs in this category include *procaine penicillin, thiazides, quinine, iodides, sulfas, and coumarins.* The bleeding ceases when the drug is withdrawn.

Minor purpuric bleeding caused by *immune complex formation* sometimes occurs with *systemic lupus, rheumatoid arthritis,* and *Sjögren's syndrome.* In *amyloidosis,* there is deposition of amyloid protein in the skin and subcutaneous tissue, which leads to vascular fragility, especially about the orbits and upper torso. The "raccoon eyes" appearance of such patients is characteristic.

Mixed Defects

A number of conditions impair the hemostatic apparatus at multiple levels. Chronic renal failure, dysproteinemias, chronic liver disease, and consumption coagulopathies are the most important examples. As noted above, *uremia* interferes with platelet function and causes deficiencies in production of clotting factors. Prolonged oozing from arterial and venipuncture sites is common. Dialysis and correction of anemia help reduce the bleeding tendency, which ranges from purpura and mucous membrane bleeding to GI hemorrhage.

Dysproteinemias (cryoglobulinemia, macroglobulinemia, myeloma) can lead to damage of the endothelial surface as immune complexes and paraproteins precipitate from the serum. The sludging and hyperviscosity commonly associated with these conditions also cause capillary anoxia. Impairment of clotting factor and platelet activity occurs in addition to endothelial damage, causing a multifactorial bleeding diathesis.

Chronic liver disease precipitates bleeding by a number of routes. Patients with severe hepatocellular failure can no longer make adequate amounts of vitamin K-dependent clotting factors, even with vitamin K administration. In addition, fibrinogen production suffers, and that which is made is defective. Patients with portal hypertension may become thrombocytopenic from platelet sequestration in the spleen, although, by itself, this rarely causes bleeding. However, varices are common in such patients, greatly increasing the risk of GI hemorrhage (see Chapter 63).

Disseminated intravascular coagulation occurs in the setting of illness that causes exposure of blood to tissue thromboplastin (eg, snake bite, extensive burn, serious infection, cancer). Activation of the extrinsic pathway in the microcirculation consumes clotting factors and platelets; it leads to bleeding that ranges from minor petechiae to hemorrhage. The condition is rarely encountered in the office setting.

DIFFERENTIAL DIAGNOSIS

The causes of a bleeding diathesis can be organized according to the subdivisions of the hemostatic apparatus: platelet function, platelet number, intrinsic pathway, extrinsic pathway, and vessels (Table 81–1). Differential diagnosis proceeds by identifying which segment of the clotting system is at fault.

WORKUP

When faced with a patient complaining of easy bruising or bleeding, the clinician needs to ascertain the likelihood of an underlying defect in hemostasis. Bleeding from multiple sites, easy bruising, spontaneous bleeding, ecchymoses greater than 3 cm in diameter, or prolonged bleeding after a surgical or dental procedure strongly suggest a bleeding diathesis. Before embarking on a detailed evaluation in the office, one should be sure there is no serious hemorrhage or major volume depletion. Inquiry is required into dyspnea, lightheadedness, marked postural fatigue, and observed quantity of blood loss. A quick check of postural signs, skin color, and skin temperature will provide added objective evi-

Table 81-1. Differential Diagnosis of Bleeding by Mechanism

Qualitative Platelet Disorders	
Defective adhesion	Von Willebrand's disease; high doses of semisynthetic penicillins and cephalosporins
Defective aggregation	Glanzmann's thrombosthenia; high doses of semisynthetic penicillins and cephalosporins
Defective activation	Nonsteroidal antiinflammatory drugs; dipyridamole; cardiopulmonary bypass
Defective acceleration	Factor V deficiency
Quantitative Platelet Disorders	
Thrombocytosis	Myeloproliferative disease
Thrombocytopenia	
Decreased production	Thiazides, alcohol, viral infection, marrow failure, megaloblastic anemia, myelophthisic process
Increased destruction	Quinidine, methyldopa, sulfa, phenytoin, barbiturates, lupus, infection, ITP, chronic lymphocytic leukemia
Increased sequestration	Hypersplenism
Intrinsic Pathway Defects	
Factor VIII deficiency	Hemophilia A
Factor IX deficiency	Hemophilia B
Factor XI deficiency	Ashkenazi Jews
Extrinsic Pathway Defects	
Vitamin K-dependent factor deficiency	Poor diet, cholestasis, hepatocellular failure, coumarin, broad-spectrum antibiotics
Vascular Defects	
Connective tissue fragility	Age, Cushing's syndrome, scurvy, purpura simplex
Hereditary defect	Marfan's syndrome, Rendu-Weber-Osler disease
Drug-induced	Procaine penicillin, sulfa, thiazides, quinine, iodides, coumarin
Paraproteinemia	Myeloma, macroglobulinemia, cryoglobulinemia
Connective tissue disease	Lupus, rheumatoid arthritis, Sjögren's syndrome
Multiple Defects	
Uremia	
Chronic hepatocellular failure	
Disseminated intravascular coagulation	
HIV infection	

Table 81-2. Differentiating Platelet, Coagulation, and Vascular Disorders

CLINICAL FEATURES	PLATELET	COAGULATION	VASCULAR
Onset	Immediate	Delayed	Immediate
Duration	Short	Prolonged	Variable
Precipitant	Trauma	Often spontaneous	Variable
Site	Skin, mucous membranes, GI	Joints, muscle, viscera	Skin, GI tract
Family history	Absent	Usually present	Usually absent
Drug related	Often	Rarely	Sometimes
Sex predominance	Often female	Usually male	Usually female
Response to focal pressure	Usually effective	Ineffective	Effective
Platelet count	Normal, low, or excessive	Normal	Normal
Prothrombin time	Normal	Abnormal in cases of factor II, VII, IX, and X deficiency	Normal
Partial thromboplastin time	Normal	Abnormal with factor VIII or IX deficiency	Normal

dence of intravascular volume status and degree of anemia. Once the presence or risk of severe hemorrhage is ruled out, the outpatient evaluation can commence.

The next task is to ascertain which segment(s) of the hemostatic system are at fault. This determination, along with an assessment of whether the condition is acquired or hereditary, can greatly help focus the evaluation (Table 81–2).

History

One needs a detailed history of the bleeding problem, including its onset, precipitants, location, clinical course, prior history, associated family history, and drug history. Inquiry into past surgery, childbirths, menses, nosebleeds (both nostrils), dental extractions, trauma, lacerations, and injections can provide important information. Especially important is a history of a transfusion requirement after minor trauma or surgery that ordinarily would not require such transfusion.

On the other hand, not all patients with a history of easy bruising have a bleeding diathesis. The complaint is common and often occurs in otherwise normal patients. Bruising that occurs on the limbs and is less than 3 cm in diameter is likely to be harmless and due to inapparent trauma in the absence of recalled injury. Likewise, minor bleeding up to 2 days after a molar extraction is within normal limits. However, ecchymoses occurring spontaneously on the trunk or measuring greater than 3 cm in diameter on the limbs are more worrisome.

As noted earlier, bleeding that is transient, superficial (confined to the skin or mucous membranes), and spontaneous or immediately posttraumatic suggests a platelet problem or vascular fragility. In contrast, patients with serious clotting-factor problems characteristically report bleeding that is deep (into tissues or viscera), delayed, and prolonged. A past medical history or family history of abnormal bleeding is strong presumptive evidence of a hereditary disorder, but its absence does not rule it out. For example, 30 percent of hemophiliacs give no family history of bleeding. In a patient with a suspected hereditary etiology, gender should be noted, because many hereditary bleeding disorders are sex-linked, especially those involving clotting factors.

A thorough review of *medications* is essential. Use of medications that are capable of interfering with platelet function (aspirin, NSAIDs, semisynthetic penicillins, cephalosporins, dipyridamole), platelet number (eg, thiazides, alcohol, quinidine, methyldopa, sulfa, phenytoin, barbiturates), or coagulation factor synthesis (warfarin) should be noted.

Presence of a recent or *concurrent illness* that might affect hemostasis ought to be given particular attention, including chronic liver disease, uremia, viral infection, connective tissue disease, myeloproliferative states, and paraproteinemias.

Physical Examination

After taking the vital signs and checking for significant volume depletion, one can proceed with a systematic examination. General appearance is noted for cushingoid habitus and marfanoid appearance. On examination of the skin, the size, number, and location of any *purpuric lesions* should be recorded, and note should be made of whether they are *petechial* (less than 3 mm) or *ecchymotic* (greater than 3 mm). Purpura represents bleeding into the skin, usually the result of vessel breakage or leakage. Petechial lesions occur with thrombocytopenia, qualitative platelet disorders, and vascular defects. Petechial rashes are also a hallmark of vasculitis, but the lesions in vasculitic cases are characteristically palpable, tender, pruritic, and surrounded by an erythematous flush. One can readily distinguish petechiae from nonpurpuric erythematous skin lesions by noting their failure to blanch when compressed with a glass slide.

Blanching lesions must not be dismissed too hastily, because they may be *telangiectasias,* which are an important clue to Rendu-Weber-Osler syndrome. Ecchymoses occurring in areas subject to trauma are a common finding in normal people; however, ecchymotic lesions greater than 6 cm in the absence of major trauma are likely to represent an underlying bleeding problem. The skin is also noted for signs of chronic liver disease (spider angiomata, jaundice).

The mucous membranes are examined for bleeding, the lymph nodes for enlargement, the abdomen for hepatosplenomegaly, and the joints and muscles for hematomas and hemarthroses. Rectal and pelvic examinations are conducted for evidence of bleeding. In a patient with thrombocytopenia, careful examination for splenomegaly is important because it may be the only clue of sequestration. Percussion of the Traube space (the area of resonance over the stomach) for dullness combined with splenic palpation in the right lateral decubitus position is the best means of detecting splenomegaly by physical examination (sensitivity 46%, specificity 97%).

Laboratory Studies

Although the history and physical examination often provide important clues regarding etiology, laboratory investigation helps to classify the cause of the bleeding more definitively. Primary hemostasis is assessed by *platelet count* and *bleeding time*. The *PT* best assays the extrinsic clotting system; the *PTT,* the intrinsic one.

Platelet Count is usually performed by an automated particle-counting machine on a sample of blood collected into a tube containing the anticoagulant ethylenediaminetetraacetic acid (EDTA). Falsely low counts occur when platelets clump on exposure to EDTA, a common phenomenon when blood is processed at low temperatures. It can be prevented by warming the blood slightly before processing, using another anticoagulant, or doing a finger-stick platelet count. The presence of a cold agglutinin in the blood will also cause clumping and a falsely low level, as will antibody that produces rosettes of platelets about white cells. A confirmatory look at the peripheral smear is always helpful. Finding platelets on examination of a peripheral smear is good presumptive of adequate quantity.

Bleeding time is a sensitive but nonspecific test of qualitative platelet function, being abnormal also in thrombocytopenia, uremia, von Willebrand's disease, and afibrinogenemia. Even anemia may produce a prolonged bleeding time, correctable by transfusion of red cells alone. The test often gives false-positive readings, as judged by a high rate of normal follow-up platelet aggregation studies.

The Ivy method is the standard technique for its performance. A cut is made in a relatively avascular area of the forearm, using a template to ensure an incision of 1 cm in length and 1 mm in depth, while venous return is obstructed with a blood-pressure cuff inflated to 40 mm Hg. Blotting paper is applied to the edge of the incision; a normal result is cessation of blotter-detected oozing by 9 minutes. Recent aspirin or current NSAID use will produce a modest prolongation in the bleeding time, although this usually does not represent a significant risk of bleeding unless there is a preexisting bleeding diathesis.

PT and PTT assay the extrinsic and intrinsic clotting factor cascades, respectively, as well as the common pathway. The PT assesses VII and common pathway factors X, V, prothrombin, and fibrinogen. The PTT reflects levels of kininogen, prekallikrein, VIII, IX, XI, XII, as well as those of the common pathway. Sensitivity is limited; clotting factor deficiency in excess of 75 percent is needed to prolong the PTT. The PT is slightly more sensitive, becoming prolonged when factor VII falls by 55 percent to 65 percent. However, bleeding is rare in the absence of such reductions. PTT prolongations unassociated with bleeding include those caused by deficiencies of factor XII, kininogen, or prekallikrein, and presence of an inhibitor.

Screening for an inhibitor is carried out by mixing equal volumes of the patient's plasma and normal donor plasma. If the prolongation in PT or PTT is corrected, then there is no inhibitor present and the workup proceeds to determine the missing clotting factor. If not corrected, then there is strong suggestive evidence of an inhibitor, and its identification is the next step. PT and PTT do not assess the final factor XIII-dependent cross-linking of fibrin; urea clot solubility testing is required. Testing for fibrinolysis also must be done separately.

Testing for a Qualitative Platelet Defect. In the setting of a bleeding complaint consistent with defective initial hemostasis (see above) and a normal platelet count, normal PT, and normal PTT, one should consider performing a bleeding time, provided there is no readily evident explanation (eg, recent aspirin or NSAID use, uremia, and so forth). An abnormal study is followed by in vitro testing of platelet function. *Aggregation testing* is conducted by adding an aggregating substance such as ADP, epinephrine, collagen, or thrombin to a platelet-rich plasma sample. If the bleeding time and the PTT are prolonged, then *ristocetin-induced agglutination* of platelets can be obtained to check for von Willebrand's disease. Aggregation is normal in von Willebrand's disease, but the platelets fail to agglutinate. Aggregation and ristocetin studies are best ordered in consultation with a hematologist.

Testing for the Cause of Thrombocytopenia. First, pseudothrombocytopenia must be ruled out. Then the task turns to differentiating increased destruction, from decreased production and sequestration. Examination of the *peripheral blood smear* is helpful in this regard. Finding a pancytopenia strongly suggests marrow failure. The presence of large immature platelets on peripheral smear in a patient with an isolated thrombocytopenia points to increased destruction. Isolated thrombocytopenia is almost always due to increased destruction. If uncertainty persists, a *bone marrow examination* can provide further clarification of mechanism. A hypocellular marrow in the setting of pancytopenia indicates marrow failure; an increase in megakaryocytes argues for increased destruction. Sequestration is best determined by examining for an enlarged spleen.

Increased destruction may be immune or nonimmune. Immune destruction is by far the more common, but before ordering elaborate tests for antibodies, one should consider a few preliminary investigations that may obviate the need for more elaborate studies. For example, simply withdrawing all potentially offending drugs and monitoring the platelet count may suffice for diagnosis of a medication-induced etiology. Testing for presence of HIV infection (enzyme-linked immunosorbent assay [ELISA] and Western blot), connective tissue disease (antinuclear antibody), or mononucleosis (heterophile) is indicated when clinical evidence is suggestive. In the absence of such common precipitants and in the setting of an otherwise normal complete blood count (CBC; mild lymphocytosis included), one should consider ITP. Whole blood is tested for presence of *platelet-bound IgG autoantibodies* (serum may contain little of the antibody). Detection is complex and controversies abound concerning the meaning of findings.

To check for consumption of platelets, a peripheral smear (examining for red cell schistocytes) is useful. Their presence suggests a microangiopathic condition such as occurs with TTP and DIC. PTT is normal in the former and abnormal in the latter.

Preoperative Screening for a Bleeding Disorder

The most important component of preoperative screening is the history. The absence of abnormal bleeding during a previous surgical procedure or trauma is strong evidence of normal hemostasis. Current medication use also needs to be carefully reviewed, especially NSAIDs, salicylates, and drugs known to precipitate thrombocytopenia. Although platelet count, PT, PTT, and bleeding time are frequently ordered, their yield is low in patients with unsuspected deficits. In particular, there is little if any correlation between bleeding time and risk of surgical bleeding. Routinely obtaining a preoperative bleeding time in a patient with no known or suspected bleeding problem is of no proven value.

PTT, PT, and platelet count continue to be ordered routinely, but their value in the absence of a condition known to compromise hemostasis remains unproven. In a study of 829 consecutive and otherwise healthy patients undergoing preoperative PT and PTT screening for orthopedic surgery, unexpected abnormalities were found in about 8 percent. None had an impact on patient management.

SYMPTOMATIC MANAGEMENT AND PATIENT EDUCATION

Patients with a clinically insignificant laboratory abnormality deserve detailed reassurance that they have adequate hemostasis. For example, the patient with a minor prolongation of bleeding time on preoperative testing yet no prior history of bleeding problems is unlikely to have anything more serious than recent salicylate exposure. Functional hemostasis will usually be preserved and no special precautions or further action (other than repeating the bleeding time) need be taken. However, the patient with a clinically important bleeding diathesis requires some basic advice, even as evaluation proceeds. The nature of the advice depends on the type of bleeding problem at hand.

Vascular Defects. Reassurance can be given to patients with purpura simplex and senile purpura. Occasionally, these patients take large doses of vitamins C and K in hopes of lessening their easy bruisability; such self-treatment measures are without proven efficacy and only add unnecessary expense. NSAIDs may exacerbate their cosmetic problem and can be withheld if the easy bruising disturbs the patient, but they ought not be avoided if there is an important indication for their use. Patients with recurrent bleeding from more serious vascular disease (eg, hereditary hemorrhagic telangiectasia) should be advised to avoid any agent that might compromise hemostasis. Bleeding episodes respond to compression if the rest of the hemostatic system is kept intact. Patients with vascular defects often suffer iron deficiency from recurrent bleeding; the resulting anemia responds well to oral iron (see Chapter 82).

Platelet Disorders. Those with a known qualitative platelet disorder and a history of bleeding should be counseled to avoid salicylates and NSAIDs. Patients who have no history of bleeding problems before nonsteroidal use can probably continue on the agent, provided the bleeding is clinically unimportant and the indication for drug use is compelling. However, the drug should be stopped in anticipation of a major surgical procedure.

Patients with platelet counts less than 50,000 are at risk for posttraumatic bleeding and should be advised to put off surgery, dental extraction, and contact sports until the problem is corrected. Use of stool softeners and a soft toothbrush is recommended. Those with counts below 20,000 are at risk for serious spontaneous bleeding and require hospitalization. While workup is in progress to identify an etiology, all but the most essential medications should be halted, with substance exposures (solvents, insecticides, alcohol) limited and NSAIDs and salicylates prohibited.

In most instances, the treatment of thrombocytopenia should be etiologic and selected in consultation with a hematologist. A few exceptions are worth noting: Thrombocytopenia associated with HIV infection is an indication for prompt initiation of antiviral therapy (see Chapter 13). That due to ITP is grounds for starting high-dose steroid therapy, especially if the patient is symptomatic. However, in both instances, hematologic consultation is still warranted and should be obtained even after starting initial therapy.

Clotting Factor Problems. Most patients on warfarin who exhibit bleeding from excessive anticoagulation need only hold their dose for a few days to allow the PT to drift back into safe therapeutic range (see Chapter 83). Vitamin K should not be used to accomplish correction of the PT, unless anticoagulation is no longer desired (it is difficult to quickly reanticoagulate a patient who has recently received large doses of vitamin K). Urgent need to correct the PT without impairing future anticoagulation efforts can be met by administering fresh frozen plasma.

Those with poor intake or malabsorption of vitamin K can be treated with oral vitamin K supplements (2.5 to 10 mg per day) or parenteral doses (10 to 25 mg, IM) in addition to attending to the underlying cause of the malabsorption (see Chapter 64). Patients with severe hepatocellular failure will not respond to vitamin K because synthetic function has been compromised (see Chapter 71).

Hemophilia. The patient and family with hemophilia face life-long problems. Detailed discussion of the management of such patients is beyond the scope of this chapter, but basic management includes specifying guidelines for permissible physical activity and teaching proper first aid. If the severity of bleeding has been only mild to moderate, then one can encourage participation in noncontact sports and other activities that have little risk of injury. The goal is to allow as much normal activity as possible. First aid treatment of an acute hemarthrosis should be learned by the family. One immobilizes the joint and applies ice packs to reduce pain and swelling. Splinting and elastic bandages can help ensure that a position of good joint function is maintained.

Pain control is important. Aspirin and related nonsteroidal agents must be avoided. Acetaminophen and codeine work well when given in adequate doses for short periods of time. The primary physician should not try to aspirate a hemarthrosis; there is high risk of further bleeding and introducing infection.

Administration of *factor VIII concentrate* has been the mainstay of therapy, used for acute bleeding episodes and before surgery and dental work. Carefully obtained and elaborately treated concentrate preparations have greatly reduced the risk of transfusion-related HIV infection, and recombinant preparations are now available, although extremely expensive. *DDAVP* is being used in place of factor VIII for treatment of patients with mild to moderate hemophilia or von Willebrand's disease and is proving effective for both acute bleeding episodes and prophylaxis. If future studies support these encouraging results, desmopressin should offer hemophiliacs an alternate means of acute treatment.

Genetic counseling is an important component of hemophiliac care. Definitive identification of women who are carriers of the hemophilia gene has been difficult, but DNA analysis techniques offer hope of improved identification to facilitate genetic counseling. Early prenatal diagnosis is also available (see above).

INDICATIONS FOR ADMISSION AND REFERRAL

Bleeding problems carry the potential for serious harm and bear very careful evaluation and monitoring. If there is any doubt as to the severity of the condition, prompt hospital admission should be considered. Patients who manifest volume depletion, gross bleeding, bleeding from multiple sites, or change in mental status require emergency admission. The otherwise well-appearing person with a dangerously low platelet count (less than 20,000), absence of platelets on smear, or a markedly prolonged bleeding time is best evaluated and monitored in the hospital. Hemophiliacs with acute bleeding require emergency factor VIII transfusion.

Referral or consultation with a hematologist can be helpful when a patient with clinical bleeding is suspected of having a qualitative platelet disorder. Proper test selection and interpretation will be facilitated. Referral is also indicated for patients with unexplained, clinically significant clotting factor deficiencies, severe thrombocytopenia, or suspected hemophilia or von Willebrand's disease.

A.H.G.

ANNOTATED BIBLIOGRAPHY

Antonarakis SE, Waber PG, Kittur SD, et al. Hemophilia A: Detection of molecular defects and of carriers by DNA analysis. N Engl J Med 1985;313:842. *(Report of DNA analysis of the factor VIII:C gene, providing an accurate method of carrier detection, which had previously been problematic.)*

Ballem PJ, Belzberg A, Devine DV, et al. Kinetic studies of the mechanism of thrombocytopenia in patients with HIV infection. N Engl J Med 1992;327:1779. *(Increased destruction, but also decreased production due to viral infection of megakaryocytes.)*

Barber A, Green D, Galluzzo T, et al. The bleeding time as a preoperative screening test. Am J Med 1985;78:761. *(Not found to be of value for routine use.)*

Barkun AN, Camus M, Green L, et al. Bedside assessment of splenic enlargement. Am J Med 1991;91:512. *(Traube-space percussion followed by palpation recommended.)*

Burns TR, Saleem A. Idiopathic thrombocytopenic purpura. Am J Med 1983;75:1001. *(Good review; includes discussion of platelet-associated IgG.)*

Bushick JB, Eisenberg JM, Kinman J, et al. Pursuit of abnormal coagulation screening tests generates modest hidden preoperative costs. J Gen Intern Med 1989;4:493. *(Routine PT and PTT added little additional cost, but impact of abnormal results was nil.)*

de la Fuente B, Kasper C, Rickles FR, et al. Response of patients with mild and moderate hemophilia A and von Willebrand's disease to treatment with desmopressin. Ann Intern Med 1985;103:6. *(Vasopressin analogue was both effective and safe in treatment and prevention of bleeding episodes.)*

Furie B, Furie BC. Molecular and cellular biology of blood coagulation. N Engl J Med 1992;326:800. *(Excellent short review for the general reader.)*

Gernsheimer T, Stratton J, Ballem PJ, et al. Mechanisms of response to treatment in autoimmune thrombocytopenic purpura. N Engl J Med 1989;320:974. *(Prednisone stimulated platelet production; splenectomy prolonged survival.)*

Kitchens CS: The anatomic basis of purpura. Prog Hemostasis Thromb 1980;5:21. *(Interesting discussion of purpura from the perspective of blood vessel structure and function.)*

Lind SE. The bleeding time does not predict surgical bleeding. Blood 1991;77:2547. *(Review of available data; finds little predictive value.)*

Petri M, Rheinschmidt M, Whiting-O'Keefe Q, et al. The frequency of lupus anticoagulant in systemic lupus erythematosus. *(Frequency 6 percent to 25 percent; good discussion of its significance.)*

Roberts HR. The treatment of hemophilia: Past tragedy and future promise. N Engl J Med 1989;321:1188. *(Editorial on new treatment options.)*

Rodgers RPC, Levin J. A critical appraisal of the bleeding time. Semin Thromb Hemost 1990;16:1. *(Detailed review of its utility and shortcomings.)*

Sinha RK, Kelton JC. Current controversies concerning the

measurement of platelet-associated IgG. Trans Med Rev 1990;4:121. *(Difficult test to perform and interpret.)*

Suchman AL, Griner PF. Diagnostic uses of the activated partial thromboplastin time and prothrombin time. Ann Intern Med 1986;104:810. *(Screening PTs and PTTs add little to screening in the absence of a history of bleeding. Normal PT and PTT rule out a clotting factor abnormality in the patient with a bleeding problem.)*

White GC, Shoemaker CB. Factor VIII gene and hemophilia A. Blood 1989;73:1. *(Excellent discussion of detection and genetic and prenatal counseling.)*

82
Management of Common Anemias

Primary Care Medicine: Office Evaluation and Management of the Adult Patient, 3rd edition, edited by Allan H. Goroll, Lawrence A. May, and Albert G. Mulley, Jr. J.B. Lippincott Company, Philadelphia

Anemias that result from deficiencies of iron, folate, and vitamin B_{12} are extremely common in primary care practice. The relative ease with which one can replace the deficient substance sometimes leads to correction of the anemia without sufficient attention to the underlying cause. Complicating the issue is inappropriate self-treatment with large doses of iron and vitamins. The primary care physician needs to be skilled in the evaluation of anemia (see Chapter 79) and the use of iron, vitamin B_{12}, and folate replacement therapies. An opportunity to treat some of the most refractory anemias (eg, those due to end-stage renal failure and other serious illnesses) has emerged with the development of recombinant erythropoietin. The primary physician should be knowledgeable about the indications for its use.

IRON DEFICIENCY ANEMIA

Iron deficiency anemia is extremely common, occurring in about 10 percent to 15 percent of premenopausal women. The condition is particularly likely to be a manifestation of underlying disease when it occurs in males and in the elderly (see Chapter 77). It helps to assess whether there is inadequate intake, poor absorption, increased loss, or a combination of factors responsible for the anemia. Knowing the most economical, effective, and best tolerated forms of supplemental iron facilitates design of an optimal replacement therapy program.

Clinical Presentation and Course

In menstruating women, the balance between dietary iron intake (1 mg per day) and loss (15 mg per month) is precarious. Low-grade anemia, especially when losses from pregnancy (approximately 500 mg) are not made up, is common. However, the many vague complaints in otherwise healthy menstruating women that are attributed to "low iron" have not been found to correlate with the severity of the anemia or to respond to its correction in controlled studies.

Iron deficiency anemia is usually slow in onset, allowing for compensatory changes such as increases in 2,3-DPG and cardiac output to minimize symptoms. When blood loss has been rapid or the anemia severe (hemoglobin below 7 g per 100 ml), patients are likely to become symptomatic, especially if cardiopulmonary reserve is limited. Replacement therapy is required in such cases, regardless of etiology.

Pica (defined as a craving for ice, starch, clay, or any other substance) is particularly common in patients with iron deficiency, but often unreported. In one study, up to 50 percent of iron-deficient patients were found to suffer from pica, with pagophagia (the craving for ice) accounting for the vast majority of cases. There was no correlation between presence of pica and etiology of the iron deficiency. Symptoms resolved with treatment.

The occasional patient with severe iron deficiency who presents with glossitis, angular stomatitis, koilonychia or esophageal web improves after correction of the deficiency. Whether the menorrhagia sometimes seen with iron deficiency is corrected by iron is a subject of debate. Patients who have undergone subtotal gastrectomy and gastrojejunostomy have up to a 60 percent chance of incurring iron deficit due to loss of acid-secreting capacity, rapid gastric emptying, and bypass of the duodenum. Pregnancy is almost certain to produce iron deficiency, because a net loss of over 500 mg of iron occurs. Iron deficiency from chronic gastrointestinal (GI) blood loss has been documented in long-distance runners.

Unless the cause of the iron deficiency is removed, recurrence rates are high, even when treatment is prescribed. In a series of 100 cases, 29 relapses were noted; in 24 instances, inadequate iron was being taken; in 12, blood loss continued in excess of iron therapy, and in 4, malabsorption was documented.

Principles of Management

As noted above, the importance of identification and treatment of the underlying etiology cannot be overemphasized, especially when the anemia is found in a man or an elderly patient. The severity of the anemia does not indicate the seriousness of the cause.

Indications for iron replacement are tempered by the fact that symptoms are often minimal and the morbidity from a mild anemia is low. Moreover, as noted previously, correction of the iron deficit is not certain to alleviate the host of vague complaints often attributed to it. Nevertheless, replacement therapy makes sense when 1) the patient is symptomatic and has a limited cardiopulmonary reserve; 2) the anemia has become moderately severe (hemoglobin 8 to 9 g per 100 ml); 3) the patient is pregnant; 4) the patient had a subtotal gastrectomy and gastrojejunostomy; 5) continued heavy blood loss is anticipated; or 6) the patient is recovering from megaloblastic anemia.

Preparations. Oral iron is preferred; the ferrous form is better absorbed than the ferric one. Absorption occurs best under conditions of low pH in the proximal small bowel. Phytates and phosphates found in food bind iron and reduce absorption. When iron tablets are taken with meals, a 40 percent drop in absorption can be demonstrated. Absorption also varies according to the severity of the deficit. About 20 percent of an oral dose is taken up initially, but absorption falls to 5 percent after 1 month of therapy, even though the anemia remains incompletely corrected.

The preparation of choice is ordinary *ferrous sulfate*. It is the least expensive and best absorbed. Slow-release and enteric-coated preparations have been touted as producing fewer side effects and requiring only once-daily administration. However, they dissolve slowly and can bypass the proximal small bowel (where most absorption takes place) before significant dissolution has occurred. There is *no* evidence they are worth the extra cost, which can be several times that of unadulterated ferrous sulfate.

Most ferrous salts (sulfate, gluconate, citrate) have equivalent rates of absorption and produce similar rates of hemoglobin replenishment. Choice is a matter of cost and side effects; the degree of GI upset is a function more of the iron content of the tablet than of the form of ferrous salt used. Some preparations contain ascorbic acid with the claim that the acid facilitates absorption, especially in patients with achlorhydria; such patients respond adequately to ferrous sulfate alone, probably because of the excess amount of iron available.

The *recommended dose* for iron deficiency is 300 mg of ferrous sulfate tid. Although taking iron with a meal reduces absorption, it also lessens disagreeable GI symptoms such as nausea and epigastric discomfort. Constipation and diarrhea are frequently reported as well, but are less a function of the amount of iron available for absorption. About 25 percent of patients report side effects.

The *response* to iron is apparent within 10 days of initiating therapy; a reticulocytosis is first noted, followed by a rise in the hemoglobin concentration of 0.1 to 0.2 g per 100 mL per day. Several weeks of therapy are required to bring the hemoglobin level back up to normal, and replenishing iron stores may take months. However, speed is not an issue unless blood loss is rapid, in which case blood transfusion rather than iron therapy is the treatment of choice. The response to parenteral iron therapy is no more rapid than that seen with oral preparations.

Iron's *effect on absorption* of other drugs needs to be kept in mind in patients taking other medications. When ingested simultaneously with iron, the absorption of levodopa, methyl dopa, tetracycline, and fluoroquinolone antibiotics (eg, norfloxacin) are reduced by up to 90 percent. A similar but more variable effect on thyroxine has been noted. Iron intake should be delayed for several hours after intake of these other medications, and monitoring of their efficacy should be stepped up during iron therapy.

Parenteral iron has a very limited role. It should be used only in patients who have had an adequate trial of oral iron and have shown a genuine intolerance to all available preparations. Patients with inflammatory bowel disease may require parenteral iron due to the irritant effect of oral iron and the need to take large doses to keep up with blood loss. Parenteral iron has also been suggested for patients with malabsorption, but most are able to absorb a sufficient amount of oral iron. Intramuscular (IM) administration has been associated with development of sarcomas at injection sites and should be avoided. Fatal anaphylactic reactions and asthma have been produced by all parenteral forms of iron administration. If parenteral iron must be used, it should be administered by the intravenous route, beginning with a very small test dose and continuing with a slow drip; a syringe with epinephrine should be drawn up at the same time and kept on hand.

Patient Education and Prevention of Iron Deficiency

To maximize compliance, patients need to be instructed on the best means of minimizing GI side effects. Starting with a small dose of ferrous sulfate (eg, 300 mg/d) and building to 900 mg per day avoids initial intolerance. Taking iron just after eating may also help. It needs to be made clear that therapy has to be continued on a regular basis for weeks and often months.

Prevention of iron deficiency is most important in those with increased needs (ie, pregnant women and young children). The average American diet contains 12 mg of iron per 2000 calories. Twenty percent is absorbed by markedly iron-deficient patients and 5 percent to 10 percent by others; thus, about 0.6 to 1.2 mg is taken up under normal circumstances each day. Daily requirement for men and postmenopausal women is 0.5 to 1.0 mg per day, indicating that dietary intake should suffice. However, 1.5 mg per day is needed by menstruating women and 2.5 mg per day is needed by pregnant women. Iron-rich foods can be used to avoid the need for iron supplements. Fish, meat (particularly liver), and iron-enriched cereals and bread are excellent sources. Eggs and green vegetables are also high in iron, but the iron is unavailable for absorption because it is bound to the phosphates and phytates present in these foods.

When diet alone seems inadequate and needs are very high, as in pregnancy, a once-daily dose of 150 to 300 mg of ferrous sulfate is recommended to avoid significant iron deficiency. It must be emphasized that most people who eat a balanced diet do not require iron supplements. Taking widely promoted supplements that contain iron, vitamins, and minerals is expensive and unnecessary in most instances. Excessive iron is associated with increased risks of malignancy and atherosclerotic disease.

VITAMIN B_{12} DEFICIENCY

Vitamin B_{12} deficiency can result from inadequate intake, impaired absorption, increased requirements, or faulty utilization. Poor intake is distinctly rare, occurring mostly in ultra-strict vegetarians who refrain from eating eggs and dairy products as well as meat. Most cases of vitamin B_{12} deficiency are due to pernicious anemia; the lack of intrinsic factor compromises absorption. Absorption can also be impaired by disease of the terminal ileum, by bacterial overgrowth from stasis, and by gastrectomy. Faulty utilization is uncommon, occurring with genetic defects in synthesis of transcobalamin, the plasma protein used for vitamin B_{12} transport.

Clinical Presentation and Course

Irrespective of etiology, vitamin B_{12} deficiency may lead to slowly evolving *megaloblastic anemia, glossitis,* and *neuropathy*. Macrocytosis is usually the first hematologic manifestation and can precede anemia by as much as 1 to 2 years. Hypersegmentation of neutrophils is another early hematologic finding. Due to the body's large vitamin B_{12} storage capacity, onset of clinical manifestations may take months to years to develop. Although megaloblastic anemia and glossitis also occur with folic acid deficiency, the neuropathy is distinctive. Traditionally, neurologic symptoms were thought to be a late development, dependent on the vitamin B_{12} level falling to less than 100 pg per mL. However, careful studies have documented vitamin B_{12}-responsive neuropsychiatric deficits in the absence of such marked vitamin B_{12} deficiency, anemia, or machine-determined macrocytosis (although hypersegmentation and macrocytosis were often noted on examination of the peripheral smear).

Classically, the neurologic syndromes include those of peripheral neuropathy and subacute combined degeneration (symmetric paresthesias in the hands and feet, progressing to ataxia from loss of vibratory and position sense as the posterior columns of the spinal cord become involved). However, cortical involvement is also prevalent and may present as memory loss (simulating dementia), disorientation, depression, hallucinations, agitation, personality change, perversions of taste and smell, irritability, or central visual scotomata. If left untreated, many neurologic deficits may become permanent.

In pernicious anemia, there may be coincident thyroid disease, rheumatoid arthritis, vitiligo, or gastric cancer. *Achlorhydria* after histamine stimulation is characteristic. Diagnosis is usually made by the Schilling test, using exogenous intrinsic factor to help document its absence (see Chapter 79).

Principles of Management

In most instances, there is no urgency to treat. However, reversibility of neurologic deficits is to some extent a function of their duration. Thus a patient with a neurologic complaint suggestive of vitamin B_{12} deficiency should be promptly diagnosed (see Chapters 79, 167, and 169) and treated. Parenteral therapy is preferred (except in the rare patient with poor intake), because most vitamin B_{12} deficiency results from malabsorption. However, use of large oral doses (in excess of 100 μg per day) may result in enough absorbed vitamin B_{12} to suffice in some cases. Cyanocobalamin is the most commonly used parenteral formulation, although hydroxocobalamin is better bound to serum proteins and less rapidly excreted, allowing less frequent administration. In practice, either form of vitamin B_{12} suffices.

Replacement Regimens. There are a host of initial replacement regimens, all of which are adequate. For example, in a commonly used program for patients with pernicious anemia, patients are initially treated with 100 to 1000 μg of IM cyanocobalamin or hydroxocobalamin daily for 1 to 2 weeks, followed by the same dose twice weekly for another month, and then once a month for the remainder of the patient's life. If neurologic symptoms are present, a twice-monthly follow-up dose is recommended for 6 months.

Some argue that 1000-μg doses are unnecessary, because only 100 μg can be effectively used at one time, with the remainder being promptly excreted in the urine. However, because of its low cost and safety, maintenance doses of 1000 μg are often given. Others note that monthly injections after initial replacement are unnecessary, finding that once every 3 to 4 months suffices for many patients. The optimal program can be individualized, although it is probably best to continue with a monthly regimen in patients with neurologic sequelae. More important than the interval of therapy is ensuring its indefinite continuation. Relapse of symptoms is common in the absence of continued therapy. Compliance with a monthly injection program is often poor; having the visiting nurse or family member give the injection is helpful and far less inconvenient than a monthly office visit.

Response to Treatment can be dramatic, with marked reticulocytosis beginning within 72 hours and rapid improvement in neurologic deficits, especially in patients with mild deficits or those of short duration. Neurologic complaints of longer duration may take 6 to 12 months to improve. However, deficits that have persisted for 12 to 18 months in spite of therapy are probably permanent, emphasizing the importance of timely diagnosis for successful therapy.

During recovery, patients who were severely vitamin B_{12} depleted can develop serious *hypokalemia* as potassium is taken up by new red cells. The serum potassium level should be monitored, and supplements should be provided if it falls below normal. There is no need for concurrent folic acid supplementation. In fact, the inappropriate use of a large pharmacologic dose of oral folate (eg, 5 mg) alone might partially and nonspecifically correct the anemia and mask an underlying vitamin B_{12} deficiency, putting the patient at risk for an acute, marked deterioration of neurologic function if vitamin B_{12} is not given. There is no harm if the patient takes folate in addition to vitamin B_{12}, but this is rarely necessary unless diet is extremely poor.

Other Treatment Modalities. Patients with vitamin B_{12} deficiency due to bacterial overgrowth or disease of the terminal ileum require treatment directed at the underlying bowel problem. Oral *antibiotic therapy* with tetracycline or amoxicillin provides temporary relief from bacterial overgrowth. More definitive treatment of inflammatory bowel disease may be indicated (see Chapter 73).

Halting Unnecessary Vitamin B_{12} Therapy. Many well-intentioned physicians have used parenteral vitamin B_{12} as a nonspecific therapy for patients bothered by fatigue or other vague symptoms. In one study of a rural health clinic, 10 percent of all patients attending the clinic were found to be receiving such treatment regularly, 6 percent in the absence of appropriate indications for its use. Many persons free of vitamin B_{12} deficiency report symptomatic benefit from monthly injections, probably as a consequence of a strong placebo effect. Even after being informed of its being unnecessary, a large proportion will remain reluctant to halt such therapy or will stop temporarily, only to seek out a physician willing to restart it. Although there is little direct risk in giving vitamin B_{12}, its use can be misleading and should be abandoned in favor of a more comprehensive and etiologic approach to the patient's underlying problems, be they those of anxiety, depression, somatization, or an underlying medical problem (see Chapters 8, 226, 227, and 230).

FOLIC ACID DEFICIENCY

Most folic acid deficiency results from inadequate intake, although occasionally increased need or impairment of absorption or utilization is encountered. *Dietary deficiency* is, in part, a consequence of limited capacity to store folate; within 3 months of assuming an inadequate diet, megaloblastic changes and anemia can develop. Foods rich in folate include green vegetables (asparagus, lettuce, spinach, broccoli), liver, yeast, and mushrooms. Excessive boiling of vegetables in water can remove a substantial amount of available folic acid. Alcoholism is responsible for many cases of inadequate intake.

Impaired absorption is seen in the context of ileal disease (eg, tropical and nontropical sprue, heavy giardial infestation), short bowel syndrome, and phenytoin use. *Increased demand* takes place in the setting of pregnancy, severe hyperthyroidism, hemolytic anemia, malignancy, and florid psoriasis. *Utilization* is *hindered* by use of methotrexate; triamterene and trimethoprim have similar although less marked effects on dihydrofolate reductase. Patients undergoing hemodialysis experience substantial folic acid *loss*, necessitating replacement therapy.

The *clinical presentation* of folic acid deficiency is one of megaloblastic anemia, sometimes accompanied by glossitis. Anemia occurs within 3 to 4 months of the onset of deficiency. Diagnostic features include a low serum folate level (less than 15 ng per mL) and a marked reticulocytosis in response to physiologic doses (200 per g) of folic acid. Response to treatment with folic acid is prompt. There are no neurologic deficits associated with folic acid deficiency.

Treatment for most patients involves orally administered pharmacologic doses of folic acid (1 to 2 mg per day). Most forms of folic acid deficiency, even malabsorptive types, can be overcome by oral therapy. Four to five weeks of treatment will usually reverse the anemia and replenish body stores. When the underlying cause persists (eg, malabsorption, malignancy, psoriasis, hemodialysis), chronic therapy is indicated. Patients taking methotrexate can be given folinic acid, which bypasses inhibition of dihydrofolate reductase. As noted above, nonspecific use of folic acid for treatment of a megaloblastic anemia is ill-advised, because it may mask an underlying vitamin B_{12} deficiency and precipitate neurologic symptoms.

ERYTHROPOIETIN DEFICIENCY

Anemias due to erythropoietin deficiency (eg, as in end-stage renal disease) have been among the most refractory. Erythropoietin replacement therapy, made possible by the advent of recombinant human erythropoietin, represents a major advance in the treatment of such anemias. Dialysis patients with regular transfusion requirements have demonstrated almost universal elimination of transfusion needs, normalization of hematocrit, and improved quality of life with thrice-weekly intravenous injections of recombinant erythropoietin (150 U per kg). Side effects are few, but include increase in blood pressure and iron deficiency. Concurrent iron supplementaton is often required. Under study is the use of erythropoietin in other situations where anemia is severe and serum erythropoietin levels are reduced (eg, AIDS, malignancy, chemotherapy). Also being investigated are anemic patients with normal erythopoietin levels (eg, those who wish to donate their own blood before surgery for autologous transfusion).

PATIENT EDUCATION

Two extremes of behavior are common in patients with common anemias. Some become overzealous in use of vitamins and iron; others continue to ignore the problem or believe that once the deficiency is corrected no further therapy is necessary. Careful patient education is essential to avoid the adverse consequences of both behaviors. Patients taking vitamin B_{12} injections unnecessarily should be counseled on the need to explore the underlying cause of their symptoms. Those taking expensive vitamin preparations should be advised that much simpler, less costly, yet equally efficacious preparations are available. Patients with folate deficiency will benefit from dietary counseling and a referral to the nutritionist. If alcoholism is the basis of the folate deficiency, then it requires a careful evaluation in its own right (see Chapter 228). Patients with chronic renal failure who have needed repeated transfusions will derive some comfort from knowing that there is an alternative available to them.

A.H.G.

ANNOTATED BIBLIOGRAPHY

Boggs DR. Fate of a ferrous sulfate prescription. Am J Med 1987;82:124. *(Most patients received an enteric-coated or slow-release form, even when not ordered; many pharmacists were unaware of this.)*

Brise H, Hallberg L. Influence of meals on iron absorption in oral iron therapy. Acta Med Scand (Suppl.) 1962;171:376. *(Absorption fell 40 percent when oral iron was taken with meals.)*

Campbell NR, Hasinoff BB. Iron supplements: A common cause of drug interactions. Br J Clin Pharmacol 1991;31:251. *(Good summary of these important interactions; most occur when tablets are taken simultaneously.)*

Campbell NR, Hasinoff BB, Stalts H, et al. Ferrous sulfate reduces thyroxine efficacy in patients with hypothyroidism. Ann Intern Med 1992;117:1010. *(Taking both at the same time reduces thyroxine efficacy; binding to iron suspected.)*

Crosby W. Who needs iron? N Engl J Med 1977;297:543. *(Terse review of iron requirements and need for supplementation.)*

Elwood P, Williams G. A comparative trial of slow-release and conventional iron preparations. Practitioner 1970;204:812. *(No therapeutic advantage found for the slow-release preparations.)*

Erslev AJ. Erythropoietin. N Engl J Med 1991;324:1339. *(Excellent review; 54 references.)*

Fry J. Clinical patterns and course of anemias in general practice. Br Med J 1961;2:1732. *(Recurrence rate of iron deficiency was 30 percent after treatment if the underlying cause was not corrected.)*

Hallberg L, Ryttinger L, Solvell L. Side effects of oral iron therapy. Acta Med Scand 1966;459(suppl):3. *(Blind controlled study documenting only 7 percent having to stop therapy because of GI intolerance.)*

Lawhorne L, Ringdahl D. Cyanocobalamin injections for patients without documented deficiency: reasons for administration and patient responses to proposed discontinuation. JAMA 1989;261:1920. *(Six percent of patients in this study of a rural clinic were getting unnecessary vitamin B_{12} injections and most wanted to continue them even after being informed they were worthless.)*

Lindenbaum J, Healton EB, Savage DG, et al. Neuropsychiatric disorders caused by cobalamin deficiency in the absence of anemia or macrocytosis. N Engl J Med 1988;318:1720. *(Emphasizes need for high index of suspicion and early treatment.)*

Oral iron. Medical Letter 1978;20:45. *(Ferrous sulfate is least expensive and no less effective or less well tolerated than other preparations.)*

Rector WG. Pica—its frequency and significance in patients with iron-deficiency anemia due to chronic gastrointestinal blood loss. J Gen Intern Med 1989;4:512. *(Found to be frequent and resolved with therapy; no relation to etiology.)*

Savage D, Lindenbaum J. Relapses after interruption of cyanocobalamin therapy in patients with pernicious anemia. Am J Med 1983;74:765. *(Emphasizes importance of ensuring indefinite provision of therapy.)*

Stevens RG, Jones DY, Micozzi MS, et al. Body iron stores and the risk of cancer. N Engl J Med 1988;319:1047. *(Just an epidemiologic reminder that too much iron can be harmful—increased risk of malignancy demonstrated.)*

Wood M, Elwood P. Symptoms of iron deficiency anemia: A community survey. Br J Prev Soc Med 1966;20:117. *(Classic study; the correlation between hemoglobin concentration and symptoms was poor. Iron therapy produced no statistically significant improvement in complaints.)*

83
Outpatient Oral Anticoagulant Therapy

ROBERT A. HUGHES, M.D.

Primary Care Medicine: Office Evaluation and Management of the Adult Patient, 3rd edition, edited by Allan H. Goroll, Lawrence A. May, and Albert G. Mulley, Jr. J.B. Lippincott Company, Philadelphia

Oral anticoagulant therapy with coumarin derivatives has become a major therapeutic tool in the prevention of fibrin thrombus formation. Approximately 300,000 patients are stricken annually by thromboembolism—over 50,000 die. A great deal of morbidity and mortality could be avoided by timely anticoagulation. It is important to know 1) indications for therapy; 2) how to initiate and maintain patients on oral anticoagulants in the outpatient setting; 3) common complications; and 4) drugs and conditions that interfere with or potentiate the anticoagulant's effect. In addition, the primary physician needs to be familiar with indications for antiplatelet therapy.

MECHANISM OF ACTION

Warfarin and other coumarin derivatives act by inhibiting the action of vitamin K in the normal carboxylation of coagulation factors II, VII, IX, and X. Noncarboxylated coagulation factors, known as PIVKAs (proteins induced by vitamin K antagonism), fail to participate effectively in the coagulation reaction. The warfarin-induced decline in active, carboxylated coagulation factors is a function of the half-life of each factor, which varies from 5 hours for factor VII to 72 hours for factor II. The prothrombin time (PT) may be prolonged after only 2 to 3 days of therapy, but this represents primarily depression of factor VII and the extrinsic clotting cascade. Full anticoagulant effect is only achieved after all factors, including the intrinsic clotting cascade, are comparably depleted after 5 to 7 days of therapy, and the partial thromboplastin time (PTT) is also prolonged.

INDICATIONS

Therapy is indicated in conditions having a high risk of thrombus formation and subsequent embolization. The traditional list of indications has been expanded by the finding of a significant reduction in stroke risk in several recent long-term, randomized, placebo-controlled studies of warfarin in patients with nonrheumatic atrial fibrillation. Consensus statements from major expert panels identify the following indications:

- rheumatic heart disease (see Chapter 33)
- prosthetic heart valves (see Chapter 33)
- atrial fibrillation with underlying heart disease (see Chapter 28)
- systemic embolization (see Chapter 171)
- congestive cardiomyopathy (see Chapter 32)
- large anterior myocardial infarction with thrombus formation
- pulmonary embolization (see Chapter 35)

Warfarin anticoagulation remains controversial in 1) secondary prevention of transient ischemic attacks; 2) ventricular aneurysm 6 months after a recent myocardial infarction; and 3) primary and secondary prevention of myocardial infarction.

Alternatives to warfarin, particularly *aspirin,* have been explored. In studies of nonrheumatic atrial fibrillation, aspirin was either found not to be effective or equivocal in effect, although study design was often not focused on the aspirin question, and more data are needed. In studies of transient ischemic attack, aspirin in doses ranging from 30 mg qd to 325 mg qid has demonstrated a reduction in stroke risk (see Chapter 171). Primary prevention of myocardial infarction has been demonstrated with use of an alternate-day aspirin program (see Chapter 30). Compared to aspirin, *dipyridamole* has been disappointing, except for preserving patency of bypass grafts after coronary bypass surgery. Gastrointestinal bleeding remains a major common complication of aspirin use (see Chapter 68).

Ticlopidine, a platelet aggregation inhibitor that inhibits ADP-induced platelet activation, has proven equal or superior to aspirin for stroke prevention. Unlike aspirin and other nonsteroidal antiinflammatory drugs (NSAIDs), it does not interfere with prostaglandin-dependent actions, but its use is associated with a small risk of reversible agranulocytosis (necessitating biweekly monitoring of complete blood count [CBC] for the first 3 months of therapy).

CONTRAINDICATIONS

Contraindications to the use of oral anticoagulants need to be considered in the context of urgency of anticoagulation, risk and seriousness of potential complications, and duration of therapy. Patients with previous *central nervous system bleeding,* recent *neurosurgery,* or *frank bleeding* should not receive warfarin. Important relative contraindications include active peptic ulcer disease, chronic alcoholism, blindness (unless in supervised situations), bleeding diathesis, and severe hypertension. When taken early in pregnancy, coumarins may cause birth defects; when they are used at delivery, fetal hemorrhage can occur. Heparin should be used in place of warfarin during early pregnancy and childbirth. Embarking on oral anticoagulant therapy is unwise when follow-up cannot be readily maintained, when laboratory facilities for accurately measuring the PT are inadequate, or when the patient is unreliable.

METHODS OF INITIATING AND MONITORING THERAPY

Initiation. Patients with acute pulmonary embolization, deep vein thrombophlebitis, or acute systemic embolization should be admitted for immediate parenteral administration of heparin, to be followed by oral warfarin therapy. Other patients are in less urgent need of immediate full anticoagulation and can be safely started on a warfarin program as outpatients. A generally accepted approach to initiating outpatient warfarin therapy is to give 5 mg daily, measure the PT at 5 to 7 days, and adjust the dose accordingly. The starting dose should be set at 2.5 mg daily in patients who weigh less than 110 lb, are older than 75 years, or are at increased risk of bleeding. It generally takes 3 to 4 months to achieve a stable dosage, and thereafter, the PT can be checked every 3 to 4 weeks. Warfarin is best taken on an empty stomach at a specific time each day. Bedtime is preferred; it allows changes to be made the same day the PT is measured.

Monitoring. The level of anticoagulation is typically expressed as the ratio of the patient's PT to the laboratory's control PT (*prothrombin-time ratio*). The therapeutic range of the ratio is 1.2 to 2.0 times control (see below). Once the desired level of anticoagulation is achieved, monitoring continues by measuring the PT once every 3 to 4 weeks. In about 75 percent of patients, dosage adjustments over time are unnecessary; in 25 percent they are. Because it is impossible to predict who will and who will not need adjustments, the PT should be checked every 3 to 4 weeks, the schedule being rigorously enforced.

Use of the PT to monitor therapy and the establishment of recommended ranges for the PT ratio for optimal safety and efficacy have been complicated by the lack of uniformity and standardization of the thromboplastin reagents used to determine PT values. It has been found that PT ratios may differ according to the reagents used and distort the monitoring of therapy. The sensitivities of commercially available reagents vary widely, but they can be measured and designated by the *International Sensitivity Index (ISI).* To compensate for these reagent-related differences in PT and ratio results, it has been proposed that the PT ratio be expressed in a manner that corrects for the ISI. This corrected ratio has been designated the *International Normalization Ratio (INR)* and is calculated by taking the PT ratio to the power of the ISI for the reagents used. Therapeutic range for INR is 2.0 to 4.5, with 2.0 to 3.0 designated for conditions in which lower-intensity therapy is appropriate, and 3.0 to 4.5 for higher-intensity conditions (see below).

Recommended Intensity of Therapy and Adjusting of Dose. After initiation, dosage should be adjusted to maintain therapeutic range. There has been extensive study supporting use of lower therapeutic ranges (PT ratio of 1.2 to 1.5 or a target INR of 2.0 to 3.0) for most groups of patients. Only those at highest risk for thromboembolization (mechanical heart valves, recent or recurrent thromboembolism) should be anticoagulated to a PT ratio of 1.5 to 2.0 (INR of 3.0 to 4.5)

There are numerous ways to adjust dose when the PT appears out of range. One that is designed to maximize safety and avoid wide swings in PT uses 10 percent changes in weekly dose, unless PT is grossly out of range. For example, if the patient is taking 7.5 mg per day, the weekly dose is 52.5 mg. If the PT is too low, the dose is increased so that on 2 of the 7 days, the patient takes 10 mg, and 7.5 mg the other 5 days. The PT is then measured weekly for the next 2 weeks.

Outpatient anticoagulation requires facilities for accurate PT measurement, reliable collection of samples, and the ability to contact patients promptly. Careful monitoring and follow-up are essential to the safety and success of any outpatient anticoagulation program. At the beginning of therapy, patients can benefit considerably from a session with a nurse who can instruct them in the use of warfarin, answer questions, test understanding, and provide informative booklets for them to take home. The importance of close monitoring and patient education cannot be overemphasized. If the patient fails to keep an appointment for a PT test, he or she should be contacted immediately. A computer system can provide reminders so that no patient is lost to follow-up. Commercial laboratory services are sometimes employed to draw samples at home for patients who have difficulty coming to the office for frequent PT determinations. Home monitoring devices are under development.

COMPLICATIONS

Reports on the incidence of *bleeding complications* in patients on long-term anticoagulant therapy have been variable. Several series have demonstrated that the incidence of hemorrhage severe enough to require hospitalization or transfusion should occur in less than 5 percent of patients who are carefully monitored. Unfortunately, the risk of serious bleeding is not always linked to excessive prolongation of the PT and can occur even with the PT in therapeutic range. Risk factors for complications include high-intensity anticoagulation, recent initiation of anticoagulation, poor patient selection, and wide fluctuation in PT. Older patients generally experience a higher incidence of complications, although old age per se is not a risk factor.

Patients with PTs in the therapeutic range who bleed from the urinary tract, rectum, or vagina while on anticoagulant therapy should be considered to have an *underlying pathologic* process until proven otherwise. In several series, a lesion responsible for the bleeding was detected in over 50 percent of patients. Often it was an occult malignancy in the bladder or colon.

In rare instances, *hemorrhagic necrosis of skin* has been reported in women and *cyanotic toes* in men—all with PTs in therapeutic range. The mechanism of this complication is believed to be a transient inhibition of endothelial vitamin K-dependent antithrombotic proteins (proteins S and C) in patients congenitally deficient in such factors.

EFFECTS OF DRUGS AND CONCURRENT ILLNESSES

Drugs that potentiate the effect of warfarin may do so by preventing synthesis or absorption of vitamin K, displacing warfarin from binding sites, inhibiting microsomal degradative enzyme activity, increasing catabolism of clotting factors, or impairing platelet function (Table 83–1). Risk of bleeding is particularly high with concurrent use of NSAIDS. In the elderly, a 13-fold increase in hemorrhagic peptic ulcer disease results from taking NSAIDS plus warfarin. Hepatocellular failure results in impaired synthesis of clotting factors and albumin; cholestasis makes for less efficient absorption of vitamin K. Both conditions are capable of prolonging the PT and potentiating the effects of warfarin.

Anticoagulant effects are decreased by agents that induce microsomal enzymes, decrease absorption of warfarin, or increase synthesis of clotting factors or binding proteins (see Table 83-1). Moreover, coumarins cause a decrease in the metabolism of tolbutamide and phenytoin by competing for the same degradative enzymes. The PT should be measured when any change in drug program is made, and it should be followed closely thereafter.

INDICATIONS FOR CONTINUATION AND TERMINATION OF THERAPY

Therapy should be continued indefinitely in patients with valvular disease, atrial fibrillation, systemic embolization, or

Table 83-1. Common Drugs That Interact with Oral Anticoagulants

EFFECT	MECHANISM	DRUG
Prolongation of PT	Inhibits clearance	Metronidazole Trimethoprim-sulfa Cimetidine* Omeprazole* sulfinpyrazone Disulfiram Anabolic steroids
	Inhibits vitamin K	Cephalosporins, 2nd, 3rd generation
	Increases metabolism of clotting factors	1-thyroxine
	Unknown	Erythromycin ? Tamoxifen ? Phenytoin ? Isoniazid ? Ketoconazole ? Piroxicam
Reduction of PT	Increases warfarin clearance	Barbiturates Carbamazepine Rifampin
	Reduces warfarin absorption	Cholestyramine
	Increases synthesis of clotting factors	Estrogens
	Unknown	Penicillins

*Causes only minimal prolongation of PT.

Adapted from Hirsh J. Oral anticoagulant drugs. N Engl J Med 1991;324:1865.

artificial heart valves. In other instances, there are few data on proper duration of therapy. In deep venous thrombosis, most experts recommend continuation of therapy for approximately 3 to 6 months; the same is true in pulmonary embolization. Deep vein thrombophlebitis or pulmonary emboli that recur after 6 months of treatment are usually followed by retreatment for a period of 12 months. If a serious bleeding problem develops in a patient on anticoagulant therapy, the PT can be corrected promptly by administration of *fresh frozen plasma*. This is the preferred mode of therapy. Parenteral administration of *vitamin K* is also effective, although it may take longer to have an effect (up to 5 hours) and can cause refractoriness to warfarin if prompt reinstitution of anticoagulant therapy is attempted. The decision to discontinue anticoagulant therapy in the context of bleeding needs to be individualized. The risk of hemorrhage has to be balanced against the risk of serious embolization.

PATIENT EDUCATION

Avoidance of unnecessary morbidity depends on thorough patient education. Before initiation of outpatient therapy, the patient and responsible family members need to learn the name of the medication, the dose, time of day to be taken, need for routine check of PT, necessity of avoiding alcohol and aspirin-containing compounds, and they must be able to recognize signs of bleeding such as melena and spontaneous ecchymoses. Teaching undertaken by the nurse, as well as distribution of helpful booklets detailing proper use of the drug, are essential components of the patient education effort. Any patient who is incapable of understanding the instructions or is deemed unreliable should not be placed on therapy, because the risks of hemorrhage probably outweigh any possible benefits. The one exception is the patient who can be closely supervised by family members or health care professionals.

The physician should know the tablet color-coding of the warfarin brand the patient is using. This helps ensure that proper doses are being taken. Constancy of brand should be advised, both to minimize dosing errors and to ensure consistency of anticoagulant effect.

ANNOTATED BIBLIOGRAPHY

American-Canadian Cooperative Study Group. Persantine-aspirin trial in cerebral ischemia. Part II: Endpoint results. Stroke 1985;16:406. *(Major study confirming the indication for aspirin in stroke prevention; the addition of persantine did not improve the efficacy of aspirin.)*

Boston Area Anticoagulation Trial for Atrial Fibrillation Investigators. The effect of low-dose warfarin on the risk of stroke in patients with nonrheumatic atrial fibrillation. N Engl J Med 1990;323:1505. *(One of several randomized trials demonstrating benefit in patients with chronic or paroxysmal AF; also shows efficacy of low-intensity therapy.)*

Bussey HI, Force RW, Bianco TW, et al. Reliance on prothrombin time ratios causes significant errors in anticoagulation therapy. Arch Intern Med 1992;152:278. *(PT ratio may be deceiving.)*

Dalen JE, Hirsch J. Second ACCP Conference on antithrombotic therapy. Chest 1989;95(suppl):15. *(Authoritative recommendations on indications for and management of oral anticoagulant therapy.)*

Dutch TIA Trial Study Group. Comparison of two doses of aspirin (30 mg versus 383 mg per day) in patients after a transient ischemic attack or minor ischemic stroke. N Engl J Med 1991;325:1261. *(Low-dose aspirin was as effective as higher doses in preventing stroke recurrence.)*

Ezekowitz MD, Bridgers SL, James KE, et al. Warfarin in the prevention of stroke associated with nonrheumatic atrial fibrillation. N Engl J Med 1992;327:1406. *(Data from the VA study further confirming that low-intensity therapy reduces risk; extends documentation of benefit to patients over 70.)*

Feder W, Auerback R. Purple toes: An uncommon sequela of oral coumarin drug therapy. Ann Intern Med 1961;55:911. *(Complication seen in 1 percent of patients, now known to be due to congenital factor S or C deficiency worsened by warfarin therapy.)*

Fihn SD, McDonell M, Martin D, et al. Risk factors for complications of chronic anticoagulation. Ann Intern Med 1993; 118:511. *(High-intensity anticoagulation, wide fluctuations in PT, recent initiation of therapy, and poor patient selection were major risk factors.)*

Gurwitz JH, Avorn J, Ross-Degnan D, et al. Aging and the anticoagulant response to warfarin therapy. Ann Intern Med 1992;116:901. *(Response increases with age and becomes particularly important to monitor closely in the elderly.)*

Hass WK, Easton JD, Adams HP Jr, et al. Randomized trial comparing ticlopidine with aspirin for the prevention of stroke in high-risk patients. N Engl J Med 1989;521:501. *(Double-blind, randomized trial of over 3000 patients with TIA or minor stroke showing a significant reduction* [approximately 10%] *in risk of stroke or death compared to aspirin.)*

Hirsh J. Oral anticoagulant drugs. N Engl J Med 1991;324:1865. *(Exhaustive, but clinically useful review; 132 references.)*

Hirsch J, Levin MN. The optimal intensity of oral anticoagulant therapy. JAMA 1987;258:2723. *(Argues that low-intensity herapy is best for most indications.)*

Lancaster TR, Singer DE, Sheehan MA, et al. The impact of long-term warfarin therapy on quality of life. Arch Intern Med 1991;151:1944. *(Quality of life well preserved.)*

Landefeld CS, Goldman L. Major bleeding in outpatients treated with warfarin: Incidence and prediction by factors known at the start of outpatient therapy. Am J Med 1989;87:144. *(Best available study; age > 65, history of stroke or GI bleeding, serious comorbid condition, and AF were predictors of risk.)*

Landefeld CS, Rosenblatt MW, Goldman L. Bleeding in outpatients treated with warfarin: Relation to the prothrombin time and important remediable lesions. Am J Med 1989;87:153. *(Companion study confirming that risk of bleeding increases with intensity of anticoagulation; also confirms value of evaluating for underlying lesions.)*

Meltzer RS, Visser CA, Fuster V. Intracardiac thrombi and systemic embolization. Ann Intern Med 1986;104:689. *(Excellent review of data justifying oral anticoagulation.)*

Petitti DB, Strom BL, Melmon KL. Duration of warfarin anticoagulant therapy and the probabilities of recurrent thromboembolism in hemorrhage. Am J Med 1986;81:255. *(Anticoagulation beyond 6 weeks associated with increased risk of hemorrhage but no apparent protection against recurrent thromboembolism.)*

Shorr RI, Ray WA, Dougherty JR, et al. Concurrent use of nonsteroidal anti-inflammatory drugs and oral anticoagulants places elderly persons at high risk of hemorrhagic peptic ulcer. Arch Intern Med 1993;153:1665. *(Risk increases 13-fold.)*

Singer DE. Randomized trials of warfarin for atrial fibrillation. N Engl J Med 1992;327:1451. *(Fine editorial tersely summarizing the known and unknown.)*

Smith P, Arneson H, Holme I. The effect of warfarin on mortality and reinfarction after myocardial infarction. N Engl J Med 1990;323:147. *(Intriguing data from Europe suggesting that warfarin may reduce rate of reinfarction.)*

Stroke Prevention in Atrial Fibrillation Investigators. Predictors of thromboembolism in atrial fibrillation. Ann Intern Med 1992;116:1,6. *(Two-part study; recent CHF, hypertension, previous embolism, LV dysfunction, and left atrial enlargement were independent predictors of stroke risk.)*

84

Approach to the Patient With Lymphoma

JERRY YOUNGER, M.D.

Primary Care Medicine: Office Evaluation and Management of the Adult Patient, 3rd edition, edited by Allan H. Goroll, Lawrence A. May, and Albert G. Mulley, Jr. J.B. Lippincott Company, Philadelphia

The lymphomas are a diverse group of malignancies, with non-Hodgkin's lymphoma about twice as common as Hodgkin's disease. Together they account for nearly 23,000 new cases of cancer per year in the United States, an incidence of 9 per 100,000 population. There are multiple subtypes, each with specific immunologic and pathologic characteristics and a distinctive clinical presentation and therapeutic response. Non-Hodgkin's lymphoma strikes much later than Hodgkin's disease; peak incidence is in the fifth decade, compared to the second decade for Hodgkin's disease (although there is a second peak in the fifth decade). Prognosis for Non-Hodgkin's lymphoma is less favorable in terms of long-term cure, although survival and responsiveness to therapy are substantial. Cure is possible for many patients with Hodgkin's disease.

Although treatment of these conditions is the province of the oncologist, the primary physician has an important role in the diagnosis and staging of the disease, coordinating plans for management, and delivering follow-up care on an outpatient basis. Because the primary physician is likely to have conducted the initial evaluation, he or she needs to be prepared to discuss with the patient and family the meaning of the findings. Even after referral, the primary physician often encounters requests for advice, being the physician the patient knows best. Consequently, a serious working knowledge of clinical presentation, prognosis, staging methods, and treatment options is important for the primary physician if the patient is to be served well.

HODGKIN'S DISEASE

Pathology, Clinical Presentation, and Course

The histology of Hodgkin's disease incorporates four categories: lymphocyte predominance, nodular sclerosis, mixed cellularity, and lymphocyte depletion. *Lymphocyte predominance* occurs in 10 percent to 15 percent of patients, *nodular sclerosis* in 20 percent to 50 percent, mixed cellularity in 20 percent to 40 percent, and *lymphocyte depletion* in 5 percent to 15 percent. In about 15 percent of cases, classification is difficult and requires expert interpretation of the histology. In all instances, the *sine qua non* of diagnosis is the pathogenic *Reed-Sternberg cell.*

The condition originates in the lymph nodes. Conceptually, Hodgkin's disease is *unicentric* in origin and progresses by contiguous extension along lymphatic pathways. Consequently, the adenopathy tends to be asymmetric. This pattern of evolution is in contrast to non-Hodgkin's lymphomas, which are multicentric and associated with more advanced stages of disease at initial presentation. Most patients present with disease above the clavicle. Less than 15 percent start out with disease initiating below the diaphragm, although any node may be involved (including those of the mediastinum, axilla, or groin). Typically, the nodes are firm and nontender; although often matted, they may be discrete and even freely movable. Subsequent spread to the spleen happens regularly and is the first manifestation of disease below the diaphragm, followed by involvement of the liver and bone marrow. Fever, weight loss, night sweats, or alcohol-induced pain may develop and almost always represents advanced disease.

The differential diagnosis of Hodgkin's disease includes infectious mononucleosis, human immunodeficiency virus (HIV) infection, and other nonbacterial adenopathies in the young (see Chapter 12). In the elderly, other malignancies are a common diagnostic consideration; they are particularly suspect in the presence of a fever of unknown origin. Excisional biopsy rather than needle aspiration is needed for diagnosis.

Classification by Stage. Because prognosis and treatment are so dependent on extent of disease, classification by stage plays a central role in Hodgkin's disease. The Ann Arbor system of classification is the one most widely referred to. In it, *stage I* is defined as disease confined to a single node-bearing area or localized involvement of a single extranodal site. *Stage II* involves two or more contiguous node-bearing areas on the same side of the diaphragm or more than one nodal region in conjunction with localized involvement of an extralymphatic organ on the same side of the diaphragm. *Stage III* is nodal involvement on both sides of the diaphragm, with or without involvement of the spleen or a local extranodal organ or site. Additional subcategories have been developed for patients with intraabdominal disease. *Stage* III_1 represents disease confined to the upper abdomen; it is generally microscopic. *Stage* III_2 designates disease extending into the pelvis with grossly involved nodes or bulky retroperitoneal tumor. *Stage IV* represents diffuse visceral disease (liver, lung parenchyma, bone marrow).

The special category designated *E* (for extranodal) was created because of data indicating that involvement of an organ contiguous to a lymph node-bearing area has a distinctly better prognosis than does visceral involvement that is hematogenous. Nonetheless, the prognosis is not as good as it would be if there were no organ involvement. *S* denotes disease in the spleen.

Approximately 20 percent of patients will have *fever, night sweats,* or *significant weight loss* (> 10%). These systemic symptoms are incorporated into the staging system because they are important determinants of prognosis. When absent, the designation is *A;* when any of the three is present, the designation is *B*. Patients with pruritus only are no longer included in the B group. Early (stages I and II) and advanced (stages III and IV) Hodgkin's disease are relatively equally distributed in terms of frequency. More sophisticated staging by pathologic as well as clinical procedures generally tends to advance the stage of disease.

Prognosis of Hodgkin's disease has improved dramatically with the advent of careful staging and improved radiation technology and chemotherapy programs. Overall 5-year survival is 80 percent; 65 percent experience 5-year relapse-free survival when all stages of disease are combined (Table 84–1). The principal determinants of outcome are stage, patient age, presence or absence of symptoms, and tumor bulk. Histology is also a factor, although not as important as others.

Staging

Staging (Table 84–2) is critical to design of a therapeutic program and estimation of prognosis. *Clinical staging* involves assessment of history, physical examination, and radiologic findings. History should ascertain presence of fever, night sweats, or weight loss. Careful palpation of all lymph nodes and assessment of liver and spleen size are important, although enlargement discovered by physical examination does not necessarily indicate involvement by the disease. One-half of patients with a palpable spleen do not have histologic splenic involvement, and one-quarter with normal-sized spleens do.

About 90 percent of patients are thought to have stage I or II disease at the time of initial clinical staging. However, most treatment decisions require *pathologic staging* (which includes biopsy), because up to a two-thirds of patients who

Table 84-2. Staging Procedures for Hodgkin's Disease

STUDY	INDICATION
Radiographic Studies	
Chest x-ray	All patients; CT if mediastinal or hilar disease
Chest CT	If x-ray abnormal or if results would change therapy
Lymphangiogram	*Only if* (a) no clinical evidence of infradiaphragmatic disease, (b) no mass or lung disease, or (c) no advanced stage signs or symptoms (B)
Abdominal CT	Complements lymphangiogram; same indications
Surgical Studies	
Laparoscopy	Preferable to laparotomy in presence of B symptoms. To identify liver pathology
Laparotomy	Strage I or II disease and no symptoms
Hematologic Studies	
Bone marrow biopsy	Only if clinical stage IIB or more

Table 84-1. Hodgkin's Disease: Stages, Relative Incidences, and Prognosis

STAGE	DEFINITION	RELATIVE INCIDENCE (%)	THERAPY	CURE (%)
Stage I	Confined to single node-bearing area	30	Radiation	70–90
Stage II	Confined to two contiguous node-bearing areas; on one side of diaphragm	25	Radiation	
Stage III	In nodal areas on both sides of the diaphragm	25	Radiation and chemotherapy	50–60
Stage IV	Visceral lesions (liver, lung) *not* in contiguity with nodes	20	Chemotherapy	
Special Categories				
E	Visceral extranodal disease in continuity with nodes. For example, lung mass extending out from hilum		Radiation +/− chemotherapy	
B	Symptoms of fever, weight loss, or sweats		Chemotherapy +/− radiation	

Adapted from DeVita VT Jr, Hellman S, Jaffee ES. Hodgkin's Disease in Cancer Principles and Practice of Oncology, 4th ed. DeVita VT Jr, Hellman S, Rosenberg SA eds. Philadelphia: JB Lippincott, 1993;1819.

present with clinical stage I or II disease turn out to have disease below the diaphragm on pathologic staging. About half of patients with B symptoms will manifest disease below the diaphragm at laparotomy, compared to 25 percent of patients with A symptoms.

The principal staging procedures include chest x-ray, computed tomography (CT), lymphangiography, and bone marrow biopsy. Staging laparotomy is indicated in selected instances. All patients should have a *chest x-ray*, because some of the most common forms of Hodgkin's disease involve the mediastinum. Even if chest x-ray is abnormal, *CT of the chest* is indicated, because it provides enhanced sensitivity for detection and definition of mediastinal, hilar, and paravertebral adenopathy. The need for chest CT in a patient with a totally normal chest film depends on whether the result will alter therapy or prognosis. CT is more sensitive than chest x-ray for detection of disease in the mediastinum and adjacent structures.

CT of the abdomen and lymphangiography provide complementary information about disease below the diaphragm. CT is best for demonstrating number and size of nodes in the retroperitoneum and pelvis. It also may show evidence of hepatic or splenic involvement, although no radiologic test (including magnetic resonance imaging [MRI] and radionuclide scanning) is sensitive enough to rule out splenic involvement. Abdominal CT provides anatomic information about nodes in areas not well visualized by lymphangiography (mesenteric, subhepatic, perisplenic, celiac, and periaortic regions). CT cannot detect microscopic disease and gives less information than the lymphangiogram about nodal architecture. MRI offers no advantage over CT.

Lymphangiography provides more detailed information on the structure of retroperitoneal nodes, capable of detecting disease in nodes that are not enlarged. By itself, lymphangiography has a low sensitivity, with a false-negative rate of 20 percent. However, when strict radiologic criteria for nodal involvement are used, specificity reaches 95 percent, with less than 5 percent false-positives noted. Thus, a positive study is helpful, but a negative lymphangiogram does not rule out disease below the diaphragm. Moreover, even if the test is positive, it does not detect involvement of the liver or spleen, which is an important determinant of therapy. The test is important to perform in patients with clinical stage I or II disease without B symptoms, particularly those patients in whom laparotomy is scheduled, to identify the lymph nodes to be removed. About 25 percent of patients classified clinically are reclassified on the basis of lymphangiogram results.

The dye load associated with lymphangiography carries a small risk of pulmonary insufficiency related to extravasation of dye into the lung parenchyma, and it should not be performed in those with severe lung disease.

Bone marrow biopsy is a useful staging procedure in patients with systemic symptoms or disease beyond stage II, being positive in up to 20 percent of such patients. Because disease in the marrow is often focal, multiple biopsies are necessary to avoid sampling error. Marrow aspiration is never useful. A positive marrow classifies the disease as stage IV and makes laparotomy unnecessary. Patients with clinical stage I or IIA disease have never been reported to have positive marrow biopsies, but stage IIB is associated with marrow involvement in 9 percent of patients.

Staging laparotomy is reserved for patients in whom the result will change the approach to therapy (eg, asymptomatic patients with clinical stage I or II disease). The procedure has the advantage of allowing more precise definition of the extent of disease and frequently results in reclassification that necessitates a different treatment program.

The procedure includes wedge biopsy of the liver, splenectomy, and examination of the lymph nodes in contiguous chains, exclusive of mesenteric nodes. The operation has a low mortality rate (0.5% to 1.0%) and negligible early morbidity. However, patients who receive radiation and chemotherapy after splenectomy are at increased risk (up to 28 percent in the first 6 years) for fulminant sepsis, with its attendant 50 percent mortality. Those who undergo splenectomy but do not receive chemotherapy appear to be much less vulnerable to serious infection. Because of the risk of infection, only those who will have their treatment program altered by the results of laparotomy should undergo the operation.

Laparoscopy has been advocated as a less invasive means of identifying liver involvement in patients with a high probability of disease below the diaphragm, for example, those with B symptoms. Liver biopsy specimens are taken from suspicious areas under direct visualization. Laparoscopy is superior to percutaneous liver biopsy (20% yield versus 5%), but its yield does not match that of open biopsy performed during staging laparotomy. Few patients with hepatic involvement are free of systemic complaints; on the other hand, neither hepatomegaly after physical examination or scan nor elevated alkaline phosphatase levels identify patients likely to have positive biopsies.

Many other tests for staging of Hodgkin's disease lack sensitivity or specificity. Such is the case for liver and spleen scans and bone scans, which are not indicated in routine staging. *Gallium scanning* may be positive in areas of disease involvement and occasionally discovers previously unknown disease. Its main use is for detection of residual disease in the mediastinum after treatment.

Complete blood count, alkaline phosphatase, and sedimentation rate are similarly nonspecific. The use of the erythrocyte sedimentation rate, serum copper, and leukocyte alkaline phosphatase as indices of disease activity and extent is promoted by various investigators, but all of these tests represent nonspecific approaches to evaluating the patient with Hodgkin's disease.

In sum, the history is reviewed for characteristic systemic symptoms; the physical examination focuses on lymph-node bearing areas. A chest x-ray is obtained, as is lymphangiography and abdominal CT in patients who are clinically in stage I or II. If the patient is clinically in stage I or II and would be treated by radiation, a staging laparotomy should be performed to identify occult disease below the diaphragm. Until it becomes possible to predict more accurately who is likely to have occult disease in the abdomen, one must rely on the laparotomy. In instances where systemic symptoms are present, a laparoscopy and bone marrow biopsy can be performed as preliminary studies; if either is positive, the need for laparotomy is obviated. Lymphangiography produces too many false-negatives to be relied on without intraabdominal evaluation and, even if positive, fails to provide information about the liver and spleen, which is necessary for selecting among radiation therapy, chemotherapy, or both.

Treatment

Although selection of treatment regimen is the responsibility of the oncologist, it is important for the primary physician to be cognizant of the major treatment regimens and their outcomes. Treatment is a function of disease stage. Therapy for Hodgkin's disease achieves a substantial cure rate in all stages (see Table 84-2).

Stages I and II. *Radiation therapy* is the treatment of choice. For patients with stage IA or IIA disease, *local and extended field radiotherapy* to contiguous node-bearing areas and adjacent regions has resulted in an 85 percent to 90 percent cure rate. *Total nodal radiation therapy* has been used in stages IB and IIB, delivered at a dose of 3500 to 4500 rads over a 3- to 4-week period through a portal referred to as the "mantle" for chest radiation and the "inverted Y" for intraabdominal lymph nodes. Stage IB and IIB patients have a 70 percent to 75 percent chance of cure with such radiation therapy. However, to be curative, radiation therapy must be done with great precision and the extent of disease must be well documented. One study found that 37 percent of treatment portals did not cover the entire extent of disease. Radiation therapy *side effects* include dental problems and increased risks of *thyroid cancer* (20-year latency), radiation *pneumonitis* (6% to 20%), accelerated *coronary artery disease,* and a *second solid tumor* (incidence approximately 1% per year). There is also an increased risk of *leukemia* in patients receiving high doses of radiation to the bone marrow.

Chemotherapy is added to radiation when there is a large mediastinal mass (greater than one-third the diameter of the chest) and substituted for it if there is a failure to respond or a relapse occurs. Some have argued that because success rates with chemotherapy are so great, all patients with early stage disease should receive chemotherapy. The debate continues, but radiation therapy remains the treatment of choice.

Stages III and IV. *Combination chemotherapy* is the cornerstone of treatment. The Mustargen, Oncovin, prednisone, procarbazine (*MOPP*) program was the prototype. Doxorubicin (Adriamycin), bleomycin, vinblastine, dacarbazine *(ABVD)* is currently in wide use. Combination regimens are designed to address issues of tumor resistance and drug toxicity. Hybrids and alternating of combinations have also proven effective. All are based on the identification of agents with individually distinctive mechanisms of antitumor activity. Their side effects are nonadditive, helping to limit the amount of drug-related morbidity. Response rates for stage III and IV disease are in the 80 percent range, and complete remission of disease is the rule. For patients with advanced disease who experience remission, there is a 50 percent chance of cure. By manipulation of dosages and schedules of drugs, most such chemotherapy can be delivered conveniently on an outpatient basis. In most instances chemotherapy is administered for 6 months, at which time restaging is carried out; in the absence of residual disease, therapy is discontinued. There is no benefit from a "maintenance program."

Choice of program remains a subject of much debate among oncologists. Of particular concern is the 20 percent rate of failure to respond, which has led to use of seven-drug and alternating four-drug regimens. There are problems with both, especially the need to prolong therapy beyond 6 months, which greatly increases risk of toxicity. Some authorities argue that the real cause of failure to respond lies with inability to administer adequate doses. Balancing response rates with treatment-related adverse effects is an art form that requires the selection of an oncologist experienced in the treatment of Hodgkin's disease.

Adverse effects of combination chemotherapy include sterility, secondary malignancy, and increased susceptibility to infection, in addition to those associated with individual drugs (see Chapter 88). MOPP produces *sterility* in almost all males. Sperm-banking is indicated before initiation of therapy. Close to 90 percent of women over age 26 become infertile, but most younger women are able to have children; however, premature menopause is common. The incidence of sterility is significantly lower with ABVD.

The risk of *leukemia* is increased for up to 10 years after chemotherapy (peak is at 5 years), especially when the program includes an alkylating agent (as in MOPP). In a comprehensive analysis of leukemia in treated Hodgkin's disease, relative risk was 9.0 over that for radiation therapy and did not increase with concomitant radiation. Risk did increase with dose and duration of chemotherapy, stage of disease, age, and splenectomy. Leukemia risk is thought to be lower with ABVD. Despite the risk of leukemia, the gain in survival afforded by combination chemotherapy greatly outweighs its adverse effects.

Other chemotherapy-related side effects include severe *emesis, bone marrow suppression,* and *neuropathy* (see Chapter 88). The risk of overwhelming *pneumococcal sepsis* associated with splenectomy can be lessened by use of polyvalent *pneumococcal vaccine.* The vaccine is often given before splenectomy but can be administered after surgery; antibody response is just as adequate after splenectomy. However, antibody production is blunted if chemotherapy is begun within 10 days of vaccination. As noted above, risk of overwhelming sepsis approaches 30 percent, with a 50 percent fatality rate.

Radiation is sometimes employed for stage III patients. Those with III_1A disease appear to do equally well with radiation or chemotherapy. Patients with stage IIIA who have a large mass of mediastinal tumor often have radiation added to their program.

Treating Relapses. Relapse occurs in 20 percent to 35 percent of patients. The probability of responding to retreatment ("salvage" therapy) is a function of the length of the initial remission and approaches 95 percent, even if the original chemotherapeutic regimen is used. A noncross-resistant regimen, such as ABVD, can be used either in place of the original program or in some form of combination with it. Relapse-free survival of 45 percent at 10 years has been noted for patients retreated after an initial remission of over 12 months; however, overall survival falls to 24 percent due to complications of retreatment (eg, second malignancy). For those with initial remission less than 12 months, the survival after retreatment is about 10 percent at 10 years.

Use of *autologous bone marrow transplantation* in drug-resistant patients has provided new options. Retreatment after transplantation produces remission in 50 percent and extended disease-free periods in a quarter to a half of those who respond.

Monitoring Therapy

Periodic examination of involved nodes is the simplest means of judging response to therapy. Many laboratory parameters have been developed but offer little advantage over physical examination and chest x-ray. The need for periodic restaging is a judgment to be made in consultation with the oncologist. Patients receiving MOPP require close surveillance (see Chapter 88). Patients being treated with radiation should be watched for bone marrow suppression and, when lung fields are involved, radiation pneumonitis and thyroid dysfunction.

The likelihood of *late relapse* (36 months or more after completion of therapy) is small, but large enough to warrant continued monitoring. Risk of late relapse is low, but patients with stage I disease show the highest rates, perhaps because of failure to irradiate all involved nodes. Also at risk for recurrence are patients presenting with a large mediastinal tumor; local recurrence is typical. Gallium scanning has proven useful in such cases, although biopsy confirmation is necessary, because false-positives do occur. Most relapses are detected by history, physical examination, or chest x-ray; abdominal CT may also help detect late disease. Careful late follow-up is warranted, even after 3 years, because response to retreatment is good.

Patient Education and Indications for Consultation and Referral

Many patients will greet the diagnosis of Hodgkin's disease with dread, equating it with a fatal outcome. Without raising false hopes, the physician can point to the excellent 5-year survival rates and the high percentage of individuals who are disease-free after 10 years. Patients who have undergone splenectomy should be advised to have polyvalent pneumococcal vaccine before undergoing chemotherapy or radiation. Because chemotherapy can cause permanent sterility, it is important to review this prospect with the patient before embarking on treatment. Pretherapy sperm storage has been advocated. Young women (under age 26) can be counseled in encouraging terms because they have been found capable of bearing phenotypically normal children.

Once the diagnosis is confirmed and clinical staging is completed, referral to the oncologist for discussion of pathologic staging and design of a treatment program is indicated. During the period of initial treatment, the patient will be followed closely by the oncologist, but the primary physician can and should serve to ensure coordination of care and provision of support to the patient and family.

NON-HODGKIN'S LYMPHOMAS

Classification, Clinical Presentation, and Prognosis

The non-Hodgkin's lymphomas represent a diverse group of malignancies originating from lymphocytes. About 85 percent arise from B cells, with the remainder deriving from T cells. The wide range of histologic appearances that characterizes the non-Hodgkin's lymphomas is believed due to maturation arrest at different stages of cellular development. Etiology remains unknown, but there is evidence of links to viral infection and deregulation of oncogenes.

Classification and Prognosis. In contrast to Hodgkin's disease, the histopathologic characteristics of non-Hodgkin lymphomas are major determinants of prognosis and response to therapy, whereas stage at time of presentation is of less importance. A host of histologic classification schemes have been put forward. The most widely accepted is that referred to as the Working Formulation (Table 84–3). It relates histology to prognosis, with nodal architecture, degree of differentiation, and cell type being the important determinants.

Three *histopathologic categories* emerge: *low-grade* or indolent, *intermediate-grade* or aggressive, and *high-grade* or highly aggressive. Survival for patients with untreated low-grade disease extends for years; for intermediate grade disease, it declines to several months; and for high-grade disease, it measures in weeks. However, response to therapy often follows an inverse pattern, with some of the many aggressive tumors responding readily to therapy and exhibiting potential for cure, whereas most low-grade lymphomas prove stubborn and typically relapse.

Clinical Presentation. Unlike Hodgkin's disease, non-Hodgkin's lymphomas are multicentric in origin and can appear in discontinuous lymph node chains. *Localized* and *regional* lymphomas (stages I and II, respectively; see below) account for less than 10 percent of cases. Most of the remainder present with *disseminated* disease (stage III or IV). Non-Hodgkin's lymphomas can occur in nodal sites, in viscera, or in both. Mediastinal disease is found in 20 percent. *Extranodal disease* is often solitary and likely to be confined to the organ of origin. Waldeyer's ring, upper gastrointestinal tract, testes, and bone are the most commonly involved extranodal sites, accounting for up to 15 percent of cases. Extranodal disease can have a favorable prognosis, particularly in the absence of nodal involvement. Five-year survival rates are as high as 30 percent to 50 percent irrespective of pathologic type. A unique site of extranodal disease is the central nervous system (CNS), especially the epidural space, leptomeninges, and cerebral hemispheres. It has a high association with HIV infection. The propensity for developing CNS lymphoma is also related to histologic type (lymphoblastic), distribution (marrow spread), and age (younger patients).

Presentation is affected by tumor grade. Patients with high-grade disease are likely to present with a rapidly growing, symptomatic mass confined to a single nodal or extranodal site. Those with low-grade disease typically report slowing enlarging nodes at multiple sites. Fever, night

Table 84-3. The Working Formulation of Non-Hodgkin's Lymphomas*

GRADE AND CELL TYPE	FREQUENCY (%)	SURVIVAL
I. Low-grade	39% total	5–7 years
A. Small lymphocytic	4	
B. Follicular, small cleaved cell	26	
C. Follicular, mixed, small cleaved cell	9	
II. Intermediate-grade	41% total	2–5 years
D. Follicular, predominantly large cell	4	
E. Diffuse small cleaved cell	8	
F. Diffuse mixed, small, large cell	7	
G. Diffuse large cell, cleaved/noncleaved	22	
III. High-grade lymphoma	20% total	0.5–2 years
H. Diffuse large cell, immunoblastic	9	
I. Lymphoblastic	6	
J. Small noncleaved cell (Burkitt's, non-Burkitt's)	5	

*Adapted from Rosenberg SA. National Cancer Institute sponsored study of classifications of non-Hodgkin lymphomas: Summary and description of a working formulation for clinical usage. Cancer 1980;45:2188.

sweats, and weight loss are more common in non-Hodgkin's lymphoma than they are in Hodgkin's disease.

Anemia is a common consequence of lymphoma. Mechanisms include immune hemolysis, hypersplenism, and marrow infiltration. In some patients, there may be sufficient numbers of lymphoma cells circulating in the blood to appear on a peripheral blood smear. In others, a *leukemic phase* may develop and account for the appearance of malignant cells on peripheral smear.

Immune dysfunction occurs in many patients, which should not be surprising given that most lymphomas are B-cell disorders. Humoral immunity is particularly impaired, leading to hypogammaglobulinemia, monoclonal gammopathies, hemolytic anemias, and immune destruction of platelets.

Principles of Management

Staging. The staging system for lymphoma is identical to that used for Hodgkin's disease, with the exception that there are no categories for symptoms or designations for contiguous visceral involvement or splenic disease. As noted above, stage is less a determinant of prognosis and treatment selection than it is for Hodgkin's disease, but it still plays some role in the selection and intensity of treatment. Pending a better staging system, the Ann Arbor scheme (see Table 84–1) continues to be used for non-Hodgkin's lymphoma, although distinctions between stages have less meaning. For patients with low-grade disease, the main issue therapeutically is whether their disease is localized or disseminated. For more aggressive forms of disease, extent of disease is less important.

Although the approach to staging is, in part, determined by the aggressiveness of the tumor's histology (see below), some generalizations are appropriate. A thorough *physical examination* of all node-bearing areas is essential, including such sites as the epitrochlear nodes, Waldeyer's ring, and the preauricular area. Liver and spleen are commonly enlarged when involved and should be carefully checked. Radiologic investigations are especially important in patients thought to have local or regional disease. *Chest x-ray* and *CT* of *chest, abdomen,* and *pelvis* are obtained. In many centers, CT of the abdomen and pelvis has replaced *lymphangiography* for nodal survey and has the added advantage of providing information on liver and spleen size. However, lymphangiogram is a reasonable alternative where CT is unavailable. CT is considerably better at detection of disease in the pelvis and retroperitoneum.

Hematologic assessment is critical and includes examination of the *peripheral smear* and *bone marrow* (aspirate plus biopsy). Bilateral or multiple bone marrow biopsies can identify occult stage IV disease. In a series of 131 patients, 27 percent had positive biopsies when more than one marrow site was sampled. Aspiration is inadequate, because the false-negative rate is 30 percent; a solid bone marrow specimen is essential.

Much of the staging workup depends on clinical or histopathologic findings. For example, patients with intermediate-grade disease found in the area of Waldeyer's ring are at increased risk of gastrointestinal involvement and need to be endoscoped if the clinical picture is suggestive. Patients with high-grade histology are almost certain to have advanced disease at the time of presentation and need not undergo extensive study. *Lumbar puncture* should be considered in patients at risk for CNS spread (ie, those with marrow involvement, lymphoblastic histology, young age, or HIV infection).

Several staging procedures are unnecessary. *Laparotomy* is *not* indicated because the yields from CT bone marrow biopsy are so high that rarely do the findings from laparotomy influence clinical decision making. Gallium scanning is also not very helpful.

Therapy

Chemotherapy is the predominant mode of treatment for non-Hodgkin's lymphoma (Table 84–4), because most patients already have widespread disease at the time of initial clinical presentation. It may be administered as a single agent or as a complex multidrug regimen. Radiation plays a role in management of localized disease. As noted, histology

Table 84-4. Treatment of Non-Hodgkin's Lymphomas

GRADE AND STAGE	TREATMENT	LONG-TERM REMISSION (%)*
Low-grade		
Early stage	Radiation	Unknown
Late stage	Controversial (single* or multiagent chemotherapy, interferon,† radiation,† watchful waiting†)	
Intermediate-grade		
Early stage	Multiagent chemotherapy +/− radiation	85–95
Late stage	Multiagent chemotherapy	60–80
High-grade		
All stages	High-dose multiagent chemotherapy, autologous marrow transplantation†	20–40

*Long-term remission is *not* synonymous with cure; cure rates actually increase with advancing grade of disease.
†Investigational method.
Adapted from Longo DL, DeVita VT Jr, Jaffee ES, et al. Lymphocytic Lymphomas in DeVita VT Jr, Hellman S, Rosenberg SA, eds. Cancer Principles and Practice of Oncology, 4th ed. Philadelphia: JB Lippincott, 1993;1859.

and stage are, respectively, the primary and secondary determinants of response to therapy. Absence of bulky disease, minimal extranodal disease, absence of B symptoms, young age, and female gender are other predictors of response to therapy and prolonged survival.

Low-Grade/Indolent Disease. The curability of low-grade indolent disease remains a subject of controversy. Most forms of therapy produce responses and remissions, but relapses are the rule. The rare patient with true early-stage disease is typically treated with radiation. For patients with *more advanced* indolent disease, treatment is controversial. Most histopathologic types appear to respond with complete remission to combination chemotherapy, high-dose single-agent therapy, radiation, or combined modality therapy, but relapse is common after 2 years. Remission after retreatment is common, but cure has never been reported (except for those with follicular mixed cell type) and the benefit of aggressive chemotherapy versus watchful waiting remains to be demonstrated. Some centers use aggressive chemotherapy plus radiation, followed by autologous bone marrow transplantation in such patients. The approach must still be considered investigational until long-term results are available, but they appear to be encouraging. Another approach is the use of *alpha-interferon* plus combination chemotherapy, which appears to give better results than chemotherapy alone.

Intermediate-Grade/Aggressive Disease. For such patients with *localized disease,* combination chemotherapy with or without local radiation to the involved area provides 5-year disease-free results in as many as 85 percent to 95 percent. Besides histopathology and stage, outcome is affected by presence of B symptoms, marrow involvement, elevations in lactate dehydrogenase (LDH), large abdominal mass, and multiple extranodal sites. In patients who fail to respond or who relapse after initial response, secondary therapy is employed, using non–cross-resistant drugs such as bleomycin and doxorubicin.

Advanced stage disease has been treated with more aggressive combination chemotherapy, providing complete remissions in 80 percent and long-term survival in up to 60 percent to 70 percent of patients who tolerate therapy. However, drug-related toxicity and serious complications are far more frequent with the more aggressive programs, often necessitating dose reductions that compromise outcomes.

High-Grade/Highly Aggressive Disease. Multidrug therapy is indicated for patients with symptomatic or rapidly progressive disease. Lymphoblastic and some Burkitt's lymphomas are treated with regimens similar to those for acute leukemia. Response rates with multidrug therapy approach 95 percent, with median survival in excess of 2 years. For some subgroups, combination chemotherapy may result in cure for 20 percent to 40 percent of patients.

Investigational therapies include use of monoclonal antibodies, autologous bone marrow transplantation, and interferon. Because most lymphomas are of B-cell origin, identification of a specific antigen allows development of a *monoclonal antibody* against the tumor cell. Monoclonal antibodies have induced remissions but are associated with development of immune responses against the immunoglobin in some patients. Another approach is to perform *autologous bone marrow transplantation* sometimes after treating the marrow with monoclonal antibodies to purge tumor cells from the marrow. The best candidates for transplantation appear to be those who are responsive to chemotherapy and are in a second remission. Five-year disease-free results have been reported in 30 percent to 60 percent of carefully selected patients, but risk is high with up to 10 percent of patients dying from complications associated with the procedure. Clinical trials with *interferon* are under way; partial remissions have been achieved.

Monitoring Therapy

Monitoring patients on chemotherapy requires close surveillance (see Chapter 88). Bone marrow suppression is the leading complication. Relapse or recurrence generally develops in the areas of previous disease (in contrast to Hodgkin's disease, where relapse is extranodal or visceral). Relapse typically occurs within 12 to 18 months of initiating treatment. Watching for development of neurologic symptoms is particularly important in those with a predisposition to CNS spread (see above).

Patient Education

The encouraging results of chemotherapy, particularly in patients with aggressive advanced disease, provide new hope. As with Hodgkin's disease, the patient can be given a fairly accurate assessment of the prognosis after careful histologic study and staging have been carried out. Often the prognosis is far better than the patient's fearful expectations and can be shared profitably. Even elderly patients are candidates for treatment of life-threatening disease.

A detailed review of possible adverse effects from therapy (eg, sterility, infection, and so forth; see Chapter 88) must be reviewed as must the experimental nature of those therapies where data on long-term outcomes are lacking. A key question remains the best approach to advanced stages of indolent disease.

Indications for Referral

These malignancies are potentially curable diseases. Referral to the oncologist should be made early when the diagnosis is first suspected. Management of the patient with Hodgkin's disease or lymphoma needs to be a cooperative venture from the start, with the primary physician working closely with the oncologist experienced in lymphoma. Selection of treatment modality requires the judgment of an oncologist who is knowledgable about available protocols, which are constantly undergoing revision. The primary physician monitors response and adverse effects, maintains continuity, and provides psychological support.

ANNOTATED BIBLIOGRAPHY

Hodgkin's Disease

Aisenberg A. The staging and treatment of Hodgkin's disease. N Engl J Med 1978;299:1288. *(One of the original studies establishing the utility of staging laparotomy; of 75 patients with clinical stage I or II disease, one-third were reclassified to stage III on the basis of a positive lymphangiogram, and another third were reclassified on the basis of a staging laparotomy.)*

Bookman MA, Longo DL. Concomitant illness in patients treated for Hodgkin's disease. Cancer Treat Rev 1986;13:77. *(Exhaustive review of medical problems associated with the illness and its treatments.)*

Buzaid AC, Lippman SM, Miller TP. Salvage therapy of advanced Hodgkin's disease. Am J Med 1987;83:523. *(Critical review of salvage regimens; 80 references.)*

Coker DD, Morris DM, Coleman JJ, et al. Infection among 210 patients with surgically staged Hodgkin's disease. Am J Med 1983;75:97. *(Overwhelming pneumococcal sepsis is uncommon in splenectomized patients in the absence of a predisposing factor, such as advanced age or advanced stage of disease.)*

Devita VT Jr, Hubbard SM. Hodgkin's disease. N Engl J Med 1993;328;580. *(Authoritative review of chemotherapy; includes discussions of treatment according to stage, program selection, and salvage therapy; 63 references.)*

Gomez GA, Reese PA, Nava H, et al. Staging laparotomy and splenectomy in early Hodgkin's disease. Am J Med 1984;77:205. *(Study that takes a critical look at the routine use of staging laparotomy for early disease and finds little.)*

Hoppe RT, Coleman CN, Cox RS, et al. The management of stage–I-II Hodgkin's disease with irradiation alone or combined modality therapy: The Stanford experience. Blood 1982;59:455. *(Radiotherapy was curative for early-stage disease, although combination with chemotherapy helped reduce the risk of relapse in patients with clinical stage IIB.)*

Horning SJ, Hoppe RT, Kaplan HS, et al. Female reproductive potential after treatment for Hodgkin's disease. N Engl J Med 1981;304:1377. *(Women under the age of 26 successfully treated for Hodgkin's disease became pregnant and delivered phenotypically normal children.)*

Kaldor JM, Day NE, Clarke EA, et al. Leukemia following Hodgkin's disease. N Engl J Med 1990;322:7. *(Case-control study of international cancer registries; risk of leukemia greatly increased by chemotherapy; not by radiation.)*

Phillips GL, Wolff SN, Herzig RH, et al. Treatment of progressive Hodgkin's disease with intensive chemoradiotherapy and autologous bone marrow transplantation in refractory Hodgkin's disease. Blood 1989;73:2086. *(Improved response achieved.)*

Rosenberg SA, Kaplan HS. The evolution and summary results of the Stanford randomized clinical trials of the management of Hodgkin's disease: 1962–1984. Int J Radiat Oncol Biol Phys 1985;11:5. *(Summary report focusing on radiation therapy; from a leading center.)*

Siber GR, Gorham C, Martin P, et al. Antibody response to pretreatment immunization and post-treatment boosting with bacterial polysaccharide vaccines in patients with Hodgkin's disease. Ann Intern Med 1986;104:467. *(Antibody response not affected by timing of immunization relative to splenectomy, but blunted if chemotherapy was begun within 10 days of immunization.)*

Wagener DJT, Burgers MV, Dekker W et al, for the EORTC Radiotherapy-Chemotherapy Cooperative Group. Sequential non–cross-resistant chemotherapy regimens (MOPP and CAVmP) in Hodgkin's disease stage IIIB and IV. Cancer 1983;52:1558. *(Alternating three- or four-drug regimens for treatment of malignancy may increase the curability potential.)*

Non-Hodgkin's Lymphoma

Aisenberg AC. Cell lineage in lymphoproliferative disease. Am J Med 1983;74:679. *(Detailed discussion of designating lymphomas on the basis of T- or B-cell origin.)*

Anderson T, Chabner BA, Young RC, et al: Malignant lymphoma. Histology and staging of 473 patients at the National Cancer Institute. Cancer 1982;50:2699. *(Review of histology and staging in a retrospective series, with emphasis on relationship to prognosis and response to therapy.)*

Armitage JO. Treatment of non-Hodgkin's lymphoma. N Engl J Med 1993;328:1023. *(Detailed, but very useful review for the generalist reader.)*

Brunning R, Bloomfield C, McKenna R et al: Bilateral trephine bone marrow biopsies in lymphoma and other neoplastic diseases. Ann Intern Med 1975;82:365. *(Reports a 37 percent yield on bilateral samples; 11 of 50 samples were positive only on one side, demonstrating the need for bilateral procedure.)*

Castillino R, Billingham M, Dorfman R. Lymphographic accuracy in Hodgkin's disease and malignant lymphoma with a note on the "reactive" lymph node as a cause of most false-positive lymphograms. Invest Radio 1974;9:155. *(False-negative rate was 8 percent, and false-positive rate was 11 percent. Most false-positives resulted from misreading a reactive lymph node.)*

Coleman M. Chemotherapy for large-cell lymphoma: Optimism and caution. Ann Intern Med 1985;103:140. *(Review of the excellent progress in treating this form of lymphoma.)*

Gordon LI, Harrington D, Andersen J, et al. Comparison of a second-generation combination chemotherapeutic regimen (m-BACOD) with a standard regimen (CHOP) for advanced diffuse non-Hodgkin's lymphoma. N Engl J Med 1992;327:1342. *(Less aggressive program provided equivalent remission and survival results, with lower rates of adverse effects.)*

National Cancer Institute. Classification of non-Hodgkin's lymphomas: Summary and description of a working formulation for clinical usage. Cancer 1982;49:2112. *(International effort to construct a new working classification scheme.)*

Simon R, Durrleman S, Hoppe RT, et al. The non-Hodgkin lymphoma pathologic classification project. Ann Intern Med 1988;109:939. *(Outcome predominantly a function of histology and stage.)*

Smalley RV, Andersoen JW, Hawkins MJ, et al. Interferon alfa combined with cytotoxic chemotherapy for patients with non-Hodgkin's lymphoma. N Engl J Med 1992;327:1336. *(Interferon improved outcome in patients with low- to intermediate-grade tumors.)*

Straus DJ, Gaynor JJ, Leiberman PH, et al. Non-Hodgkin's lymphomas: Characteristics of long-term survivors following conservative treatment. Am J Med 1987;82:247. *(Good histology, little bulk, age < 60, no B symptoms, early stage disease correlated with good outcome.)*

Surbone A, Armitage JO, Gale RP. Autotransplantation in lymphoma: Better therapy or healthier patients? Ann Intern Med 1991;114:1059. *(Editorial critically reviewing transplantation studies and discussing other treatment options.)*

Vose JM, Armitage JO, Bierman PJ, et al. Salvage therapy for relapsed or refractory non-Hodgkin's lymphoma utilizing autologous bone marrow transplantation. Am J Med 1989;87;285. *(Example of the use of bone marrow transplantation.)*

Vose JM, Armitage JO, Weisenburger DD, et al. The importance of age in survival of patients treated with chemotherapy for aggressive non-Hodgkin's lymphoma. J Clin Oncol 1988;6:1838. *(Although advancing age may reduce response rate, it does not obviate the benefit of treatment.)*

Young RC, Longo DL, Dlatstein E, et al. The treatment of indolent lymphomas: Watchful waiting vs aggressive combined modality treatment. Semin Hematol 1988;25(suppl 2):11. *(Addresses one of the key questions; interim data.)*

B
Oncology

Primary Care Medicine: Office Evaluation and Management of the Adult Patient, 3rd edition, edited by Allan H. Goroll, Lawrence A. May, and Albert G. Mulley, Jr. J.B. Lippincott Company, Philadelphia

85
Approach to the Patient With Metastatic Tumor of Unknown Origin

JERRY YOUNGER, M.D.

A malignancy is designated as a tumor of unknown origin (TUO) after meeting several criteria: 1) the tissue is histologically confirmed to be malignant and a primary tumor of the organ is ruled out; 2) routine screening fails to identify the primary source; and 3) a very late metastasis (as occurs in breast cancer, melanoma, and renal cell carcinoma) is also ruled out.

A TUO poses several problems, ranging from the utility of pursuing further workup to the efficacy of empiric therapy for disease that is already widely metastatic. Any decision to conduct a more extensive evaluation or treat empirically must include consideration of the low probability of there being a treatable cancer. Moreover, the evaluation of a TUO can prove expensive and uncomfortable. However, within this very heterogenous group are a few very responsive malignancies that could be effectively treated if recognized.

Guided by the principle of looking only for treatable disease, the primary physician should be able to conduct the major part of an effective workup in the outpatient setting and work closely with the oncologist in presentation of thoughtful treatment options to the patient.

CLINICAL PRESENTATION AND NATURAL HISTORY OF DISEASE

Clinical Presentation. Common sites of metastatic presentation are the lung, mediastinum, liver, bone, and lymph nodes. Others include the bone marrow, brain, spinal cord, peritoneum, and retroperitoneum. In the *lung*, TUO may present as a solitary nodule, multiple nodules, or recurrent pleural effusion (see Chapters 43 and 44). When a TUO presents in the mediastinum, it often does so as a catastrophic secondary complication, such as dysphagia, stridor or respiratory difficulty, or superior vena cava syndrome. In *bone*, TUO may appear as a lytic or blastic lesion of axial skeleton, long bones, or skull. Sometimes the patient reports bone pain or a pathologic fracture. Often, the finding is an incidental radiographic finding. *Bone marrow* invasion may be heralded by pancytopenia or a myelophthisic picture.

An isolated hard *lymph node* is another important presentation of a TUO. Asymmetric cervical, axillary, or inguinal disease is characteristic. Axillary nodes that histologically manifest adenocarcinoma are most commonly associated with ipsilateral breast cancer, even in the presence of a normal breast examination and normal mammogram. The presence of carcinoma in an inguinal node may represent local spread from carcinoma of the vulva, prostate, perineum, endometrium, or ovary or systemic involvement by lymphoma. Metastasis from testicular cancer usually does not present as inguinal adenopathy unless there has been previous pelvic and retroperitoneal node dissection.

Liver involvement is usually found by abnormal liver function test (eg, isolated elevation of alkaline phosphatase), detection of a hepatic nodule on physical examination, or a focal defect on abdominal ultrasound or liver scan. When a primary is discovered, the most frequent sites of origin prove to be the pancreas, liver, bowel, and stomach. Tumor that has spread to the *peritoneum* can lead to malignant ascites. Involvement of the *retroperitoneum* is usually a silent consequence of spread by lymphomas and genital cancers. *Brain* metastasis may be asymptomatic, but new onset of a focal deficit or headache is suggestive. *Spinal cord* involvement may present urgently with symptoms of cord compression (see Chapter 167).

A number of newly appreciated treatment-responsive tumors that often present as TUOs have been defined. Most manifest a poorly differentiated or undifferentiated histologic appearance. For example, *poorly differentiated carcinoma* of *neuroendocrine origin* (as determined by electron microscopy) is quite responsive to treatment (60% response rate) and typically involves the mediastinum, peripheral lymph nodes, and retroperitoneum. *Extragonadal germ-cell cancers* are another subset of the poorly differentiated carcinomas that respond to treatment. They too manifest disease of the mediastinum, retroperitoneum, or lymph nodes. Other features are patient younger than 50 years of age and elevations in serum human chorionic gonadotropin (HCG) or alpha-fetoprotein levels. *Adenocarcinoma of the peritoneum* causing malignant ascites in a woman with no known primary responds to treatment for ovarian carcinoma, even when no ovarian disease can be found; median survival increases to 23 months. Atypical presentations of *prostate cancer* may include poorly differentiated or undifferentiated histology and little clinical evidence of a primary lesion.

Natural History and Clinical Course. Because TUO represents metastatic disease, it should not be surprising that overall median survival is usually no more than 3 to 4 months; about 25 percent survive 1 year, and less than 10 percent are alive after 5 years. Overall survival is not improved by treatment when all TUO patients are considered as a group, although outcomes for responsive clinical and histopathologic subgroups can be improved considerably with treatment (see below).

DIFFERENTIAL DIAGNOSIS

Based on data from autopsy studies, pancreatic carcinoma leads the list of etiologies of cancer of unknown origin, accounting for about 25 percent of cases. Cancers of the lung, kidney, colorectum, and prostate cancer together account for another 30 percent. From the perspective of workup and management, consideration of potentially treatable cancers is most important (see Table 85–1), aided by differential diagnosis according to region of presentation (see Table 85–2). In older men, the most common treatable malignancy is prostate cancer; in younger men, it is testicular carcinoma. In women, breast and ovarian cancers lead the list. Other important etiologies are cancers of the nasopharynx, the oropharynx, and the lung (small-cell type). As noted, even patients with poorly differentiated or undifferentiated histology may have a treatable cancer, such as lymphoma, neuroendocrine carcinoma, extragonadal germ-cell cancer, peritoneal carcinomatosis, or carcinoma of the prostate. Although a number of other subtly presenting tumors (eg, pancreatic carcinoma, melanoma) are probably responsible for many TUO presentations, they are not sufficiently responsive to treatment to warrant listing.

WORKUP

Searching for Treatable Disease

When faced with a TUO, the priority is to search for treatable disease. Conducting the workup on the basis of probability rather than on responsiveness to therapy (see Table 85–3) may lead to searches that have little impact on outcome. The expense and discomfort incurred by the many diagnostic studies ordered in search of likely but poorly responsive disease can be avoided if the physician adopts the discipline of searching for malignancies that respond to treatment (see Tables 85–1, 85–2, 85–3, and 85–4).

Table 85-1. Treatable Malignancies That May Present as a Tumor of Unknown Origin

Potentially Curable, Even When Metastatic
Gestational trophoblastic tumors
Germ-cell cancer, gonadal (eg, testicular carcinoma)
Hodgkin's disease
Non-Hodgkin's lymphoma
Squamous cell carcinoma of the oropharynx
? Poorly differentiated carcinoma of neuroendocrine type*
? Poorly differentiated carcinoma of extragonadal germ-cell origin?
Very Responsive to Treatment, Although Not Curable When Metastatic
Prostate cancer
Breast cancer
Small-cell carcinoma of the lung
Ovarian carcinoma
Endometrial cancer
Thyroid cancer
Poorly differentiated carcinoma of neuroendocrine type*
Poorly differentiated carcinoma of extragonadal germ-cell origin*
Peritoneal carcinomatosis*

*Presents as TUO with poorly differentiated or undifferentiated histology.

Table 85-2. Treatable Causes of Metastatic Disease by Site of Presentation

SITE OF PRESENTATION	SOURCE OF PRIMARY
Lung and Mediastinum	Lung (small cell)
	Breast
	Hodgkin's disease
	Extragonadal germ cell
	Neuroendocrine
	Germ cell (testicular)
Bone	
Osteoblastic lesions	Prostate
	Lung (small cell)
	Hodgkin's disease
Osteolytic or mixed lesions	Breast
Liver	Breast
	Lung (small cell)
Brain	Breast
	Lung (small cell)
	Lymphoma
Bone Marrow	Breast
	Lung (small cell)
	Prostate
Lymph Nodes	
High cervical	Squamous cell cancer
	Hodgkin's disease, lymphoma
	Neuroendocrine
Axillary	Breast (ipsilateral)
	Lymphoma
	Lung (small cell)
Inguinal	Prostate
	Ovary
	Endometrium
	Lymphoma
Retroperitoneum	Lymphoma
	Hodgkin's disease
	Testes
	Prostate
	Ovarian
	Neuroendocrine
	Extragonadal germ cell

In similar fashion, once a metastatic lesion has been identified, it is *unnecessary to stage* the patient for other sites of metastases, since the incurable nature of the tumor has already been revealed. Thus, the patient who presents with a pulmonary nodule and is found to have breast cancer as a primary source does not require a liver scan to document the presence of liver disease. Treatment in patients with cancer is determined first and foremost by stage of disease, but once metastases have been identified, the tumor is sufficiently staged.

Histologic Diagnosis

The importance of *biopsy* and histologic diagnosis cannot be overstated. Before other investigations are initiated in search of a treatable cancer, a thorough *histologic assessment* of tissue from the metastatic site should be conducted. Since immunohistochemical (IH), electron-microscopic (EM), and receptor studies may need to be performed on the sample, adequate tissue must be obtained and processed properly. One portion is quick-frozen for immunohistologic study, another placed in formalin for hematoxylin and eosin staining, and a third placed in glutaraldehyde for electron microscopy. Cytologic sampling is usually insufficient, because it does not provide architectural information, which can be critical for diagnosis. Moreover, cytologic preparation may misrepresent nuclear and cytoplasmic abnormalities, which can be induced by inflammation or drugs. Therefore, in patients with serositis and pleural or peritoneal effusions, the cytologic diagnosis should be confirmed by tissue diagnosis.

The histologic assessment begins with diagnosis of the tumor by cell type (adenocarcinoma, lymphoma, small-cell carcinoma of the lung, sarcoma, squamous cell carcinoma, melanoma, undifferentiated). *Special stains*, such as the one for *mucin* (found in cancers of the prostate and kidney) may be utilized. The histologic designation *undifferentiated carcinoma* presumes a level of anaplasia which cannot be used to reliably identify the origin of the malignancy. If this is encountered, *immunohistochemical staining* is used to search for diagnostically important intracellular substances, such as prostate-specific antigen and prostatic acid phosphatase for prostate cancer, and alpha-fetoprotein and HCG for germ-cell tumors. The technique may also detect substances useful in differentiating a carcinoma from a lymphoma, melanoma, or germ-cell tumor. *Electron microscopy* may reveal subcellular structures strongly suggestive of lymphoma or neuroendocrine carcinoma. Testing for presence of *estrogen and progesterone receptors* helps to recognize breast cancer, although these receptors are also found in ovarian and endometrial cancers. *Cytogenetic studies* are a promising diagnostic technique and likely to enhance tumor identification as the methodology matures.

The histologic designation of *adenocarcinoma* does not definitively establish the primary source of the tumor. Any organ may develop a glandular malignancy. The histologic distinction between adenocarcinoma of the ovary, the stomach, the lung, or the breast is sometimes possible by pathol-

Table 85-3. Common Cancers and Their Responsiveness to Therapy

TUMOR	RESPONSE RATE
Responsive	
Breast	40%–60%
Ovary	60%–70%
Prostate	60%–70%
Head, neck	50%–70%
Testicular	80%–100%
Lymphoma	80%
Lung (small-cell)	80%
Marginally Responsive	
Neurosecretory	30%–50%
Sarcoma	30%
Colon, other GI tumors	10%–15%
Melanoma	10%–15%
Hepatoma	20%
Unresponsive	
Renal	
Lung (non–small-cell)	
Brain	

Table 85-4. Diagnosis of Some Treatable Cancers Presenting as TUO

MALIGNANCY	DIAGNOSTIC FEATURES OR STUDIES
Squamous cell, naso/oropharynx	PE (nodule, plaque), CT or MRI, blind biopsy
Lymphoma	PE (adenopathy), immunohistochemical stains
Ovarian cancer	PE (ascites or mass), pelvic CT or MRI, AFP, HCG, peritoneal implants
Prostate cancer	PE (nodule), PSA, prostate ultrasound, immunohistochemical stains
Breast	PE (breast nodule), receptor, studies
Testicular	PE (testicular nodule), ultrasound, serum AFP, HCG
Extragonadal germ-cell	PE (adenopathy), CT (lung nodules, mediastinal mass, retroperitoneal mass); immunohistochemical studies; serum AFP, HCG
Neuroendocrine carcinoma	PE (adenopathy), CT (retroperitoneal nodes, mediastinal nodes), EM

PE = physical examination
CT = computer tomography
MRI = magnetic resonance imaging
AFP = alpha-fetoprotein
HCG = human chorionic gonadotropin
PSA = prostate-specific antigen
EM = electronmicroscopy

ogy laboratory methods, but other approaches may be needed, including clinical assessment.

Clinical Assessment

All patients should undergo a careful *physical examination* that concentrates on detection of treatable malignant disease (ie, cancer of the breast, uterus, or ovaries in women; cancer of the prostate or testicles in men; lymphoma in all patients). Depending on the site of metastasis, other elements of the physical examination may also prove useful (see below and Table 85–4).

Similarly, *laboratory studies* are guided by the same principle of looking for treatable cancer rather than conducting an extensive workup for all possible primary tumors. An unfocused search can lead to the ordering of many unnecessary, uncomfortable, or expensive tests. Studies should be directed at the detection of treatable cancer (eg, *mammography* for breast cancer, *ultrasound* for a testicular or prostatic cancer, *computed tomography* [*CT*] for ovarian disease). Clinical presentation (see Table 85–2 and below) in conjunction with pathologic data can help guide the workup. Most routine blood chemistries are not helpful, although a few *serologic markers* (eg, prostate-specific antigen, alpha-fetoprotein, beta-HCG subunit) can aid in searching for treatable disease (see Table 85–4).

Pulmonary Nodules, Pleural Effusions, and Mediastinal Masses. An *open biopsy* procedure is generally necessary to obtain sufficient tissue for detailed histopathologic study and definitive diagnosis. A needle aspiration rarely suffices. Of particular importance is identification of small-cell, neuroendocrine, and extragonadal germ-cell cancers and lymphoma, which are among the more treatable malignancies that present as mediastinal or rapidly growing pulmonary mass lesions. In most other instances, identification of the primary does not affect outcome. Detailed study by the pathologist can be very useful. *EM* and *IH studies* are essential, complemented by *serologic testing* for *alpha-fetoprotein* and *beta-HCG subunit*.

Pleural effusions due to malignancy can be identified cytologically, but a *pleural biopsy* in conjunction with aspiration is more informative (see Chapter 43). A diagnosis of adenocarcinoma in cytologic fluids does not identify the primary source; one must look specifically for the source by immunohistochemical, receptor, and mammographic studies.

Mediastinal disease that produces symptoms of dysphagia, respiratory difficulty, or superior vena cava syndrome is almost invariably due to primary lung cancer, metastatic breast cancer, or lymphoma. All can be rather well managed by local radiation therapy; thus, extensive evaluation and search for the primary tumor is usually unwarranted. Clinically more silent mediastinal disease may be due to neuroendocrine or extragonadal germ-cell cancer, which can be identified by the methods noted earlier.

Osseous Metastases. The identification of an isolated bony lesion that is radiographically characteristic of neoplasia should be followed by a biopsy if tissue is not obtainable elsewhere. Note should be made of the *plain film* appearance of the lesion to determine if it is lytic, blastic, or mixed, which can help limit the differential diagnosis (see Table 85–2) and focus the evaluation. If the bony lesion is difficult to biopsy, a *bone marrow biopsy* at the iliac crest represents a reasonable alternative. The vast majority of patients with bony metastases have multiple lesions that often invade the bone marrow. Should this not prove diagnostic, one can obtain a *bone scan* to identify other sites of tumor that may be more easily accessible to biopsy. Having established a histologic diagnosis of malignancy in the bone, the search for the primary should, as always, be confined to treatable disease.

Liver metastases are usually diagnosed by ultrasound or *CT-guided needle biopsy*. Most are adenocarcinomas from gastrointestinal sources, although breast and lung are other important origins. Once a metastatic adenocarcinoma has been identified in the liver, further testing to identify the primary is usually unwarranted, because few are sufficiently responsive to justify the workup. Symptomatic patients with hepatic metastases have a life expectancy of less than 6 months, but asymptomatic persons have a significantly longer survival.

Ascites. A malignant ascitic fluid collection is most likely to derive from metastatic cancer of the pancreas, stomach, or colon involving the peritoneal surface. However, search for such cancers is of little value, because there is little that can be done to alter prognosis. However, in women, an important treatable cause of malignant ascites is diffuse peritoneal involvement by ovarian cancer. *Pelvic ultrasound*, or CT or magnetic resonance imaging (MRI), and testing for the tumor marker serum *CA125* are indicated, although peritoneal implants have been noted in patients without detectable ovarian pathology. Serologic studies (HCG, alpha-fetoprotein) and IH study of the tumor may suggest this responsive lesion.

High Cervical Lymphadenopathy. Since enlargement of a high cervical node may result from a contiguous primary site in the naso- or oropharynx or a lymphoma (two treatable cancers), intensive assessment is warranted. A careful examination of the nasopharynx, oral cavity (including base of the tongue), and larynx is essential, as is detailed examination of all lymph nodes. *CT scanning* or *MRI* is helpful in the examination of the deeper submucosal and neck structures. If node biopsy reveals squamous cell or epidermoid histology but no primary is evident, then *blind biopsies* of areas likely to harbor nasopharyngeal tumor (base of the tongue, nasopharynx) are conducted. If the histopathology is adenocarcinoma, then sinuses or the salivary glands may be the primary source. Again, careful physical examination supplemented by CT scanning or MRI may help reveal the primary. If histologic studies indicate a lymphoma or Hodgkin's disease, then the evaluation shifts to staging activities (see Chapter 84).

Axillary Adenopathy necessitates a careful breast examination and mammography. The diagnosis of breast cancer may be assisted by performing *estrogen and progesterone receptor assays* on nodal tissue obtained from the axilla. *IH study* for markers of lymphoma is also indicated. *Chest CT* may be warranted if there is the suggestion of small-cell histology.

Inguinal adenopathy is approached diagnostically in much the same manner as cervical adenopathy, emphasizing local disease and lymphoma, because they are quite responsive to treatment (see Table 85–3). Detailed pathologic study is essential and should include *IH* and *receptor studies* of the tissue obtained at biopsy. Careful pelvic and anorectal examinations are performed, complemented by ultrasound study of the pelvis. If inguinal node biopsy identifies a lymphoma, then workup proceeds for staging (see Chapter 84).

Retroperitoneal Mass. An incidentally discovered retroperitoneal mass is likely to represent advanced-stage lymphoma or metastatic prostate, germ-cell, or ovarian cancer. All are responsive to therapy and thus important to identify. Since the site is hard to biopsy, a search for a more accessible site is indicated. Careful physical examination of the peripheral nodes, prostate, and testicles in men and pelvic organs in women is indicated. Ultrasound examination may help detect a small prostatic or testicular lesion. Ultrasound may also help identify an ovarian tumor. Serum marker studies (alpha-fetoprotein, beta-HCG subunit, and prostate-specific antigen) aid the diagnostic effort.

Brain. The search focuses on breast, small-cell, and lymphomatous disease (see above). Consideration of brain biopsy is usually unnecessary unless there is no tissue available peripherally. If brain biopsy is performed, detailed IH and receptor studies should be conducted.

Bone Marrow Invasion. When pancytopenia or a myelophthisic picture with leukoerythroblastic changes is encountered, marrow invasion should be considered and confirmed by *bone marrow biopsy* (see Chapter 79). The marrow examination includes a search for clusters of malignant cells, which may help in identification. Once confirmed, a search for the several treatable tumors can commence (see Table 85–1).

TREATMENT

As emphasized above, the workup focuses intensively on identification of treatable cancers (see Tables 85–1 and 85–3). However, when the primary remains unknown (as in a substantial proportion of cases), the options for treatment become more problematic, with the choices being between empiric treatment and watchful waiting. Data on the efficacy and cost-benefit ratio of both approaches are limited. Interpretation of published outcomes data is often hindered by the absence of careful, detailed characterization of patients and their tumors. Only a few prospective, randomized, controlled trials have been done, and although responses are documented, median survival seems to improve little if at all. Many optimistic reports suffer from selection biases. Consequently, any discussion with the patient and family must address the uncertain benefit of empiric treatment and its likely adverse effects. Excluding patients with germ-cell and neuroendocrine TUOs, response rates are in the range of 25 percent to 30 percent. With certain exceptions, only those who are symptomatic ought to be considered for treatment, because response is likely to be brief, side effects prominent, and chances of long-term benefit small.

There are two basic approaches to *empiric therapy*. One is to use *"broad-spectrum" chemotherapy* (eg, Adriamycin and Mitomycin C). These are potent agents with a high potential for toxicity. Monitoring for marrow suppression is necessary. Treatment is halted if there is no response after two courses.

The other empiric approach is to treat based on a prudent estimate of the *most likely treatable tumor*, as judged by cell type, age, sex, site, and so on (see Tables 85–1, 85–2, and 85–4). If the pathologic type is undifferentiated, treatment is directed toward the most responsive tumors in this class, namely, lymphoma and germ-cell neoplasms. Metastatic adenocarcinoma in men can be treated as metastatic prostate cancer, and in women as metastatic ovarian or breast cancer, since these are the most treatable malignancies. Metastatic prostate cancer has a very high response rate to hormonal therapy. Carcinoma of the breast has a similar response rate to therapy; modalities include hormonal treatment for some patients and chemotherapy for others (see Chapter 122).

One of the more effective empiric therapies is use of *radiation* with or without node dissection in TUO patients with high cervical adenopathy and epidermoid or squamous cell histology. Treatment is conducted on the ipsilateral site, with cure rates of 20 percent to 35 percent reported. Adenocarcinoma of an inguinal node without a known primary may be treated by local radiation therapy bilaterally if there is no evidence of an anal or prostatic lesion on blind biopsy.

Radiation may also provide reasonable *palliation* for localized symptomatic disease, especially that which involves bone, mediastinum, or lymph nodes. Bony metastases are generally not treated systemically. When symptomatic, they are palliated locally by radiation therapy and, if necessary, stabilized orthopedically. In the absence of symptoms, a bony metastasis may be monitored unless a definitively responsive tumor, such as prostate or breast cancer, can be identified.

PATIENT EDUCATION AND INDICATIONS FOR REFERRAL

The finding of metastatic cancer is always very upsetting news, and even more perplexing when a source is hard to identify. However, an intelligently designed, selective search for treatable disease can provide considerable reassurance and hope. Such a diagnostic strategy should be shared with patient and family, both to provide hope and a sense of control over a difficult situation and to reduce irrational pressure to "find the cause" at all costs.

A search that proves unrevealing poses the issue of empiric therapy. Here a thoughtful and frank consultation with the oncologist is indicated to review the options. The lack of adequate data on cost and benefit often make counseling difficult, but an experienced and wise oncologist can be of great help to the patient and family. The patient suspected of having a metastatic lesion of the spinal cord requires urgent hospital admission and prompt referral to the radiation oncologist.

ANNOTATED BIBLIOGRAPHY

Bataini JP, Rodriquez J, Jaulerry C, et al. Treatment of metastatic neck nodes secondary to an occult epidermoid carcinoma of the head and neck. Laryngoscope 1987;97:1080. *(Very high rates of response and some cures.)*

Copeland EM, McBride CM. Axillary metastases from unknown primary sites. Ann Surg 1972;178:25. *(The breast is the most common primary source in a woman with an undifferentiated axillary lesion.)*

Gatter KC, Heryet A, Alcock C, et al. Clinical importance of analyzing malignant tumors of uncertain origin with immunohistological techniques. Lancet 1985;1:1302. *(Terse discussion of these important methods.)*

Gentile PS, Carloss HW, Huang T-Y, et al. Disseminated prostatic carcinoma simulating primary lung cancer. Cancer 1988;62: 711. *(The presentation of this very treatable malignancy may be quite atypical.)*

Greco FA, Vaughn WK, Hainsworth JD. Advanced poorly differentiated carcinoma of unknown primary site: recognition of a treatable syndrome. Ann Intern Med 1986;104:547. *(Patients with poorly differentiated histology and tumor in the mediastinum, retroperitoneum, and lymph nodes responded well to chemotherapy with cisplatin-based combination chemotherapy.)*

Hainsworth JD, Johnson DH, Greco FA. Poorly differentiated neuroendocrine carcinoma of unknown primary site. Ann Intern Med 1988;1090:364. *(Identification of a very treatable subgroup; electron microscopy useful.)*

Kirsten F, Chi CH, Leary JA, et al. Metastatic adeno or undifferentiated carcinoma from an unknown primary site. Q J Med 1987;62:143. *(A detailed discussion of natural history and approach to workup.)*

Le Chevalier TL, Cvitkovic E, Caille P, et al. Early metastatic cancer of unknown primary origin at presentation. Arch Intern Med 1988;148:2035. *(An autopsy study; pancreas, lung, kidney, and colon were the most common primary sites; authors recommend a workup strategy.)*

Legg MA. What role for the diagnostic pathologist? N Engl J Med 1981;305:950. *(An editorial reviewing the contributions from pathologic examination of tissue specimens.)*

Levine MN, Drummond MF, LaBelle RJ. Cost-effectiveness in the diagnosis and treatment of carcinoma of unknown primary origin. Can Med Assoc J 1985;133:977. *(Argues much diagnostic work is wasteful and treatment ineffective.)*

McMillan JH, Levine E, Stephens RH. Computed tomography in the evaluation of metastatic adenocarcinoma from an unknown primary site. Radiology 1982;143:143. *(A retrospective series comparing CT to other radiologic modalities and finding CT superior.)*

Nystrom JS, Weiner JM, et al. Identifying the primary site in metastatic cancer of unknown origin: inadequacy of roentgenographic procedures. JAMA 1979;241:381. *(Standard x-ray studies proved insensitive.)*

Sporn JR, Greenberg BR. Empiric chemotherapy in patients with carcinoma of unknown primary site. Am J Med 1990;88:49. *(Outstanding review of the entire issue, including identification of patients with responsive disease; 43 refs.)*

Primary Care Medicine: Office Evaluation and Management of the Adult Patient, 3rd edition, edited by Allan H. Goroll, Lawrence A. May, and Albert G. Mulley, Jr. J.B. Lippincott Company, Philadelphia

86
Approach to Staging and Monitoring

JERRY YOUNGER, M.D.

Staging and monitoring are essential components of cancer management. Staging is performed to assess the extent of disease, and it is used to help determine prognosis and choice of therapy. Monitoring serves to detect the reappearance or progression of cancer and contributes importantly to updating prognosis and revising treatment plans. Staging and monitoring strategies are determined by tumor type, its natural history, response to therapy, and characteristic pattern of spread. The frequency and duration of monitoring depend on the rate of disease recurrence.

The primary physician is in an ideal position to conduct much of the noninvasive staging and monitoring needed in the care of the cancer patient. To do so effectively requires an understanding of limitations of the many available laboratory tests and radiologic procedures, so that important decisions about test and procedure selection can be made effectively and unnecessary expense and discomfort can be avoided.

TERMINOLOGY, PRINCIPLES, AND PROCEDURES OF STAGING

Cancer stage is defined by the anatomic distribution of disease. The task of staging is to identify the amount and distribution of tumor. Several staging systems are used to express the extent of disease. At times, there appear to be almost as many staging schemes as there are malignancies. Some are so tumor-specific and idiosyncratic that they make for considerable confusion. However, most incorporate designations for *local disease* (confined to a visceral site), *regional extension* (with or without involvement of contiguous lymph nodes), and *distant metastasis*.

The TNM System

To standardize staging, the *TNM system* has been proposed and used with increasing frequency. The *T* refers to *tumor*, the *N* to *nodes*, and the *M metastases*. Numbers are added to designate subcategories, reflecting the size of the tumor (T1 to T5), the degree of nodal involvement (N0 to N3), and the absence or presence of distant metastases (M0 or M1).

Although varying slightly among tumors, the various subcategory designations have specific meaning. For the T categories, *Tis* refers to carcinoma *in situ*; *T1* to the smallest measurable tumor mass or to tumor confined to mucosa or submucosa; *T2* to larger tumor mass or to tumor extending directly to adjacent structures; *T3* to very large tumor or still further direct extension; *T4* to tumor of any size with very profound local tissue invasion and marked direct extension; *T5* to extension beyond adjacent organs. As regards N categories, *N0* designates no nodal metastasis; *N1* refers to ipsilateral or regional involvement or to movable regional nodes; *N2* to more extensive regional disease or fixed, matted nodes; *N3* to contralateral or distant nodal metastasis.

The TMN staging classification is increasingly preferred because of its consistency, comparability, and precision. Other staging systems commonly used for particular cancers have direct correlates to the TNM system and can be expressed in terms of it (Table 86–1).

Staging Principles and Procedures

A well-designed staging evaluation reflects the malignancy's characteristic pattern and speed of local and metastatic spread. Staging is performed both *clinically* (by means of history, physical examination, imaging procedures, and serum markers) and *pathologically* (by direct sampling of tissue). The two are complementary.

History and Physical Examination. Although much emphasis is placed on laboratory and radiologic procedures in clinical staging, the history and physical examination continue to play central roles in determination of tumor mass, local spread, and metastasis. Almost every cancer workup requires historical and physical data to intelligently stage and determine the need for additional study. Failure to conduct

Table 86-1. TNM Staging and Correlation with Conventional Staging Systems for Cancers of the Lung, Breast, and Colon

TUMOR	CONVENTIONAL STAGE/TNM DESIGNATION		COMMENTS
Lung	0	Tis, N0, M0	Carcinoma in situ
	1	T1–2, N0, M0	Local tumor ± visceral pleura involved
	2	T1–2, N1, M0	Ipsilateral hilar, peribronchial nodes
	3a	T3, N0–1, M0	Extension to chest wall, diaphragm
	3b	T1–3, N2, M0	Ipsilateral mediastinal nodes involved
	4	Any T, any N, M1	
Breast	0	Tis, N0, M0	Paget's of nipple, no palpable tumor, carcinoma in situ
	1	T1, N0–1a, M0	Tumor <2 cm, nodes feel normal
	2	T0 or T1, N1b, M0	Nodes feel diseased
	3	T2, N1a or b, M0	Tumor 2–5 cm in diameter
	3	T3, N1–2, M0	Tumor >5 cm in diameter
	4	T4, any N, any M	Direct involvement of chest wall and skin
		Any T, N3, any M	Supraclavicular nodes
		Any T, any N, M1	
Colon	0	Tis, N0, M0	
	A	T1, N0, M0	Confined to mucosa, submucosa
	B1	T2, N0, M0	Transmural disease, no extension
	B2	T3–5, N0, M0	Transmural disease plus extension
	C1	T1–2, N1, M0	Regional nodes, no direct extension
	C2	T3–4, N1, M0	Regional nodes plus extension
	D	Any T, any N, M1	

a careful history and physical runs the risk of subjecting the patient to unnecessary or misguided studies.

Imaging Procedures. If after a detailed history and physical examination it is still deemed necessary to have further noninvasive information on anatomic extent of disease, then one usually turns to consideration of imaging studies. Among the most frequently ordered are computed tomography (CT), magnetic resonance imaging (MRI), ultrasonography, and radionuclide scanning (particularly the bone scan). Even the plain film of the chest or bone can sometimes provide diagnostic information. Limitations include lack of specificity and inability to detect very early lesions.

Computed tomography and *magnetic resonance imaging* represent important advances over older contrast and radionuclide studies. They provide not only improved detection of tumor but also better quantitation of tumor burden. CT is the less expensive and more readily available of the two technologies, but MRI provides enhanced resolution in some areas, particularly the central nervous system. *Chest CT* has proven superior to conventional full-lung tomography for detection of pleural, mediastinal, and parenchymal lesions. The test is particularly useful for staging patients with lung cancer and those with sarcomas and testicular cancers, malignancies with high rates of lung and mediastinal metastasis. *CT of the abdomen* permits enhanced evaluation of the retroperitoneum, permitting identification of enlarged lymph nodes that were previously difficult to detect noninvasively. A positive scan can obviate the need for a surgical exploration. CT has also improved the search for, biopsy of, and quantitation of tumor in the pancreas, liver, adrenal gland, and kidney. Results of pelvic CT for detection and staging of early ovarian and prostate cancers have been variable, often lacking sensitivity for detection of early disease or early spread to pelvic nodes. *Head CT* has virtually eliminated invasive and radionuclide staging studies of the CNS. Conducting the study with iodinated contrast further improves sensitivity.

MRI has contributed to the staging and monitoring of cancer, particularly in the central nervous system. Compared with CT, it is more sensitive and offers better assessment of the posterior fossa and spinal cord. Its increased cost is justified when enhanced sensitivity is required. In addition, MRI is being investigated as a means of staging of pelvic malignancies. Although early results have been disappointing, methodologic advances in imaging ovarian and prostate cancers may improve sensitivity. Sensitivities have been reported in the .4 to .5 range for early disease, .6 to .7 for more advanced disease. It is too soon to recommend MRI for routine use in staging pelvic malignancies, but the literature should be followed closely.

Radionuclide scanning remains the most sensitive means of detecting metastasis to *bone*. It is far superior to plain films, except in cases of myeloma. However, bone scan results can be nonspecific, sometimes necessitating confirmation by other means. In cancers with a high propensity for spread to bone (prostate, breast, small-cell), the bone scan has become an integral part of the initial evaluation. In other instances, it is used late in the course of disease to evaluate bone pain. *Liver* scans are still frequently ordered to stage gastrointestinal cancers, but they rarely detect disease that is not predicted on the basis of abnormal liver function tests (eg, an elevated alkaline phosphatase) or clinical hepatomegaly. Furthermore, a large percentage of abnormal hepatic scans represent secondary drug effects or incidental inflammatory disease. True-positive liver scans are found in less than 1 percent of patients with otherwise operable primary breast or colon cancer; routine liver scanning for metastases is unwarranted in these conditions. As noted, CT and MRI have largely ended use of radionuclide *brain* scanning for detection of CNS disease. *Gallium scanning* suffers from inadequate sensitivity and specificity, because the radionuclide also readily enters inflamed tissue. Nevertheless, the test is recommended by some for staging melanoma and lymphoma. The discomfort of the study, which requires frequent enemas, and its high false-negative rate relegate it to infrequent use.

Ultrasonography has proven extremely useful for assessment of the prostate, ovaries, testes, liver, pancreas, kidneys, and thyroid. Ultrasonography accurately distinguishes solid masses from cystic ones, a capability of importance in evaluation of pelvic, testicular, renal, and thyroid masses. It can also help guide needle biopsy. Resolution for transabdominal studies wanes for lesions less than 1 cm in diameter. About 20 percent of such studies are inadequate due to overlying bowel gas. Transrectal ultrasound techniques have improved detection and staging of early prostate cancer. Ultrasound appears to provide results comparable to MRI for staging of early prostate disease, but at much lower cost.

Standard radiographs, such as the *metastatic series*, have a high false-negative rate and are relatively insensitive, though false-positive rates are relatively low. *Contrast studies*, such as intravenous pyelography, venography, and angiography, are infrequently applied to staging, although they may aid in planning surgery. Conventional chest tomography has been supplanted by chest CT (see above), which has a lower false-negative rate.

Lymphangiography was developed primarily for the evaluation of retroperitoneal lymph nodes in the staging of Hodgkin's disease, but it has been similarly employed for lymphoma. The usefulness of the test for staging has declined because treatment no longer depends heavily on its findings (see Chapter 84). In lymphoma, the test has been replaced by abdominal CT, but it is still used for staging in Hodgkin's disease.

Serum Chemistries and Markers. An isolated elevation in *alkaline phosphatase* (liver fraction) indicates hepatic infiltration; it may be an early sign of metastasis to liver and often precedes a radiologically detectable lesion. Marked elevations in *prostatic acid phosphatase* and *prostate-specific antigen* suggest large tumor burden and likelihood of extracapsular spread of prostate cancer.

Surgical Staging. Surgical staging is indicated when the results will alter therapeutic decision making. Clinical staging may underestimate the extent of disease by virtue of its limited ability to detect microscopic spread. However, invasive study should be conducted only when choice of therapy will be affected; otherwise the morbidity and risks incurred may not be justifiable.

Lymph node dissection was initially undertaken in patients with breast cancer, prostate carcinoma, and malignant melanoma in hope of eliminating contiguous sites of disease. However, it has been demonstrated that lymphadenectomy at the time of surgery for the primary lesion does not extend survival, although it does serve as a prognostic and therapeutic determinant in cancers of the prostate and breast. Lymph node evaluation of distant disease has become a recognized staging procedure in some tumors. For example, scalene or retroperitoneal node biopsy is sometimes performed in patients with testicular cancer. *Laparotomy* to detect intra-abdominal disease that will affect choice of therapy is central to staging of colon cancer, helpful in selected patients with Hodgkin's disease, and useful in ovarian cancer. *Mediastinoscopy* helps to determine operability for patients with lung cancer; the more invasive *Chamberlain procedure* is sometimes necessary. *Bone marrow biopsy* provides an efficient means of pathologic staging in cancers that frequently metastasize to bone marrow (eg, lymphoma, small-cell carcinoma, prostate cancer).

PRINCIPLES AND PROCEDURES OF MONITORING DISEASE

Once the extent of disease is determined and treatment initiated, monitoring begins. As noted earlier, the frequency and duration of monitoring are dependent on the rate of disease recurrence. The procedures selected are based in part on tumor type, response to therapy, stage of disease, and pattern of metastasis. Test sensitivity and specificity are also important.

Monitoring Techniques

Many of the techniques useful for staging are pertinent to monitoring. Checking for residual disease or a new primary is the objective when curative therapy is employed; monitoring for reduction in tumor burden is the goal when palliation is undertaken. Selecting a sensitive, objective marker of disease activity greatly facilitates the monitoring process.

Tumor markers have been sought with the hope of obtaining a means of tumor detection more sensitive than those provided by other clinical methods. Although initially developed to aid in early diagnosis, most markers have actually proven better suited for monitoring of disease recurrence or progression after curative or palliative therapy. Baseline and post-treatment levels are obtained and follow-up readings repeated at regular intervals.

Carcinoembryonic antigen (CEA) is present in both normal and malignant tissue; serum levels in excess of 2.5 ng/mL are suggestive of tumor, but the test is too nonspecific for screening. Its most useful application is in early detection of recurrence, especially for cancers of the colorectum, breast, and lung. The consensus is that serial CEA determinations are the best currently available noninvasive means for identifying recurrent colorectal cancer after surgery.

Alpha-fetoprotein (AFP) has been found in high serum concentrations in association with hepatomas, testicular carcinomas, and extragonadal germ-cell tumors. Although lacking sufficient specificity for diagnostic purposes, repeat AFP determinations can be used to monitor for disease recurrence and assess adequacy of treatment.

Beta subunit of human chorionic gonadotropin (HCG) is another useful tumor marker for germ-cell tumors of the testes and ovaries. Monitoring of the beta-HCG subunit provides information similar to that provided by the AFP.

Acid phosphatase elevations occur in up to 80 percent of patients with prostate cancer that has spread to bone; elevations may occur in the absence of bone metastasis. Identification of a prostatic fraction has improved the test's specificity. It is being superseded by the prostate-specific antigen.

Prostate-specific antigen is unique to prostate tissue, found in both malignant and normal cells. A concentration in excess of 10 ng/mL is strongly suggestive of cancer, being found in less than 2 percent of those with benign prostatic hypertrophy. Levels increase with degree of tumor burden and rise briefly after needle biopsy or with prostatitis, but not after a prostate examination. False-negatives occur with use of finasteride.

CA125, produced by 80 percent of epithelial ovarian cancers, correlates with the clinical course and is useful for monitoring. The specificity is high. This marker is the first of what promises to be a host of tumor-specific markers detected by monoclonal antibody methods.

Monitoring Local or Regional Disease. Patients with local or regional disease subjected to curative therapy may be monitored by history and physical examination supplemented by more detailed study of the disease site at routine intervals or as clinically indicated. Periodic evaluation of patients with regional disease who have undergone curative primary therapy should be directed less at detecting the presence of asymptomatic metastases and more at *finding new primary tumors* in the involved organ. *Endoscopy* for colorectal cancer and *mammography* for breast cancer are prime examples of this approach.

In the absence of symptoms or signs of recurrence, monitoring is conducted at 3-month intervals for the first year following operation, and at 4-month intervals for the second year. Thereafter, follow-up may be accomplished at 6-month intervals for a minimum of 5 years. In general, most tumors will recur at a maximum rate during the first 2 years following the initial operation—if in fact they are destined to recur. Three malignancies are notorious for late recurrence: breast carcinoma, melanoma, and renal-cell carcinoma. In some patients with these tumors, the lag period before the development of detectable metastases may extend beyond 10 years from initial diagnosis.

Metastatic Disease. Follow-up examinations for patients with metastatic disease who receive systemic therapy should be performed at intervals determined by the time expected for an objective clinical response. For hormonal therapy of breast cancer, clinical evidence of response may take as long as 3 months to appear. The effects of cytotoxic chemotherapy may be seen rapidly, for example, within two courses of treatment or 4 to 6 weeks. This is particularly true for exquisitely responsive tumors such as breast, testicular, ovarian, and oat-cell carcinomas.

Patients with metastatic disease receiving palliative systemic therapy should be examined for evidence of new disease. Unnecessary chemotherapy-induced morbidity can be avoided if ineffective palliative systemic therapy is discontinued at the first signs of new disease. Response to therapy may be objectively demonstrated after a predictable interval, but new growth or spread may be noted on earlier examination.

An important corollary to the monitoring of patients with metastatic disease on systemic therapeutic regimens is to define the most objective site of disease to be followed and to avoid additional staging procedures if they do not alter the therapeutic plan. For example, a patient with hepatic metastases from primary breast cancer need not endure a bone scan unless there is bone pain or fracture. The tumor is already established as being incurable, and therapy is determined by the presence of liver metastases. Alternatively, the patient with bony metastases that are difficult to monitor may undergo selective staging to identify a more measurable marker of metastatic disease, such as plasma carcinoembryonic antigen. Identification of asymptomatic metastases by radionuclide scanning is of little use, because the early detection and treatment of asymptomatic metastatic disease does not necessarily improve survival.

ANNOTATED BIBLIOGRAPHY

American Joint Committee on Cancer. Manual for staging of cancer. 2nd ed. Philadelphia: JB Lippincott, 1983. *(Basic outline of staging schema and approaches.)*

Bast RC, Jr, Klug TL, et al. Radioimmunoassay using a monoclonal antibody to monitor the course of epithelial ovarian cancer. N Engl J Med 1983;309:883. *(The development of the CA125.)*

Beard DB, Haskell CM. Carcinoembryonic antigen in breast cancer. Am J Med 1986;80:241. *(A review of CEA's role in breast cancer; especially useful in patients with advanced disease.)*

Fletcher RH. Carcinoembryonic antigen. Ann Intern Med 1986; 104:66. *(A critical review, pointing out the limitations of its usefulness.)*

Friedman MA, Resser KJ, Marcus FS, et al. How accurate are computed tomographic scans in assessment of changes in tumor size? Am J Med 1983;75:193. *(Documents the sensitivity of CT for determining changes in size; authors argue the test is the best means available.)*

Rifkin MD, Zerhouni EA, Gatsonis CA, et al. Comparison of magnetic resonance imaging and ultrasonography in staging early prostate cancer. N Engl J Med 1990;323:621. *(No difference; both found wanting in early disease, better for more advanced disease; study done before advent of rectal probe; sensitivities in the .4–.5 range for early disease, .6–.7 for more advanced disease.)*

Sears HF, Gerber FH, Sturtz DL, et al. Liver scan and carcinoma of the breast. Surg Gynecol Obstet 1975;140:409. *(Lack of usefulness found; results may be extended to other tumors.)*

Smalley RV, Malmud LS, Ritchie WGM. Preoperative scanning: evaluation for metastatic disease in carcinoma of the breast, lung, colon, bladder, and prostate. Semin Oncol 1980;7:358. *(A critical analysis of radionuclide, ultrasound, and CT scanning.)*

Stamy TA, Yang N, Hay AR, et al. Prostate-specific antigen as a serum marker for adenocarcinoma of the prostate. N Engl J Med 1987;317:909. *(The original report; more sensitive than acid phosphatase; both elevated in benign prostatic hypertrophy.)*

Van Dyke JA, Stanley RJ, Berland LL. Pancreatic imaging. Ann Intern Med 1985;102:212. *(A detailed review that discusses use of abdominal CT in documenting presence and extent of tumor.)*

Veronesi R, et al. Inefficacy of immediate node dissection in melanoma of the limbs. N Engl J Med 1977;297:627. *(A example of the failure of node dissection to alter survival, although it does aid staging.)*

Primary Care Medicine: Office Evaluation and Management of the Adult Patient, 3rd edition, edited by Allan H. Goroll, Lawrence A. May, and Albert G. Mulley, Jr. J.B. Lippincott Company, Philadelphia

87

Comprehensive Care of the Cancer Patient

JERRY YOUNGER, M.D.

The treatment of cancer is multifaceted, involving the interdigitation of physician support with surgery, radiation, cytotoxic agents, and most recently, biologic response modifiers. Comprehensive care requires a team approach, in which the primary physician plays a central role in coordinating the effort. To succeed in this role, the primary physician needs to understand the major issues of cancer management and be capable of interacting effectively with cancer specialists. The patient and family are likely to request the opinion of the primary physician, necessitating an ability to explain and assess management recommendations. Most cancer patients can remain at home with their families and receive optimal therapy on an outpatient basis when there is a primary physician working closely with a cancer center or local specialist in cancer management.

Curative treatment that focuses on the primary tumor site has traditionally been the province of surgery, with radiation and chemotherapy relegated to palliative roles. More recently, radiation and chemotherapy have been employed as adjuvants for local disease, enhancing the capability of surgery to cure. Advances in radiation therapy have effected cures of some cancers in early stages. Biologic response modifiers hold promise for achieving further improvements in outcome.

Effective care to the cancer patient begins with telling the diagnosis and strengthening the relationship between patient and physician. It also requires the establishment of a close working partnership with the cancer specialist, whose job will be to design and implement the treatment program. The primary physician can and should maintain a central role in care of the cancer patient, but to do so requires a thorough understanding of the natural history of the tumor, its staging and monitoring (see Chapter 86), and responsiveness to treatment. In addition, the patient will call on the primary physician for relief from symptoms related to the tumor or its treatment. This necessitates a thorough knowledge of measures to control pain (see Chapter 90), emesis (see Chapter 91), and related side effects of cancer therapy (see Chapters 88 and 89).

SUPPORTING THE PATIENT AND FAMILY THROUGH DIAGNOSIS AND TREATMENT

For most patients, the diagnosis of cancer evokes images of pain, suffering, mutilation, and certain death. These basic fears are so intertwined with the word "cancer" that confirmation of the diagnosis places extreme emotional stress on the patient and his family. It is in managing this anguish that the primary physician plays a most important role as the person to whom the patient and family can turn. One must be not only the source of scientific and medical expertise but also the provider of emotional support and understanding.

Giving Bad News

It is always difficult to give bad news. Physicians sometimes avoid telling the patient the diagnosis in accurate and specific terms at the outset, resorting to such euphemisms as "lump," "mass," and "lesion." Further inhibiting communication may be the ill-advised, though well-intentioned, insistence of family members that the diagnosis be kept from the patient out of fear of precipitating a severe depression. Such concerns are usually ill-conceived. It is rare that ignorance of the diagnosis or prognosis is helpful for the patient or family. Quite the contrary. Patients and their families deal better with cancer when they are well informed.

The goal in communicating the diagnosis and prognosis is to be accurate without destroying all hope. First and foremost, the words "cancer" and "malignant tumor" should be used at the outset of the interview and not avoided, although constant repetition of the terms is usually unnecessary. The term "fatal" ought to be omitted in discussions of prognosis, for it implies little hope of control. When informed of an incurable malignancy, the patient and family want to know, "How much time is left?" A rough estimate may be necessary if the patient must arrange his affairs, but, if possible, the physician should avoid indicating a specific period of time, because it is apt to be inaccurate. Preferably, the physician should direct the patient toward realistic therapeutic approaches and reinforce his role in living instead of dying.

The candor expressed by telling the diagnosis "as it is" facilitates development of trust among patient, family, and medical staff and breaks down the barrier that often isolates the cancer patient from his family. Being well informed also helps alleviate the sense of hopelessness and loss of control that can be one of the most frightening aspects of living with a malignant disease. Families are especially grateful for full and frequent reports of the patient's status and prognosis.

The consequences of not fully informing the patient and family can be considerable. The patient who is unaware of diagnosis and prognosis may fail to put affairs in order and continue to have unrealistic plans or uncomfortable relationships with other members of the family, which might otherwise be resolved if all were to understand the prognosis. Similarly, the uninformed family is unable to grieve gradually over time, and death may appear to be sudden. The resulting unresolved grief may profoundly affect the surviving family members (see Chapter 227). Both patient and family may need to grieve and resolve their own fears and anxieties. By virtue of having a long-standing relationship with the patient and family, the primary physician is in an ideal position to provide effective support and guidance.

The Patient's Response

Cancer patients have been observed to pass through a series of emotional states. These include periods of denial, hostility, anger, hope, depression, and finally acceptance. The physician can help ameliorate the more dysfunctional reactions and facilitate the patient's coping. Patient reactions at the time of presentation of the diagnosis depend on preconceived ideas about cancer and what the specter of cancer suggests to them. Common misconceptions include the certainty of death, intractable pain, and erosive, disfiguring disease. To avoid needless worry, it is essential at the outset to address these common concerns directly, even if the patient does not express them. Nonetheless, a good number of patients will respond with denial, hostility, rejection of loved ones, regression, or even withdrawal. It is important to recognize such reactions as psychological defense mechanisms and respond to them in an understanding and patient manner.

Denial of the diagnosis is generally a transient reaction. When denial is mild, the physician may need only to reinforce his remarks with re-presentation of the facts or provision of objective and tangible evidence. However, in some patients, denial is extreme and functions as a crude psychologic defense mechanism, necessary for sustaining the psyche. A constant onslaught of evidence and reinforcement of the diagnosis or prognosis may be counterproductive and is not justified.

Hostility is occasionally an early reaction to the diagnosis. Anger may be directed against the medical team for the delayed diagnosis or for inadequate attention, as well as toward family members, who may be viewed as not particularly upset and happy to finally "get their way." This phase is generally transient, receding as the patient comes to recognize the reality of the situation and the need for family and physician. Hostility is difficult for both patient and doctor and may be intense enough to lead the physician and family to reject the patient emotionally. If recognized, this reaction should be allowed to run a natural course without withdrawing support.

Regression is an accentuated response commonly occurring in the patient with a dependent personality who may have appeared overly independent before illness. If it is more than transient, the regression may turn infantile and must be mitigated by providing a parental figure who will be, on the one hand, supportive and, on the other hand, stern and demanding. Infantile regression places an inordinate burden on the family, who are called on to provide extraordinary amounts of support.

Withdrawal is an extreme form of regression, often tinged with elements of hostility. Direct confrontation is essential for the patient who withdraws; constant encouragement and the setting up of goals for achievement (such as ambulation, planning trips, or visiting friends) are critical.

Family Reactions to the Diagnosis

Reactions of the family are critical to the patient's well-being and to aiding the health care team in providing maximum support. Thus, the physician must be concerned with the family's responses to the patient and to the diagnosis. The physician is frequently obliged to deal with many members of the family, often at differing levels of need for information and support. Not uncommonly, complete families—wives, husbands, and children—may be alienated by the patient, who disallows them the opportunity to resolve their confusion. Such alienation, which may approach pathologic proportions, can be understood with the help of the physician. A frequent family reaction is to provide smothering protection in compensation for guilt over previous misunderstandings with the patient and the need to resolve such differences. Again, the physician can help alleviate such pathologic reactions.

Psychological Reactions to Cancer Treatment

The patient who enters treatment for cancer is subjected to a reinforcement of the diagnosis and a rekindling of the fears regarding threats to self-esteem and self-image. The latter may be particularly demoralizing if the cancer treatment involves bodily disfigurement or a physical limitation that is either cosmetically mutilating or functionally disabling. Thus, the patient who requires a mastectomy, jaw resection, amputation, or colostomy faces a significant and frightening change in self-image. The distortions that are incorporated into the patient's unconscious, perhaps as a result of real or imagined experiences with friends, are potentially devastating. Often these distortions are unrealistic and unsubstantiated, but, more importantly, they may be unexpressed. The physician must inquire into the patient's concerns and offer a realistic appraisal to minimize unnecessary anguish (see Chapter 1).

Patient education is a most important component of the approach to dealing with the stress of therapy. It additionally serves to cushion the stress by allowing the patient to intellectualize about the disease and its treatment. In this "demythologizing process," patient fears are identified and dealt with openly. Often the result is a more acceptable view of one's illness and treatment. Educational materials available from the American Cancer Society and the National Cancer Institute can complement the educational effort, addressing common questions that patients have about cancer therapy. Detailed explanation of the therapy in terms of its effect on the tumor as well as its potential side effects allows the patient to approach treatment realistically. Use of support groups and meditation techniques can facilitate the patient's coping with the stresses of cancer therapy.

Such supportive efforts are designed to strengthen the patient psychologically and improve quality of life. Whether they affect survival or immune function is uncertain, but they certainly can help morale and coping with illness.

APPROACHES TO TREATMENT

The approach to treatment is determined by tumor type and stage (see Chapter 86). In the earliest stages of disease, the malignancy is localized and cure is possible through locally or regionally applied therapy. Regional spread reflects more advanced disease, and the chances of cure are lessened, but not eliminated. More systemic forms of therapy are added to local measures. With important exceptions (eg, testicular cancer), distant metastasis indicates that cure is unlikely, and the goal is palliation through use of systemic therapies.

Local Tumor Control: Surgery and Radiation

Surgery has traditionally played the dominant role in the management of localized cancer. Diagnosis is established and confirmed by surgical biopsy, and cure may be effected by operation. Nonetheless, there has recently been a shift in emphasis toward minimizing surgical procedures, particularly when the prognosis is determined by factors such as distant metastases and when salvage by secondary local modalities can be accomplished. For example, lymph node dissection for malignant melanoma, limb amputation for osteogenic sarcoma, ostomy and AP resection for rectal cancer, and radical mastectomy for breast cancer have been scaled down in many cases to lesser procedures, reducing morbidity without compromising survival. The surgical approach to these lesions may be modified by the addition of local therapy (eg, radiation) or systemic therapy (eg, cytotoxic agents).

Radiation Therapy has become more effective due to development of high-energy linear accelerators and technical improvements in delivery, which have lowered rates of morbidity and increased rates of survival and local control. For example, radiation has become the therapy of choice for early stages of Hodgkin's disease (see Chapter 84). Radiati n in conjunction with surgery may be curative in some tumors when administered pre- or postoperatively. In other malignancies, the combined application of radiation and either surgery or chemotherapy may promote palliation and chances for long-term survival, although rarely achieving cure (see Chapter 89).

Regional Cancer: Surgery Plus Adjuvant or Combined Therapy

Adjuvant therapy involves the addition of chemotherapy or radiation to surgical procedures. The rationale for adding radiation therapy is primarily to promote local control of presumed residual microscopic tumor. In theory, chemotherapy functions as an adjuvant modality because of the possibility that tumor cells are released into the circulation at the time of surgery. In addition, adjuvant chemotherapy may be effective because it affects existing micrometastases at a time when they are rapidly proliferating and likely to be quite drug-sensitive.

Adjuvant therapy has been proposed or is part of ongoing trials for treatment of a number of regional cancers and is a proven and established therapy for others. For example, in breast cancer, premenopausal women with positive lymph nodes and pathologic stage II disease have benefited from the addition of chemotherapy. It has reduced the incidence of recurrence and prolonged disease-free survival. Patients with rectal cancer that extends beyond the bowel wall (so-called Duke's B2 or C lesions) have shown reduced local recurrence rates and possibly increased survival time with the use of radiation therapy. The role of preoperative radiation therapy in comparison to postoperative radiation therapy has not been definitely established.

For the vast majority of tumors, regional disease is incurable in spite of adjuvant modalities. Only 15 percent of patients with stage II malignant melanoma survive 5 years; fewer than 5 percent of patients with lung, renal cell, and pancreatic cancers that are regionally advanced show long-term survival. Thus chemotherapy, immune therapy, and radiation are not generally employed as adjuvant modalities for these tumors, unless used investigationally. For some tumors (testicular cancer, osteogenic sarcoma, Hodgkin's disease), the role of ancillary modalities is important in extending survival time and limiting morbidity of regional disease.

With the advent of more effective cytotoxic drugs, the use of radiation to sterilize local sites of tumor with minimal morbidity, and the advent of biologic response modifiers, the combined approach to local, regional, and even advanced cancers should become an increasing part of standard management. Currently, the application of forms of therapy ancillary to surgery must await the outcomes of ongoing clinical trials.

Metastatic Cancer: Cytotoxic Drugs, Biologic Response Modifiers

The management of advanced disease is largely palliative and involves systemic therapy provided by cytotoxic drugs. Biologic response modifiers may begin to play an increasingly active role as research into their efficacy advances.

Chemotherapeutic regimens have become increasingly sophisticated and complex, but they are also more effective due to development of new agents and multiple-drug regimens (see Chapter 88). Decisions concerning use and timing of cytotoxic therapy in advanced disease are difficult because of the potential morbidity associated with such therapy and the frequent lack of established benefit in promoting cure or even in prolonging survival. The decision to use chemotherapy in advanced disease is often a philosophical/psychological one, based on the feelings of patient, family, and physician.

Any decision to employ chemotherapy should involve an analysis of host tolerance as well as potential tumor responsiveness. Most important, the use of chemotherapy must be preceded by informed consent of the patient, who should be aware of the side effects as well as the potential for response. A common misconception is that the drugs invariably create morbidity and prolong life only at the cost of agonizing discomfort. In fact, when effective, chemotherapy can improve the quality of life as well as prolong it and, when it is ineffective, it will not necessarily induce more than transient morbidity.

In addition to these considerations, the primary indications for the use of chemotherapy in advanced disease include the following:

1. A probability of tumor responsiveness to chemotherapy greater than 30 percent for a partial response and greater than 5 percent for a complete response;
2. Progressive tumor growth during a period of observation (eg, pulmonary nodules doubling in fewer than 30 days);
3. Symptomatic metastatic disease (eg, pleural effusion).

Within these guidelines, cytotoxic therapy can be administered with a reasonable risk–benefit balance.

The use of *experimental drug therapy* should be reserved for the following:

1. Patients who have failed with known effective drugs (ie, those drugs with a response rate > 30% and established ability to prolong survival);
2. Patients who wish to have or insist on a new form of treatment;
3. Patients who have a measurable parameter to monitor for judging effectiveness of therapy.

Biologic response modifiers, such as the interleukins and interferons, are new forms of systemic treatment, designed to promote a generalized response that can affect tumors at any site. Although in most instances their use remains highly experimental, some have been approved for application in patients with cancer (eg, interferon-alpha for hairy-cell leukemia and Kaposi's sarcoma; levamisole for stage C colon cancer). They offer considerable promise as an adjunct to cytotoxic chemotherapy. The literature should be followed closely (see also Chapter 89).

Management of the Preterminal Phase

"Terminal cancer" is an expression commonly employed by both patients and physicians, but with distinctly different definitions. Strictly defined, "terminal cancer" means that death will ensue within a 4-week period. The physician should avoid using the term "terminal" in talking with the patient or family. Not infrequently, patients may absorb the label and yet live for months or even years. The term imposes on the family and the patient a tremendous stress, often resulting in withdrawal.

The physician's role in the terminal phase is a crucial one. It is essential to remain sensitive to all the patient's needs and, specifically, to the patient's need to know that his physician is always available. If the patient is at home, frequent home visits may be enormously appreciated. It may be helpful to allow the patient to come to the office once or twice a week, even though there are no specific medications to be administered.

It is not incumbent on the physician to reinforce the inevitability of death to patients who have entered a preterminal or terminal state and are sustaining hope for a reversal of the tumor. More important, however, during this period, the family must be apprised precisely to allow them to pass through the grieving process successfully.

The approach to preterminal care has begun to include more emphasis on comfort measures and care at home or in a hospice, where hospital routines and studies are omitted in favor of psychological and symptomatic support. Relief of pain is an essential component of effective preterminal care (see Chapter 90).

Psychotropic Drugs

Tricyclic antidepressant therapy (eg, amitriptyline starting with 25–50 mg qhs) can help with the somatic symptoms of depression, such as marked fatigue and early-morning awakening (see Chapter 227). Pain control may also be enhanced. If there is no contraindication, tricyclics should not be withheld on the basis of the common clinical misconception that "the patient is appropriately depressed, considering the diagnosis and prognosis." Checking for suicidal ideation is important because tricyclic overdose can be fatal. Asking about suicide does not suggest the act to the patient; rather, it conveys understanding of how profoundly one is suffering. *Benzodiazepines* (eg, diazepam 2 mg qhs) given for short periods can facilitate coping with particularly stressful situations and the resultant difficulty falling asleep. Patients with panic disorder may require more prolonged therapy with anxiolytics (see Chapter 226).

Nutrition and Pain Control

See Chapters 90 and 91 for discussions of nutrition and pain control.

APPROACH TO THE CARE OF CANCER SURVIVORS

Patients who survive cancer are increasing in number and are more commonly encountered than ever before in primary care practice. They present challenges in management that reflect both the psychological and physiological consequences of their disease and its therapy. An expanding appreciation of their needs is essential to helping them return to full and productive lives.

Psychological Consequences. Although surviving cancer may be expected to be a cause for joy, studies show that considerable anxiety persists. Having had cancer appears to produce a heightened *sense of vulnerability* and fear of death and a decreased feeling of control and mastery over one's life. Fear of death wanes as duration of survival increases, but *anxiety over recurrence* may persist and result in hypochondriasis or avoidance of follow-up health care. Contact with patients having active disease can be very stressful, rekindling feelings of fear and vulnerability. Conversely, some demonstrate marked anxiety over the loss of close contact with the health care team that characterized the active phase of their illness. Frank *separation anxiety* has been reported. Others begin to express feelings of *anger* and overperceived shortcomings in diagnosis and care.

Physical disabilities resulting from cancer or its treatment can have profound psychological impact, with *depression* being the most common and important. If not appreciated, it may present as fatigue or other physical complaints that generate concern in both patient and physician. Preoccupation with bodily sensations is another common manifestation of depression (see Chapter 227) that might be encountered in the surviving cancer patient. When not appreciated, symptoms due to depression may be mistaken for more serious pathology.

Interpersonal and Social Consequences. The psychosocial effects of having had cancer are equally important to keep in mind in helping the patient to adjust to survivorship. Some will miss the privileges that *the sick role* provided and may have difficulty in returning to the responsibilities of normal life. Family members and work colleagues may find it awkward to relate, not knowing whether to treat the survivor as still partially incapacitated or back to normal. A return to sexual activity may be a source of concern for the patient. Most patients with a close supportive marital relationship and no permanent loss of sexual capacity appear to do reasonably well, but preexisting marital problems or the absence of a close relationship can lead to considerable *sexual dysfunction*. Such dysfunction may result in depression. Sexual dysfunction may also be a symptom of an underlying depression unrelated to sexual issues. Of course, patients who suffered gonadal injury or bodily mutilation are prime candidates for sexual dysfunction and its interpersonal consequences. Overall, psychological distress appears to be highest in patients lacking a close, supportive relationship. Single patients are most vulnerable.

Elements of *interpersonal isolation* have been reported, especially among those who are single and reluctant to share information about their cancerous past with a potential mate. Feelings of isolation may also be triggered by difficulty discussing the cancer experience with friends, family, or coworkers. *Work difficulties* are often encountered. There are fears, real or imagined, of losing one's job. Prolonged absence and perceived inability to perform may compromise one's previous position and lead to long-term job insecurity. With job insecurity comes concern about maintaining adequate and affordable *health insurance*, especially with a past history of major illness and the tendency of insurance companies to "cherry-pick" those whom it will insure. Hopefully, insurance reform with community rating will alleviate this major worry of surviving cancer patients.

Physiological Consequences. See Chapters 88 and 89 and the chapters on specific cancers for detailed discussion of physiological consequences.

Supportive Therapy and Preparing the Patient. An understanding of the difficulties that cancer survivors may encounter helps the physician to prepare the patient for life after cancer therapy. Counseling the patient and family on the challenges and potential difficulties likely to be experienced can go a long way toward ensuring an effective return to daily life. The counseling is done in the same honest, open, and supportive manner that characterized discussions in earlier phases of the illness. The issues can be every bit as difficult for the patient and require that physician support continue unabated. Regularly scheduled office visits for a check of symptoms, physical findings, and progress in returning to normal life are greatly appreciated and extremely therapeutic. Studies suggest that it takes as long as 3 years from time of successful treatment for survivors to regain the confidence and social functioning that was lost as a result of having cancer. Many survivors also exhibit a wisdom and sense of value and proportion that comes from having faced death, an appreciation of life that benefits all whom they encounter.

ANNOTATED BIBLIOGRAPHY

Anderson BL. Sexual functioning morbidity among cancer survivors. Cancer 1985;55:1835. *(Differentiates between dysfunction due to physiologic and psychological factors.)*

Cassileth BE, Zupkis RV, Sutton-Smith K, et al. Information and participation preferences among cancer patients. Ann Intern Med 1980;92:832. *(Most patients preferred maximum amounts of information; those who were more hopeful wanted to participate in treatment decisions.)*

Cassileth BE, Walsh WP, Lusk EJ. Psychosocial correlates of cancer survival. J Clin Oncol 1988;6:1753. *(A long-term study with practical implications.)*

Cullen JW, Fox BH, Isom RN, eds. Cancer: The Behavioral Dimensions. New York: Raven Press, 1976. *(A useful introduction to the experience of patients in dealing with cancer.)*

Fauci AS, Rosenberg SA, Sherwin SA, et al. Immunomodulators in clinical medicine. Ann Intern Med 1987;106:421. *(A basic science and clinical review of biologic response modulators.)*

Gates C. Psychodynamics of the Cancer Patient. In: Lokich J, ed. Primer of Cancer Care. Boston: GK Hall, 1978. *(Based on the concept that self-esteem must be supported and maintained; assesses impact of cancer on ability to relate to surroundings, friends, and family members.)*

Goldie JH, Goldman AJ, Gudauskas GA. Rationale for the use of alternating non–cross-resistant chemotherapy. Cancer Treat Rep 1982;66:439. *(The theoretical basis for modern multi-drug regimens.)*

Krant MJ. The hospice movement. N Engl J Med 1978;299:547. *(A slightly dated but still important paper with a thoughtful presentation of the methods and issues involved in this approach to terminal care.)*

Lieberman M. The role of self-help groups for helping patients and families cope with cancer. CA 1988;38:162. *(The many pluses and some minuses reviewed.)*

Papper S. Care of patients with incurable, chronic neoplasm: one patient's perspective. Am J Med 1985;78:271. *(A deeply moving essay written by a leading clinician as he was dying of myeloma.)*

Reiser SJ. Words as scalpels: transmitting evidence in the clinical dialogue. Ann Intern Med 1980;92:837. *(A very thoughtful paper on telling the diagnosis, with a very interesting historical perspective.)*

Silberfarb PS. Psychiatric treatment of the patient during cancer therapy. CA 1988;38:133. *(Very practical advice.)*

Spiegel D, Bloom JR, Yalom I. Group support for patients with metastatic cancer. Arch Gen Psychiatry 1981;38:527. *(Documents benefits of support group interactions.)*

Welch-McCaffrey D, Hoffman B, Leigh SA, et al. Surviving adult cancers. Part 2: psychosocial implications. Ann Intern Med 1989;111:517. *(Best review to date on the subject, with an excellent review of the literature and useful discussion of key issues; 58 refs.)*

88
Principles of Cancer Chemotherapy

JERRY YOUNGER, M.D.

Primary Care Medicine: Office Evaluation and Management of the Adult Patient, 3rd edition, edited by Allan H. Goroll, Lawrence A. May, and Albert G. Mulley, Jr. J.B. Lippincott Company, Philadelphia

The availability of chemotherapy for the cancer patient represents an important contribution to patient management. However, chemotherapeutic agents are potent and relatively unselective, having adverse effects that can offset their beneficial antitumor qualities. A well-constructed chemotherapy program attempts to strike an effective balance between beneficial and adverse effects and requires the expertise of the oncologist. The primary care physician has an important supportive role, which is increasing as more cancer chemotherapy is conducted on an outpatient basis and away from cancer centers. While maintaining a close working relationship with the oncologist, the primary physician may be called on to closely monitor the effects of therapy and provide initial care for the wide range of medical and emotional problems that may arise (see Chapter 87). These responsibilities necessitate a knowledge of the general indications for chemotherapy and the major toxic and adverse side effects of the commonly employed agents. The primary care physician must know how to evaluate response to treatment and alleviate side effects.

PRINCIPLES OF THERAPY

Types of Regimens and Their Indications

Chemotherapy may be given as a preoperative (neoadjuvant) therapy, as a postoperative (adjuvant) therapy, or as palliative therapy for advanced disease. *Neoadjuvant chemotherapy* is used for preoperative treatment of *locally invasive tumors* that are moderately sensitive and responsive to drugs (eg, stage III non–small-cell *lung* cancer and stage III *breast* cancer—see Chapters 53 and 122, respectively).

The goal is to decrease tumor bulk and make possible a more conservative surgical approach, as well as to reduce the risk of systemic disease via micrometastasis. For patients with locally invasive disease, an early consultation with the medical oncologist may be helpful and even precede the surgical referral.

Postoperative adjuvant therapy has now been established as a standard form of treatment for several cancers, including stages I and II *breast* cancer (see Chapter 122) and Duke's stage C *colon* cancer (see Chapter 76). The rationale behind giving chemotherapy to patients who have had what appears to be curative surgery is the frequency of distant micrometastases and local recurrences. Chemotherapy applied just after surgery has been more successful in prolonging survival than therapy delayed until clinical evidence arises of recurrence or spread.

Chemotherapy of advanced disease has evolved from a strictly palliative modality to a *curative* one in some instances (eg, *testicular cancer*—see Chapter 143; *lymphoma*—see Chapter 84). This change has resulted from the discovery of increasingly effective chemotherapeutic agents and the development of *multidrug regimens* that have increased not only response rates but also the duration of response and the rates of complete clinical remission and cure. Nonetheless, much of chemotherapy in advanced disease remains *palliative*, designed to reduce morbidity and prolong survival without placing too heavy a burden on the patient. This is not always possible, and it takes good judgment to best decide what and when to offer and when to withhold palliative therapy. Patients who fail to demonstrate a clinically meaningful response should have their chemotherapy regimen stopped or at least changed to an alternative program.

Basic Chemotherapy Strategies

Designing combination programs and maximizing dose use are important chemotherapy strategies. *Combination chemotherapy* regimens permit increased effectiveness without greatly increasing toxicity by utilizing agents that are each active against the specific tumor but have different mechanisms of action and nonadditive side effects. Synergies are achieved, while adverse effects are minimized.

Dose intensity is essential to ensuring the effectiveness of therapy. Use of too small a dose is associated with reduced efficacy. Especially when cure is being attempted, it is better to try to maintain use of maximal doses and treat drug side effects by means other than dose reduction. Reductions in dose are among the most common causes of drug failure.

Meaningful response to therapy is usually expected within two courses of treatment. Only rarely does continued treatment in the absence of initial response result in an increased appreciation of response; usually, more therapy is unwarranted. Follow-up for assessment of response and determination of further chemotherapy is usually conducted within 2 months of initiation of the treatment program.

Adverse Effects

The principal factor limiting the usefulness of chemotherapy is its relative *lack of selectivity* for the tumor cell. Cytotoxic drugs adversely affect normal cells, especially those populations with rapid turnover (bone marrow, hair follicles, gastrointestinal mucosa). This leads to *bone marrow suppression*, *alopecia*, and *gastroenteritis* shortly after initiation of chemotherapy.

Typically, *acute marrow suppression* begins 7 to 10 days after administration of chemotherapy and may last about 1 week. Continuous cytotoxic therapy may cause a more lasting *cumulative suppression of the bone marrow*. However, most forms of adjuvant chemotherapy are usually not associated with persistent marrow suppression, although a transient fall in cellular constituents may occur.

The most serious risks of chemotherapy are *leukopenia*, leading to overwhelming sepsis, and *thrombocytopenia*, resulting in hemorrhage. In most instances, leukopenia and thrombocytopenia are dose-related and may be prevented or lessened by dose adjustment in patients who have marginal marrow reserve due to marrow invasion, age, or prior therapy. Nonetheless, the goal of most chemotherapeutic regimens is to induce some degree of leukopenia, which can serve as a measure of cytotoxic effect and as a guideline to dosage.

The *gastrointestinal (GI) toxicity* of chemotherapy can be debilitating. It includes nausea, vomiting, mucosal injury (stomatitis), and diarrhea. Although not as life-threatening as leukopenia and thrombocytopenia, GI side effects can significantly compromise quality of life, morale, and willingness to undergo further chemotherapy.

Alopecia is a consequence of most forms of chemotherapy. It is usually partial, but with doxorubicin the hair loss is generally total. It begins approximately 2 weeks after initiation of treatment and becomes complete by 4 to 6 weeks. Hair loss is almost always transient, and often some hair grows during the course of treatment; however, total restitution does not take place until chemotherapy is stopped. When hair growth returns, it usually produces darker, finer, more curly hair, but with time, hair returns to its normal texture and color.

Of concern is the increasing evidence that *secondary malignancies*, such as acute leukemia, may develop in patients treated with chemotherapy, especially with use of alkylating agents. Although the accumulating evidence grows increasingly compelling, the risk of treatment remains far outweighed by its benefits.

Cytotoxic Chemotherapeutic Agents

Cytotoxic drugs have been grouped into five categories based on their mechanism of action or the chemical derivation of the drug (Table 88–1).

The Alkylating Agents. In general, the alkylating agents have a broad spectrum of antitumor activity, chemically interacting directly with DNA. As just noted, secondary malignancy is a concern associated with their use. The most commonly used drug in this class is *cyclophosphamide*.

The antimetabolites interfere with synthesis of DNA. They have greatest effect on rapidly growing cells. The most commonly used agents in this class are *fluorouracil* and *methotrexate*. The antimetabolites are rapidly metabolized and excreted in the urine. Methotrexate is distributed

Table 88-1. Cytotoxic Chemotherapeutic Agents

CLASS	DOSE FREQUENCY	ACUTE TOXICITY			OTHER TOXICITY	ELIMINATION	PLASMA HALF-LIFE (*h*)†
		Leukocyte	*Platelet*	*Nausea/Vomiting*			
Plant Derivatives							
Taxol	q 3 wk	Moderate	Moderate	Mild	Anaphylactoid response, sensory neuropathy, alopecia	M	6–8
Vincristine	qwk	Mild	Mild	Mild	Distal neuropathy, inappropriate ADH	M	2.6
Vinblastine	qwk	Marked	Marked	Mild	Mucositis	M	3.1
VP-16	qd × 5	Moderate	Mild	Mild	Distal neuropathy	M, R	6
Antibiotics							
Dactinomycin	qd × 5	Marked	Marked	Moderate	Alopecia, mucositis	M, R	?
Doxorubicin	q 3 wk	Marked	Marked	Moderate	Alopecia, cardiomyopathy	M	3/25
Daunorubicin	3 d, q 3 wk	Marked	Marked	Moderate	Alopecia, cardiomyopathy	M	3/?
Mitomycin C	qd × 3, q 3 wk	Marked	Marked	Moderate	Renal, pulmonary	M	?
Bleomycin	qwk	Rare	Rare	Mild	Skin, pulmonary fibrosis, fever, allergic reactions	R	0.4/2
Antimetabolites							
Methotrexate (high-dose) with leucovorin	q 3 wk q 6 h × 7 doses	Mild	Mild	Moderate	Hepatic dysfunction, renal failure	R M	2/8
Methotrexate	Twice weekly	Moderate–Marked	Moderate–Marked	Mild	Stomatitis	R	2/8
5-Fluorouracil	qwk *or* qd × 5, q 4 wk	Moderate–Marked	Moderate–Marked	Mild	Cerebellar, conjunctivitis	M	0.3
5-Fluorouracil with leucovorin	qwk × 6, qd × 5 q 4 wk	Marked	Marked	Mild	Diarrhea, stomatitis	M	0.3
6-Mercaptopurine	qd × 5	Moderate–Marked	Moderate–Marked	Mild	Cholestasis	M	0.3–0.6

Cytarabine (cytosine arabinoside)	q 12 h × 5–10 d	Marked	Marked	Moderate	Cholestasis, mucositis	Moderate	0.15
Hydroxyurea	qd × 5	Marked	Moderate	Moderate	None	R, M	1.7
Fludarabine	qd × 5	Moderate	Mild	Mild	Pneumonitis, neurotoxicity	R, M	9.3
Alkylating Agents							
Cyclophosphamide	qd × 5	Marked	Mild	Moderate	Cystitis, water retention, alopecia	M	1–4
Ifosfamide	qd × 5	Moderate	Moderate	Mild	Neurotoxicity, urothelial toxicity	M	5–6
and Mesna	qd × 5.5	None	None	None	None	M	?
Melphalan	qd	Moderate	Moderate	Mild	Leukemia	M	2
Busulfan	qd	Marked	Marked	Mild	Pulmonary fibrosis	M	?
CCNU	q 6 wk	Marked	Marked	Moderate	Leukemia, pulmonary fibrosis, renal failure	M	?
BCNU	q 6 wk	Marked	Marked	Marked	Leukemia, pulmonary fibrosis, renal failure	M	1.0
Streptozocin	qd × 5 q 3–4 wk	Mild	Mild	Moderate–Marked	Renal failure, hyperglycemia, hepatic enzyme elevation	R	0.25
Chlorambucil	qd	Moderate	Moderate	Mild	Leukemia	M	1.5
cis-diamminedichloroplatinum	q 3–4 wk	Moderate	Moderate	Severe	Renal failure, Mg^{2+} wasting, peripheral neuropathy, ototoxicity	R, M	0.3
CBDCA (Carboplatin)	q 3–4 wk	Marked	Marked	Mild		R	
Miscellaneous							
DTIC (Dacarbazine)	qd × 5	Mild	Mild	Marked	Flulike syndrome, venoocclusion	M	0.65
Procarbazine	qd × 10–14 d	Moderate	Moderate	Mild	Sensitivity to amines	M	?
Mitoxantrone	q 3 wk	Moderate	Moderate	Mild	Cholestasis, cardiac	M	0.25/37

Adapted from Chabner BA. Anticancer drugs. In DeVita VT, Hellman S, Rosenberg SA, eds. Principles and Practice of Oncology, 4th ed. Philadelphia, JB Lippincott 1993; 325.

throughout total body water, making pleural effusions and ascites potential reservoirs of the drug.

The antibiotics include *doxorubicin* (Adriamycin) and *bleomycin*. Doxorubicin is an anthracycline antibiotic with a spectrum of activity comparable to that of the alkylating drugs. In combination with the alkylating drugs, doxorubicin appears to be synergistic in antitumor effect. The drug has a cumulative toxic effect on the heart that results in a *cardiomyopathy*, limiting the maximum cumulative dose to 450 to 500 mg/m^2. Periodic radionuclide scanning of the heart is indicated once the cumulative dose exceeds 300 mg/m^2. The drug is halted if a 15 percent decrease is noted in the ejection fraction. *Bleomycin*, a polypeptide antibiotic mixture, causes *pulmonary fibrosis*, an effect that may be dose-related or, occasionally, idiosyncratic. As a result, the maximum cumulative dose is 200 mg/m^2. Measurement of the pulmonary diffusion capacity is the most sensitive means of early detection. A decrease to below 40 percent of predicted capacity is a sign of lung injury (see Chapter 51).

The plant alkaloids are mitotic inhibitors and include *etoposide*, *taxol*, and *vincristine*. Taxol has the unique property of interfering with microtubular function. Much excitement has accompanied preliminary evidence for the efficacy of taxol in treatment of advanced ovarian cancer (more data are forthcoming, and the literature should be watched closely). *Allergic reactions* are common with taxol, requiring pretreatment glucocorticosteroids and H2-blockers. For vincristine and vinblastine, the chief adverse effects are cumulative *neurotoxicity* (vincristine), which recedes slowly with drug withdrawal, and marrow suppression (vinblastine). Etoposide and taxol can cause hypotension if injected rapidly.

Miscellaneous or mixed mechanism agents include two important drugs: nitrosoureas and cisplatin. The *nitrosoureas* are alkylating drugs that cross the blood–brain barrier. They have a unique, *delayed marrow-suppressive effect* that necessitates a specific drug schedule with a long hiatus between administered courses (6 weeks). *Cisplatin* can cause *renal failure* in patients who are inadequately hydrated and has been associated with *ototoxicity* and *neurotoxicity*.

Investigational Therapies

Under development are a host of new approaches to cancer therapy that expand the treatment spectrum beyond conventional chemotherapy. They include use of *monoclonal antibodies*, intensive chemotherapy with *marrow transplantation*, and biologic response modifiers (eg, *interleukin*, *interferon*). Another area of intense interest is enhancing the specificity of chemotherapy by combining it with antibody techniques. The promise of these approaches is considerable and likely to result in major advances. The reader is urged to follow the literature closely for data on efficacy, safety, and indications for use.

MANAGEMENT RECOMMENDATIONS

Administration of chemotherapy is sometimes assigned to the primary physician when the services of the oncologist are not locally available. Under such circumstances, it is particularly important to be aware of the potential hazard of *extravasation* associated with certain intravenously administered agents (eg, doxorubicin, vincristine, vinblastine, dacarbazine [DTIC], carmustine [BCNU], nitrogen mustard). The best treatment is prevention, with proper venous access being the most important element. When extravasation does occur, it results in tissue irritation and secondary inflammation leading to ulceration and necrosis. Surgical grafting and débridement are sometimes necessary. In the event of extravasation, the infusions should be stopped immediately and *ice* applied. Any accumulation of drug should be removed by aspiration. The actual inflammation and necrosis may not occur for 3 to 10 days following injection, although pain is generally present early on. Corticosteroids have been used, but there is no definitive evidence of efficacy.

Even without extravasation, repeated use of irritating intravenously administered chemotherapy drugs can lead to sclerosis and endothelial deterioration, particularly when small-caliber veins are used for infusion. Large-diameter veins in the antecubital fossa or higher are preferred. Venous access devices facilitate administration.

Suppression of Chemotherapy-Induced Nausea and Vomiting. The drugs most likely to induce severe nausea and vomiting include cisplatin, DTIC, doxorubicin, nitrogen mustard, and high doses of cyclophosphamide. Some agents cause vomiting that begins approximately 30 to 45 minutes following injection; with others, particularly cyclophosphamide and doxorubicin, the vomiting begins 4 to 5 hours after injection. Recent advances in understanding the mechanisms of chemotherapy-induced nausea and vomiting have led to the development of effective multifaceted programs (see Chapter 91).

Prevention is the best therapy and helps avoid development of anticipatory emesis. A common practice is to administer a glucocorticosteroid (eg, *dexamethasone*) in combination with a phenothiazine (eg, *prochlorperazine*) at the time of infusing chemotherapy. Because GI upset may persist hours after chemotherapy administration, the prophylactic program is continued for 12 to 24 hours. Since oral administration may not be possible in the setting of emesis, sublingual, rectal, or intravenous administration of an antiemetic may be necessary.

In many instances, sedation and steroids suffice for control of chemotherapy-induced emesis. However, curative chemotherapy regimens utilizing cisplatin and high doses of other potent agents may trigger severe emesis inadequately controlled by sedation and steroids. The serotonin-receptor blocking agent *ondansetron* has proven extremely effective for prophylaxis of the severe nausea and vomiting associated with use of cisplatin. Although expensive, the drug has proven to be of great benefit, achieving excellent control in well over 75 percent of patients. It is given parenterally hour before chemotherapy and 4 and 8 hours after, in conjunction with dexamethasone. Combination with phenothiazine use further enhances efficacy. An oral form of ondansetron is now available and should facilitate outpatient administration of chemotherapy. The drug is superior to parenteral *metoclopramide*, replacing it for use in cisplatin therapy.

An important cause of vomiting is the *conditioned vomiting response*, a learned behavior which, in time, can become more severe than that induced by the drug therapy itself. This anticipatory pattern of vomiting typically develops after two or three courses of emesis-inducing cancer treatment. It is characterized by anxiety and anorexia the day before therapy, and can be precipitated by little more than driving down the street on which the therapy center is located. The condition responds well to benzodiazepine therapy (eg, alprazolam .25–.50 mg q6h) taken orally for 24 hrs in advance of chemotherapy.

Management of bone marrow suppression requires adjustments in dose and timing of chemotherapy. Generalized marrow suppression is common. However, the advent of marrow growth factors (ie, *erythropoietin* and *granulocyte colony-stimulating factor*) have enhanced the ability to give the optimal doses of chemotherapy, which ordinarily might be limited by onset of marrow suppression. Growth factors work best when given prophylactically, rather than after marrow suppression has set in. They are expensive but can save hospitalizations and limit complications. These agents have no effect on platelet production, though other agents are under development which do.

The pattern of suppression is a function of the type of drug, its dose and schedule (Table 88–2). Dose adjustments for subsequent courses of therapy are based on the nadir levels observed. In monitoring patients on chemotherapeutic regimens, the anticipated nadir days for blood counts are the most crucial times to obtain follow-up complete blood counts. In patients who develop leukopenia, the observation period ought to be intensified, depending on the level of the count and the presence of associated fever or sepsis. Emerging data suggest that *prophylactic oral antibiotics* (such as ciprofloxacin 500 mg bid) reduce hospitalization in patients whose absolute neutrophil count falls below 1000/mm^3.

Table 88-2. Chronologic Patterns of Marrow Suppression Secondary to Chemotherapy

AGENT	NADIR DAY	DURATION
Nonsuppressive Drugs		
Bleomycin		
Vincristine		
Streptozotocin		
Corticosteroids		
DTIC		
Marrow-Suppresive Drugs		
1. *Alkylating drugs*		
Cyclophosphamide		
Nitrogen mustard	5–8	Variable
Mitomycin C	Delayed	Cumulative
2. *Antibiotics*		
Doxorubicin	12–14	5 days
Dactinomycin		
3. *Antimetabolites*		
5-Fluorouracil	5–10	<5 days
Cytosine arabinoside		
Methotrexate		
4. *Natural products*		
Vinblastine	8–12	3 days
5. *Others*		
Nitrosoureas	14–28	Cumulative
Hydroxyurea	Variable	
Procarbazine	Variable	

Table 88-3. Criteria of Response to Therapy

Survival
Measured from time of diagnosis, metastasis, or initiation of treatment in days, weeks, or months, to be compared by median (as opposed to mean) to a randomized control or historical control not receiving treatment or receiving alternative treatment. Survival as a measurement of time may also be supplemented by a time measurement of diagnosis to point of recurrence and is translated as disease-free survival.

OBJECTIVE REDUCTION IN TUMOR

Partial Response
Equals a 50% reduction in the product of the maximum perpendicular diameters of the most easily measurable lesion without increase in other lesions and with a minimum duration of 4 weeks.

Complete Response
Equals a 100% reduction in all evidence of tumor for minimum of 4 weeks without appearance of new lesions.

Stable Disease
Equals a less than 25% decrease in measurable disease without development of other lesions.

No Response (Progressive Disease)
Equals a more than 25% increase in the size of the lesion or the development of new lesions.

Improvement
Equals a 25%–50% reduction in the product of maximum perpendicular diameters lasting at least 4 weeks.

EVALUATION OF RESPONSE TO THERAPY

Monitoring patients on chemotherapeutic regimens for adverse effects is performed in concert with evaluation of the effectiveness of treatment (see also Chapter 87). Objective tumor measurements are often difficult to define, but generally the oncologist depends on them to gauge response to therapy (Table 88–3).

The criteria of response are often difficult to evaluate because partial responses may be influenced by nontumor factors. In addition, some forms of metastatic disease simply cannot be measured, such as osseous metastases and, particularly, osteoblastic lesions. There are established criteria for some metastatic patterns, such as hepatomegaly, where the criterion for response is a 30 percent decrease in the sum of measurements made below the costal margin at the midclavicular and midxiphoid lines. Peritoneal masses, pleural effusions, and skin ulcerations are not considered amenable to evaluation. Ultrasonography and computed body tomography have helped quantify lesions in the retroperitoneum.

Tumor markers (see Chapter 86) have facilitated objectively gauging response to therapy. Sequential monitoring of marker serum levels correlates well with tumor mass and often predicts recurrence before it becomes clinically evident. For example, human chorionic gonadotropin has proven useful in management of testicular cancer, and carcinoembryonic antigen in colorectal cancer. Markers derived from monoclonal antibody techniques are increasingly important, including CA19-9 for pancreatic cancer, PSA for prostate cancer, CA15-3 for breast cancer, and CA125 for ovarian cancer. Other biochemical parameters, such as alkaline phosphatase and the various hepatic enzymes, have been uniformly inadequate to evaluate the effectiveness of treatment.

PATIENT EDUCATION

The ability to tolerate chemotherapy is enhanced by a strong and trusting patient–doctor relationship. Fully educating the patient and his family about diagnosis, prognosis, and the rationale and side effects of planned treatment can greatly facilitate the development of trust and confidence (see Chapter 88). Concerns about alopecia, sterility, gastrointestinal upset, and other side effects should be elicited and directly addressed. The probability of response also deserves review. A comprehensive educational effort appropriate for the patient's level of understanding allows him to participate meaningfully in decision making and encourages a sense of partnership in the undertaking, an attitude that can help sustain the patient through this often difficult time.

INDICATIONS FOR ADMISSION AND REFERRAL

Onset of febrile neutropenia (absolute neutrophil counts below $1000/mm^3$) requires immediate hospitalization. Development of bleeding in the setting of thrombocytopenia is an indication for urgent hospitalization and consideration of platelet transfusion. The asymptomatic patient with severe thrombocytopenia (platelet count $<20,000/mm^3$) also deserves consideration for admission and platelet transfusion. Counts of 20,000 to 50,000 are an indication for close observation and warning the patient to avoid trauma.

Chemotherapy programs are in a constant state of revision as new combinations are tried and new agents developed. Each patient's treatment program must be designed in conjunction with an oncologist. When such expertise is not locally available, patients may have to travel to a regional center for therapy. Computer-based chemotherapy protocol advisory systems are now available to help provide expert input where it may not otherwise be obtainable.

ANNOTATED BIBLIOGRAPHY

Antman KS, Griffin JD, Elias A, et al. Effect of recombinant human granulocyto-macrophage colony-stimulating factor on chemotherapy induced myelosuppression. N Engl J Med 1989;319:593. *(Found effective; a major advance, facilitating ability to administer full doses of chemotherapy.)*

Comis RL, Kuppinger MS, Ginsberg SJ, et al. Role of single-breath carbon monoxide diffusing capacity in monitoring the pulmonary effects of bleomycin in germ-cell tumor patients. Cancer Res 1979;39:5076. *(A reduction to less than 40 percent of predicted suggests onset of pulmonary fibrosis.)*

Fojo AT, Ueda K, Slamon DJ, et al. Expression of a multidrug-resistant gene in human tumors and tissues. Proc Natl Acad Sci U S A 1987;84:265. *(Basic science study of the mechanism of multidrug resistance.)*

Goldie JH, Goldman AJ, Gudauskas GA. Rationale for the use of alternating noncrossresistant chemotherapy. Cancer Treat Rep 1982;66:439. *(The theoretical basis for combination chemotherapy.)*

Gottdiener JS, Mathisen DJ, Borer JS, et al. Doxorubicin cardiotoxicity: assessment of late left ventricular dysfunction by radionuclide cineangiography. Ann Intern Med 1981;94:430. *(A 15 percent reduction in ejection fraction strongly suggested onset of cardiomyopathy.)*

Herrstedt J, Sigsgaard T, Boesgaard M, et al. Ondansetron plus metopimazine compared with ondansetron alone in patients receiving moderately emetogenic chemotherapy. N Engl J Med 1993;328:1076. *(Excellent control achieved, especially when ondansetron was used with the phenothiazine.)*

Hickam DH, Shortliffe EH, Bischoff MB, et al. The treatment advice of a computer-based cancer chemotherapy protocol advisor. Ann Intern Med 1985;103:928.*(An example of care rendered through use of a computer-based advisory system.)*

Hryniuk W. Is more better? J Clin Oncol 1986;4:621. *(An editorial reviewing the issue of dose intensity.)*

Jacquillat C, Weil M, Baillet F, et al. Results of neoadjuvant chemotherapy and radiation therapy in breast conserving treatment of 250 patients with all stages of infiltrative breast cancer. Cancer 1990;66:119. *(An example of the efficacy of neoadjuvant therapy.)*

Jolivet J, Cowan KH, Curt GA, et al. The pharmacology and clinical use of methotrexate. N Engl J Med 309:1094, 1983 *(A comprehensive and clinically helpful review.)*

Loehrer PJ, Einhorn LH. Drugs five years later: cisplatin. Ann Intern Med 1984;100:704. *(Useful review for the generalist.)*

McGuire WP, Rowinsky EK, Rosenshein NB, et al. Taxol: a unique antineoplastic agent with significant activity in advanced ovarian epithelial neoplasms. Ann Intern Med 1989; 111:1778. *(An encouraging early report of efficacy.)*

Young RC, Ozols RF, Myers CE: The anthracycline antineoplastic drugs. N Engl J Med 1981;305:139. *(Detailed discussion of doxorubicin and related compounds.)*

89
Principles of Radiation Therapy

JERRY YOUNGER, M.D.

Primary Care Medicine: Office Evaluation and Management of the Adult Patient, 3rd edition, edited by Allan H. Goroll, Lawrence A. May, and Albert G. Mulley, Jr. J.B. Lippincott Company, Philadelphia

Modern radiation therapy represents an important means of achieving local and regional control of malignancy as well as providing palliation. When given with the intent of controlling disease and attempting cure, it is termed "radical"; when given for symptomatic relief, it is designated as "palliative." Although the design and implementation of such therapy is the responsibility of the radiation oncologist, the primary physician shares in the decision to use the modality, monitors and support the patient during its administration, and watches for and treats late complications. The primary care physician needs to be familiar with basic aspects of radiation therapy, its applications, and its side effects.

PRINCIPLES OF MANAGEMENT

Response to Irradiation

There is exponential killing of both tumor and normal cells after an initial sublethal accumulation of radiation. This ability to accumulate some radiation before demonstrating cell death is believed linked to *repair capacity*. The response curves of cells in culture are remarkably similar, with most of the difference in *"radiosensitivity"* due to the greater *number* of actively dividing cells in malignant tissue. Cells in the S phase of the cell cycle (when there is DNA synthesis but no mitosis) are the least sensitive to radiation, probably because of enhanced capacity for repair in this phase.

Response to irradiation is also affected by the *volume* of the tumor. Except for uniquely radiosensitive tumors (lymphomas and seminomas), the greater the tumor's volume, the more *"radioresistance"* it will show. Part of the reason for this resistance is *tissue hypoxia*. Oxygen facilitates the cytotoxic effect of x-rays. Hypoxic cells are about three times more refractory to irradiation than are cells treated in the presence of oxygen. Interior areas of large tumors can become hypoxic and relatively refractory to radiation. However, as the tumor shrinks, its hypoxic cells gain better access to oxygen, making them more susceptible to radiation if doses are given in sequential fractionated fashion (see below).

Other strategies to improve response to radiation include use of *charged particle beams* and compounds that *sensitize hypoxic tumor cells*. Charged particle beams are less dependent on oxygen for their cytotoxic action than x-rays and represent another means of treating large, poorly vascularized tumors. Compounds that will *sensitize hypoxic tumor cells* and improve their response to radiation therapy are under investigation.

The *dose of irradiation* that can be safely directed at a malignancy is limited by the tolerance of the organs surrounding it. Although the energy of the radiation determines ability to penetrate tissue, it is the amount absorbed that determines biologic effects. Cutting down on scatter to limit the amount of radiation absorbed by adjacent tissue is made possible by use of high energy beams. Radiation damage can be particularly injurious when there is absorption by cells of the heart, liver, brain, intestines, bone marrow, kidneys, or lung (see below). Usually, trade-offs must be made between therapeutic benefits and adverse effects.

The probability of radiation-induced complications depends on how narrow the difference is between the dose needed for control of the tumor and the dose that causes injury to normal tissue. (The ratio of the two doses is termed the *therapeutic ratio.*) The greater the difference in doses, the better the likelihood of beneficial effect.

Dose fractionation, shielding, and use of imaging techniques to precisely define tumor volume and location have helped limit the adverse effects of radiation therapy. *Fractionating* the dose helps to widen the margin of safety and improve selective killing of tumor cells. Normal cells repair sublethal radiation damage more effectively than do tumor cells. Most fractionation programs provide about 200 rads per treatment, applied five times per week. *Shielding* helps protect vital organs adjacent to the portal from radiation exposure. Often, custom-fabricated lead shields are made when there is risk of irradiating normal tissue abutting the tumor. *Computed tomography (CT) scanning* and *magnetic resonance imaging (MRI)* have improved delineation of the tumor volume and surrounding anatomic structures so that the target can be more precisely defined. *Simulation* reproduces the geometry of the actual radiation portal, helping to ensure that only the desired tissue is irradiated. Work is in progress to develop compounds that will preferentially protect normal cells.

Clinical Applications

There are three basic *delivery modes*. Use of external sources (teletherapy) is the most common. Encapsulated sources planted directly into the body at tumor sites (brachytherapy) has selective advantages for treating very localized disease. Systemic delivery via radionuclides is the third mode. Investigational forms entail intravenous administration of radionuclide-labelled monoclonal antibodies that are designed to selectively attack a target cancer. The theoretical attractiveness of the latter two methods is closer proximity to the tumor, limitation of area exposed, and ability to use lower doses.

Radiation is applied for cure and control as well as to achieve palliation. It may be the sole treatment, an alternative therapy, or combined with other modalities (Table 89–1).

As Sole or Alternative Therapy. Like surgery, radiation therapy is primarily a method of treating local or regional disease. The goal is to "sterilize" both the primary site and likely areas of local and regional spread. In some instances, such as stage I Hodgkin's disease or early low-grade non-Hodgkin's lymphoma (see Chapter 84), x-ray therapy is the treatment of choice. When preservation of function and appearance can be achieved with comparable survival outcome, radiation may be preferred by some patients over surgery (as in localized breast cancer or early head and neck cancers). When surgery and radiation provide similar rates of cure and control, choice depends largely on the impact of treatment on the patient.

As Combination Therapy. Radiation therapy has several qualities that make it a good complement to *surgery*. Surgery is the more effective of the two in dealing with bulk disease, whereas radiation appears better at dealing with small-volume, locally invasive disease. These qualities are the basis for the sequence of surgery of local disease followed by radiation as adjunctive therapy. Radiation can also reduce tumor bulk and destroy microscopic disease, facilitating surgical removal and local control. By allowing use of lower radiation doses and less radical surgery, combination therapy minimizes side effects. Adjuvant radiotherapy directed at regions of potential spread, such as lymph nodes, makes radical exploration unnecessary.

Table 89-1. Applications of Radiotherapy

TUMOR	COMMENTS
Radiation Therapy Alone is Curative	
Hodgkin's disease	Stages IA and IIA; 94% 10-year survival
Lymphoma	Stage I only; 90% 5-year disease-free survival
Cervical cancer	Curative for early disease; 65% 5-year disease-free survival for invasive disease
Testicular cancer	Seminomas
Head and neck cancer	Early stage disease (T1); results comparable to surgery with less functional and cosmetic loss
Radiation Combined with Another Modality is Potentially Curative	
Uterine cancer	With surgery; good results for stages I, II, and III; 70% to 90% 5-year survival
Head and neck cancer	With surgery in more advanced cases
Soft tissue sarcomas	In combination with surgery
Breast cancer	In combination with limited resection; excellent control of local recurrence
Rectal cancer	With surgery, marked improvement in survival
Radiation Therapy is Palliative	
Prostate cancer	5-year disease-free survival as high as 70% for stage B disease; drops to 36% for stage C disease
Lung cancer	For unresectable non–small-cell disease
Brain metastases	Especially as a prophylactic measure
Ovarian cancer	Exact role of radiation unsettled
Bony metastases	For painful lesions unresponsive to chemotherapy
GI cancers	For unresectable gastric, pancreatic, and esophageal cancers, results are fair; better for colon cancer when combined with surgery

Whether to give radiation before, during, or after surgery depends on several practical and theoretical issues. Favoring preoperative treatment are the need to reduce tumor size for easier resection and the desirability of sterilizing tumor cells that might be spread during surgery. Moreover, postoperative irradiation may be less effective if the vascular bed is surgically reduced and oxygen delivery impaired. Factors favoring postoperative treatment include promptness of surgery and destruction of any remaining microscopic disease. Intraoperative treatment allows one to displace normal abdominal organs (which are quite intolerant to irradiation) and better target diseased tissue.

Radiation in combination *with chemotherapy* to achieve cure is established for advanced stages of Hodgkin's disease and is being explored in other cancers. The rationale is to treat local disease with radiation and use chemotherapy for systemic coverage. The radiation can also help treat areas not readily accessible to chemotherapy, such as the brain. Although results appear promising, toxicities can be additive. Marrow suppression is the limiting problem. There are other instances of additive adverse effects: Cytoxan and radiation produce hemorrhagic cystitis; methotrexate and x-ray cause mucositis of the oral cavity; and combination chemotherapy plus radiation leads to increased risk of leukemia. Some drugs enhance radiation reactions in normal tissues, even when given up to a year after radiotherapy. Adriamycin is the most prominent example of a drug producing this "recall phenomenon."

At present, the optimal strategies for application of combined modality therapy remain unsettled. The literature should be followed for results of studies now ongoing.

As Palliative Therapy. Radiation serves an important function in providing symptomatic relief to some patients with incurable disease. For those tumors that respond to chemotherapy or hormonal therapy, radiation should be held in reserve. However, if there is localized tumor not sensitive to other modalities, palliative radiation may be an effective means of providing symptomatic relief. In most instances, treatment of asymptomatic lesions yields little benefit, though prophylactic brain irradiation appears useful in some patients with aggressive lymphoma. One of the best examples of palliative therapy is for painful *bony metastases* from such tumors as breast and prostate. Within 2 to 3 weeks of starting a relatively short course of radiotherapy (2 weeks), many patients experience welcome relief from bone pain. Radiation to bony metastases has also been used to stabilize a weight-bearing bone, but if cortical involvement is present, then surgical means of stabilizing the bone may be necessary. Radiation has an important role in urgent treatment of certain oncologic emergencies, including *spinal cord compression* and *superior vena cava syndrome* (see Chapter 92).

Table 89-2. Serious Adverse Effects of Radiotherapy

TISSUE	ADVERSE EFFECT	DOSE LIMIT (≦5%)(TOXICITY) IN RADS
Bone marrow	Marrow suppression	250
Kidneys	Nephrosclerosis	2000
Lungs	Pneumonitis	2500
Liver	Hepatitis	3000
Heart	Pericarditis	4500
Spinal cord	Infarction	4500
Intestines	Ulceration	4500
Skin	Dermatitis, sclerosis	5500
Brain	Infarction	6000

Chabner BA: Principles of cancer therapy. In: Wyngaarden JB, Smith LH, eds. Cecil's Textbook of Medicine, 16th ed. Philadelphia: WB Saunders, 1982:1034.

Adverse Effects

As noted previously, normal cells tolerate radiation better than do malignant cells. However, the degree of tolerance varies greatly (Table 89–2). Tissues having high rates of turnover and large stem cell populations are among the most vulnerable. Even organs with almost no proliferative capacity are at risk by virtue of the vulnerability of their vascular endothelium. Much radiation-induced injury is vascular in nature. Toxicity may be acute or chronic. Acute toxicity is noted in tissues with the highest rates of turnover (eg, marrow, skin, gastrointestinal mucosa). Chronic toxicity is the more serious and clinically significant.

Tolerance to radiotherapy decreases as dose is increased. The *dose limit* for a tissue can be expressed as the cumulative dose that produces a 5 percent incidence of toxicity when radiation is delivered in 200-rad fractions, 5 days per week. Beyond the dose limit, the incidence of toxicity rises quickly.

The bone marrow is the most radiosensitive tissue, with *marrow suppression* developing when exposure exceeds 250 rads. At such low doses, suppression is usually transient. Skin, gastrointestinal mucosa, and lung are of intermediate sensitivity. *Radiation pneumonitis* starts to appear when the dose surpasses 2500 rads; the incidence reaches 100 percent at doses of 4000 rads. Onset is usually within 6 to 12 weeks, characterized by dyspnea, hypoxemia, and a "ground glass" appearance on chest x-ray. Restrictive defects and chronic hypoxemia follow if fibrosis sets in, which typically takes place over the ensuing 6 to 24 months. Treatment is mainly supportive. High-dose steroids and oxygen can alleviate symptoms during the acute phase; there is no treatment once fibrosis occurs. The best approach is prevention by carefully limiting the radiation portal.

Nephrosclerosis is the renal response to doses in excess of 2000 rads. *Hepatitis* is a consequence of doses to the liver above 3000 rads. Gastrointestinal *ulceration* followed by perforation or fibrosis are complications of bowel doses exceeding 4500 rads. *Pericarditis* and *spinal cord infarction* are risks of 4500-rad doses to the heart and spinal cord, respectively. With mediastinal irradiation, pericarditis can become constrictive and valvular injury has also been noted.

Although acute reactions are common, the skin can tolerate as much as 5500 rads given over time; *dermatitis* becomes a problem at higher doses; the brain can withstand up to 6000 rads before the risk of *infarction* begins to rise. Radiation can also induce cataracts and retinal damage and can lead to blindness. Gonadal radiation is likely to induce permanent *sterility*, and pelvic irradiation during the first trimester of pregnancy is teratogenic. There is a genuine risk of *secondary malignancy* in the field of treatment; it is usually small, but in some instances may approach 1 percent per year.

The minor and temporary side effects of radiation therapy can be quite disabling unless anticipated and dealt with. *Nausea* occurs with abdominal irradiation; onset can be as soon as 1 to 2 hours after treatment. Prior administration of prochlorperazine helps to lessen gastrointestinal upset. Small, frequent feedings are better tolerated than large ones. If nausea and vomiting become problems, the daily dose can be scaled back or treatment temporarily halted. Head and neck irradiation may cause dryness in the mouth and *difficulty* with *mastication* and *swallowing*. Use of blenderized meals or liquid dietary supplements can help to maintain adequate caloric intake. *Diarrhea* resulting from bowel radiation responds to diphenoxylate (Lomotil) and loperamide. *Skin care* is commonly overlooked. Although use of megavoltage machines has cut skin exposure to 30 percent of the total dose delivered, avoidance of heat and excessive sun exposure helps preserve the integrity of irradiated skin.

PATIENT EDUCATION

Patients undergoing radiation therapy need plenty of emotional support. The fears associated with cancer are compounded by the awesome machinery and concerns about exposure to radiation. Patients who are well informed tolerate therapy better than those who are not. Answering questions and addressing concerns about the rationale for radiation therapy, the side effects to be expected, and how they will be controlled are essential to the successful conduct of a radiation therapy program. In particular, one needs to review the risk of sterility with patients of reproductive age and the chances of a second malignancy in patients considering curative radiotherapy. Such cost-benefit discussions are critical to helping the patient make an informed choice. Knowing that treatment can be adjusted to one's tolerance to therapy is also reassuring.

COORDINATION OF CARE

Conducting a radiotherapy program is the province of the radiation therapist, carried out in the context of an overall treatment plan designed by the oncologist in consultation with the primary care physician. The primary physician can ensure that the therapeutic program is well suited to the patient's needs and carefully monitored. A multidisciplinary team approach works best for the patient when there is an individual on the team to whom the patient feels he can always turn for advice and help; in many instances this important role can be best carried out by the primary care doctor.

ANNOTATED BIBLIOGRAPHY

Abe M, Takahashi M, Yabumoto E, et al. Clinical experiences with intraoperative radiotherapy for locally advanced cancers. Cancer 1980;45:40. *(Details results and limitations.)*

Coleman CN, Bump EA, Kramer RS. Chemical modifiers of cancer treatment. J Clin Oncol 1988;6:709. *(Includes a good discussion of agents used to sensitize tumors to radiation.)*

Fletcher GH. The evolution of the basic concepts underlying the practice of radiotherapy. Radiology 1978;127:3. *(The development of combination therapy utilizing radiation as one component.)*

Gottdiener JS, Katin MJ, Borer JS, et al. Late cardiac effects of therapeutic mediastinal irradiation. N Engl J Med 1983;308:569. *(Constrictive pericarditis, valvular thickening, and infarction may occur.)*

Kohn HI, Fry RJ. Radiation carcinogenesis. N Engl J Med 1984;310:504. *(A review that includes a terse, informative section on the risks associated with cancer radiotherapy.)*

Macklis RM, Kinsey BM, Kassis AI, et al. Radioimmunotherapy with alpha-particle emitting immunoconjugates. Science 1988;240:1024. *(An experimental example of systemic radiation therapy.)*

Montague ED, Fletch GH. The curative value of irradiation in the treatment of nondisseminated breast cancer. Cancer 1980;46:508. *(An example of curative radiotherapy.)*

Peschel RE, Fischer JJ. Optimization of the time-dose relationship. Semin Oncol 1981;8:38. *(A discussion of fractionation.)*

Prosnitz LR, Kapp DS, Weissberg JB: Radiotherapy. N Engl J Med 1983;309:771,834. *(A comprehensive two-part review that emphasizes recent treatment results and basic principles of radiation therapy; 157 references.)*

Tucker MA, Coleman CN, Cox RS, et al. Risk of second cancers after treatment for Hodgkin's disease. N Engl J Med 1988;318:76. *(Found to be 1 percent per year for patients undergoing curative therapy.)*

Weissberg JB. Role of radiation therapy in gastrointestinal cancer. Arch Surg 1983;118:96. *(Good overview of this difficult area.)*

90
Management of Cancer Pain

JERRY YOUNGER, M.D.

Primary Care Medicine: Office Evaluation and Management of the Adult Patient, 3rd edition, edited by Allan H. Goroll, Lawrence A. May, and Albert G. Mulley, Jr. J.B. Lippincott Company, Philadelphia

Relief of pain is an essential objective in the treatment of the cancer patient, being a direct determinant of quality of life. It is indeed a tragic situation when relentless pain is superimposed on a fatal outcome. In most instances, effective amelioration of pain can be achieved with proper use of analgesics. Unfortunately, undertreatment of pain is common.

The primary physician is the person to whom the patient most often turns for pain relief. One must know not only the appropriate treatments and their limitations but also how to support the cancer patient and minimize the emotional suffering that is invariably intertwined with the perception of pain (see Chapter 87).

PATHOPHYSIOLOGY AND CLINICAL PRESENTATIONS

The pain syndromes associated with cancer can be separated into acute and chronic clinical states, and the acute pain syndromes can be further subdivided (Table 90–1). The major pain syndromes are more often than not a prelude to the incurable stage of illness, but they may precede the terminal phase by a substantial interval.

Osseous Pain Syndromes. Metastases to the bony skeleton may cause pathologic fractures; the development of pain in a bony site is invariably secondary to interruption of the cortex, which may or may not be observed radiographically. Common sites are vertebrae, long bones, pelvis, and skull.

Another form of osseous metastasis involves the bone marrow or medullary cavity. Intramedullary tumor is characteristic of leukemia but may also be observed in some solid tumors. These produce a pain syndrome characterized by diffuse bone sensitivity in the presence of normal bone x-rays.

Thoracic Pain Syndromes. Pain associated with thoracic disease is generally a consequence of local invasion of the intercostal nerves. Pleuritic pain may develop if the malignancy spreads to involve the pleura. Direct invasion of a contiguous bony structure may result in local or referred pain.

Abdominal Pain Syndromes. Abdominal pain may develop as a consequence of intestinal obstruction; cramping pain is characteristic (see Chapter 58). Ascites can be uncomfortable as a consequence of abdominal distention. Hepatic metastases may cause pain by distending the liver capsule or irritating the peritoneal surface secondary to tumor necrosis. The latter is often associated with a friction rub.

Nerve Root Compression Syndromes. Pain originating in the back and radiating down an extremity is characteristic of root compression. When there is an associated neurologic deficit, it suggests the possibility of evolving cord compression. The tumor most commonly extends either from the retroperitoneal space or from a contiguously involved bony structure. Bone scans or radiographs often demonstrate lytic or blastic lesions. Compression syndromes may also occur as a consequence of vertebral body collapse secondary to tumor without direct tumor compression of the nerve.

Table 90-1. Classification and Types of Cancer-Related Pain

SYNDROME	CAUSES OR ANATOMIC SITE	COMMON CANCERS
Peripheral nerve compression or entrapment	Brachial plexus	Breast
	Sacral plexus	Rectum
	Paraspinal nerves	Pancreas
	Trigeminal nerve	Mouth
Nerve root compression	Paraspinal tumor or vertebral collapse	Breast
		Lung
		Myeloma
Osseous lesions	Pathologic fractures or intramedullary expansion	Breast
		Prostate
		Lung
Abdominal lesions	Obstruction	GI tumors
	Hepatic metastases	
	Ascites	
Thoracic lesions	Pleuritis or intercostal neuritis	Lung
Special pain forms		
Phantom limb	Reverberating neurocircuit	Sarcoma
Herpes zoster	Neuralgia	Hodgkin's disease
Hypertrophic pulmonary osteoarthropathy	Periarticular distal extremities	Lung Sarcoma

Peripheral Nerve Compression Syndromes. The relatively uncommon nerve compression syndromes result in pain in the shoulder or arm (brachial plexus), buttocks and perineum (sacral plexus), lumbar area (paraspinal nerves), and mouth or face (trigeminal nerve). All are secondary to nerve entrapment and, occasionally, to nerve invasion by tumor growth.

Special Pain Syndromes. The *phantom limb syndrome* characteristically develops following amputation in patients with osteogenic sarcoma, especially in those who have endured the tumor over a long period. Persistence of phantom limb pain may lead to narcotic dependence. It is only after a protracted period of time that the reverberating neural circuit is eventually exhausted.

Herpes zoster (shingles) occurs in patients with hematologic malignancies, particularly Hodgkin's disease, the non-Hodgkin's lymphomas, and chronic lymphocytic leukemia. Postherpetic pain may persist in the absence of typical skin lesions; herpes zoster should be suspected in patients complaining of pain in a dermatomal distribution (see Chapter 193).

Hypertrophic pulmonary osteoarthropathy (HPO) produces a periarticular pain syndrome that develops in patients with primary or metastatic tumors of the lung and mesotheliomas. The mechanism of the periarticular pain is unclear.

PRINCIPLES OF MANAGEMENT

Optimal selection of pain relief measures requires identification of the pathophysiologic process responsible for the discomfort. Rational therapy can then be instituted. Often a multifaceted approach is necessary. Psychological support, control of tumor, analgesics, neurosurgical procedures, and behavioral methods are among the important modalities for treatment of cancer-induced pain (Table 90–2).

Nonpharmacologic Measures

Psychological Support. The importance of psychological support from both physician and family cannot be overemphasized. The personal role of the primary physician is vital to successful control of pain. The understanding and concern given are as central to effective pain relief as are tumor control and proper use of analgesics (see Chapter 87).

Table 90-2. Approaches to Therapy of Cancer-Related Pain

1. Psychological support
2. Tumor control
3. Drug therapy
   a. Nonaddictive analgesics (anti-inflammatory drugs)
   b. Narcotic analgesics
   c. Psychotropic drugs
4. Neurosurgical ablative procedures
   a. Dorsal rhizotomy
   b. Sympathectomy
   c. Percutaneous cordotomy
   d. Chemical hypophysectomy
5. Unproven methods of pain management
   a. Hypnosis
   b. Acupuncture
   c. Behavior modification

Control of Tumor. For pain directly related to the tumor, the most important therapeutic maneuver is the introduction of *tumor-specific therapy*. Surgery and radiation therapy are the principal modalities for the treatment of localized malignancy. Adjuvant therapy, employing chemotherapy or radiation, is also being utilized. Advanced metastatic cancer can be treated with cytotoxic drugs for palliation of symptoms (see Chapter 88).

Even if disease is widespread, *local radiation* or *surgical excision* may be necessary. Cord compression responds to radiation, as does focal bony pain. Surgical excision can be used for tumors that cause pain because of size, fixation of underlying muscle, distention of the subcutaneous tissue, or localized secondary infection (eg, "toilet" mastectomy for fungating tumor). Such excision achieves a modicum of pain control and minimizes secondary infection.

Lesions of the extremities producing similar local complications (ie, pain, disfigurement, secondary infection, or poor function) may be considered for local surgical control; amputation is rarely justified or necessary. Local cryosurgery or electrocautery and, more recently, laser treatment will remove the lesion with a minimum of morbidity and permit maintenance of the limb.

Pharmacologic Measures

Aspirin, Acetaminophen, Nonsteroidals. Although narcotics are often the first drugs that come to mind in the treatment of cancer pain, there is a large degree of overlap in analgesic efficacy between the lower potency opioids and a number of non-narcotic analgesics. Even *aspirin* and *acetaminophen* can provide some relief from cancer-induced pain. Analgesic effect per dose peaks at 1300 mg, beyond which no additional analgesia is achieved. Duration of action is about 4 hours. Adding aspirin or acetaminophen to an oral opioid program boosts analgesic effect.

Aspirin's side effects include gastric mucosal irritation (see Chapter 68) and irreversible inhibition of platelet aggregation for the lifetime of the platelet (7 days—see Chapter 81). *Choline magnesium trisalicylate* is a less potent more expensive salicylate alternative, but with much less gastric irritant or platelet-inhibiting action. Overdosage of acetaminophen is injurious to the liver, but up to 4 g/d is well tolerated in patients without underlying liver disease.

Nonsteroidal anti-inflammatory agents (NSAIDS) offer analgesia that in nonprescription doses (eg, ibuprofen 200 mg) is equivalent or superior to 650 mg of either aspirin or acetaminophen and longer acting (6–12 h). Prescription preparations (eg, ibuprofen 400 mg, naproxen sodium 550 mg, ketoprofen 50 mg, ketorolac 10 mg) equal or exceed the pain relief afforded by codeine/acetaminophen preparations and last longer (6–8 h). The first *parenteral NSAID* preparation approved for acute pain control (ketorolac 30 mg IM) is comparable to 12 mg of IM morphine or 100 mg of IM meperidine. Onset of analgesia is slower, but duration of action is longer and there are no opiate risks or side effects. Repeatedly continuous parenteral use beyond 5 days is not recommended.

Chronic use of oral NSAIDS for pain control in cancer has not been as well studied as their short-term analgesic effects, but available evidence suggests quite reasonable efficacy, especially for bone pain or pain with an inflammatory component. Excellent analgesia has been demonstrated when used in *combination* with a narcotic. However, unlike narcotics, NSAIDS exhibit ceiling analgesic doses. Because there is much interpatient variation in response to individual NSAID preparations, titration of dose and trials of different preparations are often necessary to achieve the best response. (Ketorolac may have more analgesic effect than other NSAIDS, but it is expensive). Major adverse effects of NSAIDS are gastric mucosal injury, transient platelet inhibition (24–36 h), and renal impairment in patients with underlying renal insufficiency. Despite claims to the contrary, all preparations can cause significant injury to the gastric mucosa, because all inhibit gastric prostaglandin synthesis (see Chapter 68).

Narcotic Analgesics. Control of severe chronic cancer pain insufficiently responsive to the above medications is best achieved by adding an *opioid narcotic*. *Oral* therapy usually suffices, especially with use of sustained-release morphine preparations. *Parenteral* narcotic use should be reserved for treatment of severe *acute* pain. When narcotics are deemed necessary, they should be used in full pharmacologic doses as often as needed to achieve freedom from pain, an attainable and extremely important goal. Analgesics can be classified on the basis of their analgesic effectiveness (Tables 90–3 and 90–4).

Dosage requirements vary greatly among patients, necessitating careful titration of dose to degree of analgesia required. Unlike non-narcotic analgesics, there is no limit to the degree of analgesia that can be provided by increasing dose. The limiting factor is onset of adverse effects (nausea, vomiting, sedation, respiratory suppression). The degree of pain control is best and the total amount of narcotic minimized when dosing is on a *regularly scheduled* ("round-the-clock") basis, rather than on an "as needed" basis. Occasionally a between-dose administration is necessary and should be provided. To withhold narcotics until the patient is uncomfortable or to use them in subtherapeutic doses can seriously compromise provision of adequate pain control and greatly demoralize the patient.

Side effects include nausea, constipation, and sedation. Decreasing dose and increasing frequency will reduce sedation; use of sedatives, hypnotics, anxiolytics, and major tranquilizers will exacerbate it. Nausea and sedation respond to hydroxyzine and resolve rather quickly once tolerance begins to set in. However, constipation usually persists. Fluids, high fiber intake, bulk laxatives, and stool softeners can help (see Chapter 91).

Opioid tolerance may develop with regular opioid use and complicate provision of effective analgesia. Tolerance is manifested by shortening duration of pain control and an overall increase in pain complaints. Concurrent use of a non-narcotic analgesic (see above) or an adjuvant drug (see below) can delay the onset of tolerance by allowing use of lower narcotic doses and less frequent dosing. The simplest means of overcoming tolerance is to increase dose or dose frequency. Because tolerance to central nervous system (CNS) depressive effects parallels the reduction in pain relief, modestly increasing dose is not likely to risk serious

Table 90-3. Oral Analgesic Drugs

LEVEL	DRUG	SCHEDULE (STARTING)	COMMENT
I	Aspirin	600 mg q4–6h	Can enhance narcotic benefit
	Other NSAIDs*, *eg,* ibuprofen	400 mg q6h	Can enhance narcotic benefit
	Acetaminophen	600 mg q4h	Can enhance narcotic benefit
II	Codeine	30–60 mg q4–6h	Inexpensive; effective for moderate pain
	Oxycodone	5 mg q4–6h	Expensive; usually in combination preparations
III	Meperidine	100 mg q3h	Relatively ineffective orally
	Morphine	2–5 mg q3–4h	Effective; modest cost
	Sustained-release preparation	15–30 mg q12h	Prolonged analgesia
	Methadone	5 mg q4–6h	Longer half-life than morphine
	Heroin		Not available; no advantages
	Hydromorphone	2 mg q4–6h	Potent orally; expensive

*Nonsteroidal anti-inflammatory drugs.

CNS side effects. Cross-tolerance is common but not complete, making it possible to boost analgesia by switching to another narcotic, starting at half the equianalgesic dose.

Dependence presents as onset of physical abstinence symptoms (see Chapter 235) a few days after total cessation of opiate intake. As noted above, withdrawal may also occur with administration of an analgesic with opiate antagonist activity (eg, pentazocine, butorphanol) to a patient being treated with a pure opiate agonist (eg, morphine). Such dependence is a true physiologic phenomenon. Psychologic dependence (addiction) remains uncommon in cancer patients who take narcotics for pain relief. Concern about drug abuse in cancer patients is unwarranted; none has been documented among patients receiving regularly scheduled narcotics. However, "as-needed" schedules appear to encourage psychologic dependence. The risk of dependence sometimes concerns those who care for cancer patients, causing them to limit provision of effective analgesics doses to the patient. Such concern is ill-conceived in this setting and can be prevented by proper preparation of caregivers.

Codeine is the least potent opioid, with starting doses (15–30 mg) comparable in pain control to full analgesic doses of aspirin, acetaminophen, or ibuprofen. Its addiction potential is considerably less than that of morphine. Codeine in combination with acetaminophen provides effective analgesia at low cost for patients with mild to moderate pain. The related compounds *oxycodone* and *hydrocodone* are eight times more potent on an equivalent weight basis than codeine, accounting for their being preferred by patients over similar doses of codeine.

Table 90-4. Relative Potency of Narcotic Analgesics

DRUG	TRADE NAME	EQUIVALENT DOSAGES (mg)
Morphine sulfate		10
Heroin		3
Hydromorphone	Dilaudid	1–5
Oxycodone	In Percodan	15
Meperidine	Demerol	100 (orally)
Methadone	Dolophine	10
Codeine		60
Pentazocine*	Talwin	50

*Has some antagonist activity.

Morphine is the prototype opioid analgesic. It is effective orally as well as parenterally. There is considerable metabolism of an oral dose on first pass through the liver, reducing duration of analgesia to 3 to 6 hours. Use of sustained-release preparations (eg, MS Contin, Oramorph-SR) provide much more prolonged analgesia (8–12 h) with much reduction in frequency of dosing.

Some have argued that *heroin* is better than morphine and should be made available. It has a slightly shorter onset of action and is indeed more potent on a weight-for-weight basis (about 2.5 times more potent). However, it is less well suited for chronic oral use, because of its short half-life and the resultant need for frequent doses. Side effects are identical.

Hydromorphone (Dilaudid) is nearly eight times more potent on a weight basis than morphine and very effective orally. Although expensive, it is very useful in instances where morphine does not suffice. Being more potent than morphine, it also makes possible use of a smaller injected volume, an important advantage in the emaciated patient who requires parenteral analgesia.

Methadone has also proven useful and, before the advent of sustained-release morphine, was rather widely prescribed because of its oral availability and longer duration of action than plain morphine. However, with repeated dosing, its 24-hour half-life can result in excessive sedation and progressive CNS depression. Its use is declining with availability of sustained-release morphine.

Meperidine (Demerol) is commonly prescribed and available for both oral and parenteral use. Limiting its efficacy for chronic pain control is rapid inactivation of an oral dose and short duration of action. Moreover, its metabolite normeperidine causes dysphoria, tremors, and irritability. In patients taking monoamine oxidase (MAO) inhibitors, it can cause an encephalopathy.

Fentanyl, a potent opioid, is available as a transdermal preparation that provides 3 days of continuous analgesia. The drug is nearly 20 times more potent than morphine on a milligram per milligram basis and requires careful titration to avoid excessive sedation. Patch strength is a function of its surface area. The starting dose can be based on the patient's previous morphine requirement or determined empirically by starting with the lowest strength patch, which provides 25 μg/hour (the equivalent of about 90 mg of oral morphine/d or 20 mg of parenteral morphine).

Some synthetic opioids have antagonist as well as agonist activity. *Pentazocine* (Talwin) has narcotic antagonist as well as agonist qualities and is not very effective for chronic pain. Although the risk of dependence is lower with its use, its antagonist qualities can precipitate narcotic withdrawal in a patient already taking an agonist.

Butorphanol tartrate is an opioid agonist–antagonist available as a nasal spray preparation. Onset of action is within 15 minutes, peak is at 1–2 hours, and analgesia lasts 4–5 hours. The recommended dose is one spray in one nostril, with a repeat dose in 1 hour if this does not suffice. Dosing is otherwise every 4 hours as needed. Ease of administration and rapid onset of action are the principal advantages. Like other opioids with antagonist activity, it can cause withdrawal in patients who are dependent on narcotics. Consequently, it is not an optimal drug for cancer patients with long-standing narcotic requirements.

Adjuvant Agents. In conjunction with the analgesics noted above, several other agents can enhance the provision of pain relief. The *tricyclic antidepressants* (see Chapter 227) not only help to counter the reactive depression associated with cancer pain but also appear to have a separate analgesic effect, perhaps through their influence on serotonin metabolism and endorphin production. Starting doses smaller than those needed for antidepressant effect (eg, amitriptyline 10–25 mg qhs) can reduce pain, particularly that of neuropathic origin. Dose is adjusted upward as necessary. The *anticonvulsants* (carbamazepine and phenytoin) are also helpful in relieving neuropathic pain, especially that due to infiltration by tumor.

Stimulants such as *dextroamphetamine* are sometimes used to counter the somnolence associated with high-dose narcotic use. *Methylprednisolone* in patients with advanced disease has a similar stimulant effect and also lessens pain associated with inflammatory or infiltrative lesions. *Benzodiazepines* (eg, diazepam 2 mg qhs) are helpful on an occasional basis when the patient reports situational stress or increased pain with resultant difficulty falling asleep. Regular use is to be avoided (see Chapter 232). *Barbiturates* are worth consideration in terminally ill patients with intractable pain. Although not analgesic (and potentially hyperalgesic at low doses), barbiturates, when used in sufficient doses to maintain sedation, can bring relief to patients dying of terminal cancer. Large doses can be fatal, necessitating careful dose adjustment. Adding such agents to a narcotic program should be done only when necessary; they greatly increase the likelihood of adverse effects.

Neurosurgical Procedures. Occasionally, a patient with slowly growing metastatic cancer will experience chronic refractory pain in conjunction with prolonged survival. Determining the source of pain and controlling it with analgesics is sometimes difficult, leading to consideration of a neurosurgical procedure. Before such an extreme measure is utilized, it is important to characterize the pain as precisely as possible to avoid mistaking a psychogenic component for an organic one. Treating the latter while ignoring the former is bound to end in failure and unnecessary suffering.

When there is confusion as to the nature of the pain, a *nerve block* can serve an important diagnostic function. There are three types of blocks: sensory, sympathetic, and motor. By employing control solutions of normal saline in addition to titered solutions of anesthetic, the physician can determine the source of pain and, if organic, classify it into sensory, sympathetic, or motor nerve involvement.

Neurosurgical procedures are indicated only when 1) pain is uncontrolled by narcotic analgesics, 2) tumor control allows prediction of substantial longevity, 3) functional status is significantly compromised by pain, and 4) pain is localized. In properly selected patients, such procedures produce pain relief in 40 percent to 70 percent. However, there is potential for functional loss, necessitating a discussion with the patient of the risks involved. *Hypophysectomy* has been employed in a limited number of patients with disseminated pain. Pain control may be related to the opioid peptides or endorphins in the hypothalamic area and is not necessarily related to the responsiveness of the tumor to hormonal ablation.

Investigational Therapies. Behavioral therapy for pain control in cancer addresses the influence of operant conditioning on the threshold for perception and tolerance to pain. *Behavior modification* or deconditioning may, therefore, have a role in pain control. Other investigational methods are *hypnosis* and *acupuncture,* which have been demonstrated to have some effect, particularly in the relief of chronic pain syndromes. Transcutaneous nerve stimulation (TENS) delivered by a surface-held electrical source has proven to be a rather feeble and expensive, though harmless, means of controlling chronic cancer pain, although initially some benefit is usually reported.

Before resorting to such methods, one needs to be certain that specific organic causes and anatomic lesions are attended to. These therapies should never be the singular treatment, but they may help when applied in conjunction with more standard forms of pain control. They usually have a transient effect that requires reinforcement. The identification of appropriate patients is crucial. Belief in the validity of the underlying method strongly correlates with outcome.

MANAGEMENT RECOMMENDATIONS FOR SPECIFIC PAIN SYNDROMES

Peripheral Nerve Compression. The specific therapeutic approach to all such syndromes is the application of local antitumor therapy (for the most part, radiation treatment) to induce regression of the tumor. The nerve compression syndromes are, however, generally associated with a resistant tumor that has invaded along the nerve sheaths, and palliation is often only temporary.

Nerve Root Compression. The distinction between direct tumor compression and osseous impingement on the nerve is often difficult, but local radiation is the treatment of choice. The absence of improvement following radiation therapy suggests that bony compression is the major component. Structural support by orthopedic measures, including brace or corset splinting, may be salutary.

Bone Pain and Pathologic Fractures. Fractures of weight-bearing bones should be prophylactically immobilized by surgery in conjunction with radiation therapy that is instituted for therapy of bone pain. Pathologic fractures of non-weight-bearing sites with or without symptoms should be managed with radiation therapy. In either instance, rapid healing follows treatment of responsive tumors such as those of breast or prostate.

Abdominal Pain. In most instances of intra-abdominal pain, the effectiveness of the antitumor treatment is limited, making analgesic drug therapy essential. Obstruction is an indication for surgery, although intravenous fluids, stool softeners, and analgesics may palliate without operation.

Thoracic Pain. When there is invasion into a local bony structure, radiation therapy is indicated. Neurosurgical procedures may be needed later. Hypertrophic pulmonary osteoarthropathy can cause considerable discomfort, but rapid resolution of the pain is achieved with removal of the intrathoracic process either by surgery or by radiation therapy. The narcotic requirement in patients with HPO is inordinate and generally necessitates thoracic surgical intervention, regardless of the presence of metastases.

INDICATIONS FOR REFERRAL AND ADMISSION

Successful cancer management requires a team approach. As regards pain control, the primary physician has a major role in the design and implementation of an effective analgesic program and in monitoring the patient for *painful complications* of the malignancy. Should such a complication arise, prompt consultation with the oncologist, radiotherapist, or surgeon is indicated because of the likelihood of the need for further systemic treatment or additional local measures. Patients with *refractory pain* in the absence of evident focally approachable disease may benefit from consultation with a specialist in the treatment of chronic pain. In such circumstances, consideration of a patient-controlled intravenous device for administration of parenteral opioids may be indicated, as might use of ancillary methods (eg, behavioral techniques). The patient with new onset of pain suggestive of *spinal cord compression* or *pathologic fracture* needs prompt hospital admission.

PATIENT AND FAMILY EDUCATION

Patients endure their condition much better when they know that maximum pain relief is available to them. All family and health care team members need to be informed of the patient's analgesic needs to avoid underdosing. In addition, the issues of addiction, drug tolerance, and physiologic dependence should be reviewed and their significance discussed. Few patients should have to endure disabling pain, given the array of effective treatment modalities available. Many patients do best when they have an active role in their care. Enlisting their help in the design, implementation, and monitoring of the pain control program can have considerable psychologic benefit. Effective pain control is central to sustaining a reasonable quality of life and is one of the most basic requests cancer patients make of us.

ANNOTATED BIBLIOGRAPHY

American Pain Society. Principles of Analgesic Use, 3rd ed. Skokie, Illinois, American Pain Society, 1992. *(Best resource on pain medications and their proper use.)*

Brechner VL, Ferrer-Brechner T, Allen GD. Anesthetic measures in management of pain associated with malignancy. Semin Oncol 1977;4:99. *(A general and practical review of the neurosurgical and local anesthetic approaches to pain.)*

Bruera E, Roca E, Cedaro L, et al. Action of oral methylprednisolone in terminal cancer patients. Cancer Treat Rep 1985; 69:751. *(A double-blind, randomized study showing benefit in advanced disease, especially for countering sedation and inflammatory pain.)*

Cleveland CS, Rotondi A, Brechner T, et al. A model for the treatment of cancer pain. Journal of Pain Symptom Management 1986;1:209. *(A useful neuropathophysiologic overview.)*

Deyo RA, Diehl AK. Cancer as a cause for pain. J Gen Intern Med 1988;3:230. *(Age > 50, history of cancer, pain >1 month, elevated erythrocyte sedimentation rate, anemia, and failure to improve were predictors of cancer-related back pain.)*

Drugs for pain. Med Lett Drugs Ther 1993;35:1. *(Terse overview; very useful comparisons of drugs.)*

Ferrer-Brechner T, Ganz P. Combination therapy with ibuprofen and methadone for chronic cancer pain. Am J Med 1984;77:78. *(Excellent analgesia afforded; a good example of the efficacy of combination NSAID–narcotic therapy.)*

Health and Public Policy Committee, American College of Physicians. Drug therapy for severe, chronic pain in terminal illness. Ann Intern Med 1983;99:870. *(A clinically useful and wise statement on providing effective pain control.)*

Kaiko RF, Wallenstein SL, Rogers AG, et al. Analgesic and mood effects of heroin and morphine in cancer patients with postoperative pain. N Engl J Med 1981;304:1501. *(Heroin showed no unique advantages over morphine.)*

Marks RM, Sachar EJ. Undertreatment of medical inpatients with narcotic analgesics. Ann Intern Med 1973;78:173. *(Provides evidence suggesting that "refractory" pain is often due to inadequate doses and PRN use.)*

Portenoy RK. Practical aspects of pain control in the patient with cancer. CA 1988;38:327. *(Comprehensive review; 123 refs.)*

Porter J, Jick H. Addiction rare in patients treated with narcotics. N Engl J Med 1980;302:123. *(An important message to caregivers.)*

Reuler JB, Girard DE, Nardone DA. The chronic pain syndrome; misconceptions and management. Ann Intern Med 1980;93:588. *(Discusses the failure to provide adequate pain relief for terminally ill patients.)*

Truog RD, Berde CB, Mitchell C, et al. Barbiturates in the care of the terminally ill. N Engl J Med 1992;327:1678. *(A thoughtful piece on the care of the terminally ill cancer patient with refractory pain.)*

91
Managing the Gastrointestinal Complications of Cancer and Cancer Therapy

JERRY YOUNGER, M.D.

Primary Care Medicine: Office Evaluation and Management of the Adult Patient, 3rd edition, edited by Allan H. Goroll, Lawrence A. May, and Albert G. Mulley, Jr. J.B. Lippincott Company, Philadelphia

The gastrointestinal symptoms that accompany cancer and cancer therapy are among the most difficult for the patient to bear, often compromising nutritional status and quality of life. Problems may arise from primary disease, metastases, side effects of therapy, or metabolic disturbances. Successful primary care of the cancer patient necessitates attending to the anorexia, nausea, vomiting, weight loss, abdominal pain, ascites, and related gastrointestinal problems that often worsen their lives.

NAUSEA AND VOMITING

Cancer therapies are far and away the leading cause of nausea and vomiting in patients with malignancy. Treatments often have to be stopped or limited by the onset of emesis. This makes control of nausea and vomiting important not only for restoring patient comfort but also for ensuring completion of a full course of treatment. The presentation of emesis may precede, acutely follow, or follow after a short delay the application of cancer therapy; it may also become persistent.

Pathophysiology and Clinical Presentation

Much has been learned about the mechanisms of therapy-induced emesis from studies of antiemetic regimens. Current models postulate that cancer therapies trigger nausea and vomiting by acutely injuring the rapidly dividing cells of the gastric mucosa. The resultant cellular damage and accompanying inflammation cause release of serotonin from gastric enterochromaffin cells into the gastric lumen, with subsequent activation of *serotonin S3 receptors* in the gut wall. There ensues an increase in afferent vagal activity in fibers synapsing with neurons in the chemoreceptor trigger zone of the brain stem. From there, impulses travel to the vomiting center of the brain and down efferent vagal and splanchnic fibers to the gut, completing the reflex and triggering emesis. Both peripheral and central serotonin receptors are believed important to the process. A *dopaminergic pathway* is also believed to contribute to the process, though to a lesser extent.

Most treatments produce *acute*, self-limited emesis that lasts only a few hours; however, the experience can be very uncomfortable, exhausting, and demoralizing. A milder, *delayed* emesis that can occur 1 to 5 days after therapy is most commonly seen with cisplatin therapy and is believed to be related to development of gastritis and persistence of active drug metabolites. Although less severe, it is discouraging and can impede nutrition. *Anticipatory* vomiting is a psychogenic behavioral phenomenon, learned from the association between severe emesis and the administration of cancer treatment. Nausea and vomiting can come on just with anticipation of chemotherapy. *Refractory emesis* suggests a metabolic or anatomic complication of cancer or cancer therapy (see below).

Antiemetic Agents

Ondansetron, a potent serotonin S3-receptor blocking agent, has greatly facilitated the prevention and treatment of chemotherapy-induced emesis. In double-blind, randomized, prospective studies, it has proven far superior to high-dose metoclopramide (the next best antiemetic) and to placebo in preventing the severe nausea and vomiting associated with cisplatin therapy (the most emetogenic of all chemotherapeutic agents). The drug is administered intravenously at a dose of 0.15 mg/kg, over 15 minutes, starting 30 minutes before administration of chemotherapy, and repeated at 4 and 8 hours after the first dose. The approval of oral ondansetron formulations will make it easier to administer emetogenic chemotherapy on an outpatient basis. The drug is well tolerated; side effects include irritability, constipation, and headache. No serious adverse effects have been encountered. Side effects commonly seen with other antiemetic regimens (dystonia, sedation, diarrhea) do not occur. Use of ondansetron provides complete prophylaxis of cisplatin-related emesis to more than 75 percent of patients. An oral preparation is available, facilitating administration. Each dose is 8 mg.

Metoclopramide blocks both dopaminergic and serotonin receptors, which accounts for its antiemetic action and its side effects. Given parenterally in high doses just before chemotherapy, it too can suppress emesis, but considerably less so than ondansetron (42% complete suppression vs. 75%). It is frequently used in combination with other agents (see below) to achieve better results. Its dopaminergic blocking promotes gastric emptying and gastroesophageal sphincter closure but also leads to dystonia, particularly in patients younger than 30 years of age. It too is administered intravenously in a loading dose (1–3 mg/kg), 30 minutes before chemotherapy. It can be continued as a slow IV infusion, given as another dose 90 minutes after the first dose, or continued orally.

Phenothiazines, such as *prochlorperazine* (Compazine), are well established for mild nausea and vomiting due to other conditions but are less effective in chemotherapy if used alone. However, when combined with other antiemetic

Table 91-1. Chemotherapeutic Agents and Their Emetic Potential

AGENT	EMETIC POTENTIAL	AGENT	EMETIC POTENTIAL	AGENT	EMETIC POTENTIAL
Cisplatin	High	5-Fluorouracil	Low	Lumustsine	Moderate
Dacarbazine	High	Methotrexate	Low	Doxorubicin	Moderate
Dactinomycin	High	Vincristine	Low	Procarbazine	Moderate
Mechlorethamine	High	Vinblastine	Low	Daunorubicin	Moderate
Cyclophosphamide	High	Chlorambucil	Low	Cytosine arabinoside	Moderate
		Etoposide	Low	Carmustine	Moderate
		Bleomycin	Low		
		Mitomycin C	Low		

Adopted from Gralla RJ. In DeVita VT, Hellman S, Rosenberg SA (eds): Cancer: Principles and Practice of Oncology, 3rd ed, p. 2138; Philadelphia, JB Lippincott, 1989.

agents, they help provide reasonable prophylaxis. Phenothiazines act centrally, blocking serotonin and dopamine receptors in the chemoreceptor trigger zone. Sedation accompanies their use and is often desired, but extrapyramidal symptoms may also ensue. They are available in oral, suppository, and parenteral form. Route of administration has little influence on effectiveness. On the day of treatment, a prochlorperazine spansule or suppository is given 4 to 8 hours before administration of chemotherapy and continued on a regularly scheduled basis for the next 24 hours. The main drawback to phenothiazine therapy is precipitation of extrapyramidal symptoms, which are most likely to occur when daily doses exceed 50 mg/d. Their onset necessitates discontinuation of therapy. Under such circumstances, the mild antiemetic *trimethobenzamide* (Tigan) is worth a try, although it is less effective than prochlorperazine.

Haloperidol, a non-phenothiazine major tranquilizer, is similar to prochlorperazine in antiemetic and extrapyramidal effects. It blocks dopaminergic receptors. Side effects are similar to those of metoclopramide.

Benzodiazepines potentiate the activities of the central inhibitory neurotransmitter gamma-aminobutyric acid (GABA) and can enhance the antiemetic effects of other agents. They also cause a desirable degree of mild amnesia. A short-acting preparation such as *lorazepam* is commonly given before chemotherapy. It too is best used as part of a combination program. Some prescribe an *antihistamine* (eg, diphenhydramine) in place of a benzodiazepine. *Psychogenic vomiting* that occurs in anticipation of chemotherapy responds to intravenous lorazepam or oral alprazolam in conjunction with behavioral *desensitization* therapy, though the best treatment is prevention of emesis at the outset of chemotherapy.

Corticosteroids used in high doses for a brief period can lessen emesis. *Dexamethasone* is the most commonly used preparation, given its high potency. It is especially helpful in patients with delayed emesis, used orally for 2 to 5 days in doses of 4 to 16 mg in combination with metoclopramide or prochlorperazine.

Cannabinoids were transiently popular but were found to be little better than phenothiazines and have been supplanted by more effective regimens with fewer side effects.

Design of a Comprehensive Prophylactic Program

The optimal goal of antiemetic therapy is prevention of nausea and vomiting associated with cancer therapy. This eliminates the dread of undergoing therapy and prevents any behaviorally triggered emesis. Design of an effective prophylactic program requires knowing the propensity of various agents to cause emesis (Table 91–1) and the mechanisms and synergies of available antiemetic drugs (Table 91–2).

A combination strategy takes advantage of the mechanistic synergies afforded by having effective drugs with different modes of action. This makes possible more complete and extended prophylaxis, use of lower doses of individual agents, and thus fewer side effects. For example, to treat a patient with anticipatory, acute, and delayed forms of emesis, an effective program might include a benzodiazepine (lorazepam), a serotonin blocker (ondansetron), and a corticosteroid (dexamethasone). Normal food intake before chemotherapy is encouraged because it minimizes retching on an empty stomach, which produces muscle cramps and pain. The chemotherapy schedule ought to be set up so that there are no more than two to three applications per month.

Refractory Emesis. A few treatable etiologies need to be considered when a patient presents with refractory emesis. Persistent vomiting can be a manifestation of *bowel obstruc-*

Table 91-2. Combination Approach To Prophylaxis of Chemotherapy-Induced Emesis

Select

1. Neurotransmitter Blocking Agent
   a. Ondansetron (blocks serotonin S3 receptors, peripheral and central)
   b. Metoclopramide (blocks dopamine ± serotonin receptors)
   c. Phenothiazine (blocks central dopamine ± serotonin receptors)

Plus

2. Benzodiazepine or Antihistamine
   a. Lorazepam (increases central inhibitory transmission; mild amnesia)
   b. Diphenhydramine (sedates)

Plus

3. Corticosteroid
   a. Dexamethasone (mechanism unknown; ? anti-inflammatory role)
   b. Methylprednisolone (same)

tion or severe *ileus,* etiologies that respond to decompression by *nasogastric suctioning. Hypercalcemia* and *hypokalemia* may be causes as well as consequences of vomiting; monitoring of electrolytes and correction of any imbalances can help lessen the anorexia, nausea, and vomiting that sometimes accompany them.

ANOREXIA AND WEIGHT LOSS

The cachexia of cancer is one of its hallmark manifestations, characterized by anorexia, early satiety, profound weight loss, and inanition. Maintaining adequate nutrition becomes very difficult in its presence.

Pathophysiology

Although multifactorial, *cachexia* has been strongly linked to elaboration of the macrophage-derived protein *cachectin* (also referred to as *tumor necrosis factor*) that is capable of inducing a wasting syndrome in animals and mediating adverse metabolic changes in human malignancy. Increased gluconeogenesis, excessive catabolism of body protein (especially muscle), abnormal fat metabolism, and abnormal substrate use have all been observed. In addition to cachectin, tumor-induced tissue breakdown, caloric wasting, and sequestration of protein-rich ascitic fluid in the abdomen may also contribute. Further aggravating the situation are disorders of digestion and absorption that ensue from malnutrition, obstructive lesions, and surgical therapies, such as gastrectomy or intestinal bypass procedures. Abnormal caloric utilization is a consequence of tumor-related changes in the body's metabolism, with food intake and lean body mass being channeled to support the tumor's caloric demands.

The mechanisms behind *anorexia* remains incompletely understood. A paraneoplastic syndrome has been postulated, linked to a tumor-induced polypeptide that can affect the satiety center in the brain. Additionally, radiation and chemotherapeutic agents may contribute by distorting taste, causing stomatitis, and injuring the gastrointestinal mucosa and liver.

Management

The single most effective means of overcoming anorexia and cachexia is to achieve control of the underlying malignancy. In the interim, patients need practical suggestions for immediate use.

Dietary Measures. *Small frequent feedings* (about six per day) of foods high in protein and calories should be advised. *Liquid dietary supplements* in the form of milk shakes and commercial preparations are excellent if tolerated. If nausea is prominent, the patient should be advised to try foods that are *salty*, beverages that are *cool and clear*, and desserts such as *gelatin* and *popsicles*. Dry foods such as *toast* and *crackers* also help. Dietitians recommend that the food be served in a *relaxed* family or group setting, *attractively prepared* and readily available. When *altered taste* makes food unpalatable, meat should be avoided and dairy products substituted as the main source of protein. *Acidic foods* may stimulate appetite in situations where taste acuity seems to wane, as might use of *extra seasoning* and spicy foods. There are some reports of *zinc* being used to treat dysgeusia, but results are not very impressive. Foods best to *avoid* when nausea is prominent include those that are overly *sweet*, *greasy*, or *high in fat*.

Medications. *Tricyclic antidepressants* (eg, amitriptyline) have a nonspecific appetite-stimulating effect that is sometimes helpful and often independent of its antidepressant effect. *Corticosteroids* have sometimes been used to stimulate appetite, but their effect is transient and not worth the major side effects associated with the high doses and prolonged administration needed to achieve a sustained increase in appetite. *Megasterol* has been used as an anabolic steroid with some success.

Treatment of Stomatitis. Stomatitis is an often overlooked cause of weight loss resulting from a sore mouth and poor intake. The management of chemotherapy-induced stomatitis includes avoidance of smoking, alcohol, and foods that are very hot, cold, spicy, or salty. *Benadryl elixir* and *kaopectate* mixed and used as a mouth wash is often helpful and well tolerated. *Chlorhexidine gluconate* is an antimicrobial oral rinse which can be used as a preventive, but a non–alcohol-based mouthwash is better once sores occur. *Viscous xylocaine* preparations are not very helpful, because they wash away quickly and thus provide only very transient relief; paste preparations last considerably longer. Unfortunately, taste distortion can occur as a consequence of the topical anesthetic effect.

When radiation therapy to the head and neck results in *xerostomia* and *mucositis,* the dryness and thick secretions can be lessened by chewing gum or sucking on hard candy, acts that help stimulate salivation. Use of gravies and avoidance of dry foods helps deglutition in patients whose salivary glands are damaged by radiation. In refractory situations, artificial saliva preparations can be used.

MALNUTRITION

One of the most serious consequences of nausea, vomiting, and cachexia is malnutrition. A self-perpetuating and debilitating cycle of food rejection and malnutrition ensues, weakening host immune defenses and permitting further tumor growth. Moreover, host tolerance to radiation and chemotherapy is compromised, thus restricting the ability to tolerate therapeutic doses of either form of treatment.

Detection of mild to moderate malnutrition is important. Manifestations include a 10 percent weight loss, serum albumin less than 3.5 g/dL, total lymphocyte count less than 1500 cells/mm^3, and a serum creatinine level that is low for the patient's size. More severe malnutrition is characterized by further weight loss, a serum albumin less than 3.0, and a lymphocyte count less than 1000.

Treatment Strategies. The goals and methods of nutritional therapy vary according to the patient's clinical situation. In most instances where gastrointestinal function remains intact, minor dietary alterations and oral dietary supplements are sufficient. More elaborate means of nutritional support are sometimes necessary and appropriate on a temporary basis to tide the patient over a difficult period. Such therapy is rarely indicated in the very late stages of cancer.

For patients with upper alimentary discomfort but retained ability to swallow liquids, a *nutritionally complete liquid preparation* may offer a more comfortable and palatable means of keeping well nourished. These preparations are available commercially and are reasonably well tolerated. Most contain all necessary vitamins and minerals. Lactose-free formulations are available for those who might have acquired lactose intolerance. Blenderized meals are another alternative.

Hyperalimentation is worth considering for temporary nutritional support during difficult phases of cancer therapy, though evidence of cost-effectiveness is often wanting. For example, a preoperative course of intensive nutritional support can lower the risk of sepsis and surgical mortality. However, most controlled studies of hyperalimentation and other nutritional therapies have failed to demonstrate any significant improvement in response to chemotherapy or radiation, lessening of side effects from these treatment modalities, prolongation of survival, or improved tolerance to greater doses or longer periods of treatment.

Enteral hyperalimentation is utilized for nutritional support of malnourished patients with an obstructed or injured upper alimentary tract, provided the remainder of the gastrointestinal tract is intact. Such hyperalimentation is particularly well suited to patients recovering from radiation or surgery in the upper alimentary tract. A feeding tube is either passed or surgically placed beyond the point of obstruction or injury. An enteral hyperalimentation program can then commence. Long (43-inch), flexible silicon nasal feeding tubes make possible administration of feedings directly into the distal duodenum or proximal jejunum, reducing the risks of aspiration and reflux that occur with gastrostomy feedings. When a feeding tube cannot be passed nasally, feedings can be administered through a jejunostomy.

Enteral hyperalimentation utilizes milk-based and soy-based formulas, as well as less viscous formulations, although sometimes a pump is needed. The formulas are quite hypertonic and must be started at less than full strength (usually ½ strength) and increased over several days, as tolerated. Cramps, dumping syndrome symptoms (flushing, tachycardia, sweating), and diarrhea are the major manifestations of intolerance. The goal is 2000 to 3000 calories per day.

Central hyperalimentation represents a nutritional support alternative reserved for short-term use. It can be carried out *at home* so long as the patient and family are capable of mastering the procedures necessary to ensure the sterility of the line and integrity of the infusion apparatus. A visiting hyperalimentation nurse is also helpful. The access site can be maintained as a heparin lock, allowing the patient to disconnect easily from the infusion. About 12 to 14 hours per day are needed for infusions, administered in solutions containing 4.2 percent or 5.2 percent amino acids and 20 percent to 25 percent glucose. The infusion schedule provides the patient with 10 to 12 hours a day of independence and opportunity to ambulate. Careful monitoring of metabolic parameters, including glucose, calcium, phosphate, magnesium, blood urea nitrogen (BUN), and creatinine, is essential, as is close coordination with a hyperalimentation consultant.

DIARRHEA AND CONSTIPATION

Diarrhea is another gastrointestinal nemesis well known to cancer patients. When it ensues from radiation- or chemotherapy-induced enteritis, the problem is usually self-limited, resolving within the 1 to 2 weeks that it takes for the mucosal surface to reconstitute itself. If it is persistent or troublesome, low doses of *diphenoxylate* (Lomotil) or nonprescription *loperamide* (Imodium) can be prescribed for symptomatic relief (see Chapter 64). *Steatorrhea* is experienced by patients who have undergone pancreatectomy or suffer from pancreatic insufficiency; intake of several *pancreatic enzyme* tablets with each meal (see Chapter 72) usually improves the situation. The postgastrectomy patient is at risk for the symptoms of the *dumping syndrome*. Avoidance of *sweets* and large *fluid volumes* (especially those rich in sugar) helps prevent attacks, as does lying down after a meal (see Chapter 64).

Constipation can be a very troublesome, often unavoidable consequence of *narcotic use* for pain control. However, prophylactic institution of some simple measures can help prevent disabling symptoms and fecal impaction. These include a *high fiber diet*, good *fluid intake* (at least 2 L/d), use of *stool softeners* (eg, dioctyl sodium sulfosuccinate), and, if necessary, administration of a gentle *laxative* before bed (eg, milk of magnesia 15 mL). Constipation may also be a sign of *obstruction* in the lower intestinal tract or ileus, etiologies that need to be ruled out before escalating laxative therapy. *Hypokalemia* and *hypercalcemia* are two other important causes that deserve attention.

MALIGNANT ASCITES

Ascites may occur as a complication of diffuse peritoneal implantation or the combination of portal venous hypertension and hypoalbuminemia. When due to peritoneal implants and the primary is unknown, one should consider treatable malignancies such as ovarian cancer. Occasionally, the ascites will be disabling due to marked abdominal distention and pain. Only in debilitating circumstances should it be treated. The most direct means is *therapeutic paracentesis*. Recent experience with large-volume paracentesis suggests that it can be done with safety as long as care is taken to preserve intravascular volume. About 4 to 6 liters of ascitic fluid is removed slowly over 60 to 90 minutes (in conjunction with simultaneous albumin infusion in severely hypoalbuminemic patients).

Large-volume therapeutic paracentesis has reduced the need for *peritoneovenous shunting*, in which a catheter with a one-way valve is placed in the peritoneal cavity and run subcutaneously into the jugular venous system (a so-called LeVeen shunt). The LeVeen shunt may achieve good control of ascites and return otherwise lost protein and amino acids to the circulation, but it works only if fluid is free and not loculated. The complication rate can be high. Disseminated intravascular coagulation (from thromboplastin-like material in the ascitic fluid), peritonitis, sepsis, and superior vena cava syndrome are among the complications reported. Debate continues as to whether LeVeen shunt or large-volume paracentesis is best. Either should be considered only in the most refractory and disabling of cases. The use of surgical drainage for ascites is not as effective as it is for effusions of the pleural space. Similarly, intra-abdominal instillation of chemotherapeutic agents and radioisotopes has been relatively ineffective. Sclerosing drugs and irritants to seal the peritoneal space are not recommended, since an irritant effect on the bowel may result in necrosis, perforation, or secondary fibrosis and adhesions leading to obstruction.

PERITONEAL IMPLANTS, BOWEL OBSTRUCTION, AND FISTULAS

Peritoneal implants within the abdominal cavity may develop in either a diffuse miliary pattern or coalesce into large mass lesions capable of causing obstruction. A surgical *bypass* procedure or regional surgical resection (*"debulking"*) is indicated under such circumstances for palliation when there is some hope of prolonging meaningful survival. For patients with an indolent malignancy, particularly those with a localized point of obstruction, an aggressive surgical approach is worthy of consideration. Implants centered in the pelvic area may lead to formation of fistulae communicating with the bladder or skin; local *surgical excision* or *radiation* therapy can help control the problem.

OBSTRUCTIVE JAUNDICE

Surgery used to be the traditional treatment, but it is often not feasible in patients with extensive porta hepatis disease extending into the liver. More recently, endoscopic or percutaneous *placement of a stent* has provided a less invasive alternative. The procedure should only be attempted by individuals skilled in placement of such stents. Major complications do occur, particularly recurrent cholangitis. The procedure can be uncomfortable, and the stents have a tendency to become dislodged. However, if successful, significant palliation and improvement in quality of life can result for the patient willing to undergo stent placement.

Radiation therapy has also been used to treat obstructive jaundice caused by tumor in the porta hepatis. It is particularly useful in patients with radiosensitive neoplasms (eg, breast, lymphoma).

ANNOTATED BIBLIOGRAPHY

Beck TM, Ciociola A, Jones SE, et al. Efficacy of oral ondansetron in the prevention of emesis in outpatients receiving cyclophosphamide-based chemotherapy. Ann Intern Med 1993;118:407. *(Demonstrated safe and effective, with 66 percent experiencing no emetic episodes.)*

Beutler B, Cerami A. Cachectin and tumor necrosis factor: two sides of the same coin. Nature 1986;320:584. *(An interesting article on the basic science of cancer cachexia.)*

Burt ME, Gorschboth C, Brennan MF. A controlled prospective randomized trial evaluating the effects of enteral and parenteral nutrition in the cancer patient. Cancer 1982;49:1249. *(Useful data on relative benefits of each.)*

Cubeddu LX, Hoffmann IS, Fuenmayor NT, et al. Efficacy of ondansetron (GR 38032F) and the role of serotonin in cisplatin-induced nausea and vomiting. N Engl J Med 1990;322:810. *(Evidence of efficacy and the importance of the serotonin S3 receptors.)*

Epstein M. Refractory ascites. N Engl J Med 1989;321:1675. *(An editorial summarizing methods of treatment.)*

Gralla RJ, Itri LM, Pisko SE, et al. Antiemetic efficacy of high-dose metoclopramide. N Engl J Med 1981;305:905. *(A randomized, controlled study showing the drug to be effective in cisplatin-induced vomiting.)*

Kris MG, Gralla RJ, Clark RA, et al. Consecutive dose-finding trials: adding lorazepam to the combination of metoclopramide plus dexamethasone. Cancer Treat Rep 1985;69:1257. *(Evidence for the efficacy of multidrug, multimechanism therapy.)*

Kris MG, Gralla RJ, Clark RA, et al. Incidence, course, and severity of delayed nausea and vomiting following the administration of high-dose cisplatin. J Clin Oncol 1985;3:1379. *(Cisplatin is the major cause.)*

Marty M, Pouillart P, Scholl S, et al. Comparison of the 5-hydroxytryptamine (serotonin) antagonist ondansetron (GR38032) with high-dose metoclopramide in the control of cisplatin-induced emesis. N Engl J Med 1990;322:816. *(Ondansetron proved far superior, providing complete suppression in 75 percent vs. 42 percent for metoclopramide.)*

Morrow GR, Morrell C. Behavioral treatment for the anticipatory nausea and vomiting induced by cancer chemotherapy. N Engl J Med 1982;307:1476. *(Describes the phenomenon and details behavioral approaches to treatment.)*

Souter RG, Wells C, Tarin D, et al. Surgical and pathological complications associated with peritoneovenous shunting in management of malignant ascites. Cancer 1985;55:1973. *(Useful data on risks of the procedure.)*

92
Complications of Cancer: Oncologic Emergencies and Paraneoplastic Syndromes

JERRY YOUNGER, M.D.

Primary Care Medicine: Office Evaluation and Management of the Adult Patient, 3rd edition, edited by Allan H. Goroll, Lawrence A. May, and Albert G. Mulley, Jr. J.B. Lippincott Company, Philadelphia

The complications of cancer are great in number and variable in degree of urgency. They range from commonly experienced gastrointestinal difficulties and pain syndromes (see Chapters 90 and 91) to true emergencies, stubborn malignant effusions, and the uncommon, but important, paraneoplastic phenomena. Most oncologic emergencies and malignant effusions are consequences of anatomic spread. Paraneoplastic syndromes result from hormonal and immunologic disturbances. The primary care physician's important role in monitoring the cancer patient requires familiarity with the early presentations of these complications, many of which are amenable to intervention. In most instances, hospital admission for inpatient treatment will be necessary, so the emphasis is on early detection.

ONCOLOGIC EMERGENCIES AND URGENCIES

The anatomic spread of tumor is capable of causing emergent complications, including spinal cord compression, cardiac tamponade, and hypercoagulability with acute bleeding or clotting. Urgent adversities associated with malignancy ensue from a combination of tumor invasion and metabolic/immunologic effects (eg, superior vena cava syndrome, hypercalcemia, fever, infection).

Spinal Cord Compression

Extradural or epidural cord compression occurs in approximately 5 percent of patients with cancer. It is a *true emergency*, with early diagnosis and treatment essential to preventing serious, permanent neurologic damage. The majority of epidural compressions result from bony metastases in the vertebral bodies extending into the epidural space. Less frequently, metastatic tumor reaches the epidural space hematogenously or by direct extension through the intervertebral foramina. Malignancies with a propensity to spread to bone (eg, lung, breast, prostate, myeloma, lymphoma, melanoma, and renal-cell carcinoma) are associated with the greatest risk of cord compression. Lymphoma may metastasize directly to the epidural space and not produce any bony changes.

In more than 90 percent of cases, the initial symptom is *back pain,* often radicular in nature. The course is progressive; weakness and sensory deficits follow. Sphincter incontinence is a late development, unless the cauda equina is the initial site of compression. *Plain films* of the spine should be obtained in all cancer patients with back pain. If films are normal in the area of pain, the patient does not have lymphoma, and there are no neurologic deficits, no further workup need be carried out immediately, but the patient should be followed closely. If bone films are abnormal or if there are neurologic deficits, then immediate hospital admission and prompt neurologic and oncologic consultations are needed.

Imaging of the spinal cord can be performed by standard *myelography* with iodinated contrast, *computed tomography (CT) scan* with water soluble contrast, or *magnetic resonance imaging (MRI).* The frequency of abnormal myelograms in cancer patients with back pain approaches 50 percent. Use of a nonresorbable iodinated dye for the myelogram allows for convenient follow-up films without repeated dye injection, but the thick dye does not always pass an obstructing lesion. Use of a water-soluble dye (metrizamide) plus CT scan may provide better definition of an obstructing lesion. MRI appears to be the most sensitive of the imaging procedures, especially when gadolinium enhancement is used. If myelography is performed, a sample of cerebrospinal fluid should be obtained at the time of lumbar puncture and sent for cytology, cell count, protein, and glucose.

Corticosteroids and *irradiation* are mainstays of therapy, with *surgical decompression* indicated when there is rapid deterioration of neurologic function. Prognosis depends on the extent of neurologic damage at the time of presentation. Patients who are ambulatory have a 60 percent to 80 percent chance of leaving the hospital able to walk; those with paraplegia have less than a 20 percent chance of regaining their ability to walk.

Meningeal Carcinomatosis. Diffuse seeding of the meninges with malignant cells is a serious complication of a number of solid tumors (lymphoma, melanoma, breast, lung, stomach) and leukemias. Although there need not be true cord compression, the entire neuraxis may become involved, leading to meningeal, cranial nerve, and root symptoms. Diagnosis is confirmed by lumbar puncture, which typically reveals malignant cells in the cerebrospinal fluid. Corticosteroids, irradiation, and intrathecal administration of cytotoxic agents are the treatment modalities of choice.

Cardiac Tamponade

Life-threatening tamponade may arise as a complication of malignancy, either indolently or rapidly, depending on the progression of the underlying tumor. Compression may occur from tumorous encasement, malignant effusion, or scarring from radiation-induced pericarditis. Cancers associated with tamponade include breast, lung, lymphoma, leukemia, and melanoma. In some instances, symptoms and signs of pericarditis (see Chapter 20) will precede those of tamponade. The presence of *pulsus paradoxus* strongly suggests significant tamponade. Unexplained neck vein elevation, narrowed pulse pressure, inspiratory distention of neck veins, and a pericardial friction rub should raise suspicion. Unfortunately, a pericardial friction rub is often absent in cases of tamponade caused by a malignant pericardial effusion. The usual accompanying symptoms (dyspnea, weakness, chest discomfort, cough) are nonspecific. More definitive diagnosis is best made by *cardiac ultrasonography*, the most sensitive and specific noninvasive test for documenting the problem and its physiologic significance.

Strong clinical suspicion of tamponade necessitates urgent hospitalization for prompt sonography and cardiac consultation. Sometimes a right-sided heart catheterization is performed when the degree of tamponade is unclear or there is still a question about the diagnosis. *Pericardiocentesis* is the treatment of choice for urgent tamponade and may also yield positive cytology.

Hypercoagulability

A number of the natural inhibitors of clotting, many of which are endothelial in origin (protein C, protein S, tissue plasminogen factor, antithrombin III) are disrupted directly by tumor invasion or indirectly by substances elaborated by cancers. Patients with adenocarcinomas appear particularly susceptible to developing recurrent or migratory *thrombophlebitis* or even thrombotic arterial occlusions. A more disseminated consumption coagulopathy sometimes develops (*disseminated intravascular coagulation* [*DIC*]) and can present acutely as a generalized bleeding diathesis. Acute DIC is a true medical emergency. Suggestive laboratory findings include prolongations in prothrombin time, partial thromboplastin time, and thrombin time, low platelet count, and elevated concentrations of fibrin split products. The peripheral smear shows a microangiopathic picture (schistocytes). Chronic DIC is more subtle in presentation, with thrombotic end-organ damage and thrombosis being the principal manifestations. Acute DIC requires immediate hospitalization to stop the bleeding. Platelet and plasma transfusions are given to replace those blood elements that have been consumed. More definitive therapy requires treating the underlying malignancy.

Superior Vena Cava Syndrome

Obstruction of the superior vena cava is usually caused by extrinsic compression. The majority of cases are due to bronchogenic carcinoma (especially small-cell), lymphoma, and metastatic disease. The earliest manifestation is asymptomatic, unexplained *distention of the neck veins*. Late signs include swelling of the face, neck, and upper extremities, plethora, shortness of breath, and persistent headache. Though rarely fatal, increased intracranial pressure and thrombosis leading to neurologic deficits may ensue. Clinical diagnosis is reinforced by finding a mass on chest x-ray in the right superior mediastinum or hilar area. Venography and other flow studies are unnecessary in most instances.

At one time it was considered essential to treat the mass immediately with emergency *radiotherapy*. Now, the view is one of *urgency* rather than emergency. The first task is to consider obtaining a *tissue diagnosis* before instituting radiotherapy (see Chapter 44), because a host of tumors with different degrees of radiosensitivity may be responsible for the condition. Although many malignancies will respond within 1 week to radiation, some may respond better to chemotherapy, and occasionally a nonmalignant process that would not benefit from radiation is the cause (eg, tuberculous adenopathy, substernal goiter). When a tissue diagnosis will alter therapy, invasive study to obtain tissue should proceed. Finding a small-cell carcinoma or lymphoma might place *chemotherapy* ahead of radiation as the treatment of choice (see Chapters 53 and 84).

Optimal therapy depends on the underlying diagnosis, prior treatment, and overall clinical status of the patient. Diuretics and corticosteroids can occasionally diminish local symptoms, but the effect is transient and is no substitute for more definitive therapy. There is no benefit from the use of heparin. The occurrence of superior vena cava syndrome does not worsen the prognosis (if adjusted for stage of disease).

Hypercalcemia

Hypercalcemia is a accompaniment of advanced carcinomas with extensive *lytic bony involvement* (breast, myeloma, hematologic malignancies) as well as a complication of epidermoid cancers (renal cell, ovarian, bladder, head and neck, and epidermoid and squamous cell lung cancers) with little or no bony metastasis. The latter has been linked to tumor elaboration of a protein with some parathyroid hormone–like activity (*parathyroid hormone–related protein* [*PTHRP*]). Cancers that invade bone and trigger a blastic response (eg, prostate, oat cell) are rarely associated with hypercalcemia.

Monitoring the serum calcium provides the simplest means of early detection. Initially the patient is asymptomatic. Later such nonspecific symptoms as weakness, fatigue, lethargy, nausea, and constipation ensue. If the hypercalcemia progresses, it will lead to an osmotic diuresis manifested by thirst and polyuria. The electrocardiogram may undergo change, with prolongation of the PR interval, shortening of the QT interval, and widening of the T wave. Dysrhythmias become a risk at very high calcium levels. Calcium potentiates the effects of digitalis and can trigger digitalis toxicity.

Hospitalization is needed if one decides to treat the hypercalcemia. (When it occurs in the setting of terminal illness, therapy may not be indicated.) One begins with *intravenous saline*, followed by use of *furosemide* to accelerate saline diuresis. For hypercalcemia due to osteoclastic bone resorption, *mithramycin* provides good control by inhibiting the process; although effective, it must be given parenterally and refractoriness occurs. *Corticosteroids* provide some benefit in cases of myeloma, lymphoma, and metastatic breast cancer.

Long-term control can be achieved by use of *bisphosphonates*, but treatment of the underlying tumor is the most definitive. Even with control of hypercalcemia and improvement of symptoms, prognosis is poor and life expectancy limited.

Fever in the Setting of Neutropenia

Infection ranks as the leading cause of death in patients with leukemia and the cause of death in half of those with lymphoma and solid tumors.

Malnutrition, immune dysfunction, mechanical compromise, and lowered neutrophil count (mostly due to cytotoxic therapy) all contribute to the high risk of mortality from infection. Neutropenia is defined in cancer patients as granulocyte counts of less than 500/mL, the minimum needed to counter infection. Prophylactic therapy with *granulocyte colony stimulating factor* (G-CSF) is being used to prevent neutropenia and lower the attendant risk of infection.

Patients who develop a fever during periods of neutropenia should be considered infected until proven otherwise. The majority of neutropenic cancer patients with fever will have a bacterial infection (often due to a gram-negative organism). The possibility of viral, fungal, or parasitic infection is increased in those with leukemia, chronic steroid therapy, or prolonged broad-spectrum antibiotic coverage.

Often, neutropenic patients lack the usual signs of inflammation, making it hard to determine the site of infection at the time of presentation. Bacteremia without an identifiable primary site and pneumonitis lead the list of presentations. Onset of fever in the neutropenic patient is an indication for *prompt hospitalization,* regardless of whether or not there are any additional signs of infection. The mortality in such patients ranges from 18 percent to 40 percent within the first 48 hours.

Once admitted, cultures of urine, sputum, and blood samples will be needed, as will samples of material from any suspicious site (eg, cerebrospinal fluid). In the absence of an identified pathogen, broad-spectrum antibiotic therapy (usually an aminoglycoside and a broad-spectrum semisynthetic penicillin) is instituted. Studies on the use of single-agent, broad-spectrum antibiotics, such as the new generations of cephalosporins, are ongoing.

Short-term prognosis for patients treated early and aggressively is good. Sixty percent to 90 percent of neutropenic, febrile cancer patients will recover from their infection with aggressive use of antibiotics.

Malignant Effusions

Some malignant effusions can be life threatening (eg, those in the pericardium—see above). Others are an important source of discomfort and disability. For example, malignant ascites can lead to marked abdominal distention and respiratory compromise; treatment is supportive (see Chapter 91). Malignant pleural effusions from pleural implants or lymphatic obstruction can impair respiration. Lung, breast, and ovarian cancers are important causes of pleural implants; lymphomas lead to lymphatic obstruction. Optimal therapy is systemic treatment of the underlying malignancy. Repeat thoracenteses are ineffective and associated with considerable morbidity. Definitive local therapy demands placement of an indwelling chest tube for several days to allow thorough drainage and closure of the third space. Instillation of a sclerosing agent (eg, tetracycline) after drainage promotes the scarring process and helps to limit reaccumulation of exudate.

Thrombocytopenia and Bleeding

See Chapter 81.

PARANEOPLASTIC SYNDROMES

Ectopic Hormone Syndromes

Small-cell (oat cell) carcinoma of the lung is the archetypical tumor capable of ectopic hormone production. A variety of other tumors may behave in similar fashion. One or more polypeptides may issue forth from the tumor, leading to such complications as Cushing's syndrome and inappropriate antidiuretic hormone (ADH) secretion.

Cushing's Syndrome develops in approximately 5 percent of patients with small-cell carcinoma of the lung due to production of *ectopic adrenocorticotropic hormone (ACTH)*, although some degree of ectopic ACTH synthesis may take place in as many as 80 percent of patients with the tumor. The clinical syndrome can be subtle and is usually not manifested by the typical cushingoid appearance, but rather by *increased pigmentation* and metabolic and immunosuppressive effects, such as severe, recalcitrant *hypokalemia* and *impaired resistance* to infection. The hypokalemia requires extraordinary doses of supplemental potassium and use of spironolactone. Serum and urinary ketosteroids are especially abundant, with some patients demonstrating virilization. Metabolic inhibitors of adrenal hormone synthesis (metyrapone, mitotane, aminoglutethimide) have been tried; success has been variable. Prognosis is very poor; median survival is less than 2 months.

Syndrome of Inappropriate Antidiuretic Hormone (SIADH). This syndrome is not unique to cancers, but small-cell carcinomas (about 10% of cases) and a host of other cancers are capable of elaborating a polypeptide with antidiuretic hormone activity. The earliest manifestations are *hyponatremia* and renal sodium wasting. *Urine osmolality* is *inappropriately elevated.* If the serum sodium falls to very low levels, confusion and disorientation may ensue. Treatment includes use of *lithium carbonate* or *demeclocycline,* two agents that counter the action of antidiuretic hormone. *Restriction of free water* intake also helps to restore the serum sodium level. Hypertonic saline infusions are to be avoided, since these patients, although not edematous, tend to be volume overloaded. However, diuretics are contraindicated due to sodium depletion. SIADH is rapidly reversible with effective *treatment of the underlying tumor.*

Hypercalcemia associated with epidermoid cancers is, as noted above, due to ectopic production of a protein with parathyroid hormone-like activity (*PTHRP*). In contrast to hypercalcemia due to osteolytic disease, urinary cyclic AMP and serum PTHRP are elevated. Because symptoms may not develop until the serum calcium becomes markedly elevated, routine monitoring of the serum calcium is the best means of early detection and is worthwhile in tumors having a high frequency of this complication (squamous cell cancers of the head, neck, and lung, ovarian cancer, bladder cancer, hypernephroma). Diagnosis requires a high index of suspicion and testing directly for PTHRP (the protein is too structurally different to be detected by standard assays for PTH).

Symptomatic relief can be achieved acutely by lowering the serum calcium (see above and Chapter 96). Treatment of the underlying cancer is more definitive.

Hyperthyroidism and acute thyrotoxicosis have resulted from ectopic production of chorionic gonadotropin (which functions like thyroid-stimulating hormone). Choriocarcinomas are the main source of the overproduction. Patients can present with all the typical hypermetabolic manifestations of thyrotoxicosis. Beta-blockers are only modestly effective; primary treatment must be directed at the tumor.

Others. Sufficient ectopic *human chorionic gonadotropin (HCG)* is sometimes produced by testicular and lung cancers to result in *gynecomastia*. A classic manifestation of insulinoma and a rare complication of sarcoma is *fasting hypoglycemia*.

Immunologically Mediated Paraneoplastic Syndromes

A series of syndromes, mostly neurologic in nature, have been linked to aberrations in immune function. The precise identification of the mediator or immune complex has not been possible in all instances; at times, the link to an immune mechanism is merely speculative.

Myasthenic (Eaton-Lambert) Syndrome occurs most commonly in patients with small-cell carcinoma of the lung and characteristically results in *proximal muscle weakness* of the limbs. Its electromyographic pattern is distinct from that of true myasthenia, being characterized by facilitation and an increasing evoked muscle potential. Clinical management includes use of *guanidine*; the anticholinesterases used for myasthenia do not work.

Subacute Cerebellar Degeneration is another remote neurologic syndrome, with injury to the Purkinje cells of the cerebellum. Ataxia, dysarthria, dysphagia, and even dementia may comprise the clinical picture. It has been associated most commonly with small-cell carcinoma of the lung and with ovarian and breast cancers.

Peripheral Neuropathy is the most common form of neurologic deficit in cancer. Mechanism(s) are poorly defined but likely to be multifactorial. The most typical is a symmetrical sensory neuropathy seen in patients with advanced malignant disease. Motor and mixed sensory/motor neuropathies have also been described.

Paraneoplastic Syndromes of Unknown Etiology

A host of other purportedly paraneoplastic syndromes have been described, linked to malignancy by their receding with effective treatment of the underlying tumor. Identification of a tumor secretory product or other mechanism has not yet occurred.

Hypertrophic Pulmonary Osteoarthropathy presents with the findings of digital clubbing and tenderness along the distal long bones. Most commonly, the syndrome occurs in the setting of primary or metastatic lung tumors. Radiographically, x-rays of the long bones show an elevation of the periosteum, and radionuclide scanning demonstrates a distinctive pattern of increased uptake along the cortical margins. The exquisite pain accompanying these changes is relieved by removal of the tumor. The mechanism of the syndrome remains unknown.

Hyperpyrexia and Tumor-Related Fever have been observed in patients with hepatic metastases, typically from colon cancer, and also as a manifestation of the "B" syndrome associated with Hodgkin's disease. The release of pyrogens from tumor has been proposed as the cause of fever, but other possibilities include the inability to detoxify endogenous endotoxin and an alteration in metabolism of fever-producing steroids. Control can be accomplished by use of *nonsteroidal anti-inflammatory agents*, which can also serve as a diagnostic test for the condition.

Nephrotic Syndrome. Some patients with Hodgkin's disease develop massive edema with proteinuria and hypoalbuminemia. The renal lesion appears as an accumulation of immune complexes along the basement membrane. The nature of the antigen is unknown. The problem does not respond to steroid therapy but does regress with control of the malignancy.

Cachexia. See Chapter 91 for a discussion of cachexia.

Cutaneous Paraneoplastic Syndromes

Cutaneous paraneoplastic syndromes are quite rare, but they are important to recognize as clues to the presence of internal malignancy. They may be a consequence of hormone secretion, such as the hyperpigmentation or *melanosis* that occurs with ACTH-producing tumors or the *necrotizing erythema* seen with glucagon-secreting malignancies of the pancreas. Proliferation of *seborrheic keratoses* can be a sign of internal malignancy; *acanthosis nigricans* or freckling and hyperpigmentation in the axillary folds suggest neurofibromatosis and intestinal cancer. *Acquired ichthyosis* is associated with lymphomas and several other tumors.

ANNOTATED BIBLIOGRAPHY

Ahmann FR. A reassessment of the clinical implications of the superior vena cava syndrome. J Clin Oncol 1984;2:961. *(Argues that taking the time and effort to make a tissue diagnosis helps to properly select treatment.)*

Baker WF Jr. Clinical aspects of disseminated intravascular coagulation. Semin Thromb Hemost 1989;15:1. *(All you ever wanted to know about DIC.)*

Barron KD, Rodichok LD. Cancer and disorders of motor neurons. Adv Neurol 1982;36:267. *(Detailed look at the motor syndromes.)*

Burtis WJ, Brady TG, Orloff JJ, et al. Immunochemical characterization of circulating parathyroid hormone-related protein in patients with humoral hypercalcemia of cancer. N Engl J Med 1990;322:1106. *(Identifies PTHRP and links it convincingly to humoral hypercalcemia.)*

Callahan JA, Seward JB, Nishimura RA, et al. Two-dimensional echocardiographically guided pericardiocentesis. Am J Cardiol 1985;55:476. *(Ultrasound technique useful for diagnosis and treatment.)*

Chad DA, Recht LD. Neurological paraneoplastic syndromes. Cancer Invest 1988;6:67. *(Good summary and useful review of the literature.)*

Chang JC, Gross HM. Utility of naproxen in the differential diagnosis of fever of undetermined origin in patients with cancer. Am J Med 1984;76:597. *(Found to be remarkably distinguishing, though size of sample very small.)*

Fink IJ, Garra BS, Zabell A, et al. Computed tomography with metrizamide myelography to define the extent of spinal canal block due to tumor. J Comput Assist Tomogr 1984;8:1072. *(An alternative to standard myelography.)*

Hainsworth JD, Workman R, Greco A. Management of the syndrome of inappropriate antidiuretic hormone secretion in small cell lung cancer. Cancer 1983;51:161. *(Antitumor chemotherapy resulted in resolution of the SIADH.)*

Lokich JJ. The frequency and clinical biology of the ectopic hormone syndromes of small cell carcinoma. Cancer 1982;50:2111. *(The tumor most commonly associated with ectopic hormone production; still relatively infrequent.)*

Minna JD, Bunn PA. Paraneoplastic syndromes. In: DeVita VT, Hellman S, Ralston SH, Gallacher SJ, Patel U, et al. Cancer-associated hypercalcemia: morbidity and mortality. Ann Intern Med 1990;112:499. *(Prognosis poor even if corrected, but morbidity can be reduced.)*

Nussbaum SR, Younger J, VanderPol CJ, et al. Single-dose intravenous therapy with pamidronate for treatment of hypercalcemia of malignancy. Am J Med 1993;95:297.

Portenoy RK, Lipton RB, Foley KM. Back pain in the cancer patient: an algorithm for evaluation and management. Neurology 1987;37:134. *(Emphasizes the importance of a high index of suspicion for spinal metastasis and cord compression.)*

Rodichok LD, Harper GR, Ruckdeschel JC, et al. Early diagnosis of spinal epidural metastases. Am J Med 1981;70:1181. *(Early diagnosis achieved by performing myelography on known cancer patients with new back pain ± neurologic deficits and abnormal plain films of the spine.)*

Sarpel S, Sarpel C, Yu E, et al. Early diagnosis of spinal-epidural metastasis by magnetic resonance imagining. Cancer 1987;59:1112. *(Enhanced capacity for detection of early lesions.)*

7

Primary Care Medicine: Office Evaluation and Management of the Adult Patient, 3rd edition, edited by Allan H. Goroll, Lawrence A. May, and Albert G. Mulley, Jr. J.B. Lippincott Company, Philadelphia

Endocrinologic Problems

93
Screening for Diabetes Mellitus

Diabetes is, after obesity and thyroid disease, the most common metabolic disorder seen by the primary care physician. Patients' concerns about the possible need for insulin injections and about such well-known complications as blindness, kidney disease, premature vascular disease, and impotence make diabetes one of the most feared diagnoses. Detection campaigns and advertising have further heightened public awareness. Diabetes screening is commonly requested by patients, even in the absence of symptoms or risk factors. There is no question that treatment effectively reduces symptoms associated with the metabolic derangements induced by diabetes. Results of the Diabetes Control and Complications Trial (DCCT) have definitively answered longstanding questions about the reduction in complication rates that can be achieved with intensive efforts to control glucose level, at least for insulin-dependent disease. Nevertheless, the benefits of treatment initiated in the asymptomatic phase have not been demonstrated. Furthermore, labeling a patient "diabetic" on the basis of a nonspecific screening test may be harmful. Uncertainty about the natural history of the disease and its complications does not allow definitive recommendations regarding screening for, or early treatment of, diabetes.

EPIDEMIOLOGY AND RISK FACTORS

Diabetes mellitus is heterogeneous. A number of pathophysiological mechanisms cause the destruction of beta cells in the islets of Langerhans that is responsible for the clinical syndrome of type I or insulin-dependent diabetes mellitus (IDDM). The etiology and pathogenesis of type II or non–insulin-dependent diabetes mellitus (NIDDM) may be even more heterogeneous, with multiple lesions including a blunted beta cell response to insulin, a defect at the insulin receptor, and a defect in hepatic uptake of glucose contributing to glucose intolerance. Depending on the diagnostic criteria used, the prevalence of all types of diabetes in the United States is between 3 percent and 7 percent; type II diabetes is nearly ten times more common than type I diabetes.

Type I Diabetes (IDDM). Type I diabetes is generally manifest in childhood or early adulthood. Only 20 percent of patients with IDDM have a first-degree relative with diabetes. However, a predisposition to IDDM, apparently mediated through the immune system, is inherited. This pathologic predisposition to autoimmune destruction of the beta cells has been linked to the presence of certain HLA antigens, some of which are also associated with other autoimmune diseases, including Hashimoto's thyroiditis and Addison's disease. Conversely, other HLA antigens seem to be associated with protection against diabetes. Overall, the risk of eventually developing diabetes in a sibling of a patient with IDDM is between 3 percent and 6 percent. However, the risk for siblings can be defined by comparing HLA antigens with those of the index case. Although siblings who are HLA-identical to the diabetic patient face a risk of diabetes 25 times greater than the general population, relative risk for those who share no antigens or are haplo-identical is only two or three times greater. The role of autoimmune destruction of beta cells in many patients with IDDM is attested to by the presence of islet cell antibodies in a large proportion of newly diagnosed cases. Islet cell antibodies can also be detected in nondiabetic relatives of patients with IDDM.

At least in some cases, islet cell destruction is the result of viral infection, perhaps initiating the autoimmune response. Coxsackie viruses, particularly Coxsackie B4, have been most strongly implicated. Mumps, cytomegalovirus, Epstein–Barr virus (EBV), and hepatitis viruses have also been associated with IDDM. The role of viral infection has been linked to a seasonal variation in incidence of IDDM and has raised questions about a relationship between socioeconomic status and risk of IDDM, but the evidence is equivocal.

Type II Diabetes (NIDDM). Type II diabetes has a much stronger *genetic component* than IDDM; concordance in identical twins is greater than 90 percent. The genetic link is not related to HLA antigens, and islet cell antigens are no more prevalent than in the general population.

The overwhelming risk factor for NIDDM is overnutrition and resulting *obesity*. Eighty percent of adult diabetics are obese or have a history of obesity. Among adults who are at least 25 percent over their ideal body weight, one out of every five has elevated fasting blood sugar levels, and three out of every five have abnormal glucose tolerance tests. Obesity increases insulin levels and decreases the concentration of insulin receptors in tissue, including skeletal muscle and fat. The relationship between concentration of insulin receptors and glucose tolerance is modified, however, by intracellular sequences following insulin binding that are poorly understood. Exercise increases the concentration of insulin receptors, and a *sedentary lifestyle* is associated with glucose intolerance. Regular exercise has been shown to be associated with a decreased incidence of NIDDM after adjusting for body-mass index.

Steroids reduce receptor affinity for insulin, as do uremia and hepatic failure. Other drugs can impair glucose tolerance by further diminishing the sluggish response of beta cells to glucose. These include *thiazide* diuretics, beta-adrenergic blockers, alpha-adrenergic stimulants, and phenytoin. Prostaglandin inhibitors, including indomethacin and salicylate, may increase beta cell release of insulin.

Persons with *impaired glucose tolerance (IGT)* are also at greater risk of frank NIDDM (see below). Although long-term follow-up studies indicate that as many as one half of those with IGT will have normal glucose tolerance tests 5 to 10 years later, somewhere between 1 percent and 5 percent of these patients become diabetic each year.

Approximately 3 percent of previously euglycemic women develop glucose intolerance during pregnancy. The fetal hyperglycemia and hyperinsulinemia that accompany maternal diabetes results in increased neonatal morbidity and mortality and the increased birth weight common in infants of diabetic mothers. This *gestational diabetes* in the mother resolves postpartum for 90 percent, but more than half of these women will eventually develop NIDDM.

NATURAL HISTORY OF DIABETES AND EFFECTIVENESS OF THERAPY

The natural history of diabetes mellitus has been difficult to define because the condition is so heterogeneous. This problem has historically been confounded by studies that have defined diabetes using varying degrees of glucose intolerance.

The natural history of asymptomatic impaired glucose intolerance is variable; only 15 percent to 30 percent of these patients progress to frank diabetes over 10 to 15 years. Patients with impaired glucose tolerance are at increased risk for developing the macrovascular complications resulting from accelerated atherogenesis. However, unless glucose intolerance progresses to frank diabetes, they do not develop characteristic diabetic microangiopathy.

The *asymptomatic detectable period* seems to be much shorter for IDDM than it is for NIDDM. Despite some evidence for a longer period than previously estimated, the markedly lower prevalence, compared to NIDDM, makes asymptomatic IDDM a very small target for screening efforts.

The incidence of *vascular* and *neurologic complications* clearly tends to increase with the duration of clinical diabetes. However, some long-term studies of patients followed for as long as 40 years have indicated that clinical evidence of microvascular disease, atherosclerosis, or neuropathy may occur in only 20 percent to 40 percent of insulin-dependent patients.

Increased risk of vascular and neurologic complications is reflected in the relative mortality rates for diabetics. When compared with age-matched nondiabetics, diabetics' relative risk of death increases with duration of known disease. In one study of patients followed for up to 25 years, the increase in mortality risk with duration was greater after age 40 and among women. *Coronary artery disease* is the most common cause of death among diabetics. Autopsy studies indicate that coronary disease is two to three times more common among diabetics than nondiabetics. Peripheral vascular disease is also very common among diabetics; clinical studies have indicated a prevalence of about 60 percent. Diabetics in the Framingham Study were shown to be four to five times more likely to have *intermittent claudication* and two to three times more likely to suffer the morbid consequences of stroke than nondiabetics. On the other hand, the presence of peripheral vascular disease in the nondiabetic increases the risk of eventual development of NIDDM.

Retinopathy is the most common specific complication of diabetes. In general, the incidence of retinopathy increases with duration of diabetes regardless of age at onset. Prevalence ranges of 40 percent to 80 percent have been reported among patients with known diabetes lasting 20 to 30 years. In one study of patients whose diabetes began before age 30, nearly all had retinopathy 25 to 30 years later and about 50 percent had proliferative changes. Retinopathy was less prevalent among those whose diabetes began later in life and those not receiving insulin. Laser photocoagulation has been shown to decrease progression of diabetic retinopathy. However, this does not provide a basis for recommending screening of diabetes; retinopathy that warrants treatment is very rare early in the course of disease. (Once diabetes is diagnosed, screening for retinopathy is indicated.)

Renal disease has been reported in 15 percent to 80 percent of autopsies among diabetics. Renal failure is the cause of death in 6 percent to 12 percent of diabetic patients. Prevalence estimates vary widely from study to study, but it is clear that the risk of glomerulosclerosis with clinically evident functional impairment increases dramatically with the duration of the disease.

Although *duration of glucose intolerance* and associated metabolic abnormalities can be related to many of the complications of diabetes, the variability of the natural history must be kept in mind. It has been argued that all complications, including specific microangiopathic changes, have been identified in patients without evident glucose intolerance. Whether or not the morbidity and mortality associated with the complications can be influenced by therapy is a matter of long-standing debate (see Chapter 102). The DCCT provided compelling evidence that rates of microvasular complications and other consequences of diabetes could be reduced with intensive efforts to control glucose levels among patients with IDDM. Intensive therapy was associated with increased frequency of hypoglycemic episodes and considerable inconvenience and cost. Questions remain about whether these findings apply to patients with NIDDM and about whether treatment during the asymptomatic period would improve outcomes.

Gestational diabetes is a special case. As noted, it occurs in 3 percent of pregnancies, though there is considerable variation in different populations. It is associated with perinatal morbidity including macrosomia and the associated increased risk of serious birth trauma and cesarean section.

There is suggestive evidence from observational studies and randomized trials to support the contention that identification of gestational diabetes followed by management with diet and/or insulin can reduce the incidence of macrosomia and perhaps improve birth outcomes.

SCREENING AND DIAGNOSTIC TESTS

In 1979, the National Diabetes Data Group (NDDG) published criteria for the diagnosis of diabetes. By these criteria, at least one of the following conditions must be met to establish the diagnosis of diabetes in the nonpregnant adult:

1. Presence of classic symptoms of diabetes with unequivocal elevations of glycemia (*andom plasma glucose* > 200 mg/dL); or
2. *Fasting plasma glucose* >140 mg/dL or fasting venous (or capillary) whole blood glucose >120 mg/dL *on more than one occasion*; or
3. Abnormal *oral glucose tolerance test (OGTT)* performed under standardized conditions (75-g glucose load with blood measurements performed every 30 min for 2 h). Both the 2-hour level and at least one other sample must exceed 200 mg/dL.

In addition to defining these diagnostic criteria, which have since been widely accepted in the United States, the group suggested new designations for persons with glucose intolerance who do not meet criteria for frank diabetes. The term *impaired glucose tolerance* is reserved for patients with glucose tolerance between normal and frank diabetes.

In the United States, the NDDG criteria have become widely accepted as the gold standard for the diagnosis of diabetes. The World Health Organization has published similar standards that are often used in international studies. It should be remembered that any criteria for the diagnosis of diabetes based on glucose level are, by necessity, arbitrary. The sensitivity and specificity of the tests will depend on the arbitrary levels chosen. At the time of their publication, the principal effect of the NDDG criteria, which require higher levels than were commonly used previously, was to increase the specificity of the criteria at the expense of sensitivity. This trade-off reflects the judgment that little benefit can be expected from aggressive identification and treatment of early or mild degrees of glucose intolerance, *and* that the label *diabetes* can engender substantial anxiety and morbidity.

Despite widespread acceptance of these *diagnostic* tests, the indications for OGTT and for any blood glucose measurements to *screen* the asymptomatic person are controversial. Fasting glucose measurement is often used in the clinical setting to provide a quick screen for diabetes. It is more accurate than random measurement, but it has a sensitivity of only 25 percent among patients with undiagnosed diabetes. Postprandial measurement may be more convenient for patients and more sensitive, but it requires attention to scheduling. The OGTT, because of its inconvenience, is generally used as a confirmatory diagnostic test.

Screening for gestational diabetes has been widely recommended. It is generally accomplished between 24 and 28 weeks of gestation by giving 50 g of glucose orally with a measurement 1 hour later. A level of >140 mg/dL would prompt further evaluation with an OGTT (see Chapter 102).

Some have advocated the use of hemoglobin A_{1c} measurements for screening and diagnosis of diabetes. However, in population-based studies, fasting glucose levels have been found to be more sensitive and more specific.

CONCLUSIONS AND RECOMMENDATIONS

- Diabetes mellitus is a common but heterogeneous condition. The most important risk factor of IDDM is a family history with diabetes in a twin, sibling, or parent. Family history is even more predictive for NIDDM, but the most important risk factor is obesity. Persons with a history of gestational diabetes or with impaired glucose tolerance also are at risk of developing frank diabetes.
- The natural history of diabetes and the incidence of complications is highly variable. The incidence of diabetic complications increases with duration of disease. Close control of glucose levels in patients with IDDM has been shown to reduce the incidence of diabetic complications, at the expense of increased rates of hypoglycemia and substantial inconvenience and cost. However, there is no evidence that therapy of asymptomatic, nonpregnant patients with diabetes or impaired glucose tolerance offers benefit.
- Therefore, the routine measurement of blood glucose levels to screen asymptomatic, nonpregnant adults for diabetes is not recommended.

A.G.M.

ANNOTATED BIBLIOGRAPHY

Diabetes Control and Complications Trial Research Group. The effect of intensive treatment of diabetes on the development and progression of long-term complications in insulin-dependent diabetes mellitus. N Engl J Med 1993;329:977. *(Intensive therapy reduced retinopathy, proteinuria, and neuropathy in symptomatic patients.)*

Ellenberg M. Diabetic complications without manifest diabetes. JAMA 1963;183:926. *(Early review. Virtually any of the common "complications" can precede detectable abnormalities in carbohydrate metabolism.)*

Garcia MJ, McNamara PM, Gordan T, et al. Morbidity and mortality in diabetics in the Framingham populations. Diabetes 1974;23:105. *(Insulin-treated diabetic women have the greatest relative mortality. Increased mortality among diabetics is not entirely explained by associated obesity, hypertension, and hyperlipidemia.)*

Genuth SM, Houser HB, Carter JR, et al. Observations on the value of mass indiscriminate screening for diabetes mellitus based on a five-year follow-up. Diabetes 1978;27:377. *(About of nearly 2000 patients with abnormal OGTTs had normal tests 5 years later.)*

Harris MI, Hadden WC, Knowler WC, Bennett PH. Prevalence of diabetes and impaired glucose tolerance and plasma glucose levels in U.S. population aged 20–74 yr. Diabetes 1987;36: 523. *(Extrapolation of survey results provides prevalence estimate of 6.6 percent, 3.4 percent previously diagnosed and 3.2 percent undiagnosed.)*

Hirohata T, MacMahon B, Root HF. The natural history of diabetes. I. Mortality. Diabetes 1967;16:875. *(Excess mortality of* diabetes increases with age of onset and is higher in females than in males.)*

Manson JE, Nathan DM, Krolewski AS, et al. A prospective study of exercise and incidence of diabetes among U.S. male physicians. JAMA 1992;268:63. *(Relative risk was 0.77 for those who exercised once per week and 0.58 for five or more weekly exercise periods.)*

Nathan DM, Singer DE, Godine JE, Harrington CH, Perlmuter LC. Retinopathy in older type II diabetics: association with glucose control. Diabetes 1986;35:797. *(Duration of diabetes and HbA_{1C} were major predictors of presence of retinopathy among 185 type II diabetics aged 55–75.)*

National Diabetes Data Group. Classification and diagnosis of diabetes mellitus and other categories of glucose intolerance. Diabetes 1979;28:1039. *(Report of consensus panel, including diagnostic criteria.)*

O'Sullivan JB, Mahan CM. Prospective study of 352 young patients with chemical diabetes. N Engl J Med 1968;278:1038. *(Only 32 percent of those with chemical diabetes by Fajans and Conn criteria progressed to overt diabetes within 10 years.)*

Paz-Guevara AT, Hsu T-H, White P. Juvenile diabetes mellitus after 40 years. Diabetes 1975;24:559. *(Insulin-induced hypoglycemia was the most common complication. The prevalence of complications was significant visual impairment in 50 percent; nephropathy in 59 percent; neuropathy in 50 percent; peripheral vascular disease in 40 percent; and major cardiac complications in 20 percent.)*

Singer DE, Nathan DM, Fogel HA, Schachat AP. Screening for diabetic retinopathy. Ann Intern Med 1992;116:660. *(Reviews natural history of diabetic retinopathy and makes the case for screening among patients with diagnosed diabetes.)*

Singer DE, Samet JH, Coley CM, Nathan DM. Screening for diabetes mellitus. Ann Intern Med 1988;109:639. *(Well-reasoned analysis of the issues with emphasis on evidence that supports screening for gestational diabetes.)*

University Group Diabetes Program. Effects of hypoglycemic agents on vascular complications in patients with adult-onset diabetes. VIII. Evaluation of insulin therapy: final report. Diabetes 1982;31(Suppl 5):1. *(Only 15 percent of patients with variable-dose insulin had poor control, compared with 34 percent and 45 percent of those treated with fixed dose and diet, respectively. But complications were rare, and no significant differences were detected.)*

Primary Care Medicine: Office Evaluation and Management of the Adult Patient, 3rd edition, edited by Allan H. Goroll, Lawrence A. May, and Albert G. Mulley, Jr. J.B. Lippincott Company, Philadelphia

94

Screening for Thyroid Cancer

Cancer of the thyroid is a relatively rare disease with a low mortality rate. Approximately 10,000 cases are diagnosed each year in the United States; the number of deaths caused by the tumor is about 1000 annually—only 0.2 percent of cancer deaths. Nevertheless, this disease has major significance for the primary physician because of its iatrogenic relationship to childhood irradiation of the head and neck. A high prevalence of thyroid cancer, diagnosed after a long latent or asymptomatic period, has repeatedly been documented among patients exposed to such irradiation. The appropriate approach to the evaluation and management of radiation-exposed patients remains a subject of debate.

EPIDEMIOLOGY AND RISK FACTORS

Generally, the incidence of thyroid cancer increases with age. This is particularly true of tumors with anaplastic or follicular histopathologies and of the medullary carcinomas derived from the parafollicular cells. The most common tumors, with papillary histopathology, have a bimodal age-specific incidence with peaks in the thirties and late in life. Thyroid tumors occur more than twice as frequently in females. In the United States, African-Americans seem to be at lower risk than others. Wide variations in thyroid cancer prevalence at autopsy have been reported internationally, from 3 percent to more than 10 percent in nonirradiated thyroids, with the highest rates reported from Japan. Approximately 20 percent of the rare medullary carcinomas, which comprise less than 10 percent of thyroid cancers, are familial.

The major identifiable risk factor for the development of thyroid cancer is a history of *external irradiation of the head and neck.* External irradiation was used as early as 1907 to shrink an enlarged thymus in infancy. During the 1920s and subsequently until the 1950s, it was used extensively for treatment of enlarged tonsils and adenoids, cervical adenitis, mastoiditis, sinusitis, hemangiomas, tinea capitis, and acne. Concern about ill effects began to mount in 1950 when a history of neck irradiation was noted in nine of 28 cases of childhood thyroid cancer with a latency period of 5 or more years. Further documentation followed, and radiation to the neck was discontinued. In 1973, attention focused on the issue again when 40 percent of a series of adults with thyroid cancer were found to have a history of irradiation. Clearly, the latent period between exposure and diagnosis of cancer could be measured in decades. It was also clear that the exposed population at risk was substantial—estimates ranged from 1 million to 2 million individuals—and largely unidentifiable.

Successive reports focused on the risk among exposed individuals. Large studies indicated that more than 25 percent had detectable thyroid abnormalities; the prevalence of cancer was estimated at 7 percent to 9 percent. These figures must, however, be considered in light of information available regarding the prevalence of thyroid abnormalities including carcinoma in the general population.

At least one investigation has questioned the value of thyroid screening in persons with a history of radiation exposure based on the legitimate questions that can be raised about the effects of sampling bias and observer bias on results of most studies. In a small, retrospective cohort study comparing irradiated persons with siblings or patient-selected controls, the investigators found no difference in prevalence of malignant and nonmalignant thyroid abnormalities. This study has in turn been challenged, however, because of its own potential biases and limited power.

Preliminary evidence suggests that some radiation-exposed persons may be at greater risk than others. Radiation during infancy may be most carcinogenic, with cancer risk decreasing as age at the time of radiation increases. Although the threshold dose for cancer risk appears to be low, risk may be greatly increased for persons who received multiple treatments.

NATURAL HISTORY OF THYROID CANCER AND EFFECTIVENESS OF THERAPY

The prevalence of occult carcinoma of the thyroid is not well defined. Autopsy studies have indicated that prevalence ranges from 5 percent to 13 percent. An often quoted study showing an overall prevalence of 5.7 percent found highest age-specific rates in the fifth and sixth decades.

A high prevalence of asymptomatic thyroid cancer is not surprising in light of the benign clinical course of most thyroid tumors after diagnosis. Follow-up studies have determined that probability of survival depends on tissue type and age of the patient. For localized papillary carcinoma, survival approximates that of age-matched controls; in one large study, there were no deaths among patients younger than 40 years of age during 10 to 15 years of follow-up. The course of follicular cancer is only slightly more aggressive. Anaplastic tumors, on the other hand, run a rapid clinical course to death.

The relatively high prevalence of occult thyroid cancer presumed to be present, in general, raises a number of questions about the significance of tumors found during the evaluation of patients with radiation exposure. It is worth noting that in the largest study, conducted at Michael Reese Hospital in Chicago, 47 percent of the tumors were incidental findings identified after surgery was recommended because of palpable or scan abnormalities. That is, 29 of 60 cancers were not found in or near the benign nodule that prompted surgery. There is no evidence indicating that tumors found in patients with past radiation exposure are more likely to result in morbidity or mortality than occult tumors found in the general population. However, they do have a high frequency of recurrence.

SCREENING AND DIAGNOSTIC TESTS

The sensitivity of *history-taking* in identifying persons at risk is not known. Many who were irradiated during early childhood may be unaware of their exposure. *Physical examination* of the thyroid gland is often difficult, and the palpable nodule is a nonspecific finding that can be found in 4 percent to 7 percent of the adult population. *Thyroid scan* is more sensitive in detecting thyroid abnormalities but, since it fails to distinguish between benign and malignant disease, is even less specific. A number of studies indicate that physical examination itself becomes more sensitive after scanning is performed and the physician is aware of scan results.

Large studies utilizing both multiple examinations and technetium (^{99m}Tc) scanning indicate that 60 percent of thyroid abnormalities (identified by either or both modalities) will be identified by palpation alone. Scanning alone will be more than 95 percent sensitive. However, palpable abnormalities appear to be more specific for cancer. In one study of patients with palpable nodules who ultimately had thyroidectomy, the prevalence of cancer was 34 percent, compared with 19 percent among patients who went to surgery on the basis of scan abnormalities alone. Physical examination was nearly 80 percent sensitive in identifying thyroids containing cancers. Cancers found in glands with scan abnormalities alone were often incidental, unrelated to the scan abnormality.

The availability of high-resolution *ultrasonography* has increased our capacity to identify small thyroid nodules. Ultrasonography has been shown to be better than physical examination, isotope scanning, magnetic resonance imaging, and computed tomography in detecting nodules. However, no specific sonographic criteria distinguish between benign and malignant nodules. In one study, 14 percent of cystic thyroid lesions were cancers, compared with 23 percent of solid lesions.

Attempts to use measurements of serum thyroglobulin as a screening test for thyroid cancer have not been successful. Despite poor specificity, thyroglobulin abnormalities are disappointingly insensitive.

When abnormalities are detected on examination or on scan, additional diagnostic steps are indicated. The refinement of *fine-needle aspiration biopsy* and *cytologic examination* has made it the first-line diagnostic test in many centers (see Chapter 95).

When physical examination or scan findings are questionable, some physicians have used suppression of the thyroid for 3 to 6 months in an effort to shrink normal thyroid tissue, thereby increasing the sensitivity of the examination for autonomous nodules. Although this remains a reasonable approach when cancer risk is low, it must be kept in mind that regression following thyroid hormone suppression is neither perfectly sensitive nor highly specific for thyroid cancer. There are case reports of confirmed carcinomas that had apparently responded to suppression therapy; only a minority of nodules that do not respond prove to be malignant.

On the basis of animal experiments, long-term thyroid suppression as prophylaxis for thyroid cancer has also been advocated for all patients with an exposure history or, more selectively, those with questionable scans.

Patients with familial risk of medullary thyroid cancer may be tested for an exaggerated increase in serum calcitonin levels in response to calcium or pentagastrin stimulation. Such a response is reasonably sensitive, but it is not specific for medullary thyroid cancer. High resolution ultrasonography may play a role in screening of these rather rare patients.

CONCLUSIONS AND RECOMMENDATIONS

- Childhood irradiation is an important risk factor for thyroid carcinoma that may be diagnosed as long as 35 years after exposure.
- The prevalence of thyroid abnormalities among the esti-

mated 1 to 2 million patients with an exposure history is about 25 percent. The prevalence of thyroid cancer has been estimated to be 7 percent to 9 percent.

- The significance of occult thyroid cancer in exposed patients is not known. There appears to be a high prevalence of occult tumors in the general population.
- Identification of patients at risk is an important part of history-taking.
- Patients at risk should be carefully examined yearly or at least every 2 years.
- Needle biopsy may be preferred in cases where a single nodule has been identified. Multiple examinations by experienced examiners may be necessary. Thyroid suppression may increase the sensitivity of thyroid palpation. Repeat examination of patients with normal examination but abnormal scan should be performed yearly.

A.G.M.

ANNOTATED BIBLIOGRAPHY

Davis NL, Gordon M, German E, et al. Clinical parameters predictive of malignancy of thyroid follicular neoplasms. Am J Surg 1991;161:567. *(Age >50 y, nodule size >3 cm, and history of neck irradiation were associated with surgical diagnosis of cancer when needle aspiration biopsy was consistent with follicular neoplasm.)*

De los Santos ET, Keyhani-Rofagha S, Cunningham JJ, Mazzaferri EL. Cystic thyroid nodules. The dilemma of malignant lesions. Arch Intern Med 1990;150:1422. *(Of 71 cystic lesions, 14 percent were malignant, compared with 23 percent of 150 solid lesions. Sensitivity and specificity of fine-needle aspiration cytology was 88 percent and 52 percent for cystic lesions, and 100 percent and 55 percent for solid lesions.)*

Friedman M, Toriumi DM, Mafee MF. Diagnostic imaging techniques in thyroid cancer. Am J Surg 1988;155:215. *(Argues that refinement of fine-needle aspiration cytology has made radionuclide scanning and other imaging studies second-line diagnostic tools for thyroid cancer.)*

Gagel RF, Tashjian AH, Cummings T, et al. The clinical outcome of prospective screening for multiple endocrine neoplasia type 2a. N Engl J Med 1988;318:478. *(Reports 86 percent disease-free survival for 22 patients followed for mean of 11 years after screening diagnosis of medullary thyroid carcinoma.)*

Gharib H, Goeller JR. Fine-needle aspiration biopsy of the thyroid: an appraisal. Ann Intern Med 1993;118:282. *(Advocates fine-needle aspiration as the first step in diagnosis.)*

Gonzalez-Villalpando C, Frohman LA, Bekerman C, et al. Scintigraphic thyroid abnormalities after radiation. Ann Intern Med 1982;97:55. *(Palpable and nonpalpable thyroid nodules were much more common among patients with prior radiation exposure than among controls.)*

McTiernan AM, Weiss NS, Daling JR. Incidence of thyroid cancer in women in relation to previous exposure to radiation therapy and history of thyroid disease. J Natl Cancer Inst 1984;73:575. *(Relative risk for exposed women was 16.5.)*

McTiernan AM, Weiss NS, Daling JR. Incidence of thyroid cancer in women in relation to reproductive and hormonal factors. Am J Epidemiol 1984;120:423. *(Despite the impact on the production of thyroid-stimulating hormone, pregnancy and use of exogenous estrogens had little or no effect on the risk of thyroid carcinoma in this case–control study.)*

Refetoff S, Lever EG. The value of serum thyroglobulin measurement in clinical practice. JAMA 1983;250:2352. *(A review. No value in cancer screening.)*

Rojeski MT, Gharib H. Nodular thyroid disease. Evaluation and management. N Engl J Med 1985;313:428. *(An extensive, critical review.)*

Sampson RJ, Woolner LB, Bahn RC, et al. Occult thyroid carcinoma in Olmstead County, Minnesota: prevalence of autopsy compared with that in Hiroshima and Nagasaki, Japan. Cancer 1974;34:2072. *(Prevalence of 5.6 percent among 157 autopsies of clinically occult thyroid cancer. Highest age-specific prevalence between 40 and 60.)*

Schneider AB, Favus MJ, Stachura ME. Plasma thyroglobulin in detecting thyroid carcinoma after childhood head and neck irradiation. Ann Intern Med 1977;86:29. *(Thyroglobulin levels not found to be very useful.)*

Schneider AB, Recurrent W, Pinsky SM. Radiation-induced thyroid carcinoma. Ann Intern Med 1986;105:405. *(Describes the clinical course of Michael Reese cohort at 10 years' mean follow up; a high frequency of recurrent disease noted. Small nodules managed conservatively.)*

VanHerle AJ, Rich P, Ljung BE, et al. The thyroid nodule. Ann Intern Med 1982;96:221. *(An extensive review of the diagnostic value of fine needle aspiration, thyroid scanning, and ultrasonography including an analysis of alternative sequencing strategies; fine-needle aspiration followed by scan in patients with cytologically suspicious lesions is recommended.)*

Woolner LB, Beahrs OH, Black BM, et al. Classification and prognosis of thyroid carcinoma: a study of 885 cases observed in a 30-year period. Am J Surg 1961;102:354. *(Noninvasive disease without significant morbidity or mortality.)*

Primary Care Medicine: Office Evaluation and Management of the Adult Patient, 3rd edition, edited by Allan H. Goroll, Lawrence A. May, and Albert G. Mulley, Jr. J.B. Lippincott Company, Philadelphia

95
Evaluation of Thyroid Nodules

Thyroid nodules are an extremely common phenomenon, clinically, radiographically, and histologically. A palpable thyroid nodule can be detected in 4 percent to 7 percent of the adult population. The prevalence of nodules in autopsy series approaches 50 percent, a figure that is approximated by patients undergoing modern high-resolution, real-time ultrasonography of the thyroid. The incidence of thyroid nodules increases with age and neck irradiation; it is six to nine times more common in women than in men.

The principal objective in evaluating thyroid nodules is to distinguish the patient with a malignant lesion from one with a benign mass. Among patients with thyroid nodules who come to surgery, thyroid cancer is found in about 10 percent to 20 percent; the fraction increases to 30 percent to

50 percent if there has been radiation exposure. Surgery is indicated when patients have a high risk of malignant disease and avoided in those with little risk of cancer. To accomplish this task, the primary physician must be skilled in the detection of thyroid lesions by physical examination and capable of designing a cost-effective evaluation of the palpable thyroid nodule. The indications for and utilities of scanning, ultrasonography, and fine-needle aspiration are essential to the task.

PATHOPHYSIOLOGY AND CLINICAL PRESENTATION

Thyroid nodules may be single or multiple, with or without underlying disturbances of hormonal homeostasis. A solitary nodule is usually the more worrisome one, because it may represent a malignancy, although, on occasion, a multinodular gland may harbor a cancer.

Benign and malignant thyroid nodules are usually asymptomatic and discovered incidentally by the patient or examining physician. Large nodules may cause a cosmetic problem or compress an adjacent structure. The nodules are usually painless unless rapid growth, inflammation, or hemorrhage occurs and produces significant discomfort.

Solitary Nodule

Solitary thyroid nodules represent benign adenomas, carcinomas, or multinodular etiologies in which only a single nodule is palpable.

Benign Adenomas account for most nonmalignant truly solitary nodules. The majority are designated as *follicular* and have a true capsule; the remainder are labelled as *colloid* or *adenomatous nodules* and are not well encapsulated. Both behave similarly. Growth is typically slow, extending over many years. Follicular adenomas rarely become large enough to encroach on the trachea or esophagus. Thyroid-stimulating hormone (TSH) receptors are present in most, making them hormonally responsive. The majority do not produce much thyroid hormone; their radioiodine uptake on scan is also limited, sometimes giving the appearance of a "cold" nodule. Benign adenomas that outgrow their blood supply may necrose, degenerate, become fluid-filled, and appear on ultrasound as nodules with solid and cystic elements. Adenomas make up a significant proportion of such "cystic" lesions. A few follicular adenomas produce such large quantities of thyroid hormone that the patient presents with thyrotoxicosis (see Chapter 103). This is particularly true for so-called *"toxic" adenomas* that exceed 3 cm in diameter. They function autonomously, suppress TSH (which renders the rest of the gland atrophic), and appear as a *"hot" nodule* on thyroid scan. Patients with a smaller-sized hot nodule may remain euthyroid, though enough thyroid hormone is produced to suppress the rest of the gland and render it atrophic.

Thyroid Carcinomas are uncommon; the current incidence is 2.5 per 100,000 population per year, although it is higher in areas with radiation exposure. They are more frequent in women than in men. *Papillary* and *mixed papillary/follicular* carcinomas are the most common and account for 60 percent to 70 percent of all thyroid malignancies. The lesions tend to be very slow growing, spreading locally to adjacent lymph nodes but not metastasizing distantly until very late. Consequently, they have a good prognosis even after local spread. Though most are solid, some may present as mixed cystic–solid lesions due to necrosis and liquefaction. *Follicular carcinomas* are also slow growing and make up another 15 percent to 20 percent of thyroid cancers. Local spread to regional nodes may occur without invasion of the thyroid capsule, but this does not alter prognosis. However, hematogenous spread can occur early, and initial presentation is often from a metastasis to lung or bone.

Anaplastic carcinomas comprise another 10 percent to 12 percent of cases; these are very invasive, usually inoperable, and fatal within 1 year.

Medullary carcinomas, derived from the parafollicular cells of the thyroid, represent 10 percent of thyroid cancers. There are sporadic and familial forms of the disease; among the latter are familial medullary cancers unaccompanied by other conditions and *multiple endocrine neoplasia* types II and III (which occur in conjunction with pheochromocytoma and hyperparathyroidism). The malignancy often presents as a thyroid nodule located in the upper half of the thyroid gland. It can be multicentric, especially in the familial forms. At least 50 percent of medullary carcinomas of the thyroid occur sporadically. *Calcitonin*, produced by the parafollicular or "C" cells, is a unique tumor marker for medullary carcinoma.

Lymphoma may sometimes develop as a primary lesion within the thyroid of a patient with chronic lymphocytic thyroiditis. Its clinical course is a function of tissue type and stage at time of presentation (see Chapter 84). Spread to local nodes is common and prominent.

On radioiodine scan, most thyroid carcinomas present as *"cold" nodules*, failing to take up iodine, though on technetium scan a rare malignant nodule will take up the radionuclide. On ultrasonography, most cancers are solid, though a mixed cystic–solid appearance is encountered in about 20 percent, and even a purely cystic-appearing lesion may occasionally be malignant.

Multiple Nodules

Hashimoto's Thyroiditis, an autoimmune condition, is the leading cause of multinodular goiter in the United States. Evidence of the condition can be found in about 4 percent of the general population and up to 15 percent of women over the age of 65. Women patients outnumber men by a ratio of 3:1. Pathologically, there is a chronic inflammatory cell infiltrate, formation of germinal centers, fibrosis, and Hürthle cell changes involving follicular epithelial cells. Although not unique to this condition, *antimicrosomal antibodies* are found in 70 percent to 95 percent of patients. About one-third of patients manifest a multinodular goiter, though euthyroid goiter is actually the most common presentation. The immunologically mediated injury impairs thyroxine synthesis and increases leakage of hormone into the circulation. A third of patients experience progressive loss of glandular function and eventually become hypothyroid. Hyperthyroidism in uncommon but can occur in patients with a prominent lymphocytic infiltrate.

Multinodular Goiter is the second most common cause of a multinodular gland in adults. It represents an advanced stage of focal autonomous hyperplasia, which initially presents as a diffusely enlarged gland but then progresses to multinodularity as areas of focal hyperplasia undergo degenerative changes. Nodules may also develop when colloid accumulates in hyperplastic cells (*colloid cysts*). Uptake of radioiodine on scan is heterogeneous; some areas may not take up iodine and appear "cold." The thyroid gland feels less firm than it does in Hashimoto's disease. TSH may be slightly reduced, reflecting the autonomous nature of the gland's thyroxine output, but free thyroxine levels are usually within normal limits.

Cancers may arise in a multinodular gland, though this is very uncommon. Thyroid cancer and lymphoma are the leading causes. Cervical adenopathy, hoarseness (due to recurrent laryngeal nerve compression), and the continued enlargement of a "cold" nodule on thyroid scan are distinguishing features of the clinical presentation. A history of neck irradiation or family history of thyroid cancer (suggestive of hereditary disease) are risk factors. The nodule may be tender if the tumor is rapidly growing (as with lymphoma), a finding atypical of other multinodular goiters.

DIFFERENTIAL DIAGNOSIS

The vast majority of solitary nodules are benign, even those that fail to take up radionuclide on thyroid scan (see below). In the United States, Hashimoto's thyroiditis accounts for the majority of cases of multinodular goiter in the United States. Cancers account for about 10 percent to 20 percent of solitary thyroid nodules; the prevalence is lower in patients with multinodular glands. (See Table 95–1.)

Table 95-1. Differential Diagnosis of Thyroid Nodularity

CAUSE	DISTINGUISHING CHARACTERISTICS
Solitary Nodule	
Benign adenoma	Solid or mixed cystic and solid; most euthyroid and responsive to TSH; those >3 cm may become autonomous and present as a "hot" nodule on scan
Cancer	
Papillary or mixed	Single hard nodule; local adenopathy; "cold" on scan; slow growing; metastasizes very late
Follicular	Same, though metastasizes earlier; some cystic
Medullary	May be familial; multiple endocrine neoplasia; calcitonin elevated; cold nodule
Lymphoma	Primary cancer arises in patients with chronic lymphocytic thyroiditis; prominent regional nodes
Multinodular	
Hashimoto's thyroiditis	Multinodular, rubbery gland; antithyroid antibodies; 1/3 hypothyroid; heterogeneous uptake; TSH-responsive
Multinodular goiter	Multiple nodules, enlarged gland; heterogeneous uptake on scan with some areas of decreased or absent uptake; clinically euthyroid, though some with mild decrease in TSH; autonomous gland
Cancer	
Thyroid	Same as above
Lymphoma	May arise in a Hashimoto's gland

WORKUP

As noted earlier, the main objective is to differentiate a carcinoma from benign causes of nodularity. Although definitive assessment cannot be made by history and physical examination alone, these elements provide important information regarding risk and need for biopsy or excision.

History

The history is reviewed not only for the clinical presentation of the nodule and associated symptoms but also for important cancer risk factors such as history of childhood neck irradiation, exposure to excessive environmental radiation, and positive family history of thyroid cancer. Age and gender also bear noting. Patients younger than age 40 and males are at increased risk of a thyroid nodule being malignant. Symptoms suggestive of local invasion, such as hoarseness, dysphagia, and obstruction, should be noted, as should new appearance of a nodule or rapid growth of an existing one. However, bleeding into a benign cyst or subacute thyroiditis may cause a similarly abrupt change and new onset of symptoms. Conversely, many thyroid cancers are slow growing and may have been present for years; duration is not particularly useful for distinguishing benign from malignant disease. Risk factors for benign thyroid disease (living in an iodine-deficient area, goiter, or intake of goitrogens such as lithium, turnips, or beets) favors a benign lesion, as does family history of goiter (as opposed to thyroid cancer). Symptoms of hypothyroidism or hyperthyroidism argue against malignancy.

Physical Examination

The physical examination focuses on the gland and adjacent lymph nodes. The gland is noted for its overall size, consistency, and number and size of nodules. A solitary, hard nodule that is irregular and fixed (fails to move with swallowing) is suggestive of malignancy. However, finding a soft nodule does not rule out the diagnosis of cancer, because a papillary carcinoma that has undergone cystic degeneration can appear soft to the touch. Finding a single nodule increases the chances of cancer; few multinodular goiters harbor a cancer.

The adjacent lymph nodes, especially those on the ipsilateral side of the nodule, require detailed examination. A thyroid nodule with associated cervical adenopathy should be viewed with marked suspicion. A single node may be due to metastasis from the thyroid, whereas multiple nodes in a young person with a thyroid nodule raises the possibility of lymphoma. The vocal cords should be viewed in patients with hoarseness.

Laboratory Studies

Fine ("Skinny") Needle Aspiration Biopsy has become the test of choice for initial evaluation of most euthyroid patients with a thyroid nodule, supplanting the radionuclide thyroid scan and ultrasound for determining who needs surgical excision. The needle is inserted into the nodule and its contents aspirated for cytological examination. In skilled hands, the sensitivity of fine needle biopsy exceeds 95 percent. Although radionuclide scanning and ultrasound also provide high sensitivity, their specificity is poor. For fine-needle biopsy, specificity ranges from 70 percent when patients with "suspicious" readings are included in the group in need of surgery, to over 90 percent if they are not. Compared to use of ultrasound and radionuclide scan, fine-needle biopsy has reduced by half the number of patients who undergo operations needlessly, doubled the incidence of malignancy in surgically excised nodules, and reduced costs by more than 25 percent. The procedure is safe, inexpensive, and readily performed in the office setting. Fine-needle biopsy requires a skilled physician to perform the procedure and an experienced pathologist to interpret the results to minimize errors in sampling and interpretation. Failure to completely drain a cystic lesion and biopsy the residual mass is an important source of false-negative results. With only the cytologic information provided by aspiration biopsy to go on, it can be difficult for even experienced pathologists to differentiate benign Hürthle cell and follicular adenomas from their malignant counterparts. Patients with lesions labelled "suspicious" usually need to undergo surgical excision of the nodule, though sometimes malignancy can be ruled out by radionuclide scanning.

Radionuclide Scanning. As noted above, radionuclide scanning has been supplanted by fine-needle aspiration biopsy as the initial test of choice in patients with a euthyroid nodule. While it is true that most malignant disease has the appearance of a "cold" nodule on scan, only 15 percent to 20 percent of all "cold" nodules are malignant. Moreover, the occurrence of uptake in a nodule ("warm" nodule) does not entirely rule out malignancy. Thus, radionuclide scanning is best relegated to a supplemental role, following fine-needle biopsy in those with "suspicious" cytology. A "hot" nodule on scan of such patients indicates an autonomously hyperfunctioning nodule, which has a very low risk of cancer. A suspicious nodule that is "warm" or "cold" on scan has a higher probability of cancer and requires consideration of surgical excision. A radionuclide scan can also be of help in detecting multinodularity, though thyroid ultrasound is even more sensitive.

Thyroid Ultrasound has excellent sensitivity for detection of nodules (down to 1 mm), a unique ability to differentiate solid from cystic lesions, and a role in helping to localize a lesion for biopsy. However, even with the development of new, high-resolution ultrasound technology to detect ever-smaller lesions, the test still lacks diagnostic specificity because there are no clearly defined architectural criteria for differentiating benign from malignant lesions. Recently compiled combined data show that 21 percent of solid lesions, 12 percent of mixed lesions, and 7 percent of purely cystic ones are malignant. With "cystic" no longer considered synonymous with "benign," the test has fallen from use as a means of determining risk of malignancy. It is excellent for determining multinodularity, but the meaning of such multinodularity is unclear, because up to 40 percent of all patients with clinically uninodular disease are found by modern ultrasound to have multiple nodules.

Ancillary Laboratory Studies are usually of little direct help in deciding whom to biopsy, but they occasionally provide supportive information. An abnormal *TSH* is uncommon in malignant disease, as are high titers of *antimicrosomal antibodies* (useful in suspected Hashimoto's and subacute lymphocytic thyroiditis). Routine use of plain films is not cost-effective. A very high *erythrocyte sedimentation rate* in the setting of an acutely tender gland is very suggestive of subacute granulomatous thyroiditis. A serum *calcitonin* determination is indicated when there is a strong family history of thyroid cancer. There are no other markers at present for thyroid cancers. Thyroglobulin elevations do occur with cancer, but also with benign nodular thyroid disease. Response to *TSH suppression* (by administration of thyroid hormone) is not reliable for differentiating cancer from benign disease, because both may either shrink or not respond to exogenous hormone. In rare instances, a plain film of the chest may incidentally reveal punctate calcifications characteristic of the psammoma bodies of papillary carcinoma or the shell-like calcification characteristic of a benign lesion, but routinely obtaining such films is of low diagnostic yield.

Patients with Multinodular Glands usually do not require biopsy unless there is increased concern for cancer due to neck irradiation, cervical adenopathy, rapid growth of a single nodule in an otherwise stable gland, or onset of recurrent laryngeal nerve palsy. Most cases are due to Hashimoto's thyroiditis and can be diagnosed by obtaining antithyroid antibody determinations. High titers of *antimicrosomal antibodies* correlate best with biopsy-proven disease. Antithyroglobulin titers are less useful. There is an increased risk of *lymphoma* of the thyroid in patients with Hashimoto's disease, mandating *needle biopsy* of the gland if there is an enlarging tender goiter, cervical adenopathy, or a goiter markedly enlarging on thyroid hormone suppressive therapy (which should decrease nodule size in Hashimoto's disease).

Further Evaluation of the Benign Adenoma. When a lesion is found to be a benign adenoma, the question arises as to whether or not it functions autonomously and thus poses the risk of toxicity. Adenomas less than 2 cm in size rarely change much in size or function and can be followed. Those greater than 3 cm are at risk for progressing to toxicity within a few years. Diagnosis of autonomous function is achieved by performing *serial radionuclide scans* and demonstrating little change in uptake when comparing scans taken before and after *stimulation by thyrotropin releasing hormone (TRH)* or *suppression by thyroid hormone*. Observation rather than ablation is now preferred for the smaller, low-risk lesions. Annual determination of the nodule's size and hormonal output usually suffices. Every 5 years, scanning can be repeated to see if there is increasing suppression of extranodular tissue function, a sign of impending toxicity. Other signs include size greater than 3 cm, rise in serum triiodothyronine (T_3) to the upper limits of normal, and decreasing responsiveness to stimulation or suppression.

Testing Sequence. The most cost-effective testing sequence for the euthyroid patient with a single thyroid nodule on physical examination is to begin with fine-needle aspiration biopsy. If the cytology is "malignant," then surgery is indicated. If the reading is "benign," then follow-up by ultrasound and watchful waiting is sufficient. If "suspicious," then radionuclide scan for determination of nodule uptake is indicated. A "hot" nodule indicates a very low risk of cancer and requires only clinical follow-up ± treatment, depending on whether the patient is euthyroid or thyrotoxic. A "warm" or "cold" nodule in a patient with suspicious cytology raises the question of cancer and necessitates surgical excision.

SYMPTOMATIC THERAPY

Euthyroid Patients with a Benign Solitary Nodule who are otherwise healthy can be given a trial of exogenous *thyroid hormone* therapy in an attempt to decrease the size of the nodule. Approximately 10 percent to 30 percent of patients with a nontoxic solitary nodule will show a decrease in nodule size when treated with doses of levothyroxine sufficient to suppress TSH. Such treatment does not appear to work in patients with colloid nodules. The rationale for suppressive therapy is that reducing TSH stimulation should diminish nodule size in those lesions that are TSH-responsive (eg, follicular adenomas, Hashimoto's thyroiditis). The required dose of levothyroxine is in the range of 0.1 to 0.15 mg daily. One should begin with small doses (0.05 mg/d) and increase gradually until the TSH declines to 0.05 to 0.3 mU/L. More suppression increases the risk of thyroxine-induced osteoporosis (see Chapter 104). The therapy is relatively contraindicated in the elderly and those with underlying coronary disease (see Chapter 103). It is unknown whether therapy prevents increase in nodule size in patients who have not achieved a decrease.

Toxic Nodules and autonomously functioning solitary adenomas that are at high risk for becoming toxic (>3 cm in diameter, serum T_3 at upper limit of normal, increasingly unresponsive to thyroxine suppression) should be considered for *ablative therapy*. Ablation is mandatory for those with autonomous nodules that have already become toxic. One needs to choose between surgery and radioiodine. *Surgery* represents a definitive approach with low risk if done by a skilled thyroid surgeon. Young patients are the best candidates. *Radioiodine* is simpler and usually the treatment of choice in the elderly. The theoretical risk of inducing cancer in the remaining thyroid tissue makes radioiodine a less attractive option for young people, though no increase in incidence of malignancy has been reported. A palpable nodule often remains after irradiation; it is of no consequence other than cosmetic. The patient needs to be monitored for development of posttreatment hypothyroidism (see Chapter 103).

Multinodular Goiters often do not shrink much because they are composed of a great deal of fibrous tissue. Bothersome *large cysts* may require surgical removal, but smaller ones can be aspirated as necessary. Hormone therapy has no effect on recurrence of thyroid cysts after aspiration.

PATIENT EDUCATION

The primary care physician should counsel and closely follow patients with previous head or neck radiation (see Chapter 94). Regular follow-up is important in any patient with a nodule, and the patient should be instructed to call if there should be a change in size, development of lymphadenopathy, pain, dysphagia, or hoarseness.

The patient with an autonomous nodule or a multinodular goiter should be advised to avoid substances containing high concentrations of iodine (medications, kelp, radiographic contrast media), because they may precipitate thyrotoxicosis. If a contrast study is necessary, the patient should be started on a beta-blocking agent 10 days before the study.

INDICATIONS FOR REFERRAL

Detection of a solitary thyroid nodule in a clinically euthyroid patient should prompt a referral to a consultant skilled in performing fine-needle biopsy of the thyroid. Encountering a worrisome nodule (see above) in a patient with a multinodular gland represents another indication for consideration of biopsy. Patients with a toxic or large (>3 cm) autonomously functioning adenoma require consultation for discussion of ablative therapy. Those with goiters unresponsive to thyroid hormone that are causing obstruction or cosmetic discomfort may be surgical candidates.

A.H.G.

ANNOTATED BIBLIOGRAPHY

Asp AA, Georgitis W, Waldron EJ, et al. Fine needle aspiration of the thyroid: use in an average health care facility. Am J Med 1987;83:489. *(Excellent sensitivity and specificity demonstrated, indicating that the procedure can be done in the community setting, provided the physician and pathologist are well trained.)*

Baker BA, Gharib H. Correlation of thyroid antibodies and cytologic features in suspected autoimmune thyroid disease. Am J Med 1983;74:941. *(Antimicrosomal antibodies are the antibody test of choice for Hashimoto's disease.)*

Belfiori A, La Rosa GL, La Porta GA, et al. Cancer risk in patients with cold nodules: Relevance of iodine intake, sex, age and multinodularity. Am J Med 1992;93:363. *(Male sex and age <30 or >60 years were predictors of cancer, but not multinodularity.)*

De los Santos ET, Keyhani-Rofagha S, Cunningham JJ, et al. Cystic thyroid nodules: the dilemma of malignant lesions. Arch Intern Med 1990;150:1422. *(A retrospective study; 20 percent of cystic lesions were due to malignancies.)*

Fogelfeld L, Wiviott MBT, Shore-Freedman E, et al. Recurrence of thyroid nodules after surgical removal in patients irradiated in childhood for benign conditions. N Engl J Med 1989;320:835. *(A study of the utility of treatment with exogenous thyroid hormone; rate of recurrence reduced, but not risk of cancer.)*

Gharib H, James EM, Charboneau JW, et al. Suppressive therapy with levothyroxine for solitary thyroid nodules. N Engl J Med 1987;317:70. *(A double-blind, randomized study of patients with colloid nodules; no benefit.)*

Gharib H, Goellner JR, Zinsmeister AR, et al. Fine-needle aspiration biopsy of the thyroid. Ann Intern Med 1984;101:25.

(Addresses the difficult issue of what to do with the "suspicious" finding.)

Hamburger JI. The autonomously functioning thyroid adenoma. N Engl J Med 1983;309:1512. *(An editorial summarizing diagnosis and treatment.)*

Hamburger JI. Lymphoma of the thyroid. Ann Intern Med 1983;99:685. *(A clinical review drawing attention to the relation between the condition and Hashimoto's thyroiditis; provides indications for biopsy.)*

Hamburger JI. The various presentations of thyroiditis. Ann Intern Med 1986;104:219. *(Authoritative review with detailed discussions of Hashimoto's and subacute thyroiditis; 51 refs.)*

Mandel SJ, Brent GA, Larsen PR. Levothyroxine therapy in patients with thyroid disease. Ann Intern Med 1993;119:429. *(Includes use of thyroxine to reduce size of solitary nodules.)*

McCowen KD, Reed JW, Fariss BL. The role of thyroid therapy in patients with thyroid cysts. Am J Med 1980;68:853. *(Treatment with hormone did not prevent recurrence of cysts after aspiration.)*

Rallison ML, Dobyns BM, Meikle AW, et al. Natural history of thyroid abnormalities: prevalence, incidence, and regression of thyroid diseases in adolescents and young adults. Am J Med 1991;91:363. *(Data from a population exposed to high levels of environmental radiation; emphasizes the dynamic nature of these conditions.)*

Rojeski MT, Gharib H. Nodular thyroid disease. N Engl J Med 1985;313:428. *(Useful review, especially of evaluation methods; 115 refs.)*

Ross DS, Ridgeway EC, Daniels GH. Successful treatment of solitary toxic thyroid nodules with relatively low-dose iodine-131, with low prevalence of hypothyroidism. Ann Intern Med 1984;101:488. *(Reports excellent results with no hypothyroidism being induced.)*

Simpson WJ, McKinney SE, Carruthers JS, et al. Papillary and follicular thyroid cancer. Am J Med 1987;83:479. *(Extrathyroidal extension, poor differentiation, and older age were most predictive of reduced survival.)*

Van Herle AJ, Rich P, Ljung BB, et al. The thyroid nodule. Ann Intern Med 1982;96:221. *(Suggests that fine-needle biopsy supplemented by scan is the best means of evaluating thyroid nodules.)*

96
Approach to the Patient With Hypercalcemia

SAMUEL R. NUSSBAUM, M.D.

Primary Care Medicine: Office Evaluation and Management of the Adult Patient, 3rd edition, edited by Allan H. Goroll, Lawrence A. May, and Albert G. Mulley, Jr. J.B. Lippincott Company, Philadelphia

The advent of automated laboratory screening led to the increased recognition of asymptomatic individuals with hypercalcemia, rising from an annual incidence of 7.8 per 100,000 to 51 per 100,000. In addition, outpatients with nonspecific complaints, such as fatigue, weakness, abdominal discomfort, or constipation, may have hypercalcemia discovered during biochemical testing. Mild hyperparathyroidism is usually the explanation for these often inadvertently recognized calcium elevations. Hypercalcemia may also herald other important underlying diseases, such as malignancy or sarcoidosis. Asymptomatic hyperparathyroidism is not necessarily a benign condition. Long-standing action of excess parathyroid hormone on target organs, bone and kidney, may lead to skeletal loss and impairment of renal function.

The primary physician must be able to interpret an abnormal calcium value and diagnose its cause. If hyperparathyroidism is present, one must decide between surgery and medical therapy. Treatment of hypercalcemia resulting from malignancy can improve quality of life and deserves consideration.

PATHOPHYSIOLOGY AND CLINICAL PRESENTATION

The serum calcium concentration is maintained within narrow limits by parathyroid hormone. The precision of calcium homeostasis is necessitated by calcium's vital role in membrane function, hormonal secretion and action, and neuromuscular function. The free or ionized portion of serum calcium is responsible for its physiologic actions. Slightly less than 50 percent of serum calcium is in the form of free calcium ions; the remainder is bound to plasma proteins, mostly albumin. Globulins can also bind serum calcium. Calcium binding by serum proteins is pH-dependent. Increased binding occurs at alkaline pH and explains the common symptom of paresthesias that occur in conjunction with hyperventilation. The normal range for serum calcium is 8.5 to 10.4 mg/dL, or 2.12 to 2.59 mmol/L. The normal range for ionized serum calcium is 1.16 to 1.34 mmol/L. True hypercalcemia requires an increase in the ionized fraction of serum calcium. A convenient correction factor to apply to total serum calcium is to subtract or add 1 mg/dL to the calcium concentration for every 1.0 g/100 mL of serum albumin lower or higher than 4.0 g/100 mL.

Hyperparathyroidism. The hypercalcemia of hyperparathyroidism is caused by increased osteoclastic bone resorption mediated though excessive parathyroid hormone (PTH) binding to receptors on osteoblasts, as well as an increase in gut calcium absorption. PTH also increases renal tubular reabsorption of calcium and results in phosphate wasting. Pathologically, approximately 80 percent of patients are found to have a single parathyroid adenoma, whereas 20 percent have four-gland hyperplasia. Parathyroid cancer accounts for approximately 1 percent of all hypercalcemia attributed to excess parathyroid hormone secretion.

The incidence of hyperparathyroidism increases with age—peaking in the fourth through sixth decades of life—and occurs more commonly in women than men by approximately a 2:1 ratio. It is not certain whether the increased recognition of the disease relates to multiphasic biochemical screening or whether there is an increase in the disease, possibly as a result of head and neck irradiation in infancy or other environmental factors that affect parathyroid cell proliferation.

The majority of patients with hyperparathyroidism do not have symptoms. The "classic" presentation of "stones, bones, abdominal groans, and psychic moans" has been replaced by a more subtle and nonspecific presentation. *Fatigue*, *weakness*, mild gastrointestinal symptoms (*constipation*, *abdominal pain*), changes in intellectual performance, and depression may all be manifestations of hypercalcemia or excessive parathyroid hormone. Often, such nonspecific symptoms are recognized only after successful parathyroid surgery when the patient describes an improved sense of well-being.

The resultant hypercalcemia of hyperparathyroidism can lead to a renal concentrating defect and *increased urination*. Hyperparathyroidism is also associated with an increase in *calcium oxalate stones*, particularly in patients with elevated 1,25-dihydroxyvitamin D_3 levels and urinary calcium excretion in excess of 300 to 350 mg/24 h. Bone pain results from skeletal fracture and osteitis fibrosa cystica. There is a possible but somewhat controversial increase in peptic ulcer disease and pancreatitis, and a spectrum of psychiatric disease.

Hyperparathyroidism may be observed in familial settings, such as the autosomal dominant *multiple endocrine neoplasia (MEN)* type I and type II syndromes. In MEN I, parathyroid hyperplasia occurs in conjunction with adenomas of the pituitary and pancreas. In MEN II, parathyroid hyperplasia may occur with medullary cancer of the thyroid and bilateral adrenal pheochromocytoma.

Patients with *"normocalcemic hyperparathyroidism"* often have serum calcium levels at the upper limit of normal, which on repeated determinations will fluctuate into the frankly elevated range. *Thiazide diuretics* may transiently elevate serum calcium by reducing urinary calcium excretion. More sustained elevations suggest mild underlying hyperparathyroidism that is unmasked by thiazide therapy.

Familial Hypocalciuric Hypercalcemia (FHH) may cause hypercalcemia as often as multiple endocrine neoplasia type I. It is associated with an abnormality of calcium sensing by the parathyroid, leading to parathyroid gland hyperplasia. Serum PTH is not elevated. Urinary calcium excretion is often less than 100 mg/24 h.

Malignancy is the second most frequent cause of hypercalcemia and more common among hospitalized patients than outpatients. Cancers of the *breast*, *lung*, and *kidney* lead the list of malignant etiologies, accounting for 50 percent to 60 percent of such cases. The incidence of hypercalcemia during the course of breast cancer ranges from 18 percent to 42 percent; in lung cancer, from 6 percent to 16 percent. Other malignancies associated with hypercalcemia include *multiple myeloma* (incidence 30%–100%), squamous cell carcinomas of the head and neck (2%), lymphoma and leukemia (1%), and genitourinary cancer (1%).

Several *mechanisms* for the hypercalcemia of malignancy have been identified, with a common theme being increased osteoclastic bone resorption. Such resorption and resultant hypercalcemia can occur with or without bony metastasis, and many tumors that commonly metastasize to bone do not cause hypercalcemia. Squamous cell cancers produce a PTHRP, a *PTH-like peptide*, with an amino terminal structure similar to PTH and nearly identical in effect on mineral ion homeostasis. Myeloma cells produce *interleukin-1-beta* and *interleukin-6*, which stimulate osteoclast-mediated bone resorption. In some patients with lymphoma and leukemia, increased *1,25-dihydroxyvitamin* D_3 is implicated.

Hypercalcemia is rarely the sole presenting manifestation of an underlying malignancy. The presence of hypercalcemia in association with malignancy indicates a grim prognosis, as the median survival is approximately 2 months. Very high levels of serum calcium (>14 mg/dL) are most often associated with malignancy, but levels up to 20 mg/dL may be seen in acute primary hyperparathyroidism caused by large parathyroid adenomas.

Other Etiologies. In *sarcoidosis*, enhanced conversion of inactive vitamin D to its active 1,25-dihydroxy form by granulomatous tissue increases absorption of calcium from the gut and resorption of bone. *Vitamin D intoxication* and *milk-alkali syndrome* are being seen increasingly with the popularization of calcium and vitamin D supplements to avert osteoporosis. Hypercalcemia may occur when an excess of 50,000 units of vitamin D and an excess of 3 to 5 grams of calcium are consumed daily.

The *thiazide diuretics* cause a transient, mild increase in serum calcium, generally within the normal range. As noted earlier, a sustained increase in serum calcium beyond 10 days implies underlying metabolic bone disease, usually hyperparathyroidism. Some investigators have used thiazides as a provocative test for hyperparathyroidism in patients with borderline hypercalcemia. *Theophylline excess* is another pharmacologic etiology for hypercalcemia.

Hyperthyroidism is associated with mild elevations in serum calcium in approximately 20 percent of individuals due to increased skeletal turnover. *Immobilization* in young persons who have not completed skeletal growth and in patients with Paget's disease may cause severe hypercalcemia. *Lithium* therapy for manic–depressive illness is sometimes associated with hypercalcemia. Individuals taking lithium may have an altered calcium set-point for PTH secretion. *Addison's disease* and severe *liver disease* may cause hypercalcemia; mechanism(s) remain unknown.

DIFFERENTIAL DIAGNOSIS

Hyperparathyroidism is overwhelmingly the most likely etiology for hypercalcemia in the medically well, asymptomatic patient. In a Swedish population survey that yielded 95 persons with hypercalcemia, hyperparathyroidism was suspected in 88 patients and confirmed surgically in 57 of the 59 who underwent neck exploration for cure of hyperparathyroidism. Primary hyperparathyroidism accounts for more than 60 percent of hypercalcemic patients and is extremely likely to be the explanation for hypercalcemia in patients with an elevation of serum calcium dating back several years. *Malignancy*, *granulomatous disease*, *hyperthyroidism*, *Addison's disease*, and *excess* ingestion of *vitamin D* and *calcium* are the cause of most other cases. Occasionally, there is an underlying *multiple endocrine neoplasia* syndrome or *hypocalciuric hypercalcemia*.

WORKUP

Prior to a more extensive laboratory evaluation, a *repeat calcium determination* is indicated to confirm the elevation. Ordering serum albumin and globulin levels helps assure the calcium elevation is not artifactual due to elevated protein binding of calcium. Hypercalcemia that appears ephemeral may be spurious, caused by prolonged application of the tourniquet at the time of blood drawing. Should hypercalcemia be confirmed, then evaluation can proceed.

History. In the "asymptomatic" patient, subtle manifestations of hyperparathyroidism, such as fatigue, weakness, lethargy, arthralgias, nonspecific gastrointestinal complaints, impairment of intellectual performance, and depression should also be specifically sought. Associated conditions such as hypertension, gout, pseudogout, and nephrolithiasis should be recognized. A history of increased urination may indicate calcium-related defects in urine-concentrating ability. Symptoms of underlying malignancy, particularly of breast, lung, and hematologic origin, should be pursued. Review of antacids, food additives, and health food store preparations may uncover excessive ingestion of vitamin D or calcium. Symptoms of hyperthyroidism (see Chapter 103) also need to be considered.

Physical Examination in the totally asymptomatic patient is generally unrevealing. However, a careful search for signs of malignancy (breast mass, lymphadenopathy, bone tenderness) and sarcoidosis (lymph node enlargement, abnormalities on lung exam) should be undertaken. There are no readily apparent signs of hyperparathyroidism; band keratopathy is rarely visible without the slit lamp.

Laboratory Studies. After confirmation of hypercalcemia and in the absence of an obvious etiology, one should obtain a *serum parathyroid hormone (PTH)* determination. Improvements in the sensitivity and specificity of immunoradiometric assays for the intact parathyroid hormone molecule have proved to be a great advance in differentiating individuals with hyperparathyroidism from those with other causes for hypercalcemia. In virtually all patients with hyperparathyroidism, PTH 1-84 is either frankly elevated, in 90 percent, or at the upper limit of the normal range (10–60 pg/mL), in 10 percent. In hypercalcemia associated with malignancy, PTH is either undetectable or below normal in most patients. Therefore, a single laboratory test confirms the diagnosis of hyperparathyroidism.

When hyperparathyroidism is under consideration, serum *electrolytes* and *phosphate* concentrations can provide indirect evidence of the diagnosis. Fasting hypophosphatemia, hyperchloremia, and mild metabolic acidosis suggest the diagnosis. This is because parathyroid hormone induces renal phosphate and bicarbonate wasting. A normal serum phosphate does not exclude the diagnosis of hyperparathyroidism, and hypophosphatemia can be observed in malignancy. Furthermore, phosphate must be measured in the fasting state, as intake of food causes phosphate to shift into cells as glucose is phosphorylated. *Alkaline phosphatase* elevation implies increased osteoblastic activity and can be seen in malignancy, hyperparathyroidism with PTH bone disease, and Paget's disease.

Although *anemia* and an *elevated sedimentation* rate can be seen in severe hyperparathyroidism with osteitis fibrosa cystica, these laboratory findings are more suggestive of multiple myeloma, the diagnosis of which requires a serum *immunoelectrophoresis* (IEP) or, occasionally, a urine IEP for light chain excretion by myeloma. A *chest x-ray* with the findings of hilar adenopathy or pulmonary parenchymal abnormalities, in conjunction with an elevated *angiotensin converting enzyme*, is indicative of sarcoidosis. The hypercalcemia of sarcoidosis may be made more severe following an interval of sun exposure and may require more sophisticated diagnostic studies, including diffusing capacity, a hydrocortisone suppression study in which orally administered hydrocortisone (40 mg tid for 10 d) normalizes the hypercalcemia of sarcoidosis, and even bronchoscopy or mediastinoscopy with biopsy for histologic confirmation (see Chapter 48).

A *bone scan* will detect the skeletal metastases of breast cancer. *Skeletal x-rays* may show lytic or metastatic lesions. X-rays are frequently normal in hyperparathyroidism, but the finding of *subperiosteal bone resorption* is specific for and diagnostic of hyperparathyroidism. Cortical bone is lost preferentially in hyperparathyroidism. Therefore, it is important that noninvasive measurements of skeletal mass measure cortical bone, which predominates at sites such as the wrist (in contrast to trabecular bone, which predominates in the spine and is lost earliest following the menopause).

Familial hypocalciuric hypercalcemia can be considered and excluded in patients without frankly elevated serum PTH by finding a 24-hour *urinary calcium excretion* of 80 to 100 mg. *Thyroid hormone* determinations (see Chapter 103), particularly total triiodothyronine by radioimmunoassay, and measurements of serum cortisol following Cortrosyn should be performed if there is a history suggestive of hyperthyroidism or Addison's disease, respectively. A *1,25-dihydroxyvitamin* D_3 *assay* will unequivocally allay concerns of excessive vitamin D intake.

Despite the occasional usefulness of such determinations to exclude the myriad causes of hypercalcemia, the most direct approach to the workup is the measurement of PTH, utilizing the sensitive, specific PTH immunoradiometric assay that is now available. In principle, an elevated PTH concentration or an inappropriately "normal" level in the setting of hypercalcemia should indicate hyperparathyroidism. Older carboxyl-terminal and mid-region radioimmunoassays for PTH recognized PTH-like factors present in the serum in some patients with hypercalcemia of malignancy. The elevation noted by such PTH assays was minimal for the degree of hypercalcemia present. These assays do not test for PTHRP.

MANAGEMENT OF HYPERPARATHYROIDISM

A basic decision in the management of hyperparathyroidism is whether to treat definitively with surgery or follow expectantly and consider medical modalities. The decision must take into account the degree of symptomatology and the natural history of the disease. Prospective studies have attempted to ascertain the natural history of disease in asymptomatic patients. Only in rare instances does recurrent nephrolithiasis, pancreatitis, or hypercalcemic crisis develop. The major consequence of untreated disease appears to be a decrease in skeletal mass, which may predispose to fracture. There is no way to predict who will suffer these effects; monitoring is required. Routine skeletal x-rays and alkaline phosphatase measurements are insufficient for long-term follow-up of bone demineralization. *Bone densitometry* is required (see Chapter 164). Since cortical bone loss is most prominent, measurements are made in the proximal wrist. Marked *urinary calcium* elevation may predict development of nephrolithiasis.

Candidacy for Surgical Cure

Most authorities agree that the *symptomatic patient* with recurrent kidney stones or parathyroid bone disease or a serum calcium level higher than 12.5 to 13.0 mg/dL is a candidate for surgery. Less clear are the indications for surgery in *asymptomatic* or minimally or nonspecifically symptomatic patients with mild hypercalcemia. A 1990 National Institutes of Health (NIH) consensus conference to establish guidelines for the management of hyperparathyroidism in asymptomatic persons formulated a set of criteria for surgical intervention (Table 96–1). Surgical cure is warranted for all persons younger than age 40, for individuals who have a cortical bone density of two standard deviations below normal, and perhaps for patients with urinary calcium excretion greater than 350 to 400 mg in 24 hours, implying, on a restricted calcium intake, that a negative calcium balance is occurring. Cure rates for the initial neck exploration in experienced surgical centers are better than 90 percent.

As just noted, curative surgical treatment should be a serious consideration for persons with asymptomatic hyperparathyroidism who are young or middle-aged, because of the likelihood of progression of skeletal disease, particularly in women who must anticipate the synergistic effects of menopausal bone loss. The cost of medical surveillance, which includes yearly or biannual assessment of renal function and skeletal mass, may surpass the cost of surgical cure after 5 to 10 years of follow-up studies.

Table 96-1. Indications for Surgical Treatment of Hyperparathyroidism

Marked elevation of serum calcium, usually >12.5 mg/dL
History of an episode of life-threatening hypercalcemia
Reduced creatinine clearance
Presence of kidney stones detected by abdominal radiographs
Markedly elevated 24-hour urine calcium excretion
Substantially reduced bone mass as determined by direct measurement
Medical surveillance is neither desirable nor suitable:
Patient is young (<50 years old)
Patient requests surgery
Consistent follow-up is unlikely
Coexistent illness complicates management

Adapted from Proceedings of the NIH Consensus Development Conference on Diagnosis and Management of Asymptomatic Primary Hyperparathyroidism. J Bone Miner Res 1991;6 (Supp 1–2):S1.

Prior to surgery, localization of the parathyroid adenoma may be helpful even to the skilled surgeon. Ultrasonography and technetium–thallium scanning using computer programs that subtract thyroidal uptake of technetium have localized parathyroid adenomas in approximately 70 percent of patients preoperatively. Anatomic localization by selective angiography or, less commonly, by venous sampling is generally reserved for patients in whom neck exploration by an experienced parathyroid surgeon fails to cure the disease.

Medical Therapy. In patients who do not undergo surgical cure for hyperparathyroidism, several medical alternatives exist. These alternatives may help limit nonspecific symptoms of hypercalcemic parathyroidism and, more importantly, may prevent the skeletal loss.

Estrogen/progestogen therapy given to postmenopausal women may lower or even normalize serum calcium, reduce bone resorption, and increase skeletal mass. It represents a reasonable therapeutic option in older women in whom contraindications for estrogen therapy do not exist (see Chapter 164). In women with family or personal histories of breast cancer, *tamoxifen* treatment will have a beneficial effect on the skeleton and may be of therapeutic value.

Oral phosphate therapy, particularly when moderate hypophosphatemia exists, may lessen fatigue and weakness and reduce urinary calcium excretion, thereby reducing the likelihood of renal stones. Serum calcium is lowered by oral phosphate, given as 250 mg to 500 mg of neutral phosphate four times daily. The most common side effect of this therapy is dose-related frequent bowel movements, which are often preferred to the constipation of hyperparathyroidism. Phosphate should be very cautiously administered in renal insufficiency because the calcium–phosphate solubility product of 65 might be exceeded and calcium deposition might occur in skeletal and extraskeletal sites. Phosphate therapy has a potential drawback: it increases PTH secretion and, theoretically, could accelerate bone resorption.

Diuretics, such as *furosemide* or *bumetanide*, increase renal calcium excretion. *Thiazides* may actually decrease PTH secretion and urinary calcium excretion. However, risk of dehydration requires caution in the use of diuretic agents.

Calcitonin and *bisphosphonates* have *not* proven useful for long-term use in hyperparathyroidism. Tachyphylaxis develops with calcitonin therapy, and bisphosphonates result in only transient decreases in osteoclastic bone resorption and serum calcium.

Most physicians limit *dietary calcium* in patients with hyperparathyroidism. However, this restriction of dietary calcium may result in accelerated bone resorption as the body responds by maintaining the "set-point" elevation of serum calcium with increased PTH secretion. It is prudent to increase dietary calcium intake to 1 to 1.5 g daily in hyperparathyroid individuals who do not have associated nephrolithiasis.

Patients who are on phosphate or estrogen therapy or being followed expectantly for hypercalcemia for the development of skeletal or renal disease should be instructed to maintain a *fluid intake* of at least 2 liters daily and to report any illness that might lead to dehydration and worsening hypercalcemia.

INDICATIONS FOR REFERRAL AND HOSPITALIZATION

Since one cannot predict which patients with asymptomatic hyperparathyroidism will develop progressive complications of disease, recommendations for who should be referred for surgical cure cannot be rigidly applied. The decision to refer for surgery should take into account the patient's preferences, availability of skilled surgical care, and willingness to cooperate with the demands of long-term surveillance. As noted above, those who should be urged to consider surgery are younger than age 40, have a cortical bone density two standard deviations below normal, or have a urinary calcium excretion greater than 350 to 400 mg in 24 hours (which, on a restricted calcium intake, implies a negative calcium balance). Patients in whom surgical cure is planned should be referred to surgeons experienced in the complexities of parathyroid surgery, not only for cure of potential hyperplasia and discovery of the parathyroid adenoma in an unusual location, but also to avert complications of recurrent laryngeal nerve injury and hypoparathyroidism.

Hospitalization is necessary for patients with severe hypercalcemia. Hydration and bisphosphonates such as pamidronate that limit osteoclastic resorption of bone are helpful.

PATIENT EDUCATION

Several recommendations will prevent the likelihood of more severe hypercalcemia in patients with mild hyperparathyroidism. Adequacy of fluid intake and prevention of dehydration that might occur during an acute gastrointestinal illness should be encouraged. Although thiazide diuretics and calcium administration have been discouraged, thiazides may actually limit hypercalciuria and renal stone disease, and dietary calcium may decrease parathyroid hormone secretion and limit negative calcium balance. Patients should be encouraged to remain active and avoid immobilization. The necessity of surveillance for parathyroid hormone–induced skeletal disease and the delineation of symptoms that might represent manifestations of hyperparathyroidism (such as symptoms of nephrolithiasis and pancreatitis) should be carefully reviewed.

The patient who prefers to postpone surgical therapy ought to be advised that current clinical evidence suggests a 50 percent likelihood for requiring surgery over the next 5 to 10 years, often at a time of increased risk due to the development of other medical illnesses.

ANNOTATED BIBLIOGRAPHY

Bilezikian JP. Management of acute hypercalcemia. N Engl J Med 1992;326:1196. *(A current review of treatment options.)*

Broadus AD, Horst RL, Lang R, et al. The importance of circulating 1,25-dihydroxyvitamin D in the pathogenesis of hypercalciuria and renal-stone formation in primary hyperparathyroidism. N Engl J Med 1980;302:421. *(A subgroup of patients with hyperparathyroidism are likely to form renal stones because of elevated 1,25-dihydroxyvitamin D_3 levels, which increase gut absorption of calcium and produce marked degrees of hypercalciuria.)*

Christensson T, Hellstrom K, Wengle B, et al. Prevalence of hypercalcemia in a health screening in Stockholm. Acta Med Scand 1976;200:131. *(In a population of more than 15,000, 95 patients were confirmed to have hypercalcemia, with probable hyperparathyroidism in 88.)*

Heath H III, Hodgson SF, Kennedy MA. Primary hyperparathyroidism incidence, morbidity, and potential economic impact in a community. N Engl J Med 1980;302:189. *(Increased case finding with the advent of multiphasic biochemical screening and the increasing recognition of the disease in older women.)*

Insogna KL, Mitnick ME, Stewart AF, et al. Sensitivity of the parathyroid hormone 1,25-dihydroxyvitamin D axis to variations in calcium intake in patients with primary hyperparathyroidism. N Engl J Med 1985;313:1126. *(Parathyroid function may be suppressed by dietary calcium in some patients with hyperparathyroidism. Perhaps we should be encouraging increased calcium intake in nonhypercalciuric patients.)*

Marcus R, Madvig P, Crim M, et al. Conjugated estrogens in the treatment of post-menopausal women with hyperparathyroidism. Ann Intern Med 1984;100:633. *(Estrogen therapy normalized serum calcium and decreased bone turnover in 10 women with hyperparathyroidism for up to 2 years.)*

Marx SJ, Attie MF, Levine M, et al. The hypocalciuric or benign variant of familial hypercalcemia: clinical and biochemical features in fifteen kindreds. Medicine (Baltimore) 1981;60:397. *(A genetic, clinical, and physiologic review of familial hypocalciuric hypercalcemia.)*

McPherson ML, Prince SR, Atamer ER, et al. Theophylline-induced hypercalcemia. Ann Intern Med 1986;105:52. *(Documents elevations in the settings of both excess and therapeutic theophylline levels.)*

NIH Consensus Development Conference on Diagnosis and Management of Asymptomatic Primary Hyperparathyroidism. Proceedings of the Conference. J Bone Miner Res 1991; Suppl(1–2):S1. *(A scholarly compendium on the clinical spectrum and treatment options for hyperparathyroidism, especially asymptomatic disease.)*

Nussbaum SR. Pathophysiology and management of severe hypercalcemia. Endocrinol Metab Clin North Am 1993;22:343. *(A review of mechanisms of hypercalcemia with emphasis on newer inhibitors of osteoclastic bone resorption, especially bisphosphonates.)*

Nussbaum SR, Zahradnik R, Lavigne J. Highly sensitive two-site immunoradiometric assay for parathyrin and its clinical utility in evaluating patients with hypercalcemia. Clin Chem 1987; 33:1364. *(Immunoradiometric assay for intact PTH can distinguish hypercalcemic individuals with hyperparathyroidism from those with malignancy, an advantage over earlier region-specific assays.)*

Palmer M, Adami HO, Bergstrom R. Survival and renal function in persons with untreated hypercalcemia: a population-based cohort study with thirteen years of follow-up. Lancet 1987; 1:59. *(Decreased survival amongst 176 hypercalcemic individuals was largely explained by cardiovascular deaths. Are there long-term consequences of hyperparathyroidism not currently recognized?)*

Parisien M, Silverberg SJ, Shane E, et al. The histomorphometry of bone in primary hyperparathyroidism: preservation of cancellous bone structure. J Clin Endocrinol Metab 1990;70:930. *(Disproportionate loss of cortical bone in hyperparathyroidism; skeletal study must assess cortical bone.)*

Rao DS, Wilson RJ, Kleerekoper M, Parfitt AM. Lack of biochemical progression or continuation of accelerated bone loss in mild asymptomatic primary hyperparathyroidism: evidence for biphasic disease course. J Clin Endocrinol Metab 1988; 67:1294. *(Longitudinal follow-up; demonstrated unchanged calcium, PTH, and other biochemical parameters and low risk of renal or skeletal disease; larger numbers of African-Americans in the study population, with greater bone mass than whites, may explain the skeletal findings.)*

Simeone JF, Mueller PR, Ferucci JT, et al. High-resolution real-time sonography of the parathyroid. Radiology 1981;141:745. *(Ultrasonography may demonstrate the location of a parathyroid adenoma in 70%–80% of patients.)*

Stewart AF, Horst R, Deftos LJ, et al. Biochemical evaluation of patients with cancer-associated hypercalcemia. Evidence for humoral and non-humoral groups. N Engl J Med 1980;303:1377. *(The "classic" study segregating cancer patients with humoral hypercalcemia, often without bone metastases, from patients with metastatic disease.)*

Primary Care Medicine: Office Evaluation and Management of the Adult Patient, 3rd edition, edited by Allan H. Goroll, Lawrence A. May, and Albert G. Mulley, Jr. J.B. Lippincott Company, Philadelphia

97
Evaluation of Hypoglycemia

The finding of hypoglycemia raises the question of an underlying disorder of glucose homeostasis. However, the significance of a low serum glucose is not always evident, because it may occur in metabolically normal persons. Hypoglycemia is sometimes defined statistically, using a serum glucose concentration of less than 50 mg/dL (2.8 mmol/L) as the sole criterion, but this definition has been found lacking because it does not always differentiate between normals and abnormals. In fact, no quantitative definition does. This has prompted use of a clinical definition, in which hypoglycemic symptoms and prompt response to intake of sugar are added to the quantitative criterion.

The identification of hypoglycemia and its underlying causes is often made difficult by the lack of glucose measurements at the time of symptoms and the nonspecific nature of hypoglycemic symptoms (eg, tiredness, light-headedness, nervousness, irritability, palpitations, tremulousness). Compounding the diagnostic problem are the many patients with underlying psychopathology who come to physicians seeking a "hypoglycemic" explanation for their symptoms.

The primary physician needs to be able to identify patients with true hypoglycemia and differentiate postprandial from fasting pathophysiology. Postprandial hypoglycemias range in etiology from the harmless functional-reactive type to early diabetes mellitus. The fasting hypoglycemias tend to be more worrisome. One should have an effective evaluation strategy that will detect and efficiently workup the occasional patient with true hypoglycemia yet avoid unnecessary studies in the large number of patients who have no underlying disorder of glucose homeostasis.

PATHOPHYSIOLOGY AND CLINICAL PRESENTATION

Hypoglycemia can result from increased insulin secretion, enhanced glucose utilization, or inadequate functioning of one or more compensatory glucoregulatory mechanisms. When hypoglycemia occurs, the liver responds with increased glycogenolysis and glyconeogenesis, stimulated by glucagon and epinephrine, which activate hepatic phosphorylase. In addition, the pituitary secretes growth hormone, which inhibits utilization of glucose by muscle and enhances lipolysis, and adrenocorticotropic hormone (ACTH), which promotes cortisol production. The increased cortisol acts to stimulate gluconeogenesis and diminish muscle uptake of glucose.

There is *no single threshold* glucose concentration that invariably triggers hypoglycemic symptoms or characterizes patients with a disorder of glucose homeostasis. Glucose levels lower than 45 mg/dL (2.5 mmol/L) have been documented in metabolically normal men during prolonged exercise and in healthy asymptomatic women. More than 20 percent of normal patients demonstrate serum sugars below 50 mg/dL during glucose tolerance testing. Conversely, hypoglycemic thresholds may rise in poorly controlled diabetes, where levels as high as 75 mg/dL (4.3 mmol/L) may trigger symptoms. This has led to the view that onset of hypoglycemic symptoms is related to the robustness of counterregulatory responses as well as the rate of fall in serum glucose and the absolute serum glucose concentration. Patients with intensively controlled insulin-dependent diabetes have a blunted catecholamine response and may exhibit few symptoms until glucose concentrations fall to very low levels.

Hypoglycemic symptoms are typically categorized as *neuroglycopenic* (confusion, lethargy, visual disturbances, behavioral changes, impaired performance of routine tasks) or *catecholamine-mediated* (anxiety, tremulousness, headache, palpitations, sweats). Adrenergic symptoms characteristically accompany acute, rapid falls in blood sugar, especially if levels drop to concentrations below 40 mg/dL. Neuroglycopenic symptoms can develop in the absence of premonitory adrenergic complaints.

The hypoglycemias can be classified pathophysiologically as reactive (postprandial) or fasting (spontaneous). Both are characterized by the concurrence of symptoms and hypoglycemia. In the reactive variety, the fall in glucose and onset of symptoms occur within 5 hours of eating and result from an abnormal response to the intake of food. In fasting hypoglycemia, symptoms and low serum glucose levels are noted in the absence of food intake.

Reactive Hypoglycemias

Onset of hypoglycemia and symptoms *1 to 2 hours* after eating characterizes the reactive hypoglycemia of patients who have undergone *gastric surgery*. About 5 percent to 10 percent of patients having such surgery experience a reactive hypoglycemia, believed related to pyloric sphincter incompetence and the excessively rapid entry of concentrated carbohydrates into the small bowel. Unidentified gut factors are stimulated, causing the release of excessive insulin.

Symptoms should not be confused with those of the dumping syndrome (see Chapter 64), which consist of nausea, fullness, and weakness coming on within an hour of eating. An occasional patient with a *functional defect* in gastric emptying may present in similar fashion.

Functional reactive hypoglycemia designates the most common form of postprandial hypoglycemia, with onset of hypoglycemia *2 to 4 hours* after a meal in conjunction with neuroglycopenic and adrenergic symptoms. Hypotheses regarding its pathogenesis range from increased insulin sensitivity to decreased release of counterregulatory hormones; insulin secretion is normal. Concentrated sweets may precipitate symptoms, because falls in blood sugar are observed after a glucose load but not after consumption of a mixed meal. About 10 percent to 20 percent of normal persons manifest a similar fall in serum glucose 2 to 4 hours into a glucose tolerance test, but they remain asymptomatic. What differentiates them from those who become symptomatic is unclear. Some authorities warn that too many people are labelled as having functional reactive hypoglycemia. The diagnosis should be considered only when symptoms accompany a low blood sugar; an isolated low postprandial glucose concentration does not suffice.

Early *adult-onset diabetes* may result in postprandial hypoglycemia 3 to 5 hours after eating. Insulin release is found to be delayed, with levels inappropriately high for the level of serum glucose at hand. Most patients are asymptomatic, and the majority of adult-onset diabetics do not experience reactive hypoglycemia on glucose tolerance testing.

Fasting Hypoglycemias

Excessive doses of exogenous insulin or *oral hypoglycemics* account for most cases of spontaneous hypoglycemia and are usually readily apparent; however, *surreptitious administration* sometimes occurs among self-destructive persons. Patients injecting insulin secretively may have high levels of immunoreactive insulin but very low serum levels of C-reactive protein or proinsulin, because there is little endogenous insulin production. *Defects in glycogenolysis* or *gluconeogenesis* (as in advanced pituitary or adrenal insufficiency, end-stage liver disease, and severe binge-drinking in the absence of food intake) are other important precipitants of fasting hypoglycemia.

Insulinomas represent a rare but important cause of uncontrolled insulin production and account for the large majority of patients with endogenous hyperinsulinemia. More than 85 percent of insulinomas are benign islet-cell tumors. Many occur in the setting of multiple endocrine neoplasia type I, which also includes parathyroid hyperplasia and pituitary adenoma. The clinical presentation of insulinomas can be confusing and highly variable in timing and severity. The only valid generalizations are that fasting and exercise may precipitate symptoms, and profound degrees of hypoglycemia may ensue (leading to seizures in 10%). Levels of serum glucose are not always low after an overnight fast. In a series of 39 patients with proven islet-cell tumors, about half still had glucose levels above 60 mg/dL after 10 hours of fasting. Another series found symptoms equally divided between early morning, late afternoon, and several hours after a meal. Nonetheless, evidence of hyperinsulinism is evident in more than 75 percent of patients after 24 hours of fasting, and 80 percent report a combination of neuroglycopenic and adrenergic symptoms.

On occasion, a *non–islet-cell tumor* may be the cause of hypoglycemia, due to elaboration of an insulin-like growth factor (IGF-I or IGF-II); levels of immunoreactive insulin are very low.

DIFFERENTIAL DIAGNOSIS

The differential diagnosis of true hypoglycemia can be organized around whether it is fasting or postprandial (Table 97–1). The hypoglycemias most commonly encountered in the outpatient setting are postprandial and include functional reactive hypoglycemia, postgastrectomy syndrome, and early adult-onset diabetes. The most common forms of fasting hypoglycemia are caused by excessive doses of insulin or sulfonylureas. End-stage liver disease, alcoholism complicated by poor nutrition, Addison's disease, and hypopituitarism are causes of impaired glycogenolysis or gluconeogenesis that may result in hypoglycemia. Rare etiologies include insulinomas and pelvic or retroperitoneal neoplasms elaborating IGF-I or IGF-II. In an occasional case of severe hypothyroidism or chronic renal failure, there may be hypoglycemia.

Two groups of nonhypoglycemics must be differentiated from patients manifesting genuine falls in glucose in con-

Table 97-1. Important Causes of Hypoglycemia in Ambulatory Patients

CAUSE	PRINCIPAL FEATURES
Postprandial (Reactive) Hypoglycemias	
Postgastric surgery	Rapid gastric emptying; symptoms 1–2 hours after eating
Functional reactive	Onset 2–4 hours after eating; otherwise normal
Early adult-onset diabetes	Onset 3–5 hours after eating; elevated 2-h postprandial glucose
Fasting (Spontaneous) Hypoglycemias	
Insulinoma	Symptoms brought on by fasting or exercise; inappropriately high insulin and C-peptide levels; ratio of insulin to glucose >.30
Extrapancreatic neoplasm	Low insulin, high insulin-like growth factor
Surreptitious insulin use	Medical personnel; high insulin, low C-peptide
Insulin reaction	Insulin overdose; readily evident by history
Surreptitious oral agent use	High insulin, high C-peptide; high drug level
Alcohol abuse	Within 24 hours of binge; no food intake
Pituitary or adrenal insufficiency	Low cortisol
Hepatic insufficiency	End-stage disease only
Renal insufficiency	End-stage disease only

junction with symptoms. One group is composed of individuals suffering from *anxiety* or *depression* who have multiple bodily complaints of a functional or psychophysiologic nature (see Chapters 226, 227, and 230). The most common symptoms include fatigue, headache, spasms, palpitations, numbness, sweating, and mental dullness. They attribute their symptoms to "hypoglycemia" to explain their difficulties and avoid the psychosocial issues at hand. Requests for glucose tolerance testing are frequent. A second group is bothered by postprandial symptoms very similar to those experienced by patients with reactive hypoglycemia yet in the context of normal serum sugar levels. The pathophysiology of this alimentary variant is unknown.

WORKUP

It is important to keep in mind that hypoglycemia is not a diagnosis but a problem that requires investigation because it may be a manifestation of important underlying pathology. Complicating its evaluation is difficulty in proper identification of persons who require a workup.

Identifying the Truly Hypoglycemic Patient

Criteria for clinically significant hypoglycemia include 1) symptoms consistent with neuroglycopenia (blurred or double vision, confusion, odd behavior, lethargy) or adrenergic stimulation (anxiety, tremulousness, headache, palpitations, sweats); 2) low serum glucose concentration (<50 mg/dL) at the time of symptoms; and 3) relief of symptoms when glucose level is raised to normal. Simply having adrenergic symptoms or a low serum glucose in the absence of symptoms does not suffice. The objective is to document the correlation between symptoms and a low serum glucose concentration. Without such documentation, one cannot make a diagnosis of physiologically significant hypoglycemia.

A *serum glucose* determination drawn *at the time of symptoms* is essential for diagnosis and helps eliminate from consideration the large number of cases not due to hypoglycemia. In a study of patients referred with a presumptive diagnosis of reactive hypoglycemia, less than 20 percent actually had a serum glucose less than 50 mg/dL during symptoms—a finding that emphasizes the importance of a blood sugar determination at the time of symptoms.

Finger-stick methods have improved the ability to sample blood sugar at the time of symptoms, though reagent-strip techniques may be inaccurate at low glucose concentrations. Venipuncture is more accurate but less convenient. However, a sample is worth obtaining as long as symptoms are present, because the serum glucose is usually low in the presence of symptoms.

Even before hypoglycemia is confirmed by blood sugar, there are important historical clues that can help determine who needs to undergo a hypoglycemia workup. The report of neuroglycopenic or adrenergic symptoms occurring consistently before breakfast, after exertion, or postprandially suggests a possible hypoglycemic etiology, especially if symptoms abate with eating. However, neuroglycopenic symptoms may be vague and can occur in the absence of adrenergic complaints (especially in patients with fasting hypoglycemia); one should be careful not to mistake them for those of a functional or psychologic condition.

Patients not fulfilling criteria for hypoglycemia should be evaluated for other etiologies. It is essential that one avoid mislabeling then as hypoglycemic, even if symptoms follow meals. In a study of 28 patients with suspected postprandial hypoglycemia, only 20 percent had abnormal glucose levels at the time of symptoms. Patients with no correlation between their symptoms and serum glucose are unlikely to have an underlying disturbance in glucose homeostasis. For them, an alternative explanation for symptoms should be sought. Symptoms due to *anxiety* disorders, *depression*, and *hyperthyroidism* may mimic those of hypoglycemia. A story of early-morning awakening, chronic fatigue, and appetite and libido disturbances in conjunction with a history of personally significant losses provides strong presumptive evidence for depression (see Chapter 227). Paroxysms of anxiousness, palpitations, difficulty getting air in, and chest tightness unrelated to meals suggest a panic attack disorder (see Chapter 226). The presence of heat intolerance, weight loss in spite of normal food intake, constant nervousness unrelated to meals, and skin and hair changes point to hyperthyroidism (see Chapter 103).

Evaluating Hypoglycemia

History. Once hypoglycemia has been established, the evaluation proceeds to determining whether the condition is postprandial or fasting. The *timing* of symptoms should be carefully explored. Knowing the relation of symptoms to meals, fasting, and exercise helps distinguish fasting from reactive hypoglycemia and differentiates among the various postprandial etiologies.

If symptoms come on *postprandially*, then one should ascertain how soon after eating they occur and whether there is a history of *diabetes*, *gastric surgery*, or heavy use of concentrated *sweets*. In a patient with a history of gastric surgery, onset within 1 to 2 hours after eating is very strong evidence for rapid emptying as the underlying pathophysiology. Symptoms beginning 2 to 4 hours after meals suggest functional reactive disease. Onset 3 to 5 hours after eating in a patient with a family history of diabetes or recent development of polyuria/polydipsia argues for early type II diabetes.

If symptoms occur in the *fasting* state and/or after exercise, then one needs to inquire into *use of insulin* or *oral hypoglycemic agents*. As noted, intensive insulin therapy may reduce counterregulatory responses to hypoglycemia and lower the glucose level at which symptoms occur, necessitating a high index of suspicion. A person making surreptitious use of such drugs is likely to deny any intake, but a *vocational history* of medical or paramedical work should raise one's index of suspicion. A check into recent *binge drinking* in the absence of food intake identifies alcohol-induced hypoglycemia. Cases in which the fasting hypoglycemia is due to end-stage *liver* or *kidney disease*, *adrenal insufficiency*, or marked *hypopituitarism* are usually self-evident, with symptoms of the underlying condition dominating the clinical presentation (see Chapters 71, 101, and 142).

Patients with *insulinomas* or extrapancreatic neoplasms making IGF report few symptoms other than those related to their hypoglycemia, which worsens after prolonged fasting (eg, just before breakfast or late in the afternoon, especially after exercising). The occurrence of neuroglycopenic symptoms (blurred vision, diplopia, sweats, confusion, poor memory) during these periods should raise suspicion of the diagnosis. Because insulinomas often develop in the context of multiple endocrine neoplasia type I, symptoms of hypercalcemia may be evident (see Chapter 96).

Physical Examination. In most cases of reactive hypoglycemia, there are few etiologically suggestive physical findings. The exception is the upper abdominal surgical scar in a patient who has undergone gastric surgery. Patients with fasting hypoglycemia ought to be checked for postural hypotension, alcohol on the breath, needle marks at common insulin injection sites, jaundice, ecchymoses, hyperpigmentation, visual field defects, ascites, and other signs of hepatocellular failure (see Chapter 71). A careful neurologic examination is essential to rule out focal neurologic injury which would indicate a cause other than hypoglycemia.

Laboratory Studies. For years, patients suspected of having a *reactive hypoglycemia* were routinely subjected to a 5-hour *oral glucose tolerance test (OGTT)*. This was prior to appreciation of the high frequency of falsely positive serum glucose results associated with the test, especially in samples taken at 4 and 5 hours postprandially. Only blood samples manifesting hypoglycemia at time of symptoms are diagnostically valid, and they need not be obtained in the context of a formal OGTT. Consequently, the OGTT is no longer a routine part of the evaluation, though a two-hour postprandial glucose may be useful in patients suspected of having early adult-onset diabetes (see Chapter 93). In such cases, insulin levels may be obtained in search of inappropriately late insulin release.

Fasting hypoglycemias can be identified by withholding food. An *overnight fast* will suffice in many instances; extending the fast beyond 12 hours increases the diagnostic yield. Very low levels (35 mg/dL) may be encountered during a 24-hour fast. In rare instances, *72 hours of fasting* are required for demonstration of hypoglycemia. Since exercise promotes a fall in serum glucose, it may be used in conjunction with fasting to bring out hypoglycemia and precipitate symptoms. Two-thirds of the patients with insulinomas will develop hypoglycemia within 24 hours; fewer than 5 percent will have to fast for 72 hours. Concurrent measurements of *serum glucose and insulin* should be obtained when the patient is symptomatic.

Inappropriately high insulin levels suggest insulinoma, surreptitious insulin administration, or insulin antibodies. An insulin-to-glucose ratio in excess of 0.3 is consistent with insulinoma and characteristically increases as fasting progresses. When there is a question of factitious hypoglycemia due to self-administration of excess insulin, a *C-peptide* assay can be helpful, if available. In the synthesis of endogenous insulin, the C-peptide is formed as proinsulin is split. Low C-peptide levels in the presence of high serum insulin concentrations indicate exogenous insulin use. High C-peptide and plasma insulin levels suggest hyperinsulinism due to an endogenous source, but surreptitious use of oral agents can produce a similar picture. Collection of urine and serum samples to test for sulfonylurea and its metabolites can settle the issue when oral agent excess is suspected. A *C-peptide suppression test* is sometimes performed to identify an insulinoma. Insulin is infused over 1 hour, and C-peptide levels are monitored. Failure to suppress C-peptide formation strongly suggests insulinoma.

Measurement of *insulin antibodies* can help in the evaluation. High levels may cause a false-positive elevation in immunoreactive insulin, leading to hypoglycemia when insulin is released. Surreptitious insulin administration also may lead to high titers of insulin antibodies.

Need for additional studies in the patient with fasting hypoglycemia depends on the clinical context of the hypoglycemia. *Cortisol* and *ACTH* determinations are indicated if hypopituitarism or adrenal insufficiency is suspected (see Chapter 101). Extensive liver function tests may be superfluous if the patient is floridly jaundiced and ecchymotic, but the prothrombin time and serum albumin remain the best measures of hepatocellular synthetic function (see Chapter 71).

SYMPTOMATIC MANAGEMENT

Treatment of most fasting hypoglycemias requires attending directly to the underlying etiology. In the case of intensively treated insulin-dependent diabetics, symptoms may not develop until the serum glucose reaches a dangerously low concentration. Careful monitoring of glucose during such therapy is essential (see Chapter 102). Those with postprandial etiologies may respond to dietary interventions. Patients with *functional reactive hypoglycemia* have been advised to try *frequent feedings* (six per day), diets *high in protein* and *low in carbohydrate*, and reductions in consumption of concentrated sweets. Some report symptomatic improvement, although there are no controlled studies establishing the efficacy of any of these dietary manipulations. A patient who demonstrates hypoglycemia after a glucose load but not after intake of a more balanced meal might be the logical candidate for restriction of sweets.

Similar dietary advice is given to those suffering from *postgastrectomy hypoglycemia*. In addition, they have been treated with anticholinergic agents (eg, propantheline 7.5 mg before meals) to delay gastric emptying; results are fair at best. Other approaches include pre-meal use of a beta-blocking agent (eg, 10 mg propranolol), reversal of a 10 cm segment of the jejunum, and administration of pectin.

PATIENT EDUCATION

The patient who presents fearing hypoglycemia should be taken seriously, but once the diagnosis is ruled out, reassurance and a refocusing of attention to other possible etiologies should follow. A number of patients will initially refuse to accept the fact that hypoglycemia is not responsible for their symptoms, because the attribution had served as a psychologically comfortable explanation. One needs to explore their concerns and discuss other causes that might be responsible, including anxiety and depression (see Chapters 226, 227, and 230). Requests for glucose tolerance testing are common, but they are readily withdrawn when the test's lack of specificity is explained.

INDICATIONS FOR ADMISSION AND REFERRAL

Patients with fasting hypoglycemia may have serious underlying pathology and are at risk for a profound fall in serum glucose. Such patients who become very symptomatic (seizure, mental confusion) should be admitted immediately to the hospital for glucose infusion and detailed evaluation. Endocrinologic and oncologic consultations are indicated when insulinoma is a concern. Routine referral of patients with postprandial hypoglycemia for glucose tolerance testing is no longer considered necessary.

A.H.G.

ANNOTATED BIBLIOGRAPHY

American Diabetes Association. Statement on hypoglycemia. Diabetes Care 1982;5:72. *(A consensus statement of criteria for diagnosis of functional reactive hypoglycemia.)*

Boyle PJ, Schwartz NS, Shah SD, et al. Plasma glucose concentrations at the outset of hypoglycemic symptoms in patients with poorly controlled diabetes and in nondiabetics. N Engl J Med 1988;318:1487. *(Symptoms occur at higher glucose levels when the diabetes is poorly controlled.)*

Charles MA, Hofeldt F, Shackelford A, et al. Comparison of oral glucose tolerance tests and mixed meals in patients with apparent idiopathic postabsorptive hypoglycemia. Diabetes 1981;30:465. *(Mixed meals did not result in hypoglycemia; a glucose load did; provides a rationale for treatment.)*

Cryer PE, Binder C, Bolli GB, et al. Hypoglycemia in IDDM. Diabetes 1989;38:1193. *(Excellent review of the problem.)*

Fajans SS, Floyd JC. Fasting hypoglycemia in adults. N Engl J Med 1976;294:766. *(A physiologically oriented review of fasting hypoglycemia with a table of causes organized around pathophysiologic mechanisms.)*

Felig P, Cherif A, Minagawa A, Wahren J. Hypoglycemia during prolonged exercise in normal men. N Engl J Med 1982;306:895. *(A normal event during maximal exertion.)*

Gastineau CF. Is reactive hypoglycemia a clinical entity? Mayo Clin Proc 1983;58:545. *(A example of the debate surrounding the issue.)*

Kloschinsky T, Dannehl K, Gries FA. New approach to technical and clinical evaluation of devices for self-monitoring of blood glucose. Diabetes Care 1988;11:619. *(Useful critique of self-monitoring techniques.)*

Lev-Ran A, Anderson RW. The diagnosis of postprandial hypoglycemia. Diabetes 1981;30:996. *(Data and discussion on diagnosis of reactive hypoglycemia, with a focus on what is a "low" glucose level.)*

Merimee TJ, Tyson JE. Stabilization of plasma glucose during fasting—Normal variations in two separate studies. N Engl J Med 1974;291:1275. *(Fasting blood sugars in normal women may be as low as 40 mg/dL.)*

Oberg K, Skogseid B, Eriksson B. Multiple endocrine neoplasia type I: clinical, biochemical, and genetic investigations. Acta Oncol 1989;28:383. *(Comprehensive review of this syndrome, which can include insulinoma.)*

Palardy J, Havrankova J, LePage R, et al. Blood glucose measurements during symptomatic episodes in patients with suspected postprandial hypoglycemia. N Engl J Med 1989;321:1421. *(Study of a referral population indicating that postprandial hypoglycemia is infrequent and that glucose tolerance testing is of little diagnostic utility.)*

Scarlett JA, Mako ME, Ruberstein AH, et al. Factitious hypoglycemia: diagnosis by measurement of serum C-peptide and insulin-binding antibodies. N Engl J Med 1977;297:1029. *(Documents the usefulness of these measures in patients who administer insulin surreptitiously.)*

Service FJ. Hypoglycemia and the postprandial syndrome. N Engl J Med 1989;321:1472. *(An editorial emphasizing that most patients with postprandial syndrome do not have hypoglycemia.)*

Service FJ, Horwitz DL, Rubenstein AH, et al. C-peptide suppression test for insulinoma. J Lab Clin Med 1977;13:571. *(Initial description of the test.)*

Simonson DC, Tamborlane WV, DeFronzo RA, et al. Intensive insulin therapy reduces counterregulatory hormone responses to hypoglycemia in patients with type I diabetes. Ann Intern Med 1985;103:184. *(Documents risk of profound hypoglycemia in such patients.)*

Yeager J, Young RT. Nonhypoglycemia as an epidemic condition. N Engl J Med 1974;291:907. *(A succinct discussion of how to manage patients with self-diagnosed "hypoglycemia.")*

Primary Care Medicine: Office Evaluation and Management of the Adult Patient, 3rd edition, edited by Allan H. Goroll, Lawrence A. May, and Albert G. Mulley, Jr. J.B. Lippincott Company, Philadelphia

98
Evaluation of Hirsutism

SAMUEL R. NUSSBAUM, M.D.

Hirsutism in women is due to increased androgenic activity and is characterized by excessive growth of hormone-dependent pubic, axillary, abdominal, chest, and facial hair. Women are likely to present for evaluation when such hair growth is viewed as exceeding that of others in their societal, geographic, or racial environment. For a woman living in a society preoccupied with stereotyped perceptions of beauty, hirsutism may be extremely upsetting and connote loss of femininity and sexuality. For the primary physician, hirsutism raises the question of an underlying endocrinopathy, ranging in severity from minor changes in androgen metabolism to development of a hormonally active neoplasm.

When confronted with women with excessive hair growth, the primary care physician must decide whom to begin evaluating for endocrine disease and whom to reassure or treat symptomatically. Women with signs of virilization, progressive hair growth beginning after age 25, or concurrent amenorrhea should undergo endocrine evaluation (see below).

PATHOPHYSIOLOGY AND CLINICAL PRESENTATION

Hair follicles are located over the entire body except for the palms and soles. Hair growth is of two types: lanugo (neonatal) or vellus hair is soft, unpigmented, and rarely more than 2 cm long; terminal hair is coarse, pigmented, and grows in excess of 2 cm. A survey of college women revealed that one quarter had easily noticeable facial hair, one-third reported hair extending along the linea alba from the pubic area (male escutcheon) and 17 percent had periareolar hair. Three-quarters of women over age 60 have a measurable growth of facial hair. Hirsutism has familial, ethnic, and racial patterns. Eastern European women are more hirsute than Scandinavian women; white women are more hirsute than black women, who have more body hair than Asian women.

The Ferriman-Gallwey scale is used to define and grade hirsutism. Hair growth in each of nine androgen-dependent areas of the body is graded from 0 (no hair growth) to 4 (frankly virile growth). A score of 8 or more is generally accepted as indicative of hirsutism.

Hirsutism is a manifestation of excessive androgenic effect. The hormonal stimulus for hair growth is *5-alpha-dihydrotestosterone*, a potent testosterone metabolite derived from the peripheral conversion at the hair follicle of testosterone by 5-alpha-reductase. *Delta-4 androstenedione (A)*, and *dehydroepiandrosterone (DHEA)*, produced by the ovaries and adrenal glands, are the *precursors* for 50 percent to 70 percent of circulating testosterone in women; the remainder of testosterone is secreted directly by the ovaries or occasionally by the adrenals.

Hirsute women generally have *increased production* rates of the relatively weak androgens, *DHEA* and *A*, or of the more potent androgen, *testosterone*. Serum measurements of total concentrations of androgens reflect sex steroid hormone binding to sex-hormone–binding globulin: however, only the free fraction, which for testosterone is 1 percent of total testosterone, is biologically active. The source of enhanced androgen production may be the *ovary*, the *adrenal gland*, or both. *Hyperinsulinism* resulting from insulin resistance has been noted to trigger excess ovarian androgen production, providing a possible link between *obesity* and hirsutism, a common association. In addition, obesity leads to a reduction in concentration of sex-hormone–binding globulin.

Virilization (temporal hair recession, acne, deepening voice, increased muscle mass, and clitoromegaly) develops when there is autonomous androgen production originating from an adrenal or ovarian neoplasm and resulting in extremely high levels of circulating androgens.

Ovarian Sources. The majority of women with nonvirilizing hirsutism in conjunction with oligo- or amenorrhea have *polycystic ovary disease (PCO)*. Gonadotropin dynamics are abnormal, with loss of pulsatile secretion of luteinizing hormone (LH) secretion, increased LH to follicle-stimulating hormone (FSH) ratios, and elevated LH levels. In many patients, there is concurrent obesity and insulin resistance, further contributing to androgen excess. Both LH and insulin stimulate excessive secretion of ovarian testosterone and androstenedione. Large numbers of small ovarian follicles form, but follicular growth is abnormal and no preovulatory follicles develop. Menstrual abnormalities and infertility are the consequence (see Chapter 112). The ovaries may be normal-sized or enlarged and characteristically contain multiple follicular cysts.

Ovarian hyperthecosis, which may be seen in association with the syndrome of acanthosis nigricans and insulin resistance, and *ovarian tumors*, including arrhenoblastoma and hilar-cell tumors, are capable of causing *virilization* due to excess production of testosterone. The virilized patient will often have testosterone levels exceeding 200 ng/dL.

Adrenal Sources. *Late-onset congenital adrenal hyperplasia* designates a heterogeneous group of mild disorders of cortisol biosynthesis (most commonly partial deficiency of 21-hydroxylase or 3-beta-hydroxydehydrogenase) that are being increasingly recognized as an important cause of adult-onset hirsutism. The enzyme deficiencies lead to production of abnormal amounts of adrenal androgen. These conditions are inherited as an autosomal recessive trait closely linked to the HLA gene. Menstrual abnormalities are noted in conjunction with hirsutism, but clinically significant glucocorticoid deficiency does not occur.

Cushing's syndrome, especially if the underlying cause is an *adrenocortical carcinoma*, may produce virilization. Other causes of Cushing's syndrome are more likely to cause excess hair growth and typical cushingoid features without true virilization.

Androgen excess may accompany *hyperprolactinemia* as prolactin stimulates androgen production, particularly DHEA. Characteristic features are amenorrhea and galactorrhea (see Chapter 113).

Other Etiologies. Hirsute women with normal periods and normal plasma androgens are often labelled as *"idiopathic."* Although initially believed due to overproduction of testosterone, idiopathic disease is now viewed as a condition of enhanced peripheral conversion of testosterone to dihydrotestosterone by increased 5-alpha-reductase activity in hair follicles and skin.

Drugs are another important etiologic class. Most potent are anabolic steroids (methyl testosterone, oxandrolone) used surreptitiously by some women engaged in competitive body-building or athletics. Danazol, used for endometriosis, may also bring on hirsutism. In an occasional patient, oral contraceptives containing androgenic progestogens may stimulate increased hair growth (see Chapter 119), though this is not a frequent side effect. Phenytoin, glucocorticoids, cyclosporine, diazoxide, and minoxidil stimulate hair growth by poorly understood, nonandrogenic mechanisms.

DIFFERENTIAL DIAGNOSIS

The causes of hirsutism can be divided into those that do and do not cause virilization and categorized according to adrenal and ovarian sources of androgen excess (Table 98–1). In a series of 100 outpatients presenting to an endocrine unit for evaluation of true hirsutism, about 75 percent were due to polycystic ovary disease, 15 percent were labelled idiopathic, 3 percent had late-onset congenital adrenal hyperplasia, and the remainder were accounted for by Cushing's disease, ovarian tumor, drugs, or prolactinoma. In addition, some patients with anorexia nervosa report increase in body hair (see Chapter 234), and excessive tweezing (hypertrichosis) may traumatize the hair follicle and cause coarse growth of hair at the site of repeated injury.

Table 98-1. Differential Diagnosis of Hirsutism

CAUSE	MECHANISM
Hirsutism Without Virilization	
Idiopathic	Increased peripheral conversion of androgens
Late-onset congenital adrenal hyperplasia	Adrenal androgen overproduction
Cushing's syndrome (ACTH-induced)	Adrenal androgen overproduction
Polycystic ovary disease	Ovarian androgen overproduction
Insulin resistance/ obesity	Ovarian androgen overproduction
Drugs: anabolic steroids, danazol, minoxidil, phenytoin, diazoxide, glucocorticosteroids	Varies, ranging from direct androgenic activity to nonandrogenic effects
Hirsutism With Virilization	
Ovarian hyperthecosis	Autonomous ovarian androgen production
Ovarian neoplasms	Autonomous ovarian androgen production
Adrenal neoplasms, especially adrenal carcinoma	Autonomous adrenal androgen production

WORKUP

The paramount objective in the evaluation of hirsutism is to identify the women likely to have important underlying endocrine pathology.

History. Symptoms suggestive of serious endocrine disease include those of *virilization* (voice change, temporal hair recession, increased muscle mass, and acne); *rapid progression*, particularly with sudden increase in hair growth after age 25; *amenorrhea* or changes in menstruation; and *galactorrhea*. New onset of *hypertension* in the setting of hirsutism should also raise suspicion. Peripubertal onset of hirsutism is generally reassuring. A detailed *drug history* (anabolic steroids, oral contraceptives, danazol, phenytoin, corticosteroids, minoxidil, cyclosporine, diazoxide) is essential. A *family history* of southern European or Mediterranean ancestry in conjunction with hirsutism of a similar degree in mother, grandmothers, aunts, and sisters reduces the probability of serious pathology. However, a positive family history may also be found in some patients with polycystic ovary disease and partial congenital adrenal hyperplasia.

Physical Examination. It is normal to have terminal hair on the face, about the areolae, and on the lower abdomen, but new growth, especially on the upper abdomen, sternum, upper back, and shoulders suggests androgen excess and hirsutism. Virilization is indicated by temporal and vertical scalp hair loss, deep voice, acne, increase in muscle mass, and clitoromegaly. Cushing's syndrome should be suspected when centripetal obesity, muscle wasting with myopathy, and violaceous striae are encountered. Patients with oligomenorrhea require a pelvic examination for the presence of bilaterally enlarged cystic ovaries; however, a significant number of women with polycystic ovary physiology will not have palpable ovarian abnormalities. Women with virilization and amenorrhea should be examined carefully for a palpable adrenal or ovarian neoplasm. Most of these tumors are inefficient producers of androgens and do not result in high levels of circulating androgens until they become quite large.

Laboratory Studies. An abundance of costly endocrinologic hormonal assays may be performed in the evaluation of hirsutism. To avoid the expense of unnecessary testing, it is important to define the likely diagnostic considerations and the goals of therapy for hirsutism so that appropriate hormonal evaluation may be obtained rather than the indiscriminate measurement of all ovarian and androgen sex steroids and pituitary hormones. On the basis of history and physical examination, patients can be categorized as likely to have idiopathic or familial, oligomenorrheic/amenorrheic, cushingoid, or virilizing forms of disease.

Idiopathic and Familial Forms of Hirsutism. A young woman who complains of a minor increase in facial hair beginning in the peripubertal period yet has perfectly regular ovulatory menses is most likely free of serious underlying pathology and need not undergo detailed testing. The same pertains to the normally menstruating woman of southern European ancestry whose female relatives have similar degrees of facial and body hair.

Oligomenorrheic/Amenorrheic Disease. When amenorrhea or oligomenorrhea, obesity, and hirsutism occur, especially in the context of infertility, polycystic ovary disease needs to be considered. Since pelvic examination may not reveal bilaterally enlarged cystic ovaries, *pelvic ultrasound* and laboratory testing can help to confirm the clinical suspicions. Testosterone, particularly *unbound testosterone*, and *LH:FSH ratios* are increased. Because increased androgens suppress sex-hormone–binding globulin, measurement of unbound or *free serum testosterone* is more valuable than measurement of total testosterone. Free testosterone correlates best with testosterone production rates. Because testosterone secretion is episodic, *three serum samples* taken 15 minutes apart may be pooled for immunoassay.

Patients with menstrual irregularities but no evidence of polycystic disease should be evaluated for a late-onset congenital adrenal hyperplasia (most often 21-hydroxylase [21-OH] deficiency). This condition can be identified by performing an *ACTH stimulation test* and measuring *plasma 17-hydroxyprogesterone* (17-OHP) 30 to 60 minutes after intravenous administration of one ampule (25 μg) of cosyntropin (synthetic ACTH). A pretest 17-OHP level greater than 300 ng/L is suggestive, but many patients have normal levels, necessitating use of ACTH stimulation testing. A posttest level greater than 1200 ng/L at 30 minutes is diagnostic. Although these patients represent a minority of hirsute women, there are no distinguishing clinical features of this entity that set it apart from the more common PCO syndromes. *Prolactin* should be measured in women with oligo- or amenorrhea, especially if there is accompanying galactorrhea.

Cushingoid Appearance. Patients having clinical features of Cushing's syndrome should undergo screening studies with either a *24-hour determination of urinary free cortisol* or *overnight dexamethasone suppression*. Twenty-four hour urinary free cortisol, the more specific study, is greater than 100 μg in Cushing's syndrome. *Urinary 17-ketosteroids* will be elevated in adrenocortical carcinoma. For overnight dexamethasone suppression, the patient is given 1 mg of dexamethasone at midnight, and a plasma cortisol is obtained at approximately 8:00 AM the next day. Cortisol should be suppressed to less than 5 μg/dL. If the urinary free cortisol is elevated, or if suppression of elevated cortisol by dexamethasone fails to occur, more extensive dexamethasone testing to determine the likelihood and etiology of Cushing's syndrome needs to be pursued.

Virilization. When virilization is present, *serum testosterone* and *urinary 17-ketosteroids* should be measured. Serum testosterone will be greater than 200 ng/dL in women with masculinizing ovarian or adrenal neoplasms. Measurement of 17-ketosteroids will detect elevated adrenal androgens, such as androstenedione and dehydroepiandrosterone in adrenal cortical carcinoma. Although both the adrenals and ovaries can biosynthesize all androgenic steroids, the best measurement of adrenal hormonal production is *DHEA sulfate*, with more than 90 percent arising from the adrenal gland. A serum DHEA level greater than 800 μg/dL is strongly suggestive of an adrenal tumor. Androstenedione is biosynthesized equally by adrenal and ovary glands. Patients suspected of harboring one of these tumors require *ultrasound* or *computed tomography (CT) scanning*.

SYMPTOMATIC MANAGEMENT AND PATIENT EDUCATION

Alternative approaches to the management of hirsutism are based on the underlying pathophysiology. They include 1) supportive reassurance that there is no important underlying endocrine disease; 2) cosmetic manipulations such as bleaching, waxing, use of depilatories, and electrolysis; 3) medical therapy with estrogens or glucocorticoids directed at suppressing ovarian and adrenal hormone overproduction; 4) medical therapy directed at antagonizing the action of androgens at the receptor level; and 5) definitive curative therapy of underlying diseases such as Cushing's syndrome or masculinizing ovarian neoplasms.

Supportive Measures and Cosmetic Manipulations. Patients free of significant endocrine pathology can be effectively cared for with the *reassurance* that their hirsutism will not impair sexuality or fertility. If a woman is concerned about her appearance, cosmetic manipulation or medical therapy is appropriate. Hair may be bleached with 6 percent *hydrogen peroxide* solution or commercially available cream bleaches. Shaving removes unwanted hair; however, because hair grows at the rate of 1 mm/d, "stubble" appears within several days. *Epilation* with tweezers or hot wax may retard hair growth for several months but has the risk of low-grade folliculitis. *Chemical depilatories* may require the use of low concentration hydrocortisone topically to prevent irritation. *Electrolysis,* the only permanent method of hair removal, involves electrocoagulation and destruction of the hair root. It is a costly and time-consuming process and should be performed only by a licensed electrologist.

Suppression of Ovarian and Adrenal Androgen Overproduction. *Oral contraceptives* containing estrogen and progestin suppress ovarian and adrenal androgen production by decreasing FSH and LH. In addition, the estrogen increases sex-hormone–binding globulin, competes with the cytosolic receptor for dihydrotestosterone, and limits (along with progestogens) endometrial hyperplasia in hyperandrogenic *PCO* patients. Oral contraceptives also work well for patients with *idiopathic disease*, by reducing the amount of available androgenic substrate. Preparations containing at least 35 μg of ethinyl estradiol or 50 μg of mestranol are needed to reduce androgen levels; those with lower amounts of estrogen are less effective. The least androgenic progestins, such as norethindrone (1 mg) or ethynodiol acetate in combination with mestranol and ethinyl estradiol, are preferred. If androgen and clinical responses to these therapies, determined at 3 months, are inadequate, an oral contraceptive containing higher amounts of estrogen should be used. Side effects of these drugs, including increased risk of thromboembolism in smokers (see Chapter 119), must be reviewed. A decrease in hirsutism is usually not evident for 3 to 6 months; a decrease in the rate of hair growth is noted initially, followed by a transformation to lighter, finer hair.

Glucocorticoids may reduce hirsutism and lead to induction of ovulation in partial *congenital adrenal hyperplasia*, where androgens are of adrenal origin. Adrenal suppression with a concomitant decrease in androgens can best be accomplished by administration of 1 mg of dexamethasone given at bedtime. Potential concerns with this form of therapy are suppression of the hypothalamic–pituitary–adrenal axis and induction of a cushingoid appearance. Alternate-day corticosteroid therapy may suffice and may reduce the risks of such adverse effects. Following changes in the 17-OHP concentration is an effective means of monitoring therapy.

Weight reduction should be part of any program for the obese hirsute woman. Normalization of weight limits peripheral conversion of androstenedione to testosterone by fatty tissue and reduces the hyperinsulinism that may contribute to ovarian production of androgens. Impressive results are achievable.

Antagonizing Testosterone at the Target Tissue. *Spironolactone*, an antihypertensive diuretic, decreases androgen levels by decreasing testosterone biosynthesis as well as antagonizing peripheral action on the hair follicle. Doses as high as 100 mg twice daily have been shown to diminish hirsutism during a 3-month observation interval but may cause menstrual disturbances. One might begin therapy with 50 mg twice daily, given from the 4th through the 22nd day of each menstrual cycle. The drug is teratogenic and should not be used in large doses in women of child-bearing age. It is often given as an adjunct to oral contraceptives in patients with severe PCO.

Cimetidine, a histamine-2 receptor antagonist, competes with androgens for target tissue binding; it appears to be less effective than spironolactone.

Flutamide, a selective androgen receptor antagonist, and *finasteride,* a 5α reductase inhibitor, offer improved blockade of testosterone action at the target tissue. Studies are ongoing.

INDICATIONS FOR REFERRAL

Patients with virilization and elevated testosterone levels require evaluation by an endocrinologist and gynecologist, since a virilizing tumor may be present. If polycystic ovary syndrome is present and if infertility is an issue, referral for clomiphene therapy and evaluation for endometrial hyperplasia by endometrial biopsy is appropriate. Hyperprolactinemia necessitates coronal CT or magnetic resonance imaging scanning to recognize a prolactinoma or pathologic process interrupting dopaminergic inhibition of prolactin. Patients with Cushing's syndrome should be referred for endocrinologic ascertainment of its pituitary, adrenal, or ectopic ACTH origin.

ANNOTATED BIBLIOGRAPHY

Barnes R, Rosenfield RL. The polycystic ovary syndrome: pathogenesis and treatment. Ann Intern Med 1989;110:386. *(Comprehensive review of disease mechanisms, including loss of LH pulsatility, and treatment modalities based on them.)*

Cumming D, Yang JC, Rebar RW, et al. Treatment of hirsutism with spironolactone. JAMA 1984;247:1295. *(A study of 39 patients; responses observed as early as 2 months; side effects limited.)*

Ehrmann DA, Rosenfield RL. Hirsutism—beyond the steroidogenic block. N Engl J Med 1990;323:909. *(An editorial summarizing current knowledge and focusing on late-onset congenital adrenal hyperplasia.)*

Eldar-Geva T, Hurwitz A, Vecsei P, et al. Secondary biosynthetic defects in women with late-onset congenital adrenal hyperplasia. N Engl J Med 1990;323:855. *(High incidence of the condition found among Israeli women with hirsutism, menstrual disorders, and unexplained infertility; mechanisms examined.)*

Rittmaster RS, Loriaux DL. Hirsutism. Ann Intern Med 1987; 106:95. *(Very useful review, with detailed discussion of idiopathic disease; exhaustively referenced with 246 citations.)*

Siegel SF, Finegold DN, Lanes R, et al. ACTH stimulation tests and plasma dehydroepiandrosterone sulfate levels in women with hirsutism. N Engl J Med 1990;323:849. *(Basal levels were unrevealing, but those measured after ACTH testing differentiated normals from many of those with hirsutism.)*

Vigersky RA, Hehlman I, Glass AR, et al. Treatment of hirsute women with cimetidine. N Engl J Med 1980;303:1042. *(Cimetidine produced a decrease in rate of hair growth without a decrease in serum androgen.)*

Wagner RF Jr. Physical methods for the management of hirsutism. Cutis 1990;45:319. *(Useful information for advising patients.)*

Primary Care Medicine: Office Evaluation and Management of the Adult Patient, 3rd edition, edited by Allan H. Goroll, Lawrence A. May, and Albert G. Mulley, Jr. J.B. Lippincott Company, Philadelphia

99
Evaluation of Gynecomastia

Gynecomastia is defined as enlargement of the male breast due to increase in glandular tissue, which distinguishes it from simple obesity. Some patients present out of fear of loss of masculinity or onset of breast cancer. Others may not have recognized the change and come to the physician at the suggestion of friends or family. Gynecomastia is a normal transient physiologic event in 70 percent of pubertal boys; its prevalence in adults is less than 1 percent. The primary physician must be able to recognize gynecomastia and initiate an evaluation to rule out such important potential causes as adrenal and testicular cancers, cirrhosis, and hyperthyroidism. In most instances the etiology is more benign and the tasks are to allay fears and help the patient decide about treatment.

PATHOPHYSIOLOGY AND CLINICAL PRESENTATION

Pathophysiology. *Estradiol* is the growth hormone of the breast. Gynecomastia represents a phenomenon of relative estradiol excess, leading to breast tissue proliferation. Under normal circumstances most estradiol in men is derived from peripheral conversion of testosterone and adrenal estrone. The basic mechanisms of gynecomastia are a decrease in androgen production, an absolute increase in estrogen production, and increased availability of estrogen precursors for peripheral conversion to estradiol. Androgen-receptor blocking and increased androgen-binding are additional modes of reduced androgen effect.

Reduced androgen production accounts for many cases seen in older men, as well as those occurring from testicular endocrine failure, as in bilateral orchiectomy and other forms of cancer therapy. Ketoconazole inhibits testosterone production in a dose-related manner. *Reduced androgen availability* occurs in both hyperthyroidism and cirrhosis due to an increase in the serum concentration of sex-hormone–binding globulin. *Blockade of the androgen receptor* accounts for the gynecomastia associated with use of spironolactone, cimetidine, flutamide, and perhaps marijuana. *Increased estrogen production* may be seen with Klinefelter's syndrome, adrenal carcinomas, tumors producing ectopic human chorionic gonadotropin (hCG), and Leydig cell tumors of the testes. hCG-producing tumors stimulate testicular production of estradiol. Teratomas of the testes and carcinomas of the lung, pancreas, and colon are known sources of ectopic hCG. The transient gynecomastia of puberty represents a brief physiologic increase in testicular estrogen secretion and lasts 1 to 2 years before receding.

Increased estrogen precursor availability is the mechanism of gynecomastia in patients with androgen-secreting tumors, congestive heart failure, and exogenous androgen use, leading to increased conversion of testosterone and androstenedione to estradiol and estrone. Hyperthyroidism causes *increased peripheral conversion*. Much of the conversion takes place in fatty tissue. *Exogenous estrogen effect* is seen with digitalis use as well as with synthetic estrogens. *Release of free estrogen* by displacement from sex-hormone–

binding globulin occurs with ketoconazole and spironolactone.

Clinical Presentations. The most noticeable feature is an increase in breast tissue, being unilateral in a third of cases. Tenderness may also be noted in a third of patients, but actual pain is less frequent. Enlargement is usually central and symmetrical, though it is occasionally eccentric. Idiopathic and drug-induced gynecomastias are usually unilateral, while pubertal and hormonal etiologies often cause bilateral change. It may be that asymmetry is a more accurate description than unilateral enlargement, judging from the prevalence of bilaterally histologic but not clinically evident gynecomastia in autopsy series.

There are a few distinctive clinical presentations. In *Klinefelter's syndrome*, gynecomastia develops around puberty in a patient with long limbs, small, firm testes, infertility, and normal or deficient secondary sex features. In cirrhosis, patients present with loss of libido, loss of body hair, and testicular atrophy (see Chapter 71).

Recovery from *malnutrition* or *serious chronic illnesses* (severe heart failure, renal failure, liver failure) will lead to a picture resembling a second puberty, with development of transient gynecomastia.

Carcinoma of the male breast is distinct from gynecomastia; it is characterized by a unilateral, eccentrically located firm mass that may be fixed. Male breast cancer is rare; it is generally not more frequent in patients with gynecomastia, though there is a higher incidence in Klinefelter's syndrome.

DIFFERENTIAL DIAGNOSIS

In healthy pubertal males, the most likely cause is transient physiologic gynecomastia (Table 99–1). Testicular or adrenal tumors are rare in this age group, but Klinefelter's syndrome may account for a number of cases.

The two most common causes of gynecomastia in adults are drugs and alcohol-related liver disease. Estrogens, androgens, spironolactone, digitalis preparations, flutamide, ketoconazole, cimetidine, and marijuana have all been associated with gynecomastia. The association also exists but is more tenuous with use of phenothiazines, amphetamines, reserpine, methyldopa, isoniazid, imipramine, phenytoin, and heroin. In one series, 22 percent of patients had a history of taking a drug associated with gynecomastia, and 26 percent had alcoholic liver disease.

Less common causes include recovery from malnutrition or a serious chronic illness. Much rarer forms are tumor-related ectopic hCG production and feminizing adrenal, testicular, and pituitary tumors. In just under 10 percent of cases, a probable cause is not identified. Gynecomastia must be distinguished from carcinoma of the male breast.

Table 99-1. Differential Diagnosis of Gynecomastia

Inhibition of Androgen Effect
Spironolactone (at high doses only)
Cimetidine (common at high doses)
Flutamide
Decreased Androgen Availability Due to Increased Binding or Conversion
Cirrhosis (very common)
Hyperthyroidism (uncommon, except with thyrotoxicosis)
Decreased Androgen Synthesis
Testicular failure, primary (Klinefelter's syndrome) or secondary (orchiectomy, cancer drugs, ketoconazole)
Increased Estrogen Synthesis or Estrogen Effect
Estrogen-secreting tumor of the testes or adrenal gland (very rare)
Klinefelter's syndrome (about 15% of pubertal cases)
Ectopic hCG-secreting tumor of testes, lung, colon, pancreas (rare)
Digitalis (uncommon)
Exogenous estrogen (dose-related)
Increased Availability of Estrogen Substrate
Androgen-producing tumor (rare)
Exogenous androgen (common)
Congestive heart failure (common)
Physiologic
Puberty
Recovery from chronic illness or starvation
Old age

WORKUP

History. Onset, location, duration, and course deserve note. The most important aspect is a detailed inquiry into drug use, including chronic alcohol consumption, cimetidine, spironolactone, flutamide, digitalis, ketoconazole, or exogenous estrogens or androgens. Any symptoms of hyperthyroidism (see Chapter 103), heart failure (see Chapter 32), or hepatocellular failure (see Chapter 71) should be noted, as should resolution of a chronic illness and changes in libido, skin, voice, testicles, and hair quality and distribution. Any weight loss, chronic cough, hemoptysis, change in bowel habits, recovery from chronic illness, headaches, or visual field disturbances could be an important etiologic clue.

Physical Examination. Onset at puberty should trigger an examination for features of Klinefelter's syndrome (arm span greater than height, small firm testes, absence of secondary sex characteristics). In adults, one needs to look at the skin for signs of hepatocellular failure (jaundice, spider angiomata, ecchymoses, pallor, palmar erythema) and hyperthyroidism (warm, sweaty skin; fine hair). The eyes are checked for exophthalmus, and the neck is palpated for goiter.

The breast examination requires distinguishing the glandular texture of true gynecomastia from the fatty consistency of breast enlargement related to obesity and the nodularity of a carcinoma. Asymmetry and nodules deserve special note and careful palpation of the axillary nodes. The question of malignancy in the breast tissue must always be considered in gynecomastia. If the enlargement is unilateral and eccentric, the breast particularly firm or nodular, or axillary adenopathy present, then biopsy should be performed.

On cardiopulmonary examination, one checks for signs of heart failure (see Chapter 32), and on abdominal examination for signs of cirrhosis (see Chapter 71). The abdomen must be palpated for masses and the stool tested for occult blood. The testicles are examined for atrophy and nodules. The presence of a testicular nodule requires workup for a carcinoma (see Chapter 131).

Laboratory Studies. Gynecomastia not due to puberty, drugs, hyperthyroidism, hepatocellular failure, or another obvious cause requires further evaluation. Laboratory testing ought to begin with measurement of *serum gonadotropins (luteinizing hormone* [*LH*], *follicle-stimulating hormone* [*FSH*]).

High concentrations are consistent with testicular failure, Klinefelter's syndrome, and hCG-secreting tumors. Ectopic hCG production can be identified by finding elevated *serum beta-hCG subuinit* levels. This should trigger a search for the source of the ectopic gonadotropin production (see Chapter 92). To check for Klinefelter's syndrome, a buccal smear is obtained and examined for chromatin positivity (Barr bodies). If negative, the diagnosis is most likely primary testicular failure or a chromatin-negative variant of Klinefelter's syndrome.

Low gonadotropin concentrations are more worrisome, because they raise the question of autonomous androgen or estrogen production (as well as exogenous sex steroid use). Requestioning the patient regarding exogenous steroid use is critical. If the patient's responses are convincingly negative, then *free testosterone* and *estradiol* levels should be obtained, but with full cognizance of the pitfalls in their interpretation. For example, total testosterone may be affected by the concentration of sex-hormone–binding protein and not reflect the free testosterone concentration. Consequently, free testosterone must be measured. However, testosterone secretion can fluctuate greatly, necessitating the pooling of three samples obtained over 15 minutes for best results. The estradiol concentration measured may correlate poorly with the rate of estrogen production due to vagaries in peripheral uptake. Thus, normal levels do not necessarily rule out an estrogen-secreting tumor, though marked elevations are very suggestive, provided exogenous use has been ruled out. If serum estrogens are elevated, then adrenal cancer and Leydig's cell tumor of the testes should be ruled out.

Normal gonadotropin and *sex hormone levels* make serious underlying endocrinopathy unlikely and can be followed expectantly with periodic reevaluation. It is important to keep in mind that resolution of gynecomastia may trail resolution of the condition that caused it. The search for an etiology may yield few clues if the cause was transient and self-limited.

SYMPTOMATIC MANAGEMENT, PATIENT EDUCATION, AND INDICATIONS FOR REFERRAL

Removal of the offending drug usually produces regression of breast enlargement within a month or two. Gynecomastia that accompanies puberty or refeeding after starvation is a transient phenomenon that can be managed by providing reassurance. Treatment of hyperthyroidism will usually improve gynecomastia. Gynecomastia attributable to alcoholic liver disease or Klinefelter's syndrome is not likely to respond to any treatment. When hCG-secreting tumors are discovered, resection of the tumor is indicated if possible.

The persistence of gynecomastia may produce cosmetic problems. Patients who are considerably bothered by breast enlargement may elect to undergo *mastectomy*, but this should be accomplished only after the etiology has been elucidated. Experimental use of the antiestrogen *tamoxifen* has been useful in reducing breast size in patients with painful gynecomastia.

When a benign etiology such as drug-induced gynecomastia is discovered, it is comforting to reassure the patient that the condition is not a reflection of loss of maleness or a carcinomatous process. It must be remembered that some conditions that produce gynecomastia may reduce potency; this situation must be confronted and discussed with the patient. There is no evidence of carcinomatous degeneration in gynecomastia except in Klinefelter's syndrome. Pain, irritation, or social problems that may arise should be dealt with symptomatically and sympathetically.

Consultation with an endocrinologist is essential when a case of Klinefelter's syndrome is suspected, and also when ectopic hCG production is a concern or autonomous sex-hormone production is under consideration (low gonadotropin levels). Referral is also indicated when treatment of gynecomastia is being considered, be it medical therapy or surgery.

A.H.G.

ANNOTATED BIBLIOGRAPHY

Bannagan GA, Hajdu SI. Gynecomastia: clinicopathologic study of 351 cases. Am J Clin Pathol 1972;57:431. *(Idiopathic and drug-induced gynecomastias are usually discrete and unilateral, while endocrine and pubertal gynecomastias are bilateral.)*

Braunstein GD. Gynecomastia. N Engl J Med 1993;328:490. *(Comprehensive review of both pathogenesis and clinical issues.)*

Braunstein GD, Vaitukaitis JL, Carbone PP, et al. Ectopic production of human chorionic gonadotropin by neoplasms. Ann Intern Med 1973;78:39. *(One of the original reports of ectopic hCG production.)*

Cavanaugh J, Niewoehner CB, Nutall FQ. Gynecomastia and cirrhosis of the liver. Arch Intern Med 1990;150:563. *(Factors other than estrogen-testosterone ratio operative.)*

Courtiss EH. Gynecomastia: Analysis of 159 patients and current recommendations for treatment. Plast Reconstr Surg 1987; 79:740. *(The view from the plastic surgeon's perspective.)*

Feldman D. Ketoconazole and other imidazole derivatives as inhibitors of steroidogenesis. Endocr Rev 1986;7:409. *(Detailed discussion of the effects of this important class of drugs on testosterone production.)*

Jensen RT, Collen MJ, Pandol HD. Cimetidine-induced impotence and breast changes in patients with gastric hypersecretory states. N Engl J Med 1983;308:883. *(A side effect of high-dose, chronic therapy; resolves with cessation of cimetidine therapy.)*

Parker LN, Gray DR, Lai MK, et al. Treatment of gynecomastia with tamoxifen: a double-blind, crossover study. Metabolism 1986;35:705. *(An study of medical therapy for painful gynecomastia using an antiestrogen; benefit obtained.)*

Wilson JD. Gynecomastia: a continuing diagnostic dilemma. N Engl J Med 1991;324:334. *(An editorial emphasizing the difficulties in its evaluation.)*

100
Evaluating Galactorrhea and Hyperprolactinemia

Primary Care Medicine: Office Evaluation and Management of the Adult Patient, 3rd edition, edited by Allan H. Goroll, Lawrence A. May, and Albert G. Mulley, Jr. J.B. Lippincott Company, Philadelphia

Discharge of milk or colostrum from the breast in the absence of nursing is referred to as galactorrhea. When it is accompanied by disturbed menses or infertility, it suggests the possibility of hyperprolactinemia and the associated risk of pituitary neoplasm. Patients presenting with galactorrhea need careful consideration of underlying pituitary pathology.

PATHOPHYSIOLOGY AND CLINICAL PRESENTATION

Galactorrhea. Normal milk production involves the interplay of prolactin and a breast primed by estrogen and progestin. Prolactin secretion is under hypothalamic control, mediated by inhibitory dopaminergic transmission. Other hormones (eg, thyroxine, insulin) are thought to play supporting roles in facilitation of lactation. Galactorrhea can occur in the setting of a normal or elevated serum prolactin. The normal range for serum prolactin is 1 to 20 ng/mL.

Normoprolactinemic galactorrhea is believed to be a consequence of local breast stimulation or irritation in women with hormonally primed breast tissue. It is hypothesized that the breast stimulation may cause a mild transient elevation in prolactin secretion, though not a sustained one. Many cases are associated with a distant pregnancy or use of oral contraceptives. Gonadal function is preserved, with menses and fertility remaining normal. Galactorrhea in the absence of sustained hyperprolactinemia is usually noted as an isolated symptom or an incidental finding on breast examination.

Hyperprolactinemic galactorrhea develops as a consequence of excessive prolactin production, either from loss of hypothalamic inhibition of lactotrophic cells in the anterior pituitary or from development of an autonomously functioning pituitary adenoma. In rare instances, hyperprolactinemia results from decreased clearance of prolactin (as in renal failure). Even in the context of high prolactin levels, galactorrhea does not occur unless the breast is primed by estrogen, accounting for its rarity in men. Amenorrhea is a common accompaniment, caused by high prolactin levels suppressing secretion of hypothalamic gonadotropin releasing hormone (GnRH).

Hyperprolactinemia. Very high serum concentrations of prolactin are associated with autonomously functioning *prolactinomas* derived from lactotrophic cells of the anterior pituitary. The degree of hyperprolactinemia tends to correlate with tumor size. Prolactinomas greater than 10 mm in diameter ("macroadenomas") are associated with extremely high prolactin levels (>1000 ng/mL). Excluding pregnancy, serum prolactin in excess of 300 ng/mL is almost always the result of a prolactinoma. Microadenomas (<10 mm in diameter) may produce less impressive elevations.

Moderate degrees of hyperprolactinemia are characteristic of conditions which interfere with hypothalamic control of the anterior pituitary. In a study of 235 nonpregnant patients with galactorrhea, only 57 percent of those with values above 100 ng/mL had a functioning pituitary tumor; the remainder had a problem which compromised hypothalamic inhibition. Interruption of hypothalamic inhibition can occur with use of a centrally active *dopaminergic blocking agent* (eg, a phenothiazine), with *anatomic interference* by a sellar or suprasellar mass, and with *hypothyroidism* causing thyrotropin releasing hormone (TRH) stimulation of anterior pituitary lactotrophic cells. Transient prolactin elevations have been observed in patients undergoing emotional stress, physical trauma, and nipple stimulation.

Because patients with hyperprolactinemia are at risk for hypogonadism, they may experience, in addition to galactorrhea, disturbed menses, amenorrhea, infertility, and osteoporosis. In hyperprolactinemic men, galactorrhea is rare, but *impotence* is common. Those with a substantially enlarging sellar mass may complain of *headache* or a *visual field cut*.

DIFFERENTIAL DIAGNOSIS

The differential diagnosis of galactorrhea can be organized according to whether prolactin is elevated or not and according to whether an elevation in prolactin is due to decreased hypothalamic inhibition or overproduction by a functioning adenoma (Table 100–1). Only 20 percent of patients with galactorrhea have hyperprolactinemia. In patients with galactorrhea, amenorrhea, and hyperprolactinemia, prolactinoma is a leading cause. Other pituitary-area etiologies include empty sella syndrome, craniopharyngi-

Table 100-1. Differential Diagnosis of Galactorrhea

Normoprolactinemic Galactorrhea
- Local breast stimulation/irritation (suckling, trauma, inflammation)
- Oral contraceptive use
- Recent pregnancy
- Idiopathic (? transient elevation in prolactin from stress, breast stimulation)

Hyperprolactinemic Galactorrhea
- Impairment of hypothalamic pituitary inhibition
  - Drugs (phenothiazines, metoclopramide, heroin, reserpine, methyldopa, haloperidol)
  - Lesions of the pituitary stalk (nonfunctioning sellar tumors, infarction)
  - Hypothalamic disease (craniopharyngioma, infiltrative disease, infarction)
- Overproduction by a pituitary adenoma
  - Prolactinoma
  - Hypothyroidism (simulates adenoma by TRH stimulation of lactotroph cells)
- Idiopathic
  - ? Microadenoma not detectible by neuroimaging
  - ? Stress, trauma, breast stimulation

oma, pinealoma, and parasellar sarcoidosis. Nonprolactinomic pathology about and within the pituitary accounts for about one-third of patients with galactorrhea and amenorrhea. Persistent galactorrhea after childbirth accounts for just under 10 percent of cases. Drugs associated with galactorrhea include oral contraceptives and agents with central dopaminergic blocking activity (phenothiazines, haloperidol, metoclopramide) and, less commonly, reserpine, methyldopa, isoniazid, and imipramine.

WORKUP

History and Physical Examination. The workup for galactorrhea should include careful questioning about menstrual pattern, recent pregnancy, infertility, medications, change in libido, symptoms of hypothyroidism (see Chapter 104), breast stimulation, chest trauma, and presence of headache or visual complaints. A careful review of drug use, particularly oral contraceptives and drugs that block central dopaminergic transmission (see above), needs to be pursued. Physical examination ought to include detailed examination of the breasts to be sure the discharge is indeed milky and not due to local breast pathology, although no increased risk of breast cancer has been found in patients with true galactorrhea. Confrontation testing of the visual fields and funduscopic examination are important, though usually normal. Any signs of hypothyroidism (see Chapter 104) should be noted and then confirmed by obtaining a TSH.

Laboratory Testing. The development of accurate prolactin assays and the association of galactorrhea with high prolactin levels and pituitary tumors have made determination of the *serum prolactin concentration* an essential part of the diagnostic evaluation. However, caution is warranted in obtaining and interpreting a prolactin level. Prolactin concentration may be transiently elevated by stress, time of day, sleep, meals, or breast stimulation. Accuracy is enhanced by placing a catheter in the patient's vein and having the patient rest in a recumbent position for an hour before sample is drawn. The morning is the best time. The patient with galactorrhea and amenorrhea is at increased risk for a pituitary neoplasm and must be prolactin-tested unless there is an obvious explanation for both (eg, recent pregnancy, medication).

Patients with galactorrhea, menstrual irregularities, and an otherwise unexplained elevation in serum prolactin should undergo neuroimaging of the sellar region. *Magnetic resonance imaging (MRI) with gadolinium* enhancement is procedure of choice, though *computed tomography (CT)* is a reasonable alternative if MRI is unavailable. Gadolinium enhances MRI imaging of sellar structures by taking advantage of the differences in vascularity between normal pituitary tissue and adenomas. Nonetheless, microadenomas can be difficult to detect, although the absence of a visible lesion rules out an anatomically threatening neoplasm. Even patients with modest unexplained prolactin elevations (less than 200 ng/mL) should undergo neuroimaging of the pituitary region, because another type of sellar or parasellar mass could be responsible for the mild elevation. Finding a lesion in excess of 10 mm in a patient with a modest rise in prolactin necessitates consideration of other types of pituitary tumors. The prolactin rise is likely to represent compression of the pituitary stalk.

Formal visual field testing should be performed in all patients with a sellar mass or visual symptoms.

From a practical standpoint, regular menses and a normal prolactin level in a patient with galactorrhea make the likelihood of a clinically important pituitary tumor remote. Patients in whom the likelihood of tumor is low can be followed carefully with periodic determinations of prolactin, usually at 1-year intervals; if prolactin levels become elevated, neuroimaging of the sella can be pursued.

SYMPTOMATIC MANAGEMENT

No Evidence of a Mass Lesion. Patients with normal periods and normal prolactin levels need no treatment. They can be reassured and followed. Patients with galactorrhea secondary to use of a dopaminergic blocking agent can be tried on a reduced dose of the drug, though full cessation may be necessary to terminate symptoms. If hypothyroidism is the contributing factor, it should be corrected (see Chapter 104). Symptomatic patients with *idiopathic disease* (galactorrhea, abnormal periods, elevated prolactin, normal MRI, no other pathology evident) who wish an end to their symptoms can be treated as if they have a microadenoma (see below).

Prolactinoma. Treatment approach depends on the size of the lesion and its natural history. *Microadenomas* (less than 10 mm in diameter) have an excellent prognosis. Long-term studies of untreated patients demonstrate that 80 percent to 90 percent of microadenomas stay the same size or regress over time, with only 10 percent to 20 percent continuing to grow. Prolactin levels follow a similar pattern. However, among those microadenomas that grow, there may not be a close correlation between tumor size and prolactin level, necessitating close monitoring of both parameters.

Despite the favorable prognosis, many patients with stable microadenomas may be bothered by menstrual irregularities, severe galactorrhea, and infertility. As noted earlier, osteoporosis is also a risk. The treatment of choice for such symptomatic patients is the dopaminergic agonist *bromocriptine*. The drug inhibits prolactin synthesis, secretion, and cellular proliferation. In many instances, prolactin levels return to normal, galactorrhea ceases, tumor size decreases, menses resume as gonadal function returns, and osteoporosis recedes. For control of symptoms, continuous bromocriptine administration is required, though some patients will undergo spontaneous regression. A 2-year course of treatment followed by a trial of cessation is a common approach to bromocriptine therapy for patients with a symptomatic microadenoma. Doses needed to control symptoms range from 2.5 to 10 mg/d, though smaller doses often suffice for maintenance. Dopaminergic agonists with fewer side effects are under development.

Macroadenomas are also treated initially with *bromocriptine*. In many instances, the drug suffices to control symptoms and shrink the adenoma. Doses needed to establish control range from 5 to 20 mg/d. Tumor size and prolactin concentration decline substantially. Lower doses (0.625–10 mg/d) are effective for maintenance. Indefinite treatment is the rule, because spontaneous regression is rare. *Surgery* is reserved for patients with rapid progression of visual loss or refractoriness to bromocriptine therapy. Because there is a high recurrence rate with surgery, its use is limited. *Radiation therapy* is sometimes considered.

PATIENT EDUCATION AND INDICATIONS FOR REFERRAL

Patients with pituitary adenomas understandably worry about further tumor growth. Concern can be lessened by explaining the very favorable prognosis for the vast majority of microadenomas and the excellent response of most prolactinomas to bromocriptine. The patient with galactorrhea and amenorrhea should be informed that numerous options for induction of fertility are available and that these may be pursued according to the patient's wishes. By providing accurate information, moral support, and close follow-up, the primary physician can prevent a great deal of unnecessary concern.

Although the basic evaluation of galactorrhea and hyperprolactinoma can be effectively carried out by the primary physician, a consultation with the endocrinologist is indicated in a number of situations (eg, macroadenoma, suspected pituitary neoplasm other than prolactinoma, failure to respond to bromocriptine, visual loss, desire to become pregnant).

A.H.G.

ANNOTATED BIBLIOGRAPHY

Dalkin AC, Marshall JC. Medical therapy of hyperprolactinemia. Endocrinol Metab Clin North Am 1989;18:259. *(Comprehensive review with particularly detailed and useful section on use of bromocriptine.)*

Fish LH, Mariash CN. Hyperprolactinemia, infertility, and hypothyroidism. A case report and review of the literature. Arch Intern Med 1988;148:709. *(Makes the important observation that hypothyroidism may mimic prolactinoma.)*

Hooper JH, Welsh VC, Shackleford RT. Abnormal lactation associated with tranquilizing drug therapy. JAMA 1961;178:506. *(Abnormal lactation occurred in 26 of 100 women receiving major tranquilizers; the effect was dose-dependent.)*

Kleinberg DL, Noel GL, Frantz AA. Galactorrhea: a study of 235 cases, including 48 pituitary tumors. N Engl J Med 1977; 296:589. *(One of the largest reported series; 34 percent had concurrent amenorrhea; 32 percent had idiopathic galactorrhea without amenorrhea.)*

Klibanski A, Biller BMK, Rosenthal DI, et al. Effects of prolactin and estrogen deficiency in amenorrheic bone loss. J Clin Endocrinol Metab 1988:67:124. *(Bone loss results from prolactin-induced hypogonadism.)*

Koppelman MC, Jaffe MJ, Rieth KG, et al. Hyperprolactinemia, amenorrhea and galactorrhea. Ann Intern Med 1984;100:115. *(Most untreated patients experienced either no growth or spontaneous regression, with resumption of menses in some.)*

Liuzzi A, Dallabonzana D, Oppizzi G, et al. Low doses of dopamine agonists in the long-term treatment of macroprolactinomas. N Engl J Med 1985;313:656. *(Efficacy of low maintenance doses demonstrated, but therapy could not be halted.)*

Newton DR, Dillon WP, Norman D, et al. Gd-DTPA-enhanced MR imaging of pituitary adenoma. Am J Neuroradiol 1989; 10:949. *(Data on efficacy of the gadolinium-enhanced MRI for imaging of pituitary adenomas.)*

Pellegrini I, Rasolonjanahary R, Gunz G, et al. Resistance to bromocriptine in prolactinoma. J Clin Endocrinol Metab 1989;69: 500. *(Mechanisms of resistance reviewed and need to monitor therapy carefully emphasized.)*

Schlechte J, Dolan K, Sherman B, et al. The natural history of untreated hyperprolactinemia: a prospective analysis. J Clin Endocrinol Metab 1989;68:412. *(Of 30 patients, six had resumption of normal periods, normal prolactin levels, and resolution of the prolactinoma.)*

101
Evaluation for Suspected Diabetes Insipidus

Primary Care Medicine: Office Evaluation and Management of the Adult Patient, 3rd edition, edited by Allan H. Goroll, Lawrence A. May, and Albert G. Mulley, Jr. J.B. Lippincott Company, Philadelphia

When faced with a patient complaining of polyuria and polydipsia, the primary care physician needs to include diabetes insipidus (DI) in the differential diagnosis. DI is characterized clinically by the excretion of large volumes of inappropriately dilute urine. Although uncommon, DI may be a manifestation of important hypothalamic–pituitary pathology or renal tubular dysfunction. The primary care physician needs to know how to screen for DI in the patient who presents with polyuria and polydipsia and how to proceed with the basic elements of the diagnostic investigation.

PATHOPHYSIOLOGY AND CLINICAL PRESENTATION

Plasma osmolality is carefully regulated to maintain a level of 285 to 290 mOsm/kg. Any increase much above 290 mOsm/kg stimulates hypothalamic osmoreceptors, leading to release of *antidiuretic hormone (ADH, vasopressin)* from the posterior pituitary. ADH increases renal distal tubular permeability to water, resulting in enhanced water resorption. Osmoreceptor stimulation also triggers *central thirst mechanisms*. These actions serve to reestablish normal serum osmolality. A lesion in any portion of this osmoregulatory system can result in DI and its attendant water diuresis. Dehydration and hypertonicity may ensue, unless the thirst mechanism remains intact and there is access to adequate water.

Central or neurogenic DI occurs in the context of an injury to the hypothalamus or posterior pituitary. Mechanisms of central DI include idiopathic degeneration of vasopressin-secreting neurones, destruction by malignant or granulomatous disease, vascular insult, and pituitary surgery. Since the thirst center resides near the hypothalamic osmoreceptors, it too many be involved, though in many cases thirst is preserved and dehydration avoided. Anterior pituitary adenomas usually do not cause DI unless they extend posteriorly or beyond the sella.

Nephrogenic DI results from conditions or medications that damage renal tubulointerstitial function and concentrating ability (eg, hypercalcemia, hypokalemia, sickle cell disease, lithium, obstruction, pyelonephritis). ADH levels are appropriate, but renal response is impaired.

Primary polydipsia also produces polyuria, but unlike DI, the condition appears to originate with altered thirst perception. It is particularly prevalent among patients with chronic psychiatric disturbances (especially schizophrenia) but is also seen with organic brain disease (eg, multiple sclerosis). Detailed study of such patients has revealed multiple defects in osmoregulation, including problems with urinary dilution, osmoregulation of water intake, and ADH secretion. Hyponatremia may ensue.

Clinical Presentation. *Diabetes insipidus* is characterized clinically by excretion of large volumes of dilute urine in conjunction with thirst and polydipsia. A true polyuria occurs, defined as excretion of more than 3 L/24 h. Craving for ice water is common (especially with central DI). The urine is almost always colorless, even in the morning, due to its dilute nature. Urine osmolality is inappropriately low (<250 mOsm/kg). Nocturia is common. Serum osmolality may be increased, especially if the thirst mechanism is impaired.

In *primary polydipsias*, increased thirst and fluid intake are followed by polyuria, though some patients may hide this behavior. The serum osmolality may fall (<285 mOsm/kg) and may be accompanied by hyponatremia. Symptoms tend to be episodic.

DIFFERENTIAL DIAGNOSIS

The differential diagnosis for patients with polyuria/polydipsia in the outpatient setting includes *diabetes mellitus* (see Chapter 104), *diuretic use, diabetes insipidus*, and *primary polydipsia*. The differential can be organized according to 1) whether the diuresis is due to water or solute; 2) if due to water, whether it is due to DI or primary polydipsia; and 3) if due to DI, whether it is central or nephrogenic (Table 101–1). Other causes of urinary frequency unaccompanied by polydipsia (eg, *urinary tract infection, bladder dysfunction*) need to be ruled out (see Chapters 133, 134, and 140).

WORKUP

The initial diagnostic evaluation of the patient complaining of polyuria can proceed logically and efficiently by addressing a set of basic questions:

Is This True Polyuria or Just Urinary Frequency? A history of frequently voiding large volumes of dilute (colorless or pale) urine, both day and night, suggests true polyuria, whereas frequent voiding of small volumes of concentrated urine is indicative of bladder dysfunction due to infection or other local pathology. A *24-hour urine collection* provides objective confirmation of true polyuria when the volume exceeds 3 liters.

Table 101-1. Differential Diagnosis of Polyuria/Polydipsia in the Outpatient Setting

Solute Diuresis
Diabetes mellitus
Diuretics
Water Diuresis
Diabetes insipidus
Central
Idiopathic
Trauma
Tumor (local or metastatic to the sellar region)
Granulomatous disease (sarcoidosis, TB)
Postsurgical (removal of pituitary adenoma)
Vascular (Sheehan's syndrome, old stroke)
Nephrogenic
Drugs (lithium, demeclocycline, amphotericin)
Tubulointerstitial disease (pyelonephritis, polycystic kidney disease, sickle cell disease, obstructive uropathy)
Metabolic (hypercalcemia, hypokalemia)
Primary polydipsias
Psychogenic (schizophrenia)
CNS disease (multiple sclerosis)
Idiopathic

If True Polyuria, Is This a Water Diuresis or a Solute Diuresis? Measurement of the *urine osmolality* is very helpful. Those with a concentrated urine (>350 mOsm/kg) have a condition causing a solute diuresis. Those with a dilute urine (<250 mOsm/kg) suffer from a water diuresis. Patients with a urine osmolality falling between these levels may have either. To differentiate, one calculates the *total solute excretion* (urine volume/d × average urine concentration). If it is less than 1200 mOsm/d, then a water diuresis is likely. If a solute diuresis is suspected, checking the urine for glucose and electrolytes can be confirmatory.

If a Water Diuresis, Is This DI or Primary Polydipsia? Measurement of the *serum osmolality* can be helpful. If it is clearly elevated, it suggests DI, although many DI patients with an intact thirst mechanism and access to water will have a serum osmolality close to normal. If it is low, it suggests primary polydipsia. Direct measurement of serum ADH would help clarify the situation, but reliable assays are not yet widely available. Very low levels would occur with central DI; very high levels would indicate renal DI; inappropriately elevated levels would suggest primary polydipsia.

The clinical context may help suggest the etiology of the water diuresis. When it occurs in the setting of known renal tubulointerstitial disease or drug use, nephrogenic DI is the likely etiology. A central mechanism is suggested when the patient presents with other manifestations of pituitary disease or has a condition which may cause central nervous system damage (eg, cancer, granulomatous disease). Onset in a patient with mental illness raises the probability of primary polydipsia.

When the cause remains uncertain and in the absence of a reliable measure of ADH, it may be necessary to admit the patient for a *trial* of *desmovasopressin (DDAVP)*, an ADH analogue. The response to DDAVP helps clarify the underlying mechanism of the water diuresis. A decrease in urine volume, an increase in urine osmolality, and a return of serum osmolality toward normal confirms central DI. Lack of response identifies renal DI. DDAVP will also cause a decrease in polyuria and increase in urine osmolality in patients with primary polydipsias, but the serum osmolality will decrease to subnormal levels and hyponatremia may ensue. Because of such risks and the need to closely monitor fluid intake and excretion, inpatient testing is usually recommended for a DDAVP trial.

Is This Definitely Primary Polydipsia? In the patient suspected of primary polydipsia (low-normal or low serum osmolality, polyuria, low urine osmolality, concurrent psychiatric disease), an inpatient *water-restriction test* can be confirmatory, with all parameters correcting simply by restricting water. Because such dehydration testing can be very dangerous for patients with other causes of a water diuresis, it is necessary to conduct this test in a carefully supervised inpatient setting. Supervised water restriction is also made necessary by the tendency of primary polydipsic patients to be psychotic and drink surreptitiously.

SYMPTOMATIC RELIEF

The advent of *desmovasopressin* as a *nasal spray* has greatly facilitated the treatment of patients with central DI. Drugs that enhance ADH secretion (clofibrate, chlorpropamide, carbamazepine) are also helpful. Somewhat paradoxically, *thiazide diuretics* improve symptoms in patients with DI. By inducing a mild sodium diuresis, there is enhanced proximal resorption of sodium and water, reducing the amount of water that reaches the distal tubule. *Nonsteroidal anti-inflammatory agents* are sometimes helpful in patients with nephrogenic DI. By inhibiting renal prostaglandins (which are active in settings of renal disease), they reduce water delivery to the distal tubule. Treatment of the underlying psychiatric disturbance is the only treatment at present for primary polydipsia.

INDICATIONS FOR ADMISSION AND REFERRAL

As noted above, patients requiring DDAVP testing or a trial of water restriction need to be admitted. An endocrinologic consultation can be helpful in further planning the diagnostic evaluation and in interpreting its results. Patients suspected of having central DI are candidates for neuroimaging of the sella region (magnetic resonance imaging is best) and endocrinologic consultation for further testing of the hypothalamic/pituitary axis. Renal DI suggests extensive renal tubulointerstitial disease and the need for further investigation and consultation. The patient with primary polydipsia ought to have a careful psychiatric workup in search of an underlying thought disorder.

A.H.G.

ANNOTATED BIBLIOGRAPHY

Berl T. Psychosis and water balance. N Engl J Med 1988;318:441. *(An editorial summarizing disturbances of osmoregulation in psychotic persons.)*

Goldman MB, Luchins DJ, Robertson GL. Mechanisms of altered water metabolism in psychotic patients with polydipsia and hyponatremia. N Engl J Med 1988;318:397. *(Defects in osmoregulation and ADH secretion found.)*

Halperin M, Skorecki KL. Interpretation of the urine electrolytes and osmolality in the regulation of body fluid tonicity. Am J Nephrol 1986;6:241. *(Written for the subspecialist, but some very useful sections for the generalist reader.)*

Robertson GL. Differential diagnosis of polyuria. Annu Rev Med 1988;39:425. *(Comprehensive treatment of the issue.)*

Vokes TJ, Robertson GL. Disorders of antidiuretic hormone. Endocrinol Metab Clin North Am 1988. *(Authoritative review, with good section on inadequate production.)*

102
Approach to the Patient With Diabetes Mellitus

SAMUEL R. NUSSBAUM, M.D.

Primary Care Medicine: Office Evaluation and Management of the Adult Patient, 3rd edition, edited by Allan H. Goroll, Lawrence A. May, and Albert G. Mulley, Jr. J.B. Lippincott Company, Philadelphia

Diabetes mellitus is the most prevalent endocrinologic problem in primary care practice. The condition affects approximately 10 million people in the United States (3% of the population) with an annual incidence reported in community-based studies of about 130 new cases per 100,000 population. The primary physician is in the unique position to provide comprehensive care to the diabetic patient. Goals include elimination of symptomatic hyperglycemia and ketosis, the prevention of micro- and macrovascular disease, retinopathy, nephropathy and neurologic complications, and maintaining vigilance for other medical complications of diabetes including infection and the sequelae of the long-term complications of diabetes. Management requires thoughtful, skillful, and meticulous care, coupled with effective patient education.

The challenge for the primary care physician is to design a therapeutic program that is safe, practical, and acceptable to the patient. Important decisions include determining when dietary interventions have not succeeded and drug therapy is necessary, selecting between insulin and oral hypoglycemic agents, and deciding how aggressively to control the blood sugar. Practical tasks include creation of an effective means for diabetic surveillance and provision of education and encouragement that enables the patient to become a partner in management.

PATHOPHYSIOLOGY, CLINICAL PRESENTATION, AND COURSE

Definitions. Diabetes mellitus is a syndrome of diverse etiologies characterized by hyperglycemia, a relative or absolute deficiency of insulin or a resistance to the action of insulin, and a propensity to develop long-term microvascular and macrovascular disease and the clinical triopathy of retinopathy, neuropathy, and nephropathy. The *diagnosis* of diabetes is made by finding a *fasting plasma glucose of greater than 140 mg/dL* on two or more occasions in the absence of metabolic stress. If fasting blood glucose is between 100 and 140 mg/dL, the diagnosis can be made on the basis of a 75-g oral glucose tolerance test showing a *2-hour plasma glucose and one other value between 0 and 2 hours of greater than 200 mg/dL*. Impaired glucose tolerance, representing fasting plasma glucose between 115 and 140 mg/dL or 2-hour postprandial glucose between 140 and 200 mg/dL, constitutes an independent risk factor for the development of coronary artery disease and peripheral vascular disease. Approximately 1 percent to 5 percent annually of these individuals progress to type II diabetes. Those who do not progress to diabetes do not develop microvascular complications. In pregnancy, however, even minor degrees of glucose intolerance can be important (see below).

Classification. The common forms of diabetes may be classified into two broad categories, which differ in their genetic background, etiology, and clinical manifestations. *Type I diabetics* are severely *insulin deficient* and ketosis prone, and they require insulin to live; onset is typically in youth but may occur at any age. Persons with the more common *type II diabetes,* with obesity as a frequent (60%–80%) concomitant, are *neither insulin dependent nor ketosis prone* (except under severe stress of infections or surgery). These patients exhibit impaired insulin secretion at any plasma glucose concentration and "insulin resistance" (impaired insulin action at the level of the insulin receptor or signal transduction).

Pathogenesis. The pathogenesis of diabetes is incompletely understood; however, there is a genetic determinant in both type I and type II diabetes. Studies of twins demonstrate a very strong *genetic influence* in type II diabetes with 90 percent of twins exhibiting diabetes within 5 years of each other. In type I diabetes, 50 percent of twin pairs fail to develop diabetes even after intervals of 10 to 20 years, yet the concordance rate of 50 percent is greater than the approximately 6 percent concordance rate for siblings. The incidence of type I diabetes is strongly associated with a variety of markers known to be on chromosome 6, whereas type II diabetes shows no such linkage. *Beta cell autoimmunity* is present in type I, but not in type II. Defects in the insulin receptor and mutations in the glucose transporter are only rarely causes for diabetes. In patients with type II diabetes (60%–80% of whom are obese), there is considerable heterogeneity in the insulin secretory response and the degree of *insulin resistance*. Glucose intolerance in these patients may be worsened by infection, stress, thiazides, glucocorticoids, and pregnancy. Excess secretion of growth hormone, cortisol, catecholamines, or glucagon may result in glucose intolerance, as can diseases that destroy a substantial portion of the pancreas (eg, chronic pancreatitis, hemochromatosis, and cystic fibrosis).

Clinical Presentation. Type II diabetes is often discovered as an incidental finding on screening urinalysis or blood sugar. Occasionally, the diagnosis is made during the evaluation of cardiovascular, renal, neurologic, or infectious disease. A complication such as myocardial ischemia, stroke, intermittent claudication, impotence, peripheral neuropathy, proteinuria, or retinopathy may be the initial manifestation. Sometimes, fatigue is the predominant symptom. In patients with more significant hyperglycemia, polyuria, polydipsia, and polyphagia with weight loss are encountered.

Complications. The major complications of diabetes are vascular, neurologic, infectious, and ocular. Diabetic vascular disease includes both microangiopathic and large vessel atherosclerotic disease. *Premature atherosclerosis* may develop in large and medium vessels, leading to coronary ischemia, stroke, and peripheral arterial insufficiency. There appears to be synergy of smoking, hypertension, and other risk factors for vascular disease with hyperglycemia. Pathophysiology remains poorly understood. It has been suggested that *hyperinsulinemia,* attributed to impaired insulin action and compensatory beta cell hypersecretion, is the common pathway for atherosclerotic risk factors to cluster and that hyperinsulinemia leads to hypertension, low high-density lipoprotein (HDL) cholesterol, and high very low-density lipoprotein (VLDL) triglyceride. This atherogenic phenotype has been termed *syndrome X*. It is unclear to what degree this predisposition to large vessel atherosclerosis is modifiable by normalization of blood sugar. Correction of other cardiovascular risk factors, such as smoking, hypertension, and hyperlipidemia, may be more important than normalization of glucose per se to the prevention and limitation of this complication. *Microvascular disease* leads to nephropathy, retinopathy, and neuropathy.

Diabetic nephropathy, a major cause of renal failure, accounts for 25 percent of patients in end-stage renal disease. Characteristic renal changes include glomerular basement membrane thickening and mesangial proliferation. Mesangial proliferation correlates strongly with the onset of proteinuria and hypertension. Subclinical and histologic findings for diabetic nephropathy are present long before the stage of clinical proteinuria. An elevated glomerular filtration rate (GFR; hyperfiltration), genetic determinants, and hypertension contribute to progression of renal impairment. With persistent proteinuria, hypertension becomes established and glomerular filtration begins to decline at the rate of 1 mL/min/mo.

The risk of developing nephropathy correlates with duration of disease. Thirty to 50 percent of type I diabetics and 6 percent to 9 percent of type II patients will eventually develop renal failure. Tight control of the blood glucose can reduce mild proteinuria in insulin-dependent diabetics who do not yet have renal insufficiency. In the presence of significant proteinuria (>500 mg/d), near normalization of the plasma glucose may not slow the rate of renal deterioration. Bladder dysfunction and resultant urinary tract infections can also contribute to renal impairment in patients with diabetic neuropathy.

Retinopathy. The risk of *retinopathic changes* (see Chapter 209) is related to duration and severity of hyperglycemia. After 20 years of diabetes, all age groups show a 75 percent to 80 percent prevalence of retinopathy. The cumulative incidence of retinopathy can be reduced by over 50 percent with intensive insulin therapy. Reversible changes in lens configuration occur with wide fluctuations in plasma glucose and may cause transiently blurred vision. In addition, cataracts and glaucoma occur with increased frequency (see Chapters 207 and 208).

Neuropathy may lead to a peripheral sensory deficit, autonomic dysfunction, or a mononeuritis. Mechanisms include *myo*-inositol depletion in nerve cell membranes (which prolongs conduction time) and hyperglycemia-induced sorbitol accumulation in nerve tissues that have a polyol pathway for metabolism of glucose (eg, Schwann's cells). Microangiopathic changes decreasing blood supply to the myelin sheaths are believed responsible for the mononeuropathy. The *peripheral neuropathy* is predominantly sensory, reducing sensation in the lower extremities, and may progress to cause pain and dysesthesias. *Autonomic neuropathy* most commonly presents as impotence. Gastrointestinal motility disturbances, orthostatic hypotension, and urinary retention are other potential manifestations. Autonomic neuropathy is almost always seen in association with distal polyneuropathy. Its presence is an important predictor for foot and other infections. Diabetic *mononeuropathy* involves discrete cranial or peripheral nerves, singly or as a mononeuritis multiplex. The most commonly affected cranial nerves are III and VI. In contrast to other diabetic neuropathies, there is near complete resolution of mononeuropathies within 1 year of onset.

Increased susceptibility to infection in diabetics appears to result from impaired leukocyte function, compromised vascular supply, and neuropathy. Cellulitis and candidiasis occur, with infections of ischemic foot lesions especially serious because they may lead to osteomyelitis and require amputation. Overall, the occurrence of perioperative infections correlates with end-organ involvement by diabetes and to marked degrees of hyperglycemia. Recent studies show a sixfold increase in all perioperative complications (stroke, infection, and renal insufficiency) in patients with end-organ disease. Urinary tract infections are common in patients with an autonomic bladder (see Chapter 134).

PRINCIPLES OF MANAGEMENT

The goals of therapy in diabetes are normalization of carbohydrate metabolism and prevention of multisystem complications that may result from hyperglycemia. The Diabetes Control and Complication Trial (DCCT), a multicenter, randomized clinical trial comparing intensive insulin therapy with conventional insulin therapy in type I diabetics, has convincingly demonstrated that maintaining blood glucose concentrations closer to the normal range delays the onset and limits the progression of the long-term complications of diabetes—retinopathy, nephropathy, and neuropathy. Can we extrapolate the study results to the more prevalent type II (non–insulin requiring or adult onset) diabetics?

The *optimal degree of control* of blood sugar in type II diabetics remains a subject of controversy. Although tight glucose control can delay the onset and slow the progression of retinopathy, nephropathy and neuropathy, it remains unresolved whether restoration of glucose to near normal can be accomplished in persons who are not highly motivated and whether intensive insulin therapy in type II diabetics will reduce the serious large vessel consequences of diabetes (which cause death in the majority of type II diabetics).

Although normalization of blood sugars to nondiabetic postprandial and fasting levels is an ideal objective, it is difficult to achieve with available means. The risk of hypoglycemia with intensive insulin therapy is a serious concern in patients who have underlying coronary artery disease or cerebrovascular disease. More importantly for patients with severe complications, there is no evidence in humans that normalization of glucose can reverse these complications. However, the goal of safe and convenient glucose normalization may be achieved within the next decade as the technology to create small, implantable glucose sensors and insulin delivery systems is further refined.

Diet and Exercise

The cornerstone of therapy for all overweight type II diabetics is *weight reduction* through calorie restriction. Achieving ideal body weight is the single most important goal for the physician to encourage and advance to achieve metabolic control. Weight loss has been shown to enhance the sensitivity of peripheral insulin receptors to endogenous insulin and reduce requirements for administered insulin. It is not possible to predict the exact improvement in glucose control from each pound lost, but a reduction of body weight may lead to improvement in glucose tolerance.

Most type II diabetics can have hyperglycemia controlled by the achievement of ideal body weight; however, such weight reduction is often a difficult goal to sustain, requiring a permanent restriction in caloric intake. An effective *exercise program* (see Chapter 18) will enhance weight loss because of the increase in caloric consumption. Exercise can help achieve weight loss in obese individuals who may require fewer calories to maintain body weight. Rigidly developed and prescribed diets should be avoided in favor of diets adapted to the patient's lifestyle. The goal is gradual, sustained weight reduction of approximately 1 to 2 lb each week (see Chapter 233).

Diet composition for type II diabetics is less critical than achieving ideal body weight. At present, the American Diabetes Association recommends diets high in carbohydrate content, up to 60 percent, with a significant content of polyunsaturated fats. In mild glucose intolerance, isocaloric increases in carbohydrate up to 80 percent may improve glucose tolerance, particularly when complex carbohydrate, high-fiber diets are consumed. Hypertriglyceridemia secondary to the increase in carbohydrates has not been a problem, and, in several studies, triglycerides and cholesterol have fallen substantially. Recent studies in type II diabetics, however, show unchanged or worsened glycemic control on high carbohydrate diets and increases in VLDL triglyceride and cholesterol. All carbohydrates are not similar; some sources of starch, such as potato, have a greater effect on increasing blood glucose than do carbohydrates in beans or wheat. Even the inclusion of sucrose or ice cream in mixed meals does not necessarily adversely affect glucose control. Preliminary data suggest *vitamin E* and *beta-carotene* supplements may decrease the oxidation of polyunsaturated fatty acids and impact positively on preventing the accelerated atherogenesis of diabetes. (See Appendix, Chapter 27.)

High-fiber diets, generally associated with a higher intake of complex carbohydrates and decreased intake of refined carbohydrates and animal fats, are associated with low prevalence of diabetes mellitus. *Increase in fiber content* of the diet with unprocessed natural foods that include cereals, grains, fruits, and vegetables results in improved glucose tolerance in type II diabetics and decreased insulin requirements in type I diabetics. The likely mechanism for this improvement in glycemic control is delayed absorption.

Exercise has beneficial effects on glucose control in diabetes. In the well-controlled diabetic, it increases glucose consumption and improves glucose tolerance by increasing insulin receptor number and affinity. There are several precautions regarding exercise in diabetic patients. The increased absorption of insulin from an exercising limb may precipitate hypoglycemia in patients on insulin; therefore, the abdomen should be used as the site for insulin injection. Because of the possibility of underlying ischemic heart disease, an exercise electrocardiogram (ECG) should be considered before the commencement of a rigorous exercise program in a sedentary individual with more longstanding diabetes (see Chapters 18 and 36).

Patients on Insulin. For type I *insulin-requiring diabetics* who are at ideal body weight, the essential aspect of dietary therapy is the *regularity of caloric intake* and the spacing of meals. Three meals, supplemented by snacks midmorning, midafternoon, and before bed, are needed to provide a source of glucose during the sustained presence of exogenously administered insulin. The commonly used American Diabetic Association diets recommend 2/9 of calories at breakfast, 2/9 at lunch, 4/9 at dinner, and 1/9 as snacks. The timing of meals must match peak insulin effects and activity schedules; increased activity requires increased food intake or a decrease in insulin dosage to prevent hypoglycemia. *Simple sugars* are generally restricted because they worsen postprandial hyperglycemia; however, patients should carry a source of simple sugar, such as fruit juice or sugar candy, to limit an insulin reaction. Patients who are not taking insulin do not require elaborate exchange systems, careful timing of meals, or other special dietary accommodations.

Drug Therapy-Oral Agents

When reduction to ideal body weight fails to achieve reasonable control of blood sugar or amelioration of symptoms, the patient is unable to lose weight, ketosis is present, or gestational diabetes occurs, then drug therapy is indicated.

Sulfonylureas. With the introduction of potent second-generation sulfonylureas, oral hypoglycemic agents are being increasingly used in the management of diabetes. However, opinion remains divided on the effectiveness of these compounds in achieving glycemic control necessary to limit the long-term sequelae of diabetes. There is no evidence that long-term use of oral hypoglycemic agents can reduce the premature morbidity and mortality of diabetes, and there remains concern regarding their safety (see below).

The sulfonylureas acutely increase the beta cell's sensitivity to glucose and insulin release. In the long term, their hypoglycemic effects are due to increased insulin receptor binding and enhanced tissue sensitivity to insulin.

Oral agents achieve a lower blood sugar in approximately 60 percent to 70 percent of diabetics. The *University Group Diabetes Project (UGDP) study* revealed an *increased* rate of *cardiovascular death* in patients on long-term tolbutamide therapy. The UGDP report states: "The findings of the study indicate that the combination of diet and tolbutamide therapy is no more effective than diet alone in prolonging life. Moreover, the findings suggest that tolbutamide and diet may be less effective than diet alone or diet and insulin, at least in so far as cardiovascular mortality in concerned." This unanticipated result gave rise to still ongoing controversy about the design of the 12-center UGDP study, and the application of the tolbutamide findings to other first- and second-generation sulfonylureas such as chlorpropamide, glyburide, and glipizide. Independent biometric review of the UGDP study's design and data analysis has confirmed the UGDP conclusions, despite finding baseline inequalities among treatment groups after randomization, the use of standard dosages of tolbutamide that led to under- and over-treatment, and unmonitored variables, especially smoking.

Second-generation sulfonylureas are more potent. In careful side-by-side comparisons, second-generation sulfonylureas can achieve results comparable to single-dose NPH insulin in lowering hemoglobin A_{1C} (HbA_{1C}; see below). Although insulin is generally preferred to achieve glucose control, patients with symptomatic hyperglycemia who cannot take insulin because of infirmity, vision loss, or unwillingness to administer injections are candidates for an oral agent. Symptomatic, overweight patients who are entering a program of weight reduction are also reasonable candidates for therapy with sulfonylureas. If weight reduction should fail, then these drugs might best be abandoned in favor of insulin.

Glyburide (Micronase, Diabeta) and *glipizide* (Glucotrol) are the two *second-generation oral hypoglycemic sulfonylureas* available for treatment of type II diabetics. They are nonionically bound to plasma proteins and have less variation in their bioavailability than the earlier oral agents. Both are inactivated by the liver. Glyburide is excreted in bile and urine, offering a potential advantage over glipizide in patients with renal insufficiency. Sulfonylureas should be used with caution in reduced dosages in patients with liver disease. In contrast to chlorpropamide, neither glyburide nor glipizide causes the syndrome of inappropriate secretion of antidiuretic hormone, and only rarely causes disulfiram (Antabuse)-like effects. Like their predecessors, they may have their effects potentiated by sulfonamides, salicylates, and clofibrate or inhibited by coumadin. Generally, a patient can be started on 2.5 or 5.0 mg of glyburide or glipizide, respectively, once daily. Daily dose can be increased to as much as 15 mg, monitoring blood sugars and HbA_{1C} (see below). Hypoglycemia (which tends to be prolonged) occurs with increased frequency with use of glyburide (4%–6%) in comparison to glipizide (2%–4%). Occasionally, patients who have become refractory to earlier sulfonylureas may benefit by substitution with glyburide or glipizide. Doses in excess of 15 mg/day are of little additional benefit.

Drug Therapy-Insulin

Insulin is the drug therapy of choice for diabetics who develop ketosis, for symptomatic type II diabetics who cannot be controlled by diet alone, and for diabetics in whom near-normalization of blood sugar is a goal of therapy.

Preparations. *"Single peak" insulin,* prepared by chromatographic systems that result in an animal insulin preparation containing 300 to 3000 ppm of proinsulin, had been the most commonly used commercial preparation. In 1980, insulins *highly purified* by high-performance liquid chromatography and containing less than 1 ppm of proinsulin were introduced. In 1982 *human recombinant insulin* was approved by the U.S. Food and Drug Administration (FDA). The increased use of human recombinant insulin and highly purified insulins has led to decline in the incidence of local reactions, insulin allergy, immune resistance, and lipoatrophy. In some patients, human insulin may be absorbed more rapidly and have a shorter duration of action than animal insulins. Although antibody formation against human insulin is less than that against insulin from animal species, there is a measurable increase in antiinsulin antibodies in a minority of patients treated with the recombinant preparation. With more favorable pricing that makes the cost of recombinant insulin similar to animal insulins, the initiation of insulin therapy should be with human insulin.

Insulin is available in short-, intermediate-, and long-acting preparations. Intermediate types of insulin, *NPH* and *lente,* with peak action at 6 to 12 hours and 24-hour duration of insulin effect, are the most commonly used. Short-acting insulins, *CZI* and *semilente,* have an earlier onset and peak (2 to 4 hours) action. Long-acting insulins, *protamine-zinc* insulin and *ultralente* insulin, may have greatest utility in intensive insulin therapy programs to provide basal release of insulin in conjunction with multiple injections of short-acting insulin. The use of intermediate-acting lente insulin, with crystalline structures providing absorption characteristics similar to that of NPH insulin, avoids the use of a foreign protein that is used to delay the absorption of NPH insulin.

Programs. (See Table 102–1). The majority of *type II diabetics* can be reasonably controlled with a *single dose of intermediate insulin* in the morning before breakfast, although better glycemic control can be achieved with *split doses of intermediate-acting/regular-acting insulin given twice daily.* This approach limits early morning hyperglycemia, which is observed as a result of growth hormone secretion (the "dawn phenomenon").

Approximately one-third of patients have either a delayed or early response to intermediate insulins. Half are *early* or *type A responders;* they experience their peak insulin effect shortly after noon and become hypoglycemic in the early afternoon. Their insulin program consists of *splitting the dose* of intermediate insulin into two parts: two-thirds given in the morning and one-third administered before dinner. Occasionally, supplementation with a short-acting insulin is necessary in the morning and evening.

Table 102-1. Common Insulin Regimens

STANDARD REGIMENS RESPONSE TO INSULIN	REGIMEN
Early (type A)	2/3 dose intermediate insulin before breakfast
	1/3 dose intermediate insulin before dinner
Normal (type B)	Full dose of intermediate insulin before breakfast
Late (type C)	Reduced dose of intermediate insulin plus a short-acting insulin before breakfast
	Small dose of short-acting insulin before dinner, if postprandial evening hyperglycemia occurs
MORE INTENSIVE INSULIN REGIMENS DEGREE OF CONTROL	**REGIMEN**
Tight	Divide total daily intermediate insulin dose into injections before breakfast and before dinner
	Add to each of the intermediate insulin doses a small dose of short-acting insulin
Very tight*	Long-acting insulin at night Short acting insulins before each meal or more frequently based on self-monitored glucose measurements to achieve preprandial glucose between 70 and 120, postprandial glucose of <180 mg/dL and normal $HgbA_{1C}$ of <6.05%
	Pump therapy

*Intensive insulin therapy used in the DCCT.

The other half are *late* or *type C responders,* having a delayed response with the nadir of blood sugar occurring between 10 PM and 5 AM. These patients require a reduction in intermediate-acting insulin and the *addition of a short-acting insulin* to the morning dose. An additional small evening dose of short-acting insulin may be necessary if postprandial hyperglycemia is a major problem in the early evening.

For the two-thirds of patients who respond adequately to intermediate-acting insulin, *greater glucose control* may be achieved by *dividing* the total daily insulin dose into injections, one before breakfast and the other before dinner. To further improve control and minimize excursions of glycemia, this schedule is sometimes supplemented by small amounts of *short-acting insulin,* which can be mixed in the same syringe.

Intensive insulin programs to achieve near-normalization of blood sugar are increasingly emphasized as a treatment objective in motivated, carefully selected patients, facilitated by the teaching and widespread use of home blood glucose monitoring (HBGM; see below). The DCCT results have given added impetus to this more aggressive insulin therapy. Open-loop *pump therapy* represents an attempt to duplicate the normal physiologic pattern of insulin release. Insulin infusion devices (worn externally and connected to an indwelling catheter) and multiple daily injections are being widely applied in gestational diabetes and in difficult-to-control, type I diabetics. This therapeutic approach requires patient motivation and sophistication, close monitoring, and careful supervision to be safe and effective. Comparable control of glycemia can be achieved by insulin pump and conventional intensive therapy. The major advantage of insulin pumps revolves around ease of frequent insulin administration. Complications include catheter infection, inadvertent catheter displacement from the skin, and cost.

A typical *intensive insulin program* using subcutaneous injections to emulate physiologic insulin release is to administer *ultralente* insulin at 6 PM and *semilente* or *CZI* insulin before meals and before sleep. This therapy requires self-monitoring of glucose to adjust dosage schedules. Additionally, a 3 AM blood glucose would ensure that nocturnal hypoglycemia is not occurring. These therapeutic programs enable the normalization of serum HbA_{1C}, a useful indicator of long-term glucose control (see below). The major complication of intensive insulin therapy is frequent and more severe *hypoglycemia*.

Intensive therapy is indicated in pregnancy because of the proven benefit of glucose control in limiting fetal morbidity and mortality and the potential for decreasing congenital malformations, which are increased in children of diabetic mothers. Type I diabetics and younger, sophisticated, motivated patients without established complications may also be considered for this intensive therapy. Decisions regarding the expansion of intensive insulin therapies and the resources needed to apply intensive therapies across the entire diabetic population will increasingly involve discussions and decisions of broad health care and public policy.

Initiation of Insulin Therapy can be carried out safely on an ambulatory basis as long as the patient is reliable, nonketotic, and not severely hyperglycemic with intercurrent illness. Treatment should be initiated with 10 to 15 units of an intermediate-acting insulin and increased by approximately 2 units each day depending on urine, or preferably, blood sugar monitoring performed by the patient. Double-voided urine glucose determinations, commonly used in the past, have limitations (see below).

Technique and Storage. Insulin is injected subcutaneously where it is absorbed directly into the circulation. The abdomen and limbs serve as convenient injection sites, with rotation among sites used to minimize discomfort and, rarely, lipoatrophy. Rotation among multiple abdominal *injection sites* is preferable to limb injections in athletically active diabetics because of the possibility of more rapid insulin absorption from an exercising limb. Insulin, best *stored* in the refrigerator, may be left at room temperature for up to 12 hours without loss of biopotency.

Degree of Control. Most endocrinologists agree that it is desirable to achieve the best glycemic control possible. However, the vital issue is whether tight control can be accomplished safely and whether the means of insulin administration currently available are compatible with an individual's lifestyle and personal choices for therapy. Whereas an intelligent, well-motivated, reliable individual can be taught to regulate daily insulin dosages, less capable patients risk hypoglycemic reactions when tight control is attempted. Reasonable glycemic control in the latter group might be considered a fasting blood glucose of less than 150 mg/dL, and postprandial blood glucose of less than 200 mg/dL. The daily dose of insulin required to achieve euglycemia in obese, previously untreated type II diabetics can be very high, range 40 to 320 U).

Worsening Hyperglycemia (See Table 102–2). In a patient taking a previously adequate dose of insulin, hyperglycemia requires prompt attention. Although important changes in caloric intake or failure to take insulin properly may be the explanation for worsening hyperglycemia, occult infection (especially in the urinary tract), coronary ischemia, severe emotional stress, and Somogyi phenomenon (rebound hyperglycemia) must be investigated. A recently recognized phenomenon, worsening hyperglycemia in the early morning hours, is caused by the growth hormone surges that occur during sleep. An intermediate-acting insulin given at bedtime can provide excellent coverage for this early morning hyperglycemia.

The *Somogyi phenomenon* may be mistaken for inadequate control, because of the rebound hyperglycemia and possible ketosis that occurs after insulin-induced hypoglycemia. The hypoglycemia usually goes unnoticed because it occurs at night or because there is severe autonomic neuropathy. Hypoglycemia is followed by several days of poor control. Clues to recognizing nocturnal hypoglycemia include night sweats, poor sleep, nightmares, and morning headaches. Urinary monitoring reveals negative urinary glucose and ketones in the evening followed by trace urinary sugar and large ketones in the morning. The best way to recognize the Somogyi effect is to be cognizant of its potential existence and to obtain a blood glucose at a time of suspected hypoglycemia. Appropriate therapy, which involves slowly decreasing the dosage of insulin, may be commenced after documenting hypoglycemia. If detection is impractical, a diagnostic trial of reduced insulin may be used to confirm the clinical suspicion. Doses of insulin should be decreased slowly each day rather than precipitously because a dramatic decrease in insulin dosage will lead to worsening hyperglycemia.

Insulin resistance is occasionally the cause of poor control. It is arbitrarily defined as the requirement for greater than 200 units of insulin daily. Most of insulin resistance results from obesity; restoring normal weight represents the best treatment. More classic insulin resistance is immunologically mediated by antibodies directed at bovine or porcine insulin, or against protamine or protamine insulin complexes. For patients with immunologic insulin resistance, switching therapy to a lente insulin preparation or to human recombinant insulin may be advantageous. At times, high-dose glucocorticoids (80 to 100 mg of prednisone daily) may be necessary. Most patients respond, and steroid therapy can often be rapidly tapered. Immunologic insulin resistance is commonly seen in individuals who have been receiving insulin in intermittent treatment programs. In patients who will receive insulin for only limited intervals (such as during myocardial infarction or during weight reduction for obesity), human insulin represents the best choice of therapy to limit antibody development.

Hypoglycemia and Insulin Reactions. When food intake is delayed or diminished, increased physical activity is undertaken, or insulin dose is excessive, hypoglycemia may ensue. Symptoms include those of increased sympathomimetic activity: sweating, palpitations, tremor, and weakness. In addition, *neuroglycopenic symptoms* (fatigue and changes in mentation) may also be seen when there is a less precipitous decline in blood sugar. Profound hypoglycemia may lead to loss of consciousness. If autonomic neuropathy is present, or if a patient is taking a beta-adrenergic blocking drug, many hypoglycemic symptoms will be masked and mental confusion may be the paramount symptom. Patient and family education and a syringe with glucagon are important (see below).

Insulin Allergy. Represented by cutaneous reactions to insulin, this allergy occurs in approximately 5 percent of patients and only rarely manifests urticaria, angioedema, or anaphylaxis. It may be treated by a change to human insulin administered with antihistamines. Desensitization may be necessary if systemic allergic manifestations have occurred.

Insulin and Surgery. Management of the diabetic patient during surgery is to allow modest hyperglycemia and assiduously avoid hypoglycemia and ketosis. The preoperative medical evaluation is critical because the majority of perioperative complications relate not to hyperglycemia or hypoglycemia, but rather to coexisting cardiac or renal disease. Importantly, the potential for infection needs to be carefully considered and sources for fever such as pulmonary, skin, and urinary tract infection need to be investigated. Many insulin programs for operative management have been advanced. In general, the dose of insulin should be reduced by approximately one-third to one-half on the morning of surgery with carbohydrate being supplied by intravenous (IV) 5 percent dextrose at 150 mL/h. Surgery should, if possible, be performed early in the day, with postoperative monitoring of blood sugar and renal function. An ECG should be obtained because of the higher incidence of silent myocardial ischemia and infarction in diabetics. Until the patient is eating, insulin dosages may need to be decreased, unless increased secretion of counterregulatory hormones (such as growth hormone, cortisol, and catecholamines) worsens hyperglycemia and necessitates an increase in dose. Risk for infection has been found in those individuals with HbA_{1C} of 11.5 percent, indicating marked hyperglycemia in the preoperative interval.

Control of Associated Cardiovascular Risk Factors and Management of Complications

As noted earlier, controlling hyperglycemia will limit or prevent the microvascular, neurologic, and renal complications of diabetes. It is not yet proved that macrovascular disease will be altered by tight control. Consequently, it is more important that all associated risk factors for the development of coronary artery disease and renal failure be meticulously controlled. Efforts spent on cessation of smoking, control of hypertension, and reduction of hypercholesterolemia (see Chapters 26, 27, and 54) are likely to be more productive than attempting to tightly control blood sugar.

Hypertension. Treatment of hypertension in diabetics also requires attention not only to degree of control achieved but also to its effects on metabolic control, recognition of hypoglycemia, and "renal hyperfiltration." Specifically, the *thiazide* diuretics may worsen glucose intolerance, and *beta-blockers* may mask the sympathomimetic warning symptoms of hypoglycemia. On the positive side, *angiotensin-converting enzyme (ACE) inhibitors* may limit hyperfiltration and help preserve renal function (see below). Hyperkalemia needs to be watched for in the diabetic patient being treated with ACE inhibitors. Impotence and postural hypotension are features of diabetic patients that may affect the choice of antihypertensive therapy. (See Chapter 26 for a detailed discussion of alternative antihypertensive therapies.)

Renal Failure. *ACE inhibitors* reduce proteinuria and significantly slow progression of azotemia. The beneficial effect on nephropathy occurs even in normotensive patients and is independent of reduction in blood pressure. It is believed related to afferent arteriolar dilation and reduced hyperfiltration. Control of hypertension still remains important, particularly as renal function declines (see Chapter 26). *Protein restriction* (0.5 mg/kg) may also reduce hyperfiltration in early nephropathy, but ACE inhibitor therapy is likely to be more acceptable. The progression to renal failure may be inexorable once heavy proteinuria of greater than 3 g/d occurs. However, the primary care physician may still be able to prevent some forms of late renal insufficiency, such as that associated with bladder dysfunction, with pyelonephritis and acute papillary necrosis, and with contrast-induced acute renal failure that occurs in diabetics with moderate to advanced renal insufficiency. Prompt and aggressive treatment of urinary tract infections (see Chapters 133 and 140), therapy to limit urinary retention that increases the risk for infection (see Chapter 134) and avoidance of unnecessary contrast studies will help control avoidable renal insults. Necessary dye studies require maintaining hydration, using as small a dye load as possible, and administering mannitol following study. Nephrotoxic antibiotics and nonsteroidal anti-inflammatory agents (which can inhibit renal prostaglandin activity) should be avoided.

Over the past decade, the outlook for the diabetic receiving hemodialysis or renal transplantation has improved, although the mortality rate for diabetics on these treatment modalities remains higher than that of nondiabetics. Chronic ambulatory *peritoneal dialysis* has been used for diabetic patients because of concerns that the heparin used for hemodialysis may lead to a worsening of diabetic retinopathy. However, early information suggests higher infection rates in diabetic patients on chronic peritoneal dialysis.

Peripheral Vascular Disease. Lower extremity amputation is often associated with peripheral vascular disease and neuropathy in patients with diabetes. When compared to a control diabetic population, patients with amputation had greater neuropathy, vascular impairment, lower HDL levels, and less outpatient diabetic education. Surprisingly, smoking is not a statistically significant risk factor for amputation in diabetics. (See also Chapter 34 for a discussion of peripheral vascular disease.)

Foot Problems. Because of vascular insufficiency and neuropathy, diabetics have unique foot care problems. Meticulous foot care is essential for the prevention of cellulitis, osteomyelitis, and amputation. Feet must be kept clean, interdigital spaces dry, calluses pared down, and toenails carefully trimmed. Frequent inspection for skin breakdown and cellulitis by the patient needs to be stressed, as does the importance of wearing properly fitting shoes. Before bathing, the diabetic patient should use his or her hands to ascertain the water temperature to prevent scalding injuries that may occur because of loss of temperature sensation in the lower extremities. The diabetic patient who is incapable of foot care or who has had a foot infection must see a podiatrist regularly.

Neuropathy. Neuropathic *pain* has been treated with phenytoin, carbamazepine, and combinations of tricyclic antidepressants and phenothiazines, but no singularly effective treatment program has emerged. *Phenytoin* seems to have the least toxicity and should be tried first. The *postural hypotension,* impotence, and urinary retention associated with autonomic neuropathy are usually permanent. Postural hypotension may respond to the synthetic mineralocorticoid *florinef* when sexual performance is limited by *impotence*. Sexually incapacitated patients can be considered for treatment with *yohimbine* or implantation of a *prosthesis*. Anxiety and depression, which are often superimposed on neurologic dysfunction, must be excluded (see Chapters 132 and 229).

Enteropathy. Gastrointestinal motility problems, which include *gastroparesis* and *diabetic diarrhea,* can be difficult to treat. Small, frequent feedings and cholinergic drugs such as *metoclopramide* may lessen gastroparetic symptoms. Patients with diarrhea due to bacterial overgrowth of the bowel can be treated with a trial of a broad-spectrum antibiotic (eg, neomycin). *Cholestyramine* has been found to be of benefit in controlling the diarrhea of diabetic autonomic neuropathy. Fortunately, refractory nocturnal diarrhea often resolves spontaneously.

Diabetics should have regular dental examinations because of their higher incidence of *pyorrhea* and abscesses, which may also worsen diabetic control.

Ophthalmopathy. Diabetic *retinopathy* is the most important systemic disease causing blindness. Proliferative retinopathy accounts for the majority of cases of blindness among type I diabetics, whereas *macular edema* from nonproliferative retinopathy accounts for the majority of cases of blindness in type II diabetics. Photocoagulation with laser therapy can retard visual loss by 50 percent (see Chapter 209). Cataracts and glaucoma are also important complications (see Chapters 207 and 208 for management).

Glucose Intolerance and Pregnancy

Fetal hyperglycemia contributes to excessive fetal growth, which increases the risks of birth trauma, asphyxia, neonatal respiratory distress syndrome, and in utero deaths. In addition, there is an increased need for cesarean section. Maintenance of blood sugars in the physiologic range (60 to 120 mg/dL) takes on added importance during pregnancy because the complications of fetal hyperglycemia can be prevented and perinatal mortality reduced to that of nondiabetics. Even nondiabetic pregnant women who develop an otherwise insignificant degree of hyperglycemia (2-hour postprandial blood sugars in the range of 140 to 160 mg/dL) show an increased risk of macrosomia and its complications. Women with postprandial readings in excess of 165 mg/dL have an increased incidence of diabetes in later life.

The importance of glucose intolerance during pregnancy has led to the recommendation by the American Diabetic Association that all pregnant women be screened for glucose intolerance by the 24th to 28th week of gestation using a 50-g oral glucose load, which can be given at any time of day. Patients with a 1-hour serum glucose in excess of 140 mg/dL should be given a 100-g glucose tolerance test and treated if the level is greater than 165 mg/dL at 2 hours. Some argue on the basis of studies showing increased fetal risk with previously "normal" levels of glucose intolerance (120 to 160 mg/dL) that even more modest elevations are grounds for therapy, at least with dietary measures.

All patients with glucose intolerance should be treated with diets that limit simple sugars and total calories (35 to 38 calories per kilogram of ideal weight before pregnancy). Repeat testing of the blood sugar every 1 to 2 weeks until delivery is indicated. Patients showing fasting sugars in excess of 105 mg/dL or postprandial levels greater than 120 mg/dL should be considered for insulin therapy; consultation with a diabetologist is indicated.

For diabetic patients already on insulin, adjustments in dose may be necessary. During the first trimester, the type I diabetic needs a reduction in insulin because insulin requirements decrease and there is a heightened risk of hypoglycemia. In the second trimester, the type I diabetic requires more insulin as the diabetes becomes more labile and the chances of ketoacidosis (with its associated risk of fetal death) rise. Third-trimester dose requirements usually do not change, but the increase in glomerular filtration rate can lower the tubular threshold for glucose and make urine testing unreliable. Within a few hours of delivery, insulin requirements fall considerably, returning fully to prepregnancy levels within 1 to 2 weeks. Optimal control is facilitated by use of home glucose monitoring (see below).

Monitoring

Monitoring can be divided into two categories: control of glycemia and observation of signs of systemic complications.

For Control of Glycemia. The traditional means of monitoring was the double-voided urine test for glucose and ketones, usually performed before breakfast and before the evening meal in patients taking insulin. The technique requires voiding fully, then voiding again hour later and testing the urine sample by means of tape or tablets for a colorimetric response that indicates the urine glucose and ketone concentrations. At best, the correlation between urine and serum glucose concentrations is approximate. It varies from patient to patient and from time to time in the same patient because of differences and changes in renal tubular threshold for glucose, renal blood flow, and urine volume. Moreover, the test is compromised in patients with bladder dysfunction who have a postvoid residual.

Home Glucose Monitoring. The finger-stick method represents a marked improvement in monitoring. The patient obtains a finger-stick sample of capillary blood, which is tested for glucose concentration by colorimetric reading of a reagent strip to which a drop of blood is applied. Both increasingly sophisticated meters and color charts are available for making the glucose determination. Insurance companies are increasingly covering the costs. Measurements are most useful for patients on insulin therapy allowing hour-to-hour and day-to-day adjustments based on blood sugar monitoring. Frequent measurements, both fasting and at several intervals postprandially, are valuable at the time of starting or adjusting an insulin program and also during periods of illness or worsening control. Most patients can be taught the method. Numerous devices automatically perform the finger-stick. Once a stable insulin dose is achieved, a single measurement need be taken once every several days, typically before breakfast. Patients who are capable of adjusting their own insulin doses can use home monitoring to keep their sugars in the mid-100 range after a meal. Home monitoring does not obviate the need to carefully inform the patient about symptoms of hyperglycemia and hypoglycemia (see below).

Hemoglobin A_{1c} (HbA_{1C}) is the glycosylated form of hemoglobin in the red cell. The degree of glycosylation parallels the glucose concentrations encountered by the red cell over its lifespan. Measurement of the HbA_{1C} allows an assessment of overall glycemic control for the preceding 2 to 3 months. It correlates well with frequent blood glucose determinations. Levels of less than 8.0 percent indicate blood sugars of less than 200 mg/dL; values of 11 percent to 12 percent correlate with glucose levels in excess of 300 mg/dL and indicate poor carbohydrate control. This test has superseded the *random blood sugar* as the best means of assessing control over time. For the patient with mild non–insulin-dependent diabetes, a periodic HbA_{1C} will suffice for monitoring glycemia control. Patients on insulin require acute as well as chronic measurements of blood sugar.

Checking for Complications. Patients with diabetes should have at least an annual office evaluation that includes a check of the blood pressure for elevation; the skin for infection; the eyes for background retinopathy (see Chapter 209); the cardiovascular system for evidence of carotid, coronary, and peripheral vascular disease; and the feet for ischemic lesions. The evaluation should conclude with a careful neurologic examination for signs of neuropathy. Of particular importance is the need to test for and vigorously treat other risk factors for vascular disease, such as hypertension (see Chapter 14), hypercholesterolemia (see Chapter 15), and smoking (see Chapter 54). More frequent office visits are usually necessary with patients on insulin therapy and those with complications of diabetes. Laboratory monitoring should include a urinalysis for proteinuria and sediment and a BUN and creatinine for estimation of renal function. A diabetic summary sheet placed in the patient's record helps to quickly note the extent, severity, and progression of the disease and its complications.

Teaching the patient to watch for skin, eye, neurologic, and cardiovascular changes is an important part of the monitoring effort (see below).

PATIENT EDUCATION

The success of a program for metabolic control depends on patient compliance. Because *weight reduction* to ideal body weight is the most important therapy that can be offered to type II diabetics, instruction in *diet* and healthy foods should take place in a setting that includes the patient and family. Sample diets can be obtained from the American Diabetic Association. The emphasis on diet therapy for the type II diabetic should focus more on caloric restriction than actual percentages of carbohydrate or obsession with simple sugars.

The patient receiving insulin requires continuous education and encouragement, particularly as more intensive insulin treatment programs are applied to type II diabetics to limit the end-organ consequences of the hyperglycemia. Many hospital-based practices and several office practices have used a diabetes-teaching nurse to give patients careful instruction in drawing up insulin into syringes (particularly if the patient is visually impaired), to teach insulin injection techniques and the complications of excess insulin administration, and to be readily available for telephone communication with patients. Some physicians consider deliberately giving their patients mild insulin reactions so that the patient may appreciate his or her unique warning symptoms of hypoglycemia. A *syringe with glucagon* for intramuscular injection is given to the patient in the event that the patient becomes profoundly hypoglycemic. Oral administration of juices in the unconscious and obtunded patient may lead to pulmonary aspiration.

The importance of skin and foot care must be emphasized (see Chapter 29). Referral of elderly diabetics with vision loss to podiatrists for foot care is indicated.

INDICATIONS FOR ADMISSION AND REFERRAL

Patient care programs that encourage communication between patients and health care professionals reduce the need for hospitalization for dehydration, marked hyperglycemia, ketoacidosis, and infection. Acute hospitalization for IV fluids is necessary for diabetic patients with protracted nausea and vomiting who are becoming dehydrated and hyperglycemic. Often cellulitis of the foot requires IV antibiotic therapy, as does acute pyelonephritis. In general, elderly diabetic patients with pneumonia or urinary tract infections benefit from brief hospitalizations. Referral to an endocrinologist is indicated for the diabetic who has marked excursions in blood sugar with frequent hypoglycemia and hyperglycemia. When proteinuria is in the nephrotic syndrome range and creatinine is beginning to rise above 2.5, referral to a nephrologist for consideration of dialysis or transplantation is necessary. Indications for coronary artery bypass grafting are not different for the diabetic. Because of the potential severity of cholecystitis and ascending cholangitis, cholecystectomy for cholelithiasis may be a reasonable clinical course to follow, although more recent experience favors watchful waiting for asymptomatic cholelithiasis (see Chapter 69). Ophthalmologic referral is indicated when background diabetic retinopathy first becomes evident.

THERAPEUTIC RECOMMENDATIONS

- Suspect the diagnosis of diabetes mellitus and confirm by fasting plasma sugar or, if necessary, by glucose tolerance testing in individuals who a) have polyuria, polydipsia, weight loss, and visual changes that may be due to the hyperosmolar effects of hyperglycemia; b) are overweight and have a strong family history of diabetes; c) have significant risk factors for the development of coronary artery disease such as hypertension, smoking, and hypercholesterolemia; and d) have unexplained neuropathy, proteinuria, renal insufficiency, or peripheral vascular disease. Pregnant women should have fasting blood sugar determination early in pregnancy and blood sugar measured following 50 g of glucose by the 24th to 28th week of gestation, particularly if there is a family history of diabetes.
- Consider intensive insulin therapy for type I diabetics. Normalization of blood sugars and HbA_{1C} significantly decreases the development and progression of retinopathy, neuropathy, and nephropathy. Unfortunately, intensive insulin therapy places patients at greater risk for hypoglycemia and is best reserved for highly motivated patients.
- Reduce all other risk factors for the development of atherosclerosis and encourage exercise and healthful diet. Until the effectiveness of tight control in reducing macrovascular complications of diabetes is known, risk-factor reduction is more important than rigid adherence to achieving a particular blood sugar concentration.
- Emphasize weight reduction to ideal body weight as the cornerstone of therapy in type II diabetes. The composition of the diet, per se, is less important but should include a high polyunsaturated:saturated fat ratio, low cholesterol, and complex carbohydrate. Low-protein diets may be beneficial in averting diabetic nephropathy.
- Begin insulin therapy in type II patients who continue to be symptomatic despite diet therapy of diabetes, or who continue to have fasting blood sugars above 180 mg/dL. Commence with an intermediate acting insulin preparation (lente or NPH). Newly treated diabetics should receive human insulin because of less insulin allergy, insulin resistance, and antibody development.
- Consider one of the newer oral hypoglycemic sulfonylureas with the advantage of once daily administration (glyburide and glipizide) in individuals who will not consider self-injection, who cannot safely administer insulin because of visual loss, or who will only require therapy for a brief interval because of successful weight reduction.
- Teach those on insulin therapy who require daily monitoring of control how to perform home blood glucose determinations. Long-term glucose control is most accurately assessed by HbA_{1C} measurements three or four times yearly. Home blood glucose testing is an important component of the education of diabetic patients, aiding their modification of insulin schedule and dosage following exercise or change in dietary intake. Causes for worsening hyperglycemia should be carefully investigated (see Table 102–2).
- Perform a comprehensive history, physical examination, and selected laboratory studies (BUN, creatinine, HbA_{1C}, cholesterol, urinalysis) at least annually, searching for evidence of coronary artery disease, cerebrovascular disease, peripheral vascular disease, diabetic neuropathy, renal insufficiency, proteinuria, and retinopathy.
- Carefully monitor renal function if proteinuria develops. Consider tighter control of hyperglycemia and the use of an ACE inhibitor at first sign of nephropathy. When the serum creatinine reaches 3 mg/dL, obtain nephrology consultation regarding candidacy for dialysis or transplantation.
- Exercise caution in use of iodinated contrast agents, especially in the setting of renal impairment.
- Refer diabetics who have findings of background retinopathy or who have been diabetic for 5–10 years to the ophthalmologist for indirect ophthalmoscopy and, if necessary, fluorescein angiography. Regular ophthalmic examination is needed (see Chapter 209).
- Emphasize foot care in diabetics with neuropathy and vascular insufficiency. Strongly consider podiatric care in this group of patients.
- The perioperative management of diabetics undergoing surgery requires careful attention to hyperglycemia and diligent observation for infection and occult coronary artery disease, particularly in the setting of retinopathy, nephropathy, and neuropathy.

Table 102-2. Important Causes of Worsening Hyperglycemia During Insulin Therapy

Inadequate dose
Increased caloric intake
Failure to take insulin properly
Occult infection (especially urinary tract)
Coronary ischemia
Severe emotional stress
Use of corticosteroids
Somogyi phenomenon
Insulin resistance
Growth hormone surge in early morning

ANNOTATED BIBLIOGRAPHY

Arky R. Current principles of dietary therapy of diabetes mellitus. Med Clin North Am 1978;62:655. *(An overview of dietary methods of controlling diabetes.)*

Bishop JR, Moul JW, Sihelnik SA, et al. Use of glycosylated hemoglobin to identify diabetics at high risk for penile periprosthetic infections. J Urol 1992;147:386. *(All periprosthetic infections occurred in diabetic patients and most had HbA_{1C} of >11.5 percent.)*

Bojestig M, Arnqvist HJ, Hermansson G, et al. Declining incidence of nephropathy in insulin-dependent diabetes mellitus. N Engl J Med 1994;330:15. *(Probably due to improved glycemic control.)*

Brown MJ, Asbury AK: Diabetic neuropathy. Ann Neurol 1984; 15:2. *(A concise review of myriad clinical presentations of diabetic polyneuropathy.)*

Campbell PJ, Bolli G, Cryer P, et al. Pathogenesis of the dawn phenomenon in patients with insulin dependent diabetes mellitus. N Engl J Med 1985;312:1473. *(Physiologic studies implicating growth hormone, not catecholamines, in the preawakening rise in glucose.)*

DeFronzo RA, Bonadonna RC, Ferrannini E. Pathogenesis of NIDDM. A balanced overview. Diabetes Care 1992;15:315. *(A comprehensive review of hyperinsulinemia and insulin resistance in the pathogenesis of type II diabetes.)*

Diabetes Control and Complications Trial Research Group: The effect of intensive treatment of diabetes on the development and progression of long-term complications in insulin-dependent diabetes mellitus. N Engl J Med 1993;329:977. *(The multicenter, prospective, randomized trial of 1441 patients assigned to intensive versus conventional insulin therapy. The dramatic reduction in retinopathy, proteinuria, and clinical neuropathy will revolutionize the approach to the type I diabetes and, likely, to type II disease.)*

Gabbe SG: Gestational diabetes. N Engl J Med 1986;315:1025. *(An editorial reviewing the condition and the new data suggesting complications even with modest degrees of hyperglycemia.)*

Gerich JE. Oral hypoglycemic agents. N Engl J Med 1989;321: 1231. *(A general review of the pharmacology and therapeutic efficacy of the sulfonylureas in the treatment of diabetes with particular emphasis on the second-generation sulfonylureas, glipizide and glyburide.)*

Jenkins DJA, Thomas DM, Wolever MS, et al. Glycemic index of foods: A physiological basis for carbohydrate exchange. Am J Clin Nutr 1981;34:362. *(An analysis of the glycemic effects of various carbohydrates; beans lead to less hyperglycemia than potatoes or corn.)*

Jovanovic-Peterson L, Peterson CM. Pregnancy in the diabetic woman. Endocrinol Metab Clin North Am 1992;21:433. *(Comprehensive review of the evidence supporting the benefits of normalization of blood sugar and the management necessary to achieve tight control of diabetes in pregnancy.)*

Kahn CR. Insulin resistance: A common feature of diabetes mellitus. N Engl J Med 1986;315:252. *(An editorial examining the clinical significance of insulin resistance both for pathogenesis and for treatment.)*

Kahn CR, White MF. The insulin receptor and the molecular mechanism for insulin action. J Clin Invest 1988;82:1151. *(Insulin receptor defects and mutant insulins account for a small percentage of diabetics; concise discussion of the insulin receptor.)*

Lasker R. The diabetes control and complications trial. Implications for policy and practice (Editorial). N Engl J Med 1993;329:1035. *(In this editorial accompanying the DCCT study results, the public policy considerations of the implications of the extension of the DCCT to type II diabetics and the utilization of health resources is addressed.)*

Lewis EJ, et al. Effect of angiotensin-converting-enzyme inhibition on diabetic nephropathy. N Engl J Med 1993;329:1456. *(Marked reduction in proteinuria and progression to renal failure; important advance.)*

MacKenzie CR, Charlson ME. Assessment of perioperative risk in the patient with diabetes mellitus. Surg Gynecol Obstet 1988;167:293. *(End-organ consequences of diabetes rather than hyperglycemia per se predicted infectious and renal complications of surgery.)*

Miller LV, Goldstein J. More efficient care of diabetic patients in a community hospital setting. N Engl J Med 1972;286:1388. *(Demonstrates the importance of communication between patient and health care provider in reducing acute hospitalization for diabetes.)*

Nathan DM, Singer DE, Hurxthal K, et al. The clinical information value of the glycosylated hemoglobin assay. N Engl J Med 1984;310:341. *(HbA_{1C} can be used to accurately determine average mean blood sugars in a clinical population in which physicians caring for the patients were, at times, misled by other monitoring information presented by the patient.)*

Raskin P, Rosenstock J. Blood glucose control and diabetic complications. Ann Intern Med 1986;105:254. *(An extensive review of data supporting and refuting the two major hypotheses of the microvascular complications of diabetes.)*

Reaven GM. Role of insulin resistance in human disease. Diabetes 1988;37:1595. *(Syndrome X—The theory that hyperinsulinemia is etiologic in the cause of hypertension, low HDL cholesterol, and high VLDL triglyceride; an atherogenic phenotype.)*

Reiber GE, Pecoraro RE, Koepsell TD. Risk factors for amputation in patients with diabetes mellitus. A case-control study. Ann Intern Med 1992;117:97. *(Impairment in lower extremity circulation was the most powerful predictor, along with neuropathy and HDL levels. Surprisingly, smoking was not a predictor for amputation.)*

Stenmans S, Melander A, Groop PH, et al. What is the benefit of increasing the sulfonylurea dose? Ann Intern Med 1993; 118:169. *(Little benefit above the equivalent of 10–15 mg/d of glyburides.)*

Symposium on Biosynthetic Human Insulin Diabetes Care. 1981; 4:139. *(From molecular biology to clinical studies with human recombinant insulin.)*

Taguma Y, Kitamoto Y, Futaki G, et al. Effect of captopril on heavy proteinuria in azotemic diabetics. N Engl J Med 1985;313:1617. *(A reduction of proteinuria in diabetic nephropathy following captopril or enalopril therapy.)*

Tallarigo L, Giampietro O, Penno G, et al. Relation of glucose tolerance to complications of pregnancy in nondiabetic women. N Engl J Med 1986;315:989. *(Even limited degrees of glucose intolerance during pregnancy were associated with increased risks of macrosomia and its attendant complications.)*

Wilson RM, Clark P, Barkes H, et al. Starting insulin treatment as an outpatient. JAMA 1986;256:877. *(Presents data indicating this is both safe and cost effective.)*

Primary Care Medicine: Office Evaluation and Management of the Adult Patient, 3rd edition, edited by Allan H. Goroll, Lawrence A. May, and Albert G. Mulley, Jr. J.B. Lippincott Company, Philadelphia

103
Approach to the Patient With Hyperthyroidism

Hyperthyroidism is the clinical expression of a heterogeneous group of disorders that produce elevations of free thyroxine (FT_4) and/or triiodothyronine (T_3). Well-recognized causes of hyperthyroidism include diffuse toxic goiter (Graves' disease), toxic multinodular goiter, toxic uninodular goiter (toxic nodule), and excessive doses of levothyroxine. Transient hyperthyroidism has been noted in the settings of chronic lymphocytic (Hashimoto's) thyroiditis and subacute (granulomatous) thyroiditis.

Hyperthyroidism is relatively common and much more likely to occur in women than in men. Community-based studies found prevalences of 1.9 percent in women and 0.16 percent in men. Approximately 15 percent of recognized cases occur in persons over the age of 60. The clinical presentation of hyperthyroidism in the elderly is often atypical. The primary physician should be able to recognize hyperthyroidism, identify its cause, and design a therapeutic program appropriate to the patient's underlying pathophysiology, age, clinical condition, and personal preferences. The indications and limitations of surgery, radioiodine therapy, and antithyroid agents must be understood.

PATHOPHYSIOLOGY, CLINICAL PRESENTATION, AND COURSE

The pathophysiologic common denominator of hyperthyroidism is an excess of circulating thyroid hormone. The mechanisms responsible for this excess include increased production of thyroid-stimulating hormone (TSH), stimulation of thyroid TSH receptors by immunoglobulins, autonomous thyroid hormone production, increased release of thyroid hormone without increased production, and intake of exogenous hormone.

Thyroid hormone stimulates calorigenesis and catabolism and enhances sensitivity to catecholamines. Excessive amounts of the hormone lead to the classic picture of heat intolerance, nervousness, tremor, increased appetite, weight loss, excessive sweating, lid lag, stare, and muscle weakness. Diarrhea or, more precisely, frequent defecation may also ensue.

In the elderly thyrotoxic patient, the characteristic manifestations of hyperthyroidism may be absent and the clinical picture dominated instead by apathy, weight loss, and otherwise unexplained atrial fibrillation. This *apathetic hyperthyroidism of the elderly* has been mistaken for depression and occult malignancy.

Elevations in alkaline phosphatase and angiotensin-converting enzyme may accompany thyrotoxicosis and persist even after treatment. The pathophysiologic significance of these elevations remains unclear, but the findings might suggest thyroid disease and save extensive workup when other explanations for their occurrence are lacking.

Graves' Disease is an autoimmune condition in which there appears to be a deficiency of thyroid-specific suppressor T-cell lymphocytes, allowing formation of a *thyroid-stimulating IgG antibody (TSAb)*. TSAb binds to thyrotropin (TSH) receptors on the surface of thyroid cells and triggers excess thyroid hormone synthesis. Graves' disease accounts for about 90 percent of hyperthyroidism seen in those younger than age 40. Interest in an environmental precipitant such as an infectious agent has been raised by the occurrence of Graves' disease in former President Bush and his wife.

Ophthalmopathy can be a troubling accompaniment of Graves' disease, affecting about 40 percent of patients. It is believed to be a consequence of antibody-mediated inflammation and infiltration. TSAb does not appear to be directly involved, though the onset of ophthalmopathy generally parallels that of the hyperthyroidism. Antibodies to extraocular muscle and orbital fibroblasts capable of *in vitro* induction of the pathologic changes found *in vivo* have been detected. The extraocular muscles enlarge due to the inflammatory infiltrate, and cause proptosis by displacing the eye forward and orbital edema by compressing orbital veins. In general, the eye changes develop concurrently with onset of hyperthyroidism and change little once established, though up to 20 percent may experience gradual worsening with treatment (see below). Manifestations range from mild periorbital edema and conjunctival inflammation to extraocular muscle dysfunction, corneal injury, and optic nerve damage. The lid lag and stare of hyperthyroidism may exacerbate the eye appearance and make the ophthalmopathy look worse than it actually is. A host of eye complaints may occur, including pain, diplopia, proptosis, and blurred vision. The cosmetic changes may be among the most disturbing. The proptosis is a true one, differentiated from the stare, lid lag, and apparent proptosis that may accompany other forms of hyperthyroidism.

Pretibial myxedema is a less common immune-mediated infiltrative process affecting an occasional Graves' disease patient. Onset is typically years after treatment of hyperthyroidism and usually in patients with a history of ophthalmopathy. The condition is characterized by the appearance of erythematous, mildly scaly plaques limited to the skin of the ankles and pretibial area. The plaques are indurated, but nontender. They usually resolve spontaneously.

The thyroid gland in Graves' disease is diffusely enlarged, and a bruit may be heard in severe cases. The classic symptoms and signs of thyrotoxicosis are common. The skin is velvety and the hair silky. Onycholysis, vitiligo, and gynecomastia are found in some cases and may suggest the diagnosis. Cardiac complications are infrequent, due to the relative youth of the patient population, but a reversible cardiomyopathy has been identified, manifested by a fall in ejection fraction with exercise. Heart failure is rare, but impaired exercise tolerance is often reported, perhaps caused by the decrease in ejection fraction.

The clinical course of Graves' disease waxes and wanes, with exacerbations and remissions of unpredictable duration. After many years, mild hypothyroidism may ensue, especially in patients with small goiters and mild hyperthyroidism at the time of onset.

Toxic Multinodular Goiter (*Plummer's Disease*) accounts for most cases of hyperthyroidism in middle-aged and elderly persons. The condition is often associated with a long-standing simple goiter. The gland is clinically and pathologically indistinguishable from that of nontoxic multinodular goiters. Cardiovascular symptoms may dominate the clinical presentation; new onset of heart failure, atrial fibrillation, or angina is not uncommon and reflects the high prevalence of coexisting organic heart disease in this older population. In a series of 85 hyperthyroid patients between ages 60 and 82, two-thirds experienced heart failure and 20 percent reported angina. Only a minority evidenced the more typical symptoms of hyperthyroidism; for example, less than 11 percent had polyphagia. On the other hand, 33 percent suffered from anorexia, and constipation was as prevalent as diarrhea. Lid lag may be noted on occasion, but exophthalmos does not occur. Sometimes apathy and weight loss are the most prominent clinical features and can be so profound as to suggest occult malignancy or severe depression.

Elderly patients with large, nontoxic nodular goiters have demonstrated an increased risk of developing thyrotoxicosis on exposure to *iodides* (including iodinated contrast agents). The problem is most prevalent among patients who come from areas of low iodine intake (eg, Europe) but can also occur in nonendemic cases of multinodular goiter and thyroid adenoma. The mechanism involves increased release of stored hormone. The clinical course is self-limited. Laboratory findings include a low radioactive iodine (RAI) uptake and absence of antithyroid antibodies.

Single Toxic Nodule (Hot Nodule). The autonomously functioning toxic nodule presents clinically much like the toxic multinodular goiter. The principal difference is the finding of a "hot" nodule surrounded by suppressed gland on radioiodine thyroid scan. The larger the nodule, the greater its propensity to cause thyrotoxicosis, with risk quite high once the nodule reaches 3 cm in diameter. Often, onset of toxicity is first manifested by an isolated increase in serum T_3; later, T_4 levels rise. Sometimes hemorrhagic infarction terminates the overproduction of hormone and limits the progression to thyrotoxicosis.

T_3 Toxicosis is an important entity to consider when patients with clinically apparent hyperthyroidism have normal T_4 levels. The condition has been reported in association with both diffuse and nodular goiters. Clinical presentation is no different from hyperthyroidism due to elevations in T_4. Isolated elevations in T_3 concentration may also occur in euthyroid patients who have no underlying thyroid disease (see below).

Transient Hyperthyroidism may occur in association with subacute (granulomatous) or chronic (lymphocytic) thyroiditis. As noted above, the mechanism appears to be uncontrolled release of hormone from an inflamed gland. Iodine uptake is reduced during the period of hyperthyroidism. The clinical manifestations of hyperthyroidism are usually mild. The course is self-limited, and hypothyroidism often follows as intrathyroidal stores of the hormone are depleted. *Subacute thyroiditis* typically follows a viral illness, producing a tender, multinodular gland. The occasional case associated with hyperthyroidism is abrupt in onset in conjunction with thyrotoxic symptoms. The erythrocyte sedimentation rate is high, and thyroid scan characteristically shows little or no uptake of radioiodine.

Lymphocytic thyroiditis resulting in hyperthyroidism is thought to be an uncommon variant of Hashimoto's disease. In some cases, it may be due to coexisting Graves' disease. There are high titers of antibodies to microsomes and thyroglobulin. Prevalence is highest in middle-aged women and among the elderly, where it may go unrecognized. The gland feels rubbery and is enlarged, sometimes asymmetrically. Hypothyroidism eventually develops in a substantial number of cases.

Postpartum (subacute lymphocytic) thyroiditis, a previously unappreciated but surprisingly frequent problem (incidence as high as 5% in one series) can precipitate transient mild hyperthyroidism. Onset is within 3 to 6 months of delivery and often is mistaken for anxiety due to the stress of caring for a new child. The gland is nontender and may resemble that of Hashimoto's thyroiditis. RAI uptake is low and antithyroid antibodies detectable, suggesting an immunologic mechanism. The condition may persist for months before eventually resolving. A period of hypothyroidism may occur before the condition ceases. It tends to recur with subsequent pregnancies.

Overproduction of Thyroid-Stimulating Hormone. A small number of *pituitary adenomas* produce excessive TSH. The result is a diffusely enlarged gland simulating Graves' disease, but there is no ophthalmopathy. A similar clinical picture may ensue from a tumor producing human chorionic gonadotropin (hCG), such as a *hydatidiform mole* or a *choriocarcinoma*. hCG has weak thyroid-stimulating activity but when produced in massive quantities can cause hyperthyroidism.

Ectopic Thyroxine Production and Intake of Exogenous Hormone. When the source of excess thyroid hormone is extrathyroidal, the thyroid gland will appear small due to absence of TSH stimulation. A dermoid tumor of the ovary, *struma ovarii*, with elements of thyroid-like tissue, is the only neoplasm regularly capable of synthesizing excessive amounts of thyroid hormone. (Rarely thyroid cancers can cause hyperthyroidism, but only in the context of a massive tumor burden.) Intake of thyroid hormone in excess of daily requirements (>200 μg/d of levothyroxine) will make a person hyperthyroid. Sometimes the intake is surreptitious. The gland is small, and TSH is absent.

DIFFERENTIAL DIAGNOSIS

The differential diagnosis of hyperthyroidism can be organized according to pathophysiology (Table 103–1). The

Table 103-1. Causes of Hyperthyroidism

PATHOPHYSIOLOGY	ETIOLOGY
Autonomous hormone production	Toxic multinodular goiter Toxic adenoma
Increased hormone release	Subacute thyroiditis Lymphocytic (Hashimoto's) thyroiditis Iodide exposure
Increased glandular stimulation	Graves' disease (TSab) Functioning pituitary adenoma (THS) Choriocarcinoma (hCG)
Exogenous hormone intake	Intake of >200 μg/d of levothyroxine
Extraglandular production	Struma ovarii Metastatic thyroid cancer

most common cause is Graves' disease, followed by multinodular goiter, toxic adenoma, thyroiditis, and exogenous thyroid hormone. Pituitary adenoma, struma ovarii, and chorionic cancers are very rare causes.

WORKUP

Diagnosis of Hyperthyroidism

Clinical recognition of hyperthyroidism can sometimes be difficult, especially when symptoms are mild or when the condition occurs in the elderly or pregnant patient. Moreover, the correlation between symptoms and thyroid hormone levels is often poor, necessitating careful laboratory confirmation of the diagnosis and its severity.

An important biochemical hallmark of hyperthyroidism is an increase in the concentrations of serum thyroid hormones. The *free T_4* or *free T_4* index (an excellent proxy for the free T_4, calculated by multiplying the serum T_4 by the T_3 resin uptake) is the most useful determination of circulating thyroid hormone and the one most commonly obtained. Measurement of the serum *total T_3* is usually not necessary unless the patient is clinically thyrotoxic in the setting of a normal or only slightly elevated free T_4. Routinely ordering a serum T_3 is probably wasteful, because T_3 toxicosis is uncommon.

As useful as thyroid hormone levels are for diagnosis, overreliance on them can be misleading. *Euthyroid hyperthyroxemia* occurs when there is an increase in thyroid-binding globulin (eg, pregnancy, estrogen use, liver disease), which produces an increase in total T_4, while the free T_4 remains normal. More confusing are euthyroid states with increases in free T_4 as well as total T_4. Patients with autoantibodies against thyroid hormones may manifest surprisingly high free hormone levels due to interference by these immunoglobulins with the standard radioimmune assays for thyroid hormones. Acute medical, surgical, and psychiatric illnesses as well as intake of high-dose propranolol, amiodarone, and gallbladder dyes can impair peripheral conversion of T_4 to active T_3, leading to rises in free T_4 concentration in conjunction with a reduction in T_3 and an increase in reverse T_3. An unexpectedly normal or low T_3 level in a patient who is clinically euthyroid yet has elevations in T_4 and free T_4 should raise the suspicion of euthyroid hyperthyroxemia. The T_3 concentration helps in the differentiation.

The *serum TSH* determination has become an excellent means of screening for hyperthyroidism. Marked improvement in the sensitivity of the TSH assay by radioimmunologic techniques now makes it possible to diagnose hyperthyroidism solely on the basis of absence of detectable TSH. As long as the hypothalamic–pituitary axis is intact, absence of TSH represents the appropriate response to too much circulating thyroid hormone. A normal TSH level by radioimmunoassay virtually rules out hyperthyroidism, unless there is a functioning pituitary adenoma. A low TSH is a less specific finding, found in mild hyperthyroidism but also in euthyroid patients with autonomously functioning glands (thyroid adenoma, euthyroid Graves' disease), in those taking modest amounts of exogenous thyroid hormone, and in older persons without hyperthyroidism.

Thyrotropin releasing hormone (TRH) stimulation testing is sometimes used when hyperthyroidism is suspected but serum thyroxine levels are equivocal. In patients with genuine hyperthyroidism, the TSH response to TRH is minimal or absent. This reflects suppression of the pituitary by elevated levels of thyroid hormone. However, cortisol hypersecretion can also suppress TSH response to TRH, simulating the pattern seen with hyperthyroidism. With the advent of a very sensitive TSH assay, TRH stimulation testing is rarely necessary, but it remains among the most sensitive of tests for the detection of hyperthyroidism.

Identifying the Underlying Etiology

History and Physical Examination. *History* is checked for goiter, thyroid nodule, use of iodides or thyroid hormone, eye changes, recent pregnancy or viral illness, and known ovarian, pituitary, or thyroid neoplasm. Review of systems should look for symptoms of a pituitary tumor (see Chapters 100 and 101).

Physical examination focuses on the *thyroid gland*, checking for overall size and nodularity. A diffusely enlarged, nontender gland suggests Graves' disease; in rare instances, a TSH-secreting tumor may be responsible for such diffuse glandular stimulation. A bruit may accompany the diffusely enlarged gland of Graves' disease. An exquisitely tender, diffusely enlarged gland occurring in the context of a viral illness points to subacute thyroiditis. The gland in lymphocytic thyroiditis is nontender and diffusely, but only modestly, enlarged. A small gland indicates an extrathyroidal source of hormone. Multinodularity is consistent with a toxic multinodular goiter and also occurs in patients with Hashimoto's thyroiditis. An otherwise atrophic gland with a single nodule, especially if greater than 3 cm in diameter, strongly suggests toxic adenoma.

Extrathyroidal findings may have diagnostic significance and should be noted. *True proptosis* (>20 mm of eye protrusion from the orbital bone) is a hallmark of Graves' disease, as is *pretibial myxedema*. Lid lag and stare are nonspecific consequences of hyperthyroidism and may simulate proptosis. The neck nodes should be checked for adenopathy. Painless cervical lymphadenopathy raises the question of a thyroid malignancy. A pelvic examination and visual field testing are important to check for ovarian and pituitary etiologies.

Laboratory Studies. The *thyroid scan* can help differentiate among etiologies when the clinical picture remains uncertain. A toxic adenoma will be identified as a "hot nodule," with little uptake by the rest of the gland. Uptake will be low in patients with thyroiditis, exogenous hormone intake, extraglandular hormone production, and iodide exposure. Uptake will be diffusely increased in patients with Graves' disease or a functioning pituitary adenoma.

Antithyroid antibodies (including those directed against microsomal peroxidase) are increased in both Graves' disease and lymphocytic (Hashimoto's) thyroiditis, limiting their diagnostic utility. *Serum thyroglobulin* determination serves as an elegant yet simple means of detecting the patient surreptitiously taking thyroid hormone. Exogenous hormone use results in suppression of thyroglobulin synthesis. *Whole-body scanning* will identify the rare case of extrathyroidal hormone synthesis, such as a struma ovarii or a hyperfunctioning metastasis from a thyroid malignancy.

A host of nonspecific hematologic and serum chemistry abnormalities accompany hyperthyroidism, but they have little etiologic significance. They include a mild degree of anemia, granulocytosis, lymphocytosis, hypercalcemia, transaminase elevation, and alkaline phosphatase elevation.

PRINCIPLES OF THERAPY

The goals of therapy are to correct the hypermetabolic state with a minimum of side effects and with the smallest incidence of hypothyroidism. For definitive therapy, one must choose among antithyroid drugs, radioiodine, and thyroidectomy. Beta-blocking agents are useful for prompt, temporary control of hyperadrenergic symptoms. Hyperthyroidism should not go untreated, particularly in the elderly, who are at risk for cardiovascular complications. Moreover, not only are symptoms uncomfortable, but thyrotoxic crisis may ensue if the untreated patient unexpectedly encounters a severe stress such as emergency surgery or acute sepsis.

Therapeutic Modalities

Beta-Blocking Agents inhibit the adrenergic effects of excess thyroid hormone. As such, they provide excellent, prompt, symptomatic relief from many of the catecholamine-mediated manifestations of hyperthyroidism (eg, tremor, palpitations, heat intolerance, nervousness). However, beta-blockers have no intrinsic antithyroid activity, except perhaps at very high doses (where they may slow peripheral conversion of T_4 to T_3). Control of symptoms can often be achieved within a few days, making these agents an excellent choice for first-line therapy and preoperative treatment. Beta-blockers may suffice for treatment of transient hyperthyroidism, but they must be used in conjunction with other treatment modalities for definitive control of persistent disease.

Beta-blockers are particularly valuable for minimizing the major cardiac complications of hyperthyroidism (eg, atrial fibrillation—see Chapter 28; angina—see Chapter 30). Rate-related heart failure will also benefit from beta-blockade, but that due to myocardial pathology will worsen with such therapy. Consequently, beta-blockade must be applied with care in the elderly and those with preexisting heart disease (see Chapter 32).

Of the beta-blockers, propranolol remains the most widely used for control of hyperthyroidism, but other agents in this class (eg, atenolol, metoprolol, nadolol) demonstrate comparable efficacy. Those with a more sustained half-life (eg, atenolol) are particularly useful for patients who are to undergo surgery. Adequacy of dose is determined by monitoring the resting and exercise heart rates and the degree of symptomatic relief.

One important benefit from beta-blockade is the ability to proceed safely with thyroid surgery within 1 to 2 weeks. Antithyroid drugs (see below) require 6 to 8 weeks of preoperative treatment. The addition of *potassium iodide* to beta-blocker therapy produces more rapid and greater preoperative control of patients with Graves' disease who are to undergo thyroidectomy; it is especially useful in those who fail to achieve adequate control on beta-blockers alone, as defined by a resting pulse of less than 90 beats per minute and a blunting of exercise-induced tachycardia.

Antithyroid Drugs. *Methimazole* and *propylthiouracil (PTU)* are the most important antithyroid agents. PTU acts by interfering with the synthesis of thyroxine and blocking peripheral conversion of T_4 to T_3, although, at conventional doses, this latter effect does not appear to be clinically important. Methimazole does not have any peripheral effect but is more potent. Both drugs suppress thyroid autoimmunity and decrease circulating TSAb. Biochemical response to the antithyroid drugs is detectable within 1 to 2 weeks; clinical response typically takes 4 to 8 weeks.

These antithyroid agents are widely used in *young and middle-aged patients*, particularly for long-term control of *Graves' disease*, as well as for preoperative control and for therapy prior to and following radioiodine ablation. The initial dose of PTU averages 300 mg/d (100 mg q8h). For methimazole, the starting dose is 15 mg/d, which can be given as a single dose since its half-life is much longer. Therapy is adjusted as needed to attain clinical and biochemical control. Once control is achieved, the dose can be tapered to the lowest amount needed to maintain a euthyroid state. Usually, treatment is continued for 12 to 24 months and then halted to see if relapse occurs.

The chance of long-term remission in Graves' disease is enhanced by 1 to 2 years of antithyroid drug therapy. PTU induces remission in approximately 50 percent of patients with Graves' disease who are treated for 1 to 2 years, but one-third to one-half of those who respond will relapse. Reports of a remission rate of 40 percent after only 3 to 5 months of antithyroid therapy initially raised hopes that a shorter course of treatment might suffice, but longer-term follow-up revealed increased rates of relapse. The risk of inducing hypothyroidism is low. Patients who relapse or fail to achieve remission need to be considered for radioiodine or surgical therapy.

Common adverse effects include skin rash, fever, and arthralgias; these are usually not of major clinical significance. However, the rare (0.3%–0.6% of patients) but potentially fatal complication of *agranulocytosis* necessitates careful patient selection and close monitoring of therapy. The risk of agranulocytosis increases with age, (beginning at about age 40) and is independent of dose for PTU but dose-dependent for methimazole. Onset is usually within 2 months, rarely beyond 4 months. No patients taking less than 30 mg/d of methimazole have been reported to develop agranulocytosis, making this drug the safer of the two.

Close monitoring of blood counts is important, but only during the first 4 months of therapy. Mild leukopenia is common, occurring in up to 10 percent of patients; its occurrence does not require halting treatment. If the leukocyte count falls below 1500/mm^3, therapy should be withheld.

Choice of antithyroid agent has been a subject of debate. Properly monitored, either antithyroid drug is a reasonable choice. Although PTU is more widely prescribed, *methimazole* appears *preferable* in terms of cost, hematologic side effects, and ease of administration. At doses up to 30 mg/d, methimazole is about 30 percent lower in cost than a comparable dose of PTU, is much less likely to induce agranulocytosis, and need be taken only once daily. PTU might be preferable during pregnancy and breast-feeding (see below).

Radioactive Iodine (^{131}I) represents an important form of ablative therapy, first introduced in 1942 and widely used today, especially in older hyperthyroid patients, where concern for the long-term effects of radiation exposure is limited. It is indicated in Graves' disease when antithyroid drugs do not suffice, in elderly or noncompliant patients, in those with solitary toxic nodules, and in those with contraindications or a reluctance to undergo surgery. Advantages include established efficacy, relative safety, and ease of administration. Disadvantages are delay in controlling symptoms and high incidence of ensuing hypothyroidism.

Among the *side effects* of radioactive iodine therapy, the most common complication is *hypothyroidism*. High-dose radioiodine provides predictable relief but a high incidence of early hypothyroidism (70% in the first year). Low-dose regimens have a lower early risk of hypothyroidism (15% in the first year) but provide less control of the disease (50% still hyperthyroid at 1 year). Long-term follow-up studies of patients given low-dose treatment indicate a steady increase in the cumulative incidence of hypothyroidism (75% at 11 years), suggesting that its early advantages fade with time. Regardless of dose used, the risk of eventual hypothyroidism requires that patients be regularly reevaluated, typically at 6-month intervals.

Worsening ophthalmopathy is a concern and is more common with radioiodine therapy than with other forms of antithyroid treatment for Graves' disease. As noted earlier, up to 20 percent of Graves' disease patients with eye involvement predating the treatment of hyperthyroidism experience an exacerbation after treatment for their hyperthyroidism. Correction of hyperthyroidism does not appear to cause *de novo* ophthalmopathy, but treatment-induced hypothyroidism (which is common in radioiodine-treated patients) appears to increase the risk of worsening eye changes. The mechanism is unclear; a treatment-induced outpouring of antibody-stimulating antigen is hypothesized.

Prophylactic treatment with oral *prednisone* for a few months after radioiodine therapy has been shown to reduce the risk of worsening eye disease. However, the programs studied require moderately large steroid doses taken daily for several months. Although steroids are tapered after the first month, the incidence of steroid side effects (see Chapter 105) is high. Cyclosporine has also been tried. It is less effective than prednisone but has proven helpful in combination for refractory cases. At present, avoidance of hypothyroidism appears to be the best mode of prevention. The mode of therapy may also be germaine (see also Chapter 204).

The concern that radioiodine would lead to long-term *radiation injury* has not been borne out. The gonadal radiation dose from ^{131}I therapy is small, the equivalent of that from a barium enema or an intravenous pyelogram. There is no evidence of increased rates of birth defects or thyroid cancer. Available retrospective cohort studies have evaluated patients treated as long as 30 years ago.

Surgery represents the most direct ablative approach to hyperthyroidism. The objective is to reduce thyroid mass sufficiently to cure the hypermetabolic state without inducing a hypothyroid condition. Unfortunately, there is a substantial incidence of permanent hypothyroidism and smaller but perceptible risks of hypoparathyroidism and laryngeal paralysis. Moreover, hyperthyroidism may recur despite subtotal thyroidectomy in Graves' disease. Prior preparation of the patient with antithyroid drugs is required to avoid precipitating thyroid storm. Surgery is particularly useful for relieving esophageal obstruction; cosmesis and pregnancy are other indications. It is also a choice when antithyroid drugs fail or produce complications, or when patients are noncompliant or refuse radioiodine. Young patients with moderate to severe disease do particularly well. However, ^{131}I treatment is increasingly replacing surgery, because it is a less expensive and less morbid therapy.

Iodides are sometimes useful as supplemental agents, because they can block peripheral conversion of T_4 to T_3 and inhibit hormone release. *Potassium iodide* was the earliest of the iodides to be employed. The *organic iodide radiographic contrast agents* (eg, ipodate, iopanoate) have supplanted the inorganic iodides. However, control is sometimes problematic. Paradoxical increases in hormone release can occur. Thus, iodides are best utilized for preoperative control in patients who require a second drug to counter the hyperthyroidism and in those who have a contraindication to use of beta-blockers and other antithyroid medications.

Choice of Therapy

Graves' Disease. There is little consensus among thyroidologists as to the best treatment for Graves' disease, except in the case of the *elderly patient*, for whom *radioactive iodine* is considered the treatment of choice. Surveys of opinion regarding treatment of *middle-aged* and *younger patients* reveals marked diversity of opinion, split between antithyroid drugs and radioiodine, with surgery deemed best reserved for those who are not candidates for either. An initial trial of *antithyroid drug* therapy represents a reasonable starting point for treatment, supplemented by beta-blocker therapy to help establish a euthyroid state and counter-control adrenergic symptoms. Patients falling to achieve control with such therapy, unable to tolerate it, or experiencing relapse after its completion can be considered for radioiodine. Despite the absence of evidence for long-term genetic risk, concern persists about giving radioiodine to patients in their reproductive years.

Contributing to the diversity of opinion is dissatisfaction with available therapies. None appears capable of definitively halting the underlying immunopathologic process, which remains poorly understood. Recently, it was noted that adding *thyroid replacement therapy* to antithyroid drug therapy decreased the frequency of recurrence of Graves' disease and reduced the production of antibodies to TSH receptors. Perhaps this approach of letting the thyroid "rest" may open a new avenue to treatment. The reader is encouraged to follow the literature closely for more data on such new approaches to treatment.

Treatment of ophthalmopathy also remains a challenge. Etiologic therapy awaits a better understanding of the underlying disease mechanisms. Although ophthalmopathy may worsen with treatment of the hyperthyroidism, especially if hypothyroidism is induced, there is no evidence that scaling back treatment will prevent an exacerbation. However, radioiodine appears to be the modality most likely to worsen ophthalmopathy, perhaps because it is the most likely to induce hypothyroidism. This has led some to recommend thyroxine supplementation to prevent hypothyroidism. Moderately high doses of glucocorticosteroids given at the time of antithyroid treatment can reduce the risk ophthalmopathy, but such prophylactic therapy is not recommended for routine use because of the high incidence of adverse side effects, the inability to predict who will experience an exacerbation, and the low incidence (7%) of severe ophthalmopathy. However, those with moderate to marked preexisting ophthalmopathy may be reasonable candidates for such prophylactic treatment. Good eye care is also a priority.

With a host of alternative therapies available, each with its own advantages and disadvantages, it is important to individualize treatment according to the patient's needs, capabilities, and clinical status. For now, one must settle for treating the hyperthyroidism; etiologic therapy is awaited.

Toxic Nodule. Radioiodine is the treatment of choice for elderly patients with this condition. Since the rest of the gland is suppressed by the hyperfunctioning nodule, the incidence of posttreatment hypothyroidism is far less than that seen with treatment of Graves' disease. Optimal radioiodine dose remains a subject of debate. A relatively low dose of ^{131}I (5–15 mCi) appears to provide excellent results with minimal adverse effects (75% of patients euthyroid by 2 mo, >90% within 6 mo, posttreatment hypothyroidism very rare). Surgical removal may be preferable in young patients.

Hyperthyroidism in Pregnant and Nursing Patients. The choice is between antithyroid drugs and surgery, because radioiodine is contraindicated (it crosses the placenta and concentrates in the fetal thyroid). Antithyroid drug therapy is considered safer than surgery, with surgery reserved for refractory cases and patients who refuse to take their medication. Among the *antithyroid agents, PTU* is preferred; methimazole has been associated with aplasia cutis in the fetus. The risk of drug crossing into the placenta and inducing hypothyroidism in the fetus is small and not strictly dose-related, but precipitation of hypothyroidism in the mother can compromise the fetus and should be avoided. Pregnant women with Graves' disease may transfer large amounts of thyroid-stimulating antibody to the fetus and induce fetal thyrotoxicosis, even after thyroid ablation. Testing the newborn for thyrotoxicosis is essential in this setting. There is no evidence that treatment of pregnant thyrotoxic patients leads to impaired intellectual development in the offspring. The optimal antithyroid drug regimen for fetal thyroid status appears to be one that maintains maternal free T_4 levels near the upper limit of normal.

Breast-feeding mothers can transfer antithyroid medication in the milk, but the amount is small, especially with use of PTU, and not likely to induce significant hypothyroidism. However, discussions of potential risks and need for careful monitoring are important.

Short-term use of *beta-blocking agents* and/or *iodides* provide prompt, effective, and safe control of thyrotoxic symptoms. Symptoms improve within 2 to 7 days. Longer-term use of these agents is more problematic. Beta-blocking drugs have been linked to intrauterine growth retardation, small placenta, postnatal bradycardia, and hypoglycemia. Nevertheless, the complication rate is low and use during pregnancy is generally safe. Extended use of iodides is riskier, with large, obstructing fetal goiters reported.

Surgery is usually reserved for the patient who has failed or is a bad candidate for medical treatment. Operative mortality, though low, still exceeds that associated with drug therapy. Prior to subtotal thyroidectomy, preoperative medical therapy is indicated to attain control and prevent thyroid storm.

Thyroiditis. As noted above, hyperthyroidism due to thyroiditis can be managed symptomatically with *beta-blocking agents,* because spontaneous resolution is the rule. Aspirin and occasionally corticosteroids are indicated in subacute thyroiditis to control inflammatory symptoms.

Monitoring Therapy

Monitoring treatment requires attention to clinical status and indices of thyroid function. Clinical status is assessed by taking note of any changes in weight, degree of heat intolerance, tremulousness, anxiousness, appetite, level of energy, resting heart rate, ophthalmopathy, skin texture, or skin temperature. The amount of circulating thyroid hormone is assessed by monitoring change in the serum concentration of *free* T_4 (or total T_3 in the case of T_3 toxicosis). *TSH* determination provides the best measure of treatment end point (normalization of TSH) and the earliest evidence of overtreatment and development of hypothyroidism.

In patients with Graves' disease, monitoring the serum level of *antibodies to TSH receptors* also helps predict clinical course. Relapse is a strong possibility if TSAb remains elevated and less likely, though not ruled out, if it is reduced or absent.

For patients taking antithyroid drug therapy, routine monitoring of the *leukocyte count* is indicated, especially in patients taking PTU or more than 30 mg/d of methimazole. Risk is greatest during the first 4 months of therapy, necessitating more frequent monitoring (every 2–4 wk) during this period, followed by less frequent monitoring for the duration of antithyroid drug therapy.

PATIENT EDUCATION

Patients with hyperthyroidism are often relieved to know that their "nervousness" is due to an underlying medical illness rather than an emotional problem and that it will improve with therapy. Patients who are taking antithyroid agents need to be instructed on prompt reporting of symptoms suggestive of agranulocytosis (eg, fever, chills), especially during the first 4 months of therapy. Those with prominent exophthalmos should be warned to see the physician at the first sign of diplopia or visual impairment. Hyperthyroid mothers taking antithyroid drugs and eager to breastfeed their infants need not be prohibited from breast-feeding, as long as one takes the time to explain the potential risks and the importance of careful monitoring. Patients treated with radioiodine should be informed to watch for symptoms of hypothyroidism.

INDICATIONS FOR REFERRAL AND ADMISSION

Patients who are candidates for ^{131}I therapy should have a thyroid scan and be seen by the endocrinologist or radiation therapist for calculation of the dose of ^{131}I to be administered. Consultation with an endocrinologist is also indicated in the management of the pregnant or lactating hyperthyroid patient and the individual with severe ophthalmopathy of Graves' disease. Visual impairment due to severe ophthalmopathy may require hospital admission for very high-dose systemic steroid therapy or surgical decompression. Referral for consideration of surgical therapy is also indicated when the patient is pregnant, has obstruction to swallowing, desires cosmetic improvement, or fails antithyroid drug therapy. Prompt hospital admission is needed if heart failure, rapid atrial fibrillation, or angina develops.

THERAPEUTIC RECOMMENDATIONS

- For prompt control of adrenergic symptoms of hyperthyroidism regardless of underlying etiology, start treatment immediately with a *beta-blocking agent* (eg, propranolol 80 mg/d, atenolol 50 mg/d). Increase dose daily until symptoms are controlled. Use with extreme caution in patients with preexisting heart failure unrelated to thyroid disease.
- For *non-pregnant young* and *middle-aged* patients with *Graves' disease*, start *methimazole* (20–30 mg/d) in addition to the beta-blocker program. Continue both methimazole and beta-blockade for 4 to 8 weeks, and then taper the beta-blocker as the antithyroid agent takes hold. Adjust antithyroid drug dose according to clinical status and thyroid indices (TSH, FT_4). Use the lowest possible dose that maintains biochemical and biologic control. Monitor closely to avoid precipitating hypothyroidism. Monitor leukocyte count if more than 30 mg/d of methimazole is being taken or if the patient is elderly.
- If response is obtained, continue antithyroid therapy for 12 to 24 months. One can measure TSAb at 12 months. If TSAb is absent and patient appears to be in remission clinically and biochemically, then try discontinuing therapy. If relapse occurs, then consider resumption of antithyroid therapy for 12 more months or radioiodine therapy.
- For the *pregnant patient* with *Graves' disease*, consider antithyroid drug therapy, but obtain endocrinologic consultation before initiating treatment. *PTU* is preferred (starting dose 100 mg tid) and can also be used in the patient who is eager to breast-feed. Risks of such therapy should be fully explained and understood by the patient. Careful monitoring of thyroid status in both mother and baby is essential. Maintain the pregnant patient's free T_4 levels near the upper limit of normal; monitor TSH closely.
- For all patients taking antithyroid medication, *monitor the leukocyte count* every 2 to 4 weeks during the first 4 months of therapy, then every 4 to 6 months. Stop therapy if the count falls below 1500 neutrophils per milliliter. Risk of agranulocytosis and need for close monitoring are greatest in the elderly and those taking PTU or more than 30 mg/d of methimazole.
- For Graves' patients with severe symptomatic ophthalmopathy, obtain prompt endocrinologic consultation. Options include very high-dose systemic glucocorticosteroids (prednisone 120–150 mg/d), local steroid injection, surgical decompression, and radiation therapy.
- For Graves' patients with mild to moderate ophthalmopathy, minimize risk of worsening eye disease by avoiding posttreatment hypothyroidism. Routine use of systemic daily steroid therapy for prophylaxis of posttreatment exacerbation is not recommended but may be considered for patients who begin radioiodine treatment with moderately severe eye changes already established (prednisone 20–40 mg/d for the first month, followed by tapering over 3 mo). For periorbital edema, advise elevating the head of the bed and using a mild diuretic (eg, hydrochlorothiazide 50 mg/d). Prescribe methylcellulose drops to prevent corneal drying (see also Chapter 204).
- Consider *^{131}I therapy* for patients with *solitary toxic nodules*, *elderly patients with Graves' disease*, and other patients with Graves' disease who fail or cannot be maintained on antithyroid drugs (relapse, agranulocytosis). Continue beta-blockade for the 2- to 3-month period that it takes for the radioiodine to exert its full effect on the gland. Three to 6 months after onset of treatment and at 3- to 6-month intervals thereafter, monitor TSH for evidence of ensuing hypothyroidism; correct promptly by starting thyroid replacement therapy before hypothyroidism develops.
- Refer for consideration of *surgery* any patient with *neck obstruction*, *poor compliance* in taking medication, a contraindication to or failure of antithyroid drug therapy, or a *cosmetic concern*. Young patients do particularly well. If surgery is contemplated, continue antithyroid or beta-blocking therapy up to the moment of surgery. Monitor for postoperative hyperthyroidism.
- Treat patients with *transient hyperthyroidism* due to thyroiditis symptomatically with *beta-blockade* until the condition resolves on its own.

A.H.G.

ANNOTATED BIBLIOGRAPHY

Bartalena l, Marocci C, Bogazzi F, et al. Use of corticosteroids to prevent progression of Graves' ophthalmopathy after radioiodine therapy for hyperthyroidism. N Engl J Med 1989;321:1349. *(Found effective, but the moderately high daily doses needed resulted in steroid side effects.)*

Borst GC, Eil C, Burman KD. Euthyroid hyperthyroxemia. Ann Intern Med 1983;98:366. *(A detailed review of the mechanisms and syndromes causing elevation hyperthyroxemia in clinically euthyroid patients; 229 refs.)*

Burrow GN. The management of thyrotoxicosis in pregnancy. N Engl J Med 1984;313:562. *(A terse but clinically useful review; 49 refs.)*

Chopra IJ, Hershman JM, Pardridge WM, et al. Thyroid function in nonthyroidal illnesses. Ann Intern Med 1983;98:946. *(Discusses the changes in thyroid hormone levels and their consequences in nonthyroidal illness.)*

Cooper DS. Which antithyroid drug? Am J Med 1986;80:1165. *(Favors methimazole over PTU for most cases.)*

Cooper DS, Goldminz D, Levin AA, et al. Agranulocytosis associated with antithyroid drugs. Ann Intern Med 1983;98:26. *(Increasing age and dose of methimazole were associated with increased risk; the risk with use of PTU was independent of dose.)*

Forar JC, Muir AL, Sawers SA, et al. Abnormal left ventricular function in hyperthyroidism. N Engl J Med 1982;307:1165. *(Provides evidence for a reversible cardiomyopathic state directly related to excess thyroid hormone.)*

Forar JC, Miller HC, Toft AD. Occult thyrotoxicosis: a correctable cause of "idiopathic" atrial fibrillation. Am J Cardiol 1979;44:9. *(Description of the atypical presentation of hyperthyroidism of the elderly.)*

Graham GD, Burman KD. Radioiodine treatment of Graves' disease. Ann Intern Med 1986;105:900. *(Comprehensive review of potential risks; 72 refs.)*

Hashizume K, Ichikawa K, Sakurai A, et al. Administration of thyroxine in treated Graves' disease—effects on the level of antibodies to thyroid-stimulating hormone receptors and on the risk of recurrence of hyperthyroidism. N Engl J Med 1991;324:947. *(An intriguing approach in which adding thyroxine reduces TSAb levels and the risk of recurrence.)*

Ladenson PW. Treatment for Graves' disease—letting the thyroid rest. N Engl J Med 1991;324:989. *(An editorial reviewing treatment options, including the idea of adding thyroxine to antithyroid drug therapy.)*

Mariotti S, Martino E, Cupini C, et al. Low serum thyroglobulin as a clue to the diagnosis of thyrotoxicosis factitia. N Engl J Med 1982;307:410. *(An excellent way to diagnose surreptitious use.)*

Momotani N, Noh J, Oyanagi H, et al. Antithyroid drug therapy for Graves' disease during pregnancy. N Engl J Med 1986;315:24. *(The optimal antithyroid regimen for the fetus appears to be one that maintains maternal free T_4 in the mildly hyperthyroid range.)*

Ross DS. New sensitive immunoradiometric assays for thyrotropin. Ann Intern Med 1986;104:718. *(An editorial suggesting the test is very sensitive for diagnosis of hyperthyroidism and the best screening test for the condition.)*

Ross DS, Ardisson LJ, Meskell MJ. Measurement of thyrotropin in clinical and subclinical hyperthyroidism using a new chemiluminescent assay. J Clin Endocrinol Metab 1989;69:684. *(The assay's enhanced sensitivity enables one to use the TSH determination for the diagnosis of hyperthyroidism.)*

Ross DS, Ridgeway EC, Daniels GH. Successful treatment of solitary toxic thyroid nodules with relatively low dose iodine 131, with a low prevalence of hypothyroidism. Ann Intern Med 1984;101:488. *(Reports excellent efficacy and safety; argues that high doses are unnecessary.)*

Sundbeck G, et al. Clinical significance of low serum thyrotropin concentration by chemiluminometric assay in 85-year-old women and men. Arch Intern Med 1991;151:549. *(Elderly persons may have a low TSH but remain euthyroid.)*

Surks MI, Chopra IJ, Mariash CN, et al. American Thyroid Association guidelines for use of laboratory tests in thyroid disorders. JAMA 1990;263:1529. *(Recommends TSH and free T_4 as the principal tests.)*

Tajiri J, Noguchi S, Murakami T, et al. Antithyroid drug-induced agranulocytosis—the usefulness of routine leukocyte count monitoring. Arch Intern Med 1990;150:621. *(Evidence for regular monitoring.)*

Tallstedt L, Lundell G, Torring O, et al. Occurrence of ophthalmopathy after treatment for Graves' hyperthyroidism. N Engl J Med 1992;326:1733. *(A randomized, controlled trial; iodine-131 therapy was more likely to be followed by worsening ophthalmopathy than other therapies, especially in older patients.)*

Totterman TH, Karlsson FA, Bengtsson M, et al. Induction of circulating activated suppressor-like T cells by methimazole therapy for Graves' disease. N Engl J Med 1987;316:15. *(Evidence that antithyroid drugs may act in part by an immunopathologic mechanism.)*

Utiger, RD. Beta-adrenergic antagonist therapy for hyperthyroid Graves' disease. N Engl J Med 1984;310:1597. *(An editorial summarizing the use of beta-blockade as well as other modalities for treatment of Graves' disease.)*

Utiger RD. Pathogenesis of Graves' ophthalmopathy. N Engl J Med 1992;326:1772. *(Mechanisms reviewed, particularly in relation to mode of antithyroid therapy.)*

Utiger RD. Treatment of Graves' ophthalmopathy. N Engl J Med 1989;321:1403. *(An editorial reviewing the condition's natural history and commenting on prophylactic therapies.)*

Volpe R. Immunoregulation in autoimmune thyroid disease. N Engl J Med 1987;316:44. *(An editorial nicely summarizing immunopathologic mechanisms.)*

Wartofsky L, Glinoer D, Solomon B, et al. Differences and similarities in the diagnosis and treatment of Graves' disease in Europe, Japan, and the United States. Thyroid 1991;1:129. *(Notes marked diversity of opinion in treatment preferences.)*

Primary Care Medicine: Office Evaluation and Management of the Adult Patient, 3rd edition, edited by Allan H. Goroll, Lawrence A. May, and Albert G. Mulley, Jr. J.B. Lippincott Company, Philadelphia
© 1995

104
Approach to the Patient With Hypothyroidism

The development of accurate and relatively inexpensive diagnostic techniques and the availability of low-cost, high quality levothyroxine preparations have greatly facilitated diagnosis and management of hypothyroidism. Hashimoto's thyroiditis accounts for the majority of hypothyroidism seen in the United States. Other causes of thyroid injury include idiopathic thyroid atrophy, previous radioactive iodine (^{131}I) therapy, and subtotal thyroidectomy. Women are more frequently affected than men. The prevalence of hypothyroidism increases with age. As much as 5 percent of the elderly population manifests evidence of hypothyroidism, most of it resulting from thyroiditis. Less common etiologies include neck irradiation, iodide administration, and use of lithium or para-aminosalicylic acid. Pituitary insufficiency can result in secondary hypothyroidism. Rarely, hypothalamic disease is the source of difficulty. Assessment for hypothyroidism includes evaluation of the patient taking chronic thyroid hormone replacement therapy for unclear reasons. The primary physician should be able to determine when replacement therapy is indicated and to provide it with safety and precision.

PATHOPHYSIOLOGY, CLINICAL PRESENTATION, AND COURSE

Pathophysiology

The basic mechanisms of hypothyroidism can be divided into those that impair thyroid function (primary hypothyroidism) and those that principally involve hypothalamic–pituitary function (secondary hypothyroidism). In primary disease, the hypothalamus responds with an increase in output of thyrotropin releasing hormone (TRH), triggering pituitary thyrotropin (TSH) secretion, which in turn stimulates thyroid gland enlargement, goiter formation, and preferential synthesis of triiodothyronine (T_3) over thyroxine (T_4). In secondary hypothyroidism, the TSH response is inadequate, the gland is normal or reduced in size, and synthesis of both T_4 and T_3 are equally reduced.

Primary Hypothyroidism may occur as a result of blockade of thyroid TSH receptors, impaired thyroxine production, or inhibition of thyroxine release. In *Hashimoto's thyroiditis*, the most common form of hypothyroidism, *immune-mediated injury* may damage all three components of glandular function. The precipitants of excessive antibody production remain ill-defined, but TSH receptors and microsomal enzymes (eg, peroxidase) are among the targeted antigens. In fact, antimicrosomal antibodies serve as a convenient laboratory marker for the condition (see below). Pathologically, there is a lymphocytic infiltrate and glandular enlargement; frank nodularity may develop (see Chapter 95). Antibodies directed against glandular antigens can impair TSH response, hormone synthesis, and proper release. Although most Hashimoto's patients remain euthyroid, a fraction experience transient hyperthyroidism due to premature release of thyroid hormone (see Chapter 103). If hormone synthesis is sufficiently compromised, hypothyroidism may ensue and can be permanent. Most Hashimoto's patients have mild disease and remain euthyroid, though a modest goiter may develop.

Postpartum thyroiditis is believed to be a common variant of Hashimoto's thyroiditis (see Chapter 103), affecting up to 5 percent of postpartum women. Antibody production peaks 3 to 4 months after delivery and then declines. There may be a period of transient hyperthyroidism followed by hypothyroidism, but most patients return to euthyroid status. The symptoms of mild hyperthyroidism may be mistakenly attributed to "tension" and are followed by fatigue and depression resulting from onset of hypothyroidism. The symptoms resolve spontaneously over 2 to 3 months but tend to recur with subsequent pregnancies.

Radiation-induced hypothyroidism is another leading cause of thyroid injury in the United States. It is a common and permanent consequence of ^{131}I therapy and also of external neck irradiation that exceeds 2500 rads (as used for treatment of lymphoma and head and neck cancers). Onset is within 3 to 6 months of treatment.

Subacute thyroiditis following a viral upper respiratory infection is a more transient form of thyroid injury. In this condition, the gland is very tender and is enlarged, though sometimes asymmetrically so. There may be a brief period of hyperthyroidism preceding the hypofunctioning of the gland, but spontaneous remission and restoration of normal thyroid function are the rule. Pathologically, a giant-cell, granulomatous infiltrate and marked reduction in iodine uptake characterize the condition. The clinical course ranges from weeks to a few months.

Subtotal thyroidectomy will produce transient hypothyroidism in most patients and permanent hypothyroidism in about half within the first year after surgery. *Drugs* with antithyroid activity, such as *lithium*, can induce some evidence of hypothyroidism in about a fifth of cases, but only 5 percent become clinically hypothyroid. *Iodide excess* impairs thyroxine synthesis and release, especially in patients with preexisting thyroidal disease; *iodide deficiency* inhibits hormone synthesis. Drugs that have an antithyroid effect produce a rapid but reversible form of hypothyroidism.

Secondary Hypothyroidism occurs most commonly as a result of injury to thyrotrophic cells by a functioning or nonfunctioning pituitary adenoma. Many other forms of sellar or suprasellar pathology can produce the same net result, which is inadequate TSH production, an atrophic thyroid gland, and hypothyroidism. Other trophic hormone-producing cells of the pituitary may also be involved, causing a host of associated endocrinopathies (see Chapters 100 and 101).

Primary hypothyroidism can sometimes mimic secondary disease by causing pituitary enlargement, but unlike in secondary disease, the pituitary shrinks in response to exogenous thyroid hormone.

Clinical Presentation

Subclinical Hypothyroidism. Along with the ability to detect early disease (see below) comes the designation of subclinical hypothyroidism, defined as an asymptomatic elevation in serum TSH concentration (ranging from 6 mU/L to 14 mU/L, depending on the specificity desired) accompanied by thyroid hormone levels within normal limits. General population prevalences average 7 percent for women and 2.5 percent for men. About 20 percent of patients with a TSH concentration greater than 6 mU/L will develop clinically symptomatic hypothyroidism over a period of 5 years; incidence of clinical disease rises to almost 100 percent for those with a TSH greater than 14 mU/L. Patients with high titers of antithyroid antibodies are at greatest risk for becoming overtly hypothyroid, suggesting that Hashimoto's thyroiditis plays an important role. The meaning of an isolated TSH between 6 and 10 mU/L remains unclear, though there is some evidence of an increased risk of coronary artery disease due to lipid abnormalities.

Clinical Hypothyroidism. The overt symptomatic manifestations of hypothyroidism reflect the decreases in metabolic rate and sensitivity to catecholamines that result from insufficient circulating thyroid hormone. Early symptoms are gradual in onset and may occur before serum free thyroxine levels fall below normal limits, though TSH will rise as soon as circulating levels of thyroid hormone are sensed to be inappropriately low. The patient typically complains of *fatigue*, moderately *dry skin*, *heavy menstrual periods*, slight *weight gain*, or *cold intolerance*. These symptoms are followed over the next few months by reports of very dry skin, coarse hair, *hoarseness*, continued weight gain (though appetite is minimal), and slightly *impaired mental activity*. Later, *depression* may be evident.

In late stages, hydrophilic mucopolysaccharide accumulates subcutaneously, producing the *myxedematous changes* that characterize this severe form of the disease. The skin becomes doughy, the face puffy, the tongue large, expression dull, and mentation slow, even lethargic. *Muscle weakness*, *arthralgias*, *diminution in hearing*, and *carpal tunnel syndrome* are also found. Daytime sleepiness in severely myxedematous patients suggests that obstructive sleep apnea may be occurring.

On examination, a *goiter* may be evident. If due to Hashimoto's disease, the goitrous gland may feel rubbery, nontender, even nodular. In the case of subacute thyroiditis, it will be very tender and enlarged, though not always symmetrically. Diffuse enlargement also occurs with hereditary defects in thyroxine synthesis or use of iodides, para-aminosalicylic acid (PAS), or lithium. An atrophic gland is characteristic of secondary hypothyroidism.

The heart may show signs of dilatation or an effusion. Bowel sounds are diminished, and the relaxation phase of the deep tendon *reflexes* is slowed or *"hung up."*

In secondary hypothyroidism, there may be signs of accompanying ovarian and adrenal insufficiency (eg, loss of axillary and pubic hair, amenorrhea, postural hypotension) due to concurrent loss of luteinizing hormone (LH), follicle-stimulating hormone (FSH), and adrenocorticotropic hormone (ACTH) production. Myxedematous changes tend to be less marked than with primary hypothyroidism, and the gland is smaller.

Laboratory Manifestations. As noted earlier, in primary hypothyroidism, *TSH elevation* may precede clinical manifestations. The earliest development is an increase in thyrotropin releaseing hormone (TRH), followed by the TSH response. At this stage, thyroid hormone levels may still be reported as "within normal limits," although, in reality, reduced from baseline. Only later does free thyroxine fall to overtly abnormal levels. *Hypercholesterolemia* is often noted, due to an increase in low-density lipoprotein (LDL) cholesterol and a reduction in high-density lipoprotein (HDL) cholesterol. Hypothyroidism is associated with a number of *anemic states*. The most common is a mild normochromic normocytic anemia. In addition, a microcytic anemia may ensue from iron deficiency secondary to heavy menstrual bleeding. Also, a macrocytic picture that clears on administration of exogenous thyroid hormone is sometimes encountered. A true megaloblastic anemia due to vitamin B_{12} deficiency occurs in about 10 percent of hypothyroid patients with a macrocytic smear; the relation between hypothyroidism and pernicious anemia is unresolved, but an autoimmune mechanism is postulated.

In severe cases of myxedema, dilutional hyponatremia occurs as a result of inadequate renal blood flow. A warning of impending myxedema coma is a rise in arterial $PaCO_2$, which takes place as the respiratory drive weakens.

DIFFERENTIAL DIAGNOSIS

Hypothyroidism's etiologies can be listed according to whether they impair the thyroid gland (primary hypothyroidism) or the hypothalamic–pituitary axis (secondary hypothyroidism) (Table 104–1). Primary disease is far more prevalent than secondary disease. Hashimoto's thyroiditis and postirradiation disease are the leading causes in the United States.

Table 104-1. Differential Diagnosis of Hypothyroidism

Primary Hypothyroidism
Hashimoto's thyroiditis
Postpartum disease (transient)
Postirradiation disease
Subtotal thyroidectomy
Subacute thyroiditis (transient)
Antithyroid drugs (lithium, PAS, PTU, methimazole, iodide excess)
Iodide deficiency
Infiltrative disease (hemochromatosis, amyloidosis, scleroderma)
Biosynthetic defect, hereditary
Secondary Hypothyroidism
Pituitary macroadenoma
Empty sella syndrome
Infarction
Infiltrative disease (eg, sarcoidosis)
Surgery or radiation-induced injury

WORKUP

Screening for Hypothyroidism

Although screening whole populations for hypothyroidism is not warranted, certain euthyroid groups are at increased risk of developing hypothyroidism and deserved consideration for screening. These include patients with goiter, evidence of Hashimoto's thyroiditis (positive antithyroid antibodies), recent radioiodine or external neck irradiation, and recent thyroid surgery. In addition, prevalence of hypothyroidism is high among patients with mental dysfunction admitted to geriatric units and among women older than age 40 with such nonspecific complaints as fatigue.

Diagnosis of Hypothyroidism

Although history (cold intolerance, skin changes, unexplained weight gain, hoarseness, fatigue, heavy periods) and physical findings (dry skin, coarse hair, goiter, hung-up reflexes) often suggest the diagnosis, confirmation and detection of early disease require laboratory study.

The diagnosis of *primary hypothyroidism* is readily achieved by demonstrating an *increased TSH* and a *low free* T_4 (or *free* T_4 *index*). The TSH is the more sensitive indicator of primary hypothyroidism and the test of choice. The designation of *"subclinical hypothyroidism"* is given to the asymptomatic patient with a modest elevation in TSH (6–10 mU/L) and a free T_4 index remaining within normal limits. However, the range of normal for the free T_4 index is wide. A single free T_4 determination may not detect the patient who has a modest yet physiologically important decline in hormone level, because the serum concentrations may remain within normal limits. Moreover, antithyroid antibodies can interfere with the commonly used immunoassays and produce falsely high or low readings, depending on the type of assay used. Nevertheless, the free thyroxine level is a better measure of thyroid function than *total* T_4, which is affected by changes in thyroid-binding globulin independent of thyroid function.

Often, measurement of *total* T_3 is routinely ordered as part of a battery of thyroid function tests. The assay is expensive to perform, and the results correlate poorly with thyroid status, affected by such events as a fall in peripheral conversion of T_4 to T_3, which is common in the elderly and in nonthyroidal illness. Serum *cholesterol, radioactive iodine uptake*, and *thyroglobulin* are also insensitive tests that contribute little to the diagnostic evaluation.

Secondary hypothyroidism should be suspected when, in the setting of overt hypothyroidism, the TSH level is inappropriately low. Concurrent amenorrhea, galactorrhea, postural hypotension, or visual field cut also suggests pituitary–hypothalamic pathology. Imaging of the sellar region is indicated. *Computed tomography (CT) scan* is best for detection of small lesions within the sella; *magnetic resonance imaging (MRI)* is best for imaging the suprasellar region (see Chapter 100). *TRH stimulation* is sometimes used to confirm secondary hypothyroidism, but the test often fails to distinguish among secondary causes.

Evaluation of patients who are taking a thyroid preparation but lack documentation of hypothyroidism can be achieved by stopping replacement therapy. Abrupt cessation of exogenous thyroid hormone therapy is not dangerous, as long as there is no prior history of severe hypothyroidism. Prompt and adequate (though submaximal) responses of the pituitary and thyroid gland occur when hormone intake is halted. However, because it takes about 5 weeks for full functioning of the hypothalamic–pituitary–thyroid axis to return, testing for hypothyroidism should be delayed until then to avoid a false-positive diagnosis of hypothyroidism.

Identifying the Underlying Etiology

History should be checked for possible etiologic factors, such as ^{131}I exposure, neck irradiation, recent viral infection, use of medications with antithyroid activity (lithium, excess iodide), residency in an area of iodide deficiency, subtotal thyroidectomy, pituitary surgery or irradiation, and recent pregnancy.

Physical examination should include a careful look at the thyroid gland for size, consistency, and nodularity. An exquisitely tender gland suggests subacute thyroiditis. A nontender, diffusely enlarged gland is seen in early Hashimoto's disease, postpartum patients, iodide deficiency, and congenital biosynthetic defects. A rubbery, multinodular goiter suggests more advanced Hashimoto's thyroiditis. When there is clinical suspicion of secondary hypothyroidism, the blood pressure should be checked for postural hypotension and the visual fields for deficits.

Laboratory investigation is relatively limited. The *TSH* (for differentiation of primary from secondary disease) and *antimicrosomal antibodies* (strongly suggestive of Hashimoto's thyroiditis) are the most useful. In patients with a sellar mass lesion, serum levels of LH, FSH, ACTH, and prolactin may be indicated (see Chapters 100 and 101).

PRINCIPLES OF MANAGEMENT

The availability of high-quality, inexpensive preparations of levothyroxine make restoration of the euthyroid state readily achievable. The issues are when to initiate therapy, how best to do so, optimal means of monitoring, and duration of treatment.

Subclinical Hypothyroidism

There is considerable debate as to the need for replacement therapy. Favoring therapy is the opportunity to correct secondary lipid abnormalities (elevated LDL, reduced HDL) and to decrease gland size if it is enlarged. Against treatment is concern about the possibility of inducing osteoporosis in patients who are actually euthyroid. Since it is hard to predict with certainty who will progress to overt hypothyroidism, and since the beneficial and harmful effects of long-term replacement therapy in subclinical patients remain to be defined by prospective randomized study, one cannot recommend treatment of such patients at this time. However, patients with TSH elevations greater than 10 mU/L and high titers of antimicrosomal antibodies are at greatest risk of becoming clinically hypothyroid and should be monitored closely. There is no evidence that early treatment affects the natural history of the underlying etiology.

Clinical Hypothyroidism

For patients who are clinically hypothyroid, replacement therapy is indicated. Treatment of mild to moderate disease is best done gradually, because hypothyroid patients are very sensitive to the effects of thyroid hormone. (An excessive rate of replacement may cause tremor, nervousness, and palpitations.) Adequate replacement should result in resolution of fatigue, loss of excess weight, and reversal of autonomic symptoms. The first signs of response are modest loss of weight, increase in pulse rate, and resolution of constipation. Myxedematous skin changes, pleural and pericardial effusions, and elevated creatine phosphokinase levels also normalize, but require more time. Most patients feel better within 2 weeks, and clinical resolution is usually complete by 3 months. Therapy for primary hypothyroidism is continued indefinitely, except in patients with transient disease, such as those with postpartum or subacute thyroiditis.

Replacement Program. Levothyroxine is the preparation of choice (see below). A replacement dose of 100 to 125 μg/d suffices for most patients. The elderly tend to have a 20 percent lower daily requirement due to decreased T_4 clearance. Current levothyroxine replacement doses are lower than those previously cited because contemporary levothyroxine preparations are of greater potency.

Starting dose and rate of adjustment depend on age, height, weight, presence of chronic disease (especially coronary artery disease), severity and duration of symptoms, and pretreatment TSH. Young, otherwise healthy patients can be started on a nearly full dose of levothyroxine (100 μg/d). Dose can be adjusted in 25- to 50-μg increments until a euthyroid state is achieved. In patients older than age 50 (who are at increased risk for silent coronary disease) and those with known heart disease, more cautious replacement is indicated to avoid precipitating angina, arrhythmias (atrial fibrillation, sinus tachycardia), and even heart failure. In this setting, it is best to initiate therapy with 25 to 50 μg/d and build up in 25-μg steps. If angina or other cardiac symptoms occur, the dosage of thyroid hormone should be reduced. Some advocate the concurrent administration of a *beta-blocking agent* (eg, propranolol) to protect the heart from the increase in myocardial oxygen demand associated with thyroxine therapy.

The onset of effect is usually gradual, becoming evident in 2 to 4 weeks. One should allow 4 to 6 weeks between dose adjustments, because it can take that long for a given dose to become fully effective.

Preoperative management has been a subject of concern. Coronary patients found to be mildly to moderately hypothyroid can safely undergo urgent surgery (including bypass procedures) without prior replacement. The rate of complications is no greater than that for nonhypothyroid patients, and the cardiac risks are lessened compared to initiating replacement therapy preoperatively. However, careful preoperative anesthesia planning is essential, because clearance of anesthetics is reduced.

Replacement Preparations. The replacement preparation of choice is *levothyroxine* (L-T_4), based on uniform bioavailability, cost, safety, and ease of monitoring therapy (see below). Half-life is about 24 hours, allowing for convenient once-daily administration. Some of the drug is converted peripherally to T_3, making it unnecessary to use the more expensive preparations which contain so-called "physiologic" mixtures of T_4 and T_3. The use of exogenous T_3 is considered inadvisable for replacement purposes, especially in older patients, because it causes rapid increases in metabolic rate and oxygen demand and can precipitate angina. Moreover, its short half-life produces wide swings in T_3 levels and makes frequent administration necessary. For these reasons, it is best to switch patients from desiccated thyroid hormone, T_3, or T_3/T_4 preparations to levothyroxine.

Levothyroxine has its own shortcomings. In the early 1980s, there were reports of variation in biologic activity and hormonal content of some commercial preparations. Quality control efforts mandated by the Food and Drug Administration have eliminated most of this variability. Nonetheless, it is recommended that one stay with a particular levothyroxine preparation as long as it appears to provide adequate replacement and consistent performance. Absorption of levothyroxine is impaired by simultaneous ingestion of ferrous sulfate, which binds to it. Since T_3 is the pertinent feedback hormone and derives from conversion of T_4, the amount of thyroxine necessary to normalize TSH may produce serum free thyroxine levels in the high-normal to slightly elevated range.

Monitoring and Adjusting Replacement Therapy is best accomplished by measurement of serum *TSH*, using the sensitive-TSH assay, which closely correlates with physiologic measures of thyroid hormone effect. However, reliance on the TSH determination can lead to erroneous conclusions during the initial 6 to 12 months of therapy, because it can take that long for the TSH to normalize despite adequate replacement doses. *Free T_4* may also correlate poorly with physiologic status during this initial period of therapy. This makes objective monitoring difficult during the start-up phase of treatment and places increased reliance on symptoms and signs.

The role of *symptoms* and *signs* in monitoring therapy is the subject of debate. Most studies suggest the correlation between test results and clinical findings is poor, but more data are needed. For now, TSH testing appears to be the preferred method of monitoring, supplemented by correlation with clinical state during periods when TSH results may lag behind physiologic state (eg, during initiation of therapy). Thus, if the patient becomes clinically euthyroid during the early phase of replacement therapy, but the TSH is still elevated, then it is best to leave the dose unchanged and repeat the TSH in 4 to 8 weeks. If the TSH falls but remains elevated, and the patient continues to be clinically hypothyroid, then an increase in thyroxine dosage is warranted. If the hypothyroid patient has a TSH that has not changed, then poor compliance is the most likely explanation and no dose adjustment is warranted. If TSH is undetectable, then the replacement dose is excessive.

When dose excess is suggested by a very low or absent TSH, measurement of the *free T_4* (or *free T_4 index*, which is an excellent proxy for the free T_4) can help determine just how excessive the current dose is.

Once a stable replacement dosage is achieved, twice-yearly TSH determination are probably sufficient. Any upward adjustments in dosage should be made in small increments, followed by repeat TSH testing in 6 to 8 weeks.

Secondary Hypothyroidism

Treatment and monitoring must take into account the lack of TSH response and any coexisting adrenal and/or ovarian hypofunction. Because thyroid replacement and the resultant rise in metabolic rate can precipitate addisonian crisis, adrenal function should be assessed with an ACTH stimulation test before replacement therapy is prescribed in any patient suspected of having secondary hypothyroidism. Patients with inadequate ACTH response would be candidates for treatment with cortisone acetate preceding L-T_4 replacement.

MANAGEMENT RECOMMENDATIONS

- Stop any exogenous thyroid or antithyroid medication if reason for use is unclear; check TSH 4 to 6 weeks after treatment is stopped.
- Confirm the diagnosis of hypothyroidism with TSH and free T_4 or free T_4 index determinations.
- If the patient appears clinically and biochemically hypothyroid, but TSH is not appropriately elevated, test for pituitary insufficiency.

Primary Hypothyroidism

- If possible, stop all drugs with potential antithyroid effect (eg, iodides, PAS, lithium).
- Begin replacement with a once-daily morning dose of levothyroxine, initiating therapy with 50 to 100 μg/d in young, otherwise healthy patients and with 25 to 50 μg/d in older patients; size of dose is a function of patient age, weight, severity and duration of hypothyroidism, and presence of underlying heart disease. Particular caution is indicated in those with underlying coronary disease, where use of small starting doses is required.
- Monitor initial therapy by TSH determination and clinical state. The goal is normalization of the TSH, but be aware that TSH may initially require several months to normalize despite adequate thyroid hormone replacement. If patient is clinically euthyroid but TSH is still elevated, continue same dose and repeat TSH in 4 to 8 weeks. A check of the FT_4 (or free T_4 index) may be of use if TSH is low or absent. Also monitor for side effects (eg, tremor, angina, arrhythmias).
- Increase dose in increments of 25 to 50 μg, with the lower increment appropriate for the elderly and those with heart disease.
- Allow 4 to 6 weeks for a new dose to take full effect before considering another increase in dose.
- Average levothyroxine replacement dose for most adults is 100 to 125 μg/d; for the elderly, the average dose is 20 percent less.
- Avoid excessive doses of replacement therapy (TSH <0.5) because of the risk of inducing osteoporosis.
- Once the proper dose is achieved, monitor therapy every 6 to 12 months with a TSH determination.
- Levothyroxine is the thyroid replacement preparation of choice; select and stay with a particular manufacturer's preparation. Desiccated thyroid and T_3-containing preparations are not recommended.
- Patients with mild to moderate hypothyroidism and underlying coronary disease need not receive replacement therapy before urgent surgery. However, careful anesthesia planning is necessary.

Secondary Hypothyroidism

- Perform an ACTH stimulation test to assess adrenal reserve. If it is low, give cortisone acetate *before* providing thyroid replacement.
- Replace thyroid hormone as for primary hypothyroidism.
- Monitor therapy by following clinical signs and free T_4.

PATIENT EDUCATION

Euthyroid patients who are inappropriately placed on exogenous thyroid for treatment of fatigue or obesity are often reluctant to give up the medication. Documenting that their thyroid status is perfectly normal is an essential first step to taking them off the medication successfully. Often a request from the physician to temporarily halt thyroid hormone for 5 weeks to measure TSH and free T_4 is agreed to. Usually there is little change in how the patient feels, and this helps to convince the patient that exogenous hormone is unnecessary.

Hypothyroid patients need to be warned of the danger of increasing their medication too rapidly or of taking more than is prescribed. Unfortunately, some patients adjust their dosages on the basis of other symptoms they mistakenly attribute to hypothyroidism, for example, those of depression. All patients should be instructed to measure and record their weight regularly and report any unexplained change of 5 pounds or more.

It is imperative that the patient and family be instructed in the signs of worsening hypothyroidism. Hypothyroid patients have been known to stop taking their thyroid medication. The importance of continuing therapy indefinitely must be emphasized to the patient and persons close to him.

A.H.G.

ANNOTATED BIBLIOGRAPHY

Amino N, Mori H, Iwatani Y, et al. High prevalence of transient post-partum thyrotoxicosis and hypothyroidism. N Engl J Med 1982;306:849. *(The initial report of this phenomenon; incidence was 5 percent and attributed to an autoimmune thyroiditis.)*

Brown ME, Refetoff S. Transient elevation of serum thyroid hormone concentration after initiation of replacement therapy in myxedema. Ann Intern Med 1980;92:491. *(Transient elevations were noted during the first 6 months, which limited the usefulness of the T_4 and free T_4 for determining optimal replacement dosage.)*

Cooper DS. Thyroid hormone and the skeleton. JAMA 1988;259:3175. *(Osteoporosis is a risk in patients receiving excessive thyroid hormone replacement.)*

Fish LH, Schwartz HL, Cavanaugh J, et al. Replacement dose, metabolism, and bioavailability of levothyroxine in the treatment of hypothyroidism. N Engl J Med 1987;316:764. *(Detailed study of pharmacokinetics; mean replacement dose was 112 μg/d.)*

Greenspan SL, Greenspan FS, Resnick NM, et al. Skeletal integrity in premenopausal and postmenopausal women receiving long-term L-thyroxine therapy. Am J Med 1991;91:5. *(Bone loss is, at most minimal when replacement therapy is carefully treated.)*

Helfand M, Crapo LM. Screening for thyroid disease. Ann Intern Med 1990;112:840. *(Whole-population screening found to be of little value, but may be of benefit in groups where prevalence of hypothyroidism is high.)*

Krugman L, Hershman J, Chopra I, et al. Patterns of recovery of the hypothalamic-pituitary-thyroid axis in patients taken off chronic thyroid therapy. J Clin Endocrinol Metab 1975;41:70. *(Full recovery of pituitary and thyroid responsiveness to TRH occurred in euthyroid patients 5 weeks after withdrawal of chronic thyroid hormone therapy.)*

Mandel SJ, Brent GA, Larsen PR. Levothyroxine therapy in patients with thyroid disease. Ann Intern Med 1993;119:492. *(Includes detailed discussion of replacement therapy for hypothyroidism.)*

Levine HD. Compromise therapy in the patient with angina pectoris and hypothyroidism. Am J Med 1980;69:411. *(Details the difficulties in adequately controlling angina in the context of fully correcting the hypothyroidism.)*

Robuschi G, Safran M, Braverman LE, et al. Hypothyroidism in the elderly. Endocr Rev 1987;8:142. *(Comprehensive review of pathophysiology, clinical presentation, and treatment.)*

Ross DS. Monitoring L-thyroxine therapy: Lessons from the effects of L-thyroxine on bone density. Am J Med 1991;91:1. *(Outlines an approach to replacement therapy that minimizes risk of osteoporosis by carefully titrating dose and TSH response.)*

Sawin CT, Geller A, Hershman JM, et al. The aging thyroid—the use of thyroid hormone in older persons. JAMA 1990;261: 2653. *(Epidemiologic data; 10 percent prevalence of use in the elderly; in 10 percent of these patients, use was inappropriate, allowing for discontinuation of therapy.)*

Schectman JM, Pawlson LG. The cost-effectiveness of three thyroid function testing strategies for suspicion of hypothyroidism in a primary care setting. J Gen Intern Med 1990;5:9. *(A TSH-first strategy proved best.)*

Staub JJ, Althaus BU, Engler H, et al. Spectrum of subclinical and overt hypothyroidism. Am J Med 1992;92:631. *(One of the most detailed studies of subclinical hypothyroidism to date.)*

105
Glucocorticosteroid Therapy

Primary Care Medicine: Office Evaluation and Management of the Adult Patient, 3rd edition, edited by Allan H. Goroll, Lawrence A. May, and Albert G. Mulley, Jr. J.B. Lippincott Company, Philadelphia

The therapeutic potency of glucocorticosteroids has led to their widespread use. Although benefits can be substantial, adverse effects are numerous, including serious metabolic derangements and suppression of the hypothalamic–pituitary–adrenal (HPA) axis. To maximize the therapeutic response and minimize the risks, a number of questions must be addressed before steroid therapy is initiated: 1) Is the underlying disorder of such severity that the benefits of therapy outweigh the risks? 2) Will prolonged treatment be required, or will a brief, limited course suffice? 3) Have alternative, less morbid therapies been maximally utilized? 4) Does the patient have any underlying condition that will worsen on steroid therapy or predispose him to drug-induced complications? 5) Can a less suppressive regimen (eg, alternate-day therapy) be utilized?

The primary physician must decide when and how to institute steroid therapy, whether to use daily or alternate-day treatment, and how to withdraw chronic glucocorticoid treatment safely.

ADVERSE EFFECTS

Most adverse effects of glucocorticoids are a function of dosage and duration of use. A few are irreversible; fortunately, most resolve within several months of terminating therapy.

Suppression of the Hypothalamic–Pituitary–Adrenal Axis is one of the more feared consequences of steroid use. Ability to respond to a major physiologic stress (eg, surgery or injury) may be blunted, putting the patient at risk for hypotension and hypoglycemia. Symptoms and signs include *light-headedness*, *nausea*, *postural hypotension*, and *hypoglycemia*. Risk appears related to *dose*, *duration*, and *schedule* of therapy, though other, yet to be identified factors are believed operative as well. There is wide individual variation. Some patients experience clinically important HPA suppression with use of as little as 15 mg of prednisone taken daily for a few weeks, while others manifest no measurable HPA suppression despite use of higher daily doses over more prolonged periods. Thus, it is hard to predict risk of suppression in a given patient solely on the basis of dose and duration of therapy.

Scheduling of dose has some effect on degree of HPA suppression. *Daily* physiologic dosages of glucocorticosteroids (eg, 5–7.5 mg of prednisone) given in the morning do not cause suppression of any consequence, but if the same dosages are given at night, normal diurnal cortisol secretion is inhibited. Dosages just above the physiologic range are suppressive after about a month of use. *Alternate-day* therapy, utilizing short- or intermediate- acting preparations taken at 8 AM every other day, does not induce clinically significant HPA suppression. Neither does a *cyclic* program of 5 days of daily therapy followed by 2 to 4 weeks off therapy. However, cycles of 2 weeks on and 2 weeks off do lead to HPA suppression. A single, daily pharmacologic dosage of glucocorticoid produces less HPA suppression than does the same dosage divided up and given over the course of the day. *Recovery* from HPA suppression can take up to 12 months. Hypothalamic–pituitary function returns first, beginning 2 to 5 months after cessation of suppressive therapy, and is manifested by appropriate plasma adrenocorticotropic hormone

(ACTH) levels that demonstrate a normal diurnal pattern. Signs of adrenal recovery become evident at 6 to 9 months, with return of the baseline serum cortisol to normal. Maximal adrenal response to ACTH may not reappear until 9 to 12 months after cessation of therapy. There is no proven method for accelerating the restoration of normal HPA function once inhibition has occurred. The administration of ACTH does not appear to speed adrenal recovery.

As with predicting onset of HPA suppression, it is also hard to estimate how long clinically important hyporesponsiveness will persist. Again, individual variation is great, and degree of suppression cannot be reliably estimated by the basal serum cortisol concentration. In the setting of such uncertainty, *testing of the HPA axis* becomes an important adjunct to clinical decision making. Of the available stimulation tests (insulin-induced hypoglycemia, corticotropin, metyrapone, corticotropin-releasing hormone), the *corticotropin (ACTH) test* is the most widely used, producing results that correlate well with cortisol levels measured during the stress of surgery. A serum cortisol is drawn, followed by intravenous injection of a one-ampule (250-μg) bolus of synthetic ACTH *(cosyntropin)*. Additional samples of blood are drawn at 30 and 60 minutes for cortisol determinations. The test produces a few false-positives when compared to insulin-induced hypoglycemia (the "gold standard" for testing HPA function), but it is safer and more convenient to perform. Some argue that the corticotropin-releasing hormone (CRH) test combines the sensitivity and specificity of insulin-induced hypoglycemia with the convenience of corticotropin testing, but there are few direct comparisons. Basal cortisol level has shown little correlation with results of stimulation testing and is not a substitute for such testing.

Although HPA suppression is important to detect, it is not the only factor determining the ability of corticosteroid-exposed patients to respond appropriately to stress. Some patients manifest a hypotensive response to stress despite a normally responding HPA axis, and patients with a blunted HPA response may manifest no signs of clinical adrenal insufficiency. More work is needed to elucidate the mechanisms governing stress response in steroid-treated patients.

Metabolic and Endocrinologic Side Effects. *Negative nitrogen balance* (due to inhibition of protein synthesis and enhancement of protein catabolism) is believed to be partially responsible for reduced muscle mass, weakness, thinning of the skin, and striae formation. *Fat redistribution* accounts for the characteristic truncal obesity and cushingoid appearance. Both fat redistribution and negative nitrogen balance are minimized by using alternate-day therapy or no more than physiologic doses given each morning, but not by using ACTH or daily pharmacologic glucocorticoid dosages. *Acne* is seen, more often with ACTH use than with glucocorticoids, because of stimulation of adrenal androgen production.

Glucose intolerance is common. Mechanisms include increases in peripheral insulin resistance, gluconeogenesis, glucagon secretion, and substrate availability. Usually the glucose intolerance is mild, does not lead to ketosis, and resolves when therapy is stopped. In patients who develop carbohydrate intolerance, the effect appears to be dose-related.

Hypertension and *fluid retention* with peripheral edema are more common when agents with mineralocorticoid effects are used, and they are not dependent on preexistence of elevated blood pressure (Table 105–1). Again, dosage and duration of therapy are important factors. *Electrolyte derangements* are common, especially hypokalemia.

Enhanced Susceptibility to Infection results from the anti-inflammatory and immunosuppressive actions of corticosteroids. Bacterial infections are common. Candidiasis and aspergillosis sometimes result. Herpes zoster, varicella, vaccinia, and cytomegalovirus are the principal viral infections encountered in patients on steroids. Reactivation of tuberculosis is a well-recognized risk (see Chapter 49).

Osteoporosis develops when large steroid doses are used over prolonged periods. The incidence is unknown, be-

Table 105-1. Commonly Used Glucocorticoids

DURATION OF ACTION	GLUCOCORTICOID POTENCY*	EQUIVALENT GLUCOCORTICOID DOSE (mg)	MINERALOCORTICOID ACTIVITY
Short-acting			
Cortisol (hydrocortisone)	1	20	Yes†
Cortisone	0.8	25	Yes†
Prednisone	4	5	No
Prednisolone	4	5	No
Methylprednisolone	5	4	No
Intermediate-acting			
Triamcinolone	5	4	No
Long-acting			
Betamethasone	25	0.60	No
Dexamethasone	30	0.75	No

*The values given for glucocorticoid potency are relative. Cortisol is arbitrarily assigned a value of 1.

†Mineralocorticoid effects are dose-related. At dosages close to or within the basal physiologic range for glucocorticoid activity, no such effect may be detectable.

Adapted from Axelrod L: Glucocorticoid therapy. Medicine (Baltimore) 1976;55:39.

cause measuring skeletal mass accurately is difficult and expensive. The precise relation between dosage, duration of use, and risk of osteoporosis remains unclear, although there is some suggestion that alternate-day therapy minimizes the chance of serious osteoporosis. Patients with a predisposition to osteoporosis, such as menopausal women and immobilized individuals, appear to be among the most susceptible. The axial skeleton is affected more than the limbs, and vertebral compression fractures may result. *Aseptic necrosis of the femoral head* and other bones is a well-recognized and serious, but relatively rare, skeletal complication. Sometimes it may be due to the underlying illness for which corticosteroids are being given, as in rheumatoid arthritis or systemic lupus. However, risk is markedly increased with increase in steroid dose and chronicity of therapy.

Gastrointestinal Effects. Gastritis, peptic ulceration, and gastrointestinal bleeding have all been attributed to steroid use. Multiple, randomized, controlled trials have produced conflicting results, as have major meta-analyses examining pooled data from such trials (see Chapter 68). Hotly debated is the degree to which ulcer risk is a function of dosage and duration of exposure. Risk appears small until doses in excess of the equivalent of 30 mg/d of prednisone are reached and continued for over a month. Even then, the increase in rate of peptic ulceration is only in the range of 1 percent to 2 percent. Most peptic ulceration is due to concurrent use of nonsteroidal antiinflammatory agents. Antacids and food do not interfere with absorption of oral steroid preparations.

Acute pancreatitis is noted with increased frequency in patients taking corticosteroids. *Panniculitis* is unique to iatrogenic Cushing's syndrome.

Myopathy may result from chronic use of large dosages. Proximal muscle wasting and weakness of the lower extremities are characteristic. Patients complain of difficulty climbing stairs. Average time of onset is 5 months into treatment. Muscle enzymes are normal. The complication is reversible, and exercise may help minimize it.

Psychological and Behavioral Changes are particularly common in the elderly. The reported incidence is as high as 25 percent to 40 percent of patients receiving steroid therapy. Increased appetite, mild euphoria, and changes in sleep patterns are rather common at the beginning of treatment. Psychoses, which are not predictably related to dosage or duration of therapy, can occur; they slowly respond to reduction or cessation of steroid use. Some clinicians argue that the patient's premorbid personality plays a role, while others deny this. Steroid therapy can exacerbate previous psychiatric disease.

Cataracts of the posterior subcapsular type are reported in 10 percent to 35 percent of cases and are predominantly dose- and duration-dependent. A few require removal; most do not.

PRINCIPLES OF THERAPY

The challenge of glucocorticoid use is to obtain maximal therapeutic benefit with a minimum of adverse effects. In most instances, steroids do not cure disease or alter its natural history; rather, they suppress or alter the inflammatory and immunologic responses and, in doing so, reduce symptoms. Therefore, one must carefully weigh the perceived therapeutic benefit against the potential risks. Risk is negligible for a course of short-term therapy (7–14 d), even with use of high doses, which can be very effective in selected situations (eg, acute asthma, contact dermatitis). Appetite stimulation and restlessness are the principal side effects. There are no long-term consequences. The decision to initiate more prolonged steroid therapy requires greater consideration of the risks involved (see above).

Selection of Agent. Corticosteroid preparations differ principally in duration of action and degree of mineralocorticoid activity (see Table 105–1). *Short-acting agents* are less likely to cause HPA suppression, especially when prescribed for morning use, in low doses as part of an alternate-day program (see below). Long-acting agents are preferred for situations where high-dose steroid effect must be sustained (eg, increased intracranial pressure). Mineralocorticoid activity is desirable in adrenal insufficiency but not in situations of excessive inflammation or immunoreactivity. Regardless of the agent selected, it is essential to continue maximal nonsteroidal therapy, insofar as it holds down steroid requirements.

Prednisone is the most widely prescribed of the glucocorticoids. Its short half-life, low cost, and negligible mineralocorticoid effect make it useful for most immunosuppressive/anti-inflammatory indications. *Prednisolone* is the active hepatic metabolite of prednisone and is useful in the setting of liver failure. *Dexamethasone* is the long-acting glucocorticoid of choice, being about seven times more potent on a weight basis than prednisone and having a half-life of 24 hours. This potency makes the agent useful for suppressive testing of the HPA axis. *Hydrocortisone* (cortisol) is the naturally occurring glucocorticoid. It has one quarter the glucocorticoid potency of prednisone but exerts some mineralocorticoid effect when used in pharmacologic doses, making it useful for parenteral supplementation in a patient believed to be adrenally suppressed. *Florinef* (9-alpha fluorohydrocortisone), a potent mineralocorticoid with virtually no glucocorticoid effect, is used primarily for replacement in adrenal cortical insufficiency.

Theoretically, use of *ACTH* would appear attractive because it might avoid adrenal suppression, but it also induces undesirable mineralocorticoid and androgenic responses. Moreover, it must be given parenterally, and there is no way to know how much glucocorticoid effect is obtained from a given dose. These disadvantages limit its usefulness, although it is used preferentially by many neurologists for exacerbations of multiple sclerosis (see Chapter 172).

Selection of Dosing Schedule: Alternate-Day Versus Daily. Most conditions that require chronic corticosteroid treatment (eg, asthma—see Chapter 48; sarcoidosis—see Chapter 51; inflammatory bowel disease—see Chapter 73; nephrotic syndrome—see Chapter 142) can be well controlled with *alternate-day therapy*, although it is often necessary to begin with a program of daily steroids when the disease is very active and symptoms are severe. Important advantages of alternate-day treatment are avoidance of significant HPA suppression and minimization of cushingoid side effects without a substantial loss of antiinflammatory activity. It appears that the anti-inflammatory effects of glucocorticosteroids persist longer (up to 3 days) than the undesirable metabolic effects. Other adverse effects that are reduced or eliminated by an alternate-day schedule include inhibition of delayed hypersensitivity, susceptibility to infection, negative nitrogen balance, fluid retention, hypertension, and psychological and behavioral disturbances.

Alternate-day therapy by itself will not prevent HPA suppression if a long-acting steroid preparation is used (eg, dexamethasone). Moreover, therapy must be truly alternate-day, with the total dosage given first thing in the morning every other day. Intermittent therapy or doses given throughout the day every other day do not preserve HPA responsiveness.

Daily steroid therapy is indicated during acute exacerbations of disease and in the limited number of conditions that are controlled only by daily glucocorticoid administration (eg, temporal arteritis—see Chapter 161; pemphigus vulgaris). When daily therapy is necessary, HPA suppression can be minimized by having the patient take the entire daily dose first thing in the morning and by using a short-acting glucocorticoid at the lowest possible dose. Daily single-dose regimens may be as effective or nearly as effective as divided-dose regimens in controlling underlying illness. However, in contrast with alternate-day therapy, manifestations of Cushing's syndrome are not prevented.

Switching from a Daily to Alternate-Day Schedule. Most patients who experience a remission on daily therapy are candidates for a trial of alternate-day steroids (see above for exceptions). Switching allows transfer to a less morbid program without sacrificing disease control. Unlike tapering, switching continues the *same total steroid dose*. It is carried out by gradually increasing the dose on the first day and decreasing it on the second day until a double dose is taken every other day, with no drug on the in-between days.

How fast the changeover can be made varies, depending on the activity of the underlying disease, the duration of therapy, degree of HPA suppression, and the patient's cooperativeness. A rough guideline for switching to alternate-day therapy is to make changes in increments of 10 mg of prednisone (or its equivalent) when the daily prednisone dosage is greater than 40 mg, and in 5-mg increments when the daily dosage is between 20 and 40 mg. Below 20 mg/d, the change ought to be in amounts of 2.5 mg. The interval between changes ranges from 1 day to several weeks and is determined empirically, based on clinical response. It is important to keep in mind that most patients who have been on a daily steroid program for more than 2 to 4 weeks probably have some degree of HPA suppression.

Tapering and Withdrawing Therapy. The abrupt withdrawal of patients from daily steroid therapy after more than a month at dosages greater than 20 to 30 mg of prednisone per day can precipitate adrenal insufficiency, a flare-up of the underlying illness, or a withdrawal syndrome. There is no way to speed HPA recovery, nor are there specific schedules for reducing the dosage. One must monitor disease activity and decrease the dosage empirically in small amounts, watching for flare-up of disease or signs of adrenal insufficiency such as postural hypotension, weakness, and gastrointestinal distress.

One empirical approach to reducing the dosage toward physiologic levels is to make changes in decrements of 10 mg of prednisone or its equivalent every 1 to 3 weeks, as long as the dosage is above 40 mg. Below 40 mg, the decrement is 5 mg. Once a physiologic dose of prednisone is reached (5–7.5 mg/d), the patient can be switched to 1-mg prednisone tablets or the equivalent dosage of hydrocortisone, so that further reductions in dosage can be made in smaller steps than is possible using 5-mg prednisone tablets. Weekly or biweekly reductions can then be carried out in steps of 1 mg of prednisone at a time, as permitted by disease activity.

During the tapering process, some patients develop a *steroid withdrawal syndrome,* characterized by depression, myalgias, arthralgias, anorexia, headaches, nausea, and lethargy. Studies have failed to show a relationship between these symptoms and low cortisol or 17-hydroxycorticosteroid levels. In most instances, complaints are reported when levels are normal, or even elevated, but falling rapidly. HPA responsiveness has also been found to be normal in many of these patients. The mechanisms responsible for this syndrome are unknown but seem to be linked to the rapidity with which dosage is tapered.

Identification and Treatment of Steroid-Induced Adrenal Suppression. At times of anticipated stress (eg, upcoming surgery), it is important to know how responsive the HPA axis is and whether or not supplementary steroid therapy will be needed. As noted earlier, it is very difficult to predict onset and duration of HPA suppression, making testing of the HPA axis a useful adjunct for deciding who will need supplementation. In the office setting, *cosyntropin* (synthetic ACTH) administration is a convenient, safe, and effective means of testing for suppression (see above). If the serum cortisol at 60 minutes is greater than 18 μg/dL or there is an increase from baseline of at least 10 μg/dL, then adrenal responsiveness is sufficient to sustain the patient through a stress equivalent to general anesthesia. Testing can be done in similar fashion, administering 100 μg *corticotropin-releasing hormone (CRH)* as an intravenous bolus.

If the patient cannot mount an adequate cortisol response, or testing is impractical because of urgency or unavailability of agents or assays, corticosteroid supplementation should be given for acute stress. *Hydrocortisone* is usually prescribed, because it provides both glucocorticoid and mineralocorticoid effects. Depending on the severity of the stress, one administers 100 to 400 mg of hydrocortisone per day in divided doses. The lower end of the dose range is appropriate for the stress of gastroenteritis, influenza, or dental extraction. During major stress, such as trauma or surgery, the patient should be given 100 mg of hydrocortisone parenterally every 6 to 8 hours. A prepackaged syringe containing 4 mg of *dexamethasone* phosphate can be prescribed for the patient or family to carry for parenteral use in an emergency should medical care be unavailable and the patient become unconscious or so ill he cannot take steroids by mouth. The need to continue supplementation is based on the duration of the stress and the underlying state of the HPA axis.

PATIENT EDUCATION

Steroids should be used with caution in patients whose reliability or intelligence is in question because of the risk of HPA suppression and adrenocortical insufficiency. Individuals on alternate-day therapy need instruction on the importance of keeping to the every-other-day schedule and taking their medication around 8 AM so as to minimize the risk of suppression. Patients on suppressive dosage of steroid should be informed of the need for steroid supplementation when there is stress or illness and should wear an identification bracelet stating they take a corticosteroid. Patients must understand the need to contact the physician and to increase steroid dosage when subjected to physiologic stress.

Many patients are fearful or reluctant to be taken off chronic steroid therapy because of concern for recrudescence of the underlying illness or because malaise is experienced as the drug is tapered. A detailed review of the side effects of prolonged therapy is necessary so that the rationale for reducing the dosage and the desirability of eventually discontinuing corticosteroids are understood and appreciated. Any change in dosage and schedule should be written out. When chronic, daily, high-dosage therapy is required, the psychological impact of adverse effects (eg, cushingoid features) can be lessened by advising the patient of their likelihood and at least partial reversibility.

THERAPEUTIC RECOMMENDATIONS

- Use glucocorticoids only when other forms of therapy have been used in maximal dosages and proven insufficient and when the risks of steroid use are outweighed by the therapeutic benefit expected.
- To minimize the steroid dose required, always try to *add steroid therapy* to the ongoing treatment program rather than in place of it.
- In the setting of active *autoimmune* or *inflammatory disease*, initiate a full-strength program of daily glucocorticoid therapy utilizing *prednisone* (40–60 mg/d, or prednisolone if there is hepatocellular failure). When replacement therapy for adrenal cortical insufficiency is needed, use *hydrocortisone* (see below). The long-acting *dexamethasone* is reserved for testing the HPA axis and for the rare situation when very high-dose, sustained-action therapy is required (eg, increased intracranial pressure). All glucocorticosteroids can be taken with food; absorption is not impaired.
- To *minimize risk of HPA suppression*, avoid use of long-acting preparations, give the entire glucocorticoid dose in the morning or, better yet, on alternate days, and continue only for the shortest possible time.
- Try initiating therapy on an *alternate-day* basis when symptoms are not severe and the condition is not among those with an absolute requirement for daily treatment (ie, temporal arteritis, pemphigus vulgaris, severe inflammatory bowel disease).
- Once control is achieved, *taper* to the lowest dose that maintains control and terminate if possible. Tapering is done empirically, monitoring disease activity and watching for evidence of adrenal insufficiency (postural hypotension, gastrointestinal upset, fatigue, muscle weakness, hypoglycemia).
- For very brief courses of corticosteroid therapy (<7–14 d), taper rapidly over 7 to 10 days to full cessation, provided disease activity remains quiescent. When longer courses of therapy are required, taper more slowly, reducing dose in 10-mg decrements when the dosage is above 40 mg and 5-mg steps when it is below 40 mg. *Rapidity of tapering* is determined by disease activity and appearance of steroid withdrawal or adrenal insufficiency symptoms. Once the dosage is down to 5 mg of prednisone every other day, therapy can be stopped or switched to 5-mg hydrocortisone or 1-mg prednisone tablets and reduced in decrements of 2.5 mg of hydrocortisone or 1 mg of prednisone.
- If tapering is unsuccessful or prolonged therapy is deemed necessary, then ascertain and maintain the lowest effective dose and try *switching over to an alternate-day regimen*, if not already utilized.
- When switching to alternate-day therapy, begin by modestly reducing the second day's dose and adding the difference to the first day's dose. In this manner, the same total dose is maintained. If the daily dose is above 40 mg, reduce dose on the alternate day by the equivalent of 10 mg of prednisone and by 5 mg if the daily dosage is below 40 mg. Below 20 mg, the increment is 2.5 mg. The interval between changes in dosage is determined empirically, based on clinical status of the patient. The end point of switching occurs when the previous entire 2-day dosage is given once every other day.
- If withdrawal symptoms are a problem on alternate-day therapy, a small morning dose of hydrocortisone (10–20 mg) given on the off day may help alleviate symptoms without prolonging HPA suppression.
- When HPA responsiveness is in question, perform a *cosyntropin stimulation test*. Administer 250 μg parenterally and measure serum cortisol immediately before and 30 and 60 minutes after administration.
- Since 9 to 12 months of HPA suppression may begin after as little as 2 to 4 weeks of 20 to 30 mg of daily prednisone, advise patients on use of daily pharmacologic doses to supplement their steroid intake when under stress or experiencing an acute illness. In the setting of injury, surgery, or inability to take oral medication, prescribe parenteral hydrocortisone or its equivalent. Total daily stress dose is 100 to 400 mg of hydrocortisone, given in divided fashion every 6 to 8 hours. Provide a prepackaged syringe containing 4 mg of dexamethasone for intramuscular emergency use.

A.H.G.

ANNOTATED BIBLIOGRAPHY

Anatruda TT Jr, Hurst MM, D'Esposo ND. Certain endocrine and metabolic facets of the steroid withdrawal syndrome. J Clin Endocrinol Metab 1965;25:1207. *(A classic study showing that the steroid withdrawal syndrome is not due to inadequate serum levels of steroid.)*

Axelrod L. Glucocorticoid therapy. Medicine (Baltimore) 1976; 55:39. *(A superb and comprehensive review of the literature; slightly dated, but still well worth reading; 188 refs.)*

Boumpas DT, Chrousos GP, Wilder RL, et al. Glucocorticoid therapy for immune-mediated diseases: Basic and clinical correlates. Ann Intern Med 1993;119:1198. *(Excellent NIH conference on the topic; 98 refs.)*

Byyny RL. Withdrawal from glucocorticoid therapy. N Engl J Med 1976;295:30. *(Provides a very practical approach.)*

Christy NP. Pituitary-adrenal function during corticosteroid therapy: learning to live with uncertainty. N Engl J Med 1992; 326:266. *(An editorial reviewing tests for HPA suppression and the difficulty in predicting it.)*

Dale DC, Fauci AS, Wolff SM. Alternate-day prednisone, leukocyte kinetics and susceptibility to infections. N Engl J Med 1974;29:1154. *(Alternate-day steroid therapy does not reduce leukocyte count, inflammatory response, or neutrophil half-life.)*

Graeber AL, Ney RL, Nicholson WE, et al. Natural history of pituitary adrenal recovery following long-term suppression with corticosteroids. J Clin Endocrinol Metab 1965;25:11. *(Most patients on glucocorticoids for 1–10 y had full restoration of function within 1 y; hypothalamic–pituitary function returned in the first 2–5 mo; 17-hydroxycorticosteroids normalized during months 6 to 9.)*

Meikle AW, Tyler FH. Potency and duration of action of glucocorticoids. Effects of hydrocortisone, prednisone, and dexamethasone on human pituitary–adrenal function. Am J Med 1977;63:200. *(The intrinsic potency and relative rate of disappearance from plasma are the two most important factors determining the relative potency of orally administered glucocorticoids.)*

Messer J, Reithman D, Sacks HS, et al. Association of adrenocorticosteroid therapy and peptic ulcer disease. N Engl J Med 1983;309:21. *(Meta-analysis; high-dose corticosteroids do increase the risk of peptic ulcer and gastrointestinal hemorrhage; but while relative risk was 2, the absolute risk was quite small—2 percent vs. 1 percent in controls.)*

Piper JM, Ray WA, Daugherty JR, et al. Corticosteroid use and peptic ulcer disease: Role of nonsteroidal anti-inflammatory drugs. Am Intern Med 1991;114:735. *(The increased risk was due to concurrent NSAID use.)*

Rae S A, Williams IA, English J, et al. Alteration of plasma prednisolone levels by indomethacin and naproxen. Br J Clin Pharmacol 1982;14:459. *(Nonsteroidal agents may displace prednisolone from binding sites and raise the free fraction, thus augmenting effect.)*

Schlagkecke R, Kornely E, Santen RT, et al. The effect of long-term glucocorticoid therapy on pituitary-adrenal responses to exogenous corticotropin-releasing hormone. N Engl J Med 1992;326:226. *(CRH testing was nearly as accurate as insulin-induced hypoglycemia for determining HPA suppression; HPA responsiveness could not be reliably predicted from dose or duration of steroid therapy or from basal plasma cortisol level.)*

8

Primary Care Medicine: Office Evaluation and Management of the Adult Patient, 3rd edition, edited by Allan H. Goroll, Lawrence A. May, and Albert G. Mulley, Jr. J.B. Lippincott Company, Philadelphia

Gynecologic Problems

106

Screening for Breast Cancer

Breast cancer is among the most common malignancies afflicting women. Internationally, its incidence varies widely; rates in North America and northern Europe are five to six times higher than those in Asia and Africa. More than 150,000 women develop breast cancer each year in the United States, accounting for more than one in four cancer diagnoses among women. Of these, 50,000 eventually die of the disease, accounting for one in five female cancer deaths. The lifetime probability that an American woman will develop breast cancer is approximately 10 percent. As high as this rate is, many women overestimate it, probably because four out of five women have seen breast cancer in a relative or acquaintance.

Despite diagnostic and therapeutic advances, mortality rates for breast cancer have changed little in the past 30 years. The high incidence, morbidity, and mortality associated with the disease, coupled with the importance of the breasts to many women's self-image, make breast cancer one of the most feared tumors. It is also one of the rare conditions for which screening benefits have been documented, at least for some women. The primary care provider deals with breast cancer screening and diagnosis or associated fears on a daily basis.

EPIDEMIOLOGY AND RISK FACTORS

The epidemiology of breast cancer has been studied extensively. Risk factors for the disease include the following.

Age. Risk of breast cancer increases with age. Nevertheless, it is not uncommon in women younger than age 40, in whom approximately 20 percent of cases occur. The median age at the time of diagnosis is 54 years, and 45 percent of cases occur after age 65. Recent evidence suggests that decreased risk among women older than age 75 may be a result of increased use of breast cancer screening among younger women.

Reproductive History. Generally, there is an inverse relationship between breast cancer risk and parity, but maternal age at the time of first full-term pregnancy may be the most important variable. Independent of parity, an early age at first birth may reduce the risk compared with that for no pregnancy, whereas a late first birth may increase the risk. In a woman with high parity, whose first birth occurs before the age of 20, the risk of breast cancer is half that of a nulliparous woman and one-third that of the woman with one or two births after the age of 30. An aborted pregnancy does not affect cancer risk. Lactation may reduce risk, especially risk of premenopausal cancer, but the effect is disputed.

Menstrual History. Both late menarche and early natural menopause reduce breast cancer risk. Women who experienced menarche after age 16 have half the risk of those who experienced it earlier. Women in whom menopause occurred before age 45 have half the risk of those in whom menopause occurred after age 55. Women in whom early menopause is surgically induced seem to be similarly protected.

Family History. A family history of breast cancer, whether among maternal or paternal relatives, increases the risk to two to three times that of the general population. Relatives of women with bilateral disease have an even higher risk.

History of Benign Breast Disease. The relative risk of breast cancer is twofold to threefold greater in women who have a history of benign breast disease. Some researchers have estimated higher relative risks, and others have questioned whether benign breast disease confers any additional risk. The question is complicated by many issues, most of which relate to definitions of benign breast disease. Evidence indicates that a substantial majority of women with benign breast disease worrisome enough to prompt biopsy have nonproliferative changes and are not at increased risk for eventual breast malignancy. In one study, women with proliferative disease without atypical hyperplasia accounted for 26 percent of breast biopsies and had a twofold increase in risk; those with atypical hyperplasia had a fivefold increase in risk but accounted for only 4 percent of all biopsies.

Mammographic Findings. The appearance of breast tissue on mammographic examination has been related to risk of subsequent malignancy, but this association has been questioned. In 1975, Wolfe advanced a classification system that divided breasts into four categories based on mammographic appearance. The lowest-risk class included breasts that are essentially replaced by fat. The two intermediate classes included breasts with increasingly prominent ducts. Breasts in the fourth category, with evidence for extensive dysplasia, were estimated to have a 20-fold to 30-fold increased risk of cancer compared with breasts in the lowest-risk group. These findings have not been replicated. Although some investigators have found associations between mammographic density and subsequent cancer, the estimates of relative risk have been much lower and substantially affected by patient age. In a large cohort study, women who had mammographic densities in more than 65 percent of their breasts had fourfold greater risk of subsequent cancer than those who had such densities in less than 5 percent.

History of Previous Malignancy. Approximately 10 percent of women who survive for 10 years following the diagnosis of breast cancer will have a second primary malignancy, usually in the contralateral breast. Increasing popularity of breast-sparing surgery for minimal breast cancer will increase the incidence of second breast cancers; about 10 percent to 20 percent of women who choose breast-sparing surgery followed by radiation experience ipsilateral in-breast recurrences over the 10-year period following treatment of the initial tumor. Women with a history of endometrial carcinoma have slightly increased risk of breast cancer.

Diet. A number of observations suggest that breast cancer risk is influenced by diet, particularly consumption of *fats*. Unsaturated fats promote breast tumors in animal models. Geographic differences and associations between dietary intake and cancer provide supporting evidence, but the hypothesis remains unproved. Low levels of vitamin A have also been tentatively linked to small increases in risk. *Obesity* has been consistently linked to minor increases in risk. Several studies have demonstrated an association between daily moderate alcohol consumption and modest increase in breast cancer risk.

Estrogen Use. Clear association between either oral contraceptive use or postmenopausal exogenous estrogens and breast cancer has not been demonstrated. Studies that control for detection bias show no increase in relative risk. Increased risk with duration of estrogen use has been noted only in European studies, perehaps reflecting population, drug preparation, or drug use differences from American studies. Data on risk associated with use of newer estrogen–progesterone postmenopausal regimens remain sparse.

NATURAL HISTORY OF BREAST CANCER AND EFFECTIVENESS OF EARLY THERAPY

Little can be said with certainty about the natural history of breast cancer. The few observational studies of untreated breast cancer have shown widely variable tumor doubling times ranging from less than 1 week to more than 6 months. The mean duration of the preclinical phase of the disease has been estimated to be 20 months. Estimates of lead time, from the Health Insurance Plan (HIP) of Greater New York screening trial, have been 7 months at the initial screening examination and approximately 1 year for subsequent screenings at yearly intervals.

It is particularly difficult to judge the benefit of early treatment of breast cancer because of the widely variable course of the disease after diagnosis at any stage. Biologic determinism as the major influence on outcome has been widely debated. Many studies have shown that there is no clear relationship between survival rates and the length of time the patient delayed seeking medical attention after becoming aware of the tumor, despite the drop in 5-year survival rates from 85 percent to about 50 percent when there is nodal involvement.

Data from the HIP randomized breast cancer screening trial, however, suggest substantial benefits of screening. After 10 to 14 years of follow-up, breast cancer mortality was 25 percent to 30 percent lower in the study group that received yearly screening by x-ray mammography and physical examination. This reduction was evident in women older than age 50 but not in those between ages 40 and 49. In the decades since the HIP study, other randomized trials have found that screening for breast cancer among women ages 50 to 74 reduces breast cancer mortality. Among women screened in the Breast Cancer Detection and Demonstration Project (BCDDP) and followed for 4 to 10 years after diagnosis, the relative 5-, 8-, and 10-year survival rates were 88 percent, 83 percent, and 79 percent, respectively. Analyses of this data were performed in an effort to adjust for lead time and time-linked sampling biases, and to compare rates to those for women who were diagnosed in the National Cancer Institute's Surveillance, Epidemiology and End Results program. The 5- and 8-year survival rates were better for women in the BCDDP.

SCREENING METHODS

Breast Self-Examination has been a mainstay of prevention programs. Surveys have disclosed that many women perform breast self-examination but that most do not perform the procedure monthly and do not spend sufficient time to do it correctly. Age, education, marital status, having been instructed by a health professional, regular professional breast examinations, and a family history of breast cancer have all been shown to influence breast self-examination behavior.

Some still question the effectiveness of self-examination in the early detection of disease. Recent evidence supports the contention that self-examination is associated with diagnosis of smaller tumors. All agree that effectiveness depends on breast size, shape, and the density of breast tissue. Small or poorly supported pendulous breasts are most suitable. Examination of large, well-supported breasts is difficult for both patients and physicians. The effectiveness of self-examination is determined in large measure by the woman's proficiency in examining her breasts. All women should be taught systematic breast examination techniques and advised to use them on a monthly basis. Repeated episodes of brief instruction have been shown to be highly effective in increasing self-examination proficiency and frequency. Seven to 10 days after menses is the best time for premenopausal women; postmenopausal women can pick a regular calendar date, such as the first of each month. Breast self-examination should be particularly stressed for women who are at high risk and those with breasts that are anatomically suitable.

Physical Examination by the patient's clinician is extremely important and should not be neglected. It is often not appreciated that much of the benefit evident in the HIP study was derived from the physical examination rather than from mammography; only 44 percent of cancers in women aged 50 to 59, and 19 percent of those in women aged 40 to 49, were found on mammography alone. It is widely acknowledged that current mammographic techniques are much more sensitive than those used in the HIP study. Nevertheless, physical examination and mammography remain complementary procedures; a substantial proportion of cancers, particularly among younger women, will be missed by physicians who rely too heavily on mammography and thereby neglect careful, systematic inspection and palpation of the breasts. A number of studies have demonstrated that the proportion of lesions confined to stage I at the time of diagnosis is higher for tumors discovered during routine physical examination than for those presenting symptomatically or found during breast self-examination.

Mammography is a valuable aid in the diagnosis of breast masses (see Chapter 113) and as a screening test. Its precise role in general screening remains somewhat controversial. While there is general agreement about the effectiveness of routine mammographic screening among women ages 50 to 74, there are also conflicting recommendations about which women should be screened when, and about the frequency of mammography in different age groups.

The HIP study provided a rigorous test of the hypothesis that regular screening by means of physical examination and mammography can reduce breast cancer morbidity and mortality. After 14 years of follow-up, benefit has been conclusively demonstrated among women aged 50 to 59, who showed a 25 percent to 30 percent reduction in breast cancer mortality compared with women randomized to the non-screened control group. Other trials have since found mortality reductions ranging from 20 percent to 39 percent among women older than age 50. More extensive follow-up of the HIP subjects demonstrated a 25 percent reduction in mortality among women ages 40 to 49, but the statistical significance of the trend has been disputed. Questions have also been raised about the clinical significance of the finding because of the relatively low absolute risk reduction for younger women.

Data from the Breast Cancer Detection Demonstration Projects (BCDDP), derived from screening nearly 300,000 women in 29 centers in the United States, are frequently cited to support both the contribution of mammography to screening and the extension of screening to younger women. Of more than 3500 cancers detected by BCDDP examinations, 42 percent were found by mammography alone; these cancers were more likely to be stage I lesions. Approximately 32 percent of cancers were found in women younger than age 50; of these, 35 percent were detected by mammography alone. BCDDP data also provide a clear indication of how much mammographic techniques have improved since the HIP study. Whereas mammography had a sensitivity of 60 percent in the HIP program for cancers in the age 50 to 59 cohort, sensitivity for the same group was 92 percent in the BCDDP. The U.S. Preventative Services Task Force estimated the combination of clinical breast examination and mammography to have a sensitivity of 75 percent and a specificity of 94 percent to 99 percent.

Improvements in technology have also reduced risks of radiation. Although it was once asked if regular use of mammography might induce more cancers than it would detect for cure, best current estimates indicate that exposure of 1 million women to 1 rad would produce only six excess cancers after a latent period of 10 to 15 years; the risk of naturally occurring breast cancer is more than 1000-fold greater. Mammography can be performed now with considerably lower radiation exposure. Screen-film mammography requires just 0.2-rad exposure.

The findings of the BCDDP and the improved safety of mammography moved the American Cancer Society and others to modify recommendations that had previously urged annual mammography only for women older than age 50. Most recommendations now advise mammograms at intervals of 1 to 2 years between ages 40 and 49, followed by annual mammography beginning at age 50. Although these recommendations are not unreasonable, it must be kept in mind that BCDDP participants were self-selected and there were no controls. Furthermore, these recommendations are not supported by the results of a Canadian randomized trial designed to determine the benefits of mammography in younger women and to distinguish between the effects of screening mammography and screening physical examination. The Canadian National Breast Screening Study (CNBSS) enrolled 50,000 women between the ages of 40 and 49. After 7 years of follow-up, there was no evident reduction in mortality. The study has been criticized for alleged poor-quality mammography, but other, smaller trials have similarly failed to demonstrate a survival benefit among screened women after as many as 10 years of follow-up.

In approaching the controversy about routine mammography in younger women, the clinician should be mindful of evidence that breast cancer and mammography may well behave differently in young women. Evidence that, on average, breast cancer has a shorter asymptomatic detectable period in younger women may make the proposed longer screening intervals for women aged 40 to 49 an unsuitable compromise. Mammography has been shown to have a lower sensitivity and specificity among younger women, increasing the risks of false-negative and false-positive findings and their consequences. One comprehensive analysis, published before the CNBSS, estimated that addition of mammography to clinical examination of the breast would reduce a woman's risk of breast cancer death by 0.25 percent. The probability of a false-positive mammogram requiring diagnostic evaluation would be 25 percent.

CONCLUSIONS AND RECOMMENDATIONS

- Breast cancer is common. Although risk factors allow identification of subgroups at particularly high risk, women without risk factors are nonetheless at substantial risk and should receive regular, periodic screening.
- Evidence indicates that early diagnosis leads to substantial reduction in mortality.

- Self-examination should be taught to all women by the primary care provider. The technique should be emphasized when the woman is at high risk and has breasts that are suitable for effective self-examination.
- Physical examination is an important element of screening. It should be performed in all women at yearly intervals, more frequently in high-risk populations.
- Mammography has proven to be beneficial in women older than age 50. When possible, it should be performed on an annual basis in this group. Regular mammograms at 1- to 2-year intervals beginning at age 40 have also been recommended. Although this is a reasonable approach, the benefits have not been proven, and the primary physician should be mindful of the potential harm produced by an imperfect test, including overdiagnosis and false reassurance.

A.G.M.

ANNOTATED BIBLIOGRAPHY

Adami HO, Malker B, Holmberg, et al. The relation between survival and age at diagnosis in breast cancer. N Engl J Med 1986;315:559. *(Women aged 45–49 seem to have the best prognosis, with relative survival declining markedly in women whose cancer is diagnosed in later years.)*

Bains CJ, To T. Changes in breast self-examination behavior achieved by 89,835 participants in the Canadian National Breast Screening Study. Cancer 1990;66:570. *(Competence and frequency of breast self-examination increased dramatically after brief periods of instruction.)*

Bennett SE, Lawrence RS, Fleischmann KH, et al. Profile of women practicing breast self-examination. JAMA 1983;249:488. *(Breast self-examination was more common among women with a maternal history of breast disease to whom technique had been demonstrated.)*

Berg JW. Clinical implications of risk factors for breast cancer. Cancer 1984;53:589. *(Makes the important point that "low-risk" women still face substantial risk of breast cancer, that is, approximately 6 percent.)*

Brinton LA, Hoover R, Fraumeni JF Jr. Epidemiology of minimal breast cancer. JAMA 1983;249:483. *(In this case–control study, epidemiologic associations for small and larger invasive tumors were similar: family history, age at first live birth, history, oophorectomy, and obesity. In situ cancer was associated with family history and age at first childbirth but not with oophorectomy or obesity.)*

Brisson J, Merletti F, Sadowsky NL, et al. Mammographic features of the breast and breast cancer risk. Am J Epidemiol 1982;115:428. *(Did find a five fold risk of cancer in women with Wolfe's highest-risk pattern compared with those with the lowest-risk pattern. Risk was influenced by age.)*

Chu KC, Smart CR, Tarone RE. Analysis of breast cancer mortality and stage distribution by age for the Health Insurance Plan clinical trial. J Natl Cancer Inst 1988;80:1125. *(Analysis of late follow-up of the HIP study that finds evidence to support screening women in their forties.)*

Coleman EA, Feuer EJ, The NCI Breast Cancer Screening Consortium. Breast cancer screening among women 65 to 74 years of age in 1987–1988 and 1991. Ann Intern Med 1992;117:961. *(Mammography use among older women is increasing.)*

Davis DL, Love SM. Mammographic Screening. JAMA 1994; 271:152. *(An editorial summarizing the data on screening women under age 50.)*

Eddy DM. Screening for breast cancer. Center for Health Policy and Research Education, Duke University. Ann Intern Med 1989;111:389. *(A careful review and synthesis of the literature including quantitative estimates of the benefits and harms to be expected with alternative screening practices.)*

Evans JS, Wennberg JE, McNeil BJ. The influence of diagnostic radiography on the incidence of breast cancer and leukemia. N Engl J Med 1986;315:810. *(Data from a closed population and a mathematical model lead to conclusion that incidence of radiation-induced breast cancer is low.)*

Fletcher SW, Fletcher RH. The breast is close to the heart. Ann Intern Med 1992;117:969. *(Editorial reviewing the findings of the Canadian National Breast Screening Study as well as other evidence regarding the effectiveness of screening in different age groups.)*

Foster RS, Costanza MC. Breast self-examination practices and breast cancer survival. Cancer 1984;53:999. *(Women who had practiced self-examination had better survival rates following cancer diagnosis.)*

Henrick JB. The postmenopausal estrogen/breast cancer controversy. JAMA 1992;268:1900. *(A critical look at the data; finds little evidence for increased risk.)*

Helmrich SP, Shapiro S, Rosenberg L, et al. Risk factors for breast cancer. Am J Epidemiol 1983;117:35. *(A large case–control study confirming increased risk associated with age at first birth as well as independent effects of parity, a history of benign breast disease, positive family history of breast cancer, Jewish religion, and 12 or more years of education.)*

Love RR, Brown RL, Davis JE, et al. Frequency and determinants of screening for breast cancer in primary care group practice. Arch Intern Med 1993;153:2113. *(Having mammography discussed by a staff member was the strongest predictor of screening.)*

Miller AB, Baines CJ, To T, Wall C. Canadian National Breast Screening Study. 1. Breast cancer detection and death rates among women aged 40 to 49 years. Can Med Assoc J 1992; in press. *(The risk for dying of breast cancer was higher among the women randomized to the screening intervention, which included annual physical examination and mammography.)*

Miller AB, Baines CJ, To T, Wall C. Canadian National Breast Screening Study. 2. Breast cancer detection and death rates among women aged 50 to 59 years. Can Med Assoc J 1992;in press. (*Risk reduced in women randomized to screening*).

Nystrom L, Rutqvist LE, Hall S, et al. Breast cancer screening with mammography: Overview of Swedish randomized trials. Lancet 1993;341:973. (*Largest aggregate experience, helping to clarify the issue of screening those less than 40 and over 70.)*

Seidman H, Gelb SK, Silverberg E, LaVerda N, Lubera JA. Survival experience in the Breast Cancer Detection Demonstration Project. CA 1987;37:258. *(Analysis of BCDDP data focusing on comparisons between experience of women older than 50 and those aged 40–49 with conclusion that screening among the younger women was effective.)*

Shapiro S. Periodic breast cancer screening in seven foreign countries. Johns Hopkins University School of Hygiene and Public Health. Cancer 1992;69:1919. *(Reviews different approaches to the clinical and policy questions associated with the screening decision.)*

Shapiro S, Goldberg JD, Hutchinson GB. Lead time in breast cancer detection and implications for periodicity of screening. Am J Epidemiol 1974;100:357. *(Lead time estimated to be 1 year to 7 months at the initial examination and 11–13 months at subsequent screenings.)*

Shapiro S, Venet W, Strax P, et al. Ten to fourteen year effect of screening on breast cancer mortality. J Natl Cancer Inst 1982;69:349. *(Results from the randomized HIP trial.)*

Solin LJ, Fowble BL, Schultz DJ, Goodman RL. The impact of mammography on the patterns of patients referred for definitive breast irradiation. Cancer 1990;65:2464. *(Diagnosis by mammogram followed by needle localization of nonpalpable lesions leads to increased percentage of intraductal carcinomas.)*

Taber L, Fagerberg G, Duffy SW, Day NE, Gas A, Grontoft O. Update of the Swedish Two-County Program of mammographic screening for breast cancer. Radiol Clin North Am 1992;30:187. *(After 11 years of follow-up, no detectable benefit of screening for women in their forties.)*

Willett WC, McMahon B. Diet and cancer—an overview. N Engl J Med 1984;310:633. *(Reviews the relation between vitamins and trace elements and various cancers as well as the association between dietary fat and breast cancer.)*

107
Screening for Cervical Cancer

Primary Care Medicine: Office Evaluation and Management of the Adult Patient, 3rd edition, edited by Allan H. Goroll, Lawrence A. May, and Albert G. Mulley, Jr. J.B. Lippincott Company, Philadelphia

In the United States, the annual incidence of invasive cervical cancer is 13,500, and annual mortality is 6000. For an American woman, the lifetime probability of developing invasive cervical cancer is about 0.7 percent. The incidence of carcinoma in situ is more than three times that of invasive disease. There is a very long asymptomatic period during which cytologic detection of cervical neoplasia is possible. Early therapy is often curative. Appropriately, the Papanicolaou (Pap) smear is one of the most widely used cancer screening tests.

EPIDEMIOLOGY AND RISK FACTORS

Age and sexual activity are the principal risk factors for cervical cancer.

The age-specific prevalence rates for carcinoma in situ follow a bimodal distribution with the dominant, first peak of about six per 1000 women occurring in the 30-to-45 age group. A second peak of about five per 1000 occurs among women older than age 60. The highest carcinoma in situ incidence rates are in the 25-to-29 age group. The prevalence of invasive carcinoma is highest in older age groups, rising precipitously after age 50. A breakdown in host barriers at the time of menopause has been proposed as an explanation for the decreased in situ and increased invasive prevalence rates observed in these patients.

Many factors have been associated with cervical neoplasia. Most are related to sexual activity. First intercourse at a *young age* (ie, before age 18) and *multiple sexual partners* (four or more) are the factors most consistently associated with high risk. Increasing parity, poor personal hygiene, a history of venereal disease, an uncircumcised partner, and a high number of sexual partners of the husband or regular sexual partner have also been linked to cervical cancer. The extremely low risk of cervical neoplasia in women who have never had intercourse and the consistent association with variables that define sexual exposure has sparked several hypotheses about cervical cancer as a venereal disease. An association between herpes simplex type II virus and cervical cancer has been described, but more recent findings do not suggest a causal link. The strongest evidence points to *human papillomavirus (HPV)*, particularly types 16 and 18, as potential venereally transmitted oncogenic agents. It is now thought that the combination of exposure to such agents and the presence of susceptible cervical epithelium leads to cervical neoplasia. Observations that normal immature squamous epithelium in the transformation zone of the cervix is particularly sensitive to viral infections may explain some of the long-observed epidemiologic correlates of cervical cancer. Immature squamous cells are present in the developing transformation zone following menarche and during remodeling of the transformation zone following pregnancy. Women who are sexually active early in life and who have multiple pregnancies may be more likely to come in contact with oncogenic agents when their cervical epithelium is susceptible to infection. This theory would also explain the twofold to fourfold increase in risk of dysplasia and carcinoma in situ in women exposed in utero to diethylstilbestrol. Persistent susceptibility to oncogenic agents may stem from immature metaplastic squamous cells that arise in the areas of cervical and vaginal adenosis frequently found in women exposed to diethylstilbestrol (see Chapter 110).

Other factors have been associated with cervical neoplasia, but it is difficult to control for sexual exposure. The incidence of cervical cancer is decreased in Jewish women and increased in African-Americans, native Americans and Hispanics. *Socioeconomic status* may be the most important predictor, inasmuch as the racial and ethnic disparities are reduced or eliminated when socioeconomic factors are controlled. Smoking has been identified as a potentially important independent risk factor for cervical cancer in a number of studies that controlled for both sexual activity and socioeconomic status. Although the issue remains controversial, the weight of current evidence supports the association. One theory holds that smoking may make women more susceptible to the oncogenic effects of viruses. Evidence suggests that use of oral contraceptives confers a modest increase in cervical cancer risk.

The most compelling risk information comes from the Pap smear itself, in that the risk of carcinoma is 100 times greater in women with dysplasia than in those with a normal cervix.

NATURAL HISTORY OF CERVICAL CANCER AND EFFECTIVENESS OF THERAPY

Cervical cancer classically presents with *intermenstrual bleeding* prompted by coitus or douching. Symptoms invariably occur late in the course of the disease. Epidemiologic evidence indicates that the natural history of cervical neoplasia should be viewed as a progression from mild dysplasia, through carcinoma in situ, to invasive carcinoma. Only a minority of mildly dysplastic lesions progress to carcinoma. It is not clear that carcinoma in situ invariably becomes invasive, but epidemiologic data suggest that progression occurs in the vast majority of cases. Both of these premalignant lesions, which are referred to together as cervical intraepithelial neoplasia, are reliably detected by cytologic techniques.

The mean duration of the detectable asymptomatic period, as estimated from incidence and prevalence rates, is very long. The mean duration of carcinoma in situ varies with age but averages about 10 years. The duration of asymptomatic invasive carcinoma is 5 years for all age groups. It should be emphasized that these are estimated means; the proportion of cervical cancers that become invasive early in their development is not known.

There is no doubt that the earlier the clinical stage of the tumor when detected and treated, the better the prognosis. Survival for carcinoma in situ treated with hysterectomy is essentially 100 percent. However, the uncertainty about the natural course of carcinoma in situ must be kept in mind. Relative 5-year survival rates for localized and regional invasive carcinoma are about 80 percent and 40 percent, respectively. The 5-year experience of one screening program demonstrated that 86 percent of cases detected by cytologic screening were limited to regional invasion, while only 44 percent of those presenting symptomatically were in this early stage.

SCREENING METHODS AND DIAGNOSTIC TESTS

There are three techniques of cell collection for Papanicolaou staining and cytologic screening of the cervix. The easiest and least effective is aspiration from the vaginal pool. More sensitive, but requiring visualization of the cervix with a vaginal speculum, are *endocervical swabbing* and *cervical scraping*. The sensitivity of the vaginal aspirate technique has been reported in a range from 62 percent to 92 percent in the presence of invasive carcinoma and from 31 percent to 70 percent in the presence of carcinoma in situ. The range of reported sensitivities for swabbing is 82 percent to 92 percent and that for scraping, 86 percent to 100 percent. There is no consistent difference in detection rates between invasive carcinoma and carcinoma in situ with the swabbing and scraping techniques. Current recommendations suggest that two cell smears be taken for each test: one taken from the endocervical canal, with either a saline-moistened cotton swab or a cytologic brush designed specifically for the purpose, and one scraped with a spatula from the os of the cervix, which contains the squamous-columnar junction or transformation zone. Smears should be interpreted by an experienced cytopathologist.

Recent reports indicate that sensitivity in actual practice may be substantially lower because of poor cell collection technique or faulty interpretation. To roughly estimate the practical false-negative rate resulting from the combination of these potential errors, investigators have defined a smear as falsely negative if a woman subsequently developed a confirmed lesion within a defined follow-up period. In one such study, 17 percent of women developed such lesions within 2 years of a negative smear. These findings have prompted recommendations that the screening interval be kept short between the first and second smear for women regularly screened.

The *specificity* of cytologic diagnosis is very high. In a 2-year period, 151 of 25,000 cytologic examinations of the cervix performed at the Massachusetts General Hospital were read as positive. Eighty percent of these women had cervical cancer. Clearly, more than 99 percent without disease had negative smears. This high specificity limits the costs associated with false-positive results.

The *frequency* of cervical cancer screening has been controversial. Because of the usual long duration of the asymptomatic detectable period of cervical intraepithelial neoplasia, which is easily controlled and cured when detected, the American Cancer Society and others have moved away from earlier recommendations of annual Pap smears. Generally, smears are now recommended every 3 years after two successive negative smears 1 year apart at ages 20 and 21, or younger if the patient is sexually active. The purpose of the short first interval is to improve sensitivity of the first screening effort. Though women who are at high risk because of early age at first intercourse, multiple sexual partners, or other risk factors may be tested more frequently, the clinician should be mindful that the decision about test frequency depends more on the duration of the asymptomatic detectable disease rather than a woman's individual risk.

Some recommendations for more frequent screening among young women reflect concern about evidence that a greater proportion of carcinoma in situ among younger women may be rapidly progressive. For example, in 1982 the Canadian Task Force recommended that women who have had sexual intercourse should be screened annually between ages 18 and 35. Pap smears every 5 years are recommended for women ages 35 to 60. Screening is not recommended for women who have never had intercourse. Subsequent findings, however do not support the hypothesis that there is an increased frequency of lesions that move rapidly from carcinoma in situ to invasion.

Screening is recommended until age 65. The *duration* of regular screening is finite. Screening after age 65 is not cost-effective in women who have been undergoing regular screening and have had normal smears. However, those who have not been screened previously should be (cervical cancer screening is now a Medicare benefit).

Cytologic smears are not read as simply positive or negative. The original Papanicolaou system included five classes ranging from normal (class I) to suggestive of invasive cancer (class V). Subsequently, a World Health Organization committee recommended classifying specimens as "normal," "atypical," "dysplasia" (mild, moderate, or severe), "carcinoma in situ," "invasive cervical cancer," and "adenocarcinoma." In 1988, a committee of the National Cancer Institute recommended the Bethesda System, which replaces the older class II/"atypical" category with the designation "reactive and reparative change." This term is used to describe cellular changes in response to inflammation and other nonneoplastic processes. The Bethesda System also introduced the term, "squamous intraepithelial lesion," which includes two grades. Low-grade squamous intraepithelial lesions are consistent with HPV infection and mild dysplasia and correspond to the old class III/mild dysplasia category. High-grade lesions include the moderate and severe dysplasia and carcinoma in situ designations. Women whose smears show high-grade squamous intraepithelial lesions (ie, moderate to severe dysplasia) or carcinoma in situ, as well as those with smears suggestive of invasive cancer, should be referred to a gynecologist experienced in the use of the colposcope. Colposcopic examination will allow the gynecologist to select sites for biopsy and determine the limits of the lesion. This will allow informed choice between conservative measures such as electrocautery and cryotherapy, which are used increasingly frequently, and more traditional measures such as conization and hysterectomy. Such decisions will be based not only on the size, location, and histology of the lesion but also on the patient's age, parity, and reliability for follow-up.

CONCLUSIONS AND RECOMMENDATIONS

- The high prevalence, long mean duration of asymptomatic detectable disease, and availability of a highly specific screening test make cervical cancer screening an important task for all primary care providers.
- Known risk factors, including early sexual activity and high number of sexual partners, allow selection of high-risk patients and populations.
- Because of the long duration of preinvasive, detectable disease in women of reproductive age, annual screening in the absence of specific risk factors may be unnecessary. Two screens with a short interval (eg, 1 year) may be used to reduce the number of false-negative prevalence cases. The interval between subsequent screens can be lengthened for low-risk individuals. The presence of a risk factor, particularly in the menopausal or postmenopausal patient, may be an indication for more frequent (ie, yearly) screening.
- A cytologic smear positive for cancer or a high-grade squamous intraepithelial lesion is an indication for referral to a gynecologist for further evaluation, including appropriate biopsies.
- A smear suggestive of reactive or reparative changes or mild dysplasia can be further evaluated by the nongynecologist. If a concurrent infection is evident, the smear should be repeated following specific treatment of the infection. If no infection is present, the smear may be repeated after a 3- to 6-month interval. Women with repeatedly abnormal smears should be referred for colposcopy or biopsy.
- Screening can cease after age 65 in women with a history of regularly obtained, negative smears but should be performed if not done regularly before age 65 or if smear has been abnormal.

A.G.M.

ANNOTATED BIBLIOGRAPHY

Brinton LA, Fraumeni FJ Jr: Epidemiology of uterine cervical cancer. J Chronic Dis 1986;39:1051. *(Good review of epidemiology and risk factors.)*

Canadian Task Force on Cervical Cancer Screening Programs. Cervical cancer screening programs: summary of the 1982 Canadian Task Force report. Can Med Assoc J 1982;127:581. *(Recommendations for more frequent screening among younger women.)*

Crum CP, Ikenberg H, Richart RM, et al. Human papillomavirus type 16 in early cervical neoplasia. N Engl J Med 1984;310:880. *(HPV 16 virus was isolated from condylomata of the uterine cervix which contained abnormal mitotic figures and appeared to be precursors of invasive cancer of the cervix.)*

Devesa SS. Descriptive epidemiology of cancer of the uterine cervix. Obstet Gynecol 1984;63:605. *(Documents a decline in cervical cancer mortality in all age groups accompanied by a sharp rise in incidence of diagnosis of carcinoma in situ.)*

Eddy DM. Screening for cervical cancer. Ann Intern Med 1990;113:214. *(An excellent review of the literature and in-depth analysis that provides estimates of the benefits and harms of alternative screening strategies.)*

Fahs MC, Mandelblatt J, Schecter C, et al. Cost-effectiveness of cervical cancer screening for the elderly. Ann Intern Med 1992;117:520. *(Not cost-effective after age 65 if done regularly before 65 and normal smears found.)*

Kashgarian M, Dunn JE. The duration of intraepithelial and preclinical squamous cell carcinoma of the uterine cervix. Am J Epidemiol 1970;92:211. *(Detailed analysis of incidence and prevalence data from Memphis study providing estimates of preclinical duration of disease.)*

Massachusetts Department of Public Health. Papanicolaou testing—are we screening the wrong women? N Engl J Med 1976;294:223. *(Points out high frequency of screening of young women with low risk.)*

Miller AB. The cost-effectiveness of cervical cancer screening. Ann Intern Med 1992;117:529. *(An editorial supporting cessation of Pap testing after age 65 in women previously tested on a regular basis.)*

Mitchell H, Drake M, Medley G. Prospective evaluation of risk of cervical cancer after cytological evidence of human papilloma virus infection. Lancet 1986;1:573. *(Among 846 women with cytological evidence of HPV infection followed for 6 years, 30 developed carcinoma in situ, leading to a 15.6 estimate of the relative risk.)*

Richart RM, Vaillant HW. Influence of cell collection techniques upon cytological diagnosis. Cancer 1965;18:1474. *(Reviews sensitivities of endocervical swabbing, cervical scraping, and vaginal aspirate techniques.)*

Trevathan E, Layde P, Webster LA. Cigarette smoking and dysplasia and carcinoma in situ of the uterine cervix. JAMA 1983;250:499. *(A case–control study suggesting substantially increased risk of cervical cancer among young women who smoke cigarettes.)*

Van der Graaf Y, Vooijs GP. False negative rate in cervical cytology. J Clin Pathol 1987;40:438. *(Among women followed for 2 years after negative smears, 17 percent developed significant lesions.)*

Primary Care Medicine: Office Evaluation and Management of the Adult Patient, 3rd edition, edited by Allan H. Goroll, Lawrence A. May, and Albert G. Mulley, Jr. J.B. Lippincott Company, Philadelphia

108
Screening for Ovarian Cancer

Ovarian cancer is less common than breast cancer and other gynecologic malignancies; the lifetime probability is approximately one in 70. However, it has a high case-fatality rate. Each year in the United States, more than 20,000 new cases are diagnosed and more than 12,000 women die of the disease. Ovarian cancer deaths among prominent public figures, the recent availability of new diagnostic tests, and the general trend toward increased interest in disease prevention among women has focused attention on screening for ovarian cancer. The primary care provider needs to understand the epidemiology and risk factors for this disease, as well as the value and limitations of available tests, to respond appropriately to patients' questions and, when appropriate, recommend a screening intervention.

EPIDEMIOLOGY AND RISK FACTORS

Increasing age and family history are risk factors for ovarian cancer. The annual incidence of 20 per 100,000 among women ages 30 to 50 increases to 40 per 100,000 among women ages 50 to 75. The incidence among older women is even higher when one restricts the denominator to women who have not had their ovaries surgically removed.

A family history of ovarian cancer is present in about 7 percent of women with the disease. The clustering of ovarian cancer or other related cancers (breast, endometrial, or colorectal) within a kindred, or occurrence of ovarian cancer at an early age, may suggest a hereditary ovarian cancer syndrome which can confer high risk. In some families, an autosomal dominant pattern of inheritance has been demonstrated and the lifetime probability of developing ovarian cancer may be as high as 50 percent. However, it is thought that such heriditary syndromes account for less than 1 percent of ovarian cancer.

A family history of the much more common sporadic ovarian cancer also confers risk. The best estimate is that ovarian cancer in one first- or second-degree relative increases risk threefold. When two relatives have had the disease, risk is increased fivefold.

Use of the oral contraceptive pill and parity are associated with reduced risk of ovarian cancer. Any use of oral contraceptives appears to reduce risk by 35 percent, and use for 5 or more years, by 50 percent. Any pregnancy reduces risk by about 50 percent; increasing number of pregnancies is associated with decreasing risk. Other factors, including age at first pregnancy, infertility, menstrual history, hormone replacement therapy, and dietary factors, may modify risk of ovarian cancer, but evidence is inconclusive. Tubal ligation and possibly hysterectomy appear protective.

NATURAL HISTORY OF OVARIAN CANCER AND EFFECTIVENESS OF THERAPY

Mortality rates for prostate cancer have changed little over the past 3 decades. When ovarian cancer is diagnosed after clinical presentation with signs or symptoms, three out of four cases have already spread beyond the ovary. Under these circumstances, the 5-year survival rate is less than 20 percent. In contrast, 5-year survival rates of patients with tumor confined to the ovary has been greater than 70 percent in older studies and greater than 90 percent in recent case series. It is not surprising that there is great enthusiasm for using newer diagnostic modalities to advance the time of diagnosis and thereby reduce the burden of morbidity and mortality associated with ovarian cancer. It must be remembered, however, that we know little about the preclinical course of ovarian cancer, including variability in its biologic behavior. Any current estimates of screening benefit will be confounded by lead time and time-linked sampling biases. Until randomized trials of screening demonstrate reduction in population mortality rates, estimates of the benefits of screening will remain tentative.

DIAGNOSTIC TESTS

There has been little formal evaluation of the pelvic examination as a screening test for ovarian cancer among asymptomatic women. Evaluations that have been conducted comparing the physical examination with other diagnostic modalities have produced mixed results. In two studies, pelvic examination failed to detect three stage I tumors that were detected by transvaginal or abdominal ultrasound. However, in other studies, pelvic examination was able to detect early tumors. There is a general consensus that pelvic examination alone is insuffiently sensitive to be of value as a screening test.

While early use of ultrasonography to diagnose ovarian cancer used the transabdominal approach, more recent work has focusd on transvaginal ultrasonography, with the addition of color-flow Doppler techniques to improve specificity. The sensitivity of ultrasound has been estimated in studies of women with known ovarian cancer and in screening studies. In the former case, estimates of sensitivity range from 80 percent to 100 percent. Estimates are higher in the screening studies, but this may reflect failure to diagnose cancer among screened-negative study subjects. Estimates of specificity derived from screening studies range from about 75 percent to 97 percent. A recent analytic review provided summary estimates of sensitivity and specificity of 83 percent and 93 percent, respectively. Some studies have shown improvements in specificity of transvaginal ultrasound with addition of color-flow Doppler techniques, which can detect tumor neovascularization. Ultrasound is a safe diagnostic modality. Interpretations can be highly variable and depend on the skill of the operator. Cost, personnel, and patient inconvenience limit its use as a primary screening test. Furthermore, the limited specificity of the test results in low predictive values in the screening situation.

There is a great deal of interest in the use of CA125 to screen for ovarian cancer. CA125 is an antigenic determinant on a glycoprotein that is present in the serum at elevated levels in 80 percent of women with epithelial ovarian cancers. CA125 levels are also elevated in late-stage endometrial cancers and in about 60 percent of pancreatic cancers. Levels may also be elevated in patients with benign ovarian cysts, uterine leiomyoma, pregnancy, endometriosis and pelvic inflammatory disease. Estimates of sensitivity derived from women with known ovarian cancer, using a reference level of 35 U/mL, range from 61 percent to 96 percent. In the screening situation, sensitivity has been estimated at 67 percent to 100 percent. However, reported sensitivities for stage I disease have ranged from 25 percent to 75 percent. The specificity of CA125 in large screening studies, with the reference level of 35 U/mL, has been approximately 99 percent. Specificity is much lower in premenopausal women, because CA125 levels fluctuate with the menstrual cycle and because of a higher prevalence of the benign gynecologic conditions that are associated with elevated levels.

Given the sensitivity and specificity of CA125 and the prevalence of ovarian cancer in the population of women older than age 50, the expected positive predictive value of a CA125 level greater than 35 U/mL in that population would be 3 percent. If screening were restricted to women with ovarian cancer in one first-degree relative, or in two or more relatives, the positive predictive values with the same reference level would be 9 percent and 15 percent, respectively. These predictive values indicate that many screened women would have false-positive results that would require invasive diagnostic evaluation, often including laparotomy.

CONCLUSIONS AND RECOMMENDATIONS

- Women from families with a rare hereditary form of ovarian cancer are at high risk and should be screened annually with CA125 and ultrasound beginning at age 35.
- Women with a family history of sporadic ovarian cancer may benefit from screening with CA125, but because of the low predictive value and the morbidity associated with further diagnostic evaluation, *routine* screening is not recommended. However, women should be advised of the potential benefits and harms of screening. Similarly, *routine* screening is not recommended for pre- and postmenopausal women without a family history of ovarian cancer.

A.G.M.

ANNOTATED BIBLIOGRAPHY

Andolf E, Jorgensen C, Astedt B. Ultrasound examination for detection of ovarian carcinoma in risk groups. Obstet Gynecol 1990;75:106. *(Pelvic examination did not detect the ovarian cancer detected by ultrasound.)*

Bourne TH, Whitehead MI, Campbell S, Royston P, Bhan V, Collins WP. Ultrasound screening for familial ovarian cancer. Gynecol Oncol 1991;43:92. *(Women with a family history of ovarian cancer have a higher prevalence of benign ovarian abnormalities.)*

Einhorn N, Sjovall K, Knapp RC, et al. Prospective evaluation of serum CA 125 levels for the early detection of ovarian cancer. Obstet Gynecol 1992;80:14. *(Prospective cohort study of 5550 women yielding estimates of sensitivity and specificity of 67 percent to 100 percent and 99.4 percent, respectively.)*

Hankinson SE, Hunter DJ, Colditz GA, et al. Tubal ligation, hysterectomy, and risk of ovarian cancer: A prospective study. JAMA 1993;270:2813. *(Tubal ligation and possibly hysterectomy may reduce risk.)*

Hankinson SE, Colditz GA, Hunter DJ, Spencer TL, Rosner B, Stampfer MJ. A quantitative assessment of oral contraceptive use and risk of ovarian cancer. Obstet Gynecol 1992;80:708. *(Relative risk of ovarian cancer among ever-users of oral contraceptives pills was 0.65.)*

Hartge P, Schiffman MH, Hoover R, McGowan L, Lesher L, Norris HJ. A case–control study of epithelial ovarian cancer. Am J Obstet Gynecol 1989;161:10. *(One of many case–control studies which collectively provide highly variable estimates of relative risks.)*

Kerlikowske K, Brown JS, Grady DG. Should women with familial ovarian cancer undergo prophylactic oophorectomy? Obstet Gynecol 1992;80:700. *(Weighs the risks and benefits of prophylactic surgery.)*

Koch M, Gaedke H, Jenkins H. Family history of ovarian cancer patients: a case–control study. Int J Epidemiol 1989;18:782. *(One of many case–control studies which collectively provide highly variable estimates of relative risks.)*

Pittaway DE, Fayez JA. Serum CA-125 antigen levels increase during menses. Am J Obstet Gynecol 1987;156:75. *(Documents cyclic variation which could have a profound effect on sensitivity and specificity among premenopausal women.)*

Schapira MM, Matchar DB, Young MJ. The effectiveness of ovarian cancer screening: A decision analysis model. Ann Intern Med 1993;118:838. *(Found limited effect on life expectancy and not recommended for routine use.)*

Skates SJ, Singer DE. Quantifying the potential benefit of CA 125 screening for ovarian cancer. J Clin Epidemiol 1991;44:365. *(Presents a sophisticated mathematical model for estimating effects of CA125 screening.)*

Sparks JM, Varner RE. Ovarian cancer screening. Obstet Gynecol 1992;77:787. *(A good summary of the issues.)*

Van Nagell JR, DePriest PD, Puls LE, et al. Ovarian cancer screening in asymptomatic postmenopausal women by transvaginal sonography. Cancer 1991;68:458. *(Reports a sensitivity of 100 percent including all stage I cancers.)*

Primary Care Medicine: Office Evaluation and Management of the Adult Patient, 3rd edition, edited by Allan H. Goroll, Lawrence A. May, and Albert G. Mulley, Jr. J.B. Lippincott Company, Philadelphia

109
Screening for Endometrial Cancer

More than 95 percent of the cancers of the uterine corpus are adenocarcinomas arising from the endometrium. In the United States, endometrial cancer is nearly three times more common than invasive cervical cancer. There are approximately 40,000 cases and 4000 endometrial cancer deaths among American women each year. The lifetime probability of developing endometrial carcinoma is 3 percent. There is some evidence that increases in the incidence of endometrial cancer are parallel to the increased life span among American women and, until recently, to the increased use of exogenous estrogens among postmenopausal women. Most cases occur in women in whom risk factors are well defined. The tumors often present symptomatically at a time when cure is still possible. Diagnostic tests suitable for indiscriminate screening are not available. It is the responsibility of the primary care provider to be aware of the risk factors and limitations of diagnostic tests, to elicit the pertinent history, and to respond to worrisome symptoms.

EPIDEMIOLOGY AND RISK FACTORS

Advancing age is an important risk factor for endometrial cancer. Most tumors occur during the sixth and seventh decades; fewer than 5 percent occur before age 40. The risk is increased among first-degree relatives of patients with endometrial cancer. Epidemiologic studies have also shown an association with cancer of the breast and cancer of the colon. Case–control studies have also demonstrated a surprisingly high prevalence of obesity and glucose intolerance among patients with endometrial cancer. Between 20 percent and 80 percent of patients with tumors were *obese,* depending on the definition of obesity used in different studies. Up to 40 percent of patients were found to have diabetes mellitus; this relationship is less clear, partly because of varying definitions of diabetes and the likely correlation with obesity.

There is strong evidence that *estrogens,* either endogenous or exogenous, play a principal role in the etiology of endometrial carcinoma. The histologic precursor of endometrial cancer is atypical endometrial hyperplasia. Retrospective studies have indicated a progression from cystic hyperplasia through adenomatous hyperplasia to atypical hyperplasia, associated with unopposed estrogen effects. Prospective studies have demonstrated a cumulative incidence of carcinoma of 10 percent to 30 percent among patients with atypical endometrial hyperplasia.

A number of clinical syndromes that include ovarian estrogen excess have been associated with the increased risk of endometrial cancer. Postmenopausal women with estrogen-secreting tumors have been reported to have a 10 percent to 24 percent incidence of endometrial cancer. There is also a high incidence of cancer in patients with *polycystic ovary disease*; 19 percent to 25 percent of young women with endometrial carcinoma have underlying Stein-Leventhal syndrome. It is likely that less well-defined abnormalities of estrogen control explain the association of endometrial cancer with menstrual abnormalities and infertility. Approximately half of all women with endometrial carcinoma and 20 percent to 30 percent of married women with endometrial carcinoma are nulliparous.

The principal estrogen in postmenopausal women is estrone, which is peripherally converted from androstenedione produced in the adrenal glands. Peripheral conversion of androstenedione to estrone has been shown to be increased in patients with endometrial cancer, and estrone to estradiol ratios are higher. Peripheral conversion by adipose cells may be the explanatory link between obesity and endometrial cancer.

A number of retrospective case–control studies indicate that the use of *estrogens postmenopausally* substantially increases the risk of endometrial cancer. Rates of endometrial cancer among estrogen users ranged from four to 14 times those among control patients. Several studies have demonstrated a dose–response relationship, in that use of estrogen for longer periods of time was associated with greater risk. It has been argued that the association between estrogens and endometrial cancer can be explained in part by a greater likelihood of detection of preexisting tumors in women for whom estrogens are prescribed. Implications of this link between exogenous estrogens and endometrial cancer for treatment of menopausal symptoms are discussed in Chapter 118. Case–control data suggest a 50 percent decrease in risk among women who have used combination birth control pills for a minimum of 12 months, with the protective effect lasting from 8 to 15 years. A program of estrogen plus progesterone for postmenopausal hormone replacement therapy is not associated with an increased risk of endometrial carcinoma.

NATURAL HISTORY OF ENDOMETRIAL CANCER AND EFFECTIVENESS OF THERAPY

Postmenopausal bleeding, by far the most common symptom associated with endometrial cancer, must always be pursued aggressively. Clinical studies have indicated that, depending on patient selection, cancer is the explanation in from 10 percent to 70 percent of women who present with postmenopausal bleeding. In one review of more than 400 presentations of bleeding at least 2 years after menopause, 16 percent of patients had endometrial cancer. The likelihood of malignancy increased with the span of years since menopause.

In a series of more than 500 patients with endometrial cancer from the Mayo Clinic, nearly all presented with postmenopausal bleeding or similar symptoms; only 3 percent of the tumors were detected in asymptomatic women. In this series, there was little if any correlation between the duration of symptoms and the clinical stage of the tumor at the time of diagnosis. The prognosis for endometrial cancer is generally favorable. In the Mayo series, a 5-year survival rate of 75 percent was reported.

DIAGNOSTIC TESTS

Available data suggest that endometrial cancer presents with symptoms early in its natural history. There is little evidence that cytopathologic screening can appreciably advance the time of diagnosis in most patients. The diagnosis of endometrial cancer can be made on the basis of a *Papanicolaou (Pap) smear* of cells aspirated from the *vaginal pool* or scraped from the *cervical os*. However, a number of studies have indicated that the sensitivity of the Pap smear in the diagnosis of endometrial cancer is only 70 percent to 80 percent. A retrospective review of patients with endometrial cancer who had Pap smears during the year prior to diagnosis found that only 18 percent had smears that were suggestive of cancer.

Jet wash and aspiration techniques have been advocated for more direct sampling of the uterine cavity. These techniques have proved to be less painful and effective substitutes for dilation and curettage in many diagnostic situations. However, the value of using these techniques to screen asymptomatic women for premalignant and malignant lesions has not been demonstrated.

In one large reported effort to detect asymptomatic endometrial cancer, 2007 women, 80 percent of whom were postmenopausal, were screened using both vaginal pool Pap smear and an *endometrial sampling* technique. Satisfactory samples could be obtained in only 86 percent of women. Ten cancers occurred: eight were detected by endometrial samples, one was detected by vaginal pool smear, and one was missed. Endometrial sampling proved to be painful for most patients, and the authors noted difficulty in interpreting endometrial cytology. The authors were unable to conclude that such screening would be either acceptable or effective in lowering endometrial cancer morbidity and mortality.

SUMMARY AND CONCLUSIONS

Endometrial carcinoma is a source of substantial morbidity and mortality and has well-defined risk factors. Evidence indicates that endogenous and exogenous estrogen stimulation play an etiologic role. Although Pap smears potentially advance the diagnosis of cervical cancer, there are no tests as suitable for endometrial cancer screening. A prompt diagnostic workup, including endometrial biopsy, must be initiated by the primary care provider in patients presenting with postmenopausal bleeding. Endometrial sampling and other diagnostic interventions should be considered for women at risk because of hormonal therapy. Risk associated with postmenopausal estrogen therapy can be reduced by adding progesterone to the hormone replacement program (see Chapter 118).

A.G.M.

ANNOTATED BIBLIOGRAPHY

Antunes CMF, Stolley PD, Rosenshein NB, et al. Endometrial cancer and estrogen use. N Engl J Med 1979;300:9. *(Overall sixfold increased risk in estrogen users. Increased risk with dosage and duration. Stage 0 and 1 tumors are more common in estrogen users.)*

Burke JR, Lehman HF, Wolf FS. Inadequacy of Papanicolaou smears in the detection of endometrial cancer. N Engl J Med 1974;291:191. *(Only 18 percent of Pap smears taken within a year of presentation with endometrial cancer were suggestive of malignancy.)*

Centers for Disease Control Cancer and Steroid Hormone Study. Oral contraceptive use and the risk of endometrial cancer. JAMA 1983;249:1600. *(Combination pill use for more than 1 year showed a protective effect in this case–control study, particularly among nulliparous women.)*

Horwitz RI, Feinstein AR. Alternative analytic methods for case–control studies of estrogen and endometrial cancer. N Engl J Med 1978;299:1089. *(Points out the potential of bias in case finding but does not refute increased risk.)*

Koss LG, Schreiber K, Oberlander SG, Moussouris H, Lesser M. Detection of endometrial carcinoma and its hyperplasia in asymptomatic women. Obstet Gynecol 1984;64:1. *(Vaginal pool and endometrial sampling were used to screen 2586 women; 17 endometrial cancers were diagnosed.)*

Lucas WE. Causal relationships between endocrine-metabolic variables in patients with endometrial carcinoma. Obstet Gynecol Surv 1974;29:507. *(Exhaustive review with 255 refs.)*

Malkasian GD, McDonald TW, Pratt JH. Carcinoma of the endometrium. Mayo Clin Proc 1977;52:175. *(Detailed review of 523 cases with 74 percent 5-year survival rate.)*

Pachecho JC, Kempers RD. Etiology of postmenopausal bleeding. Obstet Gynecol 1968;32:40. *(Sixteen percent of 401 women with postmenopausal bleeding had endometrial cancer.)*

Pritchard KI. Screening for endometrial cancer: is it effective? Ann Intern Med 1989;110:177. *(Reviews the basis for the Canadian Task Force recommendation against screening.)*

Rodrigues MA, et al. Evaluation of endometrial jet wash technique in 303 patients in a community hospital. Obstet Gynecol 1974;43:392. *(Only three of seven cases detected; none of three focal tumors detected.)*

Smith DC, Prentice R, Thompson DJ, Hermann WL. Association of exogenous estrogen and endometrial carcinoma. N Engl J Med 1975;293:1164. *(Case–control study showing 4.5 times greater risk among exposed women.)*

Wynder EL, Escher GC, Mantel N. An epidemiological investigation of cancer of the endometrium. Cancer 1966;19:489. *(Extensive retrospective study indicating obesity is a major risk factor.)*

Ziel HK, Finkle WD. Increased risk of endometrial carcinoma among users of conjugated estrogens. N Engl J Med 1975; 293:1167. *(Case–control study showing risk increasing with duration of exposure.)*

Primary Care Medicine: Office Evaluation and Management of the Adult Patient, 3rd edition, edited by Allan H. Goroll, Lawrence A. May, and Albert G. Mulley, Jr. J.B. Lippincott Company, Philadelphia

110

Vaginal Cancer and Other Effects of Diethylstilbestrol Exposure

Vaginal cancer is a rare disease, accounting for approximately 1 percent of gynecologic malignancies. More than 90 percent of vaginal cancers are squamous cell tumors. Elderly women are at greatest risk, and because of the extensive lymphatic drainage of the vagina, the 5-year survival rate is only 20 percent to 25 percent.

Of greater concern to the primary care provider is adenocarcinoma, or clear-cell carcinoma of the vagina, which occurs in young women who were exposed to diethylstilbestrol (DES) or other synthetic estrogens in utero. Although these tumors are quite rare, the population at risk is large. The anxiety among diethylstilbestrol-exposed persons is substantial. In addition to the association with vaginal cancer, other abnormalities of the genital tract, including some that may affect reproductive function, have been reported. The primary physician must understand the risks that follow diethylstilbestrol exposure as well as the natural history of the associated conditions in order to counsel and evaluate these patients appropriately.

DIETHYLSTILBESTROL AND ABNORMALITIES OF THE GENITAL TRACT

Diethylstilbestrol is a synthetic estrogen first produced in 1938. After early studies indicated it was helpful in preventing spontaneous abortion, it and other synthetic estrogens were used extensively from the 1940s until 1971 in pregnant women at risk for miscarriage. It has been estimated that between 100,000 and 160,000 women born between 1960 and 1970 were exposed to diethylstilbestrol or similar drugs in utero. Because these agents were used more extensively in the 1940s and 1950s, well over 1 million women are estimated to have been exposed.

In 1970, a cluster of cases of the then very rare adenocarcinoma of the vagina, occurring in daughters who had been exposed to DES in utero, was reported from Massachusetts General Hospital. Since that time, the association has been confirmed, and several hundred cases of clear-cell carcinoma have been recorded and investigated. A history of DES exposure has been elicited in approximately two-thirds of all cases of malignancy.

A subsequent prospective study of 110 exposed women detailed the abnormalities of the cervix and vagina that can be found in women at risk, in addition to clear-cell carcinoma. Vaginal adenosis, the presence of glandular epithelium in the vagina, was found in 35 percent of exposed women but in only 1 percent of matched controls. Cervical erosion was present in 84 percent of exposed women and in only 38 percent of controls. Gross structural abnormalities of the cervix were found in 22 percent of exposed women but were not found among controls. No cases of carcinoma were identified in this study or in subsequent prospective studies. The cumulative incidence of carcinoma in exposed daughters is not known; many estimates cluster around one per 1000. The relative risk of vaginal clear-cell adenocarcinoma conferred by diethylstilbestrol exposure has been estimated to be approximately 400. Risk is greater for daughters exposed early during the index pregnancy. All abnormalities of the vagina and cervix identified to date occur more commonly in women who were exposed early in utero. The embryonic development of the female genital tract begins as early as the 4th week of gestation and is completed by the end of the 18th week. Patients exposed early during this period (ie, weeks 4–18) are most likely to have the epithelial changes and structural abnormalities.

While tumors have been identified in preteenage patients as young as age 7, more than 90 percent of tumors have been found in daughters age 14 or older. The peak incidence of tumors occurs between the ages of 14 and 20, suggesting that the period of greatest risk occurs when the abnormal vaginal or cervical epithelium is stimulated by ovarian hormones with the onset of puberty. It is too early to say with certainty whether the decreased incidence after age 21 indicates a true decrease in risk with age or is a result of the current age distribution of the cohort at risk.

Findings from the National Collaborative Diethylstilbestrol Adenosis (DESAD) Project indicate that women exposed to the drug in utero have a twofold to fourfold increase in risk of *cervical* and *vaginal dysplasia* over nonexposed controls. The incidence of dysplasia and carcinoma in situ was correlated with the area of *squamous metaplasia,* an immature form of normal squamous epithelium that arises in areas of adenosis. When squamous metaplasia was confined to the os or inner half of the cervix, there was no increased risk. The relative risk of dysplasia for exposed women was influenced by sexual activity; those who initiated sexual activity at an early age and those with multiple partners were at greater risk. It has been postulated that the increased risk among women exposed to diethylstilbestrol derives from the greater prevalence and extent of squamous metaplasia. It is presumed that these immature squamous cells, like the immature cells of the transformation zone (see Chapter 107), are particularly susceptible to oncogenic agents such as human papillomaviruses.

Questions have also been raised about the ability of diethylstilbestrol-exposed offspring to conceive. A high prevalence of uterine and fallopian tube abnormalities has been described in case series of exposed women who have undergone hysterosalpingography. A controlled cohort study from the DESAD Project, however, found no difference in fertility between exposed and control subjects. Subsequent studies have suggested a modest increase in risk of primary *infertility* in association with the higher prevalence of abnormal hysterosalpingograms among exposed daughters. Diethylstilbestrol-exposed women who become pregnant have been shown to be more likely to have an *unfavorable outcome* of pregnancy. Nevertheless, more than 80 percent of such women had at least one full-term live birth during the course of the DESAD study.

Genital abnormalities and infertility have also been described in male offspring of mothers who took diethylstilbestrol early in pregnancy. It is likely that these findings were influenced by selection and ascertainment biases; the only controlled study addressing this question found no differences in rates of genitourinary abnormalities, infertility, or testicular cancer in exposed and nonexposed men.

SYMPTOMS AND NATURAL HISTORY OF VAGINAL CANCER AND EFFECTIVENESS OF THERAPY

The natural history of clear-cell carcinoma is uncertain. Cases can present with *abnormal vaginal bleeding* or *discharge*, but because of increasing public and professional awareness, a substantial percentage of cases are detected in the asymptomatic stage. Adenosis has been found in proximity to adenocarcinoma in more than 95 percent of cases, and it is therefore considered a malignant precursor by some. Transitions from adenosis to carcinoma have not, however, been clearly documented.

Limited follow-up information indicates that clear-cell carcinoma is an aggressive tumor. Metastases have been found at the time of surgery in 17 percent of cases of stage 1 disease and in the majority of cases of stage 2 disease. Short-term follow-up of registry cases of clear-cell carcinoma has indicated that recurrence, death, or both occur in approximately 25 percent of patients.

It is too early to know whether cervical dysplasia and carcinoma in situ in diethylstilbestrol-exposed young women have the same natural history as in nonexposed women (see Chapter 107). However, it seems prudent to follow such patients with vigilance and yearly Papanicolaou (Pap) smears.

DIAGNOSTIC TESTS

Although the discovery of abnormal cytology has led to the detection of some cases of clear-cell carcinoma, the *Pap smear* has been shown to have a relatively low sensitivity (80%) for detecting this lesion. This may be explained by the relatively high degree of differentiation of the neoplastic cells, which may resemble endocervical cells. The cells may also be obscured by a heavy polymorphonuclear infiltration. The initial examination of a woman exposed in utero to diethylstilbestrol or similar drugs must therefore include, in addition to direct inspection of the vagina and cervix and cytologic sampling, careful *Schiller's iodine staining* and *biopsies* of areas that appear red or fail to stain with the iodine solution. *Colposcopy* is a complementary procedure. It is particularly useful in patients with abnormal iodine staining or cytology. Colposcopy should be performed by an experienced gynecologist.

Despite the poor sensitivity of the Pap smear for clear-cell cancer, Pap smears should be done yearly in all women with an exposure history. This is especially important in light of the increased risk of dysplasia and cervical cancer, particularly among women with evidence for human papillomavirus infection or other risk factors related to sexual activity.

CONCLUSIONS AND RECOMMENDATIONS

- As many as 1 million women are at risk for abnormalities of the genital tract, including clear-cell adenocarcinoma, because of in utero exposure to diethylstilbestrol or other synthetic estrogens.
- Risk of malignancy among exposed women is low. Nevertheless, because of the significant morbidity and mortality associated with these tumors, careful case finding and evaluation are indicated. Because routine screening procedures such as the Pap smear are inadequate, patients at risk must be identified by careful history-taking if they are to receive proper evaluation and counseling.
- It is recommended that exposed daughters with symptoms such as vaginal discharge or bleeding be examined promptly regardless of age. Asymptomatic daughters with a history of exposure should have an initial evaluation at age 14 with subsequent yearly examinations.
- More frequent examinations are advised when extensive epithelial changes are present. When possible, such examinations should be performed by a gynecologist experienced in the use of the colposcope.

A.G.M.

ANNOTATED BIBLIOGRAPHY

Barnes AB, Colton T, Gunderson J, et al. Fertility and outcome in pregnancy in women exposed in utero to diethylstilbestrol. N Engl J Med 1980;302:609. *(Fertility was not affected by DES exposure; there was, however, an increased risk of unfavorable outcome of pregnancy associated with DES exposure—the relative risk was 1.69.)*

Heinonen OP. Diethylstilbestrol in pregnancy: frequency of exposure and usage pattern. Cancer 1973;31:573. *(Drug utilization data for 1960s indicated that 100,000 to 160,000 women born in the United States during that decade were exposed in utero.)*

Herbst AL, Poskanzer DC, Robboy SJ, et al. Prenatal exposure to stilbestrol: a prospective comparison of exposed female offspring with unexposed controls. N Engl J Med 1975;292:332. *(Prospective examination of 110 exposed and 82 unexposed females. No cancers were found, but adenosis and other abnormalities were common among exposed individuals.)*

Johnston GA Jr. Health risks and effects of prenatal exposure to diethylstilbestrol. J Fam Pract 1983;16:51. *(Succinct review of structural and neoplastic abnormalities of the genital tract that have been linked to diethylstilbestrol.)*

Leary FJ, Resseguie LJ, Kurland LT, et al. Males exposed in utero to diethylstilbestrol. JAMA 1984;252:2984. *(Careful urologic and fertility evaluation of exposed and unexposed subjects showed no increased risk of abnormalities.)*

Melnick S, Cole P, Anderson D, Herbst A. Rates and risks of diethylstilbestrol-related clear cell adenocarcinoma of the vagina and cervix. N Engl J Med 1987;316:514. *(Risk of vaginal cancer from birth through age 34 is about one in 1000.)*

Robboy SJ, Noller KL, O'Brien P, et al. Increased incidence of cervical and vaginal dysplasia in 3980 diethylstilbestrol-exposed young women. JAMA 1984;252:2979. *(The incidence of dysplasia and carcinoma in situ was 15.7 vs. 7.9 per 1000 person-years in exposed and nonexposed women, respectively.)*

Senekjian EK, Potkul RK, Frey K, Herbst AL. Infertility among daughters either exposed or not exposed to diethylstilbestrol. Am J Obstet Gynecol 1988;158:493. *(Primary infertility in 33 percent of exposed and 14 percent of unexposed, with high prevalence of abnormal hysterosalpingograms among the exposed.)*

Sharp GB, Cole P. Vaginal bleeding and diethylstilbestrol exposure during pregnancy: relationship to genital tract clear cell adenocarcinoma and vaginal adenosis in daughters. Am J Obstet Gynecol 1990;162:994. *(The relative risks of vaginal clear-cell adenocarcinoma for in utero exposure were 366 and 459 when vaginal bleeding did and did not occur during the index pregnancy.)*

Thorp JM Jr, Fowler WC, Donehoo R, et al. Antepartum and intrapartum events in women exposed in utero to diethylstilbestrol. Ostet Gynecol 1990;75:828. *(Exposed women were more likely to be delivered abdominally.)*

Primary Care Medicine: Office Evaluation and Management of the Adult Patient, 3rd edition, edited by Allan H. Goroll, Lawrence A. May, and Albert G. Mulley, Jr. J.B. Lippincott Company, Philadelphia

111
Approach to the Woman With Abnormal Vaginal Bleeding

Abnormal vaginal bleeding is that which occurs at an inappropriate time (<21 or >36 days after last period) or in an excessive amount (clots lasting >7 days). In peri- and postmenopausal women, uterine malignancy must be ruled out. Pelvic pathology is also a possibility in younger women, but disturbances of the hypothalamic–pituitary–ovarian axis are more common precipitants of abnormal bleeding. When anovulatory and occurring in the absence of an anatomic lesion, the bleeding is sometimes referred to as "dysfunctional."

The differentiation of functional disease from anatomic pathology is the goal of the primary physician's initial evaluation and an important determinant of therapy. The problem of abnormal vaginal bleeding is particularly challenging in the perimenopausal woman, because this is a time of both normal decline in ovarian function and increased risk of endometrial cancer.

PATHOPHYSIOLOGY AND CLINICAL PRESENTATION

Normal Menstrual Bleeding

Normally, in the absence of implantation of a fertilized ovum, the ovarian corpus luteum undergoes regression within 9 to 11 days of ovulation. Estrogen and progesterone production fall and menstruation ensues. The normal menstrual cycle ranges from 23 to 39 days (mean, 29 days). Cycle length shortens as menopause approaches. The menstrual period usually lasts 2 to 7 days, with most blood lost during the first few days. Presence of clots or duration of bleeding in excess of 1 week indicates excessive blood loss. Abnormal bleeding may occur in the context of normal ovulation or in its absence.

Abnormal Bleeding in the Setting of Normal Ovulatory Cycles

In normally ovulating women, abnormal vaginal bleeding may present as *menorrhagia* (bleeding that is normal in timing but excessive in amount and duration) or *intermenstrual bleeding*. Most often the cause is an *endometrial* or *cervical lesion* (Table 111–1). However, it sometimes is the presenting symptom of a *bleeding diathesis,* most often the consequence of thrombocytopenia or a qualitative platelet disorder (see Chapter 81).

Normal ovulation may be accompanied by a small amount of midcycle vaginal staining and pelvic pain (especially on the right side). It is sometimes referred to as *"mittelschmerz,"* which occurs in the context of ovarian follicle rupture and release.

Uterine Fibroids are the most common cause and account for about one-third of cases. Their frequency is estimated at upward of 30 percent of women over the age of 35. However, only those fibroids that are submucosal in location and involve the uterine cavity lead to bleeding. Location is more important than size. Because they are so common, they may coexist with another cause of abnormal vaginal bleeding. Periods are often very heavy.

Carcinoma of the Cervix is among the more serious sources of abnormal bleeding in ovulating patients, although it accounts for only about 3 percent of cases. *Postcoital bleeding* and slight intermenstrual spotting are characteristic when there is surface ulceration, which may occur in early stages of the disease (see Chapter 123).

Endometrial carcinoma is more typically a disease of abnormal vaginal bleeding in postmenopausal women (see below), but 20 percent have the disease while still menstruating (although almost all are over the age of 40). Heavier than normal periods are noted as well as an intermenstrual watery discharge containing small amounts of blood early on.

Polyps, Erosions, and Infection. *Cervical polyps, cervical erosions,* and *vaginal lesions* present similarly, with slight spotting noted intermenstrually, especially after coitus. *Pelvic inflammatory disease,* with its fever, pelvic pain, and discharge, may lead to postcoital, intermenstrual, or heavy menstrual bleeding by causing cervicitis, endometritis, or salpingitis.

Foreign Bodies. *Intrauterine devices* (IUD) also alter the endometrial surface and can be similarly responsible for heavy menstrual bleeding or intermenstrual bleeding. Vagi-

Table 111-1. Differential Diagnosis of Abnormal Vaginal Bleeding

Ovulatory Bleeding
1. Normal variant
   a. "Mittelschmerz"
2. Anatomic lesion
   a. Uterine fibroids
   b. Cervical disease (inflammation, polyp, cancer)
   c. Endometrial carcinoma
   d. Pelvic inflammatory disease
   e. Intrauterine device
3. Concurrent disease
   a. Bleeding diathesis
   b. Foreign body

Anovulatory Bleeding
1. Hypothalamic dysfunction
   a. Puberty
   b. Perimenopausal state
   c. Situational stress, excessive exercise, weight loss
   d. Excess androgen, prolactin, cortisol; hypothyroidism
   e. Polycystic ovary syndrome
2. Oral contraceptive use
   a. Inadequate estrogen dose

Postmenopausal Bleeding
1. Endometrial pathology
   a. Fibroid
   b. Cancer
   c. Polyp
2. Cervical pathology
   a. Cancer
   b. Polyp
   c. Erosion
3. Vaginal pathology
   a. Atrophic vaginitis

Pregnancy
1. Ectopic pregnancy
2. Postabortion (retained products of gestation)
3. Failing pregnancy

nal wall irritation from *tampon* use may lead to minor vaginal bleeding.

Anovulatory Bleeding

This type of bleeding is usually a manifestation of a disturbance within the hypothalamic–pituitary–ovarian axis. *Metrorrhagia*—prolonged bleeding occurring at irregular intervals—is characteristic.

Hypothalamic Dysfunction. The pathophysiologic common denominator is *inadequate progesterone* production, most often due to *lack of a luteinizing hormone (LH) surge* at midcycle—a consequence of an alteration in the normal pattern of gonadotropin-releasing hormone (GnRH) release from the hypothalamus. This pattern is typical of patients with mild hypothalamic dysfunction, who may experience irregular menses in the context of moderate *situational stress, weight loss,* or *exercise training*. However, oligomenorrhea and amenorrhea may follow if the functional disturbance is more severe, impairing follicle-stimulating hormone (FSH) secretion and estrogen production (see Chapter 112). Those who bleed have an estrogen-withdrawal type of bleeding. The severity of the bleeding is a function of the amount of estrogen produced. The bleeding that occurs from mild hypothalamic dysfunction is sometimes referred to as "dysfunctional." *Hyperprolactinemia, hypothyroidism,* and excess production of *androgen* and *cortisol* can also disturb hypothalamic rhythmicity. Even *iron deficiency anemia* has been found to inhibit ovulation.

Histoanatomically, unruptured ovarian follicles persist, and functioning corpora lutea are absent. The endometrium shows hyperplasia resulting from unopposed estrogen effect. There is little if any secretory pattern because of the lack of progesterone. Ovulation does not occur, and anovulatory bleeding results when progesterone production returns or excessive proliferation causes sloughing of the overstimulated endometrium. There is irregularity of the menstrual interval, periods of amenorrhea, and episodes of very heavy and prolonged bleeding if there has been sufficient estrogen-induced buildup of the endometrium.

Polycystic Ovary Syndrome. This incompletely understood condition affects about 5 percent of reproductive age women and represents a leading cause of chronic anovulatory bleeding. In addition to a life-long history of irregular periods, patients may report infertility, hirsutism, obesity, and amenorrhea. Disordered hypothalamic rhythmicity is believed to cause excessive LH production without a midcycle surge, leading to ovarian overproduction of *testosterone* and *androstenedione*. Some of this androgen is converted to *estrone*, which can stimulate endometrial proliferation that ends in irregular episodes of bleeding. Serum concentrations of both estrogen and testosterone rise. *Insulin resistance* with hyperinsulinism are common and believed linked to ovarian androgen overproduction. The consequences of androgen excess range from hirsutism to frank virilization (see Chapter 98), although the latter is uncommon. Chronic unopposed endometrial estrogen stimulation can lead to adenomatous hyperplasia, cellular atypicality, and even endometrial carcinoma. Risk of cancer is increased threefold.

Puberty. The anovulatory bleeding of puberty is a consequence of immaturity of the positive-feedback mechanism responsible for the LH surge that triggers progesterone secretion. In the absence of adequate progesterone production, estrogen-withdrawal bleeding takes place. The pattern of anovulatory bleeding is irregular and may occur anytime between 22 and 45 days.

Perimenopausal Bleeding. The irregular menstrual bleeding that characterizes the perimenopausal period is also an anovulatory estrogen-withdrawal phenomenon. As the number of functioning ovarian follicles declines, insufficient estrogen is produced to cause an LH surge and ovulation. In the absence of progesterone production, an estrogen-withdrawal type of irregular bleeding occurs. Such perimenopausal bleeding can continue for months to years, but it eventually stops when estrogen production ceases.

Postmenopausal, Pregnancy-Related, and Breakthrough Types of Bleeding

Postmenopause. Here the major concern is cancer, although *uterine fibroids* still account for most cases. Women who have had chronic unopposed estrogen stimulation are at increased risk of *endometrial carcinoma*. Early on, bleeding may be subtle and little more than minor vaginal staining (see Chapter 123). Postmenopausal women with marked *atrophic vaginitis, cervical polyp,* or *cervicitis* from a prolapsed uterus may also experience some blood-stained vaginal discharge or minor spotting. Cervical carcinoma is uncommon after age 55 in women who have had Pap smears regularly but may be the cause bleeding in the early postmenopausal period.

Pregnancy. One of the most serious causes of acute abnormal vaginal bleeding in women of reproductive age is *ectopic pregnancy,* which is characterized by delay of the regular period, followed by vaginal blood spotting, often in conjunction with unilateral pelvic pain. Intraperitoneal hemorrhage can ensue if tubal rupture occurs, but this happens in fewer than 5 percent of cases. A *failing pregnancy* may be heralded by onset of bleeding. *Retained products of gestation* represents a very common cause of abnormal uterine bleeding after abortion; blood loss is often heavy.

Oral Contraceptives. If an oral contraceptive contains insufficient estrogen or if compliance is inadequate, then abnormal vaginal bleeding may occur. The characteristic pattern is one of *"breakthrough bleeding"* or staining that occurs intermenstrually (see Chapter 119).

DIFFERENTIAL DIAGNOSIS

The differential can be divided into ovulatory, anovulatory, postmenopausal, and pregnancy-related etiologies (see Table 111–1). Among postmenopausal women, endometrial cancer accounts for up to 25 percent of cases of bleeding, although most are due to submucosal uterine fibroids. In women of reproductive age, the etiology is often an anovulatory disturbance, although cancer remains a concern. Girls going through puberty and perimenopausal women who complain of irregular menses are most likely to have dysfunctional bleeding.

WORKUP

Among women of reproductive age who complain of abnormal vaginal bleeding, the initial tasks are to rule out pregnancy and determine if the bleeding is ovulatory or anovulatory. Postmenopausal bleeding has its own workup, which focuses on identifying the anatomic site of bleeding.

History

A careful and detailed menstrual history is essential. Most important is information on the patient's normal menstrual cycle (duration, frequency, intensity) and how the current bleeding pattern compares with it. If the patient is of childbearing age, then inquiry should be made into unprotected intercourse and symptoms of pregnancy (breast engorgement, morning sickness, cessation of normal menses). If menstrual regularity persists despite an increase in intensity or duration of flow or onset of intermenstrual staining, then an ovulatory etiology is likely. This is further supported by presence of premenstrual symptoms, such as breast engorgement, pelvic cramping, fluid retention, and mood swings. Anovulatory bleeding is suggested by the absence of such symptoms plus complete irregularity of menstrual periods, especially if accompanied by months of amenorrhea. Although intensity of the bleeding (eg, by number of pads or tampons used) is more useful for management than for diagnosis, the new onset of clots or duration of more than 7 days argues for abnormal bleeding.

Ovulatory Bleeding. History should include query into symptoms of a bleeding diathesis and medicines that inhibit normal clotting (see Chapter 81). Equally important is checking for dyspareunia, postcoital bleeding, vaginal discharge, pelvic pain, fever, trauma, and IUD use. Risk factors for endometrial carcinoma ought to be reviewed (see Chapter 123).

Anovulatory Bleeding. One should ask about important precipitants, such as emotional stress, weight loss, exercise, and chronic illness. If the patient is an adolescent girl, one should check for a history of irregular periods since the onset of menarche, as well as the common precipitants just noted. Review of medications for use of oral contraceptives is essential, with attention to the estrogen dose and history of breakthrough bleeding. For the perimenopausal woman, menstrual irregularity and the skipping of periods suggest a functional etiology but do not rule out cancer. Androgen excess is suggested by symptoms of hirsutism and virilization (see Chapter 98) and a history of infertility. Rapid onset of hirsutism and virilization raises the possibility of a functioning adrenal or ovarian tumor making androgens. A life-long history of irregular menses, hirsutism, infertility, and obesity suggests polycystic ovary syndrome. Inquiry into galactorrhea and development of cushingoid appearance help to check for prolactin and cortisol excess, respectively. Any symptoms of hypothyroidism (see Chapter 104) and iron deficiency (see Chapter 79) should be noted.

Postmenopausal Bleeding. Any history of bleeding, even if just minor staining, should be taken as evidence of a possible malignancy. However, inquiry into symptomatic atrophic vaginitis and uterine prolapse may provide useful clues.

Physical Examination

Regardless of presumed etiology, all patients should be checked for *postural signs* indicative of significant intravascular volume depletion. In addition, careful *speculum and bimanual pelvic examinations* are essential, with particular care taken to note any vaginal or cervical erosions, uterine or adnexal masses, focal tenderness, or purulent or bloody discharge. Signs of pregnancy (engorged breasts, pigmented aureolae, bluish cervix, enlarged uterus) should be sought in women of reproductive age.

Suspected ovulatory bleeding necessitates concentrating on the pelvic examination, but one should also check for signs of a bleeding diathesis (petechiae, ecchymoses, splenic enlargement). The patient with *suspected anovulatory bleeding* should be carefully examined for hirsutism, virilization, cushingoid appearance, milky nipple discharge, goiter, dry skin, coarse hair, and "hung-up" reflexes. Visual field testing is indicated if there is suspicion of a large pituitary adenoma. Presence of hirsutism or virilization necessitates thorough pelvic and abdominal examinations for an ovarian or adrenal mass.

On examination of the *postmenopausal woman,* particular note should be taken of the friability of the vaginal mucosa and cervix as well as the presence of any uterine or adnexal masses.

Laboratory Studies

All patients of reproductive age with abnormal vaginal bleeding should be tested for pregnancy (a *serum human chorionic gonadotropin* [*hCG*] *beta-subunit* is the most sensitive; see Chapter 112). A *complete blood count* is always useful. The *hematocrit* will help assess the severity of chronic blood loss (although not of acute hemorrhage; see Chapter 79) and a mean *red cell volume* may reveal the microcytosis of iron deficiency.

Ovulatory Bleeding. Here the goal is identification of pelvic pathology after ruling out concurrent disease that may predispose to heavy bleeding. Determinations of *BUN, creatinine,* and *platelet count* should be obtained when there is concern about a bleeding diathesis. Otherwise, one should proceed directly to *pelvic ultrasound* examination, with transvaginal study being the most sensitive noninvasive means of searching for uterine and adnexal pathology; it is superior to the standard transabdominal approach.

A *Pap smear* is indicated if the cervix appears abnormal. In women over age 40, *vaginal cytologic sampling* from the posterior cervical fornix may detect abnormal endometrial cells shed into this accessible area. Acetic acid can be added to cytology preservative if the smear sample is bloody. A *cervical culture* for gonorrhea as well as for other pathogenic organisms is needed in the patient with pain on motion of the cervix and adnexal tenderness (see Chapter 117); an elevated *sedimentation rate* suggests pelvic inflammation.

Anovulatory Bleeding. No additional studies are necessary when the etiology is evident (eg, situational stress, puberty, chronic illness, marked weight loss). If perimenopausal bleeding is suspected, an *FSH* can be confirmatory; if more than 40 IU/mL, then ovarian failure is imminent. An LH-to-FSH ratio of greater than 2:1 is characteristic of polycystic ovary syndrome. When hirsutism or virilization is noted, a serum *testosterone* is the best test. If the onset of such changes is rapid or the serum testosterone is greater than 600 nmol/L (190 ng/mL), then a functioning adrenal or ovarian neoplasm may be the source and a *17-hydroxyprogesterone* can facilitate the diagnosis. A *fasting serum insulin* level is also indicated in patients with elevated testosterone (>350 nmol/L, 100 ng/mL). A *fasting insulin* level in excess of 180 pmol/L is suggestive of insulin resistance.

Postmenopausal Bleeding. Noninvasive study for pelvic pathology is conducted as noted above. Because concern about endometrial cancer is high in this age group, consideration of an endometrial *dilation and curettage (D&C)* is appropriate, even when noninvasive study is unrevealing.

SYMPTOMATIC MANAGEMENT AND PATIENT EDUCATION

Acute Anovulatory Bleeding that is not severe can often be managed by the primary care physician in the office setting. To stop the abnormal bleeding, one can administer a course of oral *medroxyprogesterone* (Provera), 10 mg/d 10 days, or a single intramuscular injection of *progesterone,* 100 mg. These will convert a proliferative endometrium to a secretory one. Bleeding should stop within 24 to 48 hours of initiating progestin therapy, and menstrual flow should occur on its completion. If this so-called medical D&C does not stop acute bleeding, then referral for D&C and hysteroscopy is indicated.

Chronic Anovulatory Bleeding can be treated symptomatically by monthly administration of progesterone therapy. By causing regular endometrial shedding, it protects against adenomatous changes and lowers the risk of endometrial cancer associated with long-term unopposed estrogen stimulation. A course of *medroxyprogesterone* given for the last 10 to 12 days of each month will usually suffice. Cessation of further abnormal bleeding episodes argues strongly against a structural lesion, but resumption of such bleeding on progestin therapy necessitates referral for D&C.

Ovulation may resume on this program, particularly in the young person, and periodically the treatment should be halted for a month or two to observe for the return of normal cycles. If abnormal bleeding recurs despite correction of all possible precipitating factors, then maintenance hormonal therapy may be employed. In patients who do not desire pregnancy, an *estrogen–progestin* oral contraceptive preparation may be used in place of the medroxyprogesterone (see Chapter 119). Oral contraceptive therapy has the advantage of improving the hyperandrogenism that accompanies some causes of chronic anovulatory bleeding. The patient with anovulatory bleeding who desires pregnancy should be referred for consideration of clomiphene therapy. Any iron deficiency (see Chapter 82) or pelvic infection should be treated (see Chapter 117).

When anovulatory bleeding is diagnosed, it is important for the patient to know that reproductive capacity is not lost, that some causes are self-limited, and that the possibility of malignancy is very low under age 30. Addressing any contributing factors (eg, situational stress, dieting, excessive exercise, hypothyroidism [see Chapter 104], hyperprolactinemia [see Chapter 100], polycystic ovary syndrome [see Chapter 112]) is essential to successful therapy.

Perimenopausal Bleeding may be the result of anovulatory periods, but an irregular pattern may also represent intrauterine disease. When discussed openly, the concerns that most patients already harbor can be addressed and often lessened, because the majority of cases are not likely to be cancerous. Once a structural lesion has been ruled out by D&C, symptomatic therapy with monthly *medroxyprogesterone* (10 mg/d for 10 to 12 days) can commence. It will correct the irregular bleeding. Therapy is continued monthly until withdrawal bleeding stops, indicating arrival of ovarian failure and menopause. Until menopause, some ovulatory periods may still take place and cause bleeding independent of progesterone therapy. In such instances, an oral contraceptive can be used as an alternative to progesterone, provided the patient is a nonsmoker, normotensive, and not hyperlipidemic.

Breakthrough Bleeding. Patients experiencing breakthrough bleeding on low-dosage estrogen oral contraceptives need to be sure they are adhering carefully to their regimen. If they are taking the medication on schedule, switching to a preparation with a higher estrogen dose is indicated.

INDICATIONS FOR ADMISSION AND REFERRAL

Immediate hospital admission is essential for any woman who is bleeding heavily and manifests signs of intravascular volume depletion. Immediate hospital admission and gynecologic consultation are particularly important if ectopic pregnancy is a possibility, because life-threatening hemorrhage is a real, albeit slight, risk. The same applies to cases of recent abortion, because placental tissue may be retained. Bleeding in pregnancy is a definite indication for an emergency obstetric consultation.

Any patient with abnormal vaginal bleeding who has a mass lesion detected on pelvic examination, an abnormal appearing cervix, an abnormal Pap test, or risk factors for carcinoma of the cervix or endometrium (see Chapters 107 and 109) should be referred to the gynecologist. The consultation is essential for any perimenopausal or postmenopausal woman who experiences the new onset of staining or abnormal bleeding, because the risk of malignancy is greatly increased. In one retrospective series, 23 percent of women with postmenopausal bleeding were found to have endometrial carcinoma. D&C is usually required. Patients under age 30 with an otherwise normal examination are at very low risk and need not be referred. However, risk of cancer begins to increase over age 30, necessitating consideration of referral for D&C, especially in the ovulating patient with abnormal bleeding.

A.H.G.

ANNOTATED BIBLIOGRAPHY

Aksel S, Jones GS. Etiology and treatment of dysfunctional uterine bleeding. Obstet Gynecol 1974;44:1. *(A study to determine specific FSH and LH patterns associated with anovulatory uterine bleeding.)*

Barnes R. Polycystic ovary syndrome and ovarian steroidogenesis. Semin Reprod Endocrinol 1991;9:360. *(Focuses on the relation between hyperinsulinism and androgen excess in this syndrome.)*

Barnes R, Rosenfield RL. Polycystic ovary syndrome: Pathogenesis and treatment. Ann Intern Med 1989;110:386. *(Excellent review of pathophysiology; 169 refs.)*

Bayer SR, DeCherney AH. Clinical manifestations and treatment of dysfunctional uterine bleeding. JAMA 1993;269:1823. *(Helpful approach to work-up and symptomatic management.)*

Berga SL, Mortola JF, Girton L, et al. Neuroendocrine aberrations in women with functional hypothalamic amenorrhea. J Clin Endocrinol Metab 1989;68:301. *(The normal pattern of GnRH release is disturbed.)*

Coulam CB, Annegers JF, Kranz JS. Chronic anovulation syndrome and associated neoplasia. Obstet Gynecol 1983;61:403. *(Risk is increased from chronic unopposed estrogen stimulation of the endometrium.)*

Fraser IS, McCarron G, Markham R. A preliminary study of factors influencing perception of menstrual blood loss volume. Am J Obstet Gynecol 1984;149:788. *(Finds patient reports of amount of blood loss are inaccurate.)*

Goldfarb JM, Little AB. Abnormal vaginal bleeding. N Engl J Med 1980;302:666. *(Reviews pathophysiology, diagnosis, and treatment of anovulatory bleeding.)*

Isaacs JH, Ross FH. Cytologic evaluation of the endometrium in women with postmenopausal bleeding. Am J Obstet Gynecol 1978;131:410. *(A retrospective series of 143 women with postmenopausal bleeding found endometrial carcinoma in 23 percent.)*

Mischell DR, Connell E, Haney A, et al. Oral contraception for women in their 40s. J Reprod Med 1990;35(suppl):447. *(Useful in properly selected perimenopausal patients with abnormal bleeding not halted by progesterone.)*

Quick AM. Menstruation in hereditary bleeding disorders. Obstet Gynecol 1966;28:37. *(The effect of inherited hematologic pathology on menstrual bleeding.)*

Shane JM, Naftolin F, Newmark SR. Gynecologic endocrine emergencies. JAMA 1975;231:393. *(A succinct summary of gynecologic endocrine emergencies that cause uterine bleeding.)*

Shangold M, Rebar RW, Wentz AC, et al. Evaluation and management of menstrual dysfunction in athletes. JAMA 1990;263:1665. *(Useful discussion with very practical recommendations; 36 refs.)*

Weissberg SM, Dodson MG. Recurrent vaginal and cervical ulcers associated with tampon use. JAMA 1983;250:1430. *(Case reports plus review of the literature of what may be a frequent cause of minor abnormal vaginal bleeding.)*

Primary Care Medicine: Office Evaluation and Management of the Adult Patient, 3rd edition, edited by Allan H. Goroll, Lawrence A. May, and Albert G. Mulley, Jr. J.B. Lippincott Company, Philadelphia

112
Evaluation of Secondary Amenorrhea

Secondary amenorrhea is defined as cessation of menses for 3 or more months in a women with previously normal cycles. In an epidemiologic study of an unselected population, the incidence of secondary amenorrhea was 3.3 percent. The primary physician is frequently consulted by women who have missed one or more menstrual periods. Concerns about pregnancy and menopause are prominent. Knowing when and how to initiate a more extensive, systematic workup for hypothalamic dysfunction, pituitary pathology, ovarian failure, and uterine scarring is also important.

PATHOPHYSIOLOGY AND CLINICAL PRESENTATION

Amenorrhea reflects an interruption in the mechanisms of normal menstruation.

Physiology and Control of Normal Menstruation

Immediate control of the menstrual cycle resides in the *hypothalamus* and begins with release of *gonadotropin-releasing hormone (GnRH).* Normal GnRH release is pulsatile, being secreted about every 90 minutes during the *early follicular phase* of the menstrual cycle. This stimulates production and release of *follicle-stimulating hormone (FSH)* from the *anterior pituitary,* with resultant maturation of *ovarian follicles. Estradiol* production ensues, and the *uterus* responds with an increase in estrogen and progesterone *binding proteins* and *proliferation* of the endometrium. Rising levels of estradiol inhibit FSH secretion, as does the ovarian production of the hormone *inhibin.* This inhibition of FSH helps a single dominant ovarian follicle to emerge.

Late follicular phase is characterized by an increase in the frequency of GnRH release to every 60 minutes, contributing to a *midcycle surge* in release of *luteinizing hormone (LH)* and *FSH.* Estradiol levels peak just before ovulation and, together with the LH surge, they precipitate *ovulation* (rupture of the dominant ovarian follicle).

The *luteal phase* of the menstrual cycle ensues, with *luteinization* of the ovarian follicle and its production of *estradiol* and *progesterone.* The endometrium responds with *secretory* changes and the hypothalamus with a reduction in the frequency of GnRH pulses, although an increase in their amplitude. The change in GnRH release causes an increase in FSH synthesis, but its release is inhibited by estradiol and inhibin (an ovarian hormone, which peaks at the time of ovulation and continues into the luteal phase).

If there is no implantation of a fertilized ovum, then secretion of estradiol, progesterone, and inhibin fade as the *corpus luteum involutes* (usually about 14 days after ovulation). The *endometrium sheds* as the stroma becomes edematous and the blood vessels necrose. Menstrual bleeding ensues.

With the decline in progesterone in the *late luteal phase,* GnRH pulses pick up in frequency. This stimulates new secretion of FSH, no longer inhibited by estradiol and inhibin. The rise in FSH promotes new ovarian follicle development and heralds the onset of the next cycle.

In addition to the feedback controls noted above, hypothalamic GnRH secretion is also subject to both central neuronal and chemical influences and to excessive levels of several circulating hormones. *Dopaminergic* neuronal activity can inhibit GnRH release; *adrenergic* neurons facilitate it. *Endorphins* appear to exert inhibitory chemical control. Abnormally high circulating concentrations of *prolactin, androgens,* and *cortisol* appear capable of interfering with normal GnRH release. These influences help explain some of the abnormalities in hypothalamic function that characterize many cases of amenorrhea.

Pathophysiology of Secondary Amenorrhea

Cessation of normal menses may result from a disturbance at any level of this regulatory cascade or its feedback mechanisms.

Hypothalamic Amenorrhea most often represents a *functional disorder* of GnRH release, which leads to loss of LH surge and failure to ovulate. In mild forms triggered by situational stress or mild weight loss, low-normal FSH secretion and estrogen production continue, and the endometrium manifests a proliferative histology, with shedding on exposure to exogenous progesterone. More profound disturbances of GnRH release may occur in the context of *marked weight loss* (eg, anorexia nervosa; see Chapter 233), *severe emotional upset,* or *excessive exercise* (competitive athletes). GnRH release may diminish greatly in frequency and amplitude, resembling a prepubertal pattern. Estrogen levels are below normal, and there is no withdrawal bleeding after progesterone exposure. If weight falls to less than 70 percent of ideal, amenorrhea is an invariable consequence and a common accompaniment of anorexia nervosa (see Chapter 233). Restoration of weight leads to a return to normal GnRH secretion and resumption of periods. About 50 percent of competitive women long-distance runners experience secondary amenorrhea, linked closely to inhibition of normal GnRH release that can be reversed by administration of the opiate blocker naloxone, suggesting an endorphin-mediated mechanism.

A host of endocrinopathies may cause amenorrhea by interfering with normal GnRH release. Excess production of *cortisol, androgens,* and *prolactin* have been linked to impairment of GnRH release. *Hypothyroidism* may present as amenorrhea by its ability to trigger prolactin secretion.

Drugs are sometimes responsible, including oral contraceptives and agents with dopaminergic activity (eg, phenothiazines). Menses usually return within 2 months of stopping oral contraceptives, although "post-pill amenorrhea" can last up to 6 months. More prolonged amenorrhea suggests underlying pathology unrelated to oral contraceptive use.

Pituitary Pathology. Pituitary neoplasms, both functioning and nonfunctioning, are important causes of amenorrhea. Often the source of difficulty is a functioning *microadenoma* causing *hyperprolactinemia,* inhibition of GnRH release, and impairment of gonadotropin production. The classic clinical picture is one of *galactorrhea,* infertility, and amenorrhea (see Chapter 100). In addition, if there is marked impairment of gonadotropin secretion, hypoestrogenemia may ensue and put the patient at risk for bone demineralization and *osteoporosis.* The majority of prolactinomas are small (<10 mm in diameter) and designated as "microadenomas." Patients with microadenomas usually have otherwise normal pituitary function, whereas those with *"macroadenomas"* (>10 mm) may experience reduced secretion of other trophic hormones. If large enough, the tumor can impinge on the optic chiasm and cause visual field defects. In most patients with microadenomas, the tendency over time is toward a decrease in prolactin production and return of ovulation, although 10 percent of those who become pregnant may experience an enlarging lesion. Overall, only a minority of patients with prolactinomas experience a increase in tumor size.

Other forms of structural pathology are less common, but include sellar *tumors, postpartum pituitary necrosis* (Sheehan's syndrome), *empty sella syndrome,* and *granulomatous disease* (eg, sarcoidosis). Growth hormone production is the first to suffer, but usually without causing symptoms. This is followed by impairment of FSH and LH synthesis and amenorrhea, which may be the presenting complaint. Headache and visual field defects may follow later as might manifestations of panhypopituitarism. In empty sella syndrome, there appears to be herniation of the arachnoid down into the sella, compressing its contents and producing a ballooning of the bony sella on x-ray. The typical patient is female, obese, multiparous, and complaining of headache. Mild hyperprolactinemia may result from loss of normal inhibition of prolactin secretion and may lead to amenorrhea.

Ovarian Disease leading to amenorrhea is characterized by a *hypergonadotropic* response, with marked serum elevations in LH and FSH and low levels of estrogen and progesterone. *Menopause* represents the most common form of hypergonadotropic amenorrhea and results when ovarian follicles are depleted, usually between ages 45 and 55. FSH rises to greater than 35 mIU/mL, and estradiol falls to less than 5 percent of normal (about 5 pg/mL). Manifestations include hot flashes, night sweats, decreased vaginal secretions, vaginal mucosal atrophy, and eventually osteoporosis (see Chapter 118).

Menopausal symptoms in a woman under the age of 40 without evidence of other endocrine dysfunction suggest *premature menopause* due to *idiopathic ovarian failure*. Premature ovarian failure may also result from such insults as *radiation therapy* (irreversible), *chemotherapy* with alkylating agents (reversible; see Chapter 88), mumps-related *oophoritis, endometriosis,* and *autoimmune disease*. The latter is the most common cause and may be part of a polyglandular failure syndrome that presents as adrenal insufficiency and progresses to ovarian, thyroid, and pancreatic endocrine dysfunction. Myasthenia gravis or pernicious anemia sometimes accompanies the condition, which is hereditary and transmitted in autosomally recessive fashion.

Ovarian resistance to FSH is a rare condition, with premature ovarian follicles present on biopsy, but no response to FSH. In all types of ovarian failure, estrogen deficiency is marked and osteoporosis may ensue.

Polycystic ovary syndrome (formerly Stein-Leventhal syndrome) is an important ovarian cause of amenorrhea, characterized clinically by hirsutism, a life-long history of anovulatory bleeding, bilaterally enlarged ovaries, hyperinsulinism, and infertility. In addition, many of these patients are obese and manifest insulin resistance, although frank diabetes mellitus is not the rule. Infertility occurs in about 75 percent of cases, followed by hirsutism in 70 percent and amenorrhea in 50 percent. Characteristically, both ovaries are enlarged and polycystic, although not invariably. The precise pathophysiology of the condition remains incompletely understood, but appears to involve abnormally elevated *LH secretion* with loss of its normal midcycle surge, *excessive androgen production,* and *atresia of follicles*. The ratio of LH to FSH is markedly increased. The inciting event(s) remain unknown and may differ from one patient to the next, but a disturbance in hypothalamic–pituitary function is postulated. The hyperinsulinism and hyperandrogenism appear related, but the precise details of this relationship also remain incompletely defined.

Ovarian tumors rarely destroy enough ovarian tissue to cause amenorrhea, but granulosa-cell tumors, which produce excess estrogen, and arrhenoblastomas, which synthesize excess androgen, may be responsible for amenorrhea.

Uterine Pathology. Endometrial scarring may occur as a consequence of radiation therapy, septic abortion, or overly vigorous curettage. The adhesions can obliterate the uterine cavity (Asherman's syndrome). Similarly, cervical trauma can result in scarring.

DIFFERENTIAL DIAGNOSIS

The causes of secondary amenorrhea can be divided pathophysiologically into hypothalamic, pituitary, ovarian, and uterine etiologies (Table 112–1). In one representative series of patients with secondary amenorrhea, hypothalamic dysfunction accounted for 30 percent of cases, polycystic ovary syndrome for 30 percent, pituitary disease (mostly prolactinomas) for 15 percent, ovarian failure for 12 percent, and uterine problems for about 5 percent.

WORKUP

Evaluation ought to begin by first ascertaining if the patient is pregnant. History should be reviewed for recent unprotected intercourse and symptoms of early pregnancy (eg,

Table 112-1. Important Causes of Amenorrhea

1. Hypothalamic dysfunction
   a. Mild
      1. Situational stress
      2. Dieting
      3. Concurrent illness
      4. Increased exercise
      5. Drugs (phenothiazines, oral contraceptives)
      6. Idiopathic
   b. Marked
      1. Anorexia nervosa with severe weight loss
      2. Serious emotional stress or psychopathology
      3. Serious concurrent illness
      4. Competitive long-distance running
      5. Excess androgen, prolactin, or cortisol
      6. Idiopathic
2. Pituitary disease
   a. Prolactinoma
   b. Other pituitary neoplasm
   c. Empty sella syndrome
   d. Pituitary infarction (Sheehan's syndrome)
   e. Granulomatous disease (sarcoidosis)
3. Ovarian
   a. Menopause
   b. Polycystic ovary syndrome (may have hypothalamic etiology)
   c. Premature ovarian failure (idiopathic, autoimmune disease, radiation therapy, chemotherapy, endometriosis, oophoritis)
   d. FSH resistance
4. Uterine
   a. Obliteration of uterine cavity by intrauterine scarring and synechiae formation—Asherman's syndrome (overly vigorous curettage, septic abortion, radiation)
   b. Cervical scarring with resultant os closure
5. Endocrinopathies
   a. Thyroid disease
   c. Cushing's syndrome
   d. Hyperandrogenism
6. Pregnancy

morning sickness). Physical examination may reveal such suggestive findings as nipple hyperpigmentation, a bluish tint to the cervix, and uterine enlargement. Any possibility of pregnancy should lead directly to a *serum human chorionic gonadotropin (hCG) beta-subunit* determination. The test is the most sensitive and specific test for pregnancy, capable of providing a definitive answer rapidly and at a much earlier stage of pregnancy than is possible with urine testing for hCG. However, the *urine hCG-precipitation slide test* is more convenient and can be performed at home on a first morning-voided urine. It achieves 90 percent sensitivity about 6 weeks after the last menstrual period. A negative urine test requires retesting in a week or proceeding directly to serum testing. Once the question of pregnancy is settled, evaluation for other etiologies can proceed in logical, systematic fashion.

History and Physical Examination

History should begin with a detailed menstrual history and the circumstances of the amenorrhea. Age of menarche, character of normal cycles, timing of missed periods, and any prior pregnancies or abortions should be ascertained. A detailed psychosocial history may provide evidence for hypothalamic amenorrhea and should include inquiry into situational stresses (job, school, family, friends), emotional problems, excessive dieting and marked weight loss, and heavy physical training. Oral contraceptive use and intake of other medications needs to be noted.

Review of systems needs to include a check for hot flashes, skin changes of hypothyroidism (see Chapter 104), development of hirsutism, headache, visual disturbances, thyroid enlargement, breast changes or lactescent nipple discharge, increase or decrease in libido, and change in muscle mass or body habitus.

Several patterns are suggestive. Amenorrhea in the context of marked weight loss suggests anorexia nervosa (see Chapter 234). If periods were very irregular before onset of amenorrhea, then anovulatory bleeding was probably occurring and one of its etiologies is likely (see Chapter 111). Amenorrhea accompanied by galactorrhea is strongly suggestive of hyperprolactinemia, which may be due to a prolactinoma, a destructive lesion of the sella, or hypothyroidism (see Chapter 100). A history of irregular periods since menarche in conjunction with obesity and hirsutism raises the probability of polycystic ovary syndrome. Rapid onset of amenorrhea, hirsutism, and frank virilization suggests an androgen-producing neoplasm, usually of adrenal or ovarian origin.

Physical Examination starts by taking specific note of the patient's general appearance, especially for manifestations of low body weight, marked obesity, hirsutism, virilization (see Chapter 98), and Cushing's syndrome. The integument is examined for signs of hypothyroidism (see Chapter 104) and adrenal disease. Vision is checked for visual field defects, and the breasts for a lactescent nipple discharge. On pelvic examination, note should be made of any clitoromegaly, atrophy of the vaginal mucosa, scarring of the cervical os, ovarian or adnexal masses, and uterine enlargement or masses.

Laboratory Studies

As noted, When history and physical examination are unremarkable and pregnancy has been ruled out, one needs to decide whether further evaluation is indicated. An otherwise healthy appearing young woman undergoing situational stress can be followed expectantly if only one or two periods have been missed and pregnancy has been ruled out. Several modes of testing are available and often conducted in algorithmic fashion (Figure 112–1) in patients with more prolonged amenorrhea or clinical evidence suggestive of more serious underlying pathology.

Progestin Trial. Administration of either a single intramuscular 100-mg dose of *progesterone* or 5 days of oral *medroxyprogesterone* (10 mg/d) is typically the first test performed after pregnancy has been ruled out and serves as a form of bioassay for FSH secretion, estrogen synthesis, and uterine responsiveness. Onset of *withdrawal bleeding* after progestin administration indicates adequacy of these components of the menstrual cascade, but inadequate progesterone synthesis. Another way to make the same assessment is to note the pattern made by *cervical mucus* on a glass slide: the mucus from a patient with adequate estrogen secretion forms a fernlike pattern.

Patients With Withdrawal Bleeding in response to a progestin trial have a problem with proper LH release from the pituitary. It may be due to *mild hypothalamic dysfunction* disrupting normal GnRH release, which impairs the LH secretion necessary to trigger ovulation and ensure a functioning corpus luteum. Alternatively, the patient who exhibits withdrawal bleeding may be suffering from too much LH secretion, as seen in *polycystic ovary syndrome*. In both, there is no LH surge, but the former is characterized by too little circulating LH and the latter by too much. Serial serum *LH determinations* can help differentiate. Persistently high or high-normal levels without a midcycle surge are characteristic of polycystic disease. Low or low-normal levels that lack a midcycle surge are consistent with mild hypothalamic dysfunction.

The patient with withdrawal bleeding, a life-long history of menstrual irregularities, infertility, hirsutism, and an elevated LH has a high probability of polycystic ovary syndrome and is a candidate for further testing. Serum levels of *estrone, androstenedione,* and *total testosterone* may be elevated and support the diagnosis, but sometimes only the *free testosterone* level is abnormally high. The latter is a rather expensive test but may provide the only biochemical evidence of androgen excess. *Ultrasonography* for detection of enlarged polycystic ovaries can be performed for anatomic evidence of the condition, although the finding is nonspecific and its absence does not rule out the diagnosis. *Laparoscopy* and biopsy are reserved for difficult cases.

Patients Without Withdrawal Bleeding are likely to have more serious hypothalamic dysfunction, pituitary disease, or ovarian failure. In rare instances, the cause is uterine. If uterine disease is not a serious consideration, then one can proceed directly to an *FSH determination* to differentiate ovarian from pituitary and hypothalamic etiologies. The FSH is more sensitive than the LH for this purpose.

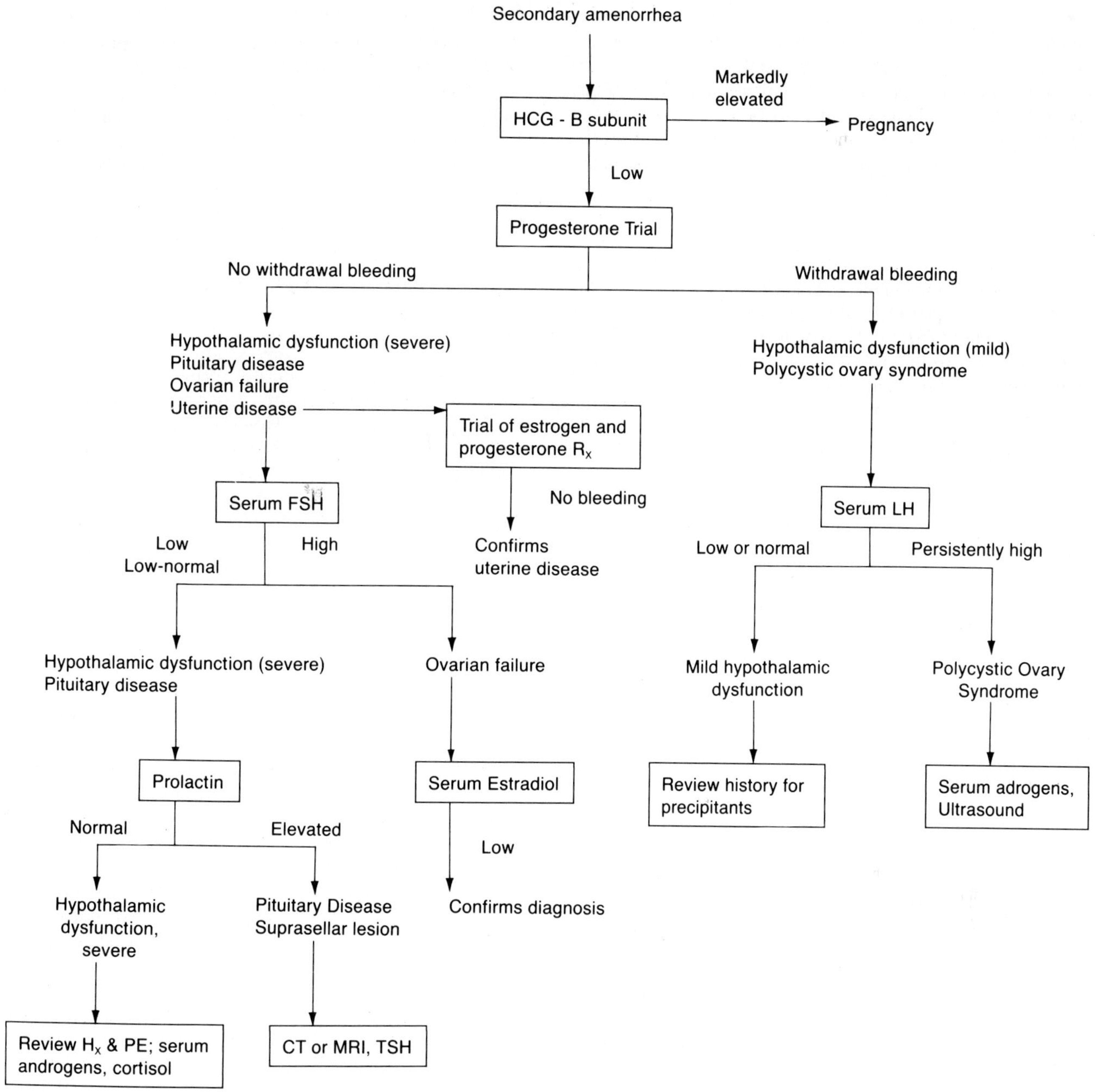

Figure 112-1. Initial testing of the patient with secondary amenorrhea.

Low or Low-Normal FSH is consistent with both severe hypothalamic dysfunction and pituitary disease. Most hypothalamic etiologies are functional and suggested by the history (eg, competitive athletics, marked weight loss, psychiatric disturbance, anorexia nervosa). Those due to excessive production of androgen, prolactin, or cortisol are usually evidenced by the clinical presentation (eg, hirsutism/virilization, galactorrhea, cushingoid appearance, respectively) and can be confirmed by serum determination of the suspected hormone (*testosterone, prolactin,* or *cortisol*). Rapid onset of hirsutism suggests a functioning ovarian or adrenal tumor, especially if accompanied by virilization and a serum testosterone in excess of 2.0 ng/mL. An overnight 1-mg dexamethasone suppression test with 8 AM serum cortisol remains the best screening test for Cushing's syndrome. A markedly elevated prolactin level suggests a pituitary prolactinoma.

Some authorities recommend that all amenorrheic patients should have a prolactin level obtained because of the frequency with which hyperprolactinemia is responsible for amenorrhea, even in the absence of galactorrhea. To avoid making a false-positive diagnosis of a hyperprolactinemic condition, the prolactin determination should be done with the patient off all medications known to stimulate prolactin secretion, including estrogens, phenothiazines, and reserpine. L-Dopa, nicotine, and ergotamine reduce prolactin output and may mask or blunt an elevation.

If prolactin is found elevated, then a search for pituitary and suprasellar pathology is indicated. *Computed tomography (CT) scan of the sella* is the most sensitive test for detection of small pituitary tumors (resolution is measured in a few millimeters). *Magnetic resonance imaging (MRI) scanning* is best for imaging larger pituitary tumors and suprasellar pathology (see Chapter 100). If an adenoma is found, it should be monitored closely if the patient becomes pregnant, because a small percentage of prolactinomas will grow.

A check for primary hypothyroidism by thyroid-stimulating hormone (TSH) determination is also indicated, because the thyrotropin-releasing hormone (TRH) elevation that develops in this condition can stimulate prolactin secretion (see Chapters 100 and 104).

Elevated FSH is a strong indicator of ovarian failure, especially in the context of a four- to fivefold increase. Confirmation can be obtained by a serum *estradiol* determination. In the absence of a readily evident cause for ovarian failure (eg, radiation therapy, chemotherapy), one should consider autoimmune disease, which is likely to involve the adrenals and thyroid as well as the ovaries. Appropriate testing of these glands (*Cortrosyn stimulation* testing [see Chapter 104]; *TSH* determination in conjunction with serum *free thyroxine* [see Chapter 104]) is indicated.

No Withdrawal Bleeding, but Normal FSH, Normal Estradiol. Patients with this profile are likely to have uterine pathology. History should be very suggestive (eg, previous endometritis from abortion or delivery, vigorous curettage). Failure of a course of conjugated *estrogens* (1.25 mg/d for 21 days) followed by *progestin* (medroxyprogesterone 10 mg per day for 5 days) to induce withdrawal bleeding is strongly supportive of the diagnosis of uterine disease and necessitates gynecologic referral for further evaluation.

SYMPTOMATIC THERAPY

Mild Hypothalamic Dysfunction—Patients with Withdrawal Bleeding. Usually, patients with mild hypothalamic amenorrhea need only advice and reassurance (see below). Their periods are likely to return quickly once the precipitant is withdrawn (be it situational stress, dieting, or exercise). There is no immediate medical need to reestablish menstrual cycles unless the patient is uncomfortable living with the uncertainty of waiting for menstrual flow to resume or the condition is chronic (eg, polycystic ovary syndrome) and associated with prolonged, unopposed estrogen stimulation of the endometrium (a risk factor for endometrial cancer). In such instances, a 5-day course of *medroxyprogesterone* (10 mg/d) will usually bring on menstrual bleeding and can be repeated as needed on a monthly or bimonthly basis. The bimonthly program allows for detection of spontaneous remission.

Polycystic ovary syndrome is also associated with infertility, androgen excess, and glucose intolerance, which may require treatment. To restore ovulation and fertility, bilateral *wedge resection* of the ovaries remains a traditional approach, although benefit is usually short-term only. *Clomiphene* administration and, more recently, preparations of *GnRH, GnRH analogues*, and *gonadotropins* are being used by fertility specialists to achieve ovulation. Excess adrenal androgen secretion can be suppressed by daily use of *prednisone* (5 mg qhs). *Oral contraceptives* will inhibit gonadotropin release and ovarian androgen overproduction. Alternatively, *spironolactone* (50 to 150 mg/d for days 1 to 25) can be used for its ability to antagonize androgen effect without causing glandular suppression. Glucose intolerance and hyperinsulinism are best treated by a program of weight loss and exercise, supplemented, if necessary, by oral hypoglycemics (see Chapter 102).

Severe Hypothalamic Dysfunction. When the cause is anorexia nervosa, menses will not resume until *weight* is *restored* to 90 percent or more of normal. Treatment can be difficult (see Chapter 234). However, if weight begins to return to normal, GnRH secretion will revert from a prepubertal pattern to a pubertal one. Competitive athletes may have to cut down on their training program to achieve restoration of menses. They sometimes exhibit excessive weight loss and eating disorders, which may also contribute to the problem and deserve attention. Those with marked hypothalamic dysfunction due to chronic illness will have to await the resolution of their underlying illness before normal menses will resume.

When severe hypothalamic amenorrhea results in inadequate secretion of both estrogen and progesterone (as evidenced by absence of withdrawal bleeding after progestin administration), then *hormonal replacement* therapy should be considered to prevent osteoporosis. A typical replacement program includes *conjugated estrogens* (0.625 to 1.25 mg/d) on days 1 to 25 plus *medroxyprogesterone* (10 mg/d) starting on day 15 and continuing for 12 days. The progesterone is added to induce adequate shedding of endometrial tissue. Some authorities recommend withholding such therapy periodically (eg, every 6 months) to see if menses have returned.

Pituitary Disease. Patients with *hyperprolactinemia* can often achieve restoration of normal GnRH release, ovulation, and menstruation with use of the dopamine agonist *bromocriptine*, which blocks excessive prolactin secretion in up to 95 percent of cases (see Chapter 100). More invasive treatment is reserved for patients with a pituitary tumor that threatens adjacent structures (eg, other areas of the pituitary or the optic chiasm).

Patients with destructive pituitary lesions (Sheehan's syndrome, tumor, granulomatous disease) may require *replacement therapy*. The program should be tailored to the deficiencies detected. Estrogen and progesterone are usually necessary; thyroid hormone and adrenal steroids are less commonly required.

Ovarian Etiologies. Patients with ovarian failure should receive *estrogen/progesterone* replacement therapy. Because some forms may be reversible, a 1- to 2-month pause every year is recommended to see if there is a return of ovarian function. Premature ovarian failure and drug-induced disease are among the reversible forms.

Uterine Disease. When the cause is granulomatous disease, treatment of the underlying disease offers the best hope for restoration of menses (see Chapters 49 and 51). Asherman's syndrome may respond to a combination of *recurettage* that severs bridging synechiae, which obliterate the uterine cavity, and *glucocorticosteroids,* which inhibit formation of new scar tissue.

PATIENT EDUCATION

Patient education occupies a central role in the management of amenorrhea. Little could be of more concern to a woman than her reproductive capacity and endocrinologic health. For the person with mild hypothalamic dysfunction, addressing fears such as pregnancy, infertility, and premature menopause, and reviewing how situational stresses can lead to the amenorrhea, comprise the principal means of treatment. The addition of simple advice regarding proper degrees of exercise and dieting and how to cope with situational stresses helps to ensure a good outcome. The competitive marathon runner with more severe hypothalamic dysfunction may care little about menses and fertility at this stage of her life, but she needs to be informed about the risk of osteoporosis and the need for hormonal replacement therapy.

Patients whose amenorrhea followed use of oral contraceptives can be reassured that they have not been rendered infertile and that normal ovulatory periods resume in more than 99 percent of patients by 6 months. If conception is not desired, the need for mechanical contraception should be stressed, because the incidence of spontaneous ovulation is high in functional amenorrhea.

Women in their late 30s and early 40s who become amenorrheic fear premature menopause and its consequences. Usually, such concerns are best met by prompt assessment for ovarian failure (see above) and communication of results, rather than by adopting a wait-and-see approach.

Patient education is no less important when the suspected etiology is more serious (eg, pituitary tumor, polycystic ovary syndrome, anorexia nervosa). Sometimes, such patients may rationalize their amenorrhea, ascribing it to a benign etiology, and delay proper evaluation and treatment.

INDICATIONS FOR REFERRAL

A very significant proportion of the initial amenorrhea evaluation can be effectively carried out by the primary physician. However, referral for more intensive study and treatment is indicated when there is evidence of serious anatomic disruption (eg, uterine synechiae), neoplasm (eg, pituitary tumor), premature ovarian failure, or marked hypothalamic dysfunction. A gynecologic endocrine consultation can be very helpful, especially in the setting of severe functional disease, hyperprolactinemia, or premature ovarian failure. Such referral is of particular importance to the woman who desires to become pregnant, because a number of therapeutic options are available. Rapid onset of hirsutism, especially if accompanied by virilization and elevations in serum androgens, suggests a functioning ovarian or adrenal tumor and necessitates prompt endocrinologic consultation. Management of a large pituitary neoplasm that threatens adjacent structures requires the advice of the endocrinologist and neurosurgeon. Patients with idiopathic hyperprolactinemia or a microadenoma (especially those desiring to become pregnant) will appreciate a gynecologic endocrine consultation for confirmation of the diagnosis, counseling, and consideration of bromocriptine therapy.

A.H.G.

ANNOTATED BIBLIOGRAPHY

Barnes R, Rosenfield RL. Polycystic ovary syndrome: Pathogenesis and treatment. Ann Intern Med 1989;110:386. *(Excellent review of pathophysiology; 169 refs.)*

Barnes R. Polycystic ovary syndrome and ovarian steroidogenesis. Semin Reprod Endocrinol 1991;9:360. *(Focuses on the relation between hyperinsulinism and androgen excess in this syndrome.)*

Berga SL, Mortola JF, Girton L, et al. Neuroendocrine aberrations in women with functional hypothalamic amenorrhea. J Clin Endocrinol Metab 1989;68:301. *(The normal pattern of GnRH release is disturbed.)*

Biller BMK, Klibanski A. Amenorrhea and osteoporosis. Endocrinologist 1991;1:294. *(Estrogen production is reduced and bony changes may ensue in women with severe hypothalamic amenorrhea.)*

Conn PM, Crowley WF. Gonadotropin-releasing hormone and its analogues. N Engl J Med 1991;324:93. *(Useful basic science review with good clinical correlations; 180 refs.)*

Davis PC, Hoffman JC Jr, Spencer T, et al. MR imaging of pituitary adenoma: CT, clinical, and surgical correlation. Am J Roentgenol 1987;148:797. *(A series of 25 patients, in which MR was best for imaging large adenomas and CT for detection of microadenomas.)*

Federman DD. Ovary. In Scientific American Medicine. Federman DD, Rubenstein E (eds.) New York: Scientific American Inc. 1993, 3III-1. *(Best exposition of normal physiology and pathophysiology for the generalist reader; includes a rational approach to workup of secondary amenorrhea, one that was adapted for use in this chapter.)*

Fries H, et al. Epidemiology of secondary amenorrhea. II. A retrospective evaluation of etiology with special regard to psychogenic factors and weight loss. Am J Obstet Gynecol 1974;118:473. *(Documents relation of secondary amenorrhea to weight loss and stressful life events.)*

Koppelman MC, Jaffe MJ, Rieth KG, et al. Hyperprolactinemia, amenorrhea and galactorrhea. Ann Intern Med 1984;100:115. *(Important data on the natural history of hyperprolactinemic conditions.)*

Loucks AB, Mortola JF, Girton L, et al. Alterations in the hypothalamic–pituitary and the hypothalamic–pituitary–adrenal axes in athletic women. J Clin Endocrinol Metab 1989;68:402. *(Heavy exercise programs can disrupt these axes and lead to amenorrhea.)*

McKenna TJ. Pathogenesis and treatment of polycystic ovary syndrome. N Engl J Med 1988;318:558. *(Terse, but very useful review; 54 refs.)*

Melmed S, Braunstein GD, Chang RJ, et al. Pituitary tumors secreting growth hormone and prolactin. Ann Intern Med 1986;105:238. *(Comprehensive discussion of pathophysiology, diagnosis, and treatment; 167 refs.)*

Molitch ME. Pregnancy and the hyperprolactinemic patient. N Engl J Med 1985;312:1364. *(Excellent paper for counseling.)*

Neufield M, MacLaren N, Blizzard R. Autoimmune polyglandular syndromes. Pediatr Ann 1980;9:154. *(A good description of these syndromes and their autoimmune pathophysiology.)*

Reindollar RH, Novak M, Tho SPT, et al. Adult onset amenorrhea. Am J Obstet Gynecol 1986;155:531. *(A series of 262 patients, providing a useful breakdown of etiologies.)*

Vance ML, Evans WS, Thorner MB. Bromocriptine. Ann Intern Med 1984;100:78. *Comprehensive review of the drug; 134 refs.)*

113
Evaluation of Breast Masses and Nipple Discharges

Primary Care Medicine: Office Evaluation and Management of the Adult Patient, 3rd edition, edited by Allan H. Goroll, Lawrence A. May, and Albert G. Mulley, Jr. J.B. Lippincott Company, Philadelphia

A solitary or dominant breast mass or an abnormal nipple discharge may be a harbinger of breast cancer, the most common malignancy among women. Because such a finding, whether discovered by the patient or by her physician, will raise legitimate fears, the primary physician must be able to proceed with deliberate speed in reaching a diagnosis that excludes carcinoma.

PATHOPHYSIOLOGY AND CLINICAL PRESENTATION

Breast Mass

Pathophysiology. A breast mass may represent proliferative changes in epithelial or mesenchymal tissue or fluid-filled cysts. The breast is a complex organ composed of epithelium that forms acini and ducts, fibrous tissue that provides support, and fat. It is exquisitely sensitive to its hormonal milieu. Estradiol stimulates proliferation of epithelial cells and accompanying increases in periductal vascularity. Progesterone induces the development of acini and opposes the mesenchymal actions of estrogens.

With each menstrual cycle, the breast exhibits its own cycle of proliferation and desquamation of duct lining. But the response of epithelium, fibrous tissue, and fat to the same hormonal stimulation is variable. Certain areas of the breast may overshoot in the monthly preparation for pregnancy, causing thickening of the breasts and lumpiness. The overgrowth may involve proliferation of fibrous tissue alone or also involve epithelial cells of the ducts and glands, leading to *fibroadenomas* or *ductal dysplasia*. Lumps can also be caused by the collection of fluids, essentially colostrum or dissolved cellular debris, which form microcysts or macrocysts.

These physiologic events may combine to produce a breast that is *fibrocystic* in quality (hence the advice by experts to drop the term *fibrocystic disease*). Fibrocystic changes can be found clinically in approximately 50 percent of women during their reproductive years and histologically in 90 percent. Most investigators believe that benign breast disease, including neoplasms such as fibroadenomas and intraductal papillomas as well as fibrocystic change, represents a spectrum of responses to normal hormonal stimulation rather than distinct diseases.

Although the variable response of breast tissue to physiologic proliferative and involutional hormonal stimuli is responsible for most benign masses, there are other causes. *Infection,* usually associated with duct obstruction, can result in an inflammatory mass. Redness, warmth, and tenderness are prominent features. *Mammary duct ectasia* can result in infection and yet may simulate cancer, because it can produce nipple discharge, nipple inversion, and a mass. Periareolar infection may ensue. Blunt trauma can lead to hematoma formation.

Approximately 20 percent of solitary or dominant breast masses are cancers. Breast cancers derive from ductal or epithelium cells. They may invade immediately or grow in situ. Breast cancer in younger women tends to be *lobular* in pathologic appearance and multicentric, but not calcifying or rapidly invading. *Ductal* carcinomas are prominent in older women. They are typically unicentric, readily calcified (producing the characteristic microcalcifications helpful in radiologic detection), and much more rapidly invasive than lobular lesions.

Growth is often associated with increasingly malignant behavior, characterized by loss of estrogen and progesterone receptors, metastasis, and more aggressive local invasion. Although metastasis can occur early, it is not an invariably early event and usually does not occur in lesions less than 1 cm in diameter (unless lymphatics have been invaded). Local growth may extend to the skin or chest wall. Axillary nodes are typically the first clinical site of spread beyond the breast.

Clinical Presentation. Cancer in the breast typically presents as a painless discrete mass. Pain is a presenting symptom in fewer than 7 percent of cases and almost always accompanied by a mass. Early on, the mass may be movable; later, it can become fixed. Nipple retraction or inversion of new onset may also herald an underlying cancer. Signs of more advanced disease include skin retraction, change in breast contour, thickening or dimpling of the skin, and fixation of the mass to the chest wall. A ductal carcinoma may present as an isolated serosanguineous nipple discharge (see below).

Benign lesions may be present in a manner clinically indistinguishable from that of cancers, but a few patterns are characteristic. In *fibrocystic change,* the breasts are diffusely lumpy and fibrous in quality. One breast may be more involved than the other. An isolated *cyst* may also be a presentation of benign disease, but those that yield blood on aspiration or recur after aspiration may be related to a malignant process.

Nipple Discharge

A nipple discharge that is unilateral, spontaneous, and localized to one duct should be considered pathologic. Nonlactescent unilateral breast discharges may reflect local inflammatory or neoplastic lesions, most of which are benign. Benign etiologies include chronic cystic mastopathy and intraductal papilloma. Many papillomas are not palpable. Approximately 5 percent of women with a breast discharge have cancer. The most worrisome nipple discharge is a bloody one, which occurs in 70 percent to 85 percent of cancers that present with a nipple discharge. However, only 25 percent of bloody discharges prove to be due to cancer. The discharge may predate onset of a clinically detectable mass. The chance of a nipple discharge being associated with cancer increases with age. Onset of a lactescent nipple discharge (galactorrhea) in a woman who is not nursing may be a sign of a prolactinoma (see Chapter 100).

DIFFERENTIAL DIAGNOSIS

The differential diagnosis of a breast mass is confusing because of lack of agreement or standardization in clinical and pathologic terminology. The category of "fibrocystic disease" has been dropped because it does not represent a pathologic state. Among lesions that come to biopsy, the most common discretely palpable solid mass is the fibroadenoma. Approximately 20 percent of solitary or dominant breast masses are cancers.

A serous or bloody discharge may occur with intraductal papillomas, ductal ectasia, and ductal carcinoma. In the largest reported series, 44 percent had papilloma or papillomatosis, 23 percent had ductal ectasia, 16 percent had fibrocystic changes, and only 11 percent had cancer.

WORKUP

Breast Mass

Physical Examination. The key finding is a *dominant nodule*. Most glandular tissue is found in the upper outer quadrant of the breast and changes with the menstrual cycle. Dominant masses are characterized by their unchanging and persistent nature throughout the cycle. Breast tenderness to examination in the absence of a dominant mass is of no pathologic significance.

Much is made of the clinical characteristics of breast masses in estimating the probability of malignant disease. Easy mobility within the breast, regular borders, and a soft or cystic feel on palpation all suggest a benign process. However, these signs are not reliable; 60 percent of cancers are freely movable, 40 percent have regular borders, and 40 percent feel soft or cystic. A "benign" physical finding reduces the probability of cancer no further than to approximately 10 percent.

The young woman with multiple nodules and diffuse thickening consistent with fibrocystic change has difficult breasts to evaluate. Reexamination at different times in the menstrual cycle is often informative and reassuring when no dominant nodule emerges. A persistent solitary or dominant nodule requires biopsy.

Examination of the lymph nodes is required in all patients with a breast lump, because it may provide important supporting evidence for a malignancy, especially if otherwise unexplained adenopathy is found in the ipsilateral axilla.

Breast Imaging. *Mammography* can be a valuable diagnostic test, especially in the woman over 30 with breast symptoms, but it must be emphasized that a negative mammogram does not obviate the need for biopsy of a clinically suspicious breast mass. Studies in which the most advanced techniques were used by the most experienced clinicians have repeatedly indicated that mammography has a false-negative rate of 8 percent to 10 percent. A mammogram should be obtained before biopsy and preoperatively for any woman undergoing breast surgery. The preoperative study can also help to delineate the mass and identify any occult lesions in the ipsilateral or contralateral breast. Mammography is used to guide needle biopsy of small lesions.

Ultrasonography can be used to differentiate a cystic from a solid palpable mass, especially in women under 30, and help guide needle aspiration. A host of improved imaging techniques are under development.

Biopsy. *Needle aspiration biopsy* of solid as well as cystic lesions, with cytologic examination of the material obtained, is sometimes a means to avoid open biopsy. It can be performed in the office or in the radiologic suite under the guidance of imaging techniques. Adequate specimens are obtained in about 60 percent to 85 percent of instances. Among adequate samples, sensitivity is in excess of 80 percent; specificity is over 99 percent. Negative cytology from a solid lesion does not rule out cancer. However, a cystic lesion that is successfully aspirated, cytologically negative, and nonrecurring requires only follow-up breast examination and mammography. Solid lesions that have negative or suspicious cytology and cystic lesions containing serosanguineous fluid require *excisional biopsy*. The procedure is usually done as an outpatient procedure.

Nipple Discharge

The patient should undergo a careful *breast examination* that includes careful palpation and noting if the discharge is unilateral or bilateral, spontaneous or expressible, and localized to one or many ducts. If unilateral and expressed only from a single duct, one should note the quadrant of the breast from which it seems to be coming. Guaiac testing helps to detect occult blood and cytologic examination may sometimes reveal abnormal cells, although sensitivity is low. These measures are followed by *mammography*, looking for dilated ducts or occult masses. Patients with nipple discharge that remains unexplained (especially if bloody) requires referral to a surgeon experienced in evaluating breast disease. The risk of cancer in such patients remains real, and *ductal exploration* may be the only means of detecting an early ductal malignancy.

SYMPTOMATIC MANAGEMENT AND PATIENT EDUCATION

The woman with painful breasts associated with fibrocystic change can be reassured that the discomfort is not a sign of cancer and that symptoms usually improve with the cyclical decrease in hormonal stimulation. Moreover, it is important to emphasize that the finding is not a risk factor for breast cancer. The physiologic nature of fibrocystic changes, their extremely high prevalence, and their favorable natural history can be reviewed. Oral contraceptives provide no benefit in treatment or prevention of the condition. Commonly recommended measures include use of a support bra, avoidance of chocolate and caffeinated beverages, and vitamin E supplements. Efficacy is variable.

The woman with a dominant breast mass or bloody discharge is more concerned with the possibility of breast cancer than with symptoms. Explaining that the likelihood of a benign etiology is still greater than that of cancer can provide a modicum of reassurance and perspective while more definitive diagnostic measures are undertaken. A prompt, efficient diagnostic evaluation is the best medicine. Reassurance can be given to the patient who fears spread of cancer from breast compression (as occurs with mammography) or needle biopsy.

A.H.G. and A.G.M.

ANNOTATED BIBLIOGRAPHY

Atkins H, Wolff B. Discharges from the nipple. Br J Surg 1964; 51:602. *(A review of 203 cases from the Breast Clinic at Guys Hospital.)*

Bell DA, Hajdu SI, Urban JA, et al. Role of aspiration cytology in the diagnosis and management of mammary lesions in office practice. Cancer 1983;51:1189. *(Data suggesting a very useful role.)*

Ernster VL. The epidemiology of benign breast disease. Epidemiol Rev 1981;3:184. *(A thoughtful review emphasizing the problem of case definition and reviewing evidence for its precipitants.)*

Kopans DB, Meyer JE, Sadowsky N. Breast imaging. N Engl J Med 1984;310:960. *(Reviews imaging techniques including mammography, ultrasonography, thermography, and MRI. Discusses reasons for limited sensitivity and specificity for each technique.)*

London RS, Sundaram GS, Goldstein PJ. Medical management of mammary dysplasia. Obstet Gynecol 1982;59:519. *(Reviews hormonal therapy, vitamin E and avoidance of methylxanthines.)*

Love SM, Gelman RS, Silen W. Fibrocystic "disease" of the breast—A nondisease? N Engl J Med 1982;307:1010. *(A critical review of clinical and histologic definitions of fibrocystic disease in a careful exploration of its role as a risk factor for breast cancer.)*

Murad, Contesso G, Mouriesse H. Nipple discharge from the breast. Ann Surg 1982;195:259. *(Provides data on etiologies, prevalences, and presentations.)*

Mushlin AI. Diagnostic tests in breast cancer. Ann Intern Med 1985;103:79. *(A superb review, logical and carefully reasoned, of test characteristics with recommendations based on diagnostic probabilities. Accompanies a position statement of the American College of Physicians in the same issue.)*

Parazzini F, Vecchia CL, Franceschi S, et al. Risk factors for pathologically confirmed benign breast disease. Am J Epidemiol 1984;120:115. *(This case–control study found identical risk factors for benign and malignant breast disease and did not detect a protective effect for oral contraceptives or body mass.)*

Preece P, Baum M, Mansel R. The importance of mastalgia in operable breast cancer. Br Med J 1982;284:1299. *(Pain was the presentation in only 7 percent of cancers and in the absence of a mass, not associated with cancer.)*

114
Evaluation of Vulvar Pruritus

ANNE W. MOULTON, M.D.
ELAINE CARLSON, M.D.

Primary Care Medicine: Office Evaluation and Management of the Adult Patient, 3rd edition, edited by Allan H. Goroll, Lawrence A. May, and Albert G. Mulley, Jr. J.B. Lippincott Company, Philadelphia

Vulvar itching can be a very annoying symptom for the patient. In the genital area, only the vulvar and perineal skin have sensory receptors that trigger the sensation of itching. However, vulvar pruritus may be secondary to a vaginal infection as well as a vulvar dermatitis or primary skin disease. In older women, it is likely to be related to declining estrogen levels and, in rare cases, may be a manifestation of a malignancy. The primary care physician should be familiar with the appearance of inflammatory, infectious, and malignant conditions of the vulva to tailor appropriate therapy and avoid delays in the detection of carcinoma.

PATHOPHYSIOLOGY AND CLINICAL PRESENTAITONS

The most common causes of vulvar pruritus are listed in Table 114–1. Patients with vaginitis often complain of itching. In *candidal vulvovaginitis,* the vulva is erythematous, often with a sharp scalloped border demarcating the area of involvement. "Satellite" lesions are characteristic, as is the cheesy discharge of the associated vaginitis (see Chapter 117). Primary cutaneous candidiasis of the vulva can also occur without evidence of vaginitis or discharge. It is more commonly seen in women with diabetes or those who are pregnant or obese. Intense vulvar inflammation also occurs with *trichomonal infection,* and, rarely, bacterial vaginosis may present with itching. *Hidradenitis suppurativa,* which is caused by inflammation or infection of the apocrine sweat glands in the vulva, can cause itching or burning and progress to fistula formation.

Lesions of *herpes genitalis* are caused in most cases by herpes simplex virus (HSV) type 2. The lesions, which begin as vesicles and progress to ulcers, cause burning, itching, and often pain and tenderness of the vulva. Vulvar lesions caused by *human papillomavirus (HPV),* also called condyloma acuminata, are generally multifocal and appear on the labia or fourchette, causing itching and often vaginal discharge. The umbilicated lesions of *molluscum contagiosum*

Table 114-1. Causes of Vulvar Pruritus

Infections	
	Candida
	Trichomonas
	Bacterial vaginosis
	Hidradenitis suppurativa
	Herpes simplex
	Human papillomavirus
	Dermatophytes
	Scabies
Dermatoses	
	Lichen sclerosis
	Lichen simplex chronicus
	Lichen planus (erosive vaginitis)
	Psoriasis
	Seborrheic dermatitis
Low Estrogen States: Atrophic Vaginitis	
	Postpartum
	Postmenopausal
Premalignant/Malignant Conditions	
	Vulvar intraepithelial neoplasia (VIN)
	Squamous cell carcinoma
	Adenocarcinoma
Irritants	
	Contact dermatitis

may also be pruritic. This infection, which is generally self-limited, is also sexually transmitted. Dermatophyte lesions (tinea cruris) are a rare cause of itching in women.

Infestation with mites or lice can cause intense pruritis. Scabies produces papular lesions and itching, which may occur in several areas on the body, including wrists, finger webs, elbows, axillae, genitals, and buttocks. *Pediculosis* is confined to areas covered by hair, since eggs are deposited on the hair shafts (see Chapter 195).

The term vulvar dystrophy has been replaced by the term *vulvar dermatoses* to describe the large group of nonneoplastic papulosquamous lesions that occur on the vulva. All of these may cause pruritus in addition to other symptoms. Any of the lesions may appear white, because they are hyperkeratotic, but less than 5 percent are premalignant. *Lichen sclerosis* presents as a symmetric, "keyhole" pattern of pale, atrophic epidermis with fine wrinkling or scaling on a whitened dermis. Chronic contact or *irritant reactions* can cause persistent scratching and lichenification (lichen simplex chronicus), which leaves the vulva thickened and furrowed. *Lichen planus,* a chronic erosive vaginitis, occurs with pruritic purple polygonal papules and plaques ("the five Ps"). *Psoriasis* may appear as moist red plaques with a silvery scale on the labia majora. *Seborrheic dermatitis* of the vulva presents with scaling erythematous lesions of the vulva.

Atrophic vaginitis occurs in low estrogen states, including postmenopause (natural and surgical) and postpartum (see Chapter 117). The mucosa is red and thin; sometimes a mild discharge is present.

Malignancy may develop in association with dermatoses such as lichen sclerosis or with infections; vulvar intraepithelial neoplasia (VIN) in association with HPV is an example. Paget's disease of the vulva, which appears as a diffuse scaling process often involving the anal region as well, is associated in 5 percent of cases with an underlying adenocarcinoma.

Squamous carcinoma of the vulva is the most ominous cause of vulvar pruritus, occurring primarily in older women: 70 percent of cases appear in women older than age 60. Delay in presentation is common; often the patient gives a history of unsuccessful trials of topical agents for symptomatic relief from itching. Squamous cell carcinoma of the vulva may present with single or multiple papules or macules, which can be confluent or discrete, usually on the labia majora or minora. The lesions can be red, white, or pigmented and may be in multiple locations on the labia. They typically arise on the vulvar skin in areas already long-involved with premalignant change. Spread is to inguinal and deep pelvic nodes. Occasionally, a patient with carcinoma complains of a lump or an ulcerated lesion. Itching may be intense, sometimes in conjunction with a slightly bloody discharge.

Vulvar intraepithelial neoplasia (VIN), which occurs in younger women (mean age 39), is akin to cervical intraepithelial neoplasia (CIN) in its relationship to previous HPV infection. A certain percentage of women who have one will have the other, necessitating a full evaluation with colposcopy. However, VIN progresses to malignancy at a much slower rate than CIN.

Vulvar irritation caused by scratching, maceration, and chemical agents is common. Deodorants, soaps, douching agents, bubble baths, and contraceptive foams may incite allergic reactions or chemical irritations, leading to itching. The vulva may appear erythematous, and edema or secondary excoriations may be present. The precipitant may be inadequate or overly aggressive genital hygiene. A warm, moist environment, which promotes infection, can occur in patients who are obese or who wear tight-fitting pants or nylon underwear. Chafing fosters maceration of the mucosa in conjunction with the itching and scratching. Elderly women, who experience urinary incontinence, may be forced to wear pads which can cause irritation. Younger women who shave their pubic hair are often bothered by pruritus from a secondary folliculitis.

DIFFERENTIAL DIAGNOSIS

In young women, vaginitis, pediculosis, scabies, chemical irritants, and allergic reactions are the major causes of vaginal itching. The same etiologies apply to older women, but atrophic vaginitis and vulvar carcinoma also become major considerations. In any woman with a persistently pruritic vulva, the possibility of a primary dermatosis should be considered.

WORKUP

It is important to inquire about vaginal discharge, any skin rashes, urinary incontinence, vulvar lesions, and other sites of itching. Possible irritants and allergies need to be identified, such as creams, soaps, bubble baths, vaginal deodorants, douches, and contraceptive foams. The sexual history or presence of genital itching in partners or roommates may suggest infection or infestation. Information related to the duration of the problem and responses to prior treatments can be useful. Presence of an ulceration or nodule that has persisted or grown should be ascertained. Any history of HPV- or HSV-associated lesions or abnormal Papanicolaou (Pap) smears should be obtained.

The vulva and perineal skin is inspected for macules, papules, scaling, erythema, ulcerations, pigmented lesions, hypopigmentation, excoriation, rash, lice, and mites. A close look at the hair shaft may reveal lice eggs (nits), which are pathognomonic of the infestation (see Chapter 195). A speculum examination helps to identify any vaginitis or discharge (see Chapter 117). Inguinal nodes should be palpated. A smear of the discharge for identification of an organism and a urinalysis for glycosuria are the major laboratory studies needed. Any suspicious lesions should be referred for biopsy.

SYMPTOMATIC MANAGEMENT, PATIENT EDUCATION, AND INDICATIONS FOR REFERRAL

The management of vulvar pruritus is most likely to be successful when a specific etiology can be identified. Self-treatments and use of potentially irritating soaps or creams ought to be stopped. Atrophic vaginitis responds well to a topical estrogen cream (see Chapter 118). Occasionally, an antihistamine may be used at night to relieve itching and break the itch–scratch cycle. In some cases, where the etiology is known, the short-term use of steroid creams may be useful to reduce inflammation.

Any persistent suspicious vulvar lesions should be referred to the dermatologist or gynecologist for biopsy.

Patients should be educated about factors that contribute to persistent vulvar irritation, including excessive hygiene or moisture (secondary to tight-fitting jeans, panty hose, nylon underwear, or exercise clothes). Women should be encouraged to perform regular vulvar self-examination. They should be taught to use a hand mirror to inspect the vulva, looking for moles, changes in pigmentation, warts, ulcers, and sores.

ANNOTATED BIBLIOGRAPHY

Brown D, Kaufman RH. Vulvovaginitis. In Glass RH (ed): Office Gynecology. Baltimore: Williams & Wilkins, 1993. *(Includes good discussion with pictures of lesions of HPV and HSV.)*

Byyny RL, Speroff L. The external genitalia. In A Clinical Guide for the Care of Older Women. Baltimore: Williams & Wilkins, 1990. *(Excellent review of vulvovaginal disorders in older women.)*

Hatch KD. Vulvovaginal human papillomavirus infections: clinical implications and management. Am J Obstet Gynecol 1991;165:1183. *(Good review of the subject.)*

McKay M. Vulvitis and vulvovaginitis: cutaneous considerations. Am J Obstet Gynecol 1991;165:1176. *(Good descriptive review of vulvar dermatoses and other vulvar lesions.)*

115
Medical Evaluation of Dyspareunia and Other Female Sexual Dysfunctions

ANNE W. MOULTON, M.D.
ELAINE CARLSON, M.D.

Primary Care Medicine: Office Evaluation and Management of the Adult Patient, 3rd edition, edited by Allan H. Goroll, Lawrence A. May, and Albert G. Mulley, Jr. J.B. Lippincott Company, Philadelphia

Dyspareunia, or painful intercourse, is more common than physicians realize, because patients often do not feel comfortable volunteering the complaint in the office. It often requires an aware and sympathetic clinician to uncover the problem. In one study, more than 60 percent of women surveyed noted that they had dyspareunia at one time in their life, and up to 30 percent of women experienced chronic dyspareunia. The majority of these women had not discussed it with their physicians. The primary care physician is often in the best position to evaluate the causes and facilitate treatment of this problem.

PATHOPHYSIOLOGY AND CLINICAL PRESENTATION

Several mechanisms may be responsible for painful intercourse (Table 115–1), depending on whether the symptoms occur with initial insertion of the penis or deep penetration. Pain is experienced in the former case because of failure of lubrication or inadequate stimulation, vaginal or vulvar irritation, and structural impediments secondary to surgery, inflammation, or anatomic variants. Deep pain can arise from friction against inflamed tissue or by jarring of inflamed parametrial structures. The psychological mechanisms of dyspareunia reflect a variety of issues.

Pain on insertion can also be caused by irritation of the vulva, which in turn is caused by multiple factors including vulvovaginal infections (see Chapters 114 and 117). A *cyst* of the *Bartholin's gland duct* occurs when mechanical irritation and the attendant inflammatory reaction obstruct the ductal lumen. Thin vulvar surface and vaginal mucosa are less resilient and more susceptible to *trauma*. These vaginal changes take place in women who are anorexic, breast-feeding, or menopausal, or who have had pelvic irradiation.

In premenopausal women, *inadequate lubrication,* because of insufficient foreplay, is among the most frequent causes of dyspareunia. Women who are postpartum may also experience short-term vaginal dryness and resultant dyspareunia, which can continue while they are breast-feeding. In postmenopausal patients, vaginal atrophy is the most important cause of inadequate lubrication. Finally, scant production of vaginal secretions may reflect fears about sexual intercourse or risk of infection, misunderstandings, or conflicts with a sexual partner.

Chronic vulvar vestibulitis, an uncommon cause of introital dyspareunia, is defined as pain of the vestibule on vaginal entry, associated with erythema of the vulva. The syndrome may be associated with subclinical human papillomavirus infection, recurrent candidiasis, or bacterial vaginosis and an

Table 115-1. Important Causes of Dyspareunia

PAIN GREATEST ON INSERTION	PAIN GREATEST ON DEEP PENETRATION
Inadequate lubrication	Pelvic inflammatory disease
Vaginitis	Ovarian cyst
Incompletely ruptured hymen	Endometriosis
Bartholin's gland cyst	Pelvic adhesions
Stricture	Relaxation of pelvic support
Inadequate episiotomy	Uterine fibroids
Vulvovaginal atrophy	
Vulvar vestibulitis	
Pudendal neuralgia	
Vaginismus	

elevated vaginal pH. A biopsy shows only chronic inflammatory changes.

Pudendal neuralgia is another cause of vulvar burning; patients with this symptom may complain of superficial burning or deep aching pain but few have physical findings. *Vaginismus* is defined as involuntary spasm of the perineal muscles induced by an attempt at physical penetration. It is an important and treatable, though uncommon, cause of dyspareunia (with a large psychogenic component).

Deep dyspareunia may occur with endometriosis, ovarian cysts, adhesions, and pelvic inflammatory disease. Penile thrusting moves the entire uterus, with resultant pulling on the peritoneum. Acute or defervescing *pelvic inflammatory disease* or *endometritis* will produce pain even on gentle motion.

DIFFERENTIAL DIAGNOSIS

All the causes of dyspareunia, listed in Table 115–1, should be considered according to the age of the patient and whether there is pain on insertion or on deep penetration.

WORKUP

In the history, one needs to determine whether dyspareunia was noticed with the first experience of sexual intercourse or has developed recently, secondary to organic change or a situational problem. The patient should be asked whether pain occurs before penetration, on penetration, or only after deep penetration. It is important to establish whether the patient can insert a tampon without pain; if she can, mechanical obstruction is unlikely. A history of recent infection, previous surgery, or pelvic pathology may suggest the etiology. The provider needs to take a complete history, including current and previous sexual experiences. Recent studies underscore a new awareness of the prevalence of sexual abuse, including incest, rape (including date rape), and domestic violence. It is not surprising that the patient may not be forthcoming with these experiences. Any history of sexual fears should be explored. An understanding of the patient's current sexual experience (circumstances, time spent on foreplay, etc.) and feelings toward the partner should be sensitively obtained (see Chapter 229). Interviewing the husband or sexual partner is essential to a complete evaluation.

The most important part of the workup is the pelvic examination. The physician inspects for signs of vulvovaginitis, atrophic vaginitis, narrowed introitus, cervicitis, and congenital abnormalities. Palpation may identify a uterine mass, a retroverted uterus, or tenderness. The cervix should be manipulated to see if pain is produced. Examination for loss of pelvic support, rectocele, or cystocele is needed. A smear should be obtained for cervical cytology to detect underlying malignancy.

A complete blood count, sedimentation rate, and cervical culture are indicated if there is evidence on physical examination suggesting pelvic inflammatory disease (see Chapter 116). Pelvic ultrasonography may be indicated to help define a suspected pelvic mass. Referral to a gynecologist for laparoscopy is indicated if endometriosis, adhesions, or an adnexal mass is under consideration.

SYMPTOMATIC MANAGEMENT, PATIENT EDUCATION, AND INDICATIONS FOR REFERRAL

The patient without organic pathology who is troubled by inadequate lubrication should be reassured that she is healthy and provided advice, which may include insisting on more prolonged foreplay and the use of a water-soluble lubricant jelly. Contraceptive creams should not be used for lubrication, because they often cause dehydration and may worsen soreness. A variety of lubricant products are available over the counter. Oral–genital foreplay, trying different positions for coitus, and guiding the man's penis for insertion are other suggestions that can be made. The postmenopausal woman with an atrophic vaginal mucosa can be given estrogen cream to use topically on an intermittent basis (see Chapter 118).

If there is an underlying vaginal or pelvic infection, it should be treated and the patient advised to refrain temporarily from intercourse (see Chapters 116 and 117). A cyst of the Bartholin's gland duct may spontaneously drain following frequent warm soaks in the bathtub, which sometimes relieves the obstruction; marsupialization by a gynecologist may be required to provide adequate drainage if the cyst is badly inflamed and infected. Patients troubled by pain from herpes simplex infection can obtain relief with use of acyclovir (see Chapter 193). Retained suture material in episiotomy scars, vulvar islands of adenosis (ectopic columnar epithelium), or nerve endings previously damaged by herpetic infection may require local excision for relief of pain.

The patient with a narrow introitus should be referred to a gynecologist for a trial of vaginal dilators. Vaginismus may be managed by education, relaxation, and Kegel exercises, all of which are usually best accomplished by an experienced therapist or sex therapy clinic. Patients bothered by pain on deep penetration may be more comfortable lying on one side during coitus so that deep penetration is limited.

Initial failure to identify or relieve dyspareunia should prompt referral to the gynecologist. This ought to be done only after a thorough evaluation has been performed, the sexual history has been elicited, any infection has been treated, advice on sexual technique has been provided, and lubricants have been tried. Referral to a psychologist or sex

Table 115-2. Secondary Causes of Sexual Dysfunction

MEDICAL	PSYCHIATRIC
Cushing's disease	Bipolar disorder
Addison's disease	Anxiety disorder
Diabetes mellitus	Major depression
Hypopituitarism	Panic disorder
Hyperprolactinemia	Somatization disorder
Degenerative joint disease	Somatiform pain disorder
Hypothyroidism	
Multiple sclerosis	
Temporal lobe lesions	
Coronary heart disease	

therapist, involving both the patient and her sexual partner, might also be considered (see Chapter 229).

EXCITEMENT AND ORGASMIC PHASE DYSFUNCTIONS

Causes of female sexual dysfunction, beyond those resulting in dyspareunia, have only recently been explored in a systematic fashion. In each case, it is important to determine whether the dysfunction is primary or secondary. The physician is most likely to encounter patients with secondary dysfunction from a variety of causes (Table 115–2). Psychiatric disorders and systemic illnesses predominate.

Excitement phase problems, beyond inadequate lubrication, are manifested by poor libido. Drug-induced decrease in sexual desire may be caused by many medications, especially antihypertensive agents and antidepressants. Fluoxetine, which is now widely prescribed, may cause both loss of libido and anorgasmia. Libido is a very sensitive indicator of general physical health, and any intercurrent illness (acute or chronic) will blunt it. There is no evidence that estrogen deficiency alone has an impact on libido, but androgen deficiency probably does, suggesting that small doses of testosterone may be helpful for postmenopausal women who experience loss of libido (see Chapter 118).

Secondary orgasmic dysfunction from medical causes is seen in patients who previously functioned normally. As with excitement phase problems, any illness can interfere with this part of sexual activity. For example, in one study, loss of orgasmic capacity occurred in 35 percent of diabetic women, and severity correlated with duration of the diabetes.

In both cases, once medical causes of dysfunction have been removed, or at least identified, referral to a sex therapist for the patient and her partner may be indicated. It is important for the primary care provider to be aware of well-trained resources in the community. Recognition of underlying psychopathology and psychosocial distress is also essential (see Chapter 229).

ANNOTATED BIBLIOGRAPHY

Byyny RL, Speroff L. Sexuality in the older years. In: A Clinical Guide for the Care of Older Women. Baltimore: Williams & Wilkins, 1993, p 109. *(A good review.)*

Drugs that cause sexual dysfunction: an update. Med Lett Drugs Ther 1992;34:73. *(The list continues to expand.)*

Glatt AE, Zinner SH, McCormack WM. The prevalence of dyspareunia. Obstet Gynecol 1990;75:433. *(Among college graduates with 10 to 20 years of sexual activity, >60 percent had had dyspareunia at some time and a third had had at least episodic pain chronically.)*

Marinoff SC, Turner MLC. Pudendal neuralgia. Am J Obstet Gynecol 1991;165:1233. *(Presents a hypothesis for basis for chronic vulvar pain.)*

Marinoff SC, Turner MLC. Vulvar vestibulitis syndrome: an overview. Am J Obstet Gynecol 1991;165:1228. *(Reviews evidence regarding etiology of syndrome involving pain on contact with the vestibule or on vaginal entry.)*

Mooradian AD, Grieff V: Sexuality in older women. Arch Intern Med 1990;150:1033. *(Good review of the changes that occur in the female sexual response with menopause and aging, as well as impact of common illnesses on sexual function.)*

116

Approach to the Patient With Menstrual or Pelvic Pain

KARYN M. MONTGOMERY, M.D.
ANNE W. MOULTON, M.D.

Primary Care Medicine: Office Evaluation and Management of the Adult Patient, 3rd edition, edited by Allan H. Goroll, Lawrence A. May, and Albert G. Mulley, Jr. J.B. Lippincott Company, Philadelphia

Pelvic pain is a major source of concern and morbidity for many women. Dysmenorrhea, or painful periods, affects approximately half of menstruating women at some time, and an estimated 10 percent of women are incapacitated by the problem. Acute episodes of pelvic pain are also common and may represent potentially serious pathology. The primary care physician should be able to distinguish pain of a functional nature from that due to infection or an anatomic lesion and know when referral to a gynecologist or urgent hospital admission is indicated. The generalist should also be able to initiate treatment and educate patients about the most common causes of pelvic pain.

PATHOPHYSIOLOGY AND CLINICAL PRESENTATION

The causes of pelvic pain can be organized into acute, chronic, and recurrent categories, with the latter group subdivided based on the relationship of the pain to the menstrual period (Table 116–1).

Table 116-1. Important Causes of Pelvic Pain

Acute Pain	
	Pelvic inflammatory disease
	Ectopic pregnancy with rupture
	Torsion of the fallopian tube, ovary, or ovarian cyst
	Ruptured ovarian cyst
	Extrapelvic disease (eg, appendicitis)
Recurrent Pain with Menstruation	
	Primary dysmenorrhea
	Secondary dysmenorrhea
	Endometriosis
	Adenomyosis
	Chronic pelvic inflammatory disease
	Intrauterine devices
Recurrent Pain Unrelated to Menstruation	
	Mittelschmerz (midcycle pain)
	Leaking ovarian cysts
	Nongynecologic pathology: adhesions, IBD, functional bowel
Chronic Pain	
	Benign neoplasms
	Malignancy
	Enigmatic or psychogenic pain

Acute Pain

Pelvic pain of acute onset may result from pelvic inflammatory disease, ectopic pregnancy, torsion of the fallopian tube or ovary, rupture of an ovarian cyst, or extra-pelvic pathology such as acute appendicitis or ureteral stones.

Pelvic Inflammatory Disease (PID) usually causes little pain until the infection has spread from the cervix through the lymphatics into the parametria and fallopian tubes. This process may not occur until weeks or even months after initial exposure to an infected partner. The consequent acute salpingitis is characteristically bilateral, though one side may be more involved than the other. Peritoneal signs may occur if infected discharge escapes from the fallopian tube and soils the overlying peritoneum. Mixed microbial infection is common. Organisms commonly implicated include alpha streptococci, *Chlamydia trachomatis*, *Escherichia coli*, *Neisseria gonorrhea*, *Mycoplasma*, and anaerobic organisms such as *Bacteroides*.

While epidemiologic reports of sexually transmitted diseases (STDs) suggest that *N. gonorrhea* infections are decreasing in incidence, antibiotic resistance appears to be increasing. All cases of PID should be treated presumptively for penicillin-resistant *N. gonorrhea*, pending cultures. The PID associated with *Chlamydia* appears to be less acute in onset (higher likelihood of asymptomatic cases) than that due to gonorrhea, but it is more likely to result in tubal damage and subsequent ectopic pregnancy and infertility. Because of the high prevalence of mixed infections, treatment regimens should always include coverage for *C. trachomatis* and *N. gonorrhea* (see Chapter 117).

Sequelae of PID include recurrent PID, ectopic pregnancy, infertility, and chronic pelvic or back pain. Twenty-five percent of patients with PID will have a subsequent pelvic infection. A prior episode of PID increases the risk of ectopic pregnancies by seven to 10 times. Recurrent pelvic infections also increase the risk of infertility: one episode is associated with a 12 percent risk of infertility, two episodes with 35 percent risk, and three episodes with a risk of 75 percent. Pelvic infection may also result in chronic pelvic pain.

Physical exam in patients with PID is notable for purulent cervical discharge, friability of the cervix, cervical motion tenderness, or adnexal tenderness. Occasionally, there may be peritoneal signs.

Ectopic Pregnancy. Ectopic pregnancy is a much-feared cause of acute pelvic pain, as catastrophic hemorrhage can result from tubal rupture. The incidence of ectopic pregnancies in the United States from 1970 to 1987 increased from 4.5 to 16.8 per 1000 pregnancies. The case-fatality rate, however, decreased dramatically, from 35.5 per 10,000 to 3.4 per 10,000 ectopic pregnancies. The drop in fatality rates was probably caused by improved diagnosis resulting from the sensitive radioimmunoassay for human chorionic gonadotropin (hCG), high resolution ultrasonography, and the frequent use of laparoscopy. In most cases of ectopic pregnancy, the menses is delayed by 1 to 2 weeks, followed by recurrent spotting. Pain is generally unilateral. Severe hemorrhage occurs in fewer than 5 percent of cases, causing sudden extreme pain and hypotension.

Patients with a prior history of PID, prior ectopic pregnancies, tubal surgery to enhance fertility, use of intrauterine devices, or ovulation-inducing drugs (which alter steroid hormone levels and affect tubal motility) may be predisposed to subsequent ectopic pregnancies.

Torsion. Torsion of the fallopian tube with or without ovarian involvement is seen most commonly in women of reproductive age. The adnexae may be normal except for the resulting ischemia, although most cases have cysts of the ovaries. Severe, acute, unilateral pain and distension are found without an elevation of white count, fever, or increased sedimentation rate, unless complicated by ischemic necrosis. The majority of patients will have an adnexal mass on ultrasound.

Ovarian Cyst. Ovarian cysts may spontaneously rupture or twist on their pedicles. Rupture can be associated with rapid blood loss, similar to a ruptured ectopic pregnancy. More commonly, only small amounts of fluid or blood are released, resulting in unilateral, often recurrent discomfort. Torsion of the pedicle of the cyst can cause ischemia and lead to extreme pain with acute peritoneal signs, fever, and leukocytosis.

Extrapelvic Pathology. Extrapelvic pathology which can cause acute pelvic pain includes appendicitis, kidney stones, urinary tract infections, bleeding from a Meckel's diverticulum, intestinal obstructions, and intestinal abscesses.

Chronic or Recurrent Pain

Conditions which result in recurrent or chronic pelvic pain are generally less urgent than those responsible for acute pain. Common etiologies include primary dysmenorrhea; secondary dysmenorrhea caused by endometriosis, adenomyosis, chronic pelvic inflammatory disease, and intrauterine devices (IUDs); uterine fibroids; ovarian cysts; nongynecologic pathology such as adhesions, inflammatory bowel disease, or irritable bowel syndrome; and psychogenic pain.

Primary Dysmenorrhea. Dysmenorrhea represents the major source of recurrent pelvic pain. It is classified as "primary" when there is no pelvic pathology and "secondary" when it occurs in the setting of an underlying gynecologic problem, such as endometriosis, PID, or IUD use. Primary dysmenorrhea affects as many as 50 percent of postpubertal women. It occurs in ovulatory cycles, therefore, beginning at the time of menarche, or soon after when the cycles become regular. The pain occurs at the onset menstrual blood flow and generally lasts for 48 to 72 hours. It is generally cramping in nature and can be located in the suprapubic region, the low back, or the inner aspect of the thighs. Dysmenorrhea which begins several years after menarche is usually secondary to gynecologic pathology.

Menstrual pain occurs because of increased prostaglandin production and release by the endometrium, which leads to abnormal uterine muscle activity. There have been several studies which show increased menstrual fluid prostaglandin levels (primarily PGF 2a), and increased circulating leukotriene and vasopressin levels in women with primary dysmenorrhea. High levels of these hormones lead to increased uterine tone and dysrhythmic contractions followed by reduction in uterine blood flow and ischemia. The pain may be either from the abnormal contractions, uterine ischemia, or stimulation of sensory pain fibers by the prostaglandins and bradykinin. Nonsteroidal anti-inflammatory agents, which reduce prostaglandin synthesis, are extremely effective at reducing menstrual pain.

Premenstrual Syndrome. There are many physiologic changes which occur in the second half of the menstrual cycle, and as a result of these changes a certain proportion of women will experience significant symptoms during this time which may seriously disrupt their lifestyles. In addition to pelvic pain, symptoms can include irritability, fatigue, bloating, food cravings, headache, inability to concentrate, breast tenderness, anxiety, and depression. Symptoms begin 7 to 10 days before the onset of menses, continue until within 4 days of blood flow, and are recurrent with each cycle. The etiology of the syndrome is unclear. However, recent reports have demonstrated decreased serotonergic activity in women with premenstrual syndrome during the luteal phase. Personality testing done during symptomatic periods does reveal abnormalities, but retesting at other stages of the menstrual cycle shows resolution of the changes, suggesting that psychologic factors may be a manifestation rather than a cause of the problem. Premenstrual syndrome is thought to be pathophysiologically distinct from dysmenorrhea, unrelated to prostaglandins, and unresponsive to nonsteroidals. The diagnosis of premenstrual syndrome is based on the history of symptoms and their correlation with the menstrual cycle. It is helpful to have patients keep a daily chart of their symptoms and their menses for two or more months to assess the pattern.

Endometriosis is a common cause of secondary dysmenorrhea. Endometriosis is caused by the presence of functioning ectopic endometrial tissue, located in such places as the ovaries, uterosacral ligaments, cul de sac, and peritoneum. It occurs in 1 percent to 5 percent of reproductive women, and approximately 30 percent of infertile women between ages 30 and 40. Pain from this condition can begin days or even a week before menstruation. It tends to subside with the onset of bleeding. It is usually bilateral and may radiate to the rectum or perineal region. There is frequently a history of infertility, dyspareunia, or menorrhagia. Symptoms of endometriosis depend on actively functioning endometrial tissue, with resolution at menopause. The frequency of dysmenorrhea has been found to be no different in patients with endometriosis compared with normal controls; however, patients with extensive endometriosis (stage III or IV by laparoscopy) were more likely to have acyclic pain. Diagnosis of endometriosis can only be made by laparoscopy or laparotomy.

Adenomyosis is caused by the presence of functioning ectopic endometrial tissue in the myometrium. It appears to be most common in women ages 41 to 50. The condition can cause menorrhagia, dysmenorrhea, and an enlarged, sometimes tender uterus. Pain may be referred to the back and rectum. There is a slightly increased rate of endometrial carcinoma in patients with adenomyosis.

Chronic Pelvic Inflammatory Disease is another source of secondary dysmenorrhea. A history of previous sexually transmitted disease, dyspareunia, menstrual irregularity, backache, rectal pressure, or pelvic pain with fever is often obtained. The physical examination typically reveals tender, thickened adnexae. Bilateral involvement is characteristic, although one side may predominate.

Intrauterine Devices are an important source of secondary dysmenorrhea. The rate of removal because of pain and bleeding ranges from 4 percent to 15 percent. Crampy menstrual pain may occur in a woman with a newly placed IUD who has never experienced dysmenorrhea. It is important to rule out concomitant PID in women with abdominal pain and an IUD.

Ovarian Cysts are usually painless unless complicated by torsion or rupture, which produces severe abdominal pain. Chronic intermittent discomfort that is worse at the time of ovulation or in the latter half of the cycle may be seen secondary to leakage of irritant contents.

Uterine Fibroids (leiomyomas) may produce a constant, chronic ache in the pelvis or back. They may also cause urinary symptoms (increased frequency and incontinence) and bleeding, particularly when they are submucosal. Significant pain and/or obstruction of the ureters is noted usually when the uterus is larger than 12 weeks gestation. Severe pelvic pain and fever, in a woman with a history of fibroids, can suggest necrosis of the tumor.

Nongynecologic Pathology may also cause chronic pelvic pain; this would include adhesions, inflammatory bowel disease, and irritable bowel syndrome. Of note, symptoms from irritable bowel syndrome such as pain, cramping, and change in bowel habits may also worsen in the second half of the menstrual cycle secondary to the effect of progestins on gastrointestinal motility.

Mittelschmerz or intermenstrual pain is not a form of dysmenorrhea, because it occurs in midcycle at the time of ovulation. It is more common on the right side than the left and may be accompanied by bleeding. There is some evidence that the ovary is the source of the blood loss. The pain, believed due to distention of the ovarian capsule, is harmless but annoying and a source of concern.

Enigmatic or Psychogenic Pain. The terms enigmatic pain and psychogenic pain are applied to chronic pelvic pain lasting more than 6 months without clear organic pathology. Approximately one-third of laparoscopies performed for long-standing symptoms fail to reveal any pathology.

Numerous theories for the pain have been proposed, including pelvic vascular congestion, retrodisplacement of the uterus, and rotation of the fundus on the cervix as a universal joint (this was felt to be secondary to lacerations of the broad and cardinal ligaments from prior obstetric procedures and to cause pain because of the hypermobility of the cervix with relation to the fundus in all directions). Surgical treatments that have been tried have included antefixation of a retroverted uterus, hysterectomy with or without salpingo-oophorectomy, and presacral neurectomy. While initial reports demonstrated some success with each of these techniques, the majority of patients continued to have pain. Studies have also reported continued symptoms in patients even with total exenteration of pelvic organs.

Because of lack of improvement with current surgical and medical regimens and the low incidence of demonstrable pathology, attention has turned to psychogenic etiologies and treatments for patients with chronic pelvic pain. Recent reports have demonstrated a significant association between a childhood history of sexual abuse and chronic pelvic pain. Women with chronic pelvic pain have also been found to have higher rates of alcohol and drug dependency, although it is unclear whether this is in response to their chronic pain.

WORKUP

In the patient with acute pain, it is important to determine the need for immediate hospitalization. Vital signs, including a rectal temperature, and postural changes in blood pressure and pulse are essential. Physical examination should determine whether there are signs of peritoneal irritation (rigidity, percussion tenderness, rebound), presence of bowel sounds, cervical motion tenderness, or abnormal masses. Laboratory evaluation should include a complete blood count (CBC), differential, sedimentation rate, urinalysis and serum beta-hCG subunit pregnancy test. Urine HCG testing is less sensitive; a negative urine hCG test within the first 6 weeks after the last menstrual period does not rule out an ectopic pregnancy. The serum hCG radioimmunoassay, on the other hand, can be positive as soon as one week post ovulation.

Any patient with a high fever, orthostatic hypotension or tachycardia, or an acute abdomen should be sent immediately to the hospital, even before laboratory studies are available. However, even if the situation is urgent, a few historical facts can help establish the diagnosis. Important questions would include any delay in the menstrual period, dyspareunia, IUD use, shaking chills, abnormal vaginal discharge or bleeding, recent abortion, and the location and radiation of the pain. Development of generalized severe pain is a worrisome symptom indicating possible peritoneal involvement, especially in conjunction with a rigid abdomen and absent bowel sounds. Unilateral pain suggests a local tubal or ovarian problem, whereas bilateral involvement is more indicative of PID or diffuse pelvic irritation. Symptoms of constipation, nausea, vomiting, diarrhea, flank pain, and dysuria need to be elicited to rule out nongynecologic etiologies such as appendicitis, acute pyelonephritis, or urethral stone.

If the pain is chronic or recurrent, a more detailed history should be obtained during the office visit, including the relationship of the pain to the menstrual cycle and a complete menstrual and obstetrical history. Onset of pain, quality and radiation of pain, and any exacerbating or ameliorating factors should be noted. Pain due to cervical, uterine, or vaginal pathology is often referred to the low back or buttock, while that due to tubal or ovarian problems is generally localized to one side and referred to the medial aspect of the thigh. A detailed pelvic and rectal exam should be done looking for adnexal thickening, cervical discharge, uterine masses, fixation of any structures, ovarian masses, and focal tenderness.

Laboratory testing should include a serum hCG, CBC, sedimentation rate, urinalysis, and culture of the cervix and rectum for gonorrhea and chlamydia. If a mass is felt, ultrasonography (possibly with transvaginal probe) is indicated to confirm the finding, better localize the mass, and distinguish a solid from a cystic lesion. Laparoscopy or D&C may be necessary to establish the diagnosis.

TREATMENT

Acute Pelvic Pain. Pelvic inflammatory disease may be treated on an outpatient basis if the patient is nontoxic and reliable. Antimicrobial regimens should include coverage for *Neisseria gonorrhea* and *Chlamydia trachomatis* (see Chapter 117). Patients and their partners should be educated about safe sexual practices and the sequelae of PID to prevent subsequent infections.

Other etiologies of severe acute pelvic pain, such as ectopic pregnancy, torsion of the fallopian tube or ovary, and ruptured ovarian cysts, are best managed by a specialist and should be referred immediately to a gynecologist.

Recurrent Pelvic Pain. *Primary dysmenorrhea* can be managed symptomatically with usage of *nonsteroidal anti-inflammatory agents* (NSAIDS). Over-the-counter formulations of ibuprofen are available in 200-mg strength. Ibuprofen (200–400 mg q4–6h) is frequently effective. Treatment is started up to a week before expected onset of menses and continued several days into it. Oral contraceptive pills are also helpful in decreasing dysmenorrhea because they suppress ovulation. Progestins also inhibit ovulation but do not appear to be as effective at reducing pain. This may be related to their effects on prostaglandin synthesis. Patient education about the mechanism of pain during menstruation may be helpful in alleviating symptoms.

Premenstrual syndrome, unlike primary dysmenorrhea, is unresponsive to NSAID therapy. Lifestyle changes such as regular aerobic exercise, daily vitamins, and the elimination of xanthines, alcohol, and salt from the diet appear helpful but offer only limited improvement. Several studies have shown dramatic reduction in both the physical and psychological symptoms of premenstrual syndrome with the use of fluoxetine. There appears to be more benefit for behavioral symptoms (75% reduction) than for the physical symptoms (40% reduction). Progesterone has not proven useful.

Endometriosis will most likely be managed by specialists, because the diagnosis is made only by laparoscopy or laparotomy. However, it is important to be aware of the medications used to treat endometriosis, as they can have some significant side effects. Oral contraceptive pills may be used continuously to achieve a "pseudo-pregnancy" effect on the endometrial tissue. Cessation of menstrual periods may decrease the painful symptoms. Danazol and gonadotropin releasing hormone (GnRH) agonists both inhibit gonadal function, leading to a pharmacologic menopause. Danazol is associated with androgenic side effects such as hirsutism, acne, and weight gain, while GnRH agonists typically have more hypoestrogenic side effects, such as hot flashes, osteoporosis, and vaginal dryness.

Other causes of recurrent pelvic pain, such as IUDs, uterine fibroids, and ovarian cysts, are best managed by a gynecologist. Indications for hysterectomy for uterine fibroids are substantial bleeding, significant pelvic pain or obstruction, or anemia refractory to iron replacement.

Chronic Pelvic Pain is best managed by a combination of psychological, behavioral and medical treatments. Primary care physicians are in a unique position to coordinate this type of therapy. Patients with chronic pain need reassurance that further diagnostic testing is unnecessary, that the physician is not abandoning them, and that there is treatment for their suffering. Psychological therapy can help pinpoint triggers for their pain and address previous sexual trauma (if any). Behavioral therapy can help decrease pain through relaxation techniques. Self-hypnosis may also be beneficial. Because of the frequency of concomitant depression and the known beneficial effects of the tricylic antidepressant amitriptyline in patients with chronic pain, it may be useful to consider an antidepressant medication in some cases.

INDICATIONS FOR REFERRAL

Patients with pelvic pain and an acute abdomen should be sent immediately to the hospital with referral to a gynecologic surgeon. Women with a pelvic mass detected by physical exam should be referred, although it may be helpful to obtain an ultrasound prior to the patient's initial visit with the gynecologist. Suspicion of chronic pelvic inflammatory disease, endometriosis, adenomyosis, ovarian cyst, or other condition best assessed by laparoscopy should prompt consultation with a gynecologist.

ANNOTATED BIBLIOGRAPHY

Barbieri RL. Endometriosis 1990. Current treatment approaches. Drugs 1990;39:502. *(Discussion of pharmacologic therapies for the treatment of endometriosis.)*

Bider D, et al. Clinical, surgical, and pathologic findings of adnexal torsion in pregnant and nonpregnant women. Surg Gynecol Obstet 1991;173:363. *(Case series of women with adnexal torsion at laparotomy.)*

Carlson KJ, et al. Indications for hysterectomy. N Engl J Med 1993;328:856. *(Discussion of the indications for hysterectomy including uterine leiomyomas, endometriosis, and chronic pelvic pain.)*

Chronic pelvic pain. Clin Obstet Gynecol 1990;33:119. *(Entire volume devoted to discussion of etiology, diagnosis, and treatment of chronic pelvic pain. Excellent section on psychogenic chronic pelvic pain.)*

Dingfelder JR. Prostaglandin inhibitors: new treatment for an old nemesis. N Engl J Med 1982;307:746. *(An editorial examining the pathophysiology and treatment of primary dysmenorrhea, with emphasis on prostaglandins.)*

Enigmatic pelvic pain (editorial). Br Med J 1978;2:1041. *(A review of the difficult problems of managing pelvic pain in the absence of detectable pathology.)*

Freeman E, Rickels K, Sondheimer SJ, et al. Ineffectiveness of progesterone suppository treatment of premenstrual syndrome: A placebo-controlled, randomized, double-blind cross-over study. JAMA 1990;264:349. *(No benefit found.)*

McCormack WM. Pelvic inflammatory disease. N Engl J Med 1994;330:115. *(Excellent review of clinical characteristics, pathogenesis, and treatment.)*

Muse KN, Cetel NS, Futterman LA, et al. The premenstrual syndrome: Effects of "medical ovariectomy." N Engl J Med 1984;311:1345. *(An intriguing double-blind, placebo-controlled study showing that use of an experimental GnRH agonist is effective in providing symptomatic relief.)*

Ory SJ. New options for diagnosis and treatment of ectopic pregnancy. JAMA 1992;267:534. *(Information on current diagnosis and treatment options.)*

Peters AAW, et al. A randomized clinical trial to compare two different approaches in women with chronic pelvic pain. Obstet Gynecol 1991;77:740. *(Study showing the efficacy of an integrated approach to patients with chronic pelvic pain by addressing psychological, dietary, and environmental factors in addition to somatic complaints.)*

Rubinow DR. The premenstrual syndrome: New views. JAMA 1992;268:1908. *(A look at the biologic triggers of the mood disturbances.)*

Trobough GE. Pelvic pain and the IUD. J Reprod Med 1977; 20:167. *(A thorough review of the role of IUDs in producing pelvic pain; 36 refs.)*

Walker E, et al. Relationship of chronic pelvic pain to psychiatric diagnoses and childhood sexual abuse. Am J Psychiatry 1988;145:75. *(Comparison study of women with chronic pelvic pain and women undergoing laparoscopy for infertility or tubal ligation for rates of sexual abuse, depression, alcohol, and drug use.)*

Wood SH, et al. Treatment of premenstrual syndrome with fluoxetine: A double-blind, placebo-controlled, crossover study. Obstet Gynecol 1992;80:339. *(A well-controlled study demonstrating significant reduction [62 percent] in both physical and psychological symptoms with fluoxetine.)*

Primary Care Medicine: Office Evaluation and Management of the Adult Patient, 3rd edition, edited by Allan H. Goroll, Lawrence A. May, and Albert G. Mulley, Jr. J.B. Lippincott Company, Philadelphia

117
Approach to the Patient With a Vaginal Discharge

ANNE W. MOULTON, M.D.
KARYN M. MONTGOMERY, M.D.

Vaginal discharge is one of the 25 most common reasons that women consult physicians in private office practice in the United States. Vaginal infections not only are extremely prevalent but also result in considerable discomfort for the patient. One should endeavor to make an accurate diagnosis and not rely on empiric therapy. A complete history, a systematic examination of the patient, and a microscopic examination of the discharge, will enable one to identify the cause in most cases and choose the appropriate therapy. Patient education can help to allay fears, encourage compliance, and reduce recurrences.

PATHOPHYSIOLOGY AND CLINICAL PRESENTATION

Normal vaginal discharge contains desquamated vaginal epithelial cells, secretions from cervical glands and from the uterus, and bacteria and bacterial products, including lactic acid. Under the microscope, the vaginal microflora of healthy asymptomatic women appear as moderate numbers of unclumped, rodlike organisms. These consist of a wide variety of anaerobic and aerobic bacterial genera and species dominated by *Lactobacillus*. The pH of a normal vagina is between 3.5 and 4.1. The vaginal environment, which is in a delicate balance, is easily altered by numerous internal and external influences. The amount or quality of vaginal discharge can be affected by normal changes in the body's hormonal milieu, such as midcycle mucus production with ovulation, menstruation, or the atrophic mucosal changes that occur after menopause.

The most common cause of an abnormal discharge is infection with bacteria, yeast, or parasites (Table 117–1). Infections with organisms such as *Trichomonas vaginalis* and *Candida albicans* generally induce an inflammatory response in the vaginal wall, which is accompanied by an increased number of leukocytes in the vaginal fluid, so-called "vaginitis." Recently, the term "nonspecific vaginitis" has been replaced by the term *bacterial vaginosis* (BV), to describe a condition of bacterial overgrowth in which inflammation is not a feature. Bacterial vaginosis is the most common form of vaginal infection (40%–50%), followed closely by vulvovaginal candidiasis (20%–25%) and finally trichomoniasis, which occurs less frequently (15%–20%). The clinical presentation, including type, amount, and odor of discharge, depends, in part, on the underlying etiologic agent.

Trichomoniasis occurs in approximately 3 million women annually. Contrary to previous belief, *Trichomonas vaginalis*, a small, mobile protozoan, is not part of normal vaginal flora. It is sexually transmitted and frequently occurs in the presence of other infections. It occurs in 13 percent to 25 percent of women attending gynecology clinics and 7 percent to 35 percent of women attending STD clinics. The belief that *T. vaginalis* is sexually transmitted is also supported by the high prevalence (30%–70%) in male partners of infected women and the improved cure rates of infected women whose partners are also treated. A substantial percentage of women with trichomoniasis (10%–50%) are asymptomatic, but one-third of asymptomatic infected women become symptomatic within 6 months.

Symptoms include vaginal discharge, pruritus, dyspareunia (caused by vulvar edema), dysuria, increased frequency of micturition, and abdominal pain. Physical examination generally reveals vulvar erythema and edema and, occasionally, characteristic petechial hemorrhages of the external genitalia and cervix (strawberry cervix is seen by the naked eye in only 1%–2% of patients). Vaginal discharge may be minimal or abundant, frothy and foul-smelling. Signs and symptoms alone are not sufficiently helpful to make the definitive diagnosis.

Candidiasis is very common in the vagina. Yeast is often recovered as a commensal organism in the vagina. In one private practice study, the incidence of candidiasis was 8.5 percent, and of these individuals, 25 percent were asymptomatic. In women with symptoms, complaints include vulvar pruritus and burning associated with a discharge. Symptoms are usually rather rapid in onset, occurring shortly before menstruation when the pH of the vagina falls. On physical examination, erythema, edema, and excoriation of the vulva are often prominent; sometimes there are pustules apparent on the skin. The discharge is typically thick, white, and adherent, often described as resembling cottage cheese.

Bacterial Vaginosis, previously referred to as gardnerella vaginitis or "nonspecific vaginitis," can be asymptomatic in up to 50 percent of women. The clinical picture tends to be one of mild discomfort, although in 10 percent to 20 percent of cases the vaginal burning and itching are more pronounced. Sometimes patients note a disagreeable odor. The discharge ranges from grayish to occasionally a yellow-green color. Wet mount of the discharge shows short, motile rods and characteristic *"clue cells"* (vaginal epithelial cells with a stippled appearance due to the adherence of bacilli on their surfaces). The diagnosis of bacterial vaginosis is made by the presence of three of the four following criteria: 1) vaginal pH greater than 4.5; 2) thin, white, homogenous discharge; 3) positive amine test; 4) clue cells on saline wet prep.

There are several other infectious etiologies that need to be considered in the differential diagnosis of a vaginal discharge. *Gonorrhea* (also covered in Chapter 137) can produce a thick, purulent, irritating discharge involving the cer-

Table 117-1. Common Causes of Vaginal Discharge

Infectious	
	Bacterial vaginosis
	Vulvovaginal candidiasis
	Trichomonas vaginitis
	Mucopurulent cervicitis (*C. trachomatis*)
	Gonorrhea
	Condyloma acuminatum
	Herpes virus type 2
	Cytolytic vaginosis
Normal discharge secondary to hormonal changes	
	Physiologic leukorrhea (midcycle cervical mucus/ postintercourse)
	Atrophic vaginitis
Other	
	Chemical/allergic vaginitis, foreign body
	Desquamative inflammatory vaginitis (erosive lichen planus)
	Chronic cervicitis
	Cervical ectropion
	Cervical polyps
	Cervical and endometrial cancer
	Collagen vascular diseases

vix, vagina, and urethra. In *type 2 herpes virus* (discussed in Chapter 192), the infection can extend to the cervix in 75 percent of cases, producing ulceration, friability, and a grayish exudate in conjunction with a profuse watery discharge. *Condyloma acuminata*, genital warts caused by papillomavirus, can cause in severe cases a profuse, irritating vaginal discharge (see Chapter 141). *Mucopurulent cervicitis* caused by *Chlamydia trachomatis* is characterized by a thick, yellow-white discharge coming from the cervical os, in conjunction with 10 or more leukocytes per microscopic field (high-power oil-immersion) on Gram-stain examination. Erythema, friability, and ectocervical ulceration may occur.

Cytolytic Vaginosis is a condition thought to be caused by an overgrowth of lactobacilli, and possibly other bacteria, which causes cytolysis of vaginal epithelium and a frothy white discharge. Symptoms, which usually increase during the second half of the menstrual cycle, include dyspareunia, vulvar pruritus, and dysuria. Physical examination is remarkable for the presence of white, frothy discharge and a pH level between 3.5 and 4.5. The four diagnostic criteria observed on wet mount are 1) absence of *Trichomonas*, bacterial vaginosis, and *Candida*; 2) few leukocytes; 3) increased lactobacilli; and 4) cytolysis of vaginal epithelial cell. Patients with cytolytic vaginosis are frequently misdiagnosed as having chronic yeast infections and treated unsuccessfully with various antifungal medications, especially when the health care provider relies on the patient's symptoms and not on a thorough examination of the wet mount.

Atrophic Vaginitis is the most common cause of vaginal discharge in older postmenopausal women. Estrogen deficiency leads to thinning of the vaginal epithelium with a decrease in the superficial layer. The vaginal pH increases to 7.0, and the potential pathogens change from those listed above to streptococci, coliform bacteria and gut anaerobes. Symptoms include vaginal and vulvar burning and soreness, occasional bleeding or itching, and dyspareunia. External burning on urination is sometimes noted, resulting from localized irritation of raw and inflamed mucosa rather than from infection of the urinary tract. Examination of the vaginal mucosa reveals a thin, erythematous surface and scant watery discharge.

Other Causes. There are a variety of other processes that cause vaginal discharge less frequently. *Lichen planus* is an idiopathic inflammatory mucocutaneous disease which causes a desquamative vaginitis. Certain *collagen vascular diseases* can also produce a type of vaginal inflammation and discharge. *Chronic cervicitis* can result from extensive chronic cervical inflammation and has been implicated in the pathogenesis of cervical eversion, squamous metaplasia, basal cell hyperplasia, leukoplakia, polyps, and carcinoma. The discharge is thick, tenacious, and yellowish-white and may be streaked with blood. Cervical inspection reveals edematous, grossly inflamed, and friable tissue. *Cervical ectropion* is found in 15 percent to 20 percent of healthy young women. It represents columnar epithelium that is found farther out on the exocervix, causing the cervix to appear granular and red. An increase in a nonirritating vaginal discharge consisting of mucus can be seen with a large ectropion.

DIFFERENTIAL DIAGNOSIS

The most common cause of an abnormal vaginal discharge in women of childbearing age is infection. If an infectious etiology is not identified, other causes must be considered, including hormonal changes, allergens, and foreign bodies. The most common irritants are intrauterine devices (IUDs); condoms; spermicidal foams, jellies, and creams; deodorants; sprays; soaps; and any chemical douches. Foreign bodies include forgotten tampons, condoms, diaphragms, and IUDs. Some vaginal discharge is expected after conization or cauterization. Cervical polyps and uterine fibroids, as well as neoplasms of the vulva, vagina, uterus, ovaries, or fallopian tubes, may produce abnormal discharge (see Table 117-1).

WORKUP

History should include the onset of the discharge, its appearance, amount, odor (if any), and any associated symptoms. The relation of the discharge to phase of menstrual cycle, coitus, and use of medication (especially antibiotics) should be noted. Details about associated symptoms such as dysuria, pruritus, pain, dyspareunia, and skin rash provide additional information. Use of a pad or tampon can be a precipitating factor or a sign of excessive discharge. Asking the patient for a detailed sexual history will aid in understanding whether she is at particular risk for any infections. Questions should be asked about possible exposure to sexually transmitted diseases and whether the patient's partner has a complaint of penile discharge or lesion. Known allergies need to be reviewed in conjunction with use of spermicidal preparations and douches. Patients should be asked about use of foreign bodies and bubble baths, soaps, or genital deodorants. A history of a previous vaginal infection, diabetes, or the recent use of antibiotics or corticosteroids needs to be considered in a search for alterations in vaginal flora or host defenses. Any self-treatment should be carefully inquired about, because antifungal medication is now readily available over-the-counter.

Physical Examination begins with careful inspection of the vulva and vaginal canal for evidence of lesions, discharge, erythema, atrophy, or prolapse. During the speculum examination, the surface of the cervix should be examined carefully, looking for any lesions, erosion, erythema, or friability. The color, consistency, pH, and odor of the discharge can provide useful clues to the etiology. On bimanual examination, the provider should check for tenderness on cervical motion and for adnexal and uterine masses.

Laboratory Studies. A wet-mount examination of the discharge is simple and potentially diagnostic. A fresh sample is placed on a microscopic slide to which a drop or two of normal saline is added, and a cover slip is placed over the suspension. The pH should be tested and the slide examined before the sample dries. Although the sensitivity of the wet mount for the detection of the motile, ovoid, trichomonads is low (25%), the finding is very specific and permits immediate diagnosis. The sample pH for *Trichomonas* is usually greater than 5.0. Although Gram's and Giemsa stains show no advantage to wet mount, cultures (which have been anaerobically incubated) have a sensitivity of up to 95 percent for the presence of trichomonads.

Saline wet mount of patients with bacterial vaginosis characteristically show few polymorphonuclear neutrophils (PMNs) and many (>20%) clue cells. Two additional diagnostic criteria for BV are a sample pH higher than 4.5 and a positive amine test (the presence of a "fishy odor" after adding potassium hydroxide [KOH] to a sample).

Adding a drop of 10 percent KOH to a sample of the discharge also aids in the recognition of *Candida*. The KOH dissolves most cellular material except for the filamentous hyphae and budding forms of *Candida*; the sensitivity of the test ranges from 40 percent to 80 percent. Gram's stain has an even higher sensitivity for detection of *Candida*. The vaginal pH with a candidal infection is closer to normal. Vaginal cultures for *Candida* are not routinely utilized but can be done on Nickerson's medium if microscopy is negative and presentation is highly suggestive of *Candida*. A wet smear of a patient's discharge that is suspected to have cytolytic vaginosis should show few leukocytes; no *Trichomonas*, clue cells, or filamentous hyphae; and an increased number of lactobacilli with evidence of epithelial cytolysis and a pH close to normal.

When other causes of vaginal discharge, such as gonorrhea and chlamydia, are being considered, a Gram's stain of the discharge can yield additional information (see Chapters 125 and 137). A Gram's stain is useful in identifying mucopurulent cervicitis due to chlamydial infection, because the presence of more than 10 leukocytes per oil-immersion field distinguishes it from other types of cervicitis. Further suspicion of *Chlamydia* infection can be followed up with direct immunofluorescent staining or culture.

A few other laboratory studies may be helpful. A complete blood count is indicated if pelvic pain or dysuria is present. Urinalysis should be obtained to check for pyuria and bacteriuria, especially if there is concurrent dysuria or flank pain. Women with poorly controlled and, occasionally, new-onset diabetes mellitus, can present with persistent or recurrent yeast infections, and a fasting blood sugar may be useful. A Papanicolaou (Pap) smear should be done, recognizing that it may be abnormal in the presence of inflammation (see Chapter 107). In some patients with obvious infection, it may be reasonable to defer the Pap test until the vaginitis or cervicitis has been treated. However, with chronic inflammation of the cervix, Pap testing and probably colposcopy are indicated.

MANAGEMENT

Trichomonal Vaginitis. *Metronidazole* is the treatment of choice for trichomoniasis (Table 117–2). This drug is probably most effective if administered orally in a dosage of 500 mg twice daily for 7 days, with cure rates up to 95 percent. A one-time oral dose of 2.0 g is less effective (80%–88%) but has better compliance rates. Efficacy for single-dose therapy is increased if the male partner is also treated. Some authorities advocate simultaneous treatment of male sexual partners in all cases; others treat the male only if the female relapses. Recommended therapy for recurrent *T. vaginalis* infections is an additional 1-week treatment with metronidazole (500 mg bid), and if symptoms persist, 2 g every day for 3 to 5 days. Patients should be instructed to avoid alcohol intake while taking the drug because of its disulfiram-like effects. Other side effects include nausea and transient neutropenia. Metronidazole is contraindicated in the first trimester of pregnancy because of the risk of fetal malformation. For patients allergic to metronidazole and for pregnant women, alternative and less effective therapies include topical clotrimazole or betadine jelly. Vinegar douches may be palliative.

Candidal Vaginitis. In considering treatment for candidal vaginitis, precipitants such as the use of broad-spectrum antibiotics, oral contraceptives, or corticosteroids or the presence of diabetes need to be addressed. First-line treatment for candidiasis is the use of topical agents. Oral agents are reserved for recurrent infections. The more common topical agents, nystatin and imidazole derivatives, act to decrease the fungal cell membrane permeability. Synthetic imidazole derivatives provide an increased cure rate of 85 percent to 90 percent when compared with nystatin (75%–80%). Generic nystatin is the least expensive of available therapies, but it must be used for longer periods than newer agents. The new agents often provide symptomatic relief within 2 days, although patients should be encouraged to complete their treatment course (3–7 d). Treatment is usually avoided during the first trimester of pregnancy because of potential risk to the developing fetus. During the second and third trimester, treatment courses are usually longer (14 days) because of decreased response rate and increased recurrence. Symptomatic relief of vulvar irritation can be obtained by using witch hazel compresses or cool water and recovery hastened by application of nystatin or a synthetic imidazole cream directly to the vulva.

For recurrent vulvovaginal candidiasis, prophylactic treatment has been achieved with 100 mg ketoconazole each day for 6 months, but the drug is very expensive, and hepatotoxicity is a concern with such prolonged use. Since *Candida* is normally found in the gastrointestinal tract, perianal

Table 117-2. Treatment for Common Vaginal Infections*

ORGANISM	MEDICATION	DOSE	APPROX. COST
Candida	butoconazole (Femstat)	suppository or cream for 3–7 days	$27.00 (28 g cream)
	clotrimazole (Mycelex)		$22.00 (vag. supp.)
	miconazole (Monistat)		$22.00 (vag. supp.)
	teraconazole (Terazol)		$33.00 (vag. supp.)
	nystatin	suppository or cream for 7–14 days	$11.00 (vag. supp.)
	ketoconazole	100 mg qd up to 6 mo (for recurrent infections and pending FDA approv. for acute infection)	$72.00 (#20 tablets)
Bacterial Vaginosis	metronidazole	2 g po single dose or	$ 9.00
		500 mg po bid for 7 days	$15.00
	metronidazole gel	suppository bid for 5 days	$28.00
	clindamycin	300 mg po bid for 7 days or	$44.00
		2% cream bid for 7 days	$42.00
Trichomonas	metronidazole	2 g po single dose or	$ 9.00
		500 mg po bid × 7 days	$15.00

*Includes treatment of initial episodes only. For recurrent infections, see text.

contamination is thought to be a possible cause of recurrent infections. Therefore, educating the patient about proper hygiene is important (see patient information section). Treatment of male partners is not usually recommended.

Bacterial Vaginosis. The best results for treatment of bacterial vaginosis have occurred with *metronidazole* therapy with a usual oral dose of 500 mg twice daily for 7 days. A single dose of 2 g metronidazole is also effective, because of increased compliance. Recently metronidazole intravaginal *gel* has been introduced for 5-day, twice-daily treatment. If there are contraindications or side effects to metronidazole use, oral or topical *clindamycin* is an alternate. Only limited success in treatment has occurred with use of ampicillin or amoxicillin, because of beta-lactamase produced by vaginal flora. Treatment of the sexual partner is not routine, since bacterial vaginosis is not sexually transmitted, but it may be indicated to reduce the recurrence rates in certain women.

Mucopurulent Cervicitis, resulting from *Chlamydia*, responds to *doxycycline* (100 mg bid for 7 d) or *erythromycin* (500 mg qid for 7 d), with treatment of the partner and follow-up culture 1 week after completed treatment. Two recently available medications, ofloxacin and azithromycin are also effective, but more expensive.

Cytolytic Vaginosis is treated with *sodium bicarbonate douches* 2 to 3 times a week, then once or twice a week as needed to increase the pH of the vagina and decrease the amount of lactobacilli. The recommended douching solution should include 30 to 60 g of sodium bicarbonate to 1 L of warm water. Commercially prepared sodium bicarbonate douches are also available.

Atrophic Vaginitis. *Estrogen cream* applied vaginally works to restore mucosal layers of squamous epithelium. Treatment is best achieved by topical use of estrogen cream for 1 to 2 weeks, followed with treatment for 1 to 2 days for occasional symptom control. Although they are less effective, oral conjugated estrogens can be prescribed (see Chapter 118).

PATIENT EDUCATION AND INDICATIONS FOR REFERRAL

Patient education is important whether the vaginal discharge is caused by normal physiologic changes, an infection, or a noninfectious process. All women should be educated about hormonal changes and their effect on the presence and appearance of normal physiologic vaginal discharge. Most infectious causes of vaginal discharge, except for bacterial vaginosis, candidiasis, and cytolytic vaginosis, are known to be sexually transmitted. Patients with discharge caused by *Trichomonas* or *Chlamydia* should be given information about the need for examination and concurrent treatment of partners and the role of barrier methods of contraception. In the prevention of these infections, women with recurrent yeast infections should be advised to avoid nylon underwear, panty hose, wet bathing suits, and tight jeans.

All patients with vaginitis, especially allergic vaginitis, should be advised to avoid douches, irritant soaps, bubble baths, and genital deodorants. Patient education about personal hygiene, including wiping from front to back after urination, is important. Often the patient's vulvar and vaginal discomfort is relieved after a few days of treatment, yet the patient should be encouraged to complete the treatment course and to abstain from intercourse during treatment, to prevent recurrence or further irritation.

Referral is needed for any patient with suspicious cervical or vaginal lesions, especially if there are erosions and ulcerations that fail to clear with treatment of a known pathogen. Colposcopy and biopsy are indicated.

ANNOTATED BIBLIOGRAPHY

Cibley L, Cibley L. Cytolytic vaginosis. Am J Obstet Gynecol 1991;165:1245. *(Review of a relatively unknown type of vaginosis.)*

Cook R, et al. Clinical, microbiological and biochemical factors in recurrent bacterial vaginosis. J Clin Microbiol 1992;30:870. *(After successful therapy, early BV recurrence represents relapse rather than reinfection.)*

Faro S. Bacterial vaginitis. Clin Obstet Gynecol 1991;34:582. *(BV has a significant impact on the number of office visits per year, a woman's psychosocial well-being, and the development of subsequent ob/gyn infections.)*

Horowitz B. Mycotic vulvovaginitis: a broad overview. Am J Obstet Gynecol 1991;165:1188. *(Mycotic vulvovaginitis is on the rise especially due to varied species.)*

Kent H. Epidemiology of vaginitis. Am J Obstet Gynecol 1991; 165:1168. *(Epidemiology of candidiasis, BV, and trichomoniasis in the U.S. and Scandinavia.)*

Krieger JN, Tam MR, Stevens CE, et al. Diagnosis of *trichomoniasis*. JAMA 1988;259:1223. *(Includes data on sensitivity and specificity of wet-mount, cytologic study, and antibody testing.)*

Lago-Miro V, Green M, Mazur L. Comparison of different metronidazole therapeutic regimens for bacterial vaginosis. JAMA 1992;268:92. *(The 2-gram oral dose as effective as any program.)*

Lossick J, Kent H. Trichomoniasis: trends in diagnosis and management. Am J Obstet Gynecol 1991;165:1217. *(Wet prep remains the first-line diagnostic tool. Also discusses metronidazole resistance and other possible treatment.)*

McCormack WM. Pelvic inflammatory disease. N Engl J Med 1994;330:115. *(Excellent review of pathogenesis, clinical presentation, and treatment.)*

Mordh P. Vaginal ecosystem. Am J Obstet Gynecol 1991;165: 1163. *(Discusses mechanism involved in vaginal flora alterations that may cause vaginitis, vaginosis, and pelvic inflammatory disease.)*

Redondo-Lopez V, et al. Emerging role of lactobacilli in the control and maintenance of the vaginal bacterial microflora. Rev Infect Dis 1990;12:856. *(Interaction between Lactobacilli and other bacterial species and the maintenance of normal vaginal flora.)*

Schaaf VM, et al. The limited value of symptoms and signs in the diagnosis of vaginal infections. Arch Intern Med 1990;150: 1929. *(Discusses the limitations of signs, symptoms, and microbiologic diagnosis.)*

Sobel JD. Vaginal infections in adult women. Med Clin North Am 1990;74:1573. *(Excellent, comprehensive review concentrating on BV, vulvovaginal candidiasis, and trichomoniasis.)*

Thomason J, et al. Bacterial vaginosis: current review with indication for asymptomatic therapy. Am J Obstet Gynecol 1991; 165:1210. *(Infection with BV is not always benign and can cause a risk for women postoperatively and during pregnancy.)*

Primary Care Medicine: Office Evaluation and Management of the Adult Patient, 3rd edition, edited by Allan H. Goroll, Lawrence A. May, and Albert G. Mulley, Jr. J.B. Lippincott Company, Philadelphia

118
Approach to the Menopausal Woman

If one uses the generally accepted definition of menopause as a full year without menstrual flow in a previously menstruating woman, then the incidence of menopause is 10 percent by age 38, 20 percent by age 43, 50 percent by age 48, 90 percent by age 54, and 100 percent by age 58. In addition, the prevalence of surgically induced menopause is estimated to be 25 percent to 30 percent of women in their mid-fifties. Despite its inevitability for the woman who lives through her sixth decade, menopause can be difficult in a society that ostensibly celebrates youthfulness. Although many of the emotional and physical changes blamed on menopause are not related to decreased estrogen levels, the cessation of menstruation has major symbolic significance, and, as a result, many symptoms and complaints are attributed to it. Hormone replacement therapy is very effective in dealing with the specific symptoms of estrogen deficiency and confers disease-prevention benefits. But hormone replacement therapy also involves potential harm, including an increased risk of cancer in some women. The primary physician can do a great deal to help women understand menopause as well as the benefits and risks of hormone replacement therapy.

PHYSIOLOGY AND CLINICAL PRESENTATION

The essential cause of menopause is decreased estrogen due to decreased responsiveness to follicle-stimulating hormone (FSH) in aging ovaries. This results in cessation of menses and rise in gonadotropins. Some estrogen production continues, but its source is primarily peripheral conversion of androstenedione. The diagnosis of menopause is confirmed by a marked increase in the gonadotropins; maximum levels of FSH and luteinizing hormone (LH) occur within 1 to 2 years of onset and remain high for 10 to 15 years. The physiologic events are similar in surgically induced menopause, but the time course is shorter, with FSH and LH rising to high levels within 20 to 30 days. Approximately 25 percent of women do not experience any symptoms, perhaps because of nonovarian sources of estrogen production.

Hot Flashes, believed to be related to rate of estrogen withdrawal and resultant vasomotor instability, are among the most specific of menopausal symptoms. An uncomfortably warm sensation radiates upward from the chest to neck and face and lasts seconds to a few minutes before subsiding. Skin temperature generally increases by about 2.5°C. The response is thought to be triggered by a hypothalamic mechanism related to catecholamine metabolism. Eating, exertion, emotional upset, and alcohol are known precipitants. As many as 20 episodes per day may occur; in most patients, the condition lasts for 2 to 3 years, but it may continue for 6 years or more. Prevalence of severe, disabling hot flashes ranges from 10 percent to 35 percent of menopausal women. No link between emotional makeup and symptoms has been demonstrated, though it is clear that the flashes can be very distracting and cause considerable misery and upset.

Other clinical manifestations of estrogen decline include *atrophy* of the *vaginal mucosa* and vulvar epithelium. The vagina becomes smaller and less compliant; lubrication decreases. Women may present with complaints of itching, discharge, bleeding, or painful intercourse. The uterus becomes smaller, but this causes no symptoms. The urethra becomes atrophic, and perineal bacteria colonize the area, increasing the risk of urethritis and dysuria. Of interest is the finding that sexually active women show less vaginal atrophy. Whether this is a cause or effect is unclear.

Sleep Disturbances occur in many menopausal women. Some are associated with nocturnal hot flashes. In addition, abnormalities in the sleep pattern, with decrease in rapid eye movement (REM) sleep, have been documented independent of hot flashes.

Cardiovascular Disease is the most common cause of morbidity and mortality among postmenopausal women. Risk of heart disease increases with age, but it is not clear that the rate of change increases in association with menopause.

Osteoporosis represents an important consequence of estrogen decline; decreased activity, inadequate nutrition, and the aging process also contribute, to varying degrees. Although irreversible, osteoporosis can be prevented by prophylactic administration of estrogen (see Chapter 164).

Various other symptoms, such as headache, nervousness, and depression, which frequently occur during the climacteric, are more a reflection of the emotional stress attending this difficult stage of life than a result of a change in hormonal milieu. Some women report feeling better emotionally on estrogen therapy, but this may represent a placebo effect. No specific psychiatric problems have been found to be linked specifically to menopause.

The cosmetic changes associated with aging have been attributed by some to a decrease in estrogens, but clinical evidence is to the contrary. Breast atrophy, loss of skin turgor, and redistribution of fat to the abdomen and thighs have not been shown to be influenced by estrogen therapy and most likely are part of the more general process of aging.

PRINCIPLES OF MANAGEMENT

Short-term objectives are to alleviate any distracting or disabling symptoms that result from estrogen deficiency and to provide support for the host of emotional and functional problems that may accompany this phase of life. The use of hormone replacement therapy to prevent disease and thereby extend and improve the quality of life is also an important consideration.

Benefits of Estrogen Replacement Therapy. Because much of the medical morbidity of menopause, including symptoms such as hot flashes, relates to estrogen deficiency, the clinician and patient are faced with the difficult decision of when to use replacement therapy. This necessitates careful consideration of benefits and risks.

Hot Flashes. Hot flashes severe enough to be a serious bother to the patient are an important indication for estrogen replacement. In most instances, the symptoms are self-limited, but relief during the year or two that symptoms are most severe can mean much and is one of the principal benefits of treatment for symptomatic women.

Atrophic Vaginitis. Atrophic vaginitis responds well to both topical and oral administration of estrogen. Even when vaginal creams are used, systemic estrogen absorption does take place and risks of adverse estrogen effects must still be considered a possibility, though probably to a lesser degree than with the use of systemic therapy. Milder symptoms (eg, mild dryness with intercourse) may respond well to use of a water-soluble vaginal lubricant and obviate the need for estrogen in the woman who wants to avoid its use.

Sleep Disorders. Sleep disorders may improve with estrogen replacement. Increases in the rate of REM sleep have been documented, regardless of whether hot flashes have been experienced.

Postmenopausal Osteoporosis. Osteoporosis can be prevented by long-term prophylactic estrogen therapy (see Chapter 164). Controlled studies have shown that rates of vertebral, wrist, and hip fractures can be reduced by 50 percent to 80 percent when estrogen replacement therapy is used for at least 5 years. Exercise and good nutrition, ensuring adequate calcium and vitamin D intake, also slow osteoporotic changes, but not as effectively as estrogen. Nevertheless, the addition of 1.0 to 1.5 g of dietary calcium carbonate per day will compensate for the intestinal malabsorption of calcium that results from estrogen deficiency and will retard bone loss, especially when combined with regular exercise. Vitamin D treatment is not beneficial unless serum levels of 25-OH vitamin D_3 are low. Small doses (400 U/d) are helpful in preventing vitamin D deficiency in elderly women; large doses are unnecessary. Risk factors for postmenopausal osteoporotic fractures include thin body build, premature surgical menopause, cigarette smoking, and heavy alcohol use. Prolonged bed rest is a potent stimulus of osteoporosis.

Since the condition is largely irreversible and resumes once therapy is stopped, treatment must be initiated prophylactically in the perimenopausal period and continued indefinitely. Ten to 15 years of therapy is not uncommon, and even more prolonged therapy is likely in the future as the average life span increases. For women willing to accept the increased risk of endometrial cancer and possible other risks in return for the best possible means of preventing osteoporosis, estrogen therapy in conjunction with exercise and modest dietary calcium supplementation offers the best option. Addition of a progestin to the long-term estrogen program is advocated as a means of limiting the risk of endometrial cancer, but it does not effect osteoporosis risk. Women who are reluctant to take estrogen should be encouraged to engage in an exercise program and maintain an adequate calcium intake (see also Chapter 164).

Cardiovascular Disease. Risk of cardiovascular disease is reduced by estrogen replacement. More than 30 published studies have evaluated the effect of estrogen replacement on risk of cardiovascular disease, and most of these have demonstrated a significant protective effect. Estimates of the relative risk of developing and dying of coronary disease among women who have ever used estrogens, compared to those who have never used them, range from 0.50 to 0.65. This 35-percent to 50-percent reduction in risk is extremely important on a population basis, because coronary heart disease is the leading cause of death among postmenopausal women. The effect of estrogen plus progestin on cardiovascular risk appears to be similar to that of estrogen alone. A feared negation of estrogen's beneficial lipoprotein effects by the addition of progesterone has not materialized. However, effect on cardiovascular morbidity and mortality remains to be determined.

Risks of Estrogen Replacement Therapy. Though relief of symptoms and disease prevention benefits have been clearly documented, so have risks of estrogen replacement therapy.

Endometrial Cancer. Endometrial cancer is the major risk associated with use of systemic estrogen. More than 35 epidemiologic studies have evaluated the association between estrogen replacement therapy and endometrial cancer, and the vast majority have found a substantial increase in risk. Relative risk of endometrial cancer among estrogen users has been estimated to be as low as 2 and as high as 15. Risk increases with dosage and duration of estrogen use. A recent analytic review calculated pooled relative risk estimates from published studies. The estimated risk for women who had ever used exogenous estrogens was 2.31; for women who used estrogens for 8 or more years, including some who were using doses that are higher than those in common use today, the relative risk estimate was 8.22. Two studies suggest that for women taking 0.625 mg for at least 5 years, risk is increased fourfold.

Estrogens cause cystic hyperplasia of the endometrium, a premalignant condition. Prolonged, continuous use makes for excessive stimulation, leading to malignant change. Fortunately, the tumors induced by estrogen therapy in postmenopausal women tend to be of low grade and in early stages when detected. Not surprisingly then, survival is better than for nonusers who develop endometrial cancer.

One way to overcome excessive endometrial stimulation is to add a *progestin* to the estrogen program. Progestins prevent the development of endometrial hyperplasia that is otherwise associated with unopposed estrogen use. At least five studies have examined the effect of estrogen plus progestin therapy on endometrial cancer risk, and none found a significant increase.

Breast Cancer. Risk of breast cancer may or may not be increased by postmenopausal estrogen therapy. Some data suggest that estrogen use raises the risk, but other studies show no such risk. A recent analytic review estimated a summary relative risk of 1.01 for women who ever used estrogens. There is some evidence to support concerns that increasing dose and duration of estrogen use may be associated with increasing risk. Recent pooled estimates of relative risk for women who have used estrogen for 8 to 15 years have been in the 1.25 to 1.30 range. The effect of estrogen plus progestin on breast cancer risk is uncertain. Both increases and decreases in risk have been hypothesized. There is now general consensus that there is no protective effect, but there is no consensus about increased risk.

Other Adverse Effects. Other effects of exogenous estrogen include fluid retention, blood pressure elevation, gallstones (due to a change in bile cholesterol content), glucose intolerance, and headaches. Often there is recurrent uterine bleeding, especially with cyclic progesterone use (see below). This complicates clinical recognition of endometrial cancer and causes inconvenience. There does not appear to be an increased risk of *thromboembolism* among menopausal women on estrogen replacement, but patients with known peripheral vascular disease who are given estrogens should be monitored closely, and a history of thromboembolism is a relative contraindication to estrogen use.

Given such a list of potentially serious adverse effects and some important risks still poorly defined, the primary physician must exert care and judgment in selecting patients for estrogen therapy. The decision to use estrogens needs to be made with full consideration of the patient's willingness to undertake the risks in exchange for specified benefits. One woman may be willing to accept the risk of endometrial cancer in return for prevention of disabling osteoporosis and decreased risk of cardiovascular disease; another might not. The addition of progestin to the hormone replacement program can reduce the risk of endometrial cancer, but other long-term effects remain to be defined.

Specific Treatment Regimens. The established dose of conjugated estrogens (Premarin) necessary to prevent osteoporosis is 0.625 mg daily. Lower doses (eg, 0.3 mg or the equivalent) may be sufficient, or higher doses (as much as 2.5 mg/d) may be necessary, to control hot flashes. Symptomatic atrophic vaginitis may be treated with vaginal estrogen cream, 1 g every 2 to 3 days, but this is not effective for prophylactic therapy.

Three approaches to oral hormone replacement are commonly used. One standard among women with intact uteri is 0.625 mg conjugated estrogens (Premarin) daily with 10 mg of medroxyprogesterone acetate (Provera) for 10 to 14 consecutive days each month. Lower doses of Provera (5 mg) may be substituted. Other regimens include unopposed estrogen (ie, 0.625 mg of Premarin or equivalent) taken daily. The practice of interrupting estrogen dosing for 5 to 7 days is not supported by current evidence. Cyclic estrogen therapy does not produce endometrial shedding, and rates of endometrial hyperplasia and endometrial cancer risk are similar in women with continuous and interrupted dosing. A third common regimen is continuous estrogen plus continuous progestin at lower doses (eg, Provera at 2.5 mg/d). The advantage of this regimen is induction of endometrial atrophy and eventual cessation of uterine bleeding. Long-term safety is yet to be established.

Transdermal estrogen is also an option. A 50-mg patch applied twice each week produces estradiol levels similar to those resulting from oral doses of 0.625 mg of Premarin daily. This approach might make most sense for the woman without a uterus who has no need for progestins. Cost is increased and beneficial effect on lipoproteins may be less than with oral therapy.

Patient Selection. Patient selection for estrogen therapy to prevent osteoporosis and cardiovascular disease remains problematic (see Chapter 158). Women who have had a hysterectomy may have the most favorable risk–benefit ratio simply because they are not subject to the greatest risk, endometrial cancer. Among women who have not had a hysterectomy, any increased risk of heart disease argues in favor of estrogen replacement. Women with increased risk of osteoporosis and hip fracture are also more likely to benefit from hormone replacement. A single measurement of bone mineral density may be useful if the decision to treat would be influenced by the threefold increase in risk associated with low bone density. Because of the uncertainty about the effect of hormones on breast cancer risk, women already at high risk may be more reluctant take estrogens with or without progestins.

Monitoring. Current evidence does not support definitive recommendations for monitoring women taking hormone replacement therapy. For women who plan to take unopposed estrogens, a baseline pelvic examination with endometrial sampling and a baseline mammogram may be well advised. An emerging alternative to routine endometrial sampling is screening with transvaginal ultrasound, with sampling reserved for women with thickened endometrium. Any vaginal bleeding should be reported by the woman taking unopposed estrogens, and the report should prompt endometrial evaluation. In the absence of bleeding, screening with transvaginal ultrasound and/or endometrial sampling should be performed on a regular basis, either every year or every 2 years. Women taking progestins as well as estrogens do not need either baseline or subsequent routine endometrial evaluations. Clinical breast examination and mammography should be performed yearly.

PATIENT EDUCATION

Since the emphasis in our society is on youth and vitality, the physician has an important supportive role to play in helping the menopausal woman to adjust psychologically and maintain her sense of self-worth and well-being. Discussion of the physiologic consequences of menopause and their clinical manifestations can give the patient a rational basis for understanding her own symptoms and properly attributing them. This might save many anxious phone calls and office visits. One can take advantage of this milestone to interest the patient in a program of regular exercise, attainment of ideal weight, and cessation of such self-destructive habits as smoking. The woman needs to know that any incapacitating symptoms due to lack of estrogen can be controlled and that many are self-limited. During the perimenopausal period, women should be reminded to use contraception because ovulation and unwanted pregnancy may occur. Reassurance that capacity for normal sexual activity will continue after menopause is often tremendously comforting. Lack of need for special vitamin supplements should be pointed out, since the lay press heavily encourages their use and this unnecessary expense can be considerable.

If estrogen therapy is being considered, the patient must share in the decision with full awareness of the potential risks and benefits. Patients with intact uteri on unopposed estrogen therapy must be reminded about the need for regular endometrial evaluation. The need for regular follow-up and prompt reporting of any abnormal vaginal bleeding, breast masses, leg swelling, and so on must be emphasized.

THERAPEUTIC RECOMMENDATIONS

- Decisions about hormone replacement therapy require careful balancing of risks and benefits. These issues should be carefully explained and discussed with the patient.
- If prescribed to control symptoms, systemic estrogen should be used in the minimal effective dose. The need for continued treatment should be reevaluated regularly.
- Atrophic vaginitis with dysuria or dyspareunia will respond to topical estrogen applied as seldom as once or twice a week. Systemic absorption occurs, but its effect is uncertain. Milder cases, with painful coitus only, can be treated with a water-soluble lubricant (eg, Lubafax), if there is a reason to avoid any estrogen exposure.
- When prescribed for disease prevention and health promotion, the risks and benefits of alternative regimens, including the need for appropriate monitoring, should be understood by patients. Oral regimens include 1) daily conjugated estrogens (eg, 0.625 mg Premarin or equivalent) with progestin (eg, 5 or 10 mg of medroxyprogesterone acetate or equivalent) added on 10 to 14 consecutive days of the month; 2) daily estrogens alone; and 3) daily estrogens combined with daily low-dose progestin (eg, 2.5 or 5 mg of medroxyprogesterone acetate or equivalent).
- Women with intact uteri should consider addition of progestin, either cyclically or continuously, to reduce risk of endometrial cancer. There is no reason to prescribe progestins for women who have had a hysterectomy.
- Estrogen therapy cannot replace lost bone, so it is not a therapy for reversing established osteoporosis. Bone loss occurs when estrogen therapy is discontinued; prolonged therapy (eg, for 10 years) is necessary to meaningfully delay the process and thereby prevent rather than simply defer complications of osteoporosis (see Chapter 164).

A.G.M.

ANNOTATED BIBLIOGRAPHY

Ballinger CG. Psychiatric morbidity and the menopause: clinical features. Br Med J 1976;1:1183. *(A description of psychiatric symptoms during the menopause.)*

Bergkvist L, Adami HO, Persson I, Hoover R, Schairer C. The risk of breast cancer after estrogen and estrogen-progestin replacement. N Engl J Med 1989;321:293. *(The relative risk for ever-users of unopposed estrogen was 1.1; for women with ≥ 9 y of unopposed estrogen use, relative risk was statistically significant at 1.8. For women with 6–9 y of estrogen and progestin use, relative risk was 4.4.)*

Boston Collaborative Drug Surveillance Program. Surgically confirmed gallbladder disease, venous thromboembolism and breast tumors in relation to postmenopausal estrogen therapy. N Engl J Med 1974;290:15. *(Postmenopausal estrogen therapy increased risk of gallstones but not of thromboembolism or breast tumor in this study.)*

Bush TL, Cowan LD, Barrett-Conner E, et al. Estrogen use and all-cause mortality. Preliminary results from the Lipid Research Clinics program follow-up study. JAMA 1983;249:903. *(A decrease in risk of cardiac mortality is found.)*

Colditz GA, Stampfer MJ, Willett WC, Hennekens CH, Rosner B, Speizer FE. Prospective study of estrogen replacement therapy and risk of breast cancer in postmenopausal women. JAMA 1990;264:2648. *(Relative risks of 1.4 and 1.2 among ever-users of unopposed estrogens and women with >15 y of use, respectively.)*

Cummings SR, Black D. Should menopausal women be screened for osteoporosis? Ann Intern Med 1986;104:817. *(Thoughtful analysis of the major issues, including excellent review of the literature; 89 refs.)*

Cummings SR, Browner WS, Grady D, Ettinger B. Should prescription of postmenopausal hormone therapy be based on the results of bone densitometry? Ann Intern Med 1990;113:565. *(Advocates single measurement of bone density if risk for osteoporosis would influence the hormone replacement decision.)*

Ditkoff EC, Crary WG, Cristo M, Lobo RA. Estrogen improves psychological function in asymptomatic postmenopausal women. Obstet Gynecol 1991;78:991. *(Estrogen therapy may improve mood and mental function, even in asymptomatic postmenopausal women.)*

Falkeborn M, Persson I, Terent A, et al. Hormone replacement therapy and risk of stroke. Arch Intern Med 1993;153:1201. *(Population study from Sweden; risk reduced 30 percent.)*

Felson DT, Zhang Y, Hannan MT, et al. The effect of postmenopausal estrogen therapy on bone density in elderly women. N Engl J Med 1993;329:1141. *(Very long-term therapy required to produce clinically meaningful benefit to women >75 years old.)*

Grady D, Ernster V. Does postmenopausal hormone therapy cause breast cancer? Am J Epidemiol 1991;134:1396. *(Commentary accompanying two case–control studies with conflicting results.)*

Grady D, Rubin SM, Petitti DB, et al. Hormone therapy to prevent disease and prolong life in postmenopausal women. Ann Intern Med 1992;117:1016. *(A comprehensive and scholarly analytic review of the literature with 265 refs; accompanied by practical recommendations for communication of risks to patients, treatment, and monitoring.)*

Henrich JB. The postmenopausal estrogen/breast cancer controversy. JAMA 1992;268:1900. *(A critical review of the available data.)*

Hillner BE, Hollenberg JP, Pauker SG. Postmenopausal estrogens in prevention of osteoporosis. Am J Med 1986;80:1115. *(A decision-analysis study that argues in favor of hormone therapy.)*

Horsman A, Jones M, Francis R, et al. The effect of estrogen dose on menopausal bone loss. N Engl J Med 1985;309:1405. *(Documents a dose-related inhibition of cortical bone resorption.)*

Jick H, Watkins RN, Hunter JR, et al. Replacement estrogens and endometrial cancer. N Engl J Med 1979;300:218. *(Long-term estrogen users in a large Seattle group practice showed an annual risk of 1 percent to 3 percent for users and a risk less than one-tenth as great for nonusers. A reduced incidence of endometrial cancer paralleled the downward trend in the use of replacement estrogens.)*

Leiblum S, Bachmann G, Kemmann E, et al. Vaginal atrophy in the postmenopausal woman. JAMA 1983;249:2195. *(Less vaginal atrophy was apparent in sexually active women compared with sexually inactive women; women with less vaginal atrophy had higher levels of estrogens and gonadotropins.)*

Lufkin EG, Wahner HW, O'Fallon W, et al. Treatment of postmenopausal osteoporosis with transdermal estrogen. Ann Intern Med 1992;117:1. *(Documents reduced risk of wrist and vertebral fractures with transdermal delivery of estrogen.)*

Myers LS, Dixen J, Morrissette D, Carmichael MJ, Davidson J. Effects of estrogen, androgen, and progestin on sexual psychophysiology and behavior in postmenopausal women. J Clin Endocrinol Metab 1990;70:1124. *(In this study, there was no improvement in libido and sexual enjoyment among estrogen-treated women.)*

Nabulisi AA, Folson AR, White A, et al. Association of hormone-replacement therapy with various cardiovascular risk factors in postmenopausal women. N Engl J Med 1993;328:1069. *(Adding progesterone does not appear to negate the beneficial effects of estrogen on cardiovascular risk factors.)*

Naessen T, Persson I, Adami HO, Bergstrom R, Bergkvist L. Hormone replacement therapy and the risk for hip fracture. A prospective, population-based cohort study. Ann Intern Med 1990;113:95. *(Cohort study showing relative risk of 0.8 for women who had ever used unopposed estrogens.)*

Padwick ML, Pryse-Davies J, Whitehead MI. A simple method for determining the optimal dosage of progestin in postmenopausal women receiving estrogens. N Engl J Med 1986;315:930. *(Adjustment of dose to induce withdrawal bleeding on or after day 11 of a 12-day progestin program was associated with a secretory endometrium.)*

Stampfer MJ, Colditz GA. Estrogen replacement therapy and coronary heart disease: a quantitative assessment of the epidemiologic evidence. Prev Med 1991;20:47. *(Good analytic overview.)*

Stampfer MJ, Colditz GA, Willett WC, et al. Postmenopausal estrogen therapy and cardiovascular disease. Ten-year follow-up from the Nurses' Health Study. N Engl J Med 1991;325:756. *(Relative risk for ever-users was 0.6.)*

Steinberg KK, Thacker SB, Smith SJ, et al. A meta-analysis of the effect of estrogen replacement therapy on the risk of breast cancer. JAMA 1991;265:1985. *(Analytic review finding no increased risk for ever-users of estrogen and relative risk of 1.3 for women who had used estrogens for at least 15 years.)*

Wenz AC. Psychiatric morbidity and menopause (editorial). Ann Intern Med 1976;84:331. *(Psychiatric symptoms are not a function of estrogen deficiency.)*

Whitehead MI, Townsend PT, Pryse-Davies J, et al. Effects of estrogens and progestins on the biochemistry and morphology of the postmenopausal endometrium. N Engl J Med 1981;305:1599. *(The original report on progestins counteracting the effects of estrogen.)*

Primary Care Medicine: Office Evaluation and Management of the Adult Patient, 3rd edition, edited by Allan H. Goroll, Lawrence A. May, and Albert G. Mulley, Jr. J.B. Lippincott Company, Philadelphia

119
Approach to Fertility Control

NANCY J. GAGLIANO, MD

The ideal contraceptive is perfectly safe, effective, inexpensive, acceptable, and available. None exists. The efficacy of individual contraceptive agents is expressed in several ways. *Theoretical effectiveness* refers to the ability of the medication, device, or procedure to prevent pregnancy if applied under ideal conditions. *Use effectiveness* combines theoretical effectiveness with inherent patient-related lapses in application. *Extended use effectiveness* adds the dimension of time. All are important aspects of evaluation of approaches to fertility control.

The primary physician should be knowledgeable about the effectiveness, difficulties, and adverse effects of available contraceptive methods to help the patient or couple intelligently select the one that suits them best.

NATURAL METHODS

Natural methods of birth control do not meet the demands of most sexually active individuals in industrialized societies. Faithfully practiced *rhythm*, with daily basal body temperature recording, usually results in one pregnancy every 2 years or at least one more child than planned by the couple by their late thirties. Rhythm practiced by abstinence according to menstrual dates is less effective. Rhythm controlled by following the cervical mucus cycle is confounded by infections, dietary changes, douching habits, oral medications, patient understanding of her anatomy, and availability of testing materials. One needs to understand reproductive anatomy and physiology and to have privacy to conduct such tests. These ingredients are unavailable to many Americans. The *amenorrhea of lactation* is useful, but the duration of ovarian inactivity in an individual is hard to predict or follow. *Withdrawal* is probably the most commonly used natural contraceptive technique. Unfortunately, sperm migration from the female perineum can occur, as does some discharging of semen prior to ejaculation.

BARRIER CONTRACEPTIVES

Condoms have extended use effectiveness. Pregnancies may occur in up to 15 per 100 couples per year using condoms, which means that, properly used, this method is 85 percent to 95 percent effective. For a few cents more than the cheapest devices, high-quality thin condoms are available, use of which is accompanied by very little loss of sensation. When used in conjunction with a spermicidal foam or jelly its effectiveness may rise to 96 percent. The condom is inexpensive and widely available. It requires no medical intervention or prescription. Failure by means of rupture is rare but easily recognized. The condom has received more attention recently due to its protective effects against infectious agents such as the human immunodeficiency virus (HIV), *Chlamydia*, gonococci, herpes simplex virus, and possibly the human papillomavirus. This effect appears to be dependent on the use of nonoxynol-9, a spermicide found in most condoms.

Diaphragms are synthetic latex barriers mounted on covered rims that deny access of sperm and penis to the anterior vaginal wall and cervical os. There are three widely used rims: all-flex, coil spring, and flat spring. These have minor differences in characteristics and provide alternatives for fitting a variety of women. The largest diaphragm that will cover the cervix and anterior vagina from the pubis symphysis to the posterior fornix, without uncomfortably stretching the rest of the vagina, should be selected. The diaphragm should be comfortable so that the women barely notices its presence, and it should not put undue pressure on the urethra. Only significant weight changes of 25 percent of body weight or more require refitting of diaphragms, despite popular belief that a 10-pound weight change should prompt refitting. Diaphragms with a small amount of spermicidal cream or jelly, properly used, are up to 96 percent effective; four pregnancies per 100 fertile women per year would be expected. The cream facilitates insertion but need not be used in the large amounts recommended by the manufacturers, as it is unpleasantly messy. Additional spermicidal cream needs to be applied intravaginally for repeated intercourse. The diaphragm is worn for 6 hours after the last coital event, since this is the length of time during which sperm motility persists. It may be worn for longer periods of time, but like all vaginal contraceptives, it will then become associated with an unpleasant odor. It may also be worn while the patient is swimming or during menstruation.

The diaphragm must be fitted to the individual woman by a physician, nurse, or trained technician. The cost of the diaphragm is reasonable, but manufacturers advocate massive use of creams, which adds to the expense. The patient must have some understanding of her anatomy and not be concerned about exploring her reproductive organs. Some adolescents reject the diaphragm because they are uncomfortable with touching themselves. Its use represents premeditated sexual intercourse, which they find less acceptable than spontaneous events. Women in their 20s seldom voice such a complaint. Some women cannot be adequately fitted with a diaphragm for anatomical reasons. The cervix may not protrude into the vagina adequately (absent pars vaginalis). The cervix may be displaced posteriorly by retroversion or extreme anteversion.

Cervical Caps fit snugly over the cervix and are slightly more difficult to insert and remove. Their use requires significant physician or nurse teaching, and they are more costly than diaphragms. Currently, four sizes are manufactured, and some women are not able to be fit. For these reasons, they are less popular than the diaphragm. For women who have recurrent urinary tract infections, however, they are particularly useful because they do not press on the urethra. Additionally, they can be worn for 48 hours, during which time intercourse may be repeated without the addition of spermicidal cream. There is evidence of a 4 percent increased incidence of abnormal Papanicolaou (Pap) tests; therefore, it is recommended that a Pap test be performed 3 months after initiating use of the cap. If the Pap smear is normal, then the woman can proceed with yearly Pap tests.

Female Condoms are now approved by the Food and Drug Administration (FDA). The condom is a lubricated polyurethane pouch that lines the vagina. One outer ring lies outside the body and a smaller inner ring is pushed up toward the cervix to hold the condom in place. It gives a woman an additional choice and freedom to protect herself from sexually transmitted diseases and pregnancy. It appears to have failure rates similar to those of the male condom. Unfortunately, it currently costs about twice as much as the male condom.

Spermicidal Creams and Jellies may have a high theoretical effectiveness, but they have lesser use effectiveness. Most contain nonoxynol-9 as the spermicidal agent. The physical nature of the creams and jellies and difficulty in their application often result in inadequately smearing the cervical os, so that sperm invasion is not prevented. Both men and women complain of the dehydrating effect of spermicidal agents and may report burning sensations. Nonoxynol-9 has the added advantage of being toxic in vitro to HIV, gonococci, *Chlamydia,* and other genital pathogens; some clinical evidence suggests an in vivo effect as well. *Foams* have better physical properties, allowing more adequate smearing of the cervical os; however, foams are effective for short periods of time only, and reapplications are necessary. This increases their cost. They also contain nonoxynol-9 and may cause irritation. Failure rates up to 75 percent are reported. However, as mentioned above, when used in conjunction with the condom, excellent pregnancy protection has been demonstrated, reaching 96 percent effectiveness. *Encapsulated foams*, compared with foams applied through applicators, are far less successful because the capsule may not be inserted deeply enough into the vagina or may not disintegrate at the appropriate interval to smear the cervical os adequately. Foams have the advantage of being readily accessible in both supermarkets and drugstores, and they do not require medical instruction or prescription.

Vaginal Contraceptive Sponges represent a more convenient, though slightly less effective, barrier method of contraception than the diaphragm. The sponge is smaller and thicker than the diaphragm, being made of hydrophilic polyurethane foam with 1 g of the spermicide nonoxynol-9 incorporated within it. Mechanisms of contraceptive action include release of spermicide, blocking of the cervical os, and absorption of semen. The sponge has an indentation on one surface to fit over the cervix. It is moistened with a few teaspoons of tap water and inserted high into the vagina. Once inserted, it is protective for 24 hours, regardless of how many episodes of intercourse occur. For maximum protection, the sponge needs to be left in at least 6 hours after intercourse. The product has a woven polyester strap attached to one side to aid in removal.

Twelve-month pregnancy rates with use of the sponge average 16 percent in the United States (range 10%–27%); this compares with 4 percent to 12 percent for use of the diaphragm. The spermicide nonoxynol-9 has been used for years as the active ingredient of most spermicidal foams, jellies, and creams. There is one report of a possible increase in congenital anomalies and spontaneous abortions in women using spermicidal agents, but other studies have failed to confirm it. No evidence exists of a significant increase in birth defects in the children of women using spermicides. Nonoxynol-9 may contain trace amounts of residues that are known carcinogens; moreover, the carcinogen 2,4-toluenediamine can form as a contaminant during the polymerization of polyurethane. Precautions have been taken to prevent formation of contaminants, and careful analyses have failed to detect any carcinogens in the sponge. If any carcinogens were present, they would be in such small concentrations as to make them unlikely to increase the risk of cancer.

Mild side effects include vaginal dryness, mild local irritation, and odor from leaving the sponge in too long. If the sponge is placed incorrectly, the strap may be hard to reach and the sponge difficult to remove. However, no episodes of toxic shock have been reported to date (only polyacrylate rayon products have been associated with the pathogenesis of toxic shock).

INTRAUTERINE DEVICES (IUDs)

The idea of inserting materials into the uterine cavity to prevent nidation is ancient. Nevertheless, the precise mechanism of IUD action remains unknown. What appears to be important is the area of surface contact. Copper enhances effectiveness. The 1-percent to 5-percent first-year pregnancy rates with IUD use are among the lowest attainable from a birth control method and are comparable to those of oral contraceptives. The lack of need for constant compliance greatly enhances efficacy. Another advantage is the lack of systemic effects, a major problem with oral contraceptives (see below). A major limitation to efficacy is expulsion, which is particularly frequent in nulliparous women. The overall expulsion rate is 19 per 100 women per year, lower with copper devices. Occasionally it is necessary to remove an IUD because of bleeding or pain, which occurs at a rate of about 11 percent per year; copper devices are better tolerated by nulliparous women.

The confirmation of a markedly increased risk of tubal infertility associated with IUD use has greatly discouraged IUD placement as a means of safe birth control, especially among nulliparous women. In 1986, sale of all IUDs, except Progestasert, was discontinued. In 1988, Paragard, a new copper IUD, was approved by the FDA. Clinical or subclinical pelvic inflammatory disease is believed to account for the tubal infertility. Risk of pelvic inflammatory disease in nulliparous sexually active women with an IUD has been found to be seven times that for similar women not using an IUD; for parous women, the risk is three times greater. In view of the infertility risk, IUD use is best confined to multiparous women and nulliparous women with a single sexual partner. The nulliparous woman considering an IUD as a means of birth control should be fully informed of the risk of tubal infertility before any decision is made regarding its use.

ORAL CONTRACEPTIVES

Combinations of synthetic estrogens and progesterones have been found to have use effectiveness rates that exceed most estimates of effectiveness of barrier methods, spermicides, and IUDs. Although some report failure rates as high as 5 percent to 10 percent, most report only one failure per 100 users per year. The combination pill appears to prevent cyclic release of follicle-stimulating hormone (FSH) and luteinizing hormone (LH), which are required for ovulation; alter the cervical mucus, thereby decreasing sperm motility; and alter the endometrial lining to inhibit implantation. At the present time, combination pills consist of an estrogen (ethinyl estradiol or mestranol) and a progestin (norethindrone, norethynodrel, norgestrel, levo-norgestrel, ethynodiol diacetate, and most recently desogestrel). Packets are made up for taking the pills from the first Sunday of the menstrual cycle, or the first day of bleeding, and continuing for the next 21 days; some packets have placebos, so that one pill is taken daily.

Preparations. More than two dozen combination preparations are available in the United States. In general, it is most useful to renew any prescription with which a patient is satisfied, as long as the patient has no new symptoms or habits that warrant discontinuation of any oral contraceptive.

Cardiovascular risks have been a significant concern when prescribing the pill. Because of the concern that these risks might increase with estrogen dosage and progestin potency, emphasis in recent years has been on use of preparations that have the lowest effective estrogen dose (20–35 μg ethinyl estradiol) and the least progestin potency. Fortunately, efficacy of 30 μg to 35 μg of estrogen for prevention of pregnancy is about the same as that of the older 50-μg estrogen pill.

It is best to begin with a pill containing 35 μg of either ethinyl estradiol or mestranol. The lowest possible progestin dosage helps minimize bothersome side effects such as increased appetite, steady weight gain, acne, and depression. Patients who have a history of symptoms suggesting hyperresponsiveness to endogenous estrogens (premenstrual breast engorgement and soreness, cyclic weight gain, heavy periods) may benefit from a preparation containing a low estrogen and a progestin with minimal estrogenic effect (eg, Ovcon with ethinyl estradiol 35 μg and norethindrone 0.4 mg). Similarly, a patient bothered by acne or hirsutism should not be given a preparation with an androgenic progestin (Table 119–1). Other side effects such as nausea seem related to estrogen content.

The disadvantages of using lower-dose agents are higher rates of spotting, breakthrough bleeding, and amenorrhea. Moreover, women who use oral contraceptives containing less than 30 μg of estrogen may experience a greater chance of pregnancy. In an attempt to improve on rates of breakthrough bleeding and pregnancy associated with low-estrogen/weak-progestin formulations, manufacturers have developed *biphasic* (eg, Ortho-Novum 10/11) and *triphasic* (eg, Ortho-Novum 7/7/7, Tri-Norinyl, Triphasil) formulations. The rationale is to more closely mimic normal ovarian patterns. Efficacy is similar to that obtained with other low-estrogen/weak-progestin preparations; no controlled evidence to date suggests that they are superior in terms of breakthrough bleeding. All low-dose preparations need to be taken religiously to be maximally effective and to minimize the chances of breakthrough bleeding.

It is helpful to become familiar with four or five pills and their minor differences, rather than use the most recently marketed combinations. Providing the patient with full, understandable information at the initiation of therapy will ward off many anxious phone calls. In particular, if one pill is missed, it can be made up by doubling the next dose. If two pills are missed, the patient should double the dose for the next 2 days, but barrier contraception is recommended for the remainder of the cycle. If three or more consecutive pills are missed, the pills should be stopped altogether, allowing withdrawal bleeding to occur, and then started 1 week after the last pill is taken. However, failure to take oral contraceptives regularly is an indication for trying another form of birth control.

Table 119-1. Effects of Synthetic Progestins*

ESTROGENIC	ANDROGENIC
Norethynodrel	Norgestrel
Ethynodiol	Norethindrone
All others have none	Norethindrone acetate
	Ethynodiol
	Norethynodrel (has none)

*In order of decreasing potency.

Breakthrough bleeding is a common side effect of the pill. If it occurs late in the cycle or in the first few months of initiation of the pill, it is usually caused by too little progesterone. If it occurs early in the cycle or after years of use, it may be caused by inadequate estrogen. This problem may be temporarily resolved by having the patient take two pills a day for 3 days. The additional pills should be obtained from a separate package of pills.

If the problem recurs monthly, then changing the pill to a stronger estrogenic or progestinal pill would be appropriate. The physician should always rule out other causes of irregular bleeding, such as infection and pregnancy.

Another common complaint is that of morning nausea. It may be improved by having the patient take the pill with her evening meal and then consume a light breakfast daily. If the symptoms persist, switching to a lower estrogen pill or a progesterone-only pill (eg, Micronor) may be indicated.

Patients require follow-up care 6 to 12 weeks after initiation of the birth control pill to check for hypertension, review proper use, and discuss side effects. The patients should then be seen yearly, checking for headaches, hypertension, breast masses, cervical abnormalities, phlebitis, and signs of cardiovascular or cerebrovascular disease.

Physicians are generally unaware of the high discontinuation rate among oral contraceptive users. Factors involved include the patient's perceptions of need and attitudes about taking medications that affect the sex organs. Oral contraceptives are expensive and require a medical prescription, important barriers for adolescents. Despite these factors and known side effects, birth control pills continue to be the most used, safest birth control method for most women younger than age 30. The pill's relative safety is most apparent in countries where the risk of dying in childbirth is high.

Adverse Effects. The major hazards of oral contraceptives are cardiovascular. The relative risks of cardiovascular events in users compared with nonusers have been reported to be four to 11 times greater for *thromboembolism,* four to 9.5 times greater for thrombotic stroke, two times greater for hemorrhagic stroke, and two to 12 times greater for myocardial infarction. These earlier studies, which demonstrated a slight increase in risk, were done on women taking 50-μg doses of estrogen. Currently, it is thought that any increased risk is due to embolic events. The Nurses Health Study demonstrated no significant differences in the rates of various cardiovascular diseases between never-users and past users of oral contraceptives. The studies consistently showed these increased risks *in smokers*. Mortality from myocardial infarction rises sixfold in women older than age 40 who are smokers. The overall excess death rate annually has been estimated to be 20 per 100,000, with risk concentrated in women older than 35, especially if they smoke cigarettes and have used oral contraceptives for 5 years or longer. Division of data at age 35 is arbitrary, and it would be prudent to assume that risk gradually increases with age. It is thought that cardiovascular risk is much lower with 35-μg estrogen pills. Progestin potency may also be associated with increased cardiovascular risk, probably because of its ability to raise low-density lipoprotein (LDL) cholesterol and lower high-density lipoprotein (HDL) cholesterol (see Chapter 15).

Any population of women provided with oral contraception will show a rise in mean blood pressure in about 3 months. Prospective studies have found that the incidence of *hypertension* increases two- to sixfold in users compared with nonusers. Patients with hypertension are at increased risk and should not use oral contraceptives. It is wise to check blood pressure before renewing a patient's prescription. The progesterone in the birth control pill, like the progesterone in the secretory phase of the menstrual cycle, increases aldosterone secretion, and estrogen increases renin substrate.

There is a twofold increase in the risk of *gallbladder disease* in users compared with nonusers, because of increased cholesterol saturation of bile. The frequency of gallstones appears to rise after 2 years' usage and to reach a plateau after 4 to 5 years' usage. This risk must be balanced against the increased risk of gallbladder disease associated with multiparity. Another hepatobiliary problem is the rare development of highly vascular *hepatic adenomas*, which can rupture spontaneously, resulting in serious hemorrhage. Isolated cases have appeared in the literature; in most cases, patients had been using the pill longer than 5 years. The actual risk is unknown. Finally, estrogen use has been associated with *cholestatic jaundice*, but oral contraceptive use does not worsen cases of mild viral hepatitis and need not be discontinued unless cholestasis or hepatocellular injury is severe.

At present, there is little evidence of increased risk of *breast cancer* from use of oral contraceptives by premenopausal women. One large, multi-center, case–control study has demonstrated that long-term oral contraceptive use in women of reproductive age confers no increased risk of breast cancer compared with other methods of delaying first pregnancy. However, a more recent study in Europe demonstrated a slightly increased risk in young, nulliparous, long-use women. The debate continues. The growth of certain cancers may be stimulated by estrogens; these include carcinoma of the breast (see Chapter 122), cervix, and endometrium (see Chapter 123). Most studies have shown diminished incidences of fibroadenomas, ovarian and endometrial cancers, and benign fibrocystic disease of the breast in pill users.

Metabolic and *endocrinologic effects* are numerous. Thyroid-binding globin levels increase, which in turn raises the serum thyroxine level. Glucose tolerance falls as circulating growth hormone rises and peripheral resistance to insulin occurs. Triglyceride levels increase, sometimes dramatically, with the concurrent boost in lipoprotein production. The estrogen component tends to result in a rise in HDL cholesterol, while the progestin may result in a rise in LDL cholesterol. There is no evidence to suggest that the oral contraceptive pill should not be prescribed in women with hypercholesterolemia. However, it may be prudent to use a pill shown to have minimal lipid-worsening effect. Such pills are those with low doses of norethindrone (Ovcon, Modicon, Brevicon) or those with a newer progestin, desogestrel (Desogen).

A few miscellaneous effects are worth noting. Birth control pills may increase the frequency of *migraine headache* in patients with prior migraine attacks. However, they are only contraindicated in the woman with neurologic symptoms associated with her migraine headache. Anecdotal reports of *exacerbation of lupus erythematosus* appear in the obstetric literature. Sensitivity to sunlight and chloasma (mask of pregnancy) are seen in some users and fade with discontinuation.

A number of gynecologic conditions are affected by use of these agents; effects may be beneficial or detrimental. Patients with menstrual irregularities prior to oral contraceptive use will have regular pill-induced periods while taking the medication. Patients should have a full evaluation of the etiology of their irregular menses prior to initiation of the oral contraceptive pill. On discontinuation of the pills, some will revert to their previous irregularity. Rarely, *amenorrhea* due to ovarian suppression will persist for several months, even a year after pill cessation (see Chapter 112). Usually, menses return promptly, and fertility rates in the first 3 months of discontinuation are increased. Occasionally, a patient will notice nipple discharge (nonpuerperal lactation) with use of oral contraceptives. The mechanism is not clear. No increased incidence of pituitary prolactinomas has been observed.

Many patients with *dysmenorrhea* find marked relief with oral contraceptives (see Chapter 116). If the dysmenorrhea is associated with endometriosis, the response is variable, with many patients complaining of exacerbation of symptoms rather than relief.

With these side effects in mind, absolute and relative contraindications can be listed (Table 119–2). Patients exposed to diethylstilbestrol have used birth control pills with no evidence to date of either beneficial or deleterious effects.

"Morning-After Pill." Large doses of estrogen (50 mg diethylstilbestrol qd for 5 days; 0.5 mg ethinyl estradiol bid for 5 days; or 100 μg ethinyl estradiol and 1.0 mg norgestrel, two

Table 119-2. Contraindications of Oral Contraceptives

Absolute Contraindications
- Thromboembolic disorders, cardiovascular disease, thrombophlebitis, or a past history of these conditions or other conditions that predipose to them
- Markedly impaired liver function from severe hepatitis, alcoholism, etc.
- Known or suspected estrogen-dependent neoplasm (cancers of the breast, endometrium, etc.)
- Undiagnosed genital bleeding
- Known or suspected pregnancy

Relative Contraindications
- Migraine headache
- Hypertension
- Familial hyperlipidemia
- Epilepsy
- Uterine leiomyoma
- History of idiopathic obstructive jaundice of pregnancy
- Smoking one-half pack or more per day
- Diabetes mellitus
- Severe heart disease
- Patient unreliability
- Age >35 years

Ovral, repeated after 12 h) will result in withdrawal bleeding, denying the conceptus an environment for nidation. This should be prescribed within 72 hours of the unprotected intercourse. Such doses usually cause nausea, and antiemetic medication may be needed. Provided that nidation has not already occurred, this approach is generally effective. However, these medications are not FDA-approved for this indication, and failures are reported, although they can be very useful in certain situations. The potent abortifacient mifepristone (RU-486) is being studied in the United States and is used widely in Europe. It is a modulator of progestin action.

SUBDERMAL AND INTRAMUSCULAR PROGESTINS

Norplant is a new method of contraception utilizing six slender Silastic tubes surgically implanted subdermally. Levo-norgestrel, a progestin, is released continuously at a very low level for 5 years and appears to suppress ovulation. Cumulative pregnancy rates over the 5 years are 0.6 percent to 4 percent and are highest among women who have regular menstrual cycles while using Norplant. The advantages are 5 years of continuous contraception and very low hormone levels, resulting in no clinically significant metabolic effects. The disadvantages are irregular bleeding (in 66%) lasting many months and a cost of hundreds of dollars.

Depo-Provera has also been FDA-approved for use as a contraceptive. Medroxyprogesterone acetate 150 mg is administered intramuscularly every 3 months. Care should be taken to ensure that the woman is not pregnant initially, and it is recommended that the drug be administered during the first 5 days of the cycle. If a patient waits longer than 14 weeks between injections, a pregnancy test should be performed before her next injection. The pregnancy rate is 1 percent if used correctly. Disadvantages include irregular bleeding and the displeasure of patients receiving injections.

ABORTION

Studies by Planned Parenthood have not found that a substantial number of American women rely on abortion as the sole method of birth control, nor has any trend to such a reliance been noted. Rather, abortion is used as a backup when other methods fail. Frequently, the necessity for an abortion initiates effective contraceptive use, particularly in those younger than age 20. No adverse effect of first-trimester induced abortion on future childbearing has been demonstrated. The effect of second-trimester abortions in rupturing cervical tissue is controversial. Rarely, an anomalous cervix may become incompetent, requiring cerclage if the patient wishes to carry future pregnancies to term. Morbidity and mortality in teenagers from induced abortion is lower than in older women.

OVERALL RISKS

Used alone by women younger than 30, condoms, diaphragms, IUDs, birth control pills, and first-trimester abortion have a mortality risk of one to two per 100,000, significantly lower than the 12 per 100,000 delivery-related risk rate. After age 30, the risk of birth control pills rises, especially in smokers, but it is still less than the morbidity and complications of childbearing without fertility control. The birth control pill may be prescribed to women in their forties, but it is contraindicated in a smoker past the age of 35. The lowest level of mortality is achieved by a combination of contraception with access to early abortion.

STERILIZATION

In 1965, one-third of the married couples in the United States used oral contraception, sterilization, or IUDs. By 1975, almost three quarters used one of these methods. Sterilization is now the most frequently used method of contraception among couples married for a decade or longer, as well as among couples who have had all the children they want.

Vasectomy is the simplest and safest means of sterilization. Only a few surgical instruments and local anesthesia are required. The procedure may be done in a clinic, doctor's office, ambulatory surgical day care unit, or hospital. The procedure does not lead to impotence; rather, men with problems associated with impotence may blame vasectomy. It takes about 90 days of average ejaculatory activity to completely empty the spermatic cord and accessory glands of residual sperm. Thus, the vasectomy subject should have a postoperative semen analysis before he is considered sterile. Alternative methods of birth control should be used in the interim. Circulating antibodies to sperm may be induced by foreign proteins as well as by sperm. The effect of elevated sperm antibodies on a man's health is not clear, but has been the subject of much concern. Retrospective cohort study of more than 10,000 vasectomized men fails to support such concerns; no serious immunopathologic consequences of vasectomy were noted. Further evidence of safety emerges from use-control and cohort studies showing no relation between vasectomy and cardiovascular disease. The only adverse effects are an increased risk of epidydimitis–orchitis and testicular changes leading to infertility (see below). Vasectomy still appears safe and effective, and it is the least expensive form of permanent sterilization. Recanalization when ends of the vas are tied too closely together may account for failures. Reanastomosis may be carried out with microsurgical techniques; however, only about one-third of patients undergoing reanastomosis father live-born children. The causes of diminished fertility are multifactorial and include damage to nerves adjacent to the vas, the development of interstitial fibrosis within the testicle, and age.

Procedures on the Fallopian Tubes. In 1975, 2 percent of women ages 25 to 34 underwent tubal sterilization. In the ensuing decade, the rate has increased markedly. Surgical division of the fallopian tubes after delivery is easily accomplished, either with normal vaginal delivery or with cesarean section. The procedure adds 1 to 2 days to the patient's hospitalization. Procedures that leave the two ends of the fallopian tubes in close proximity (Pomeroy technique, in which a suture ties a knuckle of tube and the apex of the knuckle is excised) may have a failure rate of 2 percent. Other methods that leave the two severed ends well separated have failure rates of less than 1 percent. When there is concern for the survival of the newborn, postpartum sterilization is contraindicated.

Vaginal tubal ligation is usually not done postpartum through the vagina because of the increased vascularity and the risk of sepsis. A skilled obstetrician–gynecologist can do interval sterilizations under local anesthesia, usually in a day care or hospital facility. However, leiomyoma, endometriosis, or previous infection may obstruct the approach to the tube.

The *minilaparotomy* involves a small abdominal incision of 1 to 2 inches done under local anesthesia through the peritoneum. Each fallopian tube is identified, ligated, and divided. The incision is closed with resorbable sutures, and a bandage is applied. The patient is able to go home within a few hours.

These methods have the advantage of simplicity and require commonly used instruments. They have been taught to surgical technicians in Third World countries. Such procedures may be unsuitable in an obese or anxious patient. In fact, other methods are more commonly used in the United States.

Laparoscopy requires expensive special instrumentation and an experienced gynecologist or surgeon. Although it can be done under local anesthesia, general endotracheal anesthesia is more commonly used. A fiberoptic endoscope is inserted through a subumbilical incision, and a second instrument accompanies the endoscope or is inserted through the pelvic incision. The tubes are cauterized or both cauterized and divided. Alternatively, plastic rings or clips are used to occlude them. Cauterization has the lowest failure rate; however, clips are advocated as being less likely to cause damage to bowel. In fact, complications and failures with clips are often remedied by cauterization. Furthermore, the half-life of the plastic materials used for occlusion has not been clearly defined, and very little 5-year data are available.

In experienced hands, laparoscopy is highly effective with minimal risk in a healthy woman. Laparoscopy may be accomplished on a 1-day basis or in day care facilities. The patient may be expected to continue her normal menstrual life and menopause. Anastomosis of severed fallopian tubes can be accomplished by careful surgical procedures with or without optical magnification. However, as with vasectomy, the rate of achieving patency is higher than that of live births. Motivating factors, patient age, concurrent disease, or attitudes of the partner as well as surgical technical details account for the low fertility rate.

In general, tubal sterilization should be considered irreversible. The procedure is indicated when the patient requests it. Many requests for anastomosis of divided tubes come when the procedure is initially advocated by a physician or partner. A woman of 23 with three children may be firm in her desire for sterilization, while a woman of 34 with five children may be unwilling to consider it. On the average, women are ages 28 to 30 at the time of tubal sterilization; 88 percent are married, 6 percent have never been married. Of note, risk of ovarian cancer appears to be reduced by tubal sterilization procedures. Mechanism is unknown.

The federal government will not reimburse for sterilization done at the time of abortion, because the combined procedure has been found to be more hazardous than either done separately. The rare instance in which this does not hold true is the patient in whom the risk of anesthesia is unduly high, such as a woman with myasthenia gravis. There is no federal reimbursement for sterilization of minors or mentally incompetent patients. Though awkward in individual cases, on the whole such regulations have been necessary to prevent widespread abuse of easily accomplished, low-risk surgical procedures done without due respect for the patient's understanding or desires. In addition, the government will not pay for hysterectomies done solely for the purpose of sterilization.

CHOICE OF METHOD

The choice of birth control is best viewed in terms of the patient's age and family expectations. *Unmarried adolescents and women in their early twenties* may use oral contraceptives with a high degree of safety and acceptability. Contraindications are infrequent in this age group, and the cost, in general, is not beyond their reach. Diaphragms may be as effective but often are less acceptable. Condoms and foam are an excellent choice given their effectiveness and protection from sexually transmitted diseases. Their use depends on motivation, which can be lacking at times. Though less effective and not usually recommended by physicians as a sole means of contraception, the sponge is convenient and, as such, more likely to be used by young women. IUDs are effective, but the risk of pelvic sepsis that may affect future childbearing is a concern.

For sexually active *26- to 35-year-olds*, birth control pills, diaphragms, and condoms may be equally effective, and choice is simply a matter of preference. IUDs may be a reasonable choice for parous women aware of the small risk of pelvic inflammatory disease and willing to seek help promptly at the first sign of infection. The smoker should be asked to stop tobacco use if she wants to use oral contraceptives. Many patients in this age group have completed their families and request sterilization. Nulliparous women in this age group who desire sterilization present a problem to many health care providers. If the patient is not well known to the clinic or physician, one can suggest she practice contraception for a year, then undergo sterilization if she still wants to. When such advice is given, perhaps half the patients return for the procedure. The others go elsewhere or change their minds.

For *women older than age 35*, the birth control pill may be prescribed as long as she is a nonsmoker. Diaphragms, condoms, sterilization, and more recently the pill are commonly chosen by *women older than age 40*.

PATIENT EDUCATION

There are few areas in primary care in which patient education is so important to decision making. Diagrammatic and written materials are available from most commercial distributors of contraceptive products, Planned Parenthood, many women's advocacy organizations, the American College of Obstetrics and Gynecology, and the American Medical Association. It is most important that information be clearly written in the patient's native language and that the patient be given an opportunity to ask questions and demonstrate her understanding.

The need to offer sympathetic and nonjudgmental counseling cannot be overemphasized. Regardless of the physician's personal views on abortion and birth control, the patient should be able to obtain factual information from her primary care physician or be referred to someone who is willing to provide the information and care desired.

INDICATIONS FOR REFERRAL

Patients may need or request referral for counseling on emotional responses to sexual activity and contraceptive techniques. Referral to a social worker, sex therapist, or psychiatrist with an interest in the area may be useful, but thorough discussion between the primary physician and patient usually suffices.

When a surgical procedure is being considered, the patient should meet with the gynecologist to discuss the issue in more detail. Referrals of medically uncomplicated patients may be made by phone. For patients with known medical problems, a careful history and physical examination and written referral to the specialist are helpful, so that the risks of the various procedures may be carefully discussed and therapy individualized. Patients who seem unable to use any form of birth control offered may also be referred to any of the above-named specialists, in the hope that an alternative approach will enhance motivation.

ANNOTATED BIBLIOGRAPHY

Barnes AB, Cohen E, Stoeckle JD, et al. Therapeutic abortion: Medical and social sequels. Ann Intern Med 1971;75:881. *(Summarizes impact on the patient from medical and social perspectives.)*

Burkman RT. Lipid metabolism effects with desogestrel-containing oral contraceptives. Am J Obstet Gynecol 1993;168:1033. *(A review of the studies suggests that desogestrel has minimal effect on lipoprotein metabolism.)*

Cates W, Schultz KF, Grimes DA. Risks associated with teenage abortion. N Engl J Med 1983;309:621. *(Teenagers had lower rates of morbidity or mortality from induced abortion than older women.)*

The Centers for Disease Control Cancer and Steroid Hormone Study. Oral contraceptive use and the risk of endometrial cancer. JAMA 1983;249:1600. *(A large, multi-center, case–control study detecting a significant protective effect for oral contraceptive use with a relative risk of developing endometrial cancer of 0.5; protective effect was most notable for nulliparous women.)*

The Centers for Disease Control Cancer and Steroid Hormone Study. Oral contraceptive use and the risk of ovarian cancer. JAMA 1983;249:1596. *(This multi-center, case–control study demonstrated a significant protective effect, with a relative risk of 0.6 for oral contraceptive users against ovarian cancer.)*

Collaborative Group for the Study of Stroke in Young Women. Oral contraception and increased risk of cerebral ischemia or thrombosis. N Engl J Med 1973;288:871. *(The incidence of thrombotic stroke showed a ninefold increase among women using oral contraceptives; hemorrhagic stroke showed less dramatic, but still significant, increase.)*

Collins D. Selectivity information on desogestrel. Am J Obstet Gynecol 1993;168:1010. *(Review of desogestrel's progestational effect reveals that it is weakly androgenic while retaining strong progestational activity.)*

Cramer DW, Hutchinson JB, Welch WR, et al. Factors affecting the association of oral contraceptives and ovarian cancer. N Engl J Med 1982;307:1047. *(Prior use of birth control pills appeared to provide long-lasting protection against ovarian cancer among subjects ages 40–59.)*

Edmondson HA, Henderson B, Benton B. Liver cell adenomas associated with use of oral contraceptives. N Engl J Med 1976;294:470. *(A study of 42 women with matched controls showed a dramatic rise in incidence of liver adenomas, correlated with prolonged use of pills that are more likely to contain mestranol as the synthetic estrogen.)*

Flickinger CJ. The effects of vasectomy on the testis. N Engl J Med 1985;313:1283. *(An editorial summarizing current state of knowledge; no serious adverse consequences other than infertility.)*

Gaspard UJ, Lefebvre PJ. Clinical aspects of the relationship between oral contraceptives, abnormalities in carbohydrate metabolism, and the development of cardiovascular disease. Am J Obstet Gynecol 1990;163:334. *(Low-dose oral contraceptives with reduced progestogen content have the least effect on glucose tolerance.)*

Goldacre MJ, Holford TR, Vessey MP. Cardiovascular disease and vasectomy. N Engl J Med 1983;308:805. *(A report of both a case–control study and a cohort study that did not demonstrate a relation between vasectomy and cardiovascular disease.)*

Henkinson SE, Hunter DJ, Colditz GA, et al. Tubal ligation, hysterectomy, and risk of ovarian cancer. JAMA 1993;270:2813. *(Risk is reduced significantly by tubal ligation.)*

Jarow JJ, Budin RE, Dym M, et al. Quantitative pathologic changes in the human testis after vasectomy. N Engl J Med 1985;313:1252. *(The development of interstitial fibrosis occurred with increased frequency and correlated with development of infertility.)*

Jick H, Hannan MT, Stergachis A, et al. Vaginal spermicides and gonorrhea. JAMA 1982;248:1619. *(This descriptive study suggests a protective effect against gonorrhea of vaginal spermicides.)*

Kopit S, Barnes AB. Patients' response to tubal division. JAMA 1976;236:2761. *(Of 197 patients who underwent tubal division, 93.5 percent said they would make the same choice again. Those who were regretful could not readily be identified by any preoperative characteristic such as age, parity, or marital status.)*

LeBolt SA, Grimes DA, Cates W. Mortality from abortion and childbirth. JAMA 1982;248:188. *(A pair of studies indicating that women are about seven times more likely to die from childbirth than from legal abortion and that available data are likely to be biased in the direction that overestimates abortion risks relative to the risks of childbearing.)*

Mishell DR. Contraception. N Engl J Med 1989;320:777. *(A review article discussing various contraceptive methods and their risks and benefits.)*

Rushton L, Jones DR. Oral contraceptive use and breast cancer risk: A meta-analysis of variations with age at diagnosis, parity and total duration of oral contraceptive use. Br J Obstet Gynecol 1992;99:239. *(A meta-analysis revealing a relative risk of breast cancer with oral contraceptive use of 1.16 in younger women, 1.21 in nulliparous women, and 1.27 for duration greater than 8 years.)*

Shoupe D, Mishell DR, Bopp BL, et al. The significance of bleeding patterns in Norplant implant users. Obstet Gynecol 1991;77:2:256. *(Cohort study of 234 Norplant users revealing 66.3 percent of women with irregular bleeding during the first years of use and 37.5 percent with irregular bleeding by the fifth year.)*

Spitz IM, Bardin CW. Mifepristone (RU-486)—a modulator of progestin and glucocorticoid action. N Engl J Med 1993; 329:404. *(Authoritative review of this potent abortifacient.)*

Stampfer MJ, Willet WC, Colditz GA, et al. Past use of oral contraceptives and cardiovascular disease: a meta-analysis in the context of the Nurses' Health Study. Am J Obstet Gynecol 1990;163:285. *(Large cohort study that prospectively looked at cardiovascular events and found no difference among past users as compared with never-users of the oral contraceptive.)*

Svensson L, Westrom L, Mardh P. Contraceptives and acute salpingitis. JAMA 1984;251:2553. *(Among women with the first episode of salpingitis observed through the laparoscope, women taking oral contraceptives had milder degrees of inflammation than women using IUDs or using no birth control.)*

Thomas DB. Oral contraceptives and breast cancer: review of the epidemiologic literature. Contraception 1991;43:597. *(In-depth review of studies reveals little or no overall increase in the risk of breast cancer. There may be a slight increase risk in very young women or women who use the pill for a long duration.)*

Thorogood M, Vessey MP. An epidemiologic survey of cardiovascular disease in women taking oral contraceptives. Am J Obstet Gynecol 1990;163:274. *(Review of earlier studies revealing a slight increase in cardiovascular events in women using 50-μg estrogen pill and report on early evidence showing fewer cardiovascular events in low-dose pill users.)*

Vaginal contraceptive sponge. Med Lett Drugs Ther 1983;25:78. *(Concludes it is a safe, convenient, but less effective barrier method than the diaphragm.)*

Wahl P, Walden C, Knopp R, et al. Effective estrogen/progestin potency on lipid/lipoprotein cholesterol. N Engl J Med 1983; 308:862. *(Low-estrogen/high-progestin birth control pills increase low-density lipoprotein cholesterol, but high-estrogens/low-progestin preparations, as well as estrogen use in postmenopausal women, were associated with elevated high-density lipoprotein cholesterol.)*

Primary Care Medicine: Office Evaluation and Management of the Adult Patient, 3rd edition, edited by Allan H. Goroll, Lawrence A. May, and Albert G. Mulley, Jr. J.B. Lippincott Company, Philadelphia

120
Approach to the Infertile Couple

A couple that has been engaging in regular unprotected sexual intercourse for at least a year without conceiving is deemed infertile. The primary physician is often the first to be consulted and responsible for initiating a medical evaluation of the couple. Although the usual request is to find or rule out a medical cause for the problem, there is also a need to identify any psychological or socioeconomic barriers to conception. Treatment is frequently carried out by individuals specializing in infertility, but the primary care physician should become proficient in performing the initial assessment and knowing when referral is indicated. Principal tasks include providing accurate advice and uncovering treatable etiologies.

PATHOPHYSIOLOGY AND CLINICAL PRESENTATION

Any disorder involving the male or female reproductive system may interfere with function to a degree sufficient to cause infertility.

Men

Infertility in the male can be classified in terms of gonadal, gonadotropic, obstructive, and functional etiologies and considered according to whether they present with azospermia, oligospermia, or normal sperm counts.

Azoospermic Etiologies. Patients with primary hypogonadism affecting both spermatogenesis and testosterone synthesis have azoospermia, a low testosterone, and elevations of luteinizing hormone (LH) and follicle-stimulating hormone (FSH). *Klinefelter's syndrome* is the archetype example, characterized by two X chromosomes and one Y chromosome. The extra chromatin is visible as the Barr body seen on examination of buccal mucosa cells.

Men with predominantly germinal compartment failure are also azoospermic but manifest relatively normal testosterone and normal LH, and elevated FSH. *Sertoli cell–only syndrome,* adult *mumps* orchitis, and *cancer therapy* are among the more common congenital and acquired varieties, respectively. In a study comparing childhood and adolescent cancer survivors to sibling controls, overall relative fertility was 85 percent, with radiation therapy below the diaphragm reducing it by 25 percent, and alkylating therapy alone causing a 40 percent reduction.

Hypogonadotropic hypogonadism also causes azoospermia. It too may be congenital or acquired (Table 120–1). Patients present with azoospermia and low levels of FSH, LH, and serum testosterone. Congenital disease is often associated with anosmia (*Kallmann's syndrome*). Pituitary tumors account for much of the acquired disease; a *prolactinoma* may be responsible. Large sellar tumors can lead to panhypopituitarism, with features of hypothyroidism and adrenal insufficiency dominating the clinical picture. *Drugs* (including alcohol and marijuana) can interfere with hypothalamic–pituitary function.

Azoospermia in association with normal levels of LH, FSH, and testosterone characterize *retrograde ejaculation* (due to diabetes or drugs) and *obstruction* of the ejaculatory system. There may be *congenital obstruction* of the epididymis and vas deferens or the vas may be absent. Most other types of obstruction are more proximal, giving normal testicular size and normal semen fructose.

Oligospermic Etiologies. Patients with a large *varicocele* may present with the typical "bag of worms" appearance to the testicle, but at times the only manifestation is a faint pulsation along the spermatic vein on Valsalva or coughing. The varicocele may be unilateral (usually on the left) or bilateral. There is no correlation between size of the varicocele and degree of infertility. Testicular size may be reduced, even though the scrotal contents appear enlarged. The mechanism by which varicocele results in infertility remains undetermined; some even question the association, but repair of the varicocele by spermatic vein ligation often restores normal sperm quantity and function. Effects on fertility are less clear.

Another large group of oligospermic patients with normal LH and testosterone have no detectable pathology and are labeled *idiopathic*. The condition results in a quantitative abnormality of spermatogenesis without any identifiable anatomic or endocrinologic precipitant. FSH is normal unless the sperm count falls below 20 million/mL, in which case it may begin to rise. At times, the acquired forms of selective tubular damage (*chemotherapy, irradiation*, adult *mumps*) may leave the patient oligospermic rather than azoospermic. Testosterone and LH are normal, but TSH is elevated.

In milder forms of acquired *hypothalamic–pituitary dysfunction,* some spermatogenesis may be preserved. FSH and LH are low to low normal and testosterone is low. Prolactin may be elevated due to a *microadenoma*. In *partial androgen resistance,* testosterone and LH are elevated whereas FSH remains normal. Gynecomastia develops as a result of excess estradiol production by the testicle and peripheral conversion of testosterone.

Etiologies with Normal Sperm Counts. Most patients demonstrate abnormal sperm morphology or motility and suffer from many of the same conditions as those with oligospermia (eg, varicocele). In addition, *genitourinary tract infection* may cause such qualitative sperm changes; leukocytes sometimes appear in the semen. *Antisperm antibodies* are noted in some patients, and an autoimmune mechanism may be operative in some instances, although the relationship between antibodies and infertility remains to be fully established.

Impotence ranks as a leading, although frequently overlooked, etiology. Hormone concentrations and sperm parameters are usually normal in "functional" types (although depression and situational stress can transiently reduce sperm counts). In organic etiologies of impotence, these parameters reflect the underlying pathology (see Chapters 132 and 229). Anatomic anomalies, such as proximal location of the urinary meatus, may lead to infertility because of deposition of sperm and semen too far from the cervical os.

Women

Disorders of Ovulation are among the most frequent causes of failure to conceive, comprising 20 percent to 40 percent of cases in which a female factor is responsible for the infertility. Anovulatory bleeding (irregular menses), amenorrhea, or infertility may be the presenting complaint. *Polycystic ovary syndrome* and other forms of *hypothalamic dysfunction* account for most cases (see Chapters 111 and 112). Pathophysiologically, the normal pattern of gonadotropin-releasing hormone (GnRH) release is disrupted, impairing the normal midcycle surge in luteinizing hormone (LH). The result is failure to ovulate and inadequate corpus luteum formation. Treatment can restore fertility.

Premature ovarian failure may be autoimmune or idiopathic, but an important acquired source is *cancer therapy* in children and adolescents (see above). In the study noted above comparing survivors of childhood and adolescent cancers with their siblings, overall relative fertility for women was 85 percent, with radiation therapy below the diaphragm reducing it by 25 percent but alkylating therapy having relatively little effect.

Tubal Disorders account for about 25 percent of cases. *Pelvic inflammatory disease* (particularly indolent, nongonococcal forms such as that due to *Chlamydia trachomatis* [see Chapters 116 and 117]) is the leading cause of tubal damage. In a prospective study, 12 percent of those with a single episode of salpingitis had tubal occlusion; 35 percent of those with two infections had occlusion; and 75 percent of those with three or more had occlusion. Other pelvic and abdominal infections (such as a *ruptured appendix* in childhood) may lead to tubal adhesions. Infections associated with intrauterine devices (IUDs) are a problem. *Postpartum infection* has an unusually frequent association with tubal occlusion. Infections following induced abortion, particularly if inadequately treated (eg, with inappropriately low doses of antibiotics), unrecognized, or not brought to medical attention, may lead to infertility.

Oil-based *dyes* used for uterotubograms (hysterosalpingograms) in some countries have also been associated with adhesions. Uncommon causes include *pelvic trauma* from vehicular accidents, *inflammatory bowel disease,* tuberculosis, and schistosomiasis. In general, processes that cause adhesions rather than tubal epithelial damage seem to have a better prognosis. *Endometriosis,* found in 8 percent to 15 percent of fertility clinic populations, may cause tubal obstruction as well as uterine disturbances.

Uterine Pathology represents about 5 percent of cases. *Congenital anomalies,* such as absence or duplication of the uterine fundus, often present as repeated pregnancy wastage. Complete duplication of cervix and uterus tends to diminish fertility, but less so than anomalies causing distortion of a single uterine cavity. Septate and deeply arcuate uteri may be more useful after hysteroscopic or operative repair. Urinary tract anomalies are estimated to occur with 25 percent of congenitally abnormal uteri. They are found more frequently in the completely duplicated situation or when one side of the müllerian duct is missing.

Uterine fibroids and *endometriosis* may distort or obstruct the uterine cavity. Resection and re-resection of fibroids have been surprisingly successful. The *forgotten IUD* is occasionally a cause of infertility. The role of uterine glycosaminoglycan in stimulating conversion of sperm proacrosin to acrosin, a step necessary for sperm penetration of the zona pellucida, is an area of ongoing investigation.

Cervical Factors are increasingly appreciated sources of infertility. *Cervical incompetence* may lead to repeated abortion or later trimester pregnancy losses. The incompetence can result from inadequate innervation, disturbances in synthesis or breakdown of prostaglandin, or defects in muscle and collagen fibers. Incompetence of the cervix may also compromise its role in resisting the entry of infectious agents into the sterile uterine cavity.

The precise role of *cervical mucus* is still not well understood, but normal viscosity and ferning are essential to conception and represent evidence of adequate estrogen stimulation and response. The importance of cervical mucus *antibodies* and proteins as a cause of infertility continues to be a focus of much research.

Vaginal Factors are occasionally implicated. An intact or nearly *intact hymen,* a septum, or a constricting ring in the upper vagina can limit access to the cervix. Total absence of the vagina is only rarely associated with sufficient development of the cervix and uterus to allow fertility at all. As a site of *infection,* the vagina may prove to be an important cause of pregnancy wastage. *Trichomonas, Candida albicans, Chlamydia, Mycoplasma, Gardnerella,* streptococci, and gonococci are all associated with cervical and vaginal discharge (see Chapter 117). Their role in vaginally related obstructions to conception is not clear, although their role in pregnancy wastage is established. When these organisms lead to pelvic inflammatory disease, they become more clearly accountable for infertility.

Viral *infections* of the *vulva* and *labia,* particularly herpes vaginalis and condyloma accuminata are usually only temporary impediments to fertility (see Chapter 192). Vulvar surgery per se need not cause infertility. Similarly, paralysis or hemipelvectomy may or may not be blamed for infertility; much of the impediment derives from the social and emotional impact of these conditions.

Both Partners

Interpersonal problems (see Chapter 229) are an important etiologic factor, because they may lead to sexual dysfunction. The desire for children may not be shared equally by both partners. This may be overt, with one partner seeking medical assistance to persuade the other. More often, it is covert. There may be anxiety over how family responsibilities will interfere with career development, or one partner may not want to lose the economic and social freedom of a childless couple. Sometimes one partner may be concerned about sharing the other's affection with a child. Some may feel inadequate or unwilling to assume parental duties. Such concerns can lead to sexual inactivity or frigidity. Transient situational problems arise. The young professional person may be under considerable job pressure; travel may interfere with optimal moments for insemination or lead to hypothalamic dysfunction. Acknowledged or unrecognized homosexual preference may also interfere with fertility.

Controversy surrounds the role of *genital* Mycoplasma *infection* in the genesis of infertility. In one study, if the husband was culture-positive, treatment of the infertile couple for *Mycoplasma* led to a 60 percent pregnancy rate if the infection was eradicated versus a 5 percent rate when it was not. Other studies fail to show any association between the *Mycoplasma* infection and infertility.

Table 120-1. Important Causes of Male Infertility

Hypothalamic/Pituitary
Prolactinoma
Idiopathic
Drugs (eg, alcohol, marijuana)
Testicular
Klinefelter's syndrome
Sertoli cell–only syndrome
Irradiation
Adult mumps
Alkylating agents
Anatomic/Functional
Obstruction of epididymis or vas
Impotence
Retrograde ejaculation
Infection
Antisperm antibodies
Idiopathic defects in sperm quantity or quality

DIFFERENTIAL DIAGNOSIS

In about a third of instances, a male factor is the predominant etiology. In another third, a female factor predominates. In the remainder, either the cause resides with both partners or the etiology is unknown. In the vast majority of cases attributed to a male factor, there is either a quantitative or qualitative sperm defect of unknown etiology. Among female factors, ovulatory disturbances account for up to 40 percent, tubal disorders for 10 percent to 30 percent, cervical factors for 20 percent, and uterine factors for about 5 percent. Tables 120–1 and 120–2 list some of the most important etiologies.

WORKUP

Initial Evaluation

Because the prognosis even for untreated couples is favorable (see below), an extensive "infertility workup" need

Table 120-2. Important Causes of Female Infertility

Hypothalamic/Pituitary
Hypothalamic dysfunction
Polycystic ovary syndrome
Prolactinoma
Ovarian
Primary failure (eg, premature menopause)
Irradiation
Tubal
Pelvic inflammatory disease
Endometriosis
Adhesions
Uterine
Fibroids
Scarring (Asherman's syndrome)
Anatomic abnormalities
Cervical
Poor mucus quality
Infection
Anatomic abnormalities

not be undertaken on first visit, unless the couple is older (mid- to late 30s and upward), has been unable to conceive despite trying seriously for over a year, or has a similar good reason to hasten the pace of evaluation. Otherwise, a reasonable approach to the first visit is to limit the assessment to a careful general history and physical examination, checking for such important causes as endocrinopathy, tumor, genitourinary tract infection, anatomic disorder, and interpersonal problems.

In the Male. *History* should include inquiry into drug and medication use (marijuana, alcohol, antihypertensive agents), urethral discharge, headache and other symptoms of a pituitary tumor (see Chapter 100), past history of radiation therapy or cancer chemotherapy, mumps, toxin exposure, and systemic illnesses (especially diabetes with associated retrograde ejaculation). A sexual history that reviews the marital relationship, sexual techniques, potency, and frequency of intercourse is also important.

Physical examination begins with noting general appearance and any signs of underandrogenization (decreased body hair, gynecomastia, eunuchoid proportions). The scrotum is examined for testicular size, presence of a varicocele, hypospadias, and absent vas deferens. Soft, small testes (less than 4 cm in longest diameter) are consistent with primary testicular failure and pituitary–hypothalamic insufficiency. A Valsalva maneuver performed while the patient is standing will help reveal a small varicocele. The urethra is observed for discharge, and the prostate and seminal vesicles are observed for tenderness and other signs of infection. If a pituitary condition is suspected, visual field testing by confrontation might reveal an important field defect; a normal study does not rule out a mass lesion. Testing deep tendon reflexes may uncover delay in relaxation suggestive of hypothyroidism (see Chapter 104).

In the Female. *History* focuses on the menstrual and reproductive history, including any abortions, complicated deliveries, curettages, menstrual irregularities, or episodes of amenorrhea. A life-long history of menstrual irregularities is suggestive of polycystic ovary syndrome, especially if accompanied by hirsutism and obesity. Any situational or emotional stress, marked weight loss, or excess exercise should be noted, as it can lead to hypothalamic dysfunction and impairment of ovulation (see Chapters 111 and 112). Similarly, checking for symptoms of hypothyroidism (see Chapter 104), hyperprolactinemia (see Chapter 100), Cushing's syndrome (see Chapter 100), and androgen excess (see Chapter 98) may yield clues of conditions that can impair hypothalamic function. Inquiry into headaches, visual field disturbances, galactorrhea, symptoms of pituitary insufficiency (see Chapter 100), and a history of postpartum hemorrhage helps to screen for a sella tursica lesion. Checking for a history or symptoms of pelvic inflammatory disease (vaginal discharge, pelvic pain, fever, dyspareunia) is also essential. Any malignant disease history is important to note, especially if treatment included irradiation or alkylating agents. One should also obtain a detailed psychosocial history that reviews pertinent details of the marital relationship and sexual activity. Loss of libido may signify psychosocial or hormonal dysfunction.

Physical examination focuses on checking for obesity, excessive weight loss, hirsutism, cushingoid appearance, stigmata of hypothyroidism (see Chapter 104), visual field disturbances, and goiter. Most important is a careful pelvic examination, taking special note of any ovarian, uterine, or adnexal masses, thickening, or tenderness. Examination of the cervix should include checking for erosions, discharge, polyps, masses, scarring, and pain on cervical motion. The hirsute patient is examined for clitoromegaly.

Both Partners. An empathic, supportive, nonjudgmental exploration of the marital relationship is essential; it is often best done by interviewing the couple together (to observe their interactions) as well as each partner separately.

Further Evaluation

Couples with no evidence of serious pathology on initial evaluation can be reassured and informed that more than half of such couples go on to conceive without the aid of treatment. Those who have been trying to conceive for less than 1 year can be advised to delay further evaluation until 12 months have passed, provided they are willing to do so and have no compelling reason for proceeding directly to more extensive testing. Couples who have failed to conceive after continuously trying for 12 months, or who insist on further workup at the time of initial visit, can undergo a set of basic laboratory studies to more fully define the problem and guide further evaluation and treatment.

In the Male. The first test to perform is a *semen analysis,* collecting two to three specimens over a 4- to 6-week period. Quantitative analysis includes number of sperm per milliliter of semen (counts >20 million/mL are normal) and semen volume (<1.5 mL may be inadequate to buffer vaginal acidity). Patients with normal counts should have qualitative studies of the sperm performed (motility, morphology, cervical mucus interaction), although these studies are often more useful for identifying the infertile individual than for defining a specific course of therapy (see below). In normal persons, the counts for motile forms and spermatozoa with oval heads are in excess of 50 percent.

Patients with azoospermia or oligospermia are candidates for serum gonadotropin (*LH* and *FSH*) and *testosterone* determinations, because of the possibility of an underlying disorder within the hypothalamic–pituitary–testicular axis. Proper sampling technique is important to avoid misleading results. One draws three serum samples 20 minutes apart and pools them. A primary gonadal problem is suggested by high concentrations of gonadotropins and low or low-normal testosterone. A pituitary–hypothalamic etiology is characterized by both gonadotropins and testosterone being low. Normal FSH, testosterone, and testicular size in a patient with azoospermia suggests obstruction. Normal hormone and gonadotropin concentrations in the setting of oligospermia are characteristic of patients with varicocele or idiopathic disease. Klinefelter's syndrome is suggested by small testes, gynecomastia, an elevated FSH, and a reduced testosterone. The diagnosis is confirmed by a *buccal smear* that shows the extra chromatin of a Barr body.

The patient with suspected pituitary disease needs a *prolactin level* and *computed tomography (CT) scan* of the sella turcica to search for a tumor. An elevated prolactin in the setting of a normal CT may be due to a drug-induced problem, but CT should be repeated in 6 months to be sure an early tumor has not been missed.

The utility of more elaborate studies (eg, antisperm antibodies, sperm–cervical mucus interaction, penetration testing) is best determined by the infertility specialist.

In the Female. The first task is to establish that ovulation is taking place. The time-tested approach is to use a *temperature chart.* Ovulation is accompanied by a rise in progesterone secretion, which leads to a 0.3-degree rise in basal body temperature after ovulation. Temperature is measured orally each morning before rising from bed. One uses a special thermometer graduated in tenths of degrees Fahrenheit. Absence of a rise indicates failure to ovulate. Alternatively, one can measure the *serum progesterone* on days 21 to 23 of the cycle. A level greater than 10 ng/mL indicates ovulation and a functioning corpus luteum. Endometrial biopsy may also be useful, but is more expensive, more painful, and may remove the long-awaited pregnancy. If the patient is deemed anovulatory, further testing proceeds with measurement of *serum prolactin, FSH,* and *LH* (see Chapters 111 and 112).

A *postcoital examination* is used to assess cervical mucus function and the competency of the partner. An appointment is scheduled just before the time of ovulation, and the woman is asked to come within 2 to 12 hours of coitus. A specimen of cervical mucus is obtained from the endocervical canal. Five or more motile sperm found in the specimen confirms her partner's competence. Mucus is also examined for viscosity (stretching to 6 cm is normal) and "ferning," manifestations of estrogen effect.

If after the initial history, physical examination, postcoital test, and serum progesterone, it appears that tubal or uterine disease may be responsible for infertility, then *hysterosalpingography* and *laparoscopy* deserve consideration. Choice of test should be made by the gynecologist experienced in evaluation of infertility. Hysterosalpingoscopy involves injection of a contrast agent into the uterus by way of a cervical catheter. Pretreatment doxycycline antibiotic coverage is provided. Films reveal uterine and tubal anatomy. Laparoscopy requires general anesthesia, but can detect adhesions, endometriosis, an unpalpable fibroid, and polycystic ovaries. Tubal patency and position may also be confirmed, often more accurately than by radiologic investigation. Not to be forgotten is the importance of negative findings.

PRINCIPLES OF MANAGEMENT AND INDICATIONS FOR REFERRAL

Studies from infertility clinics have shown that many couples go on to conceive without treatment (eg, 44% of those with ovulation deficiency; 61 percent of those with endometriosis, tubal defects, or seminal deficiencies; and 96 percent of those with cervical factors or idiopathic infertility). A conservative approach of watchful waiting is reasonable in such cases, provided there is no evidence of tumor, infection, anatomic defect, or serious endocrinopathy. Counseling can be a very important adjunct (see below).

When the workup suggests causative organic pathology, an appropriate referral for confirmatory testing and design of a treatment program is indicated. The continued participation of the primary physician in the care of the couple ought to remain, but the subtleties of specialized care that some types of infertility treatment require argue for referral rather than for treatment by the primary physician. Successful referral depends to a large extent on proper patient selection.

Men. A neurologic or anatomic cause of *impotence,* a suspected acquired *obstructive defect,* and *varicocele* are indications for urologic consultation. Surgical ligation of a varicocele is commonly performed, but results are often disappointing even though sperm counts may rise. Treatment of obstruction requires a urologist skilled in microsurgical techniques, as does vasectomy reversal.

Hypothalamic–pituitary disorders have a high rate of success with treatment by the reproductive endocrinologist. Those with idiopathic hypogonadotropic disease often respond successfully to gonadotropin or GnRH administration. When prolactin levels are elevated and CT scan reveals a microadenoma, bromocriptine can often restore fertility. Larger pituitary adenomas may require neurosurgical intervention.

Idiopathic oligospermia (no evidence of a varicocele; normal LH, FSH, and testosterone) has no proven therapy. Clomiphene and other antiestrogens, GnRH-releasing factor, gonadotropins, and low-doses of androgen have been tried, but without confirmed long-term benefit. There is no evidence that vitamins (A, E, C), zinc, thyroid hormone, or a host of home remedies are at all useful in men with normospermia or oligospermia. Such patients should be referred to the reproductive endocrinologist for consultation.

Men who have quantitatively and qualitatively *normal sperm* and *normal LH, FSH,* and *testosterone* pose a challenge. When *antisperm antibodies* are found in high titers in the semen, their levels can be lowered with a course of high-dose corticosteroids. However, the efficacy of this therapy is controversial. Careful patient selection by referral to the reproductive specialist is essential. In vitro fertilization is an alternative.

Artificial insemination and other assisted reproductive technologies are available for patients with otherwise *refractory qualitative sperm defects.* Patients with retrograde ejaculation might also effect pregnancy with artificial insemination, using semen recovered in the urine.

Subclinical infection, especially with *Mycoplasma,* has been suggested as a cause of infertility. Culturing both partners and treating the couple if one partner is culture-positive has produced inconsistent results. There are no known treatments for patients with gonadal failure or androgen insensitivity.

Women. Women with *hypothalamic dysfunction* have a good prognosis. Those with mild dysfunction are likely to resume ovulating without therapy and need only counseling at the time of initial evaluation. Those with moderate dysfunction often respond well to treatment, especially when FSH, thyroid function, and prolactin remain normal. Such persons have a 50 percent chance of conceiving with use of clomiphene, which is given for 3 to 5 days followed by a month of waiting for either pregnancy or an ovulatory period. Patient suffering from more severe hypothalamic dysfunction may fail clomiphene, but respond to synthetic GnRH therapy. It is more physiologic, less expensive, more comfortable, and less likely to induce multiple pregnancies and ovarian overstimulation than human menopausal gonadotropins, which had previously been used in such situations. GnRH is administered by parenteral pulse infusions, mimicking normal GnRH secretion. Careful dose adjustments are necessary to avoid multiple pregnancies. Only an experienced reproductive endocrinologist should prescribe such therapy. Those with a prolactin-secreting microadenoma require endocrinologic consultation. Bromocriptine may help restore fertility (see Chapter 100).

Gynecologic referral is indicated in patients with suspected *tubal scarring*. Microsurgical tubal reconstruction is required for successful repair, which leads to pregnancy in 10 percent to 60 percent of cases. In making the referral for tubal repair, it is important to select a gynecologist skilled in microsurgical techniques. Success rates vary considerably.

Women with *abnormal postcoital testing* may be candidates for intrauterine insemination if they are ovulating and the semen analysis is normal. Couples who have *failed other methods* may still be candidates for in vitro fertilization or gamete intrafallopian tube transfer. These are elaborate technologies that require the consultative and technical services of a specialized reproductive center. One must have adequate sperm, ovarian follicles, and a competent uterus to qualify for in vitro fertilization. These plus fallopian tube patency and accessibility are the minimum determinants for gamete intrafallopian tube transfer.

Couples. Infertility resulting from a *psychosocial problem* (eg, lack of privacy, work exhaustion, marital discord) needs to be approached with careful and understanding explanation. Some individuals may attempt to view the situation as a medical problem when there is unlikely to be a strictly medical solution. Attention needs to be directed to the home environment, work situation, and marital relation. When *sexual dysfunction* is detected, treatment is best directed toward it (see Chapter 229). However, artificial insemination is sometimes used when there is a strong desire to have a child as soon as possible.

The infertility evaluation may lead to reconsideration and redesign of treatment regimens for *underlying medical conditions* such as cancer and hypertension (see Chapters 26, 88, and 89).

PATIENT EDUCATION

Couples are eager for information about their chances of conceiving. At one end of the spectrum are men and women with permanent gonadal failure who have no chance of conceiving. At the other end are those with a transient functional deficit who are likely to conceive without any treatment other than reassurance and time. The couple that remains unsuccessful after a year of trying can be given some reassurance as they begin to undergo evaluation. Up to one-quarter of such couples achieve pregnancy within 3 months. Published findings from infertility clinics show that, overall, 25 percent to 35 percent of couples achieve conception within 1 to 2 years of registration. The percentages continue to rise over the next 4 to 5 years.

There is a slight decrease in fecundity after 30 and a marked decrease after age 35. There appears to be no difference in prognosis between infertile couples who have conceived in the past and those who have never conceived. The prognosis for women who experience recurrent spontaneous abortions is better than the approximately 20 percent live-birth rate previously estimated. Patients with ovulatory problems do reasonably well; those with tubal problems have more difficulty. As noted earlier, rates for live births after tubal repair range from 10 percent to 60 percent, depending on the severity and site of the scarring, quality of semen, age of the women, and a host of other factors. Couples whose infertility involves multiple factors do less well than those in whom only one factor is identified.

Whenever an evaluation comes out normal, it is important to reassure patients about their normality, particularly if one harbors guilt or fear about an episode of infidelity, a previous abortion, an out-of-wedlock pregnancy, or some other potentially adverse event.

The investigation of infertility provides an opportunity to educate patients about normal human reproduction and prevention of sexually transmitted disease. This area is still omitted from many school curricula and is inadequately covered in others. Education for both partners about the menstrual cycles, the best time to attempt conception, and the frequency of coitus needed to achieve pregnancy can be very helpful, sometimes even curative. The importance of using a condom to prevent spread of sexually transmitted diseases that might lead to tubal scarring cannot be overemphasized to teenagers and other patients with multiple partners. Screening such persons for chlamydial infection and treating when present may help prevent tubal infertility (see Chapter 117). A review of sexual attitudes and concerns may also be of benefit. At times, the infertility evaluation encourages couples to take better care of themselves.

A.H.G.

ANNOTATED BIBLIOGRAPHY

Aral SO, Cates W. The increasing concern with fertility. JAMA 1983;250:2327. *(An analysis of the demographics of infertility and explanations for increased demand for infertility services.)*

Barnes R, Rosenfield RL. Polycystic ovary syndrome: Pathogenesis and treatment. Ann Intern Med 1989;110:386. *(Detailed review; 169 refs.)*

Byrne J, Mulvihill JJ, Myers MH, et al. Effects of treatment on fertility in long-term survivors of childhood or adolescent cancer. N Engl J Med 1987;317:1315. *(A retrospective cohort study; fertility rates varied by sex, site of therapy, and type.)*

Collins JA, Wrixon W, Janes LB, et al. Treatment-independent pregnancy among infertile couples. N Engl J Med 1983;309:1201. *(A retrospective review indicating that the potential for a spontaneous cure is high.)*

Collins JA, Ying SO, Wilson EH, et al. The postcoital test as a predictor of pregnancy among 355 infertile couples. Fertil Steril 1984;41:703. *(Predictive value was good.)*

Diugnan NM, Jordan JA, Couglan BM, et al. One thousand consecutive cases of diagnostic laparoscopy. J Obstet Gynaecol

Br Cwlth 1972;79:1016. *(There are many series on laparoscopy; this is one of the most useful.)*

Filicori M, Flamigni C, Meriggiola MC, et al. Endocrine response determines the clinical outcome of pulsatile gonadotropin-releasing hormone ovulation induction in different ovulatory disorders. J Clin Endocrinol Metab 1991;72:965. *(Data on optimizing use of GnRH for induction of ovulation in patients with hypothalamic dysfunction.)*

Gorry GA, Pauker SG, Swartz WB. Diagnostic importance of the normal finding. N Engl J Med 1978;298:486. *(Emphasizes the value to the patient of a normal finding.)*

Gump DW, Gibson M, Ashikaga T. Lack of association between genital mycoplasmas and infertility. N Engl J Med 1984;310:937. *(Found no association between prior pelvic inflammatory disease causing infertility and presence of* Mycoplasma.*)*

Hurley DM, Brian R, Outch K, et al. Induction of ovulation and fertility in amenorrheic women by pulsatile low dose gonadotropin-releasing hormone. N Engl J Med 1984;310:1069. *(Thirteen of 14 women resistant to clomiphene therapy achieved pregnancy with subcutaneous pulses of GnRH.)*

Kaufman DG, Nagler HM. Significance and pathophysiology of the varicocele: Current concepts. Semin Reprod Endocrinol 1988;6:349. *(A review of the debate.)*

Magid MS, Cash KL, Goldstein M. The testicular biopsy in the evaluation of infertility. Semin Urol 1990;8:51. *(Especially useful in the assessment of men with normal endocrine function and suspected ductal obstruction.)*

Mueller BA, Daling JR, Moore DE, et al. Appendectomy and the risk of tubal infertility. N Engl J Med 1986;315:1506. *(Risk increased only in cases of ruptured appendix.)*

Schwartz D, Mayaux MJ. Female fecundity as a function of age. N Engl J Med 1982;306:404. *(A slight but significant decrease after age 30; more marked after age 35.)*

Seibel MM. A new era in reproductive technology. N Engl J Med 1988;318:828. *(A very useful review for the generalist reader of the technologic advances and treatment options.)*

Shepard MK, Jones RB. Recovery of *Chlamydia trachomatis* from endometrial and fallopian tube biopsies in women with infertility of tubal origin. Fertil Steril 1989;52:232. *(Provides important evidence linking chlamydial infection with tubal scarring.)*

Swerdloff RS, Overstreet JW, Sokol RZ, et al. Infertility in the male. Ann Intern Med 1985;103:906. *(A comprehensive yet practical review of the pathogenesis, evaluation, and treatment; 132 refs.)*

Primary Care Medicine: Office Evaluation and Management of the Adult Patient, 3rd edition, edited by Allan H. Goroll, Lawrence A. May, and Albert G. Mulley, Jr. J.B. Lippincott Company, Philadelphia

121
Approach to the Woman With an Unplanned Pregnancy

FLORA TREGER, M.D.
JENNIFER JEREMIAH, M.D.

The woman who suspects an unplanned or unwanted pregnancy often calls on her primary care provider to confirm a diagnosis and formulate a care plan. To provide support and assistance, the physician first must accurately diagnose the pregnancy. He or she can then inform the patient about community services available for prenatal care, abortion, and adoption. If the physician feels his or her beliefs interfere with objective counseling, then referral to another provider is necessary. Awareness of the patient's social and cultural environment is essential to lending appropriate support.

CLINICAL PRESENTATIONS

Women presenting with unplanned pregnancies have highly variable experiences. Responses to the diagnosis, coping mechanisms, and capacity to take responsibility for decision making may differ greatly from woman to woman.

A pregnancy may be untimely or unwanted because of the severe hardship a child would create. A limited single or dual income may be insufficient to support either a first or additional child. A pregnancy may hinder opportunities for education and career advancement. These factors may conflict with the woman's desire for motherhood, creating great ambivalence and frustration for her. Some women who desire children may have a partner opposed to parenting or may need family or social support to raise a child alone. They may feel pressured to terminate the pregnancy yet be unwilling to do so.

The woman who desires pregnancy but suffers from a chronic or life-threatening illness such as diabetes, systemic lupus erythematosus, or cancer endures unique stress when she faces an unplanned pregnancy. The pregnancy may jeopardize her health and her ability to care for her family, and she may face conflicting opinions regarding termination. Additionally, the impact of pregnancy on certain disease processes is not well understood.

As many as 80,000 women of childbearing age may be infected with the human immunodeficiency virus (HIV). The rate of transmission of the HIV to the fetus is estimated to be 25 percent to 50 percent. This raises new concerns for the primary care physician who must consider the welfare of both the mother and the unborn child. At this point, it is unclear whether pregnancy adversely affects the HIV disease process in the mother. Additionally, the difficult dilemma of whether to carry a potentially infected fetus to term poses many ethical questions.

Substance abuse among pregnant women continues to rise. The most significant increase is seen with cocaine, but use of heroin, methadone, and amphetamines has also grown. Cocaine use has been associated with lower birth weight and preterm labor. Heroin use during pregnancy can lead to a withdrawal syndrome in the infant. In addition to toxic drug effects, poor pregnancy outcomes may result from transmission of disease from "dirty needles," hazardous behavior to support a drug habit, malnutrition, and poor prenatal care. Often there is evidence of polysubstance abuse with additive effects. Additionally, alcohol remains a significant problem during pregnancy. The fetal alcohol syndrome, manifested by intrauterine growth retardation, microcephaly, and developmental abnormalities, occurs in approximately one in 2000 live births. Some substance abusers may respond to pregnancy with denial or indifference.

A woman with a severe, poorly controlled psychiatric illness presents many concerns. Recent data suggest that pregnant patients with psychiatric disorders may have worsening of their mental health during pregnancy. In addition, some studies suggest that patients with severe disorders may have increased birth complications resulting from poor prenatal care, concurrent substance abuse, increased incidence of homelessness, use of psychiatric medications during pregnancy, and unrecognized physical illness. The primary care physician may be asked to provide counseling and to act as a liaison between obstetric and psychiatric providers.

Some patients undergoing amniocentesis or chorionic villus sampling to identify genetic abnormalities do so on the assumption that they will consider an induced abortion. A patient may look to her primary care provider for guidance with this difficult decision-making process.

Almost 1 million adolescents in the United States become pregnant yearly. Consequences for the future of these teenagers may be immense. Pregnancy may lead to dropping out of school, limited job opportunities, and dependence on the welfare system. Adolescents may intentionally or unintentionally become pregnant for various reasons. They may exhibit risk-taking behavior in response to peer pressure, to experiment, or to test parental limits. Failure to properly use contraception may result from lack of adequate information or stem from the belief that, "It will never happen to me." Some adolescents who feel deprived of love and security from parents or partners may see a child as a companion who will provide them with unconditional love. Often, teenagers present at a later gestational age because of denial or unawareness of how to get help. This delay may result in significant negative consequences with increased morbidity and mortality from the pregnancy or termination.

A number of presentations are particularly important because of their psychosocial circumstances.

In both rural and urban areas, sexual abuse (including rape) persists to a greater extent than most professional people assume. It may occur between father and daughter, but frequently it involves another adult male in the household, such as uncle, older brother, or boyfriend. The victim may be repulsed at the thought of a baby inside her from such a traumatic experience and may not present for care until later in the pregnancy. In some states, the physician is mandated to report sexual abuse involving minors.

PRINCIPLES OF MANAGEMENT AND PATIENT EDUCATION

Diagnosis. Immunologic tests including home pregnancy kits or office slide kits that measure human chorionic gonadotropin (HCG) are commonly used for first diagnosis of pregnancy. These use urine or serum, are accurate 4 to 14 days from a missed period, and can give false-positive results because of luteinizing hormone (LH) cross-reactivity. More sensitive and specific tests include the enzyme-linked immunosorbent assay (ELISA), using serum or urine, and serum radioimmunoassay tests. These detect lower HCG levels and appear positive earlier (12 days and 7 days postconception, respectively). They are specific for the beta-HCG subunit and are not affected by LH cross-reactivity. The availability of monoclonal antibodies to the beta subunit has improved test accuracy. The half-life of HCG postdelivery is 1.5 days, so failure to normalize after pregnancy termination indicates remaining tissue, as with incomplete abortion or gestational trophoblastic disease.

Counseling. Once a diagnosis of pregnancy is confirmed, a nonjudgmental, supportive examination of the patient's feelings is needed. A thorough psychosocial history should be gathered so her options can be fully explored. Special attention to issues of rape and incest are necessary if this history is elicited or appears to be a possibility. Formal counseling is indicated in this instance. Community support groups may also be helpful.

Therapeutic Abortion. Abortion is one of the most common gynecologic procedures performed in the United States. Data regarding the use of abortion have remained fairly stable since 1980, with a 1990 national abortion ratio (number of legal abortions per 1000 live births) of 344 and a 1990 national abortion rate (number of legal abortions per 1000 women aged 15–44 years) of 24. Centers for Disease Control and Prevention (CDC) data show that, as of 1990, 92 percent of women undergoing legal abortion had the procedure in their state of residence. About 55 percent of women undergoing pregnancy termination were younger than age 25, 79 percent were unmarried, and approximately 64 percent were white. Approximately 88 percent of abortions occur within the first 12 weeks of gestation, with half occurring within 8 weeks of gestation.

When performed appropriately, pregnancy termination is safe, with less than one death per 100,000 procedures. In developed countries, legal first-trimester terminations result in lower death rates than those from pregnancy across all age groups. Termination is safest when performed earlier in gestation. Risk increases with gestational age, maternal age, and higher parity. With legalization of abortion in the United States, morbidity has decreased. There is increased physician training and expertise; increased use of the safer suction curettage procedure rather than sharp curettage, uterine instillation, and surgical procedures; and improved access, allowing earlier procedures. Service availability and practices regarding waiting periods, parental consent, and abortion funding all impact on a woman's obtaining services. Additional barriers to services include cost (earlier and nonhospital procedures are cheaper than second-trimester hospital procedures), harassment of patients at abortion facilities, and vandalism of facilities.

Preprocedure assessment includes determining any underlying medical problems that would necessitate an inpatient rather than outpatient procedure. Usual laboratory evaluation includes pregnancy testing, urinalysis, complete blood count, blood type and Rh factor determination, syphilis serologies, gonorrhea and chlamydia testing, and Papanicolaou (Pap) smear. Additional studies such as HIV testing and sonography can be considered. Contraception may also be addressed at this time, since oral contraceptives can be initiated the day following termination and IUD placement can occur with the procedure. This addresses the concern about frequent no-show rates for follow-up appointments. Rh immune globulin should be given postprocedure to Rh-negative unsensitized individuals. Postabortion instructions include no intercourse, douching, or tampons for 1 to 2 weeks.

Local anesthesia is used for first-trimester procedures. Paracervical block using lidocaine, with or without epinephrine, and preoperative analgesics or sedatives are generally safe and inexpensive. General anesthesia is most often used for procedures done later in pregnancy.

First-trimester abortions are performed at 12 weeks gestation or sooner, and 96 percent of them are performed by suction curettage. Menstrual regulation, the least invasive procedure, is performed up to 2 weeks after a first missed period in an outpatient facility, without anesthesia. A flexible plastic catheter is inserted with no more difficulty than performing endometrial biopsy or IUD placement, and suction is applied. Because the procedure is done so early in pregnancy, failure to aspirate all the tissue may occur, manifested by a persistent positive pregnancy test and absent postoperative bleeding. This may require a repeat procedure. Later first-trimester terminations involve suction curettage, commonly requiring cervical dilation with either a mechanical or osmotic dilator (synthetic laminaria or *Laminaria japonica*). Osmotic dilators may reduce the risk of cervical and uterine trauma, especially in nulliparous women. Suction using a cannula removes the pregnancy. The complication rate is two per 1000 procedures. A small percentage (3%) of pregnancy terminations use sharp curettage (D&C, the traditional dilation and curettage). These are most often later first-trimester procedures (10–12 wk) or earlier second-trimester procedures.

Second-trimester terminations are mostly dilation and evacuation (D&E) procedures involving placement of an osmotic dilator 6 to 12 hours before the procedure, which is either suction or sharp curettage. The complication rate for dilation and curettage is seven per 1000 procedures. From 16 weeks' gestation, induction terminations may be performed using intrauterine instillation of agents inducing labor. A small amount of amniotic fluid is removed and urea, prostaglandins, or rarely saline is introduced, resulting in labor and delivery over the next 12 to 24 hours. Intramuscular and vaginally-placed prostaglandin preparations are also used to induce labor. This is a hospital-based procedure, with a higher complication rate (up to 20% at some institutions) than earlier procedures, and may take several days to complete. Complications from hypertonic saline inductions include disseminated intravascular coagulation, hypernatremia, and hemorrhage from retained tissue. Prostaglandins have side effects of nausea, vomiting, diarrhea, and fever.

Hysterotomy and *hysterectomy* are rarely-performed second-trimester procedures (accounting for less than .05% of reported procedures). These have higher morbidity and mortality. Tubal sterilization can be done at the same time as hysterotomy. Hysterectomy is generally performed for an existing condition requiring hysterectomy with a coexisting pregnancy.

RU 486 (Mifepristone), a synthetic steroid widely used in France as an effective abortifacient, binds progesterone receptors, blocking normal activity and preventing implantation or inducing menstruation after implantation. Efficacy is 85 percent when used alone within 6 to 9 weeks after the last period and increases to 96 percent when progesterone is added 48 hours later. Currently, RU 486 is widely publicized in the United States, and Food and Drug Administration approval is under consideration.

Abortion related *complications* are affected by time of gestation, method of procedure, and coexisting complicating illnesses. Major complications, including uterine perforation, hemorrhage, and infection, occur at a rate of one case per 1000 procedures. The termination needs to be repeated 2.3 times per 1000 abortions. Presentations suggestive of these complications include bleeding, fever, abdominal pain or cramping, and uterine tenderness. Minor complications, including infection, cervical stenosis, cervical tear, and bleeding or incomplete abortion requiring resuctioning, occur in eight per 1000 procedures. Complication rates increase with gestational age and are estimated as follows: at 8 weeks gestation, two per 1000; at 14 weeks, six per 1000; at more than 20 weeks, 15 per 1000.

There are no conclusive data showing that serious emotional problems result after pregnancy termination in the United States. Existing data indicate that women generally experience relief as well as reduced anxiety and distress posttermination. Negative emotional reactions are more common among women with prior psychiatric illnesses, second-trimester terminations, terminations for medical or genetic reasons, or with significant ambivalence about the decision.

Women who have undergone a single first-trimester vacuum aspiration procedure are at no significant increased risk for infertility, miscarriage, ectopic pregnancy, stillbirth, or major pregnancy or delivery-associated complication. The effect of multiple abortions on future childbearing is unknown. Second-trimester D&E procedures are felt to be associated with development of an incompetent cervix which can lead to spontaneous abortion, premature delivery, and low birth weight.

Illegal abortions occur rarely today. Reasons for this choice have included financial limitations, secrecy, geographic location, knowledge deficits regarding legal termination, or choosing an ethnically familiar provider. Complication rates are unknown but are thought to be higher than those of legal procedures. In 1989, two of 20 reported abortion-related deaths followed illegal procedures. Patients may present to hospital emergency rooms with hemorrhage and sepsis.

Adoption. Placing a child for adoption is an alternative for a woman who feels it is impossible to raise a child and who would prefer not to undergo an abortion. Women choosing this option often do so with the belief that their child will have a better upbringing than they can provide. Additionally, placement may allow a woman to defer or delay parenthood, complete her education, establish economic security, or pursue goals. Adoptions, however, have declined significantly over the past decades. Fewer than 3 percent of never-married women in 1988 relinquished their infants. Societal acceptance of single motherhood, legalization of abortion, and establishment of programs offering financial assistance all contribute to this trend. If a woman decides to place her child for adoption, she may enlist a state-run or private agency. She should be encouraged to investigate an agency carefully to ensure that she is not pressured and that she agrees with its policies. Open adoption, where there is some future contact with the child, is becoming more common.

Keeping the Child. Keeping the child may emerge as a realistic option if problematic social situation is amenable to change. Identification of social supports including extended family and community agencies may facilitate this process. Adolescents need special counseling as teenage pregnancy is a serious problem resulting in poverty and child neglect.

Birth Control. Whether a patient chooses to proceed with or terminate a pregnancy, a discussion of future contraceptive options is essential (see Chapter 119).

Providing care to the woman faced with an unplanned and/or unwanted pregnancy is a challenge to the primary care provider. The provider must explore the patient's beliefs, fears, support network, and psychosocial history. Options must be thoroughly and nonjudgmentally explained. Only then can one formulate an appropriate care plan.

ANNOTATED BIBLIOGRAPHY

Adler NE, David HP, Major BN, Roth SH, Russo NF, Wyatt GF. Psychological responses after abortion. Science 1990;248:41. *(Brief review of U.S. studies examining women after legal terminations.)*

Blendon RJ, Benson JM, Donelan K. Public controversy over abortion. JAMA 1993;270:2871. *(Survey data on public attitudes about abortion.)*

Boston Women's Health Collective. Our Bodies, Ourselves. New York: Simon & Schuster, 1992; p353. *(Consumer writers.)*

Centers for Disease Control and Prevention. Abortion surveillance, 1990. MMWR 1992;41:936. *(Updated review of current information.)*

Chard T. Pregnancy tests: a review. Human Reprod 1992;7:701. *(Useful background information and review.)*

Council on Scientific Affairs, American Medical Association. Induced termination of pregnancy before and after Roe v Wade, trends in the mortality and morbidity of women. JAMA 1992;268:3231. *(Good review article.)*

Hakin-Elahi E, Tovell HMM, Burnhill MS. Complications of first-trimester abortion: a report of 170,000 cases. Obstet Gynecol 1990;76:129. *(Retrospective review of New York City Planned Parenthood cases. Letter in response in Obstet Gynecol 1990;76[6]:1145.)*

Henshaw SK, Koonin LM, Smith JC. Characteristics of U.S. women having abortions, 1987. Fam Plann Perspect 1991; 23:75. *(Resource for current data and opinion from the Alan Guttmacher Institute.)*

Miller WH, Resnick MP, Williams MH, Bloom JD. The pregnant psychiatric inpatient: a missed opportunity. Gen Hosp Psychiatry 1990;12:373 *(Study addressing the impact of psychiatric illness on pregnancy outcomes and the effects of pregnancy on psychiatric disorders.)*

Rodgers BD, Lee RV. Drug abuse. In Burrow GN, Ferris TF (eds): Medical Complications During Pregnancy, p570. Philadelphia: WB Saunders, 1988. *(Complete text for various medical issues as they relate to pregnancy.)*

Sperling RS, Stratton P. Treatment options for human immunodeficiency virus-infected pregnant women. Obstetric Gynecologic Working Group of the AIDS Clinical Trials Group of the National Institute of Allergy and Infectious Diseases. Obstet Gynecol 1992;79:443. *(Review of HIV in pregnancy, including demographics and therapeutics.)*

Spitz IM, Bardin CW. Mifepristone (RU-486)—a modulator of progestin and glucocorticoid action. N Engl J Med 1993; 329:404. *(Authoritative review of this potent abortifacient.)*

Stotland NL. The myth of the abortion trauma syndrome. JAMA 1992;268:2078. *(Commentary.)*

Streissguth AD, Grant TM, Barr HM, et al. Cocaine and the use of alcohol and other drugs during pregnancy. Am J Obstet Gynecol 1991;164:1241. *(Discusses the risks and prevalence of cocaine use in pregnancy and the likelihood of polysubstance abuse in cocaine users.)*

Sunderland MA, Handte J, Moroso G, Landesman S. The impact of human immunodeficiency virus serostatus on reproductive decisions of women. Obstet Gynecol 1992;79:1027. *(Discusses the impact of HIV status on deciding to carry or terminate a pregnancy.)*

122
Management of Breast Cancer

Primary Care Medicine: Office Evaluation and Management of the Adult Patient, 3rd edition, edited by Allan H. Goroll, Lawrence A. May, and Albert G. Mulley, Jr. J.B. Lippincott Company, Philadelphia

Breast cancer is one of the most common malignancies in the United States. About 12 percent of American women will develop breast cancer during their lifetime, more than 150,000 cases per year. Unfortunately, in spite of the expanded therapeutic armamentarium for breast cancer, survival remains relatively unchanged: 30 percent of women who develop the disease die of it.

Women with newly diagnosed breast cancer face a difficult and complex series of treatment decisions at a time when they may be least able to think rationally or bear the burden of decision-making responsibility. The breast cancer diagnosis evokes anger, a sense of isolation, irrational guilt, and, most of all, vulnerability. Clearly, this mix of emotions makes it difficult for the communication tasks necessary for the patient to be involved in decision making. Yet the most important determinants of the "right" decision for each patient are her attitudes toward the possible treatment outcomes and risks. New information about the relative effectiveness of alternative approaches to primary therapy and adjuvant therapy has added to the complexity of these decisions. The primary physician can be a critically important source of empathy and support as well as information about treatment options. After primary treatment, with or without subsequent adjuvant therapy, the primary care provider may be principally responsible for monitoring the patient's psychosocial adjustment to breast cancer and its treatment, as well as for evidence of disease recurrence. Finally, the primary care role is critically important in decision making about treatment for the woman with advanced breast cancer.

CLINICAL PRESENTATION AND COURSE

The term "early-stage breast cancer" is generally applied to stage I and stage II tumors. *Stage I* disease is defined as a primary tumor of less than 2 cm in diameter with no axillary lymph node involvement (Table 122–1). Approximately 55 percent of patients with primary breast cancer now present with stage I disease, in part because of improved screening methods. *Stage II* disease is still considered a localized disease, but it does include involvement of axillary lymph nodes. About 25 percent of patients with *clinical* stage I disease turn out to have pathologic stage II disease on sampling of the axillary nodes. Interestingly, a similar percentage of patients with clinical stage II disease (palpable axillary lymph nodes) turn out to have no tumor in the nodes on pathologic examination. In stage III disease, there is extensive tumor (>5 cm) at the primary site, and lymph nodes are larger than 2 cm with or without fixation. In stage IV disease there are distant metastases.

Because of greater use of mammographic screening, cases are increasingly identified with small lesions, including those without evidence of invasion. Noninvasive cancer, or carcinoma in situ (CIS), is characterized as ductal or lobular based on histology and location, cytologic features, and growth patterns. These two lesions behave very differently. With ductal CIS, mastectomy results in cure for 98 percent to 99 percent of women. Lobular CIS has very different treatment implications. It is not clear whether it is indeed a premalignant lesion or simply a marker for increased risk of invasive disease elsewhere in the breast(s). The incidence of invasive cancer in women with lobular CIS is about 1 percent per year.

Prognosis. For women with early-stage breast cancer, the prognosis is largely determined by the size of the tumor and the number of positive nodes. For women with negative nodes, 5-year cumulative recurrence rates for women with tumors smaller than 1 cm, 1 to 2 cm, and 2 to 5 cm in diameter are 10 percent, 20 percent, and 30 percent, respectively. Among women with one to three positive nodes, 40 percent have a recurrence within 5 years. For women with four to 10 nodes positive, the 5-year recurrence rate is 60 percent to 70 percent. For women with more than 10 nodes positive, or with stage III disease, long-term survival is less than 5 percent. Inflammatory breast cancer has a worse prognosis than noninflammatory lesions.

Table 122-1. Curability of Breast Cancer by Stage

STAGE	TUMOR EXTENT	10-YEAR DISEASE-FREE SURVIVAL (%)
I	Confined to breast	70–80
II	Involves the axillary nodes	20–40
III	Tumor >5 cm; nodes >2 cm; with or without fixation	<5
	Inflammatory	0

Table 122-2. Patterns of Recurrence and Survival in Breast Cancer

PATTERN	INCIDENCE (%)	MEDIAN TIME (MONTHS) Relapse	MEDIAN TIME (MONTHS) Survival
Multiple metastases	19	9	4
Pulmonary	12	36	18
Bone	26	15	29+
Effusions*	16	39	44
Skin and subcutaneous†	26	15	27+

*+ Minor skin nodules.
†+ Minor bone metastases.

In addition to the stage of tumor and tumor size, *estrogen receptor* and *progesterone receptor* status affect the prognosis. Patients with stage I or stage II disease whose tumors have estrogen or progesterone receptors, or both, have a better prognosis than those with the same stage of disease whose tumors are receptor-negative.

Breast cancer may metastasize to almost any site in the body, but five general categories have been distinguished by Smalley and coworkers, which are correlated with predictable response to therapy and prognosis (Table 122–2). It is evident that even in patients with metastatic disease, median survival may exceed 3 years, and there does not have to be significant change in quality of life when palliative radiation and chemotherapy or hormonal therapy are used throughout that period (see below). Today, more than 50 percent of patients with metastatic breast cancer may respond to therapy, but only a small portion (perhaps fewer than 10%) show complete regression. The median duration of response is approximately 12 to 18 months.

The clinical course of breast cancer is unique in that metastatic lesions may develop after a long period of freedom from disease, even after as long as 20 years. Thus, 5 years without evidence of metastatic spread does not indicate cure.

PRINCIPLES OF MANAGEMENT

The therapeutic options for women diagnosed by an incisional or excisional biopsy have expanded in recent years, accompanied by greater patient participation in choice of therapy. It is no longer justified to perform a biopsy and immediate mastectomy under the same anesthesia. Patients should be fully informed of the diagnosis, promptly staged, and advised of the therapeutic options.

Primary Treatment of Early-Stage Breast Cancer. Most women with early-stage breast cancer have a choice of surgical treatments. Multiple randomized trials have demonstrated that survival is the same with either *mastectomy* or *breast-sparing surgery* ("lumpectomy" or "quadrantectomy") *followed by radiation*. There are some relative contraindications to breast-sparing surgery, including tumors that are large relative to breast size, cancer that is near or involves the nipple, and tumors with extensive intraductal components within or adjacent to the primary tumor. Also, women with large breasts may fare worse cosmetically with radiation therapy. The radiation therapy is an essential component of the breast-sparing option. Without it, there is a 40 percent rate of ipsilateral breast recurrence following breast-sparing surgery. Even with radiation therapy, ipsilateral recurrences do occur, at a rate of 1 to 2 percent per year. These can usually be treated with mastectomy and, as noted, do not result in decreased survival for women who opt for the breast-sparing approach.

Adjuvant Therapy of Breast Cancer. Adjuvant therapy is administered to decrease the likelihood of, or delay, cancer recurrence and death. The most commonly used regimens are CMF (cyclophosphamide, methotrexate, and 5-FU [fluorouracil]) and other regimens that include adriamycin. The anti-estrogen tamoxifen has become the standard hormonal therapy.

The effectiveness of adjuvant therapy in decreasing rates of recurrence and breast cancer death among node-positive women has been proven for some time. More recent evidence indicates that adjuvant therapy is as effective in node-negative women. That is, the relative risk reduction afforded by either chemotherapy or hormonal therapy is the same in node-positive and node-negative women. However, the absolute risk difference is much smaller for node-negative women because their baseline risk is lower. For example, women with two positive nodes and women with negative nodes and tumors less than 1 cm might receive the same 30 percent risk-reduction benefit from adjuvant chemotherapy or hormonal therapy. For the former, that means a reduction from 40 percent to 28 percent, or an increase in disease-free survival from 60 percent to 72 percent. For the node-negative woman, the same proportional benefit means a reduction from 10 percent to 7 percent, or an increase in disease-free survival from 90 percent to 93 percent. The significant morbidity associated with adjuvant therapy may or may not be justified, depending on the absolute benefit and the woman's attitudes toward the alterative outcomes.

Adjuvant chemotherapy has become the standard of care for premenopausal women with positive nodes, regardless of hormone receptor status, and tamoxifen has become the standard for postmenopausal women with positive nodes, particularly those with positive hormone receptor levels. The relatively nontoxic response has led to increasing use of tamoxifen among node-negative, postmenopausal women. Treatment of node-negative premenopausal women has remained controversial even after the 1992 Early Breast Cancer Trialists' Collaborating Group (EBCTCG) publication of convincing evidence of effectiveness in node-negative women. The source of the continuing controversy is the question of whether the risk-reduction benefits are sufficiently great to justify the significant morbidity associated with adjuvant chemotherapy. Women who choose this option should have a clear understanding of the benefits and realistic expectations of side effects, including nausea and vomiting, alopecia, and premature menopause.

EBCTCG findings have raised new questions about adjuvant therapy regimens. There appear to be additive effects for chemotherapeutic and hormonal approaches, and trials of combined approaches will likely influence future recommendations.

Obesity has been found to be an independent predictor of poor prognosis for patients receiving adjuvant chemotherapy. The efficacy of weight reduction is being studied.

Monitoring. Following primary therapy, women with breast cancer should be seen at regular intervals. Psychosocial adjustments as well as clinical status need careful attention. A mammogram should be obtained annually. Follow-up examination of the bones should be undertaken only in patients who develop symptoms of bone pain. The crucial concern in monitoring patients with breast cancer is the increased risk of a second primary tumor, which may also be curable. The identification of early metastatic disease is less consequential, because systemic therapy should be used only in patients with either rapidly growing tumor or symptomatic disease.

Treatment of Advanced Disease. Stage III breast cancer (inoperable local disease confined to the skin, breast, or lymph nodes) may be treated either with 1) systemic therapy (either hormonal or chemotherapy) to determine the effectiveness of the systemic treatment and to reduce the bulk of tumor; or 2) with local therapy, which may be either mastectomy followed by radiation therapy or radiation therapy alone. The median length of survival after effective treatment is 18 to 24 months.

The management of stage IV (metastatic) breast cancer is determined in part by sites of metastases, menopausal status, and hormone receptor status. The decision to treat and the timing of therapy depend on the presence or absence of symptoms and the growth rate of the tumor. There are three categories of systemic therapy for advanced breast cancer: hormone therapy, chemotherapy, and combination therapy. Radiation therapy is also very effective for palliation.

Hormone therapy can be very effective for tumors that have high concentration of estrogen receptor protein (ERP) in the cytoplasm. Tumors with progesterone receptors are also more likely to be hormonally responsive. The sites of disease most often responsive to hormones are pulmonary nodules, pleural effusions, and osseous lesions. There is a much lower likelihood of response to hormonal manipulation in patients with hepatic metastases, lymphangitic pulmonary involvement, brain metastases, or skin lesions. Hormone management also depends on menopausal status. The least responsive group is perimenopausal. Following an initial response to hormonal therapy, a relapse usually occurs, but a subsequent secondary response to an alternative hormonal manipulation is not uncommon. For the most part, such secondary responses are short-lived and are not of the quality of the initial response. It is important to recognize that the effect of hormonal therapy on tumor bulk may not be observed for 1 or 2 months, even though the agent may begin working immediately. Relief of bone pain is much more rapidly achieved.

Hormonal therapy occasionally results in exacerbation of bone pain or tumor growth. The mechanism is not known. In a small percentage of these patients, the opposite hormonal maneuver (ie, ablation or supplementation) may induce an antitumor effect. In some institutions, patients are monitored in the hospital for a 10-day period to determine whether or not tumor stimulation and serious hypercalcemia occur.

The development of drugs for use in place of adrenalectomy has eased the burden of treatment for patients with advanced disease. Tamoxifen, a competitive inhibitor of endogenous estrogen, binds to estrogen receptors and achieves an antitumor effect by an unknown mechanism. The drug has a low rate of toxicity and a response rate comparable to that of other forms of hormone therapy. As a result, tamoxifen is the usual first-line hormonal therapy.

Chemotherapy should be considered in patients with advanced disease after hormonal manipulations have failed or when they are deemed inappropriate (eg, in receptor-negative patients). However, the likelihood of response is reduced when the tumor has proven resistant to other forms of treatment. The chemotherapeutic regimens most commonly used to manage advanced disease include the same regimens commonly used for adjuvant therapy. As with adjuvant therapy, combinations of hormonal manipulations and multidrug programs have been advocated on the basis of a possible synergistic interaction.

Breast cancer is particularly sensitive to radiation therapy. Metastatic bony lesions are present in more than 60 percent of patients with breast cancer, and lytic lesions are often associated with pain. Local radiation therapy at the relatively low doses of 2000 to 3500 rads may relieve pain, although persistent structural defects as a consequence of cortical bony erosion may necessitate orthopedic support and even internal fixation for weight-bearing bone structures. Another important role for radiation therapy is in palliation of patients who develop metastatic brain lesions, which occur in more than 10 percent of patients.

Autologous bone marrow transplantation in conjunction with high-dose chemotherapy remains an investigative approach, with very high cost and unproven benefits.

PATIENT EDUCATION

Whether or not a woman has had a role in decision making about breast cancer treatment can be an important determinant of her psychosocial adjustment. The primary care provider is well positioned to provide empathetic support and vital information about the benefits and harms of alternative treatment options.

A.G.M.

ANNOTATED BIBLIOGRAPHY

Bastarrachea J, Hortobagyi GN, Smith TL, et al. Obesity as an adverse prognostic factor for patients receiving adjuvant chemotherapy for breast cancer. Ann Intern Med 1994;120:18. *(Found to be an independent predictor of poor outcome.)*

Early Breast Cancer Trialists' Collaborating Group. Systemic treatment of early breast cancer by hormonal, cytotoxic, or immune therapy. Lancet 1992;339:1,71. *(Landmark overview and analysis of worldwide randomized trial experience with treatment of early breast cancer.)*

Farrow DC, Hunt WC, Samet JM. Geographic variation in the treatment of localized breast cancer. N Engl J Med 1992; 326:1097. *(Wide variations in the rates of breast-conserving surgery in different regions.)*

Fisher B, Anderson S, Fisher ER, et al. Significance of ipsilateral breast tumor recurrence after lumpectomy. Lancet 1991; 338:327. *(Ipsilateral in-breast recurrences occurred at a rate of 1.4 percent per year despite radiation following lumpectomy.)*

Fisher B, Bauer M, Margolese R, et al. Five-year results of a randomized clinical trial comparing total mastectomy and segmental mastectomy with or without radiation in the treatment of breast cancer. N Engl J Med 1985;312:665. *(A prospective, randomized study demonstrating the efficacy of segmental mastectomy plus radiation and its comparability to [if not superiority over] total mastectomy.)*

Fisher B, Redmond C, Poisson R, Margolese R, et al. Eight-year results of a randomized clinical trial comparing total mastectomy and lumpectomy with or without irradiation in the treatment of breast cancer. N Engl J Med 1989;320:822. *(Further evidence for the equivalence of the two primary treatment options in terms of distant recurrence and survival.)*

Harris JR, Hellman S, Kinne DW. Limited surgery and radiotherapy for early breast cancer. N Engl J Med 1985;313:1365. *(A report of a consensus workshop on the technical details of the surgery and radiotherapy to be used in this approach to treatment.)*

Harris JR, Lippman ME, Veronesi U, Willett W. Breast cancer. N Engl J Med 1992;327:319. *(Extensive review, first of three parts.)*

Kiang DT, Gay J, Goldman A, et al. A randomized trial of chemotherapy and hormonal therapy in advanced breast cancer. N Engl J Med 1985;313:1241. *(Evidence that combination therapy may be useful in postmenopausal patients with receptor-rich tumors.)*

McGuire WL, Clark GM. Prognostic factors and treatment decisions in axillary-node-negative breast cancer. N Engl J Med 1992;326:1756. *(Excellent review of prognostic variables among node-negative women.)*

NIH Consensus Conference. Treatment of early-stage breast cancer. JAMA 1991;265:391. *(Conclusions of the 1990 consensus conference.)*

Schover LR. The impact of breast cancer on sexuality, body image, and intimate relationships. CA 1991;41:112. *(Conflicting evidence about comparative effects of mastectomy and breast-sparing surgery. Impact of adjuvant therapy may be underappreciated.)*

123
Management of the Woman With Genital Tract Cancer

Primary Care Medicine: Office Evaluation and Management of the Adult Patient, 3rd edition, edited by Allan H. Goroll, Lawrence A. May, and Albert G. Mulley, Jr. J.B. Lippincott Company, Philadelphia

Cancers of the genital tract account for about 20 percent of cancers in women and 10 percent of cancer deaths. They range from the readily detectable and curable carcinoma of the cervix to the very problematic ovarian carcinoma, with its tendency to remain inconspicuous until very late. Endometrial carcinoma has come to be one of the most common genital cancers of the postmenopausal years. Cervical cancer is now predominantly a disease of younger women.

Treatment of the woman with genital tract cancer is usually the province of the oncologist and gynecologist, but the primary physician remains an important part of the collaborative effort. Patient counseling, monitoring, and management of ongoing medical problems are among the important responsibilities.

CARCINOMA OF THE CERVIX

The incidence of invasive cervical carcinoma peaks between the ages of 48 and 55. The peak for carcinoma in situ is between ages 25 and 40. Most women with the disease present in their 20s and 30s thanks to early detection from use of the Pap smear (see Chapter 107). Among proven risk factors are early sexual intercourse, multiple sexual partners, and infection with human papillomavirus (particularly types 16 and 18).

Principles of Management

Diagnosis. Postcoital bleeding should raise suspicion for the diagnosis. In most cases of early disease, the patient is asymptomatic and, as noted above, detection is by screening *Pap test* (see Chapter 107). Diagnosis requires biopsy confirmation of a sufficiently abnormal Pap test or a grossly suspicious-looking lesion. Patients with only mild atypia on the Pap smear (also referred to as reactive or reparative change) can be followed without biopsy, but require repeat Pap testing (usually in 3 to 6 months) to be sure there is no progression to the more serious dysplasia. If there is ongoing infection, it should be treated before the Pap smear is repeated. Patients with dysplasia seen on Pap smear are at greater risk and should be referred to the gynecologist for *colposcopy* and *biopsy*. If colposcopic examination fails to identify the area for biopsy, cervical conization is required.

Staging. Clinical staging is based on findings from biopsy, physical examination, and radiologic study. An estimate of extent of local disease can be made by *pelvic examination,* carefully palpating to see if there is lateral extension to the vagina or pelvic wall. Bimanual and rectopelvic examinations are helpful in this regard. Palpating lymph nodes may detect a distant nodal metastasis, but clinical staging for involvement of pelvic nodes and the more distant paraaortic ones requires *lymphangiography* and/or *computed tomography (CT) scan*. The latter has been especially helpful in assessment of paraaortic nodes. Studies of *magnetic resonance imaging (MRI) scanning* suggest some usefulness in delineating local extension.

Stage of disease is designated by the TMO system (Table 123–1). Prognosis worsens with advancing stage of local disease, development of regional and distant nodal metastases (especially paraaortic nodes), and histologic grade. Risk of nodal metastasis rises with growth of tumor to greater than 4 cm, lymphovascular invasion, invasion deep into the cervical stroma, and histologic grade.

Treatment and Prognosis. Early stages of carcinoma of the cervix are curable. Patients sometimes ask the opinion of their primary physician regarding the choices of therapy for early stage disease. Consequently, these choices are worth reviewing here.

For *stage 0 disease,* the treatment of choice has been *conization*. In instances where the lesion is readily visible by colposcopy and the patient can be counted on to come for regular follow-up, outpatient *cryotherapy* or *laser ablation* can serve as an alternative to conization. *Hysterectomy* is reserved for those who have intraepithelial neoplasia at the margins of the cone biopsy and do not care for future childbearing. Cure is in excess of 99 percent.

Stage IA1 is treated with *vaginal hysterectomy* when childbearing is not an issue. When it is desired, *conization* and close follow-up are the alternative if the cone margins are free of tumor. Five-year survival is over 90 percent. There is debate regarding the best approach to *stage IA2* disease. If invasion is greater than 3 mm or there is lymphovascular invasion, then these patients are usually treated like stage IB. If invasion is less than 3 mm and there is no lymphovascular involvement, then they are treated like IA1. *Intracavitary irradiation* is another curative option.

Stages IB and IIA are treated by *radical hysterectomy* plus *pelvic lymphadenectomy* or by definitive *irradiation*. Surgery is preferred in young women, because the ovarian function can be spared and the vagina is more pliable than after irradiation. Also, radiation effects on bowel and other adjacent structures are avoided. Radiation therapy spares the need for an extensive surgical procedure and its attendant complications. With either procedure, 5-year survival is equally good, with rates averaging about 85 percent for patients with no pelvic node disease. If there is involvement of pelvic nodes, 5-year survival falls to about 50 percent.

Stages IIB and beyond are treated with *irradiation*. Five-year survival averages about 60 percent for patients with IIB disease and falls to about 35 percent for stage IIIB and to 20 percent for stage IV.

The high likelihood of nodal metastasis associated with advancing stages of local disease markedly lowers the chances of cure. Clinically inapparent involvement of para-

Table 123-1. Staging of Cervical Cancer

Primary Tumor	
0	Carcinoma in situ
I	Confined to uterus
A	Preclinical invasive disease
A1	Minimal stromal invasion
A2	Invasion <5 mm
B	Invasion >5 mm
II	Invasion beyond uterus, but not to pelvic wall or lower third of vagina
A	Without parametrial invasion
B	With parametrial invasion
III	Invasion to pelvic wall, lower third of vagina, or causes hydronephrosis
A	Only invasive to lower third of vagina
B	Invasive to pelvic wall or hydronephrosis
IV	Invasion of bladder, rectum, or beyond true pelvis
Regional Lymph Nodes	
N0	No regional node metastasis
N1	Regional node metastasis
Distant Metastasis (includes paraaortic nodes)	
M0	No distant metastasis
M1	Distant metastasis

Adapted from Beahrs OH, Henson DE, Hutter RVP, Myers MH (eds): Manual for Staging of Cancer, 3rd ed, p151. Philadelphia, JB Lippincott, 1988.

aortic nodes is a particularly difficult problem, leading some to advocate surgical sampling. Prophylactic radiation to the area does not seem to improve survival.

Patient Education

Young patients need to know that carcinoma of the cervix is potentially curable and that early disease can be successfully treated without compromising childbearing capacity. Such knowledge helps to ensure that the young woman with carcinoma in situ or severe dysplasia will not refuse timely treatment out of fear. Older patients presenting with more invasive disease can still obtain some comfort from knowing the prognosis remains very favorable for most stages of this disease.

CARCINOMA OF ENDOMETRIUM

This disease continues to be the most common female genital cancer, accounting for about half of all new cases (about 33,000 per year). It predominantly strikes postmenopausal women. Peak incidence is between ages 55 and 60. Only 5 percent of cases occur in women under the age of 40. Risk factors include obesity, nulliparity, late menopause, and prolonged unopposed estrogen stimulation of the uterus (either from replacement therapy or polycystic ovary syndrome; see Chapter 111). Uninterrupted estrogen stimulation in the absence of progestin risks induction of cystic and adenomatous hyperplasia, which are considered premalignant changes. Obesity may contribute by the ability of adipose tissue to convert circulating androstenedione into estrogen. Postmenopausal bleeding (defined as uterine bleeding occurring 6 months after the onset of menopause) may be the only early clue to the development of this tumor. Occasionally, a mass is felt on routine pelvic examination.

Principles of Management

Diagnosis. Suspicion of the diagnosis mandates gynecologic referral for *fractional curettage*. When there is confusion as to whether a pelvic mass is ovarian or uterine, ordering a *pelvic ultrasound* examination can help make the distinction noninvasively, but the test is insufficient for definitive diagnosis of an intrauterine lesion. Biopsy by way of curettage is required.

Staging and Prognosis. Prognosis is a function of the extent of disease as well as of histologic type. The gynecologist will attempt to determine if the problem is confined to the uterine corpus or extends into the cervix and beyond. A careful *pelvic examination, CT scan,* and *chest x-ray* comprise the clinical staging process. Surgical staging is based on findings at the time of hysterectomy. Histologic grade, depth of myometrial penetration, and lymph node metastases influence prognosis in patients with early-stage disease. Overall survival is about 80 percent for those with stage I disease (confined to the corpus), 50 percent for stage II (involves corpus and the cervix), 27 percent for stage III (spread beyond the uterus but within the pelvis), and 9 percent for stage IV (invades bladder or rectum, extends beyond the pelvis).

Treatment. Patients with the *premalignant* change of adenomatous hyperplasia are usually advised to undergo *hysterectomy* because of the risk of developing cancer. However, a second option is *progestin therapy* followed by repeat curettage. Patients with *stage I* or *stage II* disease are curable when treated with *hysterectomy/bilateral salpingo-oophorectomy* plus *irradiation*. The addition of radiation therapy is especially useful in stage II disease. The precise type of radiation therapy depends on histologic type and degree of spread. Intracavitary as well as external beam treatments are considered. The treatment of *stage III* disease is individualized, determined by findings on laparotomy. Patients with more advanced disease are inoperable and treated with radiation, progestins, or chemotherapy for palliation.

Patient Education

Patients who are considering estrogen therapy for treatment of postmenopausal osteoporosis need to consider the risk of developing endometrial cancer. Although patients who do develop cancer from estrogen therapy are often detected early at a curable phase of illness, the disease still represents a serious consequence of an elective form of therapy. Adding a progestin to the estrogen program helps prevent unopposed endometrial proliferation and development of cystic hyperplasia (see Chapters 117 and 158).

OVARIAN CARCINOMA

Ovarian cancer ranks fourth in cancer deaths among women and leads all gynecologic cancers. Incidence increases with age, beginning shortly after menarche and continuing through the eighth decade. Risk heightens among women in their 40s, especially among those who are nulliparous. Over 80 percent of these tumors derive from the epithelial surface of the ovary, disseminating silently by surface shedding or lymph node invasion. Initial manifestations may be vague, typically nonspecific gastrointestinal complaints that seem to persist in the absence of objective evidence for bowel disease. Screening remains inadequate, despite the advent of transvaginal ultrasound for detection of an ovarian mass and monoclonal antibody techniques for detection of the tumor-associated antigen CA 125 (see Chapter 108). At the time of presentation (which might be heralded by an abdominal or pelvic mass or development of ascites), almost 70 percent of patients have already reached advanced-stage disease.

Diagnosis

Because the disease is so silent or nonspecific in its presentation, a high index of suspicion is required. Peri- and postmenopausal women with unexplained pelvic or abdominal complaints should have a thorough *pelvic examination* with emphasis on careful palpation of the adnexae for a mass. Ability to palpate the ovary in a postmenopausal woman is suspicious of pathologic enlargement, because the ovary normally involutes to less than 2 cm in size.

A *transvaginal ultrasound* can help confirm the presence of an ovarian mass and is superior to transabdominal study. The finding of a simple cyst less than 4 cm is unlikely to represent cancer but warrants further observation, especially in postmenopausal women who do not have functioning ovarian cysts. In women of reproductive age, ovarian enlargement is common and usually due to functioning follicular or corpus luteum cysts. These typically regress within one to three menstrual cycles. Finding a complex cyst increases the risk of malignancy to about 10 percent and necessitates *surgical exploration,* as does discovery of a solid mass. Spread to the opposite ovary occurs in up to 15 percent of cases, so the finding of bilateral disease should increase rather than decrease suspicion. *CT scan* helps delineate pelvic and abdominal masses, liver and pulmonary metastasis, and retroperitoneal node involvement. It can be used to assess the ovary when pelvic ultrasound study is obscured by bowel gas.

As just noted, suspicious cases require surgical exploration. Laparoscopy is not a substitute, because laparoscopically guided needle aspiration or biopsy risks spilling malignant cells into the peritoneum and washings are of insufficient sensitivity.

Use of the tumor marker *CA 125* to achieve earlier detection of ovarian cancer has proven disappointing, perhaps because only 50 percent of women with clinically detectable disease have elevated levels of the marker. In addition, many women with positive studies prove to already have advanced disease, because the frequency of marker elevation increases with tumor stage and bulk. Nonetheless, a markedly elevated CA 125 in a patient with a suspicious adnexal mass only increases the importance of proceeding with surgical exploration. A negative study does not obviate the need to refer for consideration of exploration. Combining CA 125 with transvaginal ultrasound appears to have little impact on survival when used as a screening technique (see Chapter 108).

Principles of Management

Staging and Monitoring. Staging is performed predominantly by surgical exploration. Precise staging necessitates a meticulous *laparotomy* to assess the diaphragmatic surface as well as the omentum and other intraabdominal sites to which spread is common. Disease limited to the ovaries is considered stage I; if confined to the pelvis, it is considered stage II. Stage III designates involvement of regional nodes or disseminated peritoneal seeding with spread to the upper abdomen. Stage IV signifies distant or visceral metastasis. Ascites and bulky peritoneal tumor are frequent manifestations of advanced stage disease. About 75 percent of patients present with stage III or IV disease.

The disease most commonly recurs within the abdominal cavity. Monitoring techniques include CA 125 levels, laparoscopic examination, ultrasonography, and second-look surgery. Miliary implants on the serosal surface may go undetected by imaging studies. Elevations in CA 125 are associated with residual tumor at the time of second-look surgery.

Treatment Modalities. Although the tumor is responsive to cancer treatment measures, its bulk and spread limit the results. Cure is still limited. In advanced stages of the disease, prognosis correlates with amount of residual disease after initial surgery. Those with less than 2 cm of residual disease do better than those with greater amounts of tumor remaining. Consequently, treatment often begins with *"debulking"* or tumor removal. *Omentectomy* as well as *total abdominal hysterectomy* and *bilateral salpingo-oophorectomy* are performed, in addition to the reduction of tumor masses throughout the abdominal cavity. This is believed to lessen the host–tumor burden and increase the effectiveness of ancillary or adjunctive therapeutic modalities, such as radiation or chemotherapy.

Marked improvements in response to *chemotherapy* have been achieved with use of combination regimens that make use of *cisplatin, carboplatin,* or *taxol.* Complete clinical remissions are achieved in about 40 percent of patients with advanced stage disease using cisplatin (or carboplatin) plus *cyclophosphamide.* Early studies of taxol suggest activity against otherwise refractory disease. In patients appearing to respond to chemotherapy, a *second-look operation* is performed to remove residual disease, check response, and place intraperitoneal catheters for *intraperitoneal infusion* therapy with cisplatin or etoposide. The regression of disease, confirmed by "second-look" operations, suggests that multidrug therapies should be the standard approach to ovarian cancer.

Radiation therapy to the pelvis or to the abdomen (for patients with disease that extends beyond the pelvis) has been advocated as a routine adjunct to surgery in patients with advanced stage disease, although impact on survival appears minimal. The rationale for abdominal and pelvic irradiation is based on the fact that ovarian tumors frequently cause recurrent ascites and bowel obstruction, leading to progressive inanition.

Survival. Of the 21,000 new cases discovered annually, more than two-thirds will die within a year. Prognosis correlates with amount of residual tumor after initial surgery, stage of disease, tumor grade, age, and histologic type. Those with stage I or II disease, less than 2 cm of residual disease, grade I tumor, and mucinous histology, have the best chance of achieving complete remission and long-term survival from postoperative therapy. Patients with peritoneal spread have a 5-year survival rate of about 10 percent.

Patient Education

Patients with ovarian cancer have a long and difficult clinical course. Mortality rates are high, and tumor bulk leads to considerable morbidity. Women with this disease and their families need all the support, interest, and comprehensive care that one can muster (see Chapter 87). With the advent of improved chemotherapy regimens, some hope for prolongation of survival can now be offered to those with advanced disease. However, the publicity surrounding taxol has raised some rather unrealistic expectations.

CARCINOMA OF THE VULVA

Being a disease of a readily visible area, carcinoma of the vulva lends itself to early detection and treatment. Associations between the disease and low socioeconomic class and infection with herpes simplex virus and human papillomavirus have been observed. The median age for initial presentation of carcinoma in situ is 44; for invasive disease it is 61, suggesting a slowly progressive course. Presentations include a mass or growth, vulvar pruritus, and bleeding. About 20 percent are asymptomatic. Lesions may be flat and raised or verrucal. Coloration ranges from white (leukoplakia) to brown (hyperpigmentation) to red. The term *Bowen's disease* refers to the hyperpigmented variety, and Paget's disease refers to the leukoplakial form. The best means of early diagnosis is a high index of suspicion. Surgical excision is the treatment of choice. More conservative approaches are now being used to decrease short- and long-term morbidity without sacrificing chance for cure. Cure rates in excess of 90 percent are achievable for localized disease less than 2 cm in greatest dimension. Radiation therapy is used for nonresectable disease.

CARCINOMA OF THE VAGINA

This is a relatively rare disease. Cancer found in the vagina is more likely to represent spread of disease from the cervix. Primary vaginal carcinomas are mostly squamous cell lesions, although those related to diethylstilbestrol (DES) exposure are of the clear cell variety. Prior irradiation may be a predisposing factor. The majority of lesions appear on the posterior wall and in the upper third of the vaginal vault. The tumor spreads directly and by lymphatic channels. It may present as an ulcerated lesion or as an exophytic mass extending into the vaginal vault. Preinvasive disease is asymptomatic. Invasive disease may present as postmenopausal or postcoital bleeding. Careful inspection of the posterior and distal aspects of the vagina is important in locating the lesion. Diagnosis is made by biopsy. Carcinoma in situ can be treated with local excision. Laser techniques are popular. Invasive disease is treated with radiation.

A.H.G.

ANNOTATED BIBLIOGRAPHY

Crum CP, Ikenberg H, Richart RM, et al. Human papillomavirus type 16 and early cervical neoplasia. N Engl J Med 1984; 310:880. *(Identifies one of the precursors to cervical cancer.)*

Granai CO. Ovarian cancer—Unrealistic expectations. N Engl J Med 1992;327:197. *(Feels patients may be expecting more than can be delivered.)*

Greer BE, Figgie DC, Tamimi HK, et al. Stage IA2 squamous carcinoma of the cervix: Difficult diagnosis and therapeutic dilemma. Am J Obstet Gynecol 1990;162:1406. *(Useful discussion of the key issues.)*

Gusberg SB. The changing nature of endometrial cancer. N Engl J Med 1980;302:729. *(Examines the increased incidence, clinical course, and treatment.)*

Hoskins WJ, Perez CA, Young RC. Gynecologic tumors. In DeVita VT, Hellman S, Rosenberg SA (eds): Cancer: Principles & Practice of Oncology, 4th ed, Philadelphia, JB Lippincott, 1993. pp 1153–1168. *(Excellent treatment of the topics of vulvar and vaginal cancer.)*

Lee YN, Wang KL, Lin MH, et al. Radical hysterectomy with pelvic lymph node dissection for treatment of cervical cancer. Gynecol Oncol 1989;32:135. *(Excellent results for treatment of stages IB and IIA.)*

Lovecchio JL, Averette HE, Donato D, et al. 5-Year survival of patients with periaortic nodal metastases in clinical stage IB and IIA cervical carcinoma. Gynecol Oncol 1989;34:43. *(Survival falls from 85 percent to about 50 percent with nodal positivity.)*

Mangioni C, Bolis G, Pecorelli S, et al. Randomized trial in advanced ovarian cancer comparing cisplatin and carboplatin. J Natl Cancer Inst 1989;81:1464. *(Two of the best available regimens compared.)*

McGuire WP, Rowinsky EK, Rosenshein NB, et al. Taxol: A unique antineoplastic agent with significant activity in advanced ovarian epithelial neoplasms. Ann Intern Med 1989; 111:273. *(Good overview of this promising drug.)*

National Cancer Institute. The Bethesda System for reporting cervical/vaginal cytologic diagnoses. JAMA 1989;262:931. *(An improved system that is increasingly used for designating Pap smear results.)*

Omura GA, Brady MF, Homesley HD, et al. Long-term follow-up and prognostic factor analysis in advanced ovarian carcinoma. J Clin Oncol 1991;9:1138. *(Tumor bulk, stage, and histology were among the key determinants.)*

Richart RM. The patient with an abnormal Pap smear. N Engl J Med 1980;302:332. *(A discussion of evaluation and roles for colposcopy and cryotherapy.)*

Rodriguez MH, Platt LD, Medearis AL, et al. The use of transvaginal sonography for evaluation of postmenopausal ovarian size and morphology. Am J Obstet Gynecol 1988;159:810. *(Documents its utility and enhanced sensitivity for disease detection.)*

Rubin SC, Hoskins WJ, Hakes TB, et al. Serum CA 125 levels in surgical findings in patients undergoing secondary operations for epithelial ovarian cancer. Am J Obstet Gynecol 1989; 160:677. *(Level correlates with amount of tumor found.)*

Rustin GJ, Jennings JN, Nelstrob AE, et al. Use of CA 125 to predict survival of patients with ovarian cancer. J Clin Oncol 1989;7:1667. *(Those with high levels had a worse prognosis.)*

Schapira MM, Matchar DB, Young MJ. The effectiveness of ovarian cancer screening: A decision analysis model. Ann Intern Med 1993;118:838. *(Limited effect on survival predicted by this decision-analysis study.)*

Primary Care Medicine: Office Evaluation and Management of the Adult Patient, 3rd edition, edited by Allan H. Goroll, Lawrence A. May, and Albert G. Mulley, Jr. J.B. Lippincott Company, Philadelphia

9

Genitourinary Problems

124

Screening for Syphilis

HARVEY B. SIMON, M.D.

The prevalence of syphilis in the United States began to decline with the introduction of penicillin therapy in the 1940s, falling to an all-time low of about 7000 cases in 1956. Since then, reported cases of syphilis have increased. In the 1970s, much of the increase was due to infection in homosexual men. The acquired immunodeficiency syndrome (AIDS) epidemic produced changes in sexual behavior that have reduced the incidence of syphilis in homosexual men, however, syphilis has increased dramatically in blacks, Hispanics, and inner city residents. In 1990, more than 50,000 cases of primary and secondary syphilis were reported, representing a 9 percent increase in just 1 year. Much of the increase can be attributed to drug abuse and human immunodeficiency virus (HIV) infection, factors that also account for a dramatic increase in congenital syphilis. Early detection is extremely important.

If a patient is not identified and treated during the primary or secondary stages of the disease, the infection becomes latent and is identifiable only by means of laboratory tests until late, often irreversible, clinical manifestations appear. The prevention of destructive cardiovascular and neurologic lesions by means of appropriate screening for latent syphilis is an important task for the primary physician. Because false-positive results are common and are potentially traumatic for the patient, it is critical that the sensitivities and specificities of the various serologic tests be understood.

EPIDEMIOLOGY AND RISK FACTORS

With the exception of infection in utero or, rarely, by means of blood transfusion, syphilis is transmitted exclusively by *direct sexual contact* with infectious lesions. It follows that risk increases with sexual activity. Because syphilis is readily treated with antibiotics, it is less common in populations with access to medical care. The reported incidence of syphilis in nonwhites in the United States is much higher than in whites. Rates are highest in urban areas. It must be remembered, however, when comparing incidence rates in different populations, that case reporting has been shown to be more complete in public clinics than among private practitioners.

The age-specific incidence rates parallel those of gonorrhea, with the peak incidence for both diseases occurring between ages 20 and 25. A diagnosis of gonorrhea, nongonorrheal urethritis, HIV infection, or another sexually transmitted disease should be considered a risk factor for syphilis. Drug abuse has become an important risk factor. Male homosexuals are also at high risk, presumably because of the group's tendency to have had multiple sexual contacts.

The importance of an accurate sexual history in determining risk of syphilis is obvious. Patients with early syphilis report an average of three recent sexual contacts. The probability that a known contact will develop syphilis has been shown to be approximately 30 percent, following a single exposure. Partner notification has failed to contain epidemic syphilis because infected patients tend to have relatively large numbers of anonymous sexual partners.

NATURAL HISTORY OF SYPHILIS AND EFFECTIVENESS OF THERAPY

Treponema pallidum enters the bloodstream within a few hours after inoculation through intact mucous membranes or abraded skin. A primary lesion occurs at the site of the inoculation between 10 and 90 days after contact. This incubation period depends on the size of the inoculum, but is usually less than 3 weeks. The painless chancre usually resolves within 4 to 6 weeks, ending the *primary stage*. The *secondary stage* is usually heralded by a maculopapular rash that appears approximately 6 weeks after the primary lesion has healed. When the rash subsides, after 2 to 6 weeks, the untreated patient enters the *latent stage* (arbitrarily divided into *early latent* for the first 2 years and *late latent* thereafter).

Because anorectal or vaginal chancres are not likely to be brought to medical attention, primary syphilis is usually not diagnosed among homosexual men or among women. Whereas more than 40 percent of syphilis cases are detected in the primary stage among heterosexual males, only 23 percent and 11 percent, respectively, are detected in the primary stage among homosexual males and among females.

Natural history studies from Oslo and Tuskegee indicate that approximately one-third of untreated syphilitics will develop clinically manifest tertiary disease and that autopsy evidence of cardiovascular syphilis can be found in more than half. In the retrospective Oslo study, 10 percent of patients had clinically evident cardiovascular syphilis, 7 percent had neurosyphilis, and 16 percent had gummatous disease. The incidence of cardiovascular syphilis was higher and that of neurosyphilis was lower in the prospective Tuskegee study.

Factors that influence the progression to clinical tertiary disease are incompletely understood. Congenital syphilis or disease contracted before age 15 does not predispose to cardiovascular tertiary disease. In general, late complications seem more likely to occur among untreated men than women.

The antibiotic regimens recommended in Chapter 141 are highly effective in eradicating early syphilis. If response to therapy is appropriately monitored by following the quantitative VDRL titer, the risk of late complications is virtually eliminated. Antibiotic treatment of late syphilis has less predictable results. Improvement among patients with general paresis has been reported in 40 percent to 80 percent of cases. Not surprisingly, structural cardiovascular changes caused by syphilis are not reversed by antibiotic treatment.

SCREENING AND DIAGNOSTIC TESTS

Two groups of serologic tests can be used to diagnose syphilis: nontreponemal tests and treponemal ones.

Nontreponemal tests, first introduced by Wasserman in 1906, use *cardiolipin* antigens extracted from mammalian tissues. These tests depend on cross-reactivity with antibodies against *T. pallidum.* The *rapid plasma reagin (RPR), Venereal Disease Research Laboratory (VDRL),* and the *automated reagin test (ART)* are among the most widely used. Their advantages include low cost, simplicity, and automated processing use for mass screening. Many of them can be quantified to allow serologic monitoring of response to therapy.

Nontreponemal tests are well suited for *screening* because they are highly sensitive. Virtually all patients with secondary syphilis are seropositive. Most with primary disease become positive within a week of clinical symptoms, but a minority fail to develop detectable antibodies in early infection. Patients with concomitant HIV and *T. pallidum* infections usually have positive syphilis serologies (often titers are high). Even without treatment, 25 percent of patients with syphilis become seronegative in late latent disease.

A disadvantage of nontreponemal tests is that their specificity is only about 70 percent. *Acute false-positive reactions,* which spontaneously revert to negative within 6 months, may follow many bacterial and viral infections. *Chronic false-positive reactions* occur in patients with elevated serum globulins. Such reactions are particularly common in intravenous (IV) drug abusers (about 25%), patients with systemic lupus (15%), and the healthy elderly (10%). Chronic false-positives also occur in patients with chronic liver disease, other connective tissue diseases, myeloma, and other advanced malignancies.

Treponemal Tests. All patients with positive nontreponemal tests should be retested using specific treponemal antigens. Although these tests are more sensitive and specific than the nontreponemal ones, they are better suited for diagnostic confirmation than for screening. The *microhemagglutination–T. pallidum* test *(MHA-TP)* is now the most widely used. Others include the *fluorescent treponemal antibody–absorbed test (FTA-ABS),* the *hemagglutination treponemal test for syphilis (HATTS),* and the now rarely performed *T. pallidum immobilization test (TPI).*

In general, the treponemal tests become positive earlier than nontreponemal tests and tend to remain positive throughout life. However, it has been noted that about 13 percent of patients receiving prompt treatment for primary syphilis develop negative MHA-TP tests within 3 years of therapy.

CONCLUSIONS AND RECOMMENDATIONS

- After decades of decline, syphilis is becoming more common, especially among IV drug abusers, the urban poor, and HIV-infected persons.
- Screening for latent disease is simple, and the late manifestations of syphilis are entirely preventable if treatment is instituted early.
- Many patients have been screened routinely at the time of marriage, during prenatal care, before giving blood, or on hospital admission. Frequent screening is unnecessary, but the nonreactivity of sexually active individuals, particularly those with multiple sex partners, should be documented at approximately 5-year intervals.
- Special indications for screening include contact or infection with other sexually transmitted diseases, pregnancy, IV drug abuse, and HIV infection.
- All patients with syphilis should be counseled about HIV infection and advised to accept HIV testing.
- Nontreponemal tests such as the RPR or VDRL are appropriate for screening because of their sensitivity and simplicity. MHA-TP or other treponemal tests should be reserved for confirming a diagnosis suspected on the basis of clinical presentation or positive nontreponemal tests.

ANNOTATED BIBLIOGRAPHY

Andrus JK, Fleming DW, Harger DR, et al. Partner notification: Can it control syphilis? Ann Intern Med 1990;112:539. *(The answer is no because of too many anonymous sexual contacts.)*

Centers for Disease Control and Prevention. Primary, secondary syphilis—U.S., 1981–1990. JAMA 1991;265:2940. *(Details of the changing epidemiology of the disease.)*

Clark EG, Danbold N. The Oslo study of the natural course of untreated syphilis. Med Clin North Am 1964;48:613. *(A restudy of case material of untreated syphilis collected from 1891 to 1910.)*

Hart G. Syphilis tests in diagnostic and therapeutic decision making. Ann Intern Med 1986;104:368. *(An evaluation of available tests, with consideration of their sensitivity and specificity.)*

Hutchinson CM, Hook EW. Syphilis in adults. Med Clin North Am 1990;74:1389. *(Excellent review of syphilis in adults, including serologies and treatment.)*

Rockwell DH, Yobs AR, Moore MB Jr. The Tuskegee study of untreated syphilis. Arch Intern Med 1964;114:792. *(A prospective 30-year study of untreated syphilis in 412 black males; notable for the ethical questions raised as well as the natural history of syphilis.)*

Waring GW. False-positive tests for syphilis revisited. The intersection of Bayes' theorem and Wassermann's test. JAMA 1980;243:2321. *(A reminder that as the incidence of a disease declines, so does the specificity of its screening test. The overall sensitivity of a positive STS was calculated at 85 percent.)*

Primary Care Medicine: Office Evaluation and Management of the Adult Patient, 3rd edition, edited by Allan H. Goroll, Lawrence A. May, and Albert G. Mulley, Jr. J.B. Lippincott Company, Philadelphia

125
Screening for Chlamydial Infection

Chlamydia trachomatis is responsible for close to 4 million cases of genitourinary tract infection each year in the United States. Transmission is by sexual contact. Because symptoms may be absent, mild, or nonspecific, treatment is often delayed or missed. Undetected or untreated infection can lead to pelvic inflammatory disease with such consequences as tubal scarring, infertility, and ectopic pregnancy. Over 50,000 women are rendered sterile each year. The estimated direct and indirect costs of such adverse outcomes is in excess of $2.4 billion per year. Screening for chlamydial infection should be a consideration in the provision of routine primary care to women. Key issues are whom to screen and with what method(s).

EPIDEMIOLOGY AND RISK FACTORS

Chlamydial infection is a sexually transmitted disease (STD) present in epidemic proportions. Its prevalence varies by clinical setting. Among women seen in primary care practice, the prevalence is 3 percent to 5 percent. In family planning clinics, the prevalence increases to 9 percent; in STD clinics, the rate rises to 17 percent to 28 percent. Prevalence is very high among adolescents (18%), and one study of college campus women found 50 percent were infected.

Women are at greater risk for contracting *C. trachomatis* infection than are men and also suffer more serious consequences. The risk from a single act of unprotected intercourse with an infected partner is 40 percent for women and 20 percent for men. The increased risk for women reflects their receiving an ejaculate of infected secretions from their partners' genital tract. Men do not receive such a large inoculum unless they have an intact foreskin that can serve as a reservoir for the woman's infected cervical secretions.

Among women with documented urogenital infection, the cervix is infected in 75 percent and the urethra in 50 percent. Endometritis can be demonstrated in about 33 percent; it is often clinically silent, but infection may spread to the tubes. In studies of salpingitis, *Chlamydia* are recovered from the tubes in up to 50 percent of subjects. Vaginal infection is rare.

Chlamydia may also colonize the pharynx and rectum in women engaging in oral and anal sex, respectively. Among those attending an STD clinic, the rate for oral recovery of organisms was 3.2 percent; the rectal colonization rate was 5.2 percent. Rectal involvement has been noted even in the absence of rectal intercourse.

In men, the urethra is the predominant site of infection, with over 82 percent having a symptomatic or visible urethral discharge. In 1 percent to 2 percent of infected men, the infection ascends to the epididymis, producing acute scrotal pain and discomfort. Homosexual men demonstrate even higher rates of oral and anal recovery of organisms. Lymphogranuloma strains are often present.

Age is a powerful predictor of infection. Women *younger than age 21* have the greatest risk. Other important risk factors include having a *new partner* in the last 2 months, *more than one partner* in the last 6 months, or a *partner known to have other partners*. Nonetheless, even among women who are monogamous or who have been sexually inactive in the last 2 months, prevalence can be as high as 7 percent to 10 percent.

Other significant predictors of chlamydial infection identified by multivariate analysis include *black race, low level of education, unprotected intercourse, mucopurulent cervical discharge,* and *induced mucosal bleeding* on swabbing of the cervix as significant risk factors. Among patients with *gonococcal infection,* 30 percent to 50 percent have concurrent chlamydial disease.

DIAGNOSIS

Clinical Recognition

In women, clinical recognition can be difficult because so many are asymptomatic. Although vaginal discharge, bleeding, lower abdominal discomfort, and dysuria may accompany infection, these symptoms are nonspecific and require detailed workup in their own right (see Chapters 111, 116, 117, and 133). The only features of the history that reliably suggest the problem are the risk factors identified above.

In the absence of definitive symptoms, physical findings take on additional importance. *Mucopurulent discharge, cervical ectopy, edema* in the area of ectopy, and easily *induced mucosal bleeding* have proven predictive of *C. trachomatis* infection, as has greater than 10 neutrophils per high-power field. *Uterine or adnexal tenderness* in a patient with a mucopurulent cervical discharge is suggestive of chlamydial pelvic inflammatory disease (see Chapters 116 and 117).

In men, nongonococcal *urethritis* is the most common presentation, with dysuria, penile discharge, and greater than five polys per high-power field (see Chapter 136). About a third of men with chlamydial urethritis have no symptoms or signs, although pyuria may be noted. A small number experience acute testicular pain from an ascending epididymitis (see Chapter 131).

Diagnostic Tests

Culture is the gold standard for identification. However, because chlamydia are obligate intracellular organisms, their isolation and identification require cell culture techniques similar to those used for viruses. Such cultures are technically difficult, expensive, take up to a week, and require refrigeration of the specimen and transport to the laboratory within 24 hours.

Modifications in traditional cell culture techniques have simplified isolation of the organism. Cell monolayers set up in microtiter plates are helpful in settings where titers are likely to be high (eg, STD clinics). Fluorescein-conjugated monoclonal antibodies are useful for identifying chlamydial inclusions in infected monolayers. Combining both advances provides a 14 percent increase in diagnostic yield and sensitivity, makes unnecessary second-pass testing, and shortens test time to 3 days.

Antigen Detection techniques were developed to overcome the difficulties and limitations posed by culture. *Direct immunofluorescence* staining of smears, using monoclonal antibodies, and *enzyme-linked immunoassay (ELISA)* of antigen eluted from swabs are commercially available. Using culture as the gold standard, sensitivity of the direct immunofluorescent technique in women ranges from 77 percent in intermediate prevalence populations to 90 percent in high prevalence ones. Specificity is over 95 percent in both. The ELISA has a sensitivity of 85 percent to 89 percent and a specificity in excess of 95 percent. Cost-effectiveness studies indicate that screening for *Chlamydia* with antigen detection techniques becomes cost-effective when the pretest probability of disease exceeds 7 percent. Identifying asymptomatic men for testing can be facilitated by prescreening the urine for white blood cells (WBCs).

DNA Detection techniques represent a further advance in diagnosis, making possible detection by sampling of urine as well as by the traditional urethral or cervical swab. Using a polymerase chain reaction (PCR) for detection of minute quantities of chlamydial DNA, sensitivity rises into the 90 percent range and specificity approaches 100 percent. As the test becomes available and provided its cost is not prohibitive, it should lower the pretest probability necessary to make screening cost-effective.

EFFECTIVENESS OF TREATMENT

There are several effective treatment regimens for chlamydial urogenital tract infection (see Chapters 117, 135, and 141). Urethritis and cervicitis without evidence of pelvic inflammatory disease responds well to 1 week of *doxycycline* (100 mg bid), *tetracycline* (500 qid). A single 1-g oral dose of *azithromycin* is an effective alternative and, although more expensive, ensures compliance and successful outcome of treatment, especially in persons whose compliance may be suspect. If pregnant or unable to take tetracycline or azithromycin, then *erythromycin* base 500 mg qid for 7 days is recommended.

CONCLUSIONS AND RECOMMENDATIONS

- Chlamydial genitourinary infection is worth screening for, but universal screening is not recommended in primary care practice because the prevalence of asymptomatic infection in this setting is likely to be below the threshold that makes universal screening cost-effective.
- Antigen testing becomes cost-effective in patients whose pretest risk is greater than 7 percent. Culturing becomes cost-effective in patients whose pretest risk is greater than 14 percent. DNA-based testing is likely to have the lowest pretest probability threshold for cost-efficacy, but data are incomplete.
- A policy of selective screening is recommended, based on a clinical estimate of the risk of chlamydial infection.
- Because the prevalence of chlamydial infection among sexually active teenage girls and college women under the age of 20 can be of epidemic proportion (ie, 20%–50%) and because the risk of sterility from unapparent infection is very high, annual screening should be strongly considered for these individuals.
- Sexually active women under the age of 25 coming to their primary care physician for routine gynecologic care should be considered at increased risk of chlamydial infection and screened if they report or are found to have one or more of the following risk factors: 1) new sexual partner within past 3 months; 2) more than one sexual partner in 6 months; 3) partner known to have sexual contact with others; 4) cervical friability; 5) mucopurulent cervical discharge; 6) inconsistent use of barrier contraception. Those over age 25 should be screened if they have two of the above risk factors.
- All men presenting with a urethral discharge should be screened for chlamydial infection.
- Sexually active asymptomatic young men should be prescreened by testing the urine for WBCs. Those who are positive should be screened for chlamydial infection.
- Antigen testing of a cervical or urethral swab is the most convenient and least expensive screening method. Emerging DNA-based screening technology may lower the threshold at which screening is cost-effective and make urine testing feasible (the literature should be followed closely).
- All young women coming for routine gynecologic care who do not desire pregnancy should be urged to insist on condom use during intercourse.

A.H.G.

ANNOTATED BIBLIOGRAPHY

Aronson MD, Phillips RS. Screening young men for chlamydial infection. JAMA 1993;270·2097. *(An editorial review of the data on screening young men.)*

Brunham RC, Paavonen J, Sevens CE, et al. Mucopurulent cervicitis—the ignored counterpart in women of urethritis in men. N Engl J Med 1984;311:1. *(Finding cervical mucopus and >10 PMNs/high-power field predictive of* C. trachomatis *infection.)*

Chow JM, Yonekura ML, Richwald GA, et al. The association between *Chlamydia trachomatis* and ectopic infection. JAMA

1990;263:3164. *(A case–control study finding an odds ratio of 3.0 and a relative risk of 2.4; suggests douching may increase risk.)*

Johnson BA, Poses RM, Fortner CA, et al. Derivation and validation of a clinical diagnostic model for chlamydial cervical infection in university women. JAMA 1990;264:3161. *(Identifies risk factors for chlamydial infection as a means of determining who should be screened.)*

Martin DH, et al. Controlled trial of a single dose of azithromycin for the treatment of chlamydial urethritis and cervicitis. N Engl J Med 1992;327:921. *(Found to be as effective as standard therapy.)*

Phillips RS, Aronson MD, Taylor WC, et al. Should tests for *Chlamydia trachomatis* cervical infection be done during routine gynecologic visits? Ann Intern Med 1987;107:188. *(A cost-effectiveness study indicating that if prevalence is greater than 7 percent, antigen testing is worth performing.)*

Phillips RS, Hanff PA, Holmes MD, et al. *Chlamydia trachomatis* cervical infection in women seeking routine gynecologic care: Criteria for selective testing. Am J Med 1989;86:515. *(Multivariate study; identifies low level of education, partner with other partners, sex with other partners as predictors of infection and indications for screening.)*

Sellor JW, Picard L, Gafni A, et al. Effectiveness and efficiency of selective vs universal screening for chlamydial infection in sexually active young women. Arch Intern Med 1992;152: 1837. *(Two selection rules were developed by regression analysis and tested; selective testing is preferred in low prevalence settings.)*

Shafer M-A, Schachter J, Moncada J, et al. Evaluation of urine-based screening strategies to detect *chlamydia trachomatis* among sexually active asymptomatic young males. JAMA 1993;270:2065. *(Prescreening the urine for WBCs followed by antibody testing of positive persons was most cost effective.)*

Stamm WE. Diagnosis of *Chlamydia trachomatis* genitourinary infections. Ann Intern Med 1988;108:710. *(Excellent review, with very useful discussion of clinical findings, culture, and antigen methods; 93 refs.)*

Vogels WHM, van Vooster-Vader PC, Schroder FP. *Chlamydia trachomatis* infection in a high-risk population: Comparison of polymerase chain reaction and cell culture for diagnosis and follow-up. J Clin Microbiol 1993;31:1103. *(Test characteristics of the new DNA-based methods.)*

Workanski KA, Lampe MF, Wong KG, et al. Long-term eradication of *chlamydia trachomatis* genital infection after antimicrobial therapy. JAMA 1993;270:2071. *(Treatment completely eradicates the organism.)*

Primary Care Medicine: Office Evaluation and Management of the Adult Patient, 3rd edition, edited by Allan H. Goroll, Lawrence A. May, and Albert G. Mulley, Jr. J.B. Lippincott Company, Philadelphia

126
Screening for Prostate Cancer

JOHN D. GOODSON, M.D.
MICHAEL J. BARRY, M.D.

Prostate cancer is the most commonly diagnosed serious malignancy among men in the United States. The lifetime probability that a man will be diagnosed with clinical prostate cancer is between 6 percent and 9 percent, but the probability of death due to prostatic cancer is approximately 2 percent to 3 percent. Even the patient with clinically evident disease is more likely to die of something else. Pathologic studies indicate that occult prostatic cancer is even more prevalent than these figures suggest.

The physician faces a great deal of uncertainty in making clinical decisions about prostatic cancer. These tumors are exceedingly common and have the potential to cause significant morbidity and mortality. They also have a variable, often indolent course and a higher prevalence in elderly men whose health is often more limited by coincident diseases. The clinician should be aware of the unpredictable natural history of the disease and the limitations of current knowledge about the benefits of therapy when considering the use of screening tests for prostatic cancer.

EPIDEMIOLOGY AND RISK FACTORS

The incidence of prostatic carcinoma increases with age. Reports of age-specific prevalence derived from autopsy studies range from 5 percent to 15 percent during the sixth decade, 10 percent to 30 percent during the seventh decade, and 20 percent to 50 percent or higher after age 70. Prostate cancer is rare under the age of 50. The prevalence of prostate cancer diagnosed during life has increased over the years with rising prostatectomy rates and with increasingly detailed histologic study of tissue removed at surgery for benign prostatic hyperplasia (BPH). African-Americans have about a threefold higher incidence of prostate cancer. A brother or father with prostate cancer increases risk twofold. A history of prostatitis or BPH does not confer additional risk. There is no clear etiologic relationship to environmental factors, socioeconomic status, fertility, or endogenous androgen level. Regional variations in the prevalence of prostatic cancer reflect either differences in unidentified environmental factors or, more likely, variation in case detection methods.

NATURAL HISTORY OF DISEASE AND EFFECTIVENESS OF THERAPY

Clinical Presentation and Course. Unfortunately, the biologic behavior of prostatic carcinoma varies widely, making individual cases unpredictable. In many men, early symptoms arise first from concurrent BPH (see Chapter 138) and include such symptoms of urinary tract outflow obstruction as hesitancy, frequency, nocturia, and loss of stream volume and force. In some men, prostate cancer can metastasize before symptoms prompt detection. Approximately 40 percent of patients diagnosed with prostate cancer no longer have localized disease.

An increasing number of cancers are detected in asymptomatic men or incidentally following surgery for BPH. About 10 percent of all prostatic cancers are first palpated as nodules during routine rectal examination. Another 10 percent of cases are discovered during microscopic examination of tissue removed for the treatment of BPH.

The *clinical course* after diagnosis is remarkably variable and depends more on the *degree* of *histologic* differentiation of the tumor than on the extent of the disease. Most incidentally discovered tumors have relatively well-differentiated isolated malignant foci. Even without treatment, survival in these patients is similar to age-matched controls. A minority of latent tumors have diffuse poorly differentiated histology. Prognosis in these cases is nearly as poor as those with metastases at presentation. Moderately differentiated tumors have intermediate behavior. The mean duration of the asymptomatic state of prostatic cancer has been estimated to be between 10 and 30 years, but it is apparent that patients with poorly differentiated tumors are on the short end of this distribution. It is also clear that some tumors can run a very aggressive course after they become clinically manifest. In some older series, the median survival from diagnosis to death in untreated patients was less than 2 years.

Effectiveness of Therapy. This variability in natural history complicates an assessment of therapeutic efficacy. Some have argued that early and aggressive intervention with surgical extirpation of involved tissue (radical prostatectomy) and/or radiation therapy to the pelvis may improve survival in patients in whom the tumor is isolated to the gland or is locally metastatic. However, no form of intervention applied to asymptomatic patients (whether they have latent carcinoma or carcinoma found on biopsy of a suspected malignant nodule) has as yet been shown to improve survival. In very old patients, most specialists withhold treatment until symptoms of obstruction or metastasis develop. There has been a recent trend toward more aggressive therapy in younger patients and older patients without coincident disease. This strategy may eventually prove beneficial, but it presents a higher immediate risk to the patient. Others argue that small, well-differentiated cancers are unlikely to need treatment because of their good prognosis, whereas larger, more poorly differentiated tumors are unlikely to benefit from curative treatment.

SCREENING AND DIAGNOSTIC TESTS

Digital rectal examination (DRE) of the prostate remains the most practical screening technique for prostatic carcinoma, although recent studies have called into question the efficacy of even this time-honored maneuver. The patient should be positioned so as to obtain an adequate examination. A curled lateral decubitus position, with the legs drawn to the chest, or standing, with toes together and heels apart, leaning over an examination table are the two best positions. The latter approach will work better for larger glands and for physicians with shorter fingers. The finding of a firm nodule is suspicious, whereas a stony, asymmetric prostate is highly suggestive of malignancy. Fixation to adjacent tissue and a loss of the lateral prostate sulcus suggest local spread. Unfortunately, the test characteristics of the DRE are poor for the earliest stages of prostate cancer. Compared to a multimodal screening battery including transrectal ultrasound (TRUS) and prostate-specific antigen, DRE has an estimated sensitivity of 60 percent to 70 percent. The positive predictive value (see Chapter 2) for a nodule detected on rectal examination is between 20 percent and 40 percent. As many as 60 percent to 70 percent of the cancers detected initially by rectal examination are later found to have spread beyond the capsule of the gland.

Transrectal ultrasound of the prostate is a second screening technique, identifying suspicious hypoechoic areas. Because these hypoechoic areas are frequently small and not palpable, the yield from biopsy depends on the skill of the examiner and the number of samples obtained (some biopsies are positive in areas other than the hypoechoic nodule with this approach). Unfortunately, up to 30 percent of cancers are isoechoic and would be missed by this technique. Reports of the sensitivity of TRUS range from 50 percent to as high as 90 percent, whereas the specificity is relatively low and the positive predictive value is similar to the DRE, 20 percent to 40 percent. When a rectal examination and prostate-specific antigen are both negative, the positive predictive value of ultrasound drops to 5 percent or less.

Prostate-specific antigen (PSA) is a unique glycoprotein produced by both benign and malignant prostate epithelial tissue. Its measurement can clearly improve the early detection of prostate cancer. Because there are several assays commercially available with different "normal" ranges, physicians should know which assay is used by their local laboratory. Elevations can be seen after cystoscopy, prostate trauma (such as a needle biopsy), or with infection. Vigorous rectal examination of the gland may cause a transient elevation (the half-life of the antigen is between 2 and 3 days). BPH can also produce modest PSA elevations. Using the manufacturer's normal ranges, the specificity of PSA is approximately 33 percent, too low to warrant its use as a screening test. Higher thresholds for an abnormal test improve the predictive value, but at a cost of some sensitivity. In a study using Tandem-R assay, 22 percent of men with value 4.0 to 9.9 ng/mL had prostate cancer, 67 percent with a value of 10.0 ng/mL or higher had prostate cancer. It remains to be established whether the cancers identified by PSA screening are at a lower stage and whether screening improves morbidity and mortality. Widespread PSA screening cannot be recommended until the benefits of early detection have been more clearly established.

CONCLUSIONS AND RECOMMENDATIONS

- Routine annual DRE of the prostate is recommended over age 50. If a nodule is identified in younger patients or older patients without significant comorbid disease, who would be eligible for curative treatment, a urologic referral for biopsy should be made. A normal PSA result does not exclude cancer in the presence of a palpable nodule.
- Routine TRUS screening detects relatively few cases of

prostate cancer that cannot be detected by a combination of rectal examination and PSA.

- Determination of PSA levels can be considered after the age of 50, especially in patients at higher than average risk. However, because there is no evidence that such screening reduces long-term mortality, routine screening is optional. Screening periodicity has not been established, but repeating the PSA at 1- to 2-year intervals is probably appropriate.

ANNOTATED BIBLIOGRAPHY

Catalona WJ, et al. Measurement of prostate-specific antigen in serum as a screening test for prostate cancer. N Engl J Med 1991;324:1156. *(Reports outcome of screening program involving 1653 healthy males. About a third of the cancers found in this study would not have been detected by DRE alone.)*

Chodak GW, Thisted RA, Gerber GS, et al. Results of conservative managment of clinically localized prostate cancer. N Engl J Med 1994;330:242. *(Conservative management in older men with low-grade, localized disease did not adversely affect survival.)*

Chybowski FM, Bergstahl EJ, Oesterling JE. The effect of digital rectal examination on the serum prostate specific antigen concentration. J Urol 1992;148:83. *(No effect noted; can order test on same day as examination.)*

Friedman GF, et al. Case-control study of screening for prostate cancer by digital rectal examinations. Lancet 1991;337:1526. *(A retrospective case–control study showing that the relative risk of metastatic cancer was no better among men who had received one or more rectal examinations in the preceding 10 years.)*

Garnick MB. Prostate cancer: screening, diagnosis, and management. Ann Intern Med 1993;118:804. *(A review that nicely summarizes the unresolved issues; 139 refs.)*

Gerber GS, Chodak GW. Digital rectal examination in the early detection of prostate cancer. Urol Clin North Am 1990;17:739. *(Fifty-nine percent of nodules detected by TRUS were missed on rectal examination.)*

Hudson MA, et al. Clinical use of prostate-specific antigen in patients with prostate cancer. J Urol 1989;142:1011. *(Thirty-five percent of patients with localized prostate cancer had a PSA level over 10.0 ng/L.)*

Johansson J-E, et al. Natural history of localized prostatic cancer. Lancet 1989;333:799. *(Disease-specific death was predicted most strongly by the tumor grade. The 5-year corrected survival for men with well-differentiated histology was 98.8 percent; for men with poorly differentiated histology, survival was 24.5 percent.)*

Kramer BS, Brown ML, Porok PC, et al. Prostate cancer screening: what we know and what we need to know. Ann Intern Med 1993;119:914. *(Net benefit of screening unknown, based on this analysis of available data.)*

Mettlin C, et al. The American Cancer Society National Prostate Cancer Detection Program. Cancer 1991;67:2949. *(Prospective, multicenter study of 2425 men screened with DRE, TRUS, and PSA. The positive predictive value of DRE was 25 percent, of TRUS was 15.2 percent, of DRE, TRUS, and PSA was 68 percent.)*

Oesterling JE. Prostate specific antigen: A critical assessment for adenocarcinoma of the prostate. J Urol 1991;145:907. *(Extensive review. PSA unlikely to become the sole method for prostate cancer screening because 25 percent of patients with BPH have elevated values.)*

Pienta KJ, Esper PS. Risk factors for prostate cancer. Ann Intern Med 1993;118:793. *(Comprehensive review; 178 refs.)*

Primary Care Medicine: Office Evaluation and Management of the Adult Patient, 3rd edition, edited by Allan H. Goroll, Lawrence A. May, and Albert G. Mulley, Jr. J.B. Lippincott Company, Philadelphia

127
Screening for Asymptomatic Bacteriuria and Urinary Tract Infection

Efforts to detect and treat asymptomatic bacteriuria are based on the assumption that treatment reduces the likelihood of subsequent morbidity due to symptomatic infection, sepsis, or chronic renal disease. The risk of such complications depends on the clinical situation, including the age and gender of the patient. For some, risk is well defined, and treatment is indicated; for others, the most significant morbidity may be related to the side effects of inappropriate treatment. It is therefore critical that the physician appreciate the different implications of bacteriuria in different settings.

EPIDEMIOLOGY AND RISK FACTORS

The prevalence of bacteriuria depends on age and gender. Among neonates, positive cultures are found in about 1 percent of both males and females. During school-age years, the prevalence among boys is as low as 0.03 percent, compared with 1 to 2 percent among girls. Prevalence among females increases by 1 percent of the population per decade; throughout the childbearing age, the prevalence is 2 to 4 percent, and, by age 50, it has reached 5 to 10 percent. Geriatric males are almost as likely to have bacteriuria as females because of the high incidence of prostate and other urologic disease and subsequent instrumentation in this group. Prevalence in these older age groups reaches 15 percent.

The greater susceptibility of younger women and girls can be explained anatomically in that a short urethra allows easier access to the bladder, facilitating colonization by perineal organisms. Risk increases with local trauma associated with sexual activity and the relaxation of pelvic supporting structures with age. Anatomic changes may also explain the higher prevalence of bacteriuria (4%–7%) among pregnant women. Alternatively, because users of birth control pills also have an increased risk, the higher prevalence may also reflect estrogen-mediated dilation of the urethra.

The prevalence of bacteriuria is even higher in diabetic women. The relative risk of bacteriuria among women with diabetes, compared with nondiabetic women is approximately 3. There is no increased risk among diabetic men.

It must be kept in mind that prevalence figures indicate the extent of bacteriuria at a single point in time. Because risk factors are shared by many and bacteriuria frequently resolves spontaneously as well as after therapy, the cumulative prevalence of bacteriuria is higher. By age 30, approximately 25 percent of women have experienced symptoms consistent with urinary tract infection.

Structural abnormalities, including obstruction of the urethra or ureters, significant vesicourethral reflux, neurologic lesions, and foreign bodies are important additional risk factors for bacteriuria.

NATURAL HISTORY OF ASYMPTOMATIC BACTERIURIA AND EFFECTIVENESS OF THERAPY

Asymptomatic and symptomatic urinary tract infections have the same epidemiologic correlates. Asymptomatic infections can become symptomatic; bacteriuria can persist after symptoms have resolved. Ninety percent of women with bacteriuria have had symptoms some time in the past, nearly 70 percent within the preceding year. Although both asymptomatic and symptomatic infections can resolve spontaneously, the urine is more likely to become sterile after treatment. Approximately 80 percent of women with bacteriuria have sterile urine after appropriate antibiotic treatment. However, follow-up studies indicate that only 55 percent of those treated will have sterile urine at the end of 1 year. Sterile urine developed spontaneously in fully 36 percent of untreated bacteriuric women during the same period. Significantly, women who had recurrences of infection after treatment were more likely to have associated symptoms than those who had persistent or relapsing bacteriuria. Symptomatic infection recurs within 3 years in 40 percent of women.

The importance of chronic or recurrent bacteriuria in the etiology of chronic renal failure has been deemphasized as diverse noninfectious etiologies for the pathologic findings of interstitial nephritis have been recognized. Patients with bacteriuria are more likely to be hypertensive. They are also more likely to have identifiable abnormalities on intravenous pyelogram (IVP), including small kidneys, delayed excretion, caliceal dilation and blunting, ureteral reflux, stones, and other obstructive lesions. However, chronic renal failure rarely occurs as a complication of urinary tract infection in the absence of structural abnormalities. Evidence indicates that such abnormalities predispose patients to both chronic renal failure and recurrent infection. Definitive studies that address this important question have not yet been performed.

In addition to symptomatic urinary tract infection and chronic renal disease, the clinician must also be concerned with the possibility that chronic asymptomatic infection is a potential source of disseminated infection, such as endocarditis. This danger is particularly likely in the male patient with prostate disease and infection who requires instrumentation. Bacteremia has been documented in as many as 50 percent of males whose urine is infected at the time of the procedure; it is relatively rare when the urine is sterile. In elderly populations, asymptomatic bacteriuria has been associated with increased mortality. Obviously, such increased rates may be due either to bacteriuria or to other factors that increase the risk of both bacteriuria and death. Recent evidence suggests the latter; at least one study found no difference among elderly women and men with and without bacteriuria when comorbidity such as cancer was controlled.

Special risks are associated with bacteriuria during pregnancy. Asymptomatic bacteriuria, defined by either repeated recovery of greater than 105 CFU/mL in voided urine or positive suprapubic aspirates, occurs in approximately 5 percent of pregnancies. In one study, the risk of onset of bacteriuria was greatest between the 9th and 17th weeks of gestation. Among women with bacteriuria identified early in pregnancy, there is a 40 percent incidence of acute pyelonephritis without prophylactic treatment. Women with bacteriuria are nearly twice as likely to deliver a low-birth-weight infant. Their relative risk of perinatal infant mortality has been estimated at 1.6. Randomized trials of treatment of asymptomatic bacteriuria of pregnancy have demonstrated efficacy in reducing the incidence of pyelonephritis and low-birth-weight delivery.

SCREENING AND DIAGNOSTIC TESTS

Asymptomatic bacteriuria is a laboratory diagnosis that requires careful definition. Because voided urine is easily contaminated by urethral and (in women) perineal flora during micturition, cultures of clean voided urine must be cultured quantitatively. The probability of infection in a patient whose specimen contains 105 CFU/mL is nearly 100 percent for males but only 80 percent for females. Two such positive cultures in a female increase the probability of infection to 95 percent. False-negative findings are more likely if the patient is undergoing vigorous diuresis, if the urine is unusually acidic (pH 5.5), or if the specimen was inadvertently contaminated with antibacterial detergents. Spurious positive cultures are more common because of unclean collection technique, contaminated collection equipment, or failure to promptly culture the urine.

A single culture of urine collected on urethral catheterization with 105 CFU/mL has a predictive value of infection of 95 percent. Catheterization should be limited to patients requiring relief of obstruction or those who absolutely cannot cooperate with collection techniques. The risk of introducing infection during catheterization may be as high as 5 percent. The risk of inducing bacteremia in men with an infected urinary tract approaches 50 percent. When suprapubic percutaneous bladder aspiration is used in young children or to resolve confusing problems in the adult, infection can be presumed if any bacterial growth other than that of skin contaminants occurs.

Nonquantitative approaches to diagnosis include microscopic examination for bacteria and clinical tests of bacterial activity such as the reduction of nitrate to nitrite. Dipstick nitrite testing for bacteriuria has been shown to have a sensitivity of greater than 90 percent, but specificity is limited and variable, ranging from 35 to 85 percent in different studies. This variation may be explained by differences in the prevalence of bacteria that do not reduce nitrates and variation in the time interval between collection and testing of urine. Dipstick tests for leukocyte esterase activity as a marker for pyuria are more sensitive but less specific. Reported sensitivity of the leukocyte esterase dipstick for bacteriuria range from 72 to 97 percent; the reported range for specificity is 64 to 82 percent. Dipstick tests have been shown to be less sensitive when the prior probability of infection is low based on the presence or absence of clinical findings. These and other nonspecific signs of urinary tract inflammation such as microscopic pyuria or hematuria, and proteinuria may be helpful in making a presumptive diagnosis in the symptomatic patient. They may also indicate the need for urine culture when incidental abnormalities are detected in the asymptomatic patient. Confirmation of infection with quantitative culture technology should precede a therapeutic decision in the absence of symptoms.

CONCLUSIONS AND RECOMMENDATIONS

- Bacteriuria, both symptomatic and asymptomatic, is a common phenomenon with well-defined risk factors.
- Treatment is moderately effective in the short run, but because of high rates of spontaneous recurrence and resolution, the likelihood that bacteriuria will be noted with longer follow-up is not significantly influenced by short-term therapy.
- Symptomatic infections are generally not prevented by treatment of asymptomatic bacteriuria in nonpregnant women.
- Although an association exists between bacteriuria and renal abnormalities, there is no evidence that this is an etiologic relationship. Furthermore, there is no evidence that treatment of infection in the absence of urinary tract abnormalities will prevent progressive renal disease.
- Screening for asymptomatic bacteriuria is recommended only in selected high-risk populations including 1) pregnant women; 2) elderly males with clinical prostatism or other urologic abnormalities, before and after required instrumentation; 3) all patients recently catheterized; and 4) patients with known renal calculi or other structural abnormalities of the urinary tract.

A.G.M.

ANNOTATED BIBLIOGRAPHY

Asscher AW, Sossman M, Waters WE, et al. The clinical significance of asymptomatic bacteriuria in the nonpregnant woman. J Infect Dis 1969;120:17. *(Controlled trial of treatment of asymptomatic bacteriuria. Concludes that screening for bacteriuria in nonpregnant women is unlikely to be of value.)*

Freedman LR, Seki M, Phair JP. The natural history and outcome of antibiotic treatment of urinary tract infections in women. Yale J Biol 1965;37:245. *(Short-term follow-up cultures overestimate benefits of treatment.)*

Gower PE, Haswell B, Sidaway ME, et al. Follow-up of 164 patients with bacteriuria of pregnancy. Lancet 1968;1:990. *(Fewer than 20 percent of those not treated in this study incurred pyelonephritis.)*

Kass EH, Zinner SH. Bacteriuria and renal disease. J Infect Dis 1969;120:27. *(Exhaustive review of the links between bacteriuria and renal disease. Authors conclude that a causal relationship has been demonstrated in cases of pyelonephritis in pregnancy and bacteremia postcatheterization but not in progressive renal disease among adults.)*

Kunin CM, Polyak F, Postel E. Periurethral bacterial flora in women. JAMA 1980;243:134. *(Intensively monitored small cohort of women with and without history of UTI. The most notable finding is a high frequency of asymptomatic bacteriuria with spontaneous resolution in both groups.)*

Lachs MS, Nachamkin I, Edelstein PH, et al. Spectrum bias in the evaluation of diagnostic tests: Lessons from the rapid dipstick test for urinary infection. Ann Intern Med 1992;117:135. *(Sensitivity for documented bacteriuria is much lower, approximately 50 percent, when the prior probability of infection is deemed to be low on clinical grounds.)*

Nicole LE, Mayhew WJ, Bryan L. Prospective randomized comparison of therapy and no therapy for asymptomatic bacteriuria in institutionalized elderly women. Am J Med 1987;83:27. *(There were no differences in genitourinary morbidity or mortality; antimicrobial therapy was associated with adverse effects and a higher reinfection rate.)*

Nordenstam GR, Brandberg CA, Oden AS, et al. Bacteriuria and mortality in an elderly population. N Engl J Med 1986;314: 1152. *(Nine-year cohort study finding no difference in mortality among women with and without bacteriuria; also, no difference among men when those with cancer were excluded.)*

Pels RJ, Bor DH, Woolhandler S, et al. Dipstick urinalysis screening of asymptomatic adults for urinary tract disorders. II. Bacteriuria. JAMA 1989;262:1220. *(A careful review of the literature offering estimates of sensitivity and specificity as well as recommendations.)*

Stamm WE. Prevention of urinary tract infections. Am J Med 1984;76:148. *(Thoughtful review of risk factors and preventive approaches; recommends screening only for pregnant women.)*

Stenquist K, Dahlen-Nilsson I, Lidin-Janson G, et al. Bacteriuria in pregnancy. Frequency and risk of acquisition. Am J Epidemiol 1989;129:372. *(In a study of more than 3,000 pregnancies, risk of onset of bacteriuria was greatest between the 9th and 17th weeks of gestation.)*

Takahashi M, Loveland DB. Bacteriuria and oral contraceptives. JAMA 1974;227:762. *(Fifty percent higher prevalence among oral contraceptive users.)*

128
Screening for Cancers of the Lower Urinary Tract

Primary Care Medicine: Office Evaluation and Management of the Adult Patient, 3rd edition, edited by Allan H. Goroll, Lawrence A. May, and Albert G. Mulley, Jr. J.B. Lippincott Company, Philadelphia

Lower urinary tract cancers include tumors of the renal pelves, ureters, bladder, and urethra. These lesions can logically be considered together because of similar cell types—more than 95 percent consist of transitional cells, squamous cells, or a combination of the two—and because of common epidemiologic correlates.

Cancer of the lower urinary tract is viewed by many primary physicians as a relatively benign tumor that principally affects the elderly. Nevertheless, approximately 40,000 new cases occur each year in the United States; 10,000 deaths per year can be attributed to bladder cancer. The lifetime probability of incurring cancer of the bladder is approximately 2 percent for white males and 1 percent for white females.

Risk factors, including a strong association with occupational exposure, have been well-defined. A weaker association with tobacco use has more recently been demonstrated. Screening tests are available. Although there is still insufficient understanding of the natural history of bladder cancer to allow specific screening recommendations, the physician must understand the epidemiology of these tumors as well as the potential costs and benefits of various screening practices.

EPIDEMIOLOGY AND RISK FACTORS

Cancer of the lower urinary tract is a tumor of older age groups; in the United States, the mean age at the time of diagnosis is 68 years. The incidence increases at a constant rate during adult life, varying from one per 100,000 per year at age 20 to 200 per 100,000 per year at age 80 for white males. Females have approximately one-third the risk of males. In the United States, whites are twice as likely to have bladder tumors as nonwhites. Urban dwellers, too, have consistently been shown to have a higher incidence of lower urinary tract tumors compared with people who live in rural or suburban areas.

The most notable risk factor for development of lower urinary tract cancers is *occupational exposure* to aromatic amines, first noted in England in 1895. Subsequently, dyestuff workers were shown to have a 10-fold to 50-fold increased risk of bladder carcinoma. Compounds most closely associated with bladder carcinogenesis include 2-naphthylamine and benzidine. Recent case–control studies indicate excess risk among men who worked with dyestuffs, rubber, leather, or painting or other organic chemicals. It has been estimated that these occupational exposures are responsible for 18 percent of bladder cancer cases. As little as 2 years' exposure may be sufficient to increase the risk, but the time between exposure and subsequent cancer may be as long as 45 years.

Smoking has been implicated as a risk factor for bladder cancer in many studies, most of which indicate that smokers have a twofold increase in risk over nonsmokers. Other suggested risk factors include pelvic irradiation, which was used in the past for dysfunctional bleeding, heavy coffee consumption, and abuse of phenacetin-containing analgesics.

NATURAL HISTORY OF LOWER URINARY TRACT CANCERS AND EFFECTIVENESS OF THERAPY

The natural history of lower urinary tract tumors is not well-defined. Prognosis at the time of diagnosis depends on both clinical stage, defined by depth of penetration and extent of metastases, and histologic grade of the tumor. There is often close correlation between depth of penetration and histologic grade. Urothelial tumors are grossly subdivided into papilloma, papillary carcinoma, and transitional cell carcinoma. These gross morphologic distinctions have histologic counterparts that are highly predictive of 5-year survival. Grade 1 papillary carcinoma (papilloma) has a 5-year cure or clinical control rate of approximately 95 percent. Grade 2 papillary carcinoma (papillary carcinoma) has a 5-year survival rate of only 25 percent. The outlook for grade 3 papillary and infiltrating carcinoma (transitional cell carcinoma) is worse. Prognosis for patients with squamous carcinoma is also very poor, unless the tumor is well-differentiated. Clinical staging systems that distinguish between levels of tumor penetration of the bladder have also been shown to have good prognostic value. Overall, about 50 percent of patients with treated bladder cancer survive for 5 years. However, multiple synchronous and asynchronous tumors are the rule in lower urinary tract cancer, contributing to morbidity and eventual mortality.

Hematuria is the most common presentation of lower urinary tract cancer. Other symptoms suggestive of cystitis may also occur. Although it has been claimed that 75 percent of tumors promptly diagnosed after a first episode of hematuria are localized, little data on this subject are available. The likelihood that screening tests, including urinalysis and urinary cytology, would significantly advance the time of diagnosis is likewise unproven. A progression from urothelial atypia to sessile carcinoma in situ or papilloma to higher grade malignancy has been postulated. Studies of the natural history of urothelial carcinoma in situ indicate that the majority of lesions progress to more malignant forms. Although early lesions are much less likely to be detected cytologically, 3.7 percent of detected tumors were in situ in one study. The usual synchronous and asynchronous multiplicity of such tumors makes it difficult to assess the benefits of early detection.

SCREENING TESTS

Urinary cytology is the most specific screening test for lower urinary tract cancers. Reports of the sensitivity of cytology in detecting bladder carcinoma vary from 50 percent to 90 percent. Studies have consistently demonstrated that sensitivity increases with the grade of malignancy. Although invasive transitional-cell carcinoma can regularly be detected with 90 percent or greater sensitivity, sensitivity rates for papillomas and papillary carcinomas range from 0 percent to 50 percent.

Studies of cytologic screening of high-risk populations have been conducted. In one such study, screening of 285 exposed workers produced positive results in 31, 10 of whom had the diagnosis of cancer confirmed at cystoscopy. Within 4 years, 11 additional tumors developed among the 21 cytology-positive, cystoscopy-negative patients. Cystoscopy was also performed in the 254 workers with negative cytologic findings; only one case of bladder cancer was diagnosed on that examination. In general, the specificity of urinary cytology depends on the skill of the cytologist. False-positive rates as low as 1 percent and as high as 20 percent have been reported.

The value of other urinary sediment abnormalities, particularly hematuria, has not been well-defined. In one study of cytologic detection, hematuria was absent in 50 percent of true-positive cytologic diagnoses.

Cystoscopy and radiographic procedures cannot be considered screening tools. They should be reserved for patients who present with symptoms suggestive of urinary cancer or who have positive cytologies. Frequent follow-up cystoscopies are also a part of the postoperative care of the patient with bladder cancer.

CONCLUSIONS AND RECOMMENDATIONS

- Lower urinary tract cancer is associated with significant morbidity and mortality.
- Risks of occupational exposure to dyestuffs, rubber, leather and leather products, and paint and organic chemicals have been well-defined. Smoking is associated with a smaller, but significant, increase in risk.
- Urinary cytology is an imperfect but useful screening test for high-risk groups.
- There is no evidence that screening significantly advances the time of diagnosis in an individual case or that early treatment influences the outcome. Nevertheless, because of the relatively high specificity and lack of morbidity associated with cytologic screening, identification of patients at high risk because of occupational exposure, with subsequent yearly cytologic screening, is indicated. Screening of asymptomatic smokers without risk of occupational exposure is not recommended.

A.G.M.

ANNOTATED BIBLIOGRAPHY

Cole P. Coffee-drinking and cancer of the lower urinary tract. Lancet 1971;1:1335. *(Further case–control data identifying the association between coffee drinking and cancer of the lower urinary tract, particularly among women.)*

Cole P, Hoover R, Friedell GH. Occupation and cancer of the lower urinary tract. Cancer 1972;29:1250. *(Case–control study identifying excess risk among five occupation categories: dyestuffs, rubber, leather and leather products, paint, and organic chemicals. There was no identifiable risk in those who worked with nonorganic chemicals, petroleum, or printing.)*

Cole P, Monson RR, Haning H, et al. Smoking and cancer of the lower urinary tract. N Engl J Med 1971;284:129. *(Case–control data indicating that smokers have a twofold greater risk of developing bladder cancer.)*

Foot NC, Papanicolaou GN, Holmquist ND, Seybolt JF. Exfoliative cytology of urinary sediments (a review of 2,829 cases). Cancer 1958;11:127. *(Sensitivity of 62 percent in detecting tumors of renal pelves, bladder, or ureters, 8 percent in renal tumors, and 15 percent in prostatic tumors; high specificity.)*

Heney NM, Ahmed SW, Flanagan MJ, et al. Superficial bladder cancer: Progression and recurrence. J Urol 1983;30:1083. *(Useful description of the natural history of the disease.)*

Kantor AF, Hartge P, Hoover RN, et al. Urinary tract infection risk of bladder cancer. Am J Epidemiol 1984;119:510. *(A case–control study detecting a relative risk for bladder cancer of two among those with a history of three or more urinary tract infections.)*

Matanoski GM, Elliott EA. Bladder cancer epidemiology. Epidemiol Rev 1981;3:203. *(Extensive review of descriptive epidemiology as well as risk factors including smoking, coffee drinking, use of sugar substitutes, as well as occupational exposures.)*

Melamed MR, Koss LG, Ricci A, et al. Cytohistological observations on developing carcinomas of the urinary bladder in men. Cancer 1960;13:67. *(Documents cytologic identification of latent bladder cancer in patients with occupational exposure.)*

Morrison AS, Buring JE. Artificial sweeteners and cancer of the lower urinary tract. N Engl J Med 1980;302:537. *(A case–control study that did not detect a significant association between use of artificial sweeteners and excess risk of lower urinary tract cancer.)*

129
Evaluation of the Patient With Hematuria

LESLIE S.-T. FANG, M.D., Ph.D.

Primary Care Medicine: Office Evaluation and Management of the Adult Patient, 3rd edition, edited by Allan H. Goroll, Lawrence A. May, and Albert G. Mulley, Jr. J.B. Lippincott Company, Philadelphia

Virtually every disease of the genitourinary tract can produce hematuria. The primary physician may encounter a patient complaining of gross hematuria or may find microscopic hematuria on routine examination of the urine. Sometimes the etiology is a harmless condition, especially where there is asymptomatic microscopic hematuria in an otherwise healthy, young patient. At other times, hematuria may be the only symptom of genitourinary neoplasia. Its presence demands careful consideration and often a thorough investigation to ascertain the underlying etiologic factors. One needs to be able to initiate an effective workup and decide how comprehensive and invasive it ought to be; this includes deciding when referral for urologic evaluation or renal biopsy is necessary.

PATHOPHYSIOLOGY AND CLINICAL PRESENTATION

Normally, fewer than 1000 red blood cells are excreted in the urine each minute. Microscopic hematuria ensues if the rate of excretion rises to 3000 to 4000 red blood cells per minute; two to three red blood cell per high-power field will appear on microscopic examination of the urine. If the excretion rate exceeds 1 million red blood cells per minute, macroscopic or gross hematuria will result. Definitions of clinically significant hematuria are somewhat arbitrary; however, greater than eight red blood cells per high-power field is considered a reasonable cut-off point for separating benign etiology from potentially serious pathology.

Any intrinsic lesion within the genitourinary tract involving the kidneys, ureter, bladder, prostate, or urethra can produce hematuria. Hematuria may also result from periurethral problems in the pelvis or colon, systemic diseases, bleeding diatheses, and use of certain drugs (eg, cyclophosphamide).

Symptoms associated with hematuria may provide important clues to etiology. The flank pain of renal colic is usually secondary to renal calculi but may occasionally be associated with passage of clots. Frequency, dysuria, urgency, and suprapubic pain occur with inflammatory lesions of the lower urinary tract. Dull flank pain with fever and chills may accompany pyelonephritis (see Chapter 133).

Occasionally, complaints such as fever, rash, or joint pains may indicate an underlying systemic disease. Uncommonly, hematuria occurs without any associated symptoms, although the majority of cases have a definable cause. When a thorough workup fails to reveal an etiology, the patient is said to have "essential hematuria." Renal biopsy of such patients often shows minimal glomerular or interstitial disease. Long-term prognosis of these patients is excellent.

DIFFERENTIAL DIAGNOSIS

Intrinsic genitourinary lesions involving the kidneys, ureters, bladder, prostate, and urethra can all produce hematuria (Tables 129-1 and 129-2). Gross hematuria is most commonly associated with infections and neoplasms. Microscopic hematuria is most commonly associated with infection and benign prostatic hypertrophy. The prevalence of serious underlying disease (eg, cancer, polycystic disease) in community-based study of asymptomatic microscopic hematuria is 0.1 percent comparerd to 10 percent in referred populations. Even among high-risk groups (eg, older men), community-study prevalence is only 5 percent.

Rarely, periureteral inflammatory lesions in the appendix, colon, or pelvic structures produce microscopic hematuria. On occasion, a systemic illness such as lupus erythematosus, bacterial endocarditis, or rheumatic fever is the source of hematuria. Blood dyscrasias (eg, hemophilia, sickle cell disease, polycythemia vera, and leukemia) and hemorrhagic disorders (eg, thrombocytopenic purpura and various coagulation defects) can be responsible for red cells in the urine.

Drugs such as anticoagulants, salicylates, methenamine preparations, and sulfonamides have been known to cause hematuria. Cyclophosphamide can induce hemorrhagic cystitis or microscopic hematuria (see Chapter 88). Hematuria in a patient on anticoagulants requires evaluation because an underlying urologic lesion is often found (see Chapter 83).

Fever, strenuous exercise, and long-distance running are among the harmless etiologies of microscopic hematuria in otherwise healthy patients. If a thorough workup fails to reveal an etiology, the patient is said to have "essential" hematuria.

Conditions occasionally mistaken for hematuria include menstrual bleeding and the intake of substances that can darken the urine, such as beets, rhubarb, and the drugs pyridium and rifampin.

WORKUP

The appropriate workup depends on whether the patient has macroscopic hematuria or asymptomatic microscopic hematuria, on the age and gender of the patient, and on the mode of clinical presentation. As indicated in the previous section, the likelihood of finding a significant genitourinary tract disease is higher in patients with macroscopic hematuria, particularly in the older male patients. Asymptomatic microscopic hematuria in young adults, on the other hand, carries a much lower risk. Evidence from five population-based studies indicates that 1 percent to 5 percent of children

Table 129-1. Diagnosis in 1000 Referred Cases of Gross Hematuria

DIAGNOSIS	PATIENT (%)	
Kidneys	15.0	
Tumor		3.5
Infection		3.0
Calculus		2.7
Trauma		2.0
Obstruction		1.5
Others		2.3
Ureters	6.5	
Calculus		5.3
Tumor		0.7
Others		0.5
Bladder	39.5	
Infection		22.0
Tumor		14.9
Others		2.6
Prostate	23.6	
Benign hyperplasia		12.5
Infection		9.0
Tumor		2.1
Urethra	4.3	
Stricture		1.7
Calculus		1.3
Others		1.3
Essential Hematuria	8.5	

From Lee LW, Davis E, et al. Gross urinary hemorrhage: A symptom, not a disease. JAMA 1953;153:782.

and adults would show evidence of microhematuria on routine urinalysis and fewer than 2 percent of these patients have a serious and treatable urinary tract disease. However, the incidence of urinary tract cancers rises dramatically with age and is more than twice as high in males as in females. Microscopic hematuria in the older male patient should therefore be aggressively pursued.

Table 129-2. Diagnosis in 500 Referred Cases of Asymptomatic Microscopic Hematuria

DIAGNOSIS	PATIENT (%)	
Kidneys	6.2	
Calculus		3.4
Cyst		1.2
Hydronephrosis		0.6
Tumor		0.4
Others		0.6
Ureters	0.8	
Calculus		0.4
Ureterocele		0.4
Bladder	8.6	
Infection		6.6
Tumor		1.8
Others		0.2
Prostate	23.6	
Benign hyperplasia		23.6
Urethra	23.4	
Infection		21.2
Calculus		1.8
Others		0.4
Essential Hematuria	44.0	

From Greene LF, O'Shaughnessy EJ Jr, Hendricks ED. Study of 500 patients with asymptomatic microhematuria. JAMA 1956;161:610.

History is of paramount importance in narrowing the scope of the workup. History of trauma ought to direct attention to possible renal, ureteral, or urethral injury. Massive hematuria is usually associated with bladder neoplasm, benign prostatic hypertrophy, or trauma. Passage of large bulky clots implicates the bladder as the source, whereas long shoestring-shaped clots suggest a ureteral origin. Past history of analgesic excess makes analgesic nephropathy a possibility. A prior history of nephritis requires consideration of chronic nephritis as the etiology of the hematuria. Family history of renal diseases may suggest polycystic kidney disease or hereditary nephritis. Harmless, self-limited forms of microscopic hematuria are suggested by a recent history of strenuous exercise, long-distance running, or a minor febrile illness.

Physical Examination should include observation of any fever, hypertension, rash, purpura, petechiae, friction rub, heart murmur, or joint swelling. Presence of hypertension suggests renal parenchymal disease. The abdomen has to be examined carefully for enlargement of one or both kidneys, liver, or spleen. Thorough examination of the prostate in the male and the pelvis in the female is essential.

Laboratory Testing. A repeat urinalysis is worthwhile in patients suspected of having self-limited or trivial cause for their hematuria, such as low-grade infection, menstrual period, or vigorous exercise. An entirely normal repeat study in a healthy young person requires no further investigation other than a follow-up urinalysis in a month or two. However, in an older patient, whose risk of malignancy is much greater, an abnormal number of red blood cells on a urinalysis should be taken seriously, even if a repeat urine is clear. A urinary tract malignancy may present in just this manner. The urine sediment should be carefully examined. Presence of white cells and bacteria favors a diagnosis of cystitis; white cell casts imply the presence of pyelonephritis or interstitial nephritis. Red cell casts strongly suggest glomerulonephritis. Presence of dysmorphic red cells under phase contrast microscopy is also highly suggestive of glomerular origin of the red cells. A urine specimen should be sent for routine culture when there is pyuria (see Chapter 133). Culture for urine acid-fast bacillus needs to be obtained if sterile pyuria and hematuria persist.

The need for further workup is determined by the probability of important underlying pathology. For example, a patient over age 50 is at increased risk for urinary tract cancer; it must be ruled out. On the other hand, an otherwise healthy young patient with an unremarkable history, a normal physical examination, and an otherwise benign urinary sediment need not undergo invasive testing, because the likelihood of malignancy or other serious pathology is low. In a major population study, the frequency of clinically significant microscopic hematuria was 2.3 percent with only 0.5 percent having bladder or renal cell carcinoma; malignant lesions were found almost exclusively in patients over age 50.

The *three-glass test* (see Chapter 139) can be done to attempt to identify the site of the bleeding. Initial hematuria is usually associated with anterior urethral lesions such as stenosis and urethritis. Terminal hematuria usually arises from a lesion in the posterior urethra, bladder neck, or trigone. Total hematuria is associated with lesions at the level of the bladder or above.

Renal function is checked when there is suspicion of renal parenchymal disease. In those with proteinuria, a *24-hour urine collection for creatinine and protein determinations* should be done to assess renal function and quantitatively assess the degree of proteinuria. Heavy proteinuria (greater than 3 g/24h) is usually associated with glomerular lesions (see Chapter 130). In the presence of renal colic, the urine should be strained to detect the presence of calculi or papillae. Three first-void morning urine specimens are sent for *cytology* in patients over age 40 with hematuria, because such people are at increased risk for a neoplasm. Normal cytologies do not rule out a malignancy (see Chapter 128); cystoscopy is indicated if suspicion remains. *Flat plate and upright films* of the abdomen are obtained and carefully examined to ascertain renal size and detect the presence of calcifications.

If these tests fail to define the origin of the hematuria, an *intravenous pyelogram with tomograms* should be done. Renal and ureteral abnormalities can be defined accurately. A *post-void film* should be obtained to assess the amount of postvoid residual urine to estimate the degree of bladder neck obstruction. *Ultrasonography, computed body tomography,* and *magnetic resonance imaging (MRI)* are useful to differentiate a solid mass from cystic lesion if the differentiation cannot be made on nephrotomograms. *Renal angiography* is reserved for evaluation of possible renal trauma, suspicious renal masses, and possible arteriovenous malformations.

If there is clinical evidence of glomerular disease (red cell casts, dysmorphic red cells, heavy proteinuria), *immunologic studies* should be performed and a renal biopsy should be considered. The immunologic tests of diagnostic use include ANA, anti–deoxyribonucleic acid (DNA) antibodies, and complement levels (C3, C4 and CH50) for the diagnosis of systemic lupus erythematosus (see Chapter 130); ASLO titer, antihyaluronidase, antistreptokinase, and complement levels for the diagnosis of poststreptococcal glomerulonephritis; serum and urine immunoelectrophoresis for the diagnosis of multiple myeloma; serum IgA level for patients suspected of having Berger's disease (IgA nephropathy) or Henoch-Schönlein purpura; serum antiglomerular basement membrane antibodies for patients suspected of having Goodpasture's syndrome; and antineutrophil cytoplasmic antibodies (ANCA) for pauci-immune glomerulonephritis.

INDICATIONS FOR REFERRAL

In a patient over age 50, if a distinct lesion is still not defined or there is suspicion of a bladder lesion, it is necessary to proceed to *cystoscopy* (see Chapter 128). The procedure is particularly useful during periods of active bleeding. Careful examination of the ureteral orifices for bleeding and biopsy of suspicious lesions are essential.

Referral to the nephrologist for consideration of *renal biopsy* should be carried out in patients with evidence of glomerulonephritis. Renal biopsy is indicated only for the establishment of a diagnosis that will affect the selection of therapy (see Chapter 130) and should be reserved for patients with clinical evidence of glomerular disease. Rarely, renal biopsy may be indicated if the preceding studies have not led to a diagnosis.

PATIENT EDUCAITON

It is essential to impress on the patient the necessity of a complete evaluation of hematuria. The high incidence of potentially curable neoplasms in patients over age 50 (see Chapter 143) makes thorough investigation in this group mandatory.

ANNOTATED BIBLIOGRAPHY

Bard RH. The significance of asymptomatic microscopic hematuria in women and its economic implications. Arch Intern Med 1988;148:2629. *(No bladder lesions found in 10 years; suggests cystoscopy might be unnecessary in such persons, though study population small.)*

Corwin HL, Silverstein MD. Microscopic hematuria. Clin Lab Med 1988;8:601. *(Review of methods of detection of hematuria, prevalence, etiologies, and diagnostic strategies in the patient with microscopic hematuria.)*

Mohr DN, Offord KP, Owen RA, et al. Asymptomatic microhematuria and urologic disease: A population based study. JAMA 1986;256:224. *(Community based prevalences of underlying disease.)*

Woolhandler S, Pels RJ, Bor DH, et al. Dipstick urinalysis screening of asymptomatic adults for urinary tract disorders. JAMA 1988;262:1215. *(Review of five population-based studies indicated that fewer than 2 percent of those with a positive heme dipstick have a serious and treatable urinary tract disease.)*

Primary Care Medicine: Office Evaluation and Management of the Adult Patient, 3rd edition, edited by Allan H. Goroll, Lawrence A. May, and Albert G. Mulley, Jr. J.B. Lippincott Company, Philadelphia

130
Evaluation of the Patient With Proteinuria

LESLIE S.-T. FANG, M.D., Ph.D.

Normal individuals excrete less than 150 mg of urinary protein each day; the mean is 40 to 50 mg. Excretion in excess of 150 mg/24h is classified as clinically significant proteinuria. Causes range from benign conditions, such as exercise and orthostatic proteinurias, to glomerulonephritis with rapidly deteriorating renal function. Office evaluation is frequently prompted by an incidental finding of proteinuria on routine urinalysis. The objective of the outpatient workup is to establish the presence of significant proteinuria, search noninvasively for treatable underlying conditions, and select patients who need referral for renal biopsy.

PATHOPHYSIOLOGY AND CLINICAL PRESENTATION

Small amounts of protein (2 to 8 mg/100 mL) are normally found in the urine of healthy individuals, but at a concentration below that detectable by routine methods. Two-thirds of this protein is low-molecular-weight globulin of serum origin; the remainder is albumin and nonserum protein.

Significant proteinuria can occur through a number of mechanisms:

1. Increased glomerular permeability;
2. Increased production of abnormal proteins small enough to pass freely through the glomerulus (eg, Bence Jones protein);
3. Decreased tubular reabsorption (eg, due to interstitial nephritis);
4. Lower urinary tract disease, including infection;
5. Fever, heavy exertion, congestive failure, postural changes, and surgical trauma—all believed to be related to changes in renal blood flow.

Clinical Presentations

Proteinuria can present as an isolated asymptomatic finding on urinalysis, as edema of unknown etiology, or as part of the clinical picture in a patient with known renal or systematic disease.

Isolated Proteinuria. Asymptomatic patients excreting less than 1 g of protein daily and appearing otherwise healthy, with no other evidence of renal dysfunction or systemic disease are considered to have isolated proteinuria. The urine sediment is normal. Two varieties have been described: benign, transient forms; and persistent isolated proteinuria.

Benign forms are characterized by their transient nature. A *functional* variety has been observed in the context of emotional or physical stress, an acute illness, or even a bout of congestive heart failure. The proteinuria is believed to reflect physiologic changes in renal hemodynamics. Although all forms of proteinuria worsen with standing, some persons experience proteinuria only on standing; it is absent when recumbent. The condition is common in persons under the age of 30 (especially males) and is labeled *orthostatic proteinuria.* In many individuals, the postural proteinuria resolves after a few years; in others it remains. Long-term (20-year) follow-up studies show no development of progressive renal impairment.

Other forms of benign disease in young people include *idiopathic transient proteinuria,* characterized by an occasionally positive dipstick test unrelated to posture or stress, and *intermittent proteinuria,* in which about half of dipstick tests are positive for albumin. The former is considered a physiologic variant of normal. The latter is sometimes associated with minor abnormalities on renal biopsy, but progressive disease is rare and the condition is usually self-limited. Intermittent proteinuria in older persons carries a slightly higher risk of renal impairment.

Persistent isolated proteinuria carries a worse prognosis, although the urine sediment and renal function are entirely normal. The condition is most common in healthy young men. Both mild forms of glomerular and tubular injury have been found among these patients. Long-term follow-up studies of patients with persistent isolated proteinuria reveal a 40 percent chance of developing renal insufficiency, usually secondary to glomerular disease. In some instances, nephrotic syndrome may ensue. However, even when persistent and accompanied by minor glomerular changes on biopsy, the condition has an excellent prognosis as long as there are no associated abnormalities of the urine sediment.

Proteinuria in the Setting of Renal or Systemic Disease. Proteinuria in excess of 1 g/24h suggests significant renal impairment. When it exceeds 3 g/24h, underlying *glomerular disease* is likely; lesser amounts are consistent with either glomerular or tubular dysfunction. *Obstruction* and *reflux* are important treatable causes of tubular protein leakage. Glomerular injury may be due to intrinsic renal disease or a systemic process.

Nephrotic syndrome is said to be present when more than 3.5 g/24h of protein are excreted and the serum albumin falls to less than 3.0 g/dL. Such heavy proteinuria usually indicates significant glomerular disease (either primary or secondary to systemic illness) but may occur with severe tubular injury. If the serum albumin concentration drops to less than 2 g/dL, then plasma oncotic pressure may fall sufficiently to cause *edema,* typically beginning in the medial aspect of the ankles, but, on occasion, periorbital puffiness may be the principal manifestation. *Hypercholesterolemia* is a common accompaniment reflecting increased hepatic synthesis of low-density lipoprotein (LDL) and very low-density

Table 130-1. Differential Diagnosis of Proteinuria

Asymptomatic–Transient
- Exercise
- Upright posture
- Lower urinary tract disease (eg, infection)
- Fever (occasionally)
- Congestive heart failure (occasionally)

Asymptomatic–Persistent
- Idiopathic
- Fixed postural type
- Mild glomerular injury
- Mild tubular injury

Symptomatic
- Glomerular disease
- Severe tubular disease (see Table 130-3)

lipoprotein (VLDL) cholesterol. *Lipiduria* is a diagnostic feature of the urine sediment. A *hypercoagulable* state may ensue, believed linked to reductions in protein S (an inhibitor of thrombosis). Venous thromboembolism occurs in about 20 percent. The source of embolization may be a clinically silent *renal vein thrombosis*. Risk of *bacterial infection* is increased in those with marked urinary loss of immunoglobulins. Excessive urinary loss of vitamin D may develop, causing *hypocalcemia* and secondary hyperparathyroidism. Other presenting symptoms reflect associated renal dysfunction or underlying systemic diseases.

DIFFERENTIAL DIAGNOSIS

Asymptomatic Proteinuria. Proteinuria without other abnormalities in an asymptomatic patient can be transient or persistent (Table 130–1). *Transient* forms include functional, orthostatic, idiopathic, and intermittent varieties. *Persistent isolated proteinuria* suggests underlying glomerular or tubular pathology.

Symptomatic Proteinuria. As noted above, heavy proteinuria resulting in nephrotic syndrome is usually the result of glomerular disease (either intrinsic or secondary; Table 130–2), but occasionally severe tubular injury is responsible (Table 130–3). About 50 percent to 75 percent of cases are due to intrinsic glomerular disease; the remainder are associated with systemic illnesses that cause glomerular injury (eg, long-standing diabetes mellitus, systemic lupus, amyloidosis). In adults, *membranous nephropathy* is the most common histologic abnormality seen on the biopsies of patients with nephrotic syndrome. It may be idiopathic or secondary to systemic lupus, hepatitis B, cancer (breast, lung, colon), or medication (gold, penicillamine, captopril). It accounts for close to 50 percent of patients with idiopathic disease. *Minimal change disease* is the glomerulopathy most common in children but is also seen in patients with Hodgkin's disease and hypersensitivity reactions to drugs such as nonsteroidal anti-inflammatory drugs (NSAIDs). *Focal and segmental glomerulosclerosis* is the pathologic picture in about 25 percent of those with intrinsic renal disease but is also a

Table 130-2. Important Glomerular Causes of Nephrotic Syndrome

CAUSE	PATHOLOGIC FEATURES	PROGNOSIS
Idiopathic Glomerular Injury		
Membranous nephropathy	Basement membrane thickening, granular deposits of IgG and C3	Fair–good
Minimal change disease	Normal light microscopy; no immune deposits	Excellent
Focal and segmental glomerulosclerosis	Segmental sclerosis, tubular atrophy	Fair–poor
Membranoproliferative glomerulonephritis	Hypercellular glomeruli and duplicate basement membrane; immune deposits	Poor
Secondary Glomerular Injury		
Diabetes mellitus	Nodular sclerosing	Fair–poor
Light-chain disease	Nodular sclerosing	Fair–good
Amyloidosis	Nodular sclerosing	Fair–poor
Systemic lupus	Membranoproliferative or membranous	Poor–good
Infection (endocarditis, malaria, syphilis, hepatitis B)	Membranoproliferative	Fair–poor
Non-Hodgkin's lymphoma	Membranoproliferative	Poor
Hodgkin's disease	Minimal change	Fair
Drug hypersensitivity	Minimal change	Good
Hepatitis B	Membranous	Fair–good
Cancer (lung, colon, breast)	Membranous	Fair
Nephrotoxins (gold, other heavy metals, high-dose captopril, penicillamine)	Membranous	Poor–good
Heroin	Focal glomerulosclerosis	Poor–fair
HIV infection	Focal glomerulosclerosis	Poor
Mechanical (renal vein thrombosis, IVC obstruction)		Fair–poor
Pregnancy (preeclampsia)		Good

Table 130-3. Tubular Disorders Associated with Proteinuria

Analgesic abuse
Pyelonephritis
Fanconi's syndrome
Cadmium and mercury poisoning
Balkan's nephropathy
Lowe's syndrome
Hepatolenticular degeneration

feature of human immunodeficiency virus (HIV)–infected patients and intravenous heroin abusers. *Membranoproliferative glomerulonephritis* accounts for about 15 percent of patients with idiopathic disease and also occurs in the setting of infection, non-Hodgkin's lymphoma, cryoglobulinemia, and some forms of systemic lupus.

WORKUP

Confirming Proteinuria and Its Significance

Repeat *urinalysis* that includes examination of the *urine sediment* should be the initial step when proteinuria is detected by *dipstick* on a routine random urine sample. The dipstick test is specific for albumin and can detect concentrations in excess of 30 mg/dL. A negative test does not rule out significant proteinuria, because protein excretion may be intermittent (eg, orthostatic proteinuria) or composed of a protein other than albumin (eg, light chains from myeloma). Orthostatic proteinuria can be differentiated from a more serious etiology by collecting a urine sample from the patient on arising and another after being continuously upright for 2 hours. False-positive dipstick reactions can be seen in patients with dehydration, gross hematuria, and those receiving large doses of nafcillin or cephalosporins. Note of the specific gravity should be made along with the test results.

Sediment examination is critical and should be done on a freshly collected specimen. Red cell casts indicate glomerulonephritis (although the absence of erythrocytes on one sample does not rule out glomerulonephritis). White cell casts are found in pyelonephritis and interstitial nephritis. Oval fat bodies are due to lipiduria in patients with nephrotic syndrome.

A confirmed urinalysis for protein should be followed by a *24-hour urine* collection to quantify the degree of proteinuria. In addition to measuring urinary *albumin,* the urine *creatinine* should also be noted. The latter determination enables assessment of adequacy of collection. Depending on muscle mass, the total 24-hour urine creatinine should be 15 to 24 mg/kg. In conjunction with a serum creatinine, the urine creatinine determination can also be used to calculate the *creatinine clearance*. Recent reports indicate some progress in developing quantitative estimates of heavy proteinuria using a spot urine sample. For now, 24-hour collection remains necessary.

Once significant proteinuria is established, the evaluation turns to establishing whether the patient is asymptomatic or symptomatic and, if asymptomatic, whether the proteinuria is transient or persistent. If the patient is asymptomatic, several urinalyses are performed (as described above). If the proteinuria is found to be transient (especially if orthostatic or exercise-induced), then it is likely to be benign, usually occurring in young adults with no underlying renal disease. Invasive procedures and extensive workup are unnecessary. On the other hand, persistent asymptomatic proteinuria is associated with a high incidence of renal pathology and warrants the same investigation as in patients with symptomatic proteinuria. Such patients require a careful history and physical examination, followed by selected laboratory testing.

History and Physical Examination

History should begin by focusing on risk factors for glomerular disease. These include long-standing diabetes, systemic lupus, paraproteinemia, infection (HIV, malaria, syphilis, endocarditis), medications (gold, penicillamine, NSAIDs, antibiotics, high-dose angiotensin-converting enzyme [ACE] inhibitors), hepatitis B, toxin exposure (heavy metals, heroin), allergens (bee sting, serum sickness), and malignancy (lymphoma, Hodgkin's, breast, lung, colon). Risk factors for tubular disorders also should be sought, including analgesic abuse (especially with phenacetin-containing compounds), heavy metal exposure, family history of proteinuria, and history of pyelonephritis.

Physical examination begins with a careful blood pressure determination.

Hypertension is a poor prognostic sign, raising the spectre of significant renal impairment. The patient is also checked for vasculitic skin changes, other rashes, retinopathy, lymphadenopathy, signs of right heart failure and constrictive physiology, abdominal masses, organomegaly, guaiac positivity, prostatic enlargement, peripheral edema, and joint inflammation.

Laboratory Studies

Several laboratory studies are helpful regardless of etiology:

- *Creatinine clearance* is best for determination of renal function. It approximates the glomerular filtration rate. A serum creatinine and a 24-hour urine collection for urinary creatinine levels are simultaneously obtained. Random *BUN* or *creatinine* serum levels are less accurate than a clearance determination but are useful for following the patient once the creatinine clearance is known.
- *Complete blood count* will identify any anemia resulting from severe subacute or chronic renal insufficiency. Anemia is also present at some point in all cases of myeloma.
- *The serum albumin level* is worth monitoring because it correlates inversely with the severity of proteinuria.
- *The protein selectivity index* is useful for diagnosis and therapy in patients with nephrotic syndrome. Proteinuria is considered selective when urine contains large amounts of proteins of low molecular weight. A high degree of selectivity in patients with nephrotic syndrome suggests minimal change disease, which is responsive to corticosteroids (see below).
- *KUB* can be used to judge kidney size, which may help to elucidate etiology (eg, small, shrunken kidneys suggest significant chronic, bilateral disease). *Renal ultrasound* may be more accurate and informative, being able to de-

tect cystic disease, mass lesions, and obstruction. *Intravenous pyelography* is indicated when chronic pyelonephritis is under consideration. It also gives an estimate of individual kidney function, based on how well each concentrates and excretes the contrast material. However, when creatinine clearance is reduced by more than 75 percent, the kidneys may not concentrate the contrast medium sufficiently for visualization. Contrast-induced acute renal failure is a risk in patients with preexisting renal disease, especially in those with diabetes or multiple myeloma.

Additional studies may prove useful when based on clinical findings, although they are not always necessary. The patient with long-standing diabetes mellitus accompanied by retinopathy, significant proteinuria, and azotemia is almost certain to have diabetic glomerulosclerosis and requires little additional workup other than ruling out concurrent urinary tract infection or obstruction. On the other hand, the young woman with polyarthritis, red cell casts, and heavy proteinuria should have antinuclear antibody (ANA), anti–double-stranded deoxyribonucleic acid (DNA), and serum C3 and C4 complement levels. Hepatitis serology and cryoprotein determinations are useful in the patient with a history of jaundice, hepatitis B, or its risk factors. Serum and urine electrophoreses are indicated when myeloma is under consideration (elderly patient with elevated globulins, unexplained anemia). Although occult malignancy is occasionally a possible cause, a search beyond careful breast, lymph node, abdominal, and rectal examinations, chest x-ray, mammogram, and stool guaiac has not been shown to be of sufficient yield to warrant more extensive testing. A "pan scan" for all possible etiologies of proteinuria is unlikely to be of much diagnostic value when the pretest probabilities of the conditions being tested for are low. Pan scanning is more likely to yield false-positive results (see Chapter 2).

Kidney biopsy deserves consideration when treatable disease remains a possibility, yet the etiology continues to be elusive despite careful and thorough clinical and laboratory evaluations (see below).

INDICATIONS FOR REFERRAL

A referral for consideration of renal biopsy is indicated if the result will have important therapeutic or prognostic implications. Most causes of glomerulonephritis do not respond to therapy; thus, biopsy is of academic interest only. However, at times, it will be clinically impossible to rule out a treatable form of glomerulonephritis, and either a biopsy or an empiric course of therapy may be indicated. The advice of an experienced nephrologist is essential.

Referral is also indicated when there is clinical suspicion of an etiology potentially responsive to immunosuppressive therapy (eg, membranous disease). Because the morbidity of therapy can be high, consultation is indicated for optimal design of the treatment regimen.

PRINCIPLES OF MANAGEMENT AND PATIENT EDUCATION

Asymptomatic Proteinuria. *Transient proteinuria* is, by and large, benign. Patients should be reassured; therapy is not warranted. Idiopathic and fixed orthostatic forms of proteinuria that occur as isolated findings without other associated abnormalities have been found to have excellent prognoses in prospective studies with 5 to 20 years of follow-up.

Asymptomatic patients with *persistent isolated proteinuria* can also be followed expectantly. However, they are at greater risk for eventually developing renal impairment and should be carefully followed with annual checks of blood pressure, urine, BUN, and creatinine. Referral to a nephrologist for consideration of renal biopsy and treatment is indicated if the urine sediment becomes abnormal or the blood pressure begins to rise.

Symptomatic Proteinuria/Nephrotic Syndrome. Marked proteinuria associated with systemic diseases such as multiple myeloma, diabetes, or systemic lupus erythematosus is best countered by treating the underlying disease. In addition, *ACE inhibitors* (see Chapter 26) help reduce albumin loss and preserve renal function, presumably by limiting hyperfiltration. The edema of nephrotic syndrome is aggravated by sodium retention, which can be countered by *sodium restriction* and the judicious use of loop and distal-acting *diuretics*. Modest *dietary protein restriction* (approximately 1.0 g/kg/day) may be of benefit in slowing the course of patients with progressive renal disease. Patients prescribed protein restriction require close nutritional follow-up to ensure adequate nitrogen balance. Onset of hypercholesterolemia is initially treated with a *low-saturated fat, low-cholesterol diet,* but use of a lipid-lowering agent (eg, lovastatin) may be necessary. If severe hypocalcemia or renal failure develops, *1-25 dihydroxyvitamin D* plus *calcium* supplementation can limit onset of secondary hyperparathyroidism (see Chapter 142). Due to increased risk of infection, all nephrotic patients should receive the *pneumococcal* and *influenza vaccines*.

In idiopathic nephrotic syndrome, therapy also depends on the renal pathology defined by biopsy. Minimal change disease responds to *corticosteroids* and *immunosuppressive agents,* which can enhance the already favorable rate of remission. Most patients with focal and segmental glomerulosclerosis are resistant to steroid therapy and experience renal insufficiency within 5 years of diagnosis. Some patients with idiopathic membranous nephropathy respond to high-dose alternate-day corticosteroids with partial or complete remission of proteinuria. However, 40 percent undergo spontaneous remission, and, overall, steroid treatment confers no additional improvement in long-term renal survival. Adding an alkylating agent to the steroid regimen does little to improve outcome. Membranoproliferative disease is progressive, ending in renal failure in about 50 percent of cases. Treatment appears to have little impact on renal survival.

ANNOTATED BIBLIOGRAPHY

Abuelo JG. Proteinuria: Diagnostic principles and procedures. Ann Intern Med 1983;98:186. *(A terse review with detailed discussion of patients with isolated proteinuria.)*

Bernard DB. Extrarenal complications of the nephrotic syndrome. Kidney Int 1988;33:1184. *(These include edema, hyperlipidemia, hypercoagulable state, hypocalcemia, and increased susceptibility to infection.)*

Carbone L, D'Agati VD, Cheng J-T, et al. Course and prognosis of human immunodeficiency virus-associated nephropathy. Am J Med 1989;87:389. *(More common in blacks and IV drug abusers; rapidly progressive.)*

Falk RJ, Hogan SL, Muller KE, et al. Treatment of progressive membranous glomerulopathy. Ann Intern Med 1992;116:438. *(A randomized trial comparing cyclophosphamide and corticosteroids with corticosteroids alone; no difference found.)*

Ginsberg JM, Chang BS, Matarese RA, Garella S. Use of single voided samples to estimate quantitative proteinuria. N Engl J Med 1983;309:1543. *(An attempt to identify significant proteinuria from a spot urine sample; those with a protein/creatinine ratio of greater than 3.5 were likely to have significant proteinuria.)*

Glassock RJ. Postural (orthostatic) proteinuria: No cause for concern. N Engl J Med 1981;305:639. *(An editorial summarizing the condition and arguing that reassurance and monitoring are all that are necessary.)*

Johnson RJ, Couser WG. Hepatitis B infection and renal disease. Kidney Int 1990;37:663. *(A very useful review of this increasingly appreciated association.)*

Levey AS, Lan S-P, Corwin HL, et al. Progression and remission of renal disease in the Lupus Nephritis Collaborative Study. Ann Intern Med 1992;116:114. *(Prognosis a function of initial creatinine and response to initial therapy.)*

Levey AS, Lau J, Pauker SG, et al. Idiopathic nephrotic syndrome: Puncturing the biopsy myth. Ann Intern Med 1987; 107:697. *(An alternative strategy suggested: empiric trial of alternate-day steroid therapy in lieu of biopsy.)*

Madaio MP, Harrington JT. The diagnosis of acute glomerulonephritis. N Engl J Med 1983;309:299. *(A useful guide to further evaluation, once glomerulonephritis is suspected; the role of complement levels addressed.)*

Robinson RR. Orthostatic proteinuria: Definition and prognosis. Kidney 1971;4:1. *(Review of pathogenesis and prognosis of orthostatic proteinuria.)*

Robinson RR. Idiopathic proteinuria. Ann Intern Med 1969; 71:1019. *(Short review of idiopathic benign proteinuria.)*

Springberg PD, Garrett LE, Thompson AL Jr, et al. Fixed and reproducible orthostatic proteinuria: Results of a 20-year follow-up study. Ann Intern Med 1982;97:516. *(Prognosis was excellent, with no renal impairment developing in the vast majority.)*

Primary Care Medicine: Office Evaluation and Management of the Adult Patient, 3rd edition, edited by Allan H. Goroll, Lawrence A. May, and Albert G. Mulley, Jr. J.B. Lippincott Company, Philadelphia

131
Evaluation of Scrotal Pain, Masses, and Swelling

A mass, generalized enlargement, or acute pain involving the scrotum may be noted by the patient or discovered incidentally on physical examination. Patients with scrotal complaints are often concerned about loss of sexual function and the possibility of cancer. The primary physician needs to be able to recognize torsion and epididymitis promptly and to differentiate benign masses from those suggestive of testicular malignancy, which require referral for urologic evaluation.

PATHOPHYSIOLOGY AND CLINICAL PRESENTATION

Testicular Cancer. Almost all testicular neoplasms are malignant and of germ cell origin. Fortunately, these tumors are uncommon, accounting for fewer than 1 percent of all deaths from neoplasms in men. However, testicular cancers are the most common malignancy in males aged 15 to 35, having an estimated incidence of three per 100,000. Incidence is increased in those with an undescended testicle and remains high even if orchiopexy is performed or the testicle is removed; the risk seems to be genetically determined. Peak incidence occurs between ages 20 and 40. In patients over age 60, testicular lymphoma is the most common testicular malignancy.

Typically, the tumor presents as a hard, heavy, firm, nontender testicular mass that does not transilluminate, but sometimes the lesion is smooth or even resilient in nature, leading to confusion with benign etiologies even though it blocks transmission of light. Although these lesions are usually painless, about 20 percent cause some discomfort in the scrotum, and frank pain may be reported and tenderness noted, especially if there is hemorrhage into the tumor. Metastasis to the retroperitoneum may cause vague pain in the back or abdomen. Spread to the chest can lead to dyspnea, cough, or hemoptysis. A palpable left supraclavicular node or epigastric mass may be noted. On occasion, extensive metastasis occurs with little evidence of the primary tumor. The metastatic lesion may be histologically different from the primary lesion. A few of these malignancies produce chorionic gonadotropin or estrogen, leading to gynecomastia (see Chapter 99).

Nonmalignant Testicular Disease. *Testicular torsion* presents with acute pain and a firm tender mass in a young patient. The intense pain may be associated with nausea and vomiting and may be confused with an abdominal process. The condition is mostly one of adolescent boys and young men. There is often a history of recurrent episodes of testicular pain. The testicle dangles within an abnormally enlarged tunica, likened to the clapper of a bell. An attack can come on during sleep; there need not be a history of antecedent trauma. *Testicular trauma* produces acute testicular pain and swelling similar to torsion or infection. It does not predispose to cancer. *Mumps orchitis* is usually seen 7 to 10 days after parotitis and is most often unilateral in association with fever, swelling, pain, and tenderness. On occasion parotitis is absent. The condition is more common in adults than in children.

Cystic and Vascular Scrotal Masses. Cystic masses containing fluid or sperm often develop spontaneously. They are slow-growing, usually painless, and may be large and fluctuant. *Hydroceles* are cystic accumulations of clear or straw-colored fluid within the tunica vaginalis or processus vaginalis. *Epididymal cysts* are common and benign. *Spermatoceles* are intrascrotal cysts containing sperm that derive from the small tubules of the epididymis. The space between the testicle and tunica vaginalis may also fill with fluid secondary to impaired drainage or inflammation.

Varicoceles arise from incompetent venous valves. They occur on the left in 97 percent of cases, because the left spermatic vein empties directly into the renal vein, resulting in transmission of considerable hydrostatic pressure into the scrotum when the valves are incompetent and the patient stands. A right-sided varicocele may occur in the context of venous obstruction or renal carcinoma. Varicoceles have a "bag of worms" appearance and are usually nontender; they decrease in size when the patient is recumbent.

Epididymitis. In men under age 35, epididymitis may occur as a consequence of gonococcal or chlamydial infection. *Ureaplasma* has also been implicated. Being a sexually transmitted disease, it may be accompanied by symptoms of urethritis (dysuria, discharge). In older men, the cause is more likely to be prostatitis, recent urinary instrumentation, or a structural lesion. It can occur with carcinoma of the testes. Initially, tenderness and swelling are confined to the epididymis, but as the condition progresses, the inflammation may spread to the adjacent testicle, making for a large, ill-defined, tender, scrotal mass.

Nontesticular, Intrascrotal Malignancies are rare, usually firm, and do not transilluminate, differentiating them from benign, extratesticular scrotal pathology.

Inguinal Herniation can lead to scrotal enlargement and discomfort as bowel tracks through the inguinal canal and pushes down into the scrotum.

Referred Pain. Extrascrotal sources can cause scrotal pain by stimulating one of the nerves (genitofemoral, ilio-femoral, or posterior scrotal) supplying the scrotum. Scrotal examination is unremarkable.

DIFFERENTIAL DIAGNOSIS

The differential diagnosis can be considered in terms of the clinical presentation. A clearly extratesticular, soft scrotal mass that transilluminates may be due to a hydrocele, spermatocele, epididymal cyst, or even generalized edema. A "bag of worms" presentation is characteristic of a varicocele. A tender, inflamed extratesticular mass is likely due to early epididymitis. Acutely painful testicular swelling may represent epididymitis, orchitis, torsion of the spermatic cord, trauma, or hemorrhage into a testicular cancer. A firm, nontender, nontransilluminating testicular nodule represents carcinoma until proven otherwise. A malignancy also has to be considered in the setting of a nontransilluminating extratesticular nodule, although benign etiologies are more common.

An extrascrotal source is suggested by pain in the absence of scrotal pathology. Causes include abdominal aortic aneurysm, ureteral colic, retrocecal appendix, retroperitoneal cancer, and prostatitis.

WORKUP

Because testicular cancer and testicular torsion are serious, but potentially curable diseases, they are prime, must-not-miss considerations in young men who present with a complaint referable to the scrotum or testicles. Epididymitis is similarly curable and important to recognize, because it may represent sexually transmitted disease.

History should include inquiry into acuity of symptoms, duration, clinical course, tenderness, recent trauma, urethral discharge, dysuria, fever, inguinal herniation, and concurrent infection (eg, mumps, gonorrhea, prostatitis). A complaint of scrotal heaviness is common but nonspecific, found in conditions ranging from tumor to hydrocele and epididymitis. Age is worth taking note of, because testicular cancer is a disease of men under the age of 40, and torsion is most common among adolescents and young men. A history of an undescended testicle raises the possibility of testicular cancer. Vague abdominal, back, or chest complaints should not be dismissed, because they may herald the onset of metastatic testicular cancer. Recurrent episodes in a young person suggest torsion (see below). Concurrent flank pain, abdominal pain, prostatitis, or known extratesticular cancer suggests an extrascrotal source, especially in the absence of scrotal pathology on physical examination.

Physical Examination. The key elements of the examination are careful palpation of the scrotal contents and transillumination of any palpated mass. One should try to assess whether a lesion is cystic or solid, testicular or nontesticular. Inspection should include note of any erythema, masses, hernias, or varices. To palpate the scrotal contents properly, one stands to the side and uses both hands, one to support the testicle and the other to feel and identify each structure, beginning with the uninvolved side. The head of the epididymis is usually situated above the testis; the body and tail run posteriorly. All are separately palpable from the testis. The normal testicle is freely movable and uniform in consistence. It is checked for abnormalities that may provide clues to disease on the involved side, such as the horizontal-lying "bell-clapper" mobility of a person at risk for torsion. The scrotal structures are identified and examined for tenderness, warmth, swelling, and nodularity. If a mass or nodule is found, one attempts to determine if it is testicular or extratesticular and if it feels solid or cystic. The inguinal canal is examined for a hernia.

Transillumination with a penlight in a darkened room is needed to help determine whether the lesion is cystic or solid. Cystic lesions allow transmission of light in most instances, although a bloody exudate may not. A mass that appears extratesticular and cystic is most likely benign and either a spermatocele, a cyst of the epididymis, or hydrocele. If it is hard, does not transilluminate, or is reported to be steadily growing, tumor must be considered and urologic evaluation is necessary even if the mass appears to be extratesticular.

In patients suspected of having a testicular tumor, a careful check of supraclavicular lymph nodes, chest, and abdomen is needed because more than 50 percent present with metastatic disease. In addition, the breasts are examined for gynecomastia. (Inguinal adenopathy does not suggest testicular cancer because the testicular lymphatics drain into the paraaortic nodes. Scrotal nontesticular lymphatics drain into the inguinal nodes.)

A tender scrotum in the absence of a mass, redness, increased warmth, or swelling should trigger a look for extrascrotal pathology. Careful examination of the abdomen for signs of appendicitis, aneurysm, and inguinal hernia is warranted, as is a check of the prostate and flanks for tenderness.

Laboratory Studies. When a mass is noted or uncertainty persists, a *testicular ultrasound* examination is helpful in determining whether the lesion is testicular or extratesticular, solid or cystic. Measurement human chorionic gonadotropin *(HCG)* and *alpha-fetoprotein* levels are more useful for monitoring testicular cancer than for diagnosis (see Chapter 143), but a marked elevation in either is suggestive. Unfortunately, sensitivity is low; a negative study does not rule out cancer. If metastatic disease is suspected, a *chest x-ray* and *abdominal CT* are performed as part of the staging process.

A *urinalysis* is helpful for detection of pyuria or bacteriuria in cases suggestive of an infectious process. Semen analysis should be performed only when infertility is a concurrent complaint. A right-sided varicocele or suddenly appearing left-sided varicocele requires further evaluation because of the possibility of venous obstruction or renal carcinoma. In such cases an *intravenous pyelogram* or *renal ultrasound* is indicated.

Suspected extrascrotal pathology necessitates that the workup be directed appropriately toward it (see Chapters 58 and 139).

Approach to the Patient with Acute Pain and Swelling. An acutely painful, swollen testicle requires urgent assessment because, if torsion of the testes is present, permanent damage may occur if treatment does not occur within 4 hours of onset. Acute epididymitis and torsion are the two dominant considerations. Hemorrhage into a testicular cancer is a third. In an older man with concurrent prostatitis or a younger one with urethritis (see Chapter 136), epididymitis is the more likely cause of the problem. The presence of a urethral discharge, tender prostate, pyuria, or bacteriuria further supports the diagnosis of epididymitis. A firm tender mass of acute onset in an afebrile young man with a history of prior episodes must be considered to represent torsion until proven otherwise. The diagnosis is further supported by finding a testicle with a horizontal lie on the uninvolved side. Urgent urologic consultation is necessary to determine whether the scrotum should be explored. Sometimes it can be difficult to distinguish torsion from acute epididymitis on clinical grounds, and urgent surgical exploration is mandatory.

PATIENT EDUCATION AND INDICATIONS FOR REFERRAL

It has been suggested that teaching testicular self-examination might help shorten or eliminate the delay in presentation common to patients with testicular carcinoma. The patient with a clearly extratesticular, transilluminating scrotal lesion can be reassured that cancer is virtually ruled out and that no further evaluation for cancer is necessary other than a periodic follow-up examination. On the other hand, the person with a solid testicular mass needs prompt referral to the urologist, regardless of whether the mass is tender. Testicular cancer confined to the testicle is almost 100 percent curable by orchiectomy alone (see Chapter 143).

As noted above, referral to a urologist should be swift in cases of suspected torsion, because surgical exploration must not be delayed if a viable testicle is to be preserved. Patients in whom testicular cancer is strongly suspected are also likely to require surgical evaluation, although, whenever a testicular malignancy is suspected, exploration should be conducted through an inguinal incision. Trans-scrotal biopsy may cause spillage of tumor into the scrotum and areas of lymphatic drainage. Any mass that cannot be confidently defined as cystic and separate from the testicle should be subjected to a urologist's examination.

A patient with varicocele should be referred if it does not deflate when he lies down, is painful, or is associated with infertility, although correction of the varicocele often fails to achieve conception (see Chapter 120). Referral to a general surgeon is needed for the patient with a poorly reducible hernia.

Most hydroceles and cystic lesions do not require surgical therapy, but the patient should be instructed to return if the enlargement becomes uncomfortable or interferes with intercourse. The patient should understand that surgery is an option that will not threaten virility or fertility. Patients may want a hydrocele removed for cosmetic reasons or relief of discomfort. Aspiration of a hydrocele is to be avoided. Patients with inguinal hernias that are at risk of causing bowel strangulation should be advised to have them repaired (see Chapter 67).

A.H.G.

ANNOTATED BIBLIOGRAPHY

Davis BE, Noble MJ, Weigel JW, et al. Analysis and management of chronic testicular pain. J Urol 1990;143:936. *(Very useful discussion.)*

Dilworth JP, Farrow GM, Oesterling JE. Testicular tumors of nongerm cell origin. J Urol 1991;37:399. *(Comprehensive review; 126 refs.)*

Doll DC, Weiss B. Malignant lymphoma of the testis. Am J Med 1986;81:515. *(The most common cause of testicular malignancy in men over age 60.)*

Hainsworth JD, Greco FA. Testicular germ cell neoplasms. Am J Med 1983;75:817. *(A comprehensive review of evaluation as well as therapy; 121 refs.)*

Haynes BE, Bessen HA, Haynes VE. The diagnosis of testicular torsion. JAMA 1983;249:2522. *(Emphasizes the importance of early diagnosis.)*

McGee SR. Referred scrotal pain. J Gen Intern Med 1993;8:693. *(Case reports and a review; more common than appreciated.)*

Richie JP, Birnholz J, Garnick MB. Ultrasound as a diagnostic adjunct for the evaluation of masses in the scrotum. Surg Gynecol Obstet 1982;154:695. *(Found to be a very useful test in indeterminant cases.)*

Williamson RCN. Death in the scrotum: Testicular torsion. N Engl J Med 1977;296;338. *(A succinct discussion of the problem and its clinical diagnosis.)*

Witherington R, Jarrell T. Torsion of the spermatic cord in adults. J Urol 1990;143:62. *(Presentation is usually earlier in life, but adult onset does occur.)*

132
Medical Evaluation and Management of Impotence

Primary Care Medicine: Office Evaluation and Management of the Adult Patient, 3rd edition, edited by Allan H. Goroll, Lawrence A. May, and Albert G. Mulley, Jr. J.B. Lippincott Company, Philadelphia

Most normal men have occasional episodes of erectile failure, especially at times of stress, fatigue, or distraction. Only when the rate of failure approaches 25 percent is it proper to invoke the clinical diagnosis of impotence, defined as the repeated inability to achieve or sustain an erection sufficient to engage in sexual intercourse. The condition is estimated to affect up to 10 percent of men at any given point in time. Patients sometimes mistakenly use the term "impotence" when referring to other forms of male sexual dysfunction.

In recent years, the primary physician has taken a more active role in evaluation and management of sexual problems, helped by a better understanding of sexual pathophysiology and more open discussion of sexual problems. Impotent patients who suspect their problem may have an organic basis (eg, diabetics, those taking medications, and the elderly) are especially insistent on a medical evaluation before considering psychological issues. It is estimated that up to 50 percent of impotence is organic in origin, a number that is bound to increase as the mean age of the population rises. Nonetheless, the workup of impotence requires thorough investigation from both medical and psychological perspectives (see Chapter 229) and often begins with a visit to the primary physician.

NORMAL AND PATHOLOGIC PHYSIOLOGY AND CLINICAL PRESENTATIONS

A working knowledge of both normal and abnormal erectile function is essential to conducting a proper evaluation.

Normal Physiology

Erection is predominantly a hemodynamic process, mediated by neurogenic, endothelial, endocrinologic, and cortical (psychogenic) influences. It begins when blood flow increases into the large vascular corpora cavernosa, which comprise much of the penile shaft. Flow varies according to the contractile state of smooth muscle lining the corporal arterioles and sinusoids. In the flaccid state, corporal smooth muscle tone is high and there is only basal arterial flow into the penis. In addition, venous outflow is facilitated by copious arteriovenous (A-V) shunts. On sexual stimulation, the smooth muscle relaxes, arterioles dilate, and blood flows in, engorging the corporal sinusoidal spaces. This engorgement and its restriction by the band-like tunica albuginea compress the venous plexuses and A-V shunts, impairing venous outflow. The net effect is a strong erection that may approach systemic arterial pressure. Detumescence occurs when smooth muscle tone returns, blocking arterial inflow and opening venous channels.

Mediators. In the flaccid state, penile vascular smooth muscle contraction is maintained by sympathetic *alpha-adrenergic* tone, which results in *norepinephrine* release. The vasodilation of erection can be triggered by *parasympathetic* stimulation releasing *acetylcholine* and by *nonautonomic* neurotransmission believed to involve vasoactive intestinal peptide. Vascular endothelial cells contribute to relaxation by releasing *endothelium-derived relaxing factor* (EDRF), a locally active vasodilator. *Prostaglandins* produced by corporal tissue are also capable of both smooth-muscle contraction and relaxation and may play a regulatory role. Although *androgens* have a clear effect on sexual development, behavior, and libido, their influence on erectile capacity is less well defined. Erection can occur with visual stimuli, even if circulating testosterone levels fall to castration levels. However, nocturnal erections are lost.

Control Centers. Erections may be triggered by psychic (cortical) stimulation or reflexly by tactile stimulation of the genitals. In most instances, both are operable and synergistic. A host of erotic stimuli can elicit cortical and subcortical responses, which are transmitted to the medial–anterior hypothalamus, integrated, and projected down into the spinal reflex centers. There they modulate sympathetic and parasympathetic outflow to corporal smooth muscle.

There are two spinal reflex centers. The *sympathetic* one is in the *thoracolumbar* region. It controls adrenergic tone and sustains the vasoconstriction of the flaccid state. The *parasympathetic* reflex center occupies the *midsacral* region and effects vasodilation. Tactile stimulation of the genitals produces afferent impulses carried by the internal pudendal nerve, which synapses in the reflex erectile center (sacral cord segments, 2–4). From there, efferent impulses pass over the pelvic nerves (nervi erigentes) to the parasympathetic plexuses innervating the corpora cavernosa.

Pathophysiology and Clinical Presentations

Impairment of any element of the erectile apparatus or its control can lead to impotence. Included among the major organic causes are injury to the reflex centers in the spinal cord, severance of cortical input, injury to peripheral nerves, diabetes-induced autonomic and endothelial dysfunction, and medication-induced disruption of autonomic function.

Spinal Cord Injury. The location of the injury and its severity determine the degree of sexual dysfunction. Even if the cord is functionally severed, some erectile capacity is likely to be maintained if the thoracic and sacral reflex centers are left intact. Less severe injury also increases the likelihood of an erection being possible. About 60 percent of paraplegics regain penile erections 1 to 24 months after injury. The percentage of erections is higher if the injury is above T11, lower if below. Upwards of 75 percent of all persons with cord injuries will demonstrate some erectile capacity, but only 25 percent are able to engage successfully in intercourse. The erection is reflex in nature, requiring constant penile stimulation to be maintained. Erections are totally abolished when there is complete local destruction of spinal segments *S2 to S4* or their roots. Again, the higher the location of the lesion, the better the chances of a good erection.

Ejaculation is rare when the lower thoracic and upper lumbar segments (approximately to L3) of the cord are so extensively damaged that the nearby sympathetic components are destroyed. Sexual sensation is abolished with transection anywhere above the sacral level. After tactile stimulation, a paraplegic must look to confirm that reflex erection has occurred. Ejaculation can be documented only by feeling wetness with the fingers. Orgasm must be identified by feeling for perineal muscle contractions.

Herniated intervertebral disks and metastatic cancer of the vertebral column, especially between T10 and L5, which cause local swelling and destruction of spinal cord tissue, may produce a similar clinical picture.

Surgical Procedures. Impotence results from transection of autonomic fibers. In *simple prostatectomy,* whether transurethral, suprapubic, or retropubic, erectile impotence is only occasional and is a function of age, prior potency, extent of surgical dissection, and psychological expectations. However, up to 80 percent of patients undergoing simple prostatectomy, regardless of the type of procedure performed, will develop some degree of retrograde ejaculation as a result of surgical destruction of the internal sphincter mechanism at the bladder neck. The surgically destroyed or the neurologically incompetent internal sphincter allows retrograde flow of seminal fluid into the bladder, producing a dry emission. Normal ejaculation will not occur under these circumstances because the external sphincter tightens to retain urine. Simple perineal prostatectomy has a much higher incidence of impotence because of unavoidable direct dissection of parasympathetic fibers along the posterior capsule.

Open *perineal biopsy* and posterior urethral reconstruction can result in impotence; transperineal or transrectal needle biopsy of the prostate does not. *Radical prostate, bladder,* or *colorectal surgery* can produce impotence as a result of surgical damage to the pelvic autonomic nerves, notably the nervi erigentes as they course through the perirectal, retroperitoneal tissues. Improved understanding of the course of these autonomic fibers has led to revisions of surgical technique, sparing them and lowering the risk of impotence. Good results have been achieved in younger patients undergoing radical prostatectomy. After radical *retroperitoneal lymph node dissection* for testicular tumors, young men may develop ejaculatory failure as a result of bilateral resection of the paraaortic sympathetic ganglia, but rarely erectile impotence. *Bilateral sympathectomy* of lumbar ganglia at L1 will inhibit ejaculatory capacity, but not orgasmic sensation, in more than half of cases.

Diabetes Mellitus. Impotence may be the presenting symptom and is reported in up to 50 percent of men with the disease. Parasympathetically mediated smooth muscle relaxation becomes defective, although sympathetic tone remains normal. Cholinergic transmission in corporal smooth muscle declines due to decreased synthesis of acetylcholine. In addition, EDRF becomes deficient. Occlusive disease of larger vessels plays a much less important role than was previously thought, although presence of hemodynamically significant atheromatous plaques may slow the onset of erection.

Risk of impotence appears to parallel duration and severity of the diabetes. With conventional means of achieving glucose control, the majority of diabetic men experience some degree of erectile dysfunction, with fewer than 10 percent achieving restoration of normal function. Aggressive control of type I diabetes has demonstrated a marked reduction in risk of developing autonomic neuropathy. Whether initiating tight control in an already impotent diabetic will restore erectile capacity remains to be determined. The forerunner of erectile impotence in the diabetic is most often retrograde ejaculation. The presence of dry orgasm or milky postcoital urine augurs that potency may be extinguished within a year.

Other Endocrine Disease. The common denominator of most other endocrinopathies causing impotence is decreased libido and a decline in serum testosterone. *Hypogonadism,* whether a result of chromosomal, pituitary, or testicular disorders, involves nondevelopment or regression of the secondary male sex characteristics along with feeble libido and waning potency. When the cause is testicular failure, gonadotropins will be very high; when due to a pituitary or hypothalamic etiology, gonadotropins will be low. *Hyperprolactinemia* is an important source of pituitary-derived impotence. Serum testosterone levels fall as gonadotropins decline, although impotence seems more closely related to the degree of prolactin elevation. Reduction in prolactin restores erectile function. Hyperprolactinemia may be idiopathic, the result of a functioning pituitary adenoma, or a consequence of *hypothyroidism* (stimulated by high levels of thyroid-stimulating hormone [TSH]; see Chapter 100).

Addison's disease tends to lead to loss of libido and to impotence. *Cushing's syndrome,* except when due to adrenal carcinoma, impairs libido and potency after an initial period (weeks or months) of marked increase. *Acromegaly* leads to early potency impairment and premature extinction of function. Decline in function is frequently preceded by a hyperlibidinal period.

Drugs. Although it is a common observation that drugs can interfere with sexual functioning, the precise mechanisms remain incompletely understood. Drug effects are often unpredictable and may vary from patient to patient and with dosage and duration. Most are reversible by reducing or discontinuing the medication.

Antihypertensives are frequently to blame (see Chapter 26), with methyldopa, clonidine, beta-blockers, reserpine, and diuretics leading the list. Most of these are centrally acting agents, which are believed to interfere with neurotransmitter activity. Impotence has also been observed in patients taking antihypertensives with peripheral activity (eg, hydralazine, thiazides, prazocin). On theoretical grounds, one might expect peripheral vasodilators and alpha-blockers to facilitate trabecular smooth-muscle relaxation, but clinically these antihypertensives are more likely to be the cause rather than the cure. However, agents with peripheral alpha-agonist activity (eg, clonidine) can worsen impotence by increasing trabecular smooth-muscle tone. In patients with underlying vascular insufficiency, antihypertensives may contribute to impotence by lowering perfusion pressure. Ganglionic blockers may inhibit parasympathetic activity from the sacral segments of the cord or sympathetic activity from the sympathetic chain. Although most antihypertensives have been implicated, the calcium-channel blockers and angiotensin-converting enzyme inhibitors appear to interfere the least with sexual function.

Psychotropic agents may also be responsible for unpredictable forms of sexual dysfunction. The *phenothiazines* suppress central sympathetic activity. They are capable of producing such side effects as decreased libido, impaired ejaculation, erectile impotence, and retrograde ejaculation. The anticholinergic effects of *tricyclic antidepressants* may interfere with erection, although drug treatment of depression often improves sexual function (see Chapter 227). The seratonin-reuptake inhibitors *fluoxetine* and *sertraline* have also been found to impair sexual functioning. Large doses of *alcohol* can acutely depress the sexual reflexes to the point of abolishing them. Chronic alcoholism leads to nerve damage, liver failure, and high levels of circulating estrogens (see Chapter 71). *Exogenous estrogen* therapy may have a similar effect of diminishing the libido.

Drug abuse involving barbiturates, heroin, morphine, or methadone can result in major disturbances of sexual potency. Most cases are reversible. Marijuana, amyl nitrite, hashish, and lysergic acid diethylamide may heighten the perception of the sexual experience but do not specifically increase or decrease potency. Amphetamines, in moderate users, may increase libido and delay orgasm, thus prolonging the sexual act; however, impotence often occurs with chronic, heavy use. Cocaine increases sexual excitability in males and females, but side-reactions including a flight of ideas may interfere with sustained sexual performance. Episodes of painful priapism may develop in chronic abusers.

Prostatic Disease. Impotence may be the first symptom of *prostate cancer.* Advancing centrifugal growth of neoplastic tissue in the posterior lobe of the prostate may induce local swelling and destruction of the parasympathetic fibers that run along the posterolateral aspect of the prostate. *Prostatitis* may cause painful ejaculations and even hematospermia. Premature ejaculation and postcoital fatigue occur, but impotence is not characteristic. *Benign prostatic hypertrophy* does not interfere with sexual functioning.

Compulsive vesiculoprostatitis represents a chronic congestive syndrome. It occurs in the context of habitual self-inhibited masturbation, life-long limitation of sexual activities, chronic coitus interruptus with a sexually inert partner, or habitually hastened intercourse fraught with anxiety related to threatened interruptions. Onset is gradual, and it may result in progressive weakening of erectile strength, although complete erectile impotence is not a primary feature. Other symptoms of this psychosomatic syndrome may include sacroiliac ache, irritating sensations in the glans penis, urinary urgency and frequency, minor weakness of the urinary stream, overflow prostatorrhea (especially after straining), and sometimes hematospermia.

Injury to the Penis or Urethra. *Pelvic fracture,* resulting from a crash injury in which the posterior urethra is ruptured, causes impotence in 25 to 30 percent of cases. Nonperformance may result from painful intromission associated with *Peyronie's disease, balanitis,* acute *gonorrhea, herpes genitalis,* or *phimosis.* Hypospadias with a chordee of the shaft can preclude intercourse. With *priapism,* erection may be only partial and insufficient for intercourse because irreversible fibrosis of the corpus cavernosum has occurred. A large hernia or hydrocele may mechanically interfere with coitus, although potency should remain intact.

Vascular Disease. *Arterial insufficiency* is usually listed as a leading cause of impotence in older men. Unexplained, progressive slowing of erection followed by decreased rigidity can be among the first symptoms of aortoiliac vascular disease, when plaque obstructs the iliac arteries immediately distal to the aortic bifurcation. Almost 40 percent of men with stenosis and nearly 75 percent of those with occlusion develop impotence. Symptoms of claudication in association with impotence, aortic or femoral bruits, and diminished peripheral pulses describe Leriche's syndrome. In some, there is ability to initiate erection, but inability to maintain it. Patients with hypertension, cigarette smoking, diabetes, and hypercholesterolemia are at increased risk of atheromatous disease compromising penile perfusion. Radiation therapy and pelvic trauma are other risk factors for vascular injury.

Venous dysfunction can be equally important and result from age- or lipid-induced loss of the fibroelastic compressibility. Several authorities argue that venous dysfunction may be more important than previously suspected.

Psychogenic. Anxiety is a potent precipitant of impotence. The marked sympathetic outflow that accompanies anxiety increases alpha-adrenergic tone and impedes trabecular smooth-muscle relaxation. In addition, cortical influences may inhibit sacral cord reflexes that would normally trigger erection by way of parasympathetic stimulation (see Chapter 229).

Zinc Deficiency has been touted in the lay literature as a possible cause of impotence, with health food stores promoting zinc preparations. Although zinc replacement has benefited impotent dialysis patients, the frequency of such severe zinc deficiency in most other patients is probably very low. More study of the issue is needed, especially in patients taking diuretics, which may lower zinc concentrations.

DIFFERENTIAL DIAGNOSIS

In a review of 165 men with sexual dysfunction seen at the Cleveland Clinic, 51 percent were found to have functional disorders, 47 percent had organic disorders, and 2 percent had incomplete evaluations. Peak incidence of sexual dysfunction occurred between the ages of 50 and 59. Of those suffering from organic sexual dysfunction, diabetes mellitus accounted for 41.5 percent. In 16.8 percent, sexual dysfunction was due to vascular insufficiency. Those with Peyronie's disease (15.5%) could not penetrate because of marked chordee or inability to achieve sufficient erection. In 12.9 percent, hypogonadism, resulting from low levels of serum testosterone, was a factor. In 10.3 percent, impotence followed a variety of surgical procedures. Sexual dysfunction secondary to various neurologic diseases occurred in 9 percent.

The Cleveland Clinic data represent the experience of a referral practice. Reports from primary care practice reveal higher frequencies for medications and alcohol as etiologies of sexual dysfunction, but not a substantially greater prevalence of psychological disease.

The widespread use of drugs affecting the autonomic nervous system makes pharmacologic agents an epidemiologically important source of impotence and ejaculatory disturbances. Table 132–1 provides a listing of some of the more important etiologies of secondary impotence and ejaculatory disturbances.

Many patients, especially the elderly, suffer from multifactorial sexual dysfunction. Both psychological and organic factors are often present and, in many instances, more than one medical etiology is involved.

Table 132-1. Important Organic Causes of Secondary Sexual Dysfunction

	EFFECT		
CAUSE	***Decreased Libido***	***Impotence***	***Ejaculatory Failure***
Drugs			
Alcohol	+	+	+
Amphetamines		+	
Antidepressants		+	
Antihypertensive agents (methyldopa, clonidine, beta blockers, diuretics, reserpine)		+	
Barbiturates		+	
Cocaine		Priapism with chronic abuse	
Guanethidine	+		+ (Retrograde)
H_2-blockers (cimetidine)	+	+	
Methadone		+	
Phenothiazines	+	+	+
Cord Lesions			
Well above T11	Sensation abolished		+/−
Below T11	Sensation abolished	+	+
Peripheral Autonomic Neuropathy			
Diabetes		+	+ (Retrograde)
Surgical Procedure			
Simple prostatectomy (all approaches)		Occasional	+ (Retrograde)
Perineal prostatectomy		+	
Open perineal biopsy		+	
Radical prostatectomy, bladder or rectal surgery		+	
Radical retroperitoneal node dissection			+
Bilateral sympathectomy			+
Prostatic Disease			
Benign prostatic hypertrophy		No effect on function	
Cancer of the prostate		+	
Vesiculoprostatitis		+/−	
Prostatitis			Painful
Penile and Urethral Lesions			
Pelvic fractures		+	+
Hypospadias			+
Priapism			+
Phimosis, herpes, balanitis		Painful intromission	
Peyronie's disease		Painful intromission	
Hernia or hydrocele		Interferes with coitus	
Endocrine–Metabolic Disease			
Addison's disease	+	+	
Cushing's syndrome	+	+	
Hypothyroidism	+	+/−	
Acromegaly		+	
Hypogonadism	+	+	
Hyperprolactinemia		+	
Zinc deficiency (severe, in dialysis patients)		+	
Vascular Disease			
Aortoiliac insufficiency		+	
Venous disease		+	

WORKUP

Advances in the pathophysiologic understanding of impotence have yielded an array of new diagnostic methods, many of which require referral to a specialized laboratory for their proper performance. Nonetheless, history and physical examination remain integral to proper diagnosis. A careful description of what the patient means by "impotence" is the first task and best carried out by taking a detailed sexual history. It is essential to establish that erectile function is significantly compromised before going forward with an extensive workup for impotence. Once the presence of impotence is confirmed, the evaluation shifts to differentiating psychogenic from organic disease. If psychogenic disease is deemed likely, the evaluation concentrates on its underlying etiologies (see Chapter 229). If organic disease is the more probable cause, then the search begins for historical and physical findings suggestive of an underlying precipitant.

History

Differentiating Organic from Psychogenic Disease. The condition's onset, clinical course, and effect on morning erections help differentiate psychogenic from organic mechanisms. Sudden onset and preservation of erections on awakening or masturbation are characteristic features of psychogenic disease. Gradual onset and progressive loss of duration and strength of morning erections as well as those associated with masturbation and coitus suggest organic disease. These distinctions are not absolute. For example, depression may be associated with a temporary loss of morning erections, mimicking organic disease. Inquiry into libido is also important. Its appearance in the context of impotence raises the possibility of endocrinopathy as well as psychogenic disease.

Because an intact nervous system, blood supply, and sexual apparatus are necessary to achieve an erection, any occurrence of erection and ejaculation, even if rare, suggests that the problem may be emotional rather than organic. However, it is important to recognize that, in the early phases of organically determined impotence, many patients retain some erectile function and are more likely to report a decrease in number of erections, rapid detumescence after penetration, or inability to obtain a sufficiently hard erection for intercourse. Further confusing the issue, early organic disease almost always triggers performance anxiety. Finally, the absence of an erection does not rule out a psychogenic cause, but usually one is able to elicit from patients with a psychogenic etiology a story of an occasional erection (particularly on awakening from sleep).

Inquiry into Medical Etiologies. Of primary importance are checking for symptoms of diabetes (see Chapter 102), alcohol abuse (see Chapter 228), and aortoiliac disease (see Chapter 23). As noted above, unexplained, progressive slowing of erection followed by decreased rigidity may be the presenting manifestation of aortoiliac insufficiency. Atherosclerotic risk factors (hypertension, smoking, diabetes, hyperlipidemia) should be taken note of. All medications are reviewed, especially antihypertensives, major tranquilizers, antidepressants, other drugs with anticholinergic activity, and H_2-blockers with antiandrogenic effects (eg, cimetidine). Careful inquiry into substance abuse is also indicated (see Chapter 235). If libido is reduced, it is worth checking for symptoms of thyroid disease (see Chapters 103 and 104), hyperprolactinemia (see Chapter 100), hypogonadism (see Chapter 120), and adrenal disease. Past medical history is reviewed for radical prostate or pelvic surgery, pelvic irradiation, spinal cord injury, multiple sclerosis, cancer, and pelvic fracture.

Physical Examination

The vital signs are checked for postural fall in blood pressure (indicative of autonomic or adrenal insufficiency), the general appearance for loss of secondary sexual characteristics, and the skin for spider angiomata, palmar erythema, excessive dryness, hyperpigmentation, and other dermatologic signs of endocrinopathy. The neck is noted for goiter.

The flaccid penis ought to be inspected for tumor, inflammation, discharge, phimosis of the foreskin, and the hard plaques of Peyronie's disease along the dorsolateral aspect of the shaft. If possible, assessment of the erect penis should be attempted, especially if disease of the shaft is suspected, so that precise information on degree of chordee or erectile weakness can be obtained. Testicles and prostate are checked for size, masses, nodules, and tenderness. Small soft testes suggest hypogonadism. Intrascrotal pathology such as varicocele, hydrocele, or inguinal hernia may mechanically interfere with performance and can be readily detected by a careful examination (see Chapter 131).

The aorta and femoral arteries need to be palpated and auscultated for bruits and other signs of occlusive disease, especially when there is a history of claudication (see Chapter 23). Any femoral bruits are noted. The spine is checked for focal tenderness and evidence of cord compression (see Chapter 147). Neurologic assessment includes testing for pain sensation in the genital and perianal areas and a check of the bulbocavernosus reflex, which tests the integrity of 2nd, 3rd, and 4th sacral segments of the spinal cord. This reflex is achieved when the anal sphincter contracts around the examining finger on squeezing the glans. A positive response indicates that S_2, S_3, and S_4 are intact. Other aspects of neurologic function also deserve thorough testing. Evidence of a cortical, brain stem, spinal cord, or peripheral deficit may be an important clue to etiology.

Laboratory Studies

Ordering a routine battery of "impotence" tests is rarely cost-effective. Moreover, there is no single test or set of tests that "rule out" organic disease. The best approach is to tailor the laboratory workup so it matches the patient's clinical presentation.

Chemistries. A 2-hour postprandial serum *glucose* is indicated when diabetes is suspected (see Chapter 93). Hypothyroidism is best confirmed by finding the *TSH* elevated. Serum total *testosterone* and *luteinizing hormone (LH)* are indicated when reduced libido accompanies impotence. Pooled samples of each (obtained 30 to 60 minutes apart) are necessary to avoid a sampling error from the large oscillations in serum concentration that can occur every few hours.

A consistently low testosterone confirms hypogonadism. LH and *prolactin* levels help differentiate pituitary etiologies from primary gonadal failure (see Chapter 120). Abnormally high concentrations of total testosterone are seen with hyperthyroidism and represent an indication for TSH testing. If there is evidence of peripheral vascular disease, a *cholesterol* profile can help guide therapy (see Chapter 27). The usefulness of a serum *zinc* determination is yet to be proven, except perhaps in dialysis patients. The literature should be followed to see if more widespread measurement has physiologic meaning and therapeutic implications.

Study of Nocturnal Penile Tumescence. Tumescence study serves to confirm loss of erectile function in the patient who reports total absence of erections, including those normally experienced on awakening from sleep. The physiologic basis for testing at night is the observation that 80 to 95 percent of young men experience erections during rapid eye movement (REM) sleep. Although the percentage falls with age, nocturnal monitoring represents the most sensitive available means of testing for intactness of the erectile apparatus. The absence of nocturnal tumescence indicates advanced organic disease and remains the "gold standard" for organic impotence. However, in early organic disease, some erectile function and morning episodes may persist. Thus, demonstration of tumescence does not negate the need for further medical evaluation.

Formal tumescence study is very expensive and is performed overnight in a special sleep laboratory that monitors electroencephalogram (EEG) and eye movements in addition to measures of penile tumescence. The *"postage stamp test"* is a much simpler, inexpensive method of screening for nocturnal tumescence. The patient is instructed to wrap a ring of postage stamps snugly around the flaccid penis at night before going to bed, and to moisten the overlapping stamps to seal the ring. A positive test is finding breakage along the perforations on awakening in the morning. Because sleep is not monitored, a single negative test does not rule out the capacity for nocturnal tumescence. Continued failure on repeat testing is more suggestive. Other home-monitoring devices have been developed, including plastic wires that break at different tensile strengths and a tumescence-scanning device (Rigiscan) that entails wearing two rings over three nights.

Other Studies. Most other studies are the province of the specialist in male erectile dysfunction and should be ordered only on the basis of a consultation. A few are worth mentioning because of their popularity. The vascular apparatus can be assessed by *Doppler ultrasonography,* both in the flaccid state or, more meaningfully, after an *intracavernosal injection* of a vascular smooth-muscle relaxant. Color-flow technology provides excellent images. Papaverine alone or in combination with the alpha-blocker phentolamine can be used for the inracavernosal injection. Inability to achieve a full erection within 5 to 10 minutes of injection or one that is only partial or lasts less than 1 hour strongly suggests vascular disease. However, the very anxious patient with a normal vasculature may have a false-positive result.

Patients with clinical suspicion of sacral neurologic injury can be objectively tested by measuring the *sacral nerve reflex latency time*. One applies an electrical stimulus to the penile shaft and measures the time it takes for contraction of the bulbocavernosal muscles to occur. A time in excess of 35 ms is strongly suggestive of pathology in the nerves comprising the sacral reflex arc.

SYMPTOMATIC MANAGEMENT AND PATIENT EDUCATION

Psychological Support. The deeply upsetting nature of impotence necessitates an empathic, understanding, and thorough approach to the problem. Patient education is essential to help the patient comprehend and cope with the condition. Reviewing the mechanism of erection and how it is impaired can be very useful to providing a rational basis for diagnosis, prognosis, and treatment. These informational and supportive needs are no less intense for the elderly, many of whom derive considerable self-esteem from maintaining their ability to engage in intercourse. The loss can be very demoralizing.

Most patients with organic etiologies develop performance anxieties when their ability to engage in sexual intercourse becomes impaired. The onset of anxiety can result in full loss of function in a patient who is only partially compromised physiologically. In such instances, patient and partner should come in for supportive counseling, both to remove blame and inappropriately exclusive psychological attributions and to educate as to prognosis and available therapy. Fortunately, there are many options for treatment.

Change in Medication Program. Patients taking an antihypertensive medication implicated in impotence might benefit from a trial of dose reduction, or switching to an angiotensin-converting enzyme inhibitor (eg, captopril), a calcium-channel blocker (eg, nifedipine), or a relatively selective beta-blocking agent (eg, atenolol) (see Chapter 26). The patient experiencing erectile dysfunction and loss of libido with use of cimetidine can be changed to ranitidine, which is similar in efficacy, but without the antiandrogen effect. The depressed patient whose impotence is clearly related to drug therapy can be tried on a tricyclic antidepressant with lesser anticholinergic activity (eg, nortriptyline, desipramine), but switching to a seratonin-reuptake inhibitor (eg, sertraline, fluoxetine) may not help because they too can impair sexual functioning. The psychotic patient with sexual dysfunction believed linked to the medication program should be referred to the psychiatrist for adjustment of the drug regimen.

Intracavernosal Injection Therapy. The improved understanding of erectile hemodynamics and its control has fostered attempts to reproduce erections pharmacologically. Local intracavernosal injection of smooth muscle relaxants has achieved this goal in a wide variety of patients. Diabetics, patients with neurologic injury, and even some suffering from vascular insufficiency have achieved erection by intracavernosal injection of vasoactive drugs. Among the agents used are *papaverine,* which directly relaxes trabecular smooth muscle, and *phentolamine,* a short-acting, alpha-adrenergic blocker. Most regimens use either papaverine alone or in combination with phentolamine. Other agents, such as prostaglandin E_1 analogues, are under study. They appear less likely to cause scarring.

After undergoing titration of dose, patients are set up for self-administration of the therapy at home. Insulin syringes with a very fine needle (27 to 30 gauge) are used for the intracavernosal injection. Erection usually ensues within 10 minutes of injection and lasts 30 to 60 minutes. Side effects are most common during the titration period, when excessive duration of erection and hypotension occur from doses that are too large. Patients who are cardiovascularly compromised are not good candidates for this therapy. Potential complications include ischemic injury and scarring of the corporeal tissue from erections that last longer than 4 hours, and painless fibrotic nodules. The former can lead to permanent damage and must be treated promptly by intracavernosal injection of an alpha-agonist (epinephrine, phenylephrine). The latter occurs in up to 60 percent after 1 year of treatment, with some men experiencing sufficient corporeal fibrosis to distort the penile shaft.

The optimal candidate for intracavernosal injection is one with an intact vascular apparatus and the intelligence and dexterity to self-inject properly. However, even those with concurrent vascular disease may benefit, although higher doses may be required, increasing the risk of side effects and complications. Diabetics have especially benefited, because the treatment directly addresses their underlying pathophysiology.

Penile Implants and Other Mechanical Devices. Over 30,000 prostheses are implanted annually in the United States. A prosthesis is a consideration for the patient with refractory impotence who expresses a serious need to regain his capacity to engage in coitus. Of the three types of prostheses available, the simpler ones (the semirigid and adjustable malleable types) have proven the most satisfactory. They are least likely to fail and have the fewest complications associated with their implantation and use. Although they might seem the most "natural," the inflatable prostheses have much higher breakdown and complication rates, often necessitating surgical revision. Reoperation rates range as high as 44 percent. The reservoir tends to leak, and infection is a risk on the order of 1 to 10 percent.

Overall, patient and sexual partner satisfaction with prostheses are in the range of 80 to 90 percent, with little difference reported among users of the various types. Careful counseling is required before electing implant surgery. If the cause of the impotence is a poor interpersonal relationship, then a prosthesis is going to do little for the problem.

A vacuum suction device has been advocated for use, especially in the elderly. A plastic cylinder is placed over the flaccid penis and connected to a hand-operated vacuum pump. The negative pressure in the cylinder facilitates passive blood flow into the penis. A band is placed at the base of the penis to retard venous outflow, and the cylinder is removed. The device works best in patients who respond to papaverine and is an alternative to it. Pain, ecchymoses, and difficulty ejaculating are experienced by about 10 percent. Coitus is successfully achieved in about 80 percent after 3 months of use.

Vascular Surgery. Those with vascular insufficiency have yet to achieve consistently successful results from reconstructive surgery. Correction of aortoiliac disease often meets with disappointing results because of the high frequency of coexisting distal vessel disease. Microsurgical techniques have been employed for correcting vascular disease within the penis. Success rates range from 20 to 80 percent. The best results are obtained in young men with traumatic vascular injury; the worst ones are found in older men with diffuse atherosclerotic involvement of the cavernosal artery.

Hormone Therapy. Testosterone therapy should be reserved for patients with hypogonadism, manifested by a low serum testosterone level, and not used as an all-purpose sexual stimulant. It has little effect on erections in impotent patients with normal testosterone concentrations (although it may add to frustration by raising libido). When used in such patients, particularly the elderly, testosterone has a high incidence of adverse effects. Side effects include sodium retention, prostatic enlargement, gynecomastia (from peripheral conversion to estrogens), and polycythemia. Patients with concurrent adenocarcinoma of the prostate may experience a serious flare of their testosterone-responsive disease.

Treatment is given every 3 to 4 weeks by intramuscular injection of a long-acting preparation. A period of trial and error to find the optimal dose will necessitate patience on the part of both physician and patient. Oral preparations are rapidly inactivated. A transdermal delivery system is under development.

Patients with hyperprolactinemia-induced hypogonadism may not respond to testosterone replacement therapy, because of the androgen-antagonizing effect of prolactin. Consequently, treatment of the underlying hyperprolactinemia is necessary to restore potency.

Yohimbine. This drug is an alpha-blocker touted as a medical treatment of impotence. In double-blind, randomized study of the drug in patients with organic impotence, it was found worthless. However, it did prove helpful in a similarly designed study of patients with psychological erectile dysfunction, probably due to their high level of anxiety and sympathetic tone.

Treatment of Underlying Urologic Disease. At least temporary relief from the acute discomfort of prostatosis ensues from repeated prostatic massage (see Chapter 138). Selected patients with Peyronie's disease are candidates for plaque resection and replacement with a dermal skin graft. Ability to perform sexually may return after removal of a large hydrocele or repair of an inguinal hernia. Patients recovering from routine simple prostatectomy (either transurethral or suprapubic) can be reassured that potency and ability to engage in coitus are likely to return within 4 to 8 weeks after surgery.

INDICATIONS FOR REFERRAL

Patients with urologic disease should have a urologic consultation to see if they are candidates for surgical correction. Diabetics and impotent patients with otherwise refractory disease who have a relatively well-preserved penile vascular apparatus are reasonable candidates for referral for consideration of intracavernous injection therapy. Even those with a degree of vascular insufficiency may be candidates. The risks and benefits of prosthetic surgery can also be reviewed at the same time. Referral is best made to a urologist experienced in the treatment of impotence. Patients found to have symptomatic aortoiliac disease require evaluation by a vascular surgeon (see Chapter 34). Endocrinologic advice is indicated in patients with elevated prolactin levels, primary hypogonadism (low testosterone, high LH), or evidence of pituitary–hypothalamic disease (low LH concentrations). Patients suspected of harboring a cord lesion need urgent neurologic consultation.

Psychiatric referral is essential when depression, anxiety disorder, or interpersonal conflict appear to be etiologic factors in the patient's impotence. However, premature referral to a psychiatrist before an appropriate medical evaluation is complete should be avoided because it runs the risk of inappropriately labeling the condition as purely psychological and alienating the patient. Referral may also be useful when the patient with organic disease decompensates psychologically and fails to respond to supportive psychotherapy given by the primary physician (see Chapter 229).

A.H.G.

ANNOTATED BIBLIOGRAPHY

Bennett AH, Carpenter AJ. An improved vasoactive drug combination for a pharmacologic erection program (PEP). J Urol 1991;146:1564. *(Multi-drug regimens use low doses, minimizing side effects.)*

Broderick GA, Allen GA, McClure RD. Vacuum tumescence devices: The role of papaverine in the selection of patients. J Urol 1990;145:284. *(A 94 percent positive predictive value.)*

Carter JN, Tyson JE, Tolis G, et al. Prolactin-secreting tumors and hypogonadism in 22 men. N Engl J Med 1978;299:847. *(An important report on the association of hyperprolactinemia and impotence.)*

Collins WE, McKendry JBR, Silverman M, et al. Multidisciplinary survey of erectile impotence. Can Med Assoc J 1983; 128:1393. *(Causes of impotence as seen in primary care practice.)*

Diagnostic and Therapeutic Technology Assessment. Penile implants for erectile impotence. JAMA 1988;260:997. *(Detailed critique of efficacy and acceptance; 39 refs.)*

Diagnostic and Therapeutic Technology Assessment. Intracavernous pharmacotherapy for impotence: Papaverine and phentolamine. JAMA 1990;264:752. *(Found safe and effective, but long-term use of concern due to risk of penile fibrosis.)*

Fischer C, Gross J, Zuch J. Cycle of penile erection synchronous with dreaming (REM) sleep. Arch Gen Psychiatry 1965;12:29. *(The classic report describing the association between REM sleep and nocturnal erections.)*

Frosch WA. Psychogenic causes of impotence. Med Asp Human Sexual 1978;12:57. *(Differentiates psychogenic from organic causes by history.)*

Kessler WO. Nocturnal penile tumescence. Urol Clin North Am 1988;15:1. *(A discussion of available tests.)*

Krane RJ, Goldstein I, Saenz de Tejada I. Impotence. N Engl J Med 1989;321:1648. *(Excellent review; emphasis on pathophysiology; 150 refs.)*

Mahajan SK, Abbasi AA, Prasil AS, et al. Effect of oral zinc therapy on gonadal function in hemodialysis patients. Ann Intern Med 1982;63:357. *(One of the few well-documented instances of zinc therapy proving effective.)*

Marshall PG, Morales A, Philips P, et al. Nocturnal penile tumescence with stamps: A comparative study under sleep laboratory conditions. J Urol 1983;130:88. *(A reasonable screening test, but not a gold standard.)*

Morales A, Condra MS, Owen JA, et al. Is yohimbine effective in the treatment of organic impotence? Results of a controlled trial. J Urol 1987;137:1168. *(The answer is "no" for organic disease but "yes" for psychogenic disease.)*

Mulligan T, Katz PG. Erectile failure in the aged: Evaluation and treatment. J Am Geriatr Soc 1988;36:837. *(Causes examined; use of vacuum pump suggested.)*

NIH Consensus Development Panel on Impotence. JAMA 1993; 270:83. *(Addresses impact, diagnosis, treatment modalities, and education.)*

Saenz de Tejada I, Goldstein I, Asadzoi K, et al. Impaired neurogenic and endothelium-mediated relaxation of penile smooth muscle from diabetic men with impotence. N Engl J Med 1989;320:1025. *(Mechanisms of diabetic impotence delineated; provides basis for use of intracavernosal smooth-muscle relaxant.)*

Primary Care Medicine: Office Evaluation and Management of the Adult Patient, 3rd edition, edited by Allan H. Goroll, Lawrence A. May, and Albert G. Mulley, Jr. J.B. Lippincott Company, Philadelphia

133

Approach to Dysuria and Urinary Tract Infections in Women

LESLIE S.-T. FANG, M.D.

Among adult women, urinary tract infection (UTI) is the most common of all bacterial infections. Between 20 and 30 percent of women will have a UTI in their lifetime, and 40 percent of women with one infection will have a recurrence. Thus, UTIs represent a significant source of morbidity among women. For the primary physician, evaluation should be directed at the detection of any anatomic abnormalities that may predispose the patient to recurrent infections. Therapy should be aimed at the eradication of infection to minimize morbidity.

PATHOPHYSIOLOGY AND CLINICAL PRESENTATION

Current evidence suggests that most episodes of UTI in adult women are secondary to *ascending infection*. Bacteria reach the bladder through the urethra and may then ascend to the kidneys through the ureters. Hematogenous spread has rarely been implicated in the pathogenesis of UTIs.

Bacteria that commonly cause UTI are found in the periurethral area in up to 20 percent of adult women. This *colonization* of the *vaginal introitus* has been shown to be the essential first step in the production of bacteriuria and plays an important role in recurrent UTIs. Colonization with Enterobacteriaceae occurs postmenopausally and is believed to account for much of the increase in susceptibility to UTI seen in this age group. Entry of bacteria into the bladder through the relatively short female urethra can occur spontaneously. In addition, *sexual intercourse* and use of a *diaphragm* correlate with risk of infection. Significant increases in bacteriuria follow 30 percent of intercourse episodes. Use of tampons and wiping back-to-front are not risk factors for UTI.

The establishment of a bladder infection also depends on the virulence of the bacteria introduced, the number of organisms introduced, and, most important, a lapse in the normal host defense mechanisms. A number of *host defense mechanisms* normally act together to decrease the likelihood of infection. Normal voiding eliminates some organisms. Certain chemical properties of the urine are antibacterial; urine with a high urea concentration, low pH, and high osmolarity supports bacterial growth poorly. The most important host defense mechanism resides in the ability of the bladder mucosal surface to phagocytose bacteria coming into contact with it. Vaginal epithelial cell characteristics also contribute. Susceptibility to UTI correlates with increases in cellular bacterial adhesiveness. Abnormalities in these host defense mechanisms will result in recurrent and complicated UTIs. Inability to express blood-group antigens is a risk factor.

In approximately 30 percent of cases of sustained bladder infection, further extension of the infection through the ureters into the kidneys can occur. The presence of *reflux* will increase the chance of the infection ascending. Once infected urine gains access to the renal pelvis, it can enter the renal parenchyma through the ducts of Bellini at the papillary tips, and then spread outward along the collecting ducts, leading to parenchymal infection.

Clinical Syndromes

UTIs are associated with a number of clinical syndromes, ranging from acute urethral syndrome to pyelonephritis. Most are accompanied by dysuria, frequency, urgency, and suprapubic or flank discomfort. Other features distinguish one from the other.

Acute urethral syndrome (symptomatic abacteriuria) occurs in about 10 to 15 percent of women who present with symptoms suggestive of UTI. Patients in this category have fewer than 10^5 organisms per milliliter on urine culture. In addition, urinalysis is usually unimpressive, with few white cells and no bacteria. These patients divide into two groups: approximately 70 percent have some degree of pyuria (>2 to 5 white blood cells [WBC] per high-power field in a centrifuged sample) and true infection, either with bacterial counts less than 10^5 organisms or with *Chlamydia trachomatis*. Those with bacterial counts in the 10^2 to 10^4 range may have early UTI with infection not yet established in the bladder. The remaining 30 percent have no pyuria and no infection. The etiology of their dysuria is unknown. Only those without pyuria have proven to be truly abacteriuric. A subset of truly abacteriuretic women with urinary frequency report chronic pelvic pain relieved by voiding, suprapubic tenderness, and dyspareunia. They have a normal urinalysis. Cytoscopic dilation reveals submucosal hemorrhages. The term "*interstitial cystitis*" has been used to designate the condition. Etiology is unknown; the course is chronic. Tricyclic antidepressants are sometimes helpful.

Asymptomatic bacteriuria (see Chapter 126 for a discussion of this entity).

Symptomatic bacteriuria, in the form of cystitis or pyelonephritis, is the most common of the clinical syndromes. *Cystitis* has traditionally been thought to present primarily as frequency, urgency, dysuria, and bacteriuria. *Pyelonephritis,* on the other hand, is generally believed to be associated with fever, flank pain, and systemic symptoms such as nausea and vomiting. Unfortunately, numerous investigations have shown that the ability to differentiate between bladder and kidney infection on clinical grounds alone is limited. Studies using bilateral ureteral catheterization to localize directly the site of infection have demonstrated that many patients with upper tract infection present with symptoms supposedly characteristic of lower tract infection. Moreover, patients whose infection is limited to the bladder may occasionally have fever, flank pain, and systemic symptoms usually associated with pyelonephritis. Thus, the traditional clinical clues are, at best, imprecise for identifying the site of infection.

Recurrent infections may occur in some patients. Two basic patterns of recurrences are recognized: *relapse,* in which the original organism is suppressed by antimicrobial therapy and then reappears when the antibiotic is stopped; and *reinfection,* in which the original organism is eradicated by antimicrobial therapy, and the recurrence is due to the introduction of a new bacterial strain. Approximately 80 percent of recurrences are due to reinfection. Ureteral catheterization studies have demonstrated that the majority of reinfections occur in patients in whom infection is restricted to the bladder, whereas the majority of relapses occur in patients with renal parenchymal infection.

Groups frequently bothered by recurrent infections include 1) sexually active women, who report a temporal relationship of urinary symptoms to intercourse; 2) patients with compromised host defenses because of underlying systemic illness or residual urine in the bladder; 3) patients with upper tract infections; and 4) pregnant females.

The consequences of recurrent uncomplicated infections are, for the most part, minimal and rarely result in progressive renal impairment. However, patients with infections in the setting of vesicoureteral reflux, pregnancy, or diabetes are at greater risk. *Vesicoureteral reflux* is associated with residual urine in the bladder, ascending infection, chronic pyelonephritis, and high risk of renal scarring leading to focal glomerulosclerosis, proteinuria, and progressive renal failure. Patients most likely to have vesiculoureteral reflux are those who report a long history of UTIs, beginning in childhood. UTI during pregnancy has been linked by some to increased rates of fetal complications and prematurity, especially when the infection occurs within 2 weeks of delivery. The mother has an enhanced risk of pyelonephritis. Patients with diabetes show increased susceptibility to upper tract infection.

DIFFERENTIAL DIAGNOSIS

Dysuria. The differential diagnosis of dysuria includes *UTIs, vaginitis,* and *urethritis.* Patients with vaginitis may occasionally be mistaken as having UTI. Vaginal discharge, "external" discomfort (from urinary irritation of inflamed labial tissue), absence of frequency or urgency, and negative urine cultures distinguish vaginitis from UTI. *Trichomonas vaginalis* and *Candida albicans* are the most commonly responsible organisms. Women with dysuria and absence of bacterial growth on routine urine culture may have *urethritis* due to *Neisseria gonorrhea* or *herpes simplex,* although, as previously noted, most cases will be due to *Chlamydia trachomatis* (see Chapter 125). Onset is usually gradual, dysuria is mild, and vaginal discharge may be present. Pelvic pain and vaginal or cervical discharge suggest spread of infection into the cervix and fallopian tubes, a serious development (see Chapters 116 and 117).

Pyuria typically accompanies gonococcal and trichomonal etiologies, as well as chlamydial infection. Patients with acute urethral syndrome and no pyuria may have dysuria on the basis of *local trauma* or *irritation* rather than infection, as may occur in postmenopausal women secondary to desiccation of vaginal and urethral tissue.

Flank Pain. Patients with *renal calculi* or *embolic infarction* may present with flank pain and hematuria, mimicking *pyelonephritis.* Unlike in UTI, urine cultures are sterile and no bacteria are seen on Gram's stain.

WORKUP

The pace, extensiveness, and order of the evaluation are largely dictated by the patient's clinical presentation. Candidates for outpatient evaluation include dysuric patients with no evidence of systemic toxicity or obstruction.

Acutely Ill Patients

Those presenting with fever, flank pain, and systemic symptoms require prompt evaluation for the possibility of urinary tract *obstruction* with superimposed infection. Such patients should be questioned about a history of diabetes, sickle cell anemia, and excessive analgesic use; patients with these problems are at higher risk of renal papillary necrosis and subsequent obstruction by sloughed papillae. Likewise, a history of renal calculi is cause for concern in this setting. The patient with any of these risk factors who appears toxic on examination (high temperature, prostration), restless, and markedly tender in the costovertebral angle (CVA) requires immediate hospitalization and early urologic evaluation to rule out obstruction. Infection behind an obstruction constitutes a medical and urologic emergency necessitating urgent therapeutic intervention.

Dysuric Patients

History. The acutely dysuric woman ought to be questioned about vaginal discharge, external irritation on urination, or pain on intercourse, to sort out the vaginal etiologies of dysuria from those referable to the urinary tract. Also helpful is a sexual history for risk factors of chlamydial urethritis, including new sexual partners, one with a penile discharge or recent urethritis, mucoid vaginal discharge, or gradual onset of symptoms. A recent history of gonorrhea or exposure to it should also be checked.

Physical Examination. One begins with a temperature determination, followed by percussion of the CVA to test for tenderness and palpation of the suprapubic region for discomfort and distention. The pelvic examination is essential, noting any urethral discharge, vaginal erythema, discharge, or atrophy, and any cervical discharge, erosion, vesicles, or tenderness on motion.

Laboratory Studies. *Urinalysis* and *Gram's stain* of the unspun urine are essential. Proper collection of the urine specimen is essential. The *clean-voided technique* has withstood the test of time and minimizes contamination from vaginal and labial sources. The female patient is told to straddle or squat over the toilet and to spread the labia with the nondominant hand. This position is maintained throughout collection. With the other hand, the vulva is swabbed front to back with three sterile gauze pads soaked in sterile water or with a sponge soaked in a mild nonhexachlorophene soap. A small amount of urine is then passed. This is a urethral specimen and can be saved if bacterial or protozoan urethritis is suspected. More urine is voided and collected in a sterile cup. Alternatively, the patient can be told to slide the cup into a freely flowing stream to collect a true midstream specimen. The adequacy of collection can be confirmed by examining for epithelial cells; their presence indicates vulvar or urethral contamination.

With an elderly patient, the assistance of a family member or a nurse may be needed. When repeated contamination is suspected, *straight catheterization* of the bladder can be done with relatively little risk.

Examining the urine promptly minimizes artifactual findings. The finding of *pyuria* (>2–5 WBC per high-power field on examination of a spun sediment) is indicative of UTI and predictive of a response to antibiotic therapy. The absence of pyuria suggests a vaginal cause for the dysuria or a noninfectious variant of the acute urethral syndrome. The presence of one organism on high-power field examination of a Gram-stained unspun urine sample represents clinically significant bacteriuria ($>10^5$ organisms per/mL).

Culture. The traditional criterion for infection has been a colony count of $>10^5$ oranisms per milliliter; it provides for high specificity, but poor sensitivity. Studies using suprapubic aspirates find that half of dysuric women with "negative" urine cultures by the traditional criterion are truly infected, although the colony counts were in the range of 10^2 to 10^5. Colony counts of more than 10^2 obtained on clean-voided specimens from acutely dysuric women are diagnostic of true coliform infection. Many such women who previously were labeled as having symptomatic abacteriuria fall into this category. As noted earlier, the presence of pyuria identifies those who are infected and will respond to antibiotics.

The need to obtain a urine culture on every acutely dysuric woman with mild to moderate symptoms has been challenged. The vast majority of organisms that cause infection in this group are sensitive to the antibiotic regimens commonly prescribed (see below). Even when disk-sensitivity testing designates an organism as "resistant" to an antibiotic, the resistance is only relative and the organism is usually susceptible to the much higher antibiotic concentrations found in the urine. Many authorities now recommend basing the decision to treat with antibiotics and selection of agent on the results of urine sediment examination and Gram's stain, reserving urine culture for patients with a recurrence or report of several UTIs within the past year.

At the other extreme are patients who present acutely with severe symptoms and risk of urosepsis. They require not only urine sediment examination, Gram's stain, and culture, but also at least two sets of *blood cultures* before initiation of antibiotics.

When urine culture is obtained, familiarity with important urinary pathogens facilitates interpretation of culture results. The most common urinary pathogen in community-acquired UTI is *Escherichia coli.* Occasionally, the other gram-negative rods are responsible. Of the gram-positive organisms involved in UTI, enterococci, *Staphylococcus aureus,* and Group B streptococci are common isolates. Less appreciated as a urinary pathogen is *S. saprophyticus,* a coagulase-negative staphylococcus frequently found to cause UTIs in female outpatients. Diphtheroids, lactobacilli, and alpha-hemolytic strep represent contaminants.

Intravenous Pyelography and Other Urinary Tract Investigations. Recurrent infection raises the specter of a structural lesion. However, as already noted, the vast majority of recurrences are due to reinfection in the absence of upper tract disease or other pathology. Intravenous pyelography, excretory urography, and cystoscopy in women with recurrent infection are of very low yield and are not recommended. Such radiographic and urologic evaluations should be reserved for those in whom anatomic abnormalities are suspected (eg, onset of UTIs in childhood) or in whom obstruction is likely or renal insufficiency is developing. If evidence of reflux is suggested by intravenous pyelography, a voiding cystourethrogram should be done to document the degree of reflux. Urologic evaluation is indicated when urethral meatal stenosis is strongly suspected (see Chapter 134).

PRINCIPLES OF THERAPY

The intensity and duration of therapy should match the patient's clinical presentation and risk for complications. In general, patients who are sick require consideration for hospitalization and parenteral antibiotics, especially if they are metabolically or immunologically compromised or have an anatomic or functional defect of the urinary tract.

Acutely Ill Patients—Pyelonephritis, Urosepsis. Those presenting with high fever, chills, flank pain, CVA tenderness, nausea, and vomiting may have upper tract or even bloodstream infection and should be hospitalized, especially if elderly. They require fluids, thorough evaluation for treatable precipitants (see above), and prompt initiation of parenteral antibiotics. Choice of initial antibiotic program should be consistent with the findings on urine Gram's stain, although Enterobacteriaceae account for over 90 percent of cases.

Often broad-spectrum coverage is selected in this setting because of concern for *Pseudomonas* species and other multiresistant gram-negative rods. In addition, coverage for enterococci is usually included, although the pathogen is more common in men. *Ampicillin* plus *gentamicin* is the time-honored choice for serious UTI, providing effective coverage at low cost. Expensive alternatives for initial treatment include imipenem–cilastatin, ciprofloxacin, and ceftriaxone. When culture and sensitivity results become available, the regimen can be revised to provide more focused coverage. Urosepsis requires 2 to 3 weeks of intravenous antibiotics. Pyelonephritis without bloodstream invasion can be treated parenterally until fever resolves, followed by oral antibiotics for completion of a 14-day course.

Outpatient Treatment of Pyelonephritis. Otherwise healthy patients with less severe, but still acutely incapacitating symptoms often have *uncomplicated* pyelonephritis, which can be treated entirely on an outpatient basis with 10 to 14 days of oral antibiotics, provided the patient is reliable, can take fluids, and is not seriously immunocompromised or obstructed. Choice of initial therapy is based on Gram's stain findings. For infection due to gram-negative rods, *trimethoprim–sulfamethoxazole (TMS)* or a fluoroquinolone (eg, *ciprofloxacin, norfloxacin*) is a reasonable choice. Up to 30 percent of community-acquired *E. coli* are now ampicillin-resistant, rendering this antibiotic less effective for initial outpatient treatment of pyelonephritis, although the combination preparation *amoxicillin–clavulanic acid* (Augmentin) produces cure in over 90 percent of cases. TMS resistance is also becoming more common, approaching 15 percent in some areas. With increasing TMS and ampicillin resistance among community-acquired Enterobacteriaceae, fluoroquinolone therapy may emerge as the preferred selection for outpatient treatment of pyelonephritis, with amoxicillin–clavulanic acid also assuming an increasingly important role. Gram-positive cocci seen on urine Gram's stain suggest enterococci and *S. saprophyticus*, both of which are best treated with *amoxicillin.*

Reculturing 2 to 4 days after completion of therapy is essential. Failure to respond to an appropriate antibiotic program suggests an anatomic or functional abnormality and the need for radiologic evaluation and urologic consultation (see above).

Mild to Moderate Symptoms—Uncomplicated Urinary Tract Infection. Most patients with mild to moderate symptoms have cystitis and respond well to a short course of oral antibiotics. Choice of agent is again based on urine Gram's stain. For *gram-negative rod, TMS* or *amoxicillin* should suffice for most cases of lower UTI, even those due to "resistant" strains, because of the very high bladder antibiotic concentrations achieved. For patients allergic to both sulfa and penicillin, a fluoroquinolone (eg, *ciprofloxacin*) is an effective alternative. For *gram-positive cocci, amoxicillin* is the drug of choice.

Optimal duration of therapy for uncomplicated UTI has been a subject of much interest ever since it was found that *single-dose regimens* could provide nearly the same results as conventional 7- to 10-day programs, while significantly reducing cost and the risks of vaginal candidiasis, rash, diarrhea, poor compliance, and emergence of resistant organisms. Single-dose amoxicillin (3 g orally) and TMS (two double-strength tablets) have been used successfully, with the better results reported for TMS. Ciprofloxacin (1 g) is also effective. The oral cephalosporins—cephaloridine, cefadroxil, and cefaclor—have been disappointing. A *3-day course* of antibiotics achieves a slightly higher rate of cure than does a 1-day program, yet it retains most of the advantages of single-dose therapy. Suboptimal candidates for short-course therapy include those with diabetes, a history of relapses, more than three UTIs in the past year, and immunocompromise. Such patients are best treated with a more conventional course of antibiotics (up to 2 weeks).

Failure to Respond. Failure to respond to short-course therapy has proven to be a reliable clinical criterion for upper tract disease, correlating well with results of formal localization tests. Patients may report no relief of symptoms or a relapse within days of treatment. Such patients are likely to have subclinical uncomplicated pyelonephritis and should be treated accordingly (see above).

Acute Urethral Syndrome. Patients *with pyuria,* no bacteria on Gram's stain, and no clinical evidence for chlamydial-gonococcal, or other venereal forms of urethritis can be treated with *single-dose antibiotic therapy* in the same manner as any patient with lower tract infection. Alternatively, they can be treated with *TMS* (one single-strength tablet bid for 10 days) or *doxycycline* (100 mg bid for 10 days). Doxycycline is effective against *Chlamydia* and gonococci as well as most common urinary pathogens (see Chapters 125 and 137). Recurrences are common in patients with acute urethral syndrome.

Patients *without pyuria* do not respond to antibiotics. *Symptomatic therapy* with fluids and urinary analgesics such as phenazopyridine (Pyridium) is usually prescribed.

Recurrent Infections. Patients bothered by frequent symptomatic recurrences are potential candidates for prophylactic measures. Recurrent infection should be confirmed at least once by repeat culture. The clinical setting helps determine the appropriate approach to therapy. As noted earlier, recurrences in *sexually active women* are most often reinfections. Prophylaxis at the time of intercourse with *single-tablet* therapy has proven effective in minimizing their frequency and severity. In reliable patients with fewer than three UTIs per year, a patient-initiated *1- or 3-day course* of standard antibiotic therapy for uncomplicated UTI at the first sign of symptomatic infection has proven effective. In *postmenopausal* women, a course of topical *vaginal estrogens* can prevent recurrent infection, presumably by returning the vaginal flora to its premenopausal composition of few Enterobacteriaceae. *Very elderly patients* with bladder distention, postvoid residual urine and recurrent reinfection, *continuous prophylaxis* with nightly TMS (one-half single-strength tablet qhs) usually suffices and works better than regimens using sulfisoxazole or Mandelamine and ascorbic acid. Once prophylaxis is stopped, there is no residual benefit. In patients with defined anatomic abnormalities, such as significant reflux or nephrolithiasis, surgical correction to decrease the severity and frequency of recurrences requires consideration.

Treatment of the Pregnant Patient. Treatment of symptomatic UTI in pregnancy is recommended because of an increased risk of upper tract infection in the mother and potential injury to the fetus (low birth weight, prematurity). Antibiotics proven safe for use in pregnancy include ampi-

Table 133-1. Antibiotic Regimens for Urinary Tract Infections in Women

CLINICAL SITUATION	REGIMEN
Acutely ill and toxic patient	Hospitalization; parenteral antibiotics; ampicillin plus gentamicin if urosepsis suspected; otherwise, ciprofloxacin if Gram's stain shows GNR; ampicillin if it shows GPC
Uncomplicated pyelonephritis	Oral TMS (double-strength) bid for 2 weeks or ciprofloxacin 500 mg bid for 2 weeks
Uncomplicated lower UTI	Single-dose TMS (2 double-strength tablets), ciprofloxacin (1 g) or amoxicillin (3 g) if Gram's stain shows GNR; amoxicillin if it shows GPC; 3-day course if more symptomatic using TMS (1 double-strength tablet) bid, ciprofloxacin 500 mg bid, amoxicillin 500 mg tid; 7- to 10-day course if diabetes, recurrent UTI, age >65
Relapse	Same drug as for uncomplicated UTI, but continued for at least 2 weeks
Acute urethral syndrome with pyuria	TMS as for uncomplicated UTI, or doxycycline 100 mg bid for 10 days if chlamydia suspected
Acute urethral syndrome without pyuria	No antibiotics
Recurrent infection	
Sexually active	Prophylaxis with nocturnal single-tablet dose of ampicillin, TMS, or ciprofloxacin
Elderly patient with large postvoid residual	Prophylaxis with nightly dose of TMS (half of a single-strength tablet) or ciprofloxacin (250 mg)
Pregnancy	Ampicillin, amoxicillin, and oral cephalosporins have proved safe; nitrofurantoin safe for the fetus, but potentially toxic for the mother; fluoroquinolones should be avoided

TMS = trimethorpim–sulfamethoxazole; GNR = gram-negative rod; GPC = gram-positive cocci; UTI = urinary tract infection.

cillin, amoxicillin, and oral cephalosporins. The combination preparation amoxicillin–clavulanic acid (Augmentin) is recommended for use against organisms demonstrating resistance to multiple drugs. Nitrofurantoin has also been used without evidence of fetal toxicity; however, its associated risk of inducing peripheral neuropathy, pulmonary fibrosis, and hepatic injury in adults makes it a less preferable choice. The fluoroquinolones should be avoided by pregnant patients.

Treatment of Asymptomatic Bacteriuria in the Elderly. Because there is no increased risk of urosepsis, renal failure, or mortality, there is no urgent need for antibiotics. Risk of asymptomatic infection is increased, but benefit of treatment is unclear. Antibiotics are indicated if there is obstruction or the patient is to undergo a genitourinary procedure.

THERAPEUTIC RECOMMENDATIONS

Table 133–1 summarizes therapeutic recommendations for UTIs.

INDICATIONS FOR REFERRAL OR ADMISSION

Hospitalization is indicated in patients with severe symptoms such as rigors, high fever, flank pain, nausea, and vomiting. Patients with suspected obstruction and those unable to maintain oral intake also require hospitalization. Referral to a urologist is indicated if a surgically correctable anatomic abnormality is detected or suspected.

PATIENT EDUCATION

Certain general measures are important in minimizing the possibility of recurrent infection. The patients should be instructed about increasing fluid intake during symptomatic periods and maintaining urine flow around the clock. Patients with UTIs temporally related to sexual intercourse would probably benefit from voiding after intercourse. The importance of antibiotic regimen compliance and follow-up for repeat urinalysis and culture must be impressed on patients with serious infections and relapses.

ANNOTATED BIBLIOGRAPHY

American College of Physicians. Common uses of intravenous pyelography in adults. Ann Intern Med 1989;111:83. *(A position paper recommending against routine use in women with UTI.)*

Boscid JA, Abrutyn E, Kaye D. Asymptomatic bacteriuria in elderly persons: treat or not to treat? Ann Intern Med 1987; 106:764. *(In most instances, no treatment is needed.)*

Dolan JG, Bordley DR, Polito R. Initial management of serious urinary tract infection: Epidemiologic guidelines. J Gen Intern Med 1989;4:190. *(A retrospective study; TMS was effective for young women; older women had a higher likelihood of a TMS-resistant organism; men required pseudomonal coverage.)*

Fang LST, Tolkoff-Rubin NE, Rubin RH. Efficacy of single-dose and conventional amoxicillin therapy in urinary tract infection localized by the antibody-coated bacteria technic. N Engl J Med 1978;298:413. *(Efficacy of single-dose therapy for lower UTI demonstrated.)*

Fowler JE, Pulaski ET. Excretory urography, cystography and cystoscopy in the evaluation of women with urinary tract infection. N Engl J Med 1981;304:462. *(Very low yield, even in women with two or more recent UTIs.)*

Komaroff AL. Diagnostic decision: Urinalysis and urine culture in women with dysuria. Ann Intern Med 1986;104:212. *(Urinalysis: most reliable indicator of treatable infection; urine culture: limited value except in cases of suspected upper tract infection.)*

Komaroff AL. Acute dysuria in women. N Engl J Med 1984; 310:368. *(A review; emphasizes the importance of pyuria as a sign of UTI and predictor of response to therapy; good discussion of the acute urethral syndrome; 106 refs.)*

Kunin CM. Duration of treatment of urinary tract infection. Am J Med 1981;71:849. *(Emphasizes matching duration of treatment with the natural history and consequences of the infection.)*

Kunin CM, White LV, Hua TH. A reassessment of the importance of "low-count" bacteriuria in young women with acute urinary symptoms. Ann Intern Med 1993;119:454. *(Likely to represent an early phase of UTI.)*

Latham RH, Running K, Stamm WE. Urinary tract infections in young adult women caused by *Staphylococcus saprophyticus*. JAMA 1983;250:3063. (S. saprophyticus *was the second most common cause of UTIs, accounting for 11 percent.)*

Mushin AI, Thornbury JR. Intravenous pyelography: The case against its routine use. Ann Intern Med 1989;111:58. *(Little justification for its routine use found in women with UTI.)*

National Institutes of Arthritis, Diabetes, Digestive, and Kidney Diseases. Workshop on Interstitial Cystitis. J Urol 1988; 140:203. *(A brief summary of this often overlooked condition.)*

Norrby SR. Short-term treatment of uncomplicated urinary tract infections in women. Rev Infect Dis 1990;12:458. *(A meta-analysis suggesting that 3-day regimens are generally more effective than 1-day programs.)*

Pinson AG, Philbriack JT, Lindbeck GH, et al. Oral antibiotic therapy for acute pyelonephritis: A methodologic review of the literature. J Gen Intern Med 1992;7:544. *(Critical look at available studies.)*

Raz R, Stamm WE. A controlled trial of intravaginal estriol in postmenopausal women with recurrent urinary tract infections. N Engl J Med 1993;329:753. *(Prevents recurrent UTI.)*

Safrin S, Siegel D, Black D. Pyelonephritis in adult women: Inpatient versus outpatient therapy. Am J Med 1988;85:793. *(Results are comparable; cost is greatly reduced by outpatient management.)*

Stamm WE, Counts GW, Running KR, et al. Diagnosis of coliform infection in acutely dysuric women. N Engl J Med 1982;307:463. *(10^5 organisms per milliliter is too insensitive a criterion for infection in this setting.)*

Stamm WE, Counts GW, Wagner KF, et al. Antimicrobial prophylaxis of recurrent urinary tract infections. Ann Intern Med 1980;92:770. *(All regimens proved effective and well-tolerated; no emergence of resistant strains.)*

Stamm WE, Hooton TM. Management of urinary tract infections in adults. N Engl J Med 1993;329:1328. *(Terse review of the major clinical questions; 60 refs.)*

Stamm WE, McKevitt M, Counts GW. Acute renal infection in women: Treatment with trimethoprim-sulfamethoxazole or ampicillin for two or six weeks. Ann Intern Med 1987;106:341. *(Treatment for 2 week sufficed; TMS was better.)*

Stamm WE, McKevitt M, Counts GW. Is antimicrobial prophylaxis of urinary tract infections cost effective? Ann Intern Med 1981;94:251. *(Prophylaxis became cost-effective when women had three infections per year.)*

Stamm WE, Wagner KF, Cimsel R, et al. Causes of the acute urethral syndrome in women. N Engl J Med 1980;303:409. *(Patients with pyuria had infection with coliforms,* S. saprophyticus, *or* C. trachomatis; *those without pyuria had no organism isolated.)*

Strom BL, Collins M, West SL, et al. Sexual activity, contraceptive use, and other risk factors for symptomatic and asymptomatic bacteriuria. Ann Intern Med 1987;107:816. *(Intercourse, diaphragm use, and past history of UTI were the only independent risk factors, but not tampon use or wiping improperly.)*

Wong ES, McKevsitt M, Running K, et al. Management of recurrent urinary tract infections with patient-administered single-dose therapy. Ann Intern Med 1985;102:302. *(A safe, effective, convenient, and inexpensive approach.)*

Primary Care Medicine: Office Evaluation and Management of the Adult Patient, 3rd edition, edited by Allan H. Goroll, Lawrence A. May, and Albert G. Mulley, Jr. J.B. Lippincott Company, Philadelphia

134
Approach to Incontinence and Other Forms of Lower Urinary Tract Dysfunction

JOHN D. GOODSON, M.D.

Patients with lower urinary tract dysfunction may present with incontinence, hesitancy, dribbling, loss of stream volume or force, frequency, or urgency. Such complaints are particularly prevalent among the elderly and a common problem in primary care practice. An efficient and parsimonious evaluation strategy is essential, given the large number of possible etiologies and available studies.

Incontinence can have a major impact on one's life and family. At the least, it is an embarrassment and inconvenience. Constant incontinence can predispose to local skin breakdown, serious infection, and social isolation. The primary physician must be attuned to the nature of the problem and the needs of the patient and family to design and implement an effective treatment program. Substantial progress has been made in the management of incontinence, and one should be familiar with available treatment strategies and their indications.

PATHOPHYSIOLOGY AND CLINICAL PRESENTATION

The detrusor muscle of the bladder is normally under simultaneous sympathetic and parasympathetic control. During the *filling* phase, *sympathetic* tone predominates whereas parasympathetic tone is inhibited. The internal bladder sphincter tightens under alpha-adrenergic influence, and the detrusor relaxes under beta-adrenergic influence. During *voluntary emptying, parasympathetic* stimulation produces detrusor contraction; at the same time sympathetic tone decreases, the external sphincter of the pelvic floor relaxes, and abdominal muscles tighten. Normally the urethra is oriented to the bladder so as to facilitate continence. With the initiation of *voluntary voiding,* the urethrovesicular angle changes so as to permit full drainage. Complete bladder emptying depends on unimpeded flow.

The process of voiding usually begins with a sensation of bladder fullness mediated by proprioceptive fibers in the detrusor. A reflex arc between the detrusor and the brain stem initiates and amplifies bladder contraction by parasympathetic stimulation. This arc is under cortical inhibition. Voiding occurs with the release of inhibition and voluntary relaxation of the pelvic external sphincter.

Incontinence. The pathophysiology and clinical presentations of incontinence can be divided on clinical and mechanistic grounds into categories of detrusor instability, sphincter or pelvic incompetence (stress incontinence), reflex incontinence, overflow incontinence, and functional incontinence. Clinically, two or more processes frequently coexist to varying degrees in the same patient.

Detrusor instability is characterized by reduced bladder capacity resulting from excessive and inappropriate detrusor contraction. For many, the condition appears to arise as a concomitant of *aging,* although the mechanism is unclear. In some, it seems to be the result of *decreased cortical inhibition* of detrusor contraction. Loss of cortical input can ensue from such conditions as cerebral infarction, Alzheimer's disease, brain tumor, and Parkinson's disease. For others, the detrusor overactivity is linked to *bladder irritation* from such causes as trigonitis (a common accompaniment of cystitis), chronic interstitial cystitis, postradiation fibrosis, and detrusor hypertrophy from outflow tract obstruction. Patients note a few moments of warning, frequent episodes of urgency, moderate to large volumes, and nocturnal wetting. In roughly half of patients, detrusor instability is associated with poor detrusor function. For these patients, voiding is frequent and incomplete.

Sphincter or pelvic incompetence (stress incontinence) is usually a consequence of *pelvic floor laxity* and the most common cause of urinary incontinence in women. Less frequently, it develops from *partial denervation* that reduces sphincter tone. Pelvic laxity is seen as a concomitant of normal aging and after difficult or multiple vaginal deliveries or direct perineal injury. In some cases, a cystocele forms and further impedes control. Estrogen deficiency in females reduces the competency of the internal sphincter and can also cause urethral symptoms (dysuria and frequency). In men, pelvic incompetence may result from prostatic surgery, although in most the abnormality resolves within 6 months if innervation remains largely intact. Patients complain of incontinence, which occurs predominantly at times of straining (coughing, laughing, sneezing, lifting). There is loss of small to moderate volumes of urine, very infrequent nighttime leakage, and little postvoid residual.

Reflex incontinence derives mostly from *spinal cord damage* above the sacral level. Interference with sensation and coordination of detrusor and sphincter activity due to inhibited or absent central control leads to detrusor spasticity and functional outlet obstruction. The patient is unable to sense the need to void. Spinal cord injury is the most common cause. Diabetes, multiple sclerosis, tabes dorsalis, and intrinsic or extrinsic cord compression from tumor or disk herniation are also important etiologies. Reflex incontinence takes place day and night with equal frequency and without warning or precipitating stress. Volumes are moderate, and voiding is frequent. Voluntary sphincter control and perineal sensation are reduced; sacral reflexes remain intact.

Detrusor hypotonia (overflow incontinence) results from either long-standing *outlet obstruction, detrusor insufficiency,* or *impaired sensation.* The bladder becomes hypotonic, flaccid, and distended. Voiding consists primarily of overflow spillage. In outflow tract obstruction (most often from long-standing prostatic hypertrophy), the detrusor is constantly overstretched and gradually becomes incapable of generating sufficient pressure to ensure bladder emptying. Retrograde flow of urine and increased ureteral pressures can compromise renal function if the condition is left uncorrected. Often, detrusor insufficiency is a consequence of lower motor neuron damage, as occurs with injury to the sacral cord or development of peripheral neuropathy. Importantly, numerous medications (eg, anticholinergics, antidepressants) can reduce detrusor tone. Distinguishing clinical characteristics include a palpably distended bladder and a large postvoid residual. Patients void frequently, especially after fluid loads and diuretics. A history of incomplete emptying, slow or interrupted flow, hesitancy, and need to strain are reported. Injury either to peripheral nerves (as in diabetes or vitamin B_{12} deficiency) or to the spinal cord may be accompanied by losses of perineal sensation and sacral reflexes.

Functional incontinence refers to situations in which physical or mental disability makes it impossible to void independently, even though the urinary tract may be intact. Patients with disabling illness or simply an acute change to a bedridden state may be unable to maintain sufficient control over lower urinary function to avoid incontinence. Sedating drugs in such situations may only exacerbate the problem. Patients who are aware of their condition will describe their unsuccessful attempts to maintain continence. Patients with frontal lobe dysfunction due to cortical degenerative disease or normopressure hydrocephalus may be unaware of their own voiding and, therefore, functionally incontinent. Rarely, a severely disturbed patient is deliberately incontinent.

Urinary Frequency in Conjunction with Dysuria. Frequency accompanied by dysuria is a common presentation of lower *urinary tract infection.* Inflammation of the bladder trigone and urethra are responsible for most acute symptoms. Chronic interstitial cystitis, acute urethral syndrome, and prostatosis have been implicated as causes in cases without identifiable infection, although some of these may be due to inapparent infection with *Chlamydia* (see Chapters 125, 133, 136, and 139). *Carcinoma* of the bladder trigone or urethra is a rare but important cause of dysuria, frequency, and symptoms of outflow tract obstruction.

Urinary Frequency in Conjunction with Difficulty Voiding. When associated with slow stream, hesitancy, and a sense of incomplete emptying, frequency is likely to be a manifestation of *outflow tract obstruction* (extrinsic or intrinsic). At first, the patient may notice only minor slowness of stream. If the obstruction persists, bladder instability may ensue causing frequent voiding of small volumes, followed later by chronic distention and overflow incontinence (see above). Strictures, tumor (especially prostatic enlargement), and occasionally stones are responsible for most cases of obstruction. In the setting of severe constipation, the rectal vault can become sufficiently impacted that it actually blocks the urethra and prevents bladder emptying. *Alpha-adrenergic agents* and *beta-blockers* can increase sphincter tone and impair voiding acutely, especially when used in patients with preexisting lower urinary tract dysfunction. *Drugs with anticholinergic effects* may interfere with bladder contraction.

Urinary Frequency and Polydipsia. When frequency presents in association with increased thirst, it suggests a diabetic condition leading to increased urine volume and the resultant polyuria. *Diabetes mellitus* is distinguished by significant glycosuria (see Chapter 102). *Neurogenic (idiopathic central) diabetes insipidus* is manifested by sudden onset, craving for huge volumes of cold water, and prodigious urine outputs (5 to 10 L/d). Inability to concentrate the urine after overnight fluid deprivation and response to parenteral antidiuretic hormone (ADH), with formation of a concentrated urine, characterize the condition. Patients with *nephrogenic diabetes insipidus* differ from those with the neurogenic variety in that their kidneys do not respond to intrinsic or parenteral ADH. Hypercalcemia, lithium therapy, and pregnancy are precipitants of the acquired variety. Patients with *psychogenic polydipsia* may be hard to distinguish from those with nephrogenic diabetes insipidus because they have washed out their renal concentrating system and also do not adequately respond to parenteral ADH. They do respond normally to fluid deprivation, a diagnostically useful finding, although some patients with neurogenic disease respond in a similar fashion (see Chapter 101).

Isolated Urinary Frequency may be a manifestation of reduced bladder capacity, as well as a presentation of mild diabetes mellitus, mild diabetes insipidus, a minor urinary tract infection, or bladder irritation. A large *extrinsic* or *intrinsic mass* impinging on the bladder can reduce its capacity and produce more frequent urination, usually of small volumes, distinguishing it from other forms of polyuria. Pelvic surgery, chronic interstitial cystitis, or irradiation can have a similar effect by reducing bladder capacity. Patients who surreptitiously abuse *diuretics* rarely complain of frequency, but those who take them for therapeutic purposes are often bothered by the side-effect.

DIFFERENTIAL DIAGNOSIS

The differential diagnosis of incontinence can be classified according to clinical presentation and mechanism (Table 134–1). The differential diagnosis of dysuria and frequency

Table 134-1. Important Causes of Incontinence

TYPE	MECHANISM	CHARACTERISTICS
Detrusor Instability	Unstable detrusor	Warning; frequent episodes; nocturnal wetting; small postvoid residual; intact reflexes; normal sensation
Bladder infection		
Chronic cystitis		
CNS disease (dementia, stroke)		
Detrusor hyperreflexia		
Detrusor hypertrophy		
Irradiation		
Stress Incontinence	Inadequate sphincter	Upon straining; small to moderate volumes; rarely at night; small postvoid volume
Aging		
Autonomic neuropathy		
Estrogen deficiency		
Pelvic laxity		
Perineal injury		
Urologic surgery		
Reflex Incontinence	Upper neurologic tract disease (autonomous bladder) Spinal cord injury Severe cortical disease	No warning or precipitants; severe neurologic disease; episodes can occur day and night; frequent; moderate volumes; loss of control and sensation; reflexes intact
Disk herniation		
Multiple sclerosis		
Spinal cord disease		
Tumor		
Overflow Incontinence	Bladder outlet obstruction, lower motor neuron injury, or impaired sensation; toxic impairment of detrusor contraction	Distended bladder; history of obstructive symptoms; frequent loss of small volumes; loss of reflexes and sensation if due to neurologic injury; large postvoid residual
Diabetes		
Medications		
Outflow obstruction		
Peripheral neuropathy		
Sacral cord lesion		
Tabes dorsalis		
Vitamin B_{12} deficiency		
Functional Incontinence	Inability to reach toilet in time	Functionally impaired patient
Acute illness		
Medications		
Psychiatric disease		

is that of urinary tract infection and its related syndromes (see Chapters 133 and 140). Most of those with difficulty voiding are men with prostatic enlargement (see Chapter 138). Among other causes of difficulty voiding are drugs (anticholinergics, beta-blockers, sedatives), urethral stricture, congenital valves, stone, tumor, pelvic abscess, and fecal impaction. Causes of urinary frequency in the absence of other urinary tract symptoms include diabetes mellitus, diabetes insipidus, psychogenic polydipsia, diuretics, and bladder compression.

WORKUP

The evaluation of incontinence and other lower urinary tract symptoms requires assessment of the major neuromuscular and anatomic elements involved in maintaining urinary continence and flow. Much can be gleaned from the history and physical examination, which provide important clues to the underlying pathophysiology and precipitants.

History. For the assessment of incontinence, one cannot overemphasize the importance of a detailed history, with emphasis on the circumstances, precipitants, timing, frequency, and volume of urine loss, the presence of warning symptoms, and intactness of perineal and bladder sensation. When the history is sketchy, asking the patient or family to keep a *diary* of events and contributing factors can be of considerable help.

Several clinical pictures are indicative of mechanism. Incontinence triggered only by *straining* indicates stress incontinence, although an occasional patient with overflow incontinence will report leakage under similar circumstances. Patients with overflow differ in that they also experience frequent loss of *small volumes* without warning or straining and are bothered by nocturnal episodes. A history of long-standing obstructive symptoms suggests an etiology for the overflow physiology.

In contrast to those with overflow disease, patients who suffer from frequent episodes of *urgency,* lose small amounts of urine, yet retain perineal sensation are likely to be suffering from detrusor instability. Although they may have a few moments of warning, they too report nocturnal incontinence. When this is accompanied by dysuria, a search for urinary tract infection is indicated (see Chapters 133 and 140). Frequent small voidings and urgency are also consistent with a small bladder from extrinsic compression.

Reflex incontinence is suggested by a history of spinal cord injury, diabetes, multiple sclerosis, or dementia with neurologic deficits. Severe loss of cortical function is also a precipitant of detrusor instability. The patient who reports marked distress at wetting in bed because of an inability to get to the toilet is likely to have a functional etiology, especially if there is a history of recent physical disability and confinement to bed.

Regardless of history and type of underlying pathology, the patient and family should be carefully questioned about *medications,* especially those with anticholinergic, alpha-adrenergic, beta-blocking, or tranquilizing effects (eg, tricyclic antidepressants, major and minor tranquilizers, decongestants, and antihypertensives).

Patients with isolated urinary frequency need to be asked about *increased thirst,* a feature consistent with diabetes mellitus and diabetes insipidus. Compulsive water drinkers with psychogenic polydipsia may deny their intake of water but do not report nocturia, a feature of both diabetes mellitus and diabetes insipidus. Sudden onset of intense thirst for ice-cold water is very suggestive of diabetes insipidus. Also important is inquiry into use of diuretics. Any excessive use of coffee, tea, or alcohol should be noted.

Those with symptoms of slow stream and hesitancy are likely to have outflow obstruction and should be checked for prostatism, stricture, stone, tumor, and fecal impaction.

Physical Examination. For the patient with incontinence, the examination begins by noting general appearance and any lack of attention to personal hygiene. A careful urogenital examination is essential and includes palpating and percussing the bladder suprapubically after voiding for distention and masses; one also checks the *rectum* for impaction and *prostatic enlargement.* Absence of palpable prostatic enlargement does not rule out obstruction, especially in a patient with obstructive symptoms; median lobe encroachment on the urethra is often not palpable. Moreover, the degree of prostatic enlargement does not correlate with severity of obstruction.

The woman with stress incontinence should be placed in the lithotomy position and her *pelvic motion* and continence should be noted during cough or Valsalva's maneuver. Testing for stress incontinence is best done with the bladder full, unless the problem is severe and requires little provocation. The *vaginal mucosa* is noted for presence of atrophic changes (red, thin mucosa with a watery discharge) indicative of inadequate estrogenization. A *bimanual examination* completes the evaluation, with note taken of any uterine or adnexal masses.

Neurologic control of voiding needs to be assessed to determine if there are any deficits above, within, or distal to the autonomic reflex arc. Checking the *bulbocavernosus reflex* tests the integrity of the arc. Normally squeezing the clitoris or glans penis will cause anal sphincter contraction. Lack of response suggests interruption. Another means of testing the arc is to note *anal sphincter tone.* Because control of the anal sphincter is similar to that of the bladder, the examiner can indirectly estimate its competence by checking the anal tone on rectal examination and by noting the patient's ability to contract the sphincter voluntarily. Loss of sphincter tone in a patient who retains sensation suggests a motor neuron lesion within the arc.

Perineal sensation is also tested; if it is lacking, yet sacral reflexes are preserved, reflex incontinence from a lesion above the arc is suggested, such as one due to diabetes, multiple sclerosis, or spinal cord injury. Patients with loss of both sensation and reflexes are likely to have overflow incontinence because of neurologic injury to the reflex arc. Incontinent patients who retain their reflexes and sensation suffer from detrusor instability, stress incontinence, overflow incontinence, or a functional problem.

A mental status examination is usually not necessary to detect underlying dementia in the patient with incontinence; in most cases the condition is apparent by the time incontinence occurs.

Laboratory Studies. Often a careful history and examination are sufficient to arrive at a working diagnosis of the patient with lower urinary tract symptomatology. A *urinalysis* and a few simple chemistry studies (*BUN, creatinine, and glucose*) are appropriate for most patients. Patients with overflow incontinence require a *serologic test for syphilis.* If dysuria or frequency is a problem, a clean-voided urine specimen ought to be sent for *culture.* Patients with evidence suggestive of outflow tract obstruction should have an *intravenous pyelogram* to identify the site of blockade. The test allows an estimate of postvoid residual and identifies any detrusor hypertrophy, bladder diverticula, or intravesicular prostate enlargement, useful signs of significant bladder outflow tract obstruction. *Pelvic ultrasonography* offers a noninvasive method of assessing postvoid residual and prostate size. *Straight catheterization* after voiding is a simple office technique for determining residual volume, a useful measure when overflow incontinence is in question. A volume over 50 mL is abnormal. The *voiding cystourethrogram* is indicated when urethral obstruction is suspected and ordered to document and localize the site and nature of the blockade.

The *cystometrogram* (CMG) is helpful in determining the functional characteristics of suspected neurogenic abnormalities. Normal individuals sense bladder filling between 100 and 200 mL, have a nonurgent desire to void at 250 to 350 mL, and experience detrusor contraction at 400 to 550 mL. A spastic bladder will demonstrate a small capacity and recurrent uninhibited contraction (Fig. 134–1, line *B*). An atonic bladder will show a large volume and little contractile force (see line *C*).

Measurement of *urine flow rates* provides information on outflow obstruction and aids in monitoring for progression. The normal curve (Fig. 134–2, line *A*) shows an early peak flow rate, whereas the curve of the obstructed bladder manifests a delayed and reduced flow rate (see Fig. 134–2, line *B*).

Patients with polyuria should be checked for glycosuria, hypercalcemia, and hypokalemia. Those with normal levels need a test of urine-concentrating ability by measuring *urine osmolality* after 8 hours of *fluid restriction* (usually over-

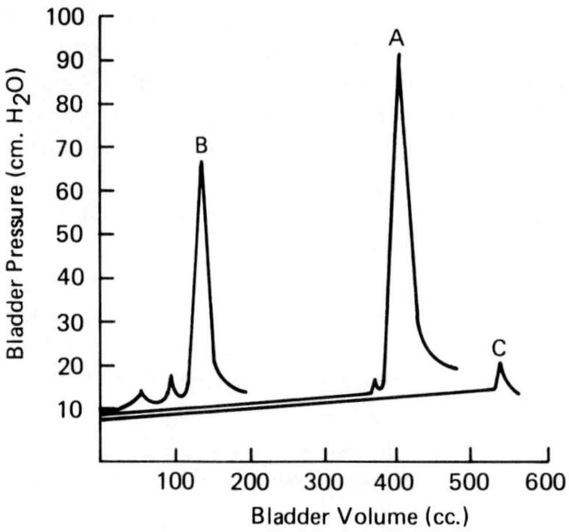

Figure 134-1. Cystometrogram findings. **(A)** Normal pressure–volume relationship; **(B)** the uninhibited neurogenic bladder; **(C)** the atonic bladder.

night). Normal persons and those with psychogenic polydipsia should be able to concentrate their urines to over 700 mOsm/L after 8 hours of fluid restriction. Inability to concentrate requires further testing that includes measurement of serum osmolality before and after water restriction and parenteral administration of ADH. Direct measurement of ADH may be helpful (see Chapter 101).

More sophisticated urodynamic testing is useful in the unusual case when the exact mechanism of detrusor, reflex, or sphincter dysfunction needs to be clarified.

MANAGEMENT OF INCONTINENCE

Management is best guided by the mechanism(s) responsible for the patient's incontinence, the patient's overall medical and mental status, and the capabilities of the family or caretakers. However, some general measures apply to all incontinent patients:

- Restrict fluid loads, coffee, tea, and alcohol.
- Limit the use of diuretics, and, if necessary, give them in the morning.
- Use of anticholinergic drugs for nonurologic purposes should be done with care and in the lowest possible dosages.
- Avoid use of indwelling catheters because of the risk of infection, exacerbation of detrusor instability, and leakage around its periphery.
- Avoid use of condom catheter, except for short, well-supervised periods.
- Advise use of an adsorbent pad for patients with refractory symptoms and recommend that it be changed frequently to prevent skin maceration.
- If long-term indwelling catheterization is unavoidable, the catheter should be inserted only by trained personnel under aseptic conditions, drained with bag always below patient's bladder, manipulated as little as possible, irrigated only if flow is reduced, changed if blocked, and removed if upper tract infection is suspected. Antibiotic prophylaxis is not recommended.

Detrusor Instability. Before initiating symptomatic therapy, one should attend to treatable etiologic factors, such as outflow obstruction or chronic bladder irritation. In most instances, the cause cannot be identified or it is not amenable to definitive treatment, making symptomatic relief the major objective. Much can be done.

- Teach the patient to void at regular, frequent intervals. Over time, the intervals can be increased.
- Provide a bedside commode or urinal for the elderly patient who may not be able to make it to the bathroom in time.

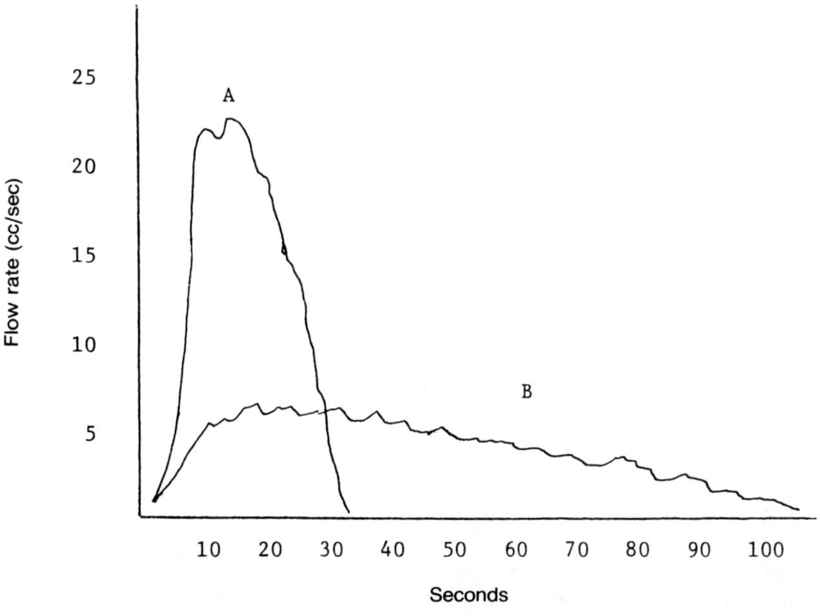

Figure 134-2. Urinary flow studies. **(A)** Normal voiding. **(B)** Obstructed voiding. The area under each curve represents the volume voided.

- Initiate a trial of a tricyclic agent such as imipramine (10 to 100 mg/d in divided doses) or an agent with both smooth-muscle relaxant and anticholinergic properties such as oxybutynin (2.5 to 5 mg tid). Lower doses can be effective in the elderly without inducing untoward central nervous system side-effects.
- A calcium-channel blocker such as nifedipine (10 mg tid) may also help and is better tolerated in the patient with coexistent coronary artery disease or hypertension. The choice of agent is determined in part by the patient's other medical problems (Table 134–2).

Detrusor Atony (Overflow Incontinence). The first priority is to treat definitively any mechanical obstruction or reversible neurologic deficit (eg, herniated disk, vitamin B_{12} deficiency), followed by efforts to reduce the postvoid residual and prevent infection. If there is a fixed obstruction, it must be removed before other therapy can proceed.

- Once the obstruction has been relieved, place an indwelling catheter or repeatedly catheterize the patient to decompress the bladder.
- If this does not restore bladder function, then teach the patient to void while performing a Credé's maneuver (suprapubic external compression) or Valsalva's maneuver.
- Add the alpha-blocker prazosin (2 to 20 mg/d in divided doses) or terazocin (1 to 2 mg/d) to reduce sphincter resistance.
- Add bethanechol (25 to 125 mg/d in divided doses) to augment bladder contraction.
- Monitor the effects of these agents by checking postvoid residuals; patients with a residual in excess of 300 mL require repeat catheterizations on an intermittent basis.
- Treat obstructed patients who cannot undergo surgery with a trial of prazosin as above.
- Initiate antibiotic prophylaxis (see Chapters 126 and 133) in patients with a significant (>100 mL) and persistent postvoid residual.

Sphincter Incompetence (Stress Incontinence) responds well to a number of simple measures, beginning with exercises to strengthen the perineal muscles that terminate the urinary stream. For postmenopausal women, estrogen cream

Table 134-2. Drugs Used to Treat Incontinence

DRUGS	DOSAGE RANGE	ACTION	SIDE-EFFECTS	POSSIBLE CONTRAINDICATIONS
Detrusor Instability				
Imipramine hydrochloride (Tofranil)	10–25 mg qd to qid	Decreases detrusor and increases internal sphincter tone	Dry mouth, blurred vision, constipation, postural hypotension, palpitations	Anatomic obstruction, cardiac arrhythmias, hyperthyroidism, glaucoma, hepatic or renal disease, pregnancy
Oxybutynin chloride (Ditropan)	2.5–5 mg qd to qid	Decrease detrusor tone	Same	Same
Detrusor Atony				
Bethanechol chloride (Urecholine)	5–25 mg bid to qid	Increases detrusor tone	Salivation, flushing, abdominal cramps, diarrhea, sweating	Anatomic obstruction, asthma, ganglionic blocker therapy (guanethidine) peptic ulcer, hyperthyroidism, age
Prazosin (Minipress)	1–5 mg bid to qid	Decreases internal sphincter tone	Lightheadedness	Postural hypotension
Terasozin (Hytrin)	1–2 mg qd	Decreases internal sphincter tone	Same	Same
Sphincter Incompetency				
Imipramine hydrochloride (Tofranil)	10–25 mg qd to qid	Decreases detrusor and increases internal sphincter tone	See above	See above
Estrogen cream (in women) (Premarin)	qd initially then biw, tiw	Increases internal sphincter tone	Uterine cancer, possibly breast cancer, hypertension, cholelithiasis, glucose intolerance, thromboembolic disease	Uterine or breast malignancy, uterine fibroid tumors
Phenylpropanolamine	25 mg qd to qid	Increases internal sphincter tone	Abdominal distress, insomnia, palpitations, nervousness	Hypertension, hyperthyroidism, glaucoma
Reflex Incontinence				
Prazosin	1–5 mg bid to qid	Decreases internal sphincter tone	See above	See above
Terasozin (Hytrin)	1–2 mg qd	Decreases internal sphincter tone	See above	See above

can also help. Surgical approaches are reserved for patients with persistently incapacitating difficulty. Purified bovine dermal *collagen* injected into suburethral tissue may provide a nonsurgical alternative.

- Instruct the male patient to exercise by voluntarily contracting the anal sphincter slowly 15 times once or twice a day.
- Instruct the female patient in the Kegel exercises.
- Advise a trial of vaginal tampon use in female patients; be sure the tampon is changed at least daily.
- If there is evidence of atrophic vaginitis, prescribe a topical estrogen cream (see Table 134–2). Apply it daily for the first 3 weeks and then once or twice weekly thereafter to maintain sufficient estrogenization to restore internal sphincter tone in postmenopausal women. Continuous use is discouraged in women with intact uteri due to increased risk of uterine cancer. This risk can be eliminated with the concurrent use of a progestin (see Chapter 118).
- Prescribe the alpha-adrenergic agonist phenylpropanolamine (50 to 100 mg/d in divided doses) for patients who need more than exercises. The agent is especially useful in the presence of weakened pelvic muscles and after surgical instrumentation of the urethra. It can be found in most over-the-counter cold remedies.
- Try a course of imipramine (10 to 100 mg/d in divided doses) for those with symptoms of both bladder irritability and stress incontinence.
- Use of Teflon injection is worth consideration in postmenopausal women who fail other therapies and in men with incontinence following prostatectomy.
- A penile clamp may be necessary in men who do not respond to other measures.

Reflex Incontinence. A major problem is a dyssynergy between bladder contraction and sphincter relaxation resulting in ureteral reflux and the potential for hydronephrosis. The bladder needs to be decompressed. An alpha-adrenergic blocking agent or mechanical maneuvers may help. For frequent urination, the mechanical measures and behavioral techniques are similar to those for detrusor instability.

- If there is bladder–sphincter dyssynergy, try pharmacologically decompressing the bladder by giving prazosin (2 to 20 mg/d in divided doses) or terazocin (1 to 2 mg/d).
- Consider an agent used for detrusor instability (see above). A sphincterotomy may be required to ensure bladder emptying.

Functional Incontinence. The prime effort is to ease the patient's access to a urinal, bed pan, or commode. Bedside placement is the obvious solution. For more disabled patients, regular use of absorbent diapers, frequent straight catheterization, or rarely condom or indwelling catheterization can be considered.

PATIENT EDUCATION

Incontinence is hard for both patient and family. The primary care physician must ensure that all understand the problem and its cause so that no one blames the patient for being incontinent. The need to provide palliative relief early in the course of the evaluation makes it important to teach symptomatic measures even before the workup is completed. Use of adult diapers, pads, and scheduled voiding times, plus elimination of xanthine-containing beverages and alcohol, and rescheduling of medication intake can do much to lessen symptoms and the stress on patient, family, and caretakers. If a penile clamp is used, teaching of proper skin care is essential to prevent breakdown. If chronic or intermittent Foley or condom catheterization is needed, a strict protocol for usage must be developed.

INDICATIONS FOR REFERRAL

The incontinent patient with a suspected cord lesion or other form of neurologic injury should be promptly referred for neurologic consultation. Urologic referral is needed in cases of outflow tract obstruction, especially those severe enough to cause a hypotonic bladder and a large postvoid residual (over 100 mL). The risk of ureteral reflux and development of hydronephrosis makes definitive therapy essential. Women with refractory stress incontinence are candidates for reconstructive surgical efforts; referral should be made to a surgeon experienced with correcting pelvic incompetence. Those with stubborn detrusor instability or hypotonia are potential candidates for some of the newer biofeedback therapies. Patients with severe sphincter dyssynergy and reflex incontinence may need a sphincterotomy if all else fails.

ANNOTATED BIBLIOGRAPHY

Brechtelsbauer DA. Care with an indwelling catheter. Postgrad Med 1992;92:127. *(Addresses the key issues of catheter use in a terse, well referenced review.)*

Burgio KL, Whitehead WE, Engel BT. Urinary incontinence in the elderly. Bladder-sphincter biofeedback and toilet training skills. Ann Intern Med 1985;104:507. *(A report of encouraging results using behavioral methods.)*

Fantl JA, Wyman JF, McClish DK, et al. Efficacy of bladder training in older women with urinary incontinence. JAMA 1991; 265:609. *(Reduced incontinent episodes by 57 percent in those with sphincter or detrusor instability.)*

Haber PA. Urinary incontinence. Ann Intern Med 1986;104:429. *(An editorial on the importance of incontinence in general internal medicine practice.)*

Hu T-W, Igou JF, Kaltreider L, et al. A clinical trial of a behavioral therapy to reduce urinary incontinence in nursing homes. JAMA 1989;261:2656. *(Behavioral methods can be very helpful.)*

Khanna OP. Disorders of micturition. Urology 1976;8:316. *(Excellent review of bladder neuropharmacology and various treatment modalities.)*

Messing EM, Stamey TA. Interstitial cystitis. Urology 1978; 12:381. *(The diagnosis should be considered in women with persistent lower urinary tract symptoms, negative cultures, and negative workup.)*

Miller-Catchpole R. Use of Teflon preparations for urinary incontinence and vesicoureteral reflux. JAMA 1993;269:2975. *(An assessment of this new technology; 44 refs.)*

National Institutes of Health Consensus Conference. Urinary incontinence in adults. JAMA 1989;261:2685. *(The conclusions of an expert panel.)*

Ouslander JG. Urinary incontinence: Out of the closet. JAMA 1989;261:2695. *(Editorial comments on the NIH consensus statement.)*

Ouslander J, Leach G, Staskin D, et al. Prospective evaluation of an assessment strategy for geriatric urinary incontinence. J Am Geriatr Soc 1989;37:715. *(A simple and inexpensive approach is tested.)*

Resnick NM, Valla SV, Laurino E. The pathophysiology of urinary incontinence among institutionalized elderly persons. N Engl J Med 1989;320:1. *(Sixty-one percent had detrusor overactivity; 50 percent had impaired contractility.)*

Resnick NM, Valla SV. Management of urinary incontinence in the elderly. N Engl J Med 1985;313:800. *(Terse, clinically useful review; 71 refs.)*

Stern P, Valtin H. Verney was right, but ... N Engl J Med 1981;305:1581. *(An editorial on the approach to workup of diabetes insipidus; underscores the pitfalls and problems.)*

135
Approach to the Patient With Nephrolithiasis

LESLIE S.-T. FANG, M.D., Ph.D.

Primary Care Medicine: Office Evaluation and Management of the Adult Patient, 3rd edition, edited by Allan H. Goroll, Lawrence A. May, and Albert G. Mulley, Jr. J.B. Lippincott Company, Philadelphia

Nephrolithiasis is a significant medical problem incurring substantial morbidity and cost. One autopsy series estimated the prevalence as 1.12 percent. In most industrialized countries, 1 percent to 3 percent of the population may be expected to have a calculus at some time and the likelihood that a white male will develop stone disease by age 70 is about 1 in 8. The annual frequency of hospitalization for nephrolithiasis is estimated at one per 1000 population. The recurrence rate without treatment for calcium oxalate renal stones is about 10 percent at 1 year, 33 percent at 5 years, and 50 percent at 10 years. In the outpatient setting, the primary physician may encounter patients with a history of renal calculi, asymptomatic nephrolithiasis, or acute colic. Others may present with hematuria or urinary tract infection. One needs to identify the nature of the stone and any precipitating factors, prevent further stone formation, and know when referral for surgical intervention or lithotripsy is needed.

PATHOPHYSIOLOGY AND CLINICAL PRESENTZTION

Two major groups of factors are important in the pathogenesis of stones: 1) changes that increase the urinary concentration of stone constituents; and 2) physicochemical changes.

Increase in concentration can occur with reductions in urinary volume or increases in excretion of concentration in calcium, oxalate, uric acid, cystine, or xanthine.

Calcium-Containing Stones. The majority of calcium-containing stones contain calcium oxalate; hypercalciuric and hyperoxaluric states promote their formation. In some instances, hyperuricemia also contributes to calcium stone formation.

Hypercalciuric states can be categorized into three groups: increased gut absorption of dietary calcium, increased resorption of calcium from bone, and the presence of a renal calcium leak. Combinations of these factors can be at play in certain clinical settings. About 50 percent of patients with calcium stones are found to be hypercalciuric.

Hyperoxaluria is less common than is hypercalciuria, but recent studies indicate that up to 30 percent of patients with calcium oxalate stones are hyperoxaluric. Hyperoxaluria may result from increased absorption of dietary oxalate, as occurs in patients with small bowel disease; from increased endogenous production of oxalate, as occurs in patients with genetic deficiency in enzymes in the glyoxalate pathway or of pyridoxine (an important cofactor in glyoxalate metabolism); or, rarely, from markedly increased ingestion of oxalate or one or its precursors.

Some patients with calcium-containing stones may be hyperuricosuric. It is believed that glutamic acid would adsorb onto a uric acid nidus and allow for growth of calcium oxalate crystals.

Magnesium Ammonium Phosphate Stones (Struvite). Struvite formation occurs in an alkaline environment and is almost invariably associated with urinary tract infection produced by a urea-splitting organism.

Uric Acid Stones. Most patients with uric acid stones have persistently acid urine, which would result in decreased solubility of uric acid. Some patients may be hyperuricosuric. Hyperuricosuric states are seen in patients with high dietary intake of protein, with primary and secondary gout. In patients with myeloproliferative disorders and during chemotherapy, significant hyperuricosuria can occur, and uric acid stones can form if adequate urine flow and alkalinization are not maintained.

Cystine Stones. Cystine stones are found exclusively in patients with cystinuria. These patients have an inherited disorder in which renal and gastrointestinal transport of cystine, ornithine, lysine, and arginine is abnormal.

Xanthine Stones. These occur in the setting of xanthinuria, an extremely rare genetic disorder of purine metabolism associated with a deficiency of xanthine oxidase. Rarely, xanthine stones may be seen in patients taking xanthine oxidase inhibitors for treatment of uric acid disorders.

Physicochemical factors that have been identified as important in stone formation include changes in *urinary pH* and urinary concentrations of potential inhibitors of stone formation, such as magnesium, citrate, sulfate, organic matrix, and pyrophosphate. As noted earlier, alkaline pH facilitates struvite formation, and acidic pH facilitates formation of uric acid and xanthine stones.

High urinary concentrations of magnesium, citrate, pyrophosphate, and certain anions are potent inhibitors of stone formation. Deficiencies in one or more of the inhibitors have been identified in some patients with recurrent stones.

Three major theories have been advanced to explain stone formation and growth. The *matrix-nucleation* theory suggests that some matrix substances (eg, uric acid) form an initial nucleus for subsequent stone growth by precipitation. The *precipitation–crystallization* theory suggests that when the urinary crystalloids are present in a supersaturated state, precipitation and subsequent growth occur. The *inhibitor-absence* theory postulates that the deficiency of one or more of numerous agents known to retard stone formation leads to nephrolithiasis. Evidence for and against each of these theories has been advanced; multiple factors may be involved in any patient.

Clinical presentation is one of pain, bleeding, or silent obstruction. *Renal "colic"* is typically a constant unilateral pain, abrupt in onset, localized to the flank when a stone sits in the upper tract, and radiating into the groin when one lodges in the lower portion of the ureter. The presentation may be mistaken for pyelonephritis and occasionally for abdominal and pelvic processes, but the initial workup should rapidly lead to the correct diagnosis.

Any *obstruction* that occurs is usually transient and of no lasting significance; however, in some instances, it persists and may be silent and progressive. Occasionally, asymptomatic calcareous calculi are detected on abdominal x-rays taken for other reasons. Calculi extending from one renal calix to another (staghorn calculi) can result in significant renal parenchymal damage, particularly in association with infection.

The *natural history* of stone formation is still a matter of some controversy. The likelihood of *recurrence* of calcium stones with time was examined prospectively in one study of patients who formed single stones. An exceedingly high incidence of recurrence was found, with a mean time to recurrence of 6.78 years. With time, the incidence of cumulative recurrence approached 100 percent. Recurrence took place early in half of the patients, but could take up to 20 years in others.

Other studies have found a more benign course. In one, a group of 101 patients was followed for an extended period (mean 7 years); additional stone formation was observed in only a third of the patients. These differences in recurrence rates undoubtedly reflect heterogeneity among patients in the respective referral groups. In any case, the incidence of recurrence is high enough to justify evaluation and consideration of preventive treatment.

Most kidney stones pass spontaneously; however, 10 percent to 30 percent do not and may cause continuing pain, infection, or obstruction.

Table 135-1. Types of Renal Calculi

Calcium oxalate	58.8%
Calcium phosphate	8.9%
Mixed calcium oxalate and phosphate	11.4%
Uric acid	10.1%
Struvite (magnesium ammonium phosphate)	9.3%
Cystine	0.7%
Miscellaneous	0.8%

DIFFERENTIAL DIAGNOSIS

In the United States, about two-thirds of all renal calculi are composed of either calcium oxalate or calcium oxalate mixed with calcium phosphate (Table 135–1). Stones of pure uric acid account for about 10 percent. Struvite or magnesium ammonium phosphate stones occur almost exclusively in patients with urinary tract infections resulting from urea-splitting organisms, and constitute about 9 percent of all stones analyzed. Other stones occur infrequently and are composed of cystine, xanthine, and salicates.

The disease states associated with nephrolithiasis are best categorized according to the type of stones formed. In many instances, stone formation is a manifestation of a systemic disease (Table 135–2).

Table 135-2. Important Conditions Associated with Nephrolithiasis

Calcium Stones

Increased gastrointestinal calcium absorption
- Primary hyperparathyroidism
- Sarcoidosis
- Vitamin D excess
- Milk-alkali syndrome
- Idiopathic nephrolithiasis

Increased bone calcium resorption
- Primary hyperparathyroidism
- Neoplastic disorders
- Immobilization
- Distal renal tubular acidosis

Renal calcium leak
- Idiopathic hypercalciuria

Hyperoxaluria
- Small bowel disease
- Enzymatic deficiency
- Pyridoxine deficiency
- Increased ingestion

Magnesium Ammonium Phosphate Stones

Alkaline environment
- Urinary tract infection due to urea-splitting organism

Uric Acid Stones

Increased uric acid production
- Primary gout
- Secondary gout (myeloproliferative disorder, chemotherapy)

Cystine Stones

Inherited disorder of amino acid transport

Xanthine Stones

Xanthine oxidase deficiency

Use of xanthine oxidase inhibitor

WORKUP

In the evaluation of the patient with recurrent nephrolithiasis, knowledge of the stone composition is essential to rational management. Obtaining the stone for analysis is the single most important study; therefore, urine should be strained for stones when renal colic is present. Ideally, studies of the stone should include the use of quantitative chemical analyses in addition to crystallographic examination.

History. When there is no stone available for analysis, certain aspects of the clinical history can be helpful in the evaluation. The *age* of the patient at onset of nephrolithiasis should be obtained because metabolic disorders such as hyperoxaluria, cystinuria, xanthinuria, and renal tubular acidosis are often associated with stones at an early age; idiopathic calcareous nephrolithiasis and primary hyperparathyroidism commonly after age 30. The *sex* of the patient can also be helpful; idiopathic nephrolithiasis is common in males, whereas primary hyperparathyroidism is more common in females. A *past history* of stones is invaluable if their composition has been previously determined. Any prior history of systemic illness (eg, sarcoidosis or cancer) and any prior urinary tract infection should be noted. *Family history* of nephrolithiasis may suggest a hereditary metabolic disorder. Careful *dietary history* should also be taken to rule out excessive protein, oxalate, or calcium intake. It is important to check for the use of *drugs* that would promote stone formation. Medications that result in an increase in risk factors for stone formation include vitamin A, C, and D, loop diuretics, acetazolamide, ammonium chloride, calcium-containing medications, alkali, and antacids. These medications may increase the urinary concentrations of calcium as in the case of vitamin D, loop diuretics, calcium-containing medications, and ammonium chloride, or they may alter urinary pH (acetazolamide, ammonium chloride, and alkali) and may decrease urinary concentrations of inhibitors (ammonium chloride, absorbable antacids, and alkali can decrease urinary citrate concentration).

Physical examination is not particularly revealing in most cases but should be checked for evidence of a systemic disease, such as sarcoidosis (lymphadenopathy, organomegaly) or cancer (adenopathy, breast mass, and so forth).

Laboratory evaluation should include *urinalysis* for determination of pH and an examination of urinary sediment for crystals. An alkaline pH suggests infection with urea-splitting organisms and struvite formation. *Urine culture* is needed. Inability to acidify the urine pH below 5.3 despite systemic acidosis suggests renal tubular acidosis. Serum should be obtained for determination of calcium, uric acid, BUN, and creatinine, and a *24-hour urine* should be collected for creatinine, calcium, uric acid, and oxalate.

Repeated determinations of *fasting serum calcium and phosphorus* are necessary if primary hyperparathyroidism is suspected. Serum albumin should be determined at the same time, because 40 percent to 45 percent of the serum calcium is protein-bound. If the serum calcium is elevated and hyperparathyroidism is suspected clinically, confirmation of the diagnosis can be made by obtaining a simultaneous *parathyroid hormone* (PTH) determination, which should reveal an inappropriately elevated level (see Chapter 96). If the clinical presentation suggests a rare cause of nephrolithiasis, such as cystinuria or xanthinuria, special 24-hour collections of urine should be sent for study.

Roentgenographic evaluation includes a plain film of the *kidneys, ureter, and bladder (KUB),* and an *intravenous pyelogram (IVP).* The flat-plate radiograph of the abdomen can provide an estimate of renal size and is important in detecting the presence of small radiopaque stones. Staghorn calculi usually denote magnesium ammonium phosphate or cystine stones. The latter usually have a more laminated appearance. *IVP* provides better details of any renal abnormalities that may be present, as well as the level of the obstruction caused by the renal calculus. *Renal ultrasound* examination is useful for detecting hydronephrosis but is not a substitute for the IVP in the initial workup of urolithiasis.

The laboratory evaluation permits identification of stones and hyperexcretory states and therefore allows rational therapy.

PRINCIPLES OF MANAGEMENT

Because of the high incidence of stone formation and its attendant morbidity, preventive therapy is indicated in all patients with nephrolithiasis.

In general, maintenance of dilute urine by means of *vigorous fluid therapy* around the clock is beneficial in *all forms of nephrolithiasis.* A number of studies have indicated that the relative probability of forming a kidney stone decreases with urinary volume. Enough fluid to maintain an output of 2 to 3 L of urine needs to be taken daily. In general, 250 mL of fluid should be taken every 4 hours, and 250 mL of fluid should be taken with meals. Specific therapy should be tailored to the type of stones involved.

Calcium-Containing Stones. Over the past decade, considerable amount of information has become available to suggest that dietary manipulation would be helpful in the management of calcium-containing stones. Increasing evidence has accumulated to indicate that *restriction of dietary protein* is helpful in preventing formation of calcium-containing stones. Population studies indicate a clear correlation between increased dietary protein and increased incidence of stone formation. Protein loading in patients would result in increase in urinary excretion of both calcium and uric acid. High dietary protein also decreases urinary concentrations of inhibitors such as citrate. These metabolic abnormalities are corrected with restriction of dietary protein. *Sodium intake* should also be restricted. Restriction of dietary sodium predictably would result in decrease in urinary calcium excretion. Oxalate is a metabolic end-product of glycine, and the bulk of the urinary oxalate is derived from metabolic pathways. However, in some patients, dietary excesses of oxalate can result in hyperoxaluria. These patients would benefit from dietary *oxalate restriction.* Considerable amount of caution has been raised about severe *calcium restriction:* severe calcium restriction would result in increased intestinal absorption of oxalate, resulting in hyperoxaluria; severe calcium restriction would also lead to mobilization of calcium from the bone because of negative calcium balance. Most investigators now advocate *modest dietary calcium restriction*. For a patient with calcium-containing stones, a reasonable diet would contain 100 mEq of sodium, 1 g per kilogram of body weight of protein, and 1000 to 1500 mg of calcium per day. The patient would be encouraged to avoid excessive oxalate intake and would be asked to drink enough fluid to maintain 2 to 3 L of urine output each day.

In the majority of cases, these dietary manipulations would be adequate to prevent further stone formation. In one series where first-time stone formers were placed on such a dietary program, there was only 27 percent recurrence of stones during a 5-year follow-up.

In patients with recurrent stone formation despite dietary therapy, every effort should be made to rule out underlying systemic conditions (see Table 135–2) before initiation of *drug therapy*. Patients with underlying primary hyperparathyroidism should be treated surgically when feasible. Drugs that can promote calcium stone formation should be stopped. Patients with sarcoidosis may benefit from steroid therapy.

Patients with *hypercalciuria* should have modest limitation of dietary calcium. *Thiazides* decrease urinary calcium excretion, and hydrochlorothiazide, 50 mg given once a day, has been found to be effective. Primary hyperparathyroidism has to be ruled out before the use of thiazides to avoid hypercalcemia.

Patients with *hyperoxaluria* should have dietary oxalates limited. Tea, rhubarb, and many leafy green vegetables should be avoided. Dietary calcium, on the other hand, should not be severely restricted, because severe calcium restriction has been shown to cause increases in urinary excretion of oxalate. In the rare patient with pyridoxine deficiency, replacement would improve the hyperoxaluric state.

Patients with *hyperuricosuria* would benefit from protein restriction and *allopurinol*. Reduction of urinary uric acid concentration would minimize the likelihood of calcium oxalate crystal growth around acid adsorbed to uric acid. Two randomized trials have shown that stone recurrence rates are lower with allopurinol treatment.

Studies in those patients with *no identifiable metabolic disorder* have demonstrated drastic reduction in new stone formation when given a *thiazide* and *allopurinol*. In one study, 30 such patients formed six stones, compared with a predicted 31.8 stones, during a 1- to 7-year follow-up period.

In addition to the therapeutic interventions outlined, several other less well-evaluated modes of therapy have been advocated. Administration of *magnesium oxide* may improve the solubility of urinary oxalate. In patients with documented hypocitraturia, *potassium citrate* may be useful in inhibition of new stone formation. These forms of therapy have not been evaluated with rigorous controlled trials.

Magnesium Ammonium Phosphate Stones. These are often very large and may have to be removed surgically. Acidification of the urine with ascorbic acid, along with a prolonged course (often, at least 2 months) of appropriate *antibiotic treatment* to eradicate any *Proteus* urinary tract infection, is essential for the prevention of recurrences of struvite.

Uric Acid Stones. *Hydration* to maintain copious urine flow, *allopurinol* therapy, and *alkalinization* of the urine are the mainstays of therapy. The solubility of uric acid is a hundred times higher at pH 7 than at pH 4.5, and every attempt should be made to maintain alkaline urine by given 100 mEq to 150 mEq of *sodium bicarbonate* every 24 hours in divided doses. In patients with myeloproliferative disorders undergoing chemotherapy, prophylactic uses of allopurinol, saline diuresis, and alkalinization should eliminate the incidence of uric acid stone formation.

Cystine Stones. Copious urine flow and maintenance of urinary pH above 7.5 are important in preventing and dissolving cystine stones. D-*Penicillamine* has also been shown to be effective, but significant side-effects may be encountered.

Xanthine Stones. Limitation of dietary purines, maintenance of urine flow, and maintenance of very high urine pH (greater than 7.6) minimize difficulties. Prophylactic alkalinization and forced diuresis should be employed in patients with myeloproliferative disorders on xanthine oxidase inhibitors.

INDICATIONS FOR ADMISSIONS AND REFERRAL

In a patient with renal colic, the needs for hospitalization and other interventions are dictated by the clinical presentation. Patients with mild to moderate pain can be managed as outpatients with oral analgesics and instructed to maintain a high fluid intake and urine output around the clock. These patients should be told to strain the urine to retrieve calculi for stone analysis.

Patients with severe pain, nausea, and vomiting need hospitalization for intravenous hydration and pain control. In these patients, KUB and IVP are indicated to localize and determine the extent of the obstruction. In the majority of cases, stones will pass spontaneously. Patients with severe symptoms and persistent obstruction beyond 3 to 4 days should be referred for urologic evaluation.

Patients presenting with fever, chills, and symptoms of renal colic require hospitalization and prompt intervention. If the presence of an infection behind an obstructed ureter is indeed confirmed, antibiotic coverage (see Chapter 133) and surgical decompression are mandatory.

Surgical intervention for nephrolithiasis has changed dramatically with the introduction of a number of new techniques: *lithotripsy* and *ureteroscopic interventions* have largely obviated the need for lithotomy in the majority of patients. In lithotripsy, the stone is shattered by subjecting it to focused ultrasonic shock waves, delivered either percutaneously through a nephrostomy or extracorporeally. *Extracorporeal shock wave lithotripsy* is an excellent choice for fragmentation and removal of simple stones in the kidneys and upper ureters. Its very low complication rate and high degree of efficacy are rapidly eliminating the need for surgical lithotomy in the centers where the lithotriptor is available. Because the equipment to perform the procedure is expensive and not widely available, *percutaneous ultrasonic lithotripsy* represents an acceptable alternative and may be the preferred initial therapy for upper tract stones lodged in the ureter for more than 4 to 6 weeks. The procedure is also indicated for larger (>2.5 cm) stones. In stones that have lodged in the ureters, *ureteroscopic* approaches have allowed for basketing of stones without having to resort to open lithotomy.

The expense and operator skill required for these technologies will limit their availability to regional centers. Patients with documented stones, especially those located in the upper tracts and kidney, causing continuous pain, infection, or obstruction, should be referred to such centers for intervention.

PATIENT EDUCATION

Meticulous care must be taken in giving dietary instructions. Instructions should also be given to help patients divide their fluid evenly to maintain a dilute urine at all times. As noted previously, a fluid intake of 2 to 3 L/d is needed to help minimize stone formation. Because there is some evidence that soft drinks acidified solely with phosphoric acid and may contribute to stone recurrence, patients might be advised to avoid them. However, most soft drinks also contain citric acid, and the combination appears to have no effect on stone recurrence. Patients who need to alkalinize their urine ought to be instructed in how to measure urinary pH with litmus test tapes. Long periods of immobilization should be avoided, and appropriate fluid intake should be prescribed if such situations are anticipated.

ANNOTATED BIBLIOGRAPHY

Goldfarb S. The role of diet in the pathogenesis and therapy of nephrolithiasis. Endocrinol Metab Clin North Am 1990;19:805. *(An excellent review of the various aspects of diet that are important to consider in the patient with nephrolithiasis including: fluid intake, protein intake, calcium and oxalate intake, and sodium intake.)*

Lingeman JE, Woods J, Toth PD, et al. The role of lithotripsy and its side effects. J Urol 1989;141:793. *(Critical examination of the technology.)*

Menon M, Koul H. Clinical review: Calcium oxalate nephrolithiasis. J Clin Endocrinol Metab 1993;74:703. *(An excellent review of the pathogenesis of calcium oxalate stones and the management options.)*

Riese RJ, Sakhaee K. Uric acid nephrolithiasis: Pathogenesis and treatment. J Urol 1992;148:765. *(A review of pathogenesis of uric acid stones and an examination of various treatment options, including allopurinol and potassium citrate therapy.)*

Shuster J, Jenkins A, Logan C, et al. Soft drink consumption and urinary stone recurrence: A randomized prevention trial. J Clin Epidemiol 1992;45:911. *(Reduction in soft drink consumption reduced risk of stone recurrence.)*

Smith LH. The pathophysiology and medical treatment of urolithiasis. Semin Nephrol 1990;10:31. *(Review of the pathogenesis of stone formation, concentrating on the medical treatment of stone disease.)*

Wilson DM. Clinical and laboratory evaluation of renal stone patients. Endocrinol Metab Clin North Am 1990;19:773. *(An in-depth review of the available tools for evaluation of the patient with renal stone.)*

136
Approach to the Male Patient With Urethritis

JOHN D. GOODSON, M.D.

Primary Care Medicine: Office Evaluation and Management of the Adult Patient, 3rd edition, edited by Allan H. Goroll, Lawrence A. May, and Albert G. Mulley, Jr. J.B. Lippincott Company, Philadelphia

A penile discharge or urethral discomfort may be the presenting manifestation of a sexually transmitted disease (STD) and, as such, requires prompt attention. Nongonococcal urethritis (NGU) has surpassed gonorrhea as the principal cause of urethral symptoms in men. Much of NGU represents chlamydial infection, which has reached epidemic proportions in sexually active adolescents and college-aged persons. It can occur as an isolated infection or in conjunction with gonorrhea or other STDs. Because chlamydial infection is fast becoming the most common STD among heterosexuals in the United States and a potential source of female infertility and infant morbidity, the primary physician needs to be especially cognizant of its clinical manifestations, epidemiologic importance, and antibiotic treatment.

PATHOPHYSIOLOGY, CLINICAL PRESENTATION, AND CLINICAL COURSE

Most penile discharges are a consequence of urethral infection or inflammation. Numerous bacterial and nonbacterial organisms can invade its mucosal lining. Organisms causing NGU are characterized by their low levels of tissue invasiveness. In older men, the discharge may result from an inflamed prostate gland or, in rare instances, a tumor.

Gonococcal Urethritis. The typical presentation of symptomatic gonococcal disease is a 2- to 4-day history of dysuria and penile discharge, with the discharge being thick and purulent. The Gram's stain reveals polymorphonuclear leukocytes (PMNs) and gram-negative intracellular diplococci. Systemic gonococcemia develops in approximately 3 percent of patients, manifested by rash, fever, and polyarthritis (see Chapter 137). *Mixed infections,* involving both gonococci and *Chlamydia* occur in up to 20 percent of patients presenting with gonococcal urethritis. Such patients complain of persistence of symptoms after being effectively treated only for gonorrhea.

Gonococcal urethritis responds well to proper antibiotic therapy, with resolution of symptoms and no sequelae. In men, even untreated disease may resolve spontaneously within a few weeks. An asymptomatic carrier state may ensue or a chronic low-grade discharge may remain. Stricture is a possible consequence of untreated disease.

Nongonococcal Urethritis (NGU). Regardless of etiology, the clinical presentation of NGU is rather stereotypical. Compared with gonococcal urethritis, NGU tends to be an indolent illness of longer duration (eg, 3 to 4 weeks). Dysuria, if present, is not as severe, and the discharge is less purulent, mucoid, sometimes scanty, or even absent. The urethral Gram's stain shows some neutrophils (by definition more than four per high-power field) and, at most, a few mixed extracellular pleomorphic organisms, helping to distinguish NGU from gonococcal infection. Only 20 percent of ambiguous Gram's stains (rare extracellular gram-negative diplococci) will be shown by subsequent culture to represent gonococcal infection. Causes range from chlamydial infection to trichomonad disease.

Chlamydia Trachomatis. Chlamydial infection of the urogenital tract has reached epidemic proportions, with 20 percent to 50 percent penetration of some populations. Prevalence is greatest among sexually active adolescents and young adults, especially those under the age of 20 with multiple partners. The condition is also concentrated among poor, inner city, African-Americans. In heterosexual men, urethritis with penile discharge and/or dysuria is the most common symptomatic clinical presentation, but 25 percent to 50 percent may manifest neither symptoms nor leukocytes on urethral swab. Proctitis can develop in homosexual men engaging in receptive anal intercourse.

In untreated cases, symptoms may wax and wane over several weeks. Spontaneous resolution can occur. Complications are rare. Prostatitis and epididymitis have been reported in untreated or poorly treated cases. Epididymitis may also be part of the initial clinical presentation. Chlamydial infection accounts for about half of the epididymitis in the United States.

Female counterparts of chlamydial NGU have been identified, including mucopurulent cervicitis and urethritis (see Chapters 117, 125, and 133). There is a very high prevalence (almost 70%) of chlamydial infection among female partners of men with chlamydial NGU (see Chapter 125).

Ureaplasma Urealyticum. This organism has finally been established as a cause of NGU after decades of debate. It accounts for 10 percent to 40 percent of NGU cases and is sexually transmitted. The related species *Mycoplasma hominis* may also be a urethral pathogen. The urethritis is indistinguishable from that of other NGU etiologies. Persistence of symptomatic urethritis after appropriate antibiotic treatment of NGU has been linked to tetracycline-resistant strains. However, most recurrent NGU is due to reinfection from an untreated sexual partner rather than from infection with a resistant organism.

Trichomonas vaginalis infection is a common cause of vaginitis in women, but also an important source of urethritis in men. A 22 percent urethral prevalence was found among male partners of women with known trichomonal infection and a 6 percent prevalence among heterosexuals attending a clinic for STDs. About 50 percent are symptomatic and have a discharge on examination. Others have symptoms, but no visible discharge. The odds ratio for trichomonal infection in patients with nongonococcal, nonchlamydial urethritis was found to be 3.8. The condition should be suspected in patients with symptoms, but little or no discharge on physical examination.

Reiter's Syndrome. The finding of genetic overlap between the histocompatibility antigen HLA-B27 (found in up to 96% of patients versus 10% of controls) and certain *Klebsiella* and *C. trachomatis* antigens suggests infection in susceptible persons may play a role in the condition's pathogenesis. It usually presents as urethritis in conjunction with a host of other mucocutaneous and musculoskeletal symptoms. Various combinations of conjunctivitis, iritis, fever, acute asymmetric polyarthritis (see Chapter 146), nonarticular bony pain (eg, of the heel), circinate balanitis, keratodermia blennorrhagica, and mucosal ulcerations may be present at any one time. The most characteristic presentation is onset of mild dysuria and a mucopurulent urethral discharge about 2 to 4 weeks after a diarrheal illness or sexual contact. Many patients present first with the urethritis, although involvement of other organ systems is frequently present in subclinical form or soon materializes within a few weeks. Most patients with Reiter's syndrome experience a self-limited illness of 6 to 12 months' duration, although a minority progress to chronic or recurrent symptoms in conjunction with bouts of arthritis.

Prostatitis. In older men, prostatic hyperplasia predisposes to obstruction and infection. Prostatitis may also represent infectious spread to the prostate. Minor penile discharge may be noted, exacerbated by prostatic massage. Symptoms of urinary outflow obstruction and perineal discomfort may dominate the clinical picture (see Chapters 138 and 139).

DIFFERENTIAL DIAGNOSIS

The differential diagnosis of a penile discharge is traditionally divided into gonococcal and nongonococcal etiologies, with NGU accounting for the majority of cases. Among the causes of NGU are chlamydial, ureaplasmal, and trichomonal infections of the urethra, Reiter's syndrome, prostatitis, and urethral malignancy. Chlamydial disease is responsible for about half of NGU. In up to a third of NGU cases, no pathogen is identified. Occasionally, urethral infection with herpes simplex virus (HSV) or human papillomavirus may be responsible for the problem.

WORKUP

History and Physical Examination

History. The duration and character of the discharge can be informative. Acute onset of a profuse purulent discharge usually suggests gonococcal infection. Several weeks of a more indolent, less profuse, mucoid discharge point toward a nongonococcal etiology. However, there is some overlap in presentations and the history is not sufficient for diagnosis. A blood-tinged discharge raises the question of prostatitis or urethral tumor. Inquiry should be made concerning number of sexual partners over the past few months and use or nonuse of barrier contraception (important considerations in assessing risk of chlamydial infection and other STDs). The history is also noted for symptoms of prostatitis (slow stream, perineal discomfort), localized or systemic gonorrheal infection (pharyngitis, proctitis, arthritis, punctate skin lesions, sepsis), and Reiter's syndrome (polyarthritis, dermatitis, conjunctivitis, bony pain). Any history of penile warts or HSV infection should be noted, as should sexual contact with a partner known to have had trichomonal infection.

Physical Examination. The temperature is taken and integument carefully examined for signs of gonococcemia (fever; punctate, centrally hemorrhagic, necrotic skin lesions; tenosynovitis, polyarthritis). Similarly, manifestations of Reiter's syndrome are sought, including conjunctivitis, iritis, oral or meatal mucosal ulcerations, circinate balanitis (ulceration and erythema on the penile glans), keratoderma blennorrhagica (pustular or hyperkeratotic lesions on the soles of the feet), inflamed joints (knees, ankles, sacroiliacs), and nonarticular bone pain (especially of the heel). The urethral meatus is examined for herpetic lesions and warts, the epididymis is palpated for tenderness and swelling, and the prostate for enlargement, bogginess, and tenderness. An acutely inflamed prostate should be examined very gingerly, because abscess is a possible concomitant.

Laboratory Studies

Gram's Stain of the urethral discharge should be the first study performed, because it helps to distinguish gonococcal from nongonococcal disease. Even if there is no visible discharge, a swab is gently inserted into the urethral meatus and a sample is obtained. A first morning sample before urination or one several hours after urination offers the best yield. Some of the sample is plated onto Thayer-Martin media for culture of *Neisseria gonorrhoeae* (see Chapter 137), whereas the remainder is placed on a glass slide and Gram-stained. The finding of PMNs with gram-negative intracellular diplococci is highly predictive of gonococcal urethritis. The sensitivity and specificity of the Gram's stain exceed 95 percent. Four or more PMNs per high-power field and mixed gram-negative and gram-positive pleomorphic extracellular organisms or leukocytes and no visible organisms are indicative of NGU. If no definite gram-negative intracellular diplococci are seen on Gram's stain, then a tentative diagnosis of NGU is appropriate. The diagnosis is confirmed by a negative gonococcal culture.

Chlamydial Testing. It is not practical to culture for *Chlamydia* or *Ureaplasma,* because of the expense, technical difficulty, and 2- to 3-day delay in obtaining results. However, antigen detection methods provide more rapid, less expensive detection of chlamydial infection. At the time of obtaining an intraurethral swab for Gram's stain, a second swabbing should also be performed and saved for chlamydial testing. Such testing can be of help even if the patient is going to be treated presumptively for chlamydial infection, because the information often helps improve compliance, facilitates counseling, and helps guide care if symptoms persist. Patients with a presumptive diagnosis of gonorrhea may also benefit from chlamydial testing, because both infections may exist concurrently.

Direct fluorescent antibody (DFA) staining of urethral smears and *enzyme immunoassay* (EIA) of secretions are the antigen detection methods most widely available. The former is more sensitive and specific; the latter is cheaper and better suited for laboratories that process large numbers of specimens. They are the preferred chlamydial testing methods for men with symptomatic urethritis. Sensitivity exceeds 70 percent and specificity approaches 99 percent in symptomatic men. Sensitivity is enhanced by obtaining a specimen several hours after the last urination. EIA testing may give a false-positive result if there is lower urinary tract infection, making the test less useful in older men with prostatic disease. Test results are available within 36 to 72 hours. If posttreatment testing is desired, it should not be done until 3 weeks after completion of treatment—sufficient time for clearing of antigen. *Rapid chlamydial testing* kits are packaged for office use and provide results within 30 minutes. They too make use of antigen detection methods and are subject to the same false-positive results. In addition, quality control problems arise because of the relatively unskilled persons performing the test. Under development is *DNA-probe* technology, which promises heightened sensitivity and specificity as well as testing of urine samples.

Other Studies. When routine cultures and Gram's stains are not diagnostic and an empiric trial of treatment for NGU is unsuccessful (see below), then reevaluation and consideration of culturing for *Ureaplasma* or *trichomonads* may be appropriate. When there is clinical suspicion of Reiter's syndrome, the patient can be checked for the presence of the *HLA-B27* histocompatibility antigen. However, its presence is not diagnostic of Reiter's syndrome, nor does its absence rule out the condition. Bloody discharge warrants referral to the urologist for consideration of *cystoscopy.*

MANAGEMENT OF NGU

Because chlamydial infection accounts for 50 percent of NGU, ranks as the most common STD among heterosexuals in the United States, and represents a potential source of morbidity to female partners and their infants, all patients with NGU should be treated, regardless of whether definite identification of *Chlamydia* has been achieved. Female partners of NGU patients should be tested; if testing is not available, they too should be treated for presumptive chlamydial infection. Male homosexual partners should be tested. Empiric treatment of asymptomatic male homosexual partners is not recommended because of the reduced incidence of *Chlamydia* infection in this population.

Initial Treatment. The Centers for Disease Control and Prevention recommendation for treatment of NGU is *doxycycline,* 100 mg bid for 7 days, or *azithromycin,* 1 g orally in a single dose. Although expensive, azithromycin provides greatly enhanced ease of use and compliance. Pregnant patients and others who should not take doxycycline or azithromycin can be treated with *erythromycin base,* 500 mg qid for 7 days. (Erythromycin estolate is contraindicated in pregnancy.) These antibiotic regimens are usually effective against *Ureaplasma* as well. Ofloxacin (500 mg bid for 7 days) is also effective for treatment of NGU, with excellent activity against both *chlamydia* and *ureaplasma.* It is superior to other fluoroquinolone antibiotics for treatment of NGU and has also proven effective against *N. gonorrhoeae* (see Chapter 137). Cost is high. *Minocycline,* a once-a-day tetracycline, appears as effective as doxycycline. At a dose of 100 mg/d, vestibular toxicity is uncommon.

Management of Recurrent NGU. Although most NGU patients experience resolution of symptoms with onset of therapy, up to 30 percent relapse. Some relapses have been attributed to tetracycline-resistant strains of *Ureaplasma*, others to poor medication compliance, reinfection, or presence of prostatitis. Because *erythromycin* is effective against tetracycline-resistant strains of *Ureaplasma* and penetrates the prostate well, it has been used as a 3-week program (500 mg qid) for treatment of recurrent disease. Such a regimen is particularly useful for patients with prostatitis as the etiology of their NGU. However, one should confirm the presence of prostatitis (see Chapter 139) as well as evaluate for reinfection before resorting to empiric antibiotics. *Chlamydia* and *Trichomonas* are often found in patients with recurrent disease. If the latter is found, treatment with *metronidazole* (250 mg tid for 1 week) may prove useful. Endoscopic urethral examination in search of intrinsic urethral pathology is of low yield and not recommended in patients with recurrent NGU.

Treatment of Reiter's Syndrome. Treatment for *Chlamydia* may shorten the duration of illness and prevent recurrences in patients who appear to have the illness on the basis of sexually transmitted chlamydial infection.

Treatment of Gonococcal Urethritis. See Chapter 137.

PATIENT EDUCATION

The most important message to patients is the importance of prevention through use of condoms. In addition, successful treatment of the disease requires contacting and treating recent sexual partners. The asymptomatic sexual partner is an important reservoir for reinfection. Treated male patients should be told to return for follow-up evaluation if symptoms return. Female partners should undergo retesting after 3 weeks to ensure eradication of chlamydial infection. There are no firm data concerning abstinence from unprotected intercourse during the treatment period, but it seems reasonable to suggest at least 7 days of treatment before sexual activity is resumed.

ANNOTATED BIBLIOGRAPHY

Centers for Disease Control and Prevention. Recommendations for the prevention and management of *Chlamydia trachomatis* infections. MMWR 1993;42:1. *(Excellent review of diagnostic methods and authoritative guidelines for treatment; essential reading; 158 refs.)*

Hooton TM, Wong ES, Barnes RC, et al. Erythromycin for persistent or recurrent nongonococcal urethritis. Ann Intern Med 1990;113:21. *(A 3-week course of treatment proved beneficial, especially in those with prostatitis.)*

Jacobs NJ, Kraus SJ. Gonococcal and nongonococcal urethritis in men. Ann Intern Med 1975;82:7. *(Sensitivity of Gram's stain was 97 percent; specificity was 98 percent for diagnosis of gonococcal urethritis; 21 percent of stains that were equivocal were gonococcal culture-positive.)*

Krieger JN, Jenny C, Verdon M, et al. Clinical manifestations of trichomoniasis in men. Ann Intern Med 1993;118:844. *(Found to be a cause of urethritis and sexually transmitted.)*

Martin DH, et al. Controlled trial of a single dose of azithromycin for the treatment of chlamydial urethritis and cervicitis. N Engl J Med 1992;327:921. *(Found to be as effective as standard therapy.)*

Martin DH, Pollack S, Kuo CC. *Chlamydia trachomatis* infections in men with Reiter's syndrome. Ann Intern Med 1984;100:207. *(Documents infection and an exaggerated immune response in some patients who go on to develop Reiter's syndrome.)*

Morris R, Metzger AL, Bluestone R, et al. HLA-B27: A clue to the diagnosis and pathogenesis of Reiter's syndrome. N Engl J Med 1974;290:554. *(A classic paper reporting 96 percent of patients with Reiter's syndrome were HLA-B27 positive.)*

Stamm WE. Diagnosis of *Chlamydia trachomatis* genitourinary infections. Ann Intern Med 1988;108:710. *(Excellent review, with very useful discussion of clinical findings, culture, and antigen methods; 93 refs.)*

Stamm WE, Koutsky LA, Benedetti JK, et al. *Chlamydia trachomatis* urethral infections in men. Ann Intern Med 1984;100:47. *(Details prevalence, risk factors, and clinical manifestations: from an STD clinic.)*

Tam MR, Stamm WE, Handsfield JJ, et al. Culture-independent diagnosis of *Chlamydia trachomatis* using monoclonal antibodies. N Engl J Med 1984;310:1146. *(Direct fluorescent antibody test for rapid diagnosis of chlamydial infection.)*

Taylor-Robinson D, McCormack WM. The genital mycoplasmas. N Engl J Med 1980;302:1003. *(A comprehensive two-part review detailing the role of* Ureaplasma *infection in NGU and other genital infections.)*

Wong ES, Hooton TM, Hill CC, et al. Clinical and microbiological features of persistent or recurrent nongonococcal urethritis in men. J Infect Dis 1988;158:1098. *(Noncompliance and reinfection were the main causes;* Chlamydia *and* Trichomonas *were often found.)*

Primary Care Medicine: Office Evaluation and Management of the Adult Patient, 3rd edition, edited by Allan H. Goroll, Lawrence A. May, and Albert G. Mulley, Jr. J.B. Lippincott Company, Philadelphia

137
Approach to the Patient With Gonorrhea

HARVEY B. SIMON, M.D.

Like other sexually transmitted diseases, gonorrhea remains a major public health problem in the United States. Although penicillinase-producing strains have become increasingly prevalent, antibiotic resistance cannot be blamed for the failure to control gonorrhea. In fact, excellent alternative drugs are available. Rather, the continued spread of gonorrhea represents the failure of "safe sex" programs to influence human behavior. Theoretically, primary prevention could control this age-old infection, but 1 million cases of gonorrhea are reported each year in the United States. Because of underreporting, it can be safely estimated that at least 3 million cases occur annually. Gonorrhea is most prevalent among teenagers and young adults, especially those belonging to minority groups and dwelling in the inner city; however, the infection crosses all age and socioeconomic barriers.

The great majority of patients with venereal disease present to an ambulatory care facility and should be diagnosed and treated in this setting. At the same time, the physician must be alert to serious systemic complications requiring hospitalization. In addition, patient education is critical to prevent inadequate treatment and recurrent infections. Finally, the responsibility of the physician must extend beyond the diagnosis and treatment of an individual patient to the identification and treatment of sexual contacts who may otherwise harbor and further disseminate these infections.

PATHOPHYSIOLOGY AND CLINICAL PRESENTATION

Gonococcal infection invariably begins with the direct infection of a mucosal surface during sexual activity. Organisms may then gain access to the bloodstream to produce bacteremia and systemic spread of infection. This is most common in women, especially at the time of menstruation, but it occurs in males as well. The clinical features of gonorrhea differ greatly in the male and female. Moreover, symptoms of the primary gonococcal infection may be absent or mistaken for another condition, making the diagnosis more difficult.

In the male, clinical symptoms usually follow within 2 to 10 days of sexual exposure. The risk that a male will acquire gonorrhea after a single exposure to an infected partner is approximately 35 percent. Absence of symptoms does not indicate absence of infection. Indeed, up to 10 percent of infected males are asymptomatic carriers of the gonococcus and are fully capable of transmitting the disease. In the male, gonorrhea is principally an infection of the anterior urethra, and hence the major symptom is purulent *urethral discharge,* often accompanied by urinary frequency and dysuria. Although spread of infection to the *prostate* or *epididymis* is uncommon in the antibiotic era, gonococci occasionally gain entry into the *bloodstream* to produce disseminated infection.

In the female, the *cervix* is the favored site of gonococcal infection. However, up to 25 percent of women with gonococcal infection are asymptomatic and must be identified through epidemiologic case finding. When symptoms do occur, cervical discharge is most common. Although the vagina is usually spared, the gonococcal infection may spread downward from the cervix to produce *urethritis,* presenting as dysuria and frequency. Infection of *Bartholin's glands* presents as labial swelling and pain, and rectal infection presents as anorectal discomfort. If, on the other hand, gonococcal infection spreads upward from the cervix, more serious processes may develop. Such upward spread is particularly likely at the time of menstruation and can produce a variety of syndromes. Gonococcal *endometritis* can cause pelvic pain and abnormal vaginal bleeding, whereas *salpingitis* characteristically leads to fever, chills, leukocytosis, and a tender adnexal mass. Both systemic and pelvic signs and symptoms are even more pronounced in frank *pelvic peritonitis,* and further intraperitoneal spread may produce gonococcal *perihepatitis* with right upper-quadrant pain and tenderness.

Primary extragenital infections are being encountered more frequently as a result of changing sexual practices. Gonococcal infection of the pharynx is usually asymptomatic but can present as an acute *exudative pharyngitis,* with fever and cervical lymphadenopathy. Gonococcal *proctitis* is also most often asymptomatic but can present as proctitis with anorectal discomfort, tenesmus, or rectal bleeding and discharge.

Gonococcal bacteremia is manifested by the *"dermatitis–arthritis syndrome."* Patients have fever, chills, and other constitutional symptoms. Skin lesions are an important clue to diagnosis; these are typically pustular, hemorrhagic, or papular, are few in number, and tend to be most common on the distal extremities. *Tenosynovitis,* especially involving the extensor surfaces of hands and feet, and *migratory polyarthritis* are typically seen. During the early stage of systemic infection, blood cultures are often positive, but joint cultures are characteristically negative. Later in the course of untreated patients, however, gonococci can produce frank *septic arthritis.* Such patients have less fever, no skin lesions, and negative blood cultures, but more impressive joint swelling and pain, often with purulent synovial fluid in which gonococci can be demonstrated by Gram's stain or culture. In rare instances, gonococci can produce *osteomyelitis* or even life-threatening bacterial *meningitis* or *endocarditis.*

DIFFERENTIAL DIAGNOSIS

The organisms besides *Neisseria gonorrhoeae* capable of producing female genital infections include *Chlamydia, Gardnerella, Trichomonas,* and *Candida* (see Chapter 117). The differential diagnosis of gonococcal salpingitis and peritonitis mainly encompasses the causes of nongonococcal pelvic inflammatory disease (PID; see Chapter 116), but other conditions, such as appendicitis, ectopic pregnancy, hemorrhagic ovarian cysts, and endometriosis, can produce similar clinical findings and often require urgent therapy very different from that of PID. In the male, the causes of nongonococcal urethritis enter the differential diagnosis (see Chapter 136). Gonococcal infection also needs to be considered among the causes of pharyngitis (see Chapter 220) and proctitis (see Chapter 66).

WORKUP

History and Physical Examination. The diagnosis of gonorrhea requires a high index of suspicion and a careful *sexual history.* Physical examination in men with urethritis is usually normal except for purulent *urethral discharge.* In asymptomatic women, the physical examination is normal, but *cervicitis* may produce cervical inflammation, discharge, and marked cervical tenderness. *Adnexal tenderness* and fullness are signs of salpingitis and may be unilateral or bilateral in women with gonorrhea. Tubal abscesses may be suspected because of a palpable mass, and rebound tenderness is a sign of pelvic peritonitis.

PID resulting from organisms other than the gonococcus may present similarly. Clinical features favoring the gonococcus include purulent cervical discharge, onset early in the menstrual cycle, no previous history of PID, and exposure to a male with urethritis.

Laboratory Studies. A properly made *Gram's stain* of the urethral discharge can be a highly reliable diagnostic tool. A Gram's stain is considered "positive" when biscuit-shaped gram-negative diplococci are seen within polymorphonuclear leukocytes; "equivocal" if diplococci are only extracellular or if intracellular organisms are morphologically atypical; and "negative" if no diplococci are found. Sensitivity of the Gram's stain is >95 percent in symptomatic men but declines to 50 to 60 percent in those with asymptomatic urethral infection. Gram's stains are much less reliable in cervical, rectal, and pharyngeal infections.

Cultures confirming the diagnosis of gonorrhea are mandatory in both sexes. *Neisseria gonorrhoeae* is a fragile and fastidious organism that requires special handling in the laboratory. The gonococcus is readily killed by drying, so all cultures must be plated promptly. Ideally, this should be done by the physician at the time of examination by streaking the swab across the surface of the culture medium in a Z-shaped pattern. Special culture media must be used. Although chocolate agar has been the traditional medium used, a modified *Thayer–Martin medium* is preferred for specimens obtained from genital, anal, or pharyngeal sites because the addition of antibiotics to this medium suppresses the growth of nonpathogenic *Neisseria* species and other bacteria. The culture medium should be at room temperature at the time of inoculation. Because the gonococcus requires a high CO_2 concentration to grow, cultures should be promptly incubated in a candle jar or CO_2 incubator. When this is not possible, the cultures should be planted on modified Thayer–Martin medium in bottles with a 10 percent CO_2 atmosphere. These bottles should be kept capped until the moment of inoculation and should be held in an upright position when open to prevent the loss of CO_2, which is heavier than air.

In the male, cultures of the anterior *urethra suffice* unless homosexual contacts are suspected, in which case cultures of the anal canal and pharynx are also indicated. In the female, the *endocervix* should be cultured by inserting a swab into the cervical os through a speculum that has been lubricated only with water. In all women, *rectal* cultures are indicated because rectal infection can result simply from direct spread of infection from the genital tract. When pharyngitis is suspected, *throat* culture is mandatory. When acute arthritis is present, *joint fluid* should be obtained by arthrocentesis and should be evaluated with cell counts, sugar and protein determinations, Gram's stain, and culture. *Blood* cultures are indicated in patients with fever, skin lesions, and tenosynovitis or arthritis.

PRINCIPLES OF MANAGEMENT AND THERAPEUTIC RECOMMENDATIONS

Overcoming Penicillin Resistance. The therapy of gonorrhea has undergone dramatic changes over the past 40 years. Penicillin has been used for decades, but during this time there has been a steady increase in penicillin resistance. The recommended dosages of penicillin are 30 times greater than those initially used with success in 1943. Until recently, this penicillin resistance was just a matter of degree, because it was based on chromosomal mutations decreasing the permeability of the cell wall to penicillin and other antibiotics. Simply increasing the dosage of penicillin sufficed.

Another form of penicillin resistance was recognized in 1975, when gonococcal strains were isolated that resisted the effects of even massive doses of penicillin by producing penicillinase. These strains were found to contain beta-lactamase–producing plasmids. In the United States, infection with a plasmid-containing strain was initially sporadic, but the number of such infections has increased dramatically and is no longer limited to a few groups of patients. More recently, very high-level, chromosomally mediated penicillin resistance has emerged. In all, about 5 percent of gonococcal strains are penicillin-resistant. A significant number of clinical isolates are also tetracycline-resistant, and heavy use of spectinomycin has led to emergence of strains resistant to it.

Unless the isolate is proven to be penicillin-sensitive, a regimen effective for resistant strains should be used. When possible, drugs that are also effective against syphilis are preferred. Because of problems with patient compliance, single-dose regimens are recommended. The parenterally administered *ceftriaxone* and the orally administered *cefixime* presently meet these requirements.

Concurrent Infection. In addition to the problem of antibiotic resistance, the management of gonorrhea is complicated by the need to treat coexisting sexually transmitted infections. Chlamydial disease is of greatest concern, coexisting with gonococci in up to 20 percent of males and 50 percent of women with sexually transmitted disease. As a result, all patients with gonorrhea should also be treated for chlamydial infection. Although much less common than *Chlamydia,* incubating syphilis can be a more serious problem and should be screened for (see Chapters 124 and 141). Confidential testing for human immunodeficiency virus (HIV) infection may be of benefit not only for case identification, but also for promotion of safer sexual practices (see below).

THERAPEUTIC RECOMMENDATIONS

Uncomplicated Gonorrhea (Including Urethral, Cervical, and Rectal Infection)

- Prescribe *ceftriaxone* (125 mg IM once), *cefixime,* ciprofloxacin (500 mg PO once), *or* ofloxacin (400 mg PO once); plus *doxycycline* (100 mg bid for 7 days).
- Prescribe *spectinomycin* (2 g IM once) for those allergic to beta-lactam antibiotics (ie, cephalosporins and penicillins), or who cannot take fluoroquinolones (eg, pregnant women).
- Prescribe *erythromycin* base (500 mg qid for 7 days) for patients who cannot take doxycycline (eg, pregnant women and those allergic to the drug).

Disseminated Gonococcal Infection

- Hospitalize initially and begin *ceftriaxone* (1 g or IM q24h for 7 days).

- Treat with higher doses for a more prolonged period if there is meningitis, endocarditis, or osteomyelitis.
- Treat with *spectinomycin* (2 g IM q12h for 7 days) those persons who are allergic to beta-lactam antibiotics.
- Discharge those who respond well to the initial 1 to 2 days of parenteral therapy, provided they return daily for IM ceftriaxone or complete a week of oral therapy with *ciprofloxacin* (500 mg bid).
- Treat also for chlamydial infection as in uncomplicated disease.

Monitoring

Because treatment failures with ceftriaxone–doxycycline are rare, immediate *follow-up cultures* are not mandatory. It may be more cost-effective to delay repeat evaluation with cultures until 1 to 2 months have passed. This allows detection of reinfection as well as treatment failures and reinforcement of patient education. Patients treated with regimens other than ceftriaxone–doxycycline do require follow-up cultures 4 to 7 days after completing therapy.

All patients with gonorrhea should have serologic *testing for syphilis*. Seronegative patients treated with ceftriaxone do not require follow-up serologies because this regimen is effective for incubating syphilis. However, patients receiving other antibiotic regimens do require repeat serologic testing in 3 months. All patients with gonorrhea should be offered confidential *testing for HIV* infection. All gonorrhea cases should be reported to the appropriate local health department. Because many patients are asymptomatic, vigorous case finding represents the only present means of controlling this epidemic.

PATIENT EDUCATION AND PREVENTION

The importance of completing a full course of therapy must be emphasized. Single-dose regimens have greatly simplified treatment of gonorrhea, but proper therapy should also include a 7-day antibiotic course directed against chlamydial infection, which is reaching epidemic proportions.

Preventive measures include attention to *case finding* and health education. When the patient is a symptomatic male, all sexual contacts within the previous 2 weeks should be notified and treated. This will result in reaching more than 90 percent of partners likely to be infected. However, if the patient is an asymptomatic male or a female, then all contacts within the previous 60 days should be notified to reach 90 percent of the people at risk.

Health education about high-risk sex (failure to use a condom, multiple partners, intercourse with a patient having a purulent discharge, or recent history of untreated gonorrhea) has not been effective over the years. However, fear of HIV infection, confidential HIV testing, and counseling on condom use do appear to encourage safer sexual activity, especially insistence by women on use of condoms. Properly used barrier methods of contraception are effective means of preventing gonorrhea. *Condoms* do not permit transmission of the gonococcus or *Chlamydia*. The diaphragm or contraceptive sponge may also offer some protection against gonorrhea, especially when used with a *vaginal spermicide* containing nonoxynol-9, the active ingredient in many preparations. *Screening* by routine office culturing of high-risk women (prostitutes, those with sexual contact with a person with gonorrhea, multiple previous episodes of gonorrhea) has the potential to be cost effective.

INDICATIONS FOR ADMISSION

Patients with disseminated disease who are febrile, who are unreliable, or who have evidence of osteomyelitis, endocarditis, or meningitis must be hospitalized. The same is true of the woman with PID who appears toxic, pregnant, unlikely to comply, or suffering from pelvic pain of unclear etiology in association with peritoneal signs.

ANNOTATED BIBLIOGRAPHY

Allen S, Serufilira A, Bogaerts J, et al. Confidential HIV testing and condom promotion in Africa: Impact on HIV and gonorrhea rates. JAMA 1992;268:3338. *(Condom use went up 300 percent, and the prevalence of gonorrhea fell by more than half.)*

Centers for Disease Control. Sexually transmitted diseases treatment guidelines. MMWR 1989;38(suppl 8):1. *(Expert committee consensus recommendations.)*

Faro S, Martens MG, Maccato M, et al. Effectiveness of oflaxacin in the treatment of *Chlamydia trachomatis* and *Neisseria gonorrhoeae* cervical infection. Am J Obstet Gynecol 1991;164:1380. *(Proved effective for both organisms.)*

Handsfield HH, Lipman TO, Harnisch JP, et al. Asymptomatic gonorrhea in men. N Engl J Med 1974;290:117. *(Asymptomatic males may be an important reservoir of infection; all sexual contacts should be cultured, whether male or female and whether symptomatic or not.)*

Handsfield HH, McCormack WM, Hook EW, et al. A comparison of single-dose cefixime with ceftriaxone as treatment for uncomplicated gonorrhea. N Engl J Med 1991;325:1337. *(Oral cefixime produced results equivalent to those of parenterally administered ceftriaxone.)*

Hook EW, Holmes KK. Gonococcal infections. Ann Intern Med 1985;102:229. *(Authoritative review: highly recommended; 157 refs.)*

Hutt DM, Judson FN. Epidemiology and treatment of oropharyngeal gonorrhea. Ann Intern Med 1986;104:655. *(Not to be forgotten as a cause of severe pharyngitis.)*

Jick H, Hannan MT, Stergachis A, et al. Vaginal spermicides and gonorrhea. JAMA 1982;248:1619. *(Suggests a protective effect against gonorrhea.)*

Judson FN. Management of antibiotic-resistant *Neisseria gonorrhoeae*. Ann Intern Med 1989;110:5. *(An editorial that succinctly reviews the options.)*

Kelaghan J, Rubin GL, Ory HW, et al. Barrier-method contraceptives and pelvic inflammatory disease. JAMA 1982;248:184. *(A relative risk of 0.6 for women using barrier methods.)*

Klein EJ, Fisher LS, Chow AW, et al. Anorectal gonococcal infection. Ann Intern Med 1977;86:340. *(A clinical review of such infections in women and homosexual males.)*

Kreiss J, Ngugi E, Holmes K, et al. Efficacy of nonoxynol 9 contraceptive sponge use in preventing heterosexual acquisition of HIV in Nairobi prostitutes. JAMA 1992;268:447. *(Rate of gonococcal infection was reduced by 60 percent, although risk of HIV infection increased by 60 percent.)*

O'Brien JP, Goldenberg DL, Rice PA. Disseminated gonococcal infection: A prospective analysis of 49 patients and a review of pathophysiology and immune mechanisms. Medicine 1983; 62:395. *(A comprehensive study of 49 patients and review of the literature.)*

Phillips RS, Safran C, Aronson M, Taylor WC. Should women be tested for gonococcal infection of the cervix during routine gynecologic visits? An economic appraisal. Am J Med 1989; 86:297. *(A decision analysis study suggesting the answer is "yes" in high-risk persons.)*

Platt R, Rice PA, McCormack WM. Risk of acquiring gonorrhea and prevalence of abnormal adnexal findings among women recently exposed to gonorrhea. JAMA 1983;250:3205. *(Risk was 50 percent, 86 percent, and 100 percent for one, two, and more than two exposures, respectively; upper genital tract spread was a common early complication.)*

Schwarcz SK, Zenilman JM, Schnell D. National surveillance of antimicrobial resistance in *Neisseria gonorrhoeae*. JAMA 1990;264:1413. *(Twenty-one percent found resistant to penicillin, tetracycline, cefoxitin, or spectinomycin; all sensitive to ceftriaxone.)*

Primary Care Medicine: Office Evaluation and Management of the Adult Patient, 3rd edition, edited by Allan H. Goroll, Lawrence A. May, and Albert G. Mulley, Jr. J.B. Lippincott Company, Philadelphia

138
Management of Benign Prostatic Hyperplasia

JOHN D. GOODSON, M.D.
MICHAEL J. BARRY, M.D.

Benign prostatic hyperplasia (BPH) is a nearly ubiquitous condition in older men and is a frequent cause of urinary tract outflow obstruction. The primary physician must distinguish BPH from the other causes of urinary symptoms (see Chapters 136, 139, and 140), determine its severity, and, when the symptoms are bothersome enough, design a therapeutic approach that provides symptomatic relief. For patients who elect a course of "watchful waiting," a monitoring strategy should be followed to preserve renal function and prevent infection.

PATHOPHYSIOLOGY AND CLINICAL PRESENTATION

Pathophysiology. BPH arises from nodular hyperplasia of prostatic stromal and glandular elements. Growth begins in the periurethral glandular tissue. As these nodules expand and coalesce over years, the true prostatic tissue is compressed outward, forming a "surgical capsule" around the adenomatous hyperplasia. The etiology of age-related prostatic hyperplasia is still unknown, although it is reasonably well established that androgenic changes at the cellular level have a major influence. A better understanding of these influences on prostatic hyperplasia is beginning to help define hormonal manipulations that may affect the natural history of the disease. As the gland enlarges, urethral resistance to urine flow increases and *muscular hypertrophy* of the bladder ensues. *Bladder instability* may develop, and emptying may become incomplete. The resulting *residual urine* predisposes to infection, which, in turn, may produce further bladder irritation. Numerous saccules or bladder herniations can form between the thickened overlapping muscular bands that compose the detrusor. These diverticula are incompletely emptied with voiding, further predisposing to infection. Ureteral dilation can be seen in advanced cases of chronic retention because of increased bladder pressure. Hydronephrosis and renal deterioration may follow thereafter.

When the detrusor is no longer able to generate sufficient pressure to overcome urethral obstruction, *bladder failure* occurs, and *urinary retention* develops. A large fluid load, impairment of the contractile function of the bladder by anticholinergics, or increased outflow resistance from sympathomimetic drugs may lead to acute urinary retention. Some proportion of acute retention may be precipitated by painless infarction in the enlarged gland. The hyperplastic prostate is highly vascular and predisposed to *bleeding;* painless hematuria occurs.

The *late-stage complications* of chronic retention caused by BPH include hydronephrosis, loss of renal concentrating ability, diminished hydrogen ion excretion (with systemic acidosis), and renal failure.

Clinical Presentation and Course. BPH is manifest clinically by symptoms of urinary tract outflow *obstruction* (see below) with or without symptoms arising from *bladder instability* and *infection*. Symptoms are unusual before age 50. Patients with clinically significant urethral obstruction due to BPH often present with hesitancy, loss of stream force, frequency, nocturia, a sense of incomplete voiding, stream interruption ("double voiding"), and dribbling. It is most common for patients to have a waxing and waning symptomatic course with very gradual deterioration over many years. Sometimes, urinary tract infection is the first indication of outlet obstruction. *Hematuria* may be an early symptom of BPH, but neoplasm must always be excluded.

The *rectal examination* of the prostate is, unfortunately, of little help in assessing the degree of obstruction resulting from gland enlargement, although it does provide a rough estimate of overall gland volume. The inability to palpate the distal margins of the gland generally indicates massive enlargement (more than three times normal size).

BPH in the elderly can have protean manifestations. It may cause so-called *silent prostatism,* which can produce a lower abdominal mass because of bladder enlargement. Confusion, anorexia, a palpable kidney, anemia, and a bleeding diathesis secondary to hydronephrosis and uremia constitute a presentation of advanced disease. Others include altered medication requirements as a consequence of diminished renal clearance and incontinence related to overflow.

PRINCIPLES OF MANAGEMENT

Assessing Severity and Significance of Symptoms

In cases of urinary outflow obstruction from BPH, the clinician must determine the extent to which the patient is bothered by his symptoms. For some, frequency and nocturia significantly interfere with a restful night of sleep, whereas for others they are a minor inconvenience. It is generally best to *monitor the patient for 3 to 6 months* to determine the stability or progression of symptoms before making any major therapeutic decisions. The elderly require special attention because their symptoms may be poorly expressed or confusing.

Primary care physicians frequently have the opportunity to identify the symptoms arising from BPH in the context of continuity care. Men over the age of 50 should be routinely asked about *urinary habits,* not only to identify the reticent patient with severe symptoms, but also to inform the patient about the relationship between certain changes in urinary habits (such as occasional nocturia or a loss in stream force) and the natural history of BPH. Prescription and nonprescription *medication use* should be reviewed because certain therapies influence urodynamic function (see above and Chapter 134). A drug change alone may relieve bothersome symptoms for some men.

The decision to proceed to prostatectomy should rarely be made quickly. It is essential that the physician understand the *importance of symptoms* to the patient and their impact on his quality of life, because the individual patient may be willing to accept a given level of symptomatology and small risk of future BPH complications to avoid surgery.

A *creatinine* and *urinalysis* should be obtained on all patients to assess renal function and check for infection or hematuria. Measurements of *postvoid residual* urine can be made by catheterization (more than 50 to 100 mL of residual urine is abnormal) or, less invasively, by transabdominal ultrasonography. However, these measurements are poorly reproducible in individual patients.

Urinary flow studies have become widely available. These tests do not require catheterization and are useful in assessing true flow rates in patients whose presentations are atypical (eg, younger patients or men with mostly irritative symptoms). A normal peak flow rate (>15 mL/s) in the setting of prostatism should prompt further evaluation for alternative explanations. However, men with true bladder outlet obstruction may maintain normal flow rates by generating high bladder pressures. Similarly, men with hypotonic bladders may have low flow rates without physiologic obstruction. A low voided volume (<150 mL) may produce a falsely low peak flow rate.

Imaging studies are not routinely necessary in typical cases of BPH. Assessment of the bladder and upper urinary tract is *optional* unless there is an elevated creatinine, hematuria, or another specific indication. Transabdominal *ultrasound* can be used to exclude hydronephrosis and assess the postvoid residual volume without the risk of a contrast reaction during an *intravenous pyelogram (IVP).* Similarly, cystourethroscopy should be done only when specifically indicated (eg, prior genitourinary instrumentation, hematuria). More sophisticated *urodynamic studies* (cystometrics and pressure-flow studies) are best reserved for patients with conflicting results on simple tests (eg, severe symptoms with a normal flow rate), neurologic disease, or prior genitourinary surgery.

Checking for Prostate Cancer. When the digital rectal examination is not suspicious for prostate cancer, a test of serum *prostate-specific antigen (PSA)* is optional for men with symptomatic BPH. The PSA is less specific for prostate cancer in men with BPH, because BPH can cause modest PSA elevations. Moreover, the "prior probability" of subclinical cancer does not seem to be appreciably elevated in the setting prostatism. Finally, no trials have documented that early detection of prostate cancer improves patient outcomes. Nevertheless, men with BPH should understand that they run a 10 percent to 15 percent risk of harboring coincidental prostate cancer and that further tests are available if the patient and his physician wish to screen for prostate cancer (see Chapter 126).

Treatment

General Measures. Most patients with urinary symptoms arising from BPH should be followed. Complicating factors, such as infections, should be treated, and medications that impair lower urinary tract function should be eliminated if possible. The patient should be told to *void frequently,* take extra time to void completely, and to avoid beverages that are likely to produce a diuresis (coffee, tea, alcohol), particularly before bed. Diuretics should be taken early in the day to avoid nocturnal bladder distention. Drugs, such as anticholinergics, mild tranquilizers, antidepressants, and the antiarrhythmic disopyramide, that can exacerbate the symptoms of bladder outflow obstruction should be used only with great care. Patients should be warned in particular about over-the-counter decongestants.

Alpha-Blockers and Hormonal Therapy. Such measures are the subject of active investigation. None of these treatments is comparable to surgery in terms of long-term effectiveness. *Alpha-blocker drugs,* used in the treatment of hypertension, have documented short-term efficacy in BPH. These agents work by relaxing detrusor and prostatic smooth muscle, thereby relieving some of the "dynamic" component of obstruction. Selective $alpha_1$-blockers (prazosin, doxazosin, terazosin) have fewer side-effects than nonselective alpha-blockers (phenoxybenzamine). These drugs can induce orthostatic hypotension, particularly after the first dose, and should be initially taken before bed (see Chapter 26). Terazocin is the only one FDA approved for use in BPH.

Hormonal manipulation is available with the advent of the 5-alpha reductase inhibitor *finasteride.* The drug blocks peripheral conversion of testosterone to its more active metabolite dihydrotestosterone, a potent stimulant of prostatic hyperplasia. The drug reduces prostate size by about 20 percent and produces mild to moderate improvements in symptoms and urinary flow rates. Results are of lesser magnitude than those achievable with *transurethral resection* of the prostate (TURP). Sexual dysfunction in the form of decreased libido, impotence, or ejaculatory difficulties occurs in about 5 percent. Chronic therapy is required (which can be very expensive), and it can take 6 to 12 months of continuous use before benefit is noted. Moreover, the drug reduces serum prostatic specific antigen, impairing PSA use for prostate cancer screening. The agent is best reserved for very symptomatic patients who refuse or cannot undergo surgery.

Surgical Approaches. Prompt surgery is indicated in patients with acute retention not due to a predisposing cause, hydronephrosis, repeated urinary tract infections, recurrent or refractory gross hematuria, or an elevated creatinine that responds to a period of bladder decompression with catheter drainage. Fortunately, such complications are rare. More commonly, the primary care physician must integrate both the symptoms reported by or elicited from the patient with an assessment of how bothered the patient is by these complaints. Surgery does provide excellent symptomatic relief in most cases but there are risks and costs associated with any procedure that some patients may not be willing to undertake. Furthermore, there are patients for whom surgery might not provide much benefit, particularly if there are concurrent detrusor abnormalities.

TURP is useful in most patients with enlarged glands and in older, debilitated patients. A *retropubic* or a *suprapubic prostatectomy* may be required if the gland is substantially enlarged. All of those operations have a low mortality rate (less than 1% for TURP). Most patients are able to maintain sexual potency regardless of the surgical approach used, although 5 percent to 20 percent of patients experience some postoperative sexual dysfunction. Complete incontinence is unusual, but up to 6 months may be required for patients to regain full sphincter control. Retrograde ejaculation and infertility are near-universal complications of prostatectomy and should be discussed with the patient before operation. A *transurethral incision* of the prostate (TUIP) may be a good choice for a younger man with a small prostate gland and carries a lower risk of retrograde ejaculation.

Prostatic operations for BPH leave a substantial amount of prostatic tissue in place. Postoperative patients have the same future risk of malignancy. Because residual prostatic tissue may continue to grow, patients may have symptom recurrence after surgery. Five percent to 10 percent of men will undergo a second prostatectomy in the 5 years after their first operation.

Balloon dilation can reduce symptoms in select patients, but relapse is common in 2 to 3 years. Newer treatments, including prostatic *stents, microwave* devices, and prostatectomy using *laser* or ultrasound energy are all being studied and becoming available to increase the range of treatment options. Data from randomized controlled clinical trials are needed.

INDICATIONS FOR REFERRAL AND ADMISSION

As noted earlier, prompt urologic consultation is needed when there is evidence of acute retention, hydronephrosis, repeated urinary tract infections, recurrent or refractory gross hematuria, or an elevated creatinine that responds to a period of bladder decompression with catheter drainage. Patients with any change in symptomatology, such as a dramatic increase in urinary frequency or the development of incontinence, must be evaluated immediately. In such cases, the bladder may be acutely distended, which can be confirmed by palpation or catheterization. In this situation, the risk of infection and renal deterioration is high, and prompt attention with hospitalization is indicated.

More commonly, the urologic consultation will be to consider options for dealing with disabling but not renally compromising disease. The urologic assessment can help to elucidate the relationship of symptoms to anatomic and physiologic changes (especially when the presentation is confusing) and to review the interventional approaches to achieving symptomatic relief. The visit can also gauge the patient's willingness to undertake an invasive procedure and its attendant risks.

PATIENT EDUCATION

One cannot overestimate the value of patient education in the effective management of BPH. When patients are provided with information about the waxing and waning natural history of symptoms and the advantages and risks of the full range of treatment options, they are likely to choose differently than if just exposed to a surgical opinion. Reviewing such information enables the primary physician and the patient to make a joint management decision. A joint management strategy ensures a therapeutic approach best suited to the patient's preferences. "Watchful-waiting" is a reasonable choice for patients free of renal impairment or recurrent infection, provided both patient and physician share a commitment to periodic review and reassessment.

TREATMENT RECOMMENDATIONS

- The primary care physician must assess the impact of obstructive symptoms on the patient's quality of life and renal function.
- All patients with prostatism should have a baseline creatinine and urinalysis.
- Routine urinary tract imaging is not necessary. Upper tract imaging, preferably by ultrasonography, is indicated if there is concern for hydronephrosis (a large postvoid residual urine volume or an elevated creatine).
- A urine flow rate measurement may be useful when symptomatology is confusing or ambiguous; it helps to identify patients with symptoms but little evidence of obstruction (peak flow rates over 15 mL/s).
- All patients should be made aware of the possible coexistence of prostate and bladder malignancy with BPH, and the availability of further evaluation for these conditions.
- Most patients can be followed expectantly, unless there is evidence of severe obstruction (hydronephrosis), recurrent or persistent infection, or deterioration in renal function. Such complications warrant prompt surgical attention. Fluid loads and drugs that affect lower urinary tract function must be avoided. Infection should be treated promptly (see Chapters 139 and 140).
- The selective alpha$_1$-blocker *terazosin* (Hytrin), 1 to 2 mg hs, can provide symptomatic relief for some patients, particularly if nocturia is prominent.
- The 5-alpha reductase inhibitor *finasteride,* 5 mg/d, is worth considering in persons with more severe symptoms who cannot or do not want to undergo surgical treatment.

The drug is expensive and may require 6 to 12 months of continuous use before benefit is noted.

- Elective urologic consultation is indicated when the diagnosis is confusing or when quality of life is sufficiently compromised to warrant consideration of an operation to achieve symptomatic relief.
- Less invasive treatments for BPH will provide an increased array of treatment options in the coming years, but *prostatectomy* remains the standard for long-term symptom relief.

ANNOTATED BIBLIOGRAPHY

Barry MJ. Epidemiology and natural history of benign prostatic hyperplasia. Urol Clin North Am 1990;17:495. *(BPH is a disease with variable symptoms; men have about a 35 percent chance of undergoing a prostatectomy in their lifetimes.)*

Barry MJ. Medical outcomes research and benign prostatic hyperplasia. Prostate 1990;3(Suppl):61. *("Watchful waiting" may be a safe strategy for men with symptomatic BPH; surprisingly few studies document the natural history of this disease.)*

Bruskewitz RC, Christensen MM. Critical evaluation of transurethral resection and incision of the prostate. Prostate 1990;3(Suppl):27. *(TUIP is an option for younger patients with small glands.)*

Christensen MM, Bruskewitz RC. Clinical manifestations of benign prostatic hyperplasia and indications for therapeutic intervention. Urol Clin North Am 1990;17:509. *(The urologist's perspective; few noncontroversial indications for a surgical intervention in patients with BPH).*

Finkle AL, Prian DV. Sexual potency in elderly men before and after prostatectomy. JAMA 1966;196:125. *(Eighty-four percent who were potent preoperatively maintained potency after prostatectomy [TURP, perineal, suprapubic]; highest level of impotency occurred with the perineal approach.)*

Gormley GJ, Stoner E, Bruskewitz RC, et al. The effect of finasteride in men with benign prostatic hyperplasia. N Engl J Med 1992;327:1185. *(Symptoms improved, flow increased; slight increase in risk of sexual dysfunction.)*

Lange PH. Is the prostate pill finally here? N Engl J Med 1992;327:1234. *(Suggests that the best finasteride candidates are those with more severe symptoms who are unwilling or unable to undergo surgery.)*

Lepor H. Role of alpha-adrenergic blockers in the treatment of benign prostatic hyperplasia. Prostate 1990;3(Suppl):75. *(Selective alpha$_1$-adrenergic blocker therapy, by reducing bladder neck and prostatic smooth muscle tone, can improve BPH symptoms.)*

McConnell JD. The pathophysiology of benign prostatic hyperplasia. J Andrology 1991;17:356. *(Symptoms of BPH arise from a complex interaction of outflow obstruction and detrusor dysfunction.)*

McConnell JD. Medical management of benign prostate hyperplasia with androgen suppression. Prostate 1990;3(Suppl):49. *(Review of antiandrogenic options for BPH therapy.)*

Mebust WK. Transurethral prostatectomy. Urol Clin North Am 1990;17:575. *(The surgical techniques and complications.)*

Miller-Catchpole R. Endoscopic balloon dilation of the prostate. JAMA 1992;267:1123. *(An assessment of this investigational method; highest success achieved among men with more moderate symptoms and less severe obstruction.)*

Neal DE, et al. Outcome of elective prostatectomy. Br Med J 1989;299:762. *(Nonrandomized cohort study of men undergoing elective prostatectomy; 79 percent had a satisfactory subjective response to surgery; unsatisfactory response to surgery could not be predicted.)*

Rittmaster RS. Finasteride. N Engl J Med 1994;330:120. *(Detailed review of the drug; 69 refs.)*

139

Management of Acute and Chronic Prostatitis

JOHN D. GOODSON, M.D.

Primary Care Medicine: Office Evaluation and Management of the Adult Patient, 3rd edition, edited by Allan H. Goroll, Lawrence A. May, and Albert G. Mulley, Jr. J.B. Lippincott Company, Philadelphia

Prostatitis is the most important cause of urinary tract infection in men. Chronic prostatitis is a common infection that can cause persistent and annoying symptoms, whereas acute prostatitis is less common but potentially much more serious. Both conditions require accurate recognition and treatment by the primary physician; prompt initiation of therapy is especially important for acute prostatitis.

CLINICAL PRESENTATION, PATHOPHYSIOLOGY, AND COURSE

Bacterial prostatitis may ensue from ascending urethral infection, reflux of infected urine, extension of rectal infection, or hematogenous spread. Gram-negative bacilli (predominantly *Escherichia coli*) and *enterococci* account for most of the single isolates obtained from culture. Occasionally, *Chlamydia, Ureaplasma,* a virus, or *Trichomonas* may be the etiologic agent.

Acute Prostatitis. The condition is readily identified by the onset of diminished urine flow, perineal pain, dysuria, and fever. On gentle rectal examination, the gland is enlarged, exquisitely tender, and boggy. Abdominal examination occasionally reveals striking bladder distention. Some patients may appear toxic at the time of presentation.

Chronic Prostatitis. In older men, the symptoms are generally those of bladder outflow obstruction. Patients complain of frequency, dribbling, loss of stream volume and force, double voiding, hesitancy, and urgency. Younger men more often complain of dysuria, dribbling and intermittent discomfort in the perineum, low back, or testicles. Some patients present initially with hematuria, hematospermia, or painful ejaculations. Rectal examination usually reveals an enlarged prostate with a variable amount of asymmetry, bogginess, and tenderness. Untreated or incompletely treated chronic prostatitis is characterized by recurrent symptomatic exacerbations, although these may be separated by long asymptomatic intervals.

Both acute and chronic prostatitis can cause urinary tract and systemic complications. The acutely infected gland may lead to renal parenchymal infection or bacteremia. Rarely, acute infection will progress to a well-defined abscess of the gland. Chronic infection can produce small prostatic stones, which may serve as a nidus for further inflammation and recurrent symptomatic bouts of infection.

Prostatosis mimics the presentation of chronic prostatitis, but cultures are negative and microscopic examination of expressed prostatic secretions shows no white cells. The term *prostatodynia* has been suggested for this condition. Detrusor/internal sphincter dyssynergy may be involved.

DIFFERENTIAL DIAGNOSIS

Acute prostatitis is readily evident by the clinical presentation and exquisitely tender prostate found on rectal examination. However, chronic prostatitis presents a more difficult diagnostic problem, often resembling, in clinical presentation, other common forms of urinary outflow tract obstruction, such as benign prostatic hypertrophy (see Chapter 138), prostatic carcinoma (see Chapter 143), and urethral stricture (see Chapter 134). The lower urinary tract irritative symptoms associated with chronic prostatitis may be seen with urethritis (see Chapter 136), bladder carcinoma (see Chapter 143), sphincter dyssynergy, and neurogenic bladder (see Chapter 134).

WORKUP

History and Physical Examination. For the patient suspected of *acute prostatitis*, history should be noted for acute onset of fever, perineal pain, dysuria, and diminished urine flow indicative of acute prostatitis. A urethral discharge is sometimes reported. Rectal examination confirms the diagnosis by revealing an exquisitely tender prostate gland, which should be examined gingerly to avoid precipitating bacteremia. If there are symptoms of urinary outflow obstruction, then abdominal examination should include checking for bladder distention.

Chronic Prostatitis. When the diagnosis is sought in young persons, inquiry is needed into recurrent perineal, back, or testicular discomfort, dribbling, slow stream, dysuria, and hematospermia. Physical examination of the prostate is done in search of an enlarged, boggy, slightly tender gland. In older men, the diagnosis is very difficult to make clinically, because symptoms are almost indistinguishable from those of prostatic hypertrophy (see Chapter 138).

Laboratory Studies. Because history and physical examination are often inadequate for making a diagnosis of prostatitis, one needs to examine *expressed prostatic secretions* (*EPS*) and may obtain *quantitative bacterial localization cultures* to garner more definitive evidence. Urines representing urethral, bladder, and postprostatic massage specimens (labeled VB_1, VB_2, and VB_3) are collected (see the Appendix), in addition to any EPS that can be obtained as a result of massage. Vigorous massage should be avoided in patients with severe acute prostatitis, because of the risk of inducing bacteremia. Gram's stain of the EPS or the spun VB_3 specimen will often demonstrate organisms or white blood cells (WBC) (>10 WBC per high-power field is abnormal). Less than 10 WBC per high-power field on EPS has an 88 percent specificity for the absence of prostatic infection. Cultures of the EPS and VB_3 should show significant growth (greater than 5000 colonies per milliliter), whereas the VB_1 and VB_2 should be sterile or have a colony count that is one order of magnitude less. Patients with >10 WBC per high-power field but no bacterial growth in the EPS may have chlamydial or ureaplasmal infection and need to be tested for it or treated empirically (see below and Chapters 125 and 136).

Older men without evidence of infection, yet bothered by lower urinary tract irritative symptoms, should have *urine cytologies* performed to help exclude a bladder malignancy. A bladder carcinoma located in the trigonal region may mimic chronic prostatitis. *Cystoscopy* may be indicated when the diagnosis is not confirmed by urine culture data. A *BUN* and *creatinine* should be obtained at the initial visit and periodically thereafter depending on the chronicity and severity of symptoms. An *intravenous pyelogram* is indicated when there is evidence of renal deterioration or symptoms of persistent outflow obstruction.

PRINCIPLES OF MANAGEMENT

Acute Prostatitis accompanied by severe pain, high fever, rigors, and marked leukocytosis requires hospitalization for intravenous antibiotic therapy. Achievement of high tissue drug levels is essential. Such patients should be examined gently for the presence of a fluctuant prostatic mass suggestive of an abscess, which may necessitate surgical drainage. Less toxic patients can be treated as outpatients with an oral antibiotic program. *Trimethoprim–sulfamethoxazole (TMS)*, ciprofloxacin, and *doxycycline* work well. Three weeks of therapy are recommended to prevent acute infection from becoming established. Most other antibiotics effective against gram-negative rods (eg, *amoxicillin*) penetrate the acutely inflamed prostate well and work satisfactorily in the acute phase of illness, but less so in subacute and chronic states.

Local measures can help reduce discomfort. Sitz baths two to three times a day for 20 minutes can relieve perineal pain. Stool softeners, antipyretics, analgesics, and bed rest are all helpful.

Chronic Prostatitis is more difficult to eradicate, partly because of the poor penetration by oral antibiotics into the prostate. Curative antibiotic therapy requires elimination of bacteria from prostatic fluid. Because the gland's secretions are normally acidic (pH 6.5 to 7.4), the most efficacious drugs are those that readily penetrate membranes (lipid-soluble) and become ionically trapped (high pH). *TMS*, the fluoroquinolones (eg, *ciprofloxacin*), and *erythromycin* have these characteristics, with good prostatic fluid levels demonstrated. Because TMS and ciprofloxacin are more effective than erythromycin against gram-negative bacteria, they are preferred. However, TMS is not effective against enterococci. *Carbenicillin* and *doxycycline* also penetrate the prostate reasonably well. The latter is especially active against *Chlamydia* and some *Ureaplasma*.

With chronicity of infection, the prostatic fluid becomes increasingly alkaline, which tends to reduce antibiotic penetration. As a result, prolonged treatment may be necessary. Some patients may not achieve cure even after 6 to 12 weeks of antibiotics. Cure rates with TMS range from 30 percent to 70 percent; slightly higher rates have been reported with 2 to 4 weeks of ciprofloxacin. To demonstrate cure, the EPS and VB_3 should be inspected and cultured after the treatment period to determine the efficacy of therapy.

Patients who achieve a partial response may be given a second extended course of treatment with the same antibiotic. Those failing to demonstrate an organism may benefit from a course of doxycycline or erythromycin (both of which are active against *Ureaplasma* and *Chlamydia*).

The relatively low cure rate achieved with antibiotics in chronic prostatitis requires that therapeutic goals be adjusted to the patient's age. When a cure is not achieved in younger patients, antibiotic therapy is directed toward *suppression* of prostatic inflammation and prevention of upper tract infection or obstruction. One *TMS* tablet daily appears to be an effective suppressive regimen. For older men, transurethral *prostatic resection* or total prostatectomy provides a surgical alternative when repeated courses of antibiotics fail. Both operations are associated with significant morbidity, including possible impotence or sterility and should be reserved for carefully selected patients. Recurrent infection associated with prostatic stones is an indication for removal of the gland.

Local measures can help reduce symptoms in patients suffering from chronic prostatitis. The patient with obstructive symptoms can try voiding while in a warm water bath with pelvic muscles relaxed. The value of *prostatic massage* is a subject of debate. Many claim that prostatic massage will relieve gland congestion in chronic cases and should be repeated every 1 to 2 weeks. (Massage of the acutely infected gland is contraindicated because it can produce bacteremia.) The patient should avoid alcohol, coffee, tea, or other beverages that might produce rapid bladder expansion. The physician should discontinue or reduce the dosage, if possible, of anticholinergics, sedatives, and antidepressants, all of which can impair bladder function (see Chapter 134).

Prostatosis. Alpha-adrenergic blockade has been applied with some success, supporting the view that motor dysfunction may be operative.

PATIENT EDUCATION

Patients should be advised of the chronic and relapsing nature of the disease and alerted to the early signs of infection in the upper urinary tract. They can also be reassured that isolated prostatitis does not cause infertility or impotence. Local symptomatic measures that can be suggested for symptomatic relief include sitz baths and voiding into a warm water bath. The importance of compliance with the prolonged antibiotic course needs to be stressed.

THERAPEUTIC RECOMMENDATIONS

- *Acute prostatitis* requires Gram's stain and culturing of EPS and VB_3, and immediate treatment.
- For the nontoxic patient, oral antibiotic therapy should suffice. Prescribe either *TMS* double-strength (160 mg trimethoprim, 800 mg sulfamethoxazole) bid or *ciprofloxacin* (500 mg bid) for 3 weeks. Amoxicillin (500 mg tid), doxycycline (100 mg bid), and carbenicillin indanyl sodium (1 g qid) are reasonable alternatives. Treatment should be continued for 21 days.
- *Chronic prostatitis* requires a prolonged antibiotic course. *TMS* (double strength bid) for 6 weeks or *ciprofloxacin* (500 mg bid) for 4 weeks is recommended. The latter is considerably more expensive. After treatment, the patient should be followed closely for return of infections. A second antibiotic course of up to 12 weeks' duration with the same or an alternative drug may be necessary in partially responsive infections. Patients who fail to respond initially can be given a 6-week trial of *doxycycline* (100 mg bid), *erythromycin* (500 mg qid), or *carbenicillin* indanyl sodium (1 g qid).
- Prostatosis/Prostatodynia may respond to a trial of an alpha-blocker (eg, terazocin 1–2 mg/d).

INDICATIONS FOR ADMISSION AND REFERRAL

Patients with high fever, leukocytosis, and severe perineal pain need intravenous antibiotics, antipyretics, and analgesics; hospitalization is indicated. In the presence of marked outflow obstruction, suprapubic bladder decompression may be necessary. A fluctuant prostatic mass suggestive of an abscess may require surgical drainage. Until culture and sensitivity data are available, treatment of the toxic patient is directed toward gram-negative bacteria and enterococci, utilizing parenteral ampicillin and gentamycin.

Patients with outflow tract obstruction or refractory chronic infection should have a urologic consultation.

ANNOTATED BIBLIOGRAPHY

Barbalias GA. Prostatodynia or painful male prostate syndrome? Urology 1990;36:146. *(A discussion of pathogenesis and possible mechanisms.)*

Brunner H, Weidner W, Schiefer HG. Studies on the role of *Ureaplasma urealyticum* and *Mycoplasma hominis* in prostatitis. J Infect Dis 1983;147:807. *(Thirteen percent had documented* Ureaplasma *infection; >80 percent responded to tetracycline.)*

Centers for Disease Control and Prevention. Recommendations for the prevention and management of *Chlamydia trachomatis* infections. MMWR;1993;42:1. *(Excellent review of diagnostic methods and authoritative guidelines for treatment; essential reading; 158 refs.)*

Childs SJ. Ciprofloxacin in the treatment of bacterial prostatitis. Urology 1990;35(suppl):15. *(Authors argue the drug is the drug of choice.)*

Drach GW, Nolan PE. Chronic bacterial prostatitis: Problems in diagnosis and therapy. Urology 1986;(Suppl)27:26. *(Using strict criteria, only 20 percent of patients referred for evaluation of prostatitis had definitely positive cultures.)*

Hooper DC, Wolfson JS. Fluoroquinolone antimicrobial agents. N Engl J Med 1991;324:384. *(Effective for many cases of pros-*

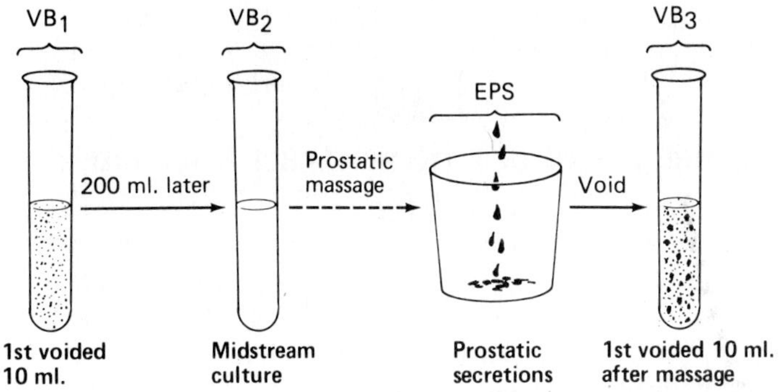

Figure 139-1. Segmented culture of the lower urinary tract in the male. (Adapted from Meares EM, Stamey T. Bacteriologic localization patterns in bacterial prostatitis and urethritis. Invest Urol 1968;5:492.)

tatitis, because they concentrate in prostatic tissue although fluid concentrations are low; ineffective against Chlamydia.*)*

Hooton TM, Wong ES, Barnes RC, et al. Erythromycin for persistent or recurrent nongonococcal urethritis. Ann Intern Med 1990;113:21. *(A 3-week course of treatment proved beneficial, especially in those with prostatitis.)*

Meares EM Jr. Long-term therapy of chronic bacterial prostatitis with trimethoprim–sulfamethoxazole. Can Med Assoc J 1975; 112:225. *(Twelve weeks produced an initially good response in 74 percent, but only 31 percent remained cured for a 30-month follow-up period.)*

Meares EM, Jr. Infected stones of the prostate gland. Urology 1974;4:560. *(Found in 13.8 percent of men; most are asymptomatic, but, where recurrent infection is demonstrated, the gland and stones must be removed.)*

Thin RN, Simmons PD. Chronic bacterial and nonbacterial prostatitis. Br J Urol 1983;55:513. *(The EPS leukocyte counts for bacterial and nonbacterial prostatitis were similar; test highly specific but poorly sensitive.)*

Appendix: Urine and Prostatic Fluid Collections in Men

Standard Clean-Voided Specimen. Specimen collection in the *male* varies with the clinical situation. When cystitis is suspected, the patient is traditionally instructed to retract the foreskin and clean the glans penis with three moist gauze pads or soap sponges. A small amount of urine is voided into the toilet and then a midstream specimen is collected. Cleansing and retraction of foreskin make no difference if a midstream specimen is obtained. However, omitting these steps does lead to contamination of initial specimens. When urethritis or prostatitis is suspected, voided bladder specimens are indicated.

Voided Bladder Specimens. The patient retracts the foreskin and cleans the glans penis. The first 10 mL is collected and labeled VB_1 (voided bladder; Fig. 139–1) and represents a urethral specimen, also useful in cases of suspected urethritis (see Chapters 125 and 136). A midstream specimen is collected in the standard fashion. This specimen is labeled VB_2. The bladder must not be completely emptied. While the patient maintains foreskin retraction with one hand, the physician massages the prostate with continuous strokes. The resulting prostatic fluid is collected in a sterile container labeled EPS (expressed prostatic secretion) and can be used for culture and Gram's or acid-fast stain. If no fluid is obtained, the patient is instructed to milk the penis, starting from the base and moving toward the tip. Finally, if there is still no fluid, the patient is told to void another 10 mL into a sterile container. This specimen is labeled VB_3 and represents roughly a 100:1 dilution of prostatic fluid; it can be cultured or spun and stained. Vigorous prostatic massage can produce a transient bacteremia and should be avoided if acute prostatitis is suspected. If the patient has chronic prostatitis and known valvular heart disease, endocarditis prophylaxis may be necessary (see Chapter 16).

The EPS and VB_3 can be inspected under the microscope for the presence of fat globules, leukocytes, and organisms. If fewer than five leukocytes are seen per high-power field, bacterial prostatic infection is unlikely. A Gram's stain should be prepared and examined, because it may aid in identifying the responsible organism. With bacterial prostatitis, growth will occur in VB_3 and EPS, but not in VB_1 and VB_2. When there is bacterial growth in both VB_2 and VB_3 samples, a prostatic infection may be masked by a bladder infection. In this situation antibiotics that sterilize the bladder contents but do not penetrate the prostate (eg, penicillin G, 500 mg four times a day orally, or Macrodantin, 100 mg three times a day orally) may be given for 2 to 3 days before specimen collection. With bacterial prostatic infection, the EPS will still grow organisms.

Urethral catheterization of the male is rarely required for culture and should be reserved for the symptomatic relief of marked outflow obstruction.

ANNOTATED BIBLIOGRAPHY

Lipsky BA, Inui TS, Plorde JJ, et al. Is the clean-catch midstream void procedure necessary for obtaining routine urine culture specimens from men? Am J Med 1984;76:257. *(Data suggesting the answer is "no.")*

Meares EM, Stamey T. Bacteriologic localization patterns in bacterial prostatitis and urethritis. Invest Urol 1968;5:492. *(Detailed description of methodology and rationale for voided bladder specimens.)*

140
Management of Urinary Tract Infection in Men

Primary Care Medicine: Office Evaluation and Management of the Adult Patient, 3rd edition, edited by Allan H. Goroll, Lawrence A. May, and Albert G. Mulley, Jr. J.B. Lippincott Company, Philadelphia

Urinary tract infection (UTI) is rare in young men, but the incidence begins to increase with age, particularly after age 50. By age 65 it equals that of women. In elderly debilitated patients confined to nursing homes, the prevalence may reach as high as 20 to 50 percent. The primary physician needs to know the clinical significance of UTI in men, what type of workup is indicated, and what modes of therapy are most cost-effective.

PATHOPHYSIOLOGY, CLINICAL PRESENTATION, AND COURSE

Young Men. UTI in young men usually represents *urethritis* or introduction of bacteria through *instrumentation* (eg, bladder catheterization for surgery). At times, a *congenital anomaly* of the urinary tract is responsible, although usually the presentation is at an earlier age. Dysuria, frequency, and urgency accompany most forms, with urethral discharge characteristic of urethritis. Most cases of urethritis are venereal in origin and respond well to treatment (see Chapter 136). Those with an anatomic defect do not improve unless the structural problem is alleviated. Patients who respond fully to a 7-day course of antibiotics are unlikely to have any serious underlying pathology.

In some young men, uncomplicated *cystitis* may develop due to exposure to uropathogenic strains of *Escherichia coli.* The exposure is seen among homosexual men engaging in anal intercourse and in heterosexual men having vaginal intercourse with a colonized partner. Lack of circumcision is a risk factor as is human immunodeficiency virus (HIV) infection with a CD4 lymphocyte count less than 200.

Middle-Aged Men. The increase in rate of UTI that occurs in men aged 50 to 65 parallels the increase in prostate size that occurs with hyperplasia of the gland. The enlargement leads to bladder outflow tract obstruction, and a postvoid residual begins to develop in the bladder. The reduced antibacterial activity of prostatic secretions among men in this age group may also contribute to infection risk. Infection of the prostate may serve as a nidus for recurrent UTI.

Elderly Men. With further prostatic enlargement, the *postvoid residual* and consequently the risk for infection continue to rise. Condom- or urethral-*catheter use,* urinary incontinence, and history of a previous UTI are other risk factors for UTI in this age group. Asymptomatic bacteriuria may occur, especially among nursing home residents. Additional contributing factors include neurogenic bladder dysfunction (see Chapter 134) and *concomitant illness* (pneumonia is a common precipitant of UTI).

Despite the high prevalence of infection with pathogenic organisms, the vast majority of infected elderly men remain asymptomatic and seem to be at low risk for serious complications. However, the usual manifestations of serious, symptomatic UTI may be absent, replaced by such vague findings as "failure to thrive" or worsening mental status. Gram-negative sepsis from a urinary tract source can be life-threatening. Debate continues as to whether bacteriuria per se increases mortality; studies controlling for comorbid conditions show no increase.

Bacteriology. In patients with infection due to a single organism, *E. coli* accounts for about 25 percent of cases, other gram-negative rods (*Proteus, Pseudomonas, Providencia*) for another 50 percent, and *enterococci* and *coagulase-negative staphylococci* for the remaining 25 percent. Those with indwelling catheters and those with recurrent infections and multiple antibiotic exposures are likely to have unusual organisms with multiple antibiotic resistances. Multiple organisms are found in as many as a third of infected nursing home patients.

WORKUP

History and Physical Examination

In men, complaints of dysuria, frequency, and urgency have a predictive value of about 75 percent for UTI. Acute onset of hesitancy, nocturia, slow stream, and dribbling have about a 33 percent predictive value for UTI. No symptoms differentiate upper- from lower-tract infection, with the possible exception of fever (which is rare in men with lower tract disease).

The temperature should be taken and a careful genitourinary tract examination performed. The urethral meatus is examined for erythema and discharge, the testes and epididymides for tenderness and swelling, and the prostate for enlargement, nodularity, and pain to palpation. In the patient with suspected acute prostatitis, palpation should be very gentle to avoid causing a bacteremia. The abdominal examination is checked for suprapubic distention and tenderness in the costovertebral angles.

Laboratory Studies

Urine Culture and Microscopic Examination. Unlike women, men require a urine culture because of the wider range of causative agents and their less predictable drug sensitivities. A diagnosis of UTI is justified on isolation of a pure culture of 10^3 colony-forming units (CFU) per milliliter of urine. A culture that grows fewer than 10^3 CFU/per milliliter or three or more organisms (without one being predominant) is suggestive of contamination. A midstream urine sample or even an initial void sample without prior cleansing of the glans suffices for most clinical situations, even if the patient is uncircumcised. Sensitivity and specificity are in excess of

97 percent. Initial and midstream urine samples correlate very well with bladder specimens ($r = 0.96$).

Both the spun and unspun urines should be examined. The spun sediment is examined for white blood cell (WBC) casts (indicative of pyelonephritis) and pyuria, and gram-stained to identify a predominant organism, if present. The unspun urine is Gram-stained. The finding of a single organism or WBC per high-power field on Gram's stain of the unspun urine has a sensitivity of 85 percent for UTI and a specificity of 0.60, about the same as other rapid diagnostic methods.

Culturing the Incontinent Patient. Those with an indwelling catheter can be cultured by first cleansing the side port of the catheter with a povidone–iodine solution and then drawing up urine through a needle attached to a sterile syringe. A positive culture for urine drawn from an indwelling catheter is the presence of 100 or more CFU per milliliter. Most patients with indwelling catheters have positive cultures.

Culturing an *incontinent patient* without resorting to catheterization can be done by cleansing the glans penis with povidone–iodine solution, applying a fresh *condom catheter* and drainage system, and collecting the first voided specimen in the drainage bag within 2 hours. The criteria for a positive study are more than 10^5 CFU/milliliter; lesser growth is considered to represent contamination.

Straight catheterization and direct bladder aspiration are alternative methods of obtaining urine for culture in incontinent patients. The former carries a slight risk of inducing a bacteremia (see Chapter 16); the latter requires skill in performing the procedure.

Measurement of Renal Function. Some UTIs and their etiologies may compromise renal function. A BUN and creatinine are reasonable determinations. A WBC usually contributes little to diagnosis but may provide confirmatory evidence in the patient who appears toxic.

Intravenous Pyelography (IVP). The dictum that all UTIs in men are complicated (ie, due to an anatomic or functional disruption of the urinary tract) has led many to routinely obtain an IVP when a UTI is detected in a male. In the absence of suspected obstruction or refractory infection, there is little evidence to support such a practice in adult males. (In bacteriuric infants and boys, the situation is different.) Although it is true that there is a high prevalence of abnormalities on IVP in men with UTIs, the contribution of these findings to management is often minimal. Pending better data on who benefits most from IVP study, many authorities recommend reserving the test for those with recurrent infection, suspected upper tract obstruction, or pyelonephritis. The IVP also provides an estimate of the postvoid residual. Renal ultrasound offers a dye-free means of checking for obstruction.

Determination of Residual Volume. In the elderly patient with recurrent UTI, assessment is often directed at identifying risk factors for recurrence. Residual volume is among the most prominent. Straight catheterization after voiding is a simple technique to determine residual volume. It entails a very low risk of infection if done after the urine is sterilized. A volume over 50 mL is abnormal. IVP also provides an estimate of residual volume. Whether reduction in residual volume by treatment of bladder outlet obstruction reduces the risks and morbidity of UTI remains to be determined.

Testing for Prostate Involvement. In the setting of recurrent or relapsing UTI, there is usually some concern that the prostate may be harboring organisms. A *three-glass test,* which includes culture and Gram's stain of the expressed prostatic secretions (see Chapter 139), may provide objective evidence for prostatic infection. However, the test is expensive (several cultures are required), and its interpretation remains uncertain (there is no gold standard test to compare it to). Under most clinical circumstances of recurrent UTI, it is assumed that there is some prostatic involvement and treatment is initiated empirically without the need for such testing (see below). However, when the results of testing for prostate infection would alter clinical decision making (eg, as in planning prostate surgery), then the test may prove worthwhile.

Localization Studies. Differentiating upper- from lower-tract infection would be helpful, because of the implications for clinical course and treatment. Clinical findings are usually nonspecific. Instrumentation (ureteral catheterization, bladder washout) is the only proven method for making such a determination. *Antibody coating* is useful as a research technique, but not in clinical practice because false positives occur in patients with prostatic involvement. The best available test has been the response to an initial course of antibiotics.

Testing for Sexually Transmitted Disease in Young Patients. Sexually transmitted diseases may present with urethral symptoms and mimic UTI. Young patients with acute urethral symptoms, even if unaccompanied by discharge, need to be tested for chlamydial infection, which has reached epidemic proportions among adolescents and young adults. Urethral swabbing is carried out (see Chapters 125 and 136). Methods that can identify chlamydial infection from a urine sample are under development. In addition, any urethral discharge should be Gram-stained, examined for gonococci and leukocytes, and plated promptly on Thayer–Martin media (see Chapter 137).

PRINCIPLES OF MANAGEMENT

Symptomatic Infection

Initial Infection. Acute onset of a symptomatic UTI in a male should be treated. In the absence of evidence for serious renal parenchymal disease or marked obstruction, one can immediately start a course of oral antibiotics. Initial choice of agent is based on Gram's-stain findings, pending culture results. If gram-negative rods are found, then one double-strength tablet of *trimethoprim–sulfamethoxazole (TMS)* twice daily usually suffices. If the organisms are gram-positive cocci, then *amoxicillin* (500 mg tid) represents a better choice. The initial program can be revised, if need be, after urine culture results and antibiotic sensitivities become available. As noted above, urine culturing is important in men because of the wide range of organisms and drug sensitivities.

Unlike women who respond well to single-dose and 3-day treatment regimens, men are customarily treated with a *7- to 10-day* course of antibiotics, based on the view that all male UTIs are at least partially "complicated." There are almost no data on abbreviated antibiotic regimens in men. If symptoms clear, no further evaluation or repeat culturing is necessary.

Refractory or Recurrent Infection. Failure to clear symptoms or quick relapse suggests persistence of the original infection. Prostatic involvement (about half of instances), obstruction, anatomic anomaly, or functional disease may be responsible, necessitating repeat urine culture and consideration of IVP, three-glass testing, and a prolonged course of therapy (6 to 12 weeks) with an antibiotic that both penetrates the prostate and is active against resistant organisms. Many authorities recommend the fluoroquinolone antibiotics in this setting (eg, *norfloxacin,* 400 mg bid). Although a third more effective than *TMS* (which is also prescribed in this setting), the fluoroquinolones are several times more expensive.

Overall, about 65 to 90 percent of men will be cured by a prolonged course of antibiotics. The variability in results depends on the frequency and severity of important underlying pathology. A patient with prostatitis and no postvoid residual has a reasonable chance for cure. But the person with a large postvoid residual is unlikely to achieve lasting benefit until the underlying etiology is addressed. Looking for and correcting any treatable precipitants of infection (obstruction, bladder dysfunction, anatomic anomaly) are likely to be more productive than depending solely on repeated or prolonged courses of increasingly potent antibiotics.

Chronic antibiotic prophylaxis against symptomatic recurrences is sometimes prescribed (eg, tablet of TMS double strength qhs). However, concerns about selecting for resistant strains, drug toxicity, and cost have limited this practice to a very small number of patients (those with frequent incapacitating episodes and those at high risk for a serious complication of infection). Because even the frail elderly have low rates of UTI complications, very few patients are treated with chronic antibiotics.

Asymptomatic Infection

Debate continues on the need to treat the debilitated elderly nursing home patient who has asymptomatic bacteriuria. The issue will remain moot so long as it continues to be virtually impossible to eradicate infection in many such patients, especially those who become incontinent and require indwelling or condom catheterization chronically. In those with an indwelling catheter of over 30 days' duration, infection becomes a near certainty. Antibiotics may temporarily clear the infection, but relapse within 4 weeks is the rule. Only those who become symptomatic derive benefit from a course of antibiotics. More important are regularly scheduled catheter changes, which reduce the risks of encrustation and obstruction. Although the incidence of bacteriuria is lower with use of a condom catheter, it still approaches 40 percent. A daily change of the collecting system apparatus helps to cut the rate of infection.

The role of antibiotic therapy is different for men with asymptomatic bacteriuria who are scheduled to undergo surgery and will require short-term urinary tract instrumentation. Preprocedure urine testing and treatment are essential to avoiding introduction of bacteria into the upper urinary tract and bloodstream. This is especially important for those scheduled to undergo urologic surgery or surgery in which a foreign body is to be introduced. A fluoroquinolone antibiotic is a reasonable choice for antibiotic therapy under these conditions, but culture and sensitivity results are the best determinants of antibiotic choice.

INDICATIONS FOR REFERRAL AND ADMISSION

Any UTI patient who appears toxic or obstructed requires immediate hospitalization. Urosepsis is a potentially life-threatening complication of UTI that necessitates high-dose parenteral antibiotics and prompt evaluation and treatment of the underlying precipitant. Symptoms of pyelonephritis and urosepsis in elderly patients may be vague (change in mental status, new onset of "failure to thrive"), so a high index of suspicion is warranted. The patient with recurrent symptomatic UTI who promptly relapses after a 6-week course of fluoroquinolone therapy should be considered for urologic evaluation, as should the person with UTI in the context of declining renal function. An infectious disease consultant can also be helpful in these difficult situations.

A.H.G.

ANNOTATED BIBLIOGRAPHY

Baldassarre JS, Kaye D. Special problems of urinary tract infection in the elderly. Med Clin North Am 1991;75:375. *(Includes the question of treating asymptomatic bacteriuria.)*

Barnes RC, Daifuku R, Roddy RE, et al. Urinary tract infection in sexually active homosexual men. Lancet 1986;1:171. *(Anal intercourse is a risk factor for cystitis.)*

Boscia JA, Abrutyn E, Kaye D. Asymptomatic bacteriuria in elderly persons: Treat or do not treat? Ann Intern Med 1987;106;764. *(The evidence seems to favor not treating.)*

Lipsky BA. Urinary tract infections in men: Epidemiology, pathophysiology, diagnosis, and treatment. Ann Intern Med 1989; 110:138. *(The best review; 107 refs.)*

Lipsky BA, Ireton RC, Fihn SD, et al. Diagnosis of bacteriuria in men: Specimen collection and culture interpretation. J Infect Dis 1987;155:1341. *(The best study of the question; initial and midstream specimens are equally valid; meatal cleansing unnecessary.)*

Nordenstam GR, Brandberg CA, Oden AS, et al. Bacteriuria and mortality in an elderly population. N Engl J Med 1986;314: 1152. *(No lowering of survival with bacteriuria when cancer is excluded.)*

Ouslander JG, Greengold BA, Silverblatt FJ, et al. An accurate method to obtain urine from culture in men with external catheters. Arch Intern Med 1987;147:286. *(A useful method in incontinent persons that avoids catheterization.)*

Saffaj, Hoagland VL, Cook T. Norfloxacin versus co-trimoxazole in the treatment of recurring urinary tract infections in men. Scand J Infect Dis 1986(suppl)48:48. *(Norfloxacin was about one-third more effective.)*

Smith JW, Jones SR, Reed WP, et al. Recurrent urinary tract infections in men. Ann Intern Med 1979;91:544. *(Half had underlying prostate infection, over 70 percent grew* E. coli *infection; most failed to respond to a standard 10-day course of therapy, whether symptomatic or not.)*

Spach DH, Stapleton AE, Stamm WE, et al. Lack of circumcision increases the risk of urinary tract infection in young men. JAMA 1992;267:679. *(A important risk factor for cystitis in young men.)*

Stamm WE, Hooton TM. Management of urinary tract infections in adults. N Engl J Med 1993;329:1328. *(Includes excellent discussion of UTI in the elderly; 60 refs.)*

Primary Care Medicine: Office Evaluation and Management of the Adult Patient, 3rd edition, edited by Allan H. Goroll, Lawrence A. May, and Albert G. Mulley, Jr. J.B. Lippincott Company, Philadelphia

141

Management of Syphilis and Other Venereal Diseases

HARVEY B. SIMON, M.D.

Syphilis

In 1943, the dramatic efficacy of penicillin treatment was established, and for the next 15 years the incidence of new cases of syphilis declined steadily to a low of about 6500 in 1956. Although *Treponema pallidum,* the spirochete that causes syphilis, has not developed resistance to penicillin, the incidence of syphilis has increased progressively in the last 25 years, largely because of a change in sexual mores, with many new cases occurring in adolescents, young adults, and homosexuals. An accelerating resurgence has been noted among inner city residents, intravenous (IV) drug abusers, and human immunodeficiency virus (HIV)–infected individuals. More than 50,000 cases are now reported each year.

PATHOPHYSIOLOGY AND CLINICAL PRESENTATION

Humans are the only natural reservoir of *T. pallidum.* Except for transplacental transmission, virtually all cases are acquired by sexual contact with persons having active infectious lesions. *T. pallidum* readily penetrates abraded skin and intact mucous membranes to multiply locally and disseminate through the lymphatics and bloodstream.

Clinical Presentation and Course. The course of syphilis can be divided into primary, secondary, latent, and tertiary phases.

Primary Syphilis. The lesion of primary syphilis is the chancre, which occurs at the site of inoculation about 3 weeks after exposure. The chancre is usually located on the genitalia, but, depending on sexual practices, it can occur in the anal canal, on oral mucosa, hands, or even more unusual locations. The lesion begins as a small papule that enlarges and undergoes superficial necrosis to produce an ulcer with a clean base and sharp margins. The chancre is typically painless, and patients are free of constitutional symptoms, although regional nodes may be enlarged. The chancre is teeming with spirochetes and is highly infectious. Even without therapy, the chancre will heal completely in 2 to 6 weeks.

Secondary Syphilis. About 2 months after the primary infection, the features of secondary syphilis may appear. Secondary syphilis is a systemic disease. A flulike syndrome is common, as is generalized lymphadenopathy. The most characteristic feature of secondary syphilis is a generalized skin eruption. Lesions may be macular, papular, or papulosquamous, but tend to be symmetric and uniform in size; typically, the palms and soles are involved. Mucous patches and split papules often occur on the mucous membranes. Secondary syphilis can involve many other organs; clinical manifestations may include aseptic meningitis, hepatitis, nephritis, or uveitis. Patients with secondary syphilis are contagious. As in primary syphilis, the manifestations of secondary syphilis resolve spontaneously even without therapy, although up to 25 percent of patients exhibit a brief relapse of secondary lesions.

Latent and Tertiary Syphilis. Untreated patients without active lesions are considered to have latent syphilis. About two-thirds of these individuals remain entirely asymptomatic, but in the remaining third, the lesions of tertiary syphilis develop, usually 10 to 40 years after primary infection. The major forms of tertiary syphilis include 1) *cardiovascular,* with aneurysmal dilation of the ascending aorta and aortic insufficiency; 2) *neurosyphilis,* which may be asymptomatic or present as general paresis with disorders of intellect and personality, or as tabes dorsalis, with ataxic gait, impaired pain and temperature sensation, autonomic dysfunction, and hypoactive reflexes; and 3) *gummas,* which are isolated, slowly progressive destructive granulomatous lesions of skin, bone, liver, or other organs.

Infection of the Central Nervous System (CNS). CNS infection may occur at any point in the natural history of untreated syphilis and is more likely in HIV-positive patients. Even in the absence of neurologic symptoms, about 25 percent of patients with primary, secondary, or latent infection have cerebrospinal fluid (CSF) abnormalities (pleocytosis, elevated protein, positive syphilis serologies). Although it is not clear how many of these patients will ultimately develop symptomatic neurosyphilis, concern is warranted. Organisms has been isolated from the CNS in 30 percent of patients with untreated primary and secondary disease.

Syphilis and HIV Disease. Patients with syphilis are at increased risk for other sexually transmitted diseases (STDs), including HIV infection. Moreover those with HIV are at increased risk of syphilis. Some studies find that HIV-infected patients have unusually high titers in their syphilis serology, whereas others find seroconversion may be delayed or blunted by concomitant HIV infection, particularly in patients with symptomatic acquired immunodeficiency syndrome (AIDS). In addition to being more common, syphilis in HIV-infected persons may be clinically atypical, unusually severe, or more difficult to treat successfully. CNS syphilis is also more likely in HIV-positive patients.

Congenital Syphilis. This form occurs as a result of transplacental transmission of spirochetes during the second or third trimester of pregnancy. Fetal loss is about 60 percent, and up to half of surviving infants have stigmata, which can result in serious permanent handicaps. Congenital syphilis can be prevented by prompt treatment of maternal infection.

DIAGNOSIS

T. pallidum cannot be cultured in vitro, but the diagnosis of syphilis can be made by direct visualization of treponemas from the chancre. This is a specialized technique that requires *dark-field or fluorescent microscopy* and very experienced observers. As a result, the diagnosis usually depends on clinical features and serologic testing.

The most widely used serologic tests for syphilis use a nontreponemal antigen (lipoidal extract of mammalian tissues). Examples include the *VDRL, Hinton,* and *RPR* tests. These are excellent screening tests, but the false-positive rate is as high as 30 percent, often as the result of unrelated infections or inflammatory diseases that produce hyperglobulinemia. More specific serologic tests use treponemal antigens and can be used to distinguish true-positive from false-positive results. The best of these treponemal tests is the *microhemagglutination*–Treponema pallidum *(MHA-TP)* test (see Chapter 124).

Some patients with primary syphilis manifest falsely negative nontreponemal and treponemal tests. False-negatives are most likely to occur for patients with infections of less than 30 days' duration. Individuals with a suspicious primary lesion should have dark-field examination performed and serologic studies repeated in 10 to 14 days. In *HIV-infected* patients with suspicious skin lesions and negative serology, skin biopsy may be necessary to rule out syphilis. The Warthin–Starry stain can be used to visualize organisms in biopsy specimens.

PRINCIPLES OF MANAGEMENT AND THERAPEUTIC RECOMMENDATIONS

The results of treatment of early syphilis are excellent. *T. pallidum* is very sensitive to *penicillin.* Because the organism multiplies slowly, the goal is to attain relatively low, but long-lasting, antibiotic levels. Present recommendations include the following:

- For early syphilis (incubating, primary, secondary, early latent stages), treat with 2.4 million units of *benzathine penicillin* intramuscularly (IM) at a single session. Penicillin-allergic patients may receive oral *tetracycline* or *erythromycin,* both 500 mg qid for 15 days, or *doxycycline*, 100 mg bid, for 15 days. *Ceftriaxone,* 250 mg IM once daily for 10 days, also appears effective, but experience with its use is limited and penicillin-allergic patients may be allergic to cephalosporins. Doxycycline and tetracycline are contraindicated in pregnancy.
- For syphilis of greater than 1 year's duration (latent or tertiary stages), treat with *benzathine penicillin,* 2.4 million units IM weekly for three consecutive weeks. Substantially higher doses of penicillin should be used for neurosyphilis, which some feel necessitates IV penicillin at so-called meningeal doses. Penicillin-allergic patients should receive oral *tetracycline* or *erythromycin,* 500 mg qid for 30 days, or *doxycycline,* 100 mg bid for 30 days.
- For HIV-positive patients with syphilis and for all HIV-negative persons with untreated syphilis of greater than 1 year's duration, strongly consider lumbar puncture with examination of the CSF for cells, protein, and syphilis serology. If CSF examination is not possible, many authorities recommend that HIV-infected patients with early syphilis be treated with the more prolonged regimens normally used for syphilis of greater than 1 year's duration. If CSF abnormalities document the presence of neurosyphilis, then treatment should be with IV penicillin G, 2 to 4 MU q4h for 10 to 14 days, or procaine penicillin, 2 to 4 MU IM daily, plus 500 mg probenecid qid for 10 to 14 days. Conventional therapy with benzathine penicillin produces only very low CSF drug levels and has failed to eradicate viable organisms in HIV-infected patients. Because there is no proven alternative treatment for neurosyphilis, desensitization should be considered for penicillin-allergic patients.

Immunity to syphilis is incomplete and reinfection may occur, especially in patients treated with penicillin within a year of infection. Follow-up of patients is essential. Quantitative nontreponemal serologies at 3, 6, and 12 months after treatment help determine adequacy of therapy. HIV-infected patients should be followed more closely. Failure to sustain a fourfold decline in titers with therapy suggests treatment failure or reinfection, and CSF examination should be considered. If lumbar puncture is not possible, retreatment with a regimen used for syphilis of greater than 1 year's duration should be considered.

All cases of syphilis should be reported to the appropriate public health authorities so that appropriate case finding can be performed. Like all patients with STDs, syphilis patients need to be screened for other venereal infections, including HIV infection, chlamydial infection, and gonorrhea (see Chapters 7, 125, and 137), and counseled about HIV infection and safer-sex practices.

Chancroid and Granuloma Inguinale

The gram-negative bacillus *Haemophilus ducreyi* causes chancroid, which presents as dirty, shaggy, painful genital ulcers often accompanied by regional adenopathy. Ceftriaxone (250 mg IM once) and erythromycin (500 mg qid for 7 days) are excellent modes of therapy. Trimethoprim–sulfamethoxazole (one double-strength tablet bid for 7 days) is also effective.

Painless, slowly progressive genital ulcers are characteristic of *granuloma inguinale,* caused by the gram-negative bacterium *Donovania granulomatis. Tetracycline* or *eryth-*

romycin is the treatment of choice. Both chancroid and granuloma inguinale are rare in temperate climates.

Lymphogranuloma Venereum

A microorganism belonging to the *Chlamydia* group of obligate intracellular parasites is the cause of lymphogranuloma venereum. In this disease, the primary genital lesion is a small, painless papule that heals spontaneously and often escapes notice. The major impact of the disease is on the regional lymphatics. Inguinal nodes enlarge and may suppurate to produce chronic draining sinuses. Scarring and lymphatic obstruction may result. Rectal fibrosis and strictures are late residua. A 21-day course of doxycycline (100 mg bid) is the treatment of choice. An alternative is erythromycin (500 mg qid for 21 days).

Other Venereal Disease

Gonorrhea. See Chapter 137.
Chlamydial Infection. See Chapters 125 and 136.
HIV Infections. See Chapters 7 and 13.
Herpes Genitalis. See Chapter 192.
Condylomata Acuminata. See Chapter 194.
Pubic Lice. See Chapter 195.

ANNOTATED BIBLIOGRPAHY

Centers for Disease Control. Primary, secondary syphilis—U.S. 1981–1990. MMWR 1991;40:314. *(The changing epidemiology of syphilis.)*

Gourevitch MC, Selwyn PA, Davenny K, et al. Effects of HIV infection on the serologic manifestations and response to treatment of syphilis in intravenous drug users. Ann Intern Med 1993;118:350. *(HIV infection did not alter the clinical presentation or course of syphilis in this cohort.)*

Hart G. Syphilis tests in diagnostic and therapeutic decision making. Ann Intern Med 1986;104:368. *(A critical look at available diagnostic tests.)*

Jackman JD. Cardiovascular syphilis. Am J Med 1989;87:425. *(A review of cardiovascular manifestations of tertiary disease.)*

Musher DM. Syphilis, neurosyphilis, penicillin, and AIDS. J Infect Dis 1991;163;1201. *(Excellent review of the need for intensive therapy in HIV-infected patients.)*

Musher DM, Hamill RJ, Baughn RE. Effect of human immunodeficiency virus (HIV) infection on the course of syphilis and on the response to treatment. Ann Intern Med 1990;113:872. *(Intensive therapy and follow-up are recommended.)*

Romanowski B, Sutherland R, Fick, et al. Serologic response to treatment of infectious syphilis. Ann Intern Med 1991;114: 1005. *(Therapeutic response must be based on illness episode and pretreatment RPR titer; seroreversion can occur after 36 months.)*

Primary Care Medicine: Office Evaluation and Management of the Adult Patient, 3rd edition, edited by Allan H. Goroll, Lawrence A. May, and Albert G. Mulley, Jr. J.B. Lippincott Company, Philadelphia

142
Management of the Patient With Chronic Renal Failure

LESLIE S-T. FANG, M.D.

Although many diseases can lead to chronic renal failure, the resulting clinical manifestations and functional derangements are remarkably constant. The primary physician is often responsible for initial conservative management. The objectives are to prevent or minimize the complications of uremia, monitor disease, and judge progression when referral to the nephrologist is indicated for consideration of dialysis or transplantation.

PATHOPHYSIOLOGY, CLINICAL PRESENTATION, AND COURSE

Pathophysiology

Chronic renal failure can result from glomerular, vascular, or tubular disease. Congenital anomalies, infection, metabolic diseases, obstructive uropathy, and collagen vascular disease can all lead to renal insufficiency. Irrespective of underlying disease, the major clinical manifestations of chronic renal failure result from disturbances in electrolyte and fluid balance, elimination of metabolic wastes and toxins, erythropoietin production, and blood pressure control. The role of urea and other toxins in the production of symptoms remains controversial.

Fluid and Electrolyte Problems. These include hyperkalemia, volume overload, hypocalcemia, hyperphosphatemia, and metabolic acidosis. With moderate renal insufficiency, *urinary concentrating ability* is impaired, so that to handle the same solute load patients have to drink and excrete more water than normal. This results in polydipsia, polyuria, and nocturia. The ability to dilute urine is compromised with further renal impairment, producing isosthenuria and obligate fluid intake. As renal function continues to decline, oliguria supervenes. The situation is similar with sodium; moderate renal failure produces mild *salt wasting*. In the later stages, sodium excretion becomes limited, *salt retention* develops, and edema supervenes.

Potassium excretion is usually preserved until late in the course, when *potassium retention* occurs as oliguria develops and the ability of the distal tubule to secrete potassium is compromised.

Decreased renal function produces *phosphate retention*, *secondary hypocalcemia*, and, consequently, *secondary hyperparathyroidism*. Decreased intestinal calcium absorption secondary to impaired hydroxylation of vitamin D also contributes to hypocalcemia.

Acidosis results from inability to excrete urinary ammonium and, with further impairment, titratable acid. Loss of bicarbonate exacerbates the problem. *Uric acid* levels increase as urate excretion falls.

Endocrine Problems. Impairment of renal endocrine function contributes to anemia, hypertension, and congestive failure, which may further compromise renal function. *Decreased erythropoietin* results in a mild to moderate normochromic normocytic anemia. Anemia also comes as a consequence of increased hemolysis and bleeding, aggravated by impaired platelet adhesiveness. *Increased renin* levels sometimes occur, causing modest hypertension and fluid retention. In addition to renal osteodystrophy, *secondary hyperparathyroidism* may lead to alterations in central nervous system (CNS) calcium, which have been implicated in some of the neurologic manifestations of renal failure.

Hematologic Problems. Anemia in the patient with chronic renal failure develops as renal production of erythropoietin declines. The anemia may be severe enough to cause symptoms, usually occurring when the patient's creatinine rises above 4 mg/dL and the hematocrit falls to less than 25%.

Clinical Presentation and Course

Early in renal failure, anorexia, lassitude, fatigability, and weakness are prominent symptoms. As renal failure worsens, the patient may complain of pruritus, nausea, vomiting, constipation, or diarrhea. Shortness of breath may occur secondary to cardiomyopathy and fluid overload. Edema, hypertension, and pericarditis are common late in the course. Neurologic manifestations include drowsiness, lethargy, peripheral myopathy, seizures, and, terminally, coma.

The course of renal failure is punctuated by periods of rapid deterioration, often precipitated by dehydration or infection. The rate of progression depends, in part, on the underlying renal disease, being more rapid for patients with diabetic nephropathy or severe hypertension and being slower for patients with polycystic kidneys. However, in patients with advanced renal failure (creatinine >10), mean survival without intervention is 100 to 150 days.

PRINCIPLES OF MANAGEMENT

Conservative management of renal failure can prolong survival and preserve quality of life by compensating for the excretory, regulatory, and endocrine functions of the kidney. The goals of therapy are to reduce symptoms, slow progression, and avoid preventable complications.

Protein Intake. The excretory function of the kidneys involves the removal of nitrogenous waste. Reduction of dietary protein intake has long been the cornerstone of therapy for uremia. Early in the course of renal disease, reduction of protein intake helps reduce the rate of progression, but the degree of benefit is actually quite modest. Late in the course of renal disease, reduction of protein intake is useful in preventing azotemia from worsening.

Restricting proteins to 0.5 g/kg/day usually allows sufficient amounts for daily requirements while lessening progression of renal failure. Foods rich in *essential amino acids* are the most effectively utilized source of nitrogen.

Blood Pressure Control. Hypertension is a common complication of renal disease. Rigid control of blood pressure is the most important of factors influencing the rate of disease progression. Blood pressure control is beneficial regardless of the antihypertensive agent or agents employed. However, the best results are associated with use of *angiotensin converting-enzyme (ACE) inhibitors,* particularly if used early. ACE inhibitors are thought to slow the rate of injury by decreasing glomerular hyperfiltration. Renal function should be monitored carefully during ACE inhibitor use because acute deterioration in renal function may be seen in some patients, particularly those with bilateral renovascular disease. Alternative antihypertensive agents include calcium channel blockers, alpha- and beta-blockers, diuretics, and vasodilators. Patients with pronounced proteinuria respond best to aggressive reduction in blood pressure.

Fluids and Electrolytes. Judicious fluid and electrolyte management is exceedingly important because patients with chronic renal failure have difficulty adjusting to variations of either excessive intake or rigid restriction of salt and fluids.

Sodium. In the early and middle stages of renal failure, salt and fluid intake must be adequate to match the excess losses that occur as tubular functions begin to deteriorate. Restriction of intake can actually accelerate renal damage by causing decreased extracellular volume and reduced renal perfusion. Concentrating ability can be measured by determining the specific gravity of a first morning urine specimenand sodium requirements can be estimated by testing a 24-hour urine collection for sodium excretion. In later stages, as excretion of sodium and water becomes limited, cautious sodium and fluid restrictions become necessary.

Potassium. Since potassium excretion is preserved until late in the course of renal failure, there is usually no need to restrict its intake until oliguria sets in. However, it is prudent to *avoid* or at least use with caution *drugs* that predispose to potassium retention, such as potassium-sparing diuretics, potassium supplements, beta-adrenergic blockers, and nonsteroidal anti-inflammatory agents (NSAIDs). Since acidosis worsens hyperkalemia, it should be corrected promptly. On the other hand, severe protracted hypokalemia can itself cause tubular damages; therefore, serum potassium should be monitored regularly and low levels corrected.

Calcium. Hypocalcemia and secondary hyperparathyroidism are best countered by reducing the elevations in serum phosphate that result from decreased renal excretion of the anion. The principle of therapy is to lower serum phosphate by reducing dietary sources, inhibiting absorption, and maintaining adequate calcium levels through pharmacologic doses of *vitamin D* and exogenous *calcium.* In patients with hypocalcemia and hyperphosphatemia, calcium citrate can be used to help with phosphate binding. It should be administered either shortly before or shortly after a meal to maximize phosphate binding. Aluminum hydroxide antacids are now used infrequently because of concern that excessive ingestion may lead to aluminum-induced osteomalacia and neuropathy.

In advanced disease, renal hydroxylation of 25-vitamin D is impaired, necessitating use of 1,25-dihydroxy vitamin D_3. This will reduce the prevalence of secondary hyperparathyroidism and the consequent metabolic bone disease. In patients with severe hyperparathyroidism, partial parathyroidectomy should be considered.

Hyperuricemia. Urate reduction is necessary only if gouty attacks develop (see Chapter 158).

Acidosis. Correction of acidosis becomes desirable when the serum bicarbonate falls below 15 mEq/L. Any external acid loads, such as aspirin, vitamin C, or excess protein intake, should be removed. *Sodium bicarbonate* is given as long as the sodium load can be tolerated. The goal is to titrate the serum bicarbonate level to 16 to 20 mEq/L.

Hematologic Problems. The advent of *recombinant erythropoietin* has greatly enhanced the management of the anemia of chronic renal failure. After patients become symptomatic (usually when the hematocrit falls below 25%), erythropoietin therapy can be started, administered either subcutaneously or intravenously three times per week in doses of 1000 to 6000 U. Patients require close monitoring of hemoglobin, reticulocyte count, and ferritin. Iron supplementation must be provided to patients who are iron deficient to maximize the efficacy of erythropoietin therapy. Most patients with symptomatic anemia respond well, with improvement in quality of life as well as in hematologic parameters. Judicious use of erythropoietin can usually raise the hematocrit to the 30 percent level and avoid the need for repeated transfusions.

Transfusion therapy is sometime used, but repeated transfusions carry the risks of hepatitis (see Chapter 70) and sensitization to leukocyte HLA antigens, which may complicate finding a compatible cadaver donor for renal transplantation.

Patients with chronic renal failure should be cautioned to avoid antiplatelet drugs. Abnormalities in platelet function can be aggravated by drugs such as aspirin and other NSAIDs (see Chapter 81). The abnormalities can be corrected by dialysis or administration of cryoprecipitates, DDAVP, or estrogens. Uremia-induced megaloblastic changes are unresponsive to folate or vitamin B_{12}.

Cardiovascular Complications. The onset of congestive heart failure poses a very difficult problem, especially late in the course of the disease when the ability to excrete sodium may be very limited. *Salt restriction* and a trial of a *loop diuretic* (eg, furosemide) may be tried but are often insufficient. *Metolazone* can be added to a loop diuretic regimen, often augmenting the diuretic effect. Renal function and electrolyte profile should be carefully monitored. Digitalization must be done with care, since renal excretion of digoxin is compromised (see Chapter 32). *Dialysis* may be the only recourse in patients with refractory fluid overload.

Uremic pericarditis is another late cardiovascular complication. Patients may have symptoms of atypical chest pain and progress to pericardial tamponade. The development of pericarditis is an indication to proceed with dialysis.

Neuromuscular Difficulties. Lethargy, inability to concentrate, and asterixis improve with *protein* restriction. However, peripheral neuropathies often progress in spite of comprehensive conservation therapy. Muscle cramping and tetany respond to correction of hypocalcemia.

Itching, Hiccups, and Nausea. These symptoms are not life-threatening but certainly contribute to the patient's misery and require attention. Pruritus can be quite stubborn, but responds to topical measures (see Chapter 178). *Prochlorperazine* is effective in lessening hiccups and nausea.

Adjustment of Medications and Avoidance of Nephrotoxic Agents. Doses of drugs and other substances that are excreted renally or are potentially nephrotoxic must be adjusted. This is one of the most crucial aspects of chronic renal failure management. *Digoxin* (see Chapter 32), *aminoglycoside* antibiotics, radiographic *contrast media*, *ACE inhibitors*, and *NSAIDs* are important examples of agents to be used with extreme care in uremic patients. Elderly azotemic patients, who are likely to have some degree of renovascular impairment, are particularly susceptible to agents that affect the renin–angiotensin system (eg, ACE inhibitors) or inhibit renal prostaglandin production (eg, NSAIDs). Diabetics with underlying renal disease may experience acute deterioration in renal function from a dye load, such as may be administered for angiography or even pyelography.

Not all drugs that cause an elevation in serum creatinine are necessarily nephrotoxic. Cimetidine and trimethoprim compete with creatinine for tubular excretion; elevations in serum creatinine may ensue, especially in patients who are azotemic. Methyldopa and cefoxitin interfere with some autoanalyzer measurements of creatinine and can give falsely elevated readings.

Aggravating Conditions. Of chief importance is early detection and correction of any condition that may further compromise renal function. Urinary tract infection, dehydration, gastrointestinal bleeding, and congestive heart failure can cause acute decompensation.

PATIENT EDUCATION AND SUPPORT

Successful therapy and good morale are strongly dependent on a well-developed doctor–patient relationship. The patient must be educated about chronic renal failure and the rationale behind therapy, because compliance is central to successful conservative management, especially if the treatment requires dietary restrictions. Renal failure is a serious chronic disease, often precipitating depression, denial, anger, and noncompliance. The physician's patience, understanding, support, and interest are powerful but sometimes underutilized elements of the treatment program.

Keeping the patient well informed enhances sense of control and facilitates compliance. Treatment alternatives must be presented honestly and completely. Discussions about diet, medications, prognosis, and therapeutic options should include the family. Psychosocial management should aim at minimizing dependence and social isolation.

INDICATIONS FOR REFERRAL AND ADMISSION

Patients can generally be managed as outpatients, but referral to a nephrologist should be made if there is continued clinical deterioration in spite of maximal supportive therapy. As the serum creatinine approaches 10 mg/dL, mean survival drops to between 100 and 150 days, warranting consideration of dialysis or transplantation. Moreover, vascular access for hemodialysis needs to be constructed with 2 to 3 months of lead time to permit maturation of the fistula and revisions. Decisions regarding dialysis and transplantation require a comprehensive evaluation of the patient's medical, psychologic, and social situation, necessitating a close working relationship among the patient, family, primary physician, and nephrologist.

Continuous ambulatory peritoneal dialysis (CAPD) and *continuous cycling peritoneal dialysis* (CCPD) have provided outpatient options with a high degree of independence for the patient and the physiologic advantage of a slow continuous dialysis process. Dialysate administrations are conducted through an indwelling abdominal catheter three to five times per day. Results are comparable to those for hemodialysis. The main disadvantage is a substantial risk of peritonitis; fortunately, most cases are mild and can be managed on an outpatient basis through self-administration of antibiotics through the catheter.

Hospitalization may be required for control of fluid overload, hypertension, hyperkalemia, or infection. In general, the multiplicity of possible metabolic disturbances in the patient with chronic renal insufficiency demands careful follow-up and constant adjustments of the treatment program.

MANAGEMENT RECOMMENDATIONS

Protein and Calories

- Restrict diet to 0.5 g/kg/day of high-quality protein if the patient is symptomatic or acidotic, 0.5 to 0.75 g/kg/day if the blood urea nitrogen (BUN) is greater than 75 but the patient is asymptomatic.
- Maintain calorie intake at 40 to 50 cal/kg/day.

Fluids

- With mild to moderate renal insufficiency, fluid restriction is not necessary unless there is concomitant hypertension or congestive heart failure.
- Restrict fluids only in the presence of oliguria. Intake should equal urine output and insensible losses.

Hypertension

- ACE inhibitors are the treatment of choice, especially in diabetics and those with marked proteinuria. Begin captopril, 25 mg tid; monitor renal function. Alternatives include alpha- and beta-blockers, calcium channel blockers, and vasodilators (see Chapter 26).
- Attempt to achieve the lowest blood pressure possible in those with marked proteinuria.

Sodium

- With mild to moderate renal insufficiency, salt restriction is not necessary.
- In patients with hypertension or congestive heart failure, salt restriction to 4 g of sodium daily may be necessary.
- Restrict sodium in the presence of oliguria or congestive heart failure.

Potassium

- In hypokalemia, administer potassium supplements in low doses and check levels frequently. Do not maintain indefinite potassium supplementation.
- Avoid potassium-sparing diuretics in patients with moderate renal insufficiency.
- Monitor potassium frequently in oliguric patients. Treat levels above 6 mEq/L and admit if electrocardiographic changes accompany levels greater than 6.5 mEq/L. Mild chronic hyperkalemia is best treated with exchange resins such as sodium polystyrene sulfonate (Kayexalate), given by mouth or instilled as an enema in sorbitol. Kayexalate exchanges sodium ion for potassium ion; therefore, be alert to possible sodium and volume overload.

Calcium and Phosphate

- Correct hyperphosphatemia with calcium citrate (667 mg tid before meals).
- Symptomatic or severe hypocalcemia despite normalization of serum phosphate requires calcium supplements (eg, calcium carbonate 600 mg bid) and/or vitamin D in pharmacologic doses (eg, calcitriol 0.25 mg qd).

Acidosis and Hyperuricemia

- Treat if serum bicarbonate concentration is less than 15 mEg/L.
- Remove external acid load.
- Treat acidosis with sodium bicarbonate, 600 mg twice daily initially, and titrate bicarbonate to the 16 to 20 mEq/L range. Follow serum potassium and calcium levels during treatment of acidosis, since both may fall.
- Treat hyperuricemia only if symptomatic gout develops; use allopurinol (see Chapter 158).

Anemia

- Treat with erythropoietin, 1000 to 6000 U subcutaneously three times per week, monitoring hemoglobin, hematocrit, reticulocyte count, and serum ferritin.
- Avoid antiplatelet drugs.
- Give oral ferrous sulfate, 325 mg per day, to patients with iron deficiency.
- Transfuse for high output failure or angina. Avoid unnecessary blood work and injections.

Congestive Heart Failure

- Treat with restriction of salt.
- Add furosemide if congestive failure persists.
- Add metolazone (2.5–5 mg) if there is refractory fluid overload; monitor renal function and electrolytes closely.
- Consider use of an ACE inhibitor, starting with captopril, 12.5 to 25 mg two or three times daily; monitor renal function closely.

- Digoxin can be used, but frequent monitoring of digoxin levels is needed.

Itching, Hiccups, and Nausea

- Minimize symptoms by reducing dietary protein intake.
- Prescribe prochlorperazine, 5 to 10 mg orally qid for nausea.
- Treat itching topically with menthol or phenol lotion or a trial of capsaicin cream; cholestyramine and ultraviolet light have also been used successfully (see Chapter 178).

Dialysis and Transplantation

- The conservative management outlined is directed toward prolongation of the symptom-free period. If dietary therapy becomes intolerable or is no longer effective, dialysis or transplantation must be considered. Referral to a nephrologist is necessary at this point. The primary physician should continue to participate in the important decisions about dialysis and transplantation.

ANNOTATED BIBLIOGRAPHY

Bennett WM, Aronoff GR, Morrison G, et al. Drug prescribing in renal failure. Am J Kidney Dis 1983;3:155. *(Extensive tables and discussion of dosing guidelines for adults with renal failure, including those on dialysis.)*

Eschback JW. The anemia of chronic renal failure. Kidney Int 1989;35:134. *(Pathophysiology and the effects of recombinant erythropoietin.)*

Evans RW, Rader B, Manninen DL, et al. The quality of life of hemodialysis recipients treated with recombinant human erythropoietin. JAMA 1990;263:825. *(Quality of life as well as hematocrit improved.)*

Fraser CL, Arieff AI. Nervous system complications of uremia. Ann Intern Med 1988;109:143. *(Intellectual dysfunction, dialysis dementia, peripheral neuropathy, and disequilibrium syndrome reviewed; 119 refs.)*

Ihle BU, Becker GJ, Whitworth JA, et al. The effect of protein restriction on the progression of renal insufficiency. N Engl J Med 1989;321:1773. *(Randomized, prospective study; efficacy most pronounced in patients with moderate to severe disease.)*

Klahr S, Levey AS, Beck G, et al. The effects of dietary protein restriction and blood-pressure control on the progression of chronic renal disease. N Engl J Med 1994;330:877. *(A small but significant benefit noted with a low-protein diet; low blood pressure was helpful in patients with pronounced proteinuria.)*

Lewis EJ, Hunsicker LG, Bain RP, et al. The effect of angiotensin-converting-enzyme inhibition on diabetic nephropathy. N Engl J Med 1993;329:1456. *(ACE inhibitor therapy slows progression of renal failure in type I diabetics; benefit found independent of blood pressure effect.)*

Mailloux LU, Bellucci AG, Mossey RT, et al. Predictors of survival in patients undergoing dialysis. Am J Med 1988;84:855. *(Advancing age and diabetes described the highest-risk group, yet these patients still benefitted.)*

Malluche HM, Faugere M-C. Renal osteodystrophy. N Engl J Med 1989;321:317. *(A terse summary of its etiology and treatment.)*

Mooradian AD, Morley JE. Endocrine dysfunction in chronic renal failure. Arch Intern Med 1984;144:351. *(A short but useful summary of the effects of chronic renal failure on endocrine function, including workup and therapy.)*

Nolph KD, Lindblad AS, Novak JW. Continuous ambulatory peritoneal dialysis. N Engl J Med 1988;318:1595. *(Terse but authoritative discussion for the general reader; includes clinical indications and complications.)*

Ravid M, Savin H, Jutrin I, et al. Long-term stabilizing effect of angiotensin-converting enzyme inhibition on plasma creatinine and on proteinuria in normotensive type II diabetic patients. Ann Intern Med 1993;118:577. *(Benefit found in type II diabetics.)*

Sherrard DJ, Andress DL. Aluminum-related osteodystrophy. Ann Intern Med 1989;39:307. *(Review of aluminum toxicity and its consequences.)*

Whelton A, Stout RL, Spilman PS, et al. Renal effects of ibuprofen, piroxicam, and sulindac in patients with asymptomatic renal failure. Ann Intern Med 1990;112:568. *(Prospective study of NSAID effects; some worsening noted, especially with ibuprofen use.)*

Primary Care Medicine: Office Evaluation and Management of the Adult Patient, 3rd edition, edited by Allan H. Goroll, Lawrence A. May, and Albert G. Mulley, Jr. J.B. Lippincott Company, Philadelphia

143
Management of Genitourinary Cancers in Men

Cancers of the genitourinary tract in men are often localized, and, if so, they can be managed by surgery or radiation. Unfortunately, advanced disease is common and requires a team approach involving the surgeon, oncologist, radiotherapist, and primary physician. The responsibilities of the primary physician include prevention, screening for early disease (see Chapter 126), counseling, support, and monitoring of patients with advanced disease. A more active role in therapy has been created by the advent of hormonally active therapy for advanced prostate cancer.

CARCINOMA OF THE PROSTATE

Epidemiology and Risk Factors

Carcinoma of the prostate has become the leading cause of cancer in men, with an estimated 100,000 new cases annually. Incidence appears to be rising, due in part to advances in detection, but perhaps also to increases in dietary, environmental, and genetic precipitants. Evidence is mounting for possible pathogenetic roles for monounsaturated fats, heavy metals, and certain oncogenes. Some familial clustering has been observed, and risk doubles among first-degree relatives. These factors may account for some of the differences in prevalence encountered across geographic and racial boundaries. Testosterone is likely to play a major role, evoked as the cause of the disease's high prevalence among African-American men and its absence among those who have been castrated. No association with benign prostatic hypertrophy or sexual activity has been found. However, age is a major determinant, with incidence and mortality rising sharply after age 50. By the ninth decade, more than 70 percent of men have at least microscopic evidence of prostate carcinoma at autopsy.

Although prostate cancer may be an almost universal affliction of very elderly men, it is far from being harmless. Over 28,000 die annually from the condition, making it the third leading cause of cancer death among men in the United States. Lifetime risk for a 50-year-old man developing clinical cancer is estimated to be 9.5 percent; lifetime risk of dying from the cancer is 2.9 percent.

Pathophysiology, Clinical Presentation, and Course

Most of the prostate cancers found at autopsy are *incidental* and have no clinical import. They are small in volume, well-differentiated, diploid, noninvasive, and originate from the transition zone; prostate-specific antigen (PSA) is normal. *Clinically important* lesions are larger, less well differentiated, invasive, nondiploid, and they originate from the peripheral zone; PSA is elevated. What converts microscopic pathology to clinically evident disease remains unknown. It is estimated that 20 percent of all prostate cancers will become clinically important. They typically progress slowly but steadily and eventually threaten survival.

In 85 percent of cases, clinically evident tumor arises in the *periphery* of the gland (posterior lobe or lamella), making detection by digital examination possible in many instances. However, only 30 percent of new cases are discovered by this means. Many now present with nonpalpable asymptomatic lesions, detected by PSA screening followed by prostate ultrasound (see Chapter 126). Others present with nonspecific symptoms of urethral obstruction (see Chapter 134). Renal insufficiency from prolonged urinary tract obstruction ensues in a small, but important fraction. About 15 percent of patients have bone pain or other manifestations of metastatic disease as the presenting complaint. Osteoblastic metastases predominate; they can be painful and are the major cause of morbidity. Metastasis to regional lymph nodes is both common and usually asymptomatic. It may occur even when disease appears clinically to be confined to the gland and before spread to bone.

Prognosis is a function of disease stage at the time of diagnosis, histologic grade of the tumor, and level of PSA. The majority of patients with prostate cancer will demonstrate metastases at the time of initial presentation, although an increasing number have localized disease due to improved means of early detection. Only a third of the new cases each year will die of the disease. Due to the advanced age of this patient population, many die of other conditions.

Staging

Staging is essential to formulating a prognosis and selecting therapy. However, clinical staging continues to underestimate the extent of disease. Metastases to regional lymph nodes often go undetected. The inadequacy of clinical staging, in part, accounts for the oft-noted poor correlation between clinical stage and response to therapy. It is also the reason for the conflicting reports of treatment results that pervade the prostate cancer literature. Attempts to compensate for the shortcomings of clinical staging and to better estimate the likelihood of metastatic disease include designation of subcategories within each stage and consideration of histologic pattern (patients with higher grade histology are more likely to harbor lymph node metastases).

Determining Extent of Local Disease. The clinical assessment begins with careful *palpation* of the prostate to establish the extent of local tumor. Emphasis is on establishing tumor size and any spread into the surrounding soft tissue. However, digital examination understages about one-third of patients thought to have disease limited to the prostate. *PSA* concentration correlates with tumor volume. Levels in excess of 15 ng/mL (Hybritech assay) suggest extension through the capsule or into the seminal vesicles. Transrectal *ultrasound* and *magnetic resonance imaging (MRI)* are often used to stage local disease, but the accuracy of such imaging studies has been disappointing (range, 58%–69%), necessitating biopsy confirmation of any positive studies. MRI adapted for transrectal use is being studied and may prove better. Computed tomography (CT) is not useful.

Determining Metastatic Involvement. Physical examination initiates the search, with careful palpation of all nodes, bones, and abdomen. *PSA* determination has become increasingly useful. If the PSA concentration exceeds 20 ng/mL (Hybritech assay), distant metastasis to bone is likely and a *bone scan* should be ordered. If the bone scan is positive, more elaborate imaging studies are unnecessary, because the disease is already stage D_2 (see below). A PSA of less than 20 ng/mL greatly reduces the likelihood of bony involvement (less than 1%) and obviates the need for bone scan, but regional metastasis still needs to be considered. *CT scan* of the pelvis and abdomen is often ordered to assess noninvasively pelvic and retroperitoneal lymph node involvement, but results have been disappointing in predicting outcome. Sensitivity is especially poor. Biopsy confirmation of a positive finding is required. *Lymphangiography* has also proven inadequate, due to poor visualization of obturator–hypogastric nodes, which are the only site of nodal disease in up to one third of patients. *Pelvic lymphadenectomy* is the only definitive means of establishing nodal disease, but its morbidity is substantial. It is typically performed when radical prostatectomy is being considered for cure.

Staging Categories and Prognosis. A typical A, B, C, and D staging system is used, based on TMO categories. In *stage A*, there is no palpable evidence of tumor. Disease at this stage consists of malignancy found incidentally during prostatectomy for treatment of benign prostatic hypertrophy. *Stage A_1* represents disease with a microscopic focus of well-differentiated malignant cells occupying less than 5 percent of tissue examined. Risk of progression is low (12%–18%), with little effect on survival of older men. *Stage A_2* denotes multiple foci or more poorly differentiated disease, with a markedly increased risk of mortality if left untreated. Pathologically, as many as 25 percent of these patients already have lymph node metastases.

In *stage B*, there is a palpable prostatic nodule noted on rectal examination. If the lesion is less than 1.5 cm in diameter and confined to one lobe, it is designated *stage B_1*. Clinical B_1 disease usually proves confined to the gland and has a very good prognosis with treatment. If the palpable lesion is greater than 1.5 cm or extends beyond one lobe, it is considered *stage B_2*. Clinical stage B_2 has a 15 to 45 percent chance of having occult metastases to lymph nodes at the time of presentation. Consequently, its prognosis is less favorable. Cure is still possible; failure to treat is potentially fatal.

In clinical *stage C*, rectal examination reveals local extension beyond the prostate to the pelvic wall, seminal vesicles, or bladder neck. In *C_1* disease, tumor is not fixed to the pelvic wall; in *C_2* disease, it is. Bone scan is normal, suggesting localized disease, but 40 to 80 percent of patients at this clinical stage will have lymph node metastases. Thus many people who are clinically stage C already have metastatic disease and a poor prognosis.

Stage D designates metastatic disease. *D_1* denotes spread to pelvic lymph nodes. *D_2* indicates distant metastasis, usually to bone. Palliation is the most that can be expected.

Histologic Grading

Histologic grading helps to overcome some of the prognostic shortcomings of clinical staging. Adenocarcinomas are scorded according to the Gleason system on a 2 to 10 scale and graded on a 1 to 3 scale. The more disrupted and undifferentiated the normal glandular architecture, the higher the grade of tumor and the poorer the prognosis.

Principles of Management

Lacking a better method, selection of treatment modality is determined largely by clinical stage, with some adjustment according to histologic grade (especially in stage A disease).

Stage A_1. Elderly patients with stage A_1 disease and low-grade histology *need not be treated*, because survival is unaffected by the disease. Such patients do require regular follow-up that includes monitoring the PSA, checking the prostate examination, and inquiring about symptoms. Patients with 10 or more years of life expectancy have a definite risk of disease progression and should undergo curative therapy (see below).

Stages A_2 and B. These patients are candidates for curative therapy, either with radical prostatectomy or radiation. The 10-year disease-specific survival rates for these patients are similar for both treatment modalities and approach 90 percent. *External beam radiation* is a relatively low-morbidity procedure and the radiation therapy procedure of choice (implants were previously popular, but associated with an unacceptable rate recurrences). It rarely causes incontinence and preserves potency in well over 50 percent. Proper technique spares permanent rectal injury, although temporary diarrhea, tenesmus, and rectal bleeding may occur. The problem of *residual tumor* after radiation therapy remains unresolved. PSA often remains detectable, and biopsy sometimes reveals residual tumor. Its importance and need for further treatment are subjects of ongoing study. The frequency of the problem is estimated to be as high as 35 percent in patients treated by radiation therapy and is an argument against use of radiation, especially in younger persons who have many years of life expectancy.

Radical prostatectomy used to cause permanent impotence in almost all patients and was shunned by many for that reason. Advances in surgical technique now spare the nerve bundles responsible for erectile function and provide a 50 to 80 percent chance of preserving erectile function. Even if impotence results, the vascular apparatus and capacity for erection via injection therapy remain intact (see Chapter 132). Although postoperative incontinence occurs in most patients, it clears by 5 weeks in over 50 percent, and is a long-term problem in only 5 to 15 percent. Most of the incontinence is mild (one to three pads per day) and of the stress variety. Bilateral pelvic lymphadenectomy is usually performed before removal of the prostate. The frozen-section findings determine candidacy for proceeding with curative surgery. Node dissection and prostatectomy increase the risks of thrombophlebitis and lymphocele. Postoperatively, PSA becomes undetectable when all tumor is removed. Surgery provides an opportunity for 15-year tumor-free survival. Factors favorable to radical prostatectomy are a small stage B lesion (less than 1.5 cm), well-differentiated histology, and the patient's willingness to put up with the adverse consequences of such surgery in return for a chance at prolonged tumor-free survival.

Stage C. Treatment remains unsatisfactory, with the optimal approach yet to be defined. Radiation is useful for local control of tumor, but fails to sterilize pelvic nodes, which have a high probability of involvement with tumor. Surgery fails for similar reasons. *Antiandrogen therapy* (see below) may represent the most effective approach. Studies are in progress.

Stage D. The mainstay of treatment for symptomatic metastatic disease is hormonal manipulation. Prostate cancers contain hormone-dependent and hormone-sensitive cells as well as hormone-independent ones. Hormone-dependent cells die a programmed death in the absence of testosterone. Hormone-sensitive cells stop dividing, but hormone-independent ones continue to grow. As a result, although prostate cancer can be halted by antiandrogen therapy, such treatment does not effect a permanent cure.

Orchiectomy. Castration is the time-honored hormonal manipulation. Bilateral removal of the testes can be done at low cost on an outpatient basis. This reduces by 95 percent total body androgen production. A small amount of adrenal androgen synthesis persists. Psychologically, orchiectomy is difficult for many patients, even the elderly. Prostheses can be placed to lessen the psychological impact.

Luteinizing Hormone–Releasing Hormone (LH-RH) Agonist. A biochemical alternative to castration is desired by many patients. Synthetic peptides that act as *LH-RH agonists* have been developed. *Leuprolide* is the first to be commercially available, packaged as a 7-mg depot preparation given intramuscularly once a month. These agents prevent the pulsatile LH release necessary for testosterone secretion and effect castration levels of testicular androgens, after causing an initial stimulative effect. The LH-RH agonists are convenient to use, effective, and well tolerated, but very expensive, costing several thousand dollars per year. Hot flashes are the main side effect. Because of the drug's initial stimulative effect, it must be used in conjunction with an antiandrogen at the outset of therapy. Some studies suggest combination use with an antiandrogen improves survival (see below).

Estrogen Therapy. The estrogen *diethylstilbestrol* has been used for decades to achieve a "chemical castration." It inhibits LH secretion and competitively blocks circulating androgens. Doses of 3 mg/d halt testosterone production, but are associated with an increased risk of thromboembolic disease. Lower doses (eg, 1 mg/d) and aspirin therapy reduce the thromboembolic risk, but lower doses do not suppress testosterone secretion as well. Gynecomastia is another side effect, which can be prevented by prophylactic low-dose irradiation of breast tissue. Their effect is comparable to orchiectomy in inducing tumor regression. The combination of orchiectomy plus estrogen fares no better than when each is used alone. Moreover, patients failing to respond to orchiectomy are unlikely to benefit from estrogen.

Antiandrogens. These agents block the effects of testosterone at the receptor level, making them useful for countering adrenal androgen secretion and the surge that accompanies early LH-RH agonist therapy. They may be steroidal (eg, megestrol acetate) or nonsteroidal (eg, flutamide). These drugs cannot be used as monotherapy, because they induce an increase in LH release that eventually stimulates sufficient testosterone secretion to overcome their blocking effect. Side effects include gynecomastia and diarrhea; a chemical hepatitis sometimes develops. Although they do not induce a hypercoagulable state or gynecomastia, they can cause impotence.

Combination Therapy. Although monotherapy with a hormonally active agent appears to provide some symptomatic relief (tumor shrinks, bony pain lessens), there is little evidence it prolongs life in patients with metastatic disease. Consequently, such therapy is reserved for onset of symptoms. However, evidence of a survival advantage has begun to emerge with use of combination programs that provide *total androgen blockade* of both of testicular and adrenal androgen sources. Total androgen blockade is a conceptually attractive option for treatment of a testosterone-responsive tumor like prostate cancer. The most widely studied is the combination of *leuprolide plus flutamide*. Significant benefit (2-year increase in survival) has been observed in those with asymptomatic bony metastasis and excellent functional status. Such findings suggest that total androgen blockade be considered early in patients with metastatic disease. Cost could be lowered by substituting orchiectomy for LH-RH agonist therapy. Combination therapy adds little to monotherapy in patients with advanced, symptomatic, metastatic disease. It is best reserved for nonpalliative use.

Secondary Hormonal Therapy. When initial hormonal monotherapy fails, flutamide is sometimes considered. Responses average 6 months and occur in only about 20 percent of patients. Hydrocortisone, aminoglutethamide, and ketoconazole have all been used to suppress adrenal androgen production. Under investigation are the 5-alpha reductase inhibitors (eg, finasteride), which block the peripheral conversion of testosterone to its more active metabolite dihydroxytestosterone.

Much can be done to make the patient with advanced disease comfortable. In addition to the above palliative measures, use of adequate analgesia (see Chapter 91) should not be overlooked.

Radiation and Chemotherapy. External beam radiation is an effective means of palliation for patients with bone pain. It can prevent fracture and is used in cases of impending spinal cord compression (see Chapter 92). Chemotherapy has been disappointing, with no agent altering survival. Response rates are on the order of less than 20 percent.

Monitoring Therapy. The serum *PSA* determination is the best means of monitoring response to therapy. Its 48-hour half-life allows it to reflect quickly changes in tumor activity and mass. The serum concentration directly correlates with tumor burden. Although prostatic procedures may transiently elevate the PSA, it quickly returns to baseline so that interpretation is usually unaffected by recent examinations or procedures.

Although the *bone scan* is sensitive for detection of bony involvement, its findings are not specific. Areas of increased uptake may reflect repair as much as damage. Thus, the test may give confusing information when used to monitor response to therapy. It is best reserved for the initial evaluation or when bone pain of unclear significance arises.

For the asymptomatic patient under no current therapy, regular inquiry into development of *symptoms* has proven an economical yet effective means of monitoring. Routine use of repeat blood tests and radiographic studies can become expensive and should be considered only when the result will substantively alter clinical decision making.

Patient Education and Indications for Referral and Admission

The primary physician has a central role in helping the patient choose among a variety of options that he is likely to face. For the patient with curable disease, the choice will be between radiation and radical prostatectomy. Risks of impotence, incontinence, and recurrence need to be reviewed. For the person with early metastatic disease, the issue of initiating total androgen blockade and whether to undergo orchiectomy or commit to a program of leuprolide therapy will need to be faced. Patients are surprised and comforted to realize they will not undergo feminization after removal of the testes.

These difficult decisions will require consultative help, but the patient will often return to the primary physician for discussion, requiring one to keep current on the options in treatment of prostate cancer. Because the patient knows the primary physician best, the patient is likely to ask his primary care doctor to select the option that would best meet his needs. Phone calls to one's consultants may be helpful in this situation.

Referral to the urologist is indicated at the time a prostate cancer is first suspected. Careful planning of the evaluation is necessary, and a tissue sample will be needed (see Chapter 126). Although most staging of the tumor can be done by the primary physician, the limitations of imaging techniques must be kept in mind. When curable disease is suspected, referrals to the urologist and radiation oncologist are indicated to help in choosing the optimal approach. When metastatic disease is encountered, an oncology consultation may facilitate design of antiandrogen therapy. Urgent hospital admission is indicated if spinal cord compression is deemed imminent (see Chapter 92).

TESTICULAR CANCER

Testicular cancer is the most common malignancy in men between ages 15 and 35 and a major cause of death in this age group. Its seriousness and curability, both in early stages and, more recently, in advanced stages, make it an important disease for the primary physician. One needs to encourage self-examination, screen young men during routine checkups (see Chapter 131), and help guide the patient with advanced disease through his illness.

Pathophysiology, Clinical Presentation, and Course

Known predisposing factors are testicular atrophy (secondary to an undescended testicle) and Klinefelter's syndrome. Suspected risk factors include natural exposure to intrapartum estrogens, exposure to insecticides, and prior history of a testicular tumor. Trauma is not a known precipitant.

Almost all testicular cancers are germ-cell tumors. *Seminomas* account for 40 to 50 percent. Most are confined to the testicle at the time of presentation. The remainder are termed *nonseminomatous germ-cell tumors* (NSGCT). These include *teratomas, choriocarcinomas, embryonal-cell carcinomas,* and *endodermal sinus tumors*. Many are of mixed cell type. Their metastases may be less differentiated than the primary.

Both groups commonly present as solid, painless, nontransilluminating testicular masses in young men (see Chapter 131). Some patients complain of "heaviness" in the scrotum. Pain is less common. These tumors are rapidly growing and spread by the lymphatics and blood. Local extension to the epididymis occurs in 10 percent. Occasionally, the tumor is occult at the primary site with metastases already established. If chorionic gonadotropin is secreted (as may occur with several of the NSGCT), gynecomastia may be an initial complaint. Disease already established in the lung may present with cough or hemoptysis.

Diagnosis and Staging

Any solid, nontransilluminating, painless testicular mass in a young man should be presumed to represent a primary testicular cancer until proven otherwise. *Testicular ultrasound* should be obtained for more definitive determination of the lesion's location. If testicular, prompt urologic consultation is required for consideration of surgical removal of the involved testicle. Testicles with suspicious lesions are subjected to *orchiectomy* through an inguinal canal approach to minimize risk of seeding the scrotum, as might occur with a transscrotal operative procedure. If the lesion is extratesticular, urologic consultation is less urgent but still advisable. Surgical removal is less likely.

Staging Procedures and Surveillance. Staging begins with *orchiectomy* findings and proceeds to *chest x-ray* and *chest CT* for metastatic disease of the chest, and *abdominal CT* for assessment of retroperitoneal lymph nodes. Circulating *tumor markers* also provide ability to detect occult disease. The *beta subunit of human chorionic gonadotropin (HCG)* is always elevated in choriocarcinoma and in about half of the other NSGCT (its elevation is rare in pure seminoma, but a number of seminomatous cases have mixed disease and elevations in HCG). *Alpha-fetoprotein* is produced by about 80 percent of patients with embryonal-cell cancer. Both markers also provide an excellent means of monitoring response to therapy (see below). *Lactic dehydrogenase (LDH)* is sometimes elevated in germ-cell tumors.

False-positive rates are low for abdominal CT, but false-negative rates are as high as 30 percent, with the poorest results in thin persons. Previously, if there was no evidence of metastatic disease by staging studies, then an ipsilateral complete *lymphadenectomy* and contralateral partial lymphadenectomy to the level of the aortic bifurcation were considered mandatory, especially for NSGCT, due to the high incidence of microscopic nodal involvement. However, lymphadenectomy is now being used less, due to advances in chemotherapy, which achieve high rates of cure even if there is delay in diagnosis of metastasis. Moreover, lymph node dissection involves extensive surgery and the risk of ejaculatory failure (a risk reduced by improvements in surgical technique). Finally, retroperitoneal lymph node dissection is unnecessary if the primary cancer is a seminoma and a course of radiation therapy to the nodes (which is highly curative) is being planned. *Lymphangiography* is sometimes useful in seminomatous patients with negative CT examinations. Abnormal paraaortic nodes are detected in 13 to 22 percent.

The decision whether to proceed with nodal dissection or opt for close surveillance using tumor markers and repeat CT scanning remains a judgment call. Factors associated with increased risk of relapse and thus favoring node dissection include high percentage of embryonal carcinoma in the primary, marked degree of local disease, and presence of vascular or lymphatic invasion. If surveillance is elected after orchiectomy, it must be done rigorously, with monthly monitoring of tumor markers, repeat CT scanning every 2 to 3 months, and periodic physical examination. Noninvasive staging may be followed by chemotherapy, with secondary surgical exploration to evaluate the retroperitoneum after treatment.

Clinical Stages. There are a host of staging systems, with one set for seminomatous disease and another for nonseminomatous disease. Common designations are stage I or stage

A for disease confined to the testis; stage II or stage B for spread to regional nodes; and stage III or stage C for spread beyond retroperitoneal nodes. Within each stage there are subcategories denoting increasing degrees of tumor burden.

Management

Treatment decisions are based on stage, histology, and tumor-marker levels.

Seminomatous Tumors. *Stage I* disease is treated with inguinal *orchiectomy* followed by retroperitoneal node *irradiation*. The cure rate is close to 100 percent. Patients who relapse are candidates for combination chemotherapy, which is extremely effective (see below). Patients with *stage IIA* disease are also treated with retroperitoneal radiation, but no longer have prophylactic mediastinal irradiation because of its morbidity and the success of chemotherapy for treatment of relapses. Cure rates are still close to 100 percent at this stage. Patients with *IIB* and stage *III* disease are treated with *cisplatin-based chemotherapy*. Cure rates exceed 90 percent.

Nonseminomatous Tumors. *Stages I and IIA* NSGCT disease are treated with *surgery only*. Surgical cure rates average 95 percent when lymph node dissection shows no regional disease. Even when retroperitoneal disease is detected, lymphadenectomy is likely to suffice for treatment as long as nodes are less than 3 cm in diameter. Patients with stage IIB disease have a high probability of relapse and thus are candidates for chemotherapy, as are patients with stage III disease.

Cisplatin-Based Chemotherapy. Multiple-agent chemotherapy based on cisplatin represented an important breakthrough in treatment of testicular cancer. Even patients with distant metastatic disease now have a high-probability of cure. The need for maintenance therapy has been eliminated. Even the severe nausea and vomiting associated with use of cisplatin has become much less problematic with the advent of *ondansetron,* a seratonin-receptor blocking agent capable of reducing cisplatin-induced emesis. Cisplatin-induced renal toxicity is preventable with good hydration.

Monitoring. Close monitoring of response to therapy is essential. *HCG* and *alpha-fetoprotein* are capable of detecting subclinical relapse and failure to respond to treatment. Resistance to therapy is suggested by an elevated serum marker level failing to decline with therapy. Its rise during follow-up indicates relapse. Patients having isolated elevations in tumor markers as the sole manifestation of relapse have nearly a 100 percent chance of cure when treated promptly with chemotherapy. In patients with advanced disease, a decline in HCG after initial chemotherapy is an excellent predictor of response to treatment. *Periodic physical examination* for development of palpable adenopathy or an abdominal mass and chest and abdominal CT scanning are additional components of the monitoring and surveillance processes (see above).

Patient Education

Although most of the details of care will be related by the oncologist, the primary physician is often consulted by the patient and needs to be familiar with some of the basic questions regarding prognosis, treatment options, and side effects. Patients are greatly relieved to know the favorable prognosis for testicular cancer, especially those with metastatic disease. Nonetheless, treatment is not without its adverse effects. Lymph node exploration is an extensive procedure and thus not without considerable morbidity. Retrograde ejaculation and subsequent infertility are still associated risks, although reduced to about 12 percent. Erection is only rarely compromised. Radiation therapy is associated with a risk of decreased spermatogenesis in the remaining normal testicle, although shielding methods have reduced the radiation exposure and, consequently, the period of infertility due to low sperm counts. Fear of chemotherapy can be lessened by reassurance that there are effective means of minimizing it. If the risk of infertility is greater than 5 percent, sperm banking should be considered prior to treatment. A pretreatment sperm count may be helpful to decison-making.

CARCINOMA OF THE BLADDER

Bladder cancer strikes about 45,000 patients annually in the United States, causing about 10,000 deaths per year. Prevalence is greatest among those aged 60 to 70. Risk factors include smoking, exposure to naphthalene or aromatic amine antioxidants, use of cyclophosphamide, and schistosomiasis. There are no long-term epidemiologic data on the relation between saccharin intake and bladder cancer, although animal studies suggest an association. The issue remains controversial.

Clinical Presentation and Course

Tumors of the bladder are usually detected when gross or microscopic hematuria is noted. In most instances, the hematuria is otherwise asymptomatic, but, in elderly men especially, there may be dysuria, urgency, frequency, or voiding of small volumes of uninfected urine. Such symptoms of vesicle irritation suggest carcinoma in situ. Because urothelial tissue extends up into the ureters and renal pelvis and down into the proximal urethra, cancer of the urothelium can present in any of these areas.

Over 90 percent of bladder cancers are transitional-cell carcinomas; squamous-cell tumors account for most of the others. A few are undifferentiated. Multiple tumors may arise simultaneously. About 80 percent are superficial and remain so; the remainder are invasive from the outset. Depth of invasion is the most important predictor of survival, although histologic grade is also a factor. Five-year survival with appropriate treatment is 95 percent for patients with carcinoma in situ, 60 percent for disease that invades the subepithelial connective tissue, 35 percent for superficial muscle invasion, 15 percent for deep muscle invasion, and nil for extension to the pelvis. Spread to the lymph nodes is common in patients with deep muscle invasion.

Diagnosis and Staging

Cystoscopy and *biopsy* of multiple sites are required for diagnosis. Urine cytology is not sensitive enough to obviate the need for invasive study, although a positive study may provide the only means of detecting an otherwise occult carcinoma in situ. *Intravenous pyelography (IVP)* is obtained for evidence of an infiltrated bladder wall, a filling defect, or a bladder diverticulum.

Staging is performed by *cystoscopy* with *biopsy* and *bimanual rectal–abdominal examination* under anesthesia to determine depth of tumor penetration and infiltration into the bladder wall. Although almost half of patients with infiltration into deep muscle have spread to lymph nodes (which carries a poor prognosis), such spread is hard to detect without resorting to pelvic lymphadenectomy. Early spread involves the hypogastric and obturator nodes. *Abdominal CT scan* is obtained to evaluate them. A chest x-ray, alkaline phosphatase, and bone scan are commonly ordered to check for distant metastases.

Prognosis has also been linked to the presence of blood-group antigens on the surface of bladder cancer cells. Patients with tumors that elaborate A, B, or H antigens have a better prognosis than those that do not. A separate T antigen correlates with invasiveness.

Treatment

Noninvasive stages of disease are often curable with local measures. *Excision* at the time of cystoscopy in conjunction with fulguration represents a most effective form of therapy for early disease. In the setting of multiple tumors, a cytotoxic agent can be instilled. *Thio-TEPA* has been widely used. More recently, *bacille Calmette-Guérin (BCG)* has emerged as superior for treatment of carcinoma in situ in patients with superficial transitional cell disease. It decreases risk of progression to invasive disease and improves survival compared to resection alone. Irradiation of the bladder can effect tumor regression, but the recurrence rate is high. Rapid recurrence of multiple lesions is an indication for combined *cystectomy* and *prostatectomy*. Diffuse carcinoma in situ with persistently positive washings despite treatment has a poor prognosis and may necessitate early cystectomy.

Infiltrative disease carries a poor prognosis due to the substantial likelihood of lymph node metastases (see above). Options include *partial bladder resection, cystectomy* with urinary diversion via an *ileal loop,* radical radiation, and combination therapy. Although partial cystectomy has the attraction of preserving some of the bladder, only a few patients are suitable candidates. *Combination therapy* consisting of *preoperative irradiation* plus *cystectomy* is often used. Complications include a surgical mortality rate of 5 percent, postoperative problems necessitating a prolonged hospitalization in about one quarter, and the possibility of need for revision of the ileal loop. Hyperchloremic metabolic acidosis sometimes occurs in these patients.

Those with *deeply invasive disease* are not candidates for surgery. External beam *megavoltage irradiation* provides a reasonable chance (50%) for local control and a small chance (no more than 25%) for cure. The rate of bowel and bladder complications is 10 to 15 percent. About half of these patients maintain sexual potency. In patients with *distant metastases, cisplatin* in conjunction with *cyclophosphamide* and *doxorubicin* have achieved substantial, but not lasting, regression. Intravesicular cisplatin is associated with anaphylaxis.

Because many patients with bladder cancer present with advanced disease, the focus of treatment is often palliative. If not previously used, radiation can provide relief from pelvic and bone pain. The onset of ureteral obstruction and subsequent uremia presents a relatively comfortable means of dying to patients with advanced disease; relief of the obstruction is rarely indicated.

Monitoring. Monitoring patients treated for early stage disease is essential. Surveillance cystoscopy and washings are conducted every 3 months during the first year and then at less frequent intervals. Monoclonal antibody staining of washings has enhanced detection of tumor cells as has use of hematoporphyrin derivatives, which stain malignant urothelium and make them more visible at cystoscopy.

Patient Education

The best treatment for bladder cancer is prevention. Risk factors such as smoking and occupational exposure should be addressed. Patients who are to undergo cystectomy need prior counseling about management of the ileal loop. Most adjust reasonably well to managing the stoma and bag. Stoma groups and teaching by a stoma nurse can be helpful.

RENAL CELL CARCINOMA (HYPERNEPHROMA)

Renal cancer is uncommon, accounting for less than 2 percent of all cancers. However, it is a potentially curable disease if detected before penetration through the capsule. There is no systemic treatment.

Clinical Presentation and Course

The disease is notorious for its protean presentations. *Painless hematuria* is the most common, found in 50 to 75 percent of cases. Aching flank pain and a palpable mass are other classic, although far less frequent manifestations and represent advanced disease. Unexplained weight loss, nausea and vomiting, fever of unknown origin, and a markedly elevated erythrocyte sedimentation rate (ESR) are sometimes systemic clues of early disease, occurring in up to a third of patients. Paraneoplastic syndromes are associated with this disease, including polycythemia and hypercalcemia secondary to production of a PTH-like substance.

The natural history of the tumor is unique, with spontaneous regression as well as long intervals before the appearance of metastases. Nevertheless, a major proportion of patients with hypernephroma present with or develop metastases.

Diagnosis

A high index of suspicion is needed to make an early diagnosis of this disease. Hematuria in the setting of a normochromic, normocytic anemia and a markedly elevated

ESR are suggestive as is the triad of fever, elevated ESR, and increased $alpha_1$ globulin.

If suspicion remains high, radiologic evaluation should begin with *IVP*. Finding a mass on IVP requires determining whether it is cystic (and therefore most likely benign) or solid. Renal *ultrasound* plus *CT* or *MRI* helps to determine local extent of disease, including perinephric involvement, renal vein obstruction, and spread to the retroperitoneal nodes. MRI has the advantage of detecting vessel invasion and caval thrombosis. Needle aspiration biopsy can be performed under imaging guidance if cytologic confirmation is desired.

Management

Tumor confined to the kidney is curable. When it extends beyond Gerota's capsule, prognosis is poor. Some authorities suggest that removal of the primary tumor may trigger regression of metastases, although the only evidence derives from case reports. Large series have failed to demonstrate such an effect or an improvement in survival. Most argue that the primary tumor in patients with metastatic disease should be removed only for control of local pain or bleeding. Metastases to lung, bone, and brain are treated with chemotherapy or irradiation.

Effective chemotherapeutic regimens are lacking for this disease. Hormonal therapies (progesterone and androgens) achieve responses in about 20 percent of patients but without prolonging survival. Interferon-alpha and interleukin-2 offer the promise of improved response rates and some prolongation of survival. Studies are ongoing.

A.H.G.

ANNOTATED BIBLIOGRAPHY

Prostate Cancer

Adolfsson J, Steineck G, Whitmore WF Jr. Recent results of management of palpable clinically localized prostatic cancer. Cancer 1993;72:310. *(Risk of death reduced by 50 percent with treatment.)*

Barzell W, Bean MA, Hilaris BS, et al. Prostatic adenocarcinoma: Relationship of grade and local extent to the pattern of metastases. J Urol 1977;118:278. *(Clinical stage often underestimates extent of disease.)*

Chodak GW, Thisted RA, Gerber GS, et al. Results of conservative management of clinically localized prostate cancer. N Engl J Med 1994;330:242. *(A pooled analysis of data from over 800 cases favoring initial conservative therapy in older patients with low-grade histology.)*

Chybowski FM, Keller JJ, Bergstraih EJ, et al. Predicting radionuclide bone scan findings in patients with newly diagnosed untreated prostate cancer. J Urol 1991;145:313. *(PSA was found to be superior to other clinical parameters.)*

Crawford ED, Eisenberger MA, McLeod DG, et al. A controlled trial of leuprolide with and without flutamide in prostatic carcinoma. N Engl J Med 1989;321:419. *(Combination therapy was superior to monotherapy in patients with advanced disease.)*

Gittes RF. Carcinoma of the prostate. N Engl J Med 1991;34:236. *(Comprehensive review; especially helpful discussions of staging and treatment; 150 refs.)*

Gittes RF. Prostate specific antigen. N Engl J Med 1987;317:954. *(The most sensitive measure of tumor burden and response to therapy.)*

Glenn JF. Subepididymal orchiectomy: An acceptable alternative. J Urol 1990;144:942. *(The procedure can be done on an outpatient basis with minimal morbidity.)*

Guinan P, Bush I, Ray V, et al. The accuracy of the rectal examination in the diagnosis of prostatic carcinoma. N Engl J Med 1980;303:499. *(It's imperfect and often underestimates the extent of disease, but remains the most important means of early detection.)*

Hanks GE, Krall JM, Pilepich MV. Comparison of pathologic and clinical evaluation of lymph nodes in prostate cancer. Int J Radiat Oncol Biol Phys 1991;21:1099. *(CT scan results were not predictive of response to therapy; lymphadenectomy results were.)*

Johansson JE, Adami HO, Andersson SO, et al. High 10-year survival rate in patients with early, untreated prostatic cancer. JAMA 1992;267:2191. *(Watchful waiting is appropriate for those with stage A_1 who are elderly.)*

Lange PH. Controversies in management of apparently localized cancer of the prostate. Urology 1989;34(suppl 4):13. *(Radiation and radical prostatectomy provide similar 10-year survival rates.)*

Miller JI, Ahmann FR, Drach GW, et al. The clinical usefulness of serum prostate specific antigen after hormonal therapy of metastatic prostate cancer. J Urol 1992;147:956. *(Found to be an excellent method of monitoring response to therapy.)*

Platt JF, Bree RL, Schwab RE. The accuracy of CT in the staging of carcinoma of the prostate. Am J Roentgenol 1987;149:315. *(Poor for local disease; better for retroperitoneal node involvement.)*

Rifkin MD, Zerhouni EA, Gatsonis CA, et al. Comparison of magnetic resonance imaging and ultrasonography in staging early prostate cancer. N Engl J Med 1990;323:621. *(Accuracy is poor for both; positive tests require biopsy confirmation.)*

Testicular Cancer

Cubeddu LX, Hoffmann IS, Fuenmayor NT, et al. Efficacy of ondansetron (GR 38032F) and the role of serotonin in cisplatin-induced nausea and vomiting. N Engl J Med 1990;322:810. *(Helps considerably.)*

Donohue JP, Foster RS, Rowland RG, et al. Nerve-sparing retroperitoneal lymphadenectomy with preservation of ejaculation. J Urol 1990;144:287. *(Advances in technique have reduced the risk of infertility.)*

Dunphy CH, Ayala AG, Swanson DA, et al. Clinical stage I nonseminomatous mixed germ cell tumors of the testis: A clinicopathologic study of 93 patients on a surveillance protocol after orchiectomy alone. Lancet 1988;62:1202. *(The use of surveillance as an alternative to lymph node dissection.)*

Einhorn LH, Donohue J. Cis-diaminedichloroplatinum, vinblastine and bleomycin combination chemotherapy in disseminated testicular cancer. Ann Intern Med 1977;87:293. *(The original report on this most important advance in treatment of testicular cancer.)*

Lange PH, McIntire R, Waldmann TA, et al. Serum alpha fetoprotein and human chorionic gonadotropin in the diagnosis and management of nonseminomatous germ-cell testicular cancer. N Engl J Med 1976;295:1237. *(The original report of the utility of these tumor markers in staging and monitoring.)*

Marks LB, Walker TG, Shipley WU, et al. The role of lymphangiography in staging testicular seminoma. Urology 1991;38:

264. *(Yield is about 15 percent in patients with a negative CT scan.)*

McLeod DG, Weiss RB, Stablein DM, et al. Staging relationships and outcome in early stage testicular cancer. J Urol 1991; 146:1178. *(Excellent outcomes achieved; in excess of 90 percent 5-year survival.)*

Picozzi VJ, Freiha FS, Hannigan JF, et al. Prognostic significance of a decline in serum human chorionic gonadotropin levels after initial chemotherapy for advanced germ-cell carcinoma. Ann Intern Med 1984;100:183. *(A fall in level was very predictive of an excellent long-term response to therapy.)*

Williams SD, Stablein DM, Einhorn LH, et al. Immediate adjuvant chemotherapy versus observation with treatment at relapse in pathological stage II testicular cancer. N Engl J Med 1987;317:1433. *(Equivalent cure rate achieved.)*

Bladder Cancer

Herr W, Laudone VP, Badalament RA, et al. Bacillus Calmette-Guérin therapy alters the progression of superficial bladder cancer. J Clin Oncol 1988;6:1450. *(An important advance in treatment of early superficial disease.)*

Raghavan D, Shipley WM, Garnick MB, et al. Biology and management of bladder cancer. N Engl J Med 1990;322:1129. *(Review of new developments; 155 refs.)*

Renal Cell Carcinoma

Figlin RA, Abi-Aad AS, Belldegrum A, et al. The role of interferon and interleukin-2 in the immunotherapeutic approach to renal cell carcinoma. Semin Oncol 1991;18:102. *(Promising results.)*

Lokich JJ, Harrison JH. Renal cell carcinoma: Natural history and chemotherapeutic experience. J Urol 1975;114:371. *(Still useful descriptions of its myriad presentations and unusual clinical course.)*

Richie JP, Garnick MB, Seltzer S, et al. Computed tomography for diagnosis and staging of renal cell carcinoma. J Urol 1983;129:1114. *(CT provides important information.)*

10

Primary Care Medicine: Office Evaluation and Management of the Adult Patient, 3rd edition, edited by Allan H. Goroll, Lawrence A. May, and Albert G. Mulley, Jr. J.B. Lippincott Company, Philadelphia

Musculoskeletal Problems

144

Screening for Osteoporosis

SAMUEL R. NUSSBAUM, M.D.

One of the major concerns of postmenopausal women is the development of osteoporosis. Osteoporotic fractures in aging women represent a major health problem in industrialized nations. In the United States, approximately 150,000 hip fractures occur annually in women over age 65, with 15 to 25 percent of these women experiencing excess mortality or needing long-term nursing home care. Current expenditures for osteoporotic fractures are well in excess of $7 billion yearly. The pathophysiologic mechanisms for postmenopausal osteoporosis are imperfectly understood, but the means to ensure maximal skeletal growth and strength, prevent loss of bone mass, and noninvasively evaluate bone mass are now available (see Chapter 164).

The frequency and import of the condition combined with capabilities to detect and treat it suggest that screening for osteoporosis might be useful. However, definitive evidence from prospective study proving the efficacy of osteoporosis screening are yet to emerge. Pending such data, the primary care physician needs to exert considerable clinical judgment in selecting candidates for osteoporosis screening. Effective advising of the perimenopausal woman requires knowledge of the epidemiology, risk factors, screening tests, and treatment modalities for osteoporosis.

EPIDEMIOLOGY AND RISK FACTORS

Epidemiology. As the life expectancy of women reaches the mid-80s, osteoporosis takes on epidemic proportions, especially among Caucasian women in industrialized societies. In the United States, incidence estimates for vertebral fracture approach 650,000 cases per year, with a prevalence of 40 percent noted by age 80 in community studies. Estimates for osteoporotic hip fractures range from 150,000 to 250,000 cases per year, and, for wrist fracture, there are an estimated 200,000 cases related to osteoporosis each year. With the aging of the population, these numbers will continue to rise. The degrees of disability and expense attributable to the consequences of osteoporosis are enormous and growing.

Risk Factors. Epidemiologic studies suggest that *inadequate calcium* intake early in life may predispose to lower bone mass and osteoporotic fractures with aging and that calcium supplementation may reduce the risk. However, significant differences in calcium intake between normal and osteoporotic women are yet to be demonstrated, although increase in calcium intake can slow the rate of bone loss in women who have inadequate daily calcium intake (see Chapter 164).

Of the other factors influencing bone mass in elderly women, it is *age, weight, muscle strength,* and *estrogen use* that are most important. A *family history* of osteoporosis, excess *alcohol* consumption, *smoking,* and *inactivity* may also play a role. Women in whom osteoporosis does not develop may have larger skeletal masses, which may be increased through physical activity.

Conditions other than aging that can lead to osteoporosis include Cushing's syndrome, exogenous glucocorticoid administration, chronic heparin therapy, thyrotoxicosis, hypogonadism, hyperprolactinemia, anorexia nervosa, and hyperparathyroidism. However, these diseases represent a small percentage of osteoporotic patients.

Unfortunately, use of clinically available osteoporosis risk factors has proven of limited value in identifying perimenopausal women with low bone mass.

NATURAL HISTORY AND EFFECTIVENESS OF THERAPY

Natural History. The resorption and formation of bone are a continuous process throughout life. Under physiologic circumstances, the rates of these processes are equal and coupled. Skeletal mass is usually maximal by age 35 and declines in women after age 40 and in men after age 50 when the rate of new bone formation does not equal the rate of bone resorption. The rate of decline in skeletal mass is most rapid in women within 2 years of menopause. The greatest loss occurs in the femoral neck and lumbar vertebrae, sites enriched in trabecular bone and subject to future fracture. Cortical bone, comprising 80 percent of skeletal bone, is lost less rapidly.

The progressive decline in skeletal mass becomes clinically manifest when fractures are sustained spontaneously or after minimal trauma. A loss of height and developing kyphosis generally indicates vertebral compression fracture. Fractures most commonly occur in the sacral and lumbar vertebrae, the hip, the humerus, and the wrist. The clinical course and the frequency of fractures in individual patients are hard to predict.

Effectiveness of Therapy (see also Chapter 164). Estrogen replacement can prevent bone loss and even lead to skeletal accretion. Observational studies have consistently noted a 35 to 50 percent reduction in hip, wrist, and vertebral fractures in women who have used estrogen for at least 5 years after menopause. However, if estrogen is discontinued, bone loss rapidly ensues, and it is difficult to reverse the significant bone loss that occurs in the first few years of menopause. Beyond age 75, the effect of as much as 7 to 10 years of estrogen therapy started at the time of menopause is barely appreciable, indicating that very prolonged estrogen therapy or a restarting in later years may be necessary.

Calcium supplementation helps preserve cortical bone mass but does not prevent bone loss to the degree that estrogen therapy does. The combination of calcium supplementation and weight-bearing exercise is more effective at stemming bone loss. Biphosphonate therapy appears promising (see also 164).

SCREENING AND DIAGNOSTIC TESTS

Noninvasive Assessments of Bone Density. Bone mineral density measurements make possible noninvasive assessment for osteoporosis. *Single photon absorptiometry (SPA)* of the *forearm* assesses cortical bone. Accuracy error is about 5 percent. Cost, time to perform study, and radiation exposure are relatively low. *Dual energy x-ray absorptiometry (DEXA)* measures both cortical and trabecular bone in the *spine* and *hip* and total body bone mineral. DEXA provides results that are more accurate and more reproducible than those derived from SPA. Cost is moderate; scanning time and radiation dose are low. *Quantitative computed tomography (QCT)* of the spine best assesses trabecular bone. It is the most costly of available tests, takes the most time, and produces the most radiation exposure.

The use of bone densitometry to predict fracture is based on the view that individuals with lower bone density are more likely to suffer a fracture, either spontaneously or with minimal trauma. Initially, bone density measurement was based on the assumption that there is a fracture threshold below which the risk of spontaneous fracture increases. The threshold concept, although useful, is not strictly correct, because there is a gradient of fracture risk with decreasing bone density. Using SPA of the forearm, the relative risk for hip fracture averages about 1.5 for each standard deviation (approximately 0.1 g/cm^2) decrease in bone mineral density. Measurements at the calcaneus, distal radius, and proximal radius are about equally predictive. Their predictive power also extends to spinal and nonspinal fractures. Preliminary data suggest that DEXA of the spine and hip is also predictive of fracture risk. Vertebral fractures are uncommon when vertebral bone density is greater than 1 g/cm^2 by dual photon absorptiometry or 100 to 110 mg/mL by quantitative CT scanning. These tests are safe and acceptable to patients, but they can be costly when serial testing is required and they involve radiation exposure.

Utility of Bone Densitometry for Osteoporosis Screening. Increasing awareness of the consequences of osteoporosis, coupled with the development of noninvasive techniques for determining bone mass, has led to enthusiasm for screening asymptomatic women for osteoporosis. However, the cost-effectiveness of such testing is the subject of ongoing debate. If bone density measurement will affect clinical decision making, then screening makes sense. The postmenopausal woman already being treated with estrogen replacement or who will be for reasons other than osteoporosis does not require routine measurement of bone mass. The woman at average risk for development of osteoporosis could be monitored for osteoporosis, if rapidly declining bone density would lead to initiation of estrogen therapy. Serial measurements would be required. In a decision-analysis study, screening asymptomatic women was found to be a reasonable cost-effective use of medical resources. However, there are still no data from prospective trials to confirm the value of screening, and widely accepted screening guidelines have yet to be established.

CONCLUSIONS AND RECOMMENDATIONS

- Osteoporosis is a common affliction of postmenopausal women that results in important morbidity. Irreversible bone loss is most rapid in the early phases of menopause, but continues indefinitely.
- Effective therapy for preventing postmenopausal bone loss is available, with estrogen replacement being the most widely used prophylactic measure.
- Clinical and epidemiologic parameters are of limited value in predicting low bone mass.
- Advances in measurement of bone density have improved test accuracy and predictive value for assessing risk of osteoporotic fracture.
- Definitive benefit from screening plus prophylactic therapy remains to be demonstrated by prospective study.
- Pending demonstration of definitive benefit, we recommend consideration of bone mass study (particularly, dual energy x-ray absorptiometry of the spine) in early menopause.
- Criteria for optimal patient selection remain to be defined. Asymptomatic women not already taking estrogen replacement, but who would if bone density were found to be markedly reduced, are reasonable candidates.
- Screening is not recommended when the results will have no effect on decision making (eg, persons already taking estrogen replacement, refusing it, or unable to take it).
- The cost-effectiveness of mass osteoporosis screening of menopausal women remains unproven and cannot be recommended.

ANNOTATED BIBLIOGRAPHY

Bauer DC, Browner WS, Cauley JA, et al. Factors associated with appendicular bone mass in older women. Ann Intern Med 1993;118:657. *(Age, weight, muscle strength, and estrogen use were the major factors.)*

Cummings SR, Black DM, Nevitt MC, et al. Appendicular bone density and age predict hip fracture in women. JAMA 1990;263;665. *(Reduction in bone density found to correlate with risk of hip fracture.)*

Grady D, Rubin SM, Petitti DB, et al. Hormone therapy to prevent disease and prolong life in postmenopausal women. Ann Intern Med 1992;117:1016. *(Includes comprehensive review of the data on costs and benefits of estrogen replacement for prevention of osteoporosis.)*

Hui SL, Slemenda CW, Johnston CC Jr. Baseline measurement of bone mass predicts fracture in white women. Ann Intern Med 1989;111:355. *(Predictive value of wrist bone density measurement demonstrated.)*

Johnston CC, Melton LJ III, Lindsay R, et al. Clinical indications for bone mass measurements. J Bone Miner Res 1989;4(suppl 2):1. *(Review of methods and indications for bone density measurement.)*

Kellie SE, AMA Council on Scientific Affairs. Measurement of bone density with dual-energy x-ray absorptiometry (DEXA). JAMA 1992;267:286. *(A promising method for assessment of bone density.)*

Melton LJ, Eddy DM, Johnston CC Jr. Screening for osteoporosis. Ann Intern Med 1990;112:516. *(A detailed review of the data; 123 refs.)*

Slemenda CW, Hui SL, Langcope C, et al. Predictors of bone mass in perimenopausal women. Ann Intern Med 1990;112:96. *(Risk factors were of limited predictive value; measurement of bone mass necessary.)*

Tosteson AN, Rosenthal DI, Melton LJ III, et al. Cost effectiveness of screening perimenopausal white women for osteoporosis: Bone densitometry and hormone replacement therapy. Ann Intern Med 1990;113:594. *(A decision analysis model that found screening to be cost-effective.)*

145
Evaluation of Acute Monoarticular Arthritis

Primary Care Medicine: Office Evaluation and Management of the Adult Patient, 3rd edition, edited by Allan H. Goroll, Lawrence A. May, and Albert G. Mulley, Jr. J.B. Lippincott Company, Philadelphia

Acute monoarticular arthritis calls for a prompt diagnostic evaluation because of the risk of bacterial infection, which can lead to rapid joint destruction and septic sequelae. Certain noninfectious causes, notably crystal-induced arthritis, also benefit from quick diagnosis and treatment. Most patients present for care on an outpatient basis, making diagnosis of monoarticular arthritis an important responsibility of the primary physician.

PATHOPHYSIOLOGY AND CLINICAL PRESENTATION

The principal mechanisms of monoarticular arthritis can be broadly categorized as inflammatory and noninflammatory, with the inflammatory etiologies subdivided into the infectious and noninfectious.

Inflammatory Disease

Septic arthritis derives predominantly from hematogenous seeding of the synovium. Occasionally it results from direct extension from a site of trauma or from osteomyelitis.

Disseminated Gonorrhea. Among previously healthy, sexually active patients, disseminated gonorrhea is the most frequent etiology of joint infection. Women account for two-thirds of cases. Pregnancy and menstruation appear to increase risk of dissemination. Dissemination occurs in about 1 to 3 percent of individuals with gonorrhea (see Chapter 137). Initially, there is a bacteremic stage with fever, polyarthralgias, transient scattered tendinitis, minimal joint effusion, necrotic skin lesions, positive blood cultures, and sterile joint fluid. This phase of the illness may be followed in several days by a septic joint stage, with monoarticular or occasionally polyarticular pain, marked joint swelling, and effusion. During the septic joint stage, gonococci can be recovered from the joint in about 50 percent of patients.

Nongonococcal Septic Arthritis. Over 80 percent of cases are monoarticular, with gram-positive organisms, especially *Staphylococcus aureus,* predominating (60% of infectious cases and most are methicillin-resistant). *Streptococcus* species account for about 18 percent. *Gram-negative Enterobacteriaceae* also cause septic arthritis, particularly in intravenous (IV) drug abusers, immunocompromised persons, and the chronically ill. Joint sepsis is more likely in patients with altered host defenses (diabetes, cirrhosis, immunodeficient states), previously damaged joints (rheumatoid arthritis), or prosthetic joints. Fever, chills, and joint inflammation are usually prominent, but the presentation may be devoid of systemic symptoms, especially if the patient is debilitated or immunosuppressed. A larger joint, such as a knee or hip, is most likely to be involved. Sternoclavicular joint infection is characteristic of IV drug abusers. Articular destruction can be rapid. Within 10 days of nongonococcal infection, radiographic evidence of cartilaginous and bony damage may appear. Joint injury from gonococcal arthritis is less precipitous, allowing more time for treatment. Permanent damage is uncommon in patients who are treated.

Lyme Disease. An acute oligoarthritis can develop months after the initial infection in untreated persons, with about 60 percent experiencing the problem (see Chapter 160). Large joints are typically involved, especially the knees. Intermittent attacks of acute arthritis lasting weeks to months are sometimes seen as is chronic erosive arthritis. Swelling may be more prominent than pain.

Mycobacterial Infection. Human immunodeficiency virus (HIV)–infected patients are at increased risk for mycobacterial joint infection, as are persons who have had recurrent glucocorticosteroid injections into a joint. Often, periarticular bony disease develops in addition to joint inflammation. A chronic picture remains more common than acute inflammation.

HIV Infection. An acute mono- or oligoarticular arthritis may be part of a syndrome accompanying the onset of HIV infection. The lower extremities are the usual site of involvement (see Chapter 13).

Noninfectious Inflammatory Disease. Acute Gout. Gout is a common cause of acute monoarticular arthritis. Sodium urate crystals in the synovium incite a brisk inflammatory response after their ingestion by polymorphonuclear leukocytes. The condition is found most commonly among middle-aged and older men. Onset is rapid, peaking within 12 to 24 hours. The metatarsophalangeal (MTP) joint of the great toe is the classic site, but midfoot, ankles, knees, wrists, and olecranon bursae are other important locations. Sodium urate crystals are found in the joint fluid. They are needlelike and negatively birefringent under the polarizing microscope. Although the likelihood of a gouty attack increases with serum uric acid, the uric acid level is a poor way to diagnose gout except at the extremes. Alcoholic binges or new use of thiazide diuretics may precipitate gouty attacks. A mild fever may even be present. Rapid response to colchicine helps differentiate crystal-induced arthritis from infection (see Chapter 158).

Pseudogout. Pseudogout results from crystals of calcium pyrophosphate inducing joint inflammation and resembles gout pathophysiologically, although clinical features differ. Knees and wrists are the most common sites. Under the polarizing microscope, synovial fluid will reveal the weakly positively birefringent rhomboid forms of calcium pyrophosphate. Chondrocalcinosis on x-ray is usually present. Pseudogout tends to occur in older patients and seems to be associated with hyperparathyroidism, hemochromatosis, and severe degenerative joint disease.

Other Inflammatory Processes. A host of conditions that typically produce polyarthritis may present initially as monoarthritis. These include rheumatoid arthritis, Reiter's syndrome, ankylosing spondylitis, psoriatic arthritis, the arthritis of inflammatory bowel disease, and the arthritis of sarcoidosis (see Chapter 144).

Noninflammatory Disease

Etiologies include acute traumatic causes such as juxtaarticular ligament or meniscus injury, frank bone fracture extending through to the joint space, or minor trauma in patients with impaired coagulation producing hemarthrosis. A variety of mechanical disorders collectively referred to as "internal derangements" of the knee may produce chronic recurrent pain and noninflammatory effusion. Osteoarthritis, characterized by articular cartilage degeneration and adjacent bony sclerosis and proliferation, often produces chronic, gradually increasing joint symptoms but may present with an acutely painful joint with a noninflammatory or mildly inflammatory effusion.

DIFFERENTIAL DIAGNOSIS

The most immediately important entities in the differential diagnosis of acute monoarthritis are infection, crystal-induced arthropathy, and trauma. The gonococcus is the leading infectious agent, followed in frequency by gram-positive organisms (staphylococci, streptococci) and in compromised hosts by gram-negative coliforms. Gout and pseudogout are the important crystal-induced etiologies.

Several polyarticular diseases may initially present with one acutely inflamed joint or with symptoms that are greatest in a single joint. These monoarticular presentations of polyarticular disease are seen in rheumatoid arthritis, Reiter's syndrome, ankylosing spondylitis, psoriatic arthritis, the arthritis of inflammatory bowel disease, and sarcoidosis.

Despite the wide range of diagnostic possibilities, it should be appreciated that recent series of monoarthritis have revealed that the most prevalent diagnoses are osteoarthritis, septic arthritis, gout, and pseudogout.

WORKUP

The first objective is to establish whether the joint is infected. Although examination of the joint fluid is the single most important diagnostic test, history and physical examination may provide useful information regarding the likelihood of infection as well as its source.

History. Onset, associated symptoms, location, risk factors, and concurrent illness are essential items to check. Abrupt onset in conjunction with fever and chills points to a septic etiology, as does a history of skin lesions, vaginal or urethral discharge, gonorrhea exposure, tick bites, diabetes, concurrent rheumatoid arthritis, joint prosthesis, immunosuppression, HIV infection, IV drug abuse, and previous trauma. Acute trauma raises the probability of periarticular injury, internal derangement, and hemarthrosis. Prior attacks are indicative of gout and pseudogout. Alcohol abuse predisposes to gout, trauma, and infection. Inflammation in the first MTP joint points to gout, especially in an elderly male; but, in diabetics, extension of osteomyelitis into the joint must be ruled out. Associated back pain and stiffness raise the possibility of one of the spondyloarthropathies. Age can be a helpful clue. Pseudogout is most common in older patients. Disseminated gonococcal infection, Reiter's syndrome, and ankylosing spondylitis are diseases of young people.

Physical Examination. All joints are carefully examined to ascertain the location and nature of the problem. Signs of inflammation are sought (increased warmth, swelling, redness, effusion). One needs to differentiate inflammation of the joint space from a periarticular process such as tendinitis, bursitis, or cellulitis, which may be mistaken for it. Sometimes this distinction is impossible to make, but preservation of range of motion despite pain in the area reduces the likelihood of true joint involvement. The probability of a periarticular process is increased by finding localized tenderness not encompassing the entire joint space. Although painful limitation of motion suggests articular disease, tendinitis and cellulitis can also cause discomfort with movement.

Once it is suspected that there is joint inflammation, the focus shifts quickly to differentiating between infectious and noninfectious etiologies. The patient's temperature should be taken. Almost all patients with septic arthritis will be febrile. Low-grade fever may also be noted in gout and rheumatoid arthritis, but a high fever suggests infection. The integument is noted for necrotic lesions on the extremities indicative of gonococcemia, the splinter hemorrhages of endocarditis, skin manifestations of HIV disease (see Chapter 13), needle tracks, tophi, rheumatoid nodules, pitting of the nails and other psoriatic manifestations, erythema nodosum (seen with sarcoidosis and inflammatory bowel disease), and the blisters of keratoderma blennorrhagicum and the circinate balanitis of Reiter's syndrome. The eyes are examined for conjunctivitis and iritis, the fundi for signs of endocarditis, the mouth for mucosal ulceration, and the heart for murmurs. The genitalia need to be checked for signs of gonococcal urethritis and cervicitis (see Chapters 136 and 137). The spine should be examined carefully for restriction of motion and tenderness indicative of spondylitis.

Laboratory Studies. Examination of Joint Fluid. Aspirating and examining joint fluid is the single most important diagnostic procedure in the evaluation of acute monoarticular arthritis. A turbid appearance to the fluid points to an inflammatory etiology, blood suggests trauma or neoplasm, and a clear, straw-colored fluid is seen with degenerative disease and minor trauma. The fluid should be *Gram-stained.* Gram-positive bacteria are seen in about 80 percent of cases where they are the responsible agent. Enterobacteriaceae show up on Gram's stain less frequently. *Neisseria gonorrhoeae* are rarely seen. It is most important to *culture* immediately the joint fluid onto proper media (including Thayer–Martin plates for detection of gonococci). Smears of the joint fluid may show organisms in the absence of a positive culture if antibiotics have already been taken. A repeat tap of the joint will improve the diagnostic yield of Gram's stain and culture if the first arthrocentesis is negative. Synovial fluid should be also be examined for *differential cell count* and *crystals.* A white blood cell (WBC) count in excess of $1000/mm^3$ is suggestive of an inflammatory process. A predominance of neutrophils confirms an inflammatory process. In gout and septic joints, the WBC count often exceeds $50,000/mm^3$. With sepsis, one may aspirate frank pus. Crystal examination using a polarizing lens provides the most rapid and sure method of diagnosing gout and pseudogout. However, urate crystals can often be seen under normal light microscopy; the crystals of pseudogout are harder to identify in this manner. *Glucose* concentration may be low in infection and rheumatoid disease.

Other Testing. Drawing *blood cultures* is indicated when sepsis is suspected. Culturing other possible foci of infection, such as skin lesions, urethral discharge, and cervix, should be considered if infection is a possibility. *Complete blood count* and *erythrocyte sedimentation rate* are moderately helpful in distinguishing inflammatory from noninflammatory disease. The serum *uric acid* level is useful only if extreme.

Serologic Studies. A host of serologic studies can be ordered. However, they are rarely diagnostic of the cause of an acute monoarticular arthritis, and false positives are common in the setting of acute inflammation. Nonetheless, they can be helpful when used carefully. Testing for *HIV antibodies* is indicated when immunocompromise is suspected. *ANA* and *rheumatoid factor* help in the diagnosis of connective tissue disease. *Lyme titers* are of variable utility, but very high levels may add weight to the diagnosis when there is other supporting evidence for the infection.

X-rays of the involved and the contralateral joints should be obtained, although an acutely inflamed joint may show little more than soft-tissue swelling. Plain films may reveal such useful findings as fracture, neoplasm, osteomyelitis, and chondrocalcinosis. The presence of osteoarthritic changes does not make the diagnosis of osteoarthritis, but their absence makes osteoarthritis unlikely. In most inflammatory monoarthritis, the early x-rays are not diagnostic, but they may serve as baseline studies for later comparison. *Magnetic resonance imaging (MRI)* is overused, but the technology is worth considering when the site of inflammation cannot be adequately ascertained clinically or when internal knee injury is suspected and confirmation is required.

Despite optimal efforts, many cases of acute monoarthritis elude diagnosis. In one study, one-third were never satisfactorily diagnosed. Reassuringly, the majority of these patients improved or, at least, did not get worse. If infection, trauma, and, less importantly, crystal-induced arthritis are ruled out, the evaluation can be approached less hurriedly.

SYMPTOMATIC MANAGEMENT

Until a diagnosis is established, the patient may feel better with rest, immobility of the joint, and ice packs. Anti-inflammatory agents should be postponed for at least 12 to 24 hours to allow for cultures to grow and repeat arthrocentesis if the first one is nondiagnostic. If pain is unbearable and a diagnosis is not yet established, an analgesic without anti-inflammatory effects (eg, codeine) may be used. After a second negative arthrocentesis, it is reasonable to institute anti-inflammatory therapy even in the absence of a specific diagnosis, provided all cultures are negative and the patient is deemed at very low risk for infection.

More definitive therapy of acute monoarticular arthritis (see Chapters 137, 156, 158, and 160) requires an etiologic diagnosis.

INDICATIONS FOR REFERRAL AND ADMISSION

Septic arthritis requires hospital admission, treatment with IV antibiotics, and consultation with an infectious disease specialist. Cases of acute monoarticular arthritis that remain undiagnosed but show high WBC counts are at risk for an infectious etiology and require infectious disease consultation for consideration of an empiric course of IV antibiotics. The more chronic case that eludes diagnosis may benefit from a rheumatologic consultation. Closed synovial biopsy or arthroscopy may be needed.

A.H.G.

ANNOTATED BIBLIOGRAPHY

Baker DG, Schumacher HR. Acute monoarthritis. N Engl J Med 1993;329:1013. *(Clinically useful review, with excellent section on analysis of the joint fluid; 60 refs.)*

Edeiken J. Arthritis: The roles of the primary care physician and the radiologist. JAMA 1975;232:1364. *(Differentiates those conditions that have mainly clinical findings from those with specific x-ray manifestations.)*

Freed JF, Nies KM, Boyer RS, et al. Acute monoarticular arthritis: A diagnostic approach. JAMA 1980;243:2314. *(Discusses the prevalence of various diagnoses and which tests were useful; one third of cases were never diagnosed.)*

Fries JF, Mitchell DM. Joint pain or arthritis. JAMA 1976;235: 199. *(Emphasis on clinical diagnosis and judicious use of the laboratory.)*

Gatter RA, Schumacher HR Jr. Joint aspiration: Indications and technique. In Gatter RA, Schumacher HR Jr (eds): A practical handbook of synovial fluid analysis, p 14. Philadelphia: Lea & Febiger, 1991. *(Best guide to joint aspiration.)*

Goldenberg DL. Infectious arthritis complicating rheumatoid arthritis and other chronic rheumatic diseases. Arthritis Rheum 1989;32:496. *(Increased risk of infection; comprehensive review of the issue.)*

Goldenberg DL, Reed JI. Bacterial arthritis. N Engl J Med 1985;312:764. *(Reviews pathophysiology, risk factors, diagnosis, and therapy; emphasizes importance of early recognition and treatment.)*

Holmes K, Counts G, Beaty H. Disseminated gonococcal infection. Ann Intern Med 1971;74:979. *(Arthritis occurred in almost 90 percent with disseminated disease; classic paper describing the syndrome; 141 refs.)*

Pascual E, Tovar J, Ruiz MT. The ordinary light microscope: An appropriate tool for provisional detection and identification of crystals in synovial fluid. Ann Rheum Dis 1989;48:983. *(One does not need a polarizing microscope to identify urate crystals.)*

Rowe IF, Forster SM, Seifert MH, et al. Rheumatic manifestations of human immunodeficiency virus infection. Am J Med 1988;85:59. *(Best description of joint involvement in HIV disease.)*

Steere AC, Schoen RT, Taylor E. The clinical evolution of Lyme arthritis. Ann Intern Med 1987;107:725. *(The multiple presentations of Lyme arthritis.)*

Weissman BN, Hussain S. Magnetic resonance imaging of the knee. Rheum Dis Clin North Am 1991;17:637. *(Good review of indications for its use.)*

Primary Care Medicine: Office Evaluation and Management of the Adult Patient, 3rd edition, edited by Allan H. Goroll, Lawrence A. May, and Albert G. Mulley, Jr. J.B. Lippincott Company, Philadelphia

146
Evaluation of Polyarticular Complaints

Polyarticular complaints are among the most frequent in primary care practice and are often associated with considerable loss of function. Although osteoarthritis accounts for many of the more obvious cases (particularly in the elderly), the differential diagnosis can encompass a bewildering array of conditions, both articular and nonarticular, inflammatory and noninflammatory (Table 146–1). Careful attention to the history and physical examination helps chart a logical course to minimize diagnostic error and cost and maximize patient benefit. In most instances, the workup can proceed in deliberate, sequential fashion, but its pace is best matched to that of the underlying illness. The initial evaluation should focus on answering the following basic questions.

1. Are the patient's complaints truly articular or nonarticular?
2. Is the arthritis inflammatory or degenerative?
3. Is the problem local or systemic?
4. How sick is the patient?

PATHOPHYSIOLOGY AND CLINICAL PRESENTATION

Pathophysiology

Polyarthritis can result from a degenerative, relatively noninflammatory process or from an inflammatory one. *Noninflammatory* forms of arthritis are, in most cases, the result of breakdown in joint cartilage and secondary mechanical disruption of the joint. This can be a primary process, or it can be associated with an underlying disease, such as hemochromatosis. Signs of inflammation are minimal, although occasionally a small joint effusion may be present. Other mechanisms of noninflammatory joint injury include synovial infiltration (amyloidosis), periosteal proliferation at the ends of long bones (hypertrophic osteoarthropathy), and ischemic injury (sickle cell disease).

Table 146-1. Differential Diagnosis of Polyarticular Pain

Inflammatory Joint Disease
Rheumatoid arthritis
Systemic lupus erythematosus
Scleroderma
Psoriatic arthritis
Reiter's syndrome
Ankylosing spondylitis
Polyarticular gout
Pseudogout
Sarcoidosis
Lyme disease
Disseminated gonococcemia
Rheumatic fever
Hepatitis B
Subacute bacterial endocarditis
Vasculitis
Noninflammatory Joint Disease
Osteoarthritis
Hypertrophic pulmonary osteoarthropathy
Myxedema
Amyloidosis
Sickle-cell disease
Inflammatory Periarticular Disease
Polymyalgia rheumatica
Dermatomyositis, polymyositis
Eosinophilia-myalgia syndrome
Noninflammatory Periarticular Disease
Fibromyalgia syndrome
Reflex sympathetic dystrophy

(Adapted from Mainardi CL. In: Kelley WN. Textbook of Internal Medicine. 2nd ed. Philadelphia: J.B. Lippincott, 1993:1002.)

Inflammatory arthritis develops as a consequence of the aggregation of inflammatory cells and their products in the joint space and synovium. Infection, gout, pseudogout, and the immunologically mediated diseases—rheumatoid arthritis (RA), lupus, the spondyloarthropathies—all produce an inflammatory type of arthritis, characterized by joint swelling, warmth, redness, effusion, and tenderness. Joint constituents may be the targets of immunologic attack or may be caught up in a more generalized inflammatory process.

Periarticular disease involving muscles and/or tendons may also present as pain referable to joints, although it is not a true arthritis. Mechanisms range from autoimmune inflammatory processes to purported vasomotor instability.

Clinical Presentation

Inflammatory Polyarthritides. The hallmark of these conditions is synovitis, with manifestations of inflammation encompassing the entire joint.

Rheumatoid Arthritis. RA typically presents in subacute fashion with symmetric polyarthritis, although atypical forms include monoarticular and asymmetric disease. The most common sites are the wrists, proximal interphalangeal (PIP) joints, and metacarpophalangeal (MCP) joints, but elbows, neck, hips, knees, ankles, and feet may also be involved. Extra-articular manifestations include vasculitis, pulmonary nodules or interstitial fibrosis, mononeuritis multiplex, Sjogren's syndrome, and Felty's syndrome (splenomegaly, anemia, thrombocytopenia). Fatigue may dominate the early clinical presentation and precede onset of joint symptoms. Other systemic symptoms (fever, weight loss) are prominent in severe cases. Women are more often affected than men. Morning stiffness is almost universal, with Raynaud's phenomenon a common accompaniment. Rheumatoid factor (RF) is found in approximately 75 percent of cases and is associated with skin nodules and more aggressive articular and extra-articular disease. Tendinous inflammation and joint destruction may ensue, producing characteristic changes (subluxation, swan-neck deformities of the fingers, ulnar deviation of the wrists). Because there is no single defining clinical feature or definitive test, diagnosis requires the presence of a constellation of findings (Table 146-2). Current criteria are believed to have a sensitivity and specificity of approximately 90 percent.

Systemic Lupus Erythematosus (SLE) usually occurs in young women, with a high prevalence in blacks. Malar rash, symmetric polyarthralgias, and nondeforming arthritis are characteristic, as is multisystem involvement, but morning stiffness and joint destruction are not as prominent as in RA. Both large and small vessel vasculitis may occur. Oral ulcers are common. Serositis leading to pleuritis, effusion, or pericarditis develops in about a third of SLE patients. Hematologic manifestations include leukopenia, immune thrombocytopenia, and hemolytic anemia. The most serious complications are glomerulonephritis and cerebritis. Testing for antinuclear antibody (ANA) by indirect immunofluorescence is positive in 95 percent to 99 percent of cases. Antibody to native double-stranded DNA (dsDNA) is specific for lupus and is found in more than 70 percent of cases, especially those with renal involvement. Antibody to the Smith (Sm) antigen is present in 30 percent and is also specific for SLE. Cardiolipin-based serologic tests for syphilis are falsely positive. As with RA, there is no single finding or test diagnostic of SLE, necessitating presence of several characteristic features for confirmation of the diagnosis (Table 146–3).

Systemic Sclerosis (Scleroderma) initially presents either as hand arthralgias, mild inflammatory hand arthritis, or Raynaud's phenomenon. Florid joint inflammation is uncommon. Skin thickening, a hallmark of the condition, follows several months later. Two clinical variants are described. One is a very slowly progressive form that does not lead to significant visceral involvement until decades of activity. It is manifested by CREST syndrome: subcutaneous *c*alcinosis of the digits, *R*aynaud's phenomenon, *e*sophageal dysmotility, *s*clerodactyly, and *t*elangiectasia. In the more aggressive form, there is rapid progression of skin thickening extending to the proximal limbs and trunk (hence the term scleroderma) and accelerated onset of visceral involvement (ie, kidneys, lung, heart, and gastrointestinal tract). The ANA is positive in most patients with diffuse organ system disease, and a speckled pattern is characteristic and disease-specific when it corresponds to antibody to the nuclear enzyme topoisomerase (Scl-70).

Vasculitis may be a consequence of rheumatoid disease (eg, RA, SLE) or an idiopathic necrotizing process that can lead to multisystem injury. Typically, vasculitis comes to attention after the appearance of palpable purpura, livedo reticularis, or skin ulceration, consequences of inflammatory injury to small dermal blood vessels (see Chapter 179).

Table 146-2. Diagnostic Criteria for Rheumatoid Arthritis*

1. Morning stiffness for more than 6 weeks
2. Arthritis involving three or more joint areas for more than 6 weeks
3. Arthritis of hand joints for more than 6 weeks
4. Symmetric arthritis for more than 6 weeks
5. Rheumatoid nodules
6. Serum rheumatoid factor in elevated titers
7. Radiologic changes (bony erosion in or adjacent to involved hand or wrist joints)

*Presence of any four or more criteria is necessary for diagnosis of definite rheumatoid arthritis.

(Adapted from Arnett FC, Edworthy SM, Block DA, et al. The American Rheumatism Association 1987 revised criteria for the classification of rheumatoid arthritis. Arthritis Rheum 1988;31:315.)

Table 146-3. Criteria for Diagnosis of Systemic Lupus Erythematosus (SLE)*

1. Malar rash
2. Discoid rash
3. Photosensitivity
4. Oral or nasopharyngeal ulceration
5. Nonerosive arthritis
6. Pleuritis or pericarditis
7. Persistent proteinuria or casts
8. Seizures or psychosis
9. Hemolytic anemia, leukopenia, or thrombocytopenia
10. Anticulear antibody
11. Anti-DNA antibody, anti-Sm antibody, or false-positive serologic test for syphilis.

*Presence of any four or more criteria is necessary for diagnosis of definite SLE, though many authorities accept fewer criteria in clinical practice, particularly if an antibody test is positive.

(Adapted from Tan EM, Cohen AS, Fries JF, et al. The 1982 revised criteria for the classification of systemic lupus erythematosus. Arthritis Rheum 1982;25:1271.)

Multisystem involvement is characteristic, heralded by neurologic deficits, hematuria/proteinuria, abdominal pain, or asymmetric polyarthritis. Diagnosis is usually made by biopsy of an affected organ; skin is the most convenient.

Mixed Connective Tissue Disease is a term sometimes used to describe an indistinct clinical syndrome that contains features of systemic sclerosis, lupus, and Sjogren's syndrome. With time, the presentation usually evolves into one of these three conditions, leading some to conclude that this is not a unique condition but rather an early, nonspecific clinical presentation.

Psoriatic Arthritis has both peripheral and axial forms. The peripheral form is asymmetric, oligoarticular, and often erosive. The distal interphalangeal (DIP) joints are most often affected, and the nails are pitted. Sausage-shaped digits and a "pencil-in-cup" radiologic appearance of the affected joints because of erosion are found in advanced disease. Psoriatic skin changes (see Chapter 187) usually predate onset of the arthritis, often by months to years, but they can be subtle. The spondylitic form of the disease (associated with HLA-B27 positivity) may resemble ankylosing spondylitis, but the extent of spinal involvement is less.

Reiter's Syndrome is primarily a disease of young men. Oligoarthritis, nongonococcal urethritis, and ocular inflammation (ie, conjunctivitis, iritis) are the defining features. The latter two may be fleeting and nonconcurrent. Dermatologic features include circinate balanitis (shallow, painless ulcers of the glans penis) and keratoderma blennorrhagia (a hyperkeratosis of the feet). Onset is sometimes associated with a recent bacillary dysentery or chlamydial urethritis. HLA-B27 positivity is common and is believed to be related to pathogenesis (shared antigenicity with the infectious agents). Joint involvement is asymmetric and of the lower extremities. Heel pain with plantar fasciitis and calcaneal periostitis is distinctive. Mild spondylitis is common. ANA is negative.

Ankylosing Spondylitis begins insidiously and affects young men most severely, producing inflammation of spinal joints and connective tissue with subsequent calcification and ossification. Characteristic x-ray findings include those of sacroiliitis and diffuse proliferation of syndesmophytes leading to spinal fusion. Peripheral arthritis does occur, more often in women. In men, it tends to develop only after spinal disease has become evident. Large proximal joints such as the hips or knees are the predominant peripheral sites. Uveitis and HLA-B27 positivity are found but are not necessary for making the diagnosis. The arthritis of inflammatory bowel disease shares many of the same features. (See also Chapter 147.)

Polyarticular Gout of an acute nature almost always occurs in patients with a prior history of mono- or oligoarticular gouty attacks, although hyperuricemia is not always present. The acute arthritis may be migratory but usually stays within the lower extremities. Diagnosis is made by finding urate crystals in synovial fluid (see Chapter 145). A chronic arthritis occurs in patients with tophaceous disease. Acute attacks may be superimposed (see Chapter 158).

Pseudogout, like gout, is mostly an acute monoarticular disease but is on occasion polyarticular. Patients are usually elderly with degenerative disease of the knees. The finding of calcium pyrophosphate crystals in the synovial fluid is diagnostic, although cartilage calcification can be seen on x-ray. A subacute form, referred to as "pseudorheumatoid arthritis," has been described, consisting of morning stiffness, synovial thickening, an elevated sedimentation rate, and low titers of RF.

Gonococcal Arthritis is the bacterial arthritis most likely to present in polyarticular fashion. Fever is usually present, and a papulovesicular rash indicative of disseminated disease develops in about two-thirds of cases. Initially, the patient may complain of diffuse polyarticular symptoms, and signs of tenosynovitis may be found in the wrists, fingers, ankles, and toes. These manifestations are followed by a purulent arthritis in a limited number of joints, usually confined to the wrists, knees, or ankles (see Chapter 137).

Acute Rheumatic Fever causes an acute migratory polyarthritis after untreated streptococcal infection. Abrupt onset of arthritis and fever are the predominant manifestations in adults. Both synovitis and periarticular inflammation occur, especially in the knees and ankles. There may be erythema of the overlying skin.

Lyme Disease may begin with migratory polyarthralgias and progress to attacks of asymmetric oligoarthritis in large joints (especially the knees) beginning about 6 months after infection in untreated patients. Later, a chronic mono- or oligoarticular arthritis may follow. The knees are a common site of chronic involvement. Erythema chronica migrans, the diagnostic annular red lesion at the site of the tick bite, occurs in about 80 percent of cases during the early phase of illness. Diagnosis of late disease can be difficult because serologic testing is imprecise (see below and also Chapter 160).

Acute Viral Hepatitis B and other viral infections may present with an immune polyarthritis, often in conjunction with urticaria. The condition is symmetric, affecting the proximal joints of the hands. Onset in hepatitis B is during the preicteric phase. The condition clears spontaneously. (See also Chapter 70.)

Subacute Bacterial Endocarditis also causes an immune-mediated polyarthritis similar to that noted with hepatitis B. Fever, petechiae, splinter hemorrhages, heart murmur, and hematuria may be seen.

Sarcoidosis can cause an acute arthritis of the knees, wrists, PIP joints, and ankles, accompanied by fever and simulating an infectious etiology. Erythema nodosum, hilar adenopathy, and periarticular involvement help to differentiate the condition from other causes. A destructive arthritis develops in a few persons; it is asymmetric and relapsing.

Noninflammatory arthritis produces joint pain with few of the manifestations of inflammation, but sometimes an effusion or even synovial thickening may ensue.

Osteoarthritis (OA) typically presents as deep, aching joint pain that is aggravated by motion and weight bearing as well as periods of inactivity. The involved joint can be enlarged as a result of osteophyte formation, but swelling is usually inconsequential, as soft tissue involvement and inflammation are minimal. In later stages, pain occurs on motion and at rest in conjunction with stiffness. Nocturnal pain after vigorous activity is common. Patients with advanced disease suffer from pain on weight bearing and joint instability. Examination often reveals crepitus and discomfort on movement of the joint. Occasionally, slight warmth is noted in severely affected weight-bearing joints, but erythema and marked warmth are absent. Limitation of motion, malalignment, and bony protuberances from spurs are frequent findings. The joints most commonly affected include the DIP joints of the hands with formation of Heberden's nodes, the carpometacarpal joint at the base of the thumb, the hips, the knees, and the cervical and lumbosacral spine.

Hypertrophic Pulmonary Osteoarthropathy may lead to diffuse bony pain in the lower extremities that is worsened by dependency. New bone formation and periostosis are the source of discomfort. Articular and periarticular complaints may be encountered. Clubbing is a hallmark, although it is not readily evident in about 25 percent of cases. Intrapulmonary pathology is an important precipitant (see Chapter 45).

Hypothyroidism severe enough to cause myxedema is associated with symmetric peripheral joint swelling that can mimic RA. The joint fluid has a low white blood cell count, and there are no clinical signs of inflammation. Nonarticular neuromuscular complaints include myalgias and hand pain related to carpal tunnel syndrome.

Amyloidosis can cause swelling of large joints secondary to synovial infiltration. Its symmetric distribution and gradual onset may simulate an immunologic etiology, but the joint fluid shows no signs of inflammation or immune hyperreactivity. Concurrent involvement of the skin, heart, liver, and peripheral nerves is characteristic. Carpal tunnel syndrome may be present.

Sickle Cell Disease sometimes produces a 2- to 3-week noninflammatory arthropathy that affects large joints and includes swelling, tenderness, and effusion. The synovial fluid is noninflammatory.

Nonarticular Disease

Inflammatory conditions affecting periarticular structures may be reported as joint discomfort even though the disease process spares the joint.

Polymyalgia Rheumatica develops gradually over weeks or months. Pain and stiffness of periarticular structures of neck and shoulders is the presentation in two-thirds of cases, with hip and thigh involvement accounting for the other third. Many complain of both shoulder and thigh involvement. Morning stiffness and pain with movement are highly characteristic; muscle strength is unimpaired. Synovitis has been documented histologically; muscle biopsies are usually normal or show minor inflammatory infiltrates. Sometimes, low-grade fever, weight loss, and fatigue precede the onset of musculoskeletal complaints. The condition is usually symmetric, but if asymmetric it may be mistaken for shoulder bursitis or hip arthritis. Most patients are elderly. The association with cranial arteritis makes this an important condition to recognize. Marked elevation of the sedimentation rate is characteristic. There are no serologic abnormalities (eee also Chapter 161).

Myositis of any type may present as musculoskeletal pain and be confused with polyarthritis, although weakness is typically more prominent than pain. *Polymyositis* is the prototypical inflammatory muscle disease, characterized by proximal muscle weakness, soreness, and elevated muscle enzymes. It may present as *dermatomyositis* in the elderly. *Eosinophilia-myalgia* syndrome is a serious myositis observed in association with ingestion of L-tryptophan preparations. Marked peripheral eosinophilia, muscle weakness and pain, and serum aldolase elevations comprise the initial presentation. Skin induration, pulmonary infiltrates, cardiac rhythm disturbances, and peripheral neuropathy may ensue.

Noninflammatory nonarticular disease accounts for a large proportion of diffuse musculoskeletal complaints in young persons.

Fibromyalgia Syndrome (Fibrositis, Fibromyositis) has been recognized, predominantly in women. Characteristic manifestations include morning stiffness worsened by changes in the weather and heavy exercise, fatigue caused by disordered sleep, and tenderness at multiple symmetric bony trigger points concentrated in the upper back and neck. The musculoskeletal discomfort is typically diffuse and poorly localized, but exacerbations caused by extremes of joint motion may produce pain referable to the joints. All hematologic and serologic parameters are normal (see also Chapter 159).

Reflex Sympathetic Dystrophy Syndrome causes diffuse musculoskeletal discomfort, swelling, weakness, and limitation of motion. A single limb is affected, usually an arm. The limb is swollen and the skin shiny, often appearing dusky and cool to the touch. Pain can be severe and burning. Periarticular structures are especially tender. Preceding trauma accounts for 50 percent of cases. A vasomotor mechanism is postulated.

DIFFERENTIAL DIAGNOSIS

The causes of polyarticular complaints can be divided into articular and nonarticular categories, and these can be subdivided into inflammatory and noninflammatory etiologies (see Table 146–1).

WORKUP

The initial assessment of the patient who presents with multiple joint complaints should ascertain 1) whether the problem is truly articular or periarticular, 2) whether the underlying disease process is inflammatory or noninflammatory, 3) whether the condition is systemic or focal, and 4) whether vital organ function or joint integrity is endangered.

In the vast majority of cases, the answers to these questions can be provided by a careful history and physical examination, supplemented by a few simple blood tests or an x-ray. Synovial fluid analysis is sometimes helpful if an accessible effusion is present. The rest of the laboratory tests that are available for rheumatologic diagnosis are best used to modify one's initial impression; they are rarely helpful as a general rheumatologic screening procedure.

One should apply official criteria for diagnosis of RA and SLE cautiously in the individual patient. Such criteria are designed more to assure uniformity in epidemiologic and therapeutic studies than to diagnose individuals. The American Rheumatism Association criteria for RA stress chronicity and symmetric polyarthritis, making them less sensitive for use in early disease. The diagnosis of SLE by official criteria poses similar problems. For the individual patient, the diagnosis of SLE must be entertained if *any* of the clinical characteristics of the disease is associated with positive serology.

History

Differentiating Articular From Nonarticular Disease. Patients complain of pain, stiffness, and loss of function and often confuse neuropathic pain, bone pain, or myalgias with arthritis. The physician should attempt to identify the anatomic basis of the symptoms by asking the patient to specify exactly where the pain is located, what aggravates it, and what functional loss has occurred. For the most part, the symptoms of joint disease are well localized to the joint and bear a logical relation to its use. Nonarticular disease rarely has a specifically articular location and does not produce loss of articular function, although some range of motion may be affected. After the location of the process has been established, the underlying disease mechanism should be elucidated.

Differentiating Inflammatory From Noninflammatory Pathology. One inquires into the characteristic hallmarks of inflammation: redness, warmth, soft tissue swelling, and tenderness. If such symptoms are localized to and encompass the entire joint, one has excellent presumptive evidence for synovitis and an inflammatory process. It is important not to mistake tenderness in a segment of the joint or a small effusion as evidence of inflammation. Response to anti-inflammatory agents is sometimes useful for differentiation, although most nonprescription agents such as aspirin and other nonsteroidal anti-inflammatory drugs (NSAIDs) also have analgesic activity that may provide nonspecific relief. Nonetheless, RA patients reach for their aspirin as soon as they awaken and clearly feel worse if they miss a dose. The response in OA patients is much less dramatic.

Elucidation of a Specific Etiology. The basic determinations of site and disease process help narrow the differential diagnosis, enabling a more focused consideration. Attention to other elements of the history, such as distribution of involved joints, associated symptoms (including those suggesting systemic disease), and age and gender, facilitate identification of the etiology.

Distribution and Temporal Pattern have considerable diagnostic value, necessitating careful inquiry into all joints affected and the sequence of involvement. Complaints that at first appear monoarticular or asymmetric may turn out to be polyarticular or symmetric on further questioning. Several patterns are quite suggestive. Symmetric noninflammatory involvement of the PIP and DIP joints, without MCP or wrist involvement and without morning stiffness, argues for OA. Asymmetric inflammatory disease of these joints points to psoriatic arthritis. Symmetric inflammatory involvement of the MCP, PIP, carpal, or MTP joints supports a diagnosis of rheumatoid disease. Bilateral heel pain suggests Reiter's syndrome and the other spondyloarthropathies, as does back pain. Hip and shoulder girdle complaints in an elderly patient with noninflammatory, nonarticular disease provide strong presumptive evidence for polymyalgia, whereas a vague distribution in conjunction with trigger points supports a diagnosis of fibromyalgia.

Temporal pattern deserves attention. A chronic, subacute, additive process is consistent with rheumatoid disease. Sudden, explosive, symmetric polyarthritis suggests an acute hypersensitivity reaction, such as that seen with early hepatitis B infection or penicillin allergy. A migratory pattern raises the possibilities of rheumatic fever, disseminated gonococcemia, Reiter's syndrome, and Lyme disease, among others.

Associated Symptoms aid diagnosis and may provide evidence for systemic involvement. A careful review of systems is essential. *Morning stiffness* is very suggestive of rheumatoid disease, which produces maximal stiffness after inactivity. In contrast, OA is characterized by maximal symptoms with use. If there is some stiffness with rest in OA, it passes quickly with activity. Acute onset of *fever* points to an infectious origin or a marked hypersensitivity reaction, whereas low-grade fever may herald the onset of rheumatoid disease. The development of a *rash* may be diagnostic for such conditions as SLE, gonococcemia, Lyme disease, and vasculitis (see later discussion). New onset of *Raynaud's phenomenon* raises the possibility of scleroderma, SLE, or RA. A history of chronic or bloody *diarrhea* suggests inflammatory bowel disease. Symptoms of *urethritis* and *conjunctivitis* are suggestive of Reiter's syndrome. *Sleep disorder* and *chronic fatigue* point to fibromyalgia. Chronically *dry mouth* and *dry eyes* suggest Sjögren's syndrome, a common accompaniment of RA. Systemic involvement with SLE is evidenced by report of nasopharyngeal ulcers, pleuritic chest pain, or mental status changes.

Age and Gender. SLE and RA are female-predominant, while Reiter's syndrome is male-predominant. Onset of rheumatic fever or ankylosing spondylitis is nearly always before age 40. Peak incidence for SLE occurs in the premenopausal period, although later onset is not rare. The incidence of RA is less dependent on age, with new onset occurring in the elderly as well as in the young. Gout in women is mainly a postmenopausal disease; in men, it occurs at all adult ages. SLE is particularly common among black women.

Severity and effect on daily activity help assess functional significance as well as etiology. Joint pain awakening the patient at night indicates severe arthritis; alternatively, it may signify a bony or neuropathic process. Marked daily fatigue, the need for afternoon naps, weight loss, and fever all suggest active systemic illness. The assessment of functional impact must take into account not only the severity of the condition but also the patient's premorbid level of activity and attitudes toward work and pain.

Past Medical History and Family History should not be overlooked. Gout may present as polyarthritis, but more often one uncovers a prior history of podagra or another form of acute lower extremity monoarthritis. A history of travel or residence in an area endemic for Lyme disease, as well as a history of recent tick bite, should be elicited. The spondyloarthropathies, gout, and the Heberden's nodes of

OA all have a familial preponderance, which should be explored.

Physical Examination

The physical examination is basically a continuation of the same approach, documenting the pattern and type of joint involvement and the nature of any extra-articular disease. The myriad of extra-articular manifestations of arthritic diseases makes a detailed general physical examination mandatory. Certain aspects deserve emphasis.

Skin and Integument. Important dermal clues to etiology include the malar rash of SLE, the annular erythema chronica migrans of Lyme disease, the necrotic-centered papulovesicular lesions of disseminated gonococcemia, the nail pitting and scaling of psoriasis, the urticarial lesions of hepatitis B infection, and the palpable purpura, ulceration, or livedo reticularis of vasculitis. The patient with suspected Reiter's syndrome should have the glans penis checked for the ulcers of circinate balanitis and the heels for the hypertrophic changes of keratodermia blennorrhagia. One should carefully palpate around the elbows, the Achilles tendons, and the pinnae searching for rheumatoid nodules and tophi, which are specific indicators of RA and gout, respectively. The nails should be examined for pitting and clubbing. Nail pitting adjacent to erosive DIP arthritis can justify the diagnosis of psoriatic arthritis in the absence of any skin psoriasis. Fingertip atrophy with healed or active ulcers suggests severe Raynaud's phenomenon and should prompt a search for the calcinosis, subungual telangiectasias, and skin tightening of scleroderma. Finding the red, tender, subcutaneous lesions of erythema nodosum raises the possibilities of sarcoidosis and inflammatory bowel disease. Dry, doughy skin and loss of the outer third of the eyebrows are signs of hypothyroidism.

HEENT, Neck, Lungs, and Heart. The anterior eye should be checked for conjunctivitis and iritis suggestive of Reiter's syndrome and spondylitis (see Chapter 199) and the posterior eye checked for retinal hemorrhages, exudates, and ischemic lesions consistent with systemic lupus and vasculitis. "Cotton-wool" exudates are the most common eye lesion in SLE. The oral and nasal mucosa should be examined for ulcers, which if painful suggest SLE and if painless suggest Reiter's syndrome. Thyroid evaluation may reveal a goiter. The chest is examined for signs of effusion, pleuritis, and pericarditis. Pleural and pericardial rubs are found in RA and SLE. Heart murmurs characterize rheumatic fever and SLE, mitral valve murmurs sometimes occur in SLE, and aortic regurgitant murmurs occur in the spondyloarthropathies. The abdominal examination includes checking for splenomegaly, which is found in a variety of rheumatic diseases, including RA and SLE.

Musculoskeletal Examination. One checks for signs of serositis, noninflammatory articular disease, and periarticular pathology. As emphasized earlier, the patient with inflammatory joint disease manifests involvement of the entire joint, with tenderness, warmth, redness, soft tissue swelling, and often an effusion. In contrast, the patient with noninflammatory disease usually shows only focal tenderness and few, if any, signs of inflammation, although there may be a small noninflammatory effusion. The distribution of disease is noted, as are any mechanical abnormalities, such as limitation of motion, instability, subluxation, or tendon injury.

A careful look at the periarticular tissues (tendons, bursa, muscles) is also indicated. Bursitis and tendinitis commonly mimic arthritis. Subacromial bursitis and bicipital tendinitis can be confused with shoulder joint disease (see Chapter 150), lateral epicondylitis (tennis elbow) and olecranon bursitis with elbow joint disease (see Chapter 153), trochanteric bursitis with hip disease (see Chapter 151), and anserine bursitis with knee disease (see Chapter 152). Muscle soreness and proximal muscle weakness raise the question of a myositis. Checking for pressure points in the upper back and neck is indicated in patients with suspected fibromyalgia syndrome.

Another important type of periarticular disease is that manifested by "frozen" joints and flexion contractures. Severe limitation of motion of a joint may occur with an intrinsically normal joint. Disuse because of neurologic disease or periarticular pain may lead to tightening of periarticular fibrous tissue and secondary contractures. The clinical presentation can be mistaken for that of arthritis, but normal joint x-rays and lack of indicators of inflammatory arthritis, plus an awareness of a predisposing illness, lead to the correct diagnosis.

If faced with stiffness or pain in the hand, a valuable screening test for finger-joint and tendinous disease is that of "*curling*." The patient is asked to extend the MCP joints and then maximally flex the PIP and DIP joints, but not to make a fist. Curling is normal if a patient can bring his fingertips into apposition with his palm. Any disease of the PIP or DIP joints interferes with curling, as does any inflammation along the dorsal extensor tendons.

For patients with a suspected spondyloarthropathy, *Schober's test* provides a useful screening test of lumbar mobility. Two marks are made on the patient's back while the patient is standing: one at the level of the posterior iliac spines and the other exactly 10 cm above the first. On bending forward maximally, the two marks should be at least 15 cm apart. An abnormal Schober's test is nonspecific, but if combined with other evidence for a spondyloarthropathy, it can advance the diagnosis.

Neurologic Examination. Motor and sensory function in the extremities is checked for evidence of peripheral neuropathy, and mental status is carefully assessed in SLE patients.

Laboratory Studies

A large number of laboratory tests, both simple and esoteric, are routinely used in the evaluation of polyarthritic complaints. Panels of tests are often offered by laboratories as a means of "screening" for common etiologies. Such panels (eg, ANA, RF, and uric acid) have been found to be costly and of little use. Diagnostic confusion that persists at the end of the physical examination is rarely resolved by such laboratory testing. More appropriate, effective test utilization derives from formulating and testing specific diagnostic hypotheses. Ordering a test when pretest probability is very low results in overutilization and a high rate of false-positives (see Chapter 2).

Suspected Inflammatory Articular Disease. In this setting, a determination of *erythrocyte sedimentation rate (ESR)* provides useful but nonspecific confirmation of inflammatory disease activity and can be followed to gauge response to therapy and clinical course. A markedly elevated reading (eg, >60 mm/h) suggests considerable inflammatory activity. A normal ESR in the setting of active joint symptoms reduces the probability of an inflammatory pathophysiology. However, the ESR is a relatively poor test for detection of inflammatory disease that is in remission. A *complete blood count* can be drawn at the same time to check for hematologic involvement by the underlying disease process.

RF testing is helpful if one's pretest probability of RA is moderately high and further supporting evidence is sought. In general, 70 percent to 80 percent of all patients meeting strict criteria for RA are RF-positive. The higher the titer of RF, the more likely the diagnosis of RA. RF negativity does not rule out RA, nor does RF positivity rule it in. RF can also be positive in other connective tissue diseases and in chronic infections, for example, SBE. Moreover, 5 to 15 percent of so-called normals (increasing with age) are RF-positive.

ANA testing is very sensitive but nonspecific for the diagnosis of inflammatory joint disease. The test remains most useful in the setting of suspected SLE. More than 95 percent of patients with definite SLE are ANA-positive. Conversely, a patient with a negative ANA and only a modest pretest probability of SLE is very unlikely to have the condition. A positive test does not necessarily confirm the diagnosis of SLE, because the test can also be positive in drug-induced lupus, RA, scleroderma, chronic hepatitis, and even in a few normal individuals. Titers of ANAs fluctuate with time but do not necessarily parallel disease activity.

Attempts to find tests more specific than the ANA have led to identification of the specific nuclear constituents functioning as autoantigens. Native dsDNA was found to be an important autoantigen in patients with SLE. *Antibody to native dsDNA* occurs in up to 70 percent of patients with SLE, is specific for the condition, and is associated with an increased risk of nephritis. Testing for antibody to dsDNA can be used to confirm the diagnosis of SLE in patients with suspected disease and a positive ANA. Antibody to Smith (Sm) antigen is similarly specific but is found in only 30 percent of SLE patients. *Antibody to Scl-70* (a nuclear topoisomerase) has proven specific for scleroderma; prevalence is only 20 percent.

Synovial fluid analysis is useful and is indicated if a joint effusion is present and the diagnosis remains undetermined. One seeks to differentiate between inflammatory and noninflammatory disease, as well as to confirm crystal-induced arthropathy and investigate any suspected infection (see Chapter 145). A white blood cell (WBC) count of more than 3000 cells per cubic millimeter supports an inflammatory etiology; less than 1000 cells/mm^3 suggests OA or a mechanical derangement. A count between 1000 and 3000 is ambiguous. Often, one obtains a synovial fluid WBC count of 5000 to 20,000 cells/mm^3 without crystals, bacteria, or other distinctive attributes, allowing little more than a designation of inflammatory arthritis, type unspecified.

Serum uric acid levels are obtained unnecessarily in most arthritis patients and too often serve as the primary basis for a diagnosis of gout. Definitive diagnosis is best made by observing urate crystals in the synovial fluid. A normal serum uric acid does not rule out the diagnosis of gout, nor does an elevated level rule it in.

X-rays are usually of minimal diagnostic value in the early stages of inflammatory polyarthritis, showing little more than soft tissue swelling. Films obtained during later stages may manifest more characteristic bony changes, but usually a diagnosis has already been established. However, early *sacroiliac films* are of value in suspected spondyloarthropathy, because they may reveal sacroiliitis, a diagnostic finding. Another early radiologic change in spondyloarthropathy is squaring of the superior and inferior margins of the vertebral bodies. Only later do prominent syndesmophytes appear.

HLA-B27 testing has not proven useful for diagnosis. Although there is a high prevalence of HLA-B27 antigen positivity in the seronegative spondyloarthropathies (90% or more), 6 percent to 8 percent of normal persons are positive for HLA-B27, negating the utility of HLA-B27 testing for diagnosis of this uncommon condition.

Blood cultures are essential if endocarditis or disseminated gonococcemia is suspected. Currently available *Lyme antibody* assays lack specificity, making their results difficult to interpret (see Chapter 160) and less useful than a careful clinical assessment. DNA-based antibody assays are under development.

Urinalysis is essential for detection of glomerular injury and is useful in screening for multisystem involvement. Routine serum chemistries are less rewarding, although assessment of renal function by *blood urea nitrogen (BUN)* and *creatinine* is indicated in patients who manifest proteinuria or hematuria. Suspected hypothyroidism can be confirmed by *thyrotropin* (TSH) determination.

Suspected Noninflammatory Polyarticular Disease. In OA, joint *x-rays* are abnormal by the time the patient becomes symptomatic and can confirm the diagnosis. However, degenerative changes are commonly found in asymptomatic joints as well. Films of long bones can be obtained to confirm hypertrophic osteoarthropathy, but the diagnosis can usually be made clinically by the presence of clubbing.

Suspected Inflammatory Nonarticular Disease. The *ESR* should be obtained in patients with clinical evidence for polymyalgia rheumatica. A high reading supports the diagnosis; a low one reduces its probability. If there is headache, jaw claudication, visual disturbance, or a tender cranial artery, then evaluation for cranial arteritis should proceed promptly (see Chapter 161). A *complete blood count* and *differential* are indicated in patients with suspected eosinophilia-myalgia, followed by referral for skin and muscle biopsy if florid peripheral eosinophilia is noted. Suspected polymyositis is evaluated by obtaining serum *creatine kinase* levels and, if markedly elevated, proceeding to consideration of *muscle biopsy*.

Suspected Noninflammatory Nonarticular Disease. The diagnosis of fibromyalgia is a clinical one. There are no abnormal laboratory findings (see Chapter 159). Similarly, the diagnosis of reflex sympathetic dystrophy is predominantly clinical. Plain films of the hand may show a nonspecific but suggestive patchy osteopenia.

INDICATIONS FOR ADMISSION AND REFERRAL

The diagnosis of polyarticular arthritis may remain uncertain for a long period. For the most part, the underlying condition is not immediately life-threatening, and the workup can take place in the outpatient setting over several visits. Short-term risk to the patient is posed primarily by extra-articular disease and infection. Any evidence of bloodstream infection, vasculitis, or involvement of the patient's eyes, lungs, heart, kidneys, or nervous system should trigger prompt consideration of hospitalization and consultation. The same pertains to persons with severe constitutional symptoms (eg, disabling fatigue, fever, weight loss). Rheumatologic consultation is also appropriate if a patient with less serious illness remains undiagnosed after completion of the initial evaluation.

SYMPTOMATIC THERAPY

Treatment should be etiologic (see Chapters 155–163), but definitive diagnosis of an inflammatory polyarthritis may take time. Pending results, and provided infection has been ruled out, the patient bothered by symptoms of joint inflammation may be given either high-dose aspirin (up to twelve 325-mg tablets qd) or a NSAID (eg, ibuprofen 400–800 mg qid).

A.H.G.

ANNOTATED BIBLIOGRAPHY

Arnett FC, Edworthy SM, Bloch DA, et al. The American Rheumatism Association 1987 revised criteria for the classification of rheumatoid arthritis. Arthritis Rheum 1988;31:315. *(A collaborative study showing sensitivity and specificity for the official criteria of approximately 90 percent.)*

Goldenberg DL. Fibromyalgia syndrome: an emerging but controversial condition. JAMA 1987;257:2782. *(Thoughtful description of the condition and its recognition.)*

Harler NM, Franck WA, Bress NM, et al. Acute polyarticular gout. Am J Med 1974;56:715. *(A study of this uncommon presentation of a very common disease.)*

Kahn MA, Kahn MK. Diagnostic value of HLA-B27 testing in ankylosing spondylitis and Reiter's syndrome. Ann Intern Med 1982;96:70. *(The test is usually unnecessary.)*

Keat A. Reiter's syndrome and reactive arthritis in perspective. N Engl J Med 1983;309:1606. *(An extensive review, including discussion of joint manifestations.)*

Kozin F. Reflex sympathetic dystrophy. Bull Rheum Dis 1986;36:1. *(Good summary of pathophysiologic hypotheses and clinical manifestations.)*

Lichtenstein MJ, Pincus T. How useful are combinations of blood tests in "rheumatic panels" in diagnosis of rheumatic diseases? J Gen Intern Med 1987;3:435. *(Positive predictive value of only .34, leading to many false-positive results.)*

Mainardi CL. Approach to the patient with pain in more than one joint. In: Kelley WN. Textbook of Internal Medicine. 2nd ed. Philadelphia: J. B. Lippincott, 1993:1000. *(Provides a useful categorization of the differential diagnosis, adapted for use in this chapter.)*

Medsger TA. Tryptophan-induced eosinophilia-myalgia syndrome. N Engl J Med 1990;322:926. *(An editorial summarizing current understanding.)*

Plotz PH, Dalakas M, Leff RL, et al. Current concepts in idiopathic inflammatory myopathies. Ann Intern Med 1989; 111:143. *(Comprehensive review that includes useful discussions of polymyositis and dermatomyositis.)*

Rahn DW, Malawista SE. Lyme disease: recommendations for diagnosis and treatment. Ann Intern Med 1991;114:472. *(Includes useful discussions of clinical manifestations and the shortcomings of serologic testing.)*

Stere AC, Schoen RT, Taylor E. The clinical evolution of Lyme arthritis. Ann Intern Med 1987;107:725. *(Attacks of asymmetric oligoarthritis begin in large joints [especially the knees] about 6 mo after infection in untreated patients.)*

Tan EM, Chan EK, Sullivan KF, et al. Antinuclear antibodies (ANAs). Clin Immunol Immunopathol 1988;47:121. *(Most comprehensive review of their diagnostic meaning and pathophysiologic significance.)*

Tan EM, Cohen AS, Fries JF, et al. The 1982 revised criteria for the classification of systemic lupus erythematosus. Arthritis Rheum 1982;25:1271. *(The official criteria, although more stringent than used in practice.)*

147
Evaluation of Back Pain

ROBERT J. BOYD, M.D.

Primary Care Medicine: Office Evaluation and Management of the Adult Patient, 3rd edition, edited by Allan H. Goroll, Lawrence A. May, and Albert G. Mulley, Jr. J.B. Lippincott Company, Philadelphia

Back pain is a common complaint in primary care practice and one of the leading causes of disability. Moreover, if a patient presents with back pain, serious underlying problems must be considered, because early recognition of tumor, infection, disc herniation, or vertebral compression fracture is essential to effective management and avoidance of permanent injury. Most back pain is caused by musculoligamentous strain, degenerative disc disease, or facet arthritis and responds to symptomatic treatment. Disc disease is often responsible for recurring mild low back discomfort and episodes of severe back pain with sciatica. Occasionally, back pain may result from problems originating outside the spinal axis. The prevalence of back pain requires that the primary physician be skilled in its assessment and conservative management and knowledgeable about the indications for referral and surgery.

PATHOPHYSIOLOGY AND CLINICAL PRESENTATION

Musculoligamentous Strain. There may be tearing of muscle fibers or distal ligamentous attachments of the paraspinal muscles, usually at the iliac crest or lower lumbar/upper sacral region. Resultant bleeding and spasm cause local swelling and marked tenderness at the site of injury. The patient typically presents after a specific episode of bending, twisting, or lifting. The strain is usually severe and is associated with a feeling of something giving way in the lower back. Onset of pain in the lower lumbar area is immediate. Pain radiates across the low back, often to the buttock and upper thigh posteriorly. Radiation of pain into the lower leg is rare, because there is usually no injury to the nerve roots.

Lumbar Disc Herniation. The pathophysiology of disc disease remains incompletely understood but involves degenerative changes in the disc. It is thought that lower lumbar disc degeneration and attritional changes are caused by the concentration of stress at the lumbosacral level. Stresses result from the enormous longitudinal and sheer forces that are a consequence of upright posture and are aggravated by bending strain. The disc annulus may become injured, inflamed, and weakened, leading to localized back pain. Pain receptors in the longitudinal ligaments probably mediate the recurring attacks of local back pain. Eventually, the disc may become so weakened that it bulges posteriorly during relatively minor stress. Compression and irritation of a lower lumbar or upper sacral nerve root result, and the radicular symptoms of *sciatica* develop.

Sciatica is the symptomatic hallmark of clinically significant disc herniation, present in 95 percent of cases. It presents as sharp or burning pain radiating down the posterior or lateral aspect of the leg to the ankle or foot (depending on the specific nerve root involved). The pain may be worsened by cough, Valsalva maneuver, or sneezing and is often accompanied by paresthesias and numbness. Weakness may also develop in the areas supplied by the irritated nerve root.

Disc herniation at the L4-5 or L5-S1 level accounts for more than 95 percent of disc ruptures, with the L5 and S1 nerve roots affected, respectively. With S1 root irritation, pain, numbness, and paresthesias involve the buttock, posterior thigh, calf, lateral aspect of the ankle and foot, and lateral toes. Calf atrophy and a diminished or absent ankle jerk can occur, as well as plantar flexion weakness. With L5 root compression, pain radiates to the dorsum of the foot and great toe, and the only neurologic deficits may be extensor weakness of the great toe and numbness of the L5 area on the dorsum of the foot at the base of the great toe (Fig. 147–1). In the rarer instance of high lumbar disc herniation, pain radiates to the anterior thigh, and the knee jerk may be diminished or absent. Quadriceps atrophy and weakness may be found.

With lower lumbar disc herniations, there is often lumbar paraspinal muscle spasm that limits lumbar motions. There may be a list away from the side of the disc herniation, so-called sciatic scoliosis, and often there is tenderness of the lower lumbar spine and sciatic notch. Straight leg raising (SLR) on the affected side is limited by back and leg pain that increases on ankle dorsiflexion at the extreme of SLR.

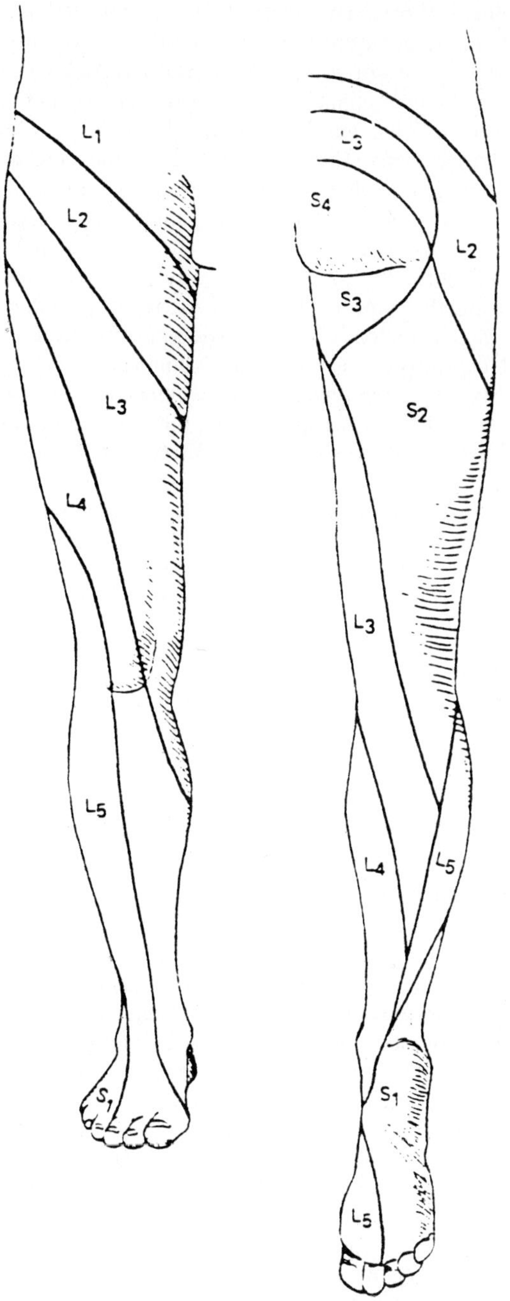

Figure 147-1. Lower extremity dermatomes. (Finneson BE: Low Back Pain. Philadelphia: JB Lippincott, 1973.)

With upper lumbar disc herniation, reverse SLR often reproduces the back and anterior thigh pain (see later discussion).

The clinical course may begin with a several-year history of recurring mild mid-low back pain related to minor back strain, with symptoms clearing spontaneously within a few days. Attacks typically increase in frequency and severity at intervals of several months to several years. Finally, an episode of persistent pain accompanied by sciatica develops, often triggered by a seemingly trivial stress (eg, bending over in the shower to pick up the soap).

Spinal stenosis has become better appreciated as an important cause of chronic low back and lower extremity complaints. It occurs in young people who have a congenitally narrowed lumbar spinal canal and also in elderly individuals with osteoarthritic spurring, chronic disc degeneration, and facet joint arthritis. These changes narrow the canal and the neuroforamina, leading to root impingement and pain.

The characteristic complaint is pain that is worsened by standing, walking, or other activities that cause spinal extension and relieved by rest, especially by sitting or lying down and flexing the spine and hips. Patients report pain in the low back, gluteal region, or lower extremities; often it is bilateral. Numbness or weakness may accompany the pain in the legs. Because symptoms are often worsened by walking and relieved by sitting down and resting, they can mimic vascular insufficiency and are sometimes referred to as "*pseudoclaudication.*"

On examination, the spine demonstrates good range of motion and little focal tenderness. SLR is usually normal. Minor neurologic deficits (eg, a diminished ankle jerk) may be present, but no pattern is characteristic.

Spondylolisthesis denotes forward subluxation of a vertebral body. In adults, the condition results from degenerative changes and arthritis of the facet joints, usually at L4-5 or L5-S1, with forward slippage of 10 percent to 20 percent of the vertebral body diameter. About 70 percent of patients with spondylolisthesis have chronic low back pain; sciatica is infrequent. The pain is caused by strain imposed on the ligaments and intervertebral joints.

Vertebral Compression Fracture. In normal bone, this fracture requires severe flexion-compression force. It is acutely painful. Spontaneous vertebral body collapse, or pathologic fracture, is most commonly seen in elderly patients with severe osteoporosis (see Chapter 164), in patients on long-term glucocorticosteroids (see Chapter 105), and in cancer patients with lytic bony metastases. Usually, there is a history of sudden back pain brought on by a minor stress. The discomfort is noted at the level of fracture, with local radiation across the back and around the trunk, but rarely into the lower extremities. The fracture is more likely to be in the middle or lower levels of the dorsal spine, which helps differentiate the problem from lumbar disc herniations, 95 percent of which occur at the L4 or L5 disc level.

Neoplasms. The most common spinal tumor is *metastatic carcinoma*, which often presents with waist-level or midback pain of insidious onset, gradually increasing in severity and aggravated by activity. About 80 percent of patients are older than 50 years of age. Although only 30 percent give a history of previous cancer, those that do have a high probability of spinal metastasis. Approximately 90 percent report night pain and pain unrelieved by lying down or bed rest. A history of prior malignancy and insidious increase in midback pain that is not relieved by lying down is highly predictive of metastatic tumor.

Breast, lung, prostate, gastrointestinal, and genitourinary neoplasms often metastasize to the spine. Purely lytic lesions, which are often caused by renal or thyroid carcinoma, are seen occasionally. The disc spaces are spared. Disc space height is usually maintained, although collapse of the vertebral body as a result of destruction and weakening of bone is common. *Myeloma* is the most common primary bone tumor involving the spine. Early in its course, the tumor may be difficult to differentiate from compression fracture because of osteoporosis.

Intraspinal tumors may present in the same manner as herniated discs. However, marked progression of neurologic deficits despite adequate conservative therapy is a clue to the existence of a tumor inside the spinal canal. *Extraspinal tumors* may eventually cause root impingement and simulate discogenic sciatica. Tumors of the retroperitoneum, pelvis, and large bowel may extend to the roots. This is a very late development; metastases may occur earlier.

Infection. Back pain resulting from infection is rare but important to detect. An identifiable source is found in 40 percent of cases; possibilities include urinary tract infection, intravenous drug abuse, skin abscess, and indwelling catheter. *Vertebral osteomyelitis* is usually hematogenous in origin but may occasionally result from a spinal procedure, such as lumbar puncture, myelography, discography, or disc surgery. It extends into the disc space as well as affecting the vertebral bodies. Dull, continuous back pain is the usual presentation, often in conjunction with low-grade fever and spasm over the paraspinous muscles. Tenderness to percussion over the involved vertebrae is common, but fever is absent in up to half of cases. A compression fracture or an epidural abscess may ensue.

Epidural abscess develops in the context of bacteremia or osteomyelitis. The infection presents as back pain, focal tenderness, and fever. Fever and spinal tenderness are present in about 85 percent of cases. If the condition is not promptly treated, it may extend to compromise the local blood supply to the spinal cord and rapidly progress from spinal ache to major motor and sensory deficits over hours to a few days.

Ankylosing Spondylitis. This seronegative spondyloarthropathy has both peripheral and axial skeleton manifestations (see also Chapter 146). Spinal involvement is most prominent in young men. Morning spinal stiffness, symptomatic improvement with exercise, gradual onset, and persistence of pain for more than 3 months are characteristic but relatively nonspecific features. The mechanism of disease is unknown, but there is a high incidence of HLA-B27 positivity, suggesting an immune pathophysiology. In some, there is a history of inflammatory bowel disease. Early clinical findings include morning back stiffness and diminished chest expansion. Spinal x-rays are often unremarkable in early phases, but films of the sacroiliac joints may show narrowing of the joint space and reactive sclerosis ("sacroiliitis"). Eventually, the sacroiliac joint space becomes obliterated, and fusion follows. Squaring of the vertebral bodies is the first spinal radiologic manifestation, followed by development of syndesmophytes. Similar though less florid changes may occur in the other seronegative spondyloarthropathies (see Chapter 146).

Psychogenic Disease. Patients with *depression* may present complaining of chronic low back pain. Often there is a history of previous back problems or onset at the time of a minor injury, with the depression amplifying the presentation and prolonging the clinical course. Mild muscle spasm may be noted on physical examination. Characteristically, the intensity of complaints and the degree of disability are much greater than the minor limitations found on examination. Multiple somatic symptoms are common (see Chapter 227). In other patients, there may be an underlying *somatization* disorder. Many of these patients appear refractory to therapy, often unwilling to take an active role in their own treatment. Some even seem to derive a sense of legitimacy and self-worth from their suffering (see Chapter 230).

Malingering implies conscious deception for the sake of obtaining gain from being ill. Inconsistencies among symptoms and physical findings typify the malingerer. These often can be brought out by distracting the patient.

Cauda Equina Syndrome. Although the spinal cord ends at the L1 level, the collection of nerve roots that make up the cauda equina are subject to injury by any process that compromises the spinal canal below the L1 level. Massive midline disc herniation is the most common cause of cauda compression and a serious, though very infrequent, event that requires prompt attention. In contrast to simple root impingement, the clinical presentation includes urinary retention in almost 90 percent of cases. Another characteristic feature is "saddle anesthesia" (reduction in sensation over the buttocks, upper posterior thighs, and perineum), reported by about 75 percent of patients. Both of these clinical findings are a consequence of sacral root compression, as is a decrease in anal sphincter tone, noted in about two-thirds of cases. Sciatica and lower extremity motor and sensory deficits are prominent and often bilateral. Patients may report falling.

DIFFERENTIAL DIAGNOSIS

The differential diagnosis of back pain can be considered in terms of whether or not there is root pain (Table 147–1).

In primary care practice, about 85 percent of patients with back pain have musculoligamentous injury or degenerative change. Up to 5 percent have a symptomatically herniated disc, with about half of those coming to surgery; 4 percent have compression fracture, 3 percent spondylolisthesis, and another 1.5 percent have either tumor, infection, or ankylosing spondylitis. The prevalence of spinal stenosis remains unknown. Herniated discs are found in up to 30 percent of asymptomatic persons who undergo a spinal imaging procedure for a reason other than back pain.

Table 147-1. Important Causes of Back Pain

Conditions Commonly Presenting With Sciatica
Disc herniation
Spinal stenosis
Compression fracture
Epidural abscess
Vertebral osteomyelitis (late)
Compression fracture
Intraspinal tumor
Spinal metastasis
Spondylolisthesis (occasionally)
Conditions Usually Presenting Without Sciatica
Musculoligamentous strain
Ankylosing spondylitis
Spondylolisthesis
Depression
Vertebral osteomyelitis (early)
Epidural abscess (very early)
Retroperitoneal neoplasm

WORKUP

Even with the advent of sophisticated spinal imaging techniques, history and physical examination remain critical to the effective evaluation and management of back pain. The findings elicited are often diagnostic, and even if they are not, they can help guide test selection and assure timely referral. Overreliance on imaging studies often results in false-positive diagnoses.

History. In elucidating the basic features of the back pain complaint (ie, quality, location, onset, radiation, etc.), one should also inquire specifically into symptoms potentially indicative of serious underlying pathology (eg, fever, progressive neurologic deficits, bilateral deficits, bladder dysfunction, saddle anesthesia, persistent pain unresponsive to bed rest). A history of recent injury and a prior history of cancer are other critical elements to be noted, as are previous therapy for back problems, recent lumbar puncture, concurrent infection, and chronic use of high-dose corticosteroids.

Presence of sciatica helps narrow the differential diagnosis (see Table 147–1).

Aggravating and alleviating factors may have diagnostic meaning. Morning stiffness in the back that is relieved by activity suggests ankylosing spondylitis or other inflammatory conditions. Worsening or onset of symptoms with standing or walking and relief with bending or sitting is characteristic of spinal stenosis, while worsening with sitting, driving, or lifting points to lumbar disc herniation.

The patient should be asked to describe the back pain's impact on daily activities. Emotional and social stressors are sought if severity and duration of symptoms appear disproportionate for the amount of organic pathology present. Under such circumstances, it is important to check for depression (see Chapter 227) and manifestations of somatization disorder (see Chapter 230).

Physical Examination. Before examining the back, one should check the abdomen, rectum, groin, pelvis, and peripheral pulses for pathology that might mimic symptoms of spinal disease. In addition, one looks for temperature elevation, skin abscess, breast mass, pleural effusion, prostate nodule, lymphadenopathy, joint inflammation, and other signs of systemic or malignant disease that may affect the spine. Thigh and calf circumferences are measured looking for evidence of atrophy, and lower extremity joint motions are tested.

The back examination begins with the patient standing and the back uncovered. One observes for any abnormalities in symmetry, muscle bulk, posture, and spinal curvature. Flexibility is assessed, noting any muscle spasm or spinal segments that do not move freely. Description of what limits back motion is more important than estimating degrees of motion, which is imprecise at best. The spine is palpated for focal tenderness suggestive of tumor, infection, fracture, and disc herniation. Lower lumbar spine and sciatic notch sensitivity usually are found with lower lumbar disc problems. Sacroiliac tenderness to deep palpation is sometimes present in ankylosing spondylitis, but the finding is nonspecific.

The SLR test is an important component of the assessment for disc disease. The maneuver serves as a sensitive indicator of lower lumbar disc herniation, particularly in patients complaining of sciatica. SLR testing is based on the observation that an L5 or S1 nerve root tethered by a herniated disc causes radicular pain if stretched. In the presence of a severely herniated disc, the additional root stretching causes impingement and pain, especially with an L5-S1 disc injury.

SLR is performed in the supine position with passive lifting of the patient's leg at the heel by the examiner while the knee is kept fully extended. The test is performed both on the side of the patient's reported sciatica (*"ipsilateral" SLR testing*) and on the opposite side (*"contralateral"* or *"crossed" SLR testing*). A positive test is one that reproduces the patient's sciatica as the leg is elevated between 30° and 70°. This should not be confused with hamstring muscle tightness, which can also cause discomfort on SLR, especially as elevation approaches 90°. (Elevation beyond 80° puts little additional stretch on the nerve root and is of little meaning.) If severe pain is reported on elevation and resistance occurs, yet the leg can be raised another 20° or 30° when the patient is distracted, the test is "negative" and other causes of the pain should be sought, such as hamstring muscle tightness. Dorsiflexion of the ankle at the extreme of SLR may exacerbate the pain of disc herniation on SLR testing and is particularly useful if the SLR test is equivocal.

The earlier the onset of pain during the test, the more specific the result and the greater the degree of disc herniation. Test sensitivity averages 80 percent for ipsilateral SLR; specificity is low (about 40%). The specificity of a positive contralateral SLR test is considerably higher (75%), but sensitivity is only 25 percent. A large disc herniation with an extruded fragment is an important cause of a positive contralateral SLR.

There is much less L4 and minimal L2 or L3 movement in SLR testing, making it less useful for detection of disc herniation above L4-5. Femoral nerve sensitivity is usually present with higher lumbar (L2, L3, or L4) root irritation. It can be tested by flexing the knee with the patient prone, which may reproduce the back and anterior thigh pain of upper lumbar disc herniation.

Neurologic examination is most efficiently performed by concentrating on the areas of compromise suggested by the history. The patient with sciatica is most likely to have deficits in the territory of the L5 and S1 roots and should be tested accordingly. The person with back pain radiating to the anterior thigh and associated quadriceps weakness should be tested for L4 function. A history of urinary retention requires a check of sacral root motor and sensory function.

Testing the *S1 root* (L5-S1 disc) involves tiptoe walking or plantar flexion against resistance, ankle deep tendon reflexes, and lateral foot sensation. Loss of plantar flexion only occurs with severe disc herniation (low sensitivity, high specificity). Assessing the *L5 root* (L4-L5 disc) includes heel walking (an imprecise test), dorsiflexing the ankle and big toe against resistance, and sensation on the anterior medial dorsal foot (see Figure 147–1). For a suspected upper lumbar disc lesion (*L4 root*), one notes the knee deep tendon reflexes, quadriceps strength, and sensation about the medial ankle.

The sensitivity of any single neurologic test for diagnosis of lumbar disc herniation is no greater than 50 percent, but it can be enhanced to almost 90 percent by considering clusters of findings. The most accurate assessment of sensory function is attained by pin-prick testing, most efficiently performed by limiting the examination to a few key distal dermatomal areas in the feet (see Figure 147–1) and noting any asymmetry of response. Responses in patients with psychological stress to neurologic testing and spinal examination may appear neuroanatomically inappropriate, but often they are diagnostically meaningful. Disturbances in strength or sensation that do not correspond to nerve root innervation patterns, inconsistency of responses to maneuvers, overreaction to palpation or passive movement, superficial or widespread tenderness, and pain on sham testing of spinal rotation (keeping arms at sides while rotating hips), are among the characteristic responses. Encountering three or more of these responses suggests considerable psychological overlay to the patient's back pain problem.

Laboratory Studies. For the majority of patients with low back pain, a careful history and physical examination usually suffice for diagnosis at the time of the initial office visit. The utility of imaging studies is limited to a few specific situations, many of which are also indications for referral or consultation (see later discussion).

Lumbosacral Spine Films. In most instances, the routine ordering of plain lumbosacral spine films in patients presenting with back pain is low in yield and neither cost-effective nor useful for decision making. Finding normal disc spaces does not rule out disc herniation, and encountering a narrowed disc space does not distinguish between disc rupture and asymptomatic degeneration. Osteophytes extending from the vertebral bodies indicates little more than long-existing disc degeneration and attempts at repair.

Nonetheless, there are situations in which early back x-rays are indicated, including suspicion of 1) malignancy (age older than 50 years, focal persistent bone pain unrelieved by bed rest, history of malignancy); 2) compression fracture (prolonged corticosteroid therapy, postmenopausal, severe trauma, focal tenderness); 3) ankylosing spondylitis (young male, limited spinal motion, sacroiliac pain); 4) chronic osteomyelitis (low-grade fever, high sedimentation rate, focal tenderness); 5) major trauma; and 6) major neurologic deficits. Back pain localized to the high lumbar or thoracic region is also an indication for prompt spinal x-rays, because compression fracture and metastatic tumor are common in these areas. Plain films may be needed for patients seeking compensation for back pain and for those who desire reassurance, but they are of little use in early osteomyelitis (in which bony changes take 10–14 days to appear).

Computed Tomography (CT) and Magnetic Resonance Imaging (MRI). If severe symptoms persist for several weeks despite conservative therapy and disc herniation or other surgically correctable pathology is suspected, then CT or MRI may be useful. They are both very sensitive, reasonably specific tests for detection of a herniated lumbar disc or spinal stenosis and can provide anatomic detail of some surgical value. The cost of CT of the lumbosacral spine is less than half the cost of MRI, but it involves radiation exposure and does not provide the visualization of the entire spine or upper vertebrae that MRI does (desirable features if the differential diagnosis includes intraspinal tumor and upper level disc herniation). Besides being costly, MRI often triggers claustrophobic responses, but there is no radiation exposure. MRI is the best available test for detection of early osteomyelitis and is also the noninvasive test of choice for spinal cord tumors, epidural abscess, and cord compression. In many instances, it obviates the need for myelography. CT provides excellent bony detail and shows changes in vertebral bodies caused by tumor and infection. MRI may reveal such pathology even earlier than CT, because it can detect marrow changes, which precede the bony ones.

MRI and CT should be limited to patients who are either sufficiently symptomatic to require consideration of a surgical intervention or suspected of having serious systemic disease. The high sensitivity of these tests for disc bulges and minor herniations can result in a false-positive rate as high as 30 percent if they are applied indiscriminately. Prospective randomized studies are needed to determine comparative cost-efficacy of CT and MRI.

Myelography usually requires hospital admission. It is best performed in conjunction with CT scan on patients with progressive neurologic deficits, especially those with findings suggestive of injury to the spinal cord (eg, loss of sphincter control, bilateral numbness and weakness). The temptation to perform myelography in the patient with chronic refractory pain is strong, but the test should be reserved for patients with objective findings that are amenable to surgery or radiation therapy.

Radionuclide Scanning. The moderately high sensitivity of the technetium bone scan for osteomyelitis and metastatic disease and its wide availability make it a reasonable consideration in the patient presenting with any combination of fever, weight loss, persistent back pain, history of malignancy, concurrent infection, and markedly elevated sedimentation rate. Gallium scanning is sometimes useful in defining soft tissue involvement by infection or abscess formation.

Immunoelectrophoresis of serum and urine samples diagnoses most cases of myeloma; crude screening with a complete blood count, ESR, and serum globulin level is probably sufficient if clinical suspicion is not high. A diagnosis of myeloma must be suspected if back pain in an older person is accompanied by unexplained anemia and a very high sedimentation rate. However, such findings are quite nonspecific and may also be due to a chronic inflammatory process.

Electromyography may be needed to document peripheral nerve deficits and help select patients who require myelography.

SYMPTOMATIC MANAGEMENT AND PATIENT EDUCATION

Acute Back Pain. Acute musculoligamentous strain, degenerative disc disease, and herniated lumbar disc with or without sciatica can usually be managed by bed rest in conjunction with analgesics, local measures, and a few carefully selected activities to prevent deconditioning.

Bed Rest and Analgesics. Approximately 98 percent of patients respond favorably. The patient may be severely incapacitated by pain at rest as well as with movement. The acute discomfort usually persists for at least several days. Symptomatic measures consist of local heat or warm baths and use of mild analgesics. Anti-inflammatory agents have been shown to be effective in randomized trials and are preferred over narcotics for all but the first night or two of symptoms. Most so-called muscle relaxants are actually minor tranquilizers; they have little direct effect on muscles but can be of help to the patient who cannot sleep. The patient should be advised to find the most comfortable position in bed. Lying supine with pillows behind the knees and a low pillow for the head usually suffices. Lying on one's side with the hips and knees flexed is sometimes quite comfortable; lying prone is usually not.

The patient with minor strain may be more comfortable after as little as 2 days in bed. Those with evidence of disc herniation may need up to 3 weeks. However, there is little evidence to support prolonged bed rest. Outcomes have not been different in randomized trials, and deconditioning with bed rest can contribute to physical and psychological morbidity.

Activity Prescription. For patients with an acutely herniated disc, a major goal is to avoid prolonged inactivity and the deconditioning that accompanies it. A reasonable activity program during the first week is to have the patient walk for about 20 minutes three times a day, interspersed with several hours of bed rest. After the spine has healed sufficiently to allow sitting without pain, the patient can ease into a program of endurance exercises that may help prevent future back problems (see later discussion).

A reasonable program of back care should be discussed after recovery from acute symptoms allows gradual mobilization and resumption of normal activities. The patient must understand that pain is a normal protective response to injury or inflammation. Discomfort should be used as a guideline to determine the pace of increasing activity. However, minor discomfort, stiffness, soreness, or mild aching should not interfere with progressive mobilization.

If symptoms recur or marked pain develops in relation to a specific activity or level of activity, the patient should temporarily limit himself or herself for several days. If pain increases within 24 hours of performing a new or greater level of activity, the activity should be halved each day until a tolerable level is reached and then gradually increased. The patient should be encouraged to progress as rapidly as symptoms permit.

Exercises and Back Care. Proper back care should become a way of life for the patient, although acute symptoms subside with rest. The patient is advised to avoid activities that cause pain as well as potentially injurious actions such as repetitive bending, heavy lifting, or snow shoveling. There is increasing evidence that physical therapy programs designed to improve muscle strength and flexibility are effective, helping to maintain good posture and reduce chances of recurrent injury. Instruction sheets are often useful (Figs. 147–2 and 147–3) to supplement instruction in the office. Controlled trials have failed to confirm any benefit from use of traction or braces in patients with disc herniation. In fact, there is concern that restriction of movement may promote muscle weakness. Mild daily exercise and more vigorous endurance exercise two to three times a week are also encouraged and appear more useful than traditional isometric exercises. Walking briskly for 20 minutes once or twice a day, supplemented by swimming twice weekly for up to 30 minutes, fulfills such an exercise requirement. Stationary bicycling or jogging can be substituted for swimming.

Spinal Manipulation by chiropractors and osteopaths may be the most common treatment for back pain. Overviews of trials suggest that there may be some benefit in acute back pain, but available evidence precludes definitive conclusions. The safety of spinal manipulation in the setting of root compression, either by disc herniation or spinal ste-

How to get along with your back

Sitting: Use a hard chair and put your spine up against it; try and keep one or both knees higher than your hips. A small stool is helpful here. For short rest periods, a contour chair offers excellent support.

Standing: Try to stand with your lower back flat. When you work standing up, use a footrest to help relieve swayback. Never lean forward without bending your knees. Ladies take note: shoes with moderate heels strain the back less than those with high heels. Avoid platform shoes.

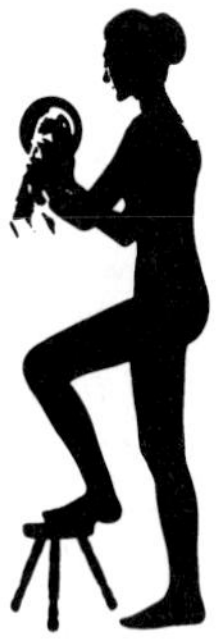

Sleeping: Sleep on a firm mattress; put a bedboard (3/4" plywood) under a soft mattress. Do not sleep on your stomach. If you sleep on your back, put a pillow under your knees. If you sleep on your side keep your legs bent at the knees and at the hips.

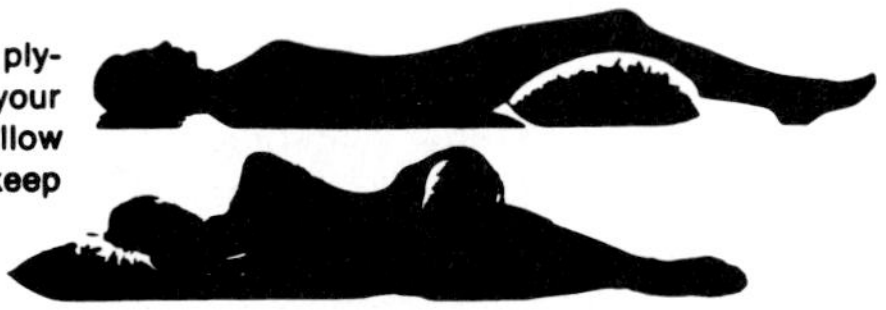

Driving: Get a hard seat for your automobile and sit close enough to the wheel while driving so that your legs are not fully extended when you work the pedals.

Lifting: Make sure you lift properly. Bend your knees and use your leg muscles to lift. Avoid sudden movements. Keep the load close to your body, and try not to lift anything heavy higher than your waist.

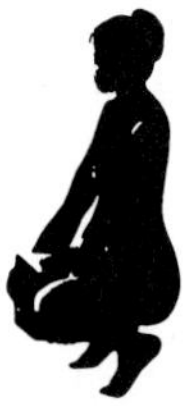

Working: Don't overwork yourself. If you can, change from one job to another before you feel fatigued. If you work at a desk all day, get up and move around whenever you get the chance.

Exercise: Get regular exercise (walking, swimming, etc.) once your backache is gone. But start slowly to give your muscles a chance to warm up and loosen before attempting anything strenuous.

See your doctor: If your back acts up, see your doctor; don't wait until your condition gets severe.

Figure 147-2. Sample instruction sheet describinig care of the back (McNeil Laboratories, Fort Washington, PA).

nosis, is not established. Most physicians advise patients with evidence of disc herniation and root impingement to avoid spinal manipulation therapy. There is no evidence to suggest that manipulation is effective in the treatment of chronic back pain.

Persistent Pain or Worsening Neurologic Deficits. Patients with evidence of lumbar disc herniation who experience 1) persistent disabling root pain despite 4 to 6 weeks of comprehensive conservative therapy; 2) progressive neurologic deficits in the lower extremities; or 3) disruption of bowel or bladder control are strong candidates for surgery. *Disc excision (discectomy)* by open operation is mandatory and urgent for patients with massive disc herniation causing a cauda equina syndrome. It is also indicated if there is major progressive neurologic deficit, calcified disc, extruded disc

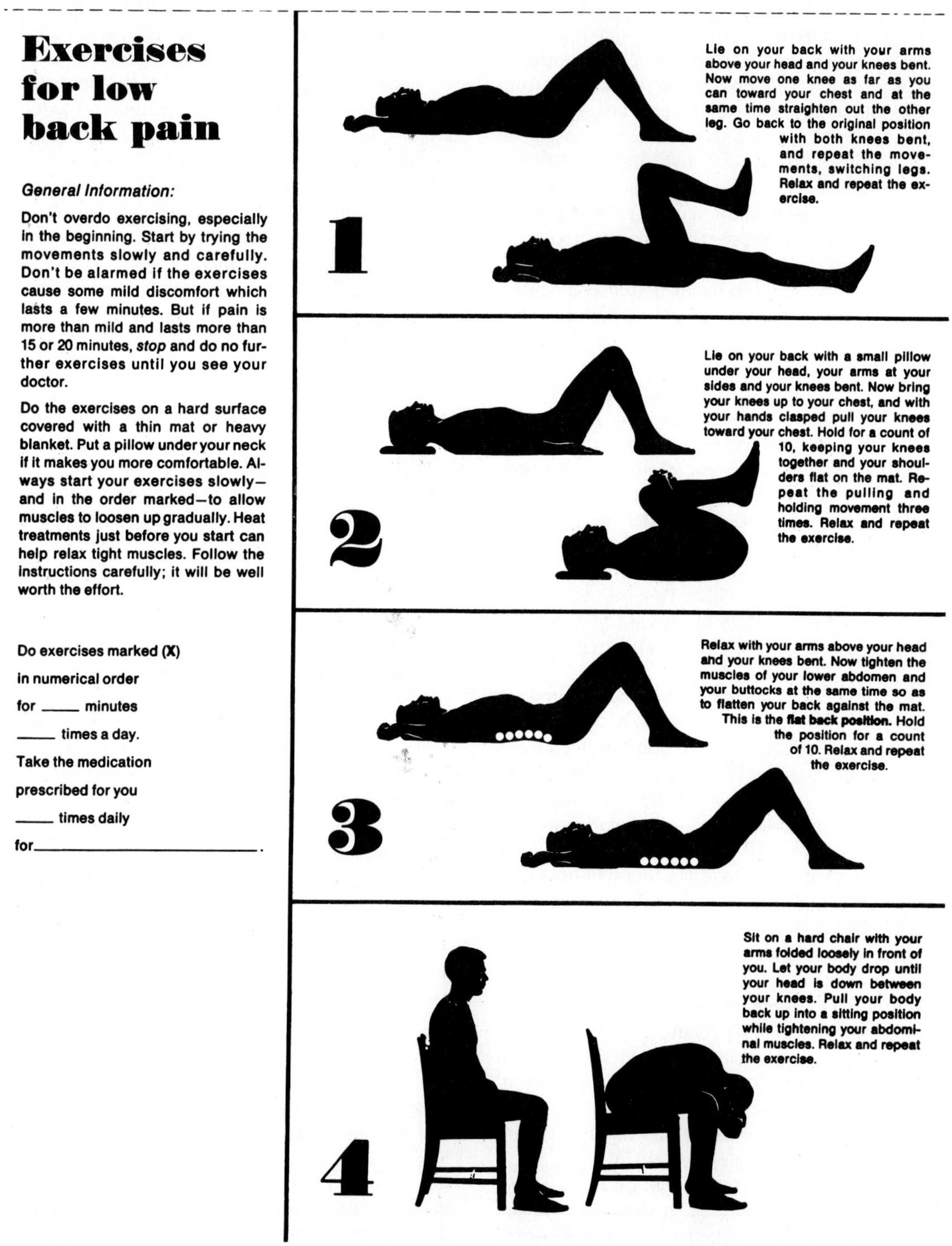

Figure 147-3. Sample instruction sheet describing exercises for low back pain (McNeil Laboratories, Fort Washington, PA).

fragments that are not in continuity with the disc space, or pain caused primarily by bony abnormalities rather than disc herniation. Relative indications for surgery include chronic disabling low back pain that persists after resolution of more acute symptoms and frequent acute recurrences of severe back pain that the patient cannot prevent by following a careful back care program.

Chymopapain disc injection is an option for patients who do not require an open procedure, although it is not indicated for backache alone. This naturally occurring enzyme acts to solubilize the nucleus pulposus, and in doing so, it decreases nerve root pressure with an effect very much like surgical disc excision. Hazards include possible nerve damage from the technique of lateral needle placement, discitis, infection, and, in 1 percent to 2 percent, an anaphylactic response. The incidence of complications is very low, and the drug is thought to be quite safe overall. However, many patients still experience back spasm and pain for several weeks after the treatment, thus prolonging the recovery period to about the same as that for surgery. Although enthusiasm for the procedure has waned, in experienced hands it still represents a less invasive means of treating disablingly painful disc herniation.

Some patients try chiropractors, acupuncturists, and other paramedical practitioners. In double-blind controlled study, *acupuncture* has proven no better than placebo for treatment of chronic back pain. There are no controlled studies on *chiropractic manipulation* for chronic back pain. *Facet joint injection* with corticosteroids has been used in some patients with chronic back pain, under the presumption that there might be a component of facet joint arthritis contributing to the patient's pain. Controlled trials have shown it to be no better than placebo. Despite initially enthusiastic reports, controlled study also found *transcutaneous electrical nerve stimulation (TENS)* ineffective.

Chronic Refractory Back Pain in the Absence of Anatomic Pathology. Patients with chronic refractory back pain and no clear anatomic deficits pose one of the most difficult long-term management problems encountered in primary care practice. Persistence of symptoms may be encouraged by social factors such as *pending litigation* or *application for disability*. At other times, the patient's amplification of symptoms and refractoriness to treatment may be manifestations of an underlying *depression* or *somatization* disorder (see Chapters 227 and 230).

There are no simple solutions to the management of these patients. Many do not take an active role in their own treatment and frustrate the well-intentioned efforts of physicians while continuing to complain of discomfort. However, some important objectives can be achieved: identification and treatment of underlying psychopathology; avoidance of inappropriate tests, addictive medications, ineffective therapies, and unnecessary surgery; and preservation of the individual's capacity to function independently.

Addressing Underlying Psychopathology and Social Factors. If depression is encountered, it should be treated (see Chapter 227) regardless of whether it is the cause or result of the patient's condition. For the person with a suspected somatization disorder, therapeutic efforts are best directed at helping the patient to find ways other than suffering to achieve a sense of self-worth. Attempting to physically "cure" such a person actually removes their one source (albeit maladaptive) of personal value. Such an effort is bound to be sabotaged by the patient, unless there is something to replace the back pain (see Chapter 230). The patient with pending legal matters should be strongly encouraged to settle them as quickly as possible. If a disability determination is needed, it should be expedited. Arranging an independent evaluation may be best. This avoids jeopardizing the patient–doctor relationship, particularly if the physician does not feel comfortable certifying that the patient is physically disabled.

Protecting the Patient from Unnecessary Procedures and Narcotics. Patients with chronic refractory back pain are at considerable risk for invasive testing (eg, myelography) and surgery, even though they may lack symptoms and signs that are considered proper indications for such procedures. The primary physician needs to protect such patients from unnecessary and potentially harmful interventions. One way to accomplish this objective is to arrange a consultation for the patient with an orthopedic surgeon or a neurosurgeon experienced in back problems, so that the patient does not feel the need to go "shopping around" for a willing surgeon.

Avoiding chronic or repeated reliance on narcotics for pain control is a key management priority. There may be repeated demands for strong analgesic agents, but unless there is an acute and reversible cause of the pain, the use of narcotics should be avoided if at all possible. Assessment for substance abuse should be considered in the back pain patient making persistent requests for narcotics (see Chapter 235).

Preserving Capacity to Function Independently. Establishing a strong doctor–patient alliance (see Chapter 1) and attending to underlying psychosocial issues are prerequisites to engaging the patient in a program of self-help. The caring, concern, and responsiveness that characterize a strong relationship help foster patient confidence and receptiveness. Even though symptoms may not disappear, it is often possible to keep the patient functioning independently through cultivation of the relationship and promulgation of a program of activity and exercise. Arranging regularly scheduled visits at intervals meaningful to the patient facilitates the sense of support and can forestall many anxious phone calls and unannounced office appearances.

PATIENT EDUCATION

The importance of patient education cannot be overemphasized in the patient with back pain. Surveys of patients with back pain find that lack of information is the greatest source of dissatisfaction with care. Patients suffering from a condition that suddenly disables them are extremely anxious and in need of detailed information about what happened, what can be done, and what lies ahead. Even if the diagnosis has not been established, a review of the working differential helps one deal with the uncertainty of the situation. The use of a model of the spine greatly simplifies explanation and helps many patients to better understand their condition. Patients with disc herniation can be reassured that the natural history of their condition is generally favorable, with most responding well to conservative therapy and very few suffering prolonged physical disability. Active patients are greatly relieved to know that jogging, stationary cycling, and swimming are not only possible but often desirable and that reemergence of mild to moderate discomfort with resumption of activity is to be expected and is not a worrisome prognostic sign. At the same time, it is important to review with the patient the symptoms of serious neurologic injury that would necessitate prompt reporting and hospital admission. The rationale and anatomic basis for back hygiene measures and exercises also need to be reviewed to assure compliance and proper implementation. A good outcome is greatly facilitated by keeping the patient well informed.

INDICATIONS FOR ADMISSION AND REFERRAL

Patients with rapidly progressive neurologic deficits require prompt neurologic and surgical consultations. Urgent admission and referral are indicated if there are symptoms suggestive of cauda equina syndrome or cord compression (eg, new bilateral neurologic deficits, urinary retention, sphincter incontinence, saddle anesthesia). The same is true for individuals with acute vertebral collapse, because spinal stability may be compromised by the fracture. Suspicion of osteomyelitis or epidural abscess is an indication for immediate hospitalization and infectious disease consultation. Particularly in patients with epidural abscess, treatment must be initiated early to be effective.

If back pain remains severe and intractable after 4 to 6 weeks of conservative therapy, or if an important neurologic deficit develops (eg, foot drop, gastroc-soleus or quadriceps weakness), then further evaluation and consideration of surgery are indicated and referral to an orthopedist or neurosurgeon with a particular interest in back problems can be helpful. Even if the patient has no sciatica or neurologic deficits and is thus not a candidate for surgery, the referral can serve to reassure the patient that a surgically correctable lesion is not being overlooked and that the efforts of the primary physician are appropriate.

ANNOTATED BIBLIOGRAPHY

Baker AS, Ojemann RG, Swartz MN, et al. Spinal epidural abscess. N Engl J Med 1975;293:463. *(An important condition to recognize. The typical progression was from spinal ache to root pain, followed by weakness and paralysis within a few days. Osteomyelitis was the cause in 38 percent and bacteremia in 26 percent.)*

Bates DW, Reuler JB. Back pain and epidural spinal cord compression. J Gen Intern Med 1988;3:191. *(Detailed review of this spinal presentation of metastatic disease; 52 refs.)*

Carette S, Marcoux S, Truchon R, et al. A controlled trial of corticosteroid injections into facet joints for chronic low back pain. N Engl J Med 1991;325:1002. *(No evidence of benefit found.)*

Deyo RA. Conservative therapy for low back pain. JAMA 1983;250:1057. *(Reviews 59 therapeutic trials; also useful for its critique of study designs.)*

Deyo RA, Bigos SJ, Maravilla KR. Diagnostic imaging procedures for the lumbar spine. Ann Intern Med 1989;111;856. *(An editorial review of available studies and need for more information on criteria for use and sequencing.)*

Deyo RA, Diehl AK. Lumbar spine films in primary care. J Gen Intern Med 1986;1:20. *(A test of criteria to limit unnecessary x-rays.)*

Deyo RA, Diehl AK, Rosenthal M. How many days of bed rest for acute low back pain? N Engl J Med 1986;315:1064. *(A randomized clinical trial showing that for patients without neurimotor deficits, 2 days of bed rest was as effective as 7.)*

Deyo RA, Loeser JD, Bigos SJ. Herniated lumbar intervertebral disk. Ann Intern Med 1990;112:598. *(Terse, critical look at diagnostic and therapeutic modalities; 41 refs.)*

Deyo RA, Rainville J, Kent DL. What can the history and physical examination tell us about low back pain? JAMA 1992;268:760. *(Required reading; summarizes available data on the diagnostic utility of historical and physical findings; many of its findings and conclusions are cited in this chapter.)*

Deyo RA, Walsh N, Martin D, et al. A controlled trial of transcutaneous electrical nerve stimulation (TENS) and exercise for chronic low back pain. N Engl J Med 1990;322:1627. *(TENS was no better than the control intervention.)*

Edelman RR, Warach S. Magnetic resonance imaging. N Engl J Med 1993;328:708. *(A major review with useful section on spinal imaging.)*

Hadler NM. Regional back pain. N Engl J Med 315:1090, 1986. *(An editorial that provides an overview of the problem and suggests that patients may be the best judge of how long to rest in bed.)*

Hall S, Bartleson JD, Onofrio BM, et al. Lumbar spinal stenosis. Ann Intern Med 1985;103:271. *(Excellent review of this often overlooked etiology.)*

Hoffman RH, Wheeler KJ, Deyo RA. Surgery for herniated discs. A literature review. J Gen Intern Med 1993;8:487. *(Finds many shortcomings in study design, but overall impression is that of some benefit from discectomy in properly selected patients.)*

Javid MJ, Nordby EJ, Ford LT, et al. Safety and efficacy of chymopapain (chymodiactin) in herniated nucleus pulposus with sciatica. JAMA 1983;249:2489. *(Useful data that helps to put the procedure in perspective.)*

Kostuik JP, Harrington I, Alexander D, et al. Cauda equina syndrome and lumbar disc herniation. J Bone Joint Surg [Am] 1986;68:386. *(Clinical features of this important syndrome are delineated.)*

Liang M, Komaroff AL. Roentgenograms in primary-care patients with acute low back pain: a cost-effectiveness study. Arch Intern Med 1982;142:1108. *(Cost is high, yield low if films are ordered on a first visit.)*

Mendelson G, Selwood T, Kranz H, et al. Acupuncture treatment of chronic back pain. Am J Med 1983;74:49. *(A double-blind, placebo-controlled study showing no difference in results.)*

Shekelle PG, Adamas AH, Chassin MP, et al. Spinal manipulation for low-back pain. Ann Intern Med 1992;117:590. *(A meta-analysis finding short-term value in those with uncomplicated acute back pain; data insufficient for determining utility in chronic back pain.)*

Waddell G, McCulloch JA, Kummel E, et al. Nonorganic physical signs in low back pain. Spine 1980;5:117. *(Describes physical findings, noted in this chapter, suggestive of persons suffering from psychological distress.)*

Weber H. Lumbar disc herniation: a controlled prospective study with ten years of observation. Spine 1983;8:131. *(The only randomized trial of medical vs surgical therapy; surgery achieved earlier relief but no difference in outcomes after 3–4 y.)*

148
Evaluation of Neck Pain

ROBERT J. BOYD, M.D.

Primary Care Medicine: Office Evaluation and Management of the Adult Patient, 3rd edition, edited by Allan H. Goroll, Lawrence A. May, and Albert G. Mulley, Jr. J.B. Lippincott Company, Philadelphia

The primary physician is often faced with the patient who complains of a stiff neck; most of the time, the problem is musculoskeletal in origin. Although the majority of musculoskeletal causes are not serious, they can result in considerable discomfort. One should be able to provide symptomatic relief to the person with a minor neck problem and to identify the patient with a serious complication of cervical spine disease, such as root compression or cord injury, that requires surgical attention.

PATHOPHYSIOLOGY AND CLINICAL PRESENTATION

Severe *neck strain* is one of the most frequent causes of neck pain and usually results from a specific injury. Tearing of muscle fibers can cause bleeding, swelling, severe muscle spasm, and pain. Symptoms increase gradually over several hours, often becoming most severe the day following the acute event. The anterior or posterior ligaments of the cervical spine may be disrupted. If the injury is not complicated by root or spinal cord compression, there are no neurologic deficits.

Neck pain from *cervical paraspinal muscle spasm* is usually secondary to neck strain or prolonged, unconscious muscle contraction associated with emotional stress. The problem is usually self-limited, although it may recur. Muscles spasm also occurs with cervical arthritis and cervical disc disease.

Trauma or degenerative changes in the intervertebral discs or joint facets can be a source of neck pain and can result in ankylosis or subluxation of the cervical spine, termed *cervical spondylosis*. Immobility and consolidation of the joint may ensue. Usually the process is localized to the lower cervical levels, such as C4-5, C5-6, or C6-7. Degenerative changes and spurring at the cervical disc spaces are prominent. The condition presents as recurring neck stiffness and mild aching discomfort, with progressive limitation of neck motion over months to years. Lateral rotation and lateral flexion of the neck toward the painful side are limited; pain is precipitated or increased by such motions.

Cervical disc degeneration can lead to narrowing of the neural foramina, causing *root impingement* and pain. Pain radiates in the distribution of the affected nerve root, and there may be associated paresthesias, numbness, and weakness. The C5, C6, and C7 nerve roots are most often affected. C5 root compression results in the development of pain, paresthesias, and numbness in the anterosuperior shoulder and anterolateral aspect of the upper arm and forearm; decreased biceps jerk and weakness of elbow flexion are found on examination. Compression of the C6 nerve root produces symptoms in the dorsoradial aspect of the forearm and thumb, while C7 impingement is denoted by altered sensation in the middle of the hand. The brachioradialis tendon reflex is affected by conditions altering C5 and C6, and the triceps jerk by injury to the C7 and C8 roots.

Whiplash is a lay term used to denote neck injury from an automobile accident. Typically, there is sudden hyperextension of the neck followed by flexion, resulting in musculoligamentous strain. Neurologic deficits are rare unless there is an accompanying cervical spine fracture leading to root or cord compression. The problem of neck pain is often complicated by concurrent legal proceedings.

DIFFERENTIAL DIAGNOSIS

The musculoskeletal causes of neck pain include muscle strain, muscle spasm, cervical spondylosis, and cervical root compression. Lymphadenopathy, thyroiditis (see Chapter 104), angina pectoris (see Chapter 20), and meningitis are important causes of cervical pain that may be mistaken for a musculoskeletal etiology.

WORKUP

History. Inquiry should focus on elucidating precipitating events, aggravating and alleviating factors (particularly specific neck movements), area of maximal tenderness, radiation of pain, presence of numbness or weakness in the extremities, course, past history of similar problems, and previous therapeutic efforts. One also should consider symptoms suggestive of coronary artery disease (see Chapter 30) or meningeal irritation.

Physical examination must include full visualization of the neck, thorax, and upper extremities. Neck motions are assessed, including flexion-extension, left and right lateral flexion, and left and right rotation. Palpation must be carefully done to identify the point of local tenderness, which gives the best indication of the structure involved. The upper extremities should also be carefully examined, including evaluation of tendon reflexes, strength, sensation, range of motion, and pulses. Every patient with fever and neck pain should be tested for meningeal signs.

Laboratory Studies. Cervical spine x-rays are mandatory if there is root pain or a neurologic deficit and should include anteroposterior, lateral, oblique, and flexion-extension views in all cases to check for fracture, subluxation, narrowing of foramina, and soft tissue abnormalities. An electrocardiogram is indicated if chest pain radiates into the neck and jaw or if the patient with isolated neck pain has risk factors for coronary disease.

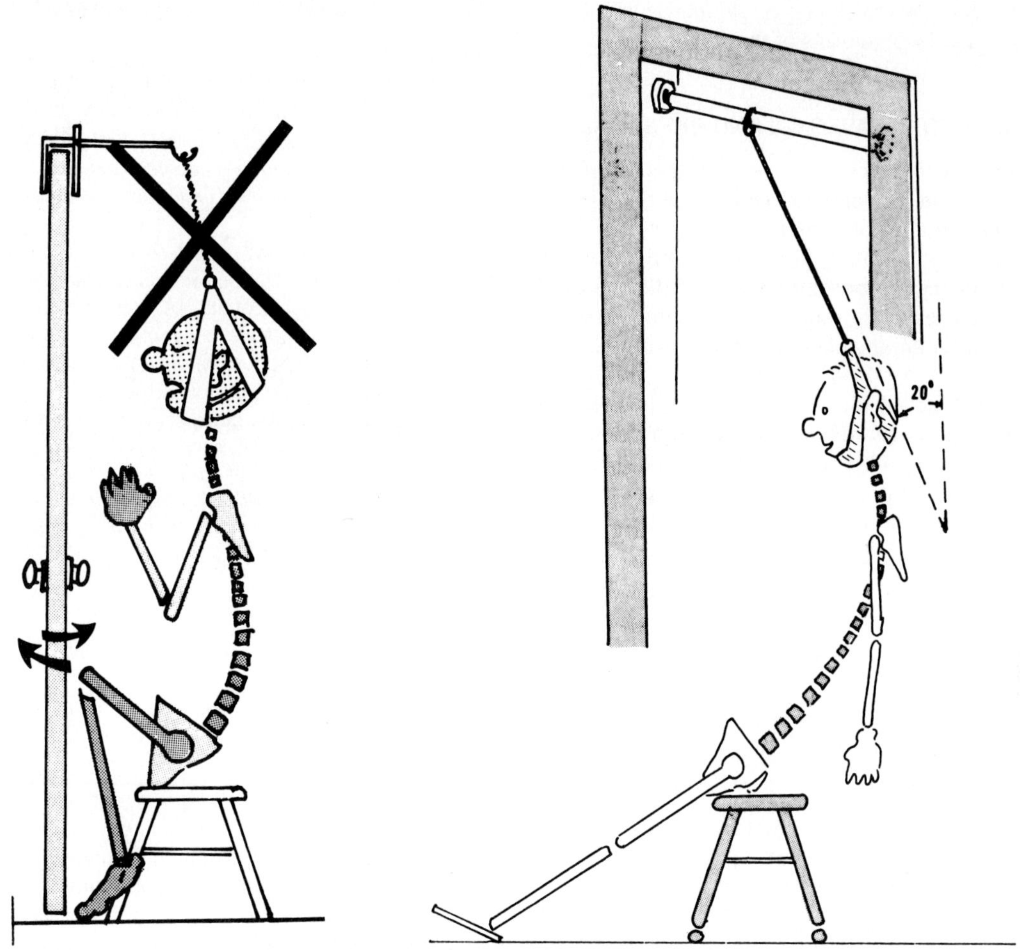

A B

Figure 148-1. (*A*), Ineffective home door cervial traction. The patient is too close to the door to get the correct neck flexion angle. The door freely opens and closes, not permitting constant traction. The patient cannot extend the legs or assume a comfortable position. This type of home traction is not recommended. (*B*) Recommended home traction from chinning bar in the sitting position. (Cailliet R: Soft Tissue Pain and Disability. Philadelphia: FA Davis, 1977:129.)

SYMPTOMATIC MANAGEMENT

Neck pain caused by minor muscle ligament strain is usually self-limited if aggravating activities are avoided. Heat and gentle massage may ease muscle spasm. There is no good evidence that injecting anesthetic into the tender body of a muscle in spasm speeds resolution of the problem, and injection may actually injure the muscle. Occasionally, a soft *cervical collar* is needed if symptoms persist. The collar should be worn for several days to a few weeks, and it should be used at all times until pain clears. After pain lessens, the collar can be worn at those times when added support may be helpful, such as at night or when riding in a motor vehicle. Most so-called *muscle relaxants* are actually minor tranquilizers marketed as relaxants. They are of limited value for prolonged use but can provide short-term help, especially for falling asleep. More useful and less expensive are therapeutic doses of a *nonnarcotic analgesic* (eg, aspirin, acetaminophen, ibuprofen), supplemented for a few days by a small nighttime dose of a generic benzodiazepine (eg, diazepam 5 mg qhs). Prolonged benzodiazepine use is to be avoided (see Chapter 226).

Home cervical traction is indicated for severe, chronic, or recurrent neck pain caused by cervical spondylosis or disc herniation associated with radiculitis. Sitting cervical traction is employed at home for 20 to 30 minutes, two to four times a day, using 6 to 10 pounds of weight. The cervical traction apparatus must be carefully aligned, pulling slightly forward at an angle of about 20° to follow the natural line in the neck (Fig. 148–1). Proper technique is essential for effective and safe use.

Spinal manipulation has proven useful for short-term relief of low back pain (see Chapter 147), and some studies suggest that it may play a role in treatment of nonspecific neck pain, but its utility, safety, and indications for use in neck pain remain to be properly defined. *Ultrasound* and *diathermy* treatments also provide subjective improvement over and above that derived from medical management, but often no more than placebo forms of these therapies.

INDICATIONS FOR ADMISSION AND REFERRAL

If pain is intractable to conservative measures, if there is significant weakness in the upper extremity, or if there is evidence of cord pressure or long tract signs, neurosurgical or orthopedic referral is indicated. Surgery may be necessary if signs of cord injury are present, unless further cervical traction in hospital results in rapid improvement. Presence of meningeal signs is an obvious indication for urgent hospitalization.

The patient with persistent neck pain is likely to request or ask about physiotherapy (eg, diathermy, ultrasound, spinal manipulation). Carefully reviewing available data on these procedures with the patient can help achieve an informed choice that is mutually satisfactory and minimizes risk and expense.

ANNOTATED BIBLIOGRAPHY

Bland JH. Disorders of the Cervical Spine: Diagnosis and Medical Management. Philadelphia: WB Saunders, 1987. *(Excellent monograph for the nonsurgical reader.)*

Cailliet R. Soft Tissue Pain and Disability. Philadelphia: FA Davis, 1977. *(Chapter 4 provides detailed discussion of soft tissue cervical problems and practical approaches to management.)*

Koes BW, Assendelft WJ, van der Heijde GJ, et al. Spinal manipulation and mobilization for back and neck pain: a blinded review. BMJ 1991;303:1298. *(A critical review; delineates the important design flaws in manipulation studies.)*

Koes BW, Bouter LM, van Mameren H, et al. The effectiveness of manual therapy, physiotherapy, and treatment by the general practitioner for nonspecific back and neck complaints. Spine 1992;17:28. *(A randomized, single-blinded, placebo controlled 3-mo trial of patients with nonspecific neck or back pain; spinal manipulation, physiotherapy, and placebo physiotherapy were superior to medical management by the general practitioner.)*

149
Approach to the Patient With Muscle Cramps

Primary Care Medicine: Office Evaluation and Management of the Adult Patient, 3rd edition, edited by Allan H. Goroll, Lawrence A. May, and Albert G. Mulley, Jr. J.B. Lippincott Company, Philadelphia

Muscle cramps are prolonged involuntary muscle contractions that can be painful and difficult to manage but rarely reflect serious underlying disease. True cramps must be differentiated from ischemic pain, contracture, tetany, and dystonia. Fluid and electrolyte disorders, medication, and endocrinologic disorders must be considered in the evaluation, although they are uncommon precipitants. Patients come in requesting symptomatic relief from these painful episodes, which can be temporarily disabling.

PATHOPHYSIOLOGY AND CLINICAL PRESENTATION

True Cramps

True muscle cramping represents motor unit hyperactivity leading to prolonged involuntary muscle contraction. Precipitants include unopposed contraction, electrolyte and volume shifts, and lower motor neuron disease. *Ordinary cramps* most commonly occur in the gastrocnemius muscle and the intrinsic muscles of the sole of the foot. Their *nocturnal* predilection appears to be related to unopposed foot plantar flexion while in bed, placing the muscles of the calves and feet in their most shortened and therefore most vulnerable position. Without modulation by opposing muscles, the sustained contraction produces the painful cramp, which is experienced as sudden severe calf pain, often with a palpable or visibly hardened muscle. In many instances, a voluntary contraction triggers the cramp. Passive stretching relieves it.

True cramps may be precipitated by *volume* and *electrolyte shifts*, accounting for their frequent occurrence during hemodialysis and their relief with hypertonic dextrose. *Heat cramps* that occur during activity are a consequence of dehydration and sodium loss and respond to their replenishment. *Hyponatremia* is a consistent feature of fluid-based muscle cramps, but hypokalemia is not, contrary to common belief. Cramps attributable to potassium-wasting diuretics are actually uncommon. Ordinary cramps are often a part of symptomatic *hypoglycemia*.

Muscle cramps are sometimes *drug-induced*, as may occur with nifedipine, beta-agonists, and, occasionally, heavy alcohol use.

The cramp is a neural or electrical phenomenon, not primarily muscular. Electromyography shows fasciculations preceding the cramp. Cramps accompanied by clinically evident fasciculations characterize those which occur in *lower motor neuron diseases*, such as recovering polio, peripheral nerve injury, nerve root compression, and amyotrophic lateral sclerosis.

Other Forms of Muscle Cramping

Contractures also represent involuntary muscle contractions, but they are electrically silent and characteristically occur during exertion, not rest. They develop in persons who have inherited metabolic defects impairing formation of adenosine triphosphate (ATP), which is needed for muscle relaxation. Most patients have McArdle's disease. Thyroid disease, both of the hyper- and hypothyroid varieties, may cause cramping. Exertional cramping has been seen with hyperthyroidism. In hypothyroidism, muscle relaxation is impaired, producing the "hung-up" reflexes that characterize the condition.

Tetany is a state of both motor and sensory hyperactivity, with muscle spasm and paresthesias. The muscles of the mouth, hands, and lower extremities are typically involved,

Table 149-1. Differential Diagnosis of Muscle Cramps

True Cramps	
	Ordinary (nocturnal)
	Heat-induced (volume depletion, hyponatremia)
	Hemodialysis (volume and electrolyte shifts)
	Lower motor neuron
	Drug-induced (nifedipine, beta-agonists)
Dystonia	
	Occupational (writer's cramp)
Tetany	
	Hypocalcemia
	Hypomagnesemia
	Respiratory alkalosis
	Hypokalemia
Contracture	
	McArdle's disease
	Thyroid disease

(Adapted from McGee SR. Muscle cramps. Arch Intern Med 1990;150:511.)

and carpopedal spasm is a characteristic manifestation, as are Chvostek's and Trousseau's signs. Hypocalcemia, hypomagnesemia, respiratory alkalosis, and hypokalemia are known precipitants. In severe cases, seizures may ensue if the condition goes uncorrected.

Occupational cramp is a form of dystonia in which muscle contractures occur in persons engaging in fine motor activities that have taken years to perfect. The typical patient is a writer or pianist whose hands curl involuntarily on attempting to begin writing or playing.

DIFFERENTIAL DIAGNOSIS

See Table 149–1 for information on the differential diagnosis of muscle cramps.

WORKUP

History. A detailed description of the cramping is essential and should include the setting in which the episodes occur. Those that develop at night or in the context of hemodialysis, hypoglycemia, or heavy sweating from prolonged exertion are likely to be true cramps, as are those coincident with use of calcium channel blockers or beta-agonists. Dystonic cramping is suggested by onset with occupation-related fine motor activity, and contracture by a lifelong onset with exercise. Associated symptoms should be reviewed for the paresthesias and carpopedal spasm of tetany, the weakness and fasciculations of lower motor neuron disease, and the cold or heat intolerance, skin changes, and related symptoms of thyroid disease (see Chapters 103 and 104). Location of the cramping is a less specific finding, but if calf pain is reported, one should include intermittent claudication in the differential diagnosis, particularly if pain is brought on by walking. Review of medications is always useful, but use of a potassium-wasting diuretic is not tantamount to an etiologic diagnosis, because hypokalemia is rarely responsible for true cramps (although it should be considered in the differential diagnosis of tetany). Also potentially pertinent in suspected tetany is any distant history of thyroidectomy (with coincident removal of the parathyroid glands).

Physical Examination. If dehydration is suspected, physical examination begins with a check of postural signs for a drop in blood pressure and rise in pulse. The skin is examined for signs of thyroid disease (see Chapters 103 and 104), the neck for evidence of thyroidectomy, the lower extremities for diminished or absent pulses, muscle wasting, and fasciculations, and the nervous system for focal weakness and absent or abnormal deep tendon reflexes. If tetany is a consideration, one can try to elicit the facial spasm of Trousseau's sign by tapping the facial nerve or the carpal spasm of Chvostek's sign by inflating the arm cuff above systolic pressure.

Laboratory determinations can be very limited. For the majority of people who present with a clinical story of nocturnal muscle cramps, laboratory testing is unlikely to provide additional information. Other situations do require a few simple tests. If the patient with ordinary cramps is diabetic and taking insulin, then testing for hypoglycemia is indicated (see Chapter 102). If severe dehydration and hyponatremia are suspected, then determinations of serum sodium, blood urea nitrogen (BUN), and creatinine can guide assessment and treatment. The patient with possible tetany needs a check of sodium, potassium, calcium, albumin (to interpret the calcium level), and magnesium. Consideration of thyroid disease is best pursued by obtaining a serum thyrotropin (TSH) determination. The patient with fasciculations and possible lower motor neuron disease may need a nerve conduction study.

PRINCIPLES OF MANAGEMENT AND INDICATIONS FOR ADMISSION

Ordinary Cramps. To relieve an established cramp, one must passively stretch the contracting muscle and gradually contract the apposing one. In some cases, this can be accomplished by simply walking around, which produces a relative dorsiflexion of the foot.

Massage of the involved muscle sometimes helps. Consciously dorsiflexing at the first sign of a leg or foot cramp might abort it. Prophylactic stretching can also prevent attacks (see Chapter 18 for stretching exercise), as might positions in bed that prevent foot dorsiflexion. Swimming-induced cramps can be avoided by sacrificing the ideal plantar-flexed kicking position and maintaining a more neutral foot position.

Patients who suffer from repeated attacks of nocturnal leg cramps seek a reduction in the frequency and severity of episodes. *Quinine sulfate* has been prescribed for decades for this purpose, but only recently have randomized, double-blind, controlled clinical trials been performed to assess its efficacy, and the number of patients studied remains small. Studies using low-to-moderate dose regimens (200–300 mg qhs) show less benefit than do those using higher doses (200 mg at supper, 300 qhs). This pattern suggests that response rates are related to serum level attained, which can vary greatly with age and preparation used. Risk of serious side effects is quite small but increases with dose and serum level. Cinchonism (nausea, vomiting, tinnitus, hearing loss), visual impairment, and ventricular arrhythmias are the most important of these adverse effects, appearing when serum levels exceed two to five times average serum concentration. An immune thrombocytopenia, occasionally fatal, has also been reported. The small, but real, risk of serious toxicity and the modest drug efficacy should temper one's uncritical use of quinine for this otherwise benign condition. The drug is available without prescription in low-dose formulations. For those who suffer disabling nocturnal cramps unresponsive to nonpharmacologic measures, a careful trial of quinine may be useful after reviewing risks and benefits with the patient. Starting with small doses (200–300 mg qhs) is best, and platelet count should be monitored periodically. Only if meaningful benefit is obtained should quinine prophylaxis be continued.

Other drugs shown to be of some benefit include methocarbamol and chloroquine. Vitamin E is promoted in health food stores for treatment of nocturnal cramps, but it has been found to be no better than placebo when tested in double-blind, placebo-controlled fashion. It may be found in combination with quinine. The calcium channel blocker verapamil has shown promise in preliminary study.

Patients with ordinary cramps related to dehydration and sodium depletion respond well to replacement therapy. Those with cramps as a consequence of hemodialysis are best treated with rapid volume expansion (hypertonic dextrose or saline infusion). If hypoglycemia is responsible, then adjustment of insulin regimen is needed (see Chapter 102). Altering the medication program may be necessary in cases in which beta-agonists or calcium channel blockers are thought to be responsible.

Occupational Cramps are difficult to treat. Rest and occupational aids can be helpful; psychotherapy is not. Minor tranquilizers provide some short-term relief but little sustained benefit. Injection of botulinum toxin has been tried with some success.

Tetany requires urgent hospital admission and careful parenteral correction of the underlying electrolyte disturbances. For patients bothered by occasional muscle cramps, medication is not a serious consideration. For those who have frequent or prolonged cramps, prophylactic medication should be considered.

L.A.M.

ANNOTATED BIBLIOGRAPHY

Baltodano N, Gallo BV, Weidler DJ. Verapamil versus quinine in recumbent nocturnal leg cramps in the elderly. Arch Intern Med 1988;148:1969. *(Open-label trial in eight elderly patients refractory to quinine, showing noteworthy improvement.)*

Connolly PS, Shirley EA, Wasson JH, et al. Treatment of nocturnal leg cramps. Arch Intern Med 1992;152:1877. *(Quinine but not vitamin E was effective; a program of 500 mg/d relieved cramps within 3–5 d.)*

Freiman JP. Fatal quinine-induced thrombocytopenia. Ann Intern Med 1990;112:308. *(An FDA report of two previously well patients who developed fatal quinine-induced thrombocytopenia.)*

Fung MC, Holbrook JH. Placebo-controlled trial of quinine therapy for nocturnal leg cramps. West J Med 1989;151:42. *(A small but well-designed study; quinine produced a statistically significant reduction in the number and severity of cramps.)*

McGee SR. Muscle cramps. Arch Intern Med 1990;150:511. *(A comprehensive review; 170 refs.)*

150

Approach to the Patient With Shoulder Pain

JESSE B. JUPITER, M.D.

The shoulder is a complex joint integrating 3 bones, 4 joints, and more than 15 muscles. The shoulder's mobility exceeds that of all other joints, subjecting it to a wide range of stresses, both in normal activity and in occupational and recreational pursuits. Shoulder pain and dysfunction are among the more common musculoskeletal complaints encountered in office practice. Successful treatment necessitates an accurate diagnosis; common nonspecific diagnoses such as "bursitis" and "tendinitis" can be misleading and delay appropriate therapeutic measures. Besides being capable of identifying an etiology, the primary physician needs to know how and when to utilize exercises, anti-inflammatory agents, and joint injection to provide safe and effective symptomatic relief.

PATHOPHYSIOLOGY AND CLINICAL PRESENTATION

Injury or degenerative change in the rotator cuff, bicipital tendon, or acromioclavicular joint can produce pain localized to the shoulder joint. Characteristically, there is focal tenderness and aggravation of pain on shoulder movement. Patients report difficulty dressing, combing their hair, or reaching up. Degenerative disease of the glenohumeral joint is uncommon; symptoms include mild stiffness, crepitus, and low-grade, aching discomfort related to vigorous or sustained use. Pain originating in or about the shoulder may be referred to the upper arm or radiate to the neck, elbow, or forearm; it does not follow a specific cervical root distribution. Although pain originating in the neck may radiate to the shoulder, it is brought on by neck motion rather than by shoulder movement and is usually not affected by shoulder position. However, there may be poorly localized sensitivity to touch extending into the shoulder, vaguely simulating shoulder pathology (see Chapter 148).

Rotator Cuff Problems. The tendons of the cuff are subjected to considerable mechanical stress. Degenerative and attritional changes take place over time in the tendons and lead to structural weakening. Tendinitis and tears may ensue. Calcific deposits develop as degenerating tendon fibers become pulverized and collections of calcium salts form. These deposits may contribute to local mechanical irritation by causing a bulge in the tendon and decreasing the clearances under the acromion and the coracoacromial ligament. Fibrous scarring with limitation of motion often occurs as part of the repair mechanism.

Calcific tendinitis is frequent and commonly affects the supraspinatus tendon. Usually, there is no major precipitating event. It can cause acute or chronic pain; initially, the pain is localized to the vicinity of the greater tuberosity and the acromion process. Pain is worsened by abduction and elevation of the shoulder joint. X-rays may demonstrate calcium deposits in the tendon.

Bursitis is rarely a primary condition; usually, it is secondary to calcific tendinitis. The subdeltoid bursa lies just above the supraspinatus tendon. The acutely inflamed and bulging tendon may irritate the overlying bursa. In addition, calcium deposits in the tendon may evacuate into the subbursal space or rupture into the bursa; if such material ruptures into the bursa, pain and tenderness may be felt in the upper third of the humerus.

A weakened rotator cuff may *tear* spontaneously as a result of minimal trauma. Most patients with tears are older than age 40 and may present with surprisingly little pain. Pain over the deltoid, especially with overhead activities, plus weakness of shoulder elevation and external rotation, are diagnostic features. Muscle atrophy is commonly present. Local sensitivity is maximal over the greater tuberosity and rotator cuff (Fig. 150–1). Passive range of motion is full. X-rays are normal or show a diminished subacromial space.

In *adhesive capsulitis*, or *frozen shoulder syndrome*, there is a characteristic symptom complex of pain and tenderness located diffusely about the anterior and posterior regions of the shoulder joint capsule. Active as well as passive motions of the glenohumeral joint are limited to a small pain-free arc. Glenohumeral motion slowly decreases over several weeks. The condition is often refractory to most forms of treatment, yet motion usually improves with time.

Biceps tendinitis of the shoulder is less common than rotator cuff tendinitis and often follows from overuse activities above the head that lead to subacromial impingement. Elbow flexion against resistance usually reproduces the pain, which is over the anterior aspect of the shoulder and upper arm. Characteristically, there is tenderness localized to the area about the long head of the biceps, in the bicipital groove over the proximal anterior margin of the humerus (see Fig. 150–1).

Glenohumeral Joint Problems. The joint is subject to considerable stress and may develop arthritis or instability.

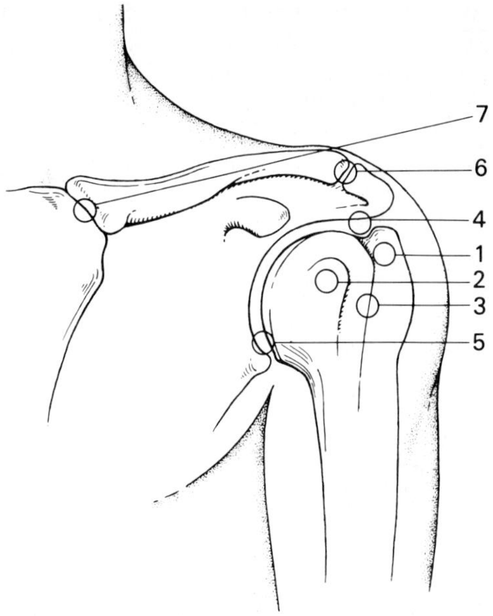

Figure 150-1. Trigger points. Palpable "trigger points" during the examination reveal the site of the pathology, corroborate the history, and indicate the type of therapy. (*1*), The greater tuberosity and the site of supraspinatus tendon insertion. (*2*), Lesser tuberosity, site of subscapularis muscle insertion. (*3*), Bicipital groove in which glides the bicipital tendon. (*4*), Site of the subdeltoid bursa. (*5*), Glenohumeral joint space. (*6*), Acromioclavicular joint. (*7*), Sternoclavicular joint. (Redrawn from Cailliet R: Shoulder Pain. Philadelphia: FA Davis, 1973.)

Instability ensues from a posttraumatic capsular tear or stretch. The patient says that the shoulder "gives out" in conjunction with discomfort and weakness. *Dislocation* usually results from trauma to the shoulder while it is hyperextended. Dislocations are most often anterior and are characterized by loss of the shoulder's rounded appearance. There is prominence of the acromion, limitation of movement by pain, and displacement of the humerus away from the trunk.

Arthritis of the joint causes symptoms at rest, exacerbated by shoulder use. The patient may note a "grinding" sound with motion. Muscle atrophy, "bone-on-bone" crepitation, and diminished motion are noted on examination. Rheumatoid disease gives a picture of symmetrical bilateral inflammatory changes.

Acromioclavicular Degenerative Lesions. Degenerative changes are seen in patients who do heavy labor or engage in contact sports. Pain arises with activities above and in front of the body and localizes to the acromioclavicular joint; tenderness is maximal over the joint and does not radiate.

Infection. The shoulder joint may become contaminated by an improperly performed injection and present with marked swelling, redness, and fever.

Referred Pain. *Shoulder-hand syndrome* (also referred to as reflex sympathetic dystrophy) follows myocardial infarction, stroke, trauma, and a host of other events. The characteristic features are persistent burning, "causalgic" pain,

Table 150-1. Important Causes of Shoulder Pain

Rotator Cuff	
	Calcific tendinitis
	Subacromial impingement
	Biceps tendinitis
	Tear
	Adhesive capsulitis
Glenohumeral Joint	
	Instability
	Dislocation
	Arthritis
	Infection
Acromioclavicular Joint	
	Arthritis
Referred	
	Cervical spondylosis
	Myocardial ischemia
	Shoulder-hand syndrome (reflex sympathetic dystrophy)
	Diaphragmatic irritation
	Thoracic outlet syndrome
	Gallbladder disease

diffuse tenderness, immobilization of the shoulder, and vasomotor changes in the hands. *Gallbladder disease* is suggested by pain at the tip of the scapula in conjunction with concurrent upper abdominal pain and tenderness. With *diaphragmatic irritation*, pain may be referred to the trapezius area running from the shoulder to the lateral aspect of the neck.

DIFFERENTIAL DIAGNOSIS

The causes of shoulder pain can be considered in terms of the structures that comprise the shoulder (Table 150–1). The vast majority of nontraumatic shoulder complaints are related to tendinitis.

WORKUP

History. One should inquire about previous trauma or an inciting event, location and radiation of pain, specific limitations of movement, associated neurologic deficits, aggravating and alleviating factors, previous history of shoulder problems, and therapies utilized. It is important to be sure there are no symptoms suggestive of angina, gallbladder disease, or diaphragmatic irritation. Pain resulting from myocardial ischemia usually originates in the precordial region but may present as shoulder or neck pain radiating into the arm. Relief with rest or nitroglycerin supports the diagnosis. An occupational history is occasionally revealing, especially if the patient has engaged in heavy labor or sports.

Complaints suggestive of shoulder disease describe a combination of pain, loss of mobility, and weakness. Pain associated with activities above the horizontal suggests subacromial impingement or acromioclavicular joint arthritis. Overuse syndromes are commonly associated with sporting activities involving throwing or racquet use. An occupational history such as wallpapering, painting, or carpentry would suggest rotator cuff pathology. A history of recent trauma may indicate a traumatic subdeltoid bursitis, whereas a past history of shoulder dislocations might suggest glenohumeral instability.

Physical Examination. Before proceeding to the examination of the shoulder, it is important to carefully check the neck, chest, heart, and abdomen for sources of referred pain. Cervical disease is often mistaken for a shoulder problem. Cervical root compression is readily distinguished from intrinsic shoulder disease by the elicitation and reproduction of pain on neck motion to the side of complaint. Brachial plexus injury causing shoulder pain is associated with tenderness on deep pressure over the neurovascular bundle and scalene muscles of the supraclavicular fossa. The chest is checked for effusion, pleural rub, and poor diaphragmatic movement. If the heart is examined during pain, one can listen for transient auscultatory signs of ischemia (eg, fourth heart sound, single second sound, mitral regurgitant murmur from papillary muscle dysfunction). The abdomen is palpated for tenderness in the right or left upper quadrant, which may signal subdiaphragmatic pathology.

For the shoulder examination, the patient is comfortably seated and sufficiently disrobed to permit evaluation and comparison of both shoulders. Close *inspection* from both front and back may demonstrate asymmetry or deformity. For example, supraspinatus muscle atrophy would suggest either rotator cuff tear or suprascapular nerve pathology. The patient is instructed to place the involved shoulder *actively* through a *full range of motion*, along with similar movements of the contralateral limb for comparison. This includes forward flexion, extension, abduction, and internal and external rotation. Internal rotation is best recorded as the level at which the patient can reach posteriorly, such as buttock or thoracolumbar junction. The scapula is observed as the patient forward flexes the shoulder against resistance. Winging of the scapula is the result of serratus anterior muscle palsy.

The patient is instructed to point out specific *sites of tenderness*. Palpation by the examiner routinely should include the anterior aspect of the acromion, the acromioclavicular joint, the bicipital groove (which is best palpated with the humerus in about 10° of internal rotation), the greater tuberosity, and the cervical spine. With the examiner's hand on the joint, the shoulder is *passively* put through a *range of motion* (Fig. 150–2). Limitations are noted, as well as any palpable crepitation.

A manual *muscle test* is helpful, in particular for comparison with the uninvolved shoulder. Inability to "shrug" the shoulder suggests trapezial muscle weakness, while weakness of forward flexion is associated with derangement of the rotator cuff (the supraspinatus, infraspinatus, and teres minor muscles). A *sensory* and *deep tendon reflex* examination of the upper extremity should be included in the routine shoulder evaluation.

Diagnostic Maneuvers. Several specific maneuvers are diagnostically helpful. *Wright's maneuver* (evaluating the radial pulse at the wrist with the shoulder in external rotation and abduction) may uncover an underlying thoracic outlet syndrome. This test is considered positive if it reproduces shoulder and arm symptoms and the radial pulse is obliterated in this shoulder position.

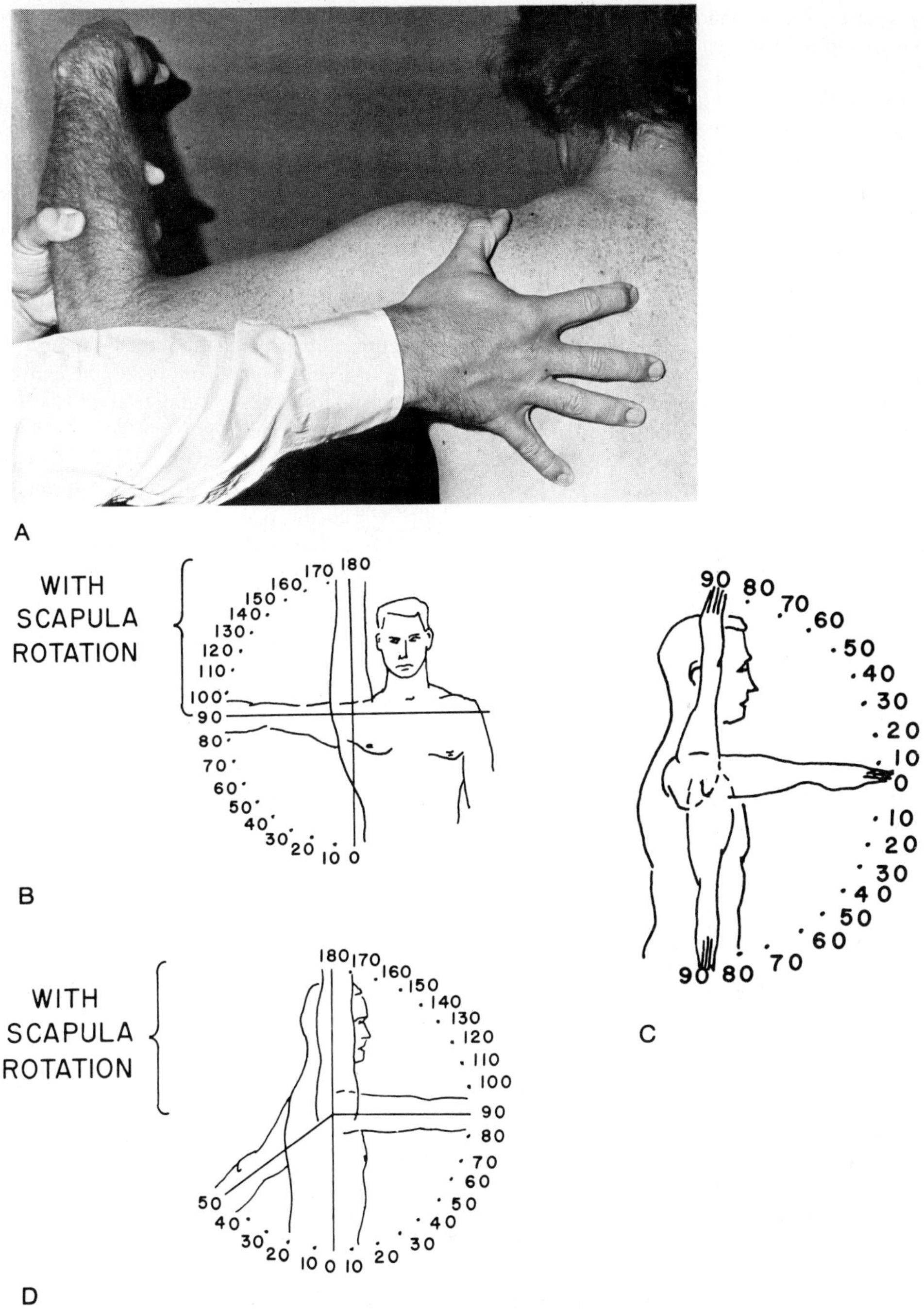

Figure 150-2. (*A*), Stabilization of the scapula while testing glenohumeral joint motion (*B*), Normal range of adduction-abduction of the shoulder with and without scapular rotation. (*C*), Normal range of external-internal rotation with upper arm at 90 degrees and elbow held at right angle. (*D*), Normal range of flexion-extension of the shoulder with and without scapular rotation. (Katz WA: Rheumatic Diseases. Philadelphia: JB Lippincott, 1977.)

The *impingement test* is performed by the examiner's standing behind the patient and bringing the involved arm to the maximum degree of forward flexion with one hand while the other functions to depress the patient's shoulder girdle. If pain is elicited in the deltoid area or beneath the acromion, impingement of the greater tuberosity of the humerus against the undersurface of the acromium is likely. This can be further confirmed if an injection of 5 mL of Xylocaine into the subacromial space relieves the symptoms. The same maneuver performed with the patient's elbow extended and the forearm supinated will accentuate the discomfort of bicipital tendinitis (Speed's sign).

A specific test for acromioclavicular joint pathology reproduces the patient's symptoms by bringing the involved arm across the body so that the *elbow touches* the *contralateral shoulder*. This can be further confirmed by repeating the maneuver after injecting the acromioclavicular joint with 1 mL of Xylocaine, using a 25-gauge needle to enter the joint.

Glenohumeral joint stability is best assessed with the patient supine. The involved arm is gently abducted, externally rotated, and held for one minute in this position. Laxity of the joint capsule causes the patient to describe a feeling of joint instability and insecurity.

Laboratory Studies. Radiographs of the shoulder are mandatory in the initial evaluation. A *standard anteroposterior view* is helpful in ruling out underlying bone tumor, infection, or arthritis of either the glenohumeral or acromioclavicular joints. The anteroposterior view with the shoulder in *internal* and *external rotation* can best identify calcification. An *axillary view* is mandatory if dislocation is suspected; it most clearly defines the relation of the humeral head to the glenoid fossa and is also helpful in assessing glenohumeral arthritis. Cervical spine films are needed if neck motion reproduces the shoulder pain or root compression symptoms are observed (see Chapter 148).

Shoulder arthrography is most helpful in identifying a suspected rotator cuff tear. Dye is injected directly into the glenohumeral joint, and the joint is then mobilized. The presence of dye extravasated from the joint is highly suggestive of disruption of the rotator cuff. *Magnetic resonance imaging (MRI)* provides a noninvasive means of assessing the integrity of the rotator cuff and in some instances obviates the need for arthrography to detect a tear. Impingement syndromes are also well imaged by MRI.

If infection is suspected in the joint or joint capsule, *aspiration*, *Gram's stain*, and *culture* are urgent so that definitive therapy can be initiated without delay (see Chapter 145). If a peripheral nerve deficit is discovered on neurologic examination, *electromyography* may help to better characterize the lesion. Testing for referred pain is indicated only in the presence of a suggestive history and corroborating physical findings.

SYMPTOMATIC THERAPY

Acute Subacromial Impingement and Calcific Tendinitis. Acute subacromial impingement and calcific tendinitis often respond to a 2- to 3-day trial of *rest*, avoidance of overhead activities, and a *nonsteroidal anti-inflammatory agent* (eg, naproxen 375 mg bid or ibuprofen 600 mg tid). *Ice packs* applied for 15- to 20-minute periods during the first few days help reduce the pain and swelling. If necessary, a *sling* is prescribed, but it should not be worn for more than 3 to 4 days to avoid the potential of adhesive capsulitis and restricted mobility.

After the acute inflammatory phase has subsided, a supervised exercise program is begun. *Pendulum exercises* aid in maintaining joint mobility. With the patient bending forward at the waist, the arm is allowed to dangle and swing in forward-to-back, side-to-side, and circular patterns (Fig. 150–3). Additional exercises, such as "wall-climbing" (Figure 150–4), are included as the pain subsides. The patient must be counseled to expect some mild discomfort with

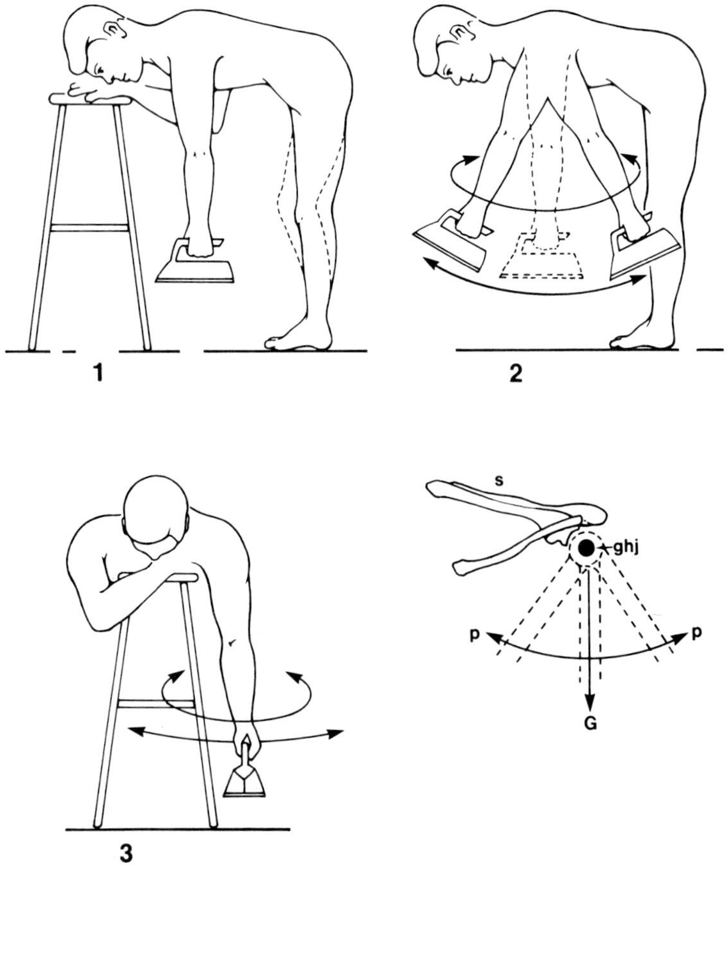

Figure 150-3. Active pendular glenohumeral exercise (so-called Codman exercises). (1) The posture to be assumed to permit the arm to "dangle" freely, with or without a weight. (2) The arm moves in forward-and-back sagittal plane, in forward and backward flexion. Circular motion in the clockwise and counterclockwise direction is also done in ever-increasing large circles. (3) The front view of the exercise showing lateral pendular movement actually in the coronal plane. The lower right diagram shows the effect of gravity, *G*, upon the glenohumeral joint, *ghj*, with an immobile scapula, *s*. The *p*-to-*p* arc is the pendular movement. (Redrawn from Cailliet R: Shoulder Pain. Philadelphia: FA Davis, 1973.)

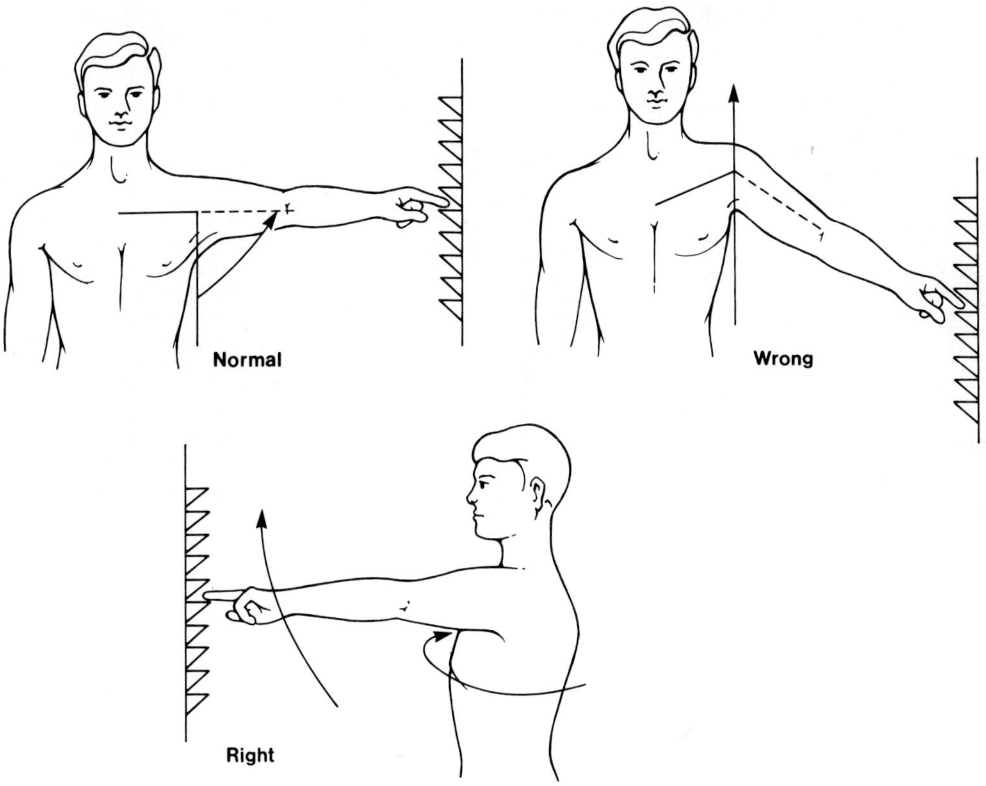

Figure 150-4. Correct and incorrect use of "wall-climbing" exercise. The wall climbing exercise frequently is done improperly. The normal arm climbs with normal scapulohumeral rhythm. If there is a pericapsulitis, the wall climb in abduction is done with "shrugging" of the scapula and accomplishes nothing. The wall climb should be started facing the wall and gradually turning the body until the patient is at a right angle to the wall. (Redrawn from Cailliet R: Shoulder Pain. Philadelphia: FA Davis, 1973.)

these exercises, as they are designed specifically to stretch the joint capsule. These exercises are performed for periods of 5 to 10 minutes, three to four times each day.

In the case of severe acute calcific tendinitis in which symptoms remain refractory after 10 to 14 days to the measures just described, a local *injection* of *corticosteroid* is often helpful. The point of maximum tenderness is carefully marked and the shoulder area prepared and draped under sterile conditions. One to two milliliters of Xylocaine is injected to determine a clinical response. If the pain is diminished, a mixture of 3 to 5 mL of Xylocaine and 40 mg of methylprednisolone (Depo-Medrol) or an equivalent steroid is injected into the same area (Fig. 150–5). Steroid injection may acutely worsen symptoms after the anesthetic wears off, but improvement is likely to follow within 48 hours. To avoid precipitating capsular atrophy, injections should be limited to no more than once every 6 to 12 months. Care must be taken not to inject into the tendon; the goal is to deliver medication into the area around it.

After joint mobility has been achieved, a program designed to strengthen the shoulder rotator muscles can be started under the supervision of a physical therapist. Orthopedic referral is appropriate if symptoms of subacromial impingement or calcific tendinitis persist beyond 2 months in spite of this therapeutic approach.

Adhesive capsulitis is difficult and often frustrating to treat; the course is prolonged, and chances for full recovery are unpredictable. The hallmark of treatment is an *active exercise program*. The patient is instructed to precede each session with the application of local heat, either by a heating pad or a warm shower, for 15 to 20 minutes. Initially, one begins by lying supine and, using the contralateral hand, brings the involved shoulder into forward flexion. External rotation exercises are also begun; one holds a broom handle in both hands and moves from internal to external rotation. The patient should be encouraged to use the shoulder as much as possible for the normal activities of daily living. It is worthwhile for a physical therapist to keep a weekly or monthly log regarding the shoulder motion, because improvement is slow and usually in small increments; these objective signs of improvement help to lessen patient frustration. *Forceful manipulation* of the shoulder is rarely indicated and, in fact, *operative caspsulotomy* may be safer. The latter is infrequently needed; most patients achieve a functional range of motion through a concerted but patiently applied exercise program.

Torn Rotator Cuff. There is little chance for spontaneous healing of a torn rotator cuff. Despite this, many patients respond to an exercise program designed to strengthen their

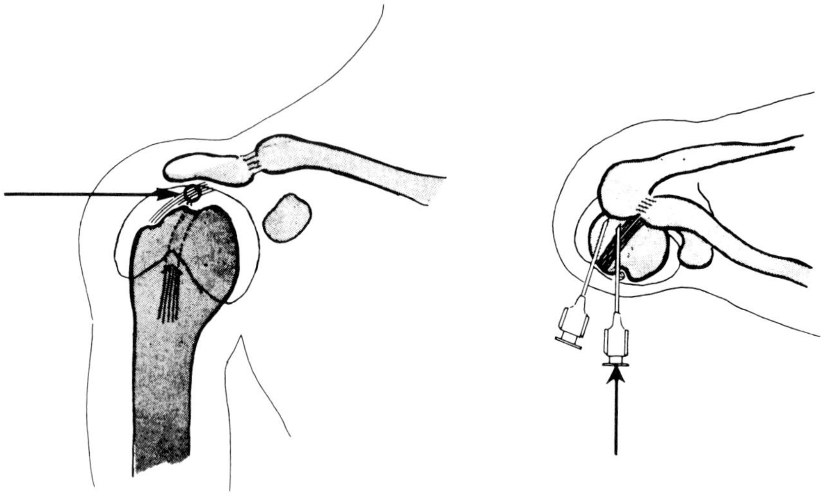

Figure 150-5. Site of injection in acute calcific tendinitis. (*A*), (*Left*) Region of supraspinatus insertion in the suprahumeral space. The region is palpable immediately below the overhanging acromion and by palpating the greater tuberosity just lateral to the bicipital groove of the humerus. (*B*), (*Right*) Insertion of needle viewed from above. Two directions of entrance are shown, with the arrow depicting that shown in the anterior view. (Cailliet R: Soft Tissue Pain and Disability. Philadelphia: FA Davis, 1977:161.)

shoulder rotator muscles. Repetitive steroid injections have no place in this disorder, because the cortisone, if anything, retards healing and leads to an increase in the deterioration of the tendons.

Glenohumeral Arthritis. Conservative treatment of glenohumeral arthritis, whether secondary to osteoarthritis or to inflammatory arthritis, employs nonsteroidal anti-inflammatory medication and exercises to maintain a functional range of motion. The same exercises as those for adhesive capsulitis can be given to the patient to do on a daily or twice-daily basis at home. Exercises directed at maximizing existing muscle strength are also prescribed, preferably with the supervision of a physical therapist. Improvements in total joint arthroplasty have offered a functional alternative to many patients refractory to medical management.

Acromioclavicular Arthritis. Anti-inflammatory medications and activity modification are often helpful in reducing the inflammatory component of acromoclavicular joint arthritis. At times, an injection of corticosteroid and Xylocaine, done preferably under fluoroscopic control, may be of help. Rarely, surgery is required, and it consists of distal clavicular excision.

INDICATIONS FOR REFERRAL

Shoulder dislocation or instability, advanced acromioclavicular or glenohumeral joint arthritis, rotator cuff pathology, and infection are best referred early to the orthopedic surgeon. Refractory subacromial impingement and associated tendinitis are indications for referral if resolution is not obtained with appropriate conservative treatment. Most of the other causes of shoulder pain can be managed, for the most part, by the primary physician.

PATIENT EDUCATION

The patient must be made to realize that thorough recovery from tendinitis requires active participation in the treatment program. Many individuals seek only relief from pain and expect oral or injectable medication to suffice. They must be told that repeated pain and limitation of function are bound to ensue if the exercise program is not taken seriously.

ANNOTATED BIBLIOGRAPHY

American Medical Association, Council on Scientific Affairs. Musculoskeletal applications of magnetic resonance imaging. JAMA 1989;262:2420. *(Critical examination of the test and comparison with other imaging methods.)*

Cailliet R. Shoulder Pain. Philadelphia: FA Davis, 1973. *(A clearly written and well-illustrated monograph that provides in-depth discussion of tendinitis.)*

Cogen L, Anderson RG, Phelps P. Medical management of the painful shoulder. Bull Rheum Dis 1982;32:54. *(Good review of therapy for the generalist.)*

151
Evaluation of Hip Pain

ROBERT J. BOYD, M.D.

Primary Care Medicine: Office Evaluation and Management of the Adult Patient, 3rd edition, edited by Allan H. Goroll, Lawrence A. May, and Albert G. Mulley, Jr. J.B. Lippincott Company, Philadelphia

Hip pain can be a major source of misery for both patient and family. The joint is essential to locomotion and weight bearing and is frequently subject to trauma and chronic mechanical stress.

Assessment of hip pain requires determinations of severity and disability as well as etiology, because surgery is now a practical therapeutic option for disabled patients refractory to conservative measures.

PATHOPHYSIOLOGY AND CLINICAL PRESENTATION

The hip is supplied by the obturator, sciatic, and femoral nerves. Pain originating in or around the hip can be felt in the groin or buttock, with radiation to the distal thigh and anteromedial aspect of the knee. Occasionally, pain from the hip may be felt only in the thigh and knee. Pain occurs in the distribution of the L2 and L3 roots and rarely is referred to the lower leg or foot. Conversely, pain caused by a problem outside the hip may be referred to the hip if the lesion irritates the femoral, sciatic, or obturator nerve or the nerve roots. Extra-hip problems include herniation of high lumbar discs, spinal stenosis (see Chapter 147), retroperitoneal or pelvic tumor, and femoral hernia; aortoiliac insufficiency may also present with hip and buttock pain (see Chapter 23).

Hip pain may be focal or diffuse, depending on the extent to which the joint and surrounding structures are involved in the pathologic process. For example, bursitis is characterized by focal pain and tenderness over the site of the bursa; synovitis is more diffuse, involving the entire joint capsule. Stiffness, limitation of motion, limp, and crepitus are frequent accompaniments of pain. Swelling is usually not evident and is difficult to detect, because the joint is buried deeply in soft tissues.

The major mechanisms of hip disease include cartilaginous degeneration, synovial inflammation, tendinitis and consequent bursitis, fracture, and ischemia.

Osteoarthritis. The hip is a major site of degenerative joint disease, with the elderly being the most affected (see Chapter 157). Obesity is also a risk factor, particularly in women. Onset is often insidious, beginning with minor aching or stiffness that may be unilateral or bilateral. Symptoms are characteristically exacerbated by prolonged standing, walking, or stair climbing. Stiffness is present on getting up after long periods of sitting. The hip begins to loosen up on first moving about but worsens with continued activity. As osteoarthritis gradually progresses, it results in decreasing hip motion, increasing stiffness, and increasing pain. A limp may develop as joint architecture is disrupted, and weight bearing becomes painful. The course of the disease is usually marked by spontaneous exacerbations and remissions.

On physical examination, the patient with substantial disease characteristically holds the leg in flexion, external rotation, and adduction. There may be an antalgic gait, positive Trendelenburg's sign (buttock falls when patient stands on opposite foot) indicative of abductor weakness, and limitation of hip motion, with or without crepitus. Pain, muscle spasm, and guarding occur when the examiner attempts to take the hip through the full range of motion. There may be buttock atrophy involving the gluteus maximus posteriorly and the gluteus medius more laterally. With severe degenerative arthritis of the hip, there may be a marked flexion deformity and pain in the hip joint even at rest.

Rheumatoid Arthritis. The hips are rarely affected in rheumatoid disease until other joints have become involved. Pain is characteristically bilateral and is associated with morning stiffness, which lessens with activity. During flares of the disease, the hip joint is tender to palpation, and capsular fullness and thickening may be felt if effusion or chronic synovitis are present. Flexion contractures occur in advanced cases.

Ankylosing Spondylitis. The disease is unique among the spondyloarthropathies in that the hip is sometimes affected. Concurrent sacroiliac and spinal involvement is usually present and in itself may cause pain radiating into the hip or buttock (see Chapters 146 and 147).

Hip Fracture. At greatest risk is the frail, elderly individual with a history of frequent falls and osteoporosis. The femoral neck and intertrochanteric region are common fracture sites. There may be loss of normal surface architecture, acute joint deformity, severe pain, guarding, and restriction of flexion and external rotation. Active straight leg raising is impaired. Competitive long-distance runners are at risk for stress fracture of the femoral neck.

Septic Arthritis. Joint infection in the hip most often follows hematogenous seeding (see Chapter 145). Because the joint is deep-seated, the ordinary signs of infection may not be readily evident. Fever, hip or knee pain (caused by pain referral), and inability to bear weight are early symptoms. The thigh is often held in flexion, and a bulging, tender joint capsule may be palpable.

Idiopathic Avascular Necrosis. Also referred to as "aseptic" necrosis of the femoral head, this condition has an ischemic pathophysiology. It occurs in patients who take high daily doses of glucocorticosteroids, alcoholics, patients with hemoglobinopathies, and those who work under conditions of increased atmospheric pressure. The mechanism of steroid-induced disease involves proliferation of intramedullary fat, tissue hypertension, and compromised perfusion of bone. Patients report gradual onset of focal pain and limitation of movement. Diagnostic x-ray changes include wedge-shaped areas of increased density and segmental collapse of the femoral head.

Bursitis. Inflammation of the bursa occurs as a consequence of trauma or spread of an inflammatory process. There is focal pain with tenderness over the bursa. *Trochanteric bursitis* is felt on the lateral aspect of the hip, posterior to the trochanter. Symptoms are increased by direct pressure or hip flexion and internal rotation. Pain may worsen at night and radiate down the leg to the knee. It may occur in runners who jog on uneven surfaces and those with one leg slightly shorter than the other. *Iliopectineal bursitis* causes pain on flexion and tenderness localized to the lateral border of Scarpa's triangle. *Ischiogluteal bursitis* presents with buttock pain that is worse on prolonged sitting, occurs at night, and occasionally radiates down the leg posteriorly, simulating sciatica.

Polymyalgia Rheumatica. A disease of the elderly and often mistaken for depression, arthritis, or bursitis, polymyalgia is characterized by bilateral aching of the hips, thighs, and shoulders in conjunction with a very high sedimentation rate. It has a strong association with cranial arteritis (see Chapter 161). Joint structures and passive range of joint motion are usually preserved.

Pigmented Villonodular Synovitis. This uncommon granulomatous disease of the synovium presents with slowly progressive pain and limitation of movement. X-rays show large cystic areas about the hip joint, distinguishing the condition from degenerative joint disease.

Referred Pain. Any pelvic, abdominal, or retroperitoneal process irritating the obturator muscle can cause pain referred to the hip that is worsened by internal rotation of the hip joint.

DIFFERENTIAL DIAGNOSIS

Hip pain is usually caused by degenerative joint disease. Other important causes include joint infection, avascular necrosis of the femoral head, bursitis, polymyalgia rheumatica, and rheumatoid arthritis. On occasion, ankylosing spondylitis or villonodular synovitis is responsible. Pain may be referred to the hip from a lumbar or pelvic problem such as high lumbar disc herniation, retroperitoneal tumor or abscess, or obturator or femoral hernia. Aortoiliac insufficiency may present with exercise-induced hip and buttock pain.

WORKUP

History. One should ascertain the onset, location, and radiation of the pain as well as inciting and alleviating factors and the presence of numbness or weakness. It is particularly important to inquire directly about trauma, involvement of other joints, morning stiffness, relation of pain to activity, response to rest, steroid or alcohol use, and current infection or fever. There are a few pitfalls regarding history. For example, stiffness by itself is a nonspecific finding, because it may occur with degenerative disease as well as with rheumatoid involvement of the hip. The response to continued activity may be of more help: stiffness usually worsens in degenerative disease and lessens in rheumatoid arthritis. Bilateral cramping hip and buttock pain that comes on with walking and is relieved by rest may actually be a sign of vascular insufficiency rather than of joint disease.

Physical Examination. The hip should be looked at for deformities such as flexion or adduction contractures, which are seen with rheumatoid disease, and for fixed external rotation, suggesting a fracture of the femoral neck. Gait is also important to check. The hip is then put through the full range of passive motion to detect crepitus, limitation of movement, flexion contracture, muscle spasm, or guarding. Normal range of hip flexion-extension is $-20°$ to $90°$ with the knee straight and $0°$ to $120°$ with the knee flexed. Normal adduction-abduction is $-20°$ to $90°$; normal internal-external rotation is $-50°$ to $+50°$. Among the earliest limitations of movement in hip disease is internal rotation with the hip hyperextended. Palpation of the joint and individual bursae for focal tenderness and swelling is important for detecting a localized inflammatory process.

Circumference measurements should be made of the thigh at a fixed distance from a bony reference point such as the tibial tubercle of the knee, the anterior superior iliac spine, or the midpatella. Atrophy is suggestive of intrinsic hip disease.

Femoral pulses should be palpated for diminution and auscultated for bruits. Pelvic and rectal examinations are helpful in searching for tumors, which may cause referred pain. The back should be examined for evidence of L1-2 or L2-3 disc herniation (see Chapter 147). Neurologic assessment of the lower extremities is needed to test for weakness, sensory loss, and reflexes.

Laboratory Studies. Hip *x-rays* are essential to the assessment of hip pain. They may be diagnostic of degenerative joint disease, rheumatoid arthritis, avascular necrosis, or fracture. Weight-bearing films help one judge the severity of degenerative hip disease by disclosing the extent of joint space narrowing. Sacroiliac and spine films are indicated if ankylosing spondylitis is under consideration (see Chapters 146 and 147). *Magnetic resonance imaging (MRI)* is the most sensitive test for avascular necrosis of the femoral head, showing expansion of intramedullary fat before bony changes become visible. It also is more sensitive than standard x-rays for detection of stress fracture of the femoral neck.

A complete blood count, sedimentation rate, and rheumatoid factor analysis may be useful if a rheumatoid disease is being considered (see Chapter 146). If a septic joint is suspected, aspiration for Gram's stain and culture is urgent (see Chapter 145).

SYMPTOMATIC THERAPY AND INDICATIONS FOR REFERRAL

Degenerative Disease. Simple treatment measures for relief of an acute exacerbation include bed rest, a nonsteroidal anti-inflammatory agent (NSAID), limitation of sitting, and crutch or cane support. After acute symptoms lessen, the patient can begin a program that includes avoidance of activities that specifically aggravate pain, rest periods of 1 hour twice daily with local heat to the hip, daily mild exercise of walking short distances as tolerated, aspirin or acetaminophen regularly, cane support, weight reduction in the obese, and specific daily range of motion and strengthening exercises, preferably outlined by a physical therapist. Acute exacerbations of hip pain can often be managed effectively by a few weeks of bed rest and several weeks' use of a partial weight-bearing crutch. If conservative measures fail to control symptoms and the patient is active, surgery may be needed. Because results of hip reconstructive procedures are now quite good and the procedure has relatively low risk, referral for consideration of surgery need not be delayed indefinitely if symptoms are disabling and not well controlled by conservative measures. The need for reconstructive surgery must be a joint decision of patient, primary physician, and orthopedic surgeon.

Bursitis. NSAID therapy (eg, naproxen 500 mg bid for 1–2 wk), in conjunction with reduced activity, often suffices. The jogger who has been running on uneven surfaces should change running surface. A heel lift may help the person with a discrepancy in leg lengths. If pain does not respond and if tenderness is well localized to a bursa, a local steroid injection can be given, using 2 mL of 2% lidocaine (Xylocaine) followed by 40 mg methylprednisolone (Depo-Medrol) in 1 mL injected into the tender area. Primary physicians who are unfamiliar with the technique of injecting a hip bursa should refer the patient to an orthopedist or rheumatologist.

Rheumatoid Disease. Polymyalgia rheumatica responds dramatically to low-dose steroids (see Chapter 161), and rheumatoid arthritis to high-dose aspirin or NSAIDs (see Chapter 151).

Hip Fracture and Septic Arthritis are indications for immediate hospitalization.

ANNOTATED BIBLIOGRAPHY

American Medical Association, Council on Scientific Affairs. Musculoskeletal applications of magnetic resonance imaging. JAMA 1989;262:2420. *(Most sensitive imaging study for avascular septic necrosis of the femoral head and stress fracture of the femoral neck.)*

Burton KE, Wright V, Richards J. Patient's expectations in relation to outcome of total hip replacement surgery. Ann Rheum Dis 1979;38:471. *(A still useful paper making the important point that expectations are often in excess of reality; preoperative counseling is important.)*

Hartz AJ, Fischer ME, Bril G, et al. The association of obesity with joint pain in osteoarthritis in the HANES data. J Chron Dis 1986;39:311. *(Finds obesity a predictor of pain and arthritis, especially in women.)*

Meyers MH. Osteonecrosis of the femoral head: pathogenesis and long-term results from treatment. Clin Orthop 1988;231:51. *(Principal mechanism is ischemic injury.)*

Paty JG. Diagnosis and treatment of musculoskeletal running injuries. Semin Arthritis Rheum 1988;18:48. *(Includes discussion of femoral neck stress fractures and hip bursitis.)*

Primary Care Medicine: Office Evaluation and Management of the Adult Patient, 3rd edition, edited by Allan H. Goroll, Lawrence A. May, and Albert G. Mulley, Jr. J.B. Lippincott Company, Philadelphia

152
Evaluation of Knee Pain

ROBERT J. BOYD, M.D.

The knee joint is frequently the site of trauma, degenerative disease, and rheumatologic conditions. Disability can be considerable because of inability to bear weight. The primary physician is called on most often for minor acute injuries or chronic knee pain that limits mobility. Occasionally, an acute monoarticular arthritis is encountered. The popularity of skiing, jogging, and long-distance running has markedly increased the prevalence of acute and recurrent knee complaints.

PATHOPHYSIOLOGY AND CLINICAL PRESENTATION

Degenerative disease, trauma-induced soft tissue derangements, and inflammatory processes are the predominant mechanisms of knee pain in the adult. The pain is characteristically worsened by weight-bearing and may radiate into the anterior thigh, posterior calf, or pretibial region. An inflamed joint capsule produces diffuse pain. The site of pain is characteristic of the underlying problem (Fig. 152–1). Locking of the joint suggests a loose body or torn meniscus. Hip disease occasionally presents as knee pain (see Chapter 151).

Degenerative Disease. Changes often originate in the medial joint compartment and patellofemoral joint, related in part to mechanical stresses. The entire joint may be painful, but often the discomfort is localized to the anterior and medial portions of the knee. Prolonged standing or walking may precipitate or worsen symptoms. Mild stiffness is common on first arising in the morning and on getting up after a long period of sitting. It initially improves on moving about, but worsens with continued activity. Symptoms gradually progress but may take many years to become disabling. Considerable degenerative change and joint destruction can occur before serious knee pain develops. Small effusions may appear after prolonged weight bearing, but few other signs or symptoms of inflammation occur.

Rheumatoid Disease. Rheumatoid arthritis commonly affects the knees. Pain, swelling, and morning stiffness are characteristic. Symmetric polyarticular involvement is the rule, with joints in the hands, feet, ankles, and wrists often affected. Symptoms wax and wane; the course is chronic (see Chapter 156). Other rheumatoid diseases can produce a similar picture (see Chapter 146).

Acute Monoarticular Arthritis. The knee is a frequent site of septic arthritis, gout, pseudogout, early rheumatoid arthritis, rheumatic fever, palindromic rheumatism, and disseminated gonorrhea. Usually there is the acute onset of unilateral swelling, pain, and generalized tenderness (see Chapter 145). Motion is limited, and muscle spasm is prominent.

Knee Sprain. Ligamentous injury caused by excessive joint strain is extremely frequent. Sprain injuries range from minor tears of a few fibers to complete tears of entire ligaments resulting in loss of joint stability. Mild sprains produce tenderness and local swelling without joint effusion or loss of joint stability. In moderate sprains, there is pain on stressing the joint, voluntary restriction of movement, some joint instability, and swelling due to an effusion. Severe sprains involve total loss of integrity and immediate swelling, marked joint instability, severe pain, and a large effusion. The collateral and cruciate ligaments are frequently injured in contact sports. Ligamentous injuries are uncommon in joggers.

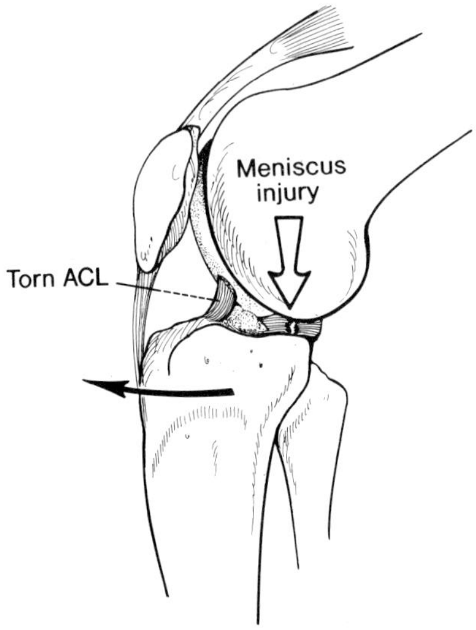

Figure 152-1. Cruciate ligament tear with associated meniscal damage.

Tearing the *anterior cruciate* ligament is a common sports-related knee injury (eg, accounting for the vast majority of sprains suffered in skiing). Typically, it occurs in the setting of sudden noncontact deceleration that causes valgus twisting of the knee. A "pop" is heard, and marked swelling ensues within a few hours due to intraarticular bleeding. The resulting subluxation of the tibia compresses the menisci between the tibia and femur, which may cause the cartilage to tear (see Figure 152–1 and below). Initially after anterior cruciate tear, the knee may function reasonably well, but instability develops on resumption of sports activity.

Degeneration or Tear of a Meniscus. An acute tear occurs as a result of excessive weight bearing, twisting, or valgus or varus stress, and may be associated with partial or complete disruption of collateral or cruciate ligaments. There is usually a history of acute trauma and immediate swelling due to tissue disruption and bleeding. A torn anterior cruciate ligament is a common precipitant of meniscal tear. If cartilaginous fragments become trapped, they will cause the knee to lock. If swelling does not develop until the next day, damage is likely to be confined to the meniscus and not involve the ligament. Such swelling is due to a reactive joint effusion. Chronic internal derangements caused by degeneration or tear of the meniscus produce recurrent pain and swelling, and a knee that gives way, catches, or locks.

Chondromalacia Patellae. Degeneration of the posterior patellar cartilage is the cause of this condition. Dessication, thinning, fissure formation, and ultimately erosion of the cartilage occur. Mechanical factors are suspected, although unproven. Chondromalacia is the most common cause of knee pain in joggers, believed related to overtraining. The patient presents with retropatellar aching that is worsened by standing up, climbing stairs, or any other form of bent-knee strain. There may be stiffness after inactivity, but there is usually no locking or giving way to the knee. Pain is reported in the peripatellar region and lateral aspect of the knee and can be elicited by applying pressure against the patella with the knee actively extended. Palpable grating can be elicited at the patellofemoral joint with flexion and extension of the knee. X-rays are normal until late stages, when the posterior surface of the patella becomes irregular and marginal osteophytes develop.

Baker's Cyst. Rupture of one of these popliteal fossa cysts can cause acute inflammation with pain, swelling, and limitation of knee flexion. The inflammation may extend down into the calf and simulate thrombophlebitis. Baker's cysts usually communicate with the knee joint space and most commonly occur in patients with osteoarthritis or rheumatoid disease. An unruptured cyst causes only mild aching and stiffness. Trauma may initiate a rupture.

Prepatellar bursitis results from repeated trauma—hence, the name "housemaid's knee." Swelling, tenderness, and occasionally erythema over the prepatellar bursae are present. Bursitis of the suprapatellar and infrapatellar bursae have similar presentations, with findings localized to the bursal site.

Villonodular synovitis is a granulomatous inflammatory condition of the synovium that lines the joints, bursae, and tendon sheaths. Etiology is unknown. It affects young adults, predominantly men, and presents with unilateral pain, persistent swelling, intermittent knee locking, and, occasionally, a palpable mass. Diagnosis requires arthroscopy or surgical exploration.

DIFFERENTIAL DIAGNOSIS

The list of conditions that can cause knee pain is extensive and includes those that cause polyarticular disease as well as those that are confined to the knee. A clinically useful classification system is to group etiologies according to whether they are acute or chronic, symmetric or asymmetric, and monoarticular or polyarticular (Table 152–1).

WORKUP

History. Besides ascertaining the pain's quality, location, alleviating and aggravating factors, and associated symptoms such as swelling, redness, and warmth, it is necessary to determine if the problem is acute or chronic, symmetric or asymmetric, and mono- or polyarticular. By combining a careful description of the problem with a characterization of its pattern and chronicity, one can quickly focus the evaluation onto a relatively limited set of conditions having similar clinical presentations (see Table 152–1).

Acute Unilateral Knee Pain. One should inquire about trauma, jogging, locking, giving out, swelling, pain on climbing stairs, concurrent fever, purulent vaginal or urethral discharge, rash, recent strep infection or sore throat, heart murmur, morning stiffness, and urethritis or conjunctivitis (see Chapter 145). Any prior history of gout, sickle cell disease, or hemophilia should be checked for. When swelling is localized, it is important to determine the exact site, because it may be a clue to bursitis or a Baker's cyst. A history of the knee locking suggests meniscal tear with lodging of cartilaginous fragments in the joint space. Reports of the knee giving out point to anterior cruciate disruption.

Table 152-1. Differential Diagnosis of Knee Pain

KNEE INVOLVEMENT							
ASYMMETRIC				SYMMETRIC			
One Knee Only		One Knee Plus Other Joints		Knees Only		Symmetric Polyarthritis	
Acute	Chronic	Acute	Chronic	Acute	Chronic	Acute	Chronic
Sprain	Osteoarthritis	See Chaps. 145, 146		Rheumatoid arthritis	Osteoarthritis	See Chap. 146	
Strain	Baker's cyst			Juvenile RA	Chondromalacia patellae		
Acute gout	Chronic gout			Early phase of other rheumatoid diseases	Bursitis		
Meniscus tear	Chondromalacia patellae			Trauma	Rheumatoid arthritis		
Early rheumatoid disease	Bursitis				Juvenile RA		
Gonococcal arthritis	Meniscal injuries				Chronic gout		
Septic arthritis					Neuropathic joints		
Reiter's syndrome					Hemophilia		
Bursitis							
Pseudogout							
Pallindromic rheumatism							
Ruptured Baker's cyst							
Hemophilia							
Sickle cell disease							
Rheumatic fever							

(Adapted from Katz WA: Rheumatic Diseases. Philadelphia, JB Lippincott, 1977)

Chronic Unilateral Knee Pain. Questioning ought to cover previous or recurrent trauma as may occur occupationally, pain in association with prolonged walking, standing or climbing stairs, knee locking, crepitus, focal swelling and recurrent acute episodes or exacerbations.

Acute Bilateral Knee Pain. When both knees are involved acutely, then the focus of inquiry should be on the symptoms of rheumatoid disease (see Chapter 146) and recent trauma.

Chronic Bilateral Knee Pain. The questioning can be similar to that for chronic unilateral disease, but there should also be consideration of rheumatoid symptoms (see Chapter 146).

Polyarticular Presentations. When other joints are also involved, inquiry into symptoms of infectious and rheumatologic conditions is essential (see Chapter 146).

Physical Examination. A complete physical examination must be performed because many systemic illnesses can present with knee pain. Skin and integument are examined for rash, clubbing, psoriatic changes, rheumatoid nodules, pallor, alopecia, and tophi. The conjunctivae are noted for erythema and petechiae; the oral cavity for aphthous ulcers; lymph nodes for enlargement; chest for signs of consolidation and effusion, heart for murmurs and rubs; abdomen for organomegaly and tenderness; pelvis for vaginal discharge and adnexal tenderness; urethra for discharge, and penis for balanitis. This is in addition to a thorough check of all joints and complete neurologic testing.

Examination of the knee should begin with a careful inspection for distortion of normal contours and irregular bony prominences at the joint margin. It is important to check for muscle atrophy. Measurements of knee, calf, and thigh circumferences can help quantitate the loss of muscle mass. Presence of an effusion needs to be determined. This is done by noting an increased knee circumference at midpatella and feeling for a distended fluctuant capsule with a fluid wave and ballotable patella. The joint line should be palpated for localized joint line tenderness suggestive of a meniscal tear. The *McMurray and Apley tests* are performed for suspected meniscal injury (Fig. 152–2). The bursal regions should be assessed for focal tenderness and swelling indicative of bursitis.

Range of motion needs to be determined. The knees normally extend symmetrically 180 degrees and may hyperextend an additional 5 or 10 degrees. Knee flexion is also symmetric and limited to 135 to 170 degrees by posterior soft tissue contact or by the heel striking the buttock. Collateral and cruciate ligaments should be examined for stability. Collateral ligaments are tested by applying mediolateral valgus-varus strain with the knee in full extension and in 15 to 20 degrees of flexion (Fig. 152–3).

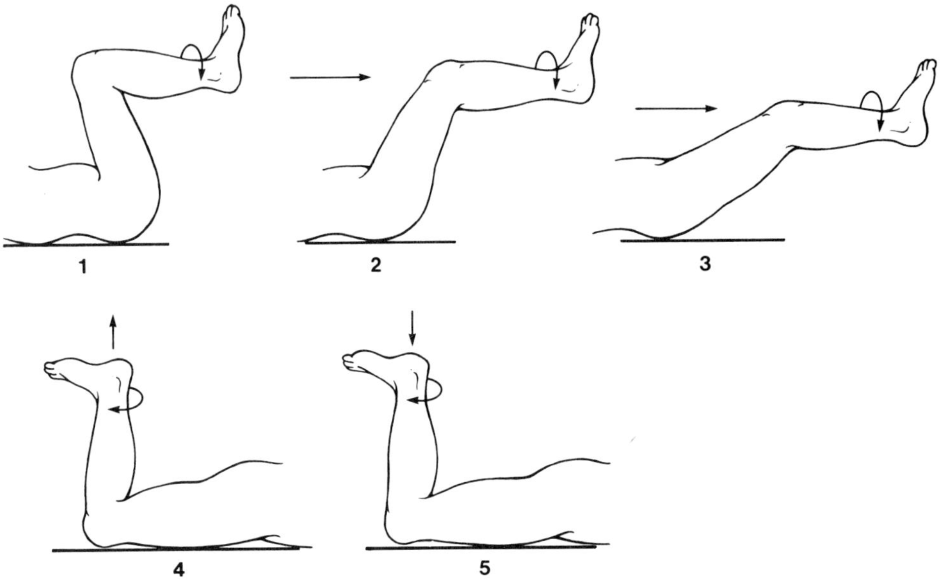

Figure 152-2. Meniscus signs (examination). (*1, 2, 3*) *McMurray test.* The patient is supine with knee flexed, heel touching the buttocks at the start. The leg is internally rotated for lateral meniscus testing or externally rotated for medial meniscus testing. Then the knee is fully extended. A painful click occurs if there is a meniscus lesion. The test is more meaningful in the first phase of knee extension. Full extension limitation does not indicate an anterior meniscus lesion. (*4, 5*) *Apley tests.* The patient is prone. Leg is internally or externally rotated with simultaneous traction. Pain indicates a capsular or ligamentous lesion. Rotation with downward pressure that causes pain indicates meniscus lesion. (Redrawn from Cailliet R: Knee Pain and Disability. Philadelphia: FA Davis, 1973.)

Anterior cruciate ligament stability is best assessed by the *anterior drawer test.* It is performed with the knee relaxed and flexed to about 25 degrees. One gently pulls the tibia anteriorly while the femur is held fixed and notes the amount of anterior displacement of the tibia relative to the femur. Patients who report their knee chronically giving out may have anterior cruciate instability, which can be assessed by testing for pivotal shift. The validity of these tests has been confirmed by arthroscopic study. They are important parts of the examination of the injured knee.

Laboratory Studies. There is no set of "routine" laboratory studies for assessment of knee pain. When there is trauma, *x-rays* are needed to rule out fracture, and stress films are indicated to determine joint stability. Knee films are also indicated for suspected degenerative or chronic rheumatoid disease. Weight-bearing films best demonstrate degree of joint obliteration. *Magnetic resonance imaging (MRI)* has enhanced diagnosis of soft tissue knee pathology. Sensitivity for detection of a meniscal tear exceeds 90 percent (better than arthography), and for cruciate tear it reaches 95 percent. However, MRI remains expensive. The test is best reserved for instances where clinical findings are not sufficient to establish a diagnosis and an invasive diagnostic procedure would otherwise be necessary. *Fiberoptic arthroscopy* remains the gold standard for diagnosis of soft tissue knee problems. Acute monoarticular effusions require prompt *arthrocentesis* for Gram's stain and cultures to rule out a septic process. Joint fluid is sent for determinations of the white cell count, differential, and glucose, and is examined for crystals (see Chapter 145). Polyarticular presentations require consideration of testing for inflammatory joint disease (see Chapter 146).

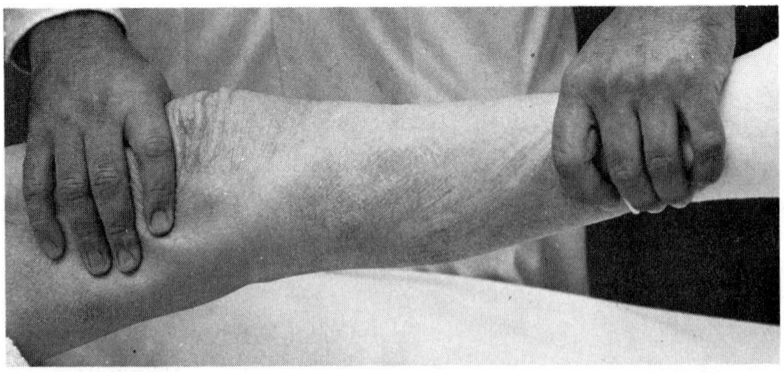

Figure 152-3. Testing for lateral instability of the knee by fixating the lower femur with one hand and forcibly abducting and adducting the joint while grasping the leg. (Katz WA: Rheumatic Diseases. Philadelphia: JB Lippincott, 1977.)

SYMPTOMATIC THERAPY AND INDICATIONS FOR REFERRAL

For the patient with a knee injury, acute pain responds best to restriction of weight-bearing activities and use of crutches. A knee brace is applied to provide support and prevent further injury by limiting range of motion. Only absolutely necessary walking is allowed, and kneeling, squatting, and stair climbing are forbidden. Aspirin may be helpful symptomatically when used in pharmacologic doses of 2 to 4 g per day. Otherwise, any one of the other nonsteroidal antiinflammatory agents is a reasonable alternative (eg, naproxen 375 mg bid or ibuprofen 400 mg tid). Once swelling subsides and full range of motion without pain returns, rehabilitation can begin. One starts with isometric quadriceps and hamstring exercises. These help prevent muscle atrophy, weakness, and thinning of ligamentous tissue. If the problem is one of acute severe injury and pain, especially if the knee gives way or locks and there is a question of joint instability or internal derangement, prompt orthopedic referral is essential. Arthroscopy may be needed.

ANNOTATED BIBLIOGRAPHY

Council on Scientific Affairs, American Medical Association. Musculoskeletal applications of magnetic resonance imaging. JAMA 1989;262:2420. *(Finds MRI sensitive for diagnosis of torn cruciate ligaments and menisci.)*

Cox JS. Chondromalacia of the patella: A review and update. Contemp Orthop 1983;6:17. *(Detailed description of the problem.)*

Paty JG. Diagnosis and treatment of musculoskeletal running injuries. Semin Arthritis Rheum 1988;18:48. *(Good description of overuse syndromes.)*

Zarins B, Adams M. Knee injuries in sports. N Engl J Med 1988;318;950. *(Authoritative review with particularly good discussions of anterior cruciate tear and resulting meniscal injury.)*

Primary Care Medicine: Office Evaluation and Management of the Adult Patient, 3rd edition, edited by Allan H. Goroll, Lawrence A. May, and Albert G. Mulley, Jr. J.B. Lippincott Company, Philadelphia

153

Approach to Minor Orthopedic Problems of the Elbow, Wrist, and Hand

JESSE B. JUPITER, M.D.

As the physician of first contact, the primary care doctor encounters a host of minor upper extremity complaints that may be causing the patient considerable discomfort. Their quick recognition and proper treatment can save the patient an unnecessary referral and allow for prompt symptomatic relief.

ELBOW PAIN

The evaluation of elbow pain requires a careful correlation of the patient's presenting symptoms with the specific anatomic site. The elbow is particularly subject to overuse syndromes, inflammatory conditions, and localized nerve entrapments. A careful history and physical examination is often all that is required to reach an accurate diagnosis and formulate a treatment plan.

Lateral Epicondylitis ("Tennis Elbow"). This condition is the result of inflammation at the common tendinous origin of the extensor muscles of the forearm, in particular the extensor carpi radialis brevis, on the humeral lateral epicondyle. It is the result of repetitive overuse, such as by tennis players making backhand strokes or by people knitting. The common denominator is a strong grasp during wrist extension. The patient complains of pain on the lateral aspect of the elbow. The physical examination reveals tenderness over the lateral epicondyle (Fig. 153–1), pain on resisted wrist extension with the elbow extended, and symptoms reproduced by resisted extension of the elbow with the forearm pronated and the wrist palmar-flexed. Radiographs are normal.

The management of epicondylitis consists of reduction of the inflammatory component, strengthening of the involved muscle, and awareness and avoidance of precipitating factors. It may take several weeks for pain to clear. Any painful activity is best avoided, including racquet sports, shaking hands, forceful use of the arm in hammering or unscrewing jars, or use of a screwdriver. There is no certain way to prevent recurrences of epicondylitis related to playing tennis, but proper stroking of shots with a firm wrist and proper elbow positioning may be helpful. Elbow bands are often tried but usually are of limited value; however, sometimes they allow play when mild pain is present.

If symptoms do not clear with avoidance, systemic antiinflammatory medication (eg, naproxen 375 mg bid or ibuprofen 600 mg tid for 1 wk) should be tried. Local steroid injection may eventually be needed, although results may not be very dramatic. Injection is best reserved for refractory cases. The area of well-localized tenderness is carefully identified and injected with 1 mL of 2% lidocaine (Xylocaine), followed by injection of 20 mg of dexamethasone.

In most cases, a program of rest, ice applications, nonsteroidal anti-inflammatory medications (NSAIDs), and a physical therapy program of friction massage, ultrasound, and exercises is successful in reducing symptoms and permitting a return to function.

Medial Epicondylitis ("Golfer's Elbow"). This is similar to "tennis elbow" but involves the common forearm flexor origin at the humeral medial epicondyle. Occasionally seen in golfers, it more commonly is associated with certain manual activities or household activities. The pain localizes to the region of the medial epicondyle and is reproduced by forcefully extending the elbow against resistance with the forearm

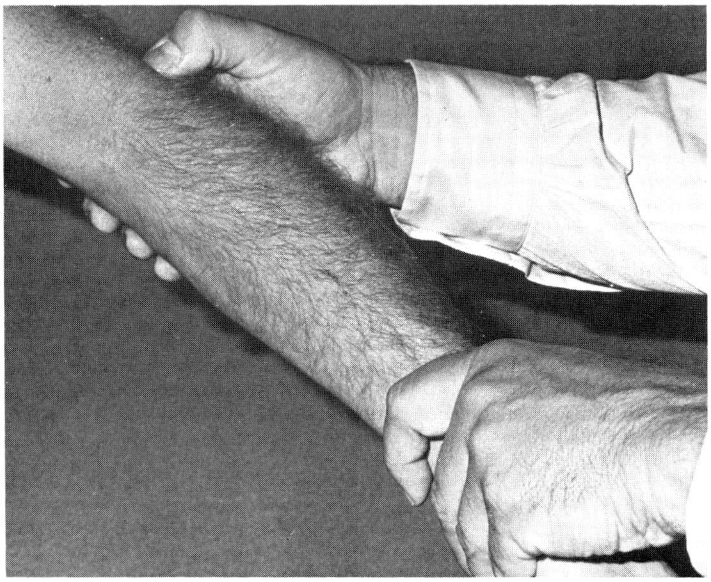

Figure 153-1. Technique of palpating the lateral epicondyle to elicit "point" tenderness typical of "tennis elbow." (Katz WA: Rheumatic Diseases. Philadelphia: JB Lippincott, 1977.)

supinated and the wrist dorsiflexed. Radiographs are normal. Treatment is the same as for lateral epicondylitis.

Calcific Periarthritis (Pseudogout). This condition is the result of an inflammatory response to a deposition of hydroxyapatite crystals adjacent to the joint. It occurs mostly in patients with degenerative joint disease and is usually not associated with trauma. The patient presents with severe pain, localized tenderness, warmth, and swelling. Radiographs demonstrate a dense, radio-opaque deposit adjacent to the joint. NSAIDs give prompt relief if taken early.

Olecranon Bursitis. The clinical presentation is a painful swelling over the posterior aspect of the elbow. The swollen bursa is usually fluctuant and transilluminates light. Localized trauma or repetitive local pressure associated with certain occupations is the most common cause, but this bursitis can also be a manifestation of such inflammatory conditions as rheumatoid arthritis, gout, or sepsis. Patients with septic bursitis commonly report a history of antecedent trauma and cellulitis of the skin, followed by localized swelling, redness, and tenderness about the elbow. Almost all cases of septic olecranon represent spread from a contiguous soft tissue infection. Gram's stain of the bursal fluid is positive for the causative organism in about 50 percent of instances. *Staphylococcus aureus* is the most common isolate, found in 80 percent of cases; streptococcal species account for most of the remainder. Presentation of septic bursitis in the immunocompromised patient is similar.

Unless sepsis is suspected, one should avoid aspiration or corticosteroid injection, because they increase the possibility of introducing sepsis. Anti-inflammatory medication, a sling as needed, and local protection to avoid pressure are the basic treatment approaches.

Nerve Entrapment Syndromes. Pain in the elbow or forearm may be secondary to compression of the ulnar nerve in the cubital tunnel, the posterior interosseous nerve in the proximal forearm, or even the median nerve in the forearm or wrist (see later discussion). With ulnar nerve compression, pain may be found beneath the medial epicondyle, and the patient may experience numbness in the little and ring fingers. Intrinsic muscle weakness is also commonly found on examination. Posterior interosseous nerve compression presents in a similar fashion as tennis elbow, but symptoms are reproduced by extension of the middle finger against resistance. Treatment of ulnar nerve compression can be as simple as avoidance of leaning on the elbow. Use of a protective pad may help. Entrapment accompanied by atrophy requires referral.

Arthritis. The elbow is not a common site for osteoarthritis, but arthritis may be found in association with prior fracture or dislocation. In contrast, elbow involvement is common in rheumatoid arthritis. On examination, limitation of motion, swelling, and pain are common findings. Radiographs demonstrate the extent of joint space involvement. Anti-inflammatory agents provide good relief (see Chapter 156).

Septic Arthritis. Most cases are the result of bloodborne infection. There is rapid onset of pain, diffuse joint swelling, and erythema. Systemic symptoms are common. It is important to rule out underlying conditions such as diabetes mellitus, steroid treatment, or rheumatoid arthritis. Suspicion of sepsis requires arthrocentesis for Gram's stain and culture of the joint fluid (see Chapter 145). Treatment includes intravenous antibiotics.

HAND AND WRIST PAIN

Carpal Tunnel Syndrome. Most commonly affecting middle-aged women, the condition typically causes nocturnal symptoms, including hand and wrist pain and paresthesias often relieved by shaking the hand. Numbness is common, affecting the middle or three radial fingers and occasionally the thumb. A number of systemic conditions are associated with carpal tunnel syndrome, including diabetes mellitus, hypothyroidism, inflammatory arthritis, and pregnancy.

Physical examination may reveal altered sensibility in the thumb, index, and long fingers and the radial side of the ring finger, although one may see changes only in one or two digits. Thenar (base of the thumb) muscle atrophy is present in prolonged or profound median nerve compression. A *Tinel's sign*, elicited by tapping over the median nerve at the wrist crease, consists of "electric shocks" or paresthesias in the median nerve distribution. *Phelan's test* is performed by having the patient palmar flex the wrist for one minute. It is considered positive and consistent with carpal tunnel syndrome if the patient's symptoms are reproduced by this test. A negative Phelan's or Tinel's sign does not necessarily rule out the presence of carpal tunnel syndrome. Definitive diagnosis can be made by *nerve conduction study* and *electromyography (EMG)*. Testing is indicated if the diagnosis is unclear or if the condition persists and some numbness or weakness appears. In a patient with the condition, the EMG and nerve conduction study demonstrate an increased motor or sensory latency, which is helpful in documenting the location and degree of nerve compression.

Conservative therapy for carpal tunnel syndrome consists of wrist splinting, control of any underlying systemic metabolic disorder, and occasional local injection of corticosteroids. A canvas mock-up or plaster wrist splint worn during sleep prevents wrist positions of extreme dorsiflexion or palmar flexion, which tend to increase the local compression within the carpal tunnel. In those patients with a significant flexor tenosynovitis, an injection of Xylocaine (1–2 mL) and dexamethasone (0.5–1 mL) directly into the carpal tunnel may be of value. The injection is placed just proximal to the transverse retinacular ligament in the wrist. If a paresthesia is elicited, a more superficial needle placement is made to avoid injecting into the nerve. Surgical intervention is considered if symptoms persist longer than 3 months, if there is associated thenar muscle atrophy, or if the motor or sensory latencies on the EMG and nerve conduction studies are extremely prolonged.

De Quervain's Tenosynovitis. On the dorsal aspect of the wrist, the extensor tendons to the hand and wrist course through six well-defined compartments. The first dorsal compartment contains the abductor pollicis longus and the extensor pollicis brevis and is located just proximal and radial to the anatomic "snuff box." A relatively common disorder is a nonspecific subacute or chronic inflammation of these tendons within the first dorsal compartment. Pain is exacerbated by use of the thumb and is reproduced by the patient's grasping the thumb with the adjacent digits and ulnarly deviating and palmar flexing the wrist (Finkelstein's test). This test differentiates tendonitis from any underlying arthritis. The usual aggravating factor is excessive repetitive handwork, such as needlepoint, knitting, or peeling vegetables.

The majority of patients respond to nonoperative treatment consisting of splinting and steroid injection. An injection preparation such as that described for carpal tunnel syndrome is carefully placed within the first dorsal extensor compartment, which is somewhat more radial and volar than one might think. Care is exercised to inject just above the abductor pollicis longus. A removable plaster or orthoplast splint holding the wrist and thumb in slight dorsiflexion and radial deviation is worn for 10 to 14 days except for bathing. Oral NSAIDs may also be of use. Failure to respond should be considered an indication for surgical referral.

Trigger Finger. Tenosynovitis is also commonly found involving the flexor tendons to the digits or thumb at the level of the metacarpophalangeal (MCP) joints just proximal to the first annular pulley of the flexor tendon sheath. Snapping of the digit (triggering) that occurs with use and locking, or inability to extend the proximal interphalangeal (PIP) joint, are the characteristic presenting complaints. Often the patient perceives the triggering to be at the level of the PIP joint. A palpable thickening of the flexor tendon may be felt at the level of the MCP joint in the palm.

Treatment consists of splinting, corticosteroid injection, and NSAIDs. The steroid-Xylocaine combination is injected just proximal to the distal palmar crease, where the first annular pulley of the flexor sheath is located. The involved digit or thumb is splinted in extension for 7 to 10 days except for bathing. Such treatment is effective in almost 90 percent of cases, and risk of serious adverse reactions is minimal.

Calcific Tendinitis. Acute inflammation involving tendons or joints within the hand or wrist may be found in association with localized deposits of calcium hydroxyapatite crystals. The clinical presentation may be so striking as to raise the specter of an acute infection. The flexor carpi ulnaris tendon on the volar, ulnar aspect of the wrist is frequently involved. Radiographs may demonstrate amorphous, calcific deposits, which may be seen to fragment and disappear on serial radiographs. Metabolic studies are normal.

Splinting and oral anti-inflammatory medications form the first-line treatments. Aspiration is advisable if concern exists regarding underlying infection or to obtain fluid for appropriate crystal analysis, including urate, calcium pyrophosphate dihydrate (CPPD), or calcium hydroxyapatite determination. If symptoms fail to improve within 2 weeks, steroid injection is advisable, with particular care taken not to inject directly into the tendon.

Ganglion Cysts. Ganglionic cysts are the most common mass occurring in the hand or wrist and may be found in a number of sites, including the dorsum of the wrist, for which the origin is the scapholunate ligament. Another common location is on the volar, radial surface of the wrist directly adjacent to and not to be confused with the radial artery. Ganglia are thought to be the result of an outpouching of the wrist capsule and contain fluid very similar to joint fluid. Their origin (stalk) is from the wrist joint, which explains the high incidence of recurrence with treatment methods such as aspiration or the traditional home remedy of striking the cyst with a heavy object, such as a Bible!

Most ganglia require no treatment. Aspiration with a large-bore (16- or 19-gauge) needle is helpful if the diagnosis is in doubt; however, even with steroid injection, the recurrence rate is high. Surgical treatment is indicated if the cyst is painful, the appearance is unsatisfactory, or concern is present regarding the exact nature of the mass.

Mucous Cysts. Associated with degenerative arthritis of the interphalangeal joints of the digits or thumb, mucous cysts are outpouchings of joint fluid similar to those of wrist ganglia. Radiographs show joint space narrowing and, often, marginal spurs or osteophytes. Osteophytes alone are the cause of the so-called Heberden's node at the distal interphalangeal joint and Bouchard's node at the PIP joint.

Arthritis. Degenerative joint disease commonly affects the carpometacarpal joint at the base of the thumb (see Chapter 157). Most often affecting women, the condition causes localized pain, decreased dexterity, and diminished grip strength. Pain and crepitation can be elicited by the examiner's grasping the thumb metacarpal and compressing it onto the trapezium (grind test). Radiographic changes may vary from mild joint space narrowing to complete joint space loss, osteophytes, and loose bodies.

Once recognized, mild to moderate arthritis of the trapeziometacarpal joint of the thumb can be effectively managed with NSAID medication and a molded splint worn 4 to 6 hours per day. The splint extends beyond the MCP joint but leaves the wrist free (a short opponens splint). It should be custom-made by a trained occupational therapist.

The hand involvement in *rheumatoid arthritis* can vary from minimal pain and swelling to extensive deformity and joint destruction. Treatment includes pharmacologic and physical therapy measures (see Chapter 156). Tendon rupture is not uncommon; its occurrence should prompt early referral.

Hand infections are potentially serious conditions, especially if they occur in a closed compartment. There are a variety of presentations. Infections around the fingernail are termed *paronychiae* and are usually caused by gram-positive organisms. Antibiotics and warm soaks suffice in mild, well-localized cases, but any spread requires referral for incisional drainage. A *felon* represents a more worrisome problem, because it is an infection in a closed compartment, the pulp space of the tip of the digit. The pulp is swollen, exquisitely tender, and erythematous. If uncorrected, the edema can compromise arterial supply and lead to necrosis of the tip. Treatment includes incision, drainage, and antibiotics. Early referral to a hand surgeon is essential for definitive treatment. A less troublesome infection seen mostly in hospital personnel is *herpetic infection* of the fingertip, which is characterized by small vesicles along the pulp. It clears spontaneously, although the patient is infectious until the vesicles clear.

Infectious flexor tenosynovitis presents with the digit symmetrically swollen, painful along the entire flexor sheath, held in a flexed posture, and tender with passive extension of the distal joint. Prompt recognition and surgical intervention are critical to preserve ultimate tendon function.

Puncture wounds, in particular human bites, may result in extremely virulent infection. Prompt and aggressive wound care, leaving the puncture site open, and antibiotic treatment may abort a more serious and destructive process. Animal bites, especially from dogs and cats, can transmit *Pasteurella multocida*, which in most instances is extremely sensitive to penicillin (see Chapter 196).

Summary

The localization of symptoms provides the keystone for evaluation. The examination should attempt to carefully localize the precise area of tenderness. A thorough functional examination, including active and passive motions of the wrist, digits, and thumb, sensory testing to light touch and pinprick, and specific flexor and extensor tendon function should be part of every hand assessment. Standard anteroposterior and lateral radiographs are generally advisable in most cases. An EMG and a nerve conduction study are part of the workup for peripheral nerve compressions.

Nonspecific tenosynovitis and mild-to-moderate degenerative arthritis generally respond to anti-inflammatory medication and simple splinting (discussed earlier). The patient with a hand infection, fracture, nerve compression, or mass should be referred to a hand specialist.

ANNOTATED BIBLIOGRAPHY

American Society for Surgery of the Hand. The Hand. Examination and Diagnosis. 2nd ed. New York: Churchill Livingstone, 1985. *(Concise, well-written, and well-illustrated; should be on the shelf of any physician who sees hand problems.)*

American Society for Surgery of the Hand. The Hand. Primary Care of Common Problems. *(A sequel to the above text; an excellent manual for anyone treating minor hand injuries.)*

Anderson B, Kaye S. Treatment of flexor tenosynovitis of the hand ("trigger finger") with corticosteroids. Arch Intern Med 1991;151:153. *(A prospective study; found to be safe and effective.)*

Bernhang AM. The many causes of tennis elbow. N Y State J Med 1979;79:1363. *(An excellent overview of the subject.)*

Flatt AE. Care of the Arthritic Hand. 4th ed. St Louis: CV Mosby, 1983. *(Presents a comprehensive overview of arthritic problems in a well-written, interesting text.)*

Roschmann RA, Bell CL. Septic arthritis in immunocompromised patients. Am J Med 1987;83:861. *(Good description of clinical findings; presentation similar to that in immunocompetent patients.)*

Primary Care Medicine: Office Evaluation and Management of the Adult Patient, 3rd edition, edited by Allan H. Goroll, Lawrence A. May, and Albert G. Mulley, Jr. J.B. Lippincott Company, Philadelphia

154

Approach to Minor Orthopedic Problems of the Foot and Ankle

JESSE B. JUPITER, M.D.

Patients often consult primary physicians for advice and help regarding foot or ankle problems. Although some patients require orthopedic referral for more detailed investigation and treatment, many can be substantially helped by the nonorthopedic physician who is knowledgeable about the diagnosis and treatment of common foot and ankle complaints. Such disorders are extremely prevalent and can incapacitate a patient. The primary care physician should be familiar with the basic types of foot and ankle complaints to effectively treat the minor conditions and appropriately refer those problems that require the skills of the orthopedic surgeon.

FOOT PROBLEMS

Foot disorders are a major cause of disability in the work force. Although often the result of normal activity, foot pain can also be precipitated by structural deformity or systemic disease. Environmental factors, such as shoe type and weight-bearing surface, add to the development and progression of symptoms.

Pathophysiology, Clinical Presentation, and Management

Anatomically, there are 26 bones in the human foot, equal to one-quarter of those in the entire human skeleton, along with 100 or more ligaments, 12 extrinsic muscle insertions, and 19 intrinsic muscles. During gait, more than two times the force of body weight is borne by the foot. In normal gait, the foot assumes several roles, including that of a shock absorber, a mobile adapter to accommodate uneven surfaces, and a rigid lever to propel the limb. Limitation or excess of these primary functions places the foot at risk for acquired mechanical trauma, with the prime candidates being the flat (pes planus) and high-arched (pes cavus) feet. Foot disorders are conveniently considered by anatomic zones: digits, forefoot, and hindfoot. Office assessment is facilitated by familiarity with the location and manifestations of common foot problems (Fig. 154–1).

Digital Problems. Complaints referable to the toes usually are related to deformities. Most digital problems present as sagittal plane deformities. There are three types: *hammer toe*, *mallet toe*, and *claw toe*. Pain with or without a "corn" (clavus) is usually the primary complaint. Toe contractures develop secondary to muscle imbalances or are shoe-induced; they can be flexible or rigid. Shoes (prescription or commercial) that allow adequate room in the toe box area are the first line of treatment. If the contractures are flexible, digital splints may be helpful. In persistent or progressive disease, surgery may be necessary if foot pain compromises daily activity.

Forefoot Problems. See Table 154–1 for a list of forefoot problems.

First Metatarsophalangeal (MTP) Joint. The most common deformity of this joint is the *hallux valgus (bunion)*. It presents as a painful swelling on the dorsomedial aspect of the first metatarsal head, associated with lateral drift of the toe. The deformity or a foot–shoe incompatibility may be the presenting complaint but, just as frequently, the patient presents with secondary problems adjacent in the forefoot, such as hammer toes or metatarsalgia. Hyperpronation (flat feet) and inappropriate shoes (high heels, pointed toe box) contribute to the development of the painful bunion, particularly in women.

On examination, a tender bursa is often present over the inner side of the head of the first metatarsal. The great toe itself may be deviated laterally and at times is not even passively reducible. Radiographs may show the underlying cause to be an increased angle between the first and second metatarsals (normal: 10°–12°). This deformity is commonly seen in patients with rheumatoid arthritis.

Properly fitted shoes (commercial or custom-made), bunion shields, and orthotic devices can afford symptomatic relief to many patients. Surgical intervention may be required to correct the structural deformity.

Hallux limitus, or hallux rigidus, is characterized by limited or total loss of dorsiflexion of the first MTP joint and a dorsal "bunion." The patient usually complains of pain on walking or problems with shoe fitting.

Physical examination reveals markedly limited mobility of the first MTP joint, especially on dorsiflexion (normal: 50°–80° passively). Pain and crepitation are usually present. Radiographs reveal changes associated with degenerative joint disease, such as joint space narrowing, osteophytes, and sclerosis. Chronic gouty arthritis may resemble this condition.

The initial treatment should be directed at limiting the stresses on the joint. An orthotic with an extension under the great toe (Morton's extension) and a shoe with extra depth should be prescribed. Limiting joint motion by stiffening the outer sole of the shoe (full-length steel shank) may also help. Surgery involving either joint resection, replacement, or fusion is indicated if conservative treatment is unsuccessful.

Sesamoid Disorders. The first MTP joint contains two sesamoid bones (medial and lateral) that articulate plantarly with the first metatarsal and serve, to some degree, as a fulcrum in normal joint mobility. Excessive or abnormal stress about this area can lead to pain and inflammation (*sesamoi-*

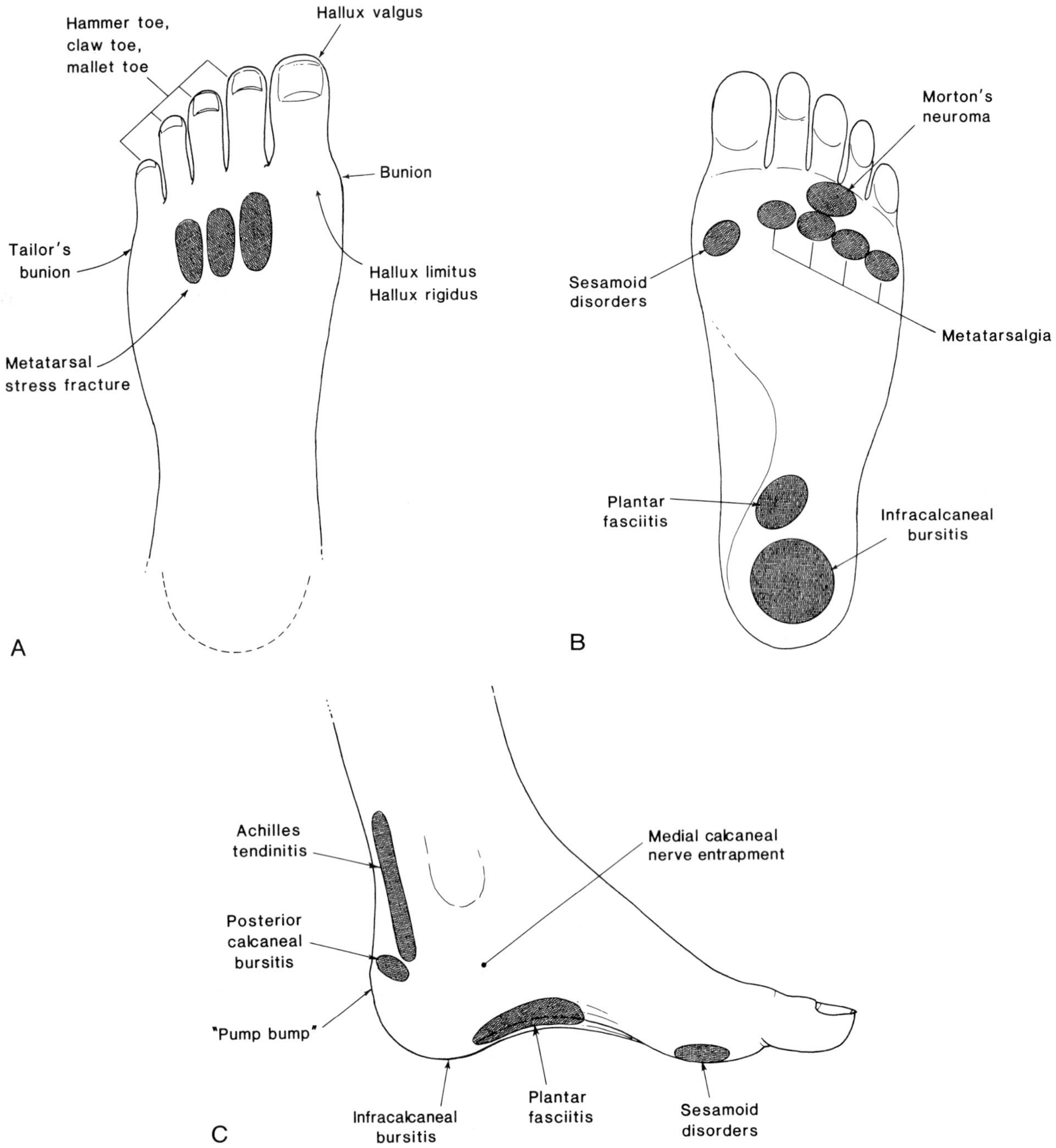

Figure 154-1. Sites of common foot problems.

ditis), *cartilage injury*, or *sesamoid fracture*. There may be no obvious history of trauma, but sesamoid injuries are not uncommon among ballet dancers, joggers, aerobic dancers, and the like.

Localized pain and swelling are present on careful examination (plantar palpation). Radiographs should include, in addition to standard anteroposterior and lateral views, a sesamoid axial view, which is crucial for an accurate diagnosis. If a fracture is suspected, one must remember that bipartite (or multipartite) sesamoids are normal variants; a bone scan may be helpful in the diagnosis of fracture.

Treatment is directed toward providing rest and reducing the weight-bearing stresses in this area. A stiff-soled, low-heeled shoe with a full-length shank and soft innersole may be all that is required to reduce stress on the sesamoids in mild cases. Orthotic devices may be of additional help. Infrequently, excision of the involved bone is required.

Lesser MTP Joints. The fifth metatarsal corollary to the bunion is the *bunionette*, which also presents as a painful deformity and foot–shoe incompatibility. The lateral aspect of the fifth metatarsal head is tender with a local bursal swelling. Radiographs may show the primary defect to be an

Table 154-1. Common Causes of Foot Pain

Digital Deformities
Hammer toe
Claw toe
Mallet toe
Forefoot Pain—Great Toe
Hallux valgus (bunion)
Hallux limitus/rigidus
Sesamoid disorders
Forefoot Pain—Other Structures
Tailor's bunion (bunionette)
Metatarsalgia
Morton's interdigital neuroma
Metatarsal stress fracture
Hindfoot Pain—Plantar
Plantar fasciitis
Infracalcaneal bursitis
Medial calcaneal nerve entrapment
Tarsal tunnel syndrome
Referred pain from subtalar arthritis or lumbosacral disc radiculopathy
Hindfoot Pain—Posterior
Posterior calcaneal bursitis
Exostosis ("pump bump")
Achilles tendinitis
Inflammatory arthritis

excessive angle between the fourth and fifth metatarsals or an enlarged fifth metatarsal head. Alteration of shoe gear (ie, wider or stretched) usually helps, although surgical correction may be necessary.

Metatarsalgia. True metatarsalgia reflects pain with weight bearing in the vicinity of the lesser metatarsal heads. Although this term is commonly used for any pain pattern in this area, it more accurately reflects an absence of other underlying conditions, such as interdigital neuroma, metatarsal stress fracture, MTP joint arthritis, or osteochondritis. The metatarsals are tender to pressure, and the plantar aspect of the foot (with the patient lying in the prone position) may reveal a protrusion in an otherwise flat forefoot surface. Hypermobility may also be found in the neighboring metatarsals. Often, a callus develops directly beneath the involved metatarsal, creating additional discomfort.

A variety of conservative methods are employed to disperse weight away from the involved metatarsal, including soft innersoles, molded shoes with innersoles, metatarsal bars, and orthotic devices. On some occasions, as in deforming rheumatoid arthritis with dorsal dislocation of the MTP joints, surgical intervention (metatarsal head resection) is necessary and most rewarding.

Interdigital (Morton's) neuroma. Burning pain and cramping, most often involving the third and fourth toes, are characteristic symptoms of this lesion. Classically, the patient is a woman who reports that symptoms are aggravated by wearing closed shoes and relieved by removal of the shoe and forefoot massage. The third intermetatarsal space is supplied by a common nerve trunk, receiving branches from both the medial and lateral plantar nerves. Compression and irritation of this trunk in a fibro-osseous ring formed by the metatarsal heads, the deep transverse intermetatarsal ligament, and the plantar weight-bearing surface are implicated in this lesion.

By compressing the forefoot and pushing up in the distal third intermetatarsal space, a "click" may be felt (Mulder's sign), with reproduction of the patient's symptoms. Relief is sometimes achieved through use of wider shoes, a metatarsal bar, soft insoles, orthotic devices, nonsteroidal anti-inflammatory agents (NSAIDs), or local anesthetic/steroid injections. Quite often, surgical excision is required.

Metatarsal stress fractures. Functional overload in a lesser metatarsal (usually the second or third metatarsal) may result in a march or fatigue fracture. The onset of symptoms is sudden and often without a history of trauma. Palpation of the metatarsal shaft elicits pain over the site of injury. Four to 6 weeks post-injury, swelling can be palpated, reflecting the presence of a healing callus. Initially, radiographs are negative, but a bone scan may confirm the diagnosis early on.

Healing is uneventful if one avoids rigorous activities and wears a stiff-soled, low-heeled shoe. Occasionally, a standard wooden postoperative shoe and an Unna boot compressive wrap are helpful in providing a more comfortable gait.

Hindfoot Problems. See Table 154–1 for a list of problems of the rear foot.

Plantar Heel Pain. Plantar heel pain is seen in both young and old patients and can be disabling. It is often mistakenly attributed to "heel spurs," most of which are asymptomatic and unrelated to the pain.

Plantar fasciitis classically causes pain with the initial step taken on getting out of bed in the morning. Pain often diminishes as the foot "stretches out," only to recur after periods of inactivity. Overuse syndromes, such as conditions caused by jogging, can contribute to small tears near the origin of the plantar fascia, with subsequent focal pain and localized inflammation. Characteristically, tenderness can be elicited along the medial plantar aspect of the foot, approximately three finger-breadths distal to the posterior heel. Pain is increased with forced dorsiflexion of the digits during the examination. Although radiographs often demonstrate a plantar spur at the anterior, inferior aspect of the calcaneus, this is usually not the cause of the symptoms.

Orthotic devices tend to be the most effective form of management, although rest, ice, tendo-Achilles stretching exercises, ultrasound, NSAIDs, and local steroid injections all have selective roles in the overall treatment. Rarely, surgical release of the plantar fascia is needed, but the operative results are not consistently good.

Intracalcaneal bursitis. In contrast to plantar fasciitis, this entity presents with an aching sensation in the direct *midplantar* aspect of the calcaneus, generally increasing with the duration of weight bearing. Symptoms are more pronounced as the day progresses. Examination reveals *point tenderness* directly under the midportion of the calcaneus. Localized warmth and swelling may be present. This localized lesion is most likely an inflamed bursa directly beneath the calcaneus. Therapy includes local modalities such as ice, massage, NSAIDs, and local steroid injections. A soft heel pad, heel cup, or appropriately fabricated orthotic device to relieve direct impact on this region should be added.

Neurologic heel pain. Local or more *proximal nerve entrapment* is an important cause of heel pain. For example, an entrapment of the medial calcaneal branch of the posterior tibial nerve in the region of the inferior calcaneus can mimic symptoms of inferior calcaneal bursitis. In this situation, however, one can elicit a proximal radiation of pain upward toward the region of the tarsal tunnel beneath the medial malleolus. A positive Tinel's sign should be sought on examination. If local steroid injection is not effective, resection of the medial calcaneal nerve branch may be required.

As the posterior tibial nerve courses behind the medial malleolus entering the fibro-osseous tarsal tunnel, local compression of the nerve because of local trauma (sprain, fracture), a space-occupying lesion (varicosity, lipoma), or repetitive hyperpronation can result. Symptoms include paresthesias, dysesthesias, and nocturnal pain along the plantar aspect of the foot or anywhere along the distribution of the medial or lateral plantar nerves. Nerve conduction studies are not consistently abnormal in this "*tarsal tunnel syndrome*." A foot surgeon should be consulted, although conservative treatment with orthotics and local steroid injections may preclude the need for surgical release.

Lastly, neurologically related heel pain can be the result of a *radiculopathy* secondary to a herniated lumbosacral disc. Careful examination of the low back and neurologic testing including sensory and reflex function should be performed, especially if the cause of the pain is not readily apparent.

Posterior Heel Pain. Two bursae are present at the posterior heel: a superficial bursa lying between the Achilles tendon and skin and a deep bursa located between the tendon and the calcaneus. *Posterior calcaneal bursitis* results from structural and functional abnormalities of the hindfoot or inappropriate shoe gear with a firm, unyielding heel counter. Pain can be elicited by compression of the heel cord just anterior to its attachment and with passive dorsal and plantar flexion of the ankle. Several systemic inflammatory conditions (rheumatoid arthritis, ankylosing spondylitis, and Reiter's syndrome) can produce a similar clinical picture, as can a tear of the Achilles tendon and posterior calcaneal exostosis (see later discussion).

The recommended treatment of acute posterior calcaneal bursitis begins with local measures such as application of ice in the first 24 hours, followed by moist heat, NSAID medication, and rest. With a more chronic condition, a heel lift or orthotic device to control heel motion and heel counter adjustments of the shoe should be considered.

Exostosis. Posterior calcaneal exostosis ("pump bump") is most commonly seen in young women, presenting as a tender enlargement about the lateral dorsal aspect of the posterior calcaneus. Pain is aggravated by a firm heel counter. A thickened bursa may overlie a true exostosis of the calcaneus, which can be seen on a lateral radiograph. The treatment of the acute, bursal inflammation parallels that of other types of heel bursitis already described. Resection of a posterior bony exostosis is reserved only for those cases in which symptoms cannot be effectively controlled conservatively.

Achilles tendinitis. A common affliction of athletes, this problem reflects inflammation or small tears near the insertion of the Achilles tendon (or paratendon). Discomfort worsens during athletic activity, with subsequent swelling and stiffness. On examination, there is tenderness to palpation of the tendon (often extending proximally), in association with a palpable fusiform swelling. In acute cases, the first line of therapy is rest, even to the point of plaster immobilization. A heel lift, ultrasound, anti-inflammatory agents, heel cord stretching, and orthotics are helpful in the chronic phase.

Systemically Related Foot Disorders. The foot can mirror systemic disease. Vascular disorders with macro- or microvascular involvement can be the underlying origin for a variety of foot problems, including ulcers and necrosis. Neurologic disorders can compromise both foot form and function. Systemic or metabolic disorders, including atherosclerosis, diabetes mellitus, gout, and rheumatoid arthritis, may all have profound effects on the foot requiring medical as well as orthopedic, vascular surgical, or podiatric treatment (see Chapters 34, 102, 156, and 158).

The Runner's Foot. The stress of repeated impact involved with athletic endeavors such as jogging predisposes the foot to significant mechanical trauma. All the specific entities discussed previously occur among runners. Just as important is the foot's biomechanical influence on the rest of the lower extremity. For example, the hyperpronated "flat" foot can cause excessive strain on the posterior tibial muscle and also increase the torque on the entire lower extremity, resulting in medial knee pain after prolonged jogging. If one does observe significant hypermobility or hyperpronation, it is best to mechanically support the foot with a molded orthotic. A rigid, cavus-type foot deformity prevents normal pronation with stance. When engaged in running, the foot may lose its capacity to act as a shock absorber. Increased shock is transmitted up the entire lower extremity, even to the lower back region. Patients with this type of foot deformity may complain of leg, knee, and hip discomfort.

ANKLE

Ankle Sprain. A sprain is the most common ankle injury. Lesions range from minor ligamentous damage to complete tear or avulsion of the bony attachment, fracture, and dislocation. A *strain* does not involve loss of joint stability or tearing of ligaments, whereas a sprain does. Sprain occurs when stress is applied while the ankle is in an unstable position, causing the ligaments to overstretch. During plantar flexion, the joint is least stable and most susceptible to eversion or inversion forces. Such stresses are encountered during running or walking over uneven surfaces. Evaluation is facilitated by early presentation, because the event producing injury is likely to be remembered and swelling is confined to the site of injury.

All too often, ankle sprains are considered minor injuries requiring little medical attention, even though experience has proven this concept to be misleading. Although many sprains heal with no residual disability, some do not. All reflect some degree of injury to one or several ligaments and may be classified as *first-degree*, involving stretching of ligamentous fibers, *second-degree*, involving a tear of some portion of the ligament with associated pain and swelling, and *third-degree*, implying complete ligamentous separation.

An *inversion injury* is the most common type of sprain, causing damage to the lateral ligaments. There is often a his-

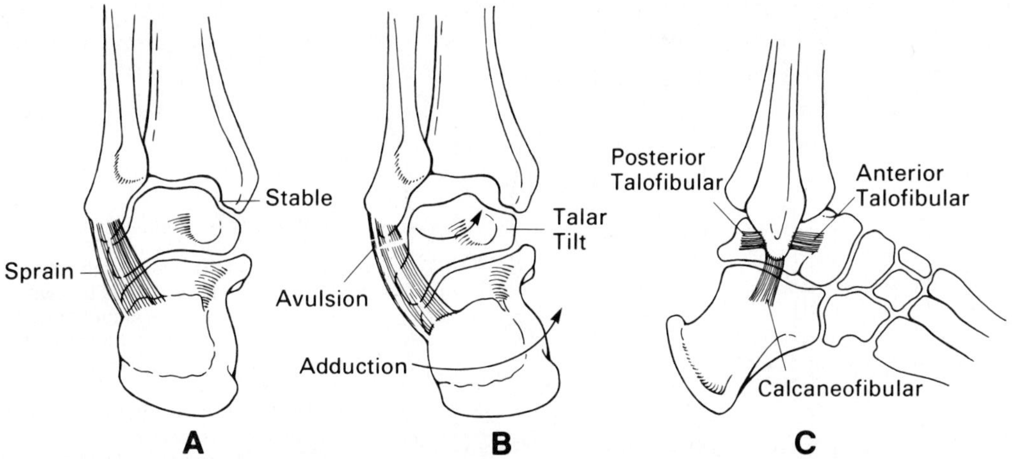

Figure 154-2. Lateral ligamentous sprain and avulsion. (*A*), Simple sprain in which the ligaments remain intact and the talus remains stable within the mortice. (*B*), Avulsion of the lateral ligaments; the talus becomes unstable and tilts within the mortice when the calcaneus is adducted. (*C*), Lateral ligaments of the ankle. The anterior talofibular and the calcaneofibular ligaments are the ligaments most frequently involved in inversion injuries. (Redrawn form Cailliet R: Foot and Ankle Pain. Philadelphia: FA Davis, 1968.)

tory of inversion during plantar flexion; a snap or tear may have been heard or felt. However, the history of injury is often inaccurate and may not be helpful in evaluating the extent of ligamentous damage. A careful physical examination is needed to identify the site and degree of injury, using one's fingertips to check the anterior capsule and medial and lateral ligaments (Fig. 154–2). Although significant edema commonly accompanies ligamentous injury, complete ligamentous and capsular disruption may produce remarkably little edema, because of extravasation into the surrounding soft tissue planes.

A useful sign of significant injury is the *anterior draw sign*. The sign maybe elicited by grasping the distal tibia in one hand and the calcaneus and heel in the other and sliding the entire foot forward. This is done both with the ankle in neutral position and with 30° of plantar flexion. Up to 2 mm of shift is normal. With disruption of the anterior or lateral ligaments, one sees 4 mm or more of anterior shift, as the fibers of the anterolateral ligaments lie in anteroposterior direction. Passive inversion of the ankle produces pain. Swelling invariably occurs, usually anterior to the lateral malleolus at the onset; ecchymoses are common. Simple strain does not result in joint instability, but with a sprain, the joint loses stability and the talus tilts if the calcaneus is adducted (see Fig. 154–2). This produces a talomalleolar gap on the lateral aspect of the ankle. If swelling or pain interferes with evaluation, an x-ray assessment after nerve block may be needed to determine joint instability.

X-rays are useful in most cases of moderate to severe injury, helping to identify any associated skeletal injury in addition to assessing degree of ligamentous damage. Three standard views are obtained: anteroposterior, lateral, and mortice (an anteroposterior view with the ankle in 20°–30° on internal rotation). In addition, a stress view is obtained (with the help of local anesthesia, if necessary) to check for talar tilt. A tilt of more than 15° is suggestive of lateral ligament injury; more than 25° of tilt is diagnostic. One must always compare the tilt of one foot to that of the other to rule out underlying ligamentous laxity.

Control of swelling is the first and immediate priority of management, because effusion and hemorrhage further stretch and distend the joint and predispose to adhesions. An elastic bandage, ice water, and elevation are often helpful in controlling edema. The ankle should be placed in ice water for 15 to 20 minutes and then elevated. An ice pack can substitute for immersion. Cold application is repeated every few hours. X-rays can be done after taping, ice water, and elevation. A bulky, conforming, nonconstricting soft dressing may be applied.

Strains and mildly to moderately severe sprains are managed by repeated ice packs, followed within 48 hours by hot soaks. The soft dressing or elastic bandage is used for 1 to 2 weeks to control swelling and provide stability. In splinting the ankle, it should be kept in neutral or slightly everted position to avoid tightening the heel cord and other posterior structures. Partial weight bearing is accomplished by using a crutch until pain subsides. Nonweight-bearing exercises are started within 2 to 3 days of injury; these include active plantar flexion, dorsiflexion, toe flexion, inversion, and eversion.

After pain subsides and swelling resolves, full weight bearing can be resumed, often with use of a functional plastic "sprain brace." A number of commercially available designs exist for these braces, and all function to support the ankle against the inversion and eversion stresses while, at the same time, allowing the ankle to dorsiflex and plantar-flex. Running should be postponed another 1 to 3 weeks depending on severity of injury. With mild ligamentous laxity of the ankle and repeated minor sprains, proper taping to support the lateral structures is indicated for athletic activity that involves contact, running, or jumping, particularly on uneven ground. Tape strips are applied from the medial aspect to the lateral aspect of the ankle (Fig. 154–3) to hold the heel and ankle in eversion and provide support. Exercises to strengthen the

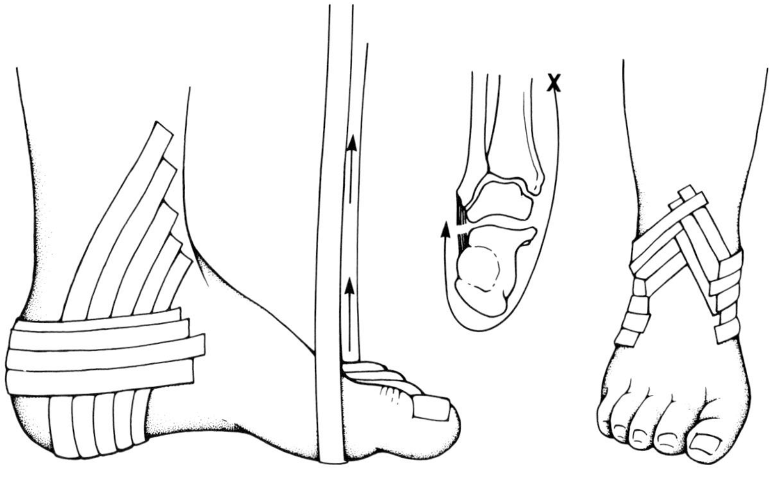

Figure 154-3. Taping a sprained ankle. The purpose of taping the ankle is to prevent further stretching of the injured ligaments until healing has occurred. The ankle must be inverted or everted to place the strained ligament at rest. The center figure depicts an avulsed lateral ligament. The tape here begins from inside and then runs under the foot to finish on the outer leg holding the heel *everted.* The horizontal strips minimize rotation of the forefoot. (Redrawn from Cailliet R: Foot and Ankle Pain. Philadelphia: FA Davis, 1968.)

ankle evertors and high-laced leather supportive shoes may also be helpful.

Ankle sprain is a serious injury; if ligaments are torn and result in marked ankle instability (determined by examination under anesthesia or stress x-rays), surgical repair or at least cast immobilization for 4 to 8 weeks is indicated. Serious sprain requires prompt orthopedic referral to maximize chances for healing and restoration of joint stability.

ANNOTATED BIBLIOGRAPHY

Cailliet R. Foot and Ankle Pain. Philadelphia: FA Davis, 1974. *(A concise, illustrated overview of foot and ankle disorders.)*

Jahss MH (ed). Disorders of the Foot. Philadelphia: WB Saunders, 1982. *(The current definitive text on foot disorders. Although comprehensive, each chapter is well illustrated and well referenced.)*

155
Approach to the Patient with Asymptomatic Hyperuricemia

Primary Care Medicine: Office Evaluation and Management of the Adult Patient, 3rd edition, edited by Allan H. Goroll, Lawrence A. May, and Albert G. Mulley, Jr. J.B. Lippincott Company, Philadelphia

Asymptomatic hyperuricemia became commonplace when physicians began using chemistry panels that routinely included measurement of the serum uric acid. Hyperuricemia is defined as a serum uric acid concentration that exceeds the mean by at least two standard deviations. The mean (as determined by colorimetric assay—the most commonly used method) is 7.5 mg/100 mL for men and 6.6 mg/100 mL for women. By statistical definition, 2.5 percent of the population is hyperuricemic. The consequences of being hyperuricemic and the need for lowering the uric acid have been subjects of debate. Some authorities have advocated prophylactic therapy in hopes of preventing acute gout, chronic tophaceous gout, stone formation, and renal failure. Others question the cost-effectiveness of such an approach and even the relationship of hyperuricemia to some of the adverse consequences attributed to it. The primary physician must decide if and when to treat the asymptomatic patient with an elevated uric acid.

PATHOPHYSIOLOGY AND CLINICAL PRESENTATION

Uric acid is the end-product of purine metabolism. In humans there is no pathway for further breakdown of uric acid; it must be excreted by the kidneys or the serum level will rise. The pathogenesis of hyperuricemia involves overproduction and/or underexcretion of urate. It is estimated that one-third of hyperuricemic patients are overproducers, that another third are underexcreters, and that the remainder have a combined deficit.

Overproduction of uric acid is especially marked in patients undergoing treatment for myeloproliferative and lymphoproliferative malignancies and in those with severe psoriasis. Rapid cellular turnover results in production of massive amounts of nucleic acid metabolites that are converted to uric acid. Overproduction may also develop from an increase in *de novo* purine synthesis, as occurs in patients with inborn errors of metabolism. Contrary to popular belief, excessive dietary intake of purine-rich foods is rarely responsible for hyperuricemia, because dietary sources of purine make up only 10 percent of the uric acid pool. However, excessive intake of alcohol (greater than 100 g/d of ethanol) results in increased urate synthesis, especially if the patient is not taking any food at the time of alcohol intake.

Underexcretion of uric acid occurs if there is an overall decrease in glomerular filtration or a defect in tubular secretion of urate, or if another substance competes with urate for tubular secretion. Hyperuricemia has been noted in hypertensive patients and viewed as a consequence of hypertensive renovascular injury. Compromise in renal blood flow due to aging and atherosclerotic disease reduces renal urate excretion. Excretion falls in patients with increased proximal tubular reabsorption of sodium, which has been linked to hyperinsulinism and might account for the oft-noted, poorly understood relation between hyperuricemia atherosclerotic cardiovascular disease. Drugs such as thiazides and low doses of aspirin reduce renal urate excretion. Fasting that results in ketosis also seems capable of transiently reducing urate excretion and raising the serum uric acid.

Well over 90 percent of hyperuricemic patients present asymptomatically. Most are individuals subjected to multiphasic screening. Half of newly discovered patients in the Framingham study were taking thiazides, and just under 3 percent had elevations secondary to a concurrent illness, such as myeloproliferative disease.

PRINCIPLES OF MANAGEMENT

Prophylactic therapy might be indicated if lowering the uric acid could prevent acute gout, chronic gouty arthritis, gouty nephropathy, or urolithiasis. For years it was assumed such complications were a direct result of untreated hyperuricemia, leading many clinicians to treat asymptomatic hyperuricemic patients with urate-lowering drugs. The statistical relationship between hyperuricemia and atherosclerotic disease was also of concern.

Prevention of Acute Gouty Arthritis. Population studies (Framingham, Normative Aging, Sudbury) confirm that the higher the serum uric acid level, the greater the chance of an attack of acute gout and that the urate concentration is the predominant determinant of risk. However, the oft-quoted 90 percent risk reported in the Framingham Study represented a 12-year cumulative incidence figure and pertained only to 10 patients who had a uric acid in excess of 9.0 mg/dL. More relevant is the average annual incidence, which was 4.0 percent in the Framingham Study and 4.7 percent in the Normative Aging Study for patients whose urate concentrations were in the top 2 percent.

To determine the utility of prophylactic therapy, one needs to consider the costs and benefits of preventing an attack of acute gout. The cost of life-long prophylactic therapy can reach thousands of dollars, because the mean age at time of detection is 35. The prevalence of adverse drug reactions has been reported to be as high as 10 percent for probenecid and 25 percent for allopurinol. These costs appear excessive when compared to the safety, efficacy, and minimal expense of promptly treating a single acute attack of gout with a short course of a nonsteroidal antiinflammatory agent (see Chapter 158). Only if gouty attacks become disabling and frequent does the cost–benefit equation shift in favor of prophylaxis. In most instances, the intervals between recurrences of acute gout are measured in years.

Prevention of Chronic Gouty Arthritis. The issue of prophylaxis for prevention of chronic gouty arthritis is of only minor importance, because almost all patients with this condition go through a stage of acute gouty attacks before developing chronic joint changes. Thus, asymptomatic patients with no evidence of clinical gout are at little if any risk for silently falling victim to chronic gouty arthritis.

Prevention of Azotemia. Despite fears to the contrary and early studies that were confounded by high lead exposures, chronic hyperuricemia does not appear to be a significant risk factor for development of azotemia, nor does hyperuricemia *due to* renal failure pose an additional threat to the kidneys. In a prospective Kaiser-Permanente study comparing 113 patients with asymptomatic hyperuricemia and 193 controls followed for 8 years, there was no difference in the incidence of azotemia (1.8% versus 2.1%, respectively). In the same study, 168 patients with clinical gout followed for 10 years showed no relation between uric acid level and risk of azotemia. In the Normative Aging Study, only 0.7 percent of the 94 patients with a uric acid in excess of 9.0 developed a creatinine greater than 2.0 mg/dL over the 15 years of follow-up. One set of investigators calculated that significant risk of renal injury from chronic hyperuricemia required a uric acid level of 13.0 mg/dL in men and 10.0 mg/dL in women sustained for 40 years. A 3-year prospective study of hyperuricemic patients with and without renal failure showed no change in renal function when allopurinol was used to normalize the serum urate concentration.

One group of hyperuricemic patients at risk for renal failure are those with myeloproliferative or lymphoproliferative malignancy who are undergoing chemotherapy. With each cytotoxic treatment comes a huge uric acid load that may trigger injurious urate crystal formation in the renal tubular cells. Acute oliguric renal failure may ensue. Such patients require pretreatment with allopurinol and vigorous hydration.

Prevention of Nephrolithiasis. The risk of nephrolithiasis in patients with asymptomatic hyperuricemia is very small. In the Kaiser study, renal calculi occurred in 3 (2.6%) of 113 hyperuricemic patients and in 2 (1.1%) of 193 controls. In two of the hyperuricemic patients with stones, the stone was composed of calcium. The risk of developing a stone attributable to hyperuricemia was calculated to be less than 1 percent per year. Among gouty patients, the control of serum uric acid was the same in those who developed stones as in those who did not.

This minimal stone risk conferred by hyperuricemia alone derives from the importance of other factors to stone formation (see Chapter 135). Family history, urinary *p*H, and level of hydration are particularly germane. Two of the three hyperuricemia patients with stones in the Kaiser study had a family history of nephrolithiasis. Urine acidity is a critical factor because the solubility of uric acid falls precipitously as the *p*H falls from 8.0 to 5.0. The amount of uric acid excreted in the urine per 24 hours has also been suggested as a cause, but careful studies have shown that the level of urinary uric acid is only a weak determinant of stone formation until extreme levels are encountered. However, dehydration is a well-established precipitant.

Urolithiasis is rarely life-threatening. In a study of 1700 patients with gout, only one patient experienced serious obstructive uropathy.

Prevention of Atherosclerotic Disease. Although there is a statistical relationship between hyperuricemia and atherosclerotic disease, it does not appear to be an etiologic one. Rather they appear to share a common pathophysiologic link. Current speculation centers on hyperinsulinism as the link. There is no evidence that treating hyperuricemia lowers the risk of atherosclerotic disease.

THERAPEUTIC RECOMMENDATIONS

- Asymptomatic hyperuricemia is associated with an increased risk of acute gouty arthritis, but the cost of prophylactic therapy in patients who have never had a single attack of gout greatly exceeds the cost of symptomatically treating an acute attack, should it occur.
- Only with development of frequent acute gouty attacks is prophylactic therapy indicated (see Chapter 158).
- Treatment to prevent chronic tophaceous gout need not be started until clinical evidence of gout develops.
- There is insufficient evidence to justify prophylaxis for prevention of renal impairment unless the patient has a myeloproliferative or lymphoproliferative disorder and is about to be treated for it. The degree of azotemia that can be attributed to hyperuricemia is mild and clinically insignificant in most other instances.
- The risk of urolithiasis is sufficiently low to justify waiting for the development of a stone before initiating prophylactic therapy, unless the patient has a strong family history of nephrolithiasis. However, dehydration should be avoided.

Although hyperuricemia is associated statistically with atherosclerotic disease, the relation is not etiologic, and there is no cardiovascular benefit from lowering the serum uric acid level.

A.H.G.

ANNOTATED BIBLIOGRAPHY

Batuman V, Maesaka JK, Haddad B, et al. The role of lead in gout nephropathy. N Engl J Med 1981;304:520. *(Detected a strong relationship between lead and nephropathy in patients with gout.)*

Berger LU, Yu TF. Renal function in gout—An analysis of 524 gouty subjects including long-term follow-up studies. Am J Med 1975;59:604. *(Follow-up for 12 years showed that hyperuricemia alone had no deleterious effect on renal function in ambulatory patients with gout.)*

Brand FN, McGee DL, Kannel WB, et al. Hyperuricemia as a risk factor of coronary heart disease: The Framingham study. Am J Epidemiol 1985;121:11. *(Finds statistical but not etiologic role in atherosclerotic disease.)*

Campion EW, Glynn RJ, DeLabry LO. Asymptomatic hyperuricemia: Risks and consequences in the Normative Aging Study. Am J Med 1987;82:421. *(A large study with 15-year follow-up; risk of gout was 4.9 percent per year for patients with a uric acid over 9 mg/dL; risk of renal failure was nil.)*

Cappuccio FP, Strazzullo P, Farinaro E, et al. Uric acid metabolism and tubular sodium handling. JAMA 1993;270:354. *(Finds hyperuricemia closely linked to excessive proximal tubular reabsorption of sodium; speculates both are manifestations of hyperinsulinemia.)*

Faller J, Fox I. Ethanol-induced hyperuricemia. N Engl J Med 1982;307:1598. *(Ethanol increases urate synthesis.)*

Fessel JW. Renal outcomes of gout and hyperuricemia. Am J Med 1979;67:74. *(A prospective study showing that the risks of renal failure and stone formation are very small and hardly justify prophylactic therapy.)*

Frohlich ED. Uric acid: A risk factor for coronary heart disease. JAMA 1993;270:378. *(Reviews the pathophysiology of hyperuricemia and its link to atherosclerotic risk factors.)*

Hall AP, Berry PE, Dawber TR, et al. Epidemiology of gout and hyperuricemia—A long-term population study. Am J Med 1967;42:27. *(The Framingham study; 19 percent of those with uric serum urates between 8 and 8.9 mg/dL and five of six patients with a uric acid* 9 mg/dL developed a gouty attack over the 12 years of follow-up.)

Liang MH, Fries JF. Asymptomatic hyperuricemia: The case for conservative management. Ann Intern Med 1978;88:666. *(A well-developed approach to asymptomatic hyperuricemia.)*

MacLaughlan MJ, Rodnan GP. Effects of food, fast, and alcohol on serum uric acid and acute attacks of gout. Am J Med 1967;42:38. *(Fasting and consumption of over 100 g of alcohol raised urate levels. Acute changes in levels precipitated gouty attacks.)*

Reif MC, Constantiner A, Levitt MF. Chronic gouty nephropathy: A vanishing syndrome. N Engl J Med 1981;304:535. *(An editorial summarizing the data on the lack of a relation between renal injury and most forms of hyperuricemia.)*

Singer JZ, Wallace SL. The allopurinol hypersensitivity syndrome: Unnecessary morbidity and mortality. Arthritis Rheum 1986;29:82. *(High incidence of adverse reactions; the drug is not harmless for prolonged use.)*

Yu TF, Berger LU. Impaired renal function in gout. Am J Med 1982;75:95. *(Hyperuricemia alone did not affect renal function; renal insufficiency correlated best with coexisting hypertension, preexisting renal disease, and ischemic heart disease.)*

Yu TF, Gutman A. Uric acid nephrolithiasis in gout: Predisposing factors. Ann Intern Med 1967;67:1133. *(A classic study of 305 gout patients correlating risk of stone formation with uric acid excretion, urine* pH*, serum urate level, and etiology.)*

156
Management of Rheumatoid Arthritis

Primary Care Medicine: Office Evaluation and Management of the Adult Patient, 3rd edition, edited by Allan H. Goroll, Lawrence A. May, and Albert G. Mulley, Jr. J.B. Lippincott Company, Philadelphia

Management of rheumatoid arthritis (RA) is a challenge because the disease is chronic, relapsing, potentially disabling, and without completely satisfactory methods of treatment. The problem is common. Population surveys indicate that 3 percent of females and 1 percent of males have definite or probable RA, based on the diagnostic criteria established by the American Rheumatism Association. Prevalence increases with age, and incidence peaks in the fourth decade. The estimated annual incidence ranges from 0.5 to 3 new cases per thousand per year. The objectives of therapy are to minimize pain and stiffness and preserve range of motion and muscle strength. The primary physician needs to implement an effective program of patient education, antiinflammatory drug therapy, exercise, and joint rest; decide when referral is needed for disease-modifying therapy; and monitor closely for disease progression and treatment side effects.

PATHOPHYSIOLOGY AND CLINICAL PRESENTATION

Pathogenesis

Rheumatoid arthritis is an immunologically mediated, chronic inflammatory disease of unknown etiology, manifested by sinovitis and destructive arthritis of the diarthrodial joints. In genetically predisposed hosts (genotype HLA-DRB1*04/04), a delayed hypersensitivity reaction to an as yet unidentified stimulus (eg, infectious agent, constituent of synovium or cartilage) appears to be the initial event. Although the precise sequence of immunologic events leading to joint injury continue to be elucidated, important cellular components of the process include CD4 helper/inducer T-cell lymphocytes, CD4 memory T cells, plasma cells, activated macrophages, and neutrophils. Cytokines (eg, interleukins, granulocyte-macrophage colony-stimulating factor, tumor necrosis factor) are released and serve as important immunomediators, stimulating B- and T-cell proliferation and differentiation and activating neutrophils and monocytes. IgG rheumatoid factor emanating from local plasma cells may form immune complexes with articular antigens and, in doing so, activate complement. The net result is elaboration of prostaglandins, vasoactive amines, oxygen-derived free radicals, activated platelets, collagenases, and other lysosomal enzymes into the joint cavity causing direct damage to articular cartilage and bone.

Pathologically, the synovium is the principal site of initial involvement. The earliest change is immunologically mediated damage to the endothelium of the microvasculature. Small vessel lumens become obliterated by thrombi and inflammatory cells, followed by new capillary formation, synovial lining cell proliferation, edema, and leukocyte infiltration. Neutrophils migrate into the joint space. As the inflammatory process progresses, the synovium becomes more hypertrophic, edematous, hypervascular, and further infiltrated by mononuclear cells. In severe cases, there is *pannus* formation, representing an invasive proliferative synovitis with lymphocytes, plasma cells, fibroblasts, and macrophages. Pannus is capable of eroding cartilage and bone, typically beginning at the joint margin, then spreading over the entire cartilaginous surface. Lysosomal enzymes released from within the pannus and latent collagenases are believed to contribute to the direct erosive capacity. Often osteopenia is seen in subchondral bone adjacent to the involved joint even before the pannus has denuded the cartilage.

Clinical Presentation

Initially, an effusion develops, distending the joint capsule. This is followed by damage to the articular surface and weakening of the capsule and periarticular ligaments. Secondary muscle atrophy results and leads to imbalance of opposing muscle groups. The net effect is an unstable, weak, swollen, subluxated joint. The synovium of tendon sheaths and bursae may also be affected by the inflammatory process, which leads to accompanying tenosynovitis and bursitis.

Clinical onset of RA is usually insidious, often beginning with vague *arthralgias, morning stiffness,* and *fatigue*. In some patients, the onset is more acute. Signs of *articular inflammation* (swelling, pain, and warmth) soon follow. The small joints of the hands and feet—the proximal interphalangeals (PIP), metacarpophalangeals (MCP), and metatarsophalangeals (MTP)—are typically among the first to be involved, but knees, ankles, wrists, or elbows may also be affected early on. *Tenosynovitis* is common. Initially, the arthritis may be asymmetric or may even present as a monoarticular arthritis, but its characteristic symmetric distribution supervenes in most instances.

In an occasional patient, RA is preceded by *palindromic rheumatism,* a condition characterized by repeated episodes of transient joint pain, swelling, and redness extending beyond the joint. The condition lasts a few hours to a few days, followed by complete resolution and no permanent joint injury. Fingers, wrists, shoulders and knees are most commonly affected. About 50 percent of these patients eventually develop typical RA.

Rheumatoid nodules appear in about 25 percent of patients with RA, usually as the disease progresses. These subcutaneous nodules are firm, nontender, and located principally along the extensor surface of the forearm and in the olecranon bursa. Their appearance is an unfavorable prognostic sign, as is persistence of acute disease for more than 1 year, high serum titers of rheumatoid factor, and age under 20 at time of presentation.

Sustained joint inflammation lasting over a year leads to permanent erosion and loss of joint function. At first, the changes are partially reversible, but as cartilage and bone erode, the injury becomes permanent.

Hands and Wrists. Characteristic hand deformities include ulnar deviation of the MCP joints, boutonnière deformities of the PIP joints, and swan-neck contractures of the fingers. In the wrists, there is often permanent loss of extension. A boggy, tender, dorsal wrist mass may result from tenosynovitis, and compression of the median nerve can occur. The subsequent *carpal tunnel syndrome* is usually reversible, but nerve damage is permanent by the time wasting of the thenar eminence is obvious.

Feet. Erosion of the metatarsal heads can lead to ventral subluxation. Increased weight-bearing on the inflamed heads and painful callus formation result. Erosive disease may be silent in the MTP joints.

Hips and Knees. Involvement of these joints can be a source of much disability, because severe pain on weight-bearing may result. Loss of internal rotation is the first change noted in the hip, followed by flexion contracture. One hip may predominate, even though the process is bilateral. In the knee, distention of the suprapatellar pouch by synovial effusion is common. If pressure rises rapidly, there can be herniation of the synovium with formation of a popliteal *Baker's cyst,* which can cause severe pain if it ruptures into the calf. Loss of full knee extension is followed by flexion contractures and gait difficulties.

Other Joints. In the *elbow,* extension may be compromised, and olecranon bursitis is often present. *Shoulder* involvement presents as a subacromial or subdeltoid bursitis or as limitation of motion. Erosion of the rotator cuff leads to painful upward subluxation of the humeral head against the acromion. In the *cervical spine,* atlantoaxial subluxation is common, but usually asymptomatic. This development is potentially serious because it can lead to direct compression of the spinal cord or of the blood supply to the brain stem; fortunately, it is a rare event. When the *temporomandibular joint* is affected, there is pain on chewing or biting and difficulty in opening the mouth. *Avascular necrosis of the femoral head* and *vertebral osteoporosis* and collapse are usually a consequence of corticosteroid therapy.

Radiographic manifestations of early disease are soft tissue swelling around the joint and periarticular osteopenia. Relatively uniform narrowing of the joint space occurs as cartilage is destroyed, a finding often noted within the first 2 years of disease. Periarticular subchondral erodes at the joint margin where pannus has developed. Finally, joint architecture is lost as the joint space is obliterated and erosion of subchondral bone progresses.

Extraarticular manifestations are most prominent in patients with persistent symptoms and high titers of rheumatoid factor (so-called seropositive disease), though up to 50 percent of RA patients may show some form of extraarticular disease. *Pulmonary* manifestations include interstitial changes, pulmonary nodules, and pleuritis. The latter is manifested by a pleural effusion, which is characteristically low in glucose (5 to 20 mg/dL), leukocyte count (< 5000 L), and complement and high in LDH. There may or may not be accompanying pleuritic pain. Asymptomatic *pericardial effusion* also may occur. Keratoconjunctivitis sicca (*Sjögren's syndrome*) has a strong association with RA, being found in up to 15 percent of patients. *Splenomegaly* is present in 5 to 10 percent of those with RA, and lymphadenopathy is not unusual. The combination of RA, splenomegaly, and neutropenia (*Felty's syndrome*) is noted in an occasional patient. Neutropenia may be severe, but the arthritis is often quiescent. Other features include chronic leg ulceration, lymphadenopathy, and cryoglobulinemia. Risk of sepsis is high.

Vasculitis is believed responsible for a number of systemic manifestations, including fever, mononeuritis multiplex, Raynaud's phenomenon, chronic leg ulcers, mucosal erosions of the gastrointestinal (GI) tract, focal ischemia of the digits, and necrotizing mesarteritis. The *anemia* of chronic disease is seen in a large percentage of RA patients.

Clinical Stages. In stage 1, there are no symptoms or signs, just the presentation of the relevant antigen to an immunologically susceptible host. In stage 2, the immune response becomes organized in the perivascular areas of the synovium. There are increasing numbers of T cells, proliferation and differentiation of B cells, antibody production, synovial cell increase, and new blood vessel formation. Morning stiffness ensues due to increased fluid about the joints. They are warm but not erythematous because superficial vessels are uninvolved. In stage 3, the same pathophysiology as in stage 2 continues, but extraarticular manifestations become evident. In stage 4, proliferating synovial membrane becomes invasive, injuring cartilage, bone, and tendons.

DIAGNOSIS

See Chapter 146.

COURSE AND PROGNOSIS

The clinical course is generally one of exacerbations and remissions. About 40 percent go on to have disability after 10 years, but outcomes are highly variable. Some patients experience a relatively self-limited disease, and others suffer a chronic progressive illness. It is difficult at the outset to predict the course of an individual case, although genotype HLA-DRB1*04/04, a high serum titer of rheumatoid factor, extraarticular manifestations, a large number of involved joints, age less than 30, female gender, and systemic symptoms all correlate with an unfavorable prognosis. Insidious onset is also an unfavorable sign. Disease that remains persistently active for over a year is likely to lead to joint deformities and disability. Cases in which there are periods of activity lasting only weeks or a few months followed by spontaneous remission have a better prognosis. Outcome is compromised when diagnosis and treatment are delayed. Other laboratory markers of poor prognosis include early radiologic evidence of bony injury, persistent anemia of chronic disease, and elevated C1q component of complement.

Overall mortality for patients with RA is reported to be 2.5 times that of the general population. In those with severe articular and extraarticular disease, mortality approaches that of three-vessel coronary disease and stage IV Hodgkin's disease. Much of the excess mortality derives from infection, vasculitis, and poor nutrition. Mortality from cancer is unchanged.

Most data on rates of disability derive from specialty units caring for referred patients with severe disease. Little information is available on patients seen in primary care community settings. Estimates suggest that over 50 percent of these patients remain fully employed, even after having disease for 10 to 15 years, with one-third having only intermittent low-grade disease, and another third experiencing spontaneous remission.

PRINCIPLES OF MANAGEMENT

The effective management of RA requires design and implementation of a comprehensive treatment program that is consistent with the patient's personality and fits well into his or her lifestyle and home environment. The goals are to relieve stiffness and pain, preserve muscle strength and range of motion, and minimize progressive disability and deformity. There is no cure.

A number of factors require consideration in design of a management program, including the patient's age, social and occupational responsibilities, emotional makeup, the activity and duration of disease, and results of prior therapies. A balanced, multifaceted approach to therapy is most likely to provide best results, because no single drug or treatment is by itself effective. The basic components of a program must include thorough patient education, adequate rest, proper exercise, and suppression of inflammation and immune-mediated articular and vascular injury.

Nonpharmacologic Measures

Exercise helps to maintain range of motion and muscle strength. The goals are to strengthen supporting muscles and minimize the chances of postinflammatory contracture. Exercises that safely put involved joints through a full range of motion are taught to the patient. When pain is too severe for active exercises, isometrics can be performed, and passive exercises can be prescribed and carried out by a physical therapist. Joints with a tense effusion should be exempted, because compression of the synovium may lead to ischemic injury. Prior application of *heat* or *cold* (either may work) will facilitate the exercise program. Hot baths, paraffin soaks, or ice packs are efficacious in loosening stiff joints for many patients. Moist heat is also useful in relieving pain and reducing the length of morning stiffness.

Exercises that use important muscle groups are prescribed to counteract the development of atrophy, strengthen periarticular tissues, and preserve joint stability. A judicious program of walking can play a similar role. Design and execution of an exercise program can be facilitated by the participation of a physical therapist. To protect the joint from damaging stress, the patient can be instructed in the use of implements that provide a mechanical advantage. Such "joint savers" are available commercially and are most helpful for tasks requiring use of the hands.

Rest and splinting can be helpful, but in the patient with mild to moderate disease, complete bedrest is not only unnecessary but potentially harmful. Prolonged rest may lead to flexion contractures, osteoporosis, and muscle atrophy. Only the patient whose acute disease is severe enough to warrant hospitalization should be put to bed, in which case there is some benefit. However, a period of rest during the day can be of considerable benefit to less ill patients with persistently active disease, most of whom are usually bothered by fatigue. Selectively resting individual joints by splinting can help relieve pain and prevent contracture of severely inflamed joints, especially those too swollen to exercise. The principle is to maintain the joint in its physiologic position, especially during periods when the joint is stressed. Splinting of the wrist at night is the best example of this form of therapy. The patient with painful tenosynovitis of the wrist can be afforded a decrease in pain and prevention of flexion deformity with its attendant loss of grip. A wrist splint applied at night places the joint in 10 to 15 degrees of extension. A cervical collar worn at night can provide similar relief when the cervical spine is involved. Deformed feet require specially constructed shoes.

Dietary Measures and Supplements. Some fatty acids have immunomodulating effects, presumably by their roles in prostaglandin and leukotriene synthesis. *Gammalinolenic acid* is a close precursor of prostaglandin E_1 and has demonstrated antiinflammatory and immunoregulating activity. Essential fatty acids may also have an immunomodulating effect independent of prostaglandin activity. The dihydro metabolite of gammalinolenic acid manifests such an effect, acting directly on T cells in vitro to suppress proliferation of interleukin-dependent T lymphocytes. Such fatty acids are essential for maintenance of cell membrane structure and function. Well-designed, small-scale prospective trials of high-dose gammalinolenic acid in RA patients have produced promising results, but further studies are warranted before such treatment can be recommended. Based on studies of fish-oil supplements, diets high in fish and plant fatty acids and low in those from animal fat may achieve a modest degree of subjective improvement.

Pharmacologic Therapy

Antiinflammatory agents. These are the first line of therapy, having both analgesic and antiinflammatory effects and often providing sufficient control of pain and inflammation; however, they do not alter the course of RA. Agents in this category include *aspirin,* other salicylates, and *nonsteroidal anti-inflammatory drugs (NSAIDs).*

Aspirin remains the cornerstone of pharmacologic therapy for many patients and is the best proven and least expensive agent for treatment of RA. Mechanism of antiinflammatory action involves inhibition of prostaglandin synthesis. In adults under age 60, serum levels of 15 to 20 mg/dL are needed to effectively suppress the inflammation of RA. No standard dose predictably achieves this level, but usually at least 3.6 to 4.8 g/d are necessary. Because of the large dose needed and the drug's short half-life (3 to 4 hours), the patient must take a large number of tablets multiple times per day. The dose can be increased to the point of tinnitus, which is a dependable and reversible sign of salicylate toxicity in adults. The most frequent adverse effect of aspirin is gastric mucosal injury, with many patients manifesting asymptomatic gastric erosions and some showing frank ulceration (see Chapter 68). Bleeding occasionally occurs from gastritis or ulceration and need not be preceded by symptoms of abdominal pain. Aspirin irreversibly inhibits platelet cyclooxygenase and impedes platelet function (see Chapter 81), causing easy bruising and a predisposition to bleeding. A single dose poisons the platelet for its entire 7-day lifespan.

Because regular aspirin is directly injurious to the gastric mucosa, additional aspirin preparations have been marketed as less "upsetting to the stomach." *Buffered* aspirin contains bicarbonate, but the amount is insufficient to overcome ambient acid and prevent aspirin-induced mucosal injury. Slightly better tolerated are preparations combining aspirin with a more potent antacid (eg, $MgAlOH_2$—Ascriptin), but cost is markedly increased. *Enteric coating* prevents aspirin's dissolution in the stomach and minimizes the risk of direct gastric mucosal injury; however, bioavailability is delayed, resulting in slower onset of pain relief, and cost is increased.

Nonacetylated salicylates (*e.g., salsalate, choline magnesium salicylate, sodium salicylate*) were developed to reduce the risks of gastric injury and platelet inhibition associated with aspirin, while preserving its analgesic and antiinflammatory effects. Lacking an acetyl moiety, they do not inhibit platelet cyclooxygenase and can be used in patients who are allergic to aspirin. However, they are still capable of causing gastric injury, and effectiveness appears no better than and in many instances less than that of aspirin for patients with RA. Cost is much increased. *Diflunisol,* a derivative of salicylic acid, does not acetylate or break down to salicylate but does act like aspirin by virtue of its ability to inhibit prostaglandin synthesis. In RA patients, it provides the analgesic and antiinflammatory effects of 2 to 4 g/d of aspirin, with a lower rate of GI side effects. However, platelet inhibition does occur and can serious GI bleeding. The drug is 15 times the cost of aspirin.

Nonsteroidal Antiinflammatory Drugs (NSAIDs). Although aspirin and its salicylate congeners are also technically NSAIDs, the term is usually reserved for the nonsalicylate nonsteroidal antiinflammatory agents. Because of their high cost and GI side effects, NSAIDs should not be used until aspirin has been tried in a program sufficient to achieve therapeutic serum levels for at least 2 to 4 weeks. Only if aspirin therapy proves inadequate or unacceptable should it be abandoned in favor of NSAIDs.

NSAIDs derive from a host of organic acids (propionic, indolacetic, phenylacetic, enolic acid, mefenamic) and share a capacity for inhibition of cyclooxygenase, a key enzyme in prostaglandin synthesis. On a millogram-per-millogram basis, they are more potent than aspirin and longer acting, permitting a marked reduction in number of tablets and frequency of doses. The degree of pain relief and antiinflammatory effect achieved is equivalent to that of full-dose aspirin therapy. Although more convenient to use, NSAIDs cost from 8 to 25 times more than aspirin.

Efficacy is partially a function of dose. No single NSAID has consistently proven more effective than another when used at full doses, but patients not responding to one preparation after 2 to 4 weeks often report benefit on trying another from a different class (Table 156–1). This may be due to individual variation in the serum level attained by taking a given dose, although differences in efficacy are usually a function of compliance with the drug regimen. Patients using tid or qid agents often fare better when switched to preparations requiring only bid or qd dosing. There is no synergy gained from using more than one NSAID at a time; mechanisms of action are similar and all bind to the same serum proteins. Evidence that NSAIDs alter the course of RA remains elusive.

Adverse Effects. Most adverse effects are related to inhibition of prostaglandins.

Gastric Ulceration and Bleeding. The integrity of the gastric mucosa depends on gastric prostaglandin activity and can be compromised by an NSAID's systemic inhibition of prostaglandin synthesis. The consequences include dyspepsia, abdominal pain, peptic ulceration, upper GI bleeding, and gastric perforation. The risk of clinically important ulceration is estimated to be 2 to 4 percent per patient-year of NSAID use. About 15 percent of chronic NSAID users demonstrate gastric ulceration at endoscopy. Risk generally increases with dose and duration of therapy, but up to one-fourth of complications have been observed within the first month of therapy. The elderly are at greatest risk (reported relative risk about 4.0), with deaths reported. NSAIDs should be used with care and at the lowest possible doses, especially in the elderly. There may be no warning symptoms preceding severe bleeding or perforation. Despite endless promotional claims to the contrary, the risk of adverse GI effects is similar for all NSAIDs, probably because they inhibit prostaglandin synthesis to a similar degree. There is no advantage to use of a prodrug preparation (eg, nabumetone), because superficial erosions are much less common than with plain aspirin. Use of NSAIDs in patients with a history of peptic ulcer disease, GI bleeding, or abdominal

Table 156-1. Nonsteroidal Antiinflammatory Drugs (NSAIDs).

Class	Duration of Action*	Relative Cost (compared to Aspirin)†
Propionic acid derivatives		
ibuprofen (generic)	Short	4×
naproxen	Medium	15×
fenoprofen (generic)	Short	9×
ketoprofen	Short	25×
flurbiprofen	Short	22×
oxaprozin	Long	22×
nabumetone	Long	18×
Indoleacetic acid derivatives		
indomethacin (generic)	Short	3×
indomethacin (extended-release)	Long	8×
sulindac (generic)	Medium	13×
tolmetin (generic)	Short	13×
Phenylacetic acid derivatives		
diclofenac	Short	21×
Enolic acid derivatives		
piroxicam (generic)	Long	20×
Mefenamic acid derivatives		
meclofenamate (generic)	Short	12×

*Short = up to 8 hours; tid to qid dosing.
Medium = up to 18 hours; bid dosing.
Long = 24 hours or more; once daily dosing.

†Based on cost of 10 cents per day for an aspirin dose of 3.6 g. Relative cost based on wholesale costs of NSAIDs from *Medical Letter* 1993;35:16. Cost to patient likely to be 10% or more higher.

pain requires careful monitoring. Use of misoprostol, an analogue of gastric prostaglandin, may help protect against NSAID-induced GI toxicity (see Chapter 68).

Platelet Inhibition. NSAIDs cause reversible inhibition of platelet cyclooxygenase. GI bleeding in the context of concurrent NSAID use can turn into life-threatening hemorrhage. However, unlike aspirin, prolongation of the bleeding time is short-lived, because inhibition quickly ceases with cessation of drug use.

Renal Injury. The normal well-perfused kidney is not dependent on renal prostaglandin activity to the extent that an injured underperfused kidney is. Under situations of hemodynamic stress, prostaglandins serve as important regulators of renal blood flow. NSAID use may lead to fluid retention and diminished sodium excretion. Azotemia may worsen, and oliguria and renal shutdown have been reported in patients with preexisting renal disease. Control of hypertension may diminish with NSAID use. Risk of renal toxicity is greatest in the setting of inadequate renal perfusion (congestive heart failure, cirrhosis, dehydration, advanced age, use of potent diuretics). Renal injury may develop after only a few days of therapy but is reversible if NSAIDs are promptly stopped. Monitoring serum creatinine is advisable, especially in high-risk patients. Sulindac may be less nephrotoxic than other preparations, because it has little effect on renal prostaglandin synthesis. NSAIDs may impair the action of antihypertensive agents. No nephrotoxicity has been reported with prolonged, high-dose aspirin use.

Mental Impairment. The elderly are particularly susceptible. There may be alterations in cognitive function, mood, or personality (especially with agents that cross the blood–brain barrier [eg, indomethacin]). Confusion, poor memory, irritability, depression, lassitude, difficulty sleeping, and even paranoid behavior are among the reactions noted. Minor neurologic side effects (eg, headache, dizziness, light-headedness) are seen in patients of all ages.

Hepatotoxicity. Mild elevation in liver enzymes is sometimes noted, but severe hepatitis is rare. Cholestatic hepatitis has been reported. Occasional monitoring of the serum aminotransferase (transaminase) will suffice; the drug is halted if levels rise above the upper limits of normal.

Selection of NSAID. Because side effects are relatively similar among NSAIDs, one can use cost, frequency of dose, and response to an empiric trial (2 to 4 weeks at maximum dosage) as the bases for selection (see Table 156–1). Inquiry into past experience with NSAIDs can help save time. If an agent from one class has not sufficed, then selecting one from another class is a reasonable approach. Aspirin remains the cheapest form of antiinflammatory therapy but requires the greatest frequency of administration and most pills per day. Generic indomethacin is also inexpensive, but frequency and severity of GI and central nervous system (CNS) side effects limit its utility, especially in the elderly. Generic ibuprofen is the most economical of the modern NSAIDs but requires tid or qid dosing. Naproxen is the least expensive of the twice-daily NSAID formulations, but it is still costly. Piroxicam offers once daily dosing but at 20 times the cost of an aspirin program.

Disease-Modifying Agents. Patients with active RA persisting for 3 to 6 months are candidates for disease-modifying therapy. Such therapy has the capacity to slow joint destruction and induce partial remissions, although drug-related toxicity can be substantial. Out of concern for such toxicity, the traditional approach has been to withhold disease-modifying therapy until symptoms become disabling or joint injury becomes evident. Data from careful radiographic studies showing disproportionate joint destruction early in the course of active disease suggest that the traditional approach might represent too slow a response. The view is supported by long-term observational studies, which find poor outcomes in patients with active disease treated in traditional fashion. Such findings have stimulated earlier application of disease-modifying therapy.

Most disease-modifying drugs are slow-acting, with clinical response taking 3 to 6 months to appear. Response rates are about 50 percent. Of the disease-modifying agents, *methotrexate* acts the most rapidly (within 6 weeks), and adverse effects are minimal when the drug is used at low dose for a limited period. These qualities have made it a popular choice among some rheumatologists for initiation of a disease-modifying program. Once control is established, they might switch to *hydroxychloroquine, sulfasalazine,* or *auranofin,* which are better tolerated for chronic use. A host of other approaches have been described, and the optimal strategy continues to be the subject of intense debate. Combination therapy is being explored. NSAIDs are commonly continued in patients taking disease-modifying drugs that have no intrinsic antiinflammatory action.

In addition to methotrexate, other cytotoxic agents with immunosuppressive activity (*e.g., azathioprine, cyclophosphamide*) have been used as solo therapy by rheumatologists for treatment of patients with aggressive refractory disease. The chelating agent *D-penicillamine* has been similarly used. The cost of disease-modifying therapy can be high, and careful monitoring for adverse effects is essential to its safe use. Some patients have to terminate treatment due to adverse drug effects. Serious toxicities include marrow suppression, nephropathy, liver damage, increased susceptibility to infection, and pulmonary fibrosis. With increasingly early and more aggressive use of disease-modifying drugs comes the need for greater expertise in their application. The principal tasks of the primary physician are to ensure proper timing of referral to the rheumatologist and monitoring for response and adverse effects.

Methotrexate. Low-dose therapy (7.5 mg/wk) is given orally once weekly or in three doses, 12 hours apart. Aspirin and NSAIDs should not be used concurrently because they slow the rate of methotrexate excretion and increase toxicity. Renal dysfunction is a contraindication to use. Short-term, low-dose therapy is well tolerated, but bone marrow suppression, hepatocellular injury, and idiosyncratic interstitial pneumonitis can occur. The latter may lead to pulmonary fibrosis and is important to recognize early. Mild, nonprogressive elevations in hepatocellular enzymes are common and not a contraindication to continued therapy, although careful monitoring is required. Longer-term therapy is often used and well tolerated, but once the cumulative methotrexate dose exceeds 1.5 g, the risk of hepatic fibrosis may begin to increase. The need for liver biopsy at this point remains unresolved.

Gold Salts. Treatment is by weekly intramuscular injection of either thiomalate (Myochrysine) or aurothioglucose (Solganal). Mechanisms of action include inhibition of mononuclear cell activity, lysozymes, and complement. Gold may temporarily halt or even partially reverse articular erosion in up to 60 percent of cases, but fewer than 2 percent of patients treated have remissions that last longer than 3 years. The effects of gold are cumulative. Decrease in inflammatory symptoms is noted in two-thirds of patients by the time the cumulative dose reaches 400 to 600 mg. Those who are going to respond do so by the time 1000 mg have been given. Adverse effects are often idiosyncratic and range from *rashes* and buccal cavity *mucosal ulcers* to *bone marrow suppression, glomerulonephritis, interstitial pneumonitis,* and *exfoliative dermatitis.* Minor toxic reactions are common. Treatment is begun slowly. Each dose is preceded by urinalysis and complete blood and platelet counts. Myochrysine may trigger an immediate postinjection vasomotor reaction of warmth, erythema, and lightheadedness. If a skin rash occurs, gold therapy is halted for a few weeks, then resumed at reduced doses. The first evidence of marrow suppression (thrombocytopenia, leukopenia) or nephropathy (hematuria, proteinuria) requires immediate cessation of therapy. Most adverse effects are reversible in the early stages.

Once the cumulative dose reaches 1 g, gold administration is cut back to every other week until 1.5 g is reached, at which point injections are given once a month. There are no clear indications as to when to stop therapy or how long to continue it.

Auranofin. is an oral gold formulation usually taken twice daily. It causes less mucocutaneous, renal, and bone-marrow toxicity than parenteral gold, but more diarrhea (which is dose-related) and sometimes colitis. Often, the GI side effects cease with continued therapy, although a lowering of the dose may be necessary. Efficacy is less than that of injectable gold but still significant in placebo-controlled studies. Auranofin's relative safety makes the drug a consideration for sustaining remissions achieved by other agents. Monitoring is similar to that for parenteral therapy, although frequency can be monthly rather than weekly. A low-dose regimen for 6 months is typical; if response is inadequate, a 3-month trial at higher dose may be considered before terminating therapy.

Hydroxychloroquine. Antimalarial therapy is not as potent as gold or methotrexate but is better tolerated and sometimes started as early as a month after onset of NSAID therapy if disease activity persists. At least 4 to 6 weeks are needed before results are detectable. The most serious toxic effect is visual impairment (even blindness) due to drug accumulation in the retina. This complication is rare but limits dosage to 200 to 400 mg/d and makes ophthalmologic examination every 6 months mandatory. Tinnitus and vertigo are sometimes noted.

Sulfasalazine is not officially approved for use in RA, but this long-standing treatment for inflammatory bowel disease has been found similar in efficacy to injectable gold and penicillamine and much less toxic. It may be superior to hydroxychloroquine. Hypersensitivity to its sulfa moiety is common, limiting use in sulfa-allergic patients. Hepatocellular injury and hematologic abnormalities sometimes occur; GI upset (anorexia, nausea, vomiting, diarrhea) is more common. Reversible oligospermia has been noted.

D-Penicillamine is a chelating agent that can slow aggressive disease. Adverse effects are similar to those of parenteral gold and best mitigated by use of low doses and slow increases in doses. Less than 50 percent of patients given the drug are able to continue with it for prolonged treatment. Fatal aplastic anemia, leukopenia, agranulocytosis, and thrombocytopenia can occur. Proteinuria is seen in 10 to 15 percent and may progress to the nephrotic syndrome. Rashes and autoimmune syndromes such as myasthenia gravis are reported. The drug is contraindicated in pregnancy. It should be reserved for those who fail to respond to all other forms of therapy and should be prescribed only under supervision of a rheumatologist skilled in its use.

Cyclophosphamide and Azathioprine. These cytotoxic immunosuppressive agents have been reserved for patients with otherwise refractory disease. Cyclophosphamide is used for treatment of systemic vasculitis. Both agents are contraindicated in pregnancy; they are teratogenic. Risk of malignancy is increased, especially with use of cyclophosphamide. Other adverse effects from cyclophosphamide include hemorrhagic cystitis, marrow suppression, and sterility. Azathioprine use is associated with GI upset, hepatitis, and marrow depression, but risk is low due to the small doses used in RA.

Corticosteroids. Although capable of rapidly suppressing sinovitis, systemic steroids are reluctantly used for treatment of RA. Well-intentioned short courses of steroid therapy invariably turn into chronic ones, associated with osteoporosis, muscle atrophy, ligamentous weakening, and aseptic necrosis of the femoral head. In extremely difficult situations, such as a flare-up of joint disease that threatens to totally disable the head of a household, very-low-dose therapy (5.0 to 7.5 mg per day of prednisone) may be started to tide the patient over until disease-modifying therapy takes hold. The only clear-cut indication for systemic steroids is life-threatening extraarticular disease, such as vasculitis, pericarditis, or alveolitis. Intraarticular injection of a long-acting steroid preparation may improve functional status when there is a single large weight-bearing joint that is disproportionately inflamed. However, repeated steroid injections into the same joint may hasten its degeneration and increase the risk of infection.

Analgesics. Those without antiinflammatory effect have little role in RA. Occasionally a narcotic analgesic is resorted to for short-term pain control. Their regular use is to be avoided because of the risk of addiction in this chronic disease.

Additional Measures

Total lymphoid irradiation and apheresis represent further attempts to inhibit the immunopathology of RA. Controlled studies of irradiation suggest some benefit in extreme situations, but risk of infection is markedly increased. The rationale behind apheresis is to remove immune complexes and other mediators of the inflammatory process. Placebo-controlled studies have failed to show significant benefit. Selective removal of lymphocytes from peripheral blood (leukopheresis) has yielded transient mild clinical improvement in refractory cases, but not of sufficient magnitude to justify the high cost.

Surgery. Arthroplasty is an important component of therapy in patients with destroyed joints and marked disability. Hip and knee procedures are most successful; hand, wrist, elbow, and ankle reconstructions are less certain in outcome, but rapid progress is being made. There is a significant risk (25%) of a loosening of the hip prosthesis, even in the absence of active disease. Conventional synovectomy is generally ineffective and results in loss of joint motion; however, arthroscopic synovectomy may permit control of particularly severe monoarticular disease involving the knee.

Unproven Modalities. A popular diet free of additives, preservatives, fruit, red meat, herbs and dairy products has been advocated as a treatment for RA. The only controlled, double-blind randomized study of this therapy failed to show any benefit in patients with long-standing, progressive active RA. Biofeedback is also without proven benefit, although it is helpful in some patients with Raynaud's phenomenon.

Monitoring

Disease activity and response to therapy are best monitored by reproducible measures such as duration of morning stiffness, sedimentation rate, number of tender swollen joints, and grip strength (which can be measured with a blood pressure cuff). Time to walk 15 m and ring size are also helpful. The titer of rheumatoid factor does not correlate with disease activity but does decrease with gold and penicillamine therapy if the patient responds. Outcomes research has emphasized the utility of additional measures of function, such as psychosocial functioning and the activities of daily living contained in the Health Assessment Questionnaire and the Arthritis Impact Measurement Scale. The patient's self-assessment and the physician's global assessment also demonstrate validity.

Detecting early disease progression is harder, yet very important if disease-modifying therapy is to be instituted in timely fashion. Joint-space narrowing is a specific, but late radiographic sign of cartilaginous erosion, which may not develop until irreversible damage has already occurred. Magnetic resonance imaging has been used experimentally to detect synovial proliferation and early pannus formation, but cost remains prohibitive for routine use. At present, one estimates the likelihood of disease progression by the duration of symptoms.

PATIENT EDUCATION AND COUNSELING

Telling the Diagnosis. For the patient with a potentially disabling disease such as RA, the act of telling the diagnosis takes on major importance. The goal is to satisfy the patient's informational needs regarding diagnosis, prognosis, and treatment without overwhelming him or her with an excessive amount of detail. This requires careful questioning and empathic listening to understand the patient's perspective, requests, and fears. Telling the patient more than he or she is intellectually or psychologically prepared to deal with (a common practice) risks making the experience so intense as to trigger withdrawal. On the other hand, failing to address issues of importance to the patient compromises the development of trust. The patient needs to know that the primary physician understands the situation and will be available for support, advice, and therapy as the situation arises. Encouraging the patient to ask questions helps to communicate interest and caring.

Discussing Prognosis and Treatment. Patients and family do best when they know what to expect and can view the illness realistically. Uncertainty contributes heavily to the "dis-ease" of RA. Many fear crippling consequences and dependency. The most common disease manifestations should be described. Without building false hopes, the physician can point out that spontaneous remissions are frequent and that over two-thirds of patients live independently without major disability. In addition, it should be emphasized that much can be done to minimize discomfort and preserve function. A review of available therapies and their efficacy helps to overcome feelings of depression stemming from an erroneous expectation of inevitable disability. Guarded optimism is appropriate at the outset in all but the most actively aggressive situations. Even the patient with a poor prognosis can derive comfort from knowing that he or she will be followed closely by the primary physician and any necessary consultants, all of whom are committed to maximizing the patient's comfort and independence. A major fear is that of abandonment.

Dealing with Misconceptions. Several common misconceptions deserve attention. A substantial proportion of patients and their families feel guilty that they have done something to cause the illness. Explaining that there are no known controllable precipitants helps to eliminate much unnecessary guilt and self-recrimination. Another frequent misconception is the view that aspirin is too weak to work in a disease as severe as RA. When prescribed, patients may scoff at its use. Sometimes, physicians select a far more expensive, although no less effective NSAID instead of aspirin because they feel it is better for patient morale. Reviewing the difference between taking sporadic low doses of aspirin and amounts sufficient to give therapeutic serum levels often suffices to convince doubters and frees the physician to prescribe the most cost-effective therapy. The active participation of the patient and family in the design and implementation of the therapeutic program helps to boost morale and ensure compliance, as does explaining the rationale for the therapies used.

Preserving a Sense of Self-Worth. A major goal is to preserve the patient's sense of worth and independence. However, when fatigue, morning stiffness, or specific joint pathology interferes with the patient's capacity to perform usual work or home responsibilities, counseling will be necessary to recommend modification of work responsibilities and perhaps retraining. By using occupational therapy, the treatment effort is geared to helping the patient maintain a meaningful work role within the limitations of the illness. The family plays an important part in striking the proper balance between dependence and independence. Household members should avoid overprotecting the patient (eg, refraining from intercourse out of fear of hurting the patient) and work to sustain the patient's pride and ability to contribute to the family. Allowing the RA patient to struggle with a task is sometimes constructive.

Supporting the Patient with Debilitating Disease. Emphasis is on comfort measures and supportive psychotherapy. Such individuals need help grieving for their disfigurement and loss of function. An accepting, unhurried, empathic manner allows the patient to express feelings. The seemingly insignificant act of touching does much to restore a sense of self-acceptance. Attending to pain with increased social support, medication, and a refocusing of attention onto function are useful. A trusting and strong patient–doctor relationship can do much to sustain a patient through times of discomfort and disability.

INDICATIONS FOR REFERRAL AND ADMISSION

Patients with evidence of persistent joint inflammation lasting more than 2 to 3 months despite antiinflammatory therapy should be referred to a rheumatologist for consideration of disease-modifying therapy, especially if they have findings suggestive of poor prognosis (genotype HLA-DRB1*04/04, high serum titer of rheumatoid factor, extraarticular manifestations, a large number of involved joints, age less than 30, female gender, systemic symptoms). The rapid evolution of disease-modifying regimens necessitates rheumatologic consultation rather than implementation by the primary physician of a more traditional approach to disease-modifying therapy (ie, single-agent therapy, onset of treatment only after symptoms become disabling or joint damage becomes evident). To be maximally effective, disease-modifying therapy should be initiated before irreversible joint injury has set in. Proper timing is best determined through consultation with the rheumatologist.

Referral to physical and occupational therapists is greatly appreciated by patients with active disease. Well-designed exercise and rehabilitation programs can greatly facilitate carrying out the activities of daily living.

The need for surgical referral is best determined by the rheumatologist, who is well trained to judge when medical therapy is insufficient. Examples of indications for surgery include carpal tunnel syndrome that persists despite corticosteroid injection, trigger finger deformity, tendon rupture with loss of manual dexterity, and refractory dorsal wrist effusions. Disabling hip or knee destruction with severe impairment of weight-bearing capacity deserves a surgical assessment regarding possible prosthetic joint replacement. Arthroscopic synovectomy may be needed for a single, very refractory joint that cannot be replaced.

When fever, floridly inflamed joints, severe pain, or marked extraarticular disease is present, hospital admission is an obvious requirement.

THERAPEUTIC RECOMMENDATIONS

- Prescribe a gentle exercise program to maintain range of motion and muscle strength, but avoid stressing a severely inflamed joint. Prior application of heat or cold (either may work) will facilitate the exercise program. Consult with a physical therapist to help design the program. Morning application of heat is particularly helpful before the patient engages in daily activity.
- Selectively rest severely inflamed individual joints that are too swollen to exercise. Maintain the joint in its physiologic position by splinting during periods when the joint is stressed (eg, at night) to support weakened joints and prevent flexion contractures. Consult the rheumatologist if splinting appears indicated.
- Advise a daily rest period for patients bothered by generalized fatigue, but avoid prolonged bedrest in outpatients.
- Prescribe aspirin as the drug of first choice. Initiate therapy in doses of 3.6 to 4.8 g per day using an enteric-coated preparation. Titrate therapeutic response against the development of toxicity. Periodically check blood levels and adjust dose to maintain a therapeutic level of 15 to 20 mg per deciliter in patients less than age 60.
- For the patient on aspirin therapy still bothered by morning stiffness, prescribe a qhs dose of an intermediate-acting NSAID (eg, naproxen 375 to 500 mg).
- Switch to NSAID therapy only if a lack of response, poor compliance, or intolerance to aspirin develops. Choose an NSAID based on cost, duration of action, and individual response (see Table 156–1). When cost is the primary concern, ibuprofen is a reasonable starting selection. Naproxen is the least expensive of the NSAIDs that allow bid administration.
- Switch to another NSAID category for a second choice if 2 weeks at full doses of the initial NSAID fails to provide symptomatic relief. Trial and error is necessary because individual responses to NSAID preparations differ.
- Use NSAIDs cautiously in the elderly and at reduced dose. Use with care in patients with impaired renal perfusion, monitoring BUN and creatinine. Also use cautiously in patients with a prior history of peptic ulcer disease or GI bleeding (see Chapter 68); monitor stool guaiacs and hematocrit.
- Refer the patient with persistently active disease of 2 to 3 months' duration to the rheumatologist for consideration of disease-modifying therapy (eg, methotrexate, gold, hydroxychloroquine, sulfasalazine). Increasingly, early rheumatologic consultation and aggressive treatment are deemed necessary if joint destruction is to be prevented, particularly in patients with findings suggestive of poor prognosis (eg, genotype HLA-DRB1*04/04, high serum titer of rheumatoid factor, extraarticular manifestations, large number of involved joints, age < 30, female gender, systemic symptoms).
- Monitor disease activity and response to therapy by checking reproducible measures such as duration of morning stiffness, sedimentation rate, number of tender swollen joints, and grip strength (squeezing a blood pressure cuff). Also monitor activities of daily living and psychosocial status.
- For patients prescribed parenteral gold therapy, monitor complete blood count (CBC), urinalysis, liver function tests, and platelet counts weekly for the first 1 to 2 months, then biweekly for 3 months; thereafter, monthly checks suffice.

- For patients prescribed oral gold therapy, monitor the same parameters as for parenteral therapy, but at monthly intervals.
- For patients prescribed hydroxychloroquine, inquire regularly about visual acuity and arrange ophthalmologic examination every 6 months.
- For patients prescribed methotrexate, follow CBC, platelet count, aminotransferase, alkaline phosphatase, BUN, and creatinine. Inquire regularly into any pulmonary symptoms, which might be the first manifestation of interstitial pneumonitis and an indication for immediate cessation of therapy.
- For patients prescribed sulfasalazine, monitor CBC, GI symptoms, and skin changes.
- For patients with a disproportionately inflamed large weight-bearing joint that is incapacitating, consider a single intraarticular injection of a long-acting corticosteroid (eg, triamcinolone acetonide 2.5 to 10 mg (depending on joint size mixed with 1 mL of xylocaine). The knee is cleansed with iodine and alcohol, and the injection is made intraarticularly under sterile conditions. Repeated injections into the same joint are to be avoided.
- Reserve systemic steroids for only the most desperate of situations and use only a short-term low-dose program (eg, prednisone 5.0 to 7.5 mg qd).
- Provide a comprehensive patient and family education program that includes psychological support and strategies for maintaining the patient's activity, independence, and self-esteem.

A.H.G.

ANNOTATED BIBLIOGRAPHY

Anderson JJ, Felson DT, Meenan RF, et al. Which traditional measures should be used in rheumatoid arthritis clinical trials? Arthritis Rheum 1989;32:1093. *(A critical look at measures of disease activity and function.)*

Arnett FC, Edworthy SM, Bloch DA, et al. The American Rheumatism Association 1987 revised criteria for the classification of rheumatoid arthritis. Arthritis Rheum 1988;31:315. *(Widely adopted diagnostic and classification criteria based on a collaborative study of over 500 patients.)*

Bardwick PA, Swezey RL. Physical therapies in arthritis. Postgrad Med 1982;72:223. *(A discussion of the standard modalities of physical therapy and when to use them.)*

Bradley LA. Psychosocial factors and disease outcomes in rheumatoid arthritis. Arthritis Rheum 1989;32:1611. *(An editorial critically reviewing outcome measures.)*

Clive DM, Stoff JS. Renal syndromes associated with nonsteroidal antiinflammatory drugs. N Engl J Med 1984;310:563. *(Risk greatest in those with impaired renal perfusion.)*

Coles LS, Fries JF, Kranines RG, et al. From experiment to experience: Side effects of nonsteroidal anti-inflammatory drugs. Am J Med 1983;74:820. *(Incidence of side effects much greater in community use settings.)*

Epstein AM, Read JL, Winickoff R. Physician beliefs, attitudes and prescribing behavior for anti-inflammatory drugs. Am J Med 1984;77:313. *(Explains the very high frequency of NSAID use compared to aspirin.)*

Fuchs HA, Kaye JJ, Callahan LF, et al. Evidence of significant radiologic damage in rheumatoid arthritis within the first two years of disease. J Rheumatol 1989;16:585. *(Disproportionate degree of joint damage found early in the course of disease.)*

Gabriel SE, Luthra HS. Rheumatoid arthritis: Can the long-term outcome be altered. Mayo Clin Proc 1988;63:58. *(A review of available studies; finds that design flaws prevent definitive conclusion, but data are suggestive of benefit.)*

Griffin MR, Ray WA, Schaffner W. Nonsteroidal antiinflammatory drug use and death from peptic ulcer in elderly persons. Ann Intern Med 1988;109:359. *(Strong correlation found, supporting cautious use in the elderly.)*

Harris ED Jr. Rheumatoid arthritis: Pathophysiology and implications for therapy. N Engl J Med 1990;322:1990. *(Excellent review that correlates disease mechanisms with clinical presentations and approaches to treatment; 160 references.)*

Jeurissen MEC, Boerbooms AMT, van de Putte LBA, et al. Influence of methotrexate and azathioprine on radiologic progression in rheumatoid arthritis: A randomized, double-blind study. Ann Intern Med 1991;114:999. *(Methotrexate halted disease progression and performed better than azathioprine.)*

Kremer JM, Jubiz W, Rynes RI, et al. Fish-oil fatty acid supplementation in active rheumatoid arthritis: A double-blinded, controlled, cross-over study. Ann Intern Med 1987;106:497. *(Subjective benefit was found as was a modest reduction in leukotriene.)*

Leventhal LJ, Boyce EG, Zurier RB. Treatment of rheumatoid arthritis with gammalinolenic acid. Ann Intern Med 1993; 119:867. *(Small-scale study, but encouraging results found with use of this dietary supplement.)*

Lorig KR, Lubeck D, Kraines RG, et al. Outcomes of self-help education for patients with arthritis. Arthritis Rheum 1985; 28:680. *(Very effective, enhancing independence.)*

Masi AT. Articular patterns in the early course of rheumatoid arthritis. Am J Med 1983;75:16. *(Patients with multijoint involvement at onset have a poorer prognosis than those with more limited disease.)*

Mills JA, Pinals RA, Ropes MW, et al. Value of bed rest in patients with rheumatoid arthritis. N Engl J Med 1971;284:453. *(Classic study; minimal benefit was obtained from enforced rest.)*

Pinals RS, Kaplan SB, Lawson JG, et al. Sulfasalazine in rheumatoid arthritis: A double-blind, placebo-controlled trial. Arthritis Rheum 1986;29:1427. *(Establishes its utility.)*

Pincus T. Rheumatoid arthritis: Disappointing long-term outcomes despite successful short-term clinical trials. J Clin Epidemiol 1988;41:1037. *(Suggests that disease-modifying therapy is being used too late to beneficially affect outcome.)*

Pincus T, Wolfe F. Treatment of rheumatoid arthritis: Challenges to traditional paradigms. Ann Intern Med 1991;115:825. *(A critical examination of basic tenets in RA therapy.)*

Rogers MP, Liang MH, Partridge AJ. Psychological care of adults with rheumatoid arthritis. Ann Intern Med 1982;96:344. *(An often overlooked area; many practical suggestions for effective personal care of both patient and family.)*

Simon LS, Mills JA. Nonsteroidal anti-inflammatory drugs. N Engl J Med 1980;302:1179,1237. *(Still useful basic review of the pharmacology and role of nonsteroidal agents in comparison to aspirin.)*

van der Heijde DM, van Riel PL, van Rijswijk MH, et al. Influence of prognostic features on the final outcome in rheumatoid arthritis: A review of the literature. Semin Arthritis Rheum 1988;17:284. *(Excellent summary of clinical and laboratory findings that predict outcome.)*

Ward JR, Williams J, Egger MJ, et al. Comparison of auranofin, gold sodium thiomalate, and placebo in the treatment of rheumatoid arthritis. Arthritis Rheum 1982;26:1303. *(Parenteral gold was the most effective, but also more likely to cause renal and mucocutaneous toxicity.)*

Weyand CM, Hicok KC, Conn DL, et al. The influence of HLA-DRB1 genes on disease severity in rheumatoid arthritis. Ann Intern Med 1992;117:801. *(HLA-DRB1 genotyping helps in early identification of patients with a poor prognosis.)*

Wilske KR, Healey LA. Remodeling the pyramid: A concept whose time had come. J Rheumatol 1989;16:565. *(Describes a more aggressive approach to use of disease-modifying therapy.)*

157
Management of Osteoarthritis

Primary Care Medicine: Office Evaluation and Management of the Adult Patient, 3rd edition, edited by Allan H. Goroll, Lawrence A. May, and Albert G. Mulley, Jr. J.B. Lippincott Company, Philadelphia

Osteoarthritis (OA), the most prevalent arthropathy, causes symptomatic discomfort in 10 percent to 20 percent of persons over age 65, and accounts for upwards of 30 percent of visits to primary care practitioners. OA remains the most common cause of disability in the elderly. Most patients have primary or idiopathic disease that is strongly associated with aging. Others present with posttraumatic and hereditary forms of the disease (eg, chondrodystrophy, hemochromatosis, inflammatory OA, chondrocalcinosis). Although many changes are irreversible, much can be done to relieve discomfort, prevent further articular damage, and keep the patient functioning independently.

PATHOPHYSIOLOGY AND CLINICAL PRESENTATION

Pathogenesis

OA is characterized by 1) degeneration of articular cartilage; and 2) reactive formation of new bone. What causes the demise of the articular cartilage remains incompletely understood. The simplistic "wear-and-tear" hypothesis has been superseded by an appreciation for the role of chondrocytes in actively remodeling cartilage. Articular damage appears to involve an interplay between cartilage metabolism and mechanical stress. Unlike rheumatoid disease, synovial inflammation appears to play only a minor role in most cases.

Histobiochemically, there is reduction in proteoglycan, a critical mucopolysaccharide component of cartilage. Monomer size and aggregation decline, leading to a decrease in resiliency. Fibrils become more readily damaged by trauma, allowing penetration of synovial collagenases. Bone elasticity, which cushions normal trauma, also appears to decline with age, allowing increased stress to be transmitted directly to the cartilage. Conditions that alter the mechanical relationships of joints further increase the likelihood that degenerative changes will develop. Eventually, the cartilage frays, shreds, and cracks. Early cartilaginous injury can be repaired by chondrocytes, but fissured hyaline cartilage is incapable of restoration.

Underlying bone responds by remodeling, which causes trabeculae to thicken. At the joint margins, hypertrophic spurs (osteophytes) develop, followed by buttressing of adjacent cortical bone (osteosclerosis). The joint space narrows in an irregular fashion. Cyst formation is also seen. There is little synovial reaction unless the degenerative process is rapid, a piece of cartilage dislodges, or calcium pyrophosphate crystals form and incite an acute inflammatory response (pseudogout).

Clinical Presentation

Radiologic evidence of OA can be found in over 80 percent of adults by age 65. The subset who are symptomatic complain of deep, aching joint pain that is aggravated by motion and weight bearing. In addition, there may be stiffness worsened by periods of inactivity. The involved joint can be enlarged due to osteophyte formation, but swelling is usually inconsequential, because soft tissue involvement and effusions are, in most instances, minimal. In later stages, pain occurs on motion and at rest in conjunction with stiffness. Nocturnal pain after vigorous activity is common. Patients with advanced disease suffer from pain on weight bearing and joint instability. Examination often reveals crepitus and discomfort on movement of the joint. Occasionally, slight warmth is noted in severely affected weight-bearing joints, but erythema and marked warmth are absent. Limitation of motion, malalignment, and bony protuberances from spurs are frequent findings.

The joints most commonly affected include the knees, hips, distal interphalangeal (DIP) joints of the hands, the carpometacarpal joint at the base of the thumb, and the cervical and lumbosacral spine.

Knees. Symptomatic knee involvement is estimated to affect as much as 10 percent of the population over age 65. OA of the knee produces pain that is localized to the joint and worsened by weight bearing. Crepitus is often marked, and range of motion is reduced. A very small effusion may be noted. The joint appears enlarged and feels bony. On occasion there may ybe very few physical findings, although pain and x-ray changes are prominent.

Hips. Degenerative hip disease arises in young patients with congenital dislocations or slipped femoral capital epiphyses, and much later from wear and tear in the elderly. Unilateral or asymmetric distribution is typical. Pain is reported deep in the hip, radiating into the anterior medial thigh, groin, or buttock. The site of radiation may be the only area of discomfort. At first, pain occurs only on weight bearing, but as OA progresses, discomfort may become continuous and especially unbearable at night. Sexual intercourse is sometimes compromised. Loss of internal rotation during flexion is the earliest change and is as reliable as x-ray for diagnosis. The Trendelenburg's test (see Chapter 151) is positive.

DIP Joints. Disease in these joints is most common in middle-aged and elderly women, and sometimes proves to be painful and tender. There appears to be a strong hereditary component in women. In some patients, a low-grade inflammatory response may accompany early rapid mucinous degenerative changes, giving the joint a tender, cystic inflammatory appearance. Later, osteophytes form, giving rise to the characteristic bony protuberances known as *Heberden's nodes*. All inflammatory activity resolves, leaving the joint nontender and with some limitation of motion. Occasionally, a similar process may affect the proximal interphalangeal joints, resulting in *Bouchard's nodes,* which may be mistaken for changes due to rheumatoid arthritis.

Thumbs. The base of the thumb, a site of much physical stress, is vulnerable to degenerative change. There is pain in the region of the thenar eminence and particularly over the carpometacarpal joint. Because the thumb is so important to manual dexterity, the development of arthritis at this site may be disabling. Grip becomes impaired, and fine movements of apposition are restricted. Osteophytes are palpable and, in rare instances, may encroach on the flexor tendon sheath, causing tenosynovitis.

Cervical Spine. Degenerative changes commonly involve the lower cervical spine (see Chapter 148). Although x-ray changes are frequent, most individuals are asymptomatic. Moreover, the correlation between symptoms and x-ray findings is often poor. The patient may complain of pain and stiffness in the neck, but sometimes only pain in the occiput, shoulder, arm, or hand is reported. In a few instances, scapular or upper anterior chest pain is produced. Osteophytes can protrude into the spinal foramina and impinge on nerve roots, causing pain that radiates into the shoulder, upper arms, hands, and fingers (brachial neuralgia). At night, the patient may awaken with paresthesias and numbness in the arms that improve on getting up and shaking them.

On examination, neck motion is restricted to some extent in all directions, and movement reproduces or aggravates symptoms. Reactive muscle spasm and tenderness are often present, and decreased sensation, weakness, and diminished reflexes occur when root compression is marked. However, even when symptoms of root compression are reported, neurologic findings may be scant and their absence does not rule out the complication.

Lumbosacral Spine. Degenerative changes in the lumbosacral spine involve the intervertebral disks and the apophyseal joints. With aging, the disk nucleus becomes brittle and less elastic. Herniation posteriorly or laterally through a defect in the disk annulus may occur and cause nerve root compression (see Chapter 147). Intervertebral spaces narrow and marginal osteophytes form. The apophyseal joints show typical secondary degenerative changes. The patient reports pain across the lower back with radiation into the buttock and posterior thigh, or down into the lower leg if root compression has occurred. Forward flexion and extension are reduced, but lateral flexion is painless. Focal areas of tenderness are common and often due to spasm of the paraspinous musculature.

Other Sites. OA may involve the great toe at the metatarsophalangeal joint, causing bony enlargement and a valgus deformity. Crepitus and pain in the temporomandibular joint are sometimes seen secondary to bruxism (grinding of the teeth because of anxiety or anger). Pain is reproduced by opening the mouth widely. Because OA is not a systemic disease, there are no extraarticular manifestations nor any serum abnormalities; the sedimentation rate is normal, as is the synovial fluid in early disease. Radiographic findings are limited to the joints and include irregular narrowing of the joint space, sclerosis of subchondral bone, bony cysts, marginal osteophytes, and buttressing of adjacent bone.

NATURAL HISTORY OF DISEASE

In large weight-bearing joints, OA tends to be a progressive condition with chronic joint pain, restricted joint motion, and resultant muscle weakness compromising mobility. Over a period of 10 to 20 years, the majority of patients with untreated symptomatic OA of the knee develop pain at rest and inability to use public transportation; disability may ensue. Early onset of symptoms and varus deformity correlate with poor prognosis. OA of the hip may follow a similar course. Obesity is a strong risk factor for progressive disease of the hips and knees (especially in women). Weight reduction reduces the risk. Progression of OA is typically limited to a few affected joints and does not become widespread. Clinical remissions do occur, especially in the hands, neck, and back.

PRINCIPLES OF MANAGEMENT

There is no cure for OA, but it helps to reduce abnormal stresses imposed on affected joints, restore joint alignment, strengthen muscles, and treat pain and muscle spasm. Pain relief is a first priority for most patients. Both pharmacologic and mechanical means are used. The progression of disease cannot be halted by available drugs, but they can offer symptomatic relief. Surgical intervention should be restricted to patients who do not respond to conservative management and are so disabled that they cannot function satisfactorily.

Analgesics. In the absence of a major inflammatory component to the disease and until etiologically acting drugs become available, analgesics remain the predominant pharmacologic approach to pain control. Pure analgesics, such as *acetaminophen,* and analgesic doses of *aspirin* are as effective as a host of more expensive alternatives. Because OA is a chronic disease, any drug selected should be both inexpensive and safe for long-term consumption. Acetaminophen and aspirin both meet these criteria. They are the least expensive of available analgesics and generally well tolerated. Acetaminophen is associated with a small risk of renal injury when used for years at very high doses. The risk of gastrointestinal (GI) bleeding and ulceration associated with aspirin is substantial, but can be reduced through use of an enteric-coated preparation (see Chapter 68). Furthermore, the doses of aspirin needed in OA are much smaller than those required in inflammatory joint disease.

Although widely prescribed, *nonsteroidal antiinflammatory drugs (NSAIDs)* provide no more relief than pure analgesics such as acetaminophen. Low, analgesic doses of NSAIDs are no better than high, antiinflammatory doses. There is theoretical concern that NSAIDs might even be injurious, because they depress proteoglycan synthesis, which is needed for cartilage repair. NSAIDs are very expensive (up to 30 times the cost of aspirin), and their risk of GI toxicity is high, especially in the elderly (see Chapter 68). The elderly are also subject to confusion and renal impairment with NSAID use (see Chapter 156). Nonetheless, an individual's response to drugs is unpredictable, and it may be necessary to try NSAID therapy if aspirin and acetaminophen prove inadequate. Intermittent use of analgesics will sometimes suffice, but continuous therapy is often needed.

Narcotic analgesics (eg, codeine, oxycodone) should be used sparingly, if at all, and only for acute disabling pain interfering with essential activity. *Propoxyphene* (Darvon), an opiate derivative, is taken by many patients with OA, but its potential for dependence is considerable—similar to that of codeine—and its analgesic properties are no greater than low doses of aspirin.

The use of *intraarticular steroids* is controversial. Although widely used, there are no controlled studies documenting their efficacy. The experimental finding of steroid suppression of cartilage catabolism has renewed interest in this form of therapy. However, repeated steroid injections may accelerate joint degeneration and weaken its supporting structures. The only time steroid injection should be considered is when there is a single disabling joint, refractory to other forms of therapy, and sufficiently inflamed to justify a trial of intraarticular steroids.

Acupuncture has produced inconsistent results in double-blind studies, sometimes working, sometimes not. Results have not been sufficiently beneficial to warrant its inclusion in a treatment program.

Antispasmodics are without effect, except for their tranquilizing action.

Exercise. Restoration of favorable mechanics is essential to minimizing damage to injured joints. Strengthening the supporting muscles may help maintain proper joint alignment. For patients with knee disease, quadriceps exercises are among the simplest, performed while sitting in a chair, extending the knee and holding the straightened leg horizontal. A program of supervised graduated isometric and isotonic quadriceps exercises can enhance distance walked and can decrease pain. Isometric and active exercises for the neck improve muscle tone and may sometimes help in cases of painful cervical spine disease (see Chapter 148). Exercises for the abdominal and paraspinous musculature are useful for preventing back problems. There is no evidence that spinal manipulation is of any use except for acute back strain (see Chapter 147).

For patients with OA of weight-bearing joints, structured aerobic exercise programs with full or partial weight bearing can greatly enhance endurance, walking distance, and sense of well-being without aggravating the arthritis. A 2-month program of supervised fitness walking combined with patient education can improve functional status by close to 40 percent in patients with symptomatic knee disease. Gentle cycling and swimming also improve endurance, benefiting the muscle groups of the hips and knees. Morale gets a great boost by participation in such conditioning programs.

As beneficial as exercise might be, excessive amounts may only exacerbate pain and cause further disruption of the joint. Excessive joint strain, such as results from stair climbing, should be reduced to the degree possible. Supervision and patient education are essential to a successful exercise program and far superior to simply telling the patient to get more exercise.

Rest and Assist Devices. Some relief can be attained by partially resting a very painfully involved joint. The objective is to reduce the mechanical stress imposed on it. However, joint rest should be alternated with exercise to prevent muscle atrophy and worsening joint alignment. Moreover, prolonged immobility greatly disturbs cartilage metabolism.

Assist devices can help rest or protect a diseased joint from excess mechanical stress. The high pressures on the hip and knee joints generated by getting up from a toilet or low seat can be lowered by installation of hand rails, grips, and a raised toilet or chair seat. An often underutilized approach to joint rest is use of a *cane* in the contralateral hand, which can reduce the mechanical stress on a weight-bearing joint by as much as 50 percent. Embarrassment and awkwardness often make patients reluctant to use a cane, but physician encouragement and a few sessions with an occupational therapist can greatly help.

A *cervical collar* can ease neck pain by supporting the spine and resting the paraspinous musculature. It may be necessary to continue use intermittently for many weeks before significant benefit is achieved. Cervical traction may also help (see Chapter 148). A *corset* or *brace* for the back may be similarly helpful but should be combined with an exercise program to avoid muscle atrophy (see Chapter 147).

Orthotics help correct malalignment. Patients with hip disease resulting from or aggravated by differences in leg length may benefit from a heal lift that equalizes leg lengths. If there is abnormal foot pronation causing varus stress on the knee joint, a shoe orthotic may reduce pain and ligamentous strain on the knee.

Weight Reduction. Weight bearing puts mechanical stresses on the hip and knee joints that can be as high as five times the patient's weight. Even modest degrees of weight loss might achieve substantial reductions in such mechanical stress. Epidemiologic studies show a strong correlation between obesity and risk of symptomatic knee arthritis as well as a 50 percent reduction in such risk with weight loss in excess of 5 kg (11 lb) over 10 years. These results suggest that the half-hearted, perfunctory advice given "to lose weight" is insufficient and passes up an important opportunity to affect outcome. A comprehensive program of mechanically sensible supervised aerobic activity combined with detailed dietary counseling should be constructed (see Chapter 233) and carried out. An assisted, supervised program is essential, because the obese person with OA is likely to feel that the advice to lose weight and exercise is otherwise beyond his or her capacity.

Heat. Moist heat can give symptomatic relief from muscle spasm, although it has no effect on the disease itself. *Diathermy* and *ultrasound* units are expensive ways to deliver heat to deep-lying tissues. Although many patients report improvement, controlled trials using sham treatments show no benefit. However, some patients derive considerable psychological benefit and a sense of well-being from coming for such therapy.

Surgery. *Osteotomy* to correct the mechanical imbalances caused by unicompartmental disease of the knee and early disease of the hip has been popular and does seem to provide at least short-term benefit. However, there are no data comparing such surgical therapy with conservative management (weight loss, orthotics, exercise), and long-term follow-up results are often disappointing. The role of such surgery may be viewed as a temporizing measure, delaying the day of total joint replacement. *Arthroscopic surgery,* entailing debridement, smoothing of joint surfaces, and washing out of debris, appears to benefit the patients who undergo the procedure, although controlled trials suggest a strong placebo effect. *Total joint replacement* represents the most extreme form of treatment, to be undertaken only after exhausting all other therapeutic options. Replacement of hip and knee joints has been particularly successful. Referral for such surgery requires comprehensive consideration of the patient's medical condition, functional status, and psychosocial state.

INDICATIONS FOR REFERRAL

Treatment of the OA patient is a team approach. *Physical and occupational therapists* are essential to the design of a successful treatment program, teaching exercises, giving suggestions on performing the tasks of daily living, and providing psychological support. Referral should be early in the course of disease to stress preventive measures, as well as later when OA begins to interfere with daily activity. Early referral to the *nutritionist* is critical to the care of the obese patient. A comprehensive program of diet and exercise is needed to effect a successful weight loss effort.

Surgical consultation deserves consideration in the significantly disabled patient who is failing conservative management. The consultation should be viewed with the patient as an opportunity to weigh treatment options, rather than as an automatic capitulation to surgical intervention. The decision to refer for surgery must be made with an understanding of the risks involved and the need to undertake a vigorous postoperative exercise program. Surgery should be considered only in patients whose limitation of motion or pain has become so severe that it prevents them from living productively. They must be mentally and physically healthy enough to tolerate surgery and sufficiently motivated to carry out the exercise program needed to ensure full rehabilitation.

PATIENT EDUCATION AND PSYCHOSOCIAL SUPPORT

Patients need to know that OA is not reversible, but also that much can be done to lessen pain, prevent further joint injury, and preserve if not enhance overall functioning. They appreciate knowing that degenerative disease is not a generalized, systemic illness. Moreover, those with cervical or lumbosacral disease can be given some hope for a spontaneous remission of their severe pain. The need to reduce weight and strengthen supporting muscles should be stressed, as well as the importance of avoiding articularly injurious activity and addicting analgesics. The teaching functions of the physical and occupational therapists and nutritionist are among the most critical components of the treatment program. It is important to avoid labeling the patient as "disabled," because active participation in the treatment program is essential to preservation of function. As noted above, surgical options should be discussed with patients who have incapacitating pain of the hips or knees.

Because a principal determinant of presenting for care is the *psychosocial state* of the OA patient, the importance of eliciting and attending to psychosocial stresses cannot be overemphasized. A careful history that includes attention to job, family, financial and interpersonal problems is likely to help in the design of an effective treatment program. If the patient reports being disabled, yet manifests only modest mechanical dysfunction, then a search for depression and somatization disorder should be sought (see Chapters 227 and 230). Prognosis is heavily influenced by how well the patient is coping psychosocially. The physician's concern and support are essential. Regularly scheduled return visits should be set up; they facilitate provision of support and communicate a sense of caring. A strong doctor–patient relationship helps many patients to tolerate the disease and remain active.

THERAPEUTIC RECOMMENDATIONS

- Begin a comprehensive, supervised program of exercise, weight loss, and patient education for patients with symptomatic disease of the hips or knees.
- Provide referrals to physical and occupational therapists for design and implementation of exercise and activity programs that strengthen quadriceps and hip muscles, increase general conditioning, avoid excessive stress on the affected joints, and ensure proper use of assist devices.
- Obtain the services of a nutritionist to help support the obese patient in a program of weight reduction.
- Inform the patient that regular aerobic exercise is beneficial and that gentle walking, swimming, and stationary cycling are permissible.
- Advise a short period (1 to 2 days) of joint rest if there is a flare of severe hip or knee pain, but continue isometric and nonweight-bearing exercises and avoid more prolonged inactivity. Limit joint stresses (eg, stair climbing) and prescribe use of a cane and other assist devices (eg, railings, hand grips, elevated toilet seat).
- Consider use of a heel lift if leg lengths are unequal and use of a shoe orthotic if there is marked foot pronation. Check with an orthopedist or podiatrist if uncertain.
- Advise those with back pain to obtain bedrest followed by exercises to strengthen supporting musculature. A corset or brace may help, but not in the absence of an exercise program (see Chapter 147).
- Prescribe a soft cervical collar to those with cervical pain. It should be worn at all times, including during the night.

Four weeks or more of use may be necessary. Cervical traction is also helpful (see Chapter 148).

- Prescribe aspirin (enteric-coated) or acetaminophen for control of pain; recommend 300 to 600 mg qid. Consider NSAIDs only for patients who fail aspirin and acetaminophen after trials at full doses. If NSAID therapy is used, use only low, analgesic doses (eg, ibuprofen 200 mg qid), unless there is an inflammatory component to the patient's arthritis.
- Elicit and address sources of psychosocial distress.
- Avoid use of narcotics, except in the setting of an acute disabling exacerbation unrelieved by maximal doses of nonnarcotic analgesics. Under such circumstances, consider no more than 1 to 2 days' worth of therapy with codeine sulfate or oxycodone.
- Consider a single intraarticular injection of corticosteroid only if there is an inflammatory component to the arthritis and a single joint is involved. Repeat injections exacerbate joint degeneration and are to be avoided. Acupuncture has not proven sufficiently beneficial to recommend its use.
- Refer for surgical consideration the patient with refractory, incapacitating disease of a major weight-bearing joint, provided the patient is well motivated and sufficiently healthy to tolerate surgery and engage in a rehabilitation program.

A.H.G.

ANNOTATED BIBLIOGRAPHY

Bradley JD, Brandt KD, Katz BP, et al. Comparison of an antiinflammatory dose of ibuprofen, an analgesic dose of ibuprofen, and acetaminophen in the treatment of patients with osteoarthritis of the knee. N Engl J Med 1991;325:87. *(No advantage for short-term antiinflammatory therapy.)*

Davis MA, Ettinger WM, Neuhous JM, et al. Knee osteoarthritis and physical functioning: Evidence from the NHANES I epidemiologic follow-up study. J Rheum 1991;18:591. *(Correlation between severity of radiologic findings and degree of functional impairment.)*

Dieppe PA, Sathapatayavong S, Jones HE, et al. Intraarticular steroids in osteoarthritis. Rheum Rehab 1980;19:212. *(A critical look at the pluses and minuses of this controversial therapy.)*

Falconer J, Hayes KW, Chang RW. Therapeutic ultrasound in the treatment of musculoskeletal conditions. Arthritis Care Res 1990;3:85. *(No benefit in controlled trials when comparison is with sham treatment.)*

Felson DT, Anderson JJ, Naimark A, et al. Obesity and knee osteoarthritis: The Framingham Study 1988;109:18. *(Strong relationship found, especially in women.)*

Felson DT, Shang Y, Anthony JM, et al. Weight loss reduces the risk for symptomatic knee osteoarthritis in women: The Framingham study. Ann Intern Med 1992;116:535. *(Epidemiologic data suggesting that 10-pound weight loss in obese women reduces the risk of developing symptomatic knee pain by over 50 percent.)*

Gaw AC, Chang LW, Shaw LC. Efficacy of acupuncture on osteoarthritic pain. N Engl J Med 1975;293:375. *(A double-blind controlled study; variable benefit.)*

Hadler NM. Knee pain is the malady—not osteoarthritis. Ann Intern Med 1992;116:598. *(Argues that psychosocial variables are the most important determinants of who presents with knee pain.)*

Hamerman D. The biology of osteoarthritis. N Engl J Med 1989; 320:1322. *(Useful basic science review; 97 refs.)*

Hernborg JS, Nilsson BE. The natural course of untreated osteoarthritis of the knee. Clin Orthop 1977;123:130. *(A natural history study of 94 joints in 71 patients showing a generally unfavorable prognosis, with pain developing at rest in the majority of patients.)*

Kovar PA, Allegrante JP, MacKenzie CR, et al. Supervised fitness walking in patients with osteoarthritis of the knee: A randomized controlled trial. Ann Intern Med 1992;116:529. *(A program of patient education and supervised walking significantly improved functional status.)*

Lane NE, Bloch DA, Hubert HB, et al. Running, osteoarthritis, and bone density: Initial 2-year longitudinal study. Am J Med 1990;88:452. *(No progression of osteoarthritic changes in this group of middle-aged patients.)*

Lawrence JS, Bremner JM, Bier F. Osteoarthrosis prevalence in the population and relationship between symptoms and x-ray changes. Ann Rheum Dis 1966;25:1. *(Prevalence of minimal disease 50 percent; more significant disease in 20 percent; x-ray changes associated with symptoms in all joints but the lumbar spine.)*

Liang MH, Cullen KE. Primary total hip or knee replacement: Evaluation of patients. Ann Intern Med 1982;97:735. *(Good review of indications, contraindications, and results.)*

Liang MH, Fortin P. Management of osteoarthritis of the hip and knee. N Engl J Med 1991;325:125. *(An overview of the approach to diagnosis and treatment.)*

Minor HA, Hewett JE, Webel RR, et al. Efficacy of physical conditioning exercise in patients with rheumatoid arthritis and osteoarthritis. Arthritis Rheum 1989;32:1396. *(Proved very beneficial and can be done without injuring involved joints.)*

Pelletier JP, Martel-Pelletier J. The therapeutic effects of NSAID and corticosteroids in osteoarthritis: To be or not to be. J Rheum 1989;16:266. *(A discussion of their effects on the underlying disease process.)*

Poss R. The role of osteotomy in the treatment of osteoarthritis of the hip. J Bone Joint Surg 1984;66:144. *(A review of indications, patient selection, and results.)*

Salaffi F, Cavalieri F, Nolli M, et al. Analysis of disability in knee arthritis: Relationship with age and psychological variables but not with radiographic score. J Rheum 1991;18:1581. *(Evidence for a strong psychosocial component.)*

158
Management of Gout

Primary Care Medicine: Office Evaluation and Management of the Adult Patient, 3rd edition, edited by Allan H. Goroll, Lawrence A. May, and Albert G. Mulley, Jr. J.B. Lippincott Company, Philadelphia

Gout is among the most common causes of acute monoarticular arthritis. Estimates of prevalence in the United States range from 0.3 percent to 2.8 percent of the population. The condition is predominantly a disease of adult men. Inborn errors in purine metabolism and abnormalities in uric acid excretion account for most cases of primary gout. The expanded use of agents that decrease uric acid excretion has markedly increased the incidence of secondary gout. In the Framingham study, almost half of new cases were associated with thiazide use.

The primary physician should be able to diagnose promptly and treat acute gout, prevent recurrences, and minimize the chance of chronic gouty arthritis developing. Patients who present with asymptomatic hyperuricemia also require attention (see Chapter 155).

PATHOPHYSIOLOGY AND CLINICAL PRESENTATION

The majority of patients with primary gout have a hereditary renal defect in uric acid excretion leading to chronic hyperuricemia (see Chapter 155). Acute gout usually occurs after many years of sustained asymptomatic hyperuricemia. The greater the uric acid concentration, the greater the risk of an acute attack, although risk remains relatively low until very high urate levels are reached (see Chapter 155). The mean duration of the asymptomatic period is about 30 years. During this time, there may be deposition of urate in synovial lining cells and possibly in cartilage as well. Acute gout develops when uric acid crystals collect in the synovial fluid as a result of precipitation from a supersaturated state or release from the synovium. Trauma, decline in temperature, fall in pH, dehydration, starvation, alcoholic binge, emotional or physical stress, and rapid change in serum uric acid concentration have all been implicated in the process. Risk is increased in renal transplantation patients undergoing cyclosporine therapy and in obese patients placed on very-low-calorie diets.

The pathogenesis of the inflammatory response appears to involve phagocytosis of crystals by leukocytes in the synovial fluid, disruption of lysosomes, release of enzymatic products, activation of the complement and kallikrein systems, and release of leukocyte chemotactic factor.

Acute Gouty Arthritis. In men, the first attack is usually during the fifth decade; in women, it tends to be after age 60. The episode is typically monoarticular and abrupt in onset, often occurring at night. Symptoms and signs of inflammation become maximal within a few hours of onset and last for a few days to a few weeks. Recovery is complete. The initial attack usually involves a joint of the lower extremity. In about half of patients the first metatarsophalangeal joint is the site of inflammation (*podagra*). The tarsal joint (located at the instep), ankle, and knee are other common sites of initial attacks. Later episodes may involve a joint of the upper extremity, such as the wrist, elbow, or finger; shoulder or hip involvement is rare. Over 80 percent of attacks occur in the lower extremity; 85 percent of patients have at least one episode of podagra. Polyarticular involvement is also noted in about 5 percent of acute gouty attacks and may be confined to the upper extremities.

Finger-joint involvement is more common in women than men and manifests a predilection for a Heberden's or Bouchard's node. In elderly patients with gout and osteoarthritis, almost half will have such nodal inflammation as the sole or initial manifestation of gout. In elderly women, the presentation of gout may be more insidious and polyarticular.

The joint involved in an attack of acute gout appears swollen and erythematous; periarticular involvement is also common. There may be a low-grade fever and leukocytosis. A substantial fraction of patients may be normouricemic at the time of the acute attack. During resolution, the skin overlying the affected joint often desquamates. The clinical presentation may simulate joint infection (see Chapter 145) or even cellulitis (see Chapter 190).

Interval gout follows the initial attack. There is an asymptomatic period that generally lasts for several years before a second episode of acute gout takes place. The original joint or another joint may be involved in subsequent attacks. Over time, the asymptomatic intervals between acute episodes shorten. In more advanced disease, polyarticular attacks are not uncommon, and resolution may be slower and less complete.

Chronic Gouty Arthritis (Tophaceous Gout) takes years to develop. *Tophi* are typically noted an average of 10 years after the initial attack of acute gout. The risk of chronic gout is a function of duration and severity of hyperuricemia. Tophi represent sodium urate collections surrounded by foreign body giant cell inflammatory reactions. They can occur in a variety of sites, including the synovium, subchondral bone, olecranon bursa, Achilles tendon, and subcutaneous tissue of the extensor surfaces of the arm. Eventually cartilage erodes, joints become deformed, and chronic arthritis ensues. The joints of the lower extremities and hands are most commonly affected. In elderly women, the fingers may be the sole site of involvement and the only manifestation of gouty disease. The process is insidious; the patient notes progressive aching and stiffness. Tumescences may develop over joints of the foot and cause difficulty with wearing shoes. Fortunately, the incidence of tophaceous gout has declined markedly with the introduction of effective antihyperuricemic agents. Less than 15 percent of patients with acute gout develop chronic gouty arthritis.

Complications. The incidence of *nephrolithiasis* among patients with clinical gout is small, with risk of new stone formation in a patient with new onset of gout less than 1 percent per year and unrelated to initial serum urate concentration or degree of uric acid control. Factors other than serum urate concentration are important to stone formation and include family history of stone formation, urine pH, hydration status, and possibly the amount of renal uric acid excretion (see Chapter 135). Stone formation is rarely dangerous; risk of obstructive uropathy is less than 0.02 percent.

Concerns about *chronic renal failure* being a complication of chronic hyperuricemia have been laid to rest by long-term studies (see Chapter 155). Lead intoxication proved to be the cause in some populations; in others, it is concurrent hypertension, diabetes, cardiovascular disease, or underlying primary renal pathology. *Acute renal failure* is a risk in patients undergoing treatment for lymphoproliferative or myeloproliferative disease. Immediately following chemotherapy, there is a massive uric acid load that may precipitate in renal tubules and elsewhere in the urinary tract, leading to acute oliguria.

DIAGNOSIS

See Chapter 145.

PRINCIPLES OF THERAPY

Acute Gouty Arthritis

Acute symptoms can be relieved by prompt institution of antiinflammatory therapy. Without treatment, an acute attack of gout usually resolves within 7 to 10 days, although severe episodes can last for weeks. Initiation of treatment at the very first sign of an acute attack produces a prompt and excellent therapeutic response. Delay of therapy is associated with less satisfactory results. Antiinflammatory therapy is usually continued until symptoms have resolved.

Nonsteroidal antiinflammatory drugs (NSAIDs) used in full doses are the treatment of choice. *Indomethacin* and *naproxen* are the best studied of the NSAIDs for use in acute gout, but almost any NSAID should suffice. Ongoing peptic ulcer disease and renal insufficiency are relative contraindications to NSAID use (see Chapter 156). Some elderly patients may experience mental confusion with indomethacin.

Colchicine is an alternative for patients unable to take NSAID therapy, but its tendency to cause gastrointestinal (GI) upset (nausea, vomiting, diarrhea) limits patient compliance. Bone marrow suppression and increased risk of myopathy and neuropathy have been reported in persons with concurrent renal or hepatic insufficiency.

Interval Gout

Although prophylactic therapy to prevent acute gouty arthritis is not necessary or cost-effective for patients with asymptomatic hyperuricemia or a first attack of gout (see Chapter 155), it may be worthwhile in patients who are having increasingly frequent, disabling attacks. Intervals between future recurrences are likely to shorten. Of the risk factors for recurrent gouty attacks, hyperuricemia is the one most amenable to treatment. Options include blocking urate production with *allopurinol* and enhancing renal excretion with *probenecid* or *sulfinpyrazone*. The goal is to lower the uric acid below 6.5 mg/dL, the level at which extracellular fluid becomes saturated with uric acid.

Allopurinol is convenient to use, relatively well tolerated, and thus widely prescribed. It inhibits the enzyme xanthine oxidase and blocks the formation of uric acid. The half-life of allopurinol is about 3 hours, but its metabolites are biologically active for up to 30 hours. As a result, the drug need be taken only once daily. Serum urate levels fall within a week of initiating therapy, but risk of gouty attacks does not decline until normouricemia has been sustained for 3 to 6 months. Interval gout patients best suited for allopurinol include those with hyperexcretion of uric acid (>1000 mg/24 h), renal insufficiency, history of nephrolithiasis, and inability to tolerate a uricosuric agent. Allopurinol has no beneficial effect on acute gouty arthritis; in fact, it may precipitate an attack during the early stages of therapy (see below).

Of the minor side effects, GI upset and rash are among the more common. The reported frequency of more serious adverse reactions is 3.5 percent. They include fever, leukopenia, hepatitis, vasculitis, and hepatocellular injury. A fulminant *hypersensitivity syndrome* characterized by desquamative rash, fever, hepatitis, eosinophilia, and renal failure is the most worrisome adverse effect. Although uncommon (prevalence <0.25%), it has a 15 percent to 25 percent mortality rate and occurs mostly in patients with concurrent renal insufficiency. Allopurinol should always be used with caution and in reduced doses in patients with renal insufficiency. Drug–drug interactions are also important. The risk of an ampicillin-induced drug rash is increased by concurrent allopurinol use, as is the activity of drugs metabolized by hepatic microsomal enzymes (eg, warfarin).

Although often preferred by patients who require urate lowering because of its convenience and low frequency of side effects, allopurinol should not be used casually. Carefully weighing the expected prophylactic benefit against the small but serious risk of a hypersensitivity reaction helps to ensure intelligent, safe use. The drug remains expensive.

Uricosuric Agents. These drugs have an excellent safety record, making them well suited for long-term prophylactic therapy. *Probenecid* and *sulfinpyrazone* are the principal uricosuric drugs, both acting to inhibit renal tubular reabsorption of uric acid. About 80 percent of patients excreting less than 700 mg/d of uric acid can be effectively managed by uricosuric therapy. A uricosuric agent is often preferred to allopurinol therapy in persons with interval gout excreting less than 700 mg/d of uric acid and having well-preserved renal function.

Their principal disadvantages are frequency of dosing and risk of precipitating nephrolithiasis. Convenience and thus compliance fall short of that for allopurinol. Probenecid must be given two to three times per day; sulfinpyrazone requires tid or qid dosing. At the onset of therapy, the uric acid excretion may reach extraordinary levels and trigger nephrolithiasis, necessitating use of modest initial doses, generous fluid intake (2 to 3 L/d), and urinary alkalinization. *Rash, autoimmune hemolytic anemia,* and *GI upset* are the most common side effects. Sulfinpyrazone has a very small risk of *marrow suppression*.

Drug–drug interactions are common. Thiazides and salicylates inhibit their uricosuric action. Probenecid blocks the renal excretion of penicillins and the hepatic uptake of rifampin, prolonging the half-lives of both.

Initiation of Antihyperuricemic Therapy. All drugs that reduce the serum uric acid can trigger an attack of acute gout during the initial 3 to 6 months of therapy. This is believed to be a consequence of their mobilizing tissue deposits of uric acid. Only after the uric acid has been normal for 3 to 6 months does the risk of a gouty attack begin to decline substantially. In the interim, low-dose antiinflammatory therapy is taken concurrently with the urate-lowering agent. Both colchicine and NSAIDs are used.

Therapy is instituted only after all manifestations of an acute attack have fully resolved. There are no definitive data on the ideal duration of concurrent antiinflammatory therapy, but most authorities recommend that it be given for 3 to 6 months or until all visible urate deposits have disappeared.

Diet. Only 10 percent of circulating purine is derived from dietary sources. Consequently, there is no need to restrict purine intake. However, reduction of excess weight (without fasting) and abstinence from excessive alcohol intake and binge drinking can help prevent future attacks. Obese, interval gout patients on a very-low-calorie diet program are at increased risk of an acute attack and may require prophylactic therapy.

Chronic Gouty Arthritis

Antihyperuricemic treatment is indicated in patients with tophaceous gout to prevent progressive articular damage. Prevention or lessening of chronic gouty arthritis requires normalizing the serum urate level. Being the more effective and more convenient antihyperuricemic, allopurinol is usually prescribed for patients with tophaceous gout. Often, tophi begin to resolve after several weeks of therapy. A uricosuric agent is a reasonable alternative, provided renal function is normal, and there is no nephrolithiasis or excessive uric acid excretion. Regardless of agent selected, concurrent antiinflammatory therapy must be given until visible urate deposits have resolved.

Renal Complications

Although the risk of a renal complication is small, there are a few instances in which attention to renal issues is required in the management of the gouty patient.

Nephrolithiasis. The gouty patient with an established uric acid stone should be treated with allopurinol and a high fluid intake; concurrent administration of a thiazide diuretic may be necessary (see Chapter 135). Allopurinol therapy for prevention of stone formation is indicated in gouty patients with a prior history of nephrolithiasis and perhaps in those with a strong family history of kidney stones. All patients should be instructed to avoid dehydration, especially if they live in warm, dry climates. Isolated hyperuricemia, per se, does not require treatment in the absence of other risk factors for nephrolithiasis (see Chapter 155).

Renal Failure. Patients undergoing chemotherapy for lymphoproliferative or myeloproliferative disease require pretreatment with allopurinol. There is no role for chronic urate-lowering therapy in the prevention of chronic renal failure in patients with gout, but avoidance of lead exposure is important, as is treatment of commonly coexisting conditions such as hypertension, diabetes, and cardiovascular disease.

PATIENT EDUCATION

Patients who suffer an acute gouty attack are highly motivated to undertake preventive measures and very receptive to advice. If obese, they should be advised to avoid starvation or very-low-calorie diets. Drinkers should be warned against binges. Maintenance of good hydration needs to be stressed to those at risk for nephrolithiasis. On the other hand, patients will find it comforting to know that severe dietary restrictions are unnecessary. However, fasting should be avoided, because it may precipitate an attack. The importance of treating an acute attack at the first sign of illness also needs to be stressed. For the patient with interval gout, a discussion of the risks and benefits of prophylactic therapy and the importance of compliance is indicated. Those taking allopurinol should be warned of the risk of a hypersensitivity reaction and advised to cease intake immediately and call at the first sign of rash, fever, or other manifestation.

THERAPEUTIC RECOMMENDATIONS

Acute Gout

- At the first sign of an attack of acute gouty arthritis, begin a nonsteroidal antiinflammatory agent (eg, naproxen 500 mg tid). Continue full-dose treatment until symptoms resolve, then taper to cessation over 72 hours. Advise the patient that delay in starting therapy may impair response.
- For patients unable to take NSAID therapy (eg, active peptic ulcer disease), consider using colchicine (0.6 mg qid), but warn that diarrhea and some upper GI upset is likely during the course of therapy; monitor blood count, liver, and renal function. Avoid if there is underlying renal or hepatic insufficiency.
- For refractory cases of definite acute gout, consider a 7- to 10-day course of oral corticosteroids, starting with prednisone at 20 to 40 mg/d and tapering as clinically indicated. Intraarticular corticosteroid therapy is another option if oral therapy is not feasible and there is just a single joint involved.
- Provide an extra supply of antiinflammatory therapy so that it will be available for prompt use in a future episode.

Interval Gout

- Determine with the patient if gouty attacks are sufficiently frequent and disabling to warrant prophylactic therapy.
- If so, determine if allopurinol or a uricosuric agent is preferred by 1) inquiring into personal or family history of kidney stones or renal dysfunction; 2) measuring renal function (BUN, creatinine); and 3) determining 24-hour urinary uric acid excretion.
- Begin allopurinol (300 mg once daily) for the patient ex-

creting more than 1000 mg/d of uric acid, having underlying azotemia, increased risk of nephrolithiasis, or allergy to or failure of uricosuric therapy. Adjust dose upward if response is inadequate. Reduce dose in the setting of renal insufficiency and use cautiously, especially when diuretics are being given concurrently. Stop at the earliest sign of a hypersensitivity reaction.

- Begin probenecid or sulfinpyrazone if the patient has normal renal function, no risk of stone disease, and a urate excretion of less than 700 mg/d. Therapy should be initiated using small doses (eg, probenecid 250 mg bid or sulfinpyrazone 50 mg bid) in conjunction with large volumes of fluid (2 to 3 L/d) to prevent precipitation of uric acid in the urinary tract. Alkalinization of the urine to a pH of 6.6 is desirable during the first week of therapy but is difficult to achieve; gram doses of sodium bicarbonate are required, supplemented by acetazolamide (250 mg) before bed.
- Advance uricosuric dose gradually to avoid triggering massive urate excretion. Continue high fluid intake during the early months of therapy. Maximum dose of sulfinpyrazone is 100 mg tid–qid; for probenecid, it is 500 to 1000 mg bid–tid. Avoid concurrent use of aspirin because it inhibits urate excretion.
- Monitor serum uric acid concentration and treat to achieve a level of less than 6.5 mg/dL, the point of supersaturation.
- To reduce the risk of an attack of gout during the first 3 to 6 months of urate-lowering treatment, prescribe concurrent antiinflammatory prophylactic therapy using either colchicine (0.6 mg qd or bid) or an intermediate-acting NSAID (eg, naproxen 250 mg qd or bid).
- Advise avoidance of precipitants such as binge drinking, fasting, and very-low-calorie diets.

Chronic Gouty Arthritis

- Treat as for interval gout. Continue concurrent antiinflammatory therapy until all visible manifestations of uric acid deposits have resolved, which might take 6 to 12 months.

Renal Complications

- Pretreat cancer patients with allopurinol if a large uric acid load is likely to result from an application of chemotherapy.
- Advise marked reduction in lead exposure (eg, home-distilled alcohol, industrial contact).
- Treat patients with urate nephrolithiasis or a strong family history of kidney stones with allopurinol (300 mg once daily) and hydration. Long-term efforts to alkalinize the urine are impractical and need not be attempted.
- Because the risk of chronic renal failure from chronic hyperuricemia is nil, there is no renal need for chronic urate-lowering therapy.

A.H.G.

ANNOTATED BIBLIOGRAPHY

Bautman V, Maesaka JK, Haddad B, et al. The role of lead in gouty nephropathy. N Engl J Med 1981;304:520. *(An important link between gout and renal injury.)*

Berger L, Yu TF. Renal function in gout—An analysis of 524 gouty subjects including long-term follow-up studies. Am J Med 1975;59:604. *(Important 12-year follow-up study which showed that hyperuricemia alone had no deleterious effect on renal function in ambulatory patients with gout.)*

Fessel JW. Renal outcomes of gout and hyperuricemia. Am J Med 1979;67:74. *(Risks of renal failure and stone formation were very small.)*

Graham R, Scott JT. Clinical survey of 354 patients with gout. Ann Rheum Dis 1976;29:461. *(Detailed look at clinical presentation and course.)*

Hadler NM, Franck WA, Bress NM, et al. Acute polyarticular gout. Am J Med 1974;56:715. *(In one-third of patients, the condition was confined to the upper extremities, and it may occur in the setting of a normal serum uric acid.)*

Hall AP, Berry PE, Dawber TR, et al. Epidemiology of gout and hyperuricemia—A long-term population study. Am J Med 1967;42:27. *(The oft-quoted Framingham study; risk of acute gout rose with uric acid level.)*

Hande KR, Noone RM, Stone WJ. Severe allopurinol toxicity. Am J Med 1984;76:47. *(A potentially fatal hypersensitivity syndrome described.)*

Lally EV, Zimmerman B, Ho G, et al. Urate-mediated inflammation in nodal osteoarthritis: Clinical and roentgenographic correlations. Arthritis Rheum 1989;32:86. *(A Heberden's or Bouchard's node was the initial or sole site of gout in almost half of elderly patients with gout and osteoarthritis.)*

Lin HY, Rocher LL, McQuillan MA, et al. Cyclosporine-induced hyperuricemia and gout. N Engl J Med 1989;321:287. *(Hyperuricemia common; gout in 7 percent.)*

Maclaughlan MJ, Rodnan GP. Effects of food, fast, and alcohol on serum uric acid and acute attacks of gout. Am J Med 1967;42:38. *(Fasting and consumption of over 100 g of alcohol raised urate levels and often precipitated attacks.)*

Meyers DC, Monteagudo FSE. Gout in females: An analysis of 92 patients. Clin Exp Rheumatol 1985;3:105. *(The presentation in women may be more an insidious polyarthritis rather than an acute monoarthritis.)*

National Task force on the Prevention and Treatment of Obesity. Very low-calorie diets. JAMA 1993;270:967. *(Risk of triggering an acute gouty attack is low, but increased in those with prior symptomatic gout.)*

Singer JZ, Wallace SL. The allopurinol hypersensitivity syndrome. Arthritis Rheum 1986;29:82. *(High mortality risk; many cases occurring in patients who did not need the drug.)*

Wallace SL, Singer JZ. Treatment of gout, in Primer on the Rheumatic Diseases, ninth edition. Edited by H. Ralph Schumacher, Jr. Atlanta: Arthritis Foundation, 1988, p 202. *(Excellent review of drug therapy.)*

Wernick R, Winkler C, Campbell S. Tophi as the initial manifestation of gout. Arch Intern Med 1992;152:873. *(Noted in the fingers of elderly women with underlying osteoarthritis, renal insufficiency, and concurrent NSAID use.)*

Yu TF, Berger LU. Impaired renal function in gout. Am J Med 1982;75:95. *(Hyperuricemia alone did not affect renal function; renal insufficiency correlated best with coexisting hypertension, preexisting renal disease, and ischemic heart disease.)*

Yu TF, Gutman A. Uric acid nephrolithiasis in gout: Predisposing factors. Ann Intern Med 1967;67:1133. *(A classic study correlating risk of stone formation with uric acid excretion, urine pH, serum urate level, and etiology.)*

159
Approach to the Patient With Fibromyalgia

Primary Care Medicine: Office Evaluation and Management of the Adult Patient, 3rd edition, edited by Allan H. Goroll, Lawrence A. May, and Albert G. Mulley, Jr. J.B. Lippincott Company, Philadelphia

Patients with chronic diffuse musculoskeletal pain but no evidence of arthritis account for a large number of office visits. Mild rheumatoid disease accounts for some cases; bony pathology, neuropathy, and myopathy are responsible for others. When no source stands out, clinicians start wondering about somatization despite protestations from the patient that the problem is "not in my head."

In recent years, a syndrome of diffuse, chronic musculoskeletal pain, stiffness, focal tenderness, disordered sleep, and fatigue has become increasingly recognized as an important clinical entity. The terms *fibromyalgia, fibrositis, and fibromyositis* have been used to designate the syndrome, although the "-itis" terminology has been discouraged because no inflammatory pathophysiology has been detected. The condition is of unknown etiology but appears to be common and estimated to have a prevalence as high as 5 percent among adult women, who account for 80 percent to 90 percent of cases.

PATHOPHYSIOLOGY, CLINICAL PRESENTATION, AND COURSE

Pathogenesis. The cause of fibromyalgia remains unknown. Although the symptoms suggest somatization, careful psychological studies reveal no relationship between symptoms and psychological status. Only an increased frequency of life stress has been found. Non-REM Stage 4 sleep is disturbed and related to symptoms, but its role in pathogenesis is unclear. Muscle biopsies and electromyographic data demonstrate no consistent or unique changes. A subset of fibromyalgia patients have antibody abnormalities, but these individuals appear to have concurrent connective tissue disease. Others have positive serology for Lyme disease, but treatment for Lyme disease usually does little to resolve symptoms. Such cases are believed to represent false-positives caused by the low specificity of Lyme serology and the high prevalence of fibromyalgia. The overlap in symptoms among patients with chronic fatigue syndrome and fibromyalgia has raised speculation about a common pathophysiology, but pathogenesis remains unknown for both conditions.

Clinical Presentation. The typical patient is a woman in her midthirties who presents complaining of chronic diffuse musculoskeletal pain, stiffness, and fatigue. The pain tends to be constant, aching, and concentrated axially (neck, shoulders, back, pelvis). Points of tenderness may also be found in the upper and lower extremities. "Stiffness" is often used to describe the discomfort, which is characteristically worse in the morning and exacerbated by change in the weather, cold, humidity, sleeplessness, and stress and helped by warmth, rest, and mild exercise. Patients awake from sleep feeling tired and unrefreshed.

Physical examination is normal except for multiple, reproducible points of exaggerated tenderness to palpation. The tender points tend to be symmetric and located in the occiput, neck, shoulder, ribs, elbows, buttocks, and knees. Eighteen characteristic locations have been identified (Fig. 159–1). Patients with fibromyositis have tenderness in at least 11 of them.

Clinical Course. Fibromyalgia is a chronic, but nonprogressive disorder. Waxing and waning with changes in the weather, degree of situational stress, and rest are characteristic. The number and location of tender points tend to be stable over time. In some patients, the condition may become disabling, at least temporarily.

DIFFERENTIAL DIAGNOSIS

Fibromyalgia must be differentiated from both regional and diffuse forms of musculoskeletal pain in which there is no arthritis. In some instances, an extraarticular source is readily evident, be it bone, bursa, tendon, muscle, ligament, or nerve. The pain of *hypertrophic osteoarthropathy* may be diffuse, but tender points are minimal, and clubbing provides a unique hallmark.

Myofascial syndromes due to overuse may be confused with fibromyalgia, in that both manifest tender points. Unlike those of fibromyalgia, the tender points of myofascial syndrome are clustered about just one area and trigger referred pain (consequently the term *trigger points*). Similarly, symptoms are focal rather than diffuse. A history of onset after excessive activity or muscle strain is typical. There is no associated fatigue or sleep disorder.

Rheumatoid disease in its early or mild forms may cause diffuse musculoskeletal discomfort, morning stiffness, fatigue, and focal tenderness on physical examination. However, the tenderness appears to be less exaggerated and serologic studies are abnormal. *Polymyalgia rheumatica* superficially resembles fibromyaglia, but onset is at a much later age, symptoms are confined to the hip and shoulder girdles, there are few tender points, and the sedimentation rate is markedly elevated. *Ankylosing spondylitis* produces axial discomfort, fatigue, and focal tenderness; however, most axially symptomatic patients are men, and sacroiliitis is a defining manifestation (see Chapter 146).

Chronic fatigue syndrome (CFS) patients have been found to share many of the clinical features of fibromyalgia, including chronic diffuse musculoskeletal pain, and tender points, making differentiation difficult at times because both are diagnosed clinically. Pain tends to be less prominent a complaint in CFS, and not all patients have tender points.

Lyme disease also enters into the differential diagnosis but is readily differentiated by the history of deer tick or en-

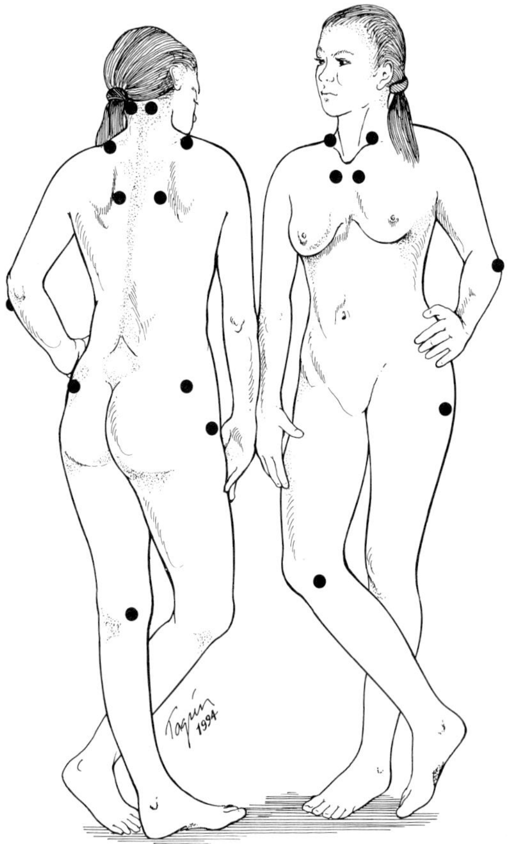

Figure 159-1. Tender points in fibromyalgia syndrome.

demic area exposure, rash, polyarthritis, and neurologic deficits (see Chapter 160).

Hypothyroidism may be accompanied by diffuse myalgias and fatigue, simulating fibromyalgia. Differentiating features include cold intolerance, unexplained weight gain, characteristic skin changes, goiter, muscle weakness and soreness, and an elevated thyrotropin (TSH) level. Similarly, *polymyositis* may produce diffuse muscle achiness, but muscles are weak, diffusely sore, and sedimentation rate and muscle enzymes are markedly elevated.

Depression and somatization disorder certainly can cause chronic musculoskeletal pain and fatigue, but they lack reproducible tender points and are accompanied by definite manifestations of underlying psychopathology (see Chapters 227 and 230).

WORKUP

Diagnosis depends entirely on the history and physical examination (Table 159–1). Laboratory studies are ordered to help rule out other conditions.

History. A careful delineation of the location of the pain is essential and helps differentiate fibromyalgia from conditions causing more localized or regional discomfort. Inquiry into associated features such as fatigue, nonrefreshing sleep, and exacerbations with changes in the weather facilitate differentiation. Pertinent negatives include other somatic and affective symptoms of depression (see Chapter 227), symptoms of hypothyroidism (see Chapter 104), frank arthritis, fever, rash, muscle weakness, and prior history of muscle injury.

Physical Examination. The skin, nails, mucous membranes, fundi, joints, spine, muscles, and bones should be examined carefully for evidence of rheumatoid disease, myopathy, osteoarthropathy, thyroid disease, and focal pathology (see Chapters 45 and Chapters 146 through 151). If no abnormalities are found, then careful palpation of the 18 tender-point sites (see Figure 159–1) is indicated. Compression should be just strong enough to cause blanching of the examining fingertip. A positive response is one that elicits exaggerated tenderness or outright pain. Tender points need to be differentiated from the trigger points of myofascial syndrome, which produce referred pain on compression. Mild discomfort to palpation is a nonspecific finding that may be elicited in a host of other musculoskeletal conditions.

Laboratory Studies. Because there are no diagnostic studies or characteristic laboratory findings, testing is conducted to rule out treatable conditions that may present in similar fashion. Among the more useful studies are an antinuclear antibody (ANA) determination, sedimentation rate, TSH, and creatine phosphokinase. Obtaining Lyme titers is not indicated unless the patient has symptoms strongly suggestive of the disease (rash, arthritis, neurologic complaints, deer tick exposure, endemic area). Patients in whom back pain is the predominant complaint may need consideration of radiologic study (see Chapter 147). When fatigue dominates the clinical picture, more extensive evaluation might be required (see Chapter 8).

PRINCIPLES OF MANAGEMENT AND PATIENT EDUCATION

Like any chronic condition with an unknown etiology, management is supportive. Among the most effective measures is treatment with a *tricyclic antidepressant* (eg, amitriptyline, which might help by its ability to restore normal sleep). Small doses may suffice (eg, 25–50 mg qhs), but larger ones are sometimes necessary. Improvements in all disease manifestations have been noted, but relapse commonly occurs with cessation of therapy. No significant improvement in symptoms is achieved with use of nonsteroidal antiinflammatory agents. Empiric parenteral antibiotic treatment for Lyme disease in patients with fibromyalgia and positive Lyme serology produces considerably more antibiotic toxicity than it does cures and is not recommended. Only patients with clinical manifestations strongly suggestive of Lyme disease (rash, arthritis, heart block, or neurologic deficits) should be considered candidates for such therapy. *Cardiovascular fitness training* raises pain thresholds and global assessment scores. No such improvement has been noted with just simple flexibility exercises.

Patient education and emotional support are essential. Patients are greatly relieved to hear that their condition is a recognized syndrome and not "imaginary." Such validation is the first step to forming a strong patient–doctor relationship, which is essential to effective management of fibromyalgia patients. Listening carefully and performing a thor-

Table 159-1. The American College of Rheumatology 1990 Criteria for the Classification of Fibromyalgia†

1. History of widespread pain.
   Definition. Pain is considered widespread when all of the following are present: pain in the left side of the body, pain in the right side of the body, pain above the waist, and pain below the waist. In addition, axial skeletal pain (cervical spine or anterior chest or thoracic spine or low back) must be present. In this definition, shoulder and buttock pain is considered as pain for each involved side. "Low back" pain is considered lower segment pain.
2. Pain in 11 of 18 tender point sites on digital palpation (see Figure 159-1).

   Definition. Pain, on digital palpation, must be present in at least 11 of the following 18 tender point sites:
   Occiput: bilateral, at the suboccipital muscle insertions.
   Low cervical: bilateral, at the anterior aspects of the intertransverse spaces at C5–C7.
   Trapezius: bilateral, at the midpoint of the upper border.
   Supraspinatus: bilateral, at origins, above the scapula spine near the medial border.
   Second rib: bilateral, at the second costochondral junctions, just lateral to the juntions on upper surfaces.
   Lateral epicondyle: bilateral, 2 cm distal to the epicondyles.
   Gluteal: bilateral, in upper outer quadrants of buttocks in anterior fold of muscle.
   Greater trochanter: bilateral, posterior to the trochanteric prominence.
   Knee: bilateral, at the medial fat pad proximal to the joint line.

   Digital palpation should be performed with an approximate force of 4 kg.
   For a tender point to be considered "positive" the subject must state that the palpation was painful. "Tender" is not to be considered "painful."

†For classification purposes, patients, will be said to have fibromyalgia if both criteria are satisfied. Widespread pain must have been present for at least 3 months. The presence of a second clinical disorder does not exclude the diagnosis of fibromyalgia.

*Adapted from Wolfe F, Smyth HA, Yunus MB, et al. Arthritis Rheum 1990;33:1.

ough physical examination conveys a sense of caring and respect for the patient's problem and helps reduce frantic demands for medically unnecessary testing and referrals to "specialists." Similarly, the patient is less apt to seek multiple evaluations and help from alternative healers when time is taken to explain current knowledge, prescribe a comprehensive treatment program, and review its rationale and the expected response. Patients receiving tricyclic therapy need to know that it is directed at the fibromyalgia (perhaps the sleep disorder) and not at depression. Knowing that the condition is chronic but not progressive or compromising of life expectancy is also appreciated, as is advice on avoidance of such aggravating factors as situational stress and sleeplessness.

A.H.G.

ANNOTATED BIBLIOGRAPHY

Dailey PA, Bishop GD, Russell IJ, et al. Psychological stress and the fibrositis/fibromyalgia syndrome. J Rheumatol 1990;17:1380. *(High level of life stress found.)*

Felson DT, Goldenberg DL. The natural history of fibromyalgia. Arthritis Rheum 1986;29:1522. *(A chronic persistent, but generally nonprogressive course noted.)*

Goldenberg DL, Simms RW, Geiger A, et al. High frequency of fibromyalgia in patients with chronic fatigue seen in a primary care practice. Arthritis Rheum 1990;33:381. *(Much overlap in the two conditions.)*

Lightfoot RW, Luft BJ, Rahn DW, et al. Empiric parenteral antibiotic treatment of patients with fibromyalgia/fatigue and a positive serologic result for Lyme disease. Ann Intern Med 1993;119:503. *(A cost-effective analysis; treatment was expensive and caused much more antibiotic toxicity than clinical cures.)*

McCain GA, Bell DA, Mai FM, et al. A controlled study of the effects of a supervised cardiovascular fitness training program on the manifestations of primary fibromyalgia. Arthritis Rheum 1988;31:1135. *(Improvement achieved with cardiovascular training, but not with simple flexibility exercises.)*

Moldofsky H, Scarisbrick P, England R, et al. Musculoskeletal symptoms and non-REM sleep disturbance in patients with "fibrositis" syndrome and healthy subjects. Psychosom Med 1975;37:341. *(The original observation of disturbed sleep.)*

Scudds RA, McCain GA, Rollman GB, et al. Improvements in pain responsiveness in patients with fibrositis after successful treatment with amitriptyline. J Rheumatol 1989;16:98. *(A double-blind, crossover study; all parameters improved.)*

Simms RW, Gunderman J, Howard G, et al. The alpha-delta sleep abnormality in fibromyalgia. Arthritis Rheum 1988;31(suppl):S100. *(The characteristic sleep disorder of fibromyalgia.)*

Wolfe F, Smythe HA, Yunus MB, et al. The American College of Rheumatology 1990 criteria for the classification of fibromyalgia: The multicenter criteria committee. Arthritis Rheum 1990;33:160. *(Consensus diagnostic criteria pending discovery of more definitive diagnostic findings.)*

Yunus MB, Ahles TA, Aldag JC, et al. Relationship of clinical features with psychological status in primary fibromyalgia. Arthritis Rheum 1991;34:15. *(No relationship found, suggesting that symptoms are independent of the patient's psychological status.)*

Yunus MB, Masi AT, Calabro JJ, et al. Primary fibromyalgia (fibrositis): Clinical study of 50 patients with matched normal controls. Semin Arthritis Rheum 1981;11:151. *(Careful delineation of clinical presentation and physical findings.)*

160
Approach to the Patient With Lyme Disease

Primary Care Medicine: Office Evaluation and Management of the Adult Patient, 3rd edition, edited by Allan H. Goroll, Lawrence A. May, and Albert G. Mulley, Jr. J.B. Lippincott Company, Philadelphia

Lyme disease is a treatable multisystem illness due to infection with the tickborne spirochete *Borrelia burgdorferi*. The condition has become the most common vectorborne disease in the United States, with over 40,000 cases reported to the Centers for Disease Control and Prevention in the past 10 years. In most instances, the acute infection can be readily diagnosed and effectively treated. The neuromusculoskeletal manifestations of later stages may be more subtle and resemble those of chronic fatigue syndrome, fibromyalgia, or depression. The nonspecificity of symptoms and shortcomings of available serologic tests lead to both underdiagnosis and overdiagnosis.

The primary physician needs to be skilled in the clinical recognition of early and late disease, clinically capable of differentiating it from other acute and chronic neuromusculoskeletal conditions, cognizant of the limitations of diagnostic methods, and capable of prescribing an effective antibiotic program.

EPIDEMIOLOGY, PATHOPHYSIOLOGY, AND CLINICAL PRESENTATION

Epidemiology

The spirochete causing Lyme disease is transmitted to humans by *Ixodes* ticks. Nymph-stage ticks feed on humans from May through July, transmitting the spirochete in the process. Endemic areas for species of the responsible tick include the northeastern coastal states, Wisconsin and Minnesota in the midwest, and along the west coast in Oregon and northern California. Outbreaks in Europe and Asia have also been reported. On the U.S. east coast and in the midwest, the deer tick *I. dammini* is the principal vector. Over a third of deer ticks carry the spirochete, accounting for outbreaks of epidemic proportion. In the western United States, the *I. pacificus* species is responsible, but the carrier rate is only 1 percent to 3 percent and human infection is much more sporadic. The condition has also been reported in Europe and Asia.

The rising frequency of Lyme disease and its geographic spread have been linked to enlarging deer populations and concurrent suburbanization. The spirochete is transmitted horizontally to field mice, which are critical to sustaining its life cycle (deer are not, but the ticks prefer them). Human infection is a biologic deadend for the spirochete.

Pathophysiology

The spirochete enters the bloodstream at the time of tick feeding. There is a short bloodstream phase, but the organism moves out of the blood and, in seemingly trophic fashion, into the skin, sinovium, heart, and nervous system. The means by which the spirochete damages tissue remains unclear, with hypotheses ranging from direct injury to production of antispirochetal antibodies that cross-react with tissue antigens. Patients with symptoms that persist after appropriate antibiotic therapy are suspected of having an exaggerated, sustained immune response. Such a response may account for the overlap in clinical manifestations with those of fibromyalgia and chronic fatigue syndromes, which are also suspected of having an immunologic pathophysiology (see Chapters 8 and 159). Patients who are HLA-DR4 positive appear to be at increased risk for such chronic illness, suggesting that severity and chronicity of disease may be related, in part, to cell surface antigens and genetic susceptibility.

Clinical Presentation and Course

The biting tick is usually no larger than the size of a pencil mark and often inapparent. Shortly after the bite, the first symptoms develop. The clinical course can be divided into three stages: 1) acute, localized disease; 2) subacute, disseminated disease; and 3) chronic disease.

Stage 1—Acute Infection. In most patients, the first clinical manifestation of *B. burgdorferi* infection is a skin reaction to the organism. About 80 percent develop a characteristic expanding erythematous rash, *erythema migrans*. It usually begins as a red macule at the site of the tick bite and spreads out to form a large annular lesion with red secondary outer rings, an intense red outer border, and some clearing toward the center, although there may be induration at the site of the bite. The lesion is large, averaging 15 cm. Minor constitutional *flulike symptoms* (a "summer flu") and regional *lymphadenopathy* may accompany the rash. The remaining 20 percent of patients have flulike symptoms without a rash or no acute-stage symptoms at all. The rash starts to fade by 3 to 4 weeks. During stage 1, the immune response is minimal.

Stage 2—Disseminated Infection. Hematogenous dissemination follows the acute phase within several days to a few weeks of the tick bite and leads to a host of symptoms, dominated by dermatologic, musculoskeletal, and neurologic complaints. Constitutional symptoms may be prominent, with patients complaining of generalized *malaise* and debilitating *fatigue*. Often, bouts of severe *headache* lasting a few hours may develop, accompanied by mild neck stiffness, as may *migratory arthralgias* and musculoskeletal pain.

Dermatologic manifestations include new *annular skin lesions*, smaller and less migratory than the initial one. Malar rash, diffuse erythema, and urticaria have also been noted.

Cardiac involvement is noted in about 5 percent to 10 percent of patients, beginning several weeks into the infection. *Transient heart block* may be a consequence, ranging from asymptomatic first-degree AV block to complete heart block with fainting. The cardiac phase lasts 3 to 6 weeks, with the most severe forms of heart block persisting for about 1 week and not requiring pacemaker placement.

Neurologic sequestration ensues weeks to months after the initial infection, affecting 15 percent to 20 percent of untreated patients. It consists of a *lymphocytic meningitis* and cranial or peripheral neuropathy. The cerebrospinal fluid (CSF) shows a pleocytosis with about 100 lymphocytes per cubic millimeter, elevated protein, normal glucose, and antibodies to the spirochete. A mild *encephalopathy* may ensue and produce mood changes, somnolence, and memory disturbances. A unilateral or bilateral *Bell's palsy* is the most common cranial nerve deficit. The *peripheral neuritis* presents as motor and/or sensory changes of the trunk or limbs in a dermatomal distribution. These neurologic manifestations can last for weeks to months.

Musculoskeletal complaints evolve into frank arthritis in up to 60 percent of untreated patients. Onset of arthritis is variable but averages 6 months from the time of initial infection. Characteristically, self-limited attacks of acute asymmetric *monoarticular* or *oligoarticular arthritis* develop. Pain and swelling are noted in one or a few large joints. The knee is the most common site. A joint effusion may form, composed of increased numbers of neutrophils (10,000 to 25,000 per cubic millimeter). No more than three joints are usually involved in the course of the illness. Symptoms and signs last several days to a few weeks. After an attack, the joint returns to normal.

Stage 3—Chronic Infection. After a latent period of several months and beginning a year from the time of original infection, symptoms of chronic infection begin to appear. Bouts of arthritis may become more prolonged, and chronic neurologic deficits may ensue.

Skin Changes. Most patients in the United States do not manifest skin changes in the late phases of Lyme disease, but in Europe, a chronic atrophic form of *acrodermatitis* unique to Lyme disease has been observed.

Arthritis. The transient form of arthritis characteristic of disseminated disease is supplanted by a more persistent one, lasting months instead of weeks. The knee remains the most common site, and the pattern continues to be oligoarticular. Joint erosion is reported but uncommon and rarely leads to permanent loss of function. A small percentage of patients experience persistence of arthritis even after a full course of antibiotic therapy. An immunologic mechanism is postulated. Over the years, the frequency of arthritic episodes declines,

Neurologic Impairment. Distal paresthesias, radicular pain, and memory loss comprise the principal neurologic manifestations of late disease, representing polyneuropathy and encephalopathy. Often, they occur concurrently. Tiredness may also be reported. In rare instances, a leukoencephalopathy with spastic paraparesis may develop. Two-thirds of patients with neurologic symptoms have elevated CSF protein, and half have Lyme antibodies in the CSF. In most patients, electrophysiologic study is abnormal, demonstrating evidence of polyaxonal degeneration.

Natural History of Disease. Untreated, about 20 percent of patients never develop disseminated disease. Attacks of oligoarthritis are common (60% to 80%) but resolve within 1 to 3 years, even without treatment. Chronic neurologic and persistent joint symptoms affect about 5 percent to 10 percent of patients. Susceptibility to late chronic disease may be genetically determined.

DIFFERENTIAL DIAGNOSIS

Acute and Early Disseminated Stages. Lyme patients with acute-phase flulike symptoms, rash, and history of tick bite may be confused with those having *Rocky Mountain spotted fever* (RMSF), which is also tickborne and produces an acute febrile illness with rash, musculoskeletal pain, headache, and gastrointestinal upset. However, the rash of RMSF is different, starting within a few days of the tick bite as an outbreak of small blanching macules on the wrists and ankles, spreading centripetally as well as to the palms and soles, and turning petechial after becoming generalized. *Summertime viral illnesses* enter into the differential diagnosis in patients who present with flulike symptoms but without erythema migrans or history of a tick bite.

Patients with symptoms and signs of meningeal irritation require careful evaluation. *Viral encephalitis* is among the summer viral illnesses that may present as headache, stiff neck, and mental changes. *Bacterial meningitis* must also be considered. The erythema migrans and concurrent Bell's palsy or radiculoneuritis of Lyme disease should help differentiate *B. burgdorferi* infection from other causes of meningeal irritation.

Late Disseminated and Chronic Stages. The presence of acute episodes of oligoarthritis raises the question of *gout, pseudogout,* and a *seronegative spondyloarthropathy* (eg, Reiter's syndrome, psoriatic arthritis, ankylosing spondylitis). At the time of the initial presentation, *infectious arthritis* also enters into the differential diagnosis. Even early *rheumatoid arthritis* may present as a monoarticular or oligoarticular disease involving a large joint. Associated clinical findings, serologic testing, and joint fluid analysis usually suffice to make the proper diagnosis (see Chapters 145 and 146).

The subtle neurologic and joint manifestations of late Lyme disease can cause considerable diagnostic confusion. *Depression, fibromyalgia,* and *chronic fatigue syndrome* have manifestations that overlap with Lyme disease. Clinicians encountering patients with these difficult conditions may overdiagnose Lyme disease, especially if too much emphasis is placed on serologic testing and too little on symptoms and signs (see below and Chapters 8, 159, and 227). Adding to the confusion is the possibility that, in some instances, Lyme disease may trigger a fibromyalgia syndrome.

WORKUP

In general, the diagnosis of Lyme disease is a clinical one, reinforced by a history of tick exposure in an endemic area and detection of antibody against *B. burgdorferi.*

Early Disease. A careful history and physical examination remain the best approach to the early diagnosis of Lyme disease. Antibody will not appear for several weeks, necessitating a clinical diagnosis at this stage of the illness. One asks about having recently been in a wooded, brushy, or grassy area of an endemic region, tick bite, rash, and a flulike illness in spring or summer. A history of tick bite is not necessary for diagnosis. (The nymph tick is very small, and its bite is easily missed.) Finding the characteristic annular lesion of *erythema migrans* is pathognomonic. It appears in 80 percent of patients. Most other clinical findings are nonspecific.

Disseminated Disease. In disseminated disease, the principal clues to the diagnosis continue to be clinical. In addition to epidemiologic inquiry, key historical features to review include new erythematous lesions, palpitations, near syncope, stiff neck, facial weakness, radicular pain, migratory musculoskeletal complaints, and later, frank oligoarticular arthritis, particularly of the knee. Physical findings of importance include the multiple annular erythematous skin lesions of *secondary erythema migrans,* irregular pulse, nuchal rigidity, facial palsy, and joint swelling with effusion. Suspicion of early disseminated Lyme disease is particularly high if the lesions of secondary erythema migrans are present.

Diagnosis can be facilitated by obtaining serum for *antibody testing,* but only in patients with clinical evidence of Lyme disease. In patients with meningeal signs, lumbar puncture should be considered. The CSF is sent for antibody testing as well as cell count, differential, and chemistries. Most patients with central nervous involvement have detectable antibody in the CSF, a pleocytosis, and elevated protein concentration. If there is a joint effusion, *arthrocentesis* is indicated. Polymerase chain reaction methods (PCR; see below) may become useful for linking *Borrelia* infection to the arthritis.

Late Disease. Diagnosis of late disease requires careful attention to the patient's musculoskeletal and neurologic symptoms. One checks for chronic oligoarticular arthritis (particularly of the knee), memory loss, spinal radicular pain, and distal paresthesias. Patients with findings suggestive of encephalopathy should have a *lumbar puncture* for antibody testing of the CSF, cell count, and chemistries. Peripheral polyneuropathy can be confirmed by *electrophysiologic study,* if necessary.

Differentiating Late Lyme Disease From Other Conditions. As noted earlier, *chronic fatigue syndrome* and *fibromyalgia* may be mistaken for Lyme disease. Tiredness and chronic neurologic and musculoskeletal complaints are common to all three. Clinical features that help to differentiate Lyme disease from the other two include 1) oligoarticular musculoskeletal complaints that include signs of joint inflammation; 2) limited and specific neurologic deficits (memory loss, distal paresthesias, radicular pain); 3) abnormalities on CSF examination and electromyography; and 4) absence of disordered sleep, chronic headache, depression, and tender points. Complicating differentiation are 1) Lyme disease's ability to trigger chronic fatigue syndrome and fibromyalgia; and 2) inadequate specificity of available diagnostic tests.

Diagnostic studies for *Borrelia* Infection. Direct confirmation of *Borrelia* infection by isolation of the spirochete remains difficult. One has had to settle for clinical findings and antibody testing. DNA detection methods are under development.

Antibody Testing. The most widely available serologic test for Lyme disease is the *enzyme-linked, immunosorbent assay (ELISA).* It detects both IgM and IgG antibodies to *B. burgdorferi.* In untreated persons, antibody titers become detectable several weeks into *Borrelia* infection and remain positive indefinitely. ELISA can also detect antibody in CSF. Hyperconcentration of antibody in the CSF is strong evidence for CNS infection.

ELISA antibody testing is sensitive, but not highly specific. Some *Borrelia* antigens are shared with other microorganisms. False-positive results have also been reported in normal persons and those with rheumatologic and neurologic diseases. Specificity can be improved by adding *Western blot* techniques to ELISA testing. Interlaboratory agreement is poor, because testing methods are not standardized. False-positives due to poor technique are common. False-negative test results are uncommon but can occur when patients are partially treated during early disease. The life-long persistence of antibodies, high test sensitivity, inadequate specificity, and lack of standardization make a positive ELISA test insufficient evidence for the diagnosis of active Lyme disease.

Minimizing False-Positive Results. One can minimize the chance of generating a false-positive ELISA result by restricting antibody testing to patients with at least an intermediate pretest probability of Lyme disease. The test is best used to confirm a clinically suspected case. Ordering a sensitive, insufficiently specific study in a person with a low pretest probability for the disease is likely to generate many more false positives than true positives (see Chapter 2). The overdiagnosis of Lyme disease has become a serious problem, leading to much unnecessary antibiotic therapy (see below). Use of a high-quality laboratory experienced in performing Lyme serology also helps to minimize false-positive results.

DNA Detection. Better diagnostic studies are needed to differentiate active from past infection in antibody-positive patients, as well as to distinguish a true-positive ELISA result from a false-positive one. Short of isolating the organism (which is difficult), one can attempt to detect its DNA. Under development is use of *polymerase chain reaction* technology to detect *Borrelia* DNA sequences in bodily fluids. Preliminary studies suggest it can be used to determine active infection in arthritic joints. Further testing is needed, but, if it proves effective, it may overcome the limitations of antibody testing.

PRINCIPLES OF MANAGEMENT

Antibiotics are effective against *B. burgdorferi.* Treatment is determined by stage of disease and type of clinical manifestation. *Doxycycline* and *amoxicillin* are preferred for oral treatment programs and *ceftriaxone* or *high-dose penicillin* when intravenous therapy is required. Optimal dose and duration of therapy continue to be the subject of study.

Table 160-1. Recommendations for Antibiotic Treatment*

Early Lyme Disease†
Doxycycline, 100 mg twice daily for 10 to 21 days
Amoxicillin, 500 mg three times daily for 10 to 21 days
Erythromycin, 250 mg four times daily for 10 to 21 days (less effective than doxycycline or amoxicillin)
Lyme Carditis
Ceftriaxone, 2 g daily intravenously for 14 days
Penicillin G, 20 million units intravenously for 14 days
Doxycycline, 100 mg orally twice daily for 14 to 21 days, may suffice‡
Amoxicillin, 500 mg orally three times daily for 14 to 21 days, may suffice‡
Neurologic Manifestations
Facial nerve paralysis
For an isolated finding, oral regimens for early disease, used for at least 21 days, may suffice.
For a finding associated with other neurologic manifestations, intravenous therapy (*see* below)
Lyme meningitis§
Ceftriaxone, 2 g daily by single dose for 14 to 21 days
Penicillin G, 20 million units daily in divided doses for 10 to 21 days
Possible alternatives for Lyme meningitis
Doxycycline, 100 mg orally or intravenously for 14 to 21 days
Chloramphenicol, 1 g intravenously every 6 hours for 10 to 21 days
Lyme Arthritis
Doxycycline, 100 mg orally twice daily for 30 days
Amoxicillin and probenecid, 500 mg each orally four times daily for 30 days
Penicillin G, 20 million units intravenously in divided doses daily for 14 to 21 days
Ceftriaxone, 2 g intravenously daily for 14 to 21 days
In Pregnant Women
For localized early Lyme disease, amoxicillin, 500 mg three times daily for 21 days
For disseminated early Lyme disease or any manifestation of late disease, penicillin G, 20 million units daily for 14 to 21 days
For asymptomatic seropositivity, no treatment necessary

These guidelines are to be modified by new findings and should always be applied with close attention to the clinical course of individual patients.

†Shorter courses are reserved for disease that is limited to a single skin lesion only.

‡Oral regimens are reserved for mild cardiac involvement (*see* text).

§Regimens for radiculononeuropathy, peripheral neuropathy, and encephalitis are the same as those for meningitis.

*From Rahn DW, Malawista SE. Lyme disease: recommendations for diagnosis and treatment. Ann Intern Med 1991;114:472.

Current recommendations are presented in Table 160-1. Response rates are excellent, but noninfectious sequelae may still develop in fully treated persons. Additional antibiotic therapy is without benefit in such persons.

Stage 1—Acute Infection

The earlier antibiotic treatment is instituted, the better the outcome and the lower the risks of dissemination and chronic disease. One should treat based on clinical findings and not wait for antibody tests to turn positive, because ELISA positivity may not occur for several weeks. Doxycycline and amoxicillin are the agents of choice. Duration of therapy ranges from 10 to 21 days, depending on severity of symptoms and rapidity of response.

Stage 2—Disseminated Disease

In disseminated disease, it is common for a host of organ systems to be involved, although treatment recommendations are by organ system and clinical presentation. If more than one is involved, then the most potent antibiotic program takes precedence.

Cardiac involvement is a potentially worrisome form of disseminated disease. Although heart block is usually self-limited, patients with a PR interval in excess of 0.4 seconds are commonly treated with intravenous antibiotics (ceftriaxone or high-dose penicillin) to prevent significant myocardial invasion. For those with a shorter PR interval, oral doxycycline or amoxicillin prescribed for 10 to 21 days suffices.

Neurologic Involvement. Although most neurologic manifestations of disseminated disease will eventually clear without treatment, antibiotic therapy is strongly recommended, both to shorten duration of symptoms and to prevent sequelae.

Facial Nerve Palsy. In the absence of evidence for meningitis, treatment can be oral with doxycycline or amoxicillin for 3 to 4 weeks.

Meningitis. Antibiotic therapy produces a prompt clinical response and shortens the clinical course substantially. Both intravenous ceftriaxone and high-dose penicillin G are curative. Ceftriaxone is much more expensive, but its once-daily schedule makes home administration possible and obviates a prolonged hospitalization. Lumbar puncture with CSF analysis is needed to confirm the diagnosis but not to assess response to treatment. Duration of therapy is best determined by clinical response. Most authorities recommend 2 weeks.

Polyneuropathy. Peripheral neuropathy and radiculopathy tend to occur in conjunction with meningitis and respond well to its treatment. When there is no clinical or CSF evidence of meningitis, an oral program of either doxycycline or amoxicillin for 3 weeks is a reasonable alternative.

Arthritis. The migratory musculoskeletal pains and brief attacks of oligoarticular arthritis are typically self-limited, but antibiotic therapy is given to halt symptoms and prevent progression to chronic arthritis. The optimal antibiotic program has not been established. The development of chronic arthritis and its persistence despite prolonged courses of antibiotics have led to antibiotic regimens of increased duration. Thirty days of oral doxycycline or amoxicillin (with probenecid to delay urinary excretion) is often recommended, with intravenous therapy reserved for more refractory chronic arthritis (see below). Intraarticular steroids are to be avoided because they increase the risk of antibiotic failure.

Stage 3—Chronic Disease. Late disease tends to be more difficult to treat, with responsiveness to antibiotics often less impressive than that for disseminated disease. This has led to prolonged and repeated courses of antibiotics. Inability to distinguish infectious from noninfectious sequelae has hindered design of treatment programs. With the advent of DNA detection techniques, it should be possible to make more pathophysiologically correct treatment recommendations. Hopefully, etiologic therapy will become available to persons with noninfectious sequelae.

Arthritis. Treatment is 30 days of oral doxycycline or amoxicillin (plus probenecid) or 2 to 3 weeks of intravenous ceftriaxone or penicillin G. Retreatment may be necessary, but only if there is objective evidence of persistent infection (eg, PCR testing of synovial fluid remains positive).

Encephalopathy. Lyme patients who develop documentable memory or cognitive deficits in conjunction with elevations in CSF protein and antibody are candidates for antibiotic therapy. The program is identical to that for meningitis. Incomplete resolution is sometimes noted, and retreatment is carried out. It is unclear whether the etiology in such cases is infectious or not. PCR testing of the CSF may prove useful in making this distinction but remains to be evaluated.

Patients with the neuropsychiatric symptoms of chronic fatigue syndrome or fibromyalgia often request treatment for Lyme disease, especially if they test antibody-positive. Those who have no clinical evidence for Lyme disease do not respond meaningfully to antibiotic therapy and should not be prescribed it, even if they are antibody-positive. Whether the occasional fibromyalgia or chronic fatigue patient whose illness appears to be directly precipitated by Lyme disease will respond is unclear, but it is unlikely if the mechanism is noninfectious.

The Pregnant Patient. Maternal–fetal transmission of infection with subsequent injury to the fetus has been reported. Antibiotic treatment should be instituted promptly in symptomatic patients. For localized early disease in which erythema migrans is the only symptom, the recommended treatment is oral amoxicillin for 3 weeks. For more disseminated disease, intravenous high-dose penicillin G is required for 2 to 3 weeks. No increased risk of fetal malformation has been found in asymptomatic women who are antibody positive. Screening asymptomatic pregnant women for Lyme antibody and treating those who test positive are not warranted.

Prophylactic Therapy After Tick Bite. Prophylactic antibiotics after a tick bite are generally not advised. It takes 24 hours from the time of tick contact with the skin to transmit the spirochete. Persons who discover a tick usually do so before that time and remove it before transmission can occur. Under such circumstances, the risk of infection is about the same as that of an adverse or hypersensitivity drug reaction. A better approach might be to wait for development of symptoms (eg, erythema migrans) and then treat promptly those who become symptomatic.

PATIENT EDUCATION AND INDICATIONS FOR REFERRAL

Patients who suspect but do not have Lyme disease require as much education about the condition as those who do. The person with depression, chronic fatigue syndrome, or fibromyalgia who insists on treatment for Lyme disease needs to know how the diagnosis is made. Those who are antibody-positive will benefit from a discussion of the minimal significance of a positive antibody test in the absence of other defining clinical manifestations. While explaining that the probability of active Lyme disease is very low, care must be taken not to deny the reality and severity of the person's symptoms. Attention should be directed to treatment of their underlying condition (see Chapters 8, 159, and 227).

Persons living or visiting in an area endemic for Lyme disease should be instructed to venture into tick-infested areas only after application of insect repellent and with skin surfaces covered by protective clothing. In addition, they should be taught to recognize the rash and other manifestations of early Lyme disease and the importance of early treatment.

Patients with Lyme disease benefit from knowing the excellent responsiveness of their condition to antibiotic therapy and its very favorable prognosis. However, those who have protracted symptoms unresponsive to antibiotic therapy and in the absence of evidence for persistent infection should be informed there is the possibility of a noninfectious pathogenesis that is usually self-limited but slow to resolve. Hopefully, more etiologic therapy will be available for such persons in the future.

Referral is indicated when the patient with strong clinical evidence of Lyme disease fails to respond to a course of appropriate antibiotic therapy. Consultation is particularly important for those with refractory neurologic deficits or debilitating arthritis.

A.H.G.

ANNOTATED BIBLIOGRAPHY

American College of Rheumatology and the Council of the Infectious Diseases Society of America. Appropriateness of parenteral antibiotic treatment for patients with presumed Lyme disease. Ann Intern Med 1993;119;518. *(A consensus statement recommending treatment for those with clinical evidence for Lyme disease and no treatment for those with nonspecific symptoms, even if accompanied by a positive serology.)*

Dinerman H, Steere AC. Lyme disease associated with fibromyalgia. Ann Intern Med 1992;117:281. *(Lyme disease often confused with fibromyalgia.)*

Lightfoot RW, Luft BJ, Rahn DW, et al. Empiric parenteral antibiotic treatment of patients with fibromyalgia and fatigue and a positive serologic result for Lyme disease. Ann Intern Med 1993;119:503. *(In most instances, antibiotic therapy is not cost-effective.)*

Logigian EL, Kaplan RF, Steere AC. Chronic neurologic manifestations of Lyme disease. N Engl J Med 1990;323:1438. *(Memory loss, radiculopathy, and leukoencephalitis described.)*

Malane MS, Grant-Kels JM, Fecer HM Jr, et al. Diagnosis of Lyme disease based on dermatologic manifestations. Ann Intern Med 1991;114:490. *(Excellent photographs and discussion of these findings, which are often pathognomonic.)*

Nocton JJ, Dressler F, Rutledge BJ, et al. Detection of *Borrelia burgdorferi* DNA by polymerase chain reaction in synovial fluid from patients with Lyme arthritis. N Engl J Med 1994;330:229. *(Use of an improved diagnostic method; suggests late arthritis is not due to persistence of organisms in the joint.)*

Rahn DW, Malawista SE. Lyme disease: Recommendations for diagnosis and treatment. Ann Intern Med 1991;114:472. *(Most useful for its discussion of antibiotic programs.)*

Steere AC, Dwyer E, Winchester R. Association of chronic Lyme arthritis with HLA-DR4 and HLA-DR2 alleles. N Engl J Med

1990;323:219. *(Evidence for genetic susceptibility to chronic arthritis unresponsive to antibiotic therapy.)*

Steere AC, Schoen RT, Taylor E. The clinical evolution of Lyme arthritis. Ann Intern Med 1987;107:725. *(Best study of the natural history of the disease; examined untreated patients.)*

Steere AC, Taylor E, McHugh GL, et al. The overdiagnosis of Lyme disease. JAMA 1993;269:1812. *(The problem results from false-positive serology.)*

Primary Care Medicine: Office Evaluation and Management of the Adult Patient, 3rd edition, edited by Allan H. Goroll, Lawrence A. May, and Albert G. Mulley, Jr. J.B. Lippincott Company, Philadelphia

161

Approach to the Patient With Polymyalgia Rheumatica or Temporal Arteritis

Polymyalgia rheumatica (PMR) is a common nonarticular rheumatoid disease characterized by neck, shoulder-girdle, and hip-girdle complaints and an elevated erythrocyte sedimentation rate (ESR). It mostly affects Caucasian patients over age 50, with a 2:1 female predominance. Annual incidence in persons over age 50 is 5 per 10,000; prevalence is 50 per 10,000. The condition is usually self-limited, but an occasional PMR patient goes on to develop temporal arteritis. The pathogenetic relationship remains unknown, but up to 40 percent of temporal arteritis patients have a prior history of PMR. Temporal arteritis (also referred to as "cranial," "giant-cell," or "granulomatous" arteritis) is a vasculitic disorder of unknown origin that can cause sudden blindness. It too is limited to persons over age 50. Incidence and prevalence are about one-fifth that of PMR. Women are more often affected than men.

The primary physician needs to be alert to these diseases, which can be subtle in presentation and easily dismissed as vague functional complaints or confused with other conditions. The associated risk of blindness makes prompt recognition and treatment of temporal arteritis especially critical. Because treatment requires chronic glucocorticosteroid therapy, it is just as important to avoid a false-positive diagnosis.

PATHOPHYSIOLOGY, CLINICAL PRESENTATION, AND COURSE

Polymyalgia Rheumatica

The pathogenesis of PMR is unknown, but a genetic susceptibility has been suggested by an association with the HLA-DR4 allele. Onset is gradual over weeks or months. Bilateral pain and stiffness of periarticular structures of *neck* and *shoulders* is the presentation in two-thirds of cases, with *hip* and *thigh* involvement accounting for the other third. Many complain of both shoulder and thigh involvement. *Morning stiffness* and pain with movement are highly characteristic. Synovitis has been documented histologically. Muscle biopsies are usually normal or show minor inflammatory infiltrates; muscle strength is unimpaired. Low-grade *fever, weight loss,* and *fatigue* may accompany the musculoskeletal symptoms. The *ESR* is almost always elevated, often markedly.

PMR tends to be either a self-limited illness of about a year's duration or a chronic persistent problem lasting several years. There are no clinical features that are predictive. An occasional patient with no evidence of cranial arteritis at initial presentation goes on to develop temporal arteritis; estimates of risk average 10 percent to 15 percent. However, a PMR patient who develops headache, jaw claudication, tender cranial artery, or visual complaints has a markedly increased probability of temporal arteritis (see below). The risk of PMR patients on corticosteroid therapy developing temporal arteritis appears to be small.

Temporal Arteritis

Temporal arteritis is a vasculitic condition of unknown origin, characterized pathologically by histiocytic, lymphocytic, and giant cell infiltrations of the walls of medium or large arteries originating from the aortic arch. Any one of these vessels can be involved, but those of the head are most often affected. The internal elastic lamina is fragmented in conjunction with proliferation. The inflammatory process tends to be segmental. Many characteristics of an autoimmune process are present, but the precise pathophysiology remains to be elucidated. Like PMR, there is an association with HLA-DR4, suggesting a genetic predisposition. Direct inflammation of the arterial wall and resultant ischemia secondary to vasculitic narrowing account for most symptoms.

Onset is gradual. Early symptoms include headache, low-grade temperature, and the aching and stiffness of PMR. *Headache* is reported in about 70 percent of cases and is the initial symptom in about 35 percent. The pain can be piercing or throbbing, often localized to the arteries of the scalp and unlike any previous headache. *Polymyalgia* symptoms may be the presenting manifestation in upward of 50 percent. *Constitutional symptoms* of fatigue, malaise, anorexia, and weight loss occur in the majority of patients.

As the condition progresses, *cranial artery tenderness* and/or enlargement may be noted. The temporal artery is most commonly affected, but any cranial artery may become involved. Ischemic symptoms such as *masseter claudication* (jaw pain with chewing) occur in one-third to one-half of patients.

Visual manifestations are due to vasculitis of the ophthalmic or posterior ciliary arteries. *Blindness* is the most dreaded manifestation, with abrupt onset and irreversible course unless treated very aggressively and very early (see below). Vision loss is sometimes preceded by transient visual symptoms, such as amaurosis fugax, flashing lights, or field defects. In untreated patients, visual loss occurs in up to 50 percent of cases. Acute *hearing loss* and *vertigo* have also been reported. An *aortic arch syndrome* may occur if there is involvement of the arch or a major branch vessel.

A *markedly increased ESR* is characteristic of the disease; a normal sedimentation rate in the absence of strongly suggestive symptoms makes the diagnosis unlikely. A low-grade *anemia of chronic disease* and mild elevations in *liver function tests* are often present as well.

Temporal arteritis is a chronic illness that may last for years. Although it tends to be self-limited, the clinical course is highly variable. Late disease complications are rare, but attempts to take patients off therapy are often met by relapses.

DIAGNOSIS

Polymyalgia Rheumatica. The diagnosis is a clinical one. Criteria include 1) bilateral pain for at least 1 month in any two of the following: neck, shoulder girdle, hip girdle, in association with morning stiffness; 2) ESR more than 40 mm per hour by the Westergren method; 3) age over 50 years; 4) exclusion of other diagnoses except for temporal arteritis; 5) marked clinical improvement in response to 1 week of less than 15 mg/d of prednisone.

Temporal Arteritis. The current American College of Rheumatology criteria for diagnosis of giant-cell (temporal) arteritis include 1) age at onset of symptoms *over 50 years*; 2) new onset or new type of localized *headache*; 3) temporal *artery tenderness* or diminished pulse; 4) *ESR more than 50 mm per hour* by the Westergren method; and 5) *temporal artery biopsy* showing mononuclear infiltration or granulomatous infiltration with giant cells. The presence of any three criteria constitutes evidence for the diagnosis of temporal arteritis (sensitivity 93.5%; specificity 91.2%). The absence of some characteristic symptoms and signs from the criteria list is due to their lack of sensitivity or specificity.

Temporal artery biopsy is the most invasive of the diagnostic criteria and sometimes a source of concern to patients. It is done under local anesthesia as an ambulatory procedure, and morbidity is very low. Best results are obtained by selecting an accessible cranial artery that feels tender or has a diminished pulse (not due to atherosclerotic disease). The temporal artery is usually selected. A 2- to 4-cm specimen is optimal because the inflammatory process may be focal and may demonstrate skip areas. A single biopsy has a sensitivity of about 90 percent. A negative first biopsy does not rule out the diagnosis.

Treatment with corticosteroids before biopsy may lower test sensitivity, but probably not by so much as to preclude immediate therapy followed by biopsy within the first 1 to 2 weeks of therapy. Some authorities suggest that biopsy can be omitted altogether when clinical evidence for temporal arteritis is compelling. However, most argue that histologic confirmation should be obtained when committing a person to such potentially morbid therapy as long-term daily corticosteroids. Biopsy is unnecessary when it will have no effect on clinical decision making.

Patients who are biopsy-negative and do not manifest sufficient clinical evidence for the diagnosis of temporal arteritis have an excellent prognosis, with fewer than 10 percent developing signs of arteritis at a later time.

Arteriography is sensitive but nonspecific and unreliable diagnostically, although helpful in choosing an area to biopsy if the first biopsy was negative.

PRINCIPLES OF MANAGEMENT

Temporal Arteritis

To establish control of the disease quickly and reduce the risk of blindness, it is necessary to begin treatment with *high-dose glucocorticosteroid* therapy. Biopsy confirmation of the diagnosis should be obtained before committing the patient to a long-term course of steroids. However, treatment can be initiated before biopsy when concern about vasculitic injury is high, provided the diagnosis is clinically evident and biopsy is obtained within 1 to 2 weeks. In most instances, response starts within 24 hours of initiating treatment.

Initiation of Therapy. The optimal starting oral program is 40 to 60 mg of *prednisone*/d. *Daily therapy* is needed; an alternate-day schedule does not control the arteritis. The initial doses can be given parenterally when there is concern about visual compromise, but parenteral treatment must be started within the first several hours of visual impairment. Ophthalmologists recommend 5 days of high-dose parenteral *methylprednisolone* (1000 mg IV q12h).

Tapering. The steroid dose is titrated against symptoms and sedimentation rate. To minimize the adverse effects of chronic daily steroid therapy (see Chapter 105), the daily prednisone dose should be tapered, starting after clinical and laboratory manifestations have normalized. Tapering can be steady but should not be precipitous. Rapid prednisone tapering to less than 20 mg/d over the first 1 to 2 months is associated with a 30 percent relapse rate. More reasonable is tapering to a daily dose of 20 to 30 mg within the first 2 months and more slowly thereafter. The goal is a maintenance dose of less than 10 mg/d, but it may take over a year to achieve it.

Monitoring and Termination of Therapy. As dose is reduced, the patient must be monitored for recurrence of *symptoms* and elevation of the *sedimentation rate*. Most patients require treatment for 2 to 3 years. Relapses occur in up to 50 percent of patients who attempt termination of therapy before that time. Nonetheless, the risk of blindness and other serious disease-related complications is minimal late in the course of disease and a trial of discontinuing therapy can be attempted every 6 to 12 months after the first year. The trial should be halted at the first sign of symptoms recurring or ESR markedly rising. Close monitoring for relapse is essential during the first 12 months off therapy. Despite tapering efforts, many patients experience steroid-related side effects because of the prolonged duration of daily steroid therapy. To minimize adrenal suppression, prednisone should be taken once daily in the morning (see Chapter 105). Efforts to limit osteoporosis should also be undertaken (see Chapter 164).

Polymyalgia Rheumatica

PMR in the absence of temporal arteritis responds quickly and well to modest doses of *prednisone* (10 to 15 mg/d). As the sedimentation rate falls and symptoms clear, one can begin tapering prednisone in small decrements (1 to 2 mg). Some patients can be switched to a *nonsteroidal antiinflammatory agent* (see Chapter 156) or alternate-day steroid therapy, but control of symptoms may not be sufficient. Months to years of daily low-dose steroid therapy may be required. To minimize adverse effects from daily steroids, the lowest possible dose of prednisone should be used (often 5–7 mg). These dosages do not protect the patient from the complications of temporal arteritis and require adjustment should vasculitic symptoms occur.

PATIENT EDUCATION

Patients with PMR in the absence of temporal arteritis can be reassured. They benefit from knowing that the risk of developing temporal arteritis is small, that there is no progression to disabling arthritis, and that their condition is self-limited, although it may take a few years to clear. They should be instructed to watch for symptoms of temporal arteritis and report them promptly. The adverse effects of corticosteroid therapy need to be reviewed so patients will use prednisone carefully and as directed.

Patients with temporal arteritis and their families must understand the rationale for daily prednisone therapy as well as its adverse side effects, both to ensure compliance and to provide an informed basis for long-term steroid use. Instruction in the means for minimizing steroid side effects is appreciated (see Chapter 105). Reassurance can be given that the serious complications of temporal arteritis can be avoided by proper therapy.

INDICATIONS FOR REFERRAL AND ADMISSION

Prompt consultation with a rheumatologist is helpful if one is considering initiation of high-dose steroid therapy for presumed temporal arteritis before temporal artery biopsy can be obtained. Urgent ophthalmologic evaluation is needed if visual impairment is reported. If it is not available, one can proceed directly to hospitalization for immediate institution of high-dose parenteral corticosteroid therapy. Rheumatologic consultation is also indicated to consider need for steroid therapy when cranial artery biopsy is negative but clinical presentation is strongly suggestive of temporal arteritis. The occasional patient with PMR or temporal arteritis who does not respond adequately to steroid therapy also requires referral for reconsideration of the diagnosis as well as use of other forms of immunosuppressive therapy (eg, azathioprine, cyclophosphamide, dapsone).

THERAPEUTIC RECOMMENDATIONS

Temporal Arteritis

- Begin therapy with daily high-dose glucocorticosteroids (eg, prednisone, 40 to 60 mg qam). Consider using intravenous methylprednisolone (1000 mg q12h × 5 days) for patients who present with visual disturbances.
- Begin reducing initial dose once the sedimentation rate has been normalized (<40 mm per hour) and symptoms have cleared, aiming after 1 to 2 months for a daily prednisone dose of 20 to 30 mg.
- Continue daily prednisone therapy, tapering slowly as tolerated over 12 to 18 months to the minimum dose sufficient to keep the sedimentation rate normal and the patient free of symptoms; a prednisone dose of less than 10 mg/d will often suffice.
- Monitor symptoms and sedimentation rate to determine rate and extent of tapering permissible. Halt tapering if ESR rises or symptoms return.
- Continue daily steroids for 18 to 24 months; consider a trial of phasing out therapy at that time and then every 6 to 12 months.
- After cessation, continue to monitor for recurrence of symptoms and rise in sedimentation rate over the next 12 months.

Polymyalgia Rheumatica

- Begin with low-dose prednisone (10–15 mg/d), provided there is no evidence of temporal arteritis.
- Taper once symptoms have resolved and the ESR has normalized; determine the lowest dose that controls symptoms and ESR (usually less than 10 mg/d).
- Consider a trial of switching within 4 to 6 weeks to a nonsteroidal antiinflammatory agent (eg, ibuprofen 400 mg tid or naproxen 375 mg bid) or to alternate-day steroids to avoid the side effects of chronic daily steroid therapy.
- If switching does not suffice, continue with the lowest possible dose of daily prednisone for 12 months, then try phasing out steroid therapy while monitoring symptoms and ESR; some patients may require prolonged treatment.
- Instruct the patient to report promptly any symptoms suggestive of temporal arteritis (eg, visual disturbances, tender cranial artery, headache).

A.H.G.

ANNOTATED BIBLIOGRAPHY

Ayoub WT, Franklin CM, Torretti D. Polymyalgia rheumatica: Duration of therapy and long-term outcome. Am J Med 1985;79:309. *(Some have a 6- to 12-month course; others require therapy for years.)*

Casselli RJ, Hunder GG, Whisnant JP. Neurologic disease in biopsy-proven giant cell (temporal) arteritis. Neurology 1988; 38:352. *(Findings include acute vertigo and hearing loss as well as visual loss.)*

Chmelewski WL, McKnight KM, Agudelo CA, et al. Presenting features and outcomes in patients undergoing temporal artery biopsy. Arch Intern Med 1992;152:1690. *(Presenting features did not always predict biopsy results; late disease complications were rare, but prolonged therapy was required.)*

Hall S, Persellin S, Lie JT et al. The therapeutic impact of temporal artery biopsy. Lancet 1983;2:1217. *(Helped in decision making; fewer than 10 percent with a negative biopsy developed signs of arteritis or required steroid therapy.)*

Hunder GG, Bloch DA, Michel BA, et al. The American College of Rheumatology criteria for the classification of giant cell arteritis. Arthritis Rheum 1990;33:1122. *(Consensus diagnostic criteria.)*

Hunder GG, Sheps SG, Allen GL, Joyce JW. Daily and alternate-day corticosteroid regimens in the treatment of giant cell arteritis. Ann Intern Med 1975;82:613. *(Alternate-day steroids do not suffice.)*

Klein RG, Hunder GG, Stanson AW, et al. Large artery involvement in giant cell (temporal) arteritis. Ann Intern Med 1975; 83:806. *(Temporal arteritis need not be limited to the cranial arteries.)*

Kyle V, Cawston TE, Hazleman BL. Erythrocyte sedimentation rate and C-reactive protein in the assessment of polymyalgia rheumatica/giant cell arteritis on presentation and during follow up. Ann Rheum Dis 1989;48:667. *(ESR closely parallels disease severity and activity in most cases.)*

Kyle V, Hazleman BL. Stopping steroids in polymyalgia rheumatica and giant cell arteritis: Treatment usually lasts for two to five years. Br Med J 1990;300:344. *(Required duration of therapy can be prolonged.)*

Kyle V, Hazleman BL. Treatment of polymyalgia rheumatica and giant cell arteritis I: Steroid regimens in the first two months. Ann Rheum Dis 1989;48:658. *(High dose required initially, then can be reduced.)*

Layfer LF, Banner BF, Huckman MS, et al. Temporal arteriography. Arthritis Rheum 1978;21:780. *(Arteriography is a highly sensitive but nonspecific.)*

Machado EB, Michet CJ, Ballard DJ, et al. Trends in incidence and clinical presentation of temporal arteritis in Olmstead County, Minnesota, 1950–1985. Arthritis Rheum 1988;31:745. *(Best epidemiologic data; clinical features changing; earlier detection.)*

Ponge T, Barrier JH, Grolleau JY, et al. The efficacy of selective unilateral temporal artery biopsy versus bilateral biopsies for diagnosis of giant cell arteritis. J Rheumatol 1988;15:997. *(Bilateral biopsy is sometimes necessary, but careful selection can obviate the need for routinely ordering biopsies of two sites.)*

Robb-Nicholson C, Chang RW, Anderson S, et al. Diagnostic value of the history and physical examination in giant cell arteritis. J Rheumatol 1988;15:1793. *(Clusters of symptoms had a high sensitivity, but specificity was lacking.)*

Rosenfeld SI, Kosmorsky GS, Klingele TG, et al. Treatment of temporal arteritis with ocular involvement. Am J Med 1986;80:143. *(High-dose intravenous steroids given acutely for 5 days offer a chance at visual recovery if started early.)*

Sox HC, Liang MW. The erythrocyte sedimentation rate. Ann Intern Med 1986;104:515. *(Useful for diagnosis and monitoring response to therapy.)*

Wong RL, Korn JH. Temporal arteritis without an elevated sedimentation rate. Am J Med 1986;80:959. *(A negative ESR does not rule out the diagnosis when other characteristic features are present.)*

162

Management of Paget's Disease

SAMUEL R. NUSSBAUM, M.D.

Primary Care Medicine: Office Evaluation and Management of the Adult Patient, 3rd edition, edited by Allan H. Goroll, Lawrence A. May, and Albert G. Mulley, Jr. J.B. Lippincott Company, Philadelphia

Paget's disease of bone, or osteitis deformans, is a focal disorder of unknown etiology characterized by deformity of the bone's external contour and internal structure that results from excessive resorption and rapid new bone formation. The incidence of Paget's disease is 3.3 percent in autopsy series and 0.1 percent to 4.0 percent in radiologic studies. The clinical presentation is variable. In the majority of cases, the diagnosis is made when the patient is asymptomatic. An elevated alkaline phosphatase is discovered on multiphasic screening, or x-rays of the pelvis, vertebrae, or skull show the hallmark radiolucent (osteolytic) areas with compensatory new bone formation. Symptomatic patients report pain in the back or lower extremities, disturbances of gait, increasing head size, hearing loss, and occasionally symptoms related to high output cardiac failure. The primary physician needs to be able to provide symptomatic relief and to know when to use agents that suppress osteoclastic activity.

PATHOPHYSIOLOGY AND CLINICAL PRESENTATION

The pathophysiologic hallmarks of Paget's disease are *excessive osteoclastic destruction* and resorption of bone, followed by *unregulated osteoblastic new bone formation*. The initial stimulus for bone resorption remains unknown, but the process culminates in an abnormal pattern of lamellar bone. There is excessive local vascularity and an increase in fibrous tissue, which extends into the marrow. Both cortical as well as cancellous bone may be involved, each with several foci at different stages. The resultant bone, which is mechanically defective, distorted, and enlarged, leads to the cardinal manifestation of Paget's disease: bone pain and pathologic fractures.

Clinical Presentation. Although any bone may become involved, the common sites are *spine, pelvis, skull, femur,* and *tibia*. Most patients are asymptomatic, with Paget's disease presenting as an incidental finding on x-ray or as an isolated elevation in alkaline phosphatase. Those who are symptomatic present with bone pain, bony deformity, fracture, or a complication of increased marrow vascularity or bony encroachment on neural structures.

Bone pain may occur from fracture or may be independent of it. In the latter instance, it is usually located over lytic areas of bone where active osteoclastic resorption is taking place. Severity does not always parallel the extent of radiographic involvement. Exacerbating factors include weight bearing, muscular activity, and cold weather.

Fractures may affect the long bones or vertebrae. The *lesser trochanter* of the femur and in the upper third of the *tibia* are characteristic sites for long bone fractures. A history of trauma can usually be elicited, but some of these fractures may occur spontaneously. Pain may result, but not always. Most vertebral fractures occur in the lumbar and sacral regions. They are usually painless, but can lead to loss of height, kyphoscoliosis, and, in rare instances, spinal cord compression.

Bony deformity and encroachment are most notable in the *skull,* which may become visibly enlarged in the frontal and occipital regions. The overlying superficial blood vessels often become prominently dilated and visibly pulsatile. *Hearing loss* can ensue from involvement of the ossicles in the middle ear, which impinge on the eighth cranial nerve in the temporal bone. Cerebellar and long-tract signs are complications of posterior fossa encroachment. Vertebral encroachment on the *spinal cord* or nerve *roots* is rare but can cause a compression syndrome, including paraplegia. Deformity of the *long bones* is manifest as anterolateral bowing; it contributes to susceptibility to fracture.

Degenerative joint disease of the hip can become a major problem in patients with long-standing subchondral bone involvement in the acetabulum and femoral head. It leads to protrusio acetabuli. Degenerative disease of the knee joint may occur in similar fashion if the distal femur or patella becomes pagetic. Extensive and severe skeletal involvement increases the risk of *osteogenic sarcoma,* a uniformly fatal cancer suffered by less than 1 percent of pagetic patients. It is heralded by localized pain and bony enlargement and occurs more frequently in the upper extremities and skull of patients over age 50.

Hyperuricemia leading to gouty arthritis and *hypercalciuria* leading to renal calculi are among the biochemical consequences of disrupted bony metabolism. *Hypercalcemia* can be precipitated by immobilization. *High output heart failure* may occur in patients with extensive Paget's disease due to the marked increase in vascular bed.

Laboratory and Radiographic Features. Serum *alkaline phosphatase,* produced by osteoblasts, is elevated, as is the *urinary hydroxyproline* excretion, an index of osteoclastic resorption of bone matrix. A technetium *bone scan* may show areas of increased uptake, even before diagnostic changes are visible on *standard x-rays.* The first radiologic bony changes occur in the lytic phase and are well-demarcated areas of decalcification (seen best in the skull). With onset of new bone formation, areas of increased density become evident, as well as expansion of bone and coarse trabeculation. In later phases there is sclerosis, enlargement, and increased bone density. Radiologic changes are most commonly evident in the pelvis, femur, and skull.

Clinical Course. Although many patients manifest slow radiologic progression, most never develop symptoms. Others are noted to have radiologic changes that remain stable; a few have rapidly progressive disease.

PRINCIPLES OF THERAPY

Most patients with Paget's disease are asymptomatic and require no specific therapy. Localized mild bone pain can be controlled with *analgesics.* Joint involvement usually responds to the *antiinflammatory agents* commonly used for arthritis (see Chapter 156). Treatment of more disabling Paget's disease is carried out using agents that specifically inhibit bone resorption. Calcitonin and etidronate have been the mainstays of specific outpatient treatment of Paget's disease. They decrease osteoclastic resorption and lead to radiographic and clinical improvement.

Indications for Specific Therapy. Although there are no universal criteria for initiation of specific therapy, indications include: 1) severe pain in pagetic areas; 2) compression of medulla, cauda equina, or auditory nerve with neurologic deficit; 3) high-output cardiac failure; 4) hypercalcemia due to immobilization; 5) marked radiographic lytic lesions in long bones and skull representing risk of fracture or brain trauma; 6) multiple fractures; 7) prevention of disfigurement when the skull is extensively involved; 8) recurrent renal calculi due to hypercalciuria; 9) severe hyperuricemia and gout; 10) prophylaxis accompanying extensive orthopedic surgery to reduce vascularity of bone; and 11) prophylaxis when disease is of early onset in an area in which disabling deformity is likely to occur.

Calcitonin. Calcitonin is most useful for patients with severe involvement that includes not only marked pain, but also nerve compression, fracture, or bony deformity. Urinary hydroxyproline starts to decline within a few days of onset of therapy followed a few weeks later by reduction in alkaline phosphatase and then clinical improvement. Biochemical and clinical remission are achieved in one-third of patients, improvement is noted in another third, and minimal or unsustained response in the balance of cases.

Synthetic salmon and human calcitonin preparations are commercially available. The salmon calcitonin preparation is the most widely used and much less expensive, differing by just one amino acid from human calcitonin. Although up to 50 percent of patients manifest neutralizing antibodies to synthetic salmon calcitonin, the risk of clinically important inactivation is small. Remission can be reestablished by switching to human calcitonin.

The major disadvantages of calcitonin are nausea (in some patients), cost, and the need for parenteral administration. Therapy is not only expensive but requires patient education and ability to learn self-injection techniques. Calcitonin dosage may be reduced when the disease is in remission. Current data suggest that a low dose needs to be continued indefinitely to prevent relapse.

Disodium Etidronate (EHDP). Etidronate is a bisphosphonate that effectively inhibits bone resorption. It is particularly useful in patients who develop pain insufficiently controlled by analgesics and antiinflammatory agents. It has the advantage of being an oral therapy that is well tolerated except for some mild diarrhea. Treatment is given until biochemical and clinical remissions occur, then it is discontinued; it is restarted if there is a relapse. Remissions achieved can last from 6 months to as long as 2 years. About 85 percent of patients have either a prolonged remission from a single course of therapy or respond well to retreatment. The remainder, who manifest more severe disease, relapse more quickly and become unresponsive to retreatment.

One disadvantage of etidronate therapy that occurs in a few patients is a temporary, paradoxical worsening of symptoms. Prolonged therapy or higher doses (10–20 mg/kg/d) induce a mineralization defect that may lead to increased fracture rates in areas of lytic bone, as well as worsening bone pain. Thus, EHDP should not be used for more than 6 consecutive months, nor at a dose greater than 5 mg/kg/d.

Newer bisphosphonates that are as effective as etidronate but do not produce a mineralization defect are being tested.

Cytotoxic Agents. *Mithramycin* and *dactinomycin* represent cytotoxic agents that potently suppress bone resorption. They are administered intravenously for patients with serious complications of Paget's disease, such as severe high-output heart failure or hypercalcemic crisis. Hospitalization and consultation are required for proper use because of the risks of acute although reversible renal, hepatic, and hematologic toxicities. Thrombocytopenia can be particularly severe.

Surgery. Neurosurgical intervention is necessary in patients with spinal cord or nerve root compression syndromes. Orthopedic procedures such as total hip replacement and tibial or femoral osteotomy may help to restore mobility.

Monitoring Therapy. Two baseline measurements of serum *alkaline phosphatase* should be obtained before therapy, followed by monthly determinations during treatment. Skeletal *x-rays* are also helpful to have at the commencement of therapy. They are not repeated routinely, but can be helpful when there is suspicion of a complication (eg, fracture, degenerative joint disease). The technetium *bone scan* provides an alternative baseline measure.

PATIENT EDUCATION AND INDICATIONS FOR REFERRAL

Patients should be instructed to drink at least 2 liters of liquid daily, especially if they are unable to keep active, because immobilization and dehydration can precipitate hypercalcemia and renal stone formation. Patients who are candidates for calcitonin therapy require detailed teaching by the nurse in the techniques of subcutaneous injection. Confirmation of proper technique should be obtained before prescribing self-administration, unless another household member is going to be administering the medication.

Hospital admission and prompt neurosurgical consultation are warranted in patients who have evidence of nerve or cord compression. Admission is also indicated for severe hypercalcemia. Orthopedic surgical consultation is indicated for the person severely limited by pagetic degenerative joint disease of the hip or knee. Consultation with an endocrinologist or rheumatologist is needed for consideration of initiating specific therapy in the asymptomatic patient with radiologic or biochemical evidence of advancing disease. Referral is beneficial when standard courses of etidronate and calcitonin fail to achieve remission and when relapse occurs.

TREATMENT RECOMMENDATIONS

- Asymptomatic patients require no treatment but should be seen at yearly intervals for clinical assessment and alkaline phosphatase measurement.
- Prescribe aspirin or another nonsteroidal antiinflammatory drug (see Chapter 156) for relief of mild to moderate pain due to localized bony involvement or degenerative joint disease.
- Begin etidronate orally (5 mg/kg/d) for the patient with bone pain inadequately controlled by NSAIDs. Continue until clinical or biochemical remission is achieved. Consider intermittent therapy if symptoms recur.
- Begin calcitonin (100 MRC units subcutaneously daily) for patients with severe bone pain, moderate high-output heart failure, mild to moderate hypercalcemia, fracture, or risk of fracture, deformity or compression. Once clinical and biochemical remissions have been achieved, reduce dose to 50 MRC units and continue therapy three times a week. Etidronate may be used in place of calcitonin for patients unable to self-administer parenteral therapy.
- Obtain two baseline measurements of alkaline phosphatase and a baseline skeletal x-ray or bone scan before therapy. Follow serum alkaline phosphatase at monthly intervals during therapy. Routine repetition of radiologic procedures is unwarranted, but x-ray may be helpful if fracture is suspected.
- Advise the patient to avoid immobilization and dehydration. Prescribe at least 2 liters of liquid per day, especially if the patient is inactive.

ANNOTATED BIBLIOGRAPHY

Altman RD. Long-term follow-up of therapy with intermittent etidronate disodium in Paget's disease of bone. Am J Med 1985;79:583. *(Eighty-five percent had a prolonged remission or responded well to retreatment.)*

Frank WA, Bries NM, Singer FR, et al. Rheumatic manifestations of Paget's disease of bone. Am J Med 1974;56:592. *(Joint disease can be an important problem for patients with Paget's disease.)*

Hosking DJ. Paget's disease of bone: an update on management. Drugs 1985;30:156. *(Detailed review that includes a good discussion of calcitonin.)*

Krane SM. Etidronate disodium in the treatment of Paget's disease of bone. Ann Intern Med 1982;96:619. *(Definitive review of the drug.)*

Nagent de Deuxchaisnes, Krane SM. Paget's disease of bone: clinical and metabolic observations. Medicine (Baltimore) 1974;43:233. *(Classic review article of clinical and biochemical manifestations.)*

Primary Care Medicine: Office Evaluation and Management of the Adult Patient, 3rd edition, edited by Allan H. Goroll, Lawrence A. May, and Albert G. Mulley, Jr. J.B. Lippincott Company, Philadelphia

163
Approach to the Patient With Raynaud's Phenomenon

Raynaud's phenomenon is strongly suggested when patients complain of bilateral blanching and discomfort in the fingers in response to cold or stress followed by purplish discoloration and reactive erythema. For some, it is an isolated problem; for others, it may represent the first manifestation of connective tissue disease, arterial occlusion, or a hematologic problem. The primary physician needs to know when to search for underlying disease and how to provide symptomatic relief.

PATHOPHYSIOLOGY AND CLINICAL PRESENTATION

Alteration in dermal blood flow is a basic mechanism of thermoregulation and also a common response to stress-induced catecholamine release. In patients with Raynaud's phenomenon, this vascular reactivity is exaggerated. It may be functional (due to *vasospasm*), anatomic (due to *arterial occlusive disease*), or rheologic (due to *alterations in blood viscosity* or red cell deformability). *Platelet activation* appears to play a role in patients with abnormal vascular anatomy. In many instances, the pathophysiology is multifactorial. The characteristic clinical sequence begins with rapid onset of digital blanching (vasospastic phase), followed by cyanosis (venospastic phase), and ending with restoration of flow and redness (reactive hyperemia).

Clinically, Raynaud's phenomenon is classified as "primary" or idiopathic (Raynaud's disease) if there is no evidence of an associated condition and as "secondary" if there is. Some have objected to this designation, because secondary causes (eg, connective tissue disease) may not become clinically evident for years.

Primary Raynaud's Phenomenon—Raynaud's Disease. Those with truly idiopathic disease appear to suffer from excessive vasospasm, with mild symptoms often precipitated by emotional stress. Peripheral adrenergic tone is especially high. The condition is most common in women, with onset often at menarche. Attacks may be frequent (several times daily), mild, precipitated by emotional stress, and present in persons with other vasomotor problems (migraine, livedo reticularis). The fingers show no edema, nailbed erythema, or ischemic changes. Prognosis is excellent in terms of ischemic injury.

A pathophysiologic relative of primary disease is that which is drug-induced. *Vasoactive drugs* used for migraine (beta-blockers, ergotamine, methysergide) have all been implicated, as has *migraine*. Whether drugs can cause the problem in the absence of an underlying vasomotor disorder remains unclear.

Secondary Raynaud's Phenomenon—Underlying Disease. Many patients with seemingly isolated Raynaud's phenomenon at the time of initial presentation eventually develop characteristic manifestations of *connective tissue disease* (especially *scleroderma* and *systemic sclerosis*), although they may not occur for several years. In some patients, subtle manifestations of connective tissue disease are already evident, including mild sclerodactyly, early calcinosis, telangiectasias, and antinuclear antibody positivity. In others, they are not, but an abnormal nailfold capillary pattern is especially predictive. Compared to patients with primary disease, men as well as women are affected, onset tends to be later (mid-twenties and older), and episodes are more severe and less precipitated by emotional stress. Loss of finger pulp and skin ulcers due to ischemia may be evident.

Raynaud's phenomenon is especially prevalent in patients with systemic sclerosis, occurring in over 90 percent of cases. In such patients, structural narrowing of digital vessels is present due to intimal fibrosis. Abnormal vascular reactivity and platelet activation have been demonstrated. Symptoms may be especially severe, and risk of digital ischemic injury is substantial. The compromise to digital blood flow is considerably less in patients with scleroderma.

A host of other conditions can cause vaso-occlusive Raynaud's phenomenon, including *atherosclerotic disease,* occupational *vibratory injury* (jackhammer operators, welders, sheet-metal workers), and *neurovascular compression* syndromes (thoracic outlet, carpal tunnel). Clinical course is a function of the underlying disease, a number of which are reversible.

DIFFERENTIAL DIAGNOSIS

The causes of Raynaud's phenomenon can be grouped according to the predominant pathophysiologic mechanism (Table 163–1), although, as noted above, multiple mechanisms may be operative. About 20 percent of patients presenting initially with idiopathic or primary Raynaud's phe-

Table 163-1. Important Causes of Raynaud's Phenomenon

Vasospastic Disease
Primary
Drug-induced (beta-blockers, ergot, methysergide)
Migraine
Arterial Occlusive Disease (+/− Platelet Activation)
Scleroderma
Systemic sclerosis
Systemic lupus erythematosus
Occupational trauma (jackhammer operator)
Atherosclerotic disease
Compression (thoracic outlet, carpal tunnel)
Hemorrhologic Disease
Paraproteinemia
Polycythemia
Cryoproteinemia

nomenon prove after 2 to 3 years to have underlying connective tissue disease.

WORKUP

History and Physical Examination

Confirming the Diagnosis. The diagnosis of Raynaud's phenomenon is a clinical one, based on a history or direct observation of the characteristic skin-color changes in response to cold or stress. If the diagnosis is uncertain, one can test the patient's response to cold by immersing his or her hands in icewater and observing for blanching, cyanosis, and reactive hyperemia. At least two of the three characteristic skin changes are needed for confirmation of the diagnosis.

Differentiating Primary From Secondary Disease. Because Raynaud's phenomenon is often the presenting manifestation of an underlying disease, it is important to consider such conditions in the early phase of the evaluation. Screening by history and physical examination can facilitate selection of patients who require more detailed testing. The differentiation is facilitated by attention to age at onset, gender, frequency and severity of attacks, distribution of skin changes, presence of ischemic skin changes, manifestations of connective tissue disease, precipitating factors, associated digital swelling, and other vasomotor phenomena such as migraine and livedo reticularis.

Primary disease is suggested by a history of teenage onset, female gender, multiple mild attacks every day, symmetric involvement, stress-precipitation, normal skin except for livedo reticularis, and migraine headaches. Secondary disease should be suspected when the patient is a male or is a female with onset in the mid-twenties or later; who reports moderate to severe attacks not necessarily occurring every day; asymmetric presentation triggered predominantly by cold; and associated finger swelling, ischemic skin ulcers, or loss of fingertip pulp.

Further Evaluation of Suspected Secondary Disease. In patients with a presentation suggestive of secondary disease, the review of systems should be checked carefully for additional symptoms of connective tissue disease (skin rash, morning stiffness, arthralgias, joint swelling, fatigue, fever; see Chapter 146) and peripheral vascular disease (claudication, angina, leg ulceration; see Chapter 23). Although less common, symptoms of thoracic outlet and carpal tunnel syndromes (see Chapter 167) and polycythemia (see Chapter 80) should also be sought if the diagnosis of underlying disease remains unclear. Occupational history is noted for any vibratory injury. Medications are reviewed for use and effects of beta-blockers, ergotamine, methysergide, and calcium-channel blockers on symptoms.

The physical examination should include a thorough check for manifestations of connective tissue disease (eg, malar flush, sclerodactyly, petechial rash, telangiectasias, calcinosis, joint redness, swelling, and effusion). The hand and arm pulses are carefully palpated, and capillary filling is noted in the digits. The fingertips are felt for loss of pulp indicative of ischemia, and the skin is observed for ischemic changes.

Laboratory Testing

Patients judged to have definite primary disease on the basis of the careful history and physical examination noted above require no additional evaluation. Those with clinical evidence suggestive of connective tissue disease are reasonable candidates for *antinuclear antibody (ANA)* testing. In ANA-positive patients, ordering an *anticentromere antibody* determination can help predict risk of developing scleroderma, but the test is expensive and its utility in clinical decision making needs to be considered before ordering it. Similarly, examining the *nailfold capillary pattern* under wide-field microscopy for asymmetry due to dropout of capillary loops helps to determine risk of progression to systemic sclerosis.

Noninvasive studies of arterial flow (*plethysmography, Doppler ultrasound*) can confirm anatomic vascular compromise; however, similar information can often be obtained by careful history and physical examination, and test data usually do not help differentiate among anatomic etiologies.

Complete blood count and *serum globulin* determinations should suffice to screen for common hematologic etiologies; *immunoelectrophoresis* is reserved for patients suspected of myeloma (elderly, markedly elevated globulin, anemia; see Chapter 79). A *cryoprotein* determination is indicated if there are other manifestations suggestive of cryoglobulinemia (arthralgias, purpura, proteinuria). A *cold-agglutinin* test is worth considering in patients with anemia and splenomegaly.

MANAGEMENT

Prevention. Regardless of etiology, keeping the trunk as well as the extremities warm on cold days is essential. Of particular importance is *truncal warmth,* because any threat to maintenance of core body temperature is a potent stimulus to reflex peripheral vasoconstriction. *Smoking cessation* and elimination of passive smoking are essential. Any drugs found to trigger episodes should be stopped or cut back.

Occupational precipitants, such as repetitive activity that leads to carpal tunnel syndrome or vibratory injury, should be reduced or eliminated. Although *pneumatic tool* operation (eg, jackhammer) is the classic occupational etiology, smaller, less inertial tools causing *high-frequency vibration* have been found to be even more capable of vascular injury. As little as 1 to 2 hours per day of working on a vibrating or rotating tool (such as used by welders, sheet-metal workers, carpenters, and painters) can inflict vascular damage. Prevention is the best approach, limiting the number of hours using such equipment, but this is often not feasible. Alternatively, at the first sign of symptoms, use should be markedly reduced or eliminated. Antivibration gloves and coated tool handles have not proven sufficient.

Symptomatic Relief. Because Raynaud's phenomenon has a strong vasoconstrictive component, it follows that vasodilators should be capable of providing symptomatic relief. *Calcium-channel blockers* have proven symptomatically useful both for patients with primary disease as well as for many with secondary disease. Mechanism of action includes vasodilation plus some platelet inhibition. The resultant improvement in perfusion sometimes helps speed the healing of skin ulcers. *Nifedipine* and its congeners (*nicardipine, isradipine,* and *felodipine)* are the most potent vasodilators. However, they can produce reflex tachycardia and cause peripheral edema secondary to venodilating effects. Occasionally, headache and flushing may be troublesome and esophageal function may worsen in patients with scleroderma. Sustained-release preparations facilitate convenience and are reasonably well tolerated. There is no evidence that vasodilator therapy alters the natural history of the underlying disease.

Alpha-blocker therapy is also capable of providing symptomatic relief. The newer preparations such as *doxazocin* are longer acting and appear less likely to cause first-dose syncope than older preparations such as prazocin. Postural lightheadedness is still a problem, especially as dose is increased above 2 to 3 mg/d.

Patients with vasospastic disease accompanied by substantial endothelial injury and platelet activation (eg, those with systemic sclerosis) may not achieve adequate symptomatic relief with sole use of vasodilator drugs. Painful episodes may persist, and ischemic skin ulcers may fail to heal. The addition of *aspirin* or *dipyridamole* to the treatment program has helped in the healing of some ulcers, but not with reduction of vasospastic symptoms. *Fish-oil supplements* rich in omega-3 fatty acids can impair platelet activation and stimulate vasodilation through prostacyclin synthesis. Paradoxically, the best responses have been noted in patients with primary disease. Intravenous *prostacyclin* and *iloprost* (a prostacylin analogue) are being studied; they are both vasodilators and inhibitors of platelet activation. Early results are encouraging, with effects lasting up to 3 months after a single 5-day course of therapy.

Sympathectomy has been used as a measure of last resort. Patients who respond to temporary ganglionic blockade with an injected anesthetic are the best candidates for sympathectomy.

PATIENT EDUCATION AND INDICATIONS FOR REFERRAL

The major elements of patient education are preventive (see above). Those with occupationally induced disease require a cost–benefit discussion of changing one's job or job activities versus the risk of developing worsening vascular compromise. Patients with strong features of primary disease can be reassured that the risk of underlying illness is low and that prognosis is excellent. Those with features of secondary disease associated with risk of developing connective tissue disease need to know their risk, but also that it may be many years before other disease manifestations ensue, if they come at all.

Referral is indicated for those with refractory symptoms, especially if accompanied by signs of ischemia.

A.H.G.

ANNOTATED BIBLIOGRAPHY

Cherniack MG. Raynaud's phenomenon of occupational origin. Arch Intern Med 1990;150:519. *(Vibratory injury is an important and common precipitant.)*

DiGiacomo RA, Kremer JM, Shah DM. Fish-oil supplementation in patients with Raynaud's phenomenon. Am J Med 1990; 86:158. *(Improved tolerance to cold exposure in patients with primary disease.)*

Fitzgerald O, Hess EV, O'Connor GT, et al. Prospective study of the evolution of Raynaud's phenomenon. Am J Med 1988; 84:718. *(A connective tissue disease developed in 19 percent of those who presented with no obvious evidence of underlying illness; nailfold capillary pattern was predictive of systemic sclerosis.)*

Malamet R, Wise RA, Ettinger WH, et al. Nifedipine in the treatment of Raynaud's phenomenon. Am J Med 1985;78:602. *(Mechanism of nifedipine action; some platelet inhibition suggested.)*

O'Keeffe ST, Tsapatsaris NP, Beethan WP Jr. Increased prevalence of migraine and chest pain in patients with primary Raynaud's disease. Ann Intern Med 1992;116:985. *(Evidence for a common pathophysiology.)*

Priollet P, Vayssairet M, Housset E. How to classify Raynaud's phenomenon: Long-term follow-up study of 73 patients. Am J Med 1987;83:494. *(Notes late onset of underlying disease; suggests means of early identification.)*

Sarkozi J, Bookman AAM, Lee P, et al. Significance of anticentromere antibody in idiopathic Raynaud's syndrome. Am J Med 1987;83:893. *(Predictive of other features of scleroderma.)*

Wigley FM, Wise RA, Seibold JR, et al. Intravenous iloprost infusion in patients with Raynaud phenomenon secondary to systemic sclerosis. Ann Intern Med 1994;120:199. *(Sustained benefit achieved with this prostacyclin analogue.)*

Primary Care Medicine: Office Evaluation and Management of the Adult Patient, 3rd edition, edited by Allan H. Goroll, Lawrence A. May, and Albert G. Mulley, Jr. J.B. Lippincott Company, Philadelphia

164
Prevention and Management of Osteoporosis

SAMUEL R. NUSSBAUM, M.D.

Osteoporotic fractures, particularly in aging women, represent a major health problem in industrialized nations. In the United States, approximately 150,000 hip fractures occur annually in women over age 65, with 15 percent to 25 percent of these women experiencing excess mortality or needing long-term nursing home care. Current expenditures for hip fractures approach $10 billion yearly. Osteoporotic vertebral crush fractures, manifested by back pain, loss of height, and decreased ambulation are present in 5 percent to 10 percent of women by age 60 and 40 percent by age 80. The pathophysiologic mechanisms for postmenopausal osteoporosis are imperfectly understood, but the means to ensure maximal skeletal growth and strength, prevent loss of bone mass, and noninvasively evaluate bone mass are now available.

The primary care physician should educate women about prevention of osteoporosis and develop personalized strategies for maximal skeletal accretion and preservation. These tasks are facilitated by knowing how to identify high-risk patients (see Chapter 144).

PATHOPHYSIOLOGY AND CLINICAL PRESENTATION

Osteoporosis is a reduction in the mass of bone per unit volume. Because a bone's strength is proportional to its density, the mechanical support of the skeleton is affected as bone mass declines. In contrast to osteoporosis, osteomalacia is characterized by a defect in the mineralization of the organic phase of bone.

Increased Osteoclastic Bone Resorption and Reduced New Bone Formation. The resorption and formation of bone is a continuous process throughout life. Under steady-state physiologic circumstances, the rates of these processes are equal and coupled. The explanations for the uncoupling of bone resorption and formation and development of osteoporosis remain speculative. Estrogen receptors exist on osteoblasts, the cells that synthesize bone matrix proteins. Communication between osteoblasts and osteoclasts (which resorb bone) occurs, but the precise mediators have not been fully identified. Cytokines in bone (eg, interleukin 1, tumor growth factor) and skeletal growth factors may act synergistically and serve as mediators of bone formation and resorption.

With onset of estrogen deficiency there is increased osteoclastic bone resorption. Later in life, there is impaired new bone formation. Fractional intestinal *absorption of calcium* in elderly persons is *decreased*. This decline in intestinal calcium absorption appears to be caused by a *decrease in formation of 1,25 dihydroxyvitamin D*, the active form of vitamin D.

Risk Factors. The most comprehensive data on risk factors for osteoporosis derive from The Study of Osteoporotic Fractures, a multicenter, prospective investigation involving nearly 10,000 postmenopausal women. Advancing *age*, *maternal fracture*, and current *smoker* were among the most important variables associated with reduced bone mass, but the strength of the associations was only moderate. Among the variables strongly associated with increased bone mass were increased weight, grip strength, and estrogen use > 2 years. Height and increased age at onset of menopause were moderate predictors of increased bone mass. Poor lifetime calcium intake had a weak association with decreased bone mass and increase in current calcium intake had a weakly positive association with increased bone mass. Other risk factors previously indentified, such as fair skin and alcohol consumption were not confirmed. Physical *inactivity* can lead to decreased bone mass as can intense exercise that results in amenorrhea. However, attempts to formulate predictive indices for vertebral osteoporosis based on such risk factors demonstrate little predictive power.

Conditions associated with osteoporosis include *Cushing's syndrome*, exogenous *glucocorticoid* administration, chronic *heparin* therapy, *thyrotoxicosis*, *hypogonadism*, *hyperprolactinemia*, *anorexia nervosa*, and *hyperparathyroidism*. However, these diseases represent a small percentage of osteoporotic patients.

Clinical Presentation. Skeletal mass is usually maximal by age 35 and declines in women after age 40 and in men after age 50 when the rate of new bone formation does not equal the rate of bone resorption. The rate of decline in skeletal mass is most rapid in women *within 2 years of menopause*. The greatest loss of trabecular bone occurs in the *femoral neck* and *lumbar vertebrae*, sites of future fracture.

The progressive decline in skeletal mass (which may approach 50%) becomes clinically manifest when fractures are sustained spontaneously or after minimal trauma. A *loss of height* and developing *kyphosis* generally indicate vertebral compression fracture. Fractures most commonly occur in the sacral and lumbar vertebrae, the hip, the humerus, and the wrist. The clinical course and the frequency of fractures in individual patients cannot be predicted.

Osteopenia is a radiologic term that indicates a reduced amount of bone and encompasses both osteomalacia and osteoporosis. The characteristic radiographic finding in osteoporosis is the loss of horizontal vertebral trabeculae, accentuating the end-plates and resulting in biconcave "codfish" vertebrae. Pseudofractures, generally occurring in weight-bearing long bones, are pathognomonic for osteomalacia.

The laboratory features of postmenopausal osteoporosis include normal serum levels of calcium, phosphate, vitamin D, parathyroid hormone, and alkaline phosphatase, although alkaline phosphatase may be elevated in the context of a healing fracture.

WORKUP

Noninvasive Assessments of Bone Density. Measurement of bone density at several skeletal sites permits stratification of fracture risk. Single-photon absorptiometry of the forearm assesses cortical bone. Dual energy x-ray absorptiometry (DEXA) of the spine and hip measures both cortical and trabecular bone and total body bone-mineral content. Quantitative computed tomography (QCT) of the spine best assesses trabecular bone.

These tests are safe, acceptable to patients, and have predictive value for the development of spinal compression fractures. If bone density measurements will affect clinical decision making, then testing should be performed. A perimenopausal woman committed to hormonal replacement therapy need not be studied. However, the untreated woman at above average risk for the development of osteoporosis can be tested if rapidly declining bone density would lead to initiation of estrogen therapy. Additionally, patients being treated for osteoporosis may require bone density measurements to determine therapeutic efficacy.

Biochemical Markers. Routine chemistries are normal and of little use. Under study are biochemical markers of bone formation (osteocalcin) and bone resorption (pyridinoline, deoxypyridinoline). It is hoped that such markers will help identify individuals who are undergoing rapid demineralization and at increased risk of becoming osteoporotic.

PRINCIPLES OF THERAPY

The goal is to reduce the risk of fracture by reducing the loss of bone mass. Prevention is more effective than treating established disease, but both require attention. Available therapies include estrogen replacement (in combination with progesterone), calcium supplementation, weight-bearing exercise, vitamin D, and bisphosphonates. If a fracture has occurred, symptomatic relief and aggressive therapy to halt further bone loss are indicated.

Estrogen

Hormone replacement therapy is the treatment of choice for postmenopausal osteoporosis. Estrogen stops bone loss and may even produce a modest degree of skeletal accretion in those with established disease. Observational studies have consistently noted a 35 percent to 50 percent reduction in hip, wrist, and vertebral fractures in women who have used estrogen for at least 5 years after menopause. In addition, the patient's lipid profile improves (HDL cholesterol rises, LDL cholesterol falls) and overall cardiovascular risk declines. The addition of progesterone does not cancel estrogen's beneficial effects, of which the cardiovascular ones are the most important overall (see Chapter 118).

Preparations. Natural estrogens (estradiol, conjugated estrogens) are preferred for replacement therapy over the synthetic ones (ethinyl estradiol), because they are shorter acting and less likely to cause adverse effects. *Estradiol* is the principal estrogen secreted by the ovary. It is available as 17-beta estradiol by *transdermal patch* or in a micronized *oral preparation*. The other natural oral formulation is *conjugated equine estrogens*. Oral preparations undergo first-pass metabolism by the liver, converting about half of estradiol to estrone. Transdermal 17-beta estradiol does not undergo hepatic first-pass metabolism; although this prolongs duration of action, it reduces the beneficial effect on hepatic lipid metabolism.

Dosage and Administration. The daily dose necessary to prevent bone loss is 0.625 mg of conjugated estrogen, 1.0 mg of estradiol, or 0.05 mg of transcutaneous estrogen. Concomitant administration of calcium may reduce the amount of estrogen required to preserve bone mass, but this remains uncertain. Estrogen is given with progesterone to avoid the risk of endometrial cancer (see below). The estrogen/progesterone program can be given cyclically or continuously. Most postmenopausal women prefer to avoid the withdrawal bleeding of cyclic therapy and opt for a continuous program (eg, 0.625 mg progesterone and 2.5 mg medroxyprogesterone daily; see Chapter 118).

Initiation and Duration of Therapy. Treatment should be at the onset of menopause if maximum prevention of bone loss is to be achieved. Once established, it is difficult to reverse the significant bone loss that occurs in the first few years of menopause. Estrogen therapy needs to be continued indefinitely, because skeletal loss will resume if treatment is halted and, after several years, the beneficial effects of estrogen will be lost. Patients over the age of 75 show little or no benefit from as much as 10 to 12 years of estrogen therapy started at the time of menopause.

Adverse Effects. For the woman with a uterus, the most serious adverse effect is a marked increase in the risk of *endometrial cancer.* The risk can be eliminated by the concurrent use of progesterone, which prevents unopposed endometrial stimulation. There is an uncertain effect of estrogen on the occurrence of *breast cancer.* Available data are conflicting; at most, the increase in risk is modest (see Chapter 122). However, the postmenopausal women with breast cancer may experience marked stimulation of tumor growth from initiation of estrogen therapy. Other adverse effects, more commonly seen with use of synthetic estrogens, include *migraine* headache, *cholelithiasis,* worsening of *endometriosis* or fibroid tumors, and acute *thrombosis*. The woman being considered for estrogen therapy needs careful breast and pelvic examinations, Pap test, and mammogram before onset of hormone replacement. Transient bloating, nausea, and breast tenderness may be noted after initiation of hormone replacement therapy.

Patient Selection. There is no universal agreement as to which patients should be considered for prophylactic therapy with estrogen at the time of menopause. The decision requires consideration not just of potential skeletal benefit, but also of cardiovascular benefit and cancer risks (see Chapter 118). From a skeletal perspective, those with known risk factors for osteoporosis (eg, maternal fracture, current smoker, small frame, lack of exercise, low calcium intake) are probably among the better candidates for prophylactic therapy, but these are not as predictive as bone density. Menopausal women who have an increased rate of decline in bone mass or an absolute reduction in bone mass that is a standard deviation greater than age-matched controls should receive estrogen therapy. Even when osteoporosis is clinically manifest by fractures or appears radiographically as osteopenia indicating at least a 30 percent to 40 percent loss of bone mass, it is still beneficial and important to initiate hormone replacement therapy, supplemented by calcium.

Calcium

Calcium carbonate in doses of 1.5 to 2.0 g/d helps preserve cortical bone mass. Although calcium therapy does not prevent bone loss to the degree that estrogen therapy does, it does represent an alternative. Its effect on bone loss falls between those of estrogen and placebo. The inadequate dietary calcium intake of most women (considerably less than the recommended 800 to 1000 mg of calcium each day) and the declining fractional absorption of calcium associated with aging makes it important to ensure a total intake of 1.5 g/d in adolescent and young women and 2 g/d in older women. Complications, such as renal stones or hypercalcemia, from intake of 1 to 2 g/d of elemental calcium have not been observed.

Dietary calcium is readily available and the most nutritious approach to adequate calcium intake. Absorption of dietary calcium is slightly better than that of calcium tablets. A cup of skim milk provides 303 mg of calcium; 8 oz of low-fat yogurt provides 345 mg; a serving of canned sardines has

354 mg. Calcium tablets provide a convenient means of supplementation. Chewable preparations are the best absorbed. The carbonate salt is the least costly. A reasonable supplemental dose of calcium is in the range of 500 to 1500 mg/d. Larger doses, particularly in conjunction with vitamin D, may predispose the patient to hypercalcemia and hypercalciuric renal stone disease. Concern about the solubilitiy and gut absorption of calcium carbonate has led to marketing of other calcium preparations (citrate, gluconate, lactate). They are often more expensive than calcium carbonate (especially the gluconate) and of little proven advantage. Taking calcium with meals increases its absorption due to the favorable action of gastric acid.

Vitamin D

Vitamin D's principal effect is on gut absorption of calcium. It also directly effects osteoblasts and osteoclasts. To date, its role in treatment of osteoporosis has been limited to patients with vitamin D deficiency, a common problem in the elderly. Its broader application is under investigation, stimulated by studies of calcitriol (1,25 dihydroxy vitamin D, the active form of vitamin D) showing prevention of spinal fractures even in persons who are not vitamin D deficient.

Exercise

An important component of the preventive therapy of osteoporosis is ensuring maximal development of skeletal mass. The amount of bone accumulated in *premenopausal women* may be critical to the appearance of osteoporosis later in life, as evidenced by the low incidence of osteoporosis in African-American women (and in men), who have a greater skeletal mass than white women. Exercise and physical activity have been shown to increase skeletal mass and increase total body calcium. Physical activity, in conjunction with a 1500-mg calcium-supplemented diet and 400 units of vitamin D daily, offers the best hope for increasing skeletal mass during skeletal growth. However, exercise programs so intensive as to induce amenorrhea and estrogen deficiency (eg, competitive marathon running) may lead to osteoporosis.

In postmenopausal women, regular weight-bearing exercise (eg, walking, low-impact aerobics, three times per week) can substantially retard bone mineral loss (down to 0.5% of the baseline value per year), especially when combined with calcium supplementation. A more ambitious program of formal exercise training (eg, 50 minutes of walking and jogging, three times per week) in combination with calcium supplementation may have even more pronounced effects (eg, increase in lumbar bone mineral content).

The efficacy of an exercise-plus-calcium program suggests an alternative to hormone replacement for treatment of postmenopausal osteoporosis in women judged not to be at high risk for fracture. An important unanswered question is the adequacy of such programs during the first postmenopausal years, when bone loss is most rapid. Available data suggest they might be insufficient during this period.

Bisphosphonates

These are synthetic compounds that bind avidly to bone mineral and can inhibit its resorption. Administration of the bisphosphonate *etidronate* increases spinal bone mineral density and decreases the rate of spinal fractures, making it a very useful treatment for patients with vertebral compression fracture. Benefits are greatest in those with low bone density and after 2 years of therapy. Because continuous use of etidronate can inhibit bone mineralization, it must be used cyclically in patients with osteoporosis. Newer, more potent bisphosphonates (pamidronate, alendronate) have shown promise in the prevention of bone loss associated with early menopause, corticosteroid use, and immobilization. Long-term effects and optimal dosing for bisphosphonate therapy remain to be determined.

Minimally Effective and Experimental Therapies

Calcitonin. Daily subcutaneous injections of 100 units of salmon calcitonin in combination with oral calcium of 1000 mg daily will increase total body calcium in postmenopausal women by several percent, presumably reflecting an increase in skeletal mass. Changes in specific bones have been too small to measure. After a year, there is no further increase in total body calcium, and it declines in parallel to untreated control patients. The high cost and minimal benefit of calcitonin make it a poor choice for treatment of osteoporosis.

Sodium fluoride therapy leads to a striking increase in trabecular bone density if given in doses ranging from 40 to 60 mg/d, but cortical bone density decreases, increasing skeletal fragility. The dense fluorotic bone is abnormal both chemically and crystallographically and has undesirable mechanical properties in vitro. Fluoride is not FDA approved for use in osteoporosis.

Parathyroid hormone stimulates new bone formation, increases trabecular bone, and improves calcium balance while producing chemically and histologically normal bone without hypercalcemia. This therapeutic approach is under active investigation.

Fractures

The risk of sustaining an osteoporotic fracture is related to the severity of bone mineral loss and chance of sustaining a fall. Attention to the former has been the focus of this chapter; prevention of falls is often overlooked.

Proper treatment of the patient who sustains a fracture is also important to subsequent outcome.

Prevention of Falls. A host of mundane, but very important steps help reduce the risk of falling. As regards the home environment, these include elimination of slippery surfaces and obstacle-laden paths, ensuring adequate illumination on stairways, installation of handrails in the bathroom, and use of seating that is easy to get up from. Personal items also require attention, such as footwear that provides good stance and stability and eyeglass prescriptions that are up to date. Patients with a neurologic or orthopedic impairment should be taught to use a cane or walker both in the house as well as outside. Also important is careful use of drugs that can cause postural hypotension or sedation and attention to conditions that impair gait and balance.

Vertebral Fractures. In patients who have sustained vertebral fractures, bedrest and adequate analgesics should be prescribed until the acute pain of the fracture subsides, often within several weeks. Thereafter, ambulation and daily exercise, such as swimming and walking, should be encouraged as tolerated. Lifting and vigorous physical activity are best avoided. Corsets and back braces, if comfortable, may facilitate ambulation in formerly bedridden patients.

Individuals who have sustained a vertebral fracture should be treated for osteoporosis. Either hormone replacement therapy or bisphosphonate should be prescribed. Both reduce the risk of new fracture. As noted earlier, the natural history of osteoporosis and compression fractures is not predictable in an individual patient. Symptomatic improvement cannot be used to measure the response to therapy because of the long fracture-free intervals. Noninvasive measurements of bone mass are needed to determine if bone loss has slowed or reversed with therapy.

Steroid-Induced Osteoporosis

Glucocorticosteroids inhibit new bone formation and calcium absorption and increase bone resorption and renal calcium excretion. Steroid-induced hypogonadism contributes to the problem in both men and women. Over 50 percent of patients on long-term steroids develop some degree of osteoporosis.

Prevention. The risk of developing steroid-induced osteoporosis can be reduced by using a short-acting preparation at the lowest possible dose in an alternate-day regimen, as well as by maintaining physical activity and ensuring adequate daily intake of calcium and vitamin D. Sodium restriction can improve calcium absorption and reduce its renal excretion.

Treatment. Bone loss from steroid use is at least partially reversible with cessation of glucocorticoid intake. The potential for recovery appears greatest in young persons. Steroid-induced osteoporosis in women who are postmenopausal or who experience steroid-induced amenorrhea (see Chapter 112) is an indication for hormone replacement therapy. Similarly, in men, any hypogonadism leading to loss of bone density can be countered by testosterone replacement. Hypercalciuria is an indication for thiazide therapy (supplemented by potassium replacement or a potassium-sparing agent). Small supplements of vitamin D can be given to those who become vitamin D deficient, but large doses are to be avoided due to risk of hypercalcemia. Bisphosphonate therapy is investigational.

Osteomalacia

When osteopenia is encountered radiologically or a hip fracture is noted, osteomalacia should be considered. Osteomalacia is defined as the inadequate deposition of calcium and phosphorus in bone tissue matrix. It is found in 10 percent to 15 percent of patients with hip fracture. *Vitamin D deficiency* is an important cause of osteomalacia in homebound elderly, who are unlikely to eat dairy products or go out in the sun. Other etiologies include *impaired vitamin D metabolism, malabsorption, systemic acidosis,* and *phosphate depletion*. Osteomalacia should be suspected in patients with hypocalcemia or hypophosphatemia. Urine pH and serum levels of 25-OH vitamin D, phosphate, calcium, and bicarbonate help detect the cause. If a 24-hour urinary calcium is greater than 100 mg/24 h, osteomalacia is unlikely.

In the absence of pseudofractures on x-ray, it is not possible to radiographically distinguish osteoporosis from osteomalacia. A bone biopsy is necessary for the definitive diagnosis of osteomalacia, but is usually reserved for patients undergoing orthopedic procedures. Osteomalacia responds dramatically to treatment with *dietary vitamin D, calcium,* and *phosphate supplements*.

PATIENT EDUCATION

The time spent educating the patient about osteoporosis is extremely well spent, because prevention and compliance are so important to effective management. Perimenopausal women are highly concerned about osteoporosis and come eager to discuss prevention and treatment. The full range of options should be reviewed and patient preferences should be elicited; failure to do so is likely to be disappointing. One should seek to design a program that is tailored to the patient's risk profile and lifestyle. The decision to initiate prophylactic hormone replacement therapy requires consideration of all risks and benefits, not just those related to osteoporosis (see Chapter 118).

THERAPEUTIC RECOMMENDATIONS

Postmenopausal Osteoporosis

- Advise young women, especially pregnant ones, to have a daily dietary intake of at least 1.0 to 1.5 g of calcium and 400 IU of vitamin D daily. Encourage a program of regular physical activity.
- For postmenopausal women, prescribe a program of weight-bearing exercise three times weekly and daily intake of 2 g of calcium and 400 IU of vitamin D.
- Supplement diet with chewable calcium carbonate tablets to achieve the 1.5 to 2 g daily total desired.
- For women who have a history of maternal osteoporotic fracture, current smoking, physical inactivity, small frame, or inadequate lifetime calcium intake, consider estrogen replacement therapy beginning in the perimenopausal period. Avoid delaying initiation of therapy, because rate of bone loss is maximal during the first few years after menopause.
- If estrogen is prescribed, consider a program of 0.625 mg of conjugated estrogens daily (in conjunction with 2.5 mg of medroxyprogesterone for the women with an intact uterus). Alternative hormone replacement regimens are available; careful monitoring is required (see Chapter 118).

- Continue hormone replacement therapy indefinitely, unless replaced by a therapy of nearly equal efficacy.
- For asymptomatic postmenopausal patients who are found to have radiographic osteopenia and no contraindications for estrogen therapy, obtain dual energy x-ray absorptiometry (DEXA) to quantify the reduction in skeletal mass, followed by treatment with estrogen, calcium, and vitamin D.
- For postmenopausal women who are not receiving hormone replacement therapy, but who are at increased risk for development of osteoporotic fracture, monitor bone loss by DEXA every 1 to 2 years and consider treatment if rate of loss is marked or absolute loss is greater than one standard deviation from the mean for age.
- Patients who have sustained fractures as a consequence of osteoporosis should be treated with bedrest and analgesics. When the pain subsides, begin ambulation, followed by mild exercise such as walking or swimming. Avoid lifting and other weight-bearing stresses. Strongly consider treatment for osteoporosis.
- For patients who have sustained a vertebral compression fracture, begin cyclic etidronate therapy (400 mg once daily, 2 hours before eating, for 2 weeks followed by no therapy for 3 months); continue indefinitely.

ANNOTATED BIBLIOGRAPHY

Aloia JF, Vaswani A, Yeh JK, et al. Calcium supplementation with and without hormone replacement therapy to prevent postmenopausal bone loss. Ann Intern Med 1994;120:97. *(Calcium produced an effect intermediate to those of estrogen and placebo.)*

Bauer DC, Browner WS, Cauley JAA, et al. Factors associated with appendicular bone mass in older women. Ann Intern Med 1993;118:657. *(Best data on risk factors for osteoporosis.)*

Dalsky GP, Stocke KS, Ehsani AA, et al. Weight-bearing exercise training and lumbar mineral content in postmenopausal women. Ann Intern Med 1988;108;824. *(An exercise program of 50 minutes, three times per week plus calcium supplementation produced an increase in lumbar bone mineral content.)*

Dawson-Hughes B, Dallal GE, Krall KA, et al. A controlled trial of the effect of calcium supplementation on bone density in postmenopausal women. N Engl J Med 1990;323:878. *(Calcium supplementation was beneficial, mostly in older women with low calcium intake—less than 400 mg/d.)*

Felson DT, Zhang Y, Hannan MT, et al. Effect of postmenopausal estrogen therapy on bone density in elderly women. N Engl J Med 1993;329:1141. *(Even as much as 10 years of prior treatment had minimal effect in women over the age of 75.)*

Holmes MM, Rovner DR, Rothert ML, et al. Women's and Physicians' utilities for health outcomes in estrogen replacement therapy. J Gen Intern Med 1987;2:178. *(Prevention of fracture was more highly valued by the women; underscores the need for eliciting the patient's views.)*

Horsman A, Jones M, Francis R, et al. The effect of estrogen dose on postmenopausal bone loss. N Engl J Med 1983;309:1405. *(Dose–response relationship noted; required dose for conjugated estrogens was 0.625 mg.)*

Johnston CC Jr, Slemenda CW, Melton LJ. Clinical use of bone densitometry. N Engl J Med 1991;324:1105. *(A review of available technologies and their utilities.)*

Lufkin EG, Wahner HW, O'Fallon WM, et al. Treatment of postmenopausal osteoporosis with transdermal estrogen. Ann Intern Med 1992;117:1. *(Found effective, but lipid changes less beneficial than with oral therapy.)*

Lukert BP, Raisz LG. Glucocorticoid-induced osteoporosis: pathogenesis and management. Ann Intern Med 1990;112;352. *(Clinically relevant discussion of disease mechanisms followed by review of treatment options.)*

Martin KA, Freeman MW. Postmenopausal hormone-replacement therapy. N Engl J Med 1993;328:1115. *(An editorial reviewing the positive effects on lipids.)*

Nabulsi et al. Association of hormone-replacement with various cardiovascular risk factors in postmenopausal women. N Engl J Med 1993;328:1069. *(Favorable estrogen effects noted, not canceled by the addition of progesterone.)*

Popcock NA, Eisman JA, Dunstan CR, et al. Recovery from steroid-induced osteoporosis. Ann Intern Med 1987;107:319. *(Reversal found in these relatively young persons.)*

Prince RL, Smith M, Dick IM, et al. Prevention of postmenopausal osteoporosis: A comparative study of exercise, calcium supplementation, and hormone-replacement. N Engl J Med 1992;325:1189. *(Bone loss was slowed or prevented by exercise plus calcium and by hormone replacement.)*

Richelson LS, Wahner HW, Melton LJ, et al. Relative contributions of aging and estrogen deficiency to postmenopausal bone loss. N Engl J Med 1984;311:1273. *(Bone loss in oophorectomized women was almost as great as that in postmenopausal women, indicating that estrogen deficiency rather than aging is the prominent cause.)*

Riggs BL, Hodgson SF, O'Fallon WM, et al. Effect of fluoride treatment on the fracture rate in postmenopausal women with osteoporosis. N Engl J Med 1990;322:802. *(Increases cancellous bone but decreases cortical bone, leading to increased skeletal fragility.)*

Sheikh MS, Santa ANA CA, Nicar MJ, et al. Gastrointestinal absorption of calcium from milk and calcium salts. N Engl J Med 1987;317:532. *(In these healthy young subjects, there were no significant differences.)*

Tilyard MW, Spears GFS, Thomson J, et al. Treatment of postmenopausal osteoporosis with calcitriol or calcium. N Engl J Med 1992;326:357. *(Continuous use reduced the rate of vertebral fractures.)*

Tosteson AN, Rosenthal DI, Melton LJ III, et al. Cost effectiveness of screening perimenopausal white women for osteoporosis: Bone densitometry and hormone replacement therapy. Ann Intern Med 1990;113:594. *(A decision analysis model that finds selective screening cost-effective.)*

Watts NB, Harris ST, Genant HK, et al. Intermittent cyclic etidronate treatment of postmenopausal osteoporosis. N Engl J Med 1990;323:73. *(Increased spinal bone mass and reduced risk of new compression fracture.)*

Primary Care Medicine: Office Evaluation and Management of the Adult Patient, 3rd edition, edited by Allan H. Goroll, Lawrence A. May, and Albert G. Mulley, Jr. J.B. Lippincott Company, Philadelphia

11

Neurologic Problems

165

Approach to the Patient With Headache

AMY A. PRUITT, M.D.

A complaint of headache raises myriad diagnostic possibilities. Fortunately, fewer than 1 percent of headaches that come to medical attention represent serious intracranial disease. Still, headache poses a diagnostic challenge for the primary physician, who must distinguish between the rare headache that represents a potentially life-threatening process and the vast majority which are harmless. Both physicians and patients worry about headaches that are persistent, severe, or sudden in onset. The primary physician's most immediate task is to efficiently identify by history and physical examination the occasional patient who requires aggressive workup. Additional priorities are to provide symptomatic relief and to systematically diagnose the headache type and its cause while formulating a long-term plan for management.

Headache can be a difficult problem to evaluate and manage. Of those who come for help, only one-third claim they are satisfied with the care received. Fortunately for neurologists and primary physicians alike, recent advances in our understanding of clinical presentation and pathophysiology have greatly facilitated diagnosis and treatment.

PATHOPHYSIOLOGY AND CLINICAL PRESENTATION

Headache pain may originate from either intracranial or extracranial structures. *Intracranial sources* of pain referable to the head include fibers of the fifth, ninth, and tenth cranial nerves and the upper cervical nerves, venous sinuses, parts of the dura at the base of the skull, the dural arteries (anterior and middle meningeal), and the large arteries at the base of the brain that give rise to the circle of Willis. Brain parenchyma is not pain-sensitive. Postulated *mechanisms* include 1) traction due to direct or indirect displacement of intracranial structures; 2) distention of intracranial arteries; 3) inflammation of pain-sensitive structures; and 4) obstruction of cerebrospinal fluid (CSF) flow by a mass lesion causing distortion of brain contents. If the intracranial source of the pain is above the tentorium, it is usually felt in the distribution of the fifth cranial nerve. Pain from a site in the posterior fossa is usually felt in the posterior half of the head, conveyed by the glossopharyngeal and vagus nerves as well as by the upper cervical spinal roots.

Extracranial sites of headache include the skin, fascia, muscles, and blood vessels of the scalp, the extracranial arteries, mucous membranes of the nasal and perinasal spaces, external and middle ear, teeth, and muscles of the scalp and facial region. Problems involving the eyes, sinuses, cervical spine, temporal mandibular joints, or cranial nerves can be important sources of headache, though some common attributions are not always correct.

Intracranial Sources

Mass Lesions. As noted above, mass lesions can cause headache by displacing a pain-sensitive structure. About one third of patients with a mass lesion have headache as an early symptom, often with the pain *localized to the side of the lesion*. There are a wide variety of presentations, with none particularly diagnostic. The headache may be mild or severe, intermittent or persistent, aching, sharp, pressure-like, or even throbbing. Characteristically, the headache remains in the *same location* but becomes *progressive*, with increases in duration and severity of pain over several months, in conjunction with subtle changes in mental status or development of focal neurologic deficits. Initially, the discomfort may be lessened by lying down, but as intracranial pressure increases, lying down may actually exacerbate the headache, as might straining at stool, coughing, or bending over. As intracranial pressure increases, a more generalized headache may develop. Nocturnal awakening is common but not diagnostic. Projectile vomiting is a late complication.

In patients with a *brain tumor*, headache may be the sole initial complaint, unaccompanied by focal neurologic deficits. However, as the condition progresses, new neurologic deficits usually ensue. *Brain abscess* may present as a mass lesion causing headache, especially in its later stages. Parenteral drug abuse, lung abscess, or parameningeal infection may serve as the source of infection. Fever and focal neurologic deficits are often absent. *Chronic subdural hematoma*, another important mass lesion, typically presents in subtle fashion, with head trauma followed by a symptom-free interval. The injury may be forgotten, but the patient begins to show mental status changes and, eventually, focal neurologic deficits.

Pseudotumor cerebri can mimic the clinical presentation of tumor. Characteristic features include onset of headache in an obese, young woman, papilledema on exam, and compressed ventricles on CT scan.

Non-Migrainous Cerebrovascular Sources. *Ischemic events* may be associated with acute headache. The pain most often occurs on the side of the lesion but may be frontal or diffuse. In some instances, the headache is a consequence of the cerebral edema that ensues. *Arteriovenous malformation* and berry *aneurysm* are much-feared causes of vascular intracranial headache. Acute rupture of an aneurysm produces sudden onset of a headache that reaches maximum intensity immediately, often accompanied by meningeal irritation. In the absence of any rupture, 10 percent to 15 percent of patients with an arteriovenous malformation may experience a chronic headache characterized by unilateral (always the same side) throbbing pain. Unlike migraine, there are no prodromal or associated symptoms. Berry aneurysms are silent until rupture, unless greater than 2 cm, in which case they may present like the headache of a mass lesion.

Migraine affects about 10 percent of adults, women more than men. Family history is present in nearly two-thirds, especially in patients with a history of migraine with aura. Migraine headaches usually begin in childhood or young adult life, though about 16 percent of women afflicted by migraine will first develop them at the time of menopause. The condition tends to get better for many women during pregnancy, though oral contraceptives have been known to precipitate migraine or convert migraine without aura to migraine with aura. Roughly one in seven women with migraine has headache confined to the first few days of menses, though many women experience an exacerbation at this time.

Migraine used to be designated as *"classic"* if it were accompanied by aural symptoms (see below) and as *"common"* if it were not. This taxonomy has been replaced by the more specific classifications of *migraine with aura* and *migraine without aura*. Both types of migraine are accompanied by nausea and photophobia. Migraine is now defined an episodic disorder manifested by headache, anorexia, nausea, vomiting, and photophobia. The new classification system requires that at least two of the following be present to establish a diagnosis of migraine headache: unilateral location, pulsating quality, moderate to severe intensity, and exacerbation by physical activity. At least one of the following must accompany the headache: nausea or vomiting, photophobia, or phonophobia. Precipitants of migraine include emotional upset, menstruation, and, in some people, ingestion of tyramine- or tryptophan-rich foods (eg, ripe cheeses, red wine, or chocolate). Headache may occur shortly after or just before a period of psychologic stress. Some patients experience a seemingly paradoxical flare-up of migraine on weekends or vacations. There is an increased risk of stroke, which may occur during a migraine attack.

Attacks may have as many as five phases: prodrome, aura, headache, termination, and postdrome. The *prodrome* is characterized by lassitude, irritability, difficulty concentrating, and nausea. Patients with *aura* often report visual complaints (scintillating scotomata, zigzag patterns, hemianopsia, diplopia), vertigo, aphasia, or even hemiplegia preceding onset of the headache. The *headache* is typically unilateral and throbbing, though it may begin as a dull sensation and take a while to reach maximum intensity. *Headache termination* usually occurs within 24 hours but sometimes not until 48 hours. The *postdrome* phase includes feelings of fatigue, sleepiness, or irritability.

There are a number of *variants*. The most common is migraine without aura. Another is *acephalgic migraine*, in which a focal neurologic deficit may evolve during an aura but is not succeeded by headache. In rare instances, the symptoms of acephalgic migraine may persist for 1 to 2 days, simulating a stroke.

A number of hypotheses have been advanced to explain migraine and account for its phases. The long-held *vascular hypothesis* for migraine fails to account for the prodrome. The *neurogenic hypothesis* views migraine as a primary neuronal event, with secondary neurotransmitter-mediated changes in vasculature and blood flow. Neuropeptides are thought to act as neurotransmitters at trigeminal nerve branches, precipitating an inflammatory process with vasodilation. *Serotonin receptors* are believed to be important in mediating these events, which can be triggered by a variety of stimuli (mechanical, electrical, or chemical). The observed decrease in blood flow during migraine is now believed to be caused by a slowly spreading cortical band of decreased neuronal function elicited by such stimuli.

Meningitis from infection or hemorrhage produces pain that is acute in onset, severe, generalized, and constant. Symptoms may be particularly intense at the base of the skull and aggravated by forward flexion of the neck or by leg raising in conjunction with knee extension and foot dorsiflexion.

Postconcussion headache occurs in cases where the wrenching and displacement of pain-sensitive central nervous system (CNS) structures from head trauma was severe enough to cause concussion. *Postconcussion syndrome* (posttraumatic nervous instability) is a complicated, poorly characterized state manifested by chronic refractory headache, neck pain, nervousness, emotional lability, crying spells, and inability to concentrate. The symptoms are suggestive of an agitated depression following trauma; the syndrome probably represents a variant of tension-type headache. The correlation between severity of symptoms and seriousness of the injury is minimal. Often legal proceedings and litigation are pending. Symptoms often tend to fade away once legal issues are settled.

Extracranial Sources

Tension-type headache ranks among the leading causes of chronic and recurrent headache. More than 90 percent are bilateral and often described as a pressure or bandlike sensation about the head. The pain is dull and steady in most instances, characteristically worsening as the day progresses and sometimes accompanied by occipital and nuchal soreness. The headache may last days, weeks, or even months. Recording of myographic potentials from head and neck muscles reveals vigorous contractions in some but not all patients with this type of headache. Vasoconstriction can also be detected and may account for the migraine-like symptoms (nausea, throbbing pain) experienced by some patients.

Precipitants include anxiety, depression, and situational stress. Patients with underlying psychopathology often describe their headache pain in vivid terms (eg, "feels like an ax," or "lightning," or "something exploding"), yet they do so without demonstrating any apparent discomfort. So psychologically engaging is the headache that many of these patients are unaware of their underlying emotional problems. Tension-type headaches may also occur secondary to muscle strain from cervical spondylosis or temporomandibular joint disease (see below).

Sinusitis. True sinusitis produces a headache that is characteristically acute in onset, worse on awakening, better on standing, only to worsen again as the day progresses. The patient reports a purulent nasal discharge, and there is a predominance of pain and skin sensitivity over the involved sinus (see Chapter 219). Many patients with other forms of headache (eg, frontal muscle-contraction headaches) misattribute their problem to "sinusitis" and self-treat with decongestants to no avail. Because the pain of sinusitis is sometimes described as throbbing in quality and can worsen on bending over, it may be mistaken for migraine or the headache of a intracranial mass lesion.

Giant cell arteritis (also referred to as *temporal arteritis* or *cranial arteritis*) is a disease of older persons (almost all are older than age 50). It affects medium and large arteries (especially those of the extracranial vasculature) and can cause blindness if it spreads to the ophthalmic artery. The headache may begin as a throbbing discomfort and progress to a dull, aching pain. Some patients complain of burning, and others note bouts of lancinating pain. Scalp tenderness (especially on hair combing) localized to the involved vessel(s) is characteristic. However, the inflamed artery may not always be tender or palpable, and although the temporal artery is commonly involved, it need not be. Jaw (masticatory muscle) claudication is often part of the clinical picture, and there is a strong association with *polymyalgia rheumatica* (see Chapter 161).

The most feared complication is *blindness*. It occurs when arteritis leads to occlusion of the ophthalmic artery, which is usually about 1 to 2 months after onset of headache. Diplopia may precede visual impairment and is predictive of it (50% risk). Once visual impairment sets in, it progresses quickly over several hours to total visual loss (see Chapter 161).

Temporomandibular joint dysfunction has received much attention in the lay press as a common, sometimes overlooked cause of chronic refractory headache. Occasionally, the problem is due to joint changes resulting from malocclusion. However, in most cases the problem is not malocclusion, but tension-induced jaw clenching and nocturnal teeth grinding (*bruxism*). Such chronic involuntary oral habits lead to masticator muscle fatigue and spasm. Chronic dull, aching, unilateral discomfort may be described about the jaw, behind the eyes and the ears, and even down the neck into the shoulders. Jaw pain, clicking sounds, and difficulty opening the mouth in the morning are characteristic. Chewing may exacerbate symptoms; locking of the jaw is common. On physical examination, masticatory muscle tenderness, mandibular hypomotility, and joint clicking and deviation on opening are noted. Molar prominences may be flat from chronic teeth grinding (see Chapter 225).

Cluster Headache. The pathophysiology of cluster headache remains obscure, though there appears to be a component of exclusively extracerebral vasodilation. Vasoactive substances are believed to be involved. The headache occurs predominantly in middle-aged men and is the only headache more common in men than in women. It is distinguished by its location, timing, and periodicity. In its most typical presentation (affecting > 50%), patients complain of an intense, nonthrobbing, unilateral headache "behind the eye" that is searing, stabbing, or burning and accompanied by ipsilateral lacrimation, nasal stuffiness, and facial flushing. In 20 percent to 40 percent, there is also ipsilateral ptosis and miosis. Headache typically begins a few hours after going to bed and lasts for 30 to 90 minutes. Attacks occur nightly for 2 to 3 months and then disappear, only to return several months to years later. About 10 percent suffer from *chronic cluster headache*, in which there are daily attacks for 1 to 2 years and no periodicity. These headaches are sometimes confused with migraine because they are unilateral and severe, but they are not throbbing and lack most of the other defining features of migraine. Stress and alcohol are believed to be precipitants, although alcohol is well tolerated between attacks.

Indomethacin-responsive headaches include chronic paroxysmal hemicrania, ice pick headache, and hemicrania continua. *Chronic paroxysmal hemicrania* is a rare cluster-variant occurring predominantly among women and characterized by a similarly severe unilateral facial pain; unlike cluster, the headaches occur in short spasms of 10 to 20 minutes up to 20 or 30 times per day. Horner's syndrome and ipsilateral tearing are often noted.

Ice pick headache occurs in patients suffering from migraine, though not exclusively. The headache is brief, sharp, and jabbing. *Hemicrania continua* differs from the others in causing continuous unilateral aching discomfort, though it is accentuated by ipsilateral jabbing pain.

Systemic infection and fever are common causes of cranial vasodilatation and diffuse, throbbing headaches. The headache that frequently accompanies a viral syndrome is typical of this type. Numerous *metabolic disturbances* and *drugs* may lead to vasodilatation and headache. A pounding headache is a prominent symptom of early carbon monoxide poisoning and a common complaint of patients who take nitrates for angina or vasodilators for other conditions.

Hypertension. Moderate to severe *hypertension* (diastolic pressures > 110 mm Hg) sometimes results in occipital headaches. The mechanism of the headache is unknown. The discomfort is worse in the morning and recedes as the day progresses. This headache resolves with correction of the hypertension. It should not be confused with the muscle contraction and psychogenic headaches that are responsible for most headaches that occur in hypertensive patients and with the headache of increased intracranial pressure that accompanies malignant hypertension.

Ocular Sources. Headaches are often attributed to eye problems, especially when they are felt about the orbit. *Eyestrain* is often blamed for headaches, though in most instances the attribution is incorrect and refraction fails to improve the problem. However, in an occasional patient, astigmatism can cause difficulty when there is prolonged use of the eyes for close work. It produces ocular muscle imbalance and sustained contraction of extraocular, frontal, and temporal muscles; aching discomfort about the orbit and the frontotemporal region results. Refraction corrects the problem. *Acute glaucoma* may produce sudden onset of an orbital headache accompanied by cloudy vision (see Chapters 201 and 207).

Cervical Radiculopathy. Headache is commonly the first symptom of cervical radiculopathy. The pain arises from mechanical irritation of an upper cervical root. Findings on radiography of the cervical spine are variable, ranging from normal to spondylosis. Pain often localizes to one side of the occiput or base of the skull, in conjunction with tenderness to palpation. It may start in the neck and at times even radiate to the forehead or eye. The discomfort is described as nagging or aching and aggravated by *neck movement*. The headache tends to be worse on awakening, perhaps related to unconscious neck motion during sleep. The mechanism of pain is believed to involve entrapment of upper cervical nerve roots as they course through toward the occiput among irritated nuchal ligaments and muscles.

Trigeminal neuralgia (*tic douloureux*) is one of the most severe pain syndromes known to man. Paroxysms of lancinating facial or cranial pain occur in middle-aged or elderly patients; these may last only a few seconds but can be excruciating and recurrent. The jaw, gums, lips, or maxillary region may be involved. Characteristically, there is a trigger zone located in the region (see Chapter 176).

DIFFERENTIAL DIAGNOSIS

The differential diagnosis of headache can be divided into acute and chronic/recurrent types (Table 165–1). Of note, the International Headache Society now subdivides migraine into *migraine headache with aura* (previously called *classical migraine*) and *migraine headache without aura* (previously referred to as *common migraine*). *Tension-type headache*, with or without associated paracranial muscle spasm, has replaced the numerous designations of *muscle contraction headache*, *psychogenic headache*, or *tension headache* previously used.

WORKUP

As noted earlier, the first priority is to distinguish the worrisome headache from the harmless one. Headaches of concern are those that are sudden in onset, severe, or persistent. Despite the advent of elaborate imaging techniques, history and physical examination remain indispensable.

Table 165-1. Important Causes of Headache

A. Acute
  1. Meningitis
  2. Intracranial hemorrhage (stroke, rupture of aneurysm)
  3. Stroke
  4. Acute increase in intracranial pressure (mostly due to cerebral edema or hemorrhage, including hypertensive encephalopathy)
  5. Acute glaucoma
  6. Acute sinusitis
  7. Acute metabolic disturbance (carbon monoxide poisoning, hypoglycemia)
  8. Acute viral illness
  9. Initial presentation of a persistent or recurrent headache

B. Persistent or Recurrent Headache
  1. Intracranial mass lesion (neoplasm, abscess, subdural hematoma, large A-V malformation)
  2. Tension-type headache
  3. Migraine, with and without aura
  4. Cluster headache
  5. Indomethacin-responsive headache (ice pick, paroxysmal hemicrania)
  6. Postconcussion syndrome
  7. Cervical spine disease
  8. Giant-cell arteritis
  9. Trigeminal neuralgia
  10. Hypertension
  11. A-V malformation
  12. Bruxism/temporomandibular joint dysfunction
  13. Medications
  14. Substance abuse

History

A careful headache history is the mainstay of evaluation. The time invested in obtaining a full description of the headache, its clinical course, associated symptoms, precipitants, aggravating and alleviating factors, and patient concerns is well worth the effort. The information obtained is often diagnostic, always critical to intelligent test selection, and essential to dealing effectively with patient worries and expectations.

Medication history is critical, because a number of agents can trigger nonspecific headaches. The list includes indomethacin, nifedipine, cimetidine, captopril, nitrates, atenolol, trimethoprim-sulfamethoxazole, and oral contraceptives. Drug-related intracranial hypertension can be seen with minocycline, isoretinoin, nalidixic acid, tetracycline, trimethoprim-sulfamethoxazole, cimetidine, corticosteroids, and tamoxifen.

The history pertinent to a new headache differs slightly from that for chronic or recurrent headache and will be discussed separately.

Headache of New Onset. History should include inquiry into any *associated neurologic deficits*, *fever*, or *neck stiffness*. The patient unaccustomed to having headaches who presents with the sudden onset of the *worst headache ever* experienced deserves prompt attention, particularly if fever, neck stiffness, ataxia, alteration in mental status, focal neurologic deficit, or visual impairment is reported. Diffuse headache in conjunction with a stiff neck and fever suggest acute meningitis. When acute headache and stiff neck occur in conjunction with ataxia of gait and profuse nausea and vomiting, a midline cerebellar hemorrhage needs to be considered. Early recognition is important because urgent surgical treatment can be life-saving. Abrupt onset of a headache that reaches maximum intensity immediately suggests rupture of a cerebral aneurysm. Hypertensive encephalopathy may be heralded by diffuse headache, nausea, vomiting, and altered mental status. Acute fever with fronto-orbital headache is suggestive of acute sinusitis. Eye pain and blurred vision raise the possibility of acute glaucoma. New onset of headache in an elderly patient requires consideration of temporal arteritis. Acute onset of a throbbing headache should trigger inquiry into migrainous epiphenomena (prodromal and aural symptoms), febrile illness, vasodilator use, carbon monoxide exposure, drug withdrawal, and hypoglycemia. A throbbing headache accompanied neurologic deficits may be migrainous, but if deficits persist beyond 24 to 36 hours, then stroke and other etiologies should be considered.

Recurrent or Persistent Headache. With migraine and tension-type headaches being the most common causes of chronic or recurrent headaches and brain tumor being the most feared, history becomes critical to the evaluation. The *clinical course* can be particularly revealing. Increases in severity and/or frequency over time raise the question of an intracranial mass lesion, whereas a headache pattern that remains constant or waxes and wanes is more typical of tension-type or migraine headache. The nightly occurrence of cluster headache followed by symptom-free intervals is among its most characteristic features.

Unlike acute headaches where severity helps to identify increased risk of serious pathology, the intensity of a chronic or recurrent headache is of little value. The headache of a brain tumor may begin as a relatively minor complaint, whereas pain due to migraine, cluster, or tension-type headache may be excruciating. Careful attention to *associated symptoms* is always essential. Inquiry into migrainous epiphenomena can be diagnostic, and eliciting a report of a new neurologic deficit strongly increases the likelihood of tumor. *Location* and *quality* are sometimes helpful, though there can be considerable overlap among etiologies. Whole-head, bandlike, and occipital-nuchal distributions suggest tension-type headache, as does tightness or pressure-like quality, but such complaints may also be reported when there is increased intracranial pressure. Unilateral location and throbbing are characteristic of migraine but sometimes are reported by patients with tension-type headache. Unilaterality and constancy of location typify the headache of tumor.

Associated symptoms are important for identification of other causes of chronic or recurrent headache. Temporomandibular pain suggests bruxism, while jaw claudication and scalp vessel tenderness indicate giant cell arteritis. Concurrent complaints of shoulder and hip-girdle discomfort provide supporting evidence. Neck pain raises the question of a cervical radiculopathy. Purulent nasal discharge is indicative of sinus disease. A history of head trauma, parameningeal infection, depression, situational stress, substance abuse, and family history of headaches should always be sought, and a careful medication history needs to be taken.

Aggravating and *precipitating factors* deserve investigation. Headache worsened by straining, coughing, or bending over is characteristic of an intracranial mass lesion; bending over may also exacerbate the headache of sinusitis. Headache brought on by taking certain foods or beverages (chocolate, cheese, red wine) is typical of migraine, which is also exacerbated by noise, odors, and bright light. Alcohol may also trigger cluster headache during a period of disease activity. Migraine can be induced or exacerbated by a host of drugs, including cimetidine, ethinyl estradiol, atenolol, indomethacin, danazol, nifedipine, selegiline, and oral contraceptives.

Physical Examination

Acute Headache. The physical examination contributes importantly to the search for serious underlying pathology. The blood pressure and temperature should be checked for elevations; the scalp for cranial artery tenderness; the sinuses for purulent discharge and tenderness; the pupils for loss of reactivity; the corneas for clouding (indicative of acute glaucoma); the disc margins for blunting; the neck for rigidity on anterior flexion; and the neurologic examination for ataxia, alteration of mental status, focal deficits, and meningeal signs.

Chronic or Recurrent Headache. The physical examination begins with a check of all elements mentioned for evaluation of acute headache and expands into other areas based on findings from the history. For example, in a patient with a headache history that includes facial pain, the oral cavity should be examined for a trigger zone indicative of trigeminal neuralgia, the teeth for signs of bruxism, the temporomandibular joint for limitation of motion and crepitus, and the neck for signs of degenerative disease (see Chapter 148) and movements that reproduce head pain. Excessively taut muscles and focal tenderness about the shoulders, neck, and occiput are noted in many patients with tension-type headache. A careful and complete neurologic examination is essential, because the finding of a fixed focal deficit is important evidence of intracranial pathology. Suspicion of a mass lesion necessitates consideration of brain abscess as well as malignancy and subdural hematoma. Under such circumstances, the nasal cavity is examined for purulent discharge, the sinuses for tenderness, and the ears for signs of chronic otitis media (see Chapter 218). Both sinusitis and chronic otitis are potential foci for parameningeal infection that could lead to brain abscess.

Laboratory Studies

Acute Headache. Patients with acute onset of the worst headache ever, especially if accompanied by meningeal signs or evidence of increased intracranial pressure, require prompt hospitalization. In such settings, an emergency *CT scan* is the test of choice for prompt detection of potentially life-threatening but treatable lesions (eg, midline cerebellar hemorrhage or CNS mass). In patients with signs of meningeal irritation, *lumbar puncture* and examination and culture of the cerebrospinal fluid should follow CT to rule out an infectious etiology, provided there is no evidence for markedly increased intracranial pressure. Plain *sinus films* can be used to confirm acute sinusitis when the diagnosis is in question. CT scan is occasionally necessary, especially when a parameningeal focus of infection is suspected (see Chapter

219). New onset of headache in an elderly patient, especially if accompanied by cranial artery or scalp tenderness, dictates the determination of an *erythrocyte sedimentation rate* to check for giant cell arteritis and consideration of a *temporal artery biopsy* (see Chapter 161).

Chronic or Recurrent Headache. Much of the controversy and discrepancies regarding proper headache evaluation result from failing to differentiate patients who present with a first headache from those who have had a chronic recurring headache. In the presence of a normal physical examination and a headache history that does not suggest intracranial disease but classifies the patient clearly into a recurring migrainous type of headache picture, ancillary studies are not likely to be useful.

A disturbing trend toward uncritical ordering of neuroimaging studies (initially *CT* and now *magnetic resonance imaging* [*MRI*]) for all patients with recurrent or chronic headache has led to escalating costs for evaluations that provide no more information than did the initial headache history and physical examination.

The probability of a chronic-headache patient with a normal neurologic examination having a positive neuroimaging study is exceedingly small. Yield is so low that in the absence of a very worrisome history or neurologic deficit on physical examination, there is no need for an imaging study. Some feel that the reassurance value of such testing can be helpful, but most patients with benign chronic headache who fear serious underlying disease can be adequately reassured if time is taken to review clinical findings and directly address patient concerns. Such steps are essential to providing meaningful reassurance and usually obviate the need for an otherwise medically unnecessary imaging procedure.

Nonetheless, there are a few instances when a neuroimaging study might still be appropriate in the absence of abnormalities on physical and neurologic examinations. These exceptions include patients with a headache of *recent onset* (< 6 mo) whose etiology is not still not apparent after thorough history and physical examination. In addition, those with a persistent headache that is *worsening* over time and does not fit the pattern of a tension-type headache should be considered for imaging study. When one uncovers a history of *aural symptoms* or *loss of consciousness* suggestive of a seizure (see Chapter 170), then a search for an intracranial mass lesion is warranted. If the patient or family member reports a *persistent personality change*, a tumor of the frontal or temporal regions might be suspected. If there is a *change in the character* of long-standing headache or if the headache fails to respond to treatment directed at a diagnosis initially suspected, such as migraine, the utility of MRI or CT scanning increases.

The efforts taken to perform a careful history and physical examination are well worth the time, for these methods remain the best means available for efficient test selection and accurate diagnosis of headache.

PRINCIPLES OF MANAGEMENT

Migraine

Migraine is the one headache disorder for which there currently exists relatively specific therapy; therefore, establishing its presence is extremely important to the patient. The neurogenic hypothesis has refocused attention from vasodilators to drugs designed to act on serotonin receptors. Several older drugs useful in the prophylaxis of migraine (*methysergide*, *cyproheptadine*) have been found to act as 5-HT_2 serotonin receptor antagonists. Drugs most useful in acute migraine attacks (*ergotamine* and its derivatives, *sumatriptan*) interact with the presynaptic serotonin 5-HT 1D and 1A receptors, inhibiting the release of neurotransmitters.

Prophylaxis. Most patients with migraine can be helped by implementing both prophylactic and abortive measures. Once the diagnosis is established by the criteria of the most recent classification system, the physician should ascertain the frequency of disabling headache. As a general rule, if headaches are interfering with work or other activities more than once per week, it is reasonable to consider prophylactic medication. Educating the migraine-prone patient to avoid precipitants such as certain foods (cheese, chocolates, citrus fruits, nuts, red wine—though not invariably in all patients), inadequate sleep, and prolonged fasting, may help prevent some headaches. Useful information on precipitants is sometimes derived by keeping a *headache diary*.

Prevention of attacks involves *nonpharmacologic measures* as well as drug treatment. Since migraine may be precipitated by emotional stress or psychologic conflict, it is important to investigate family, work, and social circumstances in designing a program of prevention. Regular *exercise* and *relaxation techniques* (see Chapter 226) may significantly decrease the frequency and severity of headaches. These activities help reduce the impact of stress. Many patients prefer to try them before attempting other forms of therapy. Patients under significant psychological stress may benefit from informal supportive psychotherapy, helping them to express their feelings and deal with their stresses. Although extensive psychotherapy may not reduce attacks, it is worth trying to determine areas of stress and search with the patient for ways to resolve them. Recommending rest or a vacation might not suffice; in fact, flare-ups are common during vacations and weekends.

Biofeedback methods are of unproven benefit and probably no better than relaxation exercises and other nonpharmacologic methods. Lack of adequately designed studies limits conclusions regarding biofeedback.

Drug therapy should be added when nonpharmacologic measures do not suffice. Several different classes of drugs have been useful in the prophylaxis of migraine. These are listed in order of the author's preference. It is often necessary to take a trial and error approach before finding the appropriate medication which is most effective with the least side effects in any individual patient. Each drug should be given at least a 2-month trial, and many patients require longer than this before full benefit is obtained. In general, *beta-blockers* are the first-line drugs for prophylaxis. Propranolol is the agent most extensively studied, though others are similarly effective. Should beta-blockers fail or should the exercise capacity of the patient preclude full beta-blockade, then a *tricyclic antidepressant* (eg, *amitriptyline*) can be tried. Another alternative is *verapamil*, the most widely prescribed calcium channel blocker for migraine prophylaxis. *Nonsteroidal antiinflammatory drugs* (eg, naproxen) have been useful, especially for patients with menstrual migraine.

They are prescribed for several days before, during, and after menstruation. *Valproate*, an anticonvulsant drug which interacts with the gamma aminobutyric acid neurotransmitter system and turns off serotoninergic raphe neurons, has also attracted interest. Additional considerations and potential side effects of each medication are listed in Table 165–2.

Abortive Therapy. For the patient with only occasional migraine headaches and for patients who are generally well controlled but have occasional severe breakthrough headaches, it is important to establish an effective abortive regimen. In general, it is best to avoid regular use of *analgesics* and *sedatives*. Popular combination analgesic/sedative formulations containing acetaminophen or aspirin, butalbital, and caffeine (eg, Fioricet and Fiorinal) are often requested by patients, having been widely prescribed in the past. While they may be helpful for occasional use, marked caution is warranted in prescribing such combination agents because of their habituation potential when used regularly in a chronic recurring condition such as migraine. In addition, Fiorinal previously contained phenacetin, which in large cumulative doses causes interstitial nephritis. Narcotic analgesics are sometimes needed, but their regular use can lead to a vicious cycle of headache, narcotic intake, drug withdrawal, more headache, and more narcotic use (see below).

Dihydroergotamine, available since the early 1940s, is highly effective when given subcutaneously, intramuscularly (IM), or intravenously (IV). Its parenteral use in emergency room settings has helped to terminate severe acute migrainous attacks. Though dihydroergotamine has minimal vasoconstrictive effects on peripheral arteries, it is contraindicated in patients with coronary disease, peripheral vascular disease, transient ischemic attacks, pregnancy, or sepsis.

Sumatriptan is the newest agent in the migraine armamentarium. It is a selective serotonin 5-HT 1D receptor agonist. A single 6-mg subcutaneous dose has proven highly effective, rapid-acting, and well tolerated for treatment of severe migraine attacks. An oral formulation is under development and has the potential for greatly improving outpatient abortive therapy.

Ergotamine tartrate is widely used for relief of acute attacks and is most useful in patients who have some warning that headache is imminent. It stimulates serotoninergic receptors and constricts the arteries of the scalp. It is believed to counteract the vasodilatation phase of migraine headache. Complete or partial relief from the headache occurs in about 70 percent of patients, but to be effective, ergotamine must be taken at the first sign of an attack, such as during the prodromal phase. The lack of a prodrome in many migraine patients means there is often little advance warning, and this limits ergotamine's usefulness.

Table 165-2. Drugs for Migraine Headache Prophylaxis

DRUG	RECOMMENDED DOSAGES	SIDE EFFECTS/SPECIAL CONSIDERATIONS
Beta-blockers		
propranolol	40–320 mg/d	Full beta-blockade required. Three months may be necessary to achieve full benefit.
nadolol	40–240 mg/d	Contraindications: congestive heart failure, asthma.
atenolol	50–150 mg/d	Side effects: drowsiness, exercise intolerance, depression.
timolol	10–30 mg/d	
Tricyclic antidepressants		
amitriptyline	10–300 mg/d	Efficacy in headache treatment is independent of antidepressant effect and may occur earlier and with lower doses than antidepressant effect.
nortriptyline	10–125 mg/d	Side effects: drowsiness, urinary retention, weight gain.
doxepin	10–150 mg/d	
Calcium channel blockers		
verapamil	240–720 mg/d	May require 1 month for perceived benefit. Contraindications: congestive heart failure, heart block, atrial fibrillation, sick sinus syndrome. Side effects: hypotension, atrioventricular block, headache, constipation, edema, congestive heart failure.
Nonsteroidal antiinflammatory drugs		
naproxen	500 mg bid	Particularly useful for women with menstrual migraine, taken for several days peri-menstruation. Side effects: gastrointestinal upset, ulcers, worsening renal function in susceptible patients. Contraindications: ulcer, aspirin sensitivity, renal failure.
Anticonvulsants		
valproate	Titration to therapeutic level from 250 mg tid	Side effects: nausea, platelet dysfunction, hair loss, hepatotoxicity.
phenytoin	Adjustment to therapeutic level, usually 200–400 mg/d	Particularly useful for children. Side effects: rash, ataxia, hepatic dysfunction, gingival hypertrophy.
Serotonin antagonist		
methysergide	2–4 mg in divided doses, usual dose 6–8 mg/day	Idiosyncratic reaction of retroperitoneal, pulmonary, or endocardial fibrosis. Cannot be given for more than 6 mo continuously. Side effects: nausea, muscle cramps, weight gain, peripheral arterial insufficiency.

The initial dose of ergotamine is 1 to 2 mg sublingually, orally, or rectally. The sublingual form is faster acting and more effective than the oral route due to reduced gastric absorption during an attack. An inhaled form is also rapid in onset of action. *Caffeine* potentiates ergotamine by increasing its absorption; as a result, some patients note even better results when using an ergot–caffeine combination preparation (eg, Cafergot). Because of nausea and vomiting, some patients prefer to use a rectal suppository preparation of ergotamine. The ergotamine should be repeated every hour if there is no relief, until a maximum 24-hour dose of 6 to 8 mg is taken. Further doses are generally not helpful and may lead to toxicity.

Ergotamine is reasonably safe when used properly. Serious reactions occur in only 0.1 percent of patients. Nausea and vomiting are common side effects which can be minimized by use of rectal suppositories, pretreatment with metoclopramide, or prochlorperazine. Adverse effects include myalgias, paresthesias, chest discomfort, peripheral ischemia, and even angina. With excessive use, rebound headache and dependency may occur. Dependency and rebound headaches are managed by discontinuing the drug and controlling the headache with other medications.

Ergotamine is contraindicated in patients with vascular disease such as Raynaud's syndrome, coronary artery disease, thromboangiitis obliterans, thrombophlebitis, and severe atherosclerosis. The drug should not be taken during pregnancy, because it causes uterine contractions as well as vasoconstriction.

For most patients, a combination of a tolerable prophylactic medication with occasional use of analgesics or abortive regimens should minimize the intrusion of this highly disabling condition into patients' daily lives. Because most prophylactic drugs require several weeks to several months to establish efficacy, it is particularly important to establish a strong and sympathetic relationship with each migraine patient.

Cluster Headache

As with migraine, both abortive and prophylactic treatments are available. One abortive treatment for an acute attack consists of *oxygen* inhalation at 5 to 8 liters per minute for 10 minutes. *Ergotamine suppositories* may be effective and can be taken at bedtime during a cluster for a patient whose symptoms all occur at night. *Dihydroergotamine* (IM or IV as outlined above) is effective, as is *sumatriptan*. A corticosteroid bolus of 8 mg of *dexamethasone* or a *prednisone* taper beginning at 20 mg three times a day and tapering over 2 weeks has also been helpful in aborting a cluster.

Prophylactic therapy for patients with chronic cluster headaches or for those with severe frequent cluster episodes includes *verapamil*, at a typical daily dose of 360 mg per day in divided doses. *Methysergide*, 2 mg three times a day, or *lithium* at doses which achieve a therapeutic level identical to that for its use in bipolar disease also are useful. A radiofrequency *trigeminal rhizotomy* is reserved for patients who are completely refractory to all the above medical therapies.

Tension-Type Headache

For the vast majority with mild or occasional tension headache, mild analgesics (aspirin, acetaminophen, nonprescription doses of nonsteroidal anti inflammatory drugs) usually suffice. Such patients usually do not consult the physician. Patients suffering from chronic or persistent tension-type headaches are candidates for evaluation of underlying anxiety and depression (see Chapters 226 and 227). Often, definitive treatment of such headaches requires addressing the underlying sources of psychological distress. *Stress reduction* measures may be of considerable help for those with an anxiety state (see Appendix, Chapter 226); *antidepressant therapy* may benefit depressed patients (see Chapter 227). Patients with chronic headache subsequent to trauma should be encouraged to conclude any pending legal proceedings.

Chronic Daily Headaches

Those with chronic daily headache are among the most difficult of headache patients encountered by primary physicians. For some, a migraine syndrome evolves into a daily headache more typical of tension-type headache with superimposed migrainous events. Depression, anxiety, and drug abuse may all complicate the picture at this stage. While counseling this group of patients about precipitating factors and lifestyle modification, it is important to elicit a history of analgesic and ergotamine use. Ergotamine or analgesic abuse can lead to a vicious headache–medication–headache cycle. As the effect of a previous dose of ergotamine or analgesic wanes, headache begins to recur, leading to more medication use. Drug-induced sleep disturbances and psychological dependence ensue, leading to a self-sustaining rhythmic headache–medication cycle. Thus, caution must be exerted to avoid prescribing large amounts of ergotamine and/or analgesics (both narcotic and non-narcotic) for patient with migraine or tension-type headache. Total elimination of analgesics and ergotamine compounds may improve the therapeutic results of other medications chosen for the prophylaxis of headache. Hospitalization for withdrawal of medication and institution of a comprehensive program may be beneficial.

Management of Other Conditions Causing Headache

For treatment of temporomandibular joint dysfunction and bruxism, see Chapter 225. See Chapter 161 for management of temporal arteritis and Chapter 219 for treatment of sinusitis.

INDICATIONS FOR ADMISSION AND REFERRAL

Urgent hospitalization is indicated for the patient with acute onset of a severe headache accompanied by signs of meningeal irritation. Intracranial hemorrhage or meningeal infection may be responsible. Evidence suggesting increased intracranial pressure is another indication for prompt admission. Severe intractable migraine may require prompt hospital admission for one of the abortive treatments outlined above.

Less urgent headache situations deserving of neurologic consultation include episodes of transient neurologic dysfunction, unilateral headache increasing in frequency and severity, change in personality, and new onset of progressive deficits suggesting an evolving process or a mass lesion. Sometimes patients with an intractable tension-type headache or severe migraine syndrome can benefit from the reassurance and suggestions provided by the neurologist. Dental consultation is indicated if temporomandibular joint problems appear refractory to conservative therapy. Surgical referral for temporal artery biopsy may be necessary in the elderly patient who is suspected of having giant cell arteritis but in need of more definitive evidence to warrant chronic steroid therapy (see Chapter 161).

The ophthalmologist needs to be consulted at once if acute glaucoma is thought to be the cause of an acute orbital headache. If prolonged close-up work is resulting in headaches, a referral is in order for a vision check and assessment of the need for refraction.

For the patient with a chronic, intractable, tension-type headache, a diagnostic consultation with a psychiatrist may serve as an important learning experience. However, many of these patients are reluctant to consider a psychological cause for their symptoms. Thus, it is important that a full medical evaluation be conducted before psychiatric referral is suggested. This obviates any misunderstanding from the patient who believes there is a medical basis for the problem and who may view the referral as an inappropriate dismissal of his symptoms.

ANNOTATED BIBLIOGRAPHY

American College of Physicians Health and Public Policy Committee. Biofeedback for headaches. Ann Intern Med 1985; 102:128. *(Concludes that there is insufficient data to recommend biofeedback for migraine and that there is no evidence suggesting it is any better than relaxation techniques.)*

Diamond S, et al. Propranolol in prophylaxis of migraine headache. Headache 1982;22:268. *(A single-blind study showing a response rate of 70 percent; no tolerance developed after 6 mo of continued use.)*

Linet MS, Cohen A. An epidemiologic study of headache among adolescents and young adults. JAMA 1989;261:2211. *(Useful information on incidence and an illustration of use of the new classification system.)*

Linet MS, Stewart WF. Migraine headache: epidemiologic perspectives. Epidemiol Rev 1984;6:107. *(Exhaustive review detailing descriptive epidemiology of migraine, genetic and physiologic predisposing factors, and factors associated with onset and frequency of attacks.)*

Mathew NT. Cluster headache. Neurology 1992;42(Suppl 2):22. *(Good overview.)*

Meyer JS. Calcium channel blockers in the prophylactic treatment of vascular headache. Ann Intern Med 1985;102:395. *(Reviews evidence for their use in prophylaxis of migraine and cluster headaches.)*

Moskowitz MA. Basic mechanisms in vascular headaches. Neurol Clin North Am 1990;8:801. *(A basic science look at an area long in need of pathophysiologic clarification.)*

Rapoport AM. The diagnosis of migraine and tension-type headache, then and now. Neurology 1992;42(Suppl 2):11. *(This article reviews the complexities of the new classification system and offers some straightforward criteria for grouping patients and for critiquing the current classification.)*

Robb-Nicholson C, Change RW, Anderson S, et al. Diagnostic value of the history and examination in giant cell arteritis. J Rheumatol 1988;15:1793. *(A retrospective study comparing clinical features with biopsy results.)*

Saper JR. Daily chronic headache. Neurol Clin North Am 1990;8:891. *(A sympathetic look at the very difficult problem of daily chronic headache with some appropriate treatment strategies.)*

Silberstein SD. Advances in understanding the pathophysiology of headache. Neurology 1992;42(Suppl 2):6. *(A brief survey of recent developments in serotonin receptor pharmacology.)*

Silberstein SD. Estrogens, progestins and headache. Neurology 1991;41:786. *(A useful review of the often contradictory evidence about hormonal influence on migraine headache.)*

Spierings EL. Clinical and experimental evidence for a role of calcium entry blockers in the treatment of migraine. Ann N Y Acad Sci 1988;522:676. *(Comprehensive and critical review of available data on efficacy.)*

Stewart WF. Prevalence of migraine headache in the United States. JAMA 1992;267:64. *(This is likely to become a classic article dispelling many previously held tenets about migraine epidemiology.)*

The Subcutaneous Sumatriptan International Study Group. Treatment of migraine attack with sumatriptan. N Engl J Med 1991;325:316. *(Double-blind, randomized, controlled, parallel study of this novel agent which appears to be highly effective both for aborting acute migraine and for cluster headache.)*

Weingarten S, Kleinman M, Elperin L, Larsen EB. The effectiveness of cerebral imaging in the diagnosis of chronic headache. Arch Intern Med 1992;152:2457. *(Cost is high; yield is exceedingly low in persons with no neurologic deficits.)*

Ziegler DK. Headache. Public health problem. Neurol Clin North Am 1990;8:781. *(This is an overview of the enormous impact of headache in the United States population.)*

Primary Care Medicine: Office Evaluation and Management of the Adult Patient, 3rd edition, edited by Allan H. Goroll, Lawrence A. May, and Albert G. Mulley, Jr. J.B. Lippincott Company, Philadelphia

166
Evaluation of Dizziness

Dizziness can be one of the more frustrating complaints to assess, a task often made difficult by a vague history and a large number of possible etiologies, ranging from psychiatric disease and cardiovascular disorders to peripheral and central defects within the nervous system. However, with a bit of patience and careful attention to the history and physical examination, the primary physician can conduct a remarkably sophisticated clinical evaluation, one that will help direct further workup and treatment. In the setting of true vertigo, the goals are to distinguish central from peripheral disease, worrisome from benign etiologies.

PATHOPHYSIOLOGY AND CLINICAL PRESENTATION

The patient complaining of "dizziness" may be suffering from vestibular dysfunction, cardiovascular insufficiency, psychiatric illness, metabolic derangement, multiple sensory deficits, cerebellar disease, or a combination of problems.

Vestibular Disease

Patients with vestibular disease experience *true vertigo*, which is defined as a head sensation of abnormal movement, be it internal or in reference to one's surroundings. Descriptive terms include not only "spinning" but also "weaving," "seasickness," "ground rising and falling," "rocking," "things moving," and "merry-go-round" sensation. Nausea, vomiting, and diaphoresis accompany severe cases. Tinnitus and hearing loss indicate associated injury to the auditory component of the eighth cranial nerve. Nystagmus is frequently found on examination (see below) or can be induced.

The vestibular problem may be central or peripheral; peripheral lesions include those which are cochlear or retrocochlear. Central lesions differ from peripheral ones in that they typically present with vertigo in association with other brainstem deficits; in peripheral disease, vertigo occurs in isolation except for accompanying tinnitus or hearing loss.

Peripheral Lesions. *Benign positional vertigo* is a common problem in the elderly, consisting of vertigo experienced only in specific positions. Onset is sudden, usually within a few seconds of assuming the triggering position. Symptoms cease after several minutes if the patient does not move, but will resume with further change in position. In most patients, the condition resolves within 6 months; recovery is usually complete. Head trauma sometimes results in this type of temporary vertigo. One suspected mechanism is development of a small fistula into the middle ear that allows changes of pressure in the middle ear to be transmitted to the inner ear, precipitating vertigo. Another possible explanation is cupulolithiasis: a piece of calcium from the internal apparatus breaks free into the endolymph and pressures the end organ. A more permanent form of positional vertigo results from vascular compression of the vestibular nerve. Patients with this condition suffer from constant positional vertigo and severe nausea; it has been labeled *"disabling positional vertigo"* to distinguish it from the more common forms of positional vertiginous disease.

Ménière's disease ensues from idiopathic endolymphatic hydrops, with damage to the hair cells from swelling of the semicircular ducts. Patients report tinnitus, pressure in the ear, and hearing loss in conjunction with vertigo. Episodes are paroxysmal, last minutes to hours, and then decrease in frequency after multiple attacks, only to recur in several months or years. Hearing loss and tinnitus usually accompany the episodes of vertigo and can be quite disabling.

Acute labyrinthitis develops as a consequence of viral infection involving the cochlea and labyrinth. The patient reports a viral upper respiratory syndrome followed by onset of vertigo, tinnitus, and hearing loss. Symptoms resolve entirely by 3 to 6 weeks, with no residual deficits. *Vestibular neuronitis* is believed to be the same illness, without any cochlear involvement; there is isolated vertigo, no hearing loss, and full clearing.

Ototoxins can injure the peripheral vestibular apparatus, although hearing impairment usually predominates. Streptomycin and gentamicin are among the toxins that are most injurious to the vestibular portion of the eighth cranial nerve.

Acoustic neuroma (benign schwannoma of the eighth cranial nerve) represents the most worrisome of the peripheral lesions, retrocochlear in location and distinguished from the others by its retrocochlear type of hearing loss (see below) and capacity to produce serious brainstem compression if untreated. Symptoms start out almost imperceptibly with mild hearing loss, tinnitus, and vague dizziness and may resemble other forms of peripheral vestibular disease. However, the clinical course is progressive, differentiating it from other peripheral etiologies. Most patients do not come to medical attention until later stages, when the expanding tumor compresses adjacent structures in the cerebellopontile (C-P) angle, causing cranial nerve and brainstem deficits to develop (eg, facial numbness, gait ataxia, weakness). A decreased corneal reflex is one of the earliest signs of damage outside the internal auditory meatus.

Central Lesions. As already noted, these are accompanied in most instances by other brainstem symptoms. In addition, the vertigo and any accompanying nystagmus can be bidirectional or vertical, which does not occur in peripheral vestibular disease.

Multiple sclerosis (MS) causing focal demyelination in the vestibular pathways of the brainstem is an important central etiology of vertigo. The often transient nature of attacks (days to weeks) and subtlety of accompanying symptoms (slight facial numbness or huskiness of voice) may at first cause one to mistake MS for one of the self-limited peripheral etiologies. Only with repeat episodes might the etiology become more evident. In the later phases of an acute attack, a central type of positional nystagmus may persist after the vertigo resolves. There are no characteristic features of the vertigo; attacks can be sudden, transient, recurrent, or persistent. Diagnosis depends on evidence of discrete central nervous system (CNS) lesions and a course of recurrent dysfunction interspersed with remissions.

Vertebrobasilar insufficiency usually produces vertigo in conjunction with diplopia, sensory loss, dysarthria, dysphagia, hemiparesis, and other brainstem deficits. Self-limited episodes are manifestations of transient ischemic attacks. In about one-quarter of cases, transient vertigo may be the initial and sole complaint; however, later episodes almost always include other brainstem symptoms.

Drugs that suppress the reticular activating system of the brainstem (eg, sedatives, anticonvulsants) can cause vertigo of a central nature, especially when taken in excess. Therapeutic doses of some drugs (eg, phenytoin) produce nystagmus.

Cardiovascular Disease

Cardiac and vascular insufficiency leading to inadequate cerebral perfusion can result in dizziness, which patients tend to describe as *"light-headedness"* or a sense of faintness (see Chapter 24). This form of dizziness is seen in patients with fixed or limited cardiac output, serious cardiac dysrhythmias, diminished vascular tone, or severe intravascular volume depletion. Symptoms typically worsen on standing and improve on lying down; postural change in blood pressure and/or pulse are characteristic.

Multiple Sensory Deficits, Cerebellar Disease, and Other Causes of Dysequilibrium

These neurologic problems produce sensations of *impaired balance* and *dysequilibrium*. Unlike other forms of dizziness, patients report the sensation to be in the feet rather than in the head. Like light-headedness, it may come on with standing; like true vertigo, it can be aggravated by walking or turning. The most common cause is multiple sensory deficits. Patients with multiple sensory deficits are usually elderly and suffer from diabetes or other conditions that impair eyesight, position sense, and motor function. Symptoms are typically worse in the dark (due to elimination of visual positional data) and improved by use of a cane or holding onto a railing. Elderly patients complaining of dysequilibrium may also suffer from degenerative cerebellar disease. Physical examination is notable for ataxia and other cerebellar signs. Acute dysequilibrium may be caused by a midline cerebellar hemorrhage and present as severe dizziness, marked gait ataxia, headache, and stiff neck.

Psychiatric Illness

Patients with psychiatric difficulties complain of ill-defined dizziness ("I just feel dizzy"), constant "light-headedness," or a "foggy" feeling. Depression, anxiety states, and psychosis, as well as the medications used to treat such conditions, are common precipitants. The precise mechanism of the light-headedness is unknown, but it is thought to be related to a confusional state induced by these illnesses or by the medications used to treat them. In the case of a panic attack leading to hyperventilation (see Chapter 226), the ensuing metabolic alkalosis usually leads to paresthesias and light-headedness, though sometimes vertigo is reported.

Metabolic Disturbances

Alteration of CNS metabolic homeostasis can cause dizziness which resembles that due to inadequate cerebral perfusion. The patient complains of light-headedness or feeling faint. Precipitants of acute symptoms include hypoglycemia, hypoxia, hypocarbia, hypercarbia, and drugs.

DIFFERENTIAL DIAGNOSIS

Conditions that cause dizziness can be grouped according to pathophysiologic mechanism (Table 166–1). Vestibular disease is divided into central and peripheral types. Central lesions are mostly caused by basilar artery disease and multiple sclerosis. Peripheral causes include acoustic neuroma, benign positional vertigo, vestibular neuronitis, Ménière's disease, and ototoxic drugs.

Table 166-1. Differential Diagnosis of Dizziness

Vestibular Disease
Benign positional vertigo
Vestibular neuronitis and ototoxic drugs
Ménière's disease
Acoustic neuroma and other tumors of the cerebellopontine angle
Basilar insufficiency
Multiple sclerosis
Cardiac and Vascular Disease
Critical aortic stenosis
Carotid sinus hypersensitivity
Volume depletion and severe anemia
Autonomic insufficiency (drugs, diabetes)
Diminished vascular reflexes of the elderly
Multiple Sensory Deficits
Diabetes mellitus
Cataract surgery
Some cases of multiple sclerosis
Cervical spondylosis
Cerebellar disease
Psychiatric Illness
Anxiety
Depression
Psychosis
Metabolic Disturbances
Hypoxia
Severe hypoglycemia
Hypo- and hypercapnia

Cardiac and vascular diseases are a second important group. Faintness on standing may be caused by critical aortic stenosis, severe volume depletion, the use of antihypertensive drugs, autonomic insufficiency, or prolonged confinement to bed. Carotid sinus hypersensitivity results in inappropriate reduction of vascular tone.

Multiple sensory deficits are most common in diabetics and others with poor vision and peripheral neuropathies. Cervical spondylosis disturbs cervical sensory input and contributes to dizziness. The thick lenses used by patients following cataract surgery distort peripheral vision and can confuse their sense of position. Cerebellar dysfunction leads to a similar clinical presentation of gait unsteadiness.

Psychiatric problems are often associated with light-headedness. Patients with anxiety, depression, and psychosis report feeling light-headed. At times, tranquilizers and antidepressants are responsible. Metabolic disturbances affecting the CNS have a similar presentation; hypoxia, hypoglycemia, hypocapnia and hypercapnia are among the most important.

In a study of 104 consecutive cases referred for evaluation of dizziness, 38 percent of patients had peripheral vestibular disease, 23 percent had hyperventilation, 13 percent had multiple sensory deficits, 9 percent had psychiatric problems, and 5 percent had cardiovascular or central neurologic illness. Many cases are multifactorial.

WORKUP

History. The most important initial step in the evaluation of dizziness is to obtain the best possible description of the patient's experience and what he means by "dizziness." A history taken without leading questions or suggested descriptions is most likely to provide meaningful clues. *True vertigo* suggests *vestibular disease*; *faintness* that is *postural* or paroxysmal implies a *cardiovascular* disorder; constant *ill-defined dizziness* or light-headedness unrelated to posture points toward a *psychogenic* etiology; a feeling of *poor balance* or disequilibrium typifies *multiple sensory deficits* and *cerebellar* causes.

If the patient complains of *vertigo,* the first task is to determine whether the lesion is *central* or *peripheral*. The most direct way of making this distinction is to inquire about brainstem symptoms (eg, diplopia, facial numbness, weakness, hemiplegia, dysphasia). Evidence of brainstem involvement rules out a peripheral lesion (with the exception of a very advanced acoustic neuroma compressing the cerebellopontile angle). The absence of brainstem symptoms does not rule out a central lesion but does make its probability very low. Even the very confusing picture of apparently isolated vertigo due to vertebrobasilar insufficiency or multiple sclerosis eventually becomes clearer as accompanying brainstem symptoms become more evident. The pattern of discrete CNS lesions and a course of recurrent episodes followed by remissions further suggest the diagnosis of MS (see Chapter 172).

In the patient with a suspected *peripheral lesion*, the focus turns to distinguishing *cochlear* from *retrocochlear* disease, that is, relatively benign etiologies from acoustic neuroma. The latter has a variable presentation and can initially mimic other peripheral types of vertigo. Episodes of vertigo, tinnitus, pressure in the ear, and hearing loss may take place, simulating Ménière's disease. However, the hearing loss is slowly and steadily progressive, rather than fluctuating or episodic. The development of brainstem symptoms (facial weakness or numbness) is a late occurrence and not very helpful for early diagnosis. When doubt still persists, physical examination and audiologic testing can be used to help make the cochlear/retrocochlear differentiation (see below).

With most other peripheral causes of vertigo, *timing* and *precipitating factors* help elucidate etiology. If symptoms occur only on change of *position* and last but a few moments, the diagnosis is benign positional vertigo, a condition mostly affecting people older than age 60. It may be a recurrent problem. A single bout of severe spontaneous vertigo, sudden in onset, sometimes after a *viral illness*, is usually vestibular neuronitis. When seen in the context of inner ear infection, it is properly called acute labyrinthitis. Some degree of positional vertigo may remain after the acute illness resolves. Ménière's disease is suggested by acute, recurrent paroxysms of vertigo that are accompanied by *tinnitus* and temporary *hearing loss*. Tinnitus, *pressure* in the ear, and hearing loss are episodic and may precede the other symptoms. Attacks can last for hours to days; residual positional vertigo occurs in 25 percent of cases.

Obtaining a thorough *drug history* is important. The ototoxic effects of the aminoglycoside antibiotics have been well documented; the diuretic ethacrynic acid also can cause eighth nerve injury, especially in patients with compromised renal function. Potent diuretics may be responsible for severe volume depletion. Vasodilators, phenothiazines, and antihypertensive agents can produce postural light-headedness. Antidepressants and minor tranquilizers cause some patients to feel dizzy.

When the complaint is light-headedness, it is worth asking if standing or turning brings on symptoms. If standing does, antihypertensive, tranquilizer, or antidepressant use should be investigated. During the examination, postural signs, carotid upstroke, and cardiac function should be evaluated, especially for signs of hemodynamically significant aortic stenosis. If turning worsens the situation, it is important to evaluate vision, search for other sensory deficits, and check for cerebellar signs (see below). If light-headedness is a constant sensation, an underlying psychiatric or metabolic disorder is likely. Anxiety and depression are frequent causes and warrant investigation (see Chapters 226 and 227).

Physical Examination. *General appearance* can be quite informative (eg, the anxious person will appear overly nervous and may hyperventilate or sigh frequently during the interview). *Blood pressure* and pulse should be taken and noted for changes between readings taken in the *supine* and *standing* positions. The skin is examined for pallor, the eyes for *nystagmus* (remembering that a few beats of nystagmus on extreme lateral gaze are normal) and the ears for tympanic membrane lesions and *hearing acuity* (see below). The carotid arteries in the neck are checked for bruits (suggestive of cerebrovascular disease) and delay in upstroke (characteristic of severe aortic stenosis). A forceful, sustained left ventricular impulse, single second heart sound, and loud ejection quality murmur on cardiac examination also support a diagnosis of significant aortic stenosis (see Chapter 21).

A thorough and careful *neurologic examination* is essential, particularly when the possibility of central vestibular disease is being considered. Most important is examination for a brainstem lesion, which suggests central pathology or extrinsic compression by an acoustic neuroma. Cranial nerves V, VII, and X can be affected by a large acoustic neuroma pressing at the cerebellopontile angle of the brainstem. Testing of sensory function, peripheral vision, and gait often reveals multiple defects in elderly patients troubled by dizziness. The *Romberg test* (standing with feet together, eyes closed) will also be abnormal in such patients, as well as in some with vestibular disease. The side to which the vertiginous patient sways has value in helping to localize the lesion. Cerebellar testing helps detect any ataxia.

Provocative maneuvers designed to trigger symptoms and reproduce the patient's complaint can be extremely useful. Asking the anxious patient to voluntarily *hyperventilate* for 30 to 120 seconds will often reproduce his "dizziness" and associated symptoms, while vestibular maneuvers (see below) will not. *Standing up* from a supine position will cause the patient with cardiac or vascular pathology to feel faint; it may trigger vertigo in the patient with vestibular disease. *Walking and turning* will cause a feeling of dysequilibrium in the patient with multiple sensory deficits, cerebellar disease, or vestibular dysfunction. The *Bárány maneuver* (also referred to as the Nylan-Bárány maneuver) and other forms of vestibular stimulation (see below) will trigger vertigo and associated symptoms.

Maneuvers which alleviate symptoms are also of diagnostic use. Getting up slowly lessens the faint feeling associated with cardiovascular causes; *paper bag rebreathing* reduces the light, giddy feeling that follows hyperventilation; *lying still* in one position may halt positional vertigo; touching the examiner's hand or using a *cane* to walk helps the patient with sensory deficits or cerebellar dysfunction. Withholding suspected drugs may be informative.

Simple office tests of hearing and stimulation of the vestibular apparatus can be very helpful in distinguishing central from peripheral disease and cochlear from retrocochlear peripheral pathology. The *Rinne test* (see Chapter 212) identifies which eighth cranial nerve is involved and helps differentiate between conductive and sensorineural hearing loss. Patients with a sensorineural hearing deficit may have a cochlear lesion or a retrocochlear one. The distinction can be made by testing *speech discrimination*, which is easily performed in the office by whispering a series of ten, two-syllable, closely linked words (eg, baseball, ice cream) into the patient's ear while making a sound in the other ear to limit its participation. The patient is asked to repeat each whispered word. Correctly identifying fewer than 20 percent of the words is very suggestive of a retrocochlear lesion (which causes a disproportionate loss of speech discrimination); a score of 70 percent or better indicates the problem is cochlear. Scores in between these are indeterminate and necessitate formal audiologic testing (see Chapter 212).

Vestibular stimulation testing serves both as a good provocative test for reproducing symptoms (useful when the description of dizziness remains unclear) and as a means of distinguishing peripheral from central vestibular disease. The *Bárány maneuver* (Fig. 166–1) is the least noxious of the standard forms of vestibular stimulation. The patient starts in a sitting position on the examination table and lies down with his head extending over the edge of the table, tilted back and turned 45° to one side. The assumption of this position need not be overly abrupt, but it should be held for at least 30 seconds. The maneuver is repeated, this time turning the head 45° to the opposite side. A final time the test is repeated without turning the head.

The Bárány maneuver provides simultaneous stimulation of all three semicircular canals. It is a useful provocative maneuver for identification of vestibular disease and potentially helpful in separating peripheral from central etiologies. One asks the patient to look straight ahead and watches for onset of nystagmus (horizontal or rotatory) and reproduction of symptoms. If symptoms occur, one asks to which side do things seem to be spinning; if nystagmus ensues, one notes to which side the slow phase moves. Combining these results with findings from Romberg and Rinne testing, one can make a diagnosis of a peripheral lesion if 1) the slow phase of nystagmus moves toward the same side as the hearing loss; 2) the patient reports the spinning is away from the side of the hearing loss; 3) the Romberg test is positive and the patient sways toward the side of the hearing deficit. Absence of any one of these findings suggests a central lesion.

Other findings of Bárány testing suggestive of central vestibular disease are immediate onset of nystagmus and vertigo (peripheral disease has a latency period of 3–40 sec), failure of nystagmus and vertigo to extinguish (symptoms usually resolve within 30 sec), and failure of the patient to adapt on repeated testing.

Laboratory Studies. *Electronystagmography* (ENG) and *audiologic testing* are indicated when clinical and provocative data are insufficient to differentiate between central and peripheral causes of vertigo (see Chapter 212). If acoustic neuroma is suspected, then one should consider *brainstem auditory evoked response* testing. It represents the best audiologic means of differentiating cochlear from retrocochlear disease. In addition, *computed tomography (CT)* or *magnetic resonance imaging (MRI)* of the internal auditory canal and C-P angle should follow if evidence of a retrocochlear lesion emerges from audiologic testing. MRI gives the best images, but CT is less expensive and more widely available. If basilar transient ischemic attacks are a concern because of transient, isolated vertiginous spells, most authorities believe it to be much safer to wait for confirmation by the appearance of accompanying brainstem symptoms than to hastily order angiography or anticoagulation.

SYMPTOMATIC THERAPY AND PATIENT EDUCATION

Dizziness can be controlled in most instances. Therapy is aimed at the underlying pathophysiology. True vertigo responds to avoidance of precipitating positions and movements, use of *meclizine* (25–50 mg q6h prn), and if nausea and vomiting are not controlled by meclizine alone, *promethazine* (25 mg q6h prn). These drugs are sedating and can cause drowsiness (which may be welcome in a patient having an acute attack but is an adverse effect in treatment of chronic disease). Low-dose meclizine (12.5 mg tid) is quite effective in elderly patients and causes less sedation.

Other drugs used to decrease vertigo include *dimenhydrinate* (Dramamine), 50 mg every 6 hours, which is more rapid in onset than meclizine, and *transdermal scopolamine*, which is longer acting (one patch lasts 3 days). Dimenhydrinate can be quite sedating, and scopolamine has considerable anticholinergic activity.

Cardiovascular faintness requires ensuring adequate hydration, standing up slowly, and discontinuing or reducing offending drugs. The patient with critical aortic stenosis should undergo evaluation for surgery (see Chapter 33).

Psychogenic light-headedness may be refractory to symptomatic therapy, though rebreathing into a *paper bag* is effective for acute hyperventilation. Treatment with an *anxiolytic* agent might help, but it can also cause symptoms (see Chapter 226). *Antidepressant* therapy is indicated when depression is the predominant etiology, though some antidepressants can cause postural light-headedness (see Chapter 227).

Patients with multiple sensory deficits or cerebellar dysfunction are aided by handrails in the home, good lighting, and use of a cane or walker. Vertigo and dysequilibrium

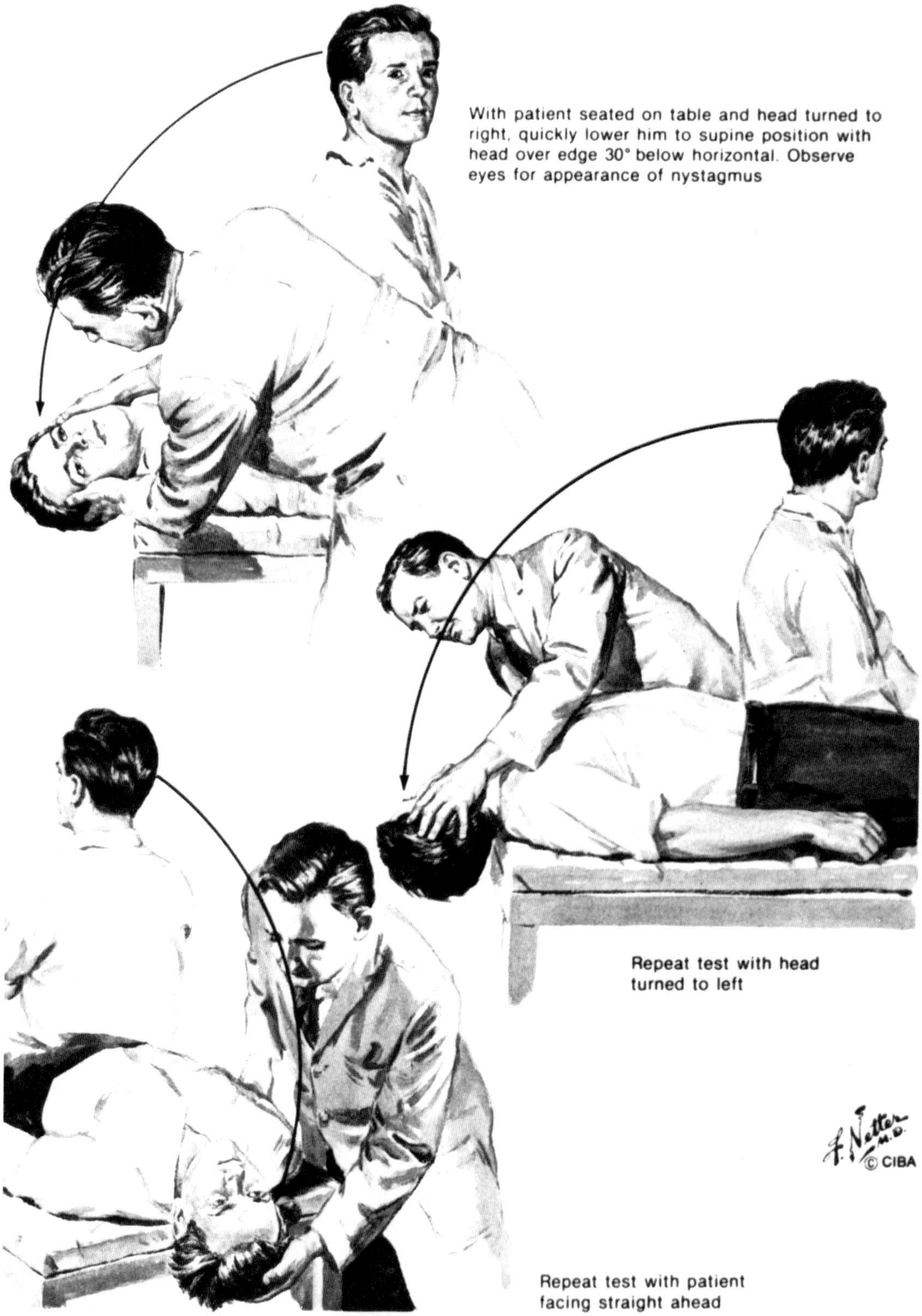

Figure 166-1. Barany test for vestibular disease. (© Copyright 1981. CIBA Pharmaceutical Company, Division of CIBA-GEIGY Corporation. Reproduced with permission from Clinical Symposia by Frank H. Netter, M.D. All rights reserved.)

caused by lesions of the cerebellum, the area about and including the vestibular nucleus, or the floor of the fourth ventricle may be associated with persistent ataxia and nausea.

Whereas patients with peripheral causes of dizziness typically recover within months, patients with central causes of dizziness may be bothered for years. *Lorazepam* (Ativan), 1 to 2 mg twice daily, may help some patients. *Gait training* and *vestibular exercises* under the supervision of a trained therapist may be beneficial. In patients with chronic vertigo, the goal is to retrain the eye and body musculature to compensate for loss of vestibular input. Benign positional vertigo is especially responsive.

The vast majority of people with dizziness have benign disorders. Symptomatic therapy combined with explanation and reassurance is always comforting. In particular, patients tolerate their problems better when they know that in most instances the symptom can be controlled or will resolve on its own. Teaching how to minimize symptoms (eg, avoiding quick change of position) is always appreciated.

INDICATIONS FOR REFERRAL

Neurologic consultation is indicated when there is concern about central vestibular disease or acoustic neuroma or when Ménière's disease appears to be progressive and disabling.

A.H.G.

ANNOTATED BIBLIOGRAPHY

Baloh RW, Honrubia V, Jacobson K. Benign positional vertigo: clinical and oculographic features in 240 cases. Neurology 1987;37:371. *(Head trauma and viral labyrinthitis were the most common causes and predated onset of symptoms by weeks to years.)*

Drachman DA, Hart CW. An approach to the dizzy patient. Neurology 1972;22:323. *(In a series of 104 patients seen in a dizziness clinic, secure diagnoses were reached in 91 percent, with peripheral vestibular disease, hyperventilation, and multiple sensory deficits making up > two-thirds of cases. Article provides details of diagnostic measures.)*

Fisher CM. Vertigo in cerebrovascular disease. Arch Otolaryngol 1967;85:85. *(Argues that unaccompanied dizziness is unlikely to be vascular in origin and that it is safe to wait and watch for developments rather than risk anticoagulation or arteriography.)*

Hart GH, Gardner DP, Howieson J. Acoustic tumors: atypical features and recent diagnostic tests. Neurology 1983;33:211. *(Excellent discussion of making this difficult diagnosis.)*

Kroenke K, Lucas CA, Rosenberg ML, et al. Causes of persistent dizziness: A prospective study of 100 patients in ambulatory care. Ann Intern Med 1992;117:898. *(Vestibular disease and psychiatric disorders were the most common causes.)*

Oosterveld WJ. Vertigo. Current concepts in management. Drugs 1985;30:275. *(A useful review of available medications.)*

Snow JB Jr. Positional vertigo. N Engl J Med 1984;310:1740. *(An editorial summarizing tests for the evaluation of vertigo.)*

Sullivan M, Clark MR, Katon WJ, et al. Psychiatric and otologic diagnoses in patients complaining of dizziness. Arch Intern Med 1993;153:1479. *(Psychiatric disease common when vestibular disease ruled out.)*

Troost BT. Dizziness and vertigo in vertebrobasilar disease. Stroke 1980;11:301,413. *(A two-part paper on central and peripheral lesions caused by vascular insufficiency.)*

Troost BT, Patton JW. Exercise therapy for positional vertigo. Neurology 1992;42:1441. *(Benign positional vertigo is especially responsive to the exercises described in this article.)*

Primary Care Medicine: Office Evaluation and Management of the Adult Patient, 3rd edition, edited by Allan H. Goroll, Lawrence A. May, and Albert G. Mulley, Jr. J.B. Lippincott Company, Philadelphia

167

Focal Neurologic Complaints: Evaluation of Nerve Root and Peripheral Nerve Syndromes

AMY A. PRUITT, M.D.

Primary physicians are frequently asked to evaluate complaints of focal numbness, tingling, weakness, pain, or some combination of these. In general, major acute neurologic disease is not at issue during an office visit. Nevertheless, the broad range of outpatient complaints encountered encompasses lesions throughout the nervous system. Disorders of nerve roots and peripheral nerves in the upper and lower extremities are especially common. Several syndromes should be analyzable by the primary physician. Identification and localization of these problems can facilitate thorough neurologic evaluation and accurately segregate those cases that must be referred to a neurologist.

PATHOPHYSIOLOGY AND CLINICAL PRESENTATION

Many peripheral nerves, because of their superficial location, are easily injured mechanically, and others are vulnerable because of specific anatomic variants or because of alterations in anatomy caused by degenerative disease.

Upper Extremity Syndromes

Cervical Radiculopathy and Myelopathy. Age-related loss of water and elasticity in cervical discs leads to increased stress on vertebral bodies. Osteophytic spurs develop and

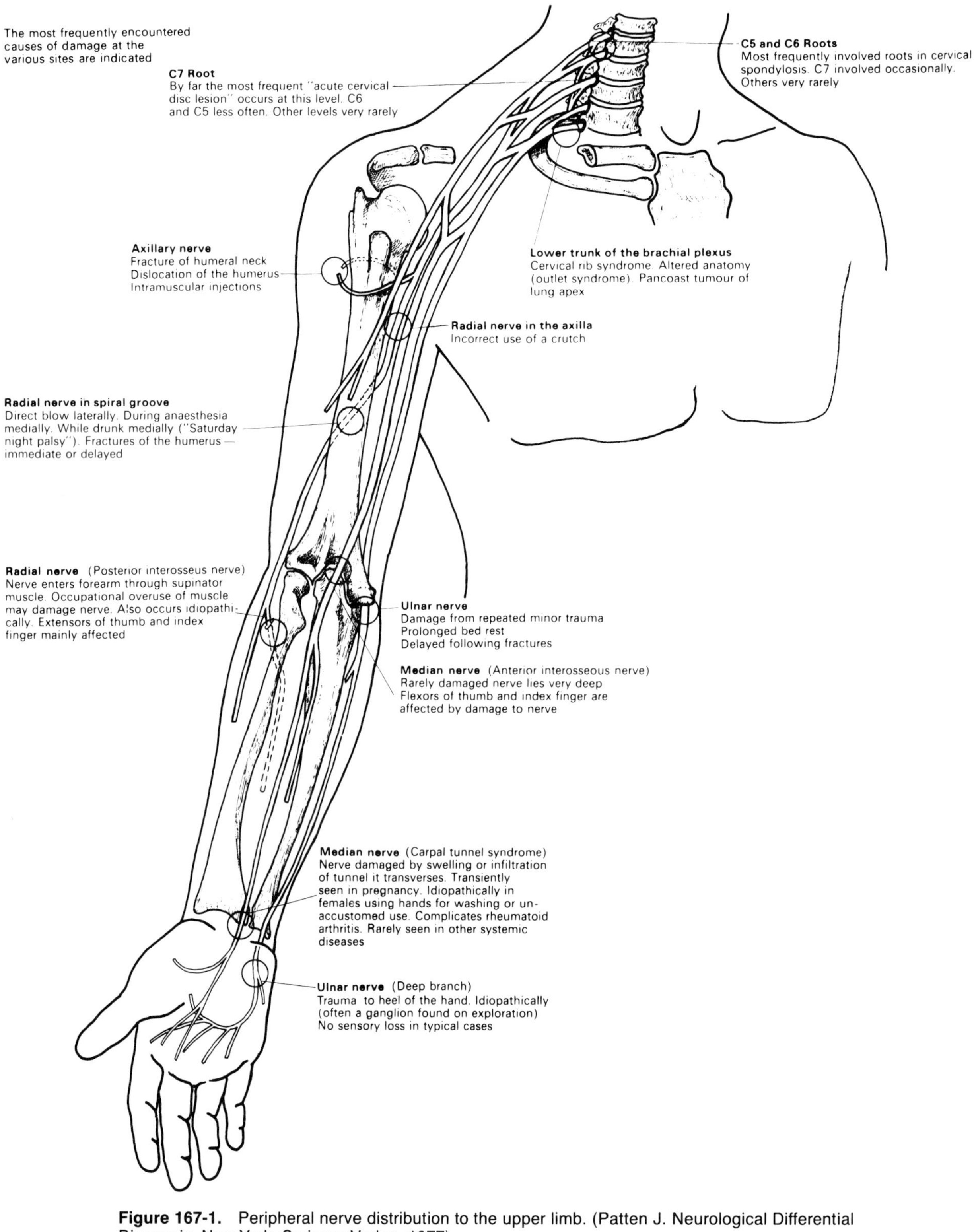

Figure 167-1. Peripheral nerve distribution to the upper limb. (Patten J. Neurological Differential Diagnosis. New York: Springer-Verlag, 1977)

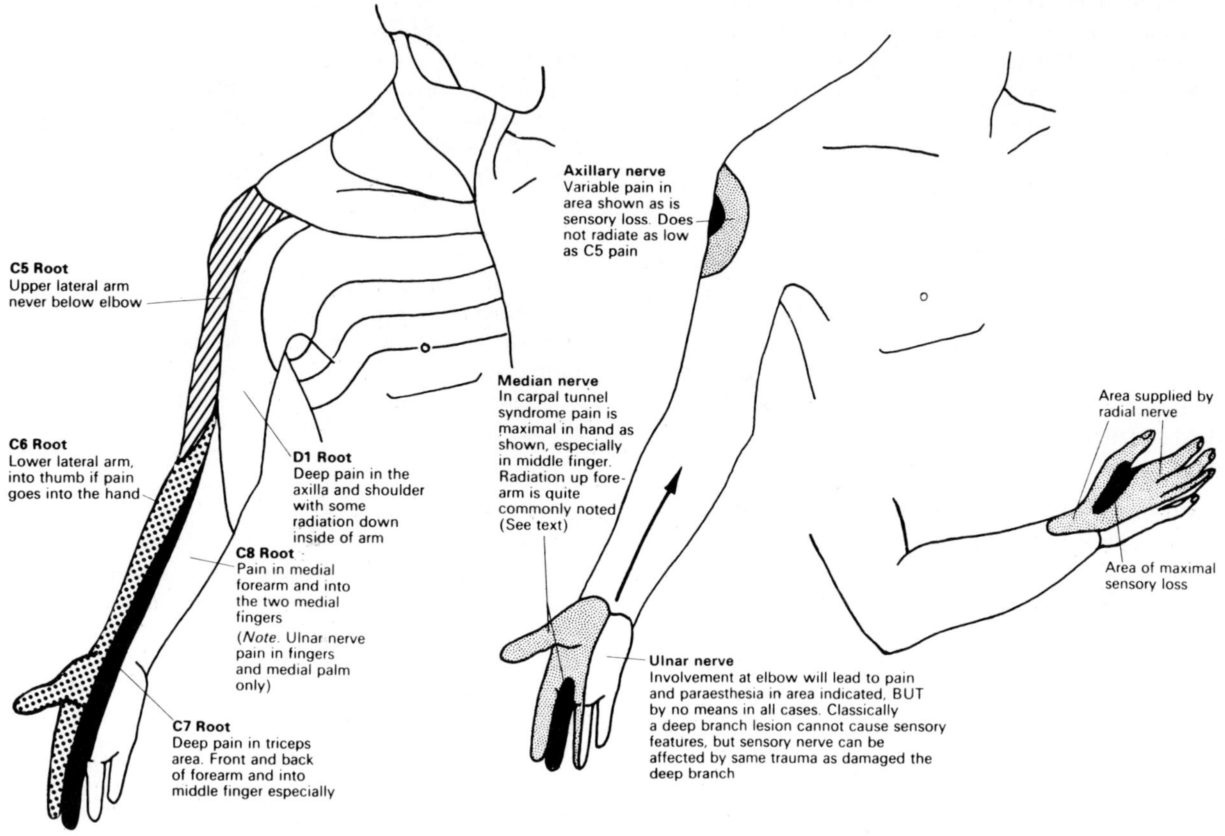

Figure 167-2. (*Left*) Distribution of root pain and paresthesia. (*Right*) Distribution of peripheral nerve pain and paresthesia. (Patten J. Neurological Differential Diagnosis. New York: Springer-Verlag, 1977)

may encroach on nerve roots. More serious but less common is encroachment on the spinal cord itself by progressive cervical spondylotic changes. Usually a combination of radiculopathy involving the C5, C6, or C7 roots (Figs. 167–1 and 167–2) and myelopathy is present. The presence of cord compression due to spondylosis is indicated by radicular pain, variable weakness, diminished reflexes, and atrophy in the arms, with spastic weakness and hyperreflexia in the lower extremities.

It may be difficult to distinguish cervical spondylotic myelopathy from other progressive myelopathies, which include multiple sclerosis, subacute combined degeneration due to vitamin B_{12} deficiency, spinal tumor, and syringomyelia. Suspicion of myelopathy should prompt referral to a neurologist.

Radiologic assessment usually includes *cervical spine films*. Unfortunately, nearly 50 percent of patients older than age 50 show degenerative cervical spine changes on x-ray, and these do not correlate well with the degree of abnormality found clinically in either radiculopathy or myelopathy. Nevertheless, plain cervical spine films with oblique views to visualize the neural foramina are often informative. *Magnetic resonance imaging (MRI)* is the best noninvasive test to assess the degree of cervical spondylosis or disc protrusion. It should be ordered when radicular pain is severe or when there is a motor or sensory deficit, reflex change, or myelopathic finding.

If the patient has only radiculopathy, a conservative trial of cervical traction is sometimes helpful (see Chapter 148). If myelopathy is suspected, myelography may be necessary to define the extent of compression, to rule out neoplastic lesions, and to assist the surgeon in a decision about decompressive laminectomy.

Brachial Plexus Neuritis. A painfully disabling condition, this syndrome develops in some patients after an immunization and presents with severe shoulder and upper arm pain followed by weakness which usually involves the upper roots of the plexus more than the lower ones. Prognosis is ultimately good, but recovery may be prolonged. Clinical examination reveals variable weakness and sensory loss in C5 to T1 root distributions (see Fig. 167–2) with diminished deep tendon reflexes. Because of the involvement of many nerve roots, confusion with a cervical disc does not usually arise. Electromyography and nerve conduction studies help to localize the abnormality. Apical lordotic views of the chest should be obtained to rule out the possibility of neoplastic invasion of the plexus from an intrathoracic tumor.

Thoracic Outlet Syndrome. A cervical rib or bony abnormality of the first rib may lead to pressure on the subclavian artery or brachial plexus as it passes through the thoracic outlet (see Fig. 167–1). Diagnosis is primarily clinical and includes the presence of pain in the arm in certain positions, color changes in the hand, and a pattern of sensory loss and weakness most pronounced in the fourth and fifth fingers. Deep tendon reflexes are usually normal. The differential diagnosis includes Raynaud's phenomenon, ulnar nerve entrapment at the elbow, and compression of the brachial plexus from neoplasm or from fibrosis due to radiation.

Cervical spine films are extremely important to demonstrate cervical ribs or elongated transverse processes of the seventh cervical vertebra. Electromyography may be entirely normal, but it will help to exclude a defect at the elbow or a carpal tunnel syndrome. Ultrasonography of the subclavian artery with the arm held in different positions may help define the extent of compression.

Most surgeons advocate removal of the potentially constricting structures (cervical rib, fascial band to first rib, or first rib). Shoulder exercises to improve posture are often advised first, and orthopedic advice should be sought in each case.

Long Thoracic Nerve Entrapment. This nerve arises from the brachial plexus and innervates the serratus anterior. It is vulnerable to injury in workers who lift or push heavy loads, occurs after direct trauma from heavy backpacks, and may evolve over several months after the injury. The patient notes a change in the appearance of the shoulder, and examination reveals winging of the scapula. Most cases have a good prognosis.

Carpal Tunnel Syndrome. In this disorder, the median nerve is entrapped at the carpal tunnel (see Fig. 167–1) because of pressure from ligamentous thickening. Most cases are idiopathic, but the disorder may be seen with rheumatoid arthritis, pregnancy, acromegaly, hypothyroidism, fractures of the carpal bones, amyloidosis, and myeloma. Occupational causes involving repetitive traumatic actions have been implicated. A combination of pain, paresthesias, and numbness in the median nerve distribution is the earliest complaint, often worse at night (see Fig. 167–2). Later, muscle weakness (particularly of thumb abduction and opposition) occurs, and thenar atrophy may be seen. Importantly, aching pain can be felt as far up as the shoulder and should not distract the examiner's attention from the wrist. Tapping on the wrist or anywhere else along the median nerve may reproduce the pain (*Tinel's sign*).

Differential diagnosis includes radiculopathy from cervical spine disease, but the exact location of the pain should conform to the median nerve rather than to just one nerve root distribution. Electromyography and *nerve conduction studies* with motor and sensory conduction latencies of the median nerve provide the most useful data. While some cases respond to conservative therapy (wrist splints, anti-inflammatory medications), surgical relief is relatively easy and effective. Failure to respond to surgical therapy should prompt rechecking of the nerve conduction studies, careful reexamination, and consideration of the possibility of coexistent cervical spine disease or of median nerve compression higher in the forearm.

Ulnar Nerve Entrapment. The most common location of ulnar entrapment is at the elbow (see Fig. 167–1). Causes include fracture deformities, arthritis, faulty positioning of the arm during surgery, or repetitive occupational or recreational trauma (eg, tennis). Sensation is usually spared in the forearm, but there is sensory loss in the fifth finger and half of the fourth (see Fig. 167–2). Wasting of the intrinsic muscles of the hand with weakness of grip occurs later. Nerve conduction studies can accurately localize the site of compression. If there is focal entrapment, repositioning of the nerve or elbow synovectomy may be necessary, but patients with trauma, diabetes, or the so-called "tardy" ulnar palsies (dysfunction developing late after injury) may not improve.

Radial Nerve Injuries. Compression of the radial nerve most often occurs in the axilla or the upper arm. It may be seen with improperly used crutches, with prolonged pressure during sleep (the Saturday night palsy), or as a result of direct injury. Wrist drop is the prominent feature. Vasomotor or atrophic changes are rarely present, and prognosis is good (recovery within 6 to 8 weeks).

Lower Extremity Syndromes

Lateral Femoral Cutaneous Nerve Compression. Also known as meralgia paresthetica, this syndrome involves a nerve formed by branches arising from the second and third lumbar roots. The nerve enters the thigh in close relation to the inguinal ligament, the anterior superior iliac spine, and the sartorius muscle insertion (Fig. 167–3). It is purely sensory and supplies the anterolateral and lateral aspects of the thigh almost as far as the knee (Fig. 167–4). Compression causes an extremely unpleasant, characteristic burning pain with increased cutaneous sensitivity. Sitting or lying usually provides relief, but standing or walking exacerbates the pain. The syndrome often occurs in obesity, in pregnancy, or when tight corsets are worn. It is more common in diabetics. Differential diagnosis includes a lesion of the second or third lumbar roots, usually associated with low back pain radiating into the lower leg. Sensory changes in this case will extend further down the leg and more medially, and there is iliopsoas or quadriceps weakness. Weakness and reflex changes do not occur in meralgia paresthetica. The neuropathy tends to regress spontaneously, but weight loss should be encouraged.

Femoral Neuropathy. The femoral nerve derives from the second, third, and fourth lumbar roots. Its posterior division is the major innervation to the quadriceps and terminates as the saphenous nerve, which supplies sensation to the medial aspect of the leg as far as the medial malleolus (see Fig. 167–3). Onset of femoral neuropathy is frequently sudden, painful, and followed quickly by wasting and weakness in the quadriceps, loss of knee jerk, and sensory impairment over the anteromedial thigh (see Fig. 167–4). If there is also marked hip flexion weakness, the site of the lesion is usually in the lumbar plexus. Sensory symptoms in the saphenous distribution are uncommon in lesions of the main trunk of the femoral nerve.

Entrapment may occur in the inguinal region and from direct retroperitoneal compression by tumor or hematoma. However, the most common cause is presumed to be nerve infarction, seen usually in diabetics. A combination of thigh pain, weakness, and sensory deficit can be a manifestation of an isolated diabetic femoral neuropathy, although electro-

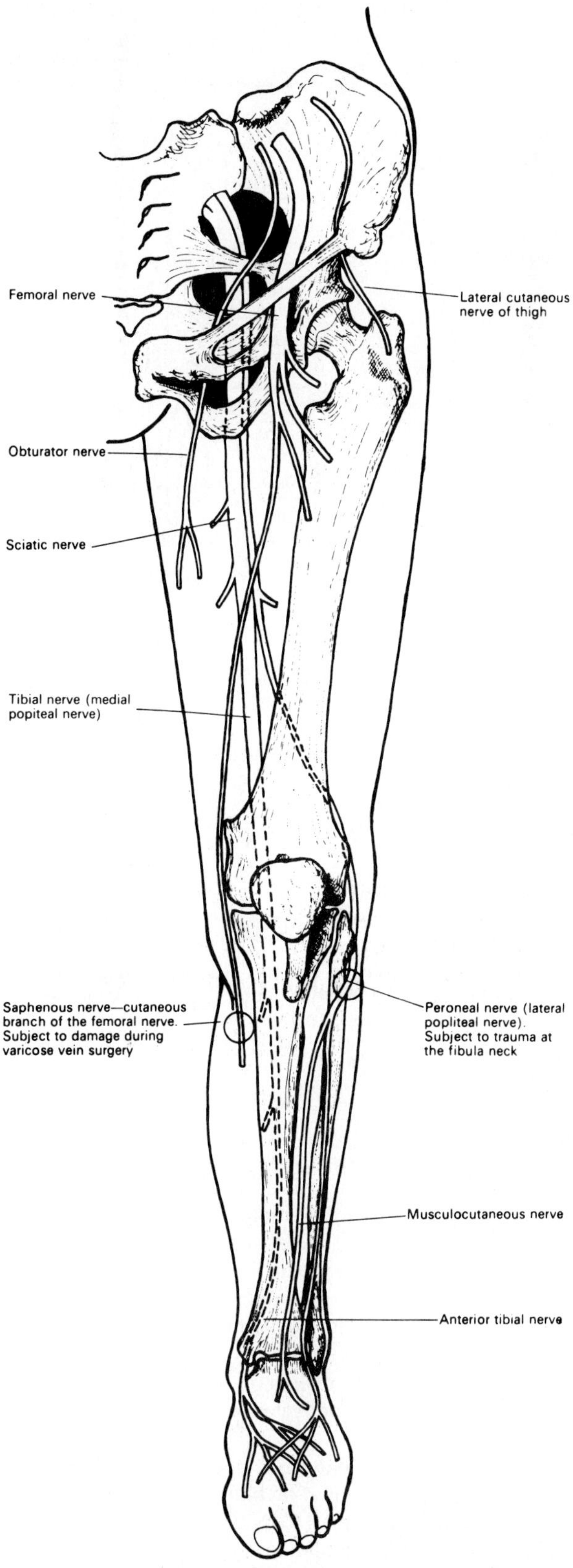

Figure 167-3. Peripheral nerve distribution to the lower limb. (Patten J. Neurological Differential Diagnosis. New York: Springer-Verlag, 1977)

myographically, the involvement in such cases is frequently more widespread. While some improvement may occur, the patient is often left quite weak.

Sciatic Nerve Syndromes. The sciatic nerve arises from the lumbosacral plexus (L4–S3) and terminates in the common peroneal and tibial nerves (see Fig. 167–3). The tibial nerve supplies gastrocnemius, plantaris, soleus, and popliteus muscles, while its extension into the calf, the posterior tibial nerve, supplies muscles of the calf. All these muscles are involved in plantar flexion. The common peroneal nerve divides into the superficial and deep peroneal nerves. The latter supplies the muscles that dorsiflex the foot and toes. The superficial peroneal nerve innervates the muscles that evert the foot.

Sciatic nerve compression may result from tumors within the pelvis or from prolonged sitting or lying on the buttocks. Gluteal abscesses and misplaced buttock injections have caused sciatic injury. Weakness of the gluteal muscles and pain in the sciatic notch area imply compression within the pelvis. Lesions just beyond the sciatic notch cause weakness in the hamstrings and in all the muscles of the lower leg.

Common peroneal compression usually occurs at the level of the fibular head (see Fig. 167–3) and is seen in cachectic patients following prolonged bedrest, in alcoholics, in diabetics, and in patients placed in tight casts. Injury leads to faulty dorsiflexion and eversion of the foot, producing a characteristic footdrop with a slapping gait. Complete or partial recovery can be expected when paralysis results from transient pressure. Treatment consists of a foot brace and careful avoidance of compressive positions.

Lumbar Disc Syndromes. Compressive neuropathies of the lower limbs must be distinguished from the very common lumbar disc syndromes. In the lumbar region, the fourth and fifth discs are most frequently affected (ie, the discs between L4 and L5 vertebral bodies and between L5 and S1 vertebrae). The most common complaint is sudden onset of severe low back pain (see Chapter 147). The inciting event is often trivial, though heavy lifting or an acute twisting motion is sometimes reported. The pain is worsened by bending forward, sneezing, or straining.

The herniated disc can compress one or more nerve roots, but a disc herniation at a particular level generally causes a distinctive picture (see Chapter 147). *L4–L5 disc herniation* usually affects the L5 root with pain over sciatic notch, lateral thigh, and leg; numbness of the web of the great toe and lateral leg; weakness of dorsiflexion of the great toe and foot; and no reflex changes (see Fig. 167–4). *L5–S1 disc herniation* catches the S1 root, producing pain down the back of the leg to the heel; numbness in the lateral heel, foot, and toe; weakness of plantar flexion; and loss of ankle jerk (see Fig. 167–4). Once the root level is defined, the usual course is a trial of bed rest and analgesia (see Chapter 147) unless there is pronounced weakness, uncontrollable pain, or bladder and bowel dysfunction. In these cases, urgent MRI or myelography may be necessary to define the extent of disc protrusion and to rule out more unusual causes of lumbar radiculopathy such as neurofibroma. MRI may be helpful in predicting the response of a patient with disc disease to conservative therapy.

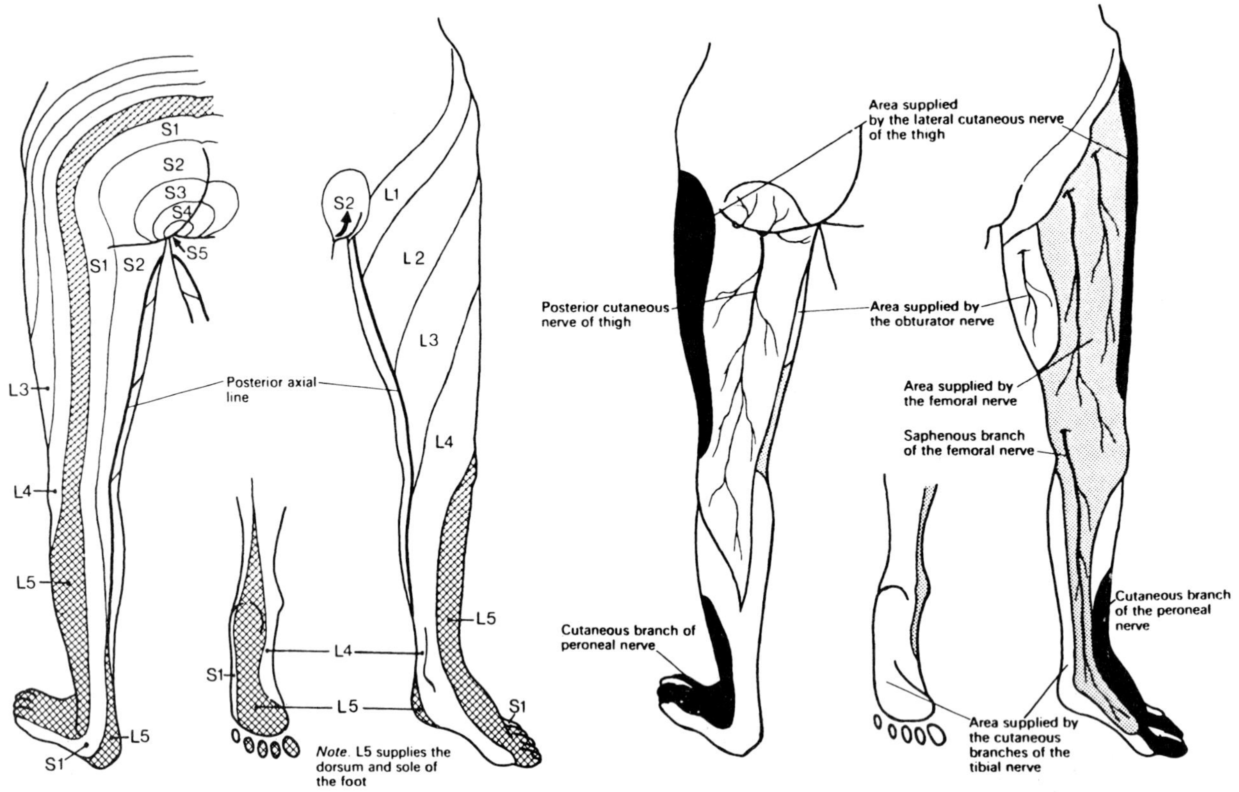

Figure 167-4. (*Left*) Lumbosacral dermatomes. (*Right*) Lower limb peripheral nerve distribution. (Patten J. Neurological Differential Diagnosis. New York: Springer-Verlag, 1977)

Peripheral Polyneuropathy. When a patient presents with distal symmetric sensorimotor or predominantly motor symptoms and is found to have diminished sensation and/or motor abnormalities in a "stocking-glove" distribution with variably hypoactive deep tendon reflexes, he is likely to have a peripheral polyneuropathy. The list of etiologies is extensive (Table 167–1). Although most produce some degree of motor and sensory dysfunction, there is usually a predominance of one component. Sensorimotor conditions present principally with sensory deficits, although a more mixed picture ensues later. Diabetes is a common source of sensorimotor polyneuropathy; symptoms respond to a tightening of glucose control (see Chapter 102). Alcoholism, B-vitamin deficiencies, renal failure, hypothyroidism, acquired immunodeficiency syndrome (AIDS), and paraneoplastic syndromes are among the other etiologies. The most dramatic of the predominantly motor polyneuropathies is the acquired autoimmune disease Guillain-Barré syndrome, with its acute onset following a viral illness and rapid progression of ascending weakness over a few days in conjunction with loss of deep tendon reflexes. Other predominantly motor polyneuropathies include those associated with monoclonal gammopathy, toxin exposure, and porphyria. A predominantly sensory polyneuropathy is seen with amyloidosis, paraneoplastic syndromes, vitamin B_6 excess, and Sjögren's syndrome.

WORKUP

Peripheral Polyneuropathy. The primary physician's objective should be to discern by history and physical examination diagnostically important variations in the peripheral polyneuropathy theme.

History includes a review of duration (years suggests a hereditary cause; weeks to months, a toxic/metabolic etiology or a paraproteinemia; days, toxin or Guillain-Barré). Distribution helps distinguish between polyneuropathy and diabetic mononeuropathy multiplex, which is more multifocal. Medication exposure is essential to review (eg, cisplatin, isoniazid, vincristine), as are habits (alcohol abuse), diet (especially as regards B-vitamin deficiencies), and concurrent medical illnesses (diabetes, renal failure, liver disease, cancer). The *physical examination* is used to clarify the relative sensory and motor components of the problem, which helps in differentiation. Signs of systemic disease may also be revealed.

Laboratory studies should include complete blood count, erythrocyte sedimentation rate, blood glucose, liver function tests, blood urea nitrogen (BUN), creatinine, immunoelectrophoresis, thyroid-stimulating hormone (TSH), and chest film. Though patients whose neuropathy is apparent from the above studies (eg, diabetic polyneuropathy) may not require *electromyography (EMG)*, this procedure helps to differen-

Table 167-1. Important Peripheral Polyneuropathies

Predominantly Motor
- A. Acute (days)
  1. Guillain-Barré syndrome
  2. Diphtheria
  3. Porphyria
  4. Toxin (organophosphate exposure)
- B. Subacute (weeks to 1–2 years)
  1. Toxin exposure (lead poisoning, glue sniffing)
  2. Paraproteinemia
- C. Chronic
  1. Hereditary (Charcot-Marie-Tooth disease)

Predominantly Sensory
- A. Acute (days)
  1. None
- B. Subacute (weeks to 1–2 years)
  1. Amyloidosis
  2. Drug toxicity (cisplatin, vitamin B_6 excess)
  3. Paraneoplastic syndrome
  4. Sjögren's syndrome
- C. Chronic (years)
  1. Hereditary sensory neuropathy

Sensorimotor
- A. Acute (days)
  1. Toxin exposure (arsenic)
- B. Subacute (weeks to 1–2 years)
  1. Diabetes
  2. Alcohol abuse
  3. B-vitamin deficiency
  4. Renal failure
  5. Hypothyroidism
  6. Connective tissue disease
  7. Paraneoplastic syndrome
  8. Drug toxicity (INH, cancer chemotherapeutic agents)
  9. AIDS
- C. Chronic (years)
  1. Charcot-Marie-Tooth disease

*Adapted from American College of Physicians Medical Knowledge Self-Assessment Program IX, 1991, 106.

tiate between demyelinating disease and axonal polyneuropathy, and between root or plexus and more distal nerve trunk involvements, distinctions that are of considerable diagnostic importance. EMG also sorts out upper from lower motor neuron weakness. *Nerve biopsy* is infrequently recommended; its main indication is in hereditary disorders or in multifocal mononeuropathy multiplex or asymmetric clinical syndromes, where it could reveal such etiologies as vasculitis, amyloidosis, or sarcoidosis. Patients with monoclonal gammopathy may profit from recently developed tests for antibody to *myelin-associated glycoprotein (anti-MAG antibody)*; it can identify those who are candidates for plasmapheresis or immunosuppressive therapy.

Other Peripheral Nerve Syndromes. Identification of the nerve root or peripheral nerve syndrome and precise localization of the neurologic lesion is possible in the office setting. Assessment is facilitated by determining 1) whether the problem is peripheral (in a nerve root or peripheral nerve) or central (in the cord or above); 2) whether the problem, if peripheral, is due to a lesion in the peripheral nerve or to nerve root injury; 3) whether there is evidence of cord compression (manifested by signs of myelopathy), particularly with upper extremity syndromes; 4) whether there is evidence (in other extremities) of more widespread peripheral neuropathy (eg, the diabetic patient with a femoral neuropathy who also has a diffuse peripheral neuropathy); and 5) whether the presence of weakness is due to a muscle or nerve lesion.

The neurologic examination should be organized to address these issues and answer the following questions:

1. Is the lesion upper motor neuron (UMN) or lower motor neuron (LMN)? Fasciculations, flaccidity, and the lack of reflexes indicate a LMN lesion and suggest that the disorder originates at the anterior horn cell or peripheral nerve level. Spasticity and increased reflexes are evidence for a lesion above the anterior horn cell that supplies the involved musculature. Thus, a cervical disc at the C6 level might decrease the biceps reflex and result in biceps weakness and atrophy, while causing increased reflexes and spasticity below that level.
2. Is the nerve dysfunction confined to one root or dermatome or to one peripheral nerve? A positive answer to this question suggests a compression neuropathy such as a radial, ulnar, or median nerve palsy. Findings of more generalized dysfunction, such as diffusely decreased deep tendon reflexes, absent vibration sense at the ankles, and a stocking-glove pattern of sensory loss, suggest a more diffuse peripheral neuropathy. Commonly seen forms of peripheral neuropathy include those associated with diabetes mellitus, excess alcohol consumption, toxin and drug exposure, and genetic diseases such as Charcot-Marie-Tooth. An electromyogram can localize the individual nerve abnormality and can confirm the presence of a generalized neuropathy.
3. Is the weakness due to nerve or to muscle disease? Weakness in conjunction with altered tendon reflexes and sensory loss suggests nerve disease. Primary muscle pathology results in preserved reflexes and normal sensation. Characteristic patterns of muscle weakness occur in the genetically determined muscular dystrophies. The toxic and metabolic myopathies produce largely proximal muscle weakness, in contrast to almost all primary nerve diseases, which affect distal musculature early and preferentially. Serum muscle enzyme elevations are seen in muscle disease, and some muscular disorders are associated with myotonia. The electromyogram, coupled with nerve conduction studies, can distinguish primary muscle disease from neuropathic processes.

Clinical identification of nerve root and peripheral nerve syndromes is often facilitated by selective use of radiologic, nerve conduction, electromyographic, and serologic studies (as detailed in discussions of each of the important syndromes). However, dependence on laboratory studies for initial assessment is usually not necessary.

INDICATIONS FOR REFERRAL AND ADMISSION

Evidence of acute spinal cord compression is an indication for immediate neurosurgical consultation and hospitalization. The patient with symptoms and signs of a slowly progressive myelopathy requires neurologic consultation and

MRI. A root or peripheral nerve compression syndrome may require surgical repair, and the patient with such a problem will need to see the neurosurgeon or orthopedist skilled in its treatment. Nevertheless, before referral, the primary physician should have localized the problem and instituted appropriate initial therapy.

ANNOTATED BIBLIOGRAPHY

Aids to the Diagnosis of Peripheral Nerve Injuries. London, Bailliere Tindal, 1986. *(A classic; lucid illustrations and diagrams of the function and examination of every clinically important peripheral nerve.)*

Asbury AK. Understanding diabetic neuropathy. N Engl J Med 1988;319:577. *(A very thorough review with good tables on this most common and important of peripheral neuropathies.)*

Dawson DM. Entrapment neuropathies of the upper extremities. N Engl J Med 1993;329:2013. *(A nice review of carpal tunnel, ulnar, and thoracic outlet syndrome.)*

Delamonte SM. Peripheral neuropathy in the acquired immune deficiency syndrome. Ann Neurol 1988;28: 485. *(A demyelinating neuropathy, this will be seen with increasing frequency by the primary physician and should be recognized.)*

Dyck PJ. The 10 P's: a mnemonic helpful in characterization and differential diagnosis of peripheral neuropathy. Neurology 1992;42:14. *(It's actually a tough mnemonic, but the paper is helpful in delineating the principles of classification and reviewing peripheral neuropathy.)*

Dyck PJ. Plasma exchange in polyneuropathy associated with monoclonal gammopathy of undetermined significance. N Engl J Med 1991;325:1482. *(This new treatment modality and the therapeutic efficacy of intravenous immunoglobulin are the reasons for pursuing a diagnosis with immunoelectrophoresis and antibody studies.)*

Katz JN, Larson MG, Sabra A, et al. The carpal tunnel syndrome: diagnostic utility of the history and physical examination. Ann Intern Med 1988;112:321. *(Very useful analysis identifying the most meaningful findings.)*

McKhann G. Guillain-Barré syndrome: clinical and therapeutic observation. Ann Neurol 1990;27(Suppl 13):110. *(A whole issue devoted to acquired autoimmune neuropathies.)*

Warmolts JR. Electrodiagnosis in neuromuscular disorders. Ann Intern Med 1981;95:599. *(A good review for the generalist of nerve conduction studies and electromyography.)*

168
Evaluation of Tremor

AMY A. PRUITT, M.D.

Primary Care Medicine: Office Evaluation and Management of the Adult Patient, 3rd edition, edited by Allan H. Goroll, Lawrence A. May, and Albert G. Mulley, Jr. J.B. Lippincott Company, Philadelphia

Tremor is best defined as a regular oscillation of a body part and must be distinguished from other rapid, involuntary movements. Many patients assume that the development of "shakiness" is a natural concomitant of aging. The physician must determine the significance of a variety of clinically similar tremors that may have widely dissimilar diagnostic, therapeutic, and prognostic implications. Workup involves differentiating the resting tremor of early parkinsonism from essential tremor and differentiating essential tremor from an exaggerated physiologic tremor. As new specific treatments are developed, accurate clinical distinction becomes increasingly valuable. Unfortunately, it may be difficult to differentiate tremors by clinical observation alone, and evaluation requires a working knowledge of simple electrophysiologic and pharmacologic characteristics.

PATHOPHYSIOLOGY AND CLINICAL PRESENTATION

The precise neural mechanisms of tremor remain unknown despite some clinicopathologic correlations, such as abolition of the parkinsonian and essential tremors by lesions in the ventrolateral nucleus of the thalamus. Drugs such as L-dopa, which are known to act centrally to increase catecholamines, may worsen essential tremor; this observation has led to the suggestion that beta-adrenergic blockers such as propranolol might exert their therapeutic action by central antagonism of beta-adrenergic receptors.

The patient most frequently reports the insidious onset of "shaking" of a limb. Very likely, he or she will have ignored the symptom's presence initially, assuming it was due to nervousness or fatigue. However, its steady progression brings the patient to see the physician. Tremors can be present during maintenance of a posture, at rest, or during an action (intention tremor).

Postural or physiologic tremors are fine tremors with a frequency of 8 to 12 Hz; they occur normally in everyone during movement and while holding a fixed position. A true physiologic tremor is defined as one that does not produce symptoms and is within the given frequency range. The movement is usually invisible to the naked eye, but may become exaggerated by anxiety, coffee ingestion, or hyperthyroidism. Drugs, notably lithium and tricyclic antidepressants, may also accentuate this tremor. Amplitude and frequency vary among different people and in the same person at different times. Physiologic tremors are unaffected by propranolol or alcohol.

Intention Tremors. The major intention tremors are those labelled *"essential"* (also referred to as *"familial"* or *"senile"*). Half of cases are transmitted as an autosomal dominant trait, and half are sporadic. The condition is characterized by an intention tremor of the hands, head, voice, and sometimes legs and/or trunk. Typically, the tremor is most prominent when the hands or head are held outstretched in a position against gravity, and least noticeable at rest (though the tremor of early parkinsonism may also be seen best in an outstretched hand). Tremor may be accentuated by tasks that require precision, such as writing, carrying full cups of liquid (also seen in some patients with parkinsonism). Many patients report that the ingestion of a small amount of alcohol will temporarily reduce their tremor. Essential tremor may begin at any age, though early and late adult life are the most common periods of onset (helping to differentiate the condition from parkinsonism, which typically begins in middle age).

A more dramatic action tremor is displayed by patients with *cerebellar diseases* and is characterized by progressively increasing amplitude of the tremor as the patient brings the limb toward a target. In younger patients, this is most frequently caused by multiple sclerosis, but similar clinical states may be produced by cerebellar infarction, by degenerative disorders of the spinocerebellar pathways, and by chronic relapsing steroid-sensitive polyneuropathy. This tremor is multiplanar, with large, irregular, and relatively slow (2–4 Hz) oscillations. The tremor often is worsened by alcohol. Propranolol has no effect, and no satisfactory therapy is available.

Rest Tremors. The most common rest tremor in a relaxed, supported limb is that due to *Parkinson's disease*. It characteristically begins in the fingers and may later involve the arm and the leg. Flexion and extension of the fingers, abduction and adduction of the thumbs, and pronation and supination of the wrist produce the well-known "pill-rolling" movement. Frequently, this is the symptom that brings parkinsonian patients to the physician, and it may occur well in advance of bradykinesia or postural difficulties characteristic of the full-blown syndrome. It is important, of course, to distinguish this tremor from essential tremor, which demands a different treatment and portends a different prognosis. The parkinsonian tremor is slow (3–8 Hz), and its electromyogram (EMG), quite unlike that of essential tremor, shows alternating discharge in antagonistic muscle groups. This EMG activity is suppressed with voluntary movement.

A few parkinsonian patients may also have a typical action (essential) tremor, and L-dopa therapy may worsen it. Phenothiazines and haloperidol worsen the tremor-at-rest (see Chapter 174).

Other Abnormal Movements. The definition of tremor as a regular oscillation of a body part serves to distinguish it from other rapid, intermittent movements that bespeak a different neurologic state. For diagnostic, therapeutic, and prognostic purposes, several categories of abnormal involuntary movements should be distinguished from tremor. All of the following involuntary movements (and most true tremors) are greatly reduced or disappear altogether with sleep.

Tics are repetitive, coordinated, usually stereotyped movements that are seen widely in the population and increase in frequency in a given patient in response to stress. They usually involve face or hand muscles, may initially be a conscious mannerism, and usually can be suppressed by voluntary effort. *Hemifacial spasm* is a kind of oscillating movement usually beginning in a middle-aged or elderly person, localized to the facial muscles. It is thought to be due to degenerative lesions of the facial nucleus or peripheral nerve, but the exact mechanism is unknown, and treatment is unsatisfactory.

Asterixis is an irregular, skeletal muscle contraction that results in flapping of the hands, electromyographically coincident with brief pauses at irregular intervals. *Chorea* is an irregular, jerking movement usually involving the fingers and often accompanied by *athetosis,* in which writhing movements of limbs or trunk may be added. *Epilepsy partialis continuens* refers to a focal seizure in which continuous seizure activity may result in a somewhat rhythmic jerking of one body part. Sudden onset of the illness is the most useful distinguishing feature here.

Dyskinesias are rhythmic, involuntary movements of the orofacial musculature resulting in tongue protrusion and chewing movements. These are important to recognize because of the frequency with which they occur as early manifestations of the tardive dyskinesia syndrome caused by use of phenothiazines and other major tranquilizers.

DIFFERENTIAL DIAGNOSIS

Tremors can be divided clinically into postural, intention, and resting types. Most postural tremors are physiologic. Among the intention tremors are the essential, senile, and cerebellar varieties. Most resting tremors are caused by Parkinson's disease. Tremors must be distinguished from other voluntary movements such as dyskinesias, tics, myoclonus, and athetosis.

WORKUP

History. Clinical assessment of tremor is greatly aided by first ascertaining the circumstances under which the tremor occurs. Some tremors are present during maintenance of a posture, some during rest, and others only during an action (the intention tremors). Careful questioning will often identify the type of tremor. Common diagnostic problems include distinguishing the resting tremor of early Parkinson's disease from an essential tremor and an essential tremor from an exaggerated physiologic one. All of these are common and some may, in fact, be present simultaneously in a given patient.

Physical examination is directed primarily at determining whether the tremor is better or worse with activity. The patient should be asked to hold out his hands, to write, to perform rapid alternating movements, and to touch finger to nose repeatedly; the objective is to detect evidence of cerebellar or extrapyramidal disease. The patient should be observed discretely during the history and during other parts of the physical examination, because calling attention to the tremor may worsen it.

Laboratory Studies. If there is some question at the end of the examination as to whether the tremor is primarily resting or primarily action, a tremor recording (EMG) may be requested. Many parkinsonian patients will have no other extrapyramidal signs at the time they present with tremor. The EMG can separate the two types, sometimes confirming that both tremors are present simultaneously.

SYMPTOMATIC MANAGEMENT

Essential Tremor. A major advance was made in 1971 when two groups independently reported the beneficial effect of *propranolol* on essential tremor. The average effective dose was 120 mg per day. The sustained release form of the drug is more convenient and equally effective as the regular preparation, which must be taken several times a day. A decade later, the anticonvulsant drug *primidone* (Mysoline) was found to be extremely effective at reducing or eliminating essential tremor in doses far smaller than those necessary for antiepileptic activity. The mechanism of primidone's action in tremor is unknown. There is no consensus on which of these two agents is the drug of choice for tremor. Since primidone is somewhat more effective for the majority of patients, starting with a low dose of 50 mg per day and working up as to as much as 250 mg per day in divided doses is a very reasonable approach to treatment. Sedation is the major side effect, but it is generally tolerated if the drug is increased slowly. Propranolol is also well tolerated in most patients, though it is relatively contraindicated in those with underlying asthma, insulin-dependent diabetes, heart block, or congestive heart failure (see Chapters 25, 32, 48, and 102). *Alprazolam* (Xanax) and other benzodiazepines have been used for essential tremor and may be effective as intermittent adjunctive agents in a patient on beta-blockers or primidone.

Physiologic Tremor. Performance anxiety sometimes exaggerates an otherwise inconsequential physiologic tremor in performers (eg, concert musicians, public speakers) and can sometimes be helped by a small pre-performance dose of a *beta-blocker* or a short-acting *benzodiazepine* (see Chapter 226). However, too large a dose of either might have an overly sedating effect and hinder performance. Moreover, regular use of benzodiazepines is associated with the risk of habituation (see Chapter 226), and beta-blockers usually have little effect on baseline physiologic tremors.

Parkinson's Disease. The tremor of Parkinson's disease, while not responding as well as bradykinesia and rigidity to dopaminergic agents, may benefit from *anticholinergic therapy* (see Chapter 174).

Cerebellar Disease. The tremor of cerebellar disease is notoriously unresponsive, though beta-blockers, primidone, baclofen, and benzodiazepines are usually tried. Wrist weights may dampen the amplitude of these tremors and make the limb more functional.

PATIENT EDUCATION AND INDICATIONS FOR REFERRAL

The etiology of the tremor and the fact that it can be controlled should be discussed with the patient. Avoidance of agents that worsen symptoms must be stressed. Patients with intention tremors and cerebellar signs must be referred to a neurologist, since demyelinating or hereditary degenerative diseases may be responsible. Disabling tremors refractory to simple therapy may benefit from neurologic consultation.

ANNOTATED BIBLIOGRAPHY

Koller WC. A new drug for treatment of essential tremor. Mayo Clin Proc 1991;66:1085. *(An editorial that is most useful for its review of treatment regimens.)*

Koller WC. Efficacy of primidone in the treatment of essential tremor. Neurology 1986;26:121. *(Established the utility of the drug in a high percentage of patients.)*

Lou JS, Jankovic J. Essential tremor: Clinical correlates in 350 patients. Neurology 1991;41:234. *(Excellent description.)*

Rajput AH, Rozdelsky B, Aug L, et al. Clinicopathologic observations in essential tremor. Neurology 1991;41:1422. *(A search for an anatomic lesion.)*

Shahani BT, Young RR. Physiological and pharmacological aids in the differential diagnosis of tremor. J Neurol Neurosurg Psychiatry 1976;39:772. *(Details key features of the various causes of tremor.)*

169
Evaluation of Dementia

AMY A. PRUITT, M.D.

Primary Care Medicine: Office Evaluation and Management of the Adult Patient, 3rd edition, edited by Allan H. Goroll, Lawrence A. May, and Albert G. Mulley, Jr. J.B. Lippincott Company, Philadelphia

Dementia is the progressive decline of intellectual ability from a previously attained level. Speech, memory, judgment, and mood may all be altered in varying proportions. Dementia in the adult population is a growing medical and social problem, occurring at all ages but increasing with advanced age. Dementia is most frequent in the population over age 75, which also is the age group increasing at the highest rate. There are an estimated 600,000 cases of advanced dementia in the United States, and milder degrees of altered mental status are very common in the elderly. The expense of long-term care at home or in a nursing facility has been estimated at 40 billion dollars a year for people age 65 and older.

When decline in mental functioning is noted, fear of Alzheimer's disease arises in patients and their families. Each patient requires careful workup for dementia and proper identification of its underlying etiology. As many as 15 percent of patients have conditions amenable to therapy. Primary physicians should know how to distinguish dementia from other, more specific cortical deficits (aphasia, agnosia, isolated memory deficit) and should be able to perform an adequate screening examination for potentially reversible disease. Prompt recognition of dementia is essential not only for initiation of a diagnostic workup but also to protect the patient from avoidable harm, such as a fall, drug overdose, fire, or inadequate nutrition.

The National Institute on Aging, in conjunction with several other National Institutes of Health agencies, convened a consensus panel in 1987 to address issues of importance in the diagnosis of dementing diseases. This group formulated a statement responding to the issues of a definition of dementia, the reversible dementing diseases, the initial evaluation of dementia, indicated diagnostic tests, and priorities for future research.

PATHOPHYSIOLOGY AND CLINICAL PRESENTATION

Definition and Description. Dementia is a syndrome characterized by a *generalized* and *sustained* decline in *intellectual functioning* from a previously attained level. It is a characteristically *progressive* disorder, measurable in months or years rather than days or weeks. The decline from a previously attained level of mental ability is broad based, usually involving *memory, cognitive capacities,* and *adaptive behavior without alteration of consciousness.* Initially, the patient may be aware of some of his or her difficulties but, later, seems mainly undisturbed by them. It is important, but not always possible, to distinguish the early stages of dementia from nonprogressive cognitive changes that occur in normal aging.

The onset of dementia is usually insidious, although it may appear to evolve rapidly. The patient initially may be noted to have slight *forgetfulness, attention* and *concentration deficits,* and increasing *repetitiousness* or *inconsistencies* in usual behavior. Later in the course of the process, the patient may display increasingly impaired judgment, inability to abstract or generalize, and *personality change* with rigidity, perseveration, irritability, and confusion as a result of minor changes in the environment. *Affective disturbances* may be prominent, and, in extreme forms, the patient loses all vestige of his or her original personality, is unable to participate in matters of personal hygiene and nutrition, and is left helpless.

Dementia is often progressive (as in degenerative diseases), but it may be static (as in a posttraumatic brain injury state). Depending on the pathologic condition that causes dementia, there may or may not be indications of disease outside the areas of the brain responsible for cognitive and behavioral change. Concomitant disorders of extrapyramidal function are particularly common.

Some conditions that result in dementia may also cause mental retardation (eg, Down's syndrome). Patients with dementia may or may not be psychotic, and a patient with psychosis may or may not have any evidence of cognitive decline consistent with dementia.

Primarily Neurologic Conditions

Alzheimer's Disease is one of the leading, if not the leading cause of dementia, accounting for well over half of cases among the elderly. Its incidence increases with advancing age. Most cases are sporadic, but there is a familial autosomal dominant form of the disease. Much attention currently centers on amyloid formation (see below).

There are no specific physical signs, although frontal lobe release signs may be present and secondarily mild extrapyramidal features may be present. Although this disease is not absolutely diagnosable with certainty during life, a high probability of the diagnosis can be obtained using the criteria established by the Alzheimer's Disease and Related Disorders Work Group of 1984. It has been reported that over 4 percent of people over 65 exhibit moderate to severe dementia and about two-thirds of these fall into the category of idiopathic senile dementia or Alzheimer's disease.

The *brain* is *atrophied,* the *ventricles* are *enlarged,* and evidence of severe vascular disease is minimal or absent. Neuropathologic study reveals *neuronal loss, neurofibrillary tangles,* and *senile plaques,* the extent of which does not clearly correlate quantitatively with the degree of dementia. Although the etiology remains unknown at present, significant accumulations of *beta-amyloid* protein in the brains of Alzheimer patients have led to new theories about the pathogenesis of this condition.

Vascular Dementia. "Hardening of the arteries" with cerebral hypoperfusion was a common, although mistaken lay view of dementia's etiology. However, multiple strokes can leave a patient with impaired cognition and produce a true dementia, often referred to as *"multi-infarct dementia."* Recent data from Scandinavia suggest that among the very elderly (over age 85), vascular dementia rivals Alzheimer's disease as the leading etiology. Although the exact contribution of vascular dementia to the overall rate of dementia remains a subject of debate, there is an increased risk among groups with a high prevalence of vascular risk factors (eg, African Americans, Japanese). An elderly patient with hypertension, diabetes, smoking, atrial fibrillation, or known carotid disease should be considered at risk. The clinical course may progress stepwise if discrete large-vessel occlusions occur, and appear more gradual if the infarctions are primarily lacunar (see Chapter 171).

Inadequately controlled *hypertension* is one of the more frequent and treatable causes of vascular dementia, causing multiple cerebral infarctions. The infarctions may be large and heralded by clear-cut episodes of neurologic injury, or present subclinically as small lacunar strokes contributing to a slow decline in intellectual function. Most patients have evidence of upper motor neuron injury. Magnetic resonance imaging (MRI) may reveal multiple lacunar infarctions and loss of periventricular white matter.

Mixed Disease. As patients age, the brain becomes increasingly vulnerable to insult. Moreover, the risks of vascular and degenerative diseases increase. For this reason, it is likely that a large percentage of cases of dementia in the very elderly are of mixed etiology, both vascular and Alzheimer's in type. The significance of this notion of mixed disease is that it focuses attention on other potential etiologies and the importance of attending to control of their risk factors (eg, improving diabetic or hypertensive control).

Normal-pressure hydrocephalus deserves special mention, both because of its reversibility and because of a tendency to overdiagnose this entity. Its name refers to slow ventricular enlargement without cortical atrophy due to poor cerebrospinal fluid (CSF) absorption. Most often there is no known precipitant, but the condition can occur when there is blockage of CSF absorption due to remote meningeal inflammation or subarachnoid hemorrhage. *Dementia* associated with *gait disturbance* and urinary and fecal *incontinence* are the classic triad. Some patients respond dramatically to ventriculoperitoneal shunting and the diagnosis is suspected clinically and radiographically. Serial lumbar punctures are undertaken to try to predict those who will respond to this maneuver.

Space-occupying lesions such as *chronic subdural hematoma* or slowly growing *tumors* of the brain produce variable dementia depending on their size and location. Those on the orbital surface of the *frontal lobe* or on the medial surface of the *temporal lobe* may present primarily with *cognitive defects* unassociated with other focal signs of cerebral tumor. The development of a progressive unilateral headache (see Chapter 165), a new neurologic deficit, or change in personality may provide a clue to the presence of a mass lesion.

Depression, when very severe, can produce the rapid onset of a true cognitive deficit that is reversible with appropriate treatment. Other symptoms of depression (hopelessness, low self-esteem, early morning awakening, fatigue, anhedonia; see Chapter 227) almost always predate the onset of the dementia and help suggest the diagnosis. However, depression also may accompany other causes of dementia, such as Alzheimer's or Parkinson's disease.

Other primary neurologic conditions associated with dementia and specific neurologic deficits include Parkinson's disease (see Chapter 174), Wilson's disease, severe multiple sclerosis (see Chapter 172), Jacob's disease, neurosyphilis, and Huntington's disease (Table 169–1). Parkinson's disease and Huntington's disease are sometimes referred to as *"subcortical dementias"* because they present with significant motor dysfunction. Proper identification is essential to initi-

Table 169-1. Neurologic Diseases Associated with Intellectual Dysfunction

DISEASE	PHYSICAL SIGNS*	CLINICAL FEATURES
Alzheimer's disease	Frontal lobe release signs; extrapyramidal signs	Enlarged ventricles *and* cortical atrophy by CT or MRI
Normal pressure hydrocephalus	Gait disorder*, incontinence	Enlarged ventricles with little or no cortical atrophy
Multi-infarct dementia	Focal deficits	Stepwise course; multiple areas of infarction, often subcortical by CT or MRI
Parkinson's disease	Extrapyramidal signs*	Usual present only after disease evident for several years
Intracranial tumor	Focal signs, papilledema	Often subacute evolution, seizures possible
Neurosyphilis	Frontal lobe signs, optic atrophy, Argyll-Robertson pupils	Positive serology serum and CSF
Human immunodeficiency virus infection	Variable systemic involvement	Positive HIV, cortical atrophy; dementia may be presenting symptom
Creutzfeldt-Jakob disease	Myoclonus*, cerebellar signs, eye movement abnormalities	Subacute course; EEG has specific abnormalities, brain biopsy diagnostic
Huntington's disease	Choreiform movements*, corticospinal signs	Often positive family history; caudate atrophy by CT or MRI
Multiple sclerosis	Brainstem signs, optic atrophy, corticospinal signs	Usually long-standing disease; episodic illness with remissions; often extensive white matter abnormalities by MRI
Wilson's disease	Extrapyramidal signs*, hepatic dysfunction, Kayser-Fleischer rings*	Onset in adolescence or young adult life, psychiatric disorders
Progressive supranuclear palsy	Failure of vertical downgaze* extrapyramidal signs*	Eye movement abnormalities; differentiate from Parkinson's disease; unresponsive or only transiently responsive to levodopa

* = invariably present; all other physical signs are neither invariably present nor pathognomonic.

ating effective treatment and providing accurate prognostic information.

Other Etiologies

Toxins, infections, metabolic disorders, and nutritional disorders may affect the brain and result in dementia (Table 169–2). Frequently more than one pathologic cause is present and this is particularly the case with *intoxications*. The patient with a progressive degenerative dementia may be taking an excess of the medication that is having a potentiating effect on the primary process or the drug itself may be causing an apparent loss of cognitive abilities. Medications capable of producing dementia in patients without other underlying conditions include *opiates* and the numerous neurotropic agents available. Less obvious but frequently used medications causing or aggravating dementia include the *anticholinergic preparations* used in movement disorders, *antihypertensives,* and *sedatives*. These agents are high on the list of causes of arrestable or reversible diseases.

Any *infection* involving the brain can produce a picture of diffuse cognitive impairment. *Neurosyphilis, human immunodeficiency virus (HIV) infection* (see Chapter 13), and *Cryptococcus* spread into the central nervous system (CNS) produce dementia, often with great regularity. Infectious agents responsible for subacute conditions like Creutzfeldt-Jakob disease and progressive multifocal leukoencephalopathy are resistant to treatment.

Endocrinologic disorders, including *hyper- and hypothyroidism, panhypopituitarism,* and *high-dose corticosteroid therapy* can cause a generally reversible loss in cognitive abilities. The metabolic derangements due to advanced renal or hepatocellular failure usually cause an encephalopathic picture that differs from true dementia because there is an alteration of consciousness. However, milder forms of metabolic disease may exacerbate an underlying dementia, as might *dehydration*.

A number of *hereditary metabolic diseases* associated with prominent cognitive alteration may appear in adult life. These include *Wilson's disease, metachromatic leukodystrophy,* and the *adrenal leukodystrophies*.

Nutritional disorders may result in prominent altered mental status. *Thiamine deficiency,* if untreated, may lead to Korsakoff's dementia, which is largely irreversible. Thiamine deficiency is a preventable deficiency seen with alcoholism, pernicious vomiting of any etiology, depression, or inadequate diet. *Pernicious anemia* may produce dementia, which may, in part, be reversible with administration of vitamin B_{12}. *Pellagra,* uncommon in developed countries, shows a dramatic response to niacin even when mental changes have been present for a long time.

Table 169-2. Systemic Conditions Associated with Intellectual Impairment

Infectious
Syphilis with CNS involvement
HIV infection with CNS involvement
Cryptococcal infection of the CNS
Endocrine
Hypothyroidism and hyperthyroidism
Panhypopituitarism
High-dose glucocorticosteroid therapy
Metabolic
Vitamin B_{12} deficiency
Thiamine deficiency
Niacin deficiency (pellagra)
Chemical Poisons
Alcohol
Metals (lead, mercury)
Aniline dyes
Drug Intoxications
Barbiturates
Opiates
Anticholinergics
Lithium
Bromides
Haloperidol
Antihypertensives

DIFFERENTIAL DIAGNOSIS

The useful way of organizing the differential diagnosis of dementia is to divide the dementing conditions into those pathologic processes that appear to be primary in the brain (see Table 169–1) and those that affect the brain secondarily such as exogenous intoxications, infections, or metabolic derangements (see Table 169-2). Diseases that are primary in the brain may be accompanied by signs of neurologic disease other than cognitive change. Diseases that affect the brain secondarily are more likely to be accompanied by signs and symptoms of medical disease and perhaps to be more reversible. Among patients presenting with dementia, Alzheimer's disease accounts for some 70 percent of cases, vascular disease with multiple infarctions for another 10 percent to 20 percent, and brain tumors for 5 percent, with 10 percent to 15 percent of cases accounted for by all other etiologies or unknown causes. Among the very old (over age 85), vascular dementia and Alzheimer's disease account for the vast majority.

WORKUP

The goal of the workup is to distinguish dementia from other causes of mental impairment and to identify the etiology as either a primary neurologic condition or a condition that secondarily affects the brain.

History

A careful history is the most important component of the initial evaluation. The help of a family member is critical to taking an adequate history, because the patient's recall may be inadequate. To differentiate dementia from other impairments of neurologic functioning requires a description by the patient or family of the specific *cognitive, memory,* and *behavioral problems* the patient is experiencing and the *consequences* of such deficits in the patient's daily life, such as difficulty with driving, work, or family relationships. Detailed questioning should define the *temporal course* of the illness, ascertaining whether the process is indeed chronic and progressive, stepwise, or static. A stepwise pattern in conjunction with focal deficits raises the question of a multi-infarct etiology. An episode of severe hypotension followed by onset of dementia points to hypoperfusion as the mechanism. A story of progressive generalized intellectual impairment without alteration of consciousness is indicative of Alzheimer's disease and other neurodegenerative etiologies, but multiple lacunar strokes may also follow this temporal pattern.

Once dementia is strongly suspected, the history should then focus on identifying potentially treatable causes, be they primarily neurologic or secondary. The search for neurologic disease includes inquiry into risk factors and specific neurologic accompaniments. For example, *cardiovascular risk factors* (smoking, hypertension, hyperlipidemia, diabetes) should be ascertained for identification of the patient at risk for vascular dementia. Questioning about *gait, incontinence*, and a prior history of *meningitis* or *subarachnoid hemorrhage* helps identify the patient at increased risk of normal pressure hydrocephalus. Prior history of *head trauma*, unexplained onset of a *focal neurologic deficit*, and unilateral *headache* worsening over time are potential clues to a mass lesion. A history of *resting tremor* and *rigidity* are likely manifestations of Parkinson's disease. Symptoms of extrapyramidal disease (dysarthria, poor coordination of voluntary movements) in a patient with hepatocellular disease and dementia are indicative of Wilson's disease. *High-risk sexual behavior* raises the probabilities of human immunodeficiency virus (HIV) infection and neurosyphilis. Any symptoms or prior history of *depression* need to be reviewed (see Chapter 227). A *family history* of dementia, Down's syndrome, or psychiatric disorders is the basis for identifying patients at risk for one of the hereditary etiologies.

History is also critical for identification of non-neurologic causes that may be the etiology or an exacerbating factor in loss of mental capacity. Concurrent illnesses and precipitating factors are reviewed. For example, one asks about previous *gastric surgery* (leading to B_{12} deficiency) and adequacy of *nutrition* (for thiamine, niacin, and B_{12} deficiency). A detailed review of *medications* (particularly opiates, sedative-hypnotics, analgesics, anticholinergics, anticonvulsants, corticosteroids, centrally acting antihypertensives, and psychotropics) should be elicited. *Alcohol* abuse and other forms of substance abuse are critical to rule out (see Chapters 228 and 235). It is important to check for symptoms of *hypothyroidism* (see Chapter 104) and *pituitary insufficiency* (see Chapter 101). *Occupational history* may reveal exposure to toxic substances (eg, aniline dyes, heavy metals).

Physical Examination

Mental Status Examination. Assessment begins with a mental status examination to confirm the presence of dementia. The complex faculties that constitute intellect are usually divided into testable, although not necessarily anatomically or pathologically exclusive, functions. This part of the examination should be geared to both the *detection of focal lesions* and to *signs of general brain dysfunction*. Mental status examination in the office can include immediate memory testing with the request to remember three objects, to recite digits forward and backward that are given by the examiner, and to recall a short story. Remote memory testing can be approached by asking about historical events of note, family milestones, or more recent happenings in the newspaper. The patient should be asked to reproduce simple drawings and to discern similarities among objects, a test that offers insight into categorizing ability. Judgment can be ascertained by presenting the patient with decision-requiring situations ("finding a stamped letter" or "seeing a fire in a theater").

General Physical and Neurologic Examinations. The physician should examine the patient to help confirm the diagnosis and uncover evidence of any coexisting abnormalities that may cause or contribute to the patient's problem. One checks for physical evidence of neurovascular risk factors (see Chapter 171) and carefully palpates and auscultates the carotid arteries. In addition, the physician notes any signs of alcoholism (see Chapter 228), hepatocellular injury (see Chapter 71), renal insufficiency (see Chapter 142), and other systemic illnesses.

Specific neurologic abnormalities, such as frontal lobe release signs (grasp, suck, snout, root), visual field cut, extraocular movement limitation, or abnormal pupillary reaction should be elicited. Nystagmus may indicate recent drug ingestion or the presence of brainstem disease. Motor examination should pay particular attention to extrapyramidal features or involuntary movements such as tardive, dyskinesias, tremors, asterixis, chorea, or myoclonus. Sensory examination may reveal evidence of peripheral neuropathy or combined system disease (B_{12} deficiency). Gait should be observed carefully; the small, rigid steps of frontal lobe gait apraxia can be distinguished from a wide-based cerebellar gait or the small steps of extrapyramidal disease.

Laboratory Studies

Standardized Mental Status Test. During the office evaluation, it is desirable to include a published *mental status test* that can be a baseline for subsequent evaluations. Examples of such tests that are appropriate for use in the primary care physician's office are the *Mini-Mental Status Test*, the Blessed Information-Memory-Concentration Test, and the Short Portable Mental Status Questionnaire. These are brief tests requiring less than 15 minutes to complete and are suitable for office use.

Diagnostic criteria for Alzheimer's disease established by the U.S. Department of Health and Human Services require the presence of dementia "established by clinical examination and documented by the Mini-Mental Test . . . or similar examination, with evidence of deficits in two or more areas of cognition; progressive worsening of memory and other cognitive function; no disturbance of consciousness; and absence of systemic disorders or other brain disease that in and of themselves could account for the deficits." No single test will establish definitive determination of dementia, and a poor score on one of these tests should not be the sole criterion for identification of dementia. The score should be considered clinically significant if it is corroborated by other components of the initial evaluation and history. Continuing observation over time may be necessary to establish the diagnosis for some patients and to identify complicating conditions.

Screening Laboratory Studies. The laboratory tests recommended should be individualized based on the patient's history and physical and mental status examinations. Because the history and physical examination will limit the differential possibilities, the patient should be spared the inconvenience and costs of overtesting. Undertesting is also hazardous, because elderly patients in whom medical diseases may have nonspecific presentations of dementia are the usual patient population.

The guidelines specified by the National Institute of Aging's Task Force on Mental Impairment in the Elderly have become the standard for investigation of patients with dementia, although they are probably more appropriate for assessment of alteration in mental functioning than they are for detecting a treatable cause of dementia. They include:

1. Complete blood count and sedimentation rate
2. Chemistry panel (electrolytes, calcium, albumin, BUN, creatinine, transaminase)
3. Thyroid-stimulating hormone (TSH)
4. VDRL test for syphilis
5. Urinalysis
6. Serum B_{12} and folate levels
7. Chest x-ray
8. Electrocardiogram
9. Head computed tomography (CT)

Because this panel was not designed to be a cost-effective workup for uncovering treatable causes of dementia, it should not be applied routinely to all patients, but rather considered a menu to select from, based on the patient's clinical presentation. Some of these tests will be useful in detection of conditions that might exacerbate mental decline in a patient with dementia. Because this list was derived before HIV infection and acquired immunodeficiency syndrome (AIDS) were appreciated as important causes of dementia, *HIV testing* should be added to it, especially in the evaluation of younger patients with a history of high-risk activity or exposure (see Chapter 13).

Neuroimaging of the brain by *CT* or *MRI* is appropriate in the presence of 1) history suggestive of a mass lesion; 2) focal neurologic signs or symptoms; 3) dementia of abrupt onset; 4) history of seizures; 5) and history of stroke. Subdural hematomas and intracranial tumors can be readily identified, especially when contrast-enhanced studies are performed, and radiologic evidence of normal pressure hydrocephalus also may be provided. MRI with gadolinium contrast enhancement is superior to CT for the diagnosis of multi-infarct dementia and for elucidation of problems referable to the posterior fossa. If clinical suspicion of tumor is high, MRI is the more sensitive test.

There is little evidence that *routine* use of neuroimaging is productive or cost-effective as a screening technique for detection of treatable occult disease in patients presenting with dementia. Use of the technology should be limited to those situations (as described above) in which clinical suspicion for potentially treatable intracranial pathology is increased.

Other Ancillary Studies. *Lumbar puncture* may be indicated when other clinical findings suggest an active infection or vasculitis and is part of the evaluation of normal pressure hydrocephalus as described above. Sugar, protein, cell count, cultures, gammaglobulin, and serology for syphilis should be obtained. There are no sufficiently well-developed markers for Alzheimer's disease, and routine lumber puncture for initial evaluation of dementia is not justified.

Electroencephalogram (EEG) may be normal even in advanced states of dementia, or nonspecific slowing of the baseline rhythm may be found. For patients who have episodic altered consciousness, and, therefore, for whom seizures may be suspected, this is an indicated procedure. Occasionally, the EEG may raise suspicion of a particular etiology: focal, delta slowing is seen with tumor, unilateral attenuation of voltage may suggest an extracranial mass such as subdural hematoma, and excessive beta activity may be consistent with drug ingestion. Finally, Creutzfeldt-Jakob disease has a highly specific EEG pattern.

Formal neuropsychologic evaluation would be appropriate for more specific information when the diagnosis is in doubt and is also helpful in providing additional information about the nature of impairment following focal brain injury. *Speech analysis* with speech therapy may improve patient and family communication. Formal *psychiatric assessment* may be desirable if depression in addition to dementia is suspected.

Studies of Limited or Uncertain Utility. *Cerebral blood flow and metabolism measurements* (positron emission tomography and single photon-emission computed tomography) have no routine use at present. Their value in predicting Huntington's and Alzheimer's disease is being investigated.

Brain biopsy for non-neoplastic and noninfectious diseases is rarely justified. Very occasionally, progressive multifocal leukoencephalopathy or Creutzfeldt-Jakob disease is diagnosed by this technique.

Noninvasive neurovascular studies (carotid ultrasound, Doppler flow studies; see Chapter 171) are not of routine value in the workup of dementia, unless the clinical course or physical examination is suggestive of cerebrovascular disease or the MRI or CT demonstrates infarction.

SYMPTOMATIC MANAGEMENT AND COUNSELING

See also Chapter 173.

Improving Mental Functioning. There is no established treatment for Alzheimer's disease or for patients with multi-infarct dementia. The findings of degeneration of cholinergic neurons and depletion of acetylcholine-synthesizing enzyme (choline-acetyl transferase) in Alzheimer's disease have led to a host of attempts at *improving cholinergic transmission*. Dietary choline repletion with lecithin supplements has produced equivocal results. Drugs that stimulate acetylcholine release are under study, as are acetylcholinesterase inhibitors and cholinergic receptor agonists. Randomized, double-blind, placebo-controlled trials involving large numbers of patients are essential to determine efficacy. In a 6-week multicenter trial of *tacrine,* a centrally active, reversible cholinesterase inhibitor, patients demonstrated a modest, but statistically significant reduction in rate of cognitive decline. However, the improvement was not clinically meaningful (no difference in scores of global functioning), and tacrine cannot be recommended as an important advance in treatment. Nonetheless, it may be worth a trial when a modest improvement in functioning might make a substantial difference in quality of life.

Other approaches under active investigation include *restorative therapy* with nerve growth factor, *protective therapy* with antioxidants, and *preventive therapy* with drugs that inhibit beta amyloid formation. There is *no* evidence to support the widely promoted use of so-called cerebral *vasodilators* (papaverine, dihydroergotoxine), although animal studies suggest that some calcium-channel blockers might improve memory.

Management of Confusion and Agitation. The chronic use of sedatives and psychoactive agents in the confused patient should be avoided unless persistent extreme agitation hampers care. If such therapy is contemplated, the lowest possible doses should be used and for the shortest time possible. Patients may respond to a small dose of *thioridazine* (10 to 25 mg qhs). *Haloperidol* is often a first choice in the setting of delusions and hallucinations. Doses in the range of 0.5 to 1 mg two or three times a day usually suffice, but one must be careful to avoid long-term use because of the risk of inducing tardive dyskinesia. Also problematic is regular use of sedative/hypnotic agents for sleep (see Chapter 226). Beta-blocking agents and anticholinergics may exacerbate confusion. Patients with depression may improve with a tricyclic compound with low anticholinergic side effects such as *desipramine* (25 to 50 mg qhs), but drugs with marked anticholinergic activity may worsen memory. A recent study of nursing home patients demonstrated substantial improvement in many patients when chronically prescribed psychotropic drugs were discontinued or reduced in dose.

Maintaining the Patient at Home. An important task is helping the family maintain and care for the patient at home. The goal is to sustain the highest level of function possible, which is facilitated by promotion of an orderly home situation and regular routine use of calendars, television, newspapers, and other means of orientation. Access to potentially dangerous appliances has to be limited. Toilet facilities should be made especially convenient. The issue of driving is discussed in the Drachman reference in the Annotated Bibliography, but early impairment of judgment and spatial concepts makes driving inadvisable for such patients, even in the early stages of disease, although regulations on the subject in most states are not clear.

Families that are willing and able to care for the demented patient at home can often find help in local support groups and social service agencies, some of which also may provide day care and group therapy services. In addition, excellent handbooks are available (see Bibliography). When care at home begins to exhaust and strain the family, sensitive counseling can do much to help a family cope with the difficult decision regarding institutionalization.

It should be remembered that some dementing diseases are infectious (eg, HIV infection) and that the bodily fluids and tissues of such patients require special handling to avoid transmission. Care in the handling of such fluids is always essential, and it is particularly important to emphasize when home care is rendered by lay persons (see Chapter 13).

Risk Factor Reduction and Attention to Underlying Etiologies. The patient with vascular dementia requires attention to control of such cerebrovascular risk factors as hypertension (see Chapter 26), diabetes mellitus (see Chapter 102), smoking (see Chapter 54), hyperlipidemia (see Chapter 27), and coronary artery disease (see Chapter 30). In addition, the question of the need for endarterectory deserves consideration when a vascular etiology is strongly suspected and a significant stenosis is found (see Chapter 171). Avoidance of toxins, correction of vitamin deficiencies, discontinuation of causative drugs, initiation of hormonal replacement therapy in cases of deficiency (see Chapters 101 and 104), and treatment of underlying infectious etiologies (see Chapters 13 and 141) are central to an effective outcome in cases where a causative factor has been identified.

INDICATIONS FOR REFERRAL AND ADMISSION

Some families will request a neurologic consultation when a diagnostic evaluation has been completed by the primary physician and no cause is apparent other than Alzheimer's disease. Such a consultation can provide reassurance to the family that a comprehensive workup was performed and that the diagnosis is correct. If the primary physician has conducted a thoughtful and complete examination as outlined above, the referral need not generate additional testing. If the means for conducting a full workup are not available to the primary physician, then a referral can be used to complete the evaluation. Additionally, patients suspected of having a potentially treatable neurologic condition (Parkinson's disease, normal pressure hydrocephalus, mass lesion, carotid artery disease) are candidates for neurologic or neurosurgical evaluation. Finally, when a suspected hereditary condition is under consideration, referral for confirmation and genetic counseling is indicated.

ANNOTATED BIBLIOGRAPHY

Avorn J, Soumerai SB, Everitt DE, et al. A randomized trial of a program to reduce the use of psychoactive drugs in nursing homes. N Engl J Med 1992;327:168. *(Reduction in unnecessary use of psychotropic drugs in this cohort with a high prevalence of dementia often led to improved functioning.)*

Clarifield AM. The reversible dementias: Do they reverse? Ann Intern Med 1988;109:476. *(Most that reversed were due to drugs or depression; comprehensive review of 32 studies.)*

Consensus Conference. Differential diagnosis of dementing diseases. JAMA 1987;258:3411. *(Lucid discussion of the differential diagnosis and appropriate diagnostic tests; consensus of physicians, psychologists, caregivers, and families of patients with Alzheimer's disease and other dementing diseases.)*

Davis KL, Thal LJ, Gamzu ER, et al. A double-blind, placebo-controlled multicenter study of tacrine for Alzheimer's disease. N Engl J Med 1992;327:1253. *(Short-term study of patients who showed some response to tacrine in a preliminary phase found statistically significant improvement in cognition, but not in global functioning or activities of daily living.)*

Drachman DA. Who may drive? Who may not? Who shall decide? Ann Neurol 1988;24:787. *(Analysis of the tricky regulation process and the physician's obligation to patients and to others.)*

Green JE. Clinical aspects of Alzheimer's disease. Current Opinion in Neurology/Neurosurgery 1988;1:479. *(Very good description of the common and not-so-common clinical features of the most common dementing illness.)*

Growdon JH. Treatment for Alzheimer's disease. N Engl J Med 1992;327:1306. *(Excellent summary of current approaches to therapy.)*

Jenkyn LR. Examining the aging nervous system. Semin Neurol 1989;9:82. *(Good overview of signs associated with normal aging.)*

Larson EB. Illnesses causing dementia in the very elderly. N Engl J Med 1993;328:203. *(Editorial summarizing available data in this fast-growing age group.)*

Larson EB, Reiffler BV, Sumi SM, et al. Diagnostic tests in the evaluation of dementia. Arch Intern Med 1986;146:1917. *(Critical look at standard tests; many not as useful as thought; others detect aggravating conditions.)*

Lindenbaum J, Healton EB, Savage DG, et al. Neuropsychiatric disorders caused by cobalamin deficiency in the absence of anemia or macrocytosis. N Engl J Med 1988;318:1720. *(Almost a third of patients with B_{12} deficiency and neuropsychiatric disease had normal hematologic findings and improved with B_{12} replacement; argues for routine B_{12} testing.)*

Mace NL. The 36 hour day: A timely guide to caring for persons with Alzheimer's disease. Baltimore, Johns Hopkins Press, 1981. *(Best book for families of patients; excellent instructional manual.)*

Petersen RC. Memory function in normal aging. Neurology 1992;42:396. *(Makes some distinctions between normal cognitive alteration with age and the pathologic changes in dementing diseases.)*

Price RW, Brew BJ. The AIDS dementia complex. J Infect Dis 1988;158:1079. *(Detailed description of this important consequence of HIV infection.)*

Siu AL. Screening for dementia and investigating its causes. Ann Intern Med 1991;115:122. *(Critical review of available studies; argues against use of a routine panel of neuroimaging and blood tests and more emphasis on clinical assessment; 102 references.)*

Skoog I, Nilsson L, Palmertz B, et al. A population-based study of dementia in 85-year-olds. N Engl J Med 1993;328:153. *(Prevalence of vascular dementia much higher than previously suspected.)*

Sudarsky L. Geriatrics, gait disorders in the elderly. N Engl J Med 1990;322:1441. *(Gives a good description, which the physician can then relay to concerned families about the common problem of altered gait and balance and falling in older people.)*

Woods BT. CPC #6-1992. N Engl J Med 1992;326:397. *(Good discussion of familial dementing diseases.)*

Yankner BA. Beta amyloid and the pathogenesis of Alzheimer's disease. N Engl J Med 1991;325:1849. *(An exciting research area.)*

Primary Care Medicine: Office Evaluation and Management of the Adult Patient, 3rd edition, edited by Allan H. Goroll, Lawrence A. May, and Albert G. Mulley, Jr. J.B. Lippincott Company, Philadelphia

170
Approach to the Patient With a Seizure

AMY A. PRUITT, M.D.

The occurrence of a convulsion is a dramatic and frightening event. One out of every 11 Americans who lives to be 80 years old will have had at least one seizure. The first experience of a seizure is likely to trigger an immediate visit to an emergency room. Retrospective clarification of a "spell" will be the diagnostic challenge in the office setting. In the context of evaluating an episode of lost or altered consciousness, the primary care physician will need to consider seizure (see Chapter 24). If a seizure is likely, then one should attempt to determine its type and plan for prevention of future episodes while conducting a diagnostic evaluation for underlying etiology.

PATHOPHYSIOLOGY AND CLINICAL PRESENTATION

A *seizure* is a paroxysmal alteration in consciousness or other cerebral cortical function and results from a synchronous activation of a population of neurons either in one focal area or generally throughout the brain. The occurrence of a single seizure does *not* constitute a diagnosis of *epilepsy,* which connotes recurrent, unprovoked seizures. Many people have a single seizure without recurrence, as can happen as a consequence of a transient metabolic disturbance (eg, severe hypoglycemia, hypoperfusion). Only about 1 percent of the U.S. population actually has epilepsy. Epileptic seizures can result from many different types of diseases, ranging from hereditary etiologies to vascular, traumatic, and neoplastic causes. Seizures can be classified as partial or generalized (Table 170–1).

Partial seizures may begin in one area of the brain and initially produce symptoms that are referable to the region of cortex involved. *Simple* partial seizures are focal neurologic events with intact consciousness, whereas *complex* partial seizures impair consciousness. Simple seizures may evolve into complex partial seizures, and both of these types of focal seizures may evolve into secondarily generalized seizures. The spread of symptoms may follow the cortical rep-

Table 170-1. Classification of Seizures

PHENOTYPE	EEG	ETIOLOGY*	PROGNOSIS	DRUG OF CHOICE IN ORDER OF PREFERENCE
Generalized				
Major Motor				
Grand mal	Normal, initially, in 20%; nonspecifically abnormal in 40%	Unknown in 85%	Age-related; overall, 25% seizure-free and off medications at 5 years	Phenytoin or carbamazepine, sodium valproate, phenobarbital
Focal onset (sensory or motor)	Focally abnormal in about 65%	Cause found in 33%	Related to etiology	Phenytoin or carbamazepine, phenobarbital
Temporal lobe onset	See below under partial seizures	Cause found in 50%	May be late result of multiple grand mal seizures; difficult to control	Phenytoin or carbamazepine *and* phenobarbital
Absence (petit mal)	80% have pathognomonic 3/second spike and wave pattern	Unknown autosomal dominant; normal EEGs in both parents in only 50%	Excellent; absences cease by age 20 in 50% but many continue to have grand mal seizures	Sodium valproate, ethosuximide, phenobarbital, trimethadione
Partial				
Simple (no loss of consciousness) motor or sensory	Focally abnormal in about 66%	Cause found in 33%	Related to etiology	Phenytoin or carbemazepine, phenobarbital
Complex (TLE with or without loss of consciousness)	Awake, 50% abnormal; asleep, 85% abnormal	Cause found in 50%; trauma, neoplasm	15% seizure free on medication; psychoses develop in 33% of idiopathic temporal lobe seizures	Phenytoin or carbamazepine *and* phenobarbital

*These figures antedate widespread use of CT scanning in evaluation.

resentation of body parts, beginning, for example, in the fingers and spreading up the arm or down the leg.

Symptoms of complex partial seizures are numerous and include coordinated, involuntary motor activity (automatisms), such as lip smacking or chewing, olfactory or gustatory hallucinations, and behavioral automatisms. Seizure activity typically begins in the temporal lobe or its connections. Premonitory symptoms include olfactory hallucinations, epigastric discomfort, and a sense of fear or deja vu. At times, the symptoms may resemble those of a psychosis. Episodes last 1 to 3 minutes, followed by a period of confusion with consciousness usually impaired but not lost.

Generalized seizures are bilaterally symmetric and without focal onset. An episode may begin with a premonitory aura that is followed by sudden loss of consciousness. A *tonic phase* of limb extension ensues, lasting 10 to 30 seconds, followed by a *clonic phase* of limb jerking of at least 30 seconds. The patient then becomes flaccid and comatose before regaining consciousness. *Postictal confusion* is characteristic and can last for hours, although 10 to 30 minutes is more typical. *Tongue biting* and *incontinence* are other characteristic features.

Important Precipitants of Seizures and Misconceptions About Them. A number of factors have been implicated in the cause of seizures, including fever, stroke, alcohol and drug use, and head trauma. Although these factors are often important, a number of misconceptions about their role are prevalent and need to be addressed:

1. Adults rarely have convulsions with *high fever;* the presence of a temperature greater than 102°F does not suffice to explain the occurrence of a seizure in an adult.
2. Seizures are rare during the initial presentation of an *embolic stroke,* although 20 percent to 25 percent of such patients may have seizures at some time after the initial stroke.
3. *Subarachnoid hemorrhage* and *lacunar strokes* rarely have seizure activity as a sequela, although *emboli* and *cortical vein thrombosis* are more likely to lead to symptomatic epilepsy.
4. *Alcohol withdrawal* seizures occur between 7 and 48 hours after cessation of drinking, with a peak at 13 to 24 hours. Usually, only one or two convulsions occur and status epilepticus is rare. Alcohol withdrawal is more likely to produce seizures in an epileptic patient than in a normal person, and less drinking is required to precipitate a seizure in patients with epilepsy who drink alcohol. *Other drugs* are associated with seizures, either when they are taken in overdose or when withdrawal occurs (Table 170–2).
5. *Trauma* is frequently invoked as a cause for seizures. However, two large studies have shown that unless the trauma was severe with loss of consciousness for more than a half hour or with a lobar hematoma or depressed skull fracture, the incidence of posttraumatic seizures was not greater than that of the general population. When there is a history of closed head trauma, epilepsy usually develops within 2 years, whereas with open head trauma,

Table 170-2. Drugs Commonly Associated with Seizures

DRUGS	OVERDOSE SEIZURES	WITHDRAWAL SEIZURES	DOSE REQUIRED TO INDUCE SEIZURE
Alcohol	−	+	Depends on previous drinking or underlying epilepsy
Meperidine (Demerol)	+	+	2–3 g/day*,†
Propoxyphene (Darvon)	+	+	Variable
Pentazocine (Talwin)	−	−	May precipitate withdrawal from other opiates with as little as 100 mg
Barbiturates	−	+	>600 mg/day (short-acting)†
Meprobamate (Miltown)	−	+	>1.2 g/day†
Chlordiazepoxide, diazepam	−	+	Unknown—may have 7-to 8-day latency period
Phenothiazines, haloperidol	− But myoclonus may occur; may cause seizures in patients with old cortical focus	−	Variable

*Overdose seizure
†Withdrawal seizure
+ = occurs
− = does not occur

seizures may develop at a greater interval from the original injury.

DIFFERENTIAL DIAGNOSIS

Conditions Mimicking Seizures. Several conditions can mimic seizures, either by causing focal deficits or producing episodic loss of consciousness. Among the former are transient ischemic attacks, migraine, and local pathology such as nerve compression. Among the latter are syncopal attacks of any etiology, including transient diminished cerebral profusion from cardiac causes and transient ischemic attacks (see Chapter 24). Psychotic episodes may resemble complex partial seizures.

Conditions Causing Seizures. The differential diagnosis of conditions responsible for a seizure is based largely on the age of the patient at the time of the first seizure and the type of seizure as determined by history, especially that obtained from observers. *Primary or idiopathic epilepsy* is the most common etiology for recurrent seizures in children, but becomes increasingly rare in the young adult population. After age 30 an *underlying cause (secondary epilepsy)* becomes increasingly likely when a patient presents with a first seizure. However, in one large retrospective study of patients with more than one documented seizure of any type, only 23 percent had a cause that became obvious after thorough investigation and a 10-year follow-up. Only 15 percent of seizures generalized from the outset had a demonstrable etiology, whereas underlying disorders could be found in over 30 percent of seizures with a focal component. In the *young adult* population (ages 18 to 45), the demonstrated causes were *drugs* (usually alcohol withdrawal), *neoplasm,* and *trauma.* In the *older adult* population, underlying pathology was divided roughly equally among *neoplasm, trauma,* and *cerebrovascular disease.* A nonepileptic convulsion may occur in the context of a transient metabolic disturbance, such as may result from cerebral hypoperfusion, hypoglycemia, a hyperosmolar state, or hyponatremia.

WORKUP

For the patient who reports a "spell," the first step is to ascertain if it was a seizure and, if so, to characterize its type. Identifying the type facilitates ascertaining whether the cause is likely to be primary (idiopathic) or secondary (underlying central nervous system [CNS] pathology; see Table 170-1). Generalized seizures with no initial focus are usually primary. Such epilepsies are often inherited, age-related, and not associated with structural lesions identified by current neuroradiographic techniques. Partial or focal seizures have a much higher prevalence of identifiable underlying disease or abnormality in the brain.

History. An effective history requires an exact description of events from witnesses as well as from the patient. Especially useful are reports from witnesses, because the patient's consciousness and recall of the event are likely to have been compromised. Questioning should include inquiry into the presence of an aura, focal onset, loss of consciousness, and observed injury during the convulsion. The occurrence of such symptoms suggests seizure rather than syncope, although there are no absolute distinguishing features.

Once it is ascertained that a seizure has occurred, it is essential to check carefully for a history of focal onset, even in patients with a history of generalized seizure. Focal onset of a witnessed seizure that became generalized may be an important clue to an underlying CNS lesion.

History is also essential for identifying precipitants and underlying disease. It should include inquiry into drugs (eg, alcohol, cocaine, amphetamines, sedatives, theophylline, insulin, diuretics), cardiac arrhythmias, valvular disease, previous malignancy, stroke, and head trauma. Symptoms of hyperglycemia and hypoglycemia (see Chapter 102) should be checked for as well as those of meningeal irritation (headache, stiff neck). A family history of convulsions should always be sought.

Physical Examination. The physician may have the opportunity to perform the neurologic examination shortly after the seizure. A focal residual abnormality such as paralysis of one arm (Todd's paralysis) may suggest a focal onset even when the witnessed event was generalized. Besides a careful neurologic examination, the physical should also include a check for postural hypotension, abnormalities in heart rate and rhythm, head trauma, carotid disease, cardiac disease, systemic infection, and signs of alcohol and drug abuse (see Chapters 228 and 235).

Laboratory Studies. *Electroencephalography (EEG)* is the most helpful laboratory diagnostic test in the diagnosis of a seizure disorder. An abnormal EEG with epileptiform features such as spikes or sharp waves supports the diagnosis of seizures and may give information about the type of seizure disorder. However, an abnormal EEG is not adequate for the diagnosis of seizures and a normal EEG can be found in up to 40 percent of patients with purely generalized seizures. The likelihood of detecting an abnormality in partial complex seizures (temporal lobe epilepsy) is increased by obtaining a *sleep EEG*. However, because the EEG concentrates on cortical disturbances, abnormalities of deep temporal lobe or diencephalic structures may not be evident on a surface EEG.

Most neurologists would agree that a *magnetic resonance imaging (MRI)* study of the brain without and then with *gadolinium* contrast enhancement would be an important part of the workup of a patient with a first seizure. This procedure is more sensitive than *computed tomography (CT)* and may be particularly useful in demonstrating abnormalities in the mesial temporal region.

Positron-emission tomography (PET) and *single photon emission computed tomography (SPECT)* are new methods of examining cerebral function in patients with seizures. They may confirm the presence of an organic abnormality and give an outline of the abnormal region that might be considered for surgical treatment of epilepsy. It is unlikely that a primary physician would refer a patient for one of these studies, but the primary physician should be aware that newer methods to differentiate generalized and partial seizures and to select patients for epilepsy surgery are available in epilepsy centers.

Unless there is evidence of infection or the patient presents in status epilepticus, it is no longer common practice to perform a *lumbar puncture* for a patient with a first seizure. If fever is present or there is a history compatible with systemic infection, lumbar puncture remains an essential part of neurologic evaluation.

PRINCIPLES OF MANAGEMENT

As precise a diagnosis as possible must be made before treatment is begun. This includes both the phenotype of the seizure, the electroencephalogram, and the identification of any underlying cause or precipitating factors. The distinction between a single seizure and epilepsy is important.

The Isolated Seizure

As noted earlier, the occurrence of an isolated convulsion does not constitute epilepsy. When a single convulsion has occurred due to a transient metabolic disturbance or drug overdose or withdrawal, it is best treated by attending to the factors that led to the disturbance. Long-term use of drugs for seizure prophylaxis in such patients is not indicated, although a short-term course may be used in the setting of alcohol or drug withdrawal (see Chapters 228 and 236). When there is no obvious self-limited etiology in a patient who presents with a single seizure, then prophylaxis is warranted, because the risk of recurrence is increased (see below).

Recurrent Epileptic Seizures

The treatment of choice for recurrent epileptic seizures is administration of a *single anticonvulsant drug* appropriate for the seizure type diagnosed (see Table 170–1). Most available antiepileptic drugs are used for the purpose of preventing recurrent seizures rather than for any specific effect on the course of established epilepsy or for the prevention of the development of seizures after trauma. As a group, generalized seizures respond best to treatment, and full seizure control is possible with monotherapy for as many as 80 percent of patients with idiopathic epilepsy.

The drug should be used in doses to control the seizures as completely as possible. If side effects become intolerable, the drug should be replaced by another medication, also used as monotherapy, until it is clear that the patient cannot be controlled with a single drug. In general, it is better initially to add rather than to substitute a second drug, thus providing seizure protection while the serum concentration of the second drug is rising. Then the patient should be tapered off the first drug, striving for monotherapy.

Side effects severe enough to necessitate a change in therapy occur in about 30 percent of patients treated with antiepileptic drugs. Drug side effects and interactions may become intolerable if more than one drug is required. A second drug should not be added until it is documented that control cannot be achieved with the dose of the first drug at either high therapeutic concentration or one that produces toxic effects.

When an antiepileptic drug is begun or the dosage of the drug is altered one must wait five drug-elimination half-lives before assessing the effect of the change. To achieve immediately a steady-state concentration equal to the usual maintenance concentration, it is usually necessary to give a loading dose of drug. Levels should be checked frequently while doses are adjusted (see Table 170–3 for appropriate intervals for antiepileptic level checks, maintenance doses, loading doses, and therapeutic levels).

Classes of Antiepileptic Agents. There are several effective drugs for treating each form of epilepsy, the drug of first choice being determined by that which has the least toxicity in any individual patient. Three types of antiepileptic drugs

Table 170-3. Pharmacokinetic Summary of Antiepileptic Drugs

DRUG (generic/brand)	INDICATIONS**	STARTING DOSE* (mg/day)	MAINTENANCE DOSE (mg/day)	ELIMINATION HALF-LIFE (hours)	TIME TO STEADY STATE PLASMA CONCENTRATION+ (days)	THERAPEUTIC RANGE OF PLASMA CONCENTRATION (μg/ml)
Phenytoin (Dilantin)	T-C,CP,SP	300	200–500	10–34	7–8	10–20
Carbamazepine (Tegretol)	T-C,CP,SP	200–400	600–1200	14–27	3–4	4–12
Phenobarbital	T-C,CP,SP	90	90–240	46–136	14–21	10–40
Primidone (Mysoline)	T-C,CP,SP	125	750–1500	6–18	4–7	5–12***
Valproic acid (Depakote)	A,M, T-C	750	1000–4000	6–15	1–2	40–100
Ethosuximide (Zarontin)	A	500	500–1500	20–60	7–10	40–120
Clonazepam (Klonopin)	A,AT, M	1.5	1.5–10	20–40	—	—
Felbamate (Felbatol)	Refractory CP	1600	1600–3600	15–20	—	—

*All doses are for adults.

**A = absence; AT = atonic; CP = complex partial; M = myoclonic; SP = simple partial; T-C = tonic-clonic

***Mysoline is metabolized to phenobarbital whose therapeutic concentrations are the same as those listed under phenobarbital. The value in this column refers to primidone concentration.

+This is the interval at which drug levels should be checked after any adjustment in dose.

are available. *Type I drugs,* which include *carbamazepine* and *phenytoin,* block sustained repetitive firing, the rapid firing of action potentials produced by an applied depolarizing current and dependent on opening of increased numbers of sodium channels. *Type II drugs,* including *phenobarbital, valproate,* and *benzodiazepines,* have dual actions to enhance gamma aminobutyric acid (GABA) inhibitory transmission and to block sustained repetitive firing. Type III is represented by *ethosuximide,* an antiepileptic drug that has no effect on either postsynaptic GABA-ergic inhibition or sustained released firing, but blocks T-calcium currents, which appear to be important in the generation of normal rhythmic activity.

Important Drug–Drug Interactions. Carbamazepine, phenobarbital, and phenytoin are *inducers* of the *hepatic microsomal cytochrome P450 enzymes.* Production of endogenous compounds such as steroids is generally compensated for by intrinsic homeostatic feedback mechanisms, but dosage increases may be necessary for medications such as steroids used in immunosuppression or cerebral edema or oral contraceptives. Table 170–4 lists selected clinically significant drug interactions for phenytoin that may be of relevance to primary care practice.

Phenytoin. For most seizure types occurring in adults, the drug of choice is phenytoin. The proprietary formulation, Dilantin (Parke-Davis), is preferable to the generic formulation. Phenytoin is well absorbed orally and has a serum half-life of 22 to 30 hours. An initial loading dose must be administered. Dose-related side effects include nystagmus, ataxia, dysarthria, and blurred vision. The presence of nystagmus can be used as a crude guide to the adequacy of dose. Duration-related side effects include osteomalacia, peripheral neuropathy, a folate deficiency anemia, and cerebellar degeneration. Idiosyncratic reactions include gingival hypertrophy, hypertrichosis, spiking fevers, exfoliative dermatitis, bone marrow depression, liver abnormalities, teratogenesis during the first trimester of gestation, and neonatal coagulation defects.

Table 170-4. Phenytoin: Side Effects and Drug Interactions

Major Side Effects

Dose related: nystagmus, ataxia, dysarthria, blurred vision, decrease in measured total T_4

Duration related: osteomalacia, peripheral neuropathy, anemia, cerebellar degeneration

Idiosyncratic: gingival hypertrophy, acne, hypertrichosis, encephalopathy

Rare, toxic: high, spiking fevers, exfoliative dermatitis, bone marrow depression, pseudo- and actual lymphoma lupus-like syndrome, teratogenesis during first trimester, neonatal coagulation defects

Interactions with Commonly Prescribed Drugs

Increased phenytoin levels with:
- Antimicrobials: chloramphenicol, INH
- Anticoagulants: coumadin
- Amphetamines (but seizure threshold decreased)
- Disulfiram (Antabuse)
- Alcohol: acute ingestion raises phenytoin levels, but see below
- Anti-inflammatory agent: phenylbutazone
- Anticonvulsants: ethosuximide; no consistent effect with simultaneous barbiturate administration
- Sedatives: chlordiazepoxide (librium), diazepam (valium, oxazepam (serax), clorazepam (clonopin)

Decreased phenytoin levels with:
- Alcohol: chronic ingestion

Phenytoin effects on levels of other drugs
- Insulin: may interfere with endogenous insulin release
- Quinidine: decreases quinidine effect at given dose
- Falsely low total T_4

Carbamazepine (Tegretol) is also an excellent first-line drug for adult-onset generalized tonic-clonic seizures and for complex partial seizures. Many patients report less fatigue and better performance on this medication than on phenytoin, but a controlled study failed to confirm that carbamazepine was clearly superior. The major disadvantages of this medication include the necessity of multiple daily dosing and the frequently required blood tests during initiation of the medication to monitor for uncommon instances of *bone marrow depression*.

Valproate. For patients allergic to phenytoin or carbamazepine, valproate (Depakote) is a good choice of medication. Many neurologists would choose this as a first-line drug for spike-and-wave or generalized tonic-clonic epilepsy even without an abnormal EEG. This drug also has to be given in multiple daily doses (see Table 170-4). Major side effects of valproate are nausea, weight gain, hair loss, platelet dysfunction, fetal anomalies (neural tube defects), and liver dysfunction.

Phenobarbital is no longer a first-line choice of drug for generalized tonic-clonic seizures, although for patients allergic to the above-mentioned three medications it provides good control usually with acceptable side effects.

New Antiepileptic Drugs. In 1993, *felbamate* (Felbatol) was approved for release. The drug is chemically similar to meprobamate, but causes less sedation. A major advantage is its lack of chemical overlap with other anticonvulsants and its low toxicity. Presently, the major indication for felbamate is as adjunctive for refractory complex partial seizures. Its usual daily dose is 1600 to 3600 mg and its half-life is 15 to 20 hours, less when co-administered with either carbamazepine or phenytoin. Addition of felbamate raises phenytoin blood levels. Several other drugs are about to be approved at the time of this writing.

Prognosis

Prognosis is a function of the underlying etiology. The prognosis of *idiopathic epilepsy* depends on both the age at onset and type of convulsion. Patients with primary generalized seizures have the best overall prognosis. Childhood-onset seizures cease by age 20 in more than half of these cases. Although statistics vary according to age at onset and type of seizure, on the average, 10 years after diagnosis over half of the patients are seizure-free with or without medication. The probability of remaining seizure-free is highest for those patients who had seizures that were generalized at the outset and were diagnosed before age 10. Eighty percent of recurrences will be within 5 years of stopping medication. The major cause of failure to control seizures is *noncompliance,* and it has been shown that as many as one-third of patients do not take their medication as prescribed.

Most neurologists would require a seizure-free interval of at least a year before considering discontinuation of medication. The EEG is of only modest help in predicting which patients may be weaned successfully from their medications in that a persistently abnormal EEG would make discontinuation of medication inadvisable, but the documentation of a normal EEG does not eliminate risk of seizure recurrence. In a large prospective study, the risk of relapse was greatest in patients with complex partial seizures with secondary generalization, an abnormal EEG before treatment that was unchanged during treatment, or a requirement for valproate.

The prognosis for recurrence of seizures after a *single convulsion* in a patient without an obvious self-limited cause (drugs, transient metabolic disturbance) has been a question of much interest. Risk of developing recurrent convulsions increases with a family history of seizures or with an EEG that shows generalized spike-and-wave activity. Most neurologists would recommend that a first seizure be treated, because likelihood of recurrence is high enough to warrant prophylaxis even for the best prognosis group of patients. New onset of seizures in a patient with a history of risk factors for HIV disease may be the first manifestation of HIV infection and its CNS consequences (see Chapter 13).

INDICATIONS FOR REFERRAL AND ADMISSION

Workup of a patient with a first seizure can be accomplished by the primary care physician with a sleep-deprived EEG and MRI. Institution of antiepileptic medication usually can be initiated in the outpatient setting, and appropriate monitoring of therapeutic levels can be planned (see Table 170–3).

For the patient who fails to respond to the first-choice medication or for whom side effects are intolerable, a second drug should be tried. If it appears that the patient may require two drugs for seizure control or if there is a question about the organic nature of all of the witnessed spells, it would be appropriate to refer the patient to a neurologic specialist comfortable with drug management and with the techniques of EEG and telemetry. Such a referral will also provide the patient access to centers in which epilepsy surgery is performed and through which newer anticonvulsant medications can be obtained.

Differentiating between an epileptic attack and other systemic disorders or psychiatric conditions can be difficult. Nonepileptic attacks and epileptic seizures can coexist in patients with seizure disorders. Monitoring with telemetry for several days in the hospital may be necessary to clarify the diagnosis. However, hospitalization is not necessary after the occurrence of a typical generalized seizure in a patient with a known seizure disorder, unless there is significant trauma or need to adjust the medication program under careful monitoring. Patients with a first generalized convulsion should be admitted for evaluation at the time of the episode, particularly to check for a cardiovascular or metabolic etiology.

PATIENT EDUCATION

Perhaps the most important obligation of the physician to the epileptic patient is in a role as counselor, educator, and, sometimes, legal advocate. This is a long-standing relationship with a patient whose chronic disease is surrounded by an enormous amount of superstition, prejudice, and misunderstanding. The diagnosis of epilepsy clearly imposes certain restrictions on the patient's life, making the certainty of diagnosis in a young healthy person imperative (see above).

Work. In addition to reviewing the prognosis with the patient, it is important to emphasize that, even if seizures are not entirely controlled, most epileptics are able to lead productive lives. Fifteen to 25 percent of the nation's four million epileptics are unemployed, a figure higher than the national average. However, only those professions that require a chauffeur's or pilot's license absolutely bar people known to suffer seizures.

Driving. Driving laws vary from state to state, but in general, states require a *seizure-free interval* of *6 months to 1 year* before reapplication for driver's license may be made. Continued supervision by a physician is mandatory.

Alcohol and Caffeine. Diagnosis of epilepsy does not make absolute abstention from alcohol mandatory, although the patient should be counseled that alcohol can lower the seizure threshold and that binge drinking is contraindicated. The relationship of seizures to the ingestion of large amounts of caffeine is less clear, but the patient should be counseled to use substances containing caffeine in moderation.

Pregnancy and Surgery. For a female epileptic considering *pregnancy,* the primary physician may be the source of much helpful information. The effect of pregnancy on a seizure disorder's severity is nil in about half of women. For the remainder, half experience slight worsening of seizures. Ideally, with well-controlled seizures, it would be possible to taper the patient off the medication before conception. However, one does not always have such luxury, and a patient may worry about teratogenesis. Risk of fetal malformations in an epileptic woman not on medication is still roughly double that of the general population. However, teratogenesis is clearly established for phenytoin (digital and craniofacial abnormalities as well as some cardiac defects), valproate (neural tube defects), and carbamazepine (facial anomalies and neural tube defects). Women on phenytoin still have a 94 percent chance of having a completely normal pregnancy outcome. Thus, the risks of continuing anticonvulsant medication must be weighed against the benefits of preventing a sustained convulsion (fetal hypoxia, mechanical injury from mother's fall). For the patient who needs to remain on antiepileptic drugs during pregnancy, monthly monitoring of her drug levels is important because the combination of decreased protein binding, decreased absorption, and increased metabolism and plasma volume result in lower drug levels.

Surgical procedures pose no special threat to the epileptic patient as long as medications are not discontinued at any time.

Breast-Feeding. Should the mother taking anticonvulsant therapy elect to breast-feed her infant, it usually poses little problem. Some sedation in the infant is sometimes seen with phenytoin, carbamazepine, or phenobarbital. However, the concentration of benzodiazepine or ethosuximide in breast milk can approach or exceed serum levels, making breast-feeding inappropriate when such agents are being taken.

Heredity of Seizures. There may be considerable worry about inheritance of seizures. Epilepsy is hereditary, although the precise genetics are not clear for all types. One-quarter to one-third of patients with idiopathic epilepsy have a family history of seizures. Three percent of children of patients of idiopathic epilepsy develop seizures. Febrile convulsions also appear to be more common in children who have afflicted relatives as do posttraumatic seizures.

Teaching First Aid. Families of patients with epilepsy should know the fundamentals of emergency management of seizures. They should be instructed in the positioning that protects the airway and cautioned against use of the time-honored tongue blade. It should be emphasized to the patient's family that few seizures last long enough to impair cardiopulmonary function.

THERAPEUTIC RECOMMENDATIONS

- Establish an etiologic diagnosis and treat the underlying cause if possible. Symptomatic therapy can begin while workup is in progress.
- To prevent further convulsions, begin with a loading dose of a drug of choice appropriate to the seizure type identified. This can often be done on an outpatient basis. Maintenance dose is then begun, and the dose is adjusted to achieve a therapeutic level with a level checked at an interval appropriate to the drug half-life.
- If seizures persist, check the serum levels of the anticonvulsants and inquire into alcohol and other drug use. Add a second drug and then taper off the first drug if seizures cannot be controlled with the drug of first choice.
- If seizures are controlled, continue the medication for at least 1 year. If the patient remains seizure-free, a cautious attempt to taper the medication can be made.
- Teach the patient how to recognize the warning signals of a seizure and what to do to minimize injury. Instruct the patient in the role of alcohol in precipitating seizures.
- Educate the patient and family about prognosis, activity, and job precautions.

ANNOTATED BIBLIOGRAPHY

Callaghan N, Garrett A, Goggin T. Withdrawal of anticonvulsant drugs in patients free of seizures for two years. N Engl J Med 1988;318:942. *(Prospective study defining the circumstances in which it is safe.)*

Drugs for epilepsy. Med Lett 1989;31:1. *(Excellent, terse summary.)*

Farwell JR, et al. Phenobarbital for febrile seizures, effects on intelligence and seizure recurrence. N Engl J Med 1990; 322:364. *(Phenobarbital should not be routinely prescribed for febrile seizures.)*

Hachinski V. Should people be treated after a first seizure? Neurology 1988;45:490. *(Decide for yourself.)*

Hauser WA. Seizure recurrence after a first unprovoked seizure and extended follow-up. Neurology 1990;40:1163. *(Again, what do the data tell you?)*

Holtzman DM, Kaku DA, So YT. New onset seizures associated with human immunodeficiency virus infection. Am J Med 1989;87:173. *(Study of 100 HIV patients with seizures; in 18 percent it was the presenting symptom; most due to infection, followed by mass lesion.)*

Mattson RH, Cramer JA, Collins JF, et al. A comparison of valproate with carbamazepine for the treatment of complex partial seizures and secondarily generalized tonic-clonic seizures in adults. N Engl J Med 1992;327:765. *(A VA multicenter randomized study; carbamazepine was found to be superior to valproate.)*

Meador HG. Comparative cognitive effects of anti-convulsants. Neurology 1990;43:91. *(All about equal, save for phenobarbital.)*

Patterson RM. Seizure disorders in pregnancy. Med Clin North Am 1989;73:661. *(Succinct summary.)*

Pedley TA. Discontinuing antiepileptic drugs. N Engl J Med 1988;318;982. *(Editorial summarizing available data and unanswered questions.)*

Scheuer M. The evaluation and treatment of seizures. N Engl J Med 1990;323:1468. *(Terse review for the generalist reader; 51 references.)*

Tempkin NR, et al. A randomized double-blind study of phenytoin for the prevention of posttraumatic seizures. N Engl J Med 1990;32:497. *(Phenytoin does not prevent the development of posttraumatic seizures.)*

171

Management of the Patient With a Transient Ischemic Attack or an Asymptomatic Carotid Bruit

AMY A. PRUITT, M.D.

Primary Care Medicine: Office Evaluation and Management of the Adult Patient, 3rd edition, edited by Allan H. Goroll, Lawrence A. May, and Albert G. Mulley, Jr. J.B. Lippincott Company, Philadelphia

Stroke is the third leading cause of death in the United States and is a major source of disability in the older population. Although medical and surgical therapies for stroke are improving, prevention is still the most effective strategy and a major responsibility of the primary care physician. Stroke prevention through risk factor management may be a major contributor to the rapid decline over the past two decades in death rates from stroke. The cornerstone of the preventive effort is the early identification and vigorous treatment of stroke risk factors (eg, hypertension, diabetes, coronary artery disease, smoking; see Chapters 26, 30, 54, and 102). Atrial fibrillation, a major risk factor for embolic stroke, also requires serious attention (see Chapters 28 and 83).

Patients who present with a transient ischemic attack or an asymptomatic carotid bruit pose the problem of stroke prevention at a more advanced stage of cerebrovascular disease. The primary physician should be able to recognize these conditions by history and physical examination, cost-effectively use appropriate noninvasive imaging and flow studies, and know when to initiate more aggressive measures, such as anticoagulant therapy or surgical intervention.

PATHOPHYSIOLOGY, CLINICAL PRESENTATION, COURSE

Transient Ischemic Attacks (TIAs)

TIAs are defined as episodes of temporary, focal cerebral dysfunction due to vascular disease that last *less than 24 hours* and *usually less than 10 minutes*. A TIA is part of a spectrum that includes ischemic events lasting more than 24 hours and partially reversible, nondisabling stroke. The distinction between TIAs, cerebral infarction with transient signs (CITS), and stroke has become less clear with the advent of computed tomography (CT) and magnetic resonance imaging (MRI), because many patients whose deficits appear to resolve completely will be found to have radiographic changes suggesting infarction. However, all of these patients fall into a group that may be at risk for further ischemic damage.

Pathogenesis. There appear to be two mechanisms for TIAs. The majority are due to *emboli* of platelets and fibrin or of atheromatous material breaking off from a vessel wall (usually the carotid) and transiently occluding a cerebral or ophthalmic artery or one of its branches. Thrombus formation distal to an atherosclerotic plaque is common in tightly stenosed (> 75% stenosis, residual lumen less than 2 mm) or even totally occluded carotid arteries and often serves as the source of emboli. The heart is the other important source of emboli. Cardiac lesions predisposing to cerebral embolism include mitral valve stenosis, mitral valve prolapse, calcified mitral annulus, ventricular aneurysm or dyskinesia, atrial or ventricular clot, valvular vegetations, and interatrial shunts. Atrial fibrillation greatly exacerbates the risk of cardiac embolization. Occasionally, the intracranial arteries are the source of emboli. This occurs with greatest frequency among African-American males and should be considered in patients with no extracranial vascular or cardiac source of emboli.

TIAs may also occur when there is *transient hypotension* in conjunction with a hemodynamically *significant carotid stenosis* (> 75% occlusion). The resulting reduction in collateral flow to the ipsilateral carotid territory can lead to transient neurologic symptoms. Blood pressure reduction rarely results in focal symptoms unless a severely stenotic lesion is already present.

In certain rare instances, TIAs may be attributable to steal phenomena (such as subclavian steal) or to hyperviscosity states such as polycythemia.

Clinical Presentation. TIAs can be divided into those that indicate disease in the carotid circulation and those that point to disease in the vertebrobasilar territory. TIA symptoms associated with *carotid disease* include transient monocular blindness, clumsiness, weakness, or numbness of the hand or disturbed speech. Transient monocular blindness is due to occlusion of the ophthalmic artery or branches ipsilateral to the carotid stenosis and classically is described by the patient as a "shade" or "curtain" that descends over the affected eye. For patients with symptoms suggestive of carotid disease, the detection of a carotid bruit on the same side as the symptomatic eye or cerebral hemisphere is suggestive but not diagnostic of high-grade carotid stenosis.

Symptoms of *vertebrobasilar disease* include binocular visual disturbance, vertigo, paresthesias, diplopia, ataxia, dysarthria, light-headedness, generalized weakness, loss of consciousness, and transient global amnesia. Each of these may be an isolated symptom of posterior circulation disease, although isolated vertigo without other brain stem symptoms is rarely due to vertebrobasilar occlusive disease (see Chapter 166).

Certain clinical features are likely to be associated with carotid or vertebrobasilar disease, but no single feature is a consistently reliable sign. In one series of 95 patients with carotid territory TIAs evaluated by arteriography, two clinical features were correlated with the arteriographic state of the artery. First, duration of hemispheric attacks over 60 minutes, whether single or multiple, was significantly associated with a normal carotid (attacks were most likely due to emboli from the heart). Second, the nonsimultaneous occurrence of both transient hemispheric episodes and transient monocular blindness was correlated with an 80 percent incidence of carotid disease. No difference between normal and diseased carotid groups was found when the cumulative number of attacks per patient was considered. Similarly, division according to pure ocular or pure hemispheric symptoms did not distinguish the two groups.

Clinical Course and Risk of Stroke. The interval since the most recent TIA appears to be the single most important factor in predicting the risk of stroke. Of those who will suffer stroke, approximately one-half will do so 1 year after the first TIA and approximately one-fifth will have their stroke during the first month after the episode. The risk of stroke cannot be predicted by the number of TIAs, the duration of symptoms, or the clinical phenomena. All patients with any type of TIA should be considered at risk for stroke, and those with recent onset (< 1 month) should be evaluated urgently (see below). About 50 percent to 75 percent of stroke patients with occlusive carotid disease have preceding TIAs.

Cardioembolic Stroke with Transient Symptoms

Patients with cardioembolic stroke who have transient symptoms tend to have symptoms lasting several hours. The neurologic disorder associated with cardioembolic infarction is maximal at onset in 80 percent of patients, and about 75 percent of emboli lodge in one of the middle cerebral arteries causing symptoms similar to those of carotid occlusive disease.

Asymptomatic Carotid Bruits

Incidental discovery on physical examination of an asymptomatic carotid bruit suggests the presence of an atherosclerotic lesion that has narrowed the lumen by at least 50 percent to less than 3 mm. The pitch of the bruit increases with severity of stenosis. Prolonged, very high-pitched bruits suggest a residual lumen of less than 1.5 mm (> 75% stenosis). Most atherosclerotic lesions causing bruits tend to be located on the posterior wall of the common carotid artery at the bifurcation, compromising flow at the origin of the internal carotid. When stenosis is tight and flow is reduced, mural thrombus may form distally in the proximal internal carotid artery, worsening occlusion and serving as a source of emboli. Plaque ulceration may also provide a nidus for mural thrombus formation.

Epidemiologic studies indicate asymptomatic bruits are associated with an increased risk of stroke, coronary disease, and death but not necessarily with increased risk of stroke on the side of the bruit. In a large prospective study of 500 patients with asymptomatic bruits followed for an average of 2 years by clinical and Doppler examinations, the overall risk of stroke in patients who remained asymptomatic was 1 percent at 1 year and 1.7 percent if those who developed TIAs were included. A major predictor of stroke was the severity of carotid stenosis, as was progression to high-grade stenosis (> 75%, residual lumen less than 2 mm). Other risk factors include hypertension, preexisting heart disease, male gender, and a positive family history.

DIFFERENTIAL DIAGNOSIS

The differential diagnosis of a TIA-like episode includes any condition that causes transient symptoms in a focal distribution and is not limited to those of vascular origin. *Focal seizures* (see Chapter 170) can produce such a picture, as can the focal aura of *migraine,* which is not always followed by headache (see Chapter 165). *Hyperventilation* can produce distal tingling and numbness. *Carpal tunnel syndrome* may present with intermittent (often nocturnal) paresthesias in a median nerve distribution. Even a protruding *cervical disc* or osteophyte may produce transient focal motor or sensory complaints (as during manipulation of the head or neck; see Chapter 167).

WORKUP

The goals in evaluating a TIA or an asymptomatic bruit are detection of significant vascular disease and assessment of stroke risk. One needs to identify those patients who require aggressive intervention. In addition, should cerebrovascular disease prove not to be the etiology, a search for other etiologies would be required. The patient with new onset of TIAs (< 30 days) has a heightened risk of stroke and should be evaluated promptly.

History. For the patient with a suspected TIA, questioning should first confirm that the transient episode was indeed a TIA, based on onset and duration. Duration of symptoms beyond 24 hours rules out TIA; cessation within 10 minutes increases its probability. An episode that lasts hours might be due to an embolic event. The onset of headache during resolution of the neurologic deficit is more suggestive of a migrainous episode (see Chapter 165). A careful description of symptoms may be helpful in distinguishing vertebrobasilar involvement from carotid disease (see above). In addition, the frequency of episodes, date of first onset, and presence of underlying heart disease and cardiovascular risk factors are important to ascertain, because they can help predict clinical course. The presence of hypertension, cardiac disease, or advanced age (> age 65) increases the risk of subsequent stroke. Patients with carotid symptoms are more likely to develop a disabling stroke than are those with vertebrobasilar dysfunction. The patient is at greatest risk for stroke in the first few months after onset of TIAs.

In the patient with an apparently asymptomatic carotid bruit found on physical examination, it is worthwhile to go back to the history and check carefully for overlooked transient neurologic events. Their presence would greatly increase the significance of the physical examination finding and indicate heightened risk of stroke. Inquiry into history of hypertension, heart disease, and family history of stroke further helps in determination of stroke risk.

Physical examination should be directed to the cardiovascular and nervous systems. One checks for hypertension, atrial fibrillation, and heart murmurs (see Chapters 21 and 33). Fundoscopic examination at the time of visual symptoms may reveal embolus in one of the retinal artery branches. Neurologic examination is likely to be normal if conducted after the TIA has passed.

Carotid arteries should be palpated and auscultated gently (so as not to dislodge any mural thrombus from a diseased vessel wall) for upstroke, volume, and presence of a bruit. As noted above, finding a bruit does not invariably herald significant stenosis (a bruit can be present with hemodynamically insignificant lesions), but in as many as 70 percent to 80 percent of cases, the bruit does identify important ipsilateral carotid disease. The pitch of the bruit and its duration should be noted, because they tend to correlate with severity of stenosis.

Palpation of facial and superficial temporal pulses with simultaneous assessment of supratrochlear and supraorbital pulses may confirm collateral flow to the latter two vessels by way of the external carotid artery and suggest occlusion of the internal carotid artery. Unfortunately, the vertebrobasilar circulation is not accessible to accurate physical examination.

Laboratory Studies. There is no entirely reliable noninvasive test for carotid or vertebrobasilar disease. In the past two decades, there have been great strides in the noninvasive evaluation of carotid and posterior circulation vessels. For assessment of suspected *carotid lesions*, the combination of *Doppler* and *B-mode ultrasound* allows determination of lumen size and visualization of the carotid arterial lesion. However, in some instances, one cannot tell if the carotid artery is completely occluded or only tightly stenosed. Use of *transcranial Doppler* techniques helps to measure flow in the ophthalmic system and assess hemodynamic significance of the carotid stenosis.

For study of the *posterior circulation, transcranial Doppler* ultrasonography provides a relatively inexpensive means of noninvasively surveying large intracranial vessels. The test measures the velocity of flow, which increases in the setting of stenosis. However, it does not provide direct anatomic information. *MRI angiography* provides the ability to image blood flow and is capable of producing angiography-like images without invasive study and iodinated contrast. However, the technology is expensive and not yet sufficiently diagnostic to obviate the need for arteriography, although it has been used to select candidates for invasive study.

CT or *MRI* of the brain should be performed to detect silent or prior infarction unsuspected hemorrhage, and nonvascular disease such as tumor.

There is no entirely reliable noninvasive test for occlusive disease, and *arteriography* remains the definitive diagnostic procedure. Using selective transfemoral catheterization or digital subtraction arteriographic techniques, arteriography should be performed only if the physician would proceed to endarterectomy in the instance of carotid disease or to anticoagulation in the case of vertebrobasilar disease. Thus, the procedure should lead to a critical management decision. The dye load involved in performing cerebrovascular angiography can be substantial, necessitating adequate hydration, particularly in patients with underlying renal disease or diabetes.

Standard B-mode echocardiography performed transthoracically makes possible identification of cardiac lesions that predispose to embolization, but the yield is low in patients over the age of 50 without evidence of cardiac disease on physical examination (see Chapter 33). *Transesophageal echocardiography* is more sensitive and specific for detecting intracardiac and aortic sources of embolization, such as left atrial thrombus and atherosclerosis of the ascending aortic arch. It should be considered when standard echocardiography is unrevealing but clinical suspicion is high for embolization. Ambulatory *Holter monitoring* is useful when there is concern about atrial fibrillation being a precipitant of embolization and the *resting electrocardiogram* is normal (see Chapters 25 and 29).

Abnormalities of blood coagulation may contribute to 4 percent of strokes in young persons. Some authorities recommend *coagulopathy workup* for stroke patients younger than age 50, those with prior venous disease, patients with a family history of abnormal clotting who have no other explanation for their stroke, and patients who have abnormal hematocrit, platelets, prothrombin time, or partial thromboplastin time.

PRINCIPLES OF MANAGEMENT

Transient Ischemic Attacks

The literature on therapeutic options in TIAs is complex and often confusing. Until recently, many studies were not well controlled, and often study populations were not well defined or characterized. Recent demographic data have clarified those patients at greatest risk for stroke. As noted earlier, the interval since the most recent TIA appears to be the most important single factor in predicting the risk of stroke. Therefore, all patients with any type of TIA should be considered at risk for stroke and those with recent onset (< 1 month) should be evaluated urgently. The physician should remember that, although TIAs are predictors of stroke, myocardial infarction is still the most common cause of death in this group (annual mortality rate is 5%) and that attention also be paid to the patient's cardiovascular status and cardiac risk factors (see Chapter 30).

Bearing in mind that optimal therapy for TIAs is an evolving therapeutic area and that new information is forthcoming regularly, the following guidelines for management are recommended.

Symptomatic patients with tight carotid stenosis, especially those with recurrent TIAs or a TIA within 4 months of the current visit, require prompt attention and consideration for *carotid endarterectomy*. If adequate radiologic support is available, these patients should have arteriography as soon as possible as well as a careful cardiovascular evaluation (see Chapter 30). Because the risk of cardiovascular mortality and morbidity from noncardiac surgery is very high in this population, a careful cardiac assessment is an essential component of the determination of surgical candidacy. (Some physicians directly admit such patients to the hospital and immediately place them on intravenous heparin until arteriography can be performed—a practice that has been the subject of several small trials; see Annotated Bibliography).

The role for surgery has recently been clarified by the North American Symptomatic Carotid Endarterectomy Trial published in 1991. This trial involved over 600 *symptomatic patients* with *high-grade (70% to 99%) stenosis* of a carotid artery in the appropriate territory for their TIA. It was terminated early when it became clear that endarterectomy (when performed by a skilled surgical team) was significantly superior to medical management (aspirin) for patients with recent hemispheric or retinal TIA or nondisabling stroke and *ipsilateral* high-grade stenosis of the *internal carotid artery*.

Symptomatic patients with less severe carotid stenosis are being studied in continuations of controlled North American and European trials comparing medical management with endarterectomy. These patients have a cardiovascular mortality risk from noncardiac surgery equal to that of patients with critical carotid stenosis, but a lower stroke risk. The reader is urged to watch the literature for reports from both of these multicenter trials for guidance on the best approach to the management of these patients.

Candidates for Medical Therapy. Medical therapy may be elected for *elderly* TIA patients, those who *cannot tolerate surgery*, patients with a *single remote TIA*, and patients seen in settings where angiographic and surgical services are unavailable. Optimal medical management of TIA is *aspirin*. Several studies have evaluated the effectiveness of aspirin in different doses for patients with threatened stroke. The Canadian cooperative study group evaluated 585 patients with TIA and showed a 19-percent overall reduced incidence of TIA, stroke, and death in male patients only. The United Kingdom study result was similar, and the recent Dutch TIA trial reported 30 mg of aspirin per day no less effective than higher doses in preventing vascular events with fewer gastrointestinal side effects. Other antiplatelet agents such as *sulfinpyrazone* and *dipyridamole* have *not* been shown to act synergistically with aspirin.

Ticlopidine, a new antiplatelet agent, appears to be effective in *reducing risk* of recurrent TIA or stroke in both men and women and is currently indicated for aspirin-intolerant male patients, for female TIA patients, or males and females with completed stroke. However, ticlopidine increases serum *cholesterol* levels and rarely has caused *neutropenia*. The neutropenia appears between 3 weeks and 3 months after initiation of therapy, and it is therefore essential to monitor complete blood count at least every 2 weeks for the first 3 months of therapy.

TIA patients with normal carotid vessels should have a thorough cardiac evaluation to rule out an embolic source from the heart. In the absence of atrial fibrillation, valvular heart disease, or carotid disease, the proper preventive treatment for future stroke is not clear. It is common practice to place such patients on *aspirin* prophylactically (325 mg per day), and there is some evidence to recommend this practice. Although aspirin may reduce the morbidity form myocardial infarction, it is unclear if it reduces stroke from noncarotid sources. In the North American trial mentioned above, there was a high rate of stroke among aspirin-treated patients, raising the question as to whether low-dose warfarin therapy might not be a better alternative. Aspirin and warfarin have yet to be compared in a well-designed, randomized study.

TIA-like episodes believed due to *cardioembolic disease* are an indication for *warfarin* therapy. Several controlled multicenter studies have demonstrated that the incidence of thromboembolic complications due to *nonrheumatic atrial fibrillation* can be significantly reduced by oral anticoagulant therapy compared to use of aspirin or placebo. Although there are some data suggesting that aspirin might provide a modicum of protection, this requires further study. Warfarin anticoagulation is currently recommended, and low-intensity therapy (prothrombin time 1.2 to 1.4 × control) has proven as efficacious and safer than standard intensity therapy for patients with nonrheumatic atrial fibrillation (see Chapter 83).

Management of the Asymptomatic Carotid Bruit

The detection of a carotid bruit in an asymptomatic patient need not be considered an invariable harbinger of stroke, but it does suggest atherosclerotic carotid disease. Stroke risk increases significantly with severity of stenosis, onset of TIAs, and progression of the lesion. The patient should have a thorough noninvasive carotid evaluation (see above) to confirm the carotid origin of the bruit, the severity of stenosis, and its hemodynamic effects.

Regardless of severity of stenosis, emphasis should be placed on recognition and *prompt reporting of any TIA symptoms* and on modification of *cardiovascular risk factors* (hypertension, smoking, lipids; see Chapters 26, 27, and 54) because myocardial infarction remains a leading cause of death in such patients. Previously asymptomatic patients with high-grade *stenosis* (70% to 99% stenosis) who subsequently experience a *TIA* are at markedly enhanced risk of stroke and should be referred promptly for consideration of *surgical intervention* (see above).

Unresolved is what to do with the *truly asymptomatic* patient with a high-grade stenosis. Stroke risk is increased in such patients. As noted earlier, such tight stenoses are important sources of emboli and may cause a serious stroke without premonitory TIAs. Estimated risk of embolic stroke is in excess of 3 percent per year. A randomized controlled Veterans study of asymptomatic patients with at least a 50 percent stenosis found a reduction in rate of ipsilateral neurologic events, but no decrease in the combined incidence of stroke and death within the first 30 days of surgery. Further randomized controlled study of this issue is needed.

Pending definitive data on medical versus surgical therapy in the truly asymptomatic patient, some authorities recommend consideration of endarterectory in those who demonstrate rapid progression to hemodynamically and anatomically critical stenosis (eg, lumen < 1 mm). In support of this view is the high risk of stroke; against it is the high cardiac risk from surgery and the absence of proven benefit. If surgery is going to be recommended, one must have access to a skilled surgical team with a proven record of low perioperative morbidity and mortality and be sure that a careful preoperative cardiac risk assessment (see Chapter 30) is carried out. There is a high risk of perioperative myocardial infarction and death in these patients. Patients who are not surgical candidates can be treated with aspirin and vigorous attention to modification of atherosclerotic risk factors.

ANNOTATED BIBLIOGRAPHY

Albers GW, et al. Stroke prevention in nonvalvular atrial fibrillation: Review of prospective randomized trials. Ann Neurol 1991;30:511. *(A meta-analysis concluding that warfarin reduces the risk of stroke.)*

American-Canadian Cooperative Study Group. Persantine-aspirin trial in cerebral ischemia. Part II: Endpoint results. Stroke 1985;16:406. *(This is the major study confirming the indication for aspirin in stroke prevention; the addition of persantine did not improve the efficacy of aspirin.)*

Aschenberg W, Schluter M, Kremer P, et al. Transesophageal two-dimensional echocardiography for the detection of left atrial appendage thrombus. J Am Coll Cardiol 1986;7:163. *(Superior to traditional echocardiography for detection of this important source of embolic stroke.)*

Barnett HJM, Haines SJ. Carotid endarterectomy for asymptomatic carotid stenosis. N Engl J Med 1993;328:267. *(Editorial arguing that benefit from endarterectomy in asymptomatic patients remains unproven.)*

Call GK, Abbott WM, MacDonald NR, et al. Correlation of continuous-wave Doppler spectral flow analysis with gross pathology in carotid stenosis. Stroke 1988;19:584. *(Close correlation found, arguing for validity of noninvasive testing.)*

Chambers BR, Norris JW. Outcome in patients with asymptomatic neck bruits. N Engl J Med 1986;315:860. *(Important natural history study; risk of stroke is greatest in those with severe stenosis, but probably does not justify surgical intervention in asymptomatic patients.)*

Davis PH, Dambrosia JM, Schoenberg BS, et al. Risk factors for ischemic stroke: A prospective study in Rochester, Minnesota. Ann Neurol 1987;22:319. *(Hypertension, coronary heart disease, and male sex were major risk factors.)*

Dutch TIA Trial Study Group. Comparison of two doses of aspirin (30 mg versus 383 mg per day) in patients after a transient ischemic attack or minor ischemic stroke. N Engl J Med 1991;325:1261. *(Low-dose aspirin was as effective as higher doses in preventing stroke recurrence.)*

Eagle KA, Boucher CA. Cardiac risk in noncardiac surgery. N Engl J Med 1989;321:1330. *(Useful discussion of risk assessment; extremely pertinent in patients with carotid disease who are being considered for surgery.)*

Gilman S. Advances in neurology. N Engl J Med 1992;26: 1608,1671. *(Excellent two-part overview of recent developments in neuroimaging, epilepsy, stroke, Parkinson's disease, and migraine with an extensive reference list.)*

Hass WK, Easton JD, Adams HP Jr, et al. Randomized trial comparing ticlopidine with aspirin for the prevention of stroke in high-risk patients. N Engl J Med 1989;521:501. *(Double-blind, randomized trial of over 3000 patients with TIA or minor stroke showing a significant reduction [approximately 10 percent] in risk of stroke or death compared to aspirin.)*

Hobson RW, Weiss DG, Fields WS, et al. Efficacy of carotid endarterectomy for asymptomatic carotid stenosis. N Engl J Med 1993;328:221. *(Randomized, controlled study showing reduction in rate of ipsilateral neurologic events, but not in the combined incidence of stroke and death.)*

Kistler JP, Buonanno FS, Gress DR. Carotid endarterectomy—specific therapy based on pathophysiology. N Engl J Med 1991;325:505. *(Excellent summary of the indications for surgical therapy of carotid disease.)*

Ley-Pozo J, Ringelstein EB. Noninvasive detection of occlusive disease of the carotid siphon and middle cerebral artery. Ann Neurol 1990;28:640. *(Description of transcranial Doppler technology.)*

Marsh EE, et al. Use of anti-thrombotic drugs in the treatment of acute ischemic stroke: Survey of neurologists and practice in the United States. Neurology 1989;39:1631. *(Sobering survey indicating the less-than-perfect rationale and lack of uniformity for the use of heparin.)*

North American Symptomatic Carotid Endarterectomy Trial Collaborators. Beneficial effect of carotid endarterectomy in symptomatic patients with high-grade carotid stenosis. N Engl J Med 1991;325:445. *(Major, multicenter, randomized study documenting the superiority of surgical over medical management in this group of patients.)*

Sauve J-S, Laupacis A, Ostbye T, et al. Does this patient have a clinically important carotid bruit? JAMA 1993;270:2843. *(Helpful discussion of the clinical examination.)*

Singer DE. Randomized trials of warfarin for atrial fibrillation. N Engl J Med 1992;327:1451. *(Terse summary of the data in support of its efficacy in prevention of embolic stroke.)*

Wolf PA. Management of risk factors. Neurol Clin North Am 1992;10:177. *(The whole issue is devoted to the treatment and prevention of cerebral ischemia and has several good review articles. This article provides the reference to the Framingham study stroke risk profile tool, which may be used in the office.)*

Wolf PA, Kannel WB, Sorlie P, et al. Asymptomatic carotid bruit and risk of stroke: The Framingham Study. JAMA 1981; 245:1442. *(Landmark epidemiologic data.)*

Primary Care Medicine: Office Evaluation and Management of the Adult Patient, 3rd edition, edited by Allan H. Goroll, Lawrence A. May, and Albert G. Mulley, Jr. J.B. Lippincott Company, Philadelphia

172
Management of Multiple Sclerosis

Multiple sclerosis (MS) is the most common demyelinating disease of the central nervous system (CNS) in young adults and a potential source of considerable disability. Prevalence is about 0.1 percent among adults. The disease's manifestations are protean, and its clinical course is highly variable from patient to patient. Although most MS patients will be under the care of the neurologist during periods of marked exacerbation, they often depend on the primary physician for close monitoring, interpretation of symptoms, and decisions regarding need for referral. Consequently, the primary physician needs to be familiar with the range of clinical presentations for MS, its natural history, and available therapeutic options. This facilitates the provision of proper primary care and ensures optimal timing of referrals.

PATHOPHYSIOLOGY, CLINICAL PRESENTATION, AND COURSE

The etiology of multiple sclerosis remains unknown, but available research suggests the interplay of genetic susceptibility, environmental exposure(s), and defective regulation of the immune response. These factors result in a series of discrete episodes of myelin-specific autoimmune injury to the CNS, separated both in time and space. Acutely, an infiltrate of lymphocytes, macrophages, and plasma cells forms in areas of involvement. T cells are thought to initiate the process, and activated macrophages to damage the myelin. There is localized edema and transient breakdown of the blood–brain barrier. Chronicity of the inflammatory process results in formation of a plaque or gliotic scar, made up of proliferated astrocytes that cluster in response to inflammatory injury of the myelin sheath. Lesions occur predominantly in the white matter of the brain and spinal cord; occasionally, there is a minor degree of gray matter involvement.

Demyelination is characteristically focal, generally sparing axons. Plaques are most commonly found in the optic nerves, spinal cord, brainstem, cerebellum, and periventricular areas. After an attack, some remyelination occurs accounting for partial resolution of symptoms. However, partially demyelinated axons are susceptible to dysfunction, particularly under conditions of heat stress but also spontaneously. Even a hot shower may cause a temporary exacerbation.

Clinical presentation is a function of the site of the inflammatory process. Attacks are by definition those that produce symptoms that last more than 24 hours. They average up to one per year and decrease in frequency over time. Transient *sensory deficits* are the most common initial presentation, affecting about 40 percent to 50 percent of patients. They include *paresthesias* or diminution of sensation in the upper or lower extremities. The sensory disturbance may be bilateral and symmetric, extending to involve the adjacent trunk. About 15 percent to 20 percent experience *acute monocular visual loss* due to *optic neuritis*. A central scotomata, transient pain on eye movement, and decreased pupillary reaction to light (Marcus-Gunn pupil) are characteristic features. *Diplopia* due to *internuclear ophthalmoplegia* or an oculomotor defect is another common symptom heralding MS. Bilateral internuclear ophthalmoplegia is very characteristic of MS and strongly suggests the diagnosis. There is failure of adduction and coarse nystagmus in the abducting eye. Other oculomotor functions remain intact. *Ataxia* and *intention tremor* are manifestations of cerebellar involvement. *Motor deficits* may occur acutely or insidiously, with the insidious variety particularly common in older patients. Legs are more likely to be involved than the arms, and initially asymmetrically. However, bilateral upgoing toes are common, even in patients with unilateral complaints. *Urinary complaints* (frequency, urgency, incontinence) are consequences of upper motor nerve injury in the spinal cord. The external sphincter fails to relax adequately, causing incomplete emptying. Such autonomic injury may also produce *constipation* and *impotence*.

Later in the course of illness, *cerebral involvement* may produce memory loss, personality change, and emotional lability. Over 60 percent of MS patients demonstrate abnormalities on formal neuropsychiatric testing, even if asymptomatic. *Paroxysmal symptoms* may result from dysfunction of partially demyelinated axons and simulate a transient ischemic attack or focal seizure, or produce an attack of tic douloureux (see Chapter 176). *Fatigue* may be prominent and may even predate exacerbations.

Clinical Course and Prognosis. The clinical course tends to follow one of three basic patterns. Younger patients manifest a *relapsing and remitting* course, characterized by attacks followed by complete or near complete remission. In later years, many such patients often develop a *chronic/progressive* course, with steady gradual worsening; spinal involvement is common. About 20 percent of patients who present with MS in later life will also have this form of disease. A still more severe form is designated *relapsing/progressive* in which patients have chronic progressive disease exacerbated by acute attacks and little remission.

After 15 years of clinical disease, about 50 percent of patients are still capable of walking and 30 percent are able to continue working. Frequent attacks early in the course of the disease increase the chances of disability, as does late onset, progressive course, or early cerebellar or pyramidal involvement.

DIAGNOSIS

The diagnosis is suggested clinically by the development of CNS symptoms and signs suggesting CNS disease separated both anatomically and in time (> 1 month). At times, symptoms suggest only a single lesion, but a careful physical examination reveals evidence of multiple lesions (bilateral upgoing toes, subtle internuclear ophthalmoplegia, mild afferent pupillary defect).

Laboratory findings help support the diagnosis, although no single test is diagnostic and clinical evidence for at least two separate neurologic lesions is still required. The most sensitive test is the *magnetic resonance imaging (MRI)* scan. Multiple periventricular plaques—presenting as areas of increased signal intensity on T2 and proton density weighted images—are characteristic and found in over 90 percent of patients with known MS. Patients with chronic progressive disease have more confluent periventricular and infratentorial lesions. However, the plaques seen on MRI are nonspecific and also occur in normal elderly patients, those with chronic uncontrolled hypertension, advanced Lyme disease, and CNS vasculitis. The *cerebrospinal fluid* examination is abnormal in 95 percent of MS patients. Nonspecific, modest increases in cell count and protein are common, but increases in *IgG* and *oligoclonal IgG bands* on electrophoresis are more specific and suggest increased risk of disseminated disease. Visual or auditory *evoked potentials* are abnormal in demyelinated tracts and may serve as additional evidence of MS when MRI results need supporting data.

PRINCIPLES OF MANAGEMENT

There is no cure for MS, but much can be done to reduce symptoms due to an acute exacerbation. More difficult is to improve the long-term course of illness. Efforts to treat MS have focused on suppressing the immunologically induced inflammatory response that characterizes the condition.

Treatment of an Acute Attack. High-dose parenteral corticosteroids appear capable of shortening an acute attack. The best available data come from The Optic Neuritis Treatment Trial, a randomized controlled study of patients presenting with isolated neuritis, comparing 3 days of high-dose *intravenous methylprednisolone* followed by several weeks of oral prednisone with oral prednisone alone or placebo. Patients with high-dose intravenous therapy demonstrated the best restoration of vision but at 12 months, showed no difference in vision from those receiving placebo. However, at 3 years, they showed a 66 percent reduction in relative risk of developing definite MS. The potential significance of this finding is great, but requires confirmation. Patients treated with oral prednisone alone did worse at 6 months than those given placebo. The worsening on oral prednisone alone is hard to account for, but such a program should not be used until more data are forthcoming. For now, a course of high-dose intravenous therapy is preferred. Whether it should be followed by a more prolonged course of oral prednisone remains unclear, because the study did not examine such a program. Additional data are needed and should be forthcoming.

Treatment of Progressive Disease. More problematic is treatment of progressive disease. Patients with rapidly progressive disease given a course of intravenous *cyclophosphamide* in conjunction with *ACTH* demonstrate stabilization over 1 year. However, remissions are often short-lived and such nonspecific immunosuppressive treatment is fraught with significant morbidity. More precise interventions using *beta interferon* (an immunomodulator) and *copolymer-1* (a stimulant of myelination) are also under study. Beta interferon has been shown capable of reducing the frequency of flares and altering the course of illness in exacerbating-remitting disease.

Treatment of Complications. *Paroxysmal symptoms* respond to *carbamazepine* (200 mg bid). Tricyclic antidepressants may help control *emotional lability*. Low doses of *amitriptyline* (25 to 75 mg per day) often suffice. Higher tricyclic doses are indicated for overt *depression* (see Chapter 227). *Spasticity* lessens with use of *baclofen* in low doses (starting at 5 to 10 mg tid). Confusion, sedation, and increased muscle weakness are its limiting side effects. Diazepam and dantrolene are alternatives. When *incontinence* is problematic, an anticholinergic (eg, proprantheline 15 mg qid PRN) will help if the cause is bladder spasm (frequency, urge incontinence); a cholinergic agent is best if there is bladder atony (see Chapter 134). Amantadine (200 mg bid) has proved useful for fatigue.

PATIENT EDUCATION

One of the most difficult aspects of MS is the uncertainty that accompanies the disease. If the diagnosis is in question, every effort should be made to confirm it or rule it out. MS patients fear becoming disabled. Providing them with as much information as possible helps them to maintain a sense of control. Even advice on handling the affairs of everyday life is greatly appreciated, such as avoiding a very hot shower that may transiently exacerbate symptoms. Although it is hard to predict future clinical course, reasonable estimates can be made on the basis of the clinical course to date.

Patients need to know that progression to disabling disease is not inevitable, that there is great variability in prognosis, and that, for many, the disease never becomes incapacitating. Patient morale appears to be an important determinant of outcome. In randomized studies, the high frequency of remission and outright clinical improvement noted among patients randomized to placebo underscores this point. It should not be surprising that a disease of immune dysfunction such as MS might be influenced by the patient's state of mind, given the well-documented finding that psychological state can affect T-cell function. Maintaining a hopeful perspective may have a remarkably positive effect and should not be overlooked. The value of establishing a close, supportive relationship cannot be overemphasized.

INDICATIONS FOR REFERRAL AND ADMISSION

When a diagnosis of MS is suspected on clinical grounds, neurologic consultation can be helpful in determining the need for further diagnostic studies (MRI scanning, lumbar puncture with immunoelectrophoresis, evoked potentials) and in selecting a treatment modality. In addition, patients experiencing an acute exacerbation of functional significance should be referred to the neurologist promptly for consideration of a course of high-dose intravenous glucocorticosteroid therapy of beta interferon treatments. Advances in home intravenous care may obviate the need for hospitalization, but neurologic consultation is still needed. Referral to an occupational therapist can greatly facilitate maintenance of daily functioning in patients with significant motor or sensory deficits.

A.H.G.

ANNOTATED BIBLIOGRAPHY

Beatty WW. Cognitive and emotional disturbances in multiple sclerosis. Neurol Clin North Am 1993;11:189. *(Mild-moderate cognitive impairment is common.)*

Beck RW, Cleary PA, Trobe JD, et al. The effect of corticosteroids for acute optic neuritis on the subsequent development of multiple sclerosis. N Engl J Med 1993;329:1764. *(Treatment found to inhibit the development of clinical MS.)*

Beck RW, Cleary PA, Anderson MM Jr, et al. A randomized, controlled trial of corticosteroids in the treatment of acute optic neuritis. N Engl J Med 1992;326:581. *(Best available evidence for efficacy of high-dose steroids.)*

Blaivas JG. Management of bladder dysfunction in multiple sclerosis. Neurology 1980;30:12. *(Use of anticholinergics for bladder spasm.)*

Bronstein MB, et al. A placebo-controlled, double-blind, randomized trial of Cop-1 in chronic progressive multiple sclerosis. Neurology 1991;41:533. *(High rates of stabilization and improvement among patients receiving Copolymer 1, but also among those receiving placebo; points out magnitude of placebo effect in these patients.)*

Ebers GC, Bulman DE, Sadovnick AD, et al. A population-based study of multiple sclerosis in twins. N Engl J Med 1986; 315:1638. *(Major degree of genetic susceptibility discovered.)*

Hauser SL, Dawson DM, Lehrich JR, et al. Intensive immunosuppression in progressive multiple sclerosis. N Engl J Med 1983;308:173. *(Randomized study showing cyclophosphamide plus ACTH best in stabilizing patients with progressive disease over 1 year.)*

IFNB Multiple Sclerosis Study Group. Interferon beta-7b is effective in relapsing-remitting multiple sclerosis. Neurology 1993;43:665. *(First report that the natural history of multiple sclerosis can be altered.)*

Lessell S. Corticosteroid treatment of acute optic neuritis. N Engl J Med 1992;326:634. *(Editorial recommending high-dose intravenous therapy for acute attacks.)*

Miller DH, Ormerod IE, Rudge P, et al. The early risk of multiple sclerosis following isolated acute syndromes of the brainstem and spinal cord. Ann Neurol 1989;26:635. *(Progression occurred in about 50 percent after 15 months and in 69 percent with an abnormal MRI at time of presentation.)*

Multiple Sclerosis Study Group. Efficacy and toxicity of cyclosporine in chronic progressive multiple sclerosis: A randomized, double-blind, placebo-controlled clinical trial. Ann Neurol 1990;27:591. *(Small, but significant improvement in slowing progression; high incidence of adverse effects and large drop-out rate; demonstrates the difficulties in studying immunosuppressive therapy.)*

Paty DW, Oger JJF, Kastrukoff MD, et al. Magnetic resonance imaging (MRI) in the diagnosis of multiple sclerosis: A prospective study with comparison of clinical evaluation, evoked potentials, oligoclonal banding and computerized tomography. Neurology 1988;38:180. *(Sensitivity found to be in excess of 90 percent.)*

Primary Care Medicine: Office Evaluation and Management of the Adult Patient, 3rd edition, edited by Allan H. Goroll, Lawrence A. May, and Albert G. Mulley, Jr. J.B. Lippincott Company, Philadelphia

173
Management of Alzheimer's Disease

MICHAEL A. JENIKE, M.D.

It is estimated that between 2 and 4 million Americans currently suffer from Alzheimer's disease, a neurodegenerative condition of unknown etiology (see Chapter 169). As more individuals survive into old age, the prevalence of this disorder will increase. About 5 to 7 percent of those over age 65 and as many as 20 percent of those over age 80 will develop Alzheimer's disease. Almost half of all nursing home patients have progressive dementing illnesses. The primary care physician who is going to manage such patients must be familiar with the course of the illness, the treatment of its psychiatric concomitants (psychosis, anxiety, depression, behavioral disturbances), the types of social services available, and approaches to family counseling.

CLINICAL PRESENTATION AND COURSE

During the earliest stages, most patients seem *mildly forgetful* and complain of such memory deficits as forgetting names or where they placed household items. The patient may seem concerned but has no social or employment problems and shows no evidence of memory deficit during a clinical interview.

The next stage of mild cognitive decline is characterized by decreased performance in demanding work or social situations. Patients complain of *poor concentration* and difficulty finding words and names, and may report that coworkers have noticed their relatively poor performance. Some patients present initially with *visuospatial deficits,* whereas others may have difficulty with *speech* early in the course of the illness. Later, patients may get lost when traveling to an unfamiliar location. Anxiety and depression are common, and many patients begin to deny symptoms.

As the illness progresses, patients become unable to travel alone and are unable to handle their personal finances. *Memory* for *recent events* will be drastically impaired, and patients display decreased knowledge of current events. Complex tasks are impossible, but patients remain well oriented to time and person and can travel to very familiar places, like the corner drugstore. Many patients are aware of their deficits and are capable of understanding what is happening to them. Patients instinctively withdraw from previously challenging situations. *Denial* may become pronounced.

During the next phase, patients can no longer survive without some assistance. They are unable to recall major relevant aspects of their current lives or even the names of close friends and family members. *Delusions* are common. For example, the spouse is accused of being an impostor or the patient talks to imaginary persons or to his or her own reflection in the mirror. *Depression, agitation,* and violent behavior may occur. Frequently patients are disoriented to time or place. However, they generally remain able to eat and use the toilet without assistance, but may have difficulty properly choosing and putting on clothing.

In the last stages of the disease, patients become totally *incapacitated* and *disoriented*. They eventually forget their own name and may not recognize their spouse. *Incontinence* is common. *Personality* and *emotional changes* become very pronounced, although these occasionally occur even in the earliest stages. Eventually all verbal abilities are lost, motor skills deteriorate, and patients require total care. Generalized cortical and focal neurologic signs and symptoms are frequently present. Death usually occurs from total debilitation or infection.

The course of Alzheimer's disease varies from 2 to as long as 20 years from onset to death. The average is around 6 to 8 years. Typically, the illness progresses at a fairly constant rate. If it has rapidly developed over the past year, it is likely to continue at that rate. A slowly progressive illness over the past 5 to 10 years suggests that the patient may survive for a number of years.

PRINCIPLES OF MANAGEMENT

Once treatable causes for dementia have been ruled out (see Chapter 169), the physician faces the challenge of caring for the Alzheimer's patient, a person with a chronic, progressively disabling illness. Management involves the skillful interplay of medication to improve cognitive function, psychopharmacologic therapy, and supportive care by family members (who often choose to maintain the patient at home) and community agencies.

Drugs for Memory Enhancement. To date, there is no treatment that has proven capable of markedly slowing or significantly improving the cognitive defects of Alzheimer's disease. Drugs that enhance cholinergic transmission have been the subject of intense study, because cholinergic neuronal degeneration and depletion of acetylcholine-synthesizing enzyme (choline-acetyl transferase) have been noted in Alzheimer's disease. Acetylcholinesterase inhibitors and cholinergic receptor agonists are being studied. One centrally active *cholinesterase inhibitor, tacrine,* has demonstrated a modest, but statistically significant reduction in rate of cognitive decline. However, the improvement was not clinically meaningful (no difference in scores of global functioning), and tacrine cannot yet be recommended as an important advance in treatment. Dietary supplements of choline precursors, such as lecithin, have not proven beneficial.

Drugs found unhelpful include cerebral vasodilators (dihydroergotoxine), central nervous system (CNS) stimulants (amphetamines), opiate antagonists (naloxone), and neuropeptides (vasopressin). *Hydergine,* a mixture of ergoloid mesylates, had been the only drug approved for treatment of Alzheimer's disease by the Federal Drug Administration. It was believed to act as a cerebral vasodilator, but it probably has some metabolic enhancer activity. Recent double-blind, controlled study failed to find it beneficial.

Other approaches under active investigation include *restorative therapy* with nerve growth factor, *protective therapy* with antioxidants, and *preventive therapy* with drugs that inhibit beta amyloid formation.

Management of Confusion and Agitation. The chronic use of sedatives and psychoactive agents in the confused patient should be avoided unless persistent extreme agitation hampers care. If such therapy is contemplated, the lowest possible doses should be used and for the shortest time possible. Patients may respond to a small dose of *thioridazine* (10 to 25 mg qhs). *Haloperidol* is often a first choice in the setting of delusions and hallucinations. Doses in the range of 0.5 to 1 mg two or three times a day usually suffice, but one must be careful to avoid long-term use because of the risk of inducing tardive dyskinesia. Also problematic is regular use of sedative/hypnotic agents for sleep (see Chapter 226). Beta-blocking agents and anticholinergics may exacerbate confusion. Patients with depression may improve with a tricyclic compound with low anticholinergic side effects such as *desipramine* (25 to 50 mg qhs), but drugs with marked anticholinergic activity may worsen memory. A recent study of nursing home patients demonstrated substantial improvement in many patients when chronically prescribed psychotropic drugs were discontinued or reduced in dose.

The safe and effective use of psychotropic medication in Alzheimer's patients necessitates adjustments in drug selection, dose, and frequency to accommodate the alterations in drug uptake and metabolism that occur in the elderly. Such adjustments are particularly important when using neuroleptics and sedative–hypnotics (see Appendix).

Management of Behavioral Disorders. Certain behaviors are particularly troublesome to family members. Among those cited most frequently are catastrophic reactions (including violent behavior), wakefulness, suspiciousness, and incontinence.

Catastrophic reactions are massive emotional overresponses typically precipitated by task failure or minor stress. Hitting and violent resistance to care are extreme forms of such reactions. Most excessive emotional responses can be minimized by teaching the family to avoid or remove the precipitating task or stress, to remain quiet and calm, and to gently change the focus of attention. Neuroleptic drugs (eg, *haloperidol,* 0.5 mg qd or bid) are sometimes helpful in difficult cases, but only as an adjunct to behavioral techniques.

Wakefulness and *night walking* often deprive the caregiver of much-needed rest. Helpful environmental interventions include placing locks on each door so that the patient will not wander out of the house at night, keeping the patient physically active during the day, and not allowing a nap.

Sedative-hypnotics, such as a short-acting benzodiazepine (eg, *lorazepam,* 1.0 mg qhs) or chloral hydrate, may be helpful (see Chapter 228). Occasionally, low doses of a neuroleptic may be needed (see Appendix).

Suspiciousness and accusatory behaviors are believed to result from the brain-injured person's efforts to explain misplaced possessions or misinterpreted events. If the family understands this, their frustration, hurt, and anger may be reduced. Simple interventions, such as keeping an orderly house or making a sign pointing to where an object is kept, may help (see below). Neuroleptics may be used as a last resort.

Incontinence is typically a late manifestation of Alzheimer's disease, but when present early, it warrants a careful search for other causes, such as urinary tract infection (see Chapter 133) and other causes of dementia such as normal pressure hydrocephalus (see Chapter 169).

Alzheimer's patients may decompensate cognitively and behaviorally when they experience a *superimposed illness.* Coexistent medical problems, such as asthma, diabetes, and congestive heart failure, should be carefully controlled. Even a minor upper respiratory tract or urinary tract infection can worsen behavior. Patients are susceptible to *medication-induced delirium;* close supervision of drug regimens is imperative.

Family members can be assured that *inappropriate sexual behavior* is very uncommon. In the rare instances where it occurs, self-stimulation is the usual form; Alzheimer's patients are not child molesters.

The Home Environment. As mentioned earlier, families need to be encouraged to maintain a *structured,* predictable environment for the patient. Any change can be devastating and stressful to a demented patient and may produce a massive emotional overresponse. A schedule in which activities such as arising, eating, taking medication, and exercise occur at the same time each day maximizes the patient's familiarity with the personal environment. At times, use of an *orientation center* in the home with pertinent information such as the date, time, schedule of household events, and pictures of relevant people is very helpful.

Of particular importance to survival and quality of life is the need to reduce the risk of *falls* in the home. It has been clearly demonstrated that falls are one of the major predictors of reduced survival. Installing hand rails, encouraging use of a walker, and eliminating throw rugs and other obstacles can be extremely important to maximizing survival and minimizing disability.

Frequently patients will want to *drive* when it is clear that they are no longer safe on the roads. If possible, it is best to avoid direct confrontation. Simple techniques such as hiding the keys, disconnecting distributor wires, or giving the patient a nonfunctional set of keys have usually been successful in discouraging patients from driving.

Any firearms should be removed from the home for obvious reasons. In addition, smoking and cooking become potentially dangerous activities. Environmental modifications, such as removing stove knobs, having a stove cut-off switch placed in an inconspicuous place, locking rooms or closets, or locking up matches, are important for safety.

Management of the Family. Some family members may well react with dread and depression to the fact that their relative has Alzheimer's disease. Those members who have a preexisting psychiatric illness may decompensate. Others will have suspected the diagnosis and are relieved to have an understanding physician who will be available and helpful over the course of the illness. Family members who are initially stunned and ask few questions should not have information forced on them. Careful explanation about any further evaluative tests should be given and a follow-up appointment should be arranged within a week. Common questions include: How long will the patient live? How rapidly will he or she deteriorate? What are the chances of other family members developing the disease—is it hereditary? Is there a treatment?

Within the first few weeks of making the diagnosis, family members should see a *social worker* who is aware of community resources such as visiting nurse services, meals-on-wheels, financial aid, and nursing homes. For the very early Alzheimer's patient, this may seem premature, but family members will be reassured by the knowledge that help will be available when needed in the future. Most families read about the illness and become acutely aware of the devastating course of the illness.

Guilt, unrealistic expectations, and assumption of excessive responsibility are common responses of families. In discussing these and similar issues, the physician should focus both on physical realities and on the family's emotional responses to the patient. One frequently encountered source of difficulty is the reversal of parent–child roles that the care of an elderly person often represents. There is no one way to handle this issue; however, in the overwhelming majority of such cases, just allowing family members to discuss these and other issues will be therapeutic.

Family members report that *lack of time for themselves* and sleep disturbances in patients are the least tolerable aspects of home care. Families do best when relatives and friends visit frequently and when provisions are made for the primary caregiver to have breaks in his or her responsibilities. Visiting nurses or day-care centers can be invaluable. Family support is the major variable in keeping the cognitively impaired elderly at home.

Even with a compassionate and empathic physician, many families feel alone with this illness and are unable to find friends who understand. Embarrassment may make them withdraw from previous social contacts. To meet the need for communication and information, families in many areas have established *volunteer organizations* that are involved in helping each other, sharing solutions to management problems, exchanging information, supporting needed legislation and research, and educating the community. These organizations welcome members who are concerned about all of the dementing illnesses, of which Alzheimer's disease is the most common. The number of such support groups is growing rapidly, and families consistently report how helpful they are. Local volunteer organizations have established a national organization, the *Alzheimer's Disease and Related Disorders Association* (ADRDA), whose goals are family support, education, advocacy, and encouraging research. The address of ADRDA is 70 E. Lake Street, Chicago, IL 60601. The national organization will give family members the addresses of local groups.

Each family member should be encouraged to read one of the available lay books on Alzheimer's disease. *The 36-Hour Day* is required reading for anyone (including the physician) who is dealing with an individual with a progressive dementing illness.

The Issue of Nursing Home Placement. It is always a difficult moment when the family considers nursing home placement. Placement represents an irrevocable loss of autonomy for the patient. The decision must be approached with careful deliberation and respect for the patient. Although the family's needs are important to consider, the physician has a special obligation to the patient. If the patient has drawn up an advance directive before becoming mentally incapacitated (see Appendix, Chapter 1), these wishes can be respected and responded to. Absent such a directive, the physician needs to act as he or she thinks the patient might have wanted. If there is a designated surrogate, this person can help in the decision making. The goal, first and foremost, is to help the patient.

Before any action is taken regarding nursing home placement, it is worth carefully reexamining the home situation to be sure all alternatives to placement have been explored. Have the use of home health aides, senior day care, and similar supports been used to relieve the family's burden?

Only after all home care resources have been exhausted or found to be insufficient is it proper to proceed with placement. An appropriate site is one that can provide emotional support, reassurance, and security. One seeks a nursing home that preserves a sense of connectedness and closeness to others. The primary physician plays a critical role in ensuring that the placement is done well and serves the best interests of the patient.

THERAPEUTIC RECOMMENDATIONS

- Once a patient has been diagnosed as having a progressive dementing illness, the primary care physician will become the main coordinator of the patient's care and advisor to the family. The physician should consciously decide whether to take on this responsibility or to refer the patient and family for care by a group specializing in the management of such patients.
- Family members should be apprised of the patient's diagnosis, and an open discussion should be part of the initial management.
- Early in the course of the illness, a social worker should meet with the family to help plan for care and provide emotional support.
- A predictable, well-structured home environment should be established, especially one that limits the risk of falls.
- All unnecessary medications, especially those that may cause cognitive impairment, should be stopped or reduced in dosage.
- When patients develop a concomitant psychiatric problem, such as depression, anxiety, behavioral disorder, or psychosis, psychopharmacologic intervention should be considered.
- For depression, begin with a low dose of a well-tolerated tricyclic agent (eg, 25 mg of desipramine qhs; see Chapter 227); for anxiety or sleep consider a low dose of a short-acting benzodiazepine (eg, 1.0 mg of lorazepam; see Chapter 226); for psychotic behavior or catastrophic reactions, a low dose of a neuroleptic may prove useful (eg, 0.5 mg haloperidol, qhs or bid; see Appendix). Drug treatment should be brief (except in depression) and with the smallest dose possible.
- Although a number of drugs are available to treat cognitive impairment, none is consistently effective and results are modest at best. *Tacrine,* a centrally active cholinesterase inhibitor, is the first drug to demonstrate in rigorous study some improvement in cognitive function, although results are modest at best. *Hydergine,* although widely used, cannot be highly recommended because results are minimal in carefully controlled studies.
- There is no evidence that vitamins or dietary supplements (eg, lecithin) have any effect, or that avoidance of aluminum-containing preparations (eg, antacids) is of any benefit.
- Family members should be advised to join the local chapter of ADRDA and to become knowledgeable about the disease and its course by reading one of the currently available books. (*The 36-Hour Day* is an excellent resource.)
- The need for nursing home placement should be approached carefully and only after maximizing home care resources. Emphasis is on providing for the emotional and physical needs of the patient, although family preferences also deserve consideration.

ANNOTATED BIBLIOGRAPHY

Albert M. Assessment of cognitive functioning in the elderly. Psychosomatics 1984;25:310. *(Discusses the cognitive changes associated with both normal aging and dementing illness.)*

American College of Physicians. Cognitively impaired subjects. Ann Intern Med 1989;111:843. *(Position paper on ethical issues regarding care.)*

Cooper JK. Drug treatment of Alzheimer's disease. Arch Intern Med 1991;151:245. *(Useful review of drugs to improve cognition and treat abnormal behavior; 78 references.)*

Davis KL, Thal LJ, Gamzu ER, et al. A double-blind, placebo-controlled multicenter study of tacrine for Alzheimer's disease. N Engl J Med 1992;327:1253. *(Short-term study of patients who showed some response to tacrine in a preliminary phase found statistically significant improvement in cognition, but not in global functioning or activities of daily living.)*

Drachman DA. Who may drive? Who may not? Who shall decide? Ann Neurol 1988;24:787. *(Analysis of the tricky regulation process and the physician's obligation to patients and to others.)*

Green JE. Clinical aspects of Alzheimer's disease. Current Opinion in Neurology/Neurosurgery 1988;1:479. *(Very good description of the common and not-so-common clinical features of the most common dementing illness.)*

Growdon JH. Treatment for Alzheimer's disease. N Engl J Med 1992;327:1306. *(Excellent summary of current approaches to therapy.)*

Larson EB, Kukull WA, Vuchner D, et al. Adverse drug reactions associated with global cognitive impairment in elderly persons. Ann Intern Med 1987;107:169. *(Adverse drug reactions were an important source of cognitive impairment, especially when more than four drugs were being taken.)*

Lipowski ZJ. Delirium in the elderly patient. N Engl J Med 1989;320:578. *(Short, very useful review; 32 references.)*

Mace NL, Rabins PV. The 36-Hour Day: A Family Guide to Caring for Persons with Alzheimer's Disease, Dementing Illness, and Memory Loss in Later Life. Baltimore, The Johns Hopkins University Press, 1991. *(Required reading for all who care for patients with dementing illnesses. Excellent for family members.)*

Meier DE, Cassel CK. Nursing home placement and the demented patient. Ann Intern Med 1986;104:98. *(A most helpful discussion of this difficult phase of care.)*

Rabins PV, Mace NL, Lucas MJ. The impact of dementia on the family. JAMA 1982;248:333. *(Interview reports from primary caregivers of 55 patients suffering from irreversible dementia. Excellent perspective on the social impact and likely problems to be encountered with dementia.)*

Thompson TL, Filley CM, Mitchell WD, et al. Lack of efficacy of hydergine in patients with Alzheimer's disease. N Engl J Med 1990;323:445. *(This drug had been widely prescribed, but never properly studied; no benefit found in this rigorously designed, controlled study.)*

Walsh JS, Welch HG, Larson EB. Survival of outpatients with Alzheimer-type dementia. Ann Intern Med 1990;113:429. *(Length of survival is more a function of severity of disease than duration; wandering, falling, and behavioral problems correlate with shortened survival.)*

Appendix: Use of Psychotropic Drugs in the Elderly

Pharmacokinetic Changes Associated with Aging. With aging, clinically important changes in drug absorption, distribution, protein binding, hepatic metabolism, and renal excretion ensue. Gastric pH increases and splanchnic blood flow decreases, altering drug solubility and absorption. Total body fat rises from 10 percent of body weight at age 20 to 24 percent at age 60, increasing the volume of distribution for lipid-soluble drugs, such as diazepam and its metabolites, and greatly prolonging drug half-life. In addition, total body water may decrease from 25 percent to 18 percent in the same period, causing water-soluble drugs, such as ethanol, to have higher concentrations due to decreased reservoir size. Serum albumin levels decline by 10 percent to 15 percent, decreasing protein-binding sites and liberating more free active drug into the circulation, thus raising the risk of toxicity. Drug metabolism slows; the activity of hepatic cytochrome P-450 decreases, as does demethylation. The result is higher levels of unmetabolized drug.

After age 40, there is a progressive decline in glomerular filtration rate and renal plasma flow. By age 70, the reduction is about 50 percent, prolonging drug action and increasing the likelihood of toxicity if dosage is not adjusted downward.

In addition to these pharmacokinetic changes, decreased CNS dopamine and acetylcholine levels, respectively, can lead to increased sensitivity to extrapyramidal and anticholinergic side effects. An increased tendency to CNS disinhibition in the elderly increases the likelihood of drug-associated confusion, sedation, and paradoxical reactions.

Neuroleptics. Violence, rage, and psychosis are common problems in patients with Alzheimer's disease. The drugs most commonly used to treat these problems are the neuroleptics. All of the neuroleptics are equally effective in treating the above symptoms. Choice of a particular drug is based on its side effects and toxicity. The main side effects of the neuroleptics are sedation, orthostatic hypotension, extrapyramidal symptoms, and anticholinergic symptoms. There is a fairly consistent relationship between potency of the neuroleptic and side effects: as the milligram potency of a neuroleptic increases, the frequency and severity of sedation, orthostatic hypotension, and anticholinergic symptoms decrease and extrapyramidal symptoms increase (Table 173–1).

Side effects can be used therapeutically. The patient who has trouble falling asleep will find sedating neuroleptics to be of more use than nonsedating agents. Sedating neuroleptics may also be used to calm an agitated patient during the day. More commonly, however, sedation is an unwanted side effect. Daytime sedation may cause or aggravate nighttime insomnia, and sedation may also increase confusion and disorientation in the demented patient. As disorientation and confusion increase, the patient typically becomes more agitated.

One of the most severe dangers when using neuroleptics is the possibility of inducing *orthostatic hypotension,* which can lead to falls and fractures, stroke, or even heart attack. Hypotensive episodes are especially apt to occur at night when the elderly patient awakens and gets up to urinate.

High-potency neuroleptics, such as *haloperidol, thiothixene,* and *fluphenazine,* are generally safe to use in the elderly, but should be started at very low doses, such as 0.5 mg of haloperidol once or twice daily. Although generally safe, these drugs are more likely than low-potency agents (such as chlorpromazine or thioridazine) to produce extrapyramidal symptoms in the elderly. As many as 50 percent of all patients between ages 60 and 80 who receive neuroleptics develop extrapyramidal symptoms, and those with brain damage, dementia, or Parkinson's disease are much more

Table 173-1. Neuroleptics

NAME (TRADE NAME)	APPROXIMATELY EQUIVALENT DAILY DOSE (MG)
High-Potency Agent	
Haloperidol (Haldol)	2
Thiothixene (Navane)	5
Trifluoperazine (Stelazine)	5
Fluphenazine (Prolixin)	2
Medium-Potency Agents	
Perphenazine (Trilafon)	10
Loxapane (Loxitane)	15
Molindone (Moban)	10
Low-Potency Agents	
Chlorpromazine (Thorazine)	100
Thioridazine (Mellaril)	100

Table 173-2. Extrapyramidal Reactions to Major Tranquilizers

REACTION	TIME INTERVAL AFTER DRUG	CHARACTERISTICS	TREATMENT
Acute dystonia	1–5 days	Spasm of muscles of neck, tongue, face, back; occasionally trismus (lockjaw)	Benzotropine 1–2 mg/day IM or Diphenhydramine 25–50 mg/day IM
Akathisia	5–60 days	Motor restlessness, jitteriness, constant pacing	Propranolol 30–80 mg/day PO or Benztropine 1–8 mg/day PO or Trihexyphenidyl 2–10 mg/day PO or Amantadine 100–200 mg/day PO
Parkinsonism	5–30 days	Bradykinesia, cogwheel rigidity, tremor	Benztropine 1–8 mg/day PO or Trihexyphenidyl 2–10 mg/day PO or Amantadine 100–200 mg/day PO
Tardive dyskinesia	Late	Involuntary, repetitive movement of face and tongue	Often irreversible; no drugs consistently effective

sensitive to these effects. The most troubling extrapyramidal symptoms are akathisia, parkinsonism, and akinesia (Table 173–2).

Akathisia is a feeling of motor restlessness associated with a subjective sensation of discomfort, often described as anxiety. Sleep is usually disturbed because the individual is unable to find a comfortable, motionless position. Sometimes this restlessness is misinterpreted as an increase in psychotic symptoms and is treated with an increase in neuroleptic dosage. A most effective treatment for akathisia is lowering the dose. Other treatments include anticholinergic agents, benzodiazepines, amantadine, and propranolol.

Neuroleptic-induced *parkinsonism* appears identical to the postencephalitic or idiopathic forms. An occasional patient will be exquisitely sensitive to this side effect and as little as one dose of a high-potency agent may precipitate the syndrome. Parkinsonism can usually be treated effectively with small doses of anticholinergic agents or with the addition of amantadine in dosages of 100 to 200 mg per day (see Chapter 174).

One of the unfortunately common and severe side effects of any neuroleptic agent is the development of *tardive dyskinesia,* manifested by a wide variety of movements, including lip smacking, sucking, jaw movements, writhing tongue movements, chorea, athetosis, dystonia, tics, and facial grimacing. In severe cases, speech, eating, walking, and even breathing can be seriously impaired. Onset is gradual, usually after long-term, high-dose administration, but on rare occasions it can occur with short-term or low-dose use. Advancing age correlates not only with increased prevalence, but also with severity. Once tardive dyskinesia has developed, it is much less likely to reverse in an elderly patient than it is in a younger one.

The best way to *prevent* tardive dyskinesia is to avoid the use of neuroleptics. Obviously, these drugs are sometimes required, but they should not be used when indications are unclear or when less potentially toxic drugs may be as efficacious. Neuroleptics should never be used for simple anxiety, uncomplicated depression, or for long periods in patients who were suffering from an *acute* psychotic episode. It is important to make a baseline examination before starting neuroleptics and to note any early signs of tardive dyskinesia, such as fine vermicular movements or restlessness of the tongue, mild choreiform finger or toe movements, and facial tics or frequent eye blinks. The patient should be monitored for the development of early tardive dyskinesia at least every 3 months. Currently, there are no consistently effective agents that are useful in the treatment of tardive dyskinesia. In view of the significant risk to the elderly patient and the ineffective treatment options, physicians should avoid the use of neuroleptic drugs in elderly patients whenever possible.

Antidepressants. See Chapter 227.

Anxiolytics. See Chapter 226.

Hypnotics. See Chapter 232.

ANNOTATED BIBLIOGRAPHY

Jenike MA. Geriatric Psychiatry and Psychopharmacology: A Clinical Approach. Chicago, IL: Year Book Medical Publishers, 1989. *(comprehensive monograph.)*

Jenike MA. Tardive dyskinesia: Special risk in the elderly. J Am Geriatr Soc 1983;31:71. *(Detailed discussion of this important complication.)*

Primary Care Medicine: Office Evaluation and Management of the Adult Patient, 3rd edition, edited by Allan H. Goroll, Lawrence A. May, and Albert G. Mulley, Jr. J.B. Lippincott Company, Philadelphia

174
Approach to the Patient With Parkinson's Disease

AMY A. PRUITT, M.D.

Of the movement disorders, the most common is Parkinson's disease, an adult-onset, neurodegenerative disease characterized by tremor at rest, rigidity, and bradykinesia. The refinement of drug therapy for Parkinson's disease has brought relief to thousands of patients suffering from this immobilizing condition. The recent development of therapy that may slow disease progression makes early diagnosis and treatment of Parkinson's disease particularly critical. Proper treatment requires careful timing and skillful utilization of drugs, because there are important difficulties associated with pharmacologic therapy. Moreover, drug efficacy declines over time and therapeutic response may be blunted by improper timing or inappropriate selection of antiparkinsonian agents.

Although the "fine tuning" of Parkinson's disease is largely in the province of the neurologist, the primary care physician is in the best position to make the diagnosis, institute therapy, and monitor the often substantial side effects associated with antiparkinsonian agents.

PATHOPHYSIOLOGY, CLINICAL PRESENTATION, AND COURSE

Pathophysiology. Parkinson's disease is a *neurodegenerative* condition. Its most characteristic pathologic feature is loss of *dopamine-containing* neurons whose nuclei reside in the pars compacta of the *substantia nigra* and whose axons terminate in the *caudate nucleus* and *putamen* (the striatum). Other pigmented and nonpigmented nuclei in the brainstem and elsewhere are affected as well. Associated with neuronal loss is the development of concentric hyalin inclusions in the cytoplasm of affected neurons called *Lewy bodies*. Symptoms are believed related to the imbalance between dopaminergic and cholinergic influences on striatal tissue created by the loss of dopamine-containing neurons. Proper striatal function depends on this balance.

Although parkinsonism may result from substance exposures, infection, and a host of other conditions (Table 174–1), idiopathic disease remains the most common form. A possible mechanism for idiopathic disease was suggested by the observation that intravenous drug abusers who injected MPTP (an analogue of meperidine) developed symptoms of parkinsonism. MPTP causes neuronal degeneration of the substantia nigra through its effects on monoamine oxidase B. Its metabolite concentrates in dopaminergic neurons, where it is bound to neuromelanin and inhibits complex 1 of the mitochondrial respiratory chain. The substantia nigra of patients with Parkinson's disease seems particularly vulnerable to *oxidative insults*. The demonstration that a toxin can produce parkinsonism led to a thus far unfruitful search for causative environmental precipitants.

Clinical Presentation. Parkinson's disease is an affliction of mid to late adult life, although 30 percent of patients report recognizable symptoms before the age of 50. Another 40 percent develop the disease between ages 50 and 60, and the remainder are greater than 60 years old at the time of diagnosis. The classic syndrome of parkinsonism includes *tremor at rest, rigidity, bradykinesia, masked face, stooped posture,* and a *shuffling gait.* Although tremor is the most obvious initial finding, it is absent in 20 percent of patients. Parkinson's disease may begin insidiously with vague, *aching pain* in the limbs, neck, or back and with *decreased axial dexterity* before tremor is noted. *Dysarthria* may be an early feature, although *dysphagia* usually occurs later. Significant *orthostatic symptoms* may predominate in some patients. Other early subtle symptoms include decreases in the caliber of *handwriting* and the volume of *voice*. *Depression* is a significant component in many patients and may be a feature of the early disease as well. The estimated frequency of *dementia* (which usually develops late) varies widely, but at least 15 to 20 percent of patients develop cognitive impairment. However, dementia is not inevitable and remediable causes of mental status changes always need to be sought.

Clinical Course. Before the introduction of levodopa, Parkinson's disease had a fairly predictable course. At 5 years from onset, 60 percent of patients were severely disabled, and at 10 years, nearly 80 percent were. The rate of progression varied widely. Death rarely was a direct consequence of parkinsonism; rather, it was a consequence of immobility (aspiration pneumonia, urinary tract infections) or of trauma. Within Parkinson's disease there are several different subgroups with specific clinical patterns. It is thought that patients who present primarily with tremor have a slower course than those for whom bradykinesia is the primary symptom. Patients who present with significant postural and gait instability are largely an older group who are more likely to be cognitively impaired and to have more rapid progression of disease.

The advent of dopaminergic agents has changed the natural history of the disease significantly. The initial benefit of levodopa therapy, as mentioned above, is one of the diagnostic criteria for the disease. Although patients with idiopathic Parkinson's disease usually will respond to levodopa, the initial benefits of therapy decline for as many as half of all patients treated after 2 or more years. Delay in onset of disability has been enhanced by use of the monoamine oxidase B inhibitor Deprenyl (see below).

DIAGNOSIS

The classic presentation of Parkinson's disease usually poses few problems in diagnosis. There are several presentations that may be more problematic. These include isolated tremor at presentation, symptoms confined to half of the body (hemiparkinsonism), and the presence of these symptoms in younger patients. Symptomatic parkinsonism can be seen in several other disorders, such as progressive supranuclear palsy and multisystem atrophy or as a side effect of numerous medications (see Table 174–1). An extrapyramidal syndrome that looks like that of parkinsonism also occurs in Alzheimer's disease and many other conditions.

The clinical diagnosis of Parkinson's disease is based on a careful examination in which the clinician looks for physical signs other than basal ganglia ones, elicits a careful drug and family history, and most likely does at least one neuroimaging study (probably magnetic resonance imaging [MRI]) to exclude significant small vessel vascular disease, which may produce a parkinsonian-like state. Table 174–2 provides a summary of inclusion and exclusion criteria, which should help the physician in this clinical diagnosis. Among the inclusion criteria is the sustained responsiveness to levodopa therapy with duration of improvement for 1 year or more. Many parkinsonian syndromes due to other causes may have a transient response to dopaminergic agents.

Table 174-1. Differential Diagnosis of Parkinsonism

Idiopathic Parkinsonism (Parkinson's disease, Lewy body disease)
Infections and Postinfectious
Postencephalitic parkinsonism (von Economo's disease)
Other viral encephalitides
Toxins
Manganese
Carbon monoxide
Carbon disulfide
Cyanide
Methanol
MPTP
Drugs
Neuroleptics
Reserpine
Metoclopramide
Lithium
Amiodarone
Alpha-methyldopa
Multisystem Degenerations
Striatonigral degeneration
Progressive supranuclear palsy
Olivopontocerebellar degeneration
Shy-Drager syndrome
Primary Dementing and Other Degenerative Disorders
Alzheimer's disease
Creutzfeldt-Jakob disease
Other CNS Disorders
Multiple cerebral infarctions (lacunar state, Binswanger's disease)
Hydrocephalus (normal pressure or high pressure)
Posttraumatic encephalopathy (pugilistic parkinsonism)
Metabolic Conditions
Hypoparathyroidism
Chronic hepatocerebral degeneration
Idiopathic calcification of basal ganglia
Hereditary Disorders
Wilson's disease
Juvenile Huntington's disease (rigid variant)

*This list is not meant to be all-inclusive. Rather, it highlights the more common disorders that may have parkinsonism as a prominent feature.

Adapted from Koller WC. How accurately can Parkinson's disease be diagnosed? Neurology 1992;42(Suppl 1):6.

Table 174-2. Criteria for the Diagnosis of Parkinson's Disease

INCLUSION CRITERIA	EXCLUSION CRITERIA
Presence for 1 year or more of two of the three cardinal motor signs: Resting or postural tremor; Bradykinesia; Rigidity	Abrupt onset of symptoms
Responsiveness to levodopa therapy with moderate to marked improvement and duration of improvement for 1 year or more	Remitting or stepwise progression
	Neuroleptic therapy within 1 year
	Exposure to drugs or toxins associated with parkinsonism
	History of encephalitis
	Oculogyric crises
	Supranuclear downward or lateral gaze palsy
	Cerebellar signs
	Unexplained upper motor neuron or lower motor neuron signs
	More than one affected relative
	Dementia from the onset of disease
	Severe autonomic symptoms

Adapted from Reich SG, DeLong M. "Parkinson's Disease" In Current Therapy in Neurologic Disease 3rd ed. Johnson R, ed. St. Louis: Mosby, 1990.

PRINCIPLES OF MANAGEMENT

There is no cure for Parkinson's disease, but advances in treatment have improved prospects for patients. The goals of therapy are to delay disease progression, relieve symptoms, and preserve functional capacity. Restoring the striatal balance between dopaminergic and cholinergic activity is at the core of efforts to achieve symptomatic relief. Inhibiting oxidative injury appears helpful in retarding disease progression. The patient and physician may tolerate many of the early signs of parkinsonism, which are sufficient to prompt medical consultation, but, aside from provoking psychological discomfort, are not disabling. The goal of therapy is to maintain the patient at maximum function with minimal medication.

Delay of Disease Progression

If degeneration of dopaminergic neurons in the substantia nigra and striatum is a consequence of oxidative injury, then might it be possible to interrupt the degenerative process and slow or halt disease progression by use of agents that inhibit oxidative activity in the central nervous system? This hypothesis led to study of the monoamine oxidase B inhibitor selegiline (Deprenyl). Convincing evidence from three double-blind, placebo-controlled studies indicate that monotherapy with Deprenyl early in the course of disease delays onset of disability and need for initiation of levodopa therapy. Although it is suspected that the mechanism of benefit is protection of striatal tissue from oxidative injury, this has yet to be proven (there may even be some direct effect on ameliorating symptoms). Nonetheless, it seems reasonable to recommend this drug as initial treatment when Parkinson's disease is first diagnosed, because it delays the requirement for levodopa therapy. It may also increase the time during which patients remain functional on levodopa and, for some patients, may decrease the levodopa requirement. This drug is given in the standard dose found to inhibit monoamine oxidase B in most patients; 5 mg are given in the morning and 5 mg at noon. Side effects of tremor and dyskinesia are common when Deprenyl is used in conjunction with levodopa. These are attributable to increased dopaminergic activity, which can be controlled by lowering the levodopa dose.

Other antioxidants have been tried. The largest and best designed of the Deprenyl studies included testing of tocopherol, a vitamin E analogue with antioxidant properties. Tocopherol showed no benefit, either alone or as an enhancer of Deprenyl activity. More study of antioxidant use and its prolonged effects is ongoing.

Symptomatic Relief

To restore the balance between cholinergic and dopaminergic influences requires either inhibition of cholinergic activity or enhancement of dopaminergic output.

Anticholinergic Therapy. Anticholinergic agents were the mainstay of parkinsonian therapy for more than a century, and they have remained important. Commonly used drugs are *trihexyphenidyl* (Artane) and *benztropine* (Cogentin). These agents may be particularly beneficial for patients with tremor as a prominent symptom. Both are muscarinic blocking agents with typical anticholinergic side effects of urine retention, dry mouth, increased intraocular pressure in patients with glaucoma, and confusion (Table 174–3).

Enhancing Dopaminergic Activity—Levodopa. Treatment with the dopamine precursor *levodopa* (in combination with a peripheral decarboxylase inhibitor) is recommended for patients who become too symptomatic to function satisfactorily despite Deprenyl and anticholinergic therapy. Prescribing only a levodopa preparation, the physician is able to offer most parkinsonian patients much benefit, although there are a number of important limitations and side effects.

One limitation is duration of action, necessitating careful consideration of when to begin levodopa therapy. At issue is the optimal time. Against early initiation of levodopa treatment is the phenomenon of a decline in its effectiveness in as many as 50 percent of patients after 2 years of use. This observation is the basis for the traditional view that onset of therapy should be delayed as long as possible. However, there are data indicating a reduction in mortality when levodopa is started within 1 to 3 years of onset of symptoms compared to delaying levodopa use until after 4 years. Clinical judgment that takes into account both of these factors is required.

Table 174-3. Drugs Used for Parkinson's Disease

DRUG	AVAILABLE PREPARATION	DOSE (MG)	SCHEDULE	STARTING DOSE (MG)	MAINTENANCE DOSE (MG)
Anticholinergic Agents (representative examples)					
Trihexyphenidyl hydrochloride (Artane)	Scored tablets	2 mg, 5 mg	3 to 4 times daily	2 mg	2–10 mg
	Elixir	2 mg/5 ml			
	Timed-release capsule	5 mg	Once daily	(Timed-release capsule may be substituted for regular Artane after maintenance dose is determined)	
Benztropine mesylate (Cogentin)	Tablets	0.5 mg, 1 mg, 2 mg	Once or twice daily	1 mg	0.5–6 mg
Dopaminergic Agents					
Carbidopa/levodopa (Sinemet)	Scored tablets 10/100, 25/100, 25/250		2 to 4 times daily	50/200 in two divided doses	400–500 mg levodopa
Sinemet CR	50/200 mg		2 times daily	50/200 mg bid	variable
Bromocriptine (Parlodel)	Scored tablets	2.5 mg	2 to 3 times daily	1.25 mg daily	7.5–30 mg
	Capsules	5.0 mg			
Pergolide mesylate (Permax)	Scored tablets	0.05 mg, 0.25 mg, 1.0 mg	3 times daily	0.05 mg daily	1–3 mg
Deprenyl (Eldepryl, selegiline hydrochloride)	Tablets	5.0 mg	2 times daily	5 mg daily	10 mg
Amantadine (Symmetrel)	Capsules	100 mg	2 times daily	100 mg daily	200 mg

Adapted from Reich SG and DeLong M: Parkinson's Disease In Current Therapy in Neurologic Disease 3rd ed. Johnson R. St. Louis: Mosby, 1990.

Levodopa is the naturally occurring precursor of dopamine, It crosses the blood–brain barrier and enhances dopaminergic activity. However, because much of the drug is converted peripherally by a decarboxylase into dopamine (which cannot cross the blood–brain barrier), levodopa is best given in combination with a peripheral decarboxylase inhibitor, such as *carbidopa*. Combination preparations containing both agents in various strengths are commonly used. A typical starting program uses the 25 mg levodopa/100 mg carbidopa combination preparation (eg, Sinemet 25/100, 2 or 3 times daily; see Table 174-3). Levodopa is rapidly absorbed after oral administration, will reach its peak effect at 30 minutes to 2 hours, and has a half-life of 1 to 3 hours. The rate of absorption is decreased by eating a protein-rich meal.

There are significant adverse reactions in many patients: *nausea, vomiting, anorexia, hypertension, dyskinesias,* and *hallucinations* can be disturbing. The nausea can be partly overcome by taking the drug with small meals. Dyskinesias include chorea, athetosis, and dystonia, which usually occur at times of peak concentrations of levodopa and are best managed by having the patient take small doses of medication at frequent intervals.

With disease progression, there appears to be a declining threshold for the development of adverse central side effects. *"Wearing off"* is the recurrence of severe symptoms hours after the most recent dose of medication and is often followed by recurrence of rigidity and bradykinesia. A *controlled-release preparation* (Sinemet CR) helps this problem for many patients.

As decline in drug efficacy develops, patients may experience the *"on/off" phenomenon* in which there is a severe fluctuation of dose–response relations with rapid onset and termination of therapeutic and adverse effects. A study of its pathophysiology revealed impaired absorption of levodopa with meals and an inhibition of levodopa transport into the brain by dietary amino acids. Treatment entails taking levodopa 1 hour before eating, adding an ergot preparation (see below), and reducing the protein content of the diet. Use of a controlled-release formulation may also help, but the development of the "on/off" state represents an advanced form of disease and a difficult one to treat. Drug "holidays" have been proposed to restore sensitivity to levodopa, but results are not impressive.

The development of a sustained-release preparation (Sinemet CR 50/200) has been a major therapeutic advance for patients afflicted with motor fluctuations. The controlled-release form can almost double the duration of effect to 5 to 6 hours. To match the effects of conventional levodopa preparations, a program of up to 25 percent more daily levodopa in the controlled-release form may be required. Doses administered after 6:00 PM can be given in the rapidly absorbed form to eliminate nocturnal side effects of the medication.

Psychiatric symptoms, including nightmares, hallucinations, and increased sexual drive, are other disturbing features of late stage disease. Paradoxically, increased mobility has in some instances led to increased disability as a result of sudden falls in previously rigid patients.

Other Dopaminergic Agents. *Amantadine,* an antiinfluenzal agent, facilitates release of dopamine from striatal nerve endings that have degenerated. It is sometimes used before levodopa, but benefit is usually short-lived, with most patients showing little response after a few months of therapy. Amantadine may transiently improve extrapyramidal symptoms when used in conjunction with levodopa. Side effects are few, but some patients are bothered by livedo reticularis, insomnia, or confusion.

Bromocriptine and *pergolide* are direct *dopamine-receptor agonists*. These agents are used to enhance the therapeutic effects of levodopa and may be particularly helpful in late stages of the disease when conversion of levodopa to dopamine is inefficient in the degenerating substantia nigra. They are less likely than levodopa to cause dyskinesias and the on/off phenomenon. In addition, they may allow use of lower doses of levodopa when used early on with levodopa as initial therapy, although this is not common practice. Side effects of the direct dopamine agonists are similar to those of levodopa. Both the direct dopamine agonists and the controlled-release preparations are likely to be prescribed by neurologists, although recognition of the necessity to move to these sorts of therapies will be in the province of the primary physician who sees the patient most frequently.

Supportive Measures

Because maintaining function is a central goal of therapy, one should not forget the value of such important adjunctive measures as *physical therapy* and *psychological support*. Physical therapy can improve functioning by helping to preserve muscle strength and flexibility. Although a central component of the supportive psychological effort involves close follow-up and detailed patient education (see below), one must also be watchful for the development of depression and the need to treat it promptly and effectively (see Chapter 227).

Experimental Therapies

Transplantation of fetal substantia nigra tissue into the striatum relieves the signs of parkinsonism in animals with experimental substantia nigra lesions. Early attempts to treat humans with Parkinson's disease with grafts of tissue, either autografts of the adrenal medulla or grafts of human fetal tissue, were disappointing, although the fetal tissue results were better than those of the adrenal medullary grafts. Adrenal medullary grafting has been abandoned, but work on fetal tissue transplantation has continued and produced increasingly beneficial results. Nonetheless, this method of therapy remains investigational at this time.

Other methods of therapy under development include new drugs to inhibit dopamine breakdown, synthesis of new dopamine-receptor agonists, and blockade of excitotoxic neurotransmitter receptors in the subthalamic nucleus. Finally, jejunal infusion of levodopa and carbidopa has been tried to improve levodopa absorption.

PATIENT EDUCATION

Patient and family education is essential to the success of therapy. The need for trial and error to obtain maximal benefit with minimal side effects must be explained. Frequent visits will be needed in the initiation period and later in the course of the disease. Although therapy can be proposed optimistically, the inevitable diminution in efficacy of therapy must be anticipated and discussed with patient and family so that they can be adequately prepared, both psychologically and practically. Patients are obviously concerned about prognosis, and a frank discussion of what is known is usually appreciated. A number of helpful guidebooks are available for patients and their families.

THERAPEUTIC RECOMMENDATIONS

- After excluding other potential causes of parkinsonism, it is appropriate to start Deprenyl (selegiline) in the early stages of disease. Daily dose is 10 mg (5 mg in the morning and 5 mg at noon). This drug may also be started in patients already on Sinemet in an attempt to lower the amount of levodopa needed.
- If symptoms progress to impair daily functioning despite use of Deprenyl, then starting the combination preparation levodopa/carbidopa (Sinemet) is indicated. Sinemet is usually begun in a dose of 25/100 mg tid, after which the dose is adjusted according to individual response.
- Combination treatment with anticholinergics, amantadine, and direct dopamine agonists (bromocriptine, pergolide) may be used to maximize effect (see Table 174–3). Anticholinergics are particularly helpful for treatment of tremor.
- Problems of long-term management and loss of efficacy include end-dose wearing off, on/off effect, drug-induced confusion, and loss of dopamine response. Appropriate consultation for adjunctive therapies can be initiated for these patients.
- The important supportive roles for physical therapy, psychological support, and recognition and treatment of depression should not be neglected in the day-to-day management of patients with Parkinson's disease.

ANNOTATED BIBLIOGRAPHY

Diamond SG, Markham CH, Hoehn MM, et al. Multi-center study of Parkinson mortality with early versus later dopa treatment. Ann Neurol 1987;22:8. *(Mortality was less in patients treated earlier than later.)*

Duvoisin RC. Parkinson's Disease: A Guide for Patient and Family, 3rd ed. New York, Raven Press, 1991. *(A sensible, very useful guide for the patient and family embarking on a course of Parkinson's treatment.)*

Fahn S. Fetal-tissue transplants in Parkinson's disease. N Engl J Med 1992;327:1589. *(Progress being made, but still an investigational therapy.)*

Goetz CG. Dopaminergic agonists in the treatment of Parkinson's disease. Neurology 1990;40:50. *(Good review of bromocriptine and pergolide.)*

Koller WC. How accurately can Parkinson's disease be diagnosed? Neurology 1992;42(suppl 1):6. *(Whole supplement deals with the use of controlled-release Sinemet, but this chapter is a particularly lucid description of the clinical diagnosis.)*

Koller WC, Hubble JP,. Levodopa therapy in Parkinson's disease. Neurology 1990;40(suppl 3):40. *(Comprehensive review.)*

Langston JW. Selegiline as neuroprotective therapy in Parkinson's disease. Neurology 1990;40 (suppl 3):61. *(A discussion of the controversy about protective versus symptomatic effects of this new drug.)*

Lieberman A. An integrated approach to patient management in Parkinson's disease. Neurol Clin North Am 1992;10:553. *(A good summary of the treatment strategies in the later stages of the disease.)*

Mayeux R, Stern Y, Mulvey K, et al. Reappraisal of temporary withdrawal ("drug holiday") in Parkinson's disease. N Engl J Med 1985;315:724. *(Ten days of withdrawal was without benefit in terms of doses needed or response.)*

Nutt JG, Woodward WR, Hammerstad JP, et al. The "on–off" phenomenon in Parkinson's disease. Relation to levodopa absorption and transport. N Engl J Med 1984;310:484. *(Absorption and transport impaired by meals and protein intake.)*

Parkinson Study Group. Effects of tocopherol and Deprenyl on the progression to disability in early Parkinson's disease. N Engl J Med 1993;328:176. *(Deprenyl, but not tocopherol, effective in delaying onset of disability and need for levodopa therapy.)*

Primary Care Medicine: Office Evaluation and Management of the Adult Patient, 3rd edition, edited by Allan H. Goroll, Lawrence A. May, and Albert G. Mulley, Jr. J.B. Lippincott Company, Philadelphia

175

Management of Bell's Palsy (Idiopathic Facial Mononeuropathy)

AMY A. PRUITT, M.D.

Bell's palsy is an idiopathic paralysis of the facial muscles innervated by the seventh cranial nerve. The condition encompasses 80 percent of all facial mononeuropathies. Satisfactory explanations for the condition are lacking, although viral infection and ischemia with subsequent edema of the facial nerve and adjacent structures have been invoked.

The primary physician should be able to distinguish Bell's palsy from other, more ominous causes of facial palsy and temper therapeutic intervention by knowledge of the disease's self-limited course and good prognosis.

CLINICAL PRESENTATION AND COURSE

The condition shows an increasing incidence with age, is slightly more common in the winter, and is associated with pregnancy, diabetes, and hypothyroidism. In patients under the age of 50, the condition is more common among women, but this gender distribution reverses in patients over the age of 50.

The distinction between Bell's palsy and other facial paralyses is usually not difficult. The onset is usually acute, with maximal deficit developing over a few hours. The motor deficit is almost always unilateral and in two-thirds of cases may be accompanied by pain in or behind the ear. Fever, tinnitus, and mild hearing diminution may be present during the first few hours. There may be some fluctuation in symptoms the first few days after onset.

Voluntary and involuntary motor responses are lost. Upper and lower parts of the face are affected, distinguishing this peripheral facial nerve lesion from a central supranuclear one, in which only lower facial muscles are affected. Patient complaints include facial muscle paresis, facial asymmetry, and drooling. The palpebral fissure appears widened, the forehead is smooth, and there is flattening of the nasolabial fold. Bell's phenomenon (the normal upward deviation of the eye with lid closure) is exaggerated because of orbicularis oculi weakness. The corneal reflex may be decreased on the involved side. Lacrimation is only rarely defective, and depending on the level of the injury, loss or perversion of taste on the anterior two-thirds of the tongue or hyperacusis may occur, causing altered taste, decreased tearing, decreased salivation, or altered sensitivity to sound.

Clinical Course. Seventy-five percent to 90 percent of cases recover to a cosmetically acceptable level without treatment. Most do so within 3 weeks. Recovery is best in children; poor prognosis has been associated with increasing age, hyperacusis, diminished taste, and severity of the initial motor deficit. Prognosis can be predicted by electromyographic (EMG) testing of the involved muscles after at least 72 hours from the clinical nadir. Patients with evidence of extensive axonal degeneration have a poorer prognosis. Those who have partial or complete preservation of the compound muscle action potential amplitude have anatomic continuity of the facial nerve, partial axonal preservation, and a better prognosis. EMG study is indicated only for patients with severe clinical involvement that has not improved 7 to 10 days after onset.

Other poor outcomes from Bell's palsy result from abnormal regeneration of damaged nerve fibers. Lacrimation with eating or "crocodile tears" result when fibers regrow and connect with lacrimal ducts instead of salivary glands. Abnormal movements (facial synkinesis) may occur if regenerating motor fibers innervate inappropriate muscles. Contracture of the involved site may be noted during voluntary movement. Seven percent of patients experience recurrent facial paralysis.

DIFFERENTIAL DIAGNOSIS

Other causes of facial paralysis involve injury to the facial nerve and include bacterial infection (from a source in the ear), herpes zoster, diabetes mellitus, sarcoidosis, Guillain-Barré syndrome, tumor (acoustic neuroma, pontine glioma, neurofibroma, cholesteatoma), trauma (fracture of the temporal bone), and Lyme disease.

WORKUP

The patient found to have a VIIth nerve mononeuropathy should be examined for evidence of an underlying etiology. One checks for zosteriform lesions (see Chapter 193) on the tympanic membrane, in the external auditory canal, and behind the ear. The skin is also examined for the characteristic truncal erythematous lesion of early Lyme disease (see Chapter 160) and for neurofibromata. The tympanic membranes are also checked for cholesteatoma and evidence of otitis media (see Chapter 218). The jaw is noted for tenderness and trauma to the temporal bone. The lymph nodes are palpated for enlargement and the chest is auscultated for signs of interstitial involvement suggestive of sarcoidosis (see Chapter 51). A careful neurologic examination completes the assessment, focusing on detection of additional neurologic deficits.

In a patient with the characteristic history and physical findings, laboratory studies are of limited value in the evaluation of this facial mononeuropathy, although they may reveal diabetes or some other medical condition associated with an increased risk of Bell's palsy. Testing for Lyme disease (see Chapter 160) may be appropriate in highly endemic areas, as suggested by a recent study in which one-fourth of summertime cases of Bell's palsy demonstrated evidence of infection with the tickborne spirochete of Lyme disease, *Borrelia burgdorferi*. The identification of Lyme disease has important consequences for management (see below and Chapter 160).

Imaging studies using computed tomography (CT) or magnetic resonance imaging (MRI) are necessary only when a posterior fossa mass is suspected as the cause of the VIIth nerve palsy. Lumbar puncture is indicated if inflammation, granuloma, or malignancy is a consideration. A mild pleocytosis of the cerebrospinal fluid has been reported in typical cases of Bell's palsy. In patients with atypical or persistent facial palsy, gadolinium-enhanced MRI can help differentiate Bell's palsy from other etiologies.

PRINCIPLES OF MANAGEMENT

Of greatest practical importance during the acute stage of the illness is the prevention of injury to the *cornea,* which is left exposed by weakness of the orbicularis muscle. When the lid is weak, methylcellulose drops should be prescribed for use twice a day and at bedtime; in addition, the lid may need to be taped shut at night. If corneal abrasion is suspected because of pain, visual impairment, or other eye complaints (see Chapter 201), then prompt referral for ophthalmic consultation and slit-lamp examination with fluorescein is indicated.

Because the prognosis for most cases of Bell's palsy is good, little or no treatment is necessary in most instances. However, if paralysis is severe and the patient is seen within a few days of onset, a short course of *corticosteroid therapy* will increase the chances for maximal recovery. One study reported full facial recovery in 88 percent of the group treated with prednisone and in 64 percent of the untreated control group. Another study found a decrease in the frequency of chronic autonomic dysfunction (from 10% to 1%) when prednisone was used early in the course of illness. Associated ear pain diminished more quickly when steroids were used. Nevertheless, the benefits from use of steroids are often difficult to demonstrate, because the disease has such a good prognosis. Steroid therapy seems to make a difference only in cases with poor prognostic signs. Patients with Lyme disease as the underlying etiology should not receive steroids, which might worsen the situation by compromising immune function.

Other treatments have been used. Based on the theory that nerve swelling contributes to the deficit, surgical decompression has been tried, but without much success. Some patients have been followed with EMG stimulation of the muscles to hasten particularly stubborn paralyses. The possible role of EMG stimulation in management is unclear; it has not been subjected to controlled study.

THERAPEUTIC RECOMMENDATIONS AND INDICATIONS FOR REFERRAL

- Ascertain that the condition is indeed Bell's palsy. Check for involvement of other cranial nerves and ear infection. Examine for zosteriform lesions on the tympanic membrane, in the external auditory canal, and behind the ear.
- In areas endemic for Lyme disease, examine the patient carefully for characteristic features and consider serologic testing (see Chapter 160).
- Explain the benign nature and good prognosis of the condition and caution the patient about corneal abrasion. Mention that altered taste, decreased tearing, decreased salivation, or altered sensitivity to sound may be experienced.
- Prescribe use of methylcellulose eyedrops twice a day and at sleep, with taping of the especially weak lid. Tarsorrhaphy may be considered when severe lid weakness exists.
- If the patient is seen within 1 week of onset of facial weakness and if there are no important contraindications to corticosteroid use (Lyme disease would be a contraindication), then a short course of prednisone may be prescribed.
- Begin with prednisone 60 mg qAM for 5 days. If improvement occurs or weakness does not progress during these 5 days, then taper and terminate over 10 more days. If improvement does not occur during the first 5 days, then continue prednisone at 60 mg qAM for a total of 10 days and taper over another 10 days. If postauricular pain recurs when the dose is tapered, then reinstitute the preceding dose.
- In the 10 percent of patients who do not achieve acceptable recovery, autografting with a hypoglossal to facial anastamosis may provide reasonable cosmetic results and afford lasting protection of the eye. Patients in this category should be referred to an otolaryngologist or to a neurosurgeon.

ANNOTATED BIBLIOGRAPHY

Adour KK. Diagnosis and management of facial paralysis. N Engl J Med 1982;307:348. *(A superb succinct clinical review not only of Bell's palsy but also of facial paralysis due to herpes zoster, trauma, otitis media, neoplasms, and other causes.)*

Adour KK, Wingerd J, Bell DN, et al. Prednisone treatment for idiopathic facial paralysis (Bell's palsy). N Engl J Med 1972;287:1268. *(Controlled part of this study stopped when authors felt pain relief and recovery were clearly aided by prednisone. However, the results for both groups were very good.)*

Halperin JJ. Lyme borreleosis in Bell's palsy. Neurology 1992; 42:1268. *(A very high incidence of Lyme seropositivity in Bell's palsy cases during summer in endemic areas.)*

Katusic SK. Incidence, clinical features, and prognosis in Bell's palsy: Rochester, MN, 1968–1982. Ann Neurol 1986;20:622. *(Best available community-based data.)*

Tien R, Dillon WP, Jackler RK. Contrast-enhanced MR imaging of the facial nerve in 11 patients with Bell's palsy. Am J Neuroradiol 1990;11:735. *(Gadolinium enhancement helpful in cases with atypical or persistent facial palsy.)*

Wolf SH, Wagner JH, Davidson S, et al. Treatment of Bell's palsy with prednisone. A prospective, randomized study. Neurology 1978;28:158. *(There was incomplete recovery in 16 percent [mild in 14 percent]. No diabetics were included.)*

Primary Care Medicine: Office Evaluation and Management of the Adult Patient, 3rd edition, edited by Allan H. Goroll, Lawrence A. May, and Albert G. Mulley, Jr. J.B. Lippincott Company, Philadelphia

176
Management of Tic Douloureux (Trigeminal Neuralgia)

AMY A. PRUITT, M.D.

Tic douloureux is among the most excruciating of pain syndromes seen in office practice. There are 15,000 new cases annually in the United States; most patients are middle-aged or elderly. Some have found the pain so intolerable that they consider suicide. The primary physician needs to know how to use available medical therapies and when to send the patient for neurosurgical consultation.

CLINICAL PRESENTATION AND NATURAL HISTORY

The illness is characterized by paroxysms of unilateral lancinating facial pain involving the jaw, gums, lips, or maxillary region (areas corresponding to branches of the trigeminal nerve). The maxillary and mandibular divisions are affected more frequently than the ophthalmic one. Attacks are often precipitated by minor, repeated contact with a trigger zone, setting off brief but fierce pain that usually lasts up to a few minutes. Repeated paroxysms may continue day and night, for several weeks. The disease is unilateral and unaccompanied by demonstrable sensory or motor deficits, which distinguishes it from other causes of trigeminal pain, such as tumor.

The condition can be chronic, although spontaneous remissions are not uncommon. Women are more often affected than men, and the incidence rises with age. The etiology of the condition remains unknown. Despite much speculation, no definitive evidence links it to herpes simplex virus. The pathologic lesion found in some electron micrographs appears to be a breakdown of myelin.

Although trigeminal neuralgia may be a symptom of multiple sclerosis, it is infrequently the initial or sole manifestation of this disease. Similarly, trigeminal neuralgia is uncommonly the isolated symptom of a cerebellopontine angle tumor. Both diseases can be demonstrated by magnetic resonance imaging (MRI), and some authors recommend MRI in all trigeminal neuralgia cases, although cost–benefit remains to be proven.

PRINCIPLES OF MANAGEMENT

Treatment is symptomatic. Because the condition may be self-limited and agents that give temporary relief are available, drug therapy should be tried before surgery is contemplated. *Carbamazepine* (Tegretol) is the drug of choice; it was initially tried because anticonvulsants were believed to be helpful in causalgic pain. Studies have shown impressive short-term effects; most patients report marked pain relief within 24 to 72 hours. The drug is so effective that some argue that failure to respond places the diagnosis in doubt. The starting dose is 100 to 200 mg bid. The maintenance dosage ranges from 400 mg to 800 mg per day and is adjusted according to serum drug level determinations—therapeutic range is 5 to 12 μg/mL. The most common side effect is sedation.

Unfortunately, by 3 years, 30 percent no longer obtain relief from carbamazepine; alternative therapy is needed. Moreover, the incidence of serious side effects (bone marrow suppression, rash, liver injury) is high (5% to 19%) and may require cessation of therapy. Fortunately, marrow suppression is often reversible if the drug is stopped early. Skin rash often precedes other serious side effects; it may be erythematous and pruritic. The onset of a skin rash is an early indication to halt therapy. Annoying side effects include nausea, diarrhea, ataxia, dizziness, and confusion. Neurologic reactions are reported most commonly and affect about 15 percent of patients. Starting carbamazepine at 200 mg daily helps to avoid many of the annoying minor side effects. During the first 2 months of therapy, complete blood and platelet counts should be obtained weekly to biweekly; later, the frequency of monitoring can be reduced to monthly. It is advisable to attempt reduction or cessation of carbamazepine therapy at least once every 2 to 3 months.

Baclofen, an agent capable of inhibiting synaptic transmission, has been used with success in a high percentage of cases. Some now consider it the drug of choice for trigeminal neuralgia. Treatment is initiated at dosages of 10 mg bid and increased slowly. The usual maintenance dose is 50 to 60 mg per day. Sedation and nausea are the most common limiting side effects. Abrupt cessation of therapy can lead to hallucinations and seizures, so discontinuation must be gradual.

Because trigeminal neuralgia tends to increase in severity, it may be necessary to use carbamazepine and baclofen in combination or either in conjunction with *phenytoin.* The usual daily dose of phenytoin that achieves therapeutic serum levels is 300 to 400 mg (see Chapter 170). Parenteral phenytoin is sometimes used emergently for patients who are having a flurry of severe attacks and cannot take medicine orally.

When drug therapy proves inadequate, *surgical approaches* can be considered. Microvascular decompression affords the best chance of long-term pain relief without sensory deficit, but because it entails more complicated surgery, it is often reserved for younger patients. The least invasive procedure producing acceptable deficits with the greatest relief of symptoms is percutaneous radiofrequency rhizotomy. The small fiber pain fibers are destroyed, whereas the more heavily myelinated touch fibers that supply the relevant zone are spared. The procedure has produced lasting relief in 90 percent of those treated once; only 5 percent have experienced undesirable loss of sensation. The late recurrence rate is 10 percent, and a repeat procedure achieves pain relief in these patients; few need further treatment.

Formerly used treatment methods include alcohol injection or partial section of the sensory root of the fifth nerve. These techniques provided pain relief, but often only for 1 to 2 years, and at the price of unacceptable permanent sensory deficits. Total tooth extraction is an ineffective and erroneous treatment method.

PATIENT EDUCATION

The patient needs to be told that the condition can be controlled and is often self-limited. This knowledge can prevent a distraught sufferer from attempting suicide. The physician must keep in mind the anguish these patients may experience; they require close support. Obvious hints, such as avoiding repetitive contacts with the trigger zone, have usually been discovered by the patient, but can be helpful and are worth mentioning. Patients treated with carbamazepine must be informed of the risk of marrow suppression and the importance of regular monitoring of the complete blood count.

THERAPEUTIC RECOMMENDATIONS AND INDICATIONS FOR REFERRAL

- Teach the patient to avoid repetitive contact with the trigger zone.
- Begin drug therapy for disabling and frequent episodes of pain with *carbamazepine* (100 mg bid); increase dosage by 200 mg per day until control of symptoms is achieved or a dosage of 800 mg per day is reached.
- During the first 2 months of carbamazepine therapy, monitor complete blood and platelet counts weekly to biweekly; thereafter, monthly checks will suffice.
- Stop carbamazepine immediately if white blood cell count falls below 3000 or if skin rash, easy bruising, fever, mouth sores, or petechiae develop.
- An alternative to carbamazepine is *baclofen,* 10 mg bid. Increase the dosage by 10 mg every 3 days until a response is achieved or a maximum of 60 mg is reached. Discontinue the medication gradually; do not withdraw it abruptly.
- If carbamazepine or baclofen alone is not sufficient to control symptoms, add *phenytoin* at a dosage of 300 mg per day.

- Avoid use of narcotics, because they are unlikely to be of help for long-term control of pain and may only lead to drug dependency.
- Refer the patient who cannot be managed by pharmacologic measures to a neurosurgeon skilled in selective radiofrequency rhizotomy or microvascular decompression.

ANNOTATED BIBLIOGRAPHY

Crill WE. Carbamazepine. Ann Intern Med 1975;79:844. *(A review of the pharmacology and use of this agent. Argues for its use as the first line of therapy in tic douloureux.)*

Fromm GH, Terrence CF, Chattha AS. Baclofen in the treatment of trigeminal neuralgia: Double-blind study and long-term follow-up. Ann Neurol 1984;15:240. *(Efficacy demonstrated.)*

Hart RG, Easton JD. Carbamazepine and hematological monitoring. Ann Neurol 1982;11:309. *(Provides guidelines for monitoring of marrow suppression.)*

Hershey R. Baclofen for neuralgia. Ann Intern Med 1984;100:905. *(An editorial discussing its use in patients with neuralgic pain.)*

Sweet WH. The treatment of trigeminal neuralgia (tic douloureux). N Engl J Med 1986;315:174. *(A concise and authoritative review of both medical and surgical approaches to treatment by a pioneer in surgical therapy for this condition.)*

12

Dermatologic Problems

Primary Care Medicine: Office Evaluation and Management of the Adult Patient, 3rd edition, edited by Allan H. Goroll, Lawrence A. May, and Albert G. Mulley, Jr. J.B. Lippincott Company, Philadelphia

177

Screening for Skin Cancers

ARTHUR J. SOBER, M.D.

Neoplasms of the skin are among the most common cancers in humans. It has been estimated that more than 700,000 new tumors occur annually in the United States. The majority are basal cell carcinomas—relatively benign, locally mutilating tumors associated with few deaths. Squamous cell carcinoma, the second most common cutaneous malignancy, causes approximately 2000 deaths annually. Malignant melanoma, of which there are more than 32,000 cases annually, is responsible for approximately 6500 deaths per year. The first two types of skin cancers derive from the epidermal keratinocytes; the third type develops from the melanocytes along the basal layer of the epidermis.

Screening for these tumors is important because they are relatively easy to diagnose in early stages when cure is possible by simple measures. This is particularly true for malignant melanoma, because we are in the midst of a striking, unexplained increase in melanoma incidence. In the past decade, the incidence of melanoma in the United States has approximately doubled. Since 1960, incidence of melanoma in the United States has increased more rapidly than that of any other cancer.

EPIDEMIOLOGY AND RISK FACTORS

Basal cell carcinomas are probably the most common malignancy in humans. They are distinctly solar-related, with risk proportional to total accumulated sun exposure. In one study of more than 800 tumors, approximately 90 percent of the lesions occurred on the head and neck. The frequency of these lesions is increased in people who work out-of-doors, such as farmers and sailors. Etiologic factors other than solar exposure are responsible for some basal cell carcinomas. For example, the basal cell nevus syndrome is a genetically transmitted autosomal-dominant disorder in which multiple basal cell carcinomas occur in relatively young persons in association with palmar pits, bone cysts, and frontal bossing. Basal cell lesions can develop in persons exposed to arsenic. Scars from radiation dermatitis and from thermal burns can also provide sites favorable to development of basal cell tumors. Previously identified disease is also a risk factor.

Once a single basal cell carcinoma has developed, there is a 20 percent chance that a second one will ensue within 1 year. After two have developed, there is a 40 percent likelihood that a third or more will occur within 1 year. This observation forms the basis of annual follow-up examinations after basal cell carcinoma has been detected.

Squamous cell carcinomas may develop from actinic keratoses and may also occur following arsenic ingestion or in areas of scarring from radiodermatitis or thermal burns. Two-thirds of squamous cell carcinomas occur on sun-exposed surfaces, with risk again proportional to total accumulated sun exposure. Those arising in sun-damaged skin usually behave biologically in a less aggressive fashion than those that occur on surfaces not exposed to the sun. It is the latter group that apparently metastasize more frequently.

Malignant melanomas, while far less common than basal cell and squamous cell cancers, account for 75 percent of the deaths caused by tumors of the skin. The incidence of malignant melanoma has been increasing rapidly over the past few decades. The current annual incidence exceeds those of Hodgkin's disease, leukemia, pancreatic cancer, carcinoma of the thyroid, and carcinoma of the pharynx and larynx. The sex ratio for melanoma in the United States is approximately 1:1. A second primary tumor develops in about 2 percent of patients; 6 percent to 10 percent have affected relatives.

Giant hairy nevus is a form of congenital nevus that has been associated with malignant degeneration in 2 percent to 40 percent of cases. Recent studies estimate the overall risk of malignancy to be about 6 percent. Melanomas may arise in these lesions at any time throughout life, but they most often do so by age 10. Malignant melanoma occasionally arises in smaller pigmented congenital nevi, but the risk is unknown.

The risk of developing skin cancer is not equal in all persons. Individuals with fair skin who tan poorly and burn easily are at greatest risk, especially those with a history of episodic, intense sun exposure. Blacks, orientals, and dark-skinned whites have a much lower risk.

Because of the rapid rise in melanoma incidence, attention has focused on melanoma precursors and risk factors. Precursor lesions include *congenital nevi* and *dysplastic nevi*. Although congenital nevi occur in approximately 1 percent of all newborns, most of these are small (<1.5 cm in diameter). Melanoma risk has been most clearly associated with medium (1.5–20 cm) and large (>20 cm) nevi.

Dysplastic nevi occur in 2 percent to 10 percent of people. They usually are recognizable early in adolescence. Among those with dysplastic nevi, the lifetime risk of melanoma has been estimated at 6 percent, or seven times that of all whites in the United States. The 8- to 12-fold risk of melanoma among first-degree relatives of persons with melanoma may be partly explained by the fact that predisposition to dysplastic nevi is inherited. In patients with dysplastic nevi and two or more first-degree relatives with cutaneous melanoma, the lifetime risk exceeds 50 percent.

NATURAL HISTORY OF SKIN CANCERS AND EFFECTIVENESS OF THERAPY

Basal cell carcinomas rarely metastasize or cause death, but they can be locally invasive and disfiguring. Metastasis is an extremely infrequent event which usually occurs in patients who have delayed therapy for many years and who have large, locally invasive, eroded lesions. Several effective forms of therapy exist, all yielding a cure rate of approximately 95 percent: *surgical excision*, *radiation* therapy, *desiccation and curettage*, and cryotherapy with *liquid nitrogen* applied by special spray apparatus.

Treatment of the 5 percent of basal cell carcinomas that recur presents a greater challenge. The cure rate of a recurrent basal cell carcinoma is about 66 percent when the above four approaches are applied. A special form of surgery, called the Mohs micrographic procedure, is used for difficult, recurrent, infiltrative basal cell carcinomas. The tissue that is excised is examined directly under the microscope to determine whether the tumor has been completely removed. Additional sections of skin are removed until all the borders are histopathologically clear of tumor. With the Mohs technique, cure rates of recurrent tumors exceed 90 percent.

The use of 5-fluorouracil (5-FU) topically and interferon-alpha intralesionally has been advocated by some physicians for the treatment of superficial basal cell carcinoma. Experience has not been sufficient to be able to place these modalities in relation to the other forms of therapy that have a clearly established track record, but they may have some role in patients with multiple lesions in whom other techniques cannot be employed.

Squamous cell carcinomas may begin as actinic keratoses, of which perhaps 1 in 1000 annually undergoes malignant change. There are several effective therapeutic modalities for actinic keratoses. Application of *5-FU* cream or solution twice daily for 2 to 4 weeks usually results in the destruction of these lesions. Some clinically inapparent lesions will also be destroyed by this therapy. The patient must be warned about the impressive inflammation that occurs when 5-FU is used. Because 5-FU is also a photosensitizing agent, treatment in late fall or winter, when solar exposure is diminished, is preferred. *Masoprocol* 10%, applied topically twice a day, is a newly introduced alternative to 5-FU. Other effective modalities include cryotherapy with *liquid nitrogen* and *light desiccation*. If a cutaneous horn is present, biopsy of the lesion may be warranted to rule out the presence of a squamous cell carcinoma. Actinic keratoses are extremely common and usually present no great threat to life. Treatment is often of cosmetic consequence only.

Bowen's disease, or squamous cell carcinoma in situ, is substantially less common than actinic keratoses. It represents the next grade of neoplasia in the keratinocytic line. *Surgical removal* of Bowen's disease lesions is probably the most effective treatment. Alternatively, this tumor can be treated satisfactorily by cryotherapy with *liquid nitrogen*. A preparation of 5% 5-FU, applied two to three times daily and covered by a plastic occlusive dressing for 6 weeks, may also be employed for treatment of Bowen's disease. Effective treatment of more advanced *squamous cell carcinomas* includes surgical *excision* and *radiation*; the latter is reserved for people older than 60 years of age.

Malignant melanomas can be divided into four primary pathologic categories. *Superficial spreading* melanoma is the most common in the United States and represents 70 percent of all malignant melanomas diagnosed. The early lesion exists 1 to 7 years before a nodule develops. The onset of a nodule indicates that deep penetration has occurred. Prior to penetration, the lesion grows superficially, and its removal during this time is associated with a 5-year survival rate approaching 100 percent.

Nodular melanoma has a poorer prognosis. It may arise de novo or within a nevus as an invasive tumor from the onset. Even with early recognition, metastasis will already have occurred in a substantial proportion of patients. This type of tumor can occur on any cutaneous surface, as can the superficial spreading melanoma. Nodular melanoma represents about 15 percent of all melanomas.

Lentigo maligna melanoma, the third type, accounts for about 5 percent of malignant melanomas and occurs on sun-damaged skin of elderly patients. It is the least aggressive of the melanomas and may be present for 5 or more years before an invasive nodule develops. Prior to nodule formation, the lesion is termed lentigo maligna. Local excision is satisfactory in the treatment of lentigo maligna. In lentigo maligna melanoma, excision with at least a 1-cm margin is advocated. Surgical outcome in this type of tumor is almost uniformly favorable, although recurrence is sometimes seen. It is unusual for a patient to die from disseminated lentigo maligna melanoma.

Acral lentiginous melanoma occurs on palms, soles, subungual areas, and mucous membranes. This is the most common type to affect blacks and orientals, but it may also occur in whites. The lesion begins as a flat, pigmented lesion that may be irregular in its border and pigment pattern. Early biopsy is essential to achieve cure before metastasis has occurred.

Prognosis. Systems for determining prognosis now exist so that the extent of surgery can be matched to the degree of severity of the lesion. The most widely used system is that of Breslow, in which measurement of the thickness of the primary tumor determines prognosis. Tumor thickness is measured with an ocular micrometer on a standard microscope from the granular cell layer down to the deepest tumor cell. Lesions thinner than 0.85 mm have nearly uniformly favorable prognosis, while those greater than 3.65 mm have a fairly poor prognosis (<0.85 mm, 99% 5-year survival; 0.85–1.69 mm, 94%; 1.70–3.64 mm, 78%; >3.65 mm, 42%).

Treatment. At present, *wide local excision* is the treatment recommended for primary melanoma. The width of excision in our institution is based on primary tumor thickness. For tumors up to 1.0 mm thick, 1.0-cm margins are recommended; 2-cm margins are recommended for tumors from 1.0 to 4.0 mm thick. As mentioned earlier, 1-cm margins are considered adequate for lentigo maligna melanoma regardless of thickness. The usefulness of elective *lymph node dissection* is still being debated; current evidence suggests that this procedure has no benefit over removal after the nodes become clinically involved. Nodal dissection is still useful as a staging procedure to identify high-risk patients, enabling meaningful stratification for adjuvant therapy studies.

The treatment of *disseminated melanoma* is at present a difficult and unrewarding problem. The most effective and widely used single agent, dacarbazine (dimethyl triazenoimidazole carboxamide DTIC), has a response rate of approximately 20 percent. The nitrosoureas have also been utilized and have approximately the same response rate. Even patients who respond usually relapse and die after a few months. Combinations of chemotherapy are currently being evaluated, as are new forms of immunotherapy. The addition of tamoxifen to dacarbazine appears to be helpful in women.

Since the prognosis in disseminated melanoma is poor, attempts are being made to use adjuvant therapy postoperatively in patients who are at high risk for recurrence. At present, none has proved beneficial.

Early surgical removal of *giant hairy nevus* (Fig. 177–1) is necessary to attempt to prevent development of malignancy. Others advocate a wait-and-see approach with regular follow-up.

SCREENING AND DIAGNOSTIC TESTS

Skin cancers are unique in their accessibility and the ease with which a tissue diagnosis can be made.

Basal cell carcinomas may take several forms. The typical appearance is that of a translucent papule with telangiectasias over the surface (Fig. 177–2) that slowly enlarges and subsequently develops a central ulceration (Fig. 177–3). This lesion has been termed the "rodent ulcer." Basal cell carcinoma may also become pigmented in darker-skinned individuals and be confused with malignant melanoma of the nodular or superficial spreading type. Superficial forms of basal cell carcinoma exist, most commonly on the back, and have the appearance of an erythematous plaque. Usually some papular elements are present at the border to assist in diagnosis. In the sclerotic form of basal cell carcinoma called the morpheaform basal cell carcinoma, nests of tumor cells are interspersed within thick fibrotic bundles. This tumor is more resistant to treatment.

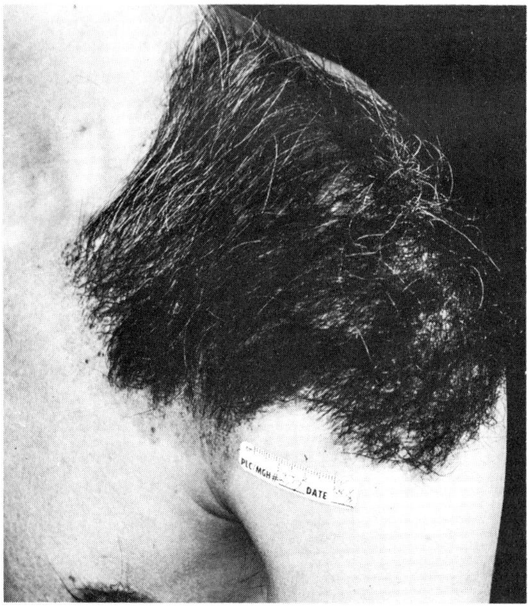

Figure 177-1. Giant hairy melanocytic nevus.

Differential diagnosis of basal cell carcinoma includes dermal nevi and other appendage tumors such as trichoepithelioma. Trichoepithelioma may be clinically indistinguishable from basal cell carcinoma. On histopathologic examination of a basal cell carcinoma, proliferation of basophilic cells is seen, usually in nests surrounded by discrete lacunae located in the upper dermis. This tumor is relatively easy for the pathologist to diagnose microscopically. Because basal cell carcinomas are more common in those who have already had one, patients should be followed on an annual basis for early detection of new lesions.

Squamous cell carcinoma is often preceded by *actinic keratosis*, which appears as flat to slightly raised, scaly erythematous patches, which may be single or multiple and occur in sun-exposed areas (Fig. 177–4). Often, this lesion is more easily felt (a sandpapery texture) than observed. It appears to go through cycles from macular erythematous le-

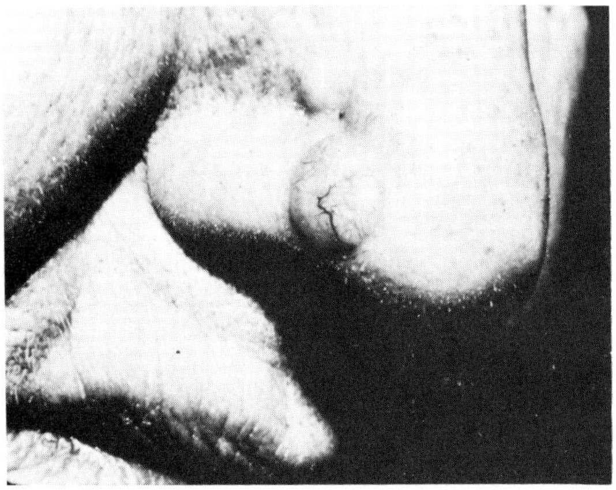

Figure 177-2. Nodular basal cell carcinoma. Note telangiectasia.

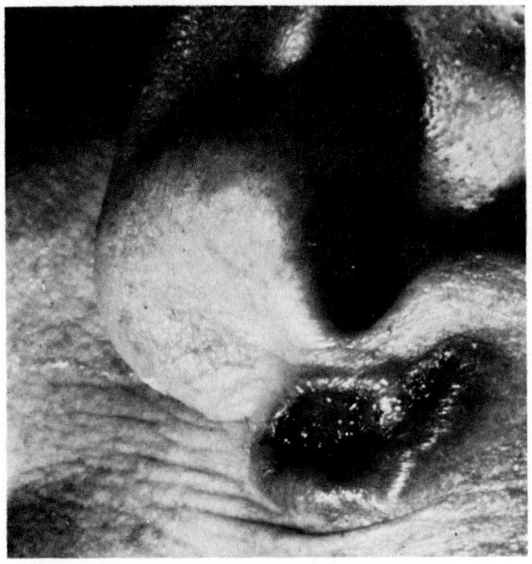

Figure 177-3. Basal cell carcinoma—"rodent ulcer."

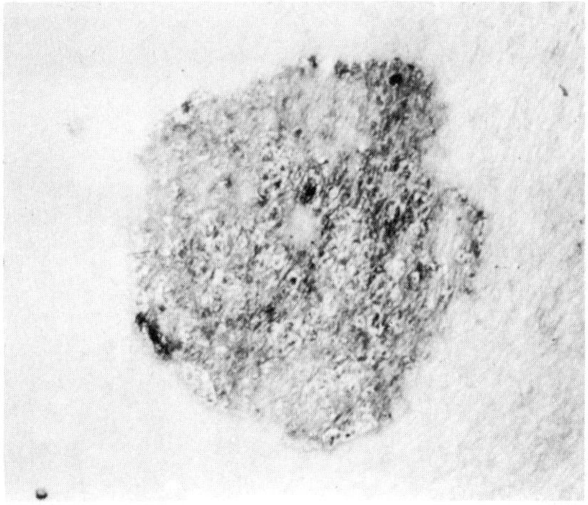

Figure 177-5. Bowen's disease—squamous cell carcinoma in situ.

sions through raised scaly lesions. In the later stages, a crusted surface, and sometimes even a horn of keratin, develop. Histopathologic examination of these lesions reveals atypical keratinocytes in the basal cell layer of the epidermis.

Bowen's disease, the carcinoma in situ stage, usually presents as a chronic, asymptomatic, nonhealing, slowly enlarging erythematous patch usually having a sharp but irregular outline. It may resemble eczematous dermatitis but does not respond to topical steroid therapy (Fig. 177–5). Within the patch, there are generally areas of crusting. The sharp borders, chronicity, and lack of symptoms are clues that suggest the necessity of performing a biopsy. In dark-skinned patients, such as those of Mediterranean descent, these lesions may have a brown to blue–gray coloration. Bowen's disease can occur on any part of the skin and on mucocutaneous sites such as the vulva. In the vulvar area, differential diagnosis includes lichen sclerosis et atrophicus, lichen simplex chronicus, squamous cell carcinoma, and, when pigmented, malignant melanoma. On histopathologic examination, atypical keratinocytes are noted throughout the epidermis. There is no invasion of keratinocytes into the dermis.

More advanced *squamous cell carcinoma* presents as a flesh-colored, asymptomatic nodule that enlarges and often undergoes ulceration and crusting (Fig. 177–6). The lesion may become keratotic and have a thickened surface. A cutaneous horn may result. Excisional biopsy with close margins is the procedure of choice for the diagnosis of this lesion. Squamous cell carcinoma may sometimes be confused with a benign keratinocytic lesion, which is dome-shaped and exhibits a prominent central plug called a keratoacanthoma (Fig. 177–7). The keratoacanthoma usually exhibits more rapid growth and often regresses spontaneously.

Under the microscope, the squamous cell carcinoma has fingers of atypical keratinocytic cells infiltrating into the dermis. The nuclei are clearly atypical; mitoses are frequently found.

Melanoma hallmarks include irregularity of the border (sometimes a notch is present; Fig. 177–8) and variegation in

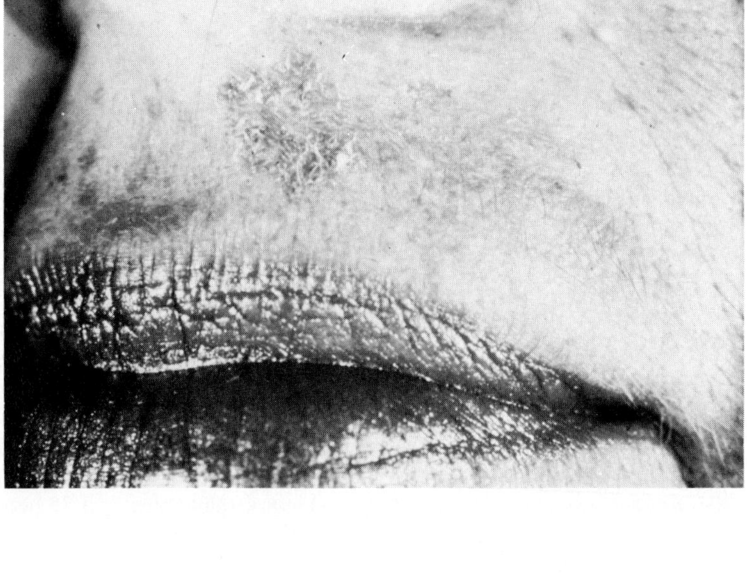

Figure 177-4. Actinic keratosis on the upper lip.

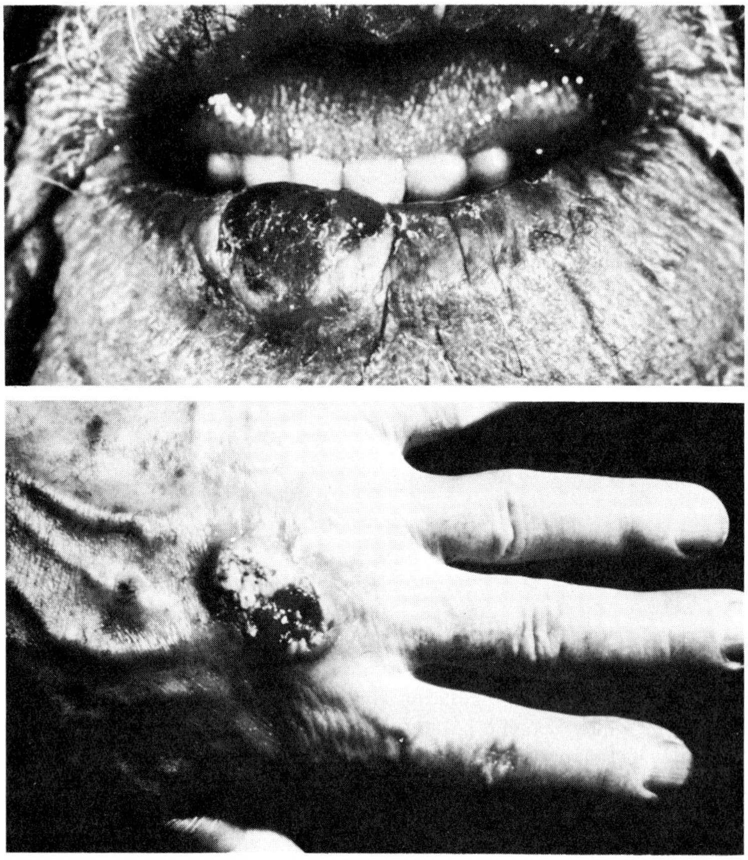

Figure 177-6. Squamous cell carcinoma in typical locations.

the color and pigmentation pattern. Colors in addition to brown and tan, such as red, white, blue, and their admixtures, grays, pinks, and purples, are of great use in distinguishing the overwhelming number of benign pigmented lesions from those that are melanomas.

The preceding characteristics are sometimes found in pigmented basal cell carcinoma and pigmented Bowen's disease lesions. In addition, odd dermal or compound nevi, irritated seborrheic keratoses, and occasionally vascular lesions are clinically confused with melanoma. The benign blue nevus also shares similar clinical features. Biopsy and histopathologic evaluation by the pathologist are warranted if a lesion meets the criteria previously noted.

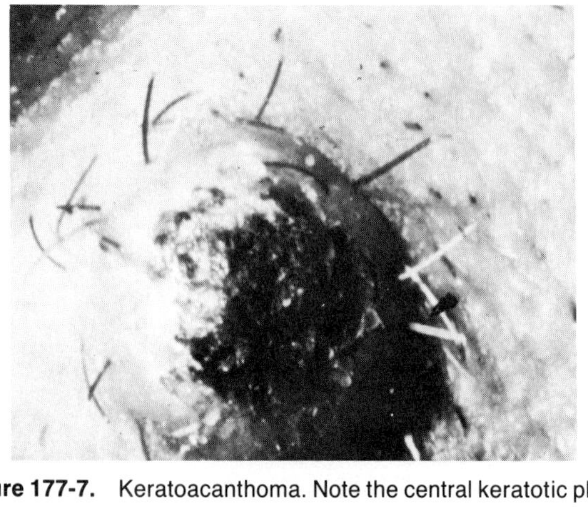

Figure 177-7. Keratoacanthoma. Note the central keratotic plug.

Each of the different types of melanoma has distinguishing features. *Superficial spreading melanomas* have some irregularity in the border and some alteration in the regularity of pigment pattern and coloration (see Figure 177–8). *Nodular melanoma*, which arises de novo or within nevi as an invasive tumor from the onset, has no radial growth component. It exists as a blue, blue-black, or gray nodule of varying size (Fig. 177–9). Most of these lesions are deeply invasive at the time of diagnosis. *Lentigo maligna* begins as a freckle-like lesion that slowly expands. It has a markedly irregular pigmentation pattern and usually an extremely irregular border. Spontaneous regression may occur; the border may advance on one side while regressing on another, so that the lesion appears to march across the skin surface. *Acral lentiginous* melanoma occurs on palms, soles, subungual areas, and mucous membranes, beginning as a flat pigmented lesion that may be irregular in its border and pigment pattern. Early biopsy is essential to achieve cure before metastasis has occurred.

Since about 2 percent of patients with melanoma develop a second primary tumor, it is worthwhile to examine the entire skin surface to look for the development of a second tumor on each encounter. In familial melanoma, as many as 30 percent of patients with melanoma may develop a second

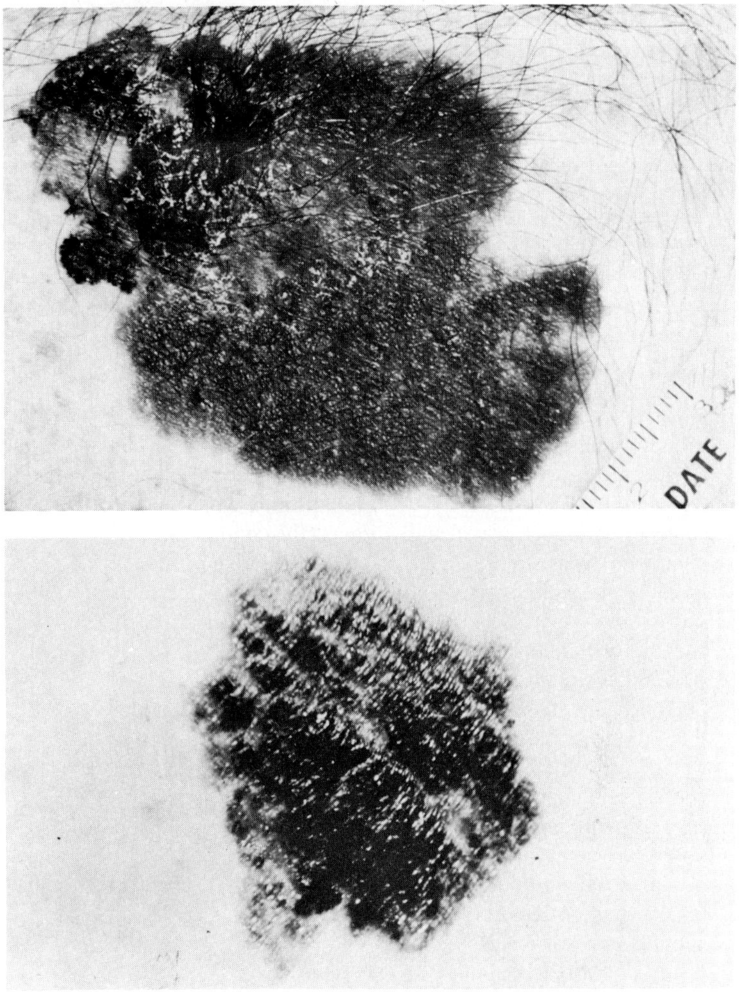

Figure 177-8. Malignant melanoma of the superficial spreading type. Note the irregularity of the border and prominent notch.

primary tumor. Because a trait favoring the development of melanoma appears to occur in families, family members of patients who have had melanoma should be examined.

Distribution of malignant melanoma across the body surface is not uniform. In both males and females, there is an aggregation on the back. In the female, the lower extremities are heavily affected, but they are spared in males, in whom the anterior torso is more likely to be involved. The bra and swim trunk areas are spared in the female, and the swim trunk area and thighs are spared in the male.

Recognition of suspicious pigmented lesions may be facilitated by the mnemonic *ABCD*: A = *asymmetry* of lesional shape; B = *border irregularity*; C = *color variegation*; D = *diameter greater than 6.0 mm* (the size of a pencil eraser tip).

CONCLUSIONS AND RECOMMENDATIONS FOR SCREENING AND PREVENTION

Screening for skin cancer represents one of the best examples of early detection leading to an improved outcome. For example, the current 5-year survival rate for malignant melanoma is 99 percent if lesions are thinner than 0.85 mm. It is estimated that by educating patients and physicians about signs of disease and the importance of early diagnosis,

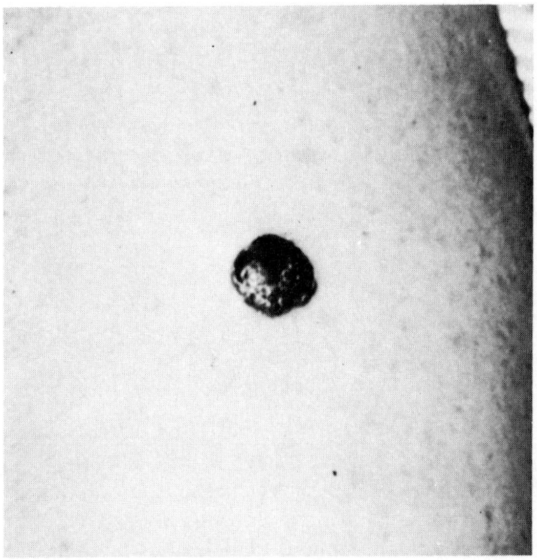

Figure 177-9. Malignant melanoma, nodular type.

the overall 5-year survival rate for malignant melanoma could approach 85 percent to 90 percent.

Every primary physician should be able to recognize the common skin cancers, and his patients should be taught to avoid risk factors and report suspicious lesions. In particular, the following precautions should be observed.

- All fair-skinned persons who sunburn easily and those in whom evidence of solar damage or skin cancer has already developed should be warned about the hazards of continued high-intensity solar exposure. They should be advised to avoid sun exposure between 11:00 AM and 2:30 PM, the period for 70 percent of harmful ultraviolet radiation.
- All persons at risk for skin cancer should be advised to use a broad-spectrum sunscreen when going out into the sun. The preparation should block some ultraviolet A (UVA) in addition to most UVB radiation and have a solar protection factor (SPF) of at least 15. Preparations which block some of the UVA wavelengths generally contain benzophenones, titanium dioxide, or dibenzoyl methane.
- Patients with a history of exposure to arsenic or previous x-ray therapy with radiation dermatitis should be watched closely for the development of cancer.
- In nonmelanomatous skin cancer, the patient should report any new, slowly growing, nodular or papular lesions that are flesh-colored or translucent and report to the physician if bleeding, ulceration, or horn formation occurs. Areas of maximum solar exposure are at greatest risk.
- In malignant melanoma, the patient is asked to see the physician about any pigmented lesion that has an irregular border or a variation in color, especially blue, gray, or black. Any growth in a pigmented lesion or change in color should also arouse suspicion.
- If any doubt exists about the benignancy of a skin lesion, the primary physician's obligation is either to biopsy the lesion or to refer the patient to an experienced specialist for an opinion. If patients and physicians work together, the incidence of skin cancer and the deaths associated with it can be greatly reduced.

ANNOTATED BIBLIOGRAPHY

Balch CM, et al (eds). Cutaneous Melanoma. 2nd ed. Philadelphia: JB Lippincott, 1992. *(Comprehensive coverage of cutaneous melanoma.)*

Cancer Manual, 8th ed. American Cancer Society, Massachusetts Division, 1990. *(Practical sections on non-melanotic and melanotic skin cancers.)*

Cocconi G, Bella M, Calabresi F, et al. Treatment of metastatic malignant melanoma with dacarbazine plus tamoxifen. N Engl J Med 1992;327:516. *(Dacarbazine plus tamoxifen was superior to dacarbazine alone in women.)*

Fitzpatrick TB, Sober AJ. Sunlight and skin cancer. N Engl J Med 1985;313:818. *(An editorial; reviews the evidence for sun exposure as the principal risk factor for skin cancer.)*

Friedman RJ, et al (eds). Cancer of the Skin. Philadelphia: WB Saunders, 1991. *(Recent compendium on all aspects of skin cancer.)*

Friedman RJ, Rigel DS, Kopf AW. Early detection of malignant melanoma: the role of physician examination and self-examination of the skin. CA Cancer J Clin 1985;35:130. *(Reprints available from the American Cancer Society. Can be used to instruct patients in self-examination of the skin.)*

Greene MH, Clark WH, Tucker MA, et al. Acquired precursors of malignant melanoma. N Engl J Med 1985;312:91. *(An important description of the natural history of both common and dysplastic nevi, including a color atlas. An accompanying editorial provides a perspective on melanoma risk associated with dysplastic nevi.)*

Koh HK. Cutaneous melanoma. N Engl J Med 1991;325;171. *(Recent review.)*

Lever WF, Schaumburg-Lever G. Tumors and cysts of the epidermis; Tumors of the epidermal appendages. In: Histopathology of the Skin. 7th ed. Philadelphia: JB Lippincott, 1990. *(Clinical and histopathologic description of cutaneous malignancies.)*

Luftman DB, Lowe NJ, Moy RL. Sunscreens: update and review. J Dermatol Surg Oncol 1991;17:744. *(Useful summary; helpful for advising patients.)*

Mihm MC, Fitzpatrick TB, Lane-Brown MM, et al. Early detection of primary cutaneous malignant melanoma: A color atlas. N Engl J Med 1973;289:989. *(Eighteen color plates illustrating typical malignant melanomas.)*

National Institutes of Health Consensus Development Panel. Precursors to malignant melanoma. JAMA 1984;251:1864. *(Consensus statement including descriptions, evidence regarding risk of melanoma, and management recommendations for both dysplastic and congenital nevi.)*

Sober AJ, Fitzpatrick TB, Mihm MC, et al. Early recognition of cutaneous melanoma. JAMA 1979;242:2795. *(Self-assessment approach to the recognition of early lesions in this color atlas.)*

Stiller MJ, Davis JC, Shupock JL. A concise guide to topical sunscreens: state of the art. Int J Dermatol 1992;31:540. *(Includes consideration of preparations blocking UVA.)*

Thompson SC, Jolley D, Marks R. Reduction of solar keratoses by regular sunscreen use. N Engl J Med 1993;329:1147. *(Study supports values of regular sunscreen use.)*

178
Evaluation of Pruritus

STEPHEN J. FRIEDMAN, M.D.

Primary Care Medicine: Office Evaluation and Management of the Adult Patient, 3rd edition, edited by Allan H. Goroll, Lawrence A. May, and Albert G. Mulley, Jr. J.B. Lippincott Company, Philadelphia

Pruritus is an unpleasant cutaneous sensation that provokes the urge to scratch. It may be localized or generalized and may occur with or without skin lesions. Itching may be caused by a dermatologic condition, systemic illness, or psychological disturbance. The complaint is particularly common among the elderly. It can pose a real challenge when the etiology remains elusive and symptoms interfere with daily functioning. The primary physician should be capable of performing a reasonably detailed evaluation and providing effective symptomatic relief.

PATHOPHYSIOLOGY AND CLINICAL PRESENTATION

Pathophysiology. The sensation of itching arises from free nerve endings of the skin. These fibers are especially concentrated in the flexor aspects of the wrist and ankles. Afferent transmission is through unmyelinated C fibers to the dorsal horn of the spinal cord, ascending to the contralateral spinothalamic tracts and terminating in the cerebral cortex. The scratch response is a spinal reflex. Many chemical mediators and modulators of itch have been suggested, including substance P, opioid and non-opioid peptides, somatostatin, neurokinin A, histamine, serotonin, kinins, and prostaglandins.

Various external stimuli decrease the threshold for itching. These include inflammation, heat, dryness, and vasodilation. Persons vary in their response to itching. There is a psychological influence on the perception of itching, which explains why a physician may experience itching after attending a patient with scabies or pediculosis.

Clinical Presentations. Pruritus may be localized or generalized and can occur with or without skin lesions. Pruritus from a systemic disease can occur with or without a primary skin lesion.

Dermatologic Disease. A host of dermatologic conditions can present with itching, including pediculosis and scabies (see Chapter 195), contact dermatitis (see Chapter 184), urticaria (see Chapter 181), psoriasis (see Chapter 187), lichen planus, and dermatitis herpetiformis. Dry skin (xerosis) is the most frequent precipitant and is particularly common in the elderly. Symptoms are worse in the winter or with use of air conditioning, which lowers indoor humidity. Tangential light reveals fine scaling and cracking. Patients with urticaria usually give a history of wheals and demonstrate dermographism (urticaria on stroking the skin with a blunt object). Scabies and dermatitis herpetiformis can be particularly subtle in presentation, with few skin manifestations at the time of initial presentation. In dermatitis herpetiformis, vesicles are characteristic, but excoriations may obliterate them. An intense burning sensation often predates appearance of skin lesions. Scabies is endemic in long-term care facilities. In persons with good hygiene, there may be fewer than 10 of the characteristic burrowing-induced skin lesions (see Chapter 195). At times, the only finding may be nonspecific papules caused by an immune skin response.

Renal Disease. Pruritus may accompany severe chronic renal failure, especially in patients receiving hemodialysis. Secondary hyperparathyroidism causing elevated levels of histamine is one suspected mechanism. Other investigations have implicated endopeptidases or kinins as substances that can accumulate in uremia.

Endocrine Disease. Generalized itching occurs among 4 percent to 11 percent of patients with Graves' disease, usually when the disease is long-standing. Increased kinin activity and slightly elevated skin temperatures are suggested mechanisms. The mechanisms for other endocrinopathies are poorly understood.

Liver Disease. Of the liver diseases, obstructive cholestatic jaundice produces the most pruritus. Itching may be especially prominent and can be the presenting manifestation in primary biliary cirrhosis. About 20 percent to 25 percent of patients with jaundice are plagued with itching, though it is rare in the absence of cholestasis. Pruritus of cholestasis has been linked to release of proteases in the skin by the bile salts. Itching during the last trimester of pregnancy has been reported in up to 1 percent to 3 percent of expectant women and is thought to be cholestatic in origin, though jaundice is uncommon.

Hematologic Disease. The itching of polycythemia vera affects 30 percent to 50 percent of patients and is exacerbated by a hot shower or bath. In mycosis fungoides, pruritus has been suggested as an adverse prognostic factor. Lymphoma and Hodgkin's disease may also cause pruritus; its role as a prognostic indicator is less than previously thought. Histamine release by an increased number of circulating basophils is a suggested pathophysiologic mechanism. Pruritus has also been found in association with iron deficiency anemia and with human immunodeficiency virus (HIV) infection. Mechanisms are unclear.

Psychiatric Disease. Patients with neurotic scratching report that they scratch even in the absence of itching. Itching is reported to occur more often at night, when other stimuli are lacking. Although the excoriations of this "neurodermatitis" may occur anywhere the patient can reach, they tend to be concentrated to the extremities. Depression and dyphoric mood are particularly common among such patients, as are serious conflict and situational stress preceding onset of pruritus.

DIFFERENTIAL DIAGNOSIS

The conditions that cause itching may be dermatologic, systemic, or psychological in origin (Table 178–1). Skin disorders account for the vast majority. The pruritus may be localized or generalized. Localized itching is usually a sign of a primary dermatologic condition, dermatophyte infection, infestation, or psychological disorder. Generalized itching raises the possibility of a systemic condition or a psychogenic etiology, though dermatologic disease still predominates. In the elderly, the most common cause of itching remains xerosis.

WORKUP

A search for a primary dermatologic disease or infestation is the first step in the evaluation of the pruritic patient. Often a careful look at the skin combined with a few clues from the history suggests the diagnosis. Skin diseases associated with recognizable lesions and characteristic distribution usually do not present significant diagnostic difficulty, unless camouflaged by excoriations, lichenification, secondary eczematizations, or infection. Systemic illnesses require a more detailed history and physical examination that extends beyond the skin, followed by selected laboratory studies.

Table 178-1. Conditions Associated with Pruritus

Dermatologic
Arthropod bites and stings
Bullous pemphigoid
Dermatitis
  Atopic dermatitis
  Contact dermatitis (allergic and irritant)
  Dermatitis herpetiformis
Dermatophytosis
Infestation
  Scabies
  Pediculosis
Lichen planus
Lichen simplex chronicus
Pityriasis rosea
Psoriasis
Urticaria and dermatographism
Varicella
Xerosis

Psychological
Neurotic excoriations
Depression
Delusions of parasitosis

Systemic
Hyperthyroidism
Renal failure, chronic
Drug reaction
Hematologic disease
  Iron deficiency anemia
  Mycosis fungoides
  Polycythemia vera
  Paraproteinemia
  Systemic mastocytosis
Hepatobiliary problems
  Intrahepatic cholestasis
  Extrahepatic obstruction
  Third trimester of pregnancy
Malignancy
  Malignant carcinoid
  Lymphoma, leukemia
  Multiple myeloma
HIV Infection
Parasitosis
  Ascariasis
  Hookworm
  Onchocerciasis
  Trichinosis

History. Location, associated symptoms, precipitants, clinical course, and severity (including effect on sleep and daily activity) should be carefully elicited. A detailed description of any skin changes or rashes should be included. If the patient reports little in the way of skin findings, clues to an underlying dermatologic condition should still be sought. For example, a history of atopy, asthma, or urticaria raises the probability of an allergic origin, while concurrent pruritus in household members is suggestive of scabies, and worsening in winter points to dry skin. Environmental factors such as sunburn, cats, fiberglass, prickly heat, and overdrying of the skin also deserve consideration. Pharmacologic exposure is important to review, because a subclinical allergic reaction may occur with almost any drug. One should also check specifically for use of opiates, amphetamines, quinidine, aspirin, B vitamins, and niacinamide.

In the setting of generalized pruritus, one should inquire about symptoms or a history of hyperthyroidism (see Chapter 103), renal failure (see Chapter 142), lymphoma (see Chapter 84), polycythemia (see Chapter 80), cholestatic liver disease (see Chapter 62), and HIV infection (see Chapter 13). Pregnancy should be suspected as the cause if the patient is a woman in her third trimester.

If the cause is not evident from the medical history, it is worth exploring psychosocial aspects of the patient's life and any relation between psychological or situational stresses and the onset of pruritus. Given the high prevalence of depression among patients with idiopathic pruritus, inquiry into symptoms of depression (see Chapter 227) may prove useful.

Physical Examination. A careful and complete inspection of the skin is essential. The presence and distribution of a rash, excoriations, lichenification, and inflammatory changes should be noted along with any evidence for xerosis (scaling and dryness). Dry skin is especially evident on the legs; tangential lighting can help reveal the scaling.

If the complaint is localized, a more detailed look at the involved area is needed. The scalp is checked for psoriasis and seborrhea; the trunk for urticaria, scabies, and the linear lesions of contact dermatitis; the inguinal area for *Candida*, pediculosis, tinea, and scabies; the hands for eczema, contact dermatitis, and the telltale interdigital lesions of scabies; the legs for neurotic excoriations, stasis dermatitis, atopic dermatitis (popliteal fossa), lichen simplex (lateral malleoli), and dermatitis herpetiformis (knees); and the feet for tinea and contact lesions.

If the pruritus is generalized and there is no evidence of primary dermatologic disease, a search for signs of a systemic condition is warranted. The skin is examined for jaundice and findings associated with HIV disease (see Chapter 13), the sclerae are checked for icterus, the lymph nodes for enlargement, the thyroid for goiter, and the liver and spleen for organomegaly.

Laboratory Studies. Test selection should be based on findings from the history and physical examination. Resorting initially to a "pan-scan" is wasteful and likely to generate false-positive results. Skin scrapings are performed to confirm a clinical diagnosis of scabies or dermatophytosis (see Chapters 191 and 195). A skin biopsy examination with special stains or direct immunofluorescence may be required to confirm a diagnosis of mastocytosis, mycosis fungoides, or one of the autoimmune bullous diseases. In the setting of suspected cholestasis, one should order serum bilirubin, alkaline phosphatase, and transaminase levels and obtain an ultrasound of the biliary tree (see Chapter 62). If there is concern for lymphoma or carcinoid, a chest x-ray or abdominal computed tomography scan may be indicated (see Chapters 44 and 84). HIV testing is indicated if the patient has a history of high-risk behavior (see Chapter 13).

If the diagnosis continues to be elusive, then a complete blood count, blood urea nitrogen (BUN), thyroid-stimulating hormone (TSH), calcium, albumin, and globulin are worth considering. Pruritus per se is not a predictor of malignancy and need not trigger a workup for occult malignancy in the absence of other clinical evidence for cancer.

SYMPTOMATIC THERAPY AND PATIENT EDUCATION

To be most effective, treatment of pruritus should be etiologic if possible. However, nonspecific symptomatic measures are sometimes needed, especially if workup is still in progress and the itching is disturbing sleep and interfering with daily life. Symptomatic treatment is also indicated for refractory conditions (eg, biliary cirrhosis). Even if little can be done for the underlying condition, relief from itching is greatly appreciated. Avoidance of provocative factors is important, complemented by simple empiric therapy of low toxicity. Teaching the patient how to overcome the itch–scratch–itch cycle is most beneficial.

Behavioral and Topical Measures. Patients should be told to trim their fingernails, to keep them clean to prevent excoriation or infection, and to rub with their palms rather than their fingers if they have an uncontrollable urge to scratch. If vasodilating drugs or foods such as coffee, spices, or alcohol precipitate itching, they should be avoided. Changing one sheet at a time helps reduce the static electricity that can precipitate itching. Rough clothing, particularly wool, should be avoided. Cotton clothing that has been doubly rinsed of detergents is preferred. Humidification of the indoor environment should be maintained when using an air conditioner and during the winter, either with humidifiers or by placing bowls of water near radiators. Frequent and prolonged showering are to be avoided because they eliminate the skin's normal oil protection, contributing to dryness. Mild soaps (Dove, Basis, Neutrogena, Purpose) are preferred to drying, antiperspirant soap products. Use of hot water is discouraged, because it worsens itching by increasing cutaneous blood flow.

Such behavioral measures can be helpful regardless of etiology and often reduce or eliminate itching without the need to resort to additional measures. Additional topical approaches include sponging the skin with cool water and lubrication before bedtime. However, only lotions and creams recommended by the physician should be used. Simple *emollient* preparations (Moisturel, Eucerin, Lubriderm) are encouraged, especially after bathing. It can be useful to add Alpha Keri or other lubricating agents to the rinse cycle when sheets are washed.

Preparations containing combinations of *menthol, phenol,* and *camphor* (eg, Sarna) applied several times daily may provide symptomatic relief. *Calamine* lotion is adequate but drying; it is most useful on weeping lesions. *Pramoxine*-containing products (Pramegel, Prax, Pramosone) also may reduce itching, but other topical anesthetics and antihistamines should be avoided because they can be potent sensitizers. *Hydrocortisone* may provide symptomatic relief of itch; however, high potency corticosteroids should be restricted to specific steroid-responsive dermatoses because prolonged use can cause dermal atrophy.

If environmental manipulation and topical agents are not effective, then systemic medications must be considered.

Systemic Measures. The systemic medications most commonly used are antihistamines, sedatives, and aspirin. By occupying the histamine receptors, the *H_1-blocker antihistamines* are very effective for allergen-mediated itch. In non-allergic itch, antihistamines are no more effective than aspirin but are often worth a try. Their sedative quality makes them useful as a bedtime medication in patients who have sleep difficulties. The choice of an ideal agent is found by trial and error on the basis of the placebo, sedative, and anticholinergic effects of the drug. *Hydroxyzine* (eg, 25 mg tid or qhs) is among the most effective of these agents. It is mildly to moderately sedating and more effective than diphenhydramine or cyproheptadine, other commonly used antihistamines. Diphenhydramine is available without prescription and is very sedating. Nonsedating antihistamines such as astemizole (Hismanal) and terfenadine (Seldane) are useful for daytime use where histamine plays a primary role, such as in urticaria, but are generally disappointing as antipruritics and do little to help the patient fall asleep. *H_2-blockers* are generally ineffective in the treatment of idiopathic pruritus, but cimetidine has been reported useful in itching associated with polycythemia or uremia.

Mild anti-inflammatory agents such as *aspirin* are occasionally useful for symptomatic relief, especially if the suspected mechanism is kinin- or prostaglandin-mediated. Systemic steroids suppress itching but should not be used for symptomatic relief.

Sedatives, especially the benzodiazepines, can be useful in acute circumstances associated with anxiety and difficulty falling asleep, but chronic use is to be avoided because of risk of habituation (see Chapter 226). *Antidepressants* are helpful in psychogenic cases in which there is evidence of concurrent depression. Doxepin, an antidepressant with antihistaminic properties, is particularly useful and may be given before bedtime. *Pimozide*, a neuroleptic, is effective for treating delusions of parasitosis.

The *chelating agents* cholestyramine and colestipol are used with benefit for cholestatic itching, including the pruritus of pregnancy. *Ultraviolet* radiation (ultraviolet B, psoralens with ultraviolet A [PUVA]) can be used for *renal* and *biliary pruritus* as well as itching associated with other systemic and primary dermatologic disorders. Recalcitrant uremic pruritus has been treated with photochemotherapy, intravenous xylocaine, activated charcoal, intravenous erythropoietin, exchange transfusion, and parathyroidectomy, with varying degrees of success. Topical *capsaicin* has been shown to be effective. The opiate antagonist *naloxone* has been shown in some studies to improve pruritus, and in others it appeared to worsen it.

INDICATIONS FOR REFERRAL

The patient with refractory or idiopathic pruritus poses a very frustrating problem that often benefits from a dermatologic consultation and consideration of skin biopsy. The consultation lets the patient know that the problem is being taken seriously and that everything is being done to address both its cause and the patient's discomfort. When pruritus represents a somatic response to psychological distress, it may be useful to consider a mental health referral with the patient.

ANNOTATED BIBLIOGRAPHY

Bernhard JD. Pruritus: Advances in treatment. Advances in Dermatology 1990;6:57. *(Comprehensive review of therapy.)*

Breneman DL, Cardone JS, Blumsack RF, et al. Topical capsaicin for treatment of hemodialysis-related pruritus. J Am Acad Dermatol 1992;26:91. *(Topical capsaicin qid relieved hemodialysis-related pruritus in 10 of 14 patients.)*

De Marchi S, Cecchin E, Villalta D, et al. Relief of pruritus and decreases in plasma histamine concentrations during erythropoietin therapy in patients with uremia N Engl J Med 1992;326:969. *(Significantly decreased pruritus and lowered plasma histamine concentrations in 20 patients with uremia.)*

Denman ST. A review of pruritus. J Am Acad Dermatol 1986; 14:375. *(A superb review emphasizing pathophysiology, workup, and treatment; 142 refs.)*

Fruensgaard K. Neurotic excoriations: a controlled psychiatric examination. Acta Psychiatr Scand 1984;69(suppl 312):3. *(High prevalence of depression; lesions often confined to the extremities.)*

Greco PJ, Ende J. Pruritus: a practical approach. J Gen Intern Med 1992;7:340. *(Very useful evaluation strategy outlined.)*

Kligman AM. Water-induced itching without cutaneous sign. Arch Dermatol 1986;122:183. *(A well-characterized subset of elderly patients with itching due to age, dry skin, and seasonal weather conditions; they respond well to local measures.)*

Lober CW. Should the patient with generalized pruritus be evaluated for malignancy? J Am Acad Dermatol 1988;19:350. *(Patients with persistent pruritus do not show increased risk for malignant disease when carefully compared with age- and sex-matched nonpruritic controls.)*

179
Evaluation of Purpura

Primary Care Medicine: Office Evaluation and Management of the Adult Patient, 3rd edition, edited by Allan H. Goroll, Lawrence A. May, and Albert G. Mulley, Jr. J.B. Lippincott Company, Philadelphia

Purpura represents bleeding into the skin. In the office setting, patients present complaining of easy bruising, spontaneous ecchymoses, or a petechial rash. Although many cases of purpura are caused by unappreciated trauma, patients who complain of easy bruising or spontaneous ecchymoses need to be evaluated for an underlying bleeding disorder (see Chapter 81). Those with petechial rashes may have a platelet problem, vasculitis, or a bacteremia. The primary physician should be able to make these distinctions and efficiently initiate the evaluation.

PATHOPHYSIOLOGY AND CLINICAL PRESENTATION

The integrity of small vessels is maintained by quantitatively and qualitatively adequate platelets and healthy connective tissue. Normally, a break in a vessel triggers prompt formation of a platelet plug followed by a fibrin clot. Purpura occurs when there is a disturbance in the integrity of the vessel wall or the mechanisms of hemostasis.

Purpura is divided in petechial and ecchymotic categories. *Petechiae* are red macules that measure less than 3 mm in diameter and reflect a defect in platelets or vessel walls. When caused by disturbances of platelets, petechiae present in dependent areas such as the ankles and lower legs (see Chapter 81). Immune-mediated inflammation of small vessels may also produce petechial macules, sometimes progressing to palpable lesions (so-called *"palpable purpura"*—see below).

Ecchymoses are purpuric lesions greater than 3 mm in diameter. They may result from trauma or a clotting factor disorder as well as from a vascular or platelet problem. Clotting factor dysfunction causes delayed but more prolonged blood loss, during which continuous oozing due to inadequate fibrin clot formation results in ecchymoses rather than petechiae (see Chapter 81).

The mechanisms of purpura can be divided into the thrombocytopenic, thrombocytopathic, coagulopathic, vascular, connective tissue, and idiopathic varieties. The first three are discussed in detail in Chapter 81. The vascular, connective tissue, and idiopathic varieties require further elaboration here.

Vascular Defects

These range from mild disruption of the endothelium to necrotizing injury. The latter are the more important.

Small vessel vasculitis of a *leukocytoclastic* variety is capable of damaging vessel walls and causing palpable purpura. It usually occurs in the context of a *hypersensitivity reaction* or *rheumatoid disease*, but causes range from dysproteinemias to immune-related gastrointestinal conditions (Table 179–1). In the hypersensitivity variety, there is immunologically mediated, necrotizing neutrophilic infiltration of arterioles, capillaries, and venules. The process can be systemic, but it is often limited to the skin. In rheumatoid disease, the postcapillary venules are the principal site of leukocytoclastic injury; systemic involvement is the rule.

The skin lesions of leukocytoclastic vasculitis typically begin as small macules that become palpable and may turn confluent or nodular. The petechial papules do not blanch; they appear in symmetric fashion and predominate in dependent areas. Urticaria, vesicles, and necrotic ulcerations may also develop. Fever, arthralgias, myalgias, arthritis, pulmonary infiltrates, effusions, pericarditis, peripheral neuropathy, abdominal pain, bleeding, and encephalopathy can occur along with the petechial rash if there is systemic

Table 179-1. Important Causes of Leukocytoclastic Vasculitis

Connective Tissue Disease
Systemic lupus erythematosus
Rheumatoid arthritis
Sjögren's syndrome
Hypersensitivity Vasculitis
serum sickness
drugs (penicillins, thiazides, aspirin, amphetamines)
Dysproteinemias
Cryoglobulinemia (mixed type)
Waldenströms' purpura
Immune-Related Gastrointestinal Disease
Ulcerative colitis
Primary biliary cirrhosis
Chronic active hepatitis
Hypocomplementemic Vasculitis

involvement. The skin commonly itches, stings, or burns. Hematuria and proteinuria are often detected.

Bacteremia can lead to vascular injury and formation of petechiae, which are sometimes palpable. Petechial lesions associated with *subacute bacterial endocarditis* are flat, do not blanch, and appear on the upper chest, neck, and extremities in addition to the mucous membranes. In *gonococcal* and *meningococcal septicemias*, petechiae develop early, become pustular, and then turn hemorrhagic and necrotic. The lower extremities are a common site for the gonococcal lesions, which resolve within 5 to 7 days. The rash of *Rocky Mountain spotted fever* begins as pink macules on the wrists, soles, ankles, and palms. The rash spreads centripetally and by the fourth day becomes petechial and papular. Hemorrhagic, ulcerated lesions may follow.

Other forms of vascular injury include *stasis dermatitis*, which causes petechial lesions in the legs resulting from capillary injury. *Scurvy* compromises the vascular endothelium, and perifollicular purpura develops because of increased capillary fragility. In *amyloidosis*, deposition of amyloid in the skin and subcutaneous tissue causes fragile vessels, with ecchymoses forming when the skin is pinched.

Connective tissue defects compromise vessel walls and supportive extravascular structures and lead to easy bruising. When caused by degeneration of dermal collagen from *age* or *corticosteroid use*, ecchymoses may develop from trivial injury and be noticed on the face, neck, dorsum of the hands, forearms, or legs. A variant is stasis or orthostatic purpura, usually occurring in the lower extremities of an elderly patient following a prolonged period of standing.

Idiopathic causes include *autoerythrocyte sensitization*, a puzzling form of purpura characterized by spontaneous, painful ecchymoses surrounded by erythema and edema. Headache, nausea, and vomiting sometimes accompany the purpura. Many patients with this condition also have pronounced psychoneurotic complaints. The mechanism is unknown, but intradermal injection of autologous red cells or DNA can reproduce the clinical picture.

Purpura simplex or *easy bruising syndrome* is an idiopathic condition of young women in otherwise good health. All platelet and bleeding parameters are normal, and there is no increased risk of hemorrhage from surgery or childbirth.

Platelet and Clotting Factor Disorders

Platelet and clotting factor disorders are discussed in Chapter 81.

DIFFERENTIAL DIAGNOSIS

The causes of purpura can be divided into thrombocytopenic, thrombocytopathic, clotting factor, vascular, connective tissue, and idiopathic categories (Table 179–2; see also Chapter 81). The most common causes are trauma, drug-induced impairment of platelet function, benign purpura simplex, and senile purpura. Vasculitis is particularly troublesome because of the wide range of potentially important causes (see Table 179–1).

WORKUP

The workup of the patient complaining of purpuric lesions must emphasize history and physical examination to avoid costly, nonproductive laboratory evaluations. The clinical findings are also essential in quickly differentiating serious hematologic, vasculitic, or infectious pathologies from more benign processes. For example, ecchymoses smaller than 6 cm, localized to such areas of trauma as the thighs, are less likely to be of pathologic significance than larger ones; palpable purpuric lesions indicate a vasculitic process; and petechial macules in dependent areas suggest a problem with platelets.

History. A careful description of the location, size, and clinical course of the purpuric lesions, along with inquiry into associated symptoms and precipitants, comprises the essence of the history. One should quickly screen for a bleeding diathesis by inquiring into blood loss from other sites, easy bruisability, bleeding into a joint, history of abnormally heavy bleeding with menstruation, surgery, or dental work, and family history of a bleeding problem. A review of medications is essential, focusing on agents that can in-

Table 179-2. Important Causes of Nonvasculitic Purpura

Connective Tissue Defects
Age (senile purpura)
Corticosteroid excess
Vascular Defects
Trauma
Venous stasis
Amyloidosis
Scurvy
Hereditary hemorrhagic telangiectasia
Idiopathic Conditions
Purpura simplex (easy bruising syndrome)
Autoerythrocyte sensitization
Quantitative Platelet Disorders (See Chapter 81)
Qualitative Platelet Disorders (See Chapter 81)
Clotting Factor Disorders (See Chapter 81)

terfere with platelet function (eg, aspirin, nonsteroidal anti-inflammatory drugs, dipyridamole, ticlopidine, sulfinpyrazone) and those that are associated with hypersensitivity reactions affecting platelets (eg, antibiotics, quinidine, phenothiazines). Any history of renal or hepatocellular failure is important to note.

Patients complaining of an early petechial rash or palpable purpura should have their systems carefully checked for fever, pruritus, joint pain, urticaria, dry mouth/dry eyes, morning stiffness, pleuritic pain, abdominal pain, melena, hematuria, lymphadenopathy, jaundice, symptoms of inflammatory bowel disease, chronic leg edema, and paresthesias. A recent streptococcal or staphylococcal infection may be responsible for a hypersensitivity vasculitis and should be noted. Medications to be reviewed include recent use of a penicillin, a thiazide, aspirin, or amphetamines. If fever is prominent, bacteremia must be considered, and the patient should be asked about recent purulent penile or vaginal discharge, pelvic pain, other recent infection, intravenous drug abuse, human immunodeficiency virus infection, and history of a heart murmur or recent dental work.

Physical examination begins with inspection of the skin lesions. If they appear petechial, it is useful to press a glass slide over them. Failure to blanch helps differentiate petechiae from nonpurpuric skin lesions. However, blanching lesions must not be dismissed too hastily, because telangiectasias and spider angiomas are signs of conditions predisposing to purpura (see Chapter 81). Shining a light tangentially to the skin is a sensitive means of detecting elevated lesions, which may be confirmed by careful palpation. The size, number, and location of purpuric lesions should be recorded and note made of whether they are palpable or macular, petechial or ecchymotic. It is sometimes helpful to circle ecchymoses so that extension or regression can be followed objectively.

If history suggests a bleeding problem or physical examination reveals petechiae in dependent areas or large ecchymoses, then the physical examination should be directed toward hematologic causes (see Chapter 81).

If palpable purpura is present, then key elements of the physical should include inspection for splinter hemorrhages, rheumatoid nodules, a separate malar rash, dry mucous membranes, jaundice, lymphadenopathy, pleural effusion, heart murmur, pericardial rub, hepatic abnormalities, purulent vaginal or urethral discharge, joint inflammation, and changes of stasis dermatitis.

If the history reveals only easy bruising and there is no evidence for hematologic or vasculitic pathology, then consideration of connective tissue and idiopathic causes is in order. Does the patient appear cushingoid or have a history of chronic corticosteroid use? Is the patient elderly with multiple small ecchymotic lesions in areas of minor everyday trauma? Are the ecchymoses tender in the absence of trauma? Is the patient an otherwise healthy young woman with easy bruising and relatively small ecchymoses?

Laboratory Studies. There is no standard battery of laboratory tests for the patient with purpura. To give meaningful information, study selection must be based on the clinical findings.

Suspected Hematologic Disease. Patients with flat petechial rashes should be checked for platelet-related pathology by ordering a *platelet count* and *bleeding time.* Those with large ecchymoses may have a clotting factor problem and are best screened by measuring the *prothrombin time (PT)* and *partial thromboplastin time (PTT).* Other hematologic testing may also be in order. (See Chapter 81 for more details of the hematologic evaluation.)

If palpable purpura is noted, the first priority is to rule out bacteremia. History and physical examination often provide important clues, but two sets of *blood cultures* should also be obtained at the outset, especially if there is fever or other manifestations of infection. If rheumatoid disease is a clinical suspicion, one can screen for *antinuclear antibodies (ANAs)* and *rheumatoid factor*, though the results may be nonspecific (see Chapter 146). Finding red cells on *urinalysis* or a positive *stool guaiac* may provide additional evidence for a systemic vasculitis, but the best means of confirming vasculitis is to perform a *skin biopsy* on one of the palpable, purpuric skin lesions. In addition to histologic processing, the biopsy specimen should also be cultured and Gram-stained.

If a leukocytoclastic vasculitis is confirmed, then more specific testing can be conducted if clinically indicated. The otherwise healthy patient with resolving skin lesions and nothing more than a recent history of using a potentially offending drug needs no further evaluation. If the lesions persist, more testing may be in order. Elderly persons are at risk for dysproteinemias; a serum *immunoelectrophoresis* should be considered. *Cryoprotein* and *serum complement* determinations may prove useful in diagnosis of a young woman with leukocytoclastic histology. Consultation with a rheumatologist is advised in optimizing test selection of the patient with vasculitis.

PATIENT EDUCATION

Detailed reassurance needs to be given to the patient with no hematologic or systemic abnormality, but only *after* thorough evaluation has been completed. In the elderly patient with senile purpura, supportive explanation that the condition is a normal concomitant of aging is often helpful. Similarly, the young woman with easy bruising syndrome can be reassured. Occasionally, such patients buy and take large doses of vitamins C and K in hopes of lessening easy bruisability. Such self-treatment is without any proven efficacy and adds an unnecessary expense. Avoidance of aspirin and nonsteroidal anti-inflammatory drugs is better advice.

For patients who require drugs that impair platelet function or compromise connective tissue integrity, it may be necessary to advise at least a reduction in dose; otherwise, they may have to accept the cosmetic unpleasantness of ecchymoses. It may be helpful to prepare those with palpable purpura for extended testing and the possibility of a skin biopsy.

INDICATIONS FOR ADMISSION AND REFERRAL

Any patient with fever and purpura requires prompt hospital admission, since bloodstream infection and systemic vasculitis are possible causes. The person who gives evidence of bleeding from multiple sites is also best hospitalized, as is the patient with severe thrombocytopenia or marked prolongation of PT or PTT.

As noted earlier, consultation with a rheumatologist is worthwhile to guide evaluation of the vasculitic patient, particularly when the cause is elusive.

A.H.G.

ANNOTATED BIBLIOGRAPHY

Gibson LE, Su WPD. Cutaneous vasculitis. Rheum Dis Clin North Am 1990;16:309. *(An important cause of purpura.)*

Goldenberg LA, Altman A. Benign skin changes associated with chronic sunlight exposure. Cutis 1984;34:33. *(Sun exposure contributes to senile purpura.)*

Hunder GG, et al. The College of Rheumatology 1990 criteria for the classification of vasculitis. Arthritis Rheum 1990;33:1065. *(Includes criteria for leukocytoclastic variety.)*

(See also Bibliography for Chapter 81, which includes papers regarding hematologic etiologies.)

Primary Care Medicine: Office Evaluation and Management of the Adult Patient, 3rd edition, edited by Allan H. Goroll, Lawrence A. May, and Albert G. Mulley, Jr. J.B. Lippincott Company, Philadelphia

180 Evaluation of Disturbances in Pigmentation

WILLIAM V. R. SHELLOW, M.D.

Disturbances in pigmentation are conspicuous and common. Patients complain about general darkening, brown spots, or depigmented areas. Pigmentary alterations may be manifestations of a genetic, endocrine, metabolic, nutritional, infectious, or neoplastic problem. Physical and chemical factors also can be important.

PATHOPHYSIOLOGY AND CLINICAL PRESENTATION

Pigmentary changes are caused by melanin being absent, increased, decreased, or abnormally placed or distributed. Hyperpigmentation may result from an increased rate of melanosome production, an increased number of melanosomes transferred to keratinocytes, or a greater size and melanization of the melanosome. Hyperpigmentation is perceived as blue when melanin is located deeply, because of the Tyndall phenomenon. The pathophysiologic mechanisms that produce hyperpigmentation through the melanocyte system include elevated adrenocorticotropic hormone (ACTH), which has a melanocyte-stimulating action, ultraviolet radiation, and certain drugs.

Hypomelanosis, or depigmentation, may result from genetic loss of melanocytes or destruction by inflammation. Inflammation may be secondary to infection or burns or associated with a variety of immunologically mediated diseases.

Hyperpigmentation

Hyperpigmentation may be circumscribed or diffuse.

Circumscribed hyperpigmentation includes freckles (ephelides), lentigines, and melasma. *Freckles* are small macular lesions seen on areas exposed to the sun. Freckles may become less dark in adults, but they darken after exposure to long-wave ultraviolet radiation. *Lentigines* are macular, and they are larger and darker than freckles. Histologically, the two are easily distinguishable. Senile lentigines appear on sun-exposed areas in older patients. They are termed "liver spots" by patients.

Melasma or *chloasma* is a blotchy hyperpigmentation that occurs on the forehead, cheeks, and upper lip, usually in women. Pregnancy, oral contraceptives, and other hormones contribute to its appearance, but exposure to sunlight appears to perpetuate the condition. During pregnancy, a physiologic darkening of the linea alba, pigmented nevi, nipples, and genitalia occurs as a result of melanocyte-stimulating hormone (MSH) and increased estrogen and progesterone.

Diffuse hyperpigmentation results from increased amounts of melanin in the epidermis. The color may be accentuated in sun-exposed areas, over pressure points or body folds, or in areas of trauma such as new scars. Increased pigmentation occurs in *Addison's disease* as a result of increased amounts of MSH and ACTH from the pituitary because of decreased cortisol levels.

Metabolic diseases such as Wilson's disease, von Gierke's hemochromatosis, biliary cirrhosis, and porphyria cutanea tarda may be accompanied by diffuse melanosis. On occasion, rheumatoid arthritis, Still's disease, and scleroderma have been associated with hyperpigmentation.

Drugs such as busulfan, cyclophosphamide, clofazimine, and zidovudine can produce diffuse melanosis, as can topical nitrogen mustard. Chronic inorganic arsenic poisoning causes diffuse hyperpigmentation with normal or lighter skin areas scattered throughout, colorfully called "rain drops in the dust." Chlorpromazine and antimalarials tend to produce a bluish-gray hyperpigmentation. Silver (argyria) and gold (chrysiasis) can accumulate in the skin, leading to hyperpigmentation depending on the dosage given.

Diffuse melanosis may be seen during *starvation*, with *hepatic insufficiency*, in *malabsorption syndromes*, and with *lymphomas and other malignancies*. *Postinflammatory hyperpigmentation* can occur secondary to a number of precipitants. For example, phytophotodermatitis occurs after contact with photosensitizing agents present in meadow grass, citrus fruits, and edible plants that cause an exaggerated sunburn. Hyperpigmentation follows the acute phase. Skin contact with organic dyes and aromatic compounds can lead to photosensitization followed by hyperpigmentation. Tar, pitch, and oils can induce similar changes.

Physical trauma, friction, and heat may also lead to postinflammatory pigmentary changes, as may inflammatory dermatoses that stimulate melanin formation.

Hypopigmentation

Hypopigmentation may be hereditary or acquired. A *hereditary* disorder may be associated with a lack or deficiency of melanin. Melanocytes that are deficient or lacking occur in the depigmented areas of partial albinism (piebaldism). A white forelock may be present. In oculocutaneous albinism, melanocytes are normal in number but unable to produce melanin secondary to defective or absent tyrosinase. Diseases involving abnormal amino acid metabolism, such as phenylketonuria and homocystinuria, have associated hypopigmentation of skin and hair. In tuberous sclerosis, elongated hypopigmented patches are seen. Certain cutaneous diseases lead to loss of melanin into the dermis, lending a gray appearance to the skin.

Vitiligo is a common, acquired disorder of hypopigmentation with an autoimmune mechanism that includes the making of antibodies to melanocytes. It may occur in the setting of pernicious anemia, Hashimoto's thyroiditis, and a host of other autoimmune endocrine disorders. Any area of the skin may be affected. Onset is usually early in adult life. Lesions may be symmetric and occur primarily on exposed skin, intertriginous areas, and bony prominences and around orifices. In involved areas, the hair may be white. The border is often sharp and hyperpigmented. Occasionally, vitiligo assumes a segmental or zosteriform pattern. Halo nevi—centrifugal areas of depigmentation that surround a pigmented nevus—accompany one-third of cases. Premature graying of the hair occurs in about 35 percent.

Partial repigmentation of vitiligo may occur in sun-exposed areas, but vitiliginous patches may burn because of the lack of protective pigmentation. Vitiligo has been associated with autoimmune diseases and endocrinopathies.

Depigmentation may be caused by a variety of *chemical agents*, most notably phenolic compounds that interfere with tyrosinase activity. Contact with rubber and antioxidants may also cause loss of pigment. Dermatitis may precede the loss of pigment, and areas remote from the inflamed sites may also lose pigment.

Dermatoses and infections may result in localized areas of pigment loss. Such areas may be more noticeable in dark-skinned persons. Small hypopigmented areas occur on women's legs and may be related to the trauma of shaving. *Tinea versicolor*, pityriasis alba, and various eczematous conditions may present as areas of hypopigmentation.

DIFFERENTIAL DIAGNOSIS

Table 180–1 lists the causes of disturbances in pigmentation.

Table 180-1. Causes of Disturbances in Pigmentation

HYPERPIGMENTATION
Circumscribed
Freckle
Lentigines
Melasma-Chloasma (pregnancy, estrogen, oral contraceptives)
Postinflammatory
Physical trauma
Diffuse
Addison's disease
Systemic conditions (Wilson's disease, hemochromatosis, hepatic insufficiency, biliary cirrhosis, porphyria cutanea tarda, rheumatoid arthritis, scleroderma)
Drugs (arsenic, antimalarials, chlorpromazine, busulfan, cyclophosphamide, clofazimine, gold, silver, zidovudine)
Nutritional (pellagra, malabsorption syndromes, starvation, folic acid deficiency)
Malignancy (lymphomas)
HYPOPIGMENTATION
Hereditary Conditions
Partial albinism
Phenylketonuria
Homocysteinuria
Vitiligo (with or without concurrent autoimmune disease, including pernicious anemia, Hashimoto's thyroiditis, male hypogonadism, diabetes mellitus)
Dermatoses
Tinea versicolor
Pityriasis alba
Eczema
Chemical Exposure
Rubber
Antioxidants
Germicides
Phenols

WORKUP

Hyperpigmentation

Evaluation of the patient with localized hyperpigmentation requires inspection of the lesions and inquiry about previous dermatoses and the use of oral contraceptives that may produce melasma. The majority of localized hyperpigmented areas are postinflammatory and of only cosmetic concern, although they should be distinguished from more worrisome pigmented lesions such as melanomas (see Chapter 177). Diffuse hyperpigmentation necessitates a careful history that specifies the time of onset and possible sun exposure. A drug history that emphasizes agents known to produce pigmentary changes should be pursued. There should be general review of systems, noting weakness associated with Addison's disease and itching and hepatic dysfunction associated with biliary cirrhosis. The physician should consider the possibility of severe vitamin deficiency or malnutrition.

The physical examination includes checking for hyperpigmentation in creases and scars (characteristic of Addison's disease) and clues to obvious underlying pathology, as may occur with malignancy, hepatic insufficiency, or malabsorption. Laboratory investigation must be based on clinical signs of underlying disease. Biopsy may be indicated if heavy metal deposition or hemosiderosis is a diagnostic consideration.

Hypopigmentation

Hypopigmentation requires a careful history of approximate time of onset and possible exposure to bleaching agents, most notably phenol-containing industrial cleaners such as those used in janitorial work. Hypopigmented areas should be scraped and a potassium hydroxide wet mount examined microscopically to diagnose tinea versicolor. The total depigmentation of vitiligo should be differentiated from partial postinflammatory hypopigmentation. Patients with vitiligo should undergo a careful general review of systems and a physical examination that seeks to identify associated conditions such as pernicious anemia, thyroid disease, diabetes, or collagen vascular disease. Ophthalmoscopic examination should be performed to detect retinal pigmentary changes. Laboratory screening for concurrent autoimmune diseases should include consideration of levels of vitamin B_{12}, thyroid-stimulating hormone (TSH), antithyroid antibodies, random glucose, and antinuclear antibodies (ANAs). Test selection is best made according to the patient's clinical presentation.

SYMPTOMATIC THERAPY AND PATIENT EDUCATION

Hyperpigmentation

In treating hyperpigmented areas, the chief symptomatic advice is strict avoidance of sunlight. Topical bleaching with *hydroquinone* cream may be effective. Strong topical corticosteroid preparations have a pigment-lightening effect, as does *retinoic acid*. A bleaching solution of retinoic acid 0.1%, hydroquinone 5%, and dexamethasone 0.1% in a hydrophilic ointment or alcohol is quite effective. Hydroquinone-sunscreen combinations such as Solaquin and Solaquin Forte are useful in treating melasma. Melanex is an alcoholic solution of hydroquinone that is cosmetically well accepted by patients. No matter what is prescribed or recommended, it is important to stress to patients that lightening of pigment which has been won after months of treatment can be undone in a single day (or less) of unprotected exposure to the sun.

Hypopigmentation

Hypopigmented areas can usually be masked by appropriate cosmetics, by bleaching normal skin, or by repigmentation with *psoralens and ultraviolet radiation (PUVA)*. Hundreds of treatments may be required. The primary physician must assess the desire for treatment and inform the patient of the alternatives. Age, sex, or duration of vitiligo does not affect the response. Lesions on the face and abdomen tend to repigment more rapidly than those on the hands, feet, and bony prominences. Treatment should probably be supervised by a dermatologist experienced in using these agents to achieve optimal cosmetic results. *PUVA* with both *oral and topical psoralens* may be effective. With oral psoralens, many months of treatments are necessary to obtain cosmetic improvements. Topical psoralen plus ultraviolet A has no systemic effects such as nausea, and eye precautions are not required. Titration is very important, however, because severe blistering can result with this method of treatment.

If careful workup reveals no accompanying hematologic or endocrinologic autoimmune disorders, the patient can be reassured that only the skin is affected. Others appreciate knowing that the condition is not contagious. The primary physician should advise the patient about cosmetic alternatives and help the patient decide on an appropriate course of treatment. Because body image may suffer in these patients, psychological support and counseling can be very helpful and should not be overlooked.

ANNOTATED BIBLIOGRAPHY

Dunston GM, Halder RM. Vitiligo is associated with HLA DR4 in black patients: a preliminary report. Arch Dermatol 1990; 126:56. *(Certain HLA antigens may be risk factors.)*

El Mofty AM, El Mofty M. Vitiligo: a symptom complex. Int J Dermatol 1980;19:237. *(Discussion of vitiligo and its association with systemic disease.)*

Fulk CS. Primary disorders of hyperpigmentation. J Am Acad Dermatol 1984;10:1. *(Good review; 135 refs.)*

Hendrix JD Jr, Greer KE. Cutaneous hyperpigmentation caused by systemic drugs. Int J Dermatol 1992;31:458. *(Best listing of offending agents.)*

Plott RT, Wagner RF. Modern treatment approaches to vitiligo. Cutis 1990;45:311. *(Current medical and surgical therapies; 64 refs.)*

Porter JR, Beuf AH, Lerner AB, et al. The effect of vitiligo on sexual relationships. J Am Acad Dermatol 1990; 22:221. *(Most felt embarrassment when showing their bodies or when meeting strangers.)*

Resnick S. Melasma induced by oral contraceptive drugs. JAMA 1967;199:601. *(A classic article; 29 percent developed melasma.)*

Tal A, Gagel RF. The diagnostic dilemma of hyperpigmentation in patients with acquired immunodeficiency syndrome. Cutis 1991;48:153. *(Both zidovudine and adrenal insufficiency may be responsible and present in similar fashion.)*

Primary Care Medicine: Office Evaluation and Management of the Adult Patient, 3rd edition, edited by Allan H. Goroll, Lawrence A. May, and Albert G. Mulley, Jr. J.B. Lippincott Company, Philadelphia

181
Evaluation of Urticaria

Urticaria (hives) is a pruritic, often immune-mediated, skin eruption of circumscribed wheals on an erythematous base. It is estimated that up to one-fifth of the population will experience an urticarial episode. There is a slight increase in prevalence among females. Angioedema is a related condition involving the deeper layers of the skin. Approximately half of patients have urticaria with angioedema, 40 percent have pure urticaria, and 10 percent have pure angioedema.

If the process occurs for less than 6 weeks, it is termed acute, but if it persists beyond 6 to 8 weeks, it is termed chronic. Most chronic urticaria resolves within a year, although persistence well beyond that occurs in approximately 10 percent of cases. The primary physician's role includes searching for precipitants and underlying causes. Eliciting the cause can be difficult and is not always possible. In the absence of an identifiable and remediable precipitant, one needs to provide symptomatic relief.

PATHOPHYSIOLOGY AND CLINICAL PRESENTATION

Urticaria results from increased vascular permeability leading to extravasation of protein-rich fluid from small blood vessels, usually post-capillary venules. The localized accumulation of fluid produces the characteristic edematous, erythematous papules which are pruritic, blanch on pressure, and range in size from a few millimeters to several centimeters, often with serpiginous borders. Individual lesions rarely persist for longer than 24 to 48 hours, and often resolve sooner.

In *angioedema*, the extravasation of fluid occurs in deeper layers of the skin, showing a preference for the periorbital, perioral, palmar and plantar surfaces of the body. The edema is more diffuse, and the overlying skin appears normal and does not itch. Systemic symptoms, which include hoarseness, shortness of breath, wheezing, nausea, vomiting, and abdominal discomfort, commonly occur in angioedema.

A host of mechanisms have been implicated, and much remains incompletely understood. There are immunologic, IgE-mediated, and nonimmunologic stimuli. Mast cell activation is the final common pathway, with release of mediators from mast cells or circulating basophils increasing vascular permeability. Histamine is one such mediator, producing a classic wheal and flare on intracutaneous injection. Transient histamine elevations occur in the extremities of patients with physical urticarias. Other mast-cell–derived mediators include eosinophilic and high molecular weight neutrophilic hemotactic factors. Prostaglandin D_2, leukotrienes, and platelet-activating factors all contribute to the pathophysiology.

Foods and Drugs. Ingested antigens trigger urticaria by an IgE-mediated reaction. The attacks tend to be brief and uncommonly cause chronic urticaria. The most commonly implicated foods include eggs, wheat, shellfish, peanuts, and milk, and the most common drugs are penicillin and sulfa-containing agents. Intravenous radiocontrast media, opiates, and amphetamines cause urticaria and angioedema by directly releasing agents from the mast cells. Aspirin and nonsteroidal anti-inflammatory agents (NSAIDs) may produce urticaria in those with an underlying abnormality in prostaglandin synthesis, which these agents block. Patients with urticarial reactions to aspirin can tolerate sodium salicylate or choline salicylate, which do not inhibit cyclooxygenase.

Physical Urticarias. These include dermatographism, cold urticaria, and cholinergic urticaria and may be due to a hyperreactivity to acetylcholine. Inadequate production of cholinesterase is suspected. Susceptible persons may show increased numbers of mast cells or elevated cutaneous levels of histamine. Substance P may contribute to the flare that surrounds urticarial wheals. Physical urticarias may also have some degree of IgE-mediated pathophysiology.

Clinical presentations include the most common form of dermatographism, in which stroking of the skin produces a wheal and flare response. In cold urticaria, application of cold produces pruritic erythematous eruptions within minutes. Cholinergic urticaria is characterized by tiny, 1- to 3-mm punctate lesions surrounded by erythema; they are intensely pruritic. Aquagenic urticaria is characterized by tiny perifollicular hives that appear after contact with water.

Hepatitis B. Urticaria during the prodrome to type B viral hepatitis may occur as a result of the formation of antigen–antibody complexes. The urticaria is complement-mediated.

Hereditary Angioedema. This is an autosomal-dominant hereditary disease characterized by reduced levels of the inhibitor of the first component of complement. Type I is characterized by marked reductions of C1 inhibitor and also low levels of C4, while type II has normal elevated C1 inhibitors but altered biologic function. The angioedema associated with angiotensin converting enzyme inhibitors appears to be mediated by bradykinins.

Other Precipitants. Certain circumstances such as heat, fever, stress, alcohol, the premenstrual period, or thyroid disorders exacerbate hives independent of the specific pathophysiology. Urticaria can occur solely because of emotional stress.

There are clearly a number of different mechanisms associated with particular forms of urticaria, and there is often a contribution of more than one mechanism. Additional precipitants and/or mediators of the urticarial reaction are constantly being identified.

DIFFERENTIAL DIAGNOSIS

Urticaria can be caused by a variety of exogenous factors, including drugs and chemicals, foods, contactants, cosmetics, physical stimuli, and, less commonly, inhalants. Endogenous sources of urticaria include infections, infestations, endocrinopathies, and certain systemic diseases (Table 181–1). Atopic persons do not have a greater prevalence of urticaria or angioedema.

WORKUP

History is the most useful component of the evaluation, yielding clues to an underlying cause or precipitant far more often than the physical examination or laboratory investigation. Consequently, the emphasis in the workup should be on the history.

History. Inquiry into recent illness, medications, foods, and inhalants that have been associated with urticaria may help to determine the proximate cause of the urticarial reaction. Patients should be encouraged to keep a food diary and alerted to include such items as toothpaste, cosmetics, food additives, and birth control pills. One should not over-

Table 181-1. Causes of Urticaria

Exogenous Causes
Foods (shellfish, peanuts, eggs, wheat, and milk, particularly in children)
Drugs (penicillin, aspirin, sulfa-containing drugs)
Food additives (penicillin in milk, yellow food dye No. 5, menthol in cigarettes, fluoride in toothpaste)
Physical factors (pressure, cold exposure, sun exposure, exercise)
Endogenous Causes
Infection, bacterial (dental abscess, sinusitis, tonsillitis, prostatitis)
Infection, viral (mononucleosis, viral hepatitis)
Infection, fungal (dermatophytosis, candidiasis)
Infection, parasitic (giardiasis, amoebiasis, trichomoniasis)
Systemic disease (juvenile rheumatoid arthritis, lymphoma, leukemia)
Idiopathic Psychological stress

look agents that may be entering through the conjunctiva, nasal mucosa, rectum, or vaginal area. One asks about intake of milk products and beer because penicillin in dairy products or yeast in beer can precipitate urticaria. One checks for parasympathetic symptoms such as abdominal cramps, diarrhea, headache, salivation, and diaphoresis. It is important to determine whether exposure to pressure, cold, light, heat, or exercise precipitates lesions. A travel history may suggest a parasitic infestation. Inquiry into agents and factors that might modulate the intensity of an urticarial reaction (eg, aspirin, alcohol, NSAIDs, heat, humidity, occlusive clothing, psychological stress) can provide clinically useful information.

The review of systems can be used to check for systemic illness that might present with urticaria. Pertinent questions include presence of night sweats; fatigue; weight loss; lymphadenopathy; jaundice; dark urine; pale stools; easy bruising; dysuria; vaginal or sinus discharge; and pain in the teeth, joints, or sinuses.

Physical Examination. Severity and occasionally etiology are revealed by the physical examination. Dermatographism is associated with linear wheals. Small lesions with erythematous flares are typical of cholinergic urticaria. Periorbital or perioral swelling is suggestive of angioedema. Careful examination of the ears, pharynx, sinuses, and teeth may help uncover a focal infection. One should check for lymphadenopathy and hepatosplenomegaly, suggestive of an underlying lymphoma or hepatocellular disease. The joints are noted for swelling, effusion, and warmth, suggestive of active rheumatoid disease.

Laboratory Studies. It is usually unproductive to attempt diagnosis through the performance of an extensive panel of laboratory tests in the absence of suggestive historic and physical examination evidence. Initial studies can be limited to a complete blood count (for infection and myeloproliferative disease), a sedimentation rate (for active connective tissue disease), and an aminotransferase (for hepatitis). Allergic skin testing has minimal value, and the costly specific IgE radioallergosorbent test (RAST) rarely reveals a cause in elusive cases. Mean serum levels of IgE are usually normal. Skin biopsy is usually not necessary to diagnose urticaria but should be considered if vasculitis is suspected. Radiologic examinations are indicated only if clinical evidence suggests a focal infection. Stool examination for ova and parasites is appropriate if recent diarrheal illness or travel to endemic areas has taken place.

Provocative tests can help ascertain the precipitants of physical urticarias. An ice cube on the skin may induce cold urticaria, while stroking can reveal dermatographism. Cholinergic urticaria may be revealed by an intradermal injection of methacholine, 0.1 mL of a 1:500 dilution. Cytotoxic food allergy testing has no scientific validity and should be firmly discouraged.

Therapeutic trials may be helpful in identifying an etiologic cause. An elimination diet that consists of lamb, rice, string beans, fresh peas, tea, and rye crackers excludes most common food allergens. A more limited approach would be to eliminate dairy products, beer, nuts, shellfish, berries, and food additives. It is often useful to stop all drugs or change preparations or brands to eliminate tartrazine dyes or the peculiar additives of particular toothpastes or cosmetics.

Chronic urticaria poses significant diagnostic and management challenges. Hospitalization for control of diet and observation is both expensive and low in diagnostic yield. Fewer than 10 percent of patients are identified as having a specific etiology, and the idiopathic designation applies even after extensive evaluation.

SYMPTOMATIC MANAGEMENT

The best treatment is identification and avoidance of etiologic agents, but in most instances this is not possible. The vast majority of patients end up being treated empirically for symptomatic relief. Half of patients with urticaria alone and 25 percent with associated angioedema are free of lesions within 1 year; 20 percent experience episodes for more than 20 years.

Available Agents

Antihistamines provide excellent symptomatic control. The *H_1-blockers* such as hydroxyzine (10–25 mg qid) and diphenhydramine (25–50 mg tid) have been the mainstay of antihistamine therapy. They are low in cost and effective but produce daytime drowsiness. The newer, nonsedating H_1-blockers (astemizole, terfenadine, loratidine) are also effective and are better tolerated for daytime use. Their disadvantages are substantial cost and, with astemizole, a tendency to stimulate appetite. It is often best to use a nonsedating antihistamine during the day and a more sedating agent at night. Chlorpheniramine and diphenhydramine are useful alternatives because they are available over the counter and are much less expensive.

In refractory cases, *H_2-blockers*, such as cimetidine or ranitidine, have been effective in combination with H_1 antihistamines. The rationale for the use of H_2-blockers is that 15 percent of the receptors in the cutaneous vasculature are H_2. *Doxepin*, a tricyclic antidepressant with antihistamine effects, has proven helpful in low doses given three times a day and may be useful adjunctively as a bedtime medication in combination with antihistamines.

Steroids and Other Drugs. For refractory cases, oral *glucocorticosteroids* have proved effective (see below), but they must be used with care if prescribed for prolonged periods (see Chapter 105). Some reports suggest that *terbutaline*, when used in fairly high doses (1.25 mg tid), can decrease itching and number of episodes, but others find little benefit, either alone or in combination with antihistamines. *Nifedipine*, a calcium channel blocker, can improve the clinical appearance of lesions by interfering with mast cell activity. *Anabolic steroids* have been used with success in hereditary angioedema (see below).

Empiric trials of broad-spectrum *antibiotics* and *antifungal agents* have been advocated in the past for treatment of patients with idiopathic urticaria, but they are *not* justified. The use of broad-spectrum antibiotics and antifungals was thought reasonable as a means of eliminating any occult infection, but data do not support this approach. Specific treatment of infections such as sinusitis or vaginitis is appropriate only if infection is confirmed.

Treatment Applications

Acute Attacks. Mild attacks can be treated with oral antihistamines. Severe attacks respond promptly to subcutaneous aqueous *epinephrine*. Intramuscular *cimetidine* was found to be more effective and less sedating than intramuscular diphenhydramine. Parenteral *corticosteroids* may be used to treat very extensive acute outbreaks.

Physical Urticaria. The physical urticarias are also treated with antihistamines. *Cyproheptadine* is an H_1-blocker that is particularly useful for aquagenic, cold-induced, and dermatographic urticaria. Topical *capsaicin* has been useful in patients with cold-induced and localized heat-induced urticaria. Antihistamines have been useful in vibratory physical urticaria. Exercise-induced urticaria can be treated by avoiding vigorous exercise, and it is important not to exercise after eating or when taking aspirins or NSAIDs.

Chronic and Refractory Urticarias. Controlling chronic urticaria requires empiricism and careful follow-up. One begins with an H_1-blocker, usually a nonsedating agent. If this fails, an H_2-blocker, such as cimetidine, is added. If the patient fails to respond, doxepin is substituted. In severe cases, a brief course of *systemic corticosteroids* (eg, prednisone 20–40 mg/d) with rapid reduction to alternate-day therapy and ultimate elimination is appropriate.

Despite optimal use of antihistamines, H_2-blockers, and doxepin, some patients remain refractory to therapy. These individuals may require more prolonged courses of corticosteroids for control of symptoms. Therapy should be administered daily at first but switched to an alternate-day regimen as soon as possible to avoid the complications associated with long-term corticosteroid use (see Chapter 105).

Hereditary Angioedema. An acute attack that threatens airway obstruction should be treated with subcutaneous *epinephrine* (0.3 mL 1/1000). Patients with known angioedema should carry an epinephrine self-administration kit. The best treatment is prevention of attacks. Danazol and stanozolol, *anabolic steroids* with reduced iatrogenic effects, have been used in cases of frequent or severe attacks. They appear to induce synthesis of normally functioning C1 esterase inhibitor. Periodic monitoring of C1 esterase inhibitor and liver function is required. A purified C1 inhibitor may become available for prophylaxis and treatment of acute attacks.

INDICATIONS FOR REFERRAL AND ADMISSION

The management of urticaria can be frustrating, and it is often useful both for the physician and the patient to enlist the aid of a specialist. Allergists can help evaluate patients with repetitive eruptions due to possible food allergies that may be detectable on testing. They may also perform penicillin skin testing, particularly with minor determinants. Their experience in seeing a large number of patients with urticaria may allow them to identify a particular additive or brand agent and help the patient in that way.

Admission for patients with acute angioedema with systemic symptoms may be necessary briefly for respiratory support or the use of epinephrine. Hospitalizations that are sometimes advocated for elimination diets are far too costly in a climate of cost-containment.

PATIENT EDUCAITON

It is important to educate the patient in advance of the workup that a cause is usually not found. Emphasize the variable natural history of hives and the high probability that lesions will disappear spontaneously. Prepare the patient for the likelihood that urticaria will recur. Instruct all patients to avoid aspirin, heat, exertion, and alcoholic beverages. Specific advice, such as the avoidance of swimming in cold water for patients with cold urticaria, can be lifesaving. Reassure the patient that the medical workup will exclude serious and/or treatable diseases and that many options are available to shorten the process and alleviate symptoms. The reduction of unrealistic expectations can reduce the disappointment that may follow a negative workup. It is important to emphasize the overall good prognosis and the high probability that remission will occur but that it may be delayed.

L.A.M.

ANNOTATED BIBLIOGRAPHY

Casale TB, Sampson HA, Hanifin J, et al. Guide to physical urticarias. J Allergy Clin Immunol 1989;82:758. *(A review of the physical urticarias.)*

Cooper KD. Urticaria and angioedema: diagnosis and evaluation. J Am Acad Dermatol 1991;25:166. *(A review of the causes and how to identify them.)*

Kennard CD, Ellis CN. Pharmacologic therapy for urticaria. J Am Acad Dermatol 1991;25:176. *(Nonsedating antihistamines in combination with antidepressants or H_2-blockers may be useful.)*

Honsinger RW Jr, Thomsen RJ. Prolonged benefit in treatment of chronic idiopathic urticaria with astemizole. Ann Allergy 1990;65:194. *(Placebo-controlled study; improvement in symptoms and lesions in 75 percent with persistent benefit after discontinuation of the drug.)*

Moscati RM, Moore GP. Comparison of cimetidine and diphenhydramine in the treatment of acute urticaria. Ann Emerg Med 1990;19:12. *(Cimetidine was more efficacious and produced less sedation.)*

Soter NA. Acute and chronic urticaria and angioedema. J Am Acad Dermatol 1991;125:146. *(History more useful than laboratory examination; half of patients with urticaria alone and 25 percent with associated angioedema are free of lesions within 1 year; 20 percent experienced episodes for more than 20 years.)*

Sussman G, Jancelewicz Z. Controlled trial of H_1 antagonists in the treatment of chronic idiopathic urticaria. Ann Allergy 1991;67:433. *(Astemizole, hydroxyzine, and diphenhydramine were compared in a double-blind, randomized study. Astemizole was more effective and produced less sedation.)*

Primary Care Medicine: Office Evaluation and Management of the Adult Patient, 3rd edition, edited by Allan H. Goroll, Lawrence A. May, and Albert G. Mulley, Jr. J.B. Lippincott Company, Philadelphia

182
Approach to the Patient With Hair Loss

WILLIAM V. R. SHELLOW, M.D.

Alopecia may be described as the lack of hair in areas where it normally grows. The most noticeable area for alopecia is the scalp, but loss of body hair may also occur. Patients may seek medical care for what is perceived as excessive hair loss even when there is no alopecia. Whether the problem is genetically induced male-pattern baldness or alopecia as a result of systemic illness, the primary care physician may be the first to whom the problem is presented and must offer the patient a rational approach to diagnosis and treatment.

PATHOPHYSIOLOGY AND CLINICAL PRESENTATION

Normal Hair Growth

Hair is a product of keratinocytes in the hair bulb. The hair shaft is made of hard keratin. Synthesis results from mitoses of cells within the hair matrix. The growth of hair is cyclical, with the length of the cycle varying with the location. Scalp hair grows from 3 to 10 years, involutes over 3 months, and rests for another 3 months. In healthy young persons, about 90 percent of all scalp hairs are in anagen, actively growing. Telogen, or resting hair, accounts for most of the remainder.

Hairs that grow for long periods and rest briefly are most susceptible to interruption of the growth cycle, and variations in the growing-to-resting ratio are most noticeable. The longer the growing period, the longer the hair. Scalp hair grows at the rate of approximately 0.35 mm per day, but there are factors that can affect the rate.

Hair Loss

The primary pathogenic mechanisms of hair loss are destruction of the hair matrix by physical agents and infectious or immunologically mediated inflammation. Hair loss may occur secondary to a slowing of hair growth from metabolic diseases, antimetabolites, or other drugs. Physiologic alterations may also produce hair loss by altering the relation between the growing and resting phases of hair follicles. During pregnancy, fewer hairs are shed, producing fewer telogen hairs. After parturition, the percentage of telogen hairs increases, and there is loss of hair. The process is diffuse and short-lived. This alteration in the relation of resting hairs to the total may also develop secondary to pharmacologic changes induced by oral contraceptives. Destructive pathogenic mechanisms often produce scarring alopecia, whereas systemic illnesses and drugs usually result in nonscarring alopecia.

Alopecia can be divided into two categories, either scarring (cicatricial) or nonscarring (noncicatricial). In the latter, the hair follicles are retained and the process is potentially reversible. In the scarring type, follicles are destroyed and hair never regrows. A few conditions that begin as nonscarring may later scar as a result of chronicity.

Scarring Alopecia. An inflammatory response to injury is often present. Physical trauma such as burns, radiation, injuries, and chronic traction are commonly responsible. Traction alopecia usually results from braiding or tight hair rollers. The pattern of hair loss is dependent on the styling. The process is initially reversible but progresses to a scarring phase with chronicity. Hot combs in combination with petrolatum used to straighten hair may result in inflammation with consequent fibrosis and hair loss. Infections—whether they be bacterial, resulting in deep cellulitis, fungal with *Trichophyton schoenleinii*, or viral, such as recurrent herpes simplex or herpes zoster—produce inflammatory change and alopecia. Dermatologic processes such as discoid lupus erythematosus, scleroderma, lichen planus, cutaneous neoplasms, and granulomas may produce scarring alopecia. There are also factitious causes and neurotic excoriations.

Nonscarring Alopecia. Most often, alopecia is nonscarring, with male- and female-pattern baldness accounting for most cases. *Male-pattern baldness* (androgenetic alopecia) is symmetrical, usually beginning in the frontoparietal scalp. Its development is related to age, genetic predisposition, and the presence of androgenic hormones. The inheritance is probably dominant, with incomplete penetrance. The process is permanent, with pigmented scalp hairs replaced by fine unpigmented vellus hairs.

The presence of a male-pattern hair loss *in a female* should provoke concern about *androgen excess*, manifested by hirsutism in mild cases and virilization in more serious ones. Polycystic ovary disease and hyperprolactinemia are common causes of mild androgen excess and hirsutism. Frank virilization occurs with androgen-producing ovarian and adrenal tumors (see Chapter 98). Dihydrotestosterone inhibits the growth of scalp hair while it stimulates the growth of facial hair and promotes a male pattern of pubic hair growth. Laboratory investigation reveals increased levels of free testosterone and/or sulfated dehydroepiandrosterone (DHEA).

Female-pattern baldness has a similar set of mechanisms to male-pattern baldness, but it is more diffuse, usually in the central and frontal areas without complete baldness. Age, family tendency, and androgenic hormones are important factors. In *postpartum alopecia*, there is resolution within 18 months, but about half of postpartum women feel they have less hair than before their pregnancy.

Nonscarring alopecia often involves systemic disease, medication, or metabolic abnormality. *Alopecia areata,* a condition of unknown etiology in which hair is rapidly lost, usually in circular patterns, is probably the second most common cause of nonscarring alopecia. *Alopecia totalis* is loss of all the scalp hair, and *alopecia universalis* includes loss of facial and body hair as well. The course of alopecia areata is unpredictable. Some persons have one episode with one or several bald spots and spontaneous regrowth. Others may develop new areas of baldness and become totally bald. Onset before puberty is associated with a poorer prognosis. Most authors believe that there is an autoimmune mechanism and an association with other autoimmune diseases.

Alopecia may follow *infectious diseases* that produce high, persistent fevers, such as typhoid or pneumonia. Secondary syphilis, superficial folliculitis, and tinea capitis also may produce nonscarring alopecia. Commonly used *medications* that can produce alopecia include beta-blockers, tricyclic antidepressants, anticonvulsants, warfarin anticoagulants, allopurinol, antithyroid medications, quinine, verapamil, indomethacin, sulfasalazine, and haloperidol, as well as excessive doses of vitamin A. Antineoplastic agents such as 5-fluorouracil, cyclophosphamide, and methotrexate predictably produce hair loss. Oral contraceptives, hyperandrogenism, and pregnancy are known to interfere with the relation between resting and growing hairs and to produce hair loss. Diffuse hair thinning may occur with *thyroid disease* and *iron deficiency*. Less commonly, hypopituitarism and parathyroid disease produce hair loss. Alopecia is a manifestation of *collagen vascular diseases*, notably systemic lupus erythematosus and dermatomyositis. Occasionally, patients have self-induced hair loss, a condition known as *trichotillomania*. These patients may not be aware that they are plucking hairs, and the condition may indicate significant psychiatric disturbance.

Hair Breakage. Hair loss must be differentiated from hair breakage, which results from physical or chemical stress to the shaft. The term proximal trichorrhexis is sometimes used to describe hair breakage that occurs within the first centimeter from the scalp, while distal trichorrhexis is that which occurs beyond this point. Hair straightening can give rise to proximal trichorrhexis. Patients often recognize distal breakage as split ends; such breakage may be accelerated by sunshine or swimming in chlorinated pools.

DIFFERENTIAL DIAGNOSIS

Table 182–1 lists the differential diagnosis of hair loss.

Table 182-1. Differential Diagnosis of Hair Loss

NON-SCARRING ALOPECIA	
Androgenetic	Antidepressants
Male-pattern	Anticonvulsants
Female-pattern	Anticoagulants
Alopecia areata	Allopurinol, probenecid
Post-febrile infection	Beta-blockers
Folliculitis (mild)	Quinine
Tinea capitis (ectothrix)	High-dose vitamin A, isotretinoin
Hypothyroidism	Oral contraceptives
Iron deficiency	Discontinuation of corticosteroids
Systemic lupus erythematosus	Psychiatric
Syphilis	Trichotillomania
Medications	Telogen effluvium
Antineoplastics	Crash diets
Antimetabolites	Postpregnancy
Propylthiouracil	
SCARRING ALOPECIA	
Physical trauma	Discoid lupus erythematosus
Burns	Morphea
Radiation	Lichen planopilaris
Chronic traction	Pseudopelade
Infection	Neoplasms
Bacterial folliculitis (severe)	Granulomatous disease
Fungal (endothrix)	Factitial

WORKUP

History. The history should begin by identifying the nature of the problem. Is the patient troubled by a specific area of hair loss or by generalized hair loss? Are there symptoms of a precipitating illness such as hypothyroidism, systemic lupus, granulomatous disease, iron deficiency, or febrile infection? Is there a history of physical trauma (eg, pulling of the hair, use of curlers, bleaching, permanent waves, straightening, hot combs)? It is helpful to review the family history for male- or female-pattern baldness and to review the medication history for antimetabolites, anticonvulsants, anticoagulants, beta-blockers, colchicine, antithyroid drugs, androgens, oral contraceptives, and excessive amounts of tretinoin (Retin-A) and vitamin A. Other precipitants worth noting include recent pregnancy, severe dieting, and skin conditions such as folliculitis and tinea.

Physical Examination. The pattern of hair loss is noted. Is it localized or diffuse? Is there an androgenetic pattern? It is essential to differentiate scarring from nonscarring alopecia. The scalp is examined carefully for areas of reduced hair growth, hair loss, and scarring. The presence of short, broken hairs suggests pulling of the hair. One examines the area surrounding the hair loss for evidence of inflammation, cellulitis, folliculitis, and fungal infection. If available, a Wood's light will produce a fluorescent glow in an area affected by fungal infection. Any area of inflammation should be scraped for microscopic examination (see Chapter 191) and culture.

It is often helpful to collect objective evidence of hair loss to differentiate perceived from genuine problems. One method is to have the patient collect the hairs lost each day in separate envelopes and count the total. Fewer than 100 hairs per day is within normal limits. Also helpful in making the differentiation between normal and excessive hair loss is the "pluck" or "pull" test. A dozen or so hairs are grasped between the thumb and index finger, and moderate traction is applied. Three areas should be tested: the vertex, the occiput, and the parietal scalp.

Extraction of two or fewer hairs per area indicates that hair loss is probably not excessive. In active androgenetic alopecia and telogen effluvium, more than six hairs will be removed. The interpretation of finding between two and six hairs is less precise, necessitating other studies which sometimes include a scalp biopsy. If the circular areas characteristic of alopecia areata are seen, light traction on the hairs at the edge of the bald area indicates whether the disease is active at that location. If hairs come out with ease, then extension of the alopecic area is to be expected.

Some dermatologists perform telogen counts by removing 100 hairs and counting how many are in the telogen phase. Telogen hair is identified by the presence of a terminal club on the hair shaft. This procedure can separate conditions resulting from telogen excess from those resulting from broken hairs, but it may be too time-consuming to be useful to the primary physician.

Evidence of systemic illness should be sought, including signs of hypothyroidism (see Chapter 104), lupus (see Chapter 146), iron deficiency (see Chapter 79), and sarcoidosis (see Chapter 51). One checks the woman with male-pattern hair loss for signs of hirsutism and virilization (see Chapter 98). It is useful to examine the nails; the presence of Beau's lines may correlate with a systemic process affecting both nail and hair growth.

Laboratory Studies. A biopsy may be helpful, particularly in cases of scarring alopecia with suspected inflammation, both to add histologic evidence and to determine areas of activity that might respond to anti-inflammatory therapy. Performance of laboratory tests for systemic disease, such as blood count, serum iron, thyroxine, antinuclear antibody, and masculinizing tumors, depends on the history and physical findings.

PRINCIPLES OF THERAPY

The primary physician can provide the patient with reassurance, advice, and, occasionally, specific therapy. The treatment of alopecia depends on identification of a probable cause. Patients with a perception of excessive hair loss that is not substantiated should be reassured, as should women with hair loss following pregnancy. Drugs associated with hair loss should be discontinued if possible and alternatives sought. Scalp infection, either bacterial or fungal, requires specific treatment (see Chapters 190 and 191), as does any underlying disease. Hair loss often resolves with successful etiologic therapy. The hair loss associated with chemotherapy is usually self-limited and is best treated with a wig and time (see Chapter 88).

Symptomatic Therapy

For the vast majority of hair-loss patients, the cause is either alopecia areata or androgenetic baldness, and treatment is symptomatic for those troubled by the cosmetic effects.

Alopecia areata is often self-limited, but if the condition is severe, it may be worth considering specific medical therapy, which should be undertaken only by a dermatologist or physician skilled in its treatment. A traditional treatment for stimulating new hair growth is irritation with *phenol* or *ultraviolet light. Topical fluorinated corticosteroids* under occlusion may be helpful, and this may be tried by the primary physician. A superpotent corticosteroid such as clobetasol solution can be used without occlusion. *Injection* of *triamcinolone acetonide* into the scalp may be considered if topical therapy fails. When made up as a dilute solution for injection, it is less likely to cause dermal atrophy than other injected steroids. Small volumes are used, and multiple injections may be necessary to cover a large area. *Systemic corticosteroids* have, on occasion, been helpful, but their effectiveness is often lost when the drugs are discontinued, and the risks of chronic therapy (see Chapter 105) outweigh the benefits. They should be used only under exceptional circumstances and only by a dermatologist experienced in treating patients with hair problems.

Approaches under investigation include use of agents that induce an immune-mediated hypersensitivity response which stimulates regrowth of hair. The response rate is approximately 70 percent, but treatment often must be repeated, and some of the agents used are potentially mutagenic. Anthralin, used in the management of psoriasis, has also been used to stimulate hair growth, but it must be applied nightly and removed in the morning. Psoralen and ultraviolet A light (PUVA) therapy has achieved some success as well.

Despite the substantial interest and literature extolling various therapies, no approach can be judged effective enough to recommend. Many experienced clinicians believe that treatment merely accelerates resolution in the approximately 50 percent of alopecia areata sufferers who would spontaneously regrow hair anyway. Some argue that, outside of a study situation, watchful waiting is the safest and most cost-effective approach.

Male-pattern baldness compromises the self-image and self-confidence of many young men. A topical 2% solution of the antihypertensive *minoxidil* (Rogaine) is widely promoted for use in such patients. The candidates most likely to respond to are those younger than 40 who have been bald for less than 10 years and have a balding area that is smaller than 4 inches in diameter. The patient needs to understand that 6 months of daily treatment may be necessary before hair growth becomes apparent and that new hair persists only as long as the twice-daily applications are continued. New growth may be lost within 2 to 6 months of stopping treatment. The only side effect is local irritation, although patients with a low systolic pressure may experience postural hypotension with dizziness.

Minoxidil may, to some extent, prevent further hair loss. Most patients feel that progression of their alopecia is halted by regular use of the medication. In one long-term study, hair growth tended to peak at 1 year, with slow decline in regrowth subsequently. After 4½ to 5 years of use, there was maintenance of nonvellus hairs above the baseline counts. The application of *tretinoin (Retin-A)* liquid or gel to the scalp several minutes before minoxidil is applied may improve the efficacy of this therapy.

Women with male-pattern hair loss may have associated hirsutism. This combination suggests androgen excess and should be treated etiologically (see Chapter 98). Symptomatically, androgen excess can be treated with *spironolactone,* 75 to 200 mg/day for at least 6 months, or by *dexamethasone,* 0.125 to 0.250 mg at bedtime for at least 6 months. The hirsutism may improve before the alopecia does.

Female-pattern hair loss is an increasingly common complaint, with 40 percent of women experiencing cosmetically significant hair loss by the sixth decade. Women who have thinning hair, even though there is no apparent baldness to the examining physician, fear that they will become bald like men with common baldness. This rarely happens, and they can be reassured concerning the prognosis. Although initially approved for use only in men, *minoxidil* can also be prescribed for women, one-third of whom also experience androgenetic alopecia. Some women initially experience increased hair loss, which makes them fearful of continuing minoxidil, but decreased shedding and stimulation of new hair growth within 12 months can be expected.

PATIENT EDUCATION

Patient education can be the most important part of the primary physician's management of the patient with alopecia. Once diagnosis is established and serious diseases are excluded, the patient can be reassured. Patients are often concerned that the hair loss will progress, and the most useful information that can be given is the actual likelihood of continued or total hair loss. Even men with genetic baldness are often reassured to know that there is no systemic disease. Success in the management of alopecia is often dependent on the physician's ability to help the patient come to terms with his or her hair loss.

Hair Care. Advice on hair care is appreciated. Patients should be advised to avoid alkaline pH shampoos and excessive toweling after washing the hair. Use of conditioner may be helpful. Combing is less injurious than brushing. If one must brush, it is useful to gently disentangle the hair from the brush and to use a natural bristle brush or a nylon brush with rounded edges. Patients should avoid bleaching, permanent waving, straightening, use of hot combs, and excessive sun exposure.

Hair Weaving and Transplants. Patients are often well aware of the option of wigs but may ask the primary physician about such issues as having their hair woven or having hair transplants. Weaving is a relatively safe procedure performed by nonphysicians. It is successful but must be repeated periodically and thereby becomes expensive and a nuisance. Hair transplants are expensive and have varying rate of success. The procedure is painful and is usually not covered by insurance. Patients with coarse, dark hair are the best candidates for hair transplants. Implants using artificial hair should be discouraged because they usually fall out or elicit a chronic foreign body reaction.

ANNOTATED BIBLIOGRAPHY

Brodland DG, Muller SA. Androgenetic alopecia (common baldness). Cutis 1991;47:173. *(A review of the clinical and endocrinologic features of pattern baldness with discussion of therapy.)*

Fiedler VC, Wendrow A, Szpunar GJ, et al. Treatment-resistant alopecia areata: response to combination therapy with minoxidil plus anthralin. Arch Dermatol 1990;126:756. *(The combination of two topical agents produced results in 11 percent of patients.)*

Kasick JM, Bergfeld WF, Steck WD, et al. Adrenal androgenic female-pattern alopecia: sex hormones and the balding woman. Cleve Clin J Med 1983;50:111. *(A discussion of endocrinologic abnormalities in women with balding and spironolactone therapy; 52 refs.)*

Modly CE, Wood CM, Burnett JW. Evaluation of alopecia: a new algorithm. Cutis 1989;43:148. *(Focuses on the presence or absence of follicular orifices.)*

Naldi L, Parazzini F, Cainelli T, et al. Role of topical immunotherapy in the treatment of alopecia areata. J Am Acad Dermatol 1990;22:654. *(A discussion of topical immunotherapy of alopecia areata with dinitrochlorobenzene, squaric acid dibutylester, and diphencyprone.)*

Olsen EA. Topical minoxidil in the treatment of androgenetic alopecia in women. Cutis 1991;48:243. *(Minoxidil 2% is effective in the treatment of female-pattern baldness.)*

Olsen EA, Weiner MS, Amara IA, et al. Five-year follow-up of men with androgenetic alopecia treated with topical minoxidil. J Am Acad Dermatol 1990;22:643. *(Hair growth tended to peak at 1 y with slow decline in regrowth subsequently, though with long-term maintenance of nonvellus hairs above the baseline counts.)*

Parkinson RW. Hair loss in women: what to say and do to ease these patients' distress. Postgrad Med 1992;91(4):417. *(A practical approach to a frequently mentioned complaint.)*

Shellow WVR, Edwards JE, Koo JYM. Profile of alopecia areata: a questionnaire analysis of patient and family. Int J Dermatol 1992;31:186. *(A strong family history in 42 percent and an association between alopecia areata and type I diabetes.)*

Primary Care Medicine: Office Evaluation and Management of the Adult Patient, 3rd edition, edited by Allan H. Goroll, Lawrence A. May, and Albert G. Mulley, Jr. J.B. Lippincott Company, Philadelphia

183
Disturbances of Skin Hydration: Dry Skin and Excessive Sweating

WILLIAM V. R. SHELLOW, M.D.

Management of Dry Skin

Dry skin, or simple xerosis, is commonly seen during the winter months and occurs more often in the elderly. The most common clinical presentation is mild to moderate itching (see Chapter 178). A related condition is mild irritant dermatitis or chapping. This is seen particularly on the hands and face. Fingertip fissuring is another common problem during winter months. Severe chronic dry skin can become eczematous and may be referred to as "asteatotic eczema." The primary physician must recognize dry skin and use simple measures and effective patient education to relieve the symptom.

PATHOPHYSIOLOGY AND CLINICAL PRESENTATION

Although the term "dry" implies that the basic defect is a lack of water, the etiology of dry skin is not fully understood. There are no significant differences in the amount of water present in the stratum corneum of "dry" compared with "normal" skin. The condition is more likely related to an increase in evaporative water loss through a defective stratum corneum.

The lipids that aid retention of water within the stratum corneum diminish with age. Xerosis in the elderly reflects a decrease in both the number and activity of sebaceous glands and a reduced rate of perspiration. Excessive use of soap, detergent, or disinfectants damages the stratum corneum and increases water loss up to 50 times the normal rate. Environmental factors such as low humidity, forced-air heat, or cold winter winds contribute to dryness. There is an unexplained familial tendency toward the development of dry skin. There are a variety of hygroscopic water-soluble chemicals, including lactic acid, urea, and sodium pyrrolidine carboxylic acid. Collectively, these substances are referred to as moisturizing agents.

Dry skin is characterized by scaling and loss of suppleness and elasticity. The clinical appearance is fine scaling of the lower portions of the legs. In severe xerosis, loss of elasticity leads to cracking and fissuring, producing a superficial appearance of "cracked porcelain," referred to as "eczema craquelé." Itching is a common concomitant and may lead to scratching and excoriation. Occasionally, dry skin is associated with systemic diseases such as hypovitaminosis A, drug reactions, hypothyroidism, or ichthyosis.

PRINCIPLES OF THERAPY

After ruling out such systemic causes as hypothyroidism (see Chapter 104), treatment is largely symptomatic. The goals are to prevent loss of water and restore hydration. The modalities available include environmental manipulations, modifications in habits, and the judicious use of agents that hold water in the skin.

Preventive Measures. It is important to humidify the indoor environment, particularly during the winter months. In cold climates, humidification can be economically achieved by leaving pails of water near radiators, but, if necessary, humidifiers may be installed into forced-air heating systems.

One should teach the patient to avoid very strong soaps and detergents, which dry the skin. Many toilet bars are essentially detergents and extremely dehydrating. Substituting a well-oilated soap is recommended. Daily bathing may also be too drying, though a brief shower is much less drying than a bath. If baths are taken, adding a bath oil is helpful. It is also wise to avoid exposure to mild irritants such as solvents and to wool clothing.

Restoring Hydration. The treatment of preexisting dryness requires the addition of water and the application of hydrophobic agents. The physician should instruct patients to soak affected areas several minutes and apply a hydrophobic substance. Basically, most of the lotions and creams contain combinations of *petrolatum* (Vaseline), *mineral oil, lanolin, glycerin,* and *water* in proprietary blends. Lotions have more water, while creams have more hydrophobic ingredients. Plain petrolatum is inexpensive and effective, but it is not as pleasant to use as many proprietary preparations. The patient should avoid lanolin-based emollients if there is an allergy to wool.

A wide variety of agents are available, and patients are subjected to multimedia advertising for many of these products. Lubriderm and Keri lotions are light and easily applied, but less occlusive than emollient creams. Lac-Hydrin V is a 5% ammonium lactate that is available over-the-counter. The prescription version, which contains a 12% concentration, is the most potent emollient available. Aquaphor and Eucerin are greasier than the above-mentioned lotions and creams. Crisco may be the most economical emollient. To avoid the greasiness felt with petrolatum-based preparations, newer formulations such as Moisturel use esterified alcohols as emollients.

The plethora of expensive skin creams do little to retain moisture in the skin. Hygroscopic agents such as urea, alpha hydroxy acids, sorbitol, and glycerol have chemical properties that hold moisture in the skin. The apparent benefit may be due as much to their ability to plasticize the stratum corneum as to any real increase in moisture. Most moisturizers contain propylene glycol. If a patient experiences irritation from use of a facial moisturizer, it may be the propylene glycol that is causing the problem.

In severe cases or in order to achieve immediate results, topical corticosteroids, often with occlusive dressing, produce effective and rapid results. The use of Lac-Hydrin or Epilyt may help fissured fingertips, but sometimes a mid-potency corticosteroid ointment is required.

Occasionally, oral antipruritic agents such as the antihistamines may be required for severe generalized itching that results from xerosis (see Chapter 178). The physician should emphasize patient education to prevent recurrence.

THERAPEUTIC RECOMMENDATIONS

- Instruct the patient on environmental modifications to increase ambient humidity. Keep room temperature as low as is compatible with comfort.
- Caution the patient to avoid dehydrating soaps, solvents, or disinfectants. Do not scrub the skin.
- Encourage the use of bath oils and well-oilated soaps. The patient should soak in the tub for 1 to 10 minutes before the bath oil is added. Warn the patient about the potential for bath oil to cause slipping.
- Emollients should be used after showering or bathing. Try a variety of agents, beginning with the cheapest, to find one that is acceptable. The newer emollients using esterified alcohols or emulsifiers are the most cosmetically acceptable and the most costly.
- Lotions or creams that contain from 2% to 20% urea or from 5% to 12% lactate help hold water in the stratum corneum and may increase the plasticity of the skin.
- In the presence of eczematous change or for a patient who insists on rapid resolution, topical corticosteroid ointments with or without occlusion may be used.
- The most important aspect of management is patient education. The physician should reinforce the adjustments that prevent the development of dryness.

ANNOTATED BIBLIOGRAPHY

Blank IH. Action of emollient creams and their additives. JAMA 1959;164:412. *(Emollients help to retain water—rather than aiding as "lubricants.")*

Ghadially R, Halkier-Sorensen L, Elias PM. Effects of petrolatum on stratum corneum structure and function. J Am Acad Dermatol 1992;26:387. *(Petrolatum does not form or act like an impermeable membrane, but permeates through the interstices of the stratum corneum, allowing normal barrier recovery.)*

Middleton JD. The effects of temperature on extensibility of isolated corneum and its relation to skin chapping. Br J Dermatol 1969;81:717. *(The suppleness of stratum corneum is reduced easily when the temperature is lowered, perhaps a mechanism in chapping.)*

Rogers RS, Callen J, Wehr R, et al. Comparative efficacy of 12% ammonium lactate lotion and 5% lactic acid lotion in the treatment of moderate to severe xerosis. J Am Acad Dermatol 1989;21:814. *(The 12% ammonium lactate lotion [Lac-Hydrin] was significantly more effective than 5% lactic acid lotion for moderate to severe xerosis.)*

Steigleder R, Raab WP. Skin protection afforded by ointments. J Invest Dermatol 1962;38:129. *(Various ointments were compared for their barrier ability; white petrolatum proved to be the best.)*

Van Scott ES, Yu RS. Hyperkeratinization, corneocyte adhesion and alpha hydroxy acids. J Am Acad Dermatol 1984;11:867. *(Humectants such as lactic acid, malic acid, and glycolic acid maintain the thickness of the stratum corneum.)*

Wehr R, Krochmal L, Bagatell F, et al. A controlled two-center study of lactate 12 percent lotion and a petrolatum-based cream in patients with xerosis. Cutis 1986;37:205. *(Lac-Hydrin was significantly more effective than Eucerin Creme in reducing the severity of xerosis during treatment and thereafter.)*

Excessive Sweating

Excessive sweating (hyperhidrosis) is a common complaint, but it rarely signifies underlying pathology. Medical consultation may be sought because of abnormal wetness, a change in the pattern or amount of sweating, sweaty palms, stained clothing, or offensive odor. There is much variation in the amount people sweat in response to the physiologic stimuli of heat, emotion, or eating. The interaction of the person, the environment, and the emotions influences the amount of sweating. The primary physician must offer scientific explanation and symptomatic management to the person who complains of excessive sweating.

PATHOPHYSIOLOGY AND CLINICAL PRESENTATION

Sweating helps maintain temperature and fluid and electrolyte homeostasis, particularly under the environmental stresses of heat. There are two kinds of sweat glands, eccrine and apocrine. Cooling results from evaporation of eccrine sweat. Eccrine glands are concentrated on the palms and soles and are present on the face, axillae, and, to a lesser extent, the back and chest. Heat causes sweating on the face, upper chest, and back. Sweating of the palms and soles is a characteristic response to stress. Gustatory sweating occurs on the face, particularly on the upper lip, often following ingestion of spicy foods. The eccrine glands have no anatomic relation to other cutaneous appendages.

Sebaceous and apocrine glands are closely associated with hair follicles. The apocrine glands are concentrated in the axillae, areolae, groin, and perineum. Apocrine secretion consists of minuscule drops, viscid and milky, that produce odor after bacteria act on them.

Eccrine sweating is controlled by neural factors or a reflex. Thermal sweating is governed by the hypothalamus, and emotional sweating by the cerebral cortex. The innervation of eccrine glands is anatomically sympathetic, but for unexplained reasons the sweat glands are under cholinergic control and are therefore mediated by acetylcholine rather than by epinephrine. Excess sweating may be induced by abnormalities of the autonomic nervous system. Autonomic overactivity of the sweat glands may occur without identifiable cause. Sweating is associated with medical diseases that increase metabolic activity, causing the need for dissipation of heat. It is well known that during defervescence sweating occurs, particularly at night. Although the eccrine glands are under cholinergic control, epinephrine stimulates excessive sweating.

Most cases of excess sweating are caused by exaggerated physiologic responses or functional variations of no pathologic consequence. Hyperhidrosis most commonly involves the palms, soles, or axillae. This may be a result of an increase in impulses from the central nervous system (CNS), or it may reflect underlying problems with the sweat glands. There is often a relation to emotional stress, and the problem is disabling if it interferes with work or social interactions. Axillary hyperhidrosis is less common than palmar or plantar and produces the need for frequent clothing changes.

DIFFERENTIAL DIAGNOSIS

The most common cause of localized hyperhidrosis is the normal physiologic response to everyday stress. Menopause is the leading cause of generalized sweats. Of the pathologic causes, *fever* is the most common. Night sweats raise the possibility of underlying *infectious disease* and *malignancy*. Central neurologic injury from *stroke* or tumor may produce hyperhidrosis. *Peripheral neuropathy* involving the autonomic nerves is associated with excess sweating, as are such medical conditions as *thyrotoxicosis* and, uncommonly, *pheochromocytoma*. *Parkinson's disease* may lead to both increased sweating and sebaceous gland activity. Various *drugs*, such as antipyretics, insulin, meperidine, emetics, alcohol, and pilocarpine, may induce sweating. Gustatory sweating, though uncommon, may be caused by compensatory diabetic neuropathy, damage to the seventh nerve during parotid surgery, the rare Frey's syndrome, or injury to the sympathetic trunk following surgery.

WORKUP

History. Is the excess sweating restricted to the axillae, palms, and soles, indicative of a normal response to everyday events, or is it more generalized, suggesting an underlying medical condition? If sweating occurs primarily at night, then inquiry into fever, fatigue, adenopathy, cough, sputum production, and other symptoms of infection and malignancy should be sought (see Chapter 11). Generalized sweating should also trigger questions regarding hyperthyroidism (see Chapter 103) and menopause (see Chapter 118). Paroxysms are consistent with panic disorder (see Chapter 226) and pheochromocytoma (see Chapter 19). A careful drug history is needed, checking for use of antipyretics, insulin, meperidine, emetics, alcohol, and pilocarpine). The physician should ask whether excess sweating began relatively recently and can be correlated with stress.

Physical Examination and Laboratory Testing. The degree of sweating and its location are noted. If fever or generalized night sweats are reported, careful examination for underlying infection and cancer is required (see Chapter 11). The patient should also be examined for signs of hyperthyroidism (see Chapter 103). The presence of a blood pressure elevation should be noted because, if it is elevated in the setting of paroxysmal flushing and sweating, then pheochromocytoma should be considered. A careful neurologic examination is needed in patients suspected of CNS disease or peripheral autonomic neuropathy.

There are no mandatory laboratory investigations. Test selection is based entirely on the findings from history and physical examination. A screening "pan-scan" is of little use and is likely to generate more false-positive results than true-positive one.

SYMPTOMATIC MANAGEMENT AND PATIENT EDUCAITON

Excessive sweating can interfere with employment and social intercourse. Many therapies have been used; several are effective, but some are associated with undesirable side effects.

Topical Therapy. The most effective topical agent for use on the hands and in the axillae is a 20% alcoholic solution of *aluminum chloride hexahydrate (Drysol)*. A preparation of 6.25% aluminum tetrachloride (Xerac) is a less potent alternative. Clinical improvement in axillary hyperhidrosis may be seen after one to three consecutive treatments per week. Maintenance can usually be obtained with only one treatment per week after dryness has been achieved. Other topical therapies include 10% formalin compresses, which work well but can induce allergic sensitization. Buffered glutaraldehyde is effective but stains the skin. *Electrical current* may be used to temporarily block sweat glands. Such topical iontophoresis using either tapwater or an anticholinergic agent and aluminum chloride can reduce sweating of the palms. Tapwater units can be used at home. Response rates are in excess of 80 percent and have been reported with an average remission of about 1 month.

Systemic Therapy. *Scopolamine* and other cholinergics decrease sweating, but can cause CNS side effects and may precipitate glaucoma or urinary obstruction in patients with underlying prostatic hypertrophy. *Phenoxybenzamine*, an - adrenergic antagonist, has been reported to be successful in several cases of generalized hyperhidrosis.

Surgery. In rare instances of genuinely incapacitating hyperhidrosis, surgery is sometimes considered. Axillary hyperhidrosis may be cured with surgical extirpation of the eccrine glands in the axillae. Studies suggest that liposuction of the axillae may remove the sweat glands without altering the normal architecture. Palmar sweating may respond to sympathectomy.

Patient Education. Patient education is crucial to the treatment of excess sweating. Providing the patient with a scientific explanation and firm understanding of sweating is helpful in relieving anxiety. Patients with night sweats should record their temperature so that any significant febrile illness can be identified. The application of topical agents should be well explained and carefully used by patients. Surgical intervention for a problem as minor as hyperhidrosis requires the patient's understanding of the risks and benefits of such a procedure and the active involvement of the primary physician in helping the patient reach a decision.

THERAPEUTIC RECOMMENDATIONS

- Reassure the patient that excess sweating is not due to a pathologic condition, once medical etiologies have been ruled out.
- For axillary sweating, recommend frequent washing and changes of clothing.
- For excess sweating of the palms or the axillae, recommend a 20% alcoholic solution of aluminum chloride hexahydrate (*Drysol*). A 6.25% aluminum tetrachloride (*Xerac*) is an effective alternative. It should be applied at bedtime and covered with a plastic food wrap; polyethylene or vinyl gloves can be worn if the palms are affected. In the morning, the treated areas should be washed with soap and water. Prescribe 1–3 consecutive treatments per week. Once dryness has been achieved, maintenance with one treatment per week should suffice.
- Electrical current may be used to temporarily block sweat glands. The device (Drionic), used daily for 1 week, may relieve sweating for up to 1 month.
- If topical therapy and reassurance fail, surgery may be considered but only if the patient's hyperhidrosis is truly incapacitating. Liposuction techniques may be useful.

ANNOTATED BIBLIOGRAPHY

Adar R, Kurchin A, Zweig A. Palmar hyperhidrosis and its surgical treatment. A report of 100 cases. Ann Surg 1977;186:34. *(Eighty-nine percent success rate for bilateral upper dorsal sympathectomy for palmar hyperhidrosis.)*

Chalmers JM, Keele CA. The nervous and chemical control of sweating. Br J Dermatol 1952;64:43. *(Classic review of the pathophysiology of eccrine sweat production.)*

Christ JE. The application of suction-assisted lipectomy for the problem of axillary hyperhidrosis. Surg Gynecol Obstet 1989;169:457. *(A single hole cannula is used to remove axillary sweat glands in the subcutaneous fat and deep dermis.)*

Elgart ML, Fuchs G. Tapwater iontophoresis in the treatment of hyperhidrosis. Int J Dermatol 1987;26:194. *(The device can be used at home by patients; provides reduction in hyperhidrosis for up to 6 weeks.)*

Manusov EG, Nadeau MT. Hyperhidrosis: A management dilemma. J Fam Pract 1989;28:4125. *(Two patients with generalized hyperhidrosis were successfully treated with phenoxybenzamine, one at 20 mg/d, the other at 80 mg/d.)*

Sato K, Kang WH, Saga K, et al. Biology of sweat glands and their disorders. II. Disorders of sweat gland function. J Am Acad Dermatol 1989;20:713. *(Definitive review with comments about therapy; 117 refs.)*

Shen J-L, Lin G-S, Li W-M. A new strategy of iontophoresis for hyperhidrosis. J Am Acad Dermatol 1990;22:239. *(Using an anticholinergic agent and aluminum chloride, these investigators achieved an 87 percent response rate and an average remission of 32 days.)*

184
Approach to the Patient With Dermatitis

Primary Care Medicine: Office Evaluation and Management of the Adult Patient, 3rd edition, edited by Allan H. Goroll, Lawrence A. May, and Albert G. Mulley, Jr. J.B. Lippincott Company, Philadelphia

Atopic and Contact Dermatitis

STEPHEN J. FRIEDMAN, M.D.

The atopic and contact dermatitides (also referred to as "eczema") are frequently encountered in medical practice and may be acute or chronic. The acute form is characterized by erythema, edema, vesiculation, oozing, crusting, and scaling. The chronic stage manifests excoriation, thickening, hyperpigmentation, and often lichenification. These conditions are defined clinically by the observable changes in the skin, which reflect a common cutaneous reaction to a variety of pathogenetic stimuli. The clinical challenges for the primary care physician are to provide symptomatic relief and identify the underlying precipitant. These tasks can be difficult, often necessitating consultation with a dermatologist.

PATHOPHYSIOLOGY AND CLINICAL PRESENTATION

Pathophysiology

Atopic Dermatitis. The pathogenesis of atopic dermatitis remains incompletely understood, but a genetic predisposition is believed to be important. Two-thirds of patients have family members with asthma, hay fever, or atopic dermatitis and often suffer from other forms of atopy themselves. Psychological stress may induce flares. Environmental factors also contribute. Certain fabrics, notably wool, may induce itching. Lesions are exacerbated by extremes of temperature and humidity. Defects in cell-mediated immunity have been noted, perhaps accounting for the observed increase in susceptibility to cutaneous viral infections. Infection may also precipitate an attack.

Contact Dermatitis. The cause is exposure of the skin to a precipitant, be it purely irritant or immunologic in effect. Irritants penetrate and disrupt the stratum corneum, injuring the underlying epidermis and causing an inflammatory reaction. Irritant effects are universal and require no previous exposure. Strong acids, alkalis, detergents, and organic solvents are among the important irritants.

Immunologically mediated contact reactions occur only in patients who have been previously sensitized to an allergen. Important sensitizing antigens include nickel; rubber;

topical anesthetics; neomycin; and the antigens of poison ivy, oak, and sumac.

Clinical Presentations

Atopic dermatitis is characterized by intense itching leading to scratching, eczematous change, and lichenification. In adults, the lesions characteristically involve the neck, wrists, the area behind the ears, and the antecubital and popliteal flexural areas. *Nummular eczema* is a variant recognized by pruritic coin-shaped lesions located on the external aspects of the extremities, the buttocks, and the posterior aspect of the trunk. The lesions may ooze, crust, and become purulent. The course varies; there may be a few constant lesions or a gradual increase in the number of lesions. The prognosis is good, with eventual clearing, although it may take years.

Contact dermatitis can affect any area of the body. Linear patterns are pathognomonic, but almost any pattern may be seen. Distribution and location of the rash may provide clues to the irritant or allergen. Patch testing can help to identify the contactant.

Chronic hand dermatitis presents a diagnostic and therapeutic challenge that can tax the most experienced dermatologist. It may be irritant in nature (eg, "housewives' hands"), pustular (chronic pustular eruption), or even vesicular (pompholyx or dyshidrosis). It can occur in the context of a fungal infection with "id" reaction, contact with household irritants, or dyshidrosis.

Regardless of cause, chronic eczematous change may lead to *lichen simplex chronicus*. Itching may be intense, and the condition may be complicated by secondary infection. Lichen simplex chronicus can also result from localized neurodermatitis and present as a circumscribed plaque of thickened skin with increased markings, some scaling, and papulation. The occipital region is a common site. Lesions may also be seen on the wrists, thighs, or lower aspects of the legs. Women are more commonly affected. The prognosis is variable, but when scratching is stopped, lesions regress.

PRINCIPLES OF MANAGEMENT

The management of eczema embodies the fundamental principles of dermatologic therapy: precipitants should be eliminated, wet lesions dried, dry lesions hydrated, and inflammation treated with corticosteroids. Resistance to treatment should be anticipated, and if basic management fails, referral to an experienced dermatologist should be prompt. A search for precipitating factors is mandatory. Topical corticosteroids are always required.

Acute eczematous dermatitis benefits from drying measures such as Burow's solution compresses. Systemic corticosteroids are sometimes used on a short-term basis for generalized or incapacitating dermatitis. Topical corticosteroids are used in milder cases. Secondary bacterial infection may require topical mupirocin ointment three times per day, or systemic antibiotics if the condition is extensive.

Chronic eczematous dermatitis usually is of an irritant nature, benefitting from identification and withdrawal of possible irritants. Detergents, gasoline, polishes, and other occupational and household products should be avoided. Frequent baths or showers, hot water, and use of drying soaps should be reduced. Although systemic corticosteroids are contraindicated in chronic eczema, topical steroids are helpful and often needed for prolonged periods.

Topical Corticosteroids

Topical steroids exert anti-inflammatory, antipruritic, and antiproliferative effects. There is a wide variation in potency of available agents as measured by vasoconstriction assays (Table 184–1). The strongest steroid is 500 times more effective in blanching the skin than is the weakest. Often, there are potency differences between generic and brand-name creams.

Preparations and Their Selection. Preparations are categorized according to strength (see Table 184–1). The halo-

Table 184-1. Topical Corticosteroid Preparations*

Group 1—Highest Potency
Betamethasone dipropionate in optimized vehicle 0.05% cream, ointment, solution (Diprolene)
Clobetasol propionate 0.05% cream, ointment, solution (Temovate)
Halobetasol propionate 0.05% cream, ointment (Ultravate)
Diflorasone diacetate 0.05% cream, ointment (Psorcon)
Group 2—High Potency
Amcinonide 0.1% ointment (Cyclocort)
Betamethasone dipropionate 0.05% ointment (Diprosone)
Desoximetasone 0.25% cream and ointment (Topicort)
Fluocinonide 0.05% cream, gel, ointment, solution (Lidex)
Halcinonide 0.1% cream, ointment (Halog)
Group 3—Medium–High Potency
Amcinonide 0.1% cream (Cyclocort)
Betamethasone dipropionate 0.05% cream (Diprosone, Maxivate)
Diflorasone diacetate 0.05% cream, ointment (Florone, Maxiflor)
Group 4—Medium Potency
Desoximetasone 0.05% cream (Topicort LP)
Flurandrenolide 0.05% ointment (Cordran)
Hydrocortisone butyrate 0.1% ointment (Locoid)
Hydrocortisone valerate 0.2% ointment (Westcort)
Mometasone furoate 0.1% cream, ointment (Elocon)
Triamcinolone acetonide 0.1% ointment (Aristocort, Kenalog)
Group 5—Low Potency
Alclometasone dipropionate 0.05% cream (Aclovate)
Betamethasone valerate 0.1% cream (Valisone)
Flurandrenolide 0.05% cream (Cordran)
Fluocinolone acetonide 0.025% cream (Synalar, Synemol, Fluonid)
Hydrocortisone butyrate 0.1% cream (Locoid)
Hydrocortisone valerate 0.2% cream (Westcort)
Triamcinolone acetonide 0.1% cream or lotion (Aristocort, Kenalog)
Group 6—Mild Potency
Desonide 0.05% cream (Tridesilon)
Fluocinolone acetonide 0.01% solution (Fluonid, Synalar)
Group 7—Lowest Potency
Dexamethasone 0.1% gel, ointment (Decadron)
Hydrocortisone 0.5%, 1%, and 2.5% cream, ointment, lotion (Hytone, Synacort, Nutracort)

*It is recommended that one become familiar with and use one agent from each category, making the selection on the basis of cost, cosmetic acceptability, and efficacy.

genated preparations are the most potent, particularly those available in ointment formulation (see below). One starts with a sufficiently potent formulation to establish control of the eczematous process and then switches to a lower potency preparation if maintenance therapy is indicated. Because of the large number of available preparations, it is recommended that the clinician become familiar with one agent from each category, making the choice on the basis of cost, cosmetic acceptability, and efficacy.

Topical hydrocortisone is available over-the-counter in strengths that cannot exceed 1%. Mild forms of dermatitis may respond, but the patient often selects the wrong vehicle—for example, an ointment when a lotion or cream would be better.

Formulations and Application. The vehicle affects potency and cosmetic acceptability. *Ointment* formulations are more potent than *creams* and are best reserved for thick, scaling lesions. Nongreasy cream formulations are quite acceptable cosmetically and easy to use on trunk, extremities, or face. *Gels* can be used in hairy areas as well as on glabrous skin, though gels are somewhat drying when used on nonhairy skin. *Lotions* may be creamy or alcohol-based, but in either case they are more drying than creams. Specialized formulations include aerosol *sprays*, which are used in the scalp or to cover large areas of skin in acute dermatitis.

Occlusion of the skin enhances penetration, with up to 100 times more vasoconstriction observed if polyethylene film is used over a given formulation than if no occlusion is used. Steroid-impregnated tape (Cordran) provides its own occlusion, but its convenience is rarely justified by its expense. Ointments are generally not occluded because folliculitis may develop.

Topical agents are normally applied two to four times daily, but retention of steroid in the stratum corneum makes one or two applications per day sufficient. Because hydration of the epidermis is salutary for healing, concomitant use of a moisturizer is beneficial.

In prescribing a topical agent, it is helpful to estimate the quantity of topical medication that will be required. A 10-day to 2-week course of therapy applied two to three times daily requires 30 g for the face, 45 g for feet or hands, 60 g for arms or legs, 60 to 90 g for the trunk, and 120 to 150 g for the whole body.

Adverse Effects. The potent halogenated corticosteroids are the most likely to cause *atrophy*, *telangiectasia*, *purpura*, *striae*, and an *acneiform eruption*. Superpotent corticosteroids have recommended restrictions for their use: no more than 45 g of medication per week and no longer than 2 weeks. Suppression of the pituitary–adrenal axis as measured by plasma cortisol levels may be demonstrable but is rarely clinically significant. Thin-skinned areas are especially susceptible to development of atrophy. Less potent formulations should also be used on areas such as the face, the dorsum of the hands, and the scrotum. Fluorinated steroids may cause *rosacea* if used on the face. Only low-potency ophthalmic preparations should be used around the eye. Low-potency products are also preferred in the groin and axillae because of the risk of striae with more potent preparations. Purpura is seen on the dorsal aspect of the forearms and hands after long-term use of potent topicals.

PATIENT EDUCATION AND INDICATIONS FOR REFERRAL

Patients must be instructed about proper use of topical steroids. They need to be specifically warned to avoid contact with eyes and eyelids (unless a low-dose ophthalmic preparation is prescribed) and to avoid use of a potent topical formulation on the face. If a brief course of oral prednisone therapy is necessary, the patient should be given a written schedule to ensure proper tapering and cessation within 10 to 14 days. For those with atopic disease, advice on substances to avoid is greatly appreciated. Simple measures such as clipping fingernails and wearing cotton gloves can reduce secondary excoriation. Early identification and treatment of eczematous exacerbations helps facilitate treatment. Those with chronic hand dermatitis need to know that prolonged treatment may be necessary.

Patients with chronic hand dermatitis often prove refractory to the basic measures prescribed by the primary physician. Referral to the dermatologist for more detailed identification of precipitants and advancement of the treatment program may be helpful.

THERAPEUTIC RECOMMENDATIONS

- Identify and remove potential contacts, allergens and irritants. Treat any skin dryness (see Chapter 183). Use of rubber gloves with cotton linings may be beneficial.
- Oozing lesions should be dried with Burow's solution compresses applied three to four times a day; colloidal oatmeal baths are indicated for more generalized lesions.
- Pruritus should be suppressed, if possible, with a topical antipruritic, (eg, Pramosone cream/lotion) or a systemic antihistamine (see Chapter 178).
- For acute dermatitis, begin with a fluorinated corticosteroid cream. Start with the highest potency steroid preparation necessary, and reduce steroid potency as soon as the acute inflammation has been controlled. If the acute process is extensive and severe, begin oral prednisone at a starting dose of 1 mg/kg/day and taper rapidly to full cessation over 10 to 14 days.
- For chronic lichenified eruptions, treat for prolonged periods with ointment formulations or, if unresponsive, steroid cream under occlusion. In refractory cases, intralesional injection or a diluted triamcinolone solution (2.0–3.0 mg/mL) given by an experienced physician may be effective.
- Refer to the dermatologist those with refractory hand dermatitis.

ANNOTATED BIBLIOGRAPHY

Epstein E. Hand dermatitis: practical management and current concepts. J Am Acad Dermatol 1984;10:395. *(Describes causes and methods of treatment.)*

Goa KL. Clinical pharmacology and pharmacokinetic properties of topically applied corticosteroids. A review. Drugs 1988; 36:51. *(A look at the drug characteristics affecting absorption, potency, and side effects; 77 refs.)*

Hanifin JM. Atopic dermatitis: new therapeutic considerations. J Am Acad Dermatol 1991;24:1097. *(Good discussion of therapeutic options.)*

Jeckler J, Larko O. Combined UVA-UVB versus UVB phototherapy for atopic dermatitis: a paired-comparison study. J Am Acad Dermatol 1990;22:49. *(Combined UVA-UVB therapy was superior to UVB therapy.)*

Stoughton RB, Cornell RC. Review of super-potent topical corticosteroids. Semin Dermatol 1987;6:72. *(Guidelines for safe and effective use of superpotent topical steroids.)*

Weidman AI, Sawicty HH. Nummular eczema. Review of the literature: survey of 516 case records and follow-up of 125 patients. Arch Dermatol 1956;73:58. *(Classic review and long-term evaluation of 125 patients.)*

STEPHEN J. FRIEDMAN, M.D.
WILLIAM V. R. SHELLOW, M.D.

Management of Seborrheic Dermatitis

Seborrheic dermatitis affects almost 5 percent of the adult population. It is a benign but chronic inflammatory skin disease that is constitutionally determined but without definite cause. Its high prevalence and incurability render it a therapeutic challenge. The primary physician must be capable of treating seborrheic dermatitis and educating the patient about chronicity and the need for continued management.

PATHOPHYSIOLOGY AND CLINICAL PRESENTATION

Pathogenesis. The cause of seborrheic dermatitis remains unknown. The anatomic localization correlates with areas of sebaceous gland concentration. The quantity or composition of sebum is not the main factor necessary for its development. Hormonal influences, fatigue, and anxiety may trigger or aggravate the condition. An etiologic relation between the yeast *Pityrosporum ovale* and seborrheic dermatitis has been postulated, supported by the finding that topical ketoconazole produces improvement or resolution in some patients. Conversely, if the number of yeast organisms increases, the problem recurs.

Clinical Presentation. Seborrheic dermatitis presents as scaly patches that are occasionally slightly papular, surrounded by minimal to moderate erythema. The borders of the lesions are ill defined, and the scales may be greasy and appear yellow. The lesion is usually asymptomatic, but pruritus may occur. More extensive disease involves the forehead at the margin of the hair, eyebrows, nasal folds, and the retroauricular and presternal area. In more severe cases, intertriginous areas, the external ear canal, and the umbilicus are involved. In these areas, erythema and exudation predominate, progressing to chronic dermatitis with scaling. The scalp is most often involved, and the condition is differentiated from common dandruff by its association with erythema. Seborrheic dermatitis can occur at any age but is most common during infancy and after the second decade of life.

Seborrheic dermatitis is associated with several conditions, such as Parkinson's disease, phenylketonuria, prior cardiac failure, zinc deficiency, and epilepsy. Cutaneous diseases such as acne vulgaris, rosacea, or psoriasis may be associated with it. Florid manifestations of seborrhea may be an early cutaneous indicator of human immunodeficiency virus (HIV) infection. The dermatitis in such patients may be very extensive and resistant to therapy.

PRINCIPLES OF MANAGEMENT

As noted earlier, the condition is chronic and persistent. The approach to treatment has evolved with the growing realization of the role of *P. ovale* in pathogenesis. Previously, treatment was strictly symptomatic, directed at removing scale, reducing oiliness and redness, and controlling itching. Now the approach is a bit more etiologic and includes reducing the yeast count on the skin. Therapy is guided by the severity, anatomic location, and relative degree of scale, erythema, and oiliness.

Ketoconazole (Nizoral) has proven to be very useful for topical use. It has both fungistatic and fungicidal action, depending on the concentration used. Its 3- to 9-day residual effect between applications is an added advantage. Cream and shampoo formulations are available. For mild to moderate facial or chest involvement, ketoconazole 2% cream to the affected areas twice a day until clear often suffices. Indefinite maintenance therapy may be required once or twice weekly. Though effective, this therapy is expensive, especially if prolonged use is required.

Shampoos for Scaling. Scaling can be prominent with scalp involvement, and it responds well to shampoo formulations. The regular use of an over-the-counter dandruff or antiseborrheic shampoo is often sufficient. To be effective, the shampoos should generate good detergent action and be allowed to remain in contact with the scalp for at least 5 to 7 minutes. Commercially available shampoos to combat seborrhea may contain selenium sulfide, zinc pyrithione, tar, salicylic acid, sulfur, or ketoconazole. Most preparations contain multiple agents but have one predominant active ingredient. Zinc pyrithione (Danex, DHS Zinc, Head & Shoulders, Sebulon, Zincon, and ZNP bar shampoos) and selenium sulfide (Selsun Blue and prescription Exsel and Selsun shampoos) have been classified as keratolytic agents. Their mode of action also appears to be fungicidal and cytostatic. The combination of sulfur and salicylic acid (Sebulex, Ionil, and Vanseb shampoos) has keratolytic, mild antifungal, and antiseptic effects. Coal tar is the prominent ingredient in Sebutone, Pentrax, T-Gel, and Zetar shampoos, which must be used cautiously, if at all, in blond or light gray-haired people because it may change the color of the hair.

The patient should be given a list of recommended antiseborrheic agents as a guide and advised to find one suitable to his preference for lather, odor, and efficacy. Many patients find that a shampoo works for a period, then becomes less effective, and a new product must be chosen.

For patients with resistant seborrheic dermatitis who have tried many over-the-counter shampoos before reaching the physician, a prescription shampoo may be of benefit: 2.5% selenium sulfide shampoo (Exel or Selsun), chloroxine shampoo (Capitrol), or ketoconazole shampoo (Nizoral) should be administered. Heavy crusts may be softened with keratolytic lotions (Sebizon, Sebucare) or oil-based agents (Derma-Smoothe F/S liquid, P & S liquid) before shampooing.

Topical Corticosteroids for Erythema. Significant erythema requires use of a topical corticosteroid preparation. In hairy areas, a lotion, spray, or gel may be applied two to four times daily. Creams should be avoided because they cause hair to become matted. Ointments are satisfactory to use at night, but they make the hair greasy and require shampooing again in the morning. On the scalp, a fluorinated corticosteroid is acceptable. Mild erythema on glabrous skin should be treated by washing with a mild soap twice a day, followed by application of hydrocortisone cream, 0.5% to 1.0%. Hydrocortisone is relatively inexpensive and has considerably less risk of causing telangiectasia and atrophy; a 1% concentration may be used for erythematous or papular lesions.

After initial success, there may be a period of tachyphylaxis, requiring increased concentrations of medium-potency, nonfluorinated steroids. Telangiectasia and other signs of dermal atrophy may occur with the long-term use of these products, and they should be avoided on the face. Topical ketoconazole produces no such adverse skin changes. Intertriginous seborrheic dermatitis may require Burow's solution compresses for exudative lesions, followed by a fluorinated corticosteroid lotion. Secondary bacterial infection may require the use of systemic antimicrobial agents.

PATIENT EDUCATION

It is reassuring for the patient to know that seborrhea is neither contagious nor progressive, but the chronic nature of the condition also needs to be noted. Its relation to stress may help explain flares. Providing the patient with a list of over-the-counter preparations is appreciated. If topical steroid therapy is needed, the patient should be cautioned about its potential adverse effects and instructed in proper application.

THERAPEUTIC RECOMMENDATIONS

- Provide the patient with a list of over-the-counter shampoos and suggest selecting one that meets personal preferences. For oily hair, advise shampooing daily for the first week, decreasing to two or three times a week for maintenance. For resistant cases, use ketoconazole shampoo every other day.
- For mild to moderate facial or chest involvement, ketoconazole 2% cream may be applied to the affected areas twice a day until clear. Maintenance therapy may be required once or twice weekly indefinitely.
- If erythema is present, prescribe a topical nonfluorinated corticosteroid preparation (eg, hydrocortisone, 1% or 2.5% cream) for the face; a fluorinated lotion is appropriate for the scalp (eg, betamethasone valerate, 0.1% lotion).
- Remove heavy crusts by softening with keratolytic lotions or oil-based agents before shampooing.
- Treat exudative intertriginous lesions with drying and a nonfluorinated topical steroid lotion.
- Blepharitis may be treated hygienically, gently rubbing the eyelashes with a coarse washcloth. Occasionally, a steroid-containing eye ointment, such as Metimyd or Blephamide solution, may be used, cautiously, because of the hazard of steroid in the eye.

ANNOTATED BIBLIOGRAPHY

Faergemann J. Treatment of seborrheic dermatitis of the scalp with ketoconazole shampoo: a double-blind study. Acta Derm Venereol (Stockh) 1990;70:171. *(Ketoconazole was superior to placebo.)*

Heng MCY, Henderson CL, Barker DC, et al. Correlation of *Pityrosporum ovale* density with clinical severity of seborrheic dermatitis as assessed by a simplified technique. J Am Acad Dermatol 1990;23:82. (P. ovale *numbers in the stratum corneum correlated with disease severity; improvement correlated with reduction in organism density.)*

Katsambas A, Antoniouu CH, Frangouli E, et al. A double-blind trial of treatment of seborrheic dermatitis with 2% ketoconazole cream compared with 1% hydrocortisone cream. Br J Dermatol 1989;121:353. (Pityrosporum *was reduced in both treatment groups, but the reduction was significantly higher for the group treated with ketoconazole.)*

Mathes BM, Douglas NC. Seborrheic dermatitis in patients with acquired immunodeficiency syndrome. J Am Acad Dermatol 1985;13:947. *(High prevalence in HIV infection; severity is greater than usual and is associated with a poor prognosis.)*

Primary Care Medicine: Office Evaluation and Management of the Adult Patient, 3rd edition, edited by Allan H. Goroll, Lawrence A. May, and Albert G. Mulley, Jr. J.B. Lippincott Company, Philadelphia

185
Management of Acne

RONALD M. REISNER, M.D.

Acne, the most common of all skin diseases, is a polygenic, multifactorial disease that, depending on the strictness of its definition, afflicts between 50 percent and 100 percent of adolescents in the United States. It ranges in severity from a few scattered whiteheads and blackheads to disfiguring, painful, deep-seated, pus-filled and bleeding nodulocystic lesions. About 15 percent of surveyed patients with acne seek medical care. The primary care physician is in a unique position to identify and treat a high proportion of acne sufferers. Properly managing acne requires a thorough understanding of the development of acne in all its phases, so that therapy appropriate to the circumstances can be selected from the available modalities. Early effective treatment minimizes the physical scarring of the disease and prevents or reduces equally important psychic trauma.

PATHOPHYSIOLOGY AND CLINICAL PRESENTATION

The pathogenesis of acne is proving to be increasingly complex. It involves the interaction of enzymatic, immunologic, and chemotactic effects of normal cutaneous microflora; hormonal influences; abnormal keratinization of the sebaceous follicular duct wall; increased sebum production; follicular fragility; and host responsiveness.

Acne is a disease of the sebaceous follicles. Each person has approximately 5000 sebaceous follicles, scattered predominantly on the face and central upper back and chest. The initial event in the pathogenesis of acne is conversion of the loose, easily shed, horny layer of the epithelium lining the follicular duct wall to a self-adhering mass that gradually obstructs the follicular duct. This has been called "retention hyperkeratosis." It takes 1 to 2 months for the accumulated mass of keratin, sebum, and bacteria to reach visible size as a closed comedo or whitehead. Whiteheads may expand the duct ("pore") opening to communicate freely with the outside. The compact, melanin-rich tip then gives the appearance and name "blackhead." The color is not caused by the oxidation of lipids in the sebum.

Chemotactic agents produced by bacteria within the duct attract leukocytes, and, in ensuing events, duct walls may rupture, releasing follicular contents into the surrounding dermis. This provokes a profound inflammatory response, leading to the development of papules, pustules, nodules, and suppurative nodules that are commonly, but mistakenly, termed "cysts." These inflammatory lesions may lead to permanent scarring.

Propionibacterium acnes, a normal inhabitant of the follicular canal in humans, may participate in the initiation and aggravation of inflammatory lesions by elaborating enzymes, including lipases, that act on sebum to release potentially irritating free fatty acids. Its hyaluronidase may increase permeability of the follicular duct wall, and its protease can damage it, increasing leakage of materials into the surrounding dermis. In addition, *P. acnes* produces chemotactic substances that contribute to the initiation and evolution of inflammatory lesions.

Clinical Presentation. Acne may most conveniently be divided into two categories, *obstructive* and *inflammatory*. The former, resulting from the impaction of horny material, bacteria, and sebum in the dilated follicular duct wall, is characterized by closed comedones (whiteheads) and open comedones (blackheads). Leakage of intrafollicular contents from comedones produces an inflammatory response. Depending on the level of leakage into the dermis and the amount of material released, lesions vary from small, erythematous papules and superficial pustules to deeper pustules and larger, persistent, and occasionally suppurative nodules. Genetic immunologic factors may contribute to an exaggerated inflammatory response and more severe cystic forms of acne.

PRINCIPLES OF THERAPY

Removal of acnegenic agents is the first principle of therapy. Some cosmetics, oils, and creams may be capable of producing comedones, and their use should be stopped. Androgens are acnegenic. Changing from an oral contraceptive containing androgenic progestins (eg, norethindrone, norgestrel) to one with more estrogenic ones can help (see Chapter 119). The physician should advise against using acnegenic drugs such as androgens, steroids, iodides, and bromides. Since there is no evidence that particular foods are acnegenic, dietary changes are not indicated.

After precipitants have been eliminated, the goals of therapy shift to treatment of existing lesions and further prevention of new ones. The modalities employed depend on the kind of lesion.

Obstructive Acne

Removal and prevention of comedones are the initial tasks. Closed comedo removal is accomplished by atraumatically nicking the covering epidermis with a No. 11 blade or blood lancet and extracting the contents with a comedo extractor. Open comedones are expressed without nicking. The expression of comedones has little influence on future inflammatory lesions but does improve appearance. Comedolytic agents are needed for prevention of future lesions.

Retinoic acid (Tretinoin, Retin-A) is the only significantly comedolytic agent currently available. It helps remove existing comedones and prevent future ones. Topical retinoic acid thins the outer horny layer of the epidermis, diminishes hyperkeratosis, and loosens existing comedones, making extraction easier. It also helps prevent formation of new lesions, both obstructive and inflammatory. Because retinoic acid thins the outer epidermis, one should advise avoiding other drying topical medications, excessive cleansing, and marked sun exposure. In addition, patients should be warned of a possible transient pustular flare after therapy is initiated.

Tretinoin is available in cream, gel, and liquid vehicle, in ascending order of dryness and irritation potential. The cream is available in 0.025%, 0.05%, and 0.1% concentrations, with the 0.025% concentration tolerated by a large proportion of all users. Most patients should start by using the 0.025% cream once daily. The gel is available at 0.01% and 0.025% concentrations and the liquid at 0.05%. The liquid would ordinarily be reserved for severe involvement of the back and chest in patients who have tolerated the cream and the gel but are not getting the desired response.

Adverse reactions to tretinoin are primarily irritation, although rare true allergic contact dermatitis has been described. Tretinoin increases the risk of sunburn. The frequency of application is adjusted to produce minimally visible erythema and desquamation.

Within 3 to 6 weeks one may add *benzoyl peroxide*, which, although minimally comedolytic, may help to reduce the formation of new comedones by reducing *P. acnes* in the follicle. Its main value, however, is in the treatment of inflammatory acne (see below). It is applied once daily, approximately 8 to 12 hours after topical retinoic acid.

Other Agents and Cleansing. Some comedolytic activity has also been suggested for the topical alpha-hydroxy acids, but this remains to be fully documented. *Cleansing* measures to remove excess oil do not affect the course of acne, although patients with acne may have oily skin and cleansing may improve an undesirable oily appearance. Gentle cleansing methods such as use of mild soap and water are well tolerated. Astringents, generally mixtures of alcohol or acetone and water, are a convenient means of removing excess oil.

Retinoic acid and benzoyl peroxide have largely replaced compounds that contain *sulfur*, *salicylic acid*, and *resorcinol*. These and other topical agents may be used concomitantly with systemic agents in more severe inflammatory acne.

Mild Inflammatory Acne

Mild inflammatory acne may be treated with topical agents used for obstructive lesions. Benzoyl peroxide is particularly useful; topical antibiotics are sometimes beneficial as well.

Benzoyl peroxide increases the rate of resorption of small erythematous papules and thin-roofed pustules. It acts primarily as a bacteriocidal agent for *P. acnes*. It is available in a variety of bases including gels, lotions, and creams, in order of decreasing drying impact of the vehicle. Concentrations commonly available are 2.5%, 5%, and 10%. For most patients, 2.5% is as effective as higher concentrations. The drying effect of topical medications of various kinds is additive and may be decreased by less frequent application, by using a less drying base (ie, a cream or a lotion rather than a gel or a hydroalcoholic solution), or by recommending a noncomedogenic moisturizer. Common side effects include irritation, which produces redness, dryness, burning, and stinging; allergic reactions, which produce a localized contact dermatitis in 1 percent to 5 percent of patients; and bleaching or discoloration of fabric and hair.

Topical antibiotics are used in mild inflammatory acne to suppress *P. acnes* and its elaboration of harmful enzymes. This is a preventive form of therapy that does little for preexisting lesions. Consequently, clinical results may take several weeks to become evident.

The topical antibiotics for acne include erythromycin, clindamycin, and meclocycline. Each of these agents is bacteriostatic for *P. acnes*. *Clindamycin* is available as a 1% solution, 1% gel, and 1% creamy lotion, in descending order of drying of the skin. Topical *erythromycin* is available in 2% solution, 2% gel, and 2% ointment.

The lotions are available with a pad applicator top. Without an applicator top, the solution can be applied with the fingertips to large areas of involvement like the back. The applicator top is a convenience but tends to become soiled after repeated use. The patient should be told that this is not harmful and that repeated use of the applicator will not "spread bacteria around the face." A convenient but more expensive way to apply erythromycin is premoistened swabs which are used once and then discarded. Fastidious patients may prefer this to the other available forms of erythromycin solution.

Adverse reactions common to the topical erythromycins and clindamycins include dryness (which is related primarily to the vehicle); irritation, characterized by redness, burning or peeling; and, occasionally, a sensation of oiliness. These preparations are, in general, irritating if they get into the eye. A few cases of severe colitis and pseudomembranous colitis have been reported to develop during or after therapy with topical clindamycin. Patients should be instructed to discontinue topical clindamycin if diarrhea develops until the problem can be identified.

Topical *meclocycline* (Meclan) is available in a cream base but is seldom used, because it has a sulfurous odor when first applied to the skin.

More severe disease is treated with systemic antibiotics (see below).

Severe Inflammatory Acne

This form of acne is characterized by large, deep papules and pustules and destructive, suppurating, nodular lesions and requires systemic therapy. Because *P. acnes* is believed to play an important role in the pathogenesis of inflammatory acne, antibiotics have become the mainstay of therapy.

Systemic antibiotic therapy is the best means of preventing new inflammatory lesions. By suppressing *P. acnes*, the risk of enzymatic injury to the gland is markedly reduced along with the rate of new lesion formation. However, because antibiotics do nothing for existing lesions, it takes as long as 6 to 8 weeks before improvement is noted. Existing papulopustular lesions may persist for 7 to 10 days, and deep, nodulocystic lesions may remain for months. Four decades of experience with systemic antibiotic therapy, including a detailed review of indications and hazards of such therapy by an ad hoc committee of the American Academy of Dermatology, has established it as rational, effective, and remarkably safe.

The usual approach to systemic antibiotic therapy is to initiate treatment with *tetracycline* or *erythromycin*, 250 mg four times daily. Therapy must be continued for at least 6 to 8 weeks to determine whether the patient is responding. Response consists of a decrease in the formation of new lesions. This is preventive therapy. After a response is observed, the dosage may gradually be decreased over a period of weeks to the lowest effective maintenance dose. To avoid the problem of poor absorption with meals, tetracycline should be given at least 1 hour before or 2 hours after meals. Because this is often difficult with teenagers who eat frequently during the day, a dosage schedule of 500 mg twice daily is often used. Generic tetracycline and generic erythromycin are the least expensive of the commonly used systemic antibiotics in acne.

Long-term systemic use of tetracycline or erythromycin may be combined with intensive topical therapy. Other members of the tetracycline family that may be preferred because their absorption is not significantly affected by food include minocycline and doxycycline. They are much more expensive than generic tetracycline. The monohydrate of doxycycline has been introduced as less irritating than the older hyclate salt. Contraindications to tetracycline include known hypersensitivity, pregnancy, and age younger than 12 years.

An occasional complication of systemic antibiotic therapy is the development of a gram-negative folliculitis with pustules around the nose and mouth spreading onto the cheeks. Culture of the lesions with identification of the organisms—usually *Klebsiella* or *Enterobacter*—is indicated. It often responds within a few days to *trimethoprim-sulpha*. More recently, 13-*cis*-retinoic acid has proved useful for gram-negative folliculitis.

Topical and Intralesional Therapies. *Benzoyl peroxide* and *retinoic acid* appear to be synergistic with antibiotic therapy, possibly increasing antibiotic concentration in the follicular duct. *Intralesional corticosteroids* may hasten involution of nodulocystic lesions, reducing the risk of permanent scarring. *Triamcinolone acetonide*, 2.0 or 2.5 mg/mL in saline injected with a 30-gauge needle directly into specific lesions, is often remarkably effective. Pseudoatrophy is a danger. The physician should avoid dosages in excess of 20 mg per week, which may suppress the pituitary–adrenal axis. Some dermatologists prefer to use cryotherapy with *liquid nitrogen*. This requires experience to avoid excessive freezing and tissue destruction.

13-*cis*-Retinoic acid (isotretinoin, Accutane) is a powerful systemic agent for the treatment of nodulocystic inflammatory acne. One or two 15- to 20-week courses often bring severe acne under complete control, with little or no further therapy. However, it is essential for the physician to recognize that this is a potent *teratogen* which has caused numerous tragic birth defects. The Guidelines of Care for Acne Vulgaris published by the American Academy of Dermatology clearly state that 13-*cis*-retinoic acid should not be therapy of first choice and that it must be demonstrated that the patient is unresponsive to other standard therapies. In the treatment of women of childbearing potential, it should be used only in patients with severe, disfiguring, cystic acne.

Guidelines for use are very well presented in a special patient use kit provided by the manufacturer. This includes a detailed informed consent protocol, which must be completed by the patient, with a copy given to the patient and a copy kept in the patient's record. The woman must use effective contraception, including abstinence, for at least 1 month before starting 13-*cis*-retinoic acne therapy and must have a negative blood test for pregnancy 2 weeks before initiating therapy. The drug should not be prescribed until the negative pregnancy test has been returned; then the patient must be instructed to initiate therapy during the second or third day of the next menstrual period. The patient should be seen monthly thereafter with suitable laboratory studies done periodically, including a recommended monthly pregnancy test. Contraceptive use must continue for at least 1 month after completion of therapy, and a blood pregnancy test should be done 1 month after completion of therapy. Should a pregnancy occur, suitable counseling must be undertaken to assist the patient in deciding on the management of the pregnancy, including possible termination.

Other side effects associated with 13-*cis*-retinoic acid include hypertriglyceridemia, pseudotumor cerebri, idiopathic skeletal hyperostosis, cheilitis, nasal mucosal dryness, nosebleeds, conjunctivitis, skin fragility, arthralgia, headaches, and transaminase elevations, but most of these effects are reversible.

Other Agents. *Spironolactone*, an anti-androgen, has been prescribed empirically for women with refractory acne. Doses of 200 mg per day are effective in two thirds of women treated, but menstrual irregularities occur in 22 percent, and some women experience breast tenderness. It should not be prescribed routinely, since there is some concern regarding its use because of reports showing the promotion of breast cancer in rats. Use is best limited to those with an underlying increase in androgen production (see Chapter 98).

Metronidazole gel is of well-established efficacy in acne rosacea (see Chapter 186). It has been found equal to systemic tetracycline therapy when applied in conjunction with 5% benzoyl peroxide cream. More data are needed to confirm these preliminary findings.

Ultraviolet light produces erythema and desquamation, enhancing resolution of inflammatory lesions. However, ultraviolet light has also been implicated in formation of new lesions and is seldom used today.

There is no evidence that *diet* has a significant effect on acne. Diuretics, vitamin A, and vaccines, which have been advocated, do not appear to have demonstrable therapeutic value. Radiation therapy is rarely if ever indicated.

Cyclic *estrogen–progestin* therapy may be considered in highly selected situations with full awareness of and careful monitoring for side effects.

INDICATIONS FOR REFERRAL AND PATIENT EDUCATION

Treatment of acne falls within the domain of the primary physician. The dermatologist should be consulted if basic topical and systemic therapies fail, and in cases of severe disfiguring lesions that may require techniques such as intralesional steroids and systemic Accutane.

Patient education and cooperation are crucial to the success of therapy. Patients must understand the chronic nature of the process and not be discouraged when lesions continue to appear. Patients who unrealistically expect cure may become discouraged, uncooperative, and finally angry.

A vast mythology about acne has developed. The patient should be assured that acne has no relation to diet, masturbation, sexual activity or inactivity, constipation, dirt, or angry feelings. The patient should be helped to gain perspective and discouraged from self-examination in brightly lit mirrors, which often produces a distorted self-image. The patient may begin to perceive himself or herself as "acne with a person attached" rather than a person with acne. Describing this process to the patient often brings an answering smile of recognition and is reassuring. Instructions for the use of topical and systemic agents must be precise and carefully followed. The patient should be reminded that therapeutic results are not achieved immediately, and treatment must be continued for 6 to 8 weeks before a response is seen.

THERAPEUTIC RECOMMENDATIONS

- Explanation to the patient is an essential part of treating acne, so that understanding and cooperation can be enlisted.
- Eliminate acnegenic drugs, such as steroids or androgens, exposure to oils, and habits such as rubbing the face.
- For obstructive acne, use retinoic acid 0.025% or 0.05% cream to a point just short of clinically visible erythema. Topical antibiotic (erythromycin or clindamycin) or benzoyl peroxide may be used if papules or pustules are present concurrently; use 8 to 12 hours after retinoic acid.
- In more severe inflammatory acne, prescribe an antibiotic, usually tetracycline or erythromycin, 1 g/day, reducing the dosage after control is achieved.
- In acne characterized by large nodules, intralesional steroids or, in the hands of experts, liquid nitrogen may be tried.
- For severe nodulocystic acne resistant to conventional therapy, systemic 13-*cis*-retinoic acid should be considered with full awareness of its risks, especially teratogenesis, and appropriate monitoring.
- For people with acne scars, dermabrasion, collagen injection, and other corrective procedures should be considered, in consultation with a dermatologist or other physician highly experienced in these procedures.

ANNOTATED BIBLIOGRAPHY

Bigby M, Stern RS. Adverse reactions to isotretinoin. J Am Acad Dermatol 1988;18:543. *(Review of the significant and less significant adverse reactions.)*

Drake LA. Guidelines of care for acne vulgaris. J Am Acad Dermatol 1990;22:676. *(A summary of the official view of the American Academy of Dermatology on the current management of acne—in outline form, including guidelines for use of 13-*cis*-retinoic acid.)*

Farrel LN. The treatment of severe cystic acne with 13-*cis*-retinoic acid. J Am Acad Dermatol 1980;3:602. *(Increased remission rate found.)*

Humbert P, Treffel P, Chapuis J-F, et al. The tetracyclines in dermatology. J Am Acad Dermatol 1991;25:691. *(A review of the tetracyclines in acne, rosacea, and other dermatological conditions; 99 refs.)*

Lammer EJ, et al. Retinoic acid embryopathy. N Engl J Med 1985;313:837. *(A detailed report of the specific fetal abnormalities produced by systemic retinoids.)*

Lucky AW, et al. Plasma androgens in women with acne. J Invest Dermatol 1983;81:70. *(A report and review of the role of circulating plasma androgens in acne in women.)*

Nielsen PG. Topical metronidazole gel use in acne vulgaris. Int J Dermatol 1991;30:662. *(Metronidazole 2% plus 5% benzoyl peroxide cream was equal to systemic tetracycline therapy.)*

Pochi PE. The pathogenesis and treatment of acne. Annu Rev Med 1990;41:187. *(An excellent summary of the pathogenesis and management of acne.)*

186

Management of Rosacea and Other Acneiform Dermatoses

STEPHEN J. FRIEDMAN, M.D.
WILLIAM V. R. SHELLOW, M.D.

Primary Care Medicine: Office Evaluation and Management of the Adult Patient, 3rd edition, edited by Allan H. Goroll, Lawrence A. May, and Albert G. Mulley, Jr. J.B. Lippincott Company, Philadelphia

The cutaneous diseases that may clinically present with acneiform lesions include rosacea, perioral dermatitis, periorbital comedones, and perlèche. Middle-aged women and men may be affected by rosacea, younger women by perioral dermatitis, and older people by periorbital comedones. These conditions occasionally cause a patient to seek medical attention but more often are noted incidentally by an examining physician seeing a patient for another reason. The primary care practitioner's responsibility involves identification of the patient with acne variants and institution of effective therapy.

PATHOPHYSIOLOGY AND CLINICAL PRESENTATION

Rosacea

Formerly known as acne rosacea, this is a chronic inflammatory condition involving the central face. Persistent erythema and flushing are prominent and may coexist with *telangiectasia*. Papules and pustules recur periodically, but comedones are rarely seen. Rosacea is more common in fair-skinned individuals in the third to fifth decades. In long-standing or severe rosacea, *rhinophyma*, a thick and lobulated overgrowth of connective tissue and sebaceous glands of the nose, may be a feature. Ocular complications commonly include blepharitis, conjunctivitis, episcleritis, and, infrequently, iritis and keratitis. A statistically significant incidence of migraine headaches accompanying rosacea has been reported.

The cause of rosacea is currently unknown. The earliest pathophysiologic change in rosacea is instability of the vasculature, which manifests with flushing and blushing and subsequently with fixed dilated vessels (telangiectasias). Flushing may be attributable to a heat-regulating reflex involving the countercurrent thermal exchange between the common carotid artery and the internal jugular vein. Aggravating factors include hot liquids, alcohol, stress, sun exposure, vasodilating drugs, and spicy foods. Ultraviolet damage may play a role in rosacea, with microscopic evidence of dermal elastotic degeneration noted in most patients with the condition.

Perioral Dermatitis

This is an erythematous, scaling, papular eruption around the mouth, chin, upper lip, and nasolabial folds, seen primarily in women ages 15 to 45. The eruption is usually bilateral and symmetrical. Occasionally, papulopustular lesions are widespread. A periocular variant has been observed.

The cause is unknown. Light sensitivity, acne rosacea, atopy, *Demodex* infection, candidiasis, overgrowth of the yeast *Pityrosporum*, and the use of fluoride or tartar control toothpaste have all been implicated as precipitating factors. The condition can be replicated by chronic use of fluorinated corticosteroid medications.

Periorbital Comedones

These are most often seen in older people. A severe variant with multiple comedones and yellowish nodular and plaque-like lesions is known as Favre-Racouchot syndrome (nodular elastosis with cysts and comedones). The condition is related to senile loss of elasticity of the skin; opened pores favor the accumulation of keratin and sebaceous materials. Senile comedones recur more slowly than comedones associated with acne vulgaris.

Perlèche (Angular Cheilitis)

Perlèche is a common inflammatory eruption restricted to the corners of the mouth. It is characterized by erythema and scaling. Fissures or pustules may be present in severe cases. The area may be secondarily infected with *Candida albicans*. The condition results from the loss of the seal at the angles of the mouth. Saliva accumulates in the area. Precipitants include underlying oral pathology such as malocclusion, wearing of braces or dentures, and frequent licking of the lips. Medications (isotretinoin), vigorous dental flossing or frequent mouth rinsing, contact dermatitis caused by lipsticks or dental hygiene products, and drying from wind and sun exposure and low humidity can also cause perlèche.

PRINCIPLES OF MANAGEMENT

Rosacea

Treatment involves removal of exacerbating conditions and the use of systemic antibiotics. Conditions that lead to flushing or vasodilation should be minimized. Some medications, including vasodilators (aminophylline, hydralazine, niacin, nitroglycerin, and papaverine), cause flushing and worsen rosacea. Exposure to sunlight, extreme heat or cold, and ingestion of hot, spicy foods should be interdicted. It is most important to caution against use of topical fluorinated corticosteroids, which produce an initial response only to result in atrophy of skin and development of permanent telangiectasia.

Topical therapy can be similar to that for acne vulgaris (see Chapter 185), using agents that enhance the turnover of skin and the restoration of normal skin. *Topical* agents such as *erythromycin*, *benzoyl peroxide*, and *retinoic acid* may be used. They are usually less effective than in acne vulgaris, and vehicles that contain alcohols or preservatives may cause irritation. *Topical metronidazole gel* is effective, but it does not reduce telangiectasia, rhinophyma, or ophthalmologic manifestations. It also does not alter the microflora of the skin, including *Demodex*. Clonidine may be helpful by suppressing menopausal flushing.

Systemic antibiotics, including the *tetracyclines* and *erythromycin*, effectively control both rosacea and the accompanying keratitis and blepharitis. They may be required for prolonged periods. *Systemic isotretinoin* or metronidazole are effective but should be reserved for severe recalcitrant cases. Surgical treatment of rhinophyma includes radiowave electrosurgery. Laser techniques may be used to treat the telangiectasia of rosacea.

Perioral Dermatitis

Patients with perioral dermatitis should avoid greasy cosmetics and cold creams. Topical acne preparations that increase turnover of skin are useful but often inadequate if used alone. *Hydrocortisone 1% cream* may promote rapid resolution of the dermatitis. Fluorinated corticosteroid creams should not be used. *Oral tetracycline* is consistently effective in controlling perioral dermatitis. If tetracycline cannot be tolerated, erythromycin may be used instead.

Periorbital Comedones

Periorbital comedones may be treated by expression of the blackheads. Redevelopment of blackheads is somewhat slow, so that periodic expression at 3- or 4-month intervals is adequate. Retinoic acid, applied judiciously, is effective in resolving the condition, but compliance may be difficult in the older population.

Perlèche

Angular cheilitis requires combined treatment, including correction of the primary oral abnormality to prevent leakage of saliva through the corners of the mouth and treatment of a possible secondary infection. Treatment with a topical anticandidal cream (*econazole*, *clotrimazole*) is usually necessary. Topical hydrocortisone cream may be applied to reduce inflammation. Dental procedures should be directed at restoring the seal at the angles of the mouth. For persistent cases, the depth of the grooves of the angles may be reduced with collagen implants, although hypersensitivity reactions are a risk.

PATIENT EDUCATION

The major element of patient education is to explain that these conditions are common and treatable but may be chronic with intermittent flares. Many patients are bothered by a single pimple, while others can sustain the disfigurement of acne rosacea without complaint. Detailed review of aggravating factors is important for prevention and helps make the patient a partner in treatment of these stubborn conditions.

THERAPEUTIC RECOMMENDATIONS

Rosacea

- Begin tetracycline, 500 mg twice a day, and continue for several weeks, followed by gradual reduction in dosage down to 250 mg every other day before considering cessation. Prolonged low-dose therapy may be necessary.
- Avoid sunlight, fluorinated steroids, fluorinated toothpaste, systemic medications, and foods known to exacerbate the condition.
- Consider topical metronidazole gel twice daily for mild cases. Continue for at least 2 months.
- Give a short-term course of a low-potency, nonfluorinated topical corticosteroid (eg, hydrocortisone 1% or 2.5% cream bid) if erythema is refractory.
- Refer for laser therapy or electrosurgery if rhinophyma or telangiectasia is disfiguring.

Perioral Dermatitis

- Treatment should begin with tetracycline, 250 mg tid, gradually reduced over a period of weeks after resolution has occurred.
- Greasy creams and cosmetics should be scrupulously avoided.
- Consider a course of hydrocortisone cream in mild cases.

Periorbital Comedones

- Periodically express the blackheads.
- Topical tretinoin cream, 0.025%, or gel, 0.01%, may be useful in patients who are concerned about their appearance and capable of compliance. Warn patients that tretinoin may cause irritation and to avoid sunlight.

Perlèche

- Use zinc oxide paste at bedtime to minimize skin contact with saliva.
- Topical anticandidal cream such as clotrimazole or econazole cream should be applied twice daily.
- Emphasize to patients to avoid licking lips.
- Consider oral or cosmetic surgery to correct malocclusion.

ANNOTATED BIBLIOGRAPHY

Beacham BE, Kurgansky D, Gould WM. Circumoral dermatitis and cheilitis caused by tartar control dentrifrices. J Am Acad Dermatol 1990;22:1029. *(A series in 20 otherwise healthy women, aged 22–51 years; probably represents an irritant contact dermatitis.)*

Chernosky ME. Collagen implant in management of perleche (angular cheilitis). J Am Acad Dermatol 1985;12:493. *(The depth of the grooves at the corners of the mouth can be reduced with collagen implants.)*

Lowe NJ, Henderson T, Millikan LE, et al. Topical metronidazole for severe and recalcitrant rosacea: a prospective open trial. Cutis 1989;43:283. *(Metronidazole was as effective as systemic antibiotics in some patients.)*

Lowe NJ, Behr KL, Fitzpatrick R, et al. Flash lamp pumped dye laser for rosacea-associated telangiectasia and erythema. J Dermatol Surg Oncol 1991;17:522. *(Use of laser to remove telangiectasia and reduce erythema.)*

Veien NK, Munkvad JM, Nielsen AO, et al. Topical metronidazole in the treatment of perioral dermatitis. J Am Acad Dermatol 1991;24:258. *(Tetracycline was significantly more effective.)*

Primary Care Medicine: Office Evaluation and Management of the Adult Patient, 3rd edition, edited by Allan H. Goroll, Lawrence A. May, and Albert G. Mulley, Jr. J.B. Lippincott Company, Philadelphia

187
Management of Psoriasis

NICHOLAS J. LOWE, M.D.

Psoriasis is a chronic skin disease that affects 2 percent to 3 percent of the U.S. adult population. It is characterized by discrete erythematous papules and plaques covered by a silvery white scale. There are also pustular and erythrodermic varieties, and arthritis sometimes complicates the condition. Patients present with concern for the cosmetic changes of their disease and also request relief from itching and pain.

The primary physician should be able to treat mild and localized forms of the disease and be knowledgeable about treatment of more severe disease to ensure appropriate referral and effect collaboration with the dermatologist.

PATHOPHYSIOLOGY AND CLINICAL PRESENTATION

Pathophysiology. The epidermal turnover time for a cell to travel from the basal cell layer of the epidermis to the granular layer is normally 14 days. In psoriatic skin, it is reduced to 2 days. Normal cell maturation cannot take place in this short time, and subsequent keratinization is faulty. Clinically, this is seen as scaling. Histologically, the epidermis is thickened, and immature nucleated cells are seen in the horny layer. An accompanying dilatation of the subepidermal blood vessels and infiltration with mononuclear cells account for erythema. Neutrophils are often seen within the stratum corneum, forming characteristic micropustules.

The exact causes of this abnormal cellular proliferation and inflammation remain unknown, but current speculation is that genetically predisposed persons experience T-cell activation in response to antigen stimulation. Affected individuals have an increased incidence of several HLA antigens, including HLA-B27 in patients with psoriatic arthritis. Psoriatic plaques are rich in activated T lymphocytes, which are capable of inducing both cell proliferation and inflammation. The search for responsible antigens is ongoing.

Drug-exacerbated psoriasis offers some insights into disease mechanisms. *Lithium* is believed to act by enhancing release of inflammatory mediators from neutrophils, *beta-blockers* by decreasing cyclic-AMP–dependent protein kinase (an inhibitor of cell proliferation), and *nonsteroidal anti-inflammatory drugs (NSAIDs)* by causing a buildup of the inflammatory mediator arachidonic acid. Antimalarials are also associated with exacerbation of the disease. Drug-induced exacerbations can be unpredictable and severe and may occur months after onset of use.

Clinical Presentation. Onset of psoriasis is usually in early adult life, but the disease may appear in childhood or old age. It typically presents with well-marginated erythematous elevated papules or plaques which, if not previously treated by the patient, also show thick, silvery scaling. Removal of this scale reveals punctate bleeding points known as Auspitz's sign. Nails often show punctate pitting and a characteristic discoloration of the surface of the nail that resembles an oil spot. Subungual collections of keratotic material are also common, with distal separation of the nail from the nailbed. Mucous membranes are rarely involved. Extensor surfaces of the arms and legs are the most common sites; the scalp is another. Skin trauma increases the risk of involvement, but any epidermal surface may become involved, even mucosa.

Other clinical types include *guttate* psoriasis, which presents with small, discrete, erythematous papular lesions. An *exfoliative* or erythrodermic form of psoriasis shows generalized erythema without any characteristic lesions. Localized *pustular* psoriasis with sterile pustules of the palms and soles may also be seen without other characteristic lesions. An uncommon but serious variant is generalized pustular disease, which is often accompanied by systemic symptoms and risk of circulatory collapse. Patients with acquired immunodeficiency syndrome (AIDS) may also develop very extensive psoriasis resistant to therapy.

The *arthritis* associated with psoriasis is often polyarticular and asymmetric, but it may be monoarticular. Classic manifestations include swelling and deformity of distal interphalangeal joints in association with the characteristic nail changes (see below). Juxta-articular inflammation produces sausage-like swelling of the fingers. Radiologic features include interphalangeal joint erosion ("pencil-in-a-cup" appearance) and erosion of the distal tuft. Arthritis occurs in about 5 percent to 10 percent of patients. The skin disease usually precedes the joint disease by months to years (see Chapter 146).

The *clinical course* of psoriasis is characterized by chronicity and seasonal fluctuations, with improvement in the summer due to sun exposure and worsening in the winter as dry skin leads to epidermal injury.

PRINCIPLES OF MANAGEMENT

The basic approaches to therapy are to directly reduce the rate of epidermal proliferation or to do so indirectly by halting the dermal inflammatory process. In addition, one seeks to protect the skin from drying and other forms of injury that may precipitate a flare.

Topical Therapy

Topical Corticosteroids. Topical corticosteroids are widely used because they are relatively easy to apply. They are worth considering in patients with mild disease involving less than 10 percent of body surface area. Plaques blanch and thin in response to treatment. The more potent steroids (see Chapter 184, Table 184–1) are usually required to produce a good response. They are sometimes effective in clearing psoriasis and helpful in treating exposed and unsightly areas. However, caution in needed in their use (see below).

The best approach is to begin with a "superpotent" corticosteroid preparation (eg, Diprolene, Psorcon, Temovate, Ultravate) and then decrease to one of lesser potency for maintenance therapy. To avoid adverse effects, the superpotent agents should be used only for a limited time and in limited amounts (see Chapter 184).

Most patients prefer creams; however, ointments are used if there is thick psoriatic scale. Topical steroid treatment used sparingly under plastic wrap occlusion may be effective if steroids applied without occlusion fail to help. Immediately before steroid application, it may be useful for patients with heavy scales to gently remove them with a soft brush during a warm bath. Hard scrubbing should be avoided, because skin trauma can exacerbate psoriasis.

Solutions are used for scalp lesions. Scalp involvement may benefit from use of a *tar shampoo* (Zetar, Sebutone, Pentrax) before steroid application. The shampoo is massaged in thoroughly and left on for 1 to 2 hours. Then water is added, and the patient shampoos gently for several minutes to remove scales. Overnight application of a moderate strength topical steroid lotion (eg, Synalar lotion) follows after rinsing and drying. Wearing a shower cap after steroid application improves results in persons with marked scalp involvement, as does use of a more potent preparation. Scalp trauma through excessive combing and scratching should be avoided.

Topical steroid therapy is not without its drawbacks. Remission times are often relatively short. *Side effects* seen with potent topical steroids include skin atrophy, rebound worsening after discontinuing use, a tendency to convert "stable" disease to "unstable" (erythrodermic or pustular) disease, significant skin absorption to produce systemic steroid effect in those with extensive disease, and the possibility of a rosacea-like syndrome after long-term facial use.

Sunlight. Exposure to sunlight improves psoriasis. A winter trip to a southern clime induces a better and more enduring remission that does use of topical steroids. In summer, topical steroid therapy can often be suspended. Although sun exposure just to the point of mild erythema is helpful, sunburn exacerbates psoriasis and must be avoided.

Ultraviolet Light Plus Coal Tar. The beneficial effect of sunlight stimulated interest in ultraviolet light therapy. In 1925, Goeckerman described the combination of ultraviolet (UV) light and coal tar ointment. Numerous modifications have followed. Coal tar appears to enhance the effects of suberythemogenic ultraviolet B (UVB). Patients with more than 10 percent of skin surface involved are reasonable candidates. The treatment is associated with an 80 percent to 90 percent remission rate and without any evidence of increased risk of skin cancer. The traditional Goeckerman program has been supplanted by modifications that allow outpatient therapy, using a less messy coal tar gel followed in 2 hours by UV treatment. Four to 6 weeks of treatment are usually necessary.

Anthralin. Anthralin is trihydroxy-anthracene, an aromatic compound with three benzene rings, used topically for psoriasis since the 19th century. It is an antimitotic capable of inhibiting DNA synthesis. Its topical application can induce remission of plaques after several weeks of use, but its tendency to irritate the skin and stain adjacent skin and clothing makes it less acceptable than other treatment options. Paradoxically, if topical steroids are added to an anthralin program, there is an earlier relapse. The application of high-concentration anthralin which is washed off after 10 to 30 minutes improves psoriasis and makes outpatient use more practical.

Calcipotriene (Doronex) is a novel vitamin D_3 analogue available as an ointment. It effects keratinocyte differentiation and proliferation, and is superior to fluocinonide (a high-potency topical steroid) for treatment of mild to moderately severe disease. It is likely to become a major alternative to topical steroid therapy for plaque-type disease.

Systemic Treatment of Psoriasis

Systemic treatment is indicated only for severe or incapacitating disease. This indication includes generalized pustular psoriasis, generalized exfoliative psoriasis, severe psoriatic arthropathy, severe uncontrolled psoriasis, and socially incapacitating disease. An additional indication is acute guttate psoriasis; use of systemic therapy may prevent this form from becoming chronic.

Methotrexate. This agent is the most widely used of the systemic antimitotic drugs. It decreases mitotic rate and DNA synthesis in the epidermis. It can control severe disease, but the risk of serious side effects limits its use to chronic refractory cases, mostly in persons past reproductive age. It is also quite effective for severe psoriatic arthritis.

Oral regimens include every-other-day and once-weekly dosing. If nausea is significant, intramuscular administration can be used. Response is usually seen within 2 to 3 weeks, at which time dose or interval is reduced.

Because of the drug's potential for hematopoietic, hepatic, and renal toxicity, close monitoring and full patient compliance are essential. Adequacy of blood cell counts (including platelets) and renal and hepatic function should be confirmed before treatment is given. The patient must be willing to have periodic blood samples taken to monitor side effects.

Monitoring begins with weekly blood samples, followed by monthly ones. Bone marrow suppression may occur, but renal and hepatic injury are uncommon at the doses used for treatment of psoriasis. Nonetheless, hepatic fibrosis may occur with prolonged use, leading some to recommend pretreatment liver biopsy. Current guidelines allow for a trial period of methotrexate before liver biopsy, as long as there is no evidence of ongoing liver disease.

Photochemotherapy. Use of the systemic photosensitizing agent *psoralen* in conjunction with long-wavelength (320–400 nm) *ultraviolet A light* (commonly referred to as "*PUVA*" therapy) has produced excellent results (80%–90%

remission) in patients with otherwise recalcitrant, severe psoriasis. However, concerns about long-term side effects (premature skin aging, carcinogenesis) remain. The risk of skin cancer is increased with both UVA and PUVA therapies, averaging about 2 percent for the latter. Squamous cell cancers are the most likely. Careful follow-up of patients who have had PUVA therapy is required. Patients at increased risk for skin cancer (fair skin, easily sunburned, previous x-ray therapy to the skin) should not receive PUVA treatment. Early and usually mild transient side effects include pruritus and phototoxic erythema. Occasionally, nausea is a problem.

At present, PUVA should be reserved for severe or recalcitrant psoriasis resistant to topical therapy. It may help some patients with generalized pustular or exfoliative psoriasis, but great care is needed to avoid worsening the condition.

Synthetic Retinoids. The aromatic retinoid *etretinate* (Tegison) has achieved significant improvement in some psoriatics. The oral dosage has to be monitored closely to control side effects (including cheilitis, itching, fragile skin, thirst, sore mouth, and peeling of the palms and soles). In 60 percent to 70 percent of patients, good responses are achieved and the benefits of treatment outweigh the side effects. Abnormalities of serum lipids may develop in some patients, and lipid levels should be monitored. Etretinate is more effective in some patients when combined with UVB or PUVA therapy.

Oral *13-*cis*-retinoic acid* (isotretinoin) was approved by the FDA in 1982 for treatment of severe pustulocystic acne. Some psoriatic patients have been treated with isotretinoin alone and also in combination with anthralin or UVB phototherapy. The drug is not effective for plaque-stage psoriasis but is useful to control generalized pustular psoriasis.

Systemic Corticosteroids. Although topical corticosteroids are helpful, systemic steroids are to be avoided, if possible, because of their tendency to convert stable disease to aggressive generalized disease on withdrawal. Occasionally, one is forced to use systemic steroids for severe, acute disease if other forms of systemic treatment are contraindicated, and some physicians use short courses of systemic steroids for treatment of acute guttate psoriasis. Nonetheless, systemic steroids are rarely prescribed. The unfortunate patient who has been treated previously with a systemic steroid and has become "steroid dependent" may require steroids indefinitely.

Investigational Treatments

Cyclosporine. Investigational use of this potent suppressor of T-cell activity has resulted in significant improvement, even total clearing, in more than two-thirds of patients treated. However, relapse within several weeks of discontinuing treatment is common. Moreover, hypertension, renal toxicity, hirsutism, and myalgias can occur on a short-term basis, and lymphoma over the longer term. The literature should be followed for further developments with use of T-cell inhibitors.

Vitamins and Fish Oil Supplements. Dietary and vitamin regimens are always popular among patients. Oral *vitamin D analogues* have been reported to be of some benefit, but prospective, controlled data are limited. Uncontrolled studies suggested that *fish oil supplements* might be beneficial. Though potentially capable of altering immune function, fish oil supplements failed to produce objective improvement in double-blind, controlled study.

PATIENT EDUCATION AND INDICATIONS FOR REFERRAL

For many, the social and psychological effects can be significant. Long-standing psoriasis can lead to loneliness and depression. Regularly scheduled visits to reinforce the details of therapy and also to render support are appreciated. Knowing that disease severity can be reduced through appropriate treatment is reassuring. Informed advice about what works and what does not is essential. Concerns about the condition being contagious or transmitted genetically need to be addressed. The chronic relapsing nature of the disease should be acknowledged so that patient expectations will be realistic. Preventive measures should be stressed, such as keeping the skin well hydrated (see Chapter 183) and avoiding sunburn and other forms of skin trauma.

The safety and efficacy of most psoriatic regimens depend on strong patient compliance. Careful teaching that includes the rationale for a given practice is helpful, as are written instructions.

Those with extensive, refractory, or acute pustular disease should be referred to the dermatologist for consideration of PUVA therapy, retinoids, antimetabolites, and immunosuppressive therapy. The development of generalized disease, especially if erythrodermal or pustular, requires hospitalization.

THERAPEUTIC RECOMMENDATIONS

- Treat localized, mild-to-moderate disease topically. Refer more extensive (> 10% skin area involvement) or refractory cases to the dermatologist.
- Emphasize the importance of keeping the skin well hydrated and avoiding sunburn and other forms of skin injury.
- Allow sun exposure if taken cautiously; avoid sunburning, and do not recommend for those at increased risk for skin cancer (fair-skinned, easily burned, history of skin irradiation).
- Review medications for potential exacerbants (lithium, beta-blockers, NSAIDs); reduce dose or substitute if possible.
- Prescribe a topical steroid program for control of bothersome visible lesions. Begin with a "superpotent" preparation (eg, Diprolene, Psorcon, Temovate, Ultravate), and change to a less potent preparation for maintenance.
- Consider calcipotriene ointment as an alternative to topical steroids. It is applied twice daily; avoid face and skin folds.

- Recommend an ointment preparation for lesions with considerable scale, although a cream may be more acceptable for daytime use and suffice for plaques with minimal scale. A twice-daily regimen of steroid application achieves best results. For unresponsive lesions, consider topical steroid treatment with plastic wrap occlusion; to avoid dermal atrophy, use sparingly.
- For patients with excessive scale, recommend gentle removal by warm bathing and soft brushing before topical steroid application. Avoid hard brushing, because skin trauma exacerbates the condition.
- For mild scalp involvement, recommend nightly use of a tar shampoo. It is rubbed in gently, left on for 1 to 2 hours, and then rinsed out gently. For more severe scalp disease, the tar shampoo is followed by gentle application of topical steroid lotion (eg, Synalar). Patients with marked scalp involvement may benefit from covering the head with a showercap after steroid application and use of a superpotent topical steroid lotion (eg, Diprolene) or a special anthralin scalp preparation.
- Refer patients who fail to respond and those with extensive disease to the dermatologist for consideration of PUVA, methotrexate, and other systemic therapies. Promptly admit to the hospital those who develop generalized pustular or erythrodermal disease.

ANNOTATED BIBLIOGRAPHY

Abel EA, Dicicco LM, Orenberg EK, et al. Drugs in exacerbation of psoriasis. J Am Acad Dermatol 1986;15:1007. *(A detailed look at this important source of exacerbation and new disease.)*

Breathnach SM. The skin immune system and psoriasis. Clin Exp Immunol 1993;91:343. *(A brief review of the evolving immunopathology.)*

Chuang T-Y, Heinrich LA, Schultz MD, et al. PUVA and skin cancer: a historical cohort study of 492 patients. J Am Acad Dermatol 1992;26:173. *(High-dose therapy associated with increased rates of squamous cell carcinoma but not of basal cell cancers.)*

Ellis CN, Fraddin MS, Mesaba JM, et al. Cyclosporine for plaque-type psoriasis. N Engl J Med 1991;324:277. *(Efficacy demonstrated.)*

Ellis CN, Kary S, Grekin RC. Etretinate therapy for psoriasis. Arch Dermatol 1985;121:877. *(Mechanism of action discussed.)*

Farber EM, Rein G, Lanigan SW. Stress and psoriasis: psychoneuroimmunologic mechanisms. Int J Dermatol 1991;30:8. *(Stress associated with exacerbations; possible mechanisms reviewed.)*

Goeckerman WH. The treatment of psoriasis. NW Med 1925; 24:229.*(The original report on coal tar plus UV.)*

Krueger GG. Psoriasis therapy—observational or rational. N Engl J Med 1993;328:1845. *(An editorial summarizing approaches to therapy.)*

Lowe NJ. New trends in topical psoriasis therapy in *Practical Psoriasis Therapy*, 2nd ed. 1993. NJ Lowe, ed. St. Louis: Mosby-Year Book, 73–76. *(Describes use of calcipotriene ointment.)*

Lowe NJ. Systemic treatment of severe psoriasis—the role of cyclosporine. N Engl J Med 1991;324:333. *(An editorial review.)*

Lowe NJ, Ashton RE, Koudsi H, et al. Anthralin for psoriasis. J Am Acad Dermatol 1984;9:69. *(Short contact therapy compared with topical steroid and conventional anthralin.)*

Lowe NJ, Wortzman MS, Breeding J, et al. Coal tar phototherapy for psoriasis reevaluated. J Am Acad Dermatol 1983;9:781. *(Useful with suberythemogenic UV therapy and mildly so when used alone.)*

Muller SA, Perry HO. The Goeckerman treatment in psoriasis: six decades of experience at the Mayo Clinic. Cutis 1984; 34:265. *(A favorable critique.)*

Parrish JH, Fitzpatrick T, Tanenbaum I. Photochemotherapy of psoriasis with oral methoxsalen and long-wave ultraviolet light. N Engl J Med 1974;291:1207. *(Efficacy of PUVA therapy in refractory disease.)*

Ramsay B, O'Reagan M. A survey of the social and psychological effects of psoriasis. Br J Dermatol 1988;118;95. *(The effects can be marked.)*

Roegnigk H, Averback R, Maibach HI. Methotrexate in psoriasis: revised guidelines. J Am Acad Dermatol 1988;19:145. *(Authoritative guidelines.)*

Soyland E, Funk J, Rajka G, et al. Effect of dietary supplementation with very-long-chain *n*-3 fatty acids in patients with psoriasis. N Engl J Med 1993;328:1812. *(Double-blind, controlled study showing no benefit.)*

Wolverton SE. Systemic drug therapy for psoriasis. The most critical issues. Arch Dermatol 1991;127:565. *(Thoughtful review.)*

188
Management of Intertrigo and Intertriginous Dermatoses

WILLIAM V. R. SHELLOW, M.D.

Primary Care Medicine: Office Evaluation and Management of the Adult Patient, 3rd edition, edited by Allan H. Goroll, Lawrence A. May, and Albert G. Mulley, Jr. J.B. Lippincott Company, Philadelphia

Intertrigo is an inflammatory condition of body folds which presents as a moist lesion with erythema and scaling. It is more common in obese people and is exacerbated by warm weather. The areas of involvement are the axillary, inguinal, and inframammary folds and the toe webs. The primary physician should be capable of distinguishing intertrigo from other body-fold eruptions such as erythrasma, seborrheic dermatitis, psoriasis, and dermatophyte infections, as well as rendering appropriate treatment.

PATHOPHYSIOLOGY AND CLINICAL PRESENTATION

Intertrigo presents as erythematous exudative inflammation in the body folds. Patients may complain of soreness and itching, and with secondary infection, overt purulence may occur. The pathogenic mechanism is mechanical. Heat, moisture, and the retention of sweat produce maceration and irritation, an environment that promotes bacterial infection.

Early intertrigo is characterized by slight maceration and erythema. The moisture initially comes from eccrine sweat that cannot evaporate in the intertriginous areas. With time, redness becomes more intense, and the epidermis becomes eroded or even denuded. Subsequent inflammation causes exudation of serous fluid. Increased moisture may lead to bacterial colonization, which accounts for the odor that may be associated with intertrigo. The groin and intergluteal areas may be colonized by gram-negative organisms. Incontinence of urine or feces may add to the maceration in the groin and gluteal areas.

DIFFERENTIAL DIAGNOSIS

Intertrigo in the groin must be differentiated from *tinea cruris* and *candidiasis*. Tinea cruris is a fungal infection characterized by small, red, scaly patches. The lesions form circinate plaques with scaly or vesicular borders and central clearing. Scraping scales, adding 20% potassium hydroxide solution, and finding hyphae under low microscopic power differentiates them from intertrigo. Candidiasis produces deep, beefy-red lesions with characteristic satellite vesicopustules outside the border of the primary lesion. Involvement of the scrotum is common; tinea usually spares the scrotum.

The groin may be affected by sexually transmitted diseases such as *condylomata*, *herpes*, *scabies*, or *pediculosis*. These cause an erythematous and pruritic eruption with characteristics that point to the underlying diagnosis (see Chapters 141, 192, 193, and 195). In severe cases of intertrigo, underlying diseases such as lichen sclerosus et atrophicus and lichen simplex chronicus should be considered.

Intertrigo in the axilla needs to be differentiated from *candidiasis*, *tinea*, *erythrasma*, and *contact dermatitis*. *Candida* presents with an erythematous eruption; tinea corporis in the axilla demonstrates an active border with scale; erythrasma has a reddish brown discoloration, and contact dermatitis usually spares the axillary vault. A condition known as benign *familial pemphigus* should also be considered. If an axillary lesion is nodular or raised, Fox-Fordyce disease and *hidradenitis suppurativa* enter the differential.

Intertrigo of the inframammary region can occur with or without *candidal infection*.

PRINCIPLES OF THERAPY

The first principle of therapy is to alter the conditions that cause maceration and irritation of closely apposed skin. The goal is to *promote drying*, which can be accomplished by exposing the intertriginous areas to air. Adding a fan or electric bulb can promote drying. A hand-held hair dryer set to a cool setting is very effective. Addition of a nonmedicated, noncornstarch, *absorbant powder* is helpful. (Cornstarch is to be avoided because it serves as a food source and stimulates growth of local bacteria). The patient should be instructed to wear loose-fitting cotton clothing. Bras that provide good support are also helpful. Hot, humid environments and clothing made of wool, nylon, or synthetic fibers can precipitate or worsen intertrigo. Nylon pantyhose is a common offender. Men with groin involvement should be encouraged to wear boxer shorts rather than briefs, and women, cotton panties rather than nylon ones. Ointments and greasy preparations retain moisture and exacerbate the condition.

There is no evidence that antibacterial soaps are more effective than ordinary toilet soaps. Medicated powders should not be used. Zeasorb powder, made from corncobs, is useful. Exudative lesions should be treated by the application of *Burow's compresses* made by adding one package or tablet to a pint of water.

Secondary infection should be treated. Pustules or scales should be examined microscopically and cultured for evidence of bacteria, yeast, and dermatophytes and appropriate therapy instituted (see Chapters 190 and 191).

In uninfected intertrigo, *topical corticosteroids* may be added to reduce inflammation. The strength of the preparation should match the severity of the condition. *Hydrocortisone cream* is an effective, safe, low-cost therapy for patients with mild-to-moderate inflammation. Fluorinated topical corticosteroids are useful when inflammation is more severe, but these should be applied only for short periods, because intertriginous striae and atrophy are common complications of more prolonged use.

Some steroid preparations promoted for use in intertrigo contain an antifungal agent (nystatin or clotrimazole) in addition to corticosteroid. The rationale is concurrent treatment or prevention of secondary candidal or dermatophyte infection. Mycolog II cream is a combination of triamcinolone (a low-potency corticosteroid) and nystatin. Its original formulation also contained sensitizing antibacterial agents and preservatives. In a randomized, controlled study comparing it with hydrocortisone, there was no difference in outcome. Lotrisone combines medium-potency betamethasone with clotrimazole. Lotions with an alcohol base are quite drying and may sting. The popular combination Vioform-Hydrocortisone (which contains the antifungal clioquinol) stains clothing yellow.

Topical medication should be used sparingly to avoid retention of moisture. Concurrent medical conditions such as diabetes or obesity should be treated.

PATIENT EDUCATION

The patient must understand the mechanical effects of skin occluding skin and be encouraged to dress accordingly to assure adequate absorption of moisture and aeration. Women with large or pendulous breasts might benefit from use of a support bra and the placement of soft cotton cloths, gauze pads, or lamb's wool between the breast and the chest wall. The patient should be taught to inspect intertriginous zones to detect the development of erythema and maceration so that effective therapy can be instituted early. In elderly immobile patients, the physician should educate the family or a friend to inspect intertriginous areas to prevent maceration and secondary infection.

THERAPEUTIC RECOMMENDATIONS

- Eliminate precipitating conditions. Carefully dry the area that separates folds with absorbent material, dust with drying powders, and recommend loose, absorbent clothing. In exudative lesions, a drying agent such as Burow's solution should be used as a compress.
- Advise avoidance of potential contactants in axillary eruptions.
- Treat mild to moderately inflamed areas with topical hydrocortisone. For more severe cases, use a low- to medium-potency fluorinated topical corticosteroid for short periods only.
- Treat secondary bacterial or fungal infection with appropriate agents (see Chapters 190 and 191).

ANNOTATED BIBLIOGRAPHY

Brophy MC, Dunagin WG. Intertriginous dermatoses. Postgrad Med 1985;78:105. *(An excellent review of differential diagnosis.)*

Epstein NN, Epstein WL, Epstein JH. Atrophic striae in patients with intertrigo. Arch Dermatol 1963;87:450. *(A hazard of treating intertrigo with potent topical corticosteroids.)*

Hedley K, Tooley P, Williams H. Problems with clinical trials in general practice—a double-blind comparison of cream containing miconazole and hydrocortisone with hydrocortisone alone in the treatment of intertrigo. Br J Clin Pract 1990;4:131. *(A well-designed study showing no difference.)*

Sarkany I, Taplin D, Blank H. Incidence and bacteriology of erythrasma. Arch Dermatol 1962;85:578. *(Concise discussion of the disease and its etiology.)*

Smith MA, Waterworth PM. The bacteriology of some cases of intertrigo. Br J Dermatol 1962;74:323. *(Brief discussion of the bacterial flora found in intertriginous areas.)*

189
Management of Corns and Calluses

WILLIAM V. R. SHELLOW, M.D.

Primary Care Medicine: Office Evaluation and Management of the Adult Patient, 3rd edition, edited by Allan H. Goroll, Lawrence A. May, and Albert G. Mulley, Jr. J.B. Lippincott Company, Philadelphia

Corns and calluses are common, vexing lesions that can interfere with daily functioning. They may not be a presenting complaint, but the primary care physician is frequently asked about them. The tasks in the primary care setting are to provide diagnosis, simple therapy, advice on prevention, and timely referral if symptoms are refractory or disabling.

PATHOPHYSIOLOGY AND CLINICAL PRESENTATION

Corns (helomas or clavi) and calluses (tylomas or tyloses) have a common pathology. Friction and pressure on the skin overlying bony prominences lead to hyperemia, hypertrophy of dermal papillae, and proliferation of keratin. Corns often have a central, hard core that is painful if the lesion is pressed. The pressure of shoes on the corn may cause pain with walking. Corns can develop at any joint, but the most common site is over the dorsum of the proximal interphalangeal joint. Hard corns show a translucent avascular core with interruption of normal skin markings. Soft corns appear macerated, resemble dermatophytosis, and are painful. The first and fourth web spaces are favored sites. Persons who do not wear shoes may develop calluses but usually do not develop corns. Calluses do not contain a central core, preserve normal skin markings, and occur preferentially across the metatarsal head area.

DIFFERENTIAL DIAGNOSIS

Calluses can be confused with plantar warts but may be distinguished by the maintenance of normal skin markings, in contrast to verrucae, in which these markings are interrupted.

PRINCIPLES OF THERAPY

The primary physician's major contribution to therapy is to encourage *prevention* through *patient education*. The elimination of friction and pressure is the essence of prevention. Shoes must fit correctly, and pressure over the toes must be evenly distributed. Softer shoe materials and sandals are often helpful. Stockings must fit properly and should cushion the foot. Keeping the feet dry by using powder and changing shoes daily also reduces friction. Careful explanation of the rationale for such measures is essential to ensuring patient compliance.

Symptomatic relief of calluses can be achieved by *paring* hyperkeratotic lesions with a No. 10 or 15 scalpel blade. Keratin should be shaved off with the blade held parallel to the skin. Repeated strokes of the blade should be made in a direction least likely to cause penetration should the patient move suddenly. Movement from proximal to distal is best. After a callus is removed, it is essential that previous weight-bearing trauma not be continued, or the callus will recur.

Patients can treat corns and calluses themselves with intermittent debridement, using *keratolytic agents*. Salicylic and lactic acid combinations and 40% salicylic acid plasters are used to reduce the thickness of tissue. The patient should cut a piece of 40% salicylic acid plaster smaller than the lesion and apply it to the skin. It may be left overnight or for as long as several days. The dressing should be removed and the foot soaked. The softened and macerated skin can be removed with a Buf-Ped or pumice stone. The plaster may be carefully reapplied as often as necessary, in order to keep the lesions flat and asymptomatic.

The treating of soft corns involves reducing excess perspiration. Use of absorbent *lamb's wool*, soaking the foot in potassium permanganate (1:4000 solution), and silver nitrate cauterization have all been successful.

Intrinsic bone problems subject the foot to uneven pressure. Any pronation, flat feet, or medial or lateral imbalances should be treated. Padding of lesions with felt moleskin or lamb's wool may prevent uneven external pressure. Foam rubber surrounding the lesion distributes pressure around the lesion rather than directly on it.

One investigational technique is the injection of medical-grade silicone under corns to cushion the skin from underlying bone. The technique has been one of the few approved uses for injectable silicone, but it is confined to only a few investigators. Other investigators have injected cross-linked collagen between the corn and the bone.

INDICATIONS FOR REFERRAL

Referral to a podiatrist or orthopedic surgeon is indicated if simple measures and advice fail to reduce symptoms or recurrences. Latex, plastic, or silicone molds can be individually adapted to prevent localized pressure from producing corns or calluses. Shoes can be constructed by a podiatrist to redistribute weight and pressure. Occasionally, surgical removal of a subjacent bony prominence eliminates the source of abnormal pressure on the skin. Diabetics and others with impaired vascular systems should receive foot care from the podiatrist.

THERAPEUTIC RECOMMENDATIONS

- Advise the patient to avoid tight, pointed-toed shoes and to obtain shoes that fit properly, changing them frequently. Socks should cushion the sensitive area.
- Corns and calluses may be treated by the patient with proprietary plasters. The physician or patient can apply a keratolytic to the lesion in the form of a 40% salicylic acid plaster for several days.
- Consider paring down a large lesion. Patients can perform this procedure on themselves, but instruct them never to pull loose skin. Protect the tender area after paring with moleskin.
- After the lesions have been removed or pared down, ensure that the foot is not subjected to the same pressures that originally produced the problem.
- Refractory lesions and those caused by underlying orthopedic disease should be referred to a podiatrist or orthopedist for definitive treatment of the structural problem. Diabetics and others with vascular insufficiency to the foot should receive regular foot care from the podiatrist.

ANNOTATED BIBLIOGRAPHY

Brainard BJ. Managing corns and plantar calluses. Physician and Sportsmedicine 1991;19:61. *(Corns and calluses arise from foot or ankle abnormalities, poor footwear selection, and overuse.)*

Collagen Podiatric Investigation Group. Subdermal collagen injections for the treatment of hyperkeratotic lesions. J Am Podiatr Med Assoc 1986;76:445. *(Discusses injectable collagen.)*

Hodgkin SE, Hoffman TJ. Minimizing corns and calluses. Physician and Sportsmedicine 1990;18:87. *(A practical approach to treatment in athletes.)*

Holmes GB Jr, Timmerman L. A quantitative assessment of the effect of metatarsal pads on plantar pressures. Foot Ankle 1990;11:141. *(Orthotic devices such as a metatarsal pad can be an inexpensive and effective method of reducing metatarsal pressures.)*

Montgomery RM. Relieving painful feet. Geriatrics 1974;29:137. *(Practical tips useful in the office.)*

Schwartz N. Callus formation. J Am Podiatr Med Assoc 1975;65:666. *(A brief discussion of some of the causes of plantar keratoma.)*

Primary Care Medicine: Office Evaluation and Management of the Adult Patient, 3rd edition, edited by Allan H. Goroll, Lawrence A. May, and Albert G. Mulley, Jr. J.B. Lippincott Company, Philadelphia

190

Approach to Bacterial Skin Infections

ELLIE J. C. GOLDSTEIN, M.D.
WILLIAM V. R. SHELLOW, M.D.

Part 1: Cellulitis

Cellulitis represents bacterial infection of the skin involving the deeper subcutaneous layers. It must be differentiated from inflammatory skin changes due to vascular insufficiency and phlebitis. Once cellulitis is identified, the primary physician has to decide who can be managed at home on oral antibiotics and who requires hospitalization.

PATHOPHYSIOLOGY AND CLINICAL PRESENTATION

Pathogenesis. Any process that causes a break in the integrity of the skin will allow normal skin bacteria to invade the underlying subcutaneous tissue and initiate an inflammatory response. Trauma, stasis ulceration, ischemia, and chronic edema are common precipitants. Contiguous or hematogenous spread from other sites occurs uncommonly.

The organisms most commonly producing cellulitis are normal skin flora, with *streptococci* and *Staphylococcus aureus* predominating. Staphylococci produce disease through their ability to multiply and produce a host of extracellular enzymes, including alpha- and beta-hemolysin, leukocidin, coagulase, hyaluronidase, and lipases. Streptococci produce more than 20 extracellular enzymes.

Conditions that impair host response may predispose to skin infection by opportunistic organisms such as *gram-negative bacteria.* Skin infections with *Escherichia coli, Pseu-*

domonas, and *Klebsiella* are seen in immunosuppressed patients, diabetics, and alcoholics. Cellulitis in the perineum may be caused by enteric aerobic and anaerobic bacteria. Injury to mucosal surfaces predisposes to infection with *anaerobic organisms*. Anaerobic bacteria can produce hyaluronidase, proteases, neuraminidase, and extracellular enzymes, and act synergistically with aerobic bacteria. Anaerobes play an important role in diabetic foot ulcers, abscesses, and traumatic wounds. Anaerobic infection also occurs in the setting of crush injuries. The degree of pain may be disproportionate to skin findings. A mixture of aerobic and anaerobic strep can lead to fasciitis and cellulitis. Once connective tissue is involved, infection spreads along fascial planes.

In certain settings, cellulitis may be caused by unusual organisms. In individuals who handle fish, poultry, or meat, cellulitic infection with *Erysipelothrix rhusiopathiae* may occur. In cases of water-related injury and sometimes in immunosuppressed patients, *Aeromonas hydrophila,* which occurs in water-related injury and sometimes in immunosuppressed patients, may produce cellulitis. Animal bites or scratches, especially from cats, produce cellulitis caused by a *Pasteurella multocida* organism. *Vibrio* species have been implicated in salt-water-related injuries. Insect bites are portals of entry for conventional strep or staph species, but one must also consider the unusual spreading cellulitis, a reaction to the toxin of a *brown recluse spider* or a *fire ant*. Another unusual cause of cellulitis simulating a septic thrombophlebitis may occur from *Campylobacter* infection, often in the context of a concurrent enteritis.

Clinical Presentation. Cellulitis presents with local redness, heat, swelling, and tenderness developing over a few days. Fever, chills, and rigors herald possible bacteremia. The clinical presentation does not allow delineation of the specific microbial etiology. Red streaks extending proximally in conjunction with tender lymph nodes indicate an associated *lymphangitis*. Crepitus indicates gas production and suggests anaerobic involvement.

Invasive strains of group A streptococcus (gm type 1 and 3) cause not only the usual forms of invasive streptococcal disease (scarlet fever, erysipelas, necrotizing fasciitis, myositis) but also a toxic-shocklike syndrome due to mucosal or cutaneous infection. Mortality is as high as 30 percent. Onset is abrupt, with fever, diarrhea, rigors, and scattered pains. Bacteremia may be detected in 60 percent; hematogenous spread is common.

WORKUP

Cellulitis first needs to be distinguished from other causes of focal erythema, swelling, and tenderness. *Superficial thrombophlebitis* may present similarly, but the inflammatory response is usually centered in the involved vein, which is tender and palpable. The dependent rubor of *arterial insufficiency* is generalized, nontender, and associated with diminished or absent pulses and a cold extremity. *Erythema nodosum* is indicated by lesions that are typically multiple, exquisitely tender, and often pretibial in location. It is a secondary phenomenon, and the cause needs to be determined. It should be remembered that cellulitis may occur concurrently with phlebitis or arterial insufficiency.

History. Once it is established that cellulitis is present, predisposing factors should be identified. The history is checked for diabetes, congestive failure, recent trauma, leg edema, claudication, previous infection, tinea pedis, and loss of sensation. One should ask about intravenous (IV) drug use, occupational exposure, recent bites and stings. A history of fever with rigors suggests bacteremia.

Physical Examination. Note is made of the temperature, area of skin involved, lymphangitic streaking, proximal lymphadenopathy, heart murmur, peripheral edema, diminished peripheral pulses, decreased sensation, and any skin atrophy, breaks, or ulceration. Marking the borders of the lesion with an indelible pen allows objective and rapid assessment of progression and resolution. Crepitus or foul odor is suggestive of anaerobic infection. One palpates for fluctuance and inspects the viability of surrounding tissue. Any tinea, dermatitis, venous insufficiency, or previous injury is noted.

Laboratory Studies. A *complete blood count* (CBC) and *differential* are always helpful in gauging severity of infection and hematologic response. Because most cellulitis is due to streptococci or staphylococci, *skin culture* is not routinely performed. Moreover, it is difficult to culture the offending organism from unbroken skin. There is no evidence that aspiration from the advancing margin is superior to sampling from any other area of involved skin. Culture is indicated in patients who have open, weeping *wounds* or infection in unusual areas such as the *perineum*. Material from such areas should be cultured both anaerobically and aerobically.

When rigors, fever, heart murmur, or lymphangitic spread is present or the patient is immunocompromised, two separate sets of *blood cultures* should be obtained before any antibiotics are administered. Blood cultures are positive in 5 to 10 percent of cellulitis cases. If crepitus, fluctuance, or devitalization is present, obtain an x-ray film to look for gas production in soft tissue, indicative of gangrene. In diabetic or immunocompromised patients, or in situations of previous injury, an x-ray is important to be sure osteomyelitis does not lurk beneath the cellulitis.

PRINCIPLES OF MANAGEMENT

The majority of patients may be treated as outpatients with oral antibiotics and supportive measures. Patients who are afebrile and in whom adenopathy and lymphangitis are absent may not even require antibiotics, but antibiotics are usually prescribed.

Antibiotics. The drugs of choice are either *penicillin* or a penicillinase-resistant *semisynthetic penicillin* preparation. There is little definitive evidence on which to base antibiotic selection. The high prevalence of streptococci, the sensitivity of some community-acquired staphylococci to penicillin, and the low cost of penicillin make it a reasonable choice. If after 24 to 48 hours the patient is still febrile or not improving, a penicillinase-resistant preparation can be substituted. The addition of probenecid as a morning dose can increase blood levels of oral penicillin. Antibiotic therapy should continue for 10 to 14 days, depending on rate of clinical resolution.

Supportive Measures. These include *elevation* of the affected part and scrupulous prevention of new trauma. *Heat* may help in resolution of cellulitis by promoting blood flow to the area. In patients with underlying conditions such as congestive failure, stasis dermatitis, or vascular insufficiency, *control of edema* and maintenance of *skin moisturization* helps prevent recurrent episodes.

In patients with open wounds, the risk of tetanus should be considered. If a booster of *tetanus toxoid* has not been obtained within 5 years, it should be given. Patients who have not had an initial tetanus series should receive both tetanus toxoid and tetanus immune globulin (see Chapter 6).

INDICATIONS FOR REFERRAL AND ADMISSION

Abscesses should be drained and necrotic tissues should be debrided, necessitating prompt surgical referral. Hospitalization and IV antibiotics are indicated for compromised hosts who are at risk for hematogenous spread of infection (eg, poorly controlled diabetics, alcoholics, IV drug abusers, human immunodeficiency virus [HIV]-infected persons). Other indications for prompt hospital admission and IV antibiotics include rapidly progressive or recurrent infection, cellulitis due to group A streptococci, subcutaneous gas or necrotizing fasciitis, and cellulitis of the orbit, face, or perineum, especially when accompanied by fever and lymphangitis. Clinical signs that suggest a need for IV therapy include high fever, systemic symptoms, and pain greater than the clinical appearance. Progression despite oral antibiotics needs reconsideration of the outpatient approach. When the patient appears unreliable and unable to care for himself at home, admission is also indicated. Services that allow home administration of IV antibiotics and professional monitoring can help shorten a hospital stay admission.

PATIENT EDUCATION

When a lower extremity is involved, the patient should be instructed to rest in bed and elevate the limb. Getting up to go to the bathroom is allowed, but bedrest is necessary. Exercises and anticoagulation may be needed to reduce the possibility of thrombophlebitis in patients at increased risk (see Chapter 35). It is crucial to protect the affected area and to insist that the patient not scratch the involved skin. The importance of taking antibiotic therapy as instructed should be emphasized. The patient should be asked to report progress by telephone and to call if cellulitis fails to resolve within 5 to 7 days.

THERAPEUTIC RECOMMENDATIONS

- Hospitalize the patient unable to care for himself at home reliably, as well as anyone with high fever, rigors, lymphangitis, rapid progression, compromised host defenses, or involvement of the face, orbit, or perineum.
- Treat the uncomplicated, mildly ill patient on an ambulatory basis, beginning with oral *phenoxymethyl penicillin,* 500 mg qid (1 hour before meals and at bedtime), and monitor closely over the next 48 hours.
- If by 48 hours inflammation and fever do not begin to resolve or if close monitoring is not possible, prescribe a penicillinase-resistant penicillin, such as *dicloxacillin,* 500 mg qid.
- In patients markedly allergic to penicillin (type I hypersensitivity), prescribe *erythromycin,* 500 mg qid. Cephalosporins, such as *cephalexin,* may be substituted if the allergy to penicillin is not anaphylactoid. The fluoroquinolones, such as *ciprofloxacin,* are effective against gram-negative cellulitis but have only moderate antistreptococcal and antistaphylococcal activity in vitro and should be used cautiously in cellulitis.
- If anaerobes are suspected, then a fluoroquinolone plus *clindamycin* or *metronidazole* is indicated.
- Patients with an open would but without a recent tetanus booster in the past 10 years should be given 0.5 mL of tetanus toxoid intramuscularly.

ANNOTATED BIBLIOGRAPHY

Baddour LM, Bisno AL. Recurrent cellulitis after coronary bypass surgery. JAMA 1984;251:1049. *(Tinea pedis was the source of bacterial entry.)*

Eron LJ. Therapy of skin and skin structure infections with ciprofloxacin: An overview. Am J Med 1987;82(Suppl 4A):224. *(The drug may have some efficacy in selected settings where gram-negative infection is likely.)*

Hook EW III, Hooton TM, Horton CA, et al. Microbiologic evaluation of cutaneous cellulitis in adults. Arch Intern Med 1986;146:295. *(Efficacy of leading margin aspirates examined; 25 percent positive culture rate.)*

Howe PM, Fajardo JE, Orcutt MA. Etiologic diagnosis of cellulitis: Comparison of aspirates obtained from the leading edge and the point of maximal inflammation. Pediatr Infect Dis 1987;6:685. *(No additional yield from leading edge site.)*

Kahn R, Goldstein EJC. Treatment of bacterial skin infections. Postgrad Med. In press. *(A review of the antimicrobial and ancillary measures required to treat a variety of common types of cellulitis.)*

Meislin HW, Lerner SA, Graves MH, et al. Cutaneous abscesses: Anaerobic and aerobic bacteriology and outpatient management. Ann Intern Med 1977;87:145. *(Incision and drainage were most important; antimicrobials played an adjunctive role.)*

Monk JP, Campoli-Richards DM. Ofloxacin: A review of its antibacterial activity, pharmacokinetics properties and therapeutic use. Drugs 33:346;1987. *(Fluoroquinolone utility in cellulitis noted.)*

Sapico FL, White JL, Canawati HN, et al. The infected foot of the diabetic patient: Quantitative microbiology and analysis of clinical features. Rev Infect Dis 1984;6(Suppl 1):171. *(The polymicrobial nature of these infections is emphasized, especially the importance of anaerobic bacteria.)*

Stevens DL. Invasive group A streptococcus infections. Clin Infect Dis 1992;14:2. *(An excellent review of the spectrum of disease encountered by these organisms.)*

Part 2: Management of Pyodermas

The common cutaneous bacterial infections include impetigo, ecthyma, folliculitis, furunculosis, and erysipelas. They demand prompt recognition by the primary physician and effective antibiotic treatment.

PATHOPHYSIOLOGY AND CLINICAL PRESENTATION

Clinical manifestations are a function of the organism, environmental factors, skin appendages, and host resistance. Primary cutaneous bacterial infections develop on normal skin and are usually initiated by a single organism such as coagulase-positive staphylococci or beta-hemolytic streptococci. Secondary infection refers to bacterial infection superimposed on diseased skin. Cutaneous bacterial infections may also be classified according to the depth of the infection and the propensity for scarring.

Impetigo, a common condition caused primarily by *Staphylococcus aureus,* begins as a small erythematous macular lesion that evolves into a vesicle beneath the stratum corneum. The thin-roofed collection of fluid ruptures easily, leaving denuded, oozing areas. A honey-colored crust forms as the fluid dries and collects. Intense erythema at the pustule's base suggests a beta-hemolytic streptococcal component to the condition. New lesions appear in the same location, and they coalesce. When the honey-colored crusts are removed, the skin appears raw. Individual lesions usually do not exceed 2 cm in size. Impetigo is seen most frequently in children, but it also occurs in adults, especially those with poor hygiene. In adults, the condition is not as contagious as it is among infants. The face is the most common site of involvement. Ordinary lesions do not produce scarring but may leave erythematous marks for a time. Untreated infections may last for weeks.

Ecthyma is a deeper version of impetigo, usually caused by *streptococci* but sometimes a sign of gram-negative or fungal sepsis. Erosion of the epidermis creates ulcerative, crusted lesions. The heaped-up crust conceals the underlying erosion. Healing is accompanied by some scarring because of the depth of the lesions. The legs are commonly involved, and children are more susceptible than adults. Antecedent conditions include eczema, scabies, arthropod bites, trauma, and hot, humid climates. The *brown recluse spider bite,* characterized by necrotizing ulcer and spreading ecthyma, is important to recognize because it requires specific therapy with dapsone.

Folliculitis is infection of the hair follicles, usually caused by coagulase-positive *staphylococci,* and may be divided into superficial and deep types. Superficial folliculitis consists of a small pustule pierced by the hair shaft. It may be seen on the scalp or other hairy portions of the body. Occupational exposure to cutting oils, coal tar products, or topical corticosteroids under occlusion may precipitate folliculitis. A fungal etiology due to *Pityrosporum* may resemble bacterial folliculitis, but it is refractory to antibiotics. Diagnosis is made by finding yeastlike organisms in a KOH wet mount, but a skin biopsy stained for fungi is sometimes required. Rarely, small pustules with surrounding erythema caused by *Propionibacterium acnes* may develop around the occiput in males. *Pseudomonas folliculitis* has been described in association with hot tubs.

Furuncles and carbuncles may develop from a preceding folliculitis and are limited to hairy areas. The erythematous lesions usually become fluctuant after 4 days. A yellowish, pointed area may be seen on the surface, and, if the lesion ruptures spontaneously, pus and necrotic tissue are extruded. The buttocks, axillae, neck, face, and waist areas are common sites of involvement. Predisposing systemic factors include diabetes, malnutrition, obesity, and hematologic disorders. Carbuncles are a coalescence of deep furuncles with multiple points of drainage.

Erysipelas, caused by *beta-hemolytic streptococci,* is characterized by a peripherally spreading, infiltrated, erythematous, sharply circumscribed plaque. The lesion is warm to touch. The face, scalp, hands, and genitals are frequently involved. Rapid evolution of the lesions is seen, and some patients have constitutional symptoms such as fever and malaise. Poor hygiene and lowered resistance promote infection. Trauma may elicit infection, and recurrent erysipelas may lead to brawny edema.

DIAGNOSIS

Lesions are usually diagnosed and treated on the basis of clinical appearance, but microscopic examination of gram-stained material is a quick and inexpensive way to confirm a diagnosis. Culture and sensitivity are usually not necessary for superficial infections but are for more destructive lesions or if the patient is not improving.

PRINCIPLES OF THERAPY

Physical measures are used to enhance resolution and make the skin surface less amenable to colonization by bacteria, whereas antibiotics are given to treat responsible pathogens and prevent recolonization.

Physical Measures. The physical measures employed differ with the pyoderma being treated. The crusts of impetigo must be debrided to expose the skin surface where bacteria are present. Furuncles and carbuncles are treated with hot compresses to enhance drainage. Fluctuant lesions may require incision. Exudative lesions require drying compresses to remove detritus and desiccate the lesion. Saline, tap water, or Burow's solution may be applied for 10 to 20 minutes, three to four times a day. Dehydration improves the appearance of the skin and destroys many organisms.

Antibiotics. *Topical antibiotics* are usually sufficient for impetigo and folliculitis, particularly when combined with cleansing and debridement. Most pyodermas are caused by gram-positive organisms and respond to topical *erythromycin* or *bacitracin. Mupirocin* (Bactroban), a creamy antibiotic ointment, is so effective it has supplanted use of systemic antibiotics in many cases. It is cosmetically well tolerated, although slightly shiny on the skin. Washing with *chlorhexidine* (Hibiclens) is a valuable adjunct because of its bactericidal properties. Patients should wash the areas with the liquid two or three times daily before mupirocin is applied. Antibiotic creams and ointments containing *neomycin* can be used, although neomycin is a known contact sensitizer. However, sensitization usually develops only after long-term use on areas that are denuded.

Reducing colonization is particularly important in the treatment of recurrent furunculosis. Frequent cleansing with soap, particularly chlorhexidene, is useful. Nails should be clipped and vigorously scrubbed. *Mupirocin* ointment should be instilled into the anterior nares. It can be used in the nares on a long-term basis to reduce bacterial carriage in patients who repeatedly develop pyoderma. Additional preventive measures include soaking the beard with hot water for 5 minutes before shaving, and discarding blades after each use. The razor should be soaked in alcohol. Separate towels, sheets, and clothing should be used, and everything should be laundered and changed frequently. If vigorous reduction of colonization is unsuccessful, consideration should be given to replacement of pathogenic staphylococci with a less pathogenic strain.

Systemic antibiotics are indicated when there are constitutional symptoms or if the patient is uncooperative. Phenoxymethyl *penicillin* is sufficient for streptococcal infection; oral *erythromycin* is effective against most staphylococcal and streptococcal species that cause pyodermas. Resistant staph species may require *dicloxacillin* or *cephalexin*. There is no evidence that antibiotic therapy prevents poststreptococcal glomerulonephritis. As noted, antibiotic selection may be based on clinical appearance, but microscopic examination of gram-stained material is quick and inexpensive. Culture and sensitivity are reserved for more destructive lesions or if the patient is not improving.

PATIENT EDUCATION AND INDICATIONS FOR REFERRAL

A primary consideration in the therapy of all pyodermas is patient education. Teaching aggressive and regular use of cleansing and debridement is central to the successful resolution of the infection. In addition, careful review of preventive measures and antibiotic use are essential.

If aggressive hygienic measures and attempts to eliminate the staphylococcal carrier state fail to prevent recurrent infection, consider referral for replacement with nonpathogenic staphylococci or treatment with rifampin, which is effective for eradicating nasal carriage of pathogenic staphylococci.

THERAPEUTIC RECOMMENDATIONS

Impetigo

- Apply Burow's compresses for 20 minutes, two to four times daily, followed by gentle debridement using a washcloth and cleansing with a chlorhexidene-containing agent.
- Lightly apply mupirocin to the area after drying. A nighttime application is also advised.
- Advise the patient not to cover the lesions and the family to avoid using the same towel or washcloth; keep children away from the patient with impetigo.

Folliculitis

- Treat with debridement and topical antibiotics as for impetigo.

Furuncles and Carbuncles

- Treat with hot compresses until the lesions are fluctuant and spontaneous drainage occurs. Larger lesions may require removal of the core with a 4-mm biopsy punch to facilitate drainage.
- Treat furuncles or carbuncles associated with cellulitis, fever, or facial location with oral antistaphylococcal antibiotics, either erythromycin (333 mg tid for 10 days), or dicloxacillin (250 qid for 10 days).
- Treat recurrent infection with a 10- to 14-day course of a systemic antibiotic, combined with removal of bacteria from potential sources such as the skin, nares, nails, razor, and other fomites.

Erysipelas

- Treat with cool compresses and phenoxymethyl penicillin (500 mg qid) for 7 to 10 days.

Recurrent Pyodermas

- Eradicate the staphylococcal nasal carrier state. Prescribe oral dicloxacillin (500 mg qid) for 10 to 14 days in combination with topical mupirocin applied twice daily for at least 5 days.

ANNOTATED BIBLIOIGRAPHY

Bisno AL. Cutaneous infections: Microbiologic and epidemiologic considerations. Am J Med 1984;76:172. *(Important review.)*

Demidovichy CW, Wittler RR, Ruff ME, et al. Impetigo: Current etiology and comparison of penicillin, erythromycin, and cephalexin therapies. Am J Dis Child 1990;144:1313. *(Treatment failures found with penicillin.)*

Duncan WC, Dodge BG, Knox JM. Prevention of superficial pyogenic skin infections. Arch Dermatol 1969;99:465. *(The regular use of an antibacterial soap reduced the incidence of superficial bacterial infections.)*

Heskel NS, Siepman NC, Pichotta PJ, et al. Erythromycin versus cefadroxil in the treatment of skin infections. Int J Dermatol 1992;31:131. *(The two antibiotics were equally effective.)*

McLinn S. A bacteriologically controlled, randomized study comparing the efficacy of 2% mupirocin (Bactroban) with oral erythromycin in the treatment of patients with impetigo. J Am Acad Dermatol 1990;22:883. *(2% mupirocin was as effective as oral erythromycin.)*

Reagan DR, Doebbeling BN, Pfaller MA, et al. Elimination of coincident *Staphylococcus aureus* nasal and hand carriage with intranasal application of mupirocin calcium ointment. Ann Intern Med 1991;114:101. *(At 3 months, 71 percent of subjects remained free of nasal staphylococci; positive hand cultures were reduced to 2.9 percent.)*

191
Management of Superficial Fungal Infections

WILLIAM V. R. SHELLOW, M.D.

Primary Care Medicine: Office Evaluation and Management of the Adult Patient, 3rd edition, edited by Allan H. Goroll, Lawrence A. May, and Albert G. Mulley, Jr. J.B. Lippincott Company, Philadelphia

Though neither dangerous nor life-threatening, superficial fungal infections are prevalent, irritating, and often recurrent. They are easily diagnosed but commonly confused with nonfungal dermatoses such as impetigo (see Chapter 184). The primary physician should be capable of definitive diagnosis, cost-effective therapy, and prevention through patient education.

PATHOPHYSIOLOGY AND CLINICAL PRESENTATION

Why some people resist these ubiquitous pathogens while others cannot remains unknown. Sometimes a systemic disease such as diabetes is responsible. Hereditary factors may be involved. Dampness, darkness, and friction leading to skin maceration are important local precipitants.

Fungal infection occurs when one of these ubiquitous organisms invades the superficial layers of the skin. Dermatophytes do not invade below the level of keratin because a potent antifungal factor prevents deeper infection. Candidal infection produces inflammatory change through elaboration of an endotoxin-like substance.

Clinical Presentations

Dermatophytic and candidal infections produce scaly, erythematous lesions with defined margins, occurring in characteristic areas of the body that promote the growth of fungi.

Tinea versicolor (pityriasis versicolor) is characterized by brown, pink, red, or white scaly patches that occur on the chest, back, and shoulders. During the summer, it may present as hypopigmented areas, sometimes erroneously interpreted as vitiligo. The organism appears to prevent pigment transfer from melanocytes to epidermal cells. The diagnosis can be suspected if scratching a macular area raises a small amount of fine scale. Examination of the skin with a Wood's light reveals gold or orange-brown fluorescence. The infection is diagnosed by scraping a scaly lesion and examining it with a drop of 20% potassium hydroxide (KOH) for characteristic short hyphae and spores, sometimes referred to as "*spaghetti and meatballs*."

Dermatophyte infections are defined by the area of the body they affect. The most common are *tinea cruris*, which involves the groin and inner thighs and sometimes extends onto the abdomen and buttocks. *Tinea pedis* is characterized by blisters and inflammation on the soles and interdigital areas of the feet. *Tinea corporis* affects other areas of the body, including the trunk and extremities. If there is involvement of the face, it may be called *tinea faciei*. *Tinea capitis*, or scalp ringworm, occurs almost exclusively in children. *Tinea barbae* involving the bearded area has become very uncommon. *Onychomycosis* is characterized by the accumulation of subungual keratin, which produces a thickened, distorted, crumbling nail. *Trichophyton rubrum*, *Trichophyton mentagrophytes*, and *Epidermophyton floccosum* are the most common infecting organisms. *Microsporum canis*, which is acquired by contact with infected pet cats and dogs, is another pathogenic fungus.

***Candida* infections** of the skin occur principally in *intertriginous* locations such as the axillae, groin, intergluteal folds, inframammary area, or interdigital web spaces. Crusted involvement of the labial commissures, known as perlèche, and involvement of the glans penis also occur. The presence of erythema on the glans penis and scrotum suggest a candidal rather than a dermatophyte infection. Lesions are pustular and thin-walled, on a red base, often producing burning and itching. Candidiasis may be clinically suspected as a result of the presence of characteristic *satellite pustules* outside of the margin of the primary lesion.

DIAGNOSIS

The finding of scaly, erythematous lesions with defined margins occurring in characteristic areas of the body that promote the growth of fungi should raise suspicion of a superficial fungal infection. Satellite pustules suggest a candidal involvement. In intertriginous areas, fungal infection must be differentiated from intertrigo and erythrasma. Asymptomatic, slightly erythematous to light brown finely scaling patches in the groin and upper thigh with little or no central clearing are characteristic of erythrasma (a corynebacterial infection). Early intertrigo is characterized by slight maceration and erythema. With time, redness becomes more intense, and the epidermis becomes eroded or even denuded.

The KOH Preparation. Suspicion of dermatophyte infection requires microscopic examination of scrapings from an involved area of skin. To prepare a specimen for microscopic examination, the border of the lesion is scraped lightly using a No. 15 scalpel blade or the side of a microscope slide. The scale is collected onto a clean microscope slide, using a coverslip to push all the scale into a small mound. One or, at most, two drops of 20% KOH solution or KOH with dimethyl sulfoxide (DMSO) are placed in the center of the mound of scale, and a coverslip is laid over it. If the KOH solution does not contain DMSO, the slide must be heated lightly to improve "clearing" of the epithelial cells. If DMSO is present, heating is not required.

Under 40x power with reduced light, thread-like hyphae can be seen crossing cell walls. If budding spores and pseudohyphae are found, the diagnosis is candidal infection. Branched, septate hyphae can be confirmed using higher power (100x). This second step is necessary to make sure that artifacts are not being mistaken for hyphae. Occasionally, a scraping must be planted on Sabouraud's agar for culturing in order to identify fungal infection.

If candidal infection is identified or topical fungal infection is recurrent or extensive, one should check for conditions associated with immune compromise (human immunodeficiency virus [HIV] infection, diabetes, cirrhosis, lymphoma, steroid use, chemotherapy, etc.).

PRINCIPLES OF MANAGEMENT

Effective management requires attention to predisposing factors as well as proper use of antifungal agents. For example, on a systemic scale, diabetes control should be tightened and use of immunosuppressive agents cut back. Locally, the *elimination of moisture* and *prevention of maceration* are priorities (see below and Chapter 188). Further drying of inflammatory or weeping lesions can be achieved with the application of compresses containing an astringent such as aluminum acetate, available as *Burow's* tablets or packets.

After predisposing factors have been reduced and the lesions dried, specific antifungal medication is appropriate. There are a host of effective agents available. One should identify and use the least expensive, most effective agent that produces the fewest side effects. Patients with fungal infections have invariably tried over-the-counter remedies before they visit the physician. It is important to find out what they have used before prescribing the same product in its prescription version.

Antifungal Agents

There are four classes of topical antifungal agents currently available. Costs to patients are similar for most of these agents, with the over-the-counter preparations the least expensive (though not necessarily inexpensive).

The largest class of agents is the *azoles*, with the older ones (miconazole, clotrimazole, tolnaftate) available without prescription. Others include econazole (Spectazole), oxiconazole (Oxistat), sulconazole (Exelderm), and ketoconazole (Nizoral). The second class is the ethanolamines, with ciclopirox olamine (Loprox) the only example available. The third class is the allylamines, which includes naftifine (Naftin) and terbinafine. These agents are unrelated to the azoles and are unique in being fungicidal rather than fungistatic. However, cure rate is similar to that of other agents. The fourth class is the polyene antibiotics, with topical amphotericin and nystatin, which are anticandidal.

New topical antifungal agents seem to appear monthly. Claims of unique efficacy are made for each one, but all have a similar cure rate of approximately 85 percent for acute infections and much less for chronic ones. Some preparations have special properties that make them useful in particular circumstances. For example, ciclopirox is best at penetrating the nail plate, making it useful for treatment of onychomycosis. Topical lotions are more drying, less messy, and more useful for daytime application; a cream should be used at night.

If marked improvement of clinical lesions and symptoms is not seen within 3 weeks, it may help to try combination therapy, using an antifungal agent from one class during the day and another from a different class at night. *Systemic antifungal therapy* with griseofulvin or ketoconazole may also deserve consideration if the patient is immunocompromised (eg, because of HIV, lymphoma, chemotherapy, cirrhosis, etc.) and refractory to topical therapy. However, the systemic antifungal agents are potentially toxic to bone marrow and liver and must be used with care, especially if prolonged courses of therapy are needed. Rapid clearing is likely to follow, but relapses are common and intermittent therapy may be necessary indefinitely.

Treatment of Specific Conditions

Tinea Versicolor. For effectiveness, convenience, and least expense, a 2.5% suspension of *selenium sulfide* (Selsun) or a *zinc pyrithione* shampoo (Zincon, Head & Shoulders) can be applied with a rough washcloth. It should be allowed to remain on the affected areas for 10 minutes and then rinsed off. Daily application for 1 week is recommended. An 87 percent success rate at the end of 4 weeks was found with use of this program. In refractory cases, selenium sulfide suspension can be left on the skin overnight. The topical antifungal agents are much more expensive but are useful in treating recalcitrant involvement of small areas. *Ketoconazole shampoo* may prove to be quite effective for treating tinea versicolor.

After treatment, patients should be reexamined for continued scaling, which suggests persistent activity. Patients with no signs of persistence or relapse should be advised that depigmentation may persist until they go back into the sun.

For immunocompromised patients with infection too widespread for topical therapy, systemic *ketoconazole* is worth consideration. A dose of 200 mg is prescribed daily for 7 to 10 days, with close monitoring of liver function. For best results, ketoconazole should be taken with an acidic fruit juice or followed by exercise-induced sweating. The patient is advised not to shower until the next day. This regimen is repeated 1 week later and can also be repeated monthly to prevent recurrences. There is no evidence that a course of ketoconazole shorter than 14 days in duration is associated with the idiosyncratic hepatotoxicity that may be seen in 1 of 15,000 patients taking the drug for longer periods.

Other Diffuse Tineas. In moist intertriginous areas, the patient should dry oozing lesions by applying compresses soaked in Burow's solution for 30 to 60 minutes one to three times daily. A nonmedicated or antifungal powder may be used to absorb moisture. In very inflamed pruritic lesions of the groin and other intertriginous areas, adding a topical corticosteroid can help relieve the inflammatory component, and this is often prescribed in conjunction with topical antifungal therapy (see Chapter 188). Topical treatment suffices for involvement of glabrous skin, but systemic drugs should be considered if hair sheaths are involved, widespread involvement exists, or associated folliculitis occurs.

Tinea Pedis. Athlete's foot is sometimes difficult to treat. The patient must be instructed to wear nonocclusive leather footwear or sandals and absorbent cotton socks, and to dry the feet frequently without rubbing, perhaps by using a hair dryer. Topical antifungals alone often suffice. Naftifine cream used once daily for tinea pedis is effective and may yield better results than clotrimazole used twice daily. If widespread scaling with hyperkeratosis occurs (so-called "moccasin-type" tinea pedis), keratolytic agents are required. The nightly application of Keralyt gel under occlusion, with antifungal creams used two to three times daily, may successfully treat this difficult problem.

Onychomycosis. Nailbed involvement by fungus is extremely refractory to treatment, although fingernail infections usually respond better than do toenail infections. Most topical agents cannot penetrate the nail plate, but topical *ciclopirox* (Loprox) may, and it can be tried nightly with applications under occlusion. Weeks to months of treatment may be necessary before improvement is noted. Often, topical therapy is insufficient, and the question of employing systemic antifungal therapy comes up. The value of the cosmetic benefit must be weighed against the cost and risks of prolonged systemic treatment. Even with successful therapy, relapse is common.

The standard oral program is *griseofulvin* (250 mg bid–qid) for 6 to 12 months. A polyethylene glycol griseofulvin preparation facilitates absorption. Griseofulvin must be taken until the infected portion of the nail has grown out to the end of the nail, accounting for the extended duration of therapy required. Because leukopenia has been observed, periodic blood counts are advised, and liver function is monitored as well. It may be necessary to remove the affected nail. Even if a cure is obtained, reinfection is common. *Ketoconazole* has been used in patients who do not respond to griseofulvin or who cannot tolerate it, but risk of hepatotoxicity is greatly increased by the need for prolonged treatment, leading some authorities not to recommend its use for this condition. Baseline liver function tests should be documented and then laboratory studies repeated at least monthly. Fluconazole is an effective but safer systemic antifungal. It is very expensive and has not been tested for use in onychomycosis.

Patients should be given the option to live with their toenail infections. Women may choose to use nail polish to cover cosmetic unsightliness. Reducing the hyperkeratotic nail with filing helps the appearance.

Candidiasis. Treatment begins with attention to predisposing factors such as use of systemic corticosteroids, birth control pills, tetracycline, and other antibiotics, as well as diabetes, Cushing's syndrome, and HIV infection. One proceeds to meticulous drying of the area, adequate exposure to air, and specific anticandidal therapy. Gentian violet or Castellani's paint are time-proven but quite messy and have largely been abandoned. *Imidazole* creams or lotions (eg, clotrimazole) should be used two or three times daily, but ointments should be avoided because they maintain a moist local environment. In highly inflamed infections, initiating therapy with a topical *corticosteroid* cream in combination with clotrimazole (Lotrisone) applied lightly is useful. Oral ketoconazole is recommended for difficult candidal infections in immunocompromised patients, although fluconazole (Diflucan) is gaining popularity because of its superior safety profile.

Paronychial infection is difficult to treat. Therapy consists of avoiding exposure to water and using rubber gloves with cotton lining whenever water contact is unavoidable. Nystatin or amphotericin B (Fungizone) lotion should be applied two to four times daily to the affected area. In highly inflamed conditions, nystatin or clotrimazole with steroids may be applied overnight under a fingercot. Nails grow out normally after the paronychia has healed. Ketoconazole should be given orally if local therapy fails. Fluconazole is also effective but is quite costly for the patient.

INDICATIONS FOR REFERRAL

Referral to the dermatologist should be considered if a fungal infection proves refractory to conventional topical treatment and prolonged or repeated systemic therapy is being contemplated. Consultation for consideration of the risks and benefits can be quite worthwhile, as can a second look at the problem. Short courses of systemic therapy (<2 wk) are of little risk and often do not require dermatologic referral.

PATIENT EDUCATION

At the time of the first incident, patients with fungal infection should be instructed about appropriate measures to prevent recurrence.

Maintaining Dryness. Instructing the patient about how to keep the skin dry and prevent maceration is critical to both successful treatment and prophylaxis. Dryness is particularly important in tinea pedis, tinea cruris, and candidal infections. Preventive measures should be taken in areas that have shown a tendency to become infected. In addition, the patient should be told to apply powder liberally to naturally moist areas of the body and to wear cotton clothing and loose-fitting underwear. Also, patients with tinea pedis should always wear socks and avoid sneakers and rubber-soled shoes, and the physician should encourage exposure of feet to the air as often as possible. Last, people who sweat profusely should change clothing more frequently, shower, and apply nonmedicated talcum powder.

Other Advice. Fungal infections may be slow to clear. To assure compliance, it is essential to instruct the patient carefully on appropriate application and duration of treatment. Patients should be instructed to call at the first sign of recurrence and to institute appropriate drying measures and specific therapy after physician consultation.

THERAPEUTIC RECOMMENDATIONS

- Prescribe a topical preparation approved for once-a-day use. This is both cost-effective and likely to improve patient compliance.
- Avoid creams for intertriginous areas, because patients may use too much medication and thereby increase maceration. Prescribe a lotion or solution instead.
- If there is incomplete clearing after 2 to 3 weeks, the short-term use of a systemic antifungal should be considered.

ANNOTATED BIBLIOGRAPHY

Borelli D, Jacobs PH, Nall L. Tinea versicolor: epidemiologic, clinical and therapeutic aspects. J Am Acad Dermatol 1991; 25:300. *(An in-depth discussion of tinea versicolor with emphasis on treatment considerations.)*

Cohn MS. Superficial fungal infections. Topical and oral treatment of common types. Postgrad Med 1992;91:239. *(A practical discussion of diagnosis and treatment, including the more recently approved antifungal agents.)*

Hay RJ, Logan RA, Moore MK, et al. A comparative study of terbinafine versus griseofulvin in "dry-type" dermatophyte infections. J Am Acad Dermatol 1991;24:243. *(After 12 wk of therapy, 100 percent of the terbinafine-treated group were clear compared with only 45 percent in the group treated with griseofulvin.)*

Jacobs P. Treatment of fungal infections: state of the art. J Am Acad Dermatol 1990;23:549. *(Discusses ketoconazole regimens for tinea versicolor, tinea corporis, and tinea pedis.)*

Jones HE, Reinhardt JH, Rinaldi MG. A clinical, mycological and immunological survey of dermatophytosis. Arch Dermatol 1973;108:61. *(The pathophysiology of dermatophyte infections.)*

Korting HC, Schäfer-Korting M. Is tinea unguium still widely incurable? Arch Dermatol 1992;28:243. *(A discussion of various strategies to successfully treat onychomycosis and to prevent recurrences.)*

Macura, AB. Fungal resistance to antimycotic drugs: a growing problem. Int J Dermatol 1991;30:181. *(Some antifungal agents are only fungistatic at lower concentrations while at high ones they are fungicidal.)*

Maibach HI, Kligman AM. The biology of experimental human cutaneous moniliasis (*Candida albicans*). Arch Dermatol 1962;85:233. *(Still the definitive monograph.)*

Sanchez JL, Torres VM. Double-blind efficacy study of selenium sulfide in tinea versicolor. J Am Acad Dermatol 1984;11:235. *(Daily 10-min application of 2.5% selenium sulfide for 1 wk proved an effective, convenient treatment, with 87 percent success at the end of 4 wk.)*

Smith EB, Wiss K, Hanifin JM, Jordon RE, et al. Comparison of once- and twice-daily naftifine cream regimens with twice-daily clotrimazole in the treatment of tinea pedis. J Am Acad Dermatol 1990;22:1116. *(Naftifine cream used once daily for tinea pedis is effective and may be more effective than clotrimazole used twice daily.)*

Primary Care Medicine: Office Evaluation and Management of the Adult Patient, 3rd edition, edited by Allan H. Goroll, Lawrence A. May, and Albert G. Mulley, Jr. J.B. Lippincott Company, Philadelphia

192
Management of Cutaneous and Genital Herpes Simplex

JEFFREY E. GALPIN, M.D.

Herpes simplex virus (HSV) is a ubiquitous virus that clinically affects man. *HSV type 1* is the prototype for cutaneous disease of the upper body; *HSV type 2* generally produces genital and lower body infections. The two types share 50 percent common genetic material and may be interchangeable clinically. They differ in sensitivity to viral drugs and in their ability to cause specific disease in other organs.

Many patients seek help to confirm the herpes infection they suspect or because they have frequent or recurrent rashes and symptoms. The primary care physician must seek a prompt diagnosis, know how to utilize the approaches to treatment, and address the concerns and negative social stigma that often accompany genital infection.

PATHOPHYSIOLOGY AND CLINICAL PRESENTATION

Primary Infection

Primary HSV-1 infection usually goes unnoticed but may present as severe exudative pharyngitis or gingivostomatitis, with high fevers and tender lymphadenopathy. The illness often is mistaken for streptococcal disease, other bacterial infections of the oropharynx, or mononucleosis. Systemic manifestations of the illness may outweigh the local presentation.

Primary HSV-2 infection also may be missed or misdiagnosed. In its most overt form, an exudative, painful vulvovaginitis is seen in the female and penile ulceration with tender inguinal nodes in the male. The genital lesions are painful in 95 percent of men and 99 percent of women. Local symptoms increase during the first 6 to 7 days of illness and peak between days 8 and 10, gradually decreasing during the next week. Lymph nodes are enlarged, firm, and tender. Although suppurative lymphadenopathy does not occur, superimposed bacterial infections can produce this finding. Primary genital infection usually takes place in adolescence, but it may be contracted at the time of birth. Fever and malaise occur in 67 percent of patients, dysuria in 63 percent, and tender adenopathy in 80 percent.

Complications of primary infection by HSV-2 include extragenital lesions in 20 percent, secondary yeast infections in 11 percent, aseptic meningitis in 8 percent, and sacral autonomic nerve dysfunction in 2 percent. Many studies of patients with cervical cancer demonstrate a high association with HSV-2 antibodies or HSV-2 presence, although no study or series has directly found HSV genetic material within these cancer cells. The risk of cervical cancer secondary to HSV may be an epidemiologic relation and not etiologic.

An unusual form of primary infection results from implantation of virus into broken skin, producing a *herpetic whitlow* characterized by pain, swelling, and erythema of the fingers with pronounced adenopathy. Wrestlers may develop *herpes gladiatorum*, a primary herpes infection on exposed parts of the body that are inoculated during the rough activity of wrestling.

Recurrent Infection

The most common form of HSV disease is recurrent infection. After acute infection, the virus resides in the associated dorsal root ganglion and circulates along the endoneural sheath to the skin if there is a breakdown in host defenses. Loss of cytotoxic killer cell activity or other cytotoxic T-cell function, cytokine abnormalities, a decrease in local secretory IgA, or local skin damage permits reactivation. The result is a localized, self-limited form of illness. It may begin with a prodrome of tingling or discomfort as well as more generalized symptoms such as nausea, fatigue, or even fever.

Although some patients develop pain without rash, most experience the characteristic *maculopapular-vesicular* eruption. The lesions become turbid as interferon is produced in the vesicles and as lymphocytes stimulated by interleukin-2, interleukin-6, and other cytokines begin controlling the infection. During the initial 3 to 4 days, some patients autoinoculate themselves in other areas, but secondary infections are usually brief, mild, self-limited, and incapable of establishing disease in new regions. Recurrent infections can occur in different distributions along the same ganglia, and there is heterogeneity in the illness.

Eventually, there is re-epithelialization of the skin, usually without scarring. Secondary bacterial infections (caused by streptococci or staphylococci) can lead to cellulitis and lymphangitis and must be watched for. The risk of transmission is greatest in the first 96 hours after the appearance of the rash. Even without evidence of disease, silent shedding occurs in 2 percent to 5 percent of patients, particularly those with recurrent genital disease.

Chronic pain syndromes associated with infection without lesions are being identified more frequently. Post-herpetic neuralgia due to HSV-1 is described as a recurrent syndrome without clinical evidence of skin lesions. Vulvar burning alone may be an expression of HSV-2 infection. Elsberg's syndrome with radiculomyelopathy and acute urinary retention may also be secondary to clinically inapparent disease. *Hemorrhagic cystitis* and dyspareunia can both be the result of herpes simplex disease. Finally, HSV has been associated with acute *retinal necrosis* syndrome presenting as eye pain and visual loss.

Complications of local recurrent infections are few. Sacral or perirectal disease can lead to *proctitis* or colitis. Sacral disease is also associated with risk of recurrent *aseptic meningitis*. Recurrent disease sometimes takes the form of *erythema multiforme* without evidence of vesicles. In atopic individuals, HSV can produce a devastating generalized *eczema herpeticum*. The incidence of neonatal HSV caused by retrograde spread of HSV-2 from maternal infection or during passage of the infant through the birth canal is estimated at 10 percent in women with recurrent or primary infection at 32 weeks and several-fold higher if infection is present at term. Congenital HSV is often multisystemic and devastating, but it is fortunately rare.

DIFFERENTIAL DIAGNOSIS AND WORKUP

The diagnosis of herpes simplex infection is important, especially identification of type 2 disease, because of its social and psychological significance. Approximately 50 percent of ulcerative lesions in the genital area are herpetic. Herpes infection, however, may overlap with *syphilis* or *chancroid* (see Chapter 141). Ulcerations may also occur from noninfectious causes such as Behçet's syndrome, inflammatory bowel disease, or simply as a result of excoriations and secondary bacterial infections caused by vigorous sexual activity. Syphilis serology should always be performed if genital HSV is suspected.

WORKUP

In most instances, the diagnosis is a clinical one, based on the finding of the characteristic lesions. Unroofing a vesicle and performing a *Tzanck preparation* (see Chapter 193) can be helpful, but it is less specific than *viral culture*. *Antigen detection techniques* are of limited sensitivity. *DNA probes* may provide a more sensitive, specific, and much more rapid approach to viral isolation. The use of polymerase chain reaction (PCR) assays for presence of specific DNA or RNA sequences offers the best and most sensitive means for diagnosing active disease; cost is a consideration. Promising monoclonal and oligoclonal detection methods are under development. *Serology* can confirm prior infection and type but is less useful in documenting the origin of an ongoing episode, because titers often do not rise sufficiently and there is cross-reactivity between HSV types 1 and 2. Serology also has the disadvantage of not producing data within the period that the patient is clinically affected, and patients, once exposed, carry titers forever whether they ever reactivate. High IgE levels seem to occur during active recurrences. This may be responsible for the associated presentation of erythema multiforme in these cases.

Genital herpes is a major cause of types 2 and 3 Pap smear abnormalities and should be routinely sought if these changes are seen. It is important to differentiate this benign inflammatory abnormality from real metaplastic or anaplastic disease.

PRINCIPLES OF THERAPY

Herpes infection is self-limited. The goals of therapy are to increase the speed of healing and reduce the duration of symptoms, the frequency and severity of recurrences, and the risk of complications.

Acyclovir. The mainstay of treatment is acyclovir, a purine analogue substrate for viral thymidine kinase. The kinase is uniquely activated in cells that are infected with HSV. Acyclovir is effective against both types of HSV, although HSV-1 is the more sensitive. Oral acyclovir shortens viral shedding time and reduces the time to healing and crusting of lesions. The earlier the treatment is instituted, the better. Continuous use of acyclovir in patients with frequent recurrences reduces the number and severity of repeat episodes. Unfortunately, once the drug is discontinued, its effect on recurrences ceases. Long-term use is associated with slow adaptation of the virus to the drug, but clinically important resistance has not been reported. Cessation of use results in reversion to original sensitivity. One can readily treat for 12 months at a time without adverse effect.

The use of acyclovir for genital herpes in *pregnancy* appears to dramatically decrease the chance of fetal transmission in the last trimester, but safety remains to be established. Often a cesarean section is advocated in these cases.

Intravenous acyclovir is indicated in *immunocompromised hosts* and in disseminated disease such as meningoencephalitis. Intravenous acyclovir produces higher, more consistent blood levels than oral acyclovir, which is only 15 percent absorbed. The oral vehicle is acceptable for mucocutaneous manifestations in immunocompetent hosts.

There is little place for *topical acyclovir*, although it has some limited efficacy in primary infection. Topical acyclovir is also of little use in keratoconjunctivitis, a dangerous illness; trifluorothymidine ointment plus oral or intravenous acyclovir should be used.

Adjuncts. Good local skin care and the use of drying agents to speed the transition from active vesicle to crusting are the essence of adjunctive therapy. Topical surfactants such as ether or chloroform seems to give some additional relief. Some have advocated, with little evidence, the associated use of cimetidine because of research evidence suggesting that histamine$_2$ antagonists have antiherpes activity. Vidarabine, ribavirin, bromodeoxyuridine, and ganciclovir sodium (DHPG) have some promise of antiviral activity. Care of skin lesions is especially important in the immunocompromised or eczematous host, in whom dissemination and autoinoculation can lead to serious consequences.

Some clinicians use *topical corticosteroids* to abort progression of herpetic lesions. This empiric approach often works, though it lacks scientific evidence and raises a theoretical concern about spread. No evidence has been published to document this danger.

Over-the-counter preparations such as Blistex, Campho-Phenique, or Anbesol may provide some minimal symptomatic relief but do not affect the course of the eruption. Considering the long history of ineffective therapy, physicians should remain skeptical about new remedies offered.

Vaccines. There is growing evidence that long-term modulation of the immune system by vaccines is capable of maintaining benign latency. The in vivo stimulation of natural killer cells, interferon, interleukin-2, and other lymphokines by several vaccines is being studied in this country and in Europe. Initial results have been encouraging.

PATIENT EDUCATION

Genital Herpes. Reassurance of the frightened patient with genital herpes is critical. Herpes has acquired an unjustifiably vicious reputation in the media. The only substantial danger with HSV infection is during childbirth. Risk of infection of the fetus can be reduced by frequent culture and the use of cesarean section if there is a question of active lesions or culturable infection. The stigma associated with this disease must be reduced. The patient must be made to understand that herpes infection is common and is not a badge of disgrace, nor is the patient a constant threat for transmission to other people. Guilt should be assuaged, and the patient should be educated to know the probable signs of disease and to recognize that asymptomatic recurrence does occur and that it is occasionally difficult to prevent recurrences.

Nonetheless, educate patients about transmissibility. It is important that they know what constitutes high-risk activity. The concept of silent spreading must also be appreciated by the patient. Transmission is less likely with the use of condoms but is still possible. By confirming the presence of antibody in a sexual partner, anxiety surrounding sexual relations can be reduced.

Pamphlets about the disease are available through the Centers for Disease Control, the National Institutes of Health, and the American Social Health Association. These are superior sources to many of the lay-initiated hotlines, which may overplay the emotional problems. It should be emphasized that recurrent infections are far less likely to produce discomfort or pain than primary infection.

Facial Involvement. The presence of facial lesions is always annoying and is embarrassing to some. Protection from sunburn and trauma should be urged, as should good local care, with use of drying agents to speed the transition from active vesicle to crusting. Patients are reassured knowing the risk for scarring is very small and that there is effective oral therapy for shortening severe episodes and reducing risk of recurrences.

INDICATIONS FOR REFERRAL AND ADMISSION

Consult with an obstetrician regarding safety and advisability of using of acyclovir treatment in the third trimester versus cesarean section at the time of delivery to prevent the risk of fetal HSV transmission. Patients with suspected eye involvement should be referred urgently to the ophthalmologist for eye examination and treatment with trifluorothymidine and acyclovir. The immunocompromised person who appears to be disseminating requires prompt admission for intravenous therapy.

THERAPEUTIC RECOMMENDATIONS

- Treat symptomatic lesions with oral acyclovir, 200 mg five times a day, beginning at the first sign of infection. Provide enough medication for the patient to restart therapy at the first suspicion of reactivation. Titrate the dosage according to response to treatment. Oral acyclovir in 800-mg doses is now available and can be used two to four times per day, if required, with little additional evidence of intolerance.

- Consider chronic acyclovir prophylaxis for patients who have more than six to eight recurrences per year. Titrate dose to the lowest level possible without reactivation and continue for up to 12 months at a time.
- Educate patients about transmissibility of genital herpes. Recommend use of condoms, but also help keep the problem in perspective.
- Watch for secondary bacterial infection and disseminated HSV disease. In patients who are immunosuppressed, dissemination may present as gangrenous ulcers or deep-seated eschars.
- Follow genital infections closely during pregnancy.

ANNOTATED BIBLIOGRAPHY

Bierman SM. Recurrent genital herpes simplex infection. A trivial disorder. Arch Dermatol 1985;121:173. *(A good normative statement placing this illness in perspective.)*

Corey L, Spear PG. Infection with herpes simplex viruses. N Engl J Med 1986;314:686,749. *(A two-part state-of-the-art review.)*

Dahm C, Elgas M, Kuhn JE, et al. The diagnostic significance of the polymerase chain reaction and isoelectric focusing in herpes simplex virus encephalitis. J Med Virol 1992;36:147. *(Use of PCR for diagnosis HSV infection.)*

Douglas JM, Critchlow C, Benedetti J, et al. A double-blind study of oral acyclovir for suppression of recurrences of genital herpes simplex virus infection. N Engl J Med 1984;310:1551. *(Oral acyclovir given for 4 mo markedly reduced but did not eliminate recurrences. The natural history of recurrences was not affected.)*

Gonzales GR. Postherpes simplex type 1 neuralgia simulating postherpetic neuralgia. J Pain Symptom Manage 1992;7:320. *(Gives evidence of HSV presenting much like post-herpetic neuralgia caused by herpes zoster.)*

Koutsky LA, Stevens CE, Holmes KK, et al. Underdiagnosis of genital herpes by current clinical and viral-isolation procedures. N Engl J Med 1992;326:1533. *(Sensitivity is low; new strategies for diagnosis reviewed.)*

Luby ED, Klinge V. Genital herpes: a pervasive psychosocial disorder. Arch Dermatol 1985;121:494. *(An article emphasizing the adverse effect of herpes on intimate sexual relationships.)*

Maccato ML, Kaufman RH. Herpes genitalis. Dermatol Clin 1992;10:415. *(Review of HSV genitalis with attention to silent shedding.)*

Mckay M. Vulvodynia. Diagnostic patterns. Dermatol Clin 1992; 10:423. *(Defines multiple causes, including HSV, of vulvar burning.)*

Mertz GJ, Critchlow CW, Benedetti J, et al. Double-blind placebo controlled trial of oral acyclovir in first-episode genital herpes simplex virus infection. JAMA 1984;252:1147. *(Acyclovir treatment shortened the duration of viral shedding, symptoms, and lesions but did not reduce subsequent recurrences.)*

Solomon A, Rasmussen JE, Varani J. The Tzanck smear in the diagnosis of cutaneous herpes simplex. JAMA 1984;251:633. *(Viral culture was superior, but Tzanck prep is still a useful, cost-effective aid in early diagnosis.)*

193
Management of Herpes Zoster

JEFFREY E. GALPIN, M.D.

Primary Care Medicine: Office Evaluation and Management of the Adult Patient, 3rd edition, edited by Allan H. Goroll, Lawrence A. May, and Albert G. Mulley, Jr. J.B. Lippincott Company, Philadelphia

Herpes zoster (shingles) is a common viral cutaneous eruption estimated to affect 300,000 persons a year in the United States. Most cases represent reactivation of the varicella-zoster virus (VZV). Incidence increases with age and degree of host immunosuppression. A community-based study found 100 cases per 100,000 person-years among those ages 15 to 35, rising with each decade to reach 450 cases per 100,000 by age 75. The seasonal variation seen with varicella does not occur with zoster; shingles is rarely an epidemic illness. Shingles may present as a pain syndrome without vesicles and pose a diagnostic problem. The primary physician must recognize zoster, make the patient comfortable, and prevent complications.

PATHOPHYSIOLOGY AND CLINICAL PRESENTATION

Varicella, the chickenpox virus, usually affects people early in life and then lies dormant in a nerve ganglion in a genomic state until reactivation occurs. The nerve root changes consist of necrotization and sometimes cyst formation. A decrease in *cellular immunity* may allow the latent virus to reactivate and spread along the nerve, resulting in clinical zoster. Helper T cells and several lymphokines produced by other T-cell subsets usually protect the host from reactivation. The disorder occurs with increased frequency among immunocompromised patients and the elderly, probably as a consequence of defects in cellular immunity. Humoral immunity does not appear to be an important factor; even severely infected patients show significantly elevated antibody titers to zoster, and fewer than 5 percent of persons born in the United States do not possess varicella antibody. It has been suggested that every person who has had chickenpox harbors latent virus, that 50 percent of all people who live to the age of 85 will have an attack of zoster, and that approximately 10 percent will have at least two attacks. Occasional outbreaks may result from trauma to a nerve in which the virus is latent.

There is no evidence of an increased *risk of latent cancer* in those with herpes zoster. Relative cancer risk is only 1.1 times that of the general population, although there is a tenuous suggestion of a somewhat higher than average risk of colon cancer. The *risk of transmission* is low despite the fact that zoster skin lesions contain large amounts of virus. However, immunosuppressed patients and those who have never had chickenpox are at risk from patients with zoster. Reactivation on exposure to zoster has even been observed in a few patients with a previous history of chickenpox.

The clinical presentation is one of radicular pain followed by the appearance of tense, grouped vesicles on an erythematous base ("dew drops on a rose petal") in a dermatomal distribution. The pain too is dermatomal and may begin as an itch or tenderness that precedes the cutaneous lesion by 1 to 7 days. Patients describe burning, tingling, sharp knifelike pricking, or deep boring discomfort. More than half of patients have unilateral involvement of one or more of the thoracic dermatomes. The cranial dermatomes account for approximately 15 percent of cases, while cervical and lumbar dermatomes each account for approximately 10 percent. Vesicles on the tip of the nose were thought to indicate nasociliary involvement (putting the eye at risk), but a recent review of ophthalmic zoster does not confirm the validity of this clinical saw.

The cutaneous eruption becomes pustular within a few days, followed by crusting and healing over the course of 14 to 21 days. The crust is often dark, almost black. Scarring and atrophy can occur if the lesions are deep.

Malaise, low-grade fever, and adenopathy accompany severe eruptions. The total course is related to the time of new vesicle development: several days of vesicles usually means a 2- to 4-week course, whereas vesicles that persist over a week predict a longer course.

About one in eight patients experiences at least one complication. Major complications include postherpetic neuralgia, uveitis, motor deficits, infection, and systemic involvement such as meningoencephalitis, pneumonia, deafness, or dissemination. *Post-herpetic neuralgia* occurs most frequently in patients older than age 50. The pain is often excruciating and does not respond well to conventional methods of pain control.

The presence of more than 10 lesions outside a single dermatome of distribution is early evidence of *dissemination*. Acquired immunodeficiency syndrome (AIDS) patients may have VZV infections as part of the AIDS-related complex. In most cases, it presents as typical dermatomal illness; occasionally, it is disseminated and can be complicated by hepatitis, pneumonia, meningitis, or proctitis. In immunocompromised hosts, VZV and herpes simplex infections may present in similar and atypical fashion, sometimes without vesicles, or in unusual distributions.

DIAGNOSIS

Diagnosis is generally not difficult if the characteristic dermatomal rash and pain are present. The most serious diagnostic problem occurs during the prodromal days when patients present with a pain syndrome. Periorbital headache, unexplained back pain, or chest wall pain may represent the prodromal period of herpes zoster. Prodromal zoster pain has been mistaken for myocardial infarction, cholecystitis, and appendicitis. The characteristic eruption may not appear until 2 to 5 days later.

In patients with the characteristic rash, a positive *Tzanck preparation* demonstrating *multinucleated giant cells* provides strong supportive evidence of zoster. Tzanck prep has proven superior to viral isolation for obtaining positive results in early lesions. Culture, though slow to report, allows for confirmation. The diagnosis may also be confirmed by demonstrating *rising antibody titer*, which requires two separate determinations, or by immunofluorescence. More rapid diagnosis is afforded by use of *polymerase chain reaction (PCR) assays*, which detects VZV DNA sequences. Herpes zoster can also be recognized by host T-cell recognition of an immediate early integument protein (IE62) or glycoprotein I of VZV. Such rapid molecular diagnostic assays are expensive and best reserved for prompt diagnosis of severely ill persons who present acutely but nonspecifically (eg, the person with meningeal infection).

PRINCIPLES OF THERAPY

The goals of therapy are to dry the vesicles, relieve pain, and prevent secondary infection and complications. Lesions are kept clean and dry by the application of a wet-to-dry compress soaked with *Burow's solution* three to four times a day. If purulence or erythema suggesting secondary infection develops, antibiotics are indicated. There are no data to support the use of prophylactic antibiotics.

Relief of Discomfort. Pain relief can usually be achieved with a mild analgesic such as *aspirin* or *acetaminophen*, but one should not hesitate to use *codeine* if need be. The pain of thoracic zoster may be reduced by splinting the affected area with a *tight wrap*. Trunk lesions are covered with a nonadherent dressing, and then the area is wrapped with an elastic bandage. Malaise reflects viremia and should be treated with rest. Severe local pain can be ameliorated with *intralesional* injections of *triamcinolone,* 2 mg/mL in lidocaine. There is little evidence to suggest that pain or the rate of healing can be ameliorated by use of *systemic corticosteroids*; however, such treatment may reduce the incidence of post-herpetic neuralgia (see below). Pruritus may be relieved by oral *antihistamines* (see Chapter 178) or by *calamine lotion*, which both reduces itching and dries the rash.

Topical therapies have been studied. *Topical capsaicin* has been tried, but with only minimal success. Investigational use of topically applied aspirin and diethyl ether shows promising results.

Shortening Clinical Course and Reducing Risk of Complications. Use of the antiviral agent *acyclovir* can shorten the course of VZV infection and reduce the incidence of postherpetic neuralgia. Therapy must begin early in the syndrome. Because VZV is much more resistant to acyclovir than herpes simplex virus is, double-dose therapy is required (800 mg qid for 10 d). There is growing acceptance of acyclovir treatment in adults who develop zoster. A 6-deoxy prodrug of acyclovir is under development and may prove more efficacious.

The severity of post-herpetic neuralgia pain, its refractoriness to treatment, and reports of responsiveness to early use of *systemic glucocorticosteroids* have stimulated prescribing of steroids prophylactically, particularly in patients older than age 50. Data on efficacy are limited but suggest that early therapy with high doses for a short period can both shorten the duration of pain and prevent its chronicity. Therapy typically begins during the acute phase of illness with 60 to 80 mg/day of prednisone taken orally with food or antacid and tapered over 7 to 10 days.

Several varicella *vaccines* have completed trials and should soon be available for adults who have not had chickenpox and for those at high risk for reactivation. It is hoped that the vaccine will stimulate T-cell subsets and cytotoxic T killer cells and make reactivation less likely. In studies of immunosuppressed persons, *interferon* and *vidarabine* have proven to be promising.

Treatment of Post-herpetic Neuralgia. Nonnarcotic methods such as *antidepressants*, transcutaneous *nerve stimulation*, and the anticonvulsive drug *carbamazepine* have also been used with some efficacy. Success has also been reported with repeated *triamcinolone* injections into symptomatic areas or as a sympathetic ganglion block. Other clinicians have found that *chlorprothixene* (Taractan) in doses of 25 to 50 mg or *Triavil* four times per day reduces pain. Recent work has suggested possible roles for L-*dopa* and *cimetidine* in the management of post-herpetic neuralgia. Adenosine monophosphate injections into the area of pain were dramatic in one study.

INDICATIONS FOR REFERRAL

If there is any suggestion of compromise of vision or other *ocular involvement*, prompt ophthalmologic consultation for herpetic eye care is essential to avoid scarring and permanent visual impairment. *Otic* involvement can lead to severe pain and otic nerve damage, making referral to an ear, nose, and throat specialist important. The patient with herpetic skin lesions and signs of meningeal irritation requires prompt hospitalization.

ANNOTATED BIBLIOGRAPHY

Balfour HH Jr. Acyclovir therapy for herpes zoster: advantages and adverse effects. JAMA 1986;255:387. *(An editorial position on using acyclovir for zoster.)*

Crooks RJ, Jones DA, Fiddian AP. Zoster-associated chronic pain: an overview of clinical trials with acyclovir. Scand J Infect Dis Suppl 1991;80:62. *(Evidence is suggestive of benefit.)*

Eaglestein WH, Katz R, Brown JS. The effects of early corticosteroid therapy on the skin eruption and pain of herpes zoster. JAMA 1970;211:1681. *(The duration of post-herpetic neuralgia was decreased by oral triamcinolone therapy begun early in the disease course.)*

Gershon AA, LaRussa P, Hardy I, et al. Varicella vaccine: the American experience. J Infect Dis 1992;166(Suppl 1):S63. *(Use of varicella vaccines in healthy and immunocompromised hosts.)*

Liesegang TJ. The varicella-zoster virus: systemic and ocular features. J Am Acad Dermatol 1984;11:165. *(A superb review with emphasis on ophthalmic disease.)*

Ragozzino MW, Melton LJ, Kurland LT, et al. Risk of cancer after herpes zoster. N Engl J Med 1982;307:393. *(No increased risk found.)*

Sklar SH, Blue WH, Alexander EJ, et al. Herpes-zoster. The treatment and prevention of neuralgia with adenosine monophosphate. JAMA 1985;253:1427. *(Encouraging results found for both acute zoster and postherpetic neuralgia; many side effects, however.)*

Solomon AR, Rasmussen JE, Weiss JS. A comparison of the Tzanck smear and viral isolation in varicella-herpes zoster. Arch Dermatol 1986;122:282. *(Tzanck prep was superior to viral isolations in obtaining positive results in early lesion.)*

Taub A. Relief of post-herpetic neuralgia with psychotropic drugs. J Neurosurg 1973;39:235. *(Guidance for treatment of the difficult problem.)*

Weller TH. Varicella and herpes zoster. N Engl J Med 1983; 309:1362,1434. *(A two-part review, best for epidemiology and natural history.)*

Whitley RJ. Therapeutic approaches to varicella-zoster virus infections. J Infect Dis 1992;166(Suppl 1):S51. *(Review of therapeutic options in treating the presentations of varicella-zoster infections.)*

194
Management of Warts

WILLIAM V. R. SHELLOW, M.D.

Primary Care Medicine: Office Evaluation and Management of the Adult Patient, 3rd edition, edited by Allan H. Goroll, Lawrence A. May, and Albert G. Mulley, Jr. J.B. Lippincott Company, Philadelphia

Warts result from skin infection with human papillomavirus (HPV). Though a relatively harmless affliction, warts can be cosmetically bothersome and occasionally a source of pain. The primary care physician should be able to distinguish warts from other skin tumors, select effective treatment, and educate the patient in proper self-care and prevention.

PATHOPHYSIOLOGY, CLINICAL PRESENTATION, AND COURSE

HPV is a DNA virus, with more than 60 types identified. It is epitheliotropic and causes tumors of the epidermis. At least five types are potentially oncogenic, with two implicated in cervical carcinoma (see Chapter 107) and three in squamous cell carcinoma (see Chapter 177). Warts can be transmitted by direct contact or by autoinoculation. Young people have a high frequency of warts. Healing can occur spontaneously, presumably through immunologic mechanisms. Approximately two-thirds of warts disappear spontaneously within 2 years of their appearance, but if they are left untreated, additional warts may develop from the original ones.

Clinical presentations vary according to site and viral strain involved. The *common wart (verruca vulgaris)* is associated with HPV-2 and HPV-4 infection and appears flesh-colored or grayish white with a papillated hyperkeratotic surface. It may be punctuated with black dots due to thrombosis of superficial capillaries, which are present in large numbers. It may be seen anywhere but commonly affects the elbows, knees, fingers, and palms. Filiform warts are more delicate and threadlike. *Flat warts (verruca plana)*, caused by HPV-3, are smaller than common warts and have a smoother surface. Great numbers of them may appear on the hand, on the beard area, and on the shaved legs of women.

The *plantar wart (verruca plantaris)* results from HPV-1 or HPV-4 infection of the plantar surface of the foot and appears as a small skin nodule that produces grayish or yellow interruptions in the skin lines of the foot. It is less elevated than other warts because weight bearing presses it inward. These warts may be solitary, multiple, or confluent; if confluent, the term "mosaic wart" is used.

Anogenital warts (condylomata acuminata) result from sexual transmission of HPV-6 and HPV-16 and grow on mucous membranes. They range in size from pinpoint to cauliflower-like. Coexistent venereal disease is common. Mucocutaneous warts may become refractory despite appropriate therapy.

Most warts are asymptomatic; however, plantar warts may be the source of considerable foot pain, acting as a foreign body during weight bearing. Anogenital warts may become friable, bleed, and cause discomfort. Periungual lesions may become fissured.

DIFFERENTIAL DIAGNOSIS

Verrucae vulgaris should be differentiated from *squamous cell carcinoma* and also from a *cutaneous horn* arising from an actinic keratosis (see Chapter 177). Multiple verrucae planae on the face should be differentiated from trichoepitheliomas, syringomas, and the cutaneous lesions of sarcoidosis. Anogenital warts must be differentiated from the *condylomata lata* of syphilis and *squamous cell carcinoma*. Bowenoid papulosis (associated with HPV-16) appears as wartlike lesions on the male and female genitalia and is a form of carcinoma in situ; it has little biologic tendency to become malignant.

WORKUP

Appearance is usually sufficient for diagnosis, but early genital warts can be difficult to identify. Typically, a patient comes for evaluation because warts have been found in a sexual partner. In the male, the penis and upper portion of the scrotum should be carefully examined under magnification. If there are no visible lesions, acetic acid can be used. Soaking the penis with a gauze moistened with 5% acetic acid (vinegar) for 5 minutes demonstrates early lesions not readily evident under hand lens magnification, but magnification alone usually suffices. For the gynecologic examination, there is no better way to demonstrate early verrucae than to make them white with acetic acid. The colposcope provides still higher magnification. In using acetic acid, one must remember that it is a very nonspecific test: any disease or lesion that alters the stratum corneum will test acetowhite.

PRINCIPLES OF MANAGEMENT

Not all warts need to be removed. The primary care physician should observe the basic principle that warts are benign tumors that often regress spontaneously. Treatment should not be so aggressive as to produce permanent scarring. Simple and safe treatments should be employed.

Location, discomfort, cosmetic effect, and therapies available influence the decision to treat. Larger warts of long duration and those involving the plantar, perianal, or periungual area are the most difficult to treat but among those patients most desire to have removed. The patient's occupation, skin pigmentation, and body area should be considered when designing therapy. The goal is to destroy the epidermal tumor while minimizing damage to the underlying dermis. The greater the dermal injury, the greater is the risk of scar formation. Only minimal scarring should be expected or considered acceptable.

A host of measures are available; choice is based on efficacy, patient acceptability, and scarring potential of the therapy as well as on location, size, and type of lesion. Physicians will most likely be seeing a self-selected group of patients for whom over-the-counter remedies have failed.

Common Warts. Freezing the lesion with cotton-swab application of *liquid nitrogen* is convenient, well tolerated, often effective, and associated with a low risk of serious scarring. Solid freezing of the lesion is usually achieved by 5 to 10 minutes of repeated application of the liquid nitrogen from a cotton swab dipped into a Styrofoam cup containing the supercold liquid. The freezing injury leads to the wart's separating from the underlying dermis. The successfully treated wart will fall off within 2 weeks. Before freezing, the thickened keratin should be pared off, but care should be taken not to cut into the profuse collection of capillaries within the wart. It is best to freeze a few millimeters of the surrounding normal tissue to facilitate separation from the underlying dermis. The patient should be warned that the area may hurt for several hours after treatment, and occasionally hemorrhagic blistering develops, especially with vigorous treatment. If not completely gone, the wart can be retreated within 2 to 3 weeks. In difficult areas or on large lesions, several treatments may be necessary. Liquid nitrogen has the advantage of being quick, bloodless, and not too painful, but the liquefied gas evaporates quickly and requires storage in special containers. Commercial kits generating sticks of "dry ice" from compressed carbon dioxide gas are available, but because the sticks are not as cold as liquid nitrogen, they are not as effective and require more pressure and a longer duration of application.

Curettage with or without *electrodesiccation* is effective but time consuming, and substantial scarring can result if treatment is too vigorous. *Chemical cautery* with *nitric acid* or *mono-, bi-,* or *trichloroacetic acid* is an older alternative to liquid nitrogen.

Plantar Warts. Nonsurgical methods are preferred to surgical removal because scarring in this location can cause permanent discomfort. The lesion should be pared and then treated with application of 40% *salicylic acid plasters*, taped in place for 1 to 3 days, followed by scraping off of the macerated skin. This procedure is used for 2 to 3 weeks and can be performed by the patient. A salicylic acid preparation suspended in a karaya gum that promotes absorption (Trans-Ver-Sal) is a convenient way to apply the medication. The pad containing the suspension is cut to size after the wart is pared down with an emery board. A drop of water is placed on the wart and the pad is applied and left in place for 8 hours each day. A larger salicylic acid patch (Trans Plantar) is indicated for treating large plantar warts. The convenience of this method is offset by the expense, but it is appreciated by some patients. *Liquid nitrogen* can be used on plantar warts in nonweight-bearing areas.

Daily 10% *formalin* or 25% *glutaraldehyde compresses* are sometimes used for mosaic plantar warts. Occlusal-HP is a prescription salicylic acid–lactic acid combination that contains salicylic acid in a polyacrylic vehicle. It is quite effective for plantar warts but has also been used successfully for verrucae on the hands.

Flat Warts. Topical *5-fluorouracil* cream or solution and *retinoic acid* cream or gel are used effectively for flat warts, especially those on the face. With both of these topical agents, patients will probably experience irritation characterized by erythema, scaling, and burning. Patients must be counseled that irritation will occur. Men should switch to an electric razor if they are using a blade razor, as cutting facial warts spreads them throughout the beard area. Similarly, women with flat warts on their legs must switch to an electric razor or use depilatory creams. Alternatively, 6% salicylic acid gel (Keralyt) is sometimes effective in treating multiple flat warts on the legs.

Genital Warts. A preparation of 20% to 40% *podophyllin* in compound tincture of benzoin is used to treat *macerated genital warts*. It must be applied sparingly, only to the wart, and allowed to dry thoroughly before the patient dresses. The medication is washed off by the patient 1 to 4 hours after application. Repeat treatment is the rule. Podophyllin is contraindicated in pregnancy. *Podofilox* 0.2% (Condylox) is available for the treatment of external genital warts in both men and women. It is a purified fraction of podophyllin resins and is the first prescription product for treatment of warts safe for self-application at home. It is applied for 3 consecutive days, followed by 4 days of no treatment, and repeated if the warts persist.

The *carbon dioxide laser* is quite useful in destroying large numbers of verrucae in the vagina or around the anus. The procedure is carried out in an operating-room environment. The postoperative morbidity is much less than when conventional methods are used.

As noted earlier, evaluation for concurrent venereal disease is mandatory in patients presenting with genital warts (see Chapters 125 and 126).

Refractory Warts. Sublesional *bleomycin*, diluted to 10 U/mL, has a distinct role in the treatment of refractory warts, both those on the hands and the plantar variety. Usually one or two units injected beneath the verruca is sufficient. Blanching occurs immediately, followed by blackening of the wart with subsequent clean sloughing. It is less painful than liquid nitrogen for the most part, and there are no systemic effects.

Interferon-alpha (both type 2a and type 2b) has been approved for treatment of refractory genital warts. Lesions are injected intralesionally three times a week for 3 weeks. Fewer than 50 percent of patients show clearance of lesions, and it has the disadvantage of being both painful and expensive.

Immunostimulation is sometimes tried. *Dinitrochlorobenzene* (DNCB) sensitization followed by repeated applications of diluted DNCB has been used to treat resistant warts. This form of immunotherapy is sometimes effective, but DNCB has been shown to be a potential carcinogen in some studies. Autogenous wart *vaccines* appear no more effective than placebos.

The *carbon dioxide laser* has become an increasingly popular method for treating warts, although in many instances it is little more than an expensive method of causing tissue destruction. It is best reserved for specialized situations such as extensive vaginal or anal warts or refractory periungual lesions.

PATIENT EDUCATION

Prevention entails avoiding others with warts and removing warts from the patient so that the viral reservoir is reduced. Although warts may initially have come from contact with others, biting and picking at warts may result in additional lesions. Patients with periungual warts should be cautioned that biting the warts or pulling hangnails may result in the spread of lesions. Patients with genital warts can be reassured that not everyone develops warts on exposure, but condom use should be urged.

Treatment of warts can be both time consuming and expensive. Recurrences are seen in about one-third of instances. The patient must be made to understand that warts are caused by a virus and that treatment usually does not eliminate the virus. Nonetheless, reassurance can be given that in most instances the immune system will eventually prevent HPV from causing warts despite the continued presence of the virus. The length of treatment, cost, discomfort, risk of scarring, and possible failure of therapy should be candidly discussed before treatment is initiated.

INDICATIONS FOR REFERRAL

A Papanicolaou (Pap) smear showing cervical dysplasia and evidence of HPV requires referral to a gynecologist for consideration of cervical biopsy. Women with extensive involvement by vaginal warts are also candidates for gynecologic consultation and possible laser therapy. Patients with truly refractory lesions who still insist on their removal may benefit from a dermatologic or surgical consultation. If topical treatment proves ineffective, electrocoagulation or surgical excision deserves consideration. Excision of large venereal warts that do not respond to podophyllin is indicated to rule out malignancy.

THERAPEUTIC RECOMMENDATIONS

- Use liquid nitrogen for initial treatment of common warts. Apply with a cotton swab to an area that includes a small rim of surrounding skin.
- Treat plantar warts by first paring them down carefully with a scalpel and then applying a piece of 40% salicylic acid plaster cut to the shape of, but slightly smaller than, the wart. Cover with occlusive adhesive tape and leave in place for 24 to 72 hours. Continue treatment at home, with gentle paring and reapplication of salicylic acid plaster as needed. Check progress regularly.
- Treat flat warts with topical 5-fluorouracil, retinoic acid, or Keralyt, a 6% salicylic acid gel.
- Treat moist anogenital warts with topical podophyllin; remind the patient to remove the medication after 4 to 6 hours. Consider topical podofilox for patient administration at home if repeated treatment is needed.
- If these topical treatments prove ineffective or if the patient has extensive anal or genital involvement, then refer for consultation and consideration of more aggressive therapy.

ANNOTATED BIBLIOGRAPHY

Bart BJ, Biglow J, Vance JC, et al. Salicylic acid in karaya gum patch as treatment for verruca vulgaris. J Am Acad Dermatol 1989;20:74. *(A 69 percent cure rate achieved.)*

Carne CA, Dockerty G. Genital warts: need to screen for coinfection. BMJ 1990;300:459. *(High percentage of coexisting venereal disease.)*

Cobb MW. Human papillomavirus infection. J Am Acad Dermatol 1990;22:547. *(Comprehensive review covering virology, epidemiology, pathogenesis, immunology, clinical manifestations, and treatment; 138 refs.)*

Crum CP, et al. Human papilloma virus type 16 and early cervical neoplasia. N Engl J Med 1984;310:880. *(Association of type 16 subtype of papilloma virus with cervical neoplasia.)*

Kirby P, Dunne A, King, DH, et al. Double-blind randomized clinical trial of self-administered podofilox solution versus vehicle in the treatment of genital warts. Am J Med 1990;88:465. *(Very effective and safe when applied by patients themselves.)*

Ling MR. Therapy of genital human papillomavirus infections. Int J Dermatol 1992;31:682,769. *(Excellent two-part review, including rationale and methods for treatment; 96 refs.)*

Massing AM, Epstein WL. Natural history of warts. Arch Dermatol 1963;87:306. *(One thousand children observed for 2 years; without treatment there was a net increase.)*

Parish LC, Monroe E, Rex IH Jr. Treatment of common warts with high-potency (26%) salicylic acid. Clin Ther 1988;10:462. *(Eighty-one percent improved or cured after 2 weeks of treatment for warts on the hands.)*

Street ML, Roenigk RK. Recalcitrant periungual verrucae: the role of carbon dioxide laser vaporization. J Am Acad Dermatol 1990;23:115. *(Seventy-one percent cured after one or two treatments.)*

Primary Care Medicine: Office Evaluation and Management of the Adult Patient, 3rd edition, edited by Allan H. Goroll, Lawrence A. May, and Albert G. Mulley, Jr. J.B. Lippincott Company, Philadelphia

195
Management of Scabies and Pediculosis

STEPHEN J. FRIEDMAN, M.D.
WILLIAM V. R. SHELLOW, M.D.

Parasitic diseases of the skin include scabies and lice. Although accurate diagnosis, effective and safe treatment, and preventive measures are available, infestations with scabies and lice have been pandemic, affecting millions of people worldwide. The primary physician must quickly recognize the various manifestations of ectoparasitic infestation and treat them effectively.

PATHOPHYSIOLOGY, CLINICAL PRESENTATION, AND DIAGNOSIS

Scabies

Scabies is caused by an infestation with the human skin mite, *Sarcoptes scabiei var hominis*. The condition is transmitted by close personal contact and affects all socioeconomic levels, both sexes, and all age groups. Inanimate objects (fomites) are unimportant in its transmission. Once contracted, scabies usually persists until specific therapy is instituted.

The scabies mite is 1/60 inch in length. The adult female attaches to skin and digs into the horny layer where it is thin. Copulation with a wandering male renders the female fertile for life. The female mite remains within her burrow for the rest of her 1-month life, laying two or three eggs a day. These eggs hatch within 3 to 4 days. Mature adults develop over the next 10 to 14 days. While in her burrow, the female chews on epidermal cells and feeds on liquid oozing from them. The average number of female mites on the body is 11.

A cardinal symptom is *nocturnal itching*. Itching also occurs when patients remove their clothing or become overheated. Eighty-five percent of infested individuals have *burrows* on the fingers, interdigital areas, and wrists. Other common sites are extensor aspects of the elbows, feet and ankles, penis and scrotum, buttocks, and axillae. Vigorous scratching may make the scabetic rash eczematous, crusted, excoriated, or secondarily infected.

In adults, infestation rarely extends above the neck, but in infants, young children, or the elderly, lesions may occur on the head and neck. Atypical (crusted or Norwegian) scabies may occur in patients with human immunodeficiency virus (HIV) infection. Failure to scratch or failure to develop hypersensitivity allows the mites to proliferate profusely. It is highly contagious because of the myriad of mites in the exfoliating scales.

The *rash* seen in patients does not necessarily correspond to places where the mite is found. The itch and eruption reflect sensitization to the organism or scybala (fecal droppings). In patients who have never been infested, the pruritic rash develops after 2 to 4 weeks. The initial phase of infestation is asymptomatic. Treatment kills the mite and ova but does not remove the sensitizing material from the burrow. Pruritus may continue for a few weeks after treatment, until the contents of the burrow are shed with the natural turnover of skin. Persistent post-scabetic papules may occur, especially on the penis, which may require intralesional injection of corticosteroids.

Pediculosis

Human lice are wingless, dorsoventrally flattened, bloodsucking insects of two types: *Pediculus humanus*, which infests the head and body, and *Phthirus pubis*, which infests the pubic area. These are elongated insects, 3 to 4 mm in length, which are transmitted by contact with infested clothing, combs, or bedding. Body lice are most common in people with poor personal hygiene or in indigent populations. Vertical excoriations on the trunk are characteristic. The adult louse lives and lays eggs in clothing, often in the seams, and travels onto the skin for a blood meal. The head louse typically infests the occipital portion of the scalp and sometimes the postauricular region. Although there are few adults, there are many oval eggs (nits) cemented to the hair. Head lice are a public health problem among school children.

Pediculosis pubis is usually a sexually transmitted infestation caused by the crab louse. This organism has a more rounded body, 3 to 4 mm in length, with the second and third pairs of legs serving as claws that clasp hairs tightly. The nits hatch and evolve into adults within 2 or 3 weeks. Lice live for about a month, requiring blood meals to survive. Without blood meals, they die within a few days. They affect primarily the pubic hairs; however, eyelashes, axillary, chest, and thigh hairs can be involved. Itching is the cardinal symptom, caused by the lice injecting saliva, digestive juices, and feces into the skin.

DIAGNOSIS

Scabies

The diagnosis is suggested by finding topical grayish-white burrows, 1 to 2 mm long, perhaps with a black speck (the mite) at the end. Burrows should be sought on hand, wrist, ankle, and genital areas, where the recovery rate is highest. The roof of the burrow is shaved off with a scalpel, and the base is scraped to remove its contents. The material is placed on a microscope slide, and a drop of light mineral oil and a cover slip are added. In mineral oil, but not in potassium hydroxide, movement of the mite is seen. The lowest power objective should be used. The presence of adult mites, immature mites, ova, or tan–brown scybala confirms the diagnosis. Presumptive diagnosis can be made based on the symptoms, the appearance of the rash, and the history of contacts who are also itching.

Few adult lice are found at the bases of the hair, but many nits are typically seen. Often the patient's underwear is speckled with blood. Characteristic asymptomatic, macular, blue discolorations called maculae ceruleae are sometimes seen on the trunk and thighs.

Pediculosis

Diagnosis is made by direct examination of the involved area and finding egg cases (nits) and active forms of the organism. They are usually visible to the naked eye, but a hand lens and light may help. The examination should be done with gloves and other precautions to avoid infestation. Identification of head lice is facilitated by plucking a few hairs and identifying the full or empty egg cases about 7 to 10 mm up the hair shaft. Organisms may be found in the nape of the neck and behind the ears. Pyoderma of the nape or the occiput requires that pediculosis capitis be ruled out. Vertical excoriations on the trunk are a cardinal sign of body lice.

PRINCIPLES OF MANAGEMENT AND PATIENT EDUCATION

Relief of itching and elimination of the infestation are the goals of treatment.

Scabies

Because infection is person-to-person, close contacts of a scabies patient should be treated even if free of symptoms. Treatment kills the mite and ova but does not remove the sensitizing material from the burrow. Pruritus may continue for a few weeks after treatment, until the contents of the burrow are shed with the natural turnover of skin. During this time, it may be necessary to use topical corticosteroids and oral antihistamines to help control the rash and pruritus. Occasionally, systemic steroids are required (see Chapter 105).

Permethrin 5% cream is currently the first-line medication for scabies. It is a combination of synthetic pyrethroids and has low mammalian toxicity because of minimal absorption and quick reduction to inactive metabolites. *Lindane* 1% (gamma benzene hexachloride—Qwell) lotion had been the agent of choice for the treatment of scabies. Because of reports of organism resistance and neurotoxicity in infants and persons with a extensively compromised epidermal barrier, lindane has been relegated to alternative treatment status. It also can induce a mild, dry, irritant dermatitis.

Crotamiton 10% lotion is antipruritic but is usually less successful as a scabicide than lindane. The cure rate after five consecutive days of therapy is only about 55 percent. Precipitated *sulfur* ointment, 5% to 10%, has been recommended occasionally for treatment in young children. However, sulfur causes staining, is absorbed from the skin, and has an unpleasant odor. *Malathion lotion* 0.5% is one of the least toxic organophosphorus insecticides available. It inhibits cholinesterase in insects but is rapidly detoxified in humans and vertebrates. Two topical applications may be required 1 or 2 weeks apart.

To prevent reinfestation, bed linens and underwear of all household members should be washed thoroughly in hot water with detergent or dry cleaned. Treatment of scabies is generally effective, provided all close contacts are treated simultaneously.

Pediculosis

Permethrin 1% cream rinse shampoo is the treatment of choice for pediculosis. Less than 2 percent is absorbed, and the drug is quickly reduced to inactive metabolites. The 1% preparation is effective for treatment of pediculosis capitis. Over-the-counter shampoos for pediculosis contain natural pyrethrins and piperonyl butoxide (synergized pyrethrins). They derive from chrysanthemum flowers and are approved for use in pediculosis capitis and pubis. The synergized pyrethrins have a wide safety margin because they are minimally absorbed through the skin.

Lindane shampoo has long been in use and is regarded by many to be safe and effective if used properly. The potential for neurotoxicity has led to more stringent Food and Drug Administration guidelines concerning the treatment of infants, children, and pregnant women with lindane. *Malathion lotion* 0.5% is pediculocidal and ovicidal. The lotion has a potentially drying effect on hair and has an unpleasant odor.

Eyelash involvement may be treated with nonirritating, nontoxic *petrolatum*. The lice either suffocate or slip off the greased hairs.

To prevent reinfestation, asymptomatic close contacts should be treated simultaneously. Bedsheets and all clothing worn in the past 3 days should be laundered in hot soapy water or dry cleaned. Brushes and combs should be washed in hot water for 10 to 20 minutes. Floors, furniture, and play areas should be thoroughly vacuumed to remove hairs that may have been shed with viable eggs attached.

On occasion, there may be secondary bacterial infection, which can be treated with topical mupirocin 2% ointment applied three times daily or by appropriate oral antibiotics.

PATIENT EDUCATION

Patient education is essential. Treatment failure is usually the result of poor patient compliance. Written instructions are helpful. Preventive measures are very important to review.

THERAPEUTIC RECOMMENDATIONS

Scabies

- Prescribe 5% permethrin cream, applied from the neck down (including all body folds and creases) and left on overnight for 8 to 12 hours. About 30 g is sufficient for the average adult. One treatment is usually adequate.
- Advise changing and cleaning of underwear and bed linen.
- Treat all household members.
- Only if reinfestation has occurred should a second course of treatment be necessary.
- Prescribe topical corticosteroids and oral antihistamines if rash and pruritus are bothersome; if severe, oral steroids can be considered.

Pediculosis

- Have the patient routinely shampoo without medication, followed by application of sufficient permethrin 1% cream rinse to thoroughly wet the hair. It is left on for 10 minutes and then rinsed out.
- Alternatively, recommend synergized pyrethrins shampoo, applied undiluted until the infested areas are entirely wet. After 10 minutes, the areas are washed thoroughly with warm water and then dried. Because it is less effective as an ovicide, this treatment should be repeated in 7 to 10 days to kill any newly hatched lice.
- Remove nits from the hair shaft to reduce the chance of reinfestation.
- Advise drying the hair after treatment with a pediculocide, using a clean towel and removing any remaining nits with a fine-toothed comb.
- Treat eyelash involvement with petrolatum jelly up to five times a day for 5 to 7 days. Alternately, recommend physostigmine ophthalmic ointment 0.25%, applied to the lashes four times daily for three consecutive days.

ANNOTATED BIBLIOGRAPHY

Burkhart CG. Scabies: an epidemiologic reassessment. Ann Intern Med 1983;98:498. *(Reviews epidemiology, clinical manifestations, treatment, and prevention.)*

Friedman SJ. Lindane neurotoxic reaction in nonbullous congenital ichthyosiform erythroderma. Arch Dermatol 1987;124: 638. *(Neurotoxicity noted in patients with extensive rashes that compromise epidermal barrier function.)*

Meinking T, Taplin D, Kalter DC, et al. Comparative efficacy of treatment for pediculosis capitis infestations. Arch Dermatol 1986;122:267. *(Evaluates various treatments for pediculosis and questions widespread use of lindane.)*

Purvis RS, Tyring SK. An outbreak of lindane-resistant scabies treated successfully with permethrin 5% cream. J Am Acad Dermatol 1991;25:1015. *(Lindane-resistant scabies cured by a single treatment with permethrin.)*

Schultz MW, Gomez M, Hansen RC, et al. Comparative study of 5% permethrin cream and 1% lindane lotion for the treatment of scabies. Arch Dermatol 1990;126:167. *(Permethrin 5% cream and lindane 1% lotion were equally effective.)*

Taplin D, Meinking TL. Pyrethrins and pyrethroids in dermatology. Arch Dermatol 1990;126:213. *(Development of natural pyrethrins and synthetic pyrethroids.)*

Taplin D, Meinking TL, Chen JA, et al. Comparison of crotamiton 10% cream (Eurax) and permethrin 5% cream (Elimite) for the treatment of scabies in children. Pediatr Dermatol 1990;7:67. *(Low toxicity and high efficacy of permethrin in scabies therapy.)*

Primary Care Medicine: Office Evaluation and Management of the Adult Patient, 3rd edition, edited by Allan H. Goroll, Lawrence A. May, and Albert G. Mulley, Jr. J.B. Lippincott Company, Philadelphia © 1995

196
Management of Skin Trauma: Bites and Burns

Animal and Human Bites
ELLIE J. C. GOLDSTEIN, M.D.

Animal bites are common. Patients often present to the primary physician for advice and therapy. Patients may appear shortly after injury concerned about rabies, tetanus, or repair of a disfiguring tear. Sometimes they delay seeking care, only to present later with infection. The primary physician must provide first aid and tetanus prophylaxis, decide whether antibiotics are necessary, and estimate the risk of rabies. Human bites are less common but potentially more serious. Particularly treacherous are clenched-fist injuries which result from striking the teeth. Occlusional bites and paronychial infections may also result in infection.

PATHOPHYSIOLOGY AND CLINICAL PRESENTATIONS

Most bites are minor. It is estimated that about 80 percent of patients neither need nor seek medical care. Bite wounds that produce a break in the skin allow inoculation of bacteria that normally inhabit the skin or, more usually, the oral cavity. Once the protective barrier of the skin is compromised, conditions favoring infection have been established, especially if there is a crush injury or the bite involves the hand. The longer the wound is left unattended, the greater the risk of the patient's presenting with infection. Bites initially thought to be trivial may become infected hours or days later. Women who have undergone radical or modified mastectomy with resultant edema of the limb are at risk for more severe infections.

The most serious bite wounds are caused by *clenched-fist injuries*. Damage occurs when the tendons and other tissues of the exterior area of the finger are stretched to full length, the skin is broken, and the tendon and possibly the joint are exposed. As the fingers are straightened, the damaged parts relax, and infecting organisms are carried into the tissues, producing infection in wounds that may initially appear minor. If the joint capsule is penetrated, there is a risk of septic arthritis or osteomyelitis.

Bacteriology. In animal bites, the infecting organisms are usually the normal oral flora of the biting animal. *Pasteurella multocida* is present in 50 percent of animal oral cavities and in 20 percent of dog and 50 percent of cat bite wounds. Bites from animals who ingest feces may be infected with enteric organisms. Cat bites are more prone to infection than are dog bites and may lead to severe cellulitis. Cat-scratch disease is caused by *Afipia felis*, a fastidious gram-negative rod; it often presents with fever and lymphadenopathy and is more frequently seen in the cold weather months. Any patient with splenectomy or alcoholic liver disease is prone to sepsis with *Capnocytophaga canimorsus* (formerly DF-2).

The mouth flora of humans is more abundant than in most animals and includes *Streptococcus viridans, Hemophilus influenza, Eikenella corrodens, Bacteroides* species, anaerobic diphtheroids, fusobacteria, and spirochetes. Wounds may also be infected by *skin flora* such as a group A beta-streptococcus (*Streptococcus pyogenes*) or staphylococcus (*Staphylococcus aureus*). If anaerobic bacteria are present, the infection is more severe and may lead to abscess formation. Human bites are responsible for most severe bite wound infections because of the heavy bacterial inoculum.

PRINCIPLES OF THERAPY

Principles of therapy include characterization of the injury, vigorous cleansing, tetanus prophylaxis, and appropriate antibiotics.

Animal Bites

It is important to elicit a history of the circumstances surrounding the injury. If an animal bite occurred, the type of animal and the animal's behavior need to be detailed, as well as whether the animal had been vaccinated and whether the attack was provoked or unprovoked. The wound should be diagrammed in the chart, noting proximity to bones or joints. Minor animal puncture wounds should be cleansed with *soap and water* and treated expectantly without antibiotics. Copious *irrigation* of wounds with normal saline is an important therapeutic adjunct. Animal puncture wounds that are small and clean require no other treatment.

Rabies. Since 1967, there have been only one or two cases of rabies in humans each year in the United States. There have been no cases of rabies in New York City or Los Angeles for many years. In 1990, 4826 animals in the United States were reported to have rabies. Two recent outbreaks of raccoon rabies occurred in the mid-Atlantic states and the southeastern states. In most other states, skunks and bats are the most common rabid animals. Rabies is more prevalent in cats than in dogs in the United States. Rabies is a concern if the attack is unprovoked, occurs in a rural setting, or involves a raccoon, a bat, a skunk, or an animal that is behaving in a peculiar manner. The local health department provides data regarding the local incidence of rabies and should be notified for follow-up and statistical reasons. If rabies is considered a possibility, *human diploid cell vaccine* should be given along with *rabies immune globulin* without delay (see Chapter 6 and Table 6–4). If a person is bitten by a pet, the animal should be watched at home by the owner for 2 weeks and reported to the local health department.

Tetanus. It is important to determine if the patient has had an initial series of tetanus shots and a booster within the past 5 years. Those who have not had an initial series should be given both *tetanus toxoid* and *tetanus immune globulin* (see Chapter 6). In those who have had the initial series but no booster in 5 years, 0.5 mL of *tetanus toxoid* should be administered intramuscularly.

Tear Wounds. Therapy for tear wounds is problematic. There have been no controlled trials of closure versus nonclosure, with or without antibiotics. The principles of therapy are to cleanse and debride the wound. After the wound is left open for 24 hours, the edges can be approximated with Steri-strips or sutured, and *phenoxymethyl penicillin*, 250 to 500 mg four times a day, is given for 3 to 5 days. Secondary closures may be done if it is apparent that no infection is present. Facial wounds may be closed and antibiotics given. It is useful to refer these patients to a plastic surgeon.

Infected Wounds. Patients who present after 24 hours with infection should receive debridement, drainage, cleansing, delayed closure of the wound, and antibiotics. *Penicillin* is the drug of choice because it is effective against *P. multocida,* some staphylococci, streptococci, anaerobes, and *E. corrodens*. In penicillin-allergic patients, *doxycycline* is preferred, because *P. multocida* is often resistant to erythromycin and cephalexin. *Amoxicillin/clavulanic acid* (Augmentin) is an effective but more expensive alternative. Only anecdotal clinical data exist regarding the use of quinolones or oral second generation cephalosporins for animal bites.

Human Bites

Human bites are usually located on an extremity. Wounds of the hand are the most serious. The same principles of cleansing, drainage, and debridement apply. Human bites should not be closed primarily, though edges may be approximated if the tear is severe. Antibiotics should be instituted after wound cultures are taken. *Penicillin* plus a *penicillinase-resistant penicillin* or *amoxicillin/clavulanic acid* should be administered pending culture results to cover beta-lactamase–producing oral anaerobes and gram-positive cocci, particularly *S. aureus*. Infrequently, a gram-negative organism may be present, necessitating a change in antibiotic regimen. *Tetanus toxoid* 0.5 mL should be administered to all those previously immunized who have not had a booster in 5 years. Follow-up is essential because of the potential of late serious infection.

Clenched-Fist Injuries. These usually require specialized care. Radiographs should be taken to rule out fractures and to provide a baseline for future assessment of osteomyelitis. Extension and flexion of digits should be carefully checked and sensation tested. The third metacarpophalangeal joint is most often affected. The integrity of the joint capsule must be determined, and this may require an experienced surgeon. If the capsule is intact, the hand is cleaned, debrided, immobilized, and elevated. *Penicillin* plus a *penicillinase-resistant penicillin* or *ampicillin/sulbactam* or *cefoxitin* are started and *tetanus toxoid* administered. Patients seen within 8 hours of injury with intact joint capsules may be managed as outpatients with careful follow-up. Those with torn capsules need to be admitted for surgery and treatment with intravenous antibiotics. Patients who present after 8 hours should be admitted for observation whether the capsule is intact or interrupted.

THERAPEUTIC RECOMMENDATIONS AND PATIENT EDUCATION

- Clean all wounds vigorously with soap and water. Copiously irrigate with normal saline. A needle and syringe may be used to generate a high pressure jet to cleanse puncture wounds.
- Immunize against tetanus with 0.5 mL of tetanus toxoid intramuscularly in those who have previously been immunized but have not had a booster in the past 5 years.

Animal Bites

- Animal puncture wounds that are trivial and clean, without crush injury, and do not involve the hand, require no other treatment.
- Treat moderate or severe fresh, uninfected animal tear wounds with cleansing, debridement, and phenoxymethyl penicillin (250 mg qid), followed by secondary closure in 24 to 48 hours if there are no signs of infection.
- Treat infected animal bite wounds with debridement, drainage, and cleansing. Culture the wound, delay wound closure until infection subsides, and begin penicillin (500 mg qid). Add a penicillinase-resistant penicillin (eg, dicloxacillin 500 mg qid) if erythema appears to be spreading or if *S. aureus* is suspected. Amoxicillin/clavulanic acid may be used as a single agent. If the patient is allergic to penicillin, use doxycycline 500 mg twice a day for initial antibiotic therapy.
- Treat for 7 to 10 days for an uncomplicated cellulitis.

Human Bites

- Treat all human bites initially with both penicillin and a penicillinase-resistant agent (eg, dicloxacillin). Delay closure of the wound.
- Elevate affected limb until the swelling declines, usually 3 to 5 days.
- Immobilize clenched-fist injuries and obtain hand-surgery consultation promptly.
- Instruct the patient to watch the wound for signs of infection, such as pain, redness, warmth, swelling, or purulent exudate.

ANNOTATED BIBLIOGRAPHY

Chuinard RG, D'Ambrosia RD. Human bite infections of the hand. J Bone Joint Surg 1977;59:416. *(A classic paper outlining early and aggressive surgical management; stresses the need for the determination of capsule integrity.)*

Fallouji MA. Traumatic love bites. Br J Surg 1990;77:100. *(The underreported problem of "love" bites.)*

Goldstein EJC. Bite wounds and infection. Clin Infect Dis 1992; 14:633. *(A review of the current literature and a guide to proper management.)*

Goldstein EJC, Citron DM, Richwald GA. Lack of *in-vitro* efficacy of oral forms of certain cephalosporins, erythromycin, and oxacillin against *Pasteurella multocida.* Antimicrob Agents Chemother 1988;32:213. *(Notes that many strains of* P. multocida *isolated from human wounds causing bite infections are resistant to cephalexin, erythromycin, and oxacillin.)*

Goldstein EJC, Citron DM, Wield B, et al. Bacteriology of human and animal bite wounds. J Clin Microbiol 1978;8:667. *(Stresses the broad range of bacteria, both aerobic and anaerobic, found in bite wounds.)*

Hicklin H, Verghese A, Alvarez S. Dysgonic fermenter 2 septicemia. Rev Infect Dis 1987;9:884. *(Can cause fatal sepsis in splenectomied patients and those with alcoholic liver disease.)*

Mann RJ, Hoffeld TA, Farmer CB. Human bites of the hand: twenty years of experience. J Hand Surg 1977;2:97, *(*S. viridans *was the most common aerobic pathogen; 44 percent of wounds had* S. aureus. *The use of penicillinase-resistant penicillin is recommended.)*

Taylor GA. Management of human bite injuries of the hand. Can Med Assoc J 1985;133:191, *(A well-conceived approach.)*

Weber DJ, Wolfson JS, Swarz MN, et al. *Pasteurella multocida* infections: report of 34 cases and review of the literature. Medicine (Baltimore) 1984;63:133. *(Comprehensive review.)*

Management of Minor Burns

Accidental minor burns are common. The majority of the estimated 2 million annual burn victims can be treated as outpatients. The primary physician is often asked for advice about immediate care and should render definitive treatment for localized partial-thickness burns.

PATHOPHYSIOLOGY AND CLINICAL PRESENTATION

Burns represent direct thermal injury to the cells of the skin and underlying structures. The clinical presentation is dependent on the degree of damage, which is a direct function of the intensity of heat and duration of exposure.

First-Degree Burns. These involve just the superficial layers of the epidermis. The skin is painful, red, and swollen. It blanches with pressure and shows little or no edema. Ultraviolet radiation, scalding, low-intensity exposure to steam, or brief contact with a hot object are common causes. Complete recovery usually occurs within a week, often with peeling and sometimes with postinflammatory hyperpigmentation.

Second-Degree Burns. Second-degree burns involve the epidermis and dermis; a broad distinction is made between superficial and deep burns, based on the amount of dermis involved. Deep second-degree burns involve the entire papillary dermis, with penetration to some or all of the reticular dermis. Second-degree burns present as painful red blisters or broken epidermis exposing a weeping edematous surface. They are most often caused by scalds or brief exposure to a flame. Recovery requires 2 to 3 weeks; sometimes scarring occurs.

Third-Degree Burns. These involve all layers of the epidermis and dermis, with penetration into underlying fat and muscle. They usually result from prolonged contact with steam, hot objects, or flames and present with ulceration and tissue necrosis. They are painless because nerve tissue in the area has been destroyed. Deep tissue destruction can occur in electrical or chemical burns that may not become evident for several days.

Sunburn and Photosensitivity Reactions. Sunburn is one of the most common types of burns presenting to the office-based physician. It has two phases: an immediate, initial, erythematous phase, which generally fades within 30 minutes after exposure, and a delayed response—what patients call sunburn—occurring 3 to 6 hours after the exposure to the sun and peaking in 12 to 24 hours. Sunburn is characterized by erythema, pruritus, and tenderness but may proceed to edema, vesiculation, and even blistering.

Sun-related eruptions may also occur as a result of photosensitizing medications. The primary culprits are thiazide diuretics, sulfa-containing agents, tetracyclines (particularly demeclocycline), griseofulvin, phenothiazines, and nalidixic acid. Topical substances, particularly furocoumarins (found in parsley, celery, carrots, certain perfumes, and aftershave lotions) are also photosensitizing.

PRINCIPLES OF THERAPY

The first task is to assess depth and extent of injury. Treatment of burn wounds is based on the depth and surface area of skin involved. The surface area of burns has traditionally been based on the "rule of nines." Each arm is considered 9 percent of the body surface area, each leg is 18 percent, the anterior and the posterior trunk are each 18 percent, the head is 9 percent, and the perineum/genitalia is 1 percent.

Using these classifications, the treatment of burns can proceed in an organized fashion. All second-degree burns greater than 5 percent to 10 percent, all third-degree burns, any burns associated with electrical current, and all burns of the ears, eyes, face, hands, feet, or perineum should be immediately referred to a major hospital familiar with burn care. A history of prolonged contact with scalding liquids, flaming clothing, or high-voltage electrical current portends full-thickness damage and need for referral, as does dry, parchment-like skin with loss of hair follicles and sensation.

The remaining first-degree burns and second-degree burns involving less than 5 percent of body surface can be cared for on an outpatient basis by the primary physician with adequate wound care and follow-up, provided the patient is reliable and the home situation amenable.

The goals of therapy are to reduce inflammation, prevent infection, relieve pain, and promote healing.

First-Degree Burns

First aid to minor burns involves immediate application of *ice packs* or *cold compresses* of water, milk, or oatmeal.

Cold reduces discomfort, edema, and hyperemia and may diminish the extent of injury. The application of cold should continue until the burn is pain-free. *No dressing* is required, just skin lubricant and instructions to return if blistering occurs. Prophylactic antibiotics appear to have little or no effect.

Pain can usually be relieved with aspirin or acetaminophen. Aspirin has the advantage of suppressing inflammation and is particularly helpful in sunburn.

In cases of extensive sunburn, a topical corticosteroid lotion or spray may provide symptomatic relief. Systemic corticosteroids do not reduce the edema associated with sunburn and are not indicated.

Second-Degree Burns

If the skin is broken, the wound requires protection so that healing may occur without infection. This involves gently *washing* the area of the burn with water and a mild antiseptic soap, such as one containing chlorhexidine. Washing is followed by gentle *irrigation* with sterile isotonic saline and application of a sterile *occlusive dressing*. For chemical burns, the involved area is placed under running water for at least 15 to 30 minutes before cleansing or debridement is started. A syringe or water pick can be used to help irrigate and remove embedded debris. Devitalized tissue should be debrided (see Appendix to Section 12). Patients complaining of pain or displaying anxiety should be given an analgesic or a sedative before manipulation of the injured area. Adherent tar can be removed after being hardened by the application of ice or softened by use of a topical antibiotic such as polysporin or mupirocin (Bactroban) ointment. *Tetanus prophylaxis* is indicated and includes administering tetanus toxoid booster to previously immunized patients (see Chapter 6).

Management of blisters is somewhat controversial. Some argue that blisters provide an excellent burn dressing and protective barrier, while other evidence suggests that the trapped fluid can become a culture medium for bacteria. Small, thick-walled blisters probably should be left intact, while those that are larger, thin-walled, located on hairy skin that is prone to infection, or located in areas of movement that are more likely to cause rupture should be removed. Removal should be complete, because needle aspiration simply negates the protective barrier while retaining the potential culture medium for infection.

Prophylaxis against infection is provided by the topical antibiotic preparation *silver sulfadiazine* (Silvadene). The cream is easy to apply and provides softening as well as antibacterial effect. It is contraindicated in those with allergies to sulfa and in pregnant and nursing women. The agent should be applied in a layer thick enough to prevent the burn from being visible, using a tongue depressor or glove. Pain can be minimized by keeping the cream refrigerated. Silver sulfadiazine should be removed daily or every other day and reapplied. *Systemic antibiotics* are indicated only for established infection and are not appropriate for prophylaxis or outpatient use.

Dressings are prepared by applying a nonadherent fine mesh gauze soaked in sterile saline to the burn and covering this with a bulky dressing that allows drainage into but not through it (see Appendix to Section 12). The patient should be examined in 2 days for pain, adenopathy, and fever, and the dressing should be checked. If no evidence of infection is seen, the dressing may remain for 5 to 7 days, after which the area is re-examined to determine the need for a dressing change.

Pain relief is an essential part of management, and usually aspirin or a nonsteroidal agent such as ibuprofen suffices. Short courses of agents containing codeine or oxycodone are appropriate for painful burns. Topical anesthetics may provide symptomatic relief but are not justified because of the risk of sensitization. In cases of extensive sunburn, topical corticosteroid sprays may provide modest symptomatic relief, but a short course of systemic steroids may be more effective.

Moisturization is important but often overlooked. After healing of the burn, the new epithelial layer may tend to dry and crack, and this problem can be reduced by the application of a moisturizing cream such as Eucerin or aloe vera for 4 to 8 weeks after apparent resolution.

INDICATIONS FOR REFERRAL AND ADMISSION

Referral for surgical consultation and/or hospitalization is indicated if burns exceed 10 percent to 15 percent of body area or full-thickness burns exceed 3 percent. Prompt admission and surgical consultation should be considered for circumferential or full-thickness burns; involvement of the eyes, ears, other organs of sensation, the hands, or perineum; evidence of inhalation injury; or serious concurrent medical conditions such as diabetes or immunosuppression. Patients who are unreliable or unable to care for themselves may also require inpatient treatment.

PATIENT EDUCATION

Patient education is critical to successful recovery from a burn. The patient and caretaker should be instructed to keep the wound clean and note erythema or inflammation, which are signs of infection. Instruct the patient to note numbness, tingling, or change in skin color or temperature, which may suggest that the dressing is too tight and circulation is being impaired. Explicit, often written instructions on the removal of dressings, the cleansing of the wound, reapplication of topical sulfadiazine, and treatment of dried skin are important. Patients with healed burns should be instructed to avoid exposure to direct sunlight because of increased sensitivity during the year following a burn injury. A burn is a good opportunity to reinforce the importance of sunscreens.

The occurrence of a burn, even a minor one, is a good opportunity to reinstruct patients on the importance of burn prevention. The obvious caveats are against smoking and for keeping flammable material and matches away from children. Specific instructions on the use of pot holders, careful puncturing and removal of plastic wraps from microwaved food, and reduction of the temperature at the hot water tap are all helpful. Reminders about the importance of smoke detectors and maintaining an approved fire extinguisher are important. A written burn-prevention checklist is a useful aid.

THERAPEUTIC RECOMMENDATIONS

- For first-degree burns, immediately apply cold and maintain it until the area is free of pain even after the cold is withdrawn.
- If the skin is broken, cleanse with a mild soap and water before applying cold water or ice.
- No dressing or antibiotic is indicated for first-degree burns. Emollients such as Eucerin or aloe vera should be used if blistering does not occur after several days.
- For severe sunburn, prescribe a gentle topical corticosteroid lotion for symptomatic relief. Aspirin or ibuprofen provides analgesia and helps limit inflammation. Consider a brief course of systemic steroids for extensive sunburn.
- For second-degree burns, spread silver sulfadiazine (Silvadene) over the involved area in a thickness sufficient to prevent the burn's showing through. Refrigerated sulfadiazine is less painful. Wrap the area with six or seven layers of gauze for protection.
- Prescribe systemic antibiotics, usually dicloxacillin, for any secondary cellulitis. Prophylactic oral antibiotics should not be used for fear of selecting out resistant gram-negative organisms.

L.A.M.

ANNOTATED BIBLIOGRAPHY

Deitch EA. The management of burns. N Engl J Med 1990;323:1249. *(A comprehensive discussion, including the approach to more serious burns.)*

Herbert K, Lawrence JC. Chemical burns. Burns 1989;15:381. *(A good review of this important category of burn injury.)*

Peate WF. Outpatient management of burns. Am Fam Physician 1992;45:1321. *(Well-referenced discussion of outpatient management.)*

Rockwell WB, Ehrlich HP. Should burn blister fluid be evacuated? J Burn Care Rehabil 1990;11:93. *(The authors argue for removal of even intact blisters because the fluid can be a good culture medium for bacteria.)*

Waymack JP, Pruitt BA Jr. Burn wound care. Adv Surg 1990;23:261. *(Focuses on surgical management and indications for admission.)*

197
Management of Skin Ulceration

STEPHEN J. FRIEDMAN, M.D.

Primary Care Medicine: Office Evaluation and Management of the Adult Patient, 3rd edition, edited by Allan H. Goroll, Lawrence A. May, and Albert G. Mulley, Jr. J.B. Lippincott Company, Philadelphia

Skin ulceration can be a troublesome, disabling, and potentially dangerous skin problem. Cutaneous ulcers commonly encountered in medical practice include leg and pressure ulcerations. Approximately 1 percent of the population is affected by venous leg ulcers. Diabetics and others with arterial insufficiency are at increased risk for ischemic ulceration and limb-threatening infection. About 20 percent of geriatric patients have pressure ulcers, with an associated fourfold increase in mortality. The primary physician who recognizes and effectively treats the early skin changes can prevent many of the debilitating consequences.

PATHOPHYSIOLOGY AND CLINICAL PRESENTATION

Skin ulceration most commonly results from venous or arterial insufficiency or from prolonged, excessive pressure. Infectious and malignant etiologies are also encountered, especially in immunocompromised persons.

Venous Insufficiency. The initial manifestation of venous insufficiency is edema, usually absent on arising and severe at the end of the day. Venous valves become incompetent with age, thrombophlebitis, and the hereditary tendency to develop venous varicosities. All three mechanisms cause abnormally high venous pressure during ambulation and encourage fibrinogen to leak from the engorged capillary bed. A precapillary fibrin layer develops and interferes with oxygen and nutrient exchange. Pigmentation, induration, dermatitis (*stasis dermatitis*), and finally ulceration may develop. The rupture of delicate venules releases hemoglobin, which changes to hemosiderin, producing pigmentation. Scaling and oozing develop when the skin is scratched. Vesicles may indicate a contact dermatitis from a topical medication. Secondary bacterial invasion occurs and may lead to cellulitis.

Stasis ulcerations develop within areas of dermatitis or indurated cellulitis. They occur most often above the medial malleolus because of its poor vascular supply and sparse subcutaneous tissue. Minor trauma can precipitate ulceration. The size of the stasis ulcers varies from small erosions to a size that encircles the ankle. They may or may not be painful. The base of the ulcer is usually moist with exuberant granulation tissue. Purulence indicates secondary infection.

Arterial Insufficiency. The most common cause of arterial insufficiency is *atherosclerotic disease*. The leg is cold and appears pale or cyanotic (though there may be dependent rubor), and peripheral pulses are lost or reduced. The ulcers are initially small, punctate, and superficial but, with worsening ischemia, become larger and deeper. Typically, they occur on the sides of the feet, the heels, the toes, and the nailbeds.

Ischemic ulcers are also associated with *hypertensive disease* and *vasculitis*. Those occurring in the context of hypertension characteristically develop over the lateral malleoli. They begin as painful, blue–red plaques which soon ulcerate. A purpuric halo may surround the ulceration. Vasculitic ulcers occur in the context of connective tissue disease, hematologic and malignant conditions, and hypersensitivity reactions, beginning as palpable purpuric lesions or hemorrhagic vesicles (see Chapter 179).

Decubitus Ulcer

The pressure sore or decubitus ulcer is common in bedridden or semiambulatory patients. They may present as nonblanchable erythema, soft tissue loss, blisters, or eschar over bony prominences. Pressure ulcer severity is reflected by the stage of the lesion. Stage 1 lesions are manifested by nonblanchable erythema of intact skin. Stage 2 ulcers involve only the epidermis and dermis. Stage 3 ulcers extend into the subcutaneous tissues and undermine the surrounding skin. Stage 4 lesions extend through deep fascia involving muscle and may extend to the bone.

Factors contributing to the development of pressure sores include shearing forces, friction, and moisture. Decubiti usually occur over bony prominences. The pressure gradient occludes lymphatic vessels and overloads the microvascular system, leading to the accumulation of waste products and ultimately to necrosis. The lower part of the body and sacrococcygeal area are the predominate sites, with the hip, malleolus, and heel being the other important areas.

Pressure sores can lead to cellulitis, bacteremia, osteomyelitis, and even meningitis. The microbiota of decubiti is polymicrobial, and the organisms that cause the most problems, including life-threatening bacteremias, are *group A streptococci*, *Staphylococcus aureus*, *Escherichia coli*, and *Bacteroides fragilis*.

PRINCIPLES OF MANAGEMENT

Many of the principles of ulcer management are similar, independent of cause or location. Important objectives are to restore circulation (see Chapters 34 and 35), improve local factors, reduce pressure, remove necrotic tissue, maintain cleanliness, and prevent further injury.

Leg Ulcers

Regardless of cause, treatment of the leg ulcer begins with washing the leg and ankle with a mild soap. Emollients are used to prevent drying (xerosis). In leg ulcers with a clean base, application of an Unna paste boot or an occlusive wound dressing may encourage healing and re-epithelialization. An *Unna boot* is a flesh-colored gauze roll bandage impregnated with zinc oxide, calamine, glycerin, and gelatin. Topical enzymes and hydrophilic beads are sometimes useful adjunctive agents in leg ulcers or pressure ulcers.

The bewildering array of commercially available *occlusive wound dressings* includes polyurethane films (Opsite, Tegaderm, Bioclusive), polyethylene oxide hydrogel (Vigilon, Spenco 2nd Skin), foam dressings (Lyofoam, Allevyn), laminate dressings (Biobrane), alginate dressings (Sorbsan, Kaltostat), and hydrocolloid dressings (DuoDerm). The dressing is replaced every 3 to 7 days, or sooner if it begins to leak. The patient must be warned to expect an unpleasant odor, caused by a buildup of fluid, when the dressing is removed. The optimal occlusive dressing for wound healing remains to be developed. DuoDerm is readily available and convenient to use.

Occlusive dressings are promoted as capable of shortening the healing time, although they often prove no better than simple *wet-to-wet dressings*. Wet-to-wet dressings, along with cleaning and gentle debridement with gauze sponges several times daily, are useful. Dilute hydrogen peroxide can be used to clean the ulcerated area. Occlusive dressings do offer greater convenience and some pain relief. Occlusive dressings should not be used on wounds complicated by cellulitis.

Treatment of Stasis Dermatitis. Any stasis dermatitis must be attended to, because it can lead to further ulceration. Venous insufficiency and edema should be treated (see Chapter 35). *Topical corticosteroids*, creams or ointments, are useful to reduce the inflammatory component and itching. Corticosteroids should not be applied near an ulcer since they may delay wound healing. Oozing dermatitis requires wet dressings and bed rest. Acute exudative dermatitis can be soothed and dried with cool *Burow's compresses*. Scratching, use of over-the-counter medications, and adhesive tape on the dermatitic areas should be avoided and warned against.

Secondarily infected dermatitis should be treated with *oral antibiotics* active against staphylococcal infection, such as dicloxacillin, amoxicillin/clavulanate (Augmentin), or erythromycin. *Topical antibiotics* may be used in mild cases. Topical mupirocin is effective against a wide range of staphylococci, including methicillin-resistant organisms. However, it should not be continued beyond 14 days because of the risk of resistant species' emerging with longer use. Neomycin should be avoided because of its tendency to induce contact sensitization and dermatitis.

External *compressive bandages* or *stockings* may be used to reduce venous pressure in the lower extremities. Graduated compressive surgical stockings are expensive but can be helpful (see Chapter 35). The patient should apply the compression in the morning before getting out of bed. Prolonged standing should be avoided, weight loss emphasized, and periods of leg elevation encouraged. Intermittent pneumatic compression has been used successfully as an alternative to elastic compression in refractory cases to speed ulcer healing.

Decubitus Ulcer

Nutritional repletion is important to reverse catabolism and to correct all factors that affect the oxygenation of tissue, such as anemia, edema, and vascular problems. *Reducing pressure* on the affected area is critical. In some cases, an alternating-pressure air mattress may be indicated. The basic principle of debridement is to use *wet-to-wet dressings* or an occlusive dressing. A variety of biochemical agents that dissolve debris are purported to promote healing, though double-blind evidence for their efficacy is generally lacking. Occasionally, grafts are required to close the ulceration.

If decubiti are complicated by infection, the antibiotic program should include anaerobic as well as aerobic coverage. Even a shallow ulcer may hide a deep infective sinus or a tunnel to an osteomyelitis. A roentgenogram may be useful for detection of chronic osteomyelitis.

Further measures include use of laser sterilization, growth factors, allografts, and platelet aggregation inhibitors. The best treatment remains primary prevention.

PATIENT EDUCATION

In most ulcers, prevention is the key. Patients and family must be educated to look for the preulcerative changes in stasis dermatitis and use compensatory measures before ulceration occurs. In patients with chronic vascular disease, advice about nail cutting, treating sores early, and seeking medical care at the first sign of a break in skin is important. For people confined to beds or chairs, educate the family to prevent prolonged pressure on a bony prominence.

INDICATIONS FOR REFERRAL AND ADMISISON

Failure of ulcers to heal after good management with a compliant patient indicates the need for surgical consultation. Surgical debridement and split-thickness or full-thickness skin grafting may be necessary. If fever or other signs of bacteremia develop, then intravenous antibiotics and prompt hospitalization are needed. Mortality risk is high, especially with associated anemia and hypoalbuminemia.

THERAPEUTIC RECOMMENDATIONS

Venous Insufficiency and Stasis Dermatitis

- In all patients with stasis changes, control edema by rest, elevation, diuretics, avoidance of dependency, and external compression with stockings or bandages.
- Treat any concurrent nutritional deficiency, hypertension, diabetes, or congestive heart failure.
- Treat pruritus with application of midrange-potency topical corticosteroids (eg, 0.1% triamcinolone acetonide). Ointments are indicated if the area is dry and scaly, and creams should be used if the area is moist. Avoid application near or on an ulcer, since corticosteroids may delay wound healing.
- Treat acute exudative dermatitis with cool Burow's compresses (1:40 dilution) two to three times daily for 30 to 60 minutes.
- Scratching and use of over-the-counter medicaments should be discouraged.

Cutaneous Ulceration

- Prescribe wet-to-wet dressings, followed by cleaning and gentle debridement with gauze sponges several times daily. Dilute hydrogen peroxide can be used to clean the ulcerated area.
- Occlusive dressings are worth a trial because they may ease pain, debride ulcers, and lead to healing without need for surgical intervention.
- In the clinical setting of secondary infection, culture for aerobic and anaerobic bacteria, and treat accordingly with oral or intravenous antibiotics.
- In cases of mild skin infection, topical antibiotic creams such as mupirocin can be considered for short-term use (< 2 wk), but preparations that contain neomycin should be avoided.
- Persistent deep ulcers of long duration require consideration of underlying osteomyelitis. A roentgenogram may be useful.
- Refer for surgical consultation patients whose ulcers prove refractory to proper conservative management. Surgical debridement and split-thickness or full-thickness skin grafting may be necessary.

ANNOTATED BIBLIOGRAPHY

Allman RM. Pressure ulcers among the elderly. N Engl J Med 1989;320:850. *(Good discussion of risk factors.)*

Falanga V. Occlusive wound dressings. Arch Dermatol 1988;124:872. *(Reviews commercially available occlusive dressings.)*

Falanga V, Eaglestein WH. A therapeutic approach to venous ulcers. J Am Acad Dermatol 1986;14:777. *(A systematic approach, emphasizing the usefulness of newer and more effective occlusive dressings.)*

Friedman SJ, Su D. Management of leg ulcers with hydrocolloid occlusive dressing. Arch Dermatol 1984;120:1329. *(Convenience of management and relief of pain were major advantages, but wound healing was no faster than with wet-to-wet dressings.)*

Mol MAE, Nanninga PB, van Eendenburg J-P, et al. Grafting of venous leg ulcers. J Am Acad Dermatol 1991;24:77. *(Indications and success of skin grafting of leg ulcers.)*

Phillips TJ, Dover JS. Leg ulcers. J Am Acad Dermatol 1991;25:965. *(Comprehensive review; 211 refs.)*

Yarkony GM, Kirk PM, Carlson C, et al. Classification of pressure ulcers. Arch Dermatol 1990;126:1218. *(Pathophysiology and updated classification of pressure ulcers.)*

Primary Care Medicine: Office Evaluation and Management of the Adult Patient, 3rd edition, edited by Allan H. Goroll, Lawrence A. May, and Albert G. Mulley, Jr. J.B. Lippincott Company, Philadelphia

Appendix to Section 12 Minor Surgical Office Procedures for Skin Problems

ERIC KORTZ, M.D.
CHARLES J. McCABE, M.D.

SIMPLE LACERATIONS

Treatment of simple lacerations is one of the most commonly performed outpatient surgical procedures. All lacerations should be evaluated for the extent of injury to surrounding structures, particularly nerves. This is most important with lacerations of the face, hand, and wrist. All injuries involving peripheral nerves should be referred to an emergency room; digital nerve branches can be approximated with excellent long-term benefit. All tendon injuries should receive the attention of a hand surgeon. Those lacerations complicated by bone fracture should be treated by an orthopedic surgeon.

In uncomplicated wounds, foreign material around and within the wound, including devitalized tissue, should be removed before definitive closure.

The following materials are used to treat simple lacerations:

Anesthetic

1. 1% or 2% Xylocaine without epinephrine
2. 5-mL to 10-mL syringes
3. 19-G to 22-G needles

Prep Solution

1. Gentle soap solution
2. Betadine
3. Normal saline

Drapes

1. Three or four sterile towels

Instruments

1. Adson forceps
2. Needle holders (plastic)
3. Hemostat
4. Irrigation bulb syringe
5. Suture scissors
6. Suture material (Table 1)
7. Six to 12 sterile gauze pads
8. Sterile gloves

Dressings

1. Xeroform gauze
2. Two gauze pads
3. Tape or gauze roll

Anesthesia

- Infiltration of the wound edges may either precede or follow wound cleansing and debridement, depending on the patient and the wound.
- The path of the injecting needle should proceed from clean, prepped areas to deeper tissue levels. The interior of the wound should be avoided.
- Aspiration should precede infiltration of anesthetic to prevent intravascular injection.

Skin-Wound Preparation and Draping

- Copiously irrigate the wound with normal saline under moderate pressure. Foreign material and devitalized tissue are removed at this time. The wound and surrounding skin are then cleansed with a gentle detergent, followed by an antiseptic such as Betadine applied to the surrounding skin only.
- Sterile drapes are placed to isolate the wound completely, including enough surrounding skin to allow easy approach and a working surface area.

Wound Closure

- Hemostasis is obtained. Bleeding is usually minimal. Closure proceeds in one or several layers, depending on the depth of the wound. Subcutaneous sutures are of the absorbable type, either 3-0 or 4-0 Dexon or chromic. These sutures should be simple, interrupted stitches secured with minimal tension.
- Skin closure for minor lacerations is best achieved with a nonabsorbable monofilament suture. Nylon is an inexpen-

Table 1. Suture Selection and Removal Time

LOCATION	SUTURES	REMOVAL TIME (DAYS)
Scalp	3-0	10–14
Face	5-0, 6-0	4–5
Neck	3-0, 4-0	7–10
Trunk	3-0	7–10
Extremities	3-0	8–12
Hands	4-0, 5-0	8–12
Feet	3-0, 4-0	8–12
Oral mucosa	4-0, 3-0 chromic	10–14

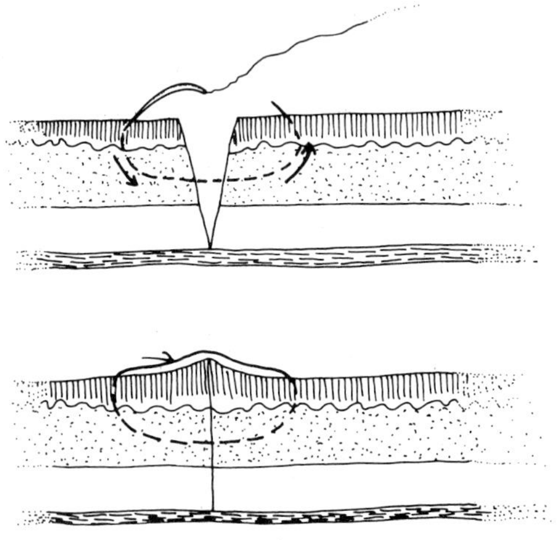

Side views

Figure 1. Simple interrupted stitch for skin closure. Notice the path of the needle; the needle enters and leaves the skin at acute angles, which allows eversion of the skin edges. (Grossman JA: Minor Injuries and Disorders: Surgical and Medical Care, p 52. Philadelphia, JB Lippincott, 1984)

sive and excellent choice. The suture placement technique should be simple, interrupted, and allow for approximation of the wound edges without inducing ischemia. As Figure 1 demonstrates, the curved needle should enter the skin at an acute angle. Advancement is then with the natural curve of the needle and includes all layers (epidermis, dermis, and the upper subcutaneous tissue). Care should be taken to maintain equal depth and width from the wound edge with each stitch. A good technique is to sequentially divide the wound in half. The first stitch is placed directly in the center of the laceration. Subsequent sutures subdivide the remaining open surface. Corresponding parts of an irregular wound should be approximated first.

Dressings

- After the entire wound is closed, normal saline or a gauze sponge can be used to clean the skin of dried blood and Betadine.
- The wound is then covered with a strip of xeroform gauze and dry sterile dressing.
- Lacerations involving the fingers, palm, or wrist should be immobilized.
- Follow-up for patients with minor lacerations can be done at the time of suture removal. A convenient schedule for suture removal is presented in Table 1.

SIMPLE PARONYCHIA

Paronychia (Fig. 2) represents a soft tissue infection and abscess formation along the nail border. The patient usually complains of pain, and the area surrounding the nail base is red, swollen, and tender.

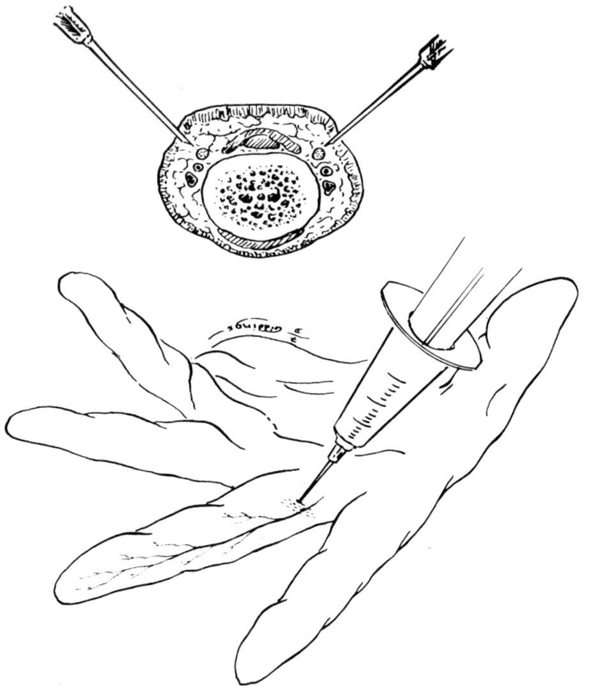

Figure 2. Metacarpal block. Entrance of needle is at the palmar base of finger, medial and lateral. The needle path is then toward the palmar metacarpal head. (Van Way CW III, Buerk CA (eds): Surgical Skills in Patient Care, p 55. St Louis, CV Mosby, 1978)

The following materials are used to treat simple paronychia:

Anesthetic

1. 1% or 2% Xylocaine without epinephrine
2. 5-mL to 10-mL syringes
3. 19-G to 22-G needles

Prep Solution

1. Gentle soap solution
2. Betadine or alcohol
3. Normal saline

Drapes

1. Three or four sterile towels

Instruments

1. Adson forceps
2. Pediatric suture scissors
3. Kelly clamps
4. No. 15 scalpel blade
5. Scalpel handle
6. Sterile gloves

Dressings

1. Nu-Gauze ¼ inch
2. Two gauze pads
3. Tape or gauze roll

Anesthesia

Complete anesthesia of the finger may be accomplished with a metacarpal block (Fig. 3). After alcohol preparation of the skin over the metacarpophalangeal joint is performed, points for needle entrance are selected on the medial and lateral palmar surface of the metacarpal head. Care is taken to aspirate each time before the infiltration of 1 to 2 mL of Xylocaine.

Preparation of Skin

The entire digit, including the metacarpal head, may be washed with a gentle soap solution, followed by application of a uniform layer of Betadine.

Draping

Placement of sterile towels must achieve isolation of the digit involved and exposure of the metacarpal area. Additional anesthesia is sometimes necessary.

Incision and Drainage

Treatment of the laterally based infection (see Figure 2) involves incising the skin along the lateral edge of the nail; a small incision is made directly over the swollen, fluctuant area. After drainage of purulent material, a wick is used to prevent premature wound closure. The wick is removed after 24 to 36 hours and soaking of the digit is begun on a twice-daily schedule.

Occasionally, a portion of the nail must be removed to establish adequate drainage, particularly if the infection has established penetration of the subungual space. A small scissors is used to separate the nail from the underlying matrix. This dissection is carried out from the tip of the nail to the base in a vertical strip involving ⅙ to ¼ inch of the nail surface. The nail is then incised with a No. 15 blade or a scissors along this vertical line. A Kelly clamp is then used to grasp the portion of nail to be removed and tease the nail from beneath the eponychium.

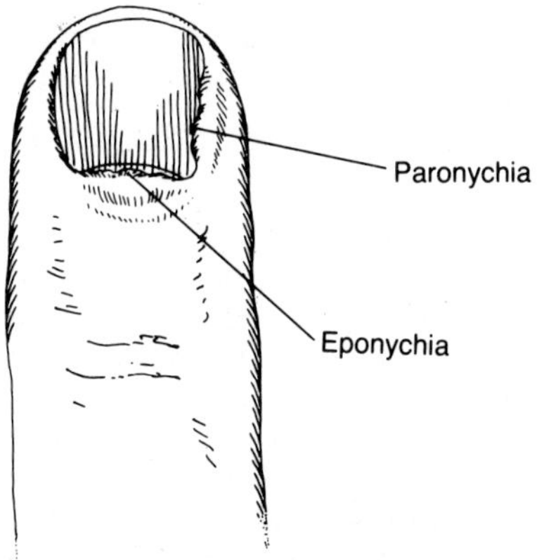

Figure 3. Simple paronychia. (Grossman JA: Minor Injuries and Disorders: Surgical and Medical Care, p 253. Philadelphia, JB Lippincott, 1984)

Dressing

Xeroform or Vaseline-impregnated gauze is placed within the wound created by nail removal, taking care to place a layer between the matrix and the eponychium to ensure that nail growth can occur in the area of resection. A gauze pad covers this dressing, which is secured in place. Routine administration of antibiotics is unnecessary; however, those patients with diabetes should be placed on antistreptococcal and antistaphylococcal coverage for 7 days.

ABSCESS

A subcutaneous abscess is often seen. The patient usually complains of pain and swelling. Abscesses commonly occur in the perianal region. If fluctuance is present, incision and drainage should be performed.

The following materials are used to treat abscesses:

Anesthetics

1. 1% to 2% Xylocaine without epinephrine
2. 5-mL to 10-mL syringes
3. 19-G to 22-G needles

Prep Solution

1. Betadine

Drapes

1. Three or four sterile towels

Instruments

1. No. 11 or 15 scalpel blade
2. Scalpel handle
3. Kelly clamps
4. Adson forceps
5. Five or six gauze pads
6. Sterile gloves

Dressing

1. ¼- to ½-inch Nu-Gauze strip

Anesthesia

After alcohol preparation of the skin, superficial skin infiltration is carried out in a linear course across the abscess. A second linear course is then traversed directly perpendicular to the first. Care is taken to remain superficial to the abscess cavity.

Skin Preparation

A single layer of Betadine is applied to the abscess and sufficient surrounding skin for adequate exposure.

Drapes

Placement of drapes ensures isolation of the abscess and the prepared surrounding skin.

Incision and Drainage

A linear incision is made through the skin, entering the abscess cavity. The cavity is opened widely across the entire abscess dimension. If more drainage is desired, a second incision is made perpendicular to the first, forming a cruciate design.

Dressing

After complete drainage of the cavity, placement of strip gauze within the wound is necessary to maintain drainage and ensure secondary healing of the wound. Although antibiotics are not necessary for most, those patients with diabetes or accompanying cellulitis may benefit from 24 to 48 hours of gram-positive coverage. Continued packing of the wound should proceed with daily changes until healthy closure of the defect occurs.

BURNS

Burns of the skin can result from many sources: flame, steam, scald, electrical, and chemical. These agents cause variable cellular damage to the layers of epidermis, dermis, and subcutaneous fat, depending on the depth. Classification, and therefore treatment, of burn wounds is based on the depth and surface area of skin involved. *First-degree burns* are those that involve just the superficial layers of the epidermis (Fig. 4). *Second-degree burns* involve the epidermis and dermis; a broad distinction is made between superficial and deep burns, based on the amount of dermis involved. Deep second-degree burns involve the entire papillary dermis, with penetration to some or all of the reticular dermis. *Third-degree burns* involve all layers of the epidermis and dermis, with penetration into underlying fat and muscle.

The surface area of burns has traditionally been based on the rule of nines. Each arm is considered 9 percent of the body surface area, each leg is 18 percent, the anterior and the posterior trunk are each 18 percent, the head is 9 percent, and perineum/genitalia is 1 percent.

Using these classifications, the treatment of burns can proceed in an organized fashion. All second-degree burns covering more than 5 percent to 10 percent of the body, all third-degree burns, any burns associated with electrical current, and all burns of the ears, eyes, face, hands, feet, or perineum should be immediately referred to a major hospital familiar with burn care. The remaining first-degree burns and second-degree burns covering less than 5 percent of the body can be cared for on an outpatient basis with adequate wound care and follow-up.

The following materials are used to treat burns:

Prep Solution

1. pHisoHex, gentle soap
2. Normal saline

Drapes

1. Three or four sterile drapes

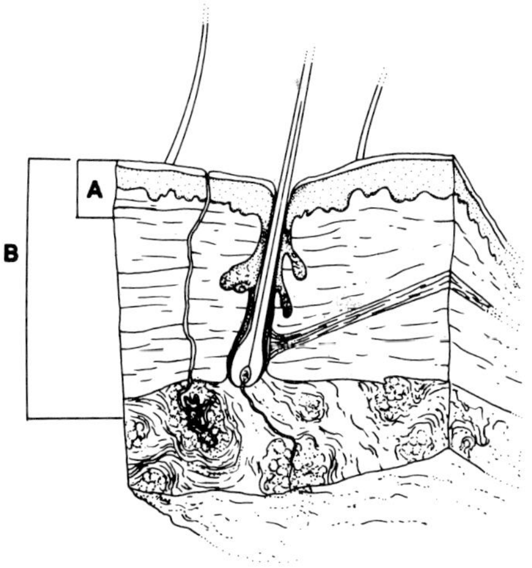

Figure 4. Anatomy of the skin demonstrating (*A*) epidermis, (*B*) epidermis and dermis (ie, full thickness). (Grossman JA: Minor Injuries and Disorders: Surgical and Medical Care, p 71. Philadelphia, JB Lippincott, 1984)

Instruments

1. Adson forceps
2. Suture scissors
3. Silvadene cream
4. Sterile gloves

Dressings

1. Sterile gauze pads
2. Roll gauze

Skin Preparation

Chemical burns should first receive generous lavage with normal saline to dilute the irritant. First- and second-degree burns should be washed with a gentle soap solution. For second-degree burns with ruptured bullae, all free skin should be debrided.

Draping

The cleansed, debrided area of a burn is isolated on a sterile field.

Dressing

Silvadene cream is applied to the surface of the burn in a thin, even layer. Application with a tongue depressor works nicely. Silvadene is subsequently covered with dry gauze pads, which are secured with rolled gauze. Complete dressing change should then be done twice daily, with complete cleansing of the wound before a new dressing is applied. Healing for first-degree burns can be expected in 3 to 4 days; second-degree burns require 10 to 20 days. Although controversial, treatment with oral penicillin at moderate dosages, 250 mg four times a day for 3 days, may help to prevent deepening of the burn wound secondary to strep infection.

SKIN BIOPSY

The following materials are used in skin biopsies:

Anesthesia

1. 1% or 2% Xylocaine without epinephrine
2. 5-mL syringe
3. 22-G needle

Prep Solutions

1. Gentle soap solution
2. Betadine

Drapes

1. Three or four drapes

Instruments

1. No. 15 scalpel blade and handle
2. Sterile skin biopsy punch
3. Adson forceps
4. Suture scissors
5. Needle holders
6. Nylon suture
9. Five or six sterile gauze pads
10. Pathology specimen container
11. Sterile gloves

Dressings

1. Xeroform gauze
2. Gauze pad
3. Tape or gauze roll

Anesthesia

After alcohol preparation of the skin is done, complete superficial skin infiltration is accomplished, including the lesion of interest.

Skin Preparation

After the area is cleansed with a gentle soap, a single layer of Betadine is applied.

Draping

The entire prepared area is isolated from surrounding skin and environment.

Biopsy

If a scalpel blade is to be used, an ellipse, surrounding the lesion in question, is created. The entire depth of the epidermis and dermis should be penetrated. Care is taken in the creation of the ellipse to ensure sufficient local skin mobility to allow edge approximation after skin excision has been done. Skin excision is accomplished by elevating one of the corners and sharply separating it from underlying subcutaneous tissue with sharp scissors. Hemostasis is easily obtained by gentle pressure for 1 to 2 minutes. Wound closure then follows, as described for lacerations.

Alternatively, skin biopsy can be performed by using a skin punch. After anesthesia and skin preparation, the circular punch is pressed against the skin, and cutting is achieved with a gentle twisting motion. Once the entire depth of skin has been traversed, it is separated from underlying subcutaneous tissue with sharp scissors. Wound closure is accomplished with several simple sutures. The specimen is then placed in the proper pathology container and solution.

Dressing

The sutured wound should be covered with a strip of Vaseline-impregnated gauze. A dry sterile gauze pad is placed and held securely with tape or gauze roll.

Primary Care Medicine: Office Evaluation and Management of the Adult Patient, 3rd edition, edited by Allan H. Goroll, Lawrence A. May, and Albert G. Mulley, Jr. J.B. Lippincott Company, Philadelphia

13

Ophthalmologic Problems

198

Screening for Glaucoma

CLAUDIA U. RICHTER, M.D.

Glaucoma affects more than 1 million Americans and is the cause of 11 percent of the cases of blindness in the United States. The condition represents a group of diseases characterized by damage to the optic nerve and loss of visual field caused primarily by abnormally high intraocular pressure. Among adults, primary open-angle glaucoma is the most frequent type, presenting asymptomatically until visual loss is advanced. Although the underlying disease process is neither preventable nor curable, visual loss can be prevented or minimized if the patient is identified early and the intraocular pressure is controlled.

EPIDEMIOLOGY AND RISK FACTORS

The prevalence of glaucoma increases with age. For patients aged 50 to 54 years, prevalence is 0.2 percent; it rises to 2.0 percent for those aged 70 to 74 years. The condition is more common among African Americans than whites.

Elevated intraocular pressure is the principal risk factor for glaucomatous visual loss. However, the majority of people with elevated pressure do not develop visual loss. The reported incidence of visual loss within a 5-year period among those with an elevated intraocular pressure ranges from 1.5 percent to 5.0 percent. In people initially classified as having normal intraocular pressure, the incidence of glaucomatous visual loss is about 0.6 percent.

There is a genetic predisposition to the development of primary open-angle glaucoma, manifested by a prevalence among first-degree relatives of approximately 6 percent. The other principal risk factor is advancing age.

PATHOPHYSIOLOGY, NATURAL HISTORY, AND EFFECTIVENESS OF EARLY THERAPY

The pathophysiology of visual loss in glaucoma remains incompletely understood, but a number of factors appear to contribute. Raised intraocular pressure increases vascular resistance, causing decreased vascular perfusion of the optic nerve and ischemia. Axoplasmic flow in the ganglion cell axons becomes compromised, leading to cell dysfunction and death. Compression of the lamina cribrosa (the sieve-like structure through which axons pass when leaving the eye) may ensue and interfere with axonal function. These mechanisms vary in importance in different patients, but the end result is that elevated intraocular pressure causes optic nerve damage and loss of vision.

The relationship between intraocular pressure and visual loss (as manifested by field defects) is highly variable among individuals. The mean duration of intraocular pressure elevation before development of field defects has been estimated to be 18 years. The annual incidence of glaucomatous field defects among patients with ocular hypertension is about 1 percent.

Glaucomatous visual field loss is irreversible. Although incurable, the underlying disease process can be controlled by lowering intraocular pressure. Medical, laser, and surgical approaches are available (see Chapter 207). Early diagnosis and treatment are important. Once damage has occurred, the optic nerve becomes increasingly vulnerable to any increase in intraocular pressure. Lower pressure must be maintained to prevent progression, especially in more advanced cases.

SCREENING METHODS

Tonometry. In areas with readily available ophthalmologic services, measurement of intraocular pressure is usually performed by the eye specialist using applanation tonometry. In areas where such services and equipment are not available, Schiotz tonometry is the most feasible method for measuring intraocular pressure. Applanation tonometry is generally agreed to be both more accurate and more precise, but the equipment is expensive and the technique demands considerable skill. Newer tonometers using an air jet to measure pressure are not available to most primary physicians.

Sensitivity and specificity of screening for glaucoma by measurement of intraocular pressure depends on the pressure elevation used to designate abnormality and the number of readings taken. Depending on the cutoff used for a single reading, sensitivity ranges from 50 percent to 70 percent and specificity from 60 percent to 90 percent.

The predictive value of a positive test is a function of disease prevalence and is affected by the uncertain relationship between intraocular pressure and risk of glaucomatous visual loss. About 7 percent of the older adult population has an intraocular pressure in excess of 21 mm Hg, but only 2 percent actually have glaucomatous physiology, meaning that many without the disease will be referred for evaluation based on a single intraocular pressure reading.

Ophthalmoscopy. Changes in the contour of the optic cup in the center of the optic disc provide the first definitive evidence of glaucomatous damage. The usual cup has a round, regular contour. The cup in early glaucoma becomes notched on the superotemporal or inferotemporal rim. Later changes include an increase in the depth and width of the physiologic cup, nasal displacement of the central retinal vessels, and progressive pallor of the optic nerve head. Other disc changes associated with glaucoma are asymmetric discs and disc hemorrhages.

There is some disagreement about the value of ophthalmoscopy in detecting early glaucoma. Assessment of disc pathology is not as simple as measurement of intraocular pressure. It requires greater skill, but it improves sensitivity to as much as 85 percent, which is especially helpful in detection of early disease. Performing pupillary dilation greatly facilitates the evaluation. Such specificity is unattainable by other screening methods before the onset of manifest visual field defects.

Visual Field Testing. Traditional manual visual field testing is inadequate for mass glaucoma screening because of the time and technical difficulty in performing an adequate examination. In addition, early glaucomatous visual field defects are usually nonspecific and subtle. Manual perimetry is often insensitive to such changes, but automated perimetry is sensitive, demonstrating 92 percent sensitivity (and 46% specificity) in one study. This compared to 72 percent sensitivity and 64 percent specificity for ophthalmoscopy, and 72 percent sensitivity and 60 percent specificity for tonometry. Automated perimetry is still being investigated as a screening tool but is not practical due to its high cost.

CONCLUSIONS AND RECOMMENDATIONS

- Glaucoma is highly prevalent in the older adult population and is a major cause of blindness.
- Risk factors for glaucomatous visual loss include elevated intraocular pressure, a family history of glaucoma, advancing age, and African-American heritage.
- Treatment early in the course of the disease is more effective and more likely to prevent visual loss than that which is delayed until onset of symptoms. Early treatment necessitates detection of the asymptomatic patient.
- Individuals over 40 years of age should have their intraocular pressure measured periodically. Pressure measurement every 3 to 5 years is sufficient after a stable baseline is established for the individual patient.
- In the absence of readily available ophthalmologic services, screening for ocular hypertension can be performed by the primary physician using a Schiotz tonometer. Individuals with elevated intraocular pressures (> 21.9 mm Hg) and/or asymmetry of pressures (> 4 mmHg) should be referred for examination by an ophthalmologist.
- Funduscopic examination, with attention to the appearance of the optic cup, is an important component of the screening evaluation and should be performed by all primary care physicians.
- Automated perimetry may be a valuable screening adjunct in the future, but cost is too great to recommend it at present.

ANNOTATED BIBLIOGRAPHY

Gottlieb LK, Schwartz B, Pauker SG. Glaucoma screening. A cost-effectiveness analysis. Surv Ophthalmol 1983;28:206. *(Examines the cost-effectiveness of tonometry, ophthalmoscopy, and perimetry.)*

Kass AM, Gordon MO, Hoff MR, et al. Topical timolol administration reduces the incidence of glaucomatous damage in ocular hypertensive individuals. Arch Ophthalmol 1989;107:1590. *(Evidence that lowering intraocular pressure reduces the incidence of glaucomatous damage in ocular hypertensive individuals.)*

Keltner JL, Johnson CA. Screening for visual field abnormalities with automated perimetry. Surv Ophthalmol 1983;28:175. *(An expensive but sensitive screening method.)*

Levi L, Schwartz B. Glaucoma screening in the health care setting. Surv Ophthalmol 1983;28:164. *(A review of available data concluding that physicians should use ophthalmoscopy in screening.)*

Margolis KL, Money BE, Kopietz LA, et al. Physician recognition of ophthalmoscopic signs of open-angle glaucoma. J Gen Intern Med 1989;4:296. *(An educational program that includes good photographs of the key findings.)*

Mundorf TK, Zimmerman TJ, Nardin GF, et al. Automated perimetry, tonometry, and questionnaire in glaucoma screening. Am J Ophthalmol 1989;108:505. *(Tonometry alone much less sensitive than perimetry.)*

Perkins ES. The Bedford glaucoma survey. I. Long-term follow-up of borderline cases. Br J Ophthalmol 1973;57:179. *(Four percent of 141 patients followed for 5 to 7 years because of ocular hypertension, suspicious discs, or a positive family history developed glaucoma.)*

Pollack IR. The challenge of glaucoma screening. Surv Ophthalmol 1968;13:4. *(Notes the rise in pressure with age and recommends age-specific screening levels.)*

Steinmann WC, Millstein ME, Sinclair SH. Pupillary dilation with tropicamide 1% for funduscopic screening. Ann Intern Med 1987;107:181. *(An approach to pupillary dilation in primary care practice.)*

199
Evaluation of the Red Eye
ROGER F. STEINERT, M.D.

Primary Care Medicine: Office Evaluation and Management of the Adult Patient, 3rd edition, edited by Allan H. Goroll, Lawrence A. May, and Albert G. Mulley, Jr. J.B. Lippincott Company, Philadelphia

The red eye is the most common eye problem encountered by the primary care physician. Most cases represent benign self-limited disorders that can be expeditiously diagnosed and treated by the primary physician; however, because redness of the eye may signal serious disease that threatens vision, the physician must be aware of the differential diagnosis and able to conduct a proper initial evaluation.

PATHOPHYSIOLOGY AND CLINICAL PRESENTATION

Redness of the eye and the periocular tissues reflects inflammation or hemorrhage. Causes of inflammation include bacterial, viral, chlamydial, and fungal infections, allergic responses, immune disorders, elevated intraocular pressure, environmental and pharmacologic irritants, foreign bodies, and trauma. Hemorrhage may be due to laceration, contusion, coagulopathy, or concomitant infection.

The pattern of conjunctival injection provides important clues in differential diagnosis. Corneal or intraocular inflammation produces "ciliary flush," dilatation of the fine capillaries around the corneal border producing a red–violet halo. Larger, deep episcleral vessels may also be engorged. Primary conjunctivitis induces diffuse vessel engorgement on the palpebral as well as bulbar conjunctiva, without a ciliary flush. The clinical presentations of various causes of red eye are distinctive (Table 199–1).

A red eye may be due to pathology in the conjunctiva, cornea, uveal tract, eyelids, or orbit.

Conjunctival Pathology

Conjunctivitis is the most common cause of a red eye. Discharge, conjunctival erythema (especially of the peripheral bulbar segment), normal vision, lids stuck together in the morning, and absence of photophobia are the major manifestations. The etiology may be infectious, allergic, or chemical.

Bacterial conjunctivitis is characterized by a mucopurulent discharge and usually occurs unilaterally without preauricular adenopathy. The eyelids have a thick crust on them after a night's sleep. *Pneumococcus* is most commonly the infectious agent in temperate zones, and *Haemophilus aegyptius* in tropical climates. Grossly purulent conjunctivitis suggests *Neisseria infection,* which may scar or perforate the cornea or lead to systemic dissemination. Chronic conjunctivitis is often due to *Staphylococcus aureus* or *Moraxella lacunata*. Concomitant sterile marginal corneal ulcers are common with chronic staph infection.

Chlamydial conjunctivitis, transmitted from the genitourinary tract, occurs as bilateral "inclusion conjunctivitis" in sexually active young adults. Exudate is profuse, and preauricular adenopathy is common.

Trachoma is a major cause of blindness worldwide but is rare in the United States except among American Indians in the Southwest. However, the rapidly increasing rate of chlamydial cervicitis (see Chapter 115) among young women raises the risk of trachoma in a much wider population of newborns.

Viral conjunctivitis is characterized by watery, sometimes mucoid discharge, often beginning in one eye but spreading to the other eye several days later. Preauricular adenopathy is common. It may be associated with fever and pharyngitis (pharyngoconjunctival fever), particularly in children. Epidemic keratoconjunctivitis (EKC) is a highly contagious adenoviral infection that may be accompanied by corneal epithelial defects in the first week and subepithelial infiltrates in the second week, with some diminution of vision. Pseudomembranes or scarring of the conjunctiva may occur and sometimes is painful.

Allergic conjunctivitis may be associated with seasonal allergies and atopic dermatitis and is characterized by bilateral itching and clear tears. Vernal keratoconjunctivitis is a

Table 199-1. Some Important Causes of Red Eye

Conjunctival Disease
Infection (bacterial, viral, chlamydial)
Allergy
Foreign body
Subconjunctival hemorrhage
Pinguecula
Pterygium
Episcleritis
Scleritis
Abrasion
Corneal Disease
Herpes simplex
Adenovirus
Herpes zoster
Keratoconjunctivitis sicca
Exposure keratopathy
Chemical trauma
Corneal ulceration (with or without concomitant infection)
Uveal Tract Disease
Primary iritis and choroiditis
Secondary iritis (infection, trauma)
Systemic diseases (collagen vascular)
Diseases of the Eyelid and Orbit
Blepharitis
Chalazion
Hordeolum
Dacryocystitis
Cellulitis
Hemorrhage
Intraocular Disease
Acute glaucoma

chronic recurrent hypersensitivity reaction that may lead to the formation of corneal ulcers.

Bilateral sterile conjunctival inflammation occurs in acne rosacea, Reiter's syndrome, and Stevens-Johnson syndrome.

Hypersensitivity to eye medications may cause erythema of the external lids, especially at the lateral canthus. *Angioneurotic edema* of the lids may occur bilaterally as an allergic response to a systemic allergen, often food, or unilaterally secondary to exposure to local allergens such as topical chemicals, poison ivy, and insect bites; it develops rapidly and resolves in 1 to 2 days. Edema without erythema suggests allergy.

Pinguecula is a yellow harmless nodule of the scleral conjunctiva, usually found on the nasal side, causing only mild discoloration. However, a related disorder, *pterygium,* is vascularized. It causes redness and encroaches on the cornea. The condition is most common in patients heavily exposed to strong sunlight.

Subconjunctival hemorrhage usually occurs secondary to trauma, although the patient may be unaware of the minor trauma involved. In patients receiving anticoagulant medications, spontaneous subconjunctival hemorrhage may be a sign of overdosage. Massive subconjunctival hemorrhage accompanied by proptosis and limited extraocular movements, usually after trauma, signals orbital hemorrhage, which may compromise the optic nerve and retinal circulation.

Foreign body on the bulbar conjunctiva or under either the upper or lower lid may result in copious tearing, conjunctival injection, and a sensation that something has gotten "into" the eye. On occasion, the foreign body may be well tolerated, with the eye remaining white and quiet.

Episcleritis is usually a benign inflammation of superficial episcleral vessels. The conjunctiva manifests areas of circumscribed nodular inflammation, seen in association with collagen disease, gout, allergic conditions, and such skin diseases as psoriasis. The patient complains of tender irritated eyes. Vision and lids are normal, the corneas are clear, and the conjunctivae show local raised areas of redness.

Scleritis, often associated with rheumatoid arthritis and other immune disorders, is a potentially destructive inflammation of the collagen in the deep episcleral vessels and the sclera. The eye is sometimes painful. Fortunately, scleritis is rare. An experienced observer is required to make the diagnosis.

Corneal Disease

Keratitis presents with a perilimbal ciliary flush, accompanied by clear tears and photophobia. Corneal ulcers detected by fluorescein staining may be sterile or caused by bacteria, viruses, or fungi. Particularly distinctive is the "dendritic" figure of herpes simplex keratitis, in which the epithelium stains in a fine, branching pattern. Herpes simplex and zoster may also cause broader, "geographic" defects. *Staphylococcus aureus* may cause a sterile infiltrate in the corneal limbus.

Corneal abrasions stain with fluorescein but have no infiltrate unless they are untreated for several days. *Hyphema* (blood layering in the anterior chamber) indicates severe trauma and requires ophthalmologic consultation. *Recurrent erosion* presents as an epithelial defect at the site of an abrasion that occurred months or years before and was often caused by organic material (eg, tree branch, fingernail). It may also occur in corneal dystrophies. In both instances, it is due to a defect in epithelial adherence to the underlying stroma. A *corneal foreign body* may cause tearing and hyperemia with little sensation of a foreign body. This is particularly true of rust rings left by ferrous foreign bodies. Dry eyes can cause intense reactions secondary to superficial keratitis, as does overwearing of contact lenses (corneal hypoxia) and ultraviolet keratitis. *Corneal laceration* with perforation is suggested by a shallow or absent anterior chamber, markedly decreased intraocular pressure, and eccentric pupil with iris prolapse into the wound.

Chemical keratoconjunctivitis is a common industrial injury due to a splash of an irritant solution. The conjunctiva is uniformly red, the pupil constricted, vision decreased, the cornea hazy, and the eye painful because of spasm of the iris.

Uveal Tract Disease

Uveitis refers to inflammation of the uveal tract, including the iris, ciliary body, and choroid. The diagnosis is suggested by pain, photophobia, redness, and ciliary flush. Iritis presents with eye pain, photophobia, redness, and pupillary contraction. It may be unilateral or bilateral; if unilateral, the pupil is smaller than that of the other eye because of spasm. Flashlight examination shows a slightly cloudy anterior chamber. Slit lamp examination discloses cells in the anterior chamber and "flare," representing increased aqueous humor protein. Inflammatory cells, called "keratic precipitates," may collect in clusters on the posterior cornea.

Iritis and uveitis are usually idiopathic, but may be associated with a large number of systemic and ocular diseases. *Ankylosing spondylitis, sprue, granulomatous colitis, tuberculosis, sarcoidosis,* and *juvenile rheumatoid arthritis* are sometimes associated with uveitis. The HLA-B27 tissue antigen is strongly associated with iritis, often accompanied by ankylosing spondylitis or *Behçet's disease*. Secondary iritis occurs in response to blunt trauma or corneal inflammation.

Eyelid and Orbital Disease

Blepharitis connotes inflammation involving the structures of the lid margin with redness, scaling, and crusting. Examination of the lid margin may reveal inspissated sebaceous material. Staphylococcal blepharitis causes dry scales, lash loss, and sometimes conjunctivitis and corneal limbal infiltrates. Seborrheic blepharitis is associated with greasy scales and less redness. Blepharitis tends to be chronic with acute flare-ups and is more common in fair-skinned people.

Hordeolum is an acute staphylococcal infection of the meibomian glands (internal hordeolum) or of the glands of Zeis or Moll around the lashes (external hordeolum or sty). It may present as diffuse redness, tenderness, and edema, localized only by an inspissated meibomian gland. An internal hordeolum may point either to the skin or conjunctival side of the lid, whereas an external hordeolum always points to the skin. Hordeolum may produce a diffuse superficial lid infection known as "preseptal cellulitis."

Chalazion is a sterile granulomatous inflammation of the meibomian gland, which may be tender and mildly inflamed or a quiet, discrete mass.

Acute dacryocystitis is a tender, warm, localized infection of the tear ducts over the lateral nose; purulent material may be expressed from the tear duct on the application of pressure.

Hemorrhage in the lids or forehead, either spontaneous or traumatic, may rapidly dissect along the tissue planes of the lids and cause an impressive generalized ecchymosis, greatly alarming the patient.

Orbital cellulitis is usually caused by gram-positive organisms that enter the orbit either directly from the sinuses or through venous channels. It presents as swollen, red eyelids with chemosis, exophthalmos, pain, fever, and leukocytosis. If it progresses, it may lead to paresis of the third, fourth, and sixth cranial nerves, or the ophthalmic division of the fifth, signs of the very serious complication *cavernous sinus thrombosis*.

Intraocular Disease

Acute glaucoma is an ocular emergency that presents as a painful, red eye with prominent ciliary flush. The pupil is mid-dilated and fixed, and the cornea is cloudy secondary to edema. Intraocular pressure exceeds 40 mm Hg and may reach 70 to 80 mm Hg. The patient reports cloudy vision, colored rings around lights (due to corneal edema), and unilateral headache, often accompanied by nausea and vomiting, occasionally leading the physician to consider an acute abdomen. Acute glaucoma is usually due to closure in eyes with narrow angles but may be due to inflammatory cells or red blood cells in the anterior chamber, neovascularization of the iris (rubeosis iridis), or peripheral anterior synechiae.

DIFFERENTIAL DIAGNOSIS

The causes of red eye can be divided anatomically into the categories of conjunctival, corneal, uveal, eyelid–orbital, and intraocular disease (see Table 199–1). Differentiation can usually be made on clinical grounds (Table 199–2).

WORKUP

History is directed toward ascertaining the duration of redness, rapidity of onset, the patient's activity at the time, and the degree and quality of symptoms. Ophthalmologic history and medications should be noted. Key symptoms include visual changes, pain, itching, crusting in the morning, tearing, mucoid or purulent discharge, photophobia, and foreign body sensation. Although usually helpful, the history can be misleading, because viral conjunctivitis may be accompanied by itching or a foreign body sensation, or the patient may ascribe the symptoms of herpes simplex keratitis to a "chemical in the eye" because she first noted the symptoms after a home hair permanent.

Table 199-2. The Red Eye

	CONJUNCTIVITIS			CORNEAL INJURY OR INFECTION	IRITIS	ACUTE GLAUCOMA
	Bacterial	*Viral*	*Allergic*			
Vision	–	–	–	↓ or ↓↓	↓	↓↓
Pain	–	–	–	+	+	+++
Photophobia	–	±	–	+	++	–
Foreign body sensation	–	±	±	+	–	–
Itch	±	±	++	–	–	–
Tearing	+	++	+	++	+	–
Discharge	Mucopurulent	Mucoid	–	–	–	–
Preauricular adenopathy	–	+	–	⋆	–	–
Pupils	–	–	–	NL or small†	Small	Mid-dilated and fixed
Conjunctival hyperemia	Diffuse	Diffuse	Diffuse	Diffuse and ciliary flush	Ciliary flush	Diffuse and ciliary flush
Cornea	Clear	Sometimes faint punctate staining or infiltrates	Clear	Depends on disorder	Clear or lightly cloudy	Cloudy
Intraocular pressure	NL	NL	NL	NL‡	↓, NL or ↑	↑↑

⋆In herpes keratitis.
†Indicates secondary iritis.
‡Very low in perforating trauma.

Physical Examination. Accurate measurement of visual acuity, preferably at a distance, is essential. If it is abnormal, it is important to check for uncorrected optical abnormality by use of a pinhole. Any patient with reduced vision not readily explained by a preexisting or obviously harmless condition needs immediate referral to an ophthalmologist. Mucus and tearing may reduce vision one or two lines at most. Corneal lesions may further reduce vision, with only partial improvement on pinhole testing; a central epithelial abrasion typically maintains vision at about 20/100 or better. Preauricular nodes should be palpated. A complete examination of the eye and fundus is important. The lid margins should be inspected for crusting, ulceration, inspissations, and masses, and the conjunctiva for distribution of redness, ciliary flush, foreign bodies (including lid eversion), and, if a slit lamp is available, follicles and papillae. Corneal clarity is noted with a flashlight, and a direct ophthalmoscope set at about +15 diopters can be used to magnify corneal details.

If fluorescein stain is available, it can be used in conjunction with a blue filter to visualize the cornea for infection and other injury. However, if there is any suspicion of corneal injury, referral is needed quickly for slit lamp examination.

Intraocular pressure should be determined if glaucoma is suspected. Depth of the anterior chamber of the other eye can be assessed by a flashlight aimed parallel to the iris (coronal plane) from the temporal side. A shallow anterior chamber is usually convex and will cast a shadow on the nasal iris.

Laboratory studies are usually the responsibility of an ophthalmologist. The primary practitioner may attempt conjunctival smears, which show polymorphonuclear leukocytes in acute bacterial conjunctivitis, lymphocytes in viral or late bacterial conjunctivitis, and eosinophils in allergic reactions. This is time-consuming and generally not necessary. Purulent discharges should be cultured on blood agar and, if *Neisseria* is suspected, plated on chocolate agar and Gram stained. Scrapings for inclusion bodies in suspected chlamydial or viral disease are usually unrewarding, and scraping and culture of an infected corneal ulcer require an ophthalmologist.

White blood cell and differential counts are indicated, as are blood cultures, in suspected cellulitis. Clotting studies for subconjunctival hemorrhage are not indicated unless other evidence of coagulopathy is present or the patient is being treated with anticoagulants (see Chapter 85).

PRINCIPLES OF MANAGEMENT AND INDICATIONS FOR REFERRAL

Red eye problems associated with eye pain, visual disturbance, or corneal damage require immediate referral, as does acute glaucoma. In most other situations, the primary physician can provide symptomatic relief or at least first aid. A nonophthalmologist should never prescribe topical steroid or steroid–antibiotic combination drops, because infection may worsen and a corneal ulcer may rapidly form and cause perforation.

Conjunctival Disease. Conjunctivitis, in the absence of photophobia, eye pain, or change in visual acuity, can be managed by the primary physician. *Viral conjunctivitis* is contagious, and live virus is shed in the tears for up to 2 weeks. The patient should be instructed to refrain from rubbing the eye and transmitting infection to the other eye or to another person. Treatment is expectant, because the condition is self-limited, usually clearing within 2 to 3 weeks. Cases that fail to improve spontaneously should be referred to the ophthalmologist.

Bacterial conjunctivitis responds well to erythromycin ophthalmic ointment (prescribed qid) or polymyxin/trimethoprim (Polytrim) drops (prescribed qid). Improvement is usually noted in several days. Bacitracin ophthalmic ointment and sodium sulfacetamide are alternative antibiotics. Neomycin causes allergic keratitis in 5 percent of patients treated topically and should be avoided if possible. More potent topical antibiotics such as the aminoglycosides and fluoroquinolones should not be used for routine conjunctivitis.

Allergic conjunctivitis in seasonal allergies is relieved by cool compresses and decongestant–antihistamine drops (Vasocon-A, Naphcon-A, Albalon-A) four times daily. However, long-term use of these drops is not recommended, because marked rebound vasodilation may develop. Ketorolac ophthalmic drops (a nonsteroidal antiinflammatory agent) may help alleviate allergic symptoms. Oral antihistamines are another alternative. Severe allergic conditions may require topical steroid therapy instituted by an ophthalmologist.

Subconjunctival hemorrhage usually requires only reassurance; compresses (initially cool, then warm) and erythromycin ophthalmic ointment or a lubricating ointment may reduce discomfort in cases with marked swelling.

Conjunctival foreign bodies are usually easily removed with a cotton swab or fine forceps; erythromycin ointment tid for 2 days is adequate for healing.

Eye Lid and Orbital Disease. *Blepharitis* usually responds to lid hygiene measures and topical antibiotics. One can instruct the patient to dilute Johnson's baby shampoo 50:50 with water and use a cotton ball to scrub the lids well with the eyes closed. After rinsing with water, a hot compress is applied to the closed lids for 5 to 10 minutes, and then erythromycin or bacitracin ophthalmic ointment is instilled in the inferior fornix. The excess is rubbed into the eyelash base. Carrying out this procedure as many as three to four times daily will improve most cases. After improvement is obtained, the lids can be maintained by nightly lid hygiene and warm compresses. An occasional stubborn case will require nightly antibiotic ointment as prophylaxis.

A *hordeolum* may respond to this treatment or, like *chalazia,* may require incision and curettage by an ophthalmologist. *Mild cellulitis* of the lid margin (preseptal cellulitis) responds to topical treatment plus oral antibiotics. Dicloxacillin (250 mg qid) is a good first choice. Erythromycin (250–500 mg PO tid) is an effective alternative for patients who are penicillin allergic. Warm compresses and oral antibiotics are also indicated for *acute dacryocystitis,* but persistent localized abscess requires incision and drainage by an ophthalmologist. Orbital cellulitis and cavernous sinus thrombosis are medical emergencies that require immediate hospitalization for intravenous therapy.

Mild hypersensitivity reactions of the lids respond rapidly to discontinuation of the offending agent and application of cool compresses. Systemic antihistamines are useful in moderate reactions, and steroids are useful in severe reactions.

Traumatic lid ecchymoses are minimized by cool compresses and ice packs applied early. Later, warm compresses speed resolution.

Corneal Disease. *Corneal ulcers* require intensive emergency evaluation and treatment by an ophthalmologist. Patients with typical herpes simplex dendritic keratitis may be started on idoxuridine drops or vidarabine ointment five times daily and erythromycin ointment twice daily if an ophthalmologist is not available. *Corneal abrasions* heal rapidly with erythromycin ointment and a tight sterile patch that prevents lid motion for 24 to 48 hours. If the initial abrasion was sizable (roughly 25% of the cornea or more), healing should be checked after removal of the patch. Lesions of this size also require cycloplegia for relief of painful secondary iritis during healing (see iritis treatment). After reepithelialization occurs, ointment applied three times daily for 4 days helps complete the healing process.

Cases involving *foreign bodies* are treated with vigorous irrigation. Rust rings are treated like abrasions once the foreign body has been washed away. Foreign bodies that do not wash away with irrigation can be removed with a cotton swab, a sterile "golf stick," or an 18-gauge needle with a syringe as a handle, but such removal should not be attempted by the nonophthalmologist unless specifically trained to do so. Rust on the surface is easily debrided, but scraping is prohibited because it will damage Bowman's membrane and cause permanent scarring. Left untreated, rust may be irritating but will surface and slough in 1 or 2 weeks.

Contact lens overwear and *ultraviolet keratitis* respond to brief cycloplegia, erythromycin ointment, and sterile pressure patching for 24 hours. The associated pain often requires codeine.

Suspected *corneal laceration* and *perforation* is an ophthalmic emergency. A protective metal shield ("Fox shield") should be placed over the eye; no medication should be instilled.

Uveal Tract Disease. An ophthalmologist must evaluate and treat *primary iritis*, but initial cycloplegia by tropicamide 1% qid or cyclopentolate 1% qid will prevent posterior synechia formation and relieve pain. *Iritis* secondary to corneal abrasion may be treated with these medications or, in an eye that will be patched for 1 or 2 days, several drops of scopolamine 0.25% will provide longer cycloplegia. The nonophthalmologist should avoid atropine because its effects persist for 1 to 2 weeks.

Intraocular Disease. *Acute glaucoma* should be treated by immediate administration of acetazolamide, 500 mg IV, and glycerol, 120 cc orally in orange juice. Pilocarpine 2% should be begun with instillation as frequently as every 15 minutes to break the attack. Immediate attention by an ophthalmologist is necessary because the only definitive treatment is laser or surgical iridotomy.

ANNOTATED BIBLIOGRAPHY

Bienfang DC, Kelly LD, Nicholson DH, et al. Ophthalmology. N Engl J Med 1990;323:956. *(Excellent review and overview for the general reader; 115 refs.)*

Rosenbaum JT, Nozik RA. Uveitis: Many diseases, one diagnosis. Am J Med 1985;79:545. *(Terse review of the differential diagnosis.)*

Shingleton BJ, Hersh PS, Kenyon KR. Eye Trauma. Philadelphia: Mosby; 1991. *(The definitive text on the subject; includes detailed sections on management of foreign bodies and abrasions.)*

Steinert RF. Current therapy for bacterial ketatitis and bacterial conjunctivitis. Am J Ophthalmology 1991;112:10S-14S. *(Treatment options and indications.)*

Thoft RA. Corneal disease. N Engl J Med 1978;298:1239. *(Remains a very good summary for the generalist reader.)*

Vaughan D, Asbury T. General Ophthalmology. Ed 12. Los Alto: Lange; 1989. *(A practical and inexpensive reference that includes useful photographs of conditions causing a red eye.)*

200
Evaluation of Impaired Vision

CLAUDIA U. RICHTER, M.D.

Primary Care Medicine: Office Evaluation and Management of the Adult Patient, 3rd edition, edited by Allan H. Goroll, Lawrence A. May, and Albert G. Mulley, Jr. J.B. Lippincott Company, Philadelphia

Patients with decreasing or blurred vision often refer themselves directly to an eye specialist, but at times they first present to their primary physician. Sudden visual loss is a medical emergency. Gradual diminution of sight raises the specter of eventual blindness and inability to function independently. Paradoxically, some elderly patients may not volunteer that their vision is decreasing because they consider it a natural part of aging. Consequently, the primary physician needs to screen elderly patients for treatable causes of decreased vision. In addition, one should be capable of distinguishing visual impairment due to refractive error, cataracts, glaucoma, retinal disease, and trauma to provide proper initial care and appropriate referral.

PATHOPHYSIOLOGY AND CLINICAL PRESENTATION

Vision is impaired when there is a change in the refracting surfaces of the eye, opacification of the transparent ocular media, damage to the photoreceptor cells of the retina, or a lesion of the optic nerve, its radiations, or the visual cortex. Anatomic orientation provides a framework for considering the pathophysiology of visual difficulties, beginning with the cornea and working inward.

Refractive error remains the most common cause of decreased visual acuity. It results from the inability of the eye to focus light precisely on the retina and may be due to an abnormality in the cornea, lens, or size of the globe. Myopic patients commonly present during their teens and early 20s. Patients in their 40s may report decreased visual acuity but, in fact, simply cannot accommodate to near distances and require reading glasses. Early cataracts can increase myopia before they opacify and block transmission of light. Uncontrolled diabetes mellitus can produce swelling of the lens and myopia, which resolves with control of the blood sugar. Sulfonamides, thiazides, and anticholinergic agents may cause blurred vision.

Eyelid and Corneal Disease. Occasionally, sudden visual loss results from eyelids being closed by *swelling* due to trauma, insect bites, cellulitis, or angioneurotic edema. Acute *blepharospasm* secondary to ocular surface pain may be described as inability to see.

The cornea is the major refracting surface of the eye, and any change in it can lead to visual disturbances. A *corneal abrasion,* herpes simplex virus keratitis, or ulcer causes irregularity of the corneal epithelium and opacity of the normally clear cornea. *Acute glaucoma* causes sudden visual loss by producing corneal edema. Corneal dystrophies or degenerations result in a more gradual reduction in visual acuity, often progressing over a period of years.

The *anterior chamber* may be opacified by inflammatory cells resulting from iritis or red blood cells resulting from a *hyphema.*

Cataracts, opacifications of the lens, are a leading cause of gradual vision loss in older patients. The usual history is one of a painless, slow deterioration of eyesight. However, a traumatic cataract may develop over a period of hours to days.

Vitreous opacification occurs most often from *hemorrhage,* less commonly from inflammation or infection. Proliferative diabetic retinopathy, a retinal hole or detachment, trauma, sickle cell retinopathy, hypertension, and clotting abnormalities may cause vitreous hemorrhage. A vitreous *floater* may transiently blur vision or be called a blind spot.

Glaucoma may damage nerve fibers at the optic disk and cause visual field defects. Four types of visual field defects occur: paracentral scotomas occurring along the distribution of the arcuate nerve fiber bundle, arcuate scotomata, sector-shaped defects, and nasal steps. As the disease progresses, these visual field defects enlarge. Central vision remains intact until late in the disease, but even this may be lost. The optic cup becomes enlarged and irregular (see Chapter 198). Acute angle-closure glaucoma produces a red eye, fixed pupil, hazy cornea, eye pain, and acute impairment of vision. Acute angle-closure glaucoma accounts for less than 5 percent of all glaucoma cases. Most visual loss due to glaucoma is gradual and progressive (see Chapter 207).

Retinal Injury. The retina may be compromised by degeneration, inflammation, trauma, detachment, or ischemia.

Senile macular degeneration occurs in patients over age 55 and is a leading cause of legal blindness. Central vision is impaired whereas peripheral vision remains intact. Fundoscopic examination may show loss of the foveal reflex, macular drusen, atrophy of the retinal pigment epithelium with prominent choroidal vessels, subretinal edema or hemorrhage, or a central fibrous scar. Some 15 percent of patients with senile macular degeneration have treatable disease, presenting with early visual symptoms and a subretinal neovascular net that can be obliterated with laser photocoagulation. They need to be seen promptly to maximize their chances of effective treatment. Those at particular risk of developing exudative senile macular degeneration have drusen or a disciform scar in one macula. They should screen their central vision daily with an Amsler grid (see Chapter 206).

A host of other retinal problems may lead to loss of vision. *Central serous retinopathy* is an idiopathic, spontaneous *detachment* of the retina in the macular area. Patients range in age from 20 to 50 years old. Central vision is reduced, but recovery is usually spontaneous within a few months. *Inflammation* of the retina and choroid, such as histoplasmosis, toxoplasmosis, cytomegalovirus, or herpes virus infections, can involve the macula or produce a vitritis, decreasing vision.

Cytomegalovirus (CMV) retinitis is of concern in HIV-infected patients and important to recognize because it is treatable. Spread to the eye is hematogenous. Initially, eye involvement may be asymptomatic, followed later by losses of visual acuity and visual fields. Fundoscopic manifestations include perivascular yellow-white retinal lesions presenting as a focal white granular infiltrate with or without hemorrhage, expanding in a "brush-fire" pattern.

Trauma may cause retinal edema and decreased visual acuity when it occurs in the macular region. This edema resolves within a few days.

Retinal detachment may be extensive and cause decreased visual acuity or be small and noted as a minor field defect. Flashing lights and a *shower of vitreous floaters* may presage a retinal detachment. As a detachment extends, the patient may note that the visual field defect progresses like a shade being drawn. A detached retina appears ballooned forward with undulating folds.

Systemic diseases may involve the retina and cause decreased vision. Vascular injury is the most common mechanism, as occurs with hypertension, diabetes mellitus, and systemic lupus erythematosus. Infiltrative disease may also affect the retina.

Optic Nerve Damage. The *vasculature* of the *retina* or *optic nerve* may be compromised, leading to sudden visual loss. The vascular diseases involving the arteries include central retinal artery occlusion, giant-cell arteritis, and anterior ischemic optic neuropathy. In *central retinal artery occlusion,* there is sudden, painless loss of ability to perceive light or hand movements. The patient may have had previous episodes of amaurosis fugax with fleeting blindness lasting 10 to 15 minutes. Ophthalmoscopy reveals a pale optic disk, attenuated arterioles, "boxcar" veins, hazy edematous retina, and a *cherry-red spot* in the macula. Occasionally, an *embolus* may be seen at a bifurcation of a retinal arteriole.

The most common embolic source is an atheromatous plaque in the ipsilateral carotid artery.

Giant-cell or *temporal arteritis,* a granulomatous inflammation of the medium and large arteries in elderly people, may cause sudden visual loss (see Chapter 161). These patients may have premonitory visual symptoms similar to amaurosis fugax and may have symptoms of polymyalgia rheumatica. The fundus examination may reveal a swollen optic disk, a normal optic disk, or a central retinal artery occlusion.

Anterior ischemic optic neuropathy is produced by ischemia to the anterior portion of the optic nerve. The patient notes decreased visual acuity or a visual field defect, usually involving the superior or inferior visual field and the macula. The optic disk initially appears edematous, sometimes in just one portion, with a few flame-shaped hemorrhages. Optic atrophy follows the disk edema. The most common etiology is *thrombosis* of an arteriosclerotic vessel. The patients tend to be younger than those affected by giant-cell arteritis and have hypertension or diabetes mellitus.

Central or branch *retinal vein occlusions* cause a sudden painless decrease in visual acuity. In central retinal vein occlusion, the *fundus* has a classic *"blood and thunder"* appearance: the veins are tortuous and dilated and the retina is edematous and covered with flame-shaped hemorrhages. The optic disk margin is blurred. The fundus changes in branch retinal vein occlusion are similar, but limited to the distribution of the involved vein. Decreased visual acuity is due to macular edema and ischemia. In central retinal vein occlusion, 20 percent of patients have preexisting chronic open-angle glaucoma, and 50 percent of men have preexisting hypertension. In branch retinal vein occlusion, 75 percent have preexisting hypertension.

Optic neuritis, inflammation of the optic nerve, presents with a relatively acute impairment of vision in young persons (ages 15 to 40). It is usually idiopathic, but 20 percent to 50 percent eventually develop clinical *multiple sclerosis.* Clinically, there is progressive loss of vision over hours to days, typically unilateral, with pain on eye motion and improved visual function in the second to third week. Examination reveals an afferent pupillary defect, globe tenderness, visual field defects, and impairment of color vision.

Infiltrative or compressive lesions of the optic nerve, such as pituitary adenomas, meningiomas, gliomas, or internal carotid artery aneurysms, cause gradual visual field loss. It is unusual for lesions posterior to the optic chiasm to present with decreased visual acuity because of the decussation of fibers in the optic chiasm. Unilateral lesions, such as a tumor or a cerebrovascular accident, cause a homonymous hemianopsia or related visual field defect. Bilateral central nervous system lesions may cause profound visual loss.

Many patients complain of blurred vision at night. Rarely, these patients may be found to have true *night blindness* caused by retinitis pigmentosa or vitamin A deficiency. More commonly, no etiology is found; a slight decrease in visual acuity at night is common and normal.

Psychogenic pathology sometimes presents as visual loss or compromise. Characteristically, the eye examination and objective measures of visual function that do not require the patient's report are intact. Hysteria and malingering account for most psychogenic cases.

DIFFERENTIAL DIAGNOSIS

The causes of visual impairment can be logically considered in terms of anatomic site affected (Table 200–1). The leading causes of blindness include cataracts, open-angle glaucoma, and macular degeneration.

WORKUP

History is most important in evaluating a complaint of visual loss. It is essential to establish the onset, duration, clinical course, and pattern of visual loss. Any associated visual phenomena should be ascertained as well as any pain. The presence of premonitory symptoms is helpful. Acute loss is suggestive of a vascular event or retinal detachment. Preceding episodes of amaurosis fugax indicate central retinal artery occlusion or giant-cell arteritis. A sudden flurry of flashes of light (photopsia) and vitreous floaters may herald a retinal detachment. Scintillating scotomata may herald mi-

Table 200-1. Causes of Impaired Vision

Eyelids
Edema
Blepharospasm
Cornea
Abrasion
Edema
Degeneration
Infection
Anterior Chamber
Inflammatory cells (from iritis)
Hyphema
Lens
Cataract
Swelling (as in poorly controlled diabetes)
Vitreous
Hemorrhage
Floaters
Retina
Senile macular degeneration
Central serous retinopathy
Inflammation
Trauma
Detachment
Diabetes
Hypertension
Infection (CMV retinitis)
Vasculature
Central retinal artery occlusion
Giant-cell (cranial or temporal) arteritis
Anterior ischemic optic neuropathy
Retinal vein occlusion
Optic Nerve
Compression (glaucoma, tumor)
Psychiatric
Hysteria
Malingering
Refractive error

graine. Progressive visual loss points to a chronic disturbance, such as cataract, macular degeneration, or glaucoma. Previous episodes of decreased visual acuity with halos around lights and pain indicate angle-closure glaucoma. A foreign body sensation indicates a corneal abrasion, foreign body, or herpes simplex keratitis. The presence of other diseases such as diabetes mellitus, hypertension, heart disease, or sickle cell anemia may be contributory. A history of trauma is important to note.

Physical Examination and Laboratory Studies. *Visual acuity testing* should be done formally, one eye at a time. If the patient complains of pain, a topical anesthetic such as proparacaine should be used to allow testing. If the lids are tightly swollen, it may be necessary to pry them apart forcibly. The patient should wear his or her glasses. A Snellen eye chart with its standardized letter sizes is most convenient, but if one is not available any printed material can be used. One notes the size of the smallest print the patient can read and the distance at which he or she can read it. If letters cannot be read, the distance at which the patient can accurately count fingers or identify hand motions is noted. If targets cannot be seen, it is important to determine whether the eye can perceive light. Vision is rechecked with the patient looking through a pinhole to eliminate any residual refractive error.

The *pupils* should be examined carefully, noting size, direct and consensual reactions to light, and presence of any afferent pupillary defect. An afferent pupillary defect may be found in optic neuritis, central retinal artery occlusion, giant-cell arteritis, and extensive retinal diseases. A fixed pupil in conjunction with a red eye is indicative of acute angle-closure glaucoma.

The *conjunctiva* is examined to determine whether the eye is red and inflamed or white and quiet. With the exception of trauma, acute glaucoma, and infection, the diseases that cause sudden visual loss do not cause a red eye (see Chapter 199). The *cornea* normally is clear with a crisp light reflex and no fluorescein stain. If a tonometer is available, the *intraocular pressure* should be measured.

Ophthalmoscopy is important; it should first be noted whether the *fundus* can be visualized or if a dense cataract or vitreous opacity is present. If the fundus can be visualized, the optic disk is examined for papilledema or atrophy. The *macula* is examined, looking for a cherry-red spot, hemorrhages, and scars. The *fundoscopic vessels* are examined, with attention paid to the caliber and the presence of visible emboli. Patients over age 50 with sudden visual loss should have a careful check for temporal arteritis, which includes palpation of the *cranial arteries* for tenderness, enlargement, and loss of pulsation and determination of the *erythrocyte sedimentation rate* for marked elevation (see Chapter 161).

If a patient is a malingerer or hysterical, the examination of the eye will be normal, including opticokinetic responses, stereoscopic vision, and visual fields. One can quickly check *opticokinetic responses* by passing the front page of a newspaper before the eyes of the patient.

Vision Screening in Primary Care Practice. Often, adults with gradual onset of visual impairment do not recognize or complain of their deficit. In addition, many patients being cared for by primary care physicians (especially hypertensives, diabetics, and the elderly) are at increased risk for potentially serious eye disease that may compromise vision. Yield for detection of important eye pathology can be high when persons at increased risk are screened by a brief ophthalmologic history complemented by Snellen chart testing of visual acuity. Findings indicative of benefit from ophthalmologic referral include age over 65 years; history of diabetes, glaucoma, eye trauma, eye infection, or other eye problem; and best eye worse than 20/40 by Snellen testing or a difference of greater than two Snellen lines between eyes. Diabetics are particularly well served by referral for a screening opthalmologic examination.

SYMPTOMATIC MANAGEMENT AND INDICATIONS FOR REFERRAL

Patients with sudden visual loss need immediate ophthalmologic consultation. If an ophthalmologist is not immediately available, appropriate emergency measures should be taken.

If a *central retinal artery occlusion* exists that is less than 24 hours old, it is reasonable to attempt heroic measures to salvage vision. The goal is to encourage the embolus to break apart or at least to move distally. First, one can gently *massage the globe* with the fingers to attempt to dislodge the embolus. Next, have the patient *breathe* a *mixture* of *5%* CO_2 and *95%* O_2; this will cause the retinal vessels to vasodilate and allow delivery of a high PO_2 to any viable retinal cells. If this mixture is not available, have the patient *breathe into a paper bag*. Next, give the patient *500 mg intravenous acetazolamide* to decrease the production of aqueous humor and to lower intraocular pressure.

If *giant-cell arteritis* is suspected, the patient should be started at once on high-dose glucocorticosteroids (eg, *prednisone* 60 mg/d) and considered for temporal artery biopsy. Some vision may be salvaged in the affected eye, and the other eye is protected (see Chapter 161).

Acute angle-closure glaucoma should be treated at once with *topical pilocarpine 2%* in both eyes and *acetazolamide 500 mg intravenously*. The pilocarpine acts therapeutically in the involved eye and prophylactically in the uninvolved eye. Pain medication and antiemetics are appropriate. If available, osmotic agents such as intravenous *mannitol* or oral *glycerol* should be used. All patients with acute angle-closure glaucoma need a laser iridotomy or peripheral iridectomy to prevent further attacks.

INDICATIONS FOR REFERRAL

All patients with acute loss of vision should be seen immediately by an ophthalmologist. Individuals suspected of having glaucoma, macular degeneration, retinal vein occlusion, or an infectious etiology as well as those in whom the cause of impaired vision is unclear, should have early ophthalmologic consultation. Diabetics should be referred, even if asymptomatic, because screening can prevent vision loss. Type 1 diabetics require annual ophthalmologic examination starting 5 years after onset of disease. At the time of diagnosis, type 2 diabetics should be referred for a detailed retinal examination and then every 4 years if no abnormalities are found on the first examination. Patients with refractive error should be referred to an eye specialist for proper refraction. Only myopic patients who fail or cannot wear either eyeglasses or contact lenses should be considered for correction by *surgical laser.*

ANNOTATED BIBLIOGRAPHY

Bienfang DC, Kelly LD, Nicholson DH, et al. Ophthalmology. N Engl J Med 1990;323:956. *(Good overview for the general reader.)*

Bloom JN, Palestine AG. The diagnosis of cytomegalovirus retinitis. Ann Intern Med 1988;109;963. *(Required reading for those caring for HIV patients.)*

Margolis KL, Money BE, Kopietz LA, et al. Physician recognition of ophthalmoscopic signs of open-angle glaucoma. J Gen Intern Med 1989;4:296. *(An educational program that includes good photographs of the key findings.)*

Singer DE, Nathan DM, Fogel HA, et al. Screening for diabetic retinopathy. Ann Intern Med 1992;116:660. *(Finds screening beneficial.)*

Strahlman E, Ford D, Whelton P, et al. Vison screening in a primary care practice. Arch Intern Med 1990;150:2159. *(High yield in high-risk persons.)*

Tielsch JM, Sommer A, Witt K, et al. Blindness and visual impairment in an American urban population. Arch Ophthalmol 1990;108:286. *(Important epidemiologic data.)*

201
Evaluation of Eye Pain

ROGER F. STEINERT, M.D.

Primary Care Medicine: Office Evaluation and Management of the Adult Patient, 3rd edition, edited by Allan H. Goroll, Lawrence A. May, and Albert G. Mulley, Jr. J.B. Lippincott Company, Philadelphia

Pain in the eye is most often produced by conditions that do not threaten vision. However, at times, the discomfort may result from corneal or intraocular pathology that is capable of compromising eyesight. The first responsibility of the primary physician is to determine promptly if there is an immediate threat to vision that requires urgent therapy or quick referral to the ophthalmologist; minor problems can be treated symptomatically in the office.

Ocular pain is usually not the only presentation of injury or disease. Several distinct pain categories can be identified that, when combined with assessment of inflammation (see Chapter 199) and vision (see Chapter 200), allow the primary physician to categorize the nature of the problem and make appropriate disposition.

PATHOPHYSIOLOGY AND CLINICAL PRESENTATION

The external ocular surfaces (lid, conjunctiva, and cornea) and the uveal tract are richly innervated to detect pain. Localization within these structures is relatively less precise. The orbit and sinuses may give rise to pain localized to the eye. Pathology confined to the vitreous, retina, or optic nerve is rarely a source of pain.

Eyelids. Inflammation of the eyelid causes tenderness and foreign body sensation. Common causes are hordeolum (stye), trichiasis (inturned lashes), and tarsal foreign bodies. Redness and edema may accompany the pain.

Conjunctiva. Viral and bacterial conjunctivitis cause mild burning and foreign body sensation, whereas allergic conjunctivitis primarily elicits itching (see Chapter 199). Toxic, chemical, and mechanical injuries are commonly responsible for unilateral disease.

Cornea. The cornea is densely innervated by pain fibers, so that even a minor injury may result in considerable discomfort. Pain arises from exposure of nerve endings in the epithelium; the patient complains of a burning or foreign body sensation. Reflex photophobic lacrimation may accompany the discomfort. Blinking exacerbates the pain, which is generally relieved by a pressure patch holding the lid shut.

Keratitis (inflammation of the cornea) occurs with trauma, infection, exposure, vascular disease, or decreased lacrimation. Contact lens use has become an important source of microbial keratitis. Cellular infiltration and loss of corneal luster ensue. If blood vessels invade the normally avascular corneal stroma, vision may become cloudy. Severe pain is a prominent symptom; movement of the lid typically exacerbates symptoms. Fluorescein stain reveals the epithelial defects quite well and allows identification with a penlight.

Sclera. Compared to disease of the eyelids, scleral problems are more likely to cause dull, deep pain. If the condition involves the anterior sclera, it may be readily visible as an area of redness. The blood supply to the sclera is not extensive and its metabolism is relatively inactive. Consequently, inflammatory conditions of the sclera tend to be rather torpid; many are associated with connective tissue disease.

Uveal Tract. Anterior uveitis or iritis is accompanied by a dull ache and photophobia due to the irritative spasm of the pupillary sphincter. Posterior uveitis without anterior involvement may be painless or cause deep-seated aching. Profound ocular and orbital pain radiating to the frontal and temporal regions accompanies sudden elevation of pressure, as in acute angle-closure glaucoma. Vagal stimulation with high pressure may result in nausea and vomiting. Often the patient gives a history of mild intermittent episodes of blurred vision preceding the onset of an attack of throbbing pain, nausea, vomiting, and decreased visual acuity; halos about lights are sometimes noted. A fixed, midposition pupil, redness, and a hazy cornea may be present (see Chapter 207).

Orbit. Inflammation and rapidly expanding mass lesions may cause deep pain. Displacement of the globe and diplopia may ensue. One important etiology is *optic neuritis,* a condition of younger patients (age 15 to 40 years). Onset is acute. Eye movement may cause sharp pain due to meningeal inflammation (the extraocular rectus muscles insert along the dura of the nerve sheath at the orbital apex). Most cases are idiopathic, but 10 percent to 15 percent are associated with multiple sclerosis. As many as 20 percent to 50 percent eventually develop multiple sclerosis. Symptoms include pain on eye movement, abnormal color vision, and some loss of central vision. In most instances, the optic disk appears normal, but occasionally there is edema. A central scotoma may be found.

Sinusitis may also cause secondary orbital inflammation and tenderness on extremes of eye movement. In orbital cellulitis there is proptosis, limitation of extraocular movement, injection, and diminished vision.

Other Sources. Mild headache referred to the orbit is associated with refractive error, ocular muscle imbalance, sinusitis, and other causes of nonocular headache, such as tension headache, temporal arteritis, and the prodromal phase of herpes zoster. Severe aches in the eye cannot be attributed to refractive error, nor can aches about the eye that are noted on awakening in the morning.

DIFFERENTIAL DIAGNOSIS

The causes of eye pain can be considered anatomically (Table 201-1).

Table 201-1. Important Causes of Eye Pain

Extraocular Causes
Lid
Hordeolum (a small abscess of the lid)
Acute dacryocystitis
Cellulitis
Chalazion
Conjunctival
Irritant exposure (prolonged sun exposure, pollution, occupational irritants, aerosol propellants, wind, dust)
Infection (viral or bacterial)
Lack of sleep
Corneal
Incipient zoster
Abrasions
Foreign bodies
Ulcers
Ingrown lashes
Contact lens abuse
Excessive exposure to sun or other forms of UV radiation
Infection (bacterial or viral)
Scleral
Episcleritis
Scleritis (connective tissue disease)
Intraocular Conditions
Anterior Eye
Acute angle-closure glaucoma
Acute anterior uveitis (idiopathic, connective tissue disease, sarcoidosis, inflammatory bowel disease)
Refractive error (mild pain only)
Posterior Eye
Posterior uveitis
Orbital Disease
Tumor
Inflammatory disease
Retrobulbar optic neuritis
Referred Pain from Extraocular Sources
Sinusitis
Tooth abscess
Tension headache
Temporal arteritis
Prodrome of herpes zoster
Ocular muscle imbalance

WORKUP

The initial task is to be sure that there is no threat to vision. Most intraocular conditions that cause eye pain may compromise vision and should be carefully checked for, as should corneal injuries.

History. The quality of the pain needs to be considered. Deep pain is suggestive of an intraocular problem; a foreign body sensation makes it likely that the problem is on the surface of the eye. The patient should be asked about any change in visual acuity or color vision, because any report of deteriorating vision requires urgent ophthalmologic consultation. A history of diplopia and displacement of the eye raises the possibility of an orbital problem. Ascertaining the aggravating and alleviating factors can aid diagnosis. Pain exacerbated by lid movement and relieved by cessation of lid motion is suggestive of a foreign body or corneal lesion. Pain worsened by eye motion may be due to retrobulbar optic neuritis, especially if accompanied by loss of central vision and a normal appearing optic disc. Photophobia is often prominent in acute anterior uveitis. Localization of a extraocular lesion by history is often difficult, because most of the time the foreign body sensation is felt in the outer portion of the upper lid, regardless of the lesion's location. In considering causes of conjunctival irritation, it is important to ask about occupational exposures, trauma, sun, sun lamp, and other forms of ultraviolet radiation (eg, arc welding), as well as foreign body contact. History of sinusitis and headaches should be noted.

Physical Examination. An ophthalmoscope, penlight, ability to perform lid eversion, and use of fluorescein stain can be very helpful for assessment. First, visual acuity, color vision, and extraocular movements should be tested and recorded. The eye, lid, and conjunctiva are inspected for masses and redness, the pupil for reactivity, the cornea for clarity, and the fundus for any abnormalities of the disc. A cloudy cornea in conjunction with a fixed, midposition pupil is consistent with acute glaucoma; the eye may be red. A constricted pupil in the presence of an eye that is tearing excessively suggests anterior uveitis; in severe cases, the eye also may be reddened and the anterior chamber hazy. Finding a central scotoma should raise suspicion of retrobulbar neuritis; a normal appearing disk supports the diagnosis. The upper lid should be inverted with a cotton-tipped applicator to check for a foreign body or chalazion. The penlight can then be used to survey the cornea for gross injury; examination is facilitated by use of a small hand lens. The iris ought to be examined for evidence of dilated vessels around the limbus; this ciliary flush is characteristic of intraocular inflammation and occurs in anterior uveitis. Often the flush cannot be seen without the aid of a slit lamp.

Fluorescein Staining. All but very small corneal epithelial lesions can be detected without the use of a slit lamp if fluorescein staining and a cobalt blue filtered light are employed in the eye examination. Because of the ease of bacterial (particularly pseudomonal) contamination of the fluorescein, it must be instilled by means of either a single-dose container or sterile fluorescein strips wetted with sterile saline. The strip is touched to the inferior cul de sac while the patient looks upward; the patient is then asked to blink once. The fluorescein stains into denuded areas of corneal epithelium, producing a bright green color when viewed by normal light. The intensity of staining is enhanced if the eye is illuminated with a cobalt blue light. Among the lesions that can be identified by fluorescein staining are the dendritic ulcers of herpes keratitis, abrasions, small foreign bodies, and punctate defects caused by irradiation.

Intraocular Pressure. If pain is not clearly related to the external eye or adnexa, the intraocular pressure should be measured to rule out glaucoma, provided there is no infection and the globe is intact without external or penetrating foreign bodies.

INDICATIONS FOR REFERRAL

Significant loss of vision always requires prompt ophthalmic evaluation. Progressive pain, redness, or discharge that fails to respond to conservative treatment must be evaluated. Care must be taken not to mistake penetrating trauma for a simple abrasion. An eccentric pupil or shallow chamber may indicate loss of aqueous humor. One should never instill antibiotic ointment if there is a possibility of a perforation. Under such circumstances, patch the eye with a metal or plastic shield, which protects the eye, and arrange referral; do not place any pressure on the globe.

SYMPTOMATIC MANAGEMENT

Most serious causes of eye pain require prompt ophthalmologic referral, but some foreign bodies and abrasions can be managed in the office setting.

Foreign Bodies. Irrigation with normal saline from a squirt bottle, syringe without a needle, or intravenous tubing may flush out foreign material. If irrigation fails, no further attempt should be made by the nonophthalmologist to remove the foreign body if it is firmly embedded in the cornea. Use of a dry cotton-tipped applicator will only remove much normal corneal epithelium. Use of a cotton-tipped applicator or needle for foreign body removal requires topical anesthesia, good visualization, and specific training.

Abrasions. Superficial epithelial abrasions usually heal well with prophylactic antibiotic medication (eg, erythromycin ointment) and a tight pressure patch for 24 to 48 hours.

Conjunctivitis; Glaucoma. See Chapters 199 and 207, respectively.

ANNOTATED BIBLIOGRAPHY

Bienfang DC, Kelly LD, Nicholson DH, et al. Ophthalmology. N Engl J Med 1990;323:956. *(Excellent review and overview for the general reader; 115 refs.)*

Shingleton BJ, Hersh PS, Kenyon KR. Eye Trauma. Philadelphia: Mosby; 1991. *(The definitive text on the subject; includes detailed sections on management of foreign bodies and abrasions.)*

202
Evaluation of Dry Eyes

DAVID A. GREENBERG, O.D., M.P.H.

Primary Care Medicine: Office Evaluation and Management of the Adult Patient, 3rd edition, edited by Allan H. Goroll, Lawrence A. May, and Albert G. Mulley, Jr. J.B. Lippincott Company, Philadelphia

The normal tear film provides important protection to the eye. Defects in tear production are uncommon, but often occur in conjunction with systemic disease. The primary physician must decide if systemic disease does exist, provide symptomatic relief, and know when referral is needed.

PATHOPHYSIOLOGY AND CLINICAL PRESENTATION

The ocular tear film performs a host of functions, including maintenance of the corneal and conjunctival epithelium, lubrication of lid motion, delivery of oxygen and uptake of CO_2 from the cornea, carriage of antimicrobial defenses, clearance of foreign matter and tissue debris, and smoothing of the anterior ocular surface for clear vision. The tear film is inherently unstable, depending on the interaction of its three components for stability.

The outermost layer of the tear film is lipid, excreted by the lid meibomian glands. This layer retards evaporation and counters gravitational forces on the aqueous layer. The middle layer is aqueous, secreted by the lacrimal glands and accounting for most of the tear film. The innermost layer is mucinous, primarily secreted by conjunctival goblet cells and attaching to the corneal epithelium. This converts the corneal surface from a hydrophobic to a hydrophilic one. Each blink redistributes and replenishes the tear film. Dry eyes ensue from a defect in maintenance of the tear film.

Aqueous Deficiency. A defect in production of the aqueous phase by lacrimal glands causes dry eyes or *keratoconjunctivitis sicca*. The condition most often occurs as a physiologic consequence of *aging,* commonly exacerbated by the desiccating effect of dry environmental conditions. It also may develop in the setting of *connective tissue disease, anticholinergic drug* use (eg, phenothiazines, tricyclic antidepressants, antihistamines), and neurologic disease.

In *Sjögren's syndrome,* the lacrimal glands become involved in immune-mediated inflammation. The condition may occur in the context of other rheumatoid diseases or as an isolated event. Characteristic features include the triad of dry eyes, dry mouth, and arthritis. Facial telangiectasias, parotid enlargement, Raynaud's phenomenon, and dental caries are associated features. Patients complain first of burning and a sandy, gritty, foreign body sensation, particularly later in the day. Increased eye debris and mucus are noted. Secondary bacterial infection develops in severe cases.

Mucin Deficiency. Mucin production may decline in the setting of *vitamin A deficiency,* which causes primary goblet cell deficiency. When this is combined with protein deficiency (as occurs in underdeveloped parts of the world), *keratomalacia* results. Secondary loss of goblet cells and mucin deficiency follows chemical *burns,* benign ocular *pemphigoid,* and *trachoma.* With loss of main and accessory lacrimal production, a combined mucin-aqueous deficiency ensues. Dry eyes linked to problems in mucin production have been noted in patients using the antiacne preparation *isotretinoin* (Accutane).

Eyelid Defects. Compromised lid function may affect the entire tear film, because of impaired rewetting. Incomplete blinking, 5th or 7th cranial nerve palsy, exophthalmos, and exposure during sleep are among the conditions that result in drying of the inferior interpalpebral cornea. Lid movement may also be hindered by scar formation.

Neurogenic Hyposecretion is a potential consequence of such uncommon conditions as basal skull fracture or the Ramsay-Hunt syndrome.

Patients with dry eyes are more likely to report grittiness, itching, burning, soreness, difficulty in moving the eyelids, or the sensation of a foreign body present with that complaint. When ocular irritation stimulates excess reflex tearing, the patient may present paradoxically with watery eyes. In rare instances, a corneal ulcer or red eye may ensue.

Table 202-1. Principal Causes of Dry Eyes

Lacrimal Gland Dysfunction
Age
Systemic disease (Sjögren's syndrome, sarcoidosis, Hodgkin's disease)
Anticholinergic drugs (atropine, antihistamines, tricyclics)
Compromised Eyelid Function
5th or 7th nerve palsy
Exophthalmos
Scar formation
Mucin Deficiency
Chemical burns
Hypovitaminosis A
Isotretinoin (Accutane)
Benign ocular pemphigoid
Trachoma
Environmental Factors
Excessive dryness
Excessive exposure (e.g., exophthalmos, Bell's palsy)
Lipid Abnormalities
Chronic blepharitis
Meibomitis

DIFFERENTIAL DIAGNOSIS

The differential diagnosis of dry eyes can be organized pathophysiologically (Table 202-1). As noted, the most common cause is the generalized diminution of lacrimal secretion associated with aging, followed by systemic conditions and anticholinergic drugs. Keratoconjunctivitis sicca secondary to a mucin or lipid abnormality is less common. Environmental factors contribute.

WORKUP

History. The workup should begin by noting the duration and frequency of symptoms and particularly if onset is related to dry environmental conditions. Symptoms of keratoconjunctivitis sicca are usually more pronounced as the day progresses and are frequently exacerbated by tobacco smoke. The physician should ask if tears are produced with crying and if the patient finds himself removing strands of mucus from the inner canthi on awakening (a very suggestive symptom). It is important to note any associated dry mouth, joint pains, prior ocular disease, infection, or surgery. A drug history is helpful.

Physical Examination. Attention is paid to frequency and completeness of blinking and note taken of any lid pathology. Blepharitis and meibomitis are evident as lid margin crusting and engorgement of the meibomian glands, respectively. Other physical findings may include thick yellow mucous strands in the lower fornix, hyperemic and edematous bulbar conjunctiva, and corneal dullness. It is mandatory to check for completeness of lid closure as well as position of eyelashes. The corneal reflex is checked if there is concern about a neuroparalytic keratitis or facial nerve palsy. Skin and joints should be examined for signs of rheumatoid disease (see Chapter 146).

Studies. The *Schirmer test* diagnoses aqueous deficiency by measuring the wetting of a filter paper strip (Whatman No. 41 filter paper, 5 mm by 35 mm). A folded end is hooked over the lower lid nasally and the patient is instructed to keep the eyes lightly closed during the test. In the Schirmer I test, wetting is measured after 5 minutes; less than 5 mm is usually abnormal. A basal Schirmer test using topical anesthetic to prevent reflex tearing caused by the paper strip is sometimes performed; its need is debated.

SYMPTOMATIC MANAGEMENT AND INDICATIONS FOR REFERRAL

As long as there are no signs of ocular disease, the primary physician may attempt symptomatic relief. The first step is to reduce any environmental dryness that exacerbates the aqueous deficiency of aging. Often this can be accomplished by use of a room humidifier. A 2-week trial of one of the many commercially available *artificial tear substitutes* may also be helpful. Of the commercially available preparations, methylcellulose (Visulose, 0.5% or 1%), polyvinyl alcohol (Liquifilm Tears, 1.4%, or Liquifilm Forte, 3%), and hydroxypropyl methylcellulose, 1% (Ultra Tears, Tears Naturale and Adsorbotear) have been used successfully. These nonprescription drops are soothing and, through a variety of formulations, provide aqueous replacement and sometimes mucomimetic substances.

Drops may be instilled as often as desired. Topical application of one to two drops, four times a day, is a useful starting dosage. The patient may increase the frequency of application to as often as hourly to achieve comfort; a bland ointment can be used at night. Toxicity is uncommon, but topical sensitivity or corneal epithelial damage may occur. More severe cases may warrant a trial of slow-release methylcellulose inserts (Lacrisert); acceptance of these has been limited. Steroids and antibiotics should not be prescribed for uncomplicated disease.

The patient should be instructed to seek immediate ophthalmologic attention in the event of a red eye, visual disturbance, or eye pain. An eye specialist should be consulted when simple symptomatic treatment does not give rapid relief.

PATIENT EDUCATION

It is critical for the primary physician to be certain that the patient knows how to instill the drops into the eye. Instructions should include the careful instillation of the drop into the lower fornix without contact occurring between the dropper and the eye and the utilization of digital pressure in the punctal or inner region of the lower lid to reduce drainage and prolong contact. The patient should also be educated that the instillation of more than one drop at a time exceeds the physical capacity of the inferior fornix and is wasteful.

ANNOTATED BIBLIOGRAPHY

Barsam PC, et al. Treatment of the dry eye and related problems. Ann Ophthalmol 1972;4:122. *(Subjective relief provided by artificial tear substitute in patients with idiopathic ocular discomfort and dry eye.)*

Holly FJ, Lemp MA. Tear physiology and dry eyes. Surv Ophthalmol 1977;22:69. *(Classic review.)*

Jones DB. Prospects in the management of tear deficiency states. Trans Am Acad Ophthalmol Otolaryngol 1977;83:OP692. *(Includes comprehensive listing of the causes by mechanism.)*

Sjögren H, Block KJ. Keratoconjunctivitis sicca and Sjögren's syndrome. Surv Ophthalmol 1971;16:143. *(Classic paper.)*

Primary Care Medicine: Office Evaluation and Management of the Adult Patient, 3rd edition, edited by Allan H. Goroll, Lawrence A. May, and Albert G. Mulley, Jr. J.B. Lippincott Company, Philadelphia

203
Evaluation of Common Visual Disturbances: Flashing Lights, Floaters, and Other Transient Phenomena

CLAUDIA U. RICHTER, M.D.

Flashes of light, specks, halos, and discolorations are among the transient visual phenomena reported by patients. Flashes of light (*photopsia*) and dark moving lines and specks (*floaters*) are particularly common, usually benign occurrences, but on occasion, they herald a retinal tear or detachment. Visual distortion (*metamorphopsia*) can be the presenting symptom of age-related macular degeneration. Other short-lived disturbances accompany such diverse conditions as migraine, digitalis toxicity, and acute glaucoma. The primary physician needs to know the significance of these visual phenomena and when they presage a serious ophthalmologic or systemic event that requires prompt ophthalmological attention.

PATHOPHYSIOLOGY AND CLINICAL PRESENTATION

Vitreoretinal traction is the principal cause of retinal tears and detachments, which can lead to sudden onset of flashes and floaters. As the vitreous gel liquefies with age, its fibrous matrix contracts and pulls away from the retina. Because the vitreous is attached to the retina at several sites (including the optic nerve), any traction can cause tearing that leads to a retinal hole and/or detachment. Detachment may be exacerbated by flow of vitreous through the hole in the retina and up behind it. If the tearing involves a superficial retinal vessel, then hemorrhage into the vitreous may follow and compromise vision.

Floaters are vitreous opacities that cast a shadow on the retina. They can be single or multiple, characteristically moving across the visual field and transiently blurring vision if they cross the macula. Their presence is most notable when gazing at a clear blue sky or blank white wall. New onset of floaters may occur as a consequence of *vitreous detachment*, a *retinal tear* or *detachment,* or an intraocular hemorrhage. Acute or chronic intraocular inflammation and/or infection is sometimes the cause, as in the immunocompromised patient with *cytomegalovirus (CMV) retinitis*. The sudden appearance of one or more floaters suggests onset of serious underlying pathology. Floaters that are multiple and long-standing are associated with *myopia* and *aging* with or without a vitreous detachment.

Flashes (photopsia) are perceptions of bright, small flickering lights or lightninglike flashes of light. They are most vividly seen in the dark and usually occur with mechanical stimulation of the retina. They account for "seeing stars" when one suffers head trauma or coughs very hard. New onset may be a consequence of vitreous traction on the retina leading to *retinal tear* or *detachment*. Just rubbing the eyes can cause similar symptoms. *Migraine* pathophysiology accounts for recurrent episodes.

Distortion (metamorphopsia) refers to the curvilinear distortion of straight lines or patterns. This visual disturbance is the consequence of an altered shape of the retinal surface, either from the collection of fluid beneath the retina or scarring on the surface. Metamorphopsia is seen with age-related *macular degeneration,* epiretinal fibrosis, and a variety of ocular diseases that cause traction on the retinal surface and/or retinal scarring. Macular edema, as occurs in *diabetic retinopathy,* may be responsible.

Zig-Zag Lines. *Migraine* can produce a complex set of prodromal visual phenomena that include zig-zag lines (sometimes referred as *fortification phenomena*) and flashes of light with transient blind spots (*scintillating scotomata*). These may present with or without a subsequent headache. Typically, the zig-zag lines occur adjacent to a grey area of shaded darkness. Both the grey area and the zig-zag lines slowly expand. The visual phenomena typically end in 20 to 30 minutes with the onset of the headache and leave no residual visual deficit (see also Chapter 165).

Halos, Discolorations, and Visual Hallucinations. The first clinical manifestations of *digitalis toxicity* may be visual (see Chapter 32) and include lightning flashes, yellow discoloration, halos, and the appearance of frost over objects. *Acute glaucoma* (see Chapter 207) also produces colored halos around lights, but not lightning flashes. *Visual hallucinations* caused by *seizure* activity in the occipital cortex and the adjacent association area produce static light and stars. Hallucinations from the parastriate area 18 cause luminous sensations or colored flashes and rings.

DIFFERENTIAL DIAGNOSIS

The sudden onset of a visual phenomenon may be the first sign of important underlying ophthalmic or systemic pathology. Causes can be listed according to clinical presentation (Table 203-1).

Table 203-1. Important Causes of Flashes, Floaters, and Other Visual Phenomena

Floaters
Myopia
Aging
Vitreous
Detachment
Retinal tear
Retinal detachment
Intraocular inflammation (uveitis, retinitis)
Vitreous hemorrhage
Flashing Lights
Vitreoretinal traction
Retinal detachment
Mechanical stimulation (cough, rubbing the eyes, head trauma)
Migraine
Seizure in the visual cortex
Distorted Vision
Macular degeneration, age-related
Macular edema due to diabetes
Other causes of retinal scarring or traction
Halos
Digitalis toxicity
Acute glaucoma
Colored Flashes or Rings
Acute glaucoma
Seizure activity

WORKUP

History. A complete and detailed description of the patient's symptoms uninfluenced by leading questions is the most important part of the history, followed by information regarding their onset, course, and presence of any associated symptoms (eg, headache, decreased visual acuity). The sudden onset of flashing lights and/or floaters is highly suggestive of vitreoretinal traction, possibly in association with a vitreous detachment, retinal tear, or retinal detachment. New onset in an immunocompromised patient should suggest CMV retinitis. Flashes of light on waking and rubbing the eyes are usually harmless, as are floaters that have been present for an extended time without marked increase in number. The patient who complains of halos needs to be checked for glaucoma (see Chapter 198). A report of lightning flashes, yellow discoloration, or frost over objects in a patient taking a digitalis preparation requires consideration of digitalis toxicity. Visual distortion should lead to a search for a subretinal fluid accumulation.

Physical examination should include visual acuity testing, measurement of the intraocular pressure (see Chapter 198), and careful examination of the fundus. One looks for hemorrhage in the vitreous, a ballooning white area suggestive of a retinal detachment, areas of retinal inflammation, and abnormalities in the appearance of the macula suggestive of macular degenerative disease. In the immunocompromised patient, funduscopic examination should include a look for the manifestations of CMV retinitis (eg, focal, granular, perivascular yellow-white lesions with or without hemorrhage in a "brush-fire" pattern). Detection of retinal tears and small retinal detachments requires indirect ophthalmoscopy or diagnostic contact lens examination performed by the ophthalmologist. Patients with migraine will have a normal ophthalmologic examination.

Studies. The most important study in patients with new flashes and/or floaters is indirect ophthalmoscopy and scleral depression done by the ophthalmologist. Patients with metamorphopsia need fluorescein angiography. The patient with halos needs to be checked for glaucoma (see Chapter 198). The patient taking a digitalis preparation who reports visual disturbances should have a serum drug level measured (see Chapter 32).

PATIENT EDUCATION AND INDICATIONS FOR REFERRAL

New onset of unexplained flashes or floaters requires urgent referral to an ophthalmologist because of the possibility of a retinal tear, retinal detachment, or an inflammatory/infectious process (eg, CMV retinitis). Vision is best preserved when treatment of such conditions is prompt. If a field loss is detected by the patient or examiner, referral is even more urgent. Metamorphopsia is also an indication for urgent referral, because age-related macular degeneration has a better visual prognosis when subretinal neovascularization is treated with early macular photocoagulation. A report of halos should lead to referral for evaluation of glaucoma. Visual hallucinations require workup for seizure activity and visual cortex pathology.

Patients with chronic flashes and floaters should have a complete ophthalmologic examination, including indirect ophthalmoscopy, but it is not urgent. All patients with flashes and floaters need to be warned that a sudden onset of new floaters or flashes or the appearance of a peripheral visual field defect may represent a retinal hole or detachment necessitating prompt ophthalmologic attention. The patient with chronic floaters in the absence of ocular disease can be reassured; prognosis is excellent, as it is for the person with visual phenomena associated with migraine. Flashes that occur with minor mechanical stimulation (cough, rubbing of the eyes) require only reassurance and explanation, as long as there is no evidence of more serious pathology.

ANNOTATED BIBLIOGRAPHY

Aring CD. The scintillating scotoma. JAMA 1972;220:519. *(A detailed discussion of these migrainous visual phenomena.)*

Bienfang DC, Kelly LD, Nicholson DH, et al. Ophthalmology. N Engl J Med 1990;323;956. *(A succinct review of recent improvements in ophthalmological care, including CMV retinitis.)*

Morris PH, Scheie HG, Aminlari A. Light flashes as a clue to retinal disease. Arch Ophthalmol 1974;91:179. *(In this series, 23 percent had demonstrable vitreoretinal disease; of these, 16 percent had retinal breaks.)*

204

Evaluation of Exophthalmos

CLAUDIA U. RICHTER, M.D.

Primary Care Medicine: Office Evaluation and Management of the Adult Patient, 3rd edition, edited by Allan H. Goroll, Lawrence A. May, and Albert G. Mulley, Jr. J.B. Lippincott Company, Philadelphia

Exophthalmos is defined as protrusion of the eye. It may be a variation of normal physiognomy or a sign of systemic or orbital disease. The primary physician must be able to recognize it and evaluate the patient for a possible endocrinologic, neoplastic, or vascular cause and decide on the need for further study or referral.

PATHOPHYSIOLOGY AND CLINICAL PRESENTATION

Pathologic forms of exophthalmos may result from inflammation, infiltration, a mass lesion, or a vascular abnormality.

Graves' Disease. The ophthalmopathy of Graves' disease occurs as a consequence of an autoimmune inflammatory process leading to infiltration of the soft tissues of the orbit. Pathologically, there is an inflammatory infiltrate of lymphocytes, mucopolysaccharides, and edema, followed by proliferation of fibroblasts and increase in the volume of orbital connective tissue. The proliferation of orbital fibroblasts and their fibrotic restriction of extraocular-muscle movement account for the clinical picture of Graves' ophthalmopathy.

In its mildest form, there is minor lid retraction, stare, lid lag, and mild protrusion of the eye (proptosis). A particularly severe form, "malignant" exophthalmos, causes edema of the lids and conjunctiva, marked proptosis, limitation of extraocular movements, exposure keratopathy, and optic nerve compression. Although it is usually a bilateral disease, it may present unilaterally or asymmetrically.

The relatively close clinical relationship between ophthalmopathy of Graves' disease, pretibial dermopathy, and hyperthyroidism suggests a common pathophysiologic mechanism. However, the ophthalmopathy can occur in the absence of thyroid dysfunction or pretibial dermopathy, and it may worsen with some treatments for thyrotoxicosis. Its precise mechanism remains to be elucidated (see Chapter 103).

Primary orbital neoplasms, such as *meningiomas,* produce exophthalmos by mass effect. Some vascular lesions, such as *hemangiomas,* produce only a mass effect, whereas a *carotid-cavernous sinus fistula* may present with a diffusely congested orbit with exophthalmos, prominent episcleral vessels, and elevated intraocular pressure. Mass lesions and vascular abnormalities are unilateral processes. They may lead to diplopia, ocular irritation, and photophobia (secondary to corneal exposure). Stretching or compression of the optic nerve impairs visual acuity.

Orbital cellulitis is an extremely serious, although rare cause of proptosisis. Because the orbit is bordered on three sides by paranasal sinuses, orbital infection can result from sinusitis extending directly through the lamina papyracea. Lid edema, ptosis, proptosis, chemosis, and diminished ocular movements make for a dramatic clinical presentation. Retrograde extension can lead to *cavernous sinus thrombosis*.

DIFFERENTIAL DIAGNOSIS

Bilateral exophthalmos is usually caused by Graves' disease, but occasionally it occurs with Cushing's syndrome, acromegaly, lithium ingestion, metastatic tumor, and orbital lymphoma.

Unilateral exophthalmos is most often due to tumor (predominantly hemangioma, meningioma, or optic nerve glioma), but occasionally the cause is an inflammatory or infectious condition. Orbital pseudotumor mimics a mass lesion. Tumors extending into the orbit include those originating in the eye, lids, and paranasal sinuses. Among inflammatory etiologies are sarcoidosis, orbital cellulitis, foreign body, orbital thrombophlebitis, and ruptured dermoid cyst. Hemangioma, aneurysm, varices, carotid-cavernous sinus fistula, and cavernous sinus thrombosis constitute the important vascular etiologies. Skeletal abnormalities (eg, Paget's disease) may produce exophthalmos. Asymmetry of the orbits, severe unilateral myopia, facial nerve paresis, eyelid retraction, and congenital glaucoma may give the appearance of exophthalmos. Ptosis or enophthalmos of the opposite eye can mimic exophthalmos.

WORKUP

The first task is to determine if the condition is unilateral or bilateral. Bilateral disease has a limited differential diagnosis, with Graves' disease accounting for most cases. Attention is directed toward its confirmation (see Chapter 103). The broader differential of unilateral disease necessitates a more extensive workup.

History should include inquiry into the time course of the exophthalmos. Old photographs are helpful in determining if the problem is new in onset or simply a long-standing anatomic variant. Associated symptoms are also important to note. Change in visual acuity, diplopia, pain, excessive lacrimation, photophobia, and foreign body sensation are indications of adverse effects from the exophthalmos. A prior history or current symptoms of trauma to the orbit, thyroid disease, cancer, severe sinus infection, or worsening headache should be noted.

Physical examination begins with documenting the degree of exophthalmos. The distance to be measured is from the lateral orbital rim to the apex of the cornea with the patient looking straight ahead. The upper limit of normal is 21 to 22 mm; a difference between both eyes of 2 mm is also considered significant. Visual acuity, intraocular pressure, and extraocular muscle function should also be tested. The conjunctiva and cornea are observed for signs of drying, aided by fluorescein or rose bengal dye if available. Color vision, pupillary reactivity, and visual fields are assessed to investigate possible optic nerve compression, which may also produce a pale or swollen optic nerve head on ophthalmoscopic examination. The globe and orbit need to be auscultated for bruits and pulsation suggestive of vascular fistula. The sinuses are checked for tenderness and discharge. In the setting of bilateral disease, the neck should be checked for goiter and bruit, the pretibial region for dermopathy, and the remainder of the examination for signs of thyroid hormone excess (see Chapter 103).

Laboratory Studies. Thyroid indices should be ordered in the patient with bilateral disease, but the absence of hyperthyroidism does not rule out Graves' disease. Even in patients without evidence of thyrotoxicosis, antibodies to thyrotropin receptors and peroxidase can be detected (see Chapter 103).

Patients with unilateral exophthalmos are candidates for orbital imaging. At present, axial and coronal computed tomography is the study of choice in the evaluation of orbital abnormalities. It provides good definition of both bony and soft orbital tissues. Ultrasound is sometimes used to screen for a mass lesion. Orbital magnetic resonance imaging (MRI) may be helpful in the noninvasive evaluation of certain vascular and neoplastic disorders. Invasive study is the province of the ophthalmologist.

SYMPTOMATIC MANAGEMENT AND INDICATIONS FOR REFERRAL

The primary physician must be cognizant of potential ocular complications of exophthalmos and give advice for relief of minor symptoms. Periorbital and lid edema may be reduced by elevating the head of the bed at night. Exposure keratopathy causes a foreign body sensation, which can be relieved by use of artificial tear lubricants and taping the eyelids closed at night. If such simple measures are inadequate, referral to the ophthalmologist for consideration of eyelid or orbital surgery may be necessary.

There is no means of preventing Graves' ophthalmopathy. Treatment is undertaken only when symptoms become severe or vision is threatened. Likelihood of progression is hard to determine and available therapies have their own adverse effects. Inflammatory symptoms such as periorbital edema and ocular discomfort are treated with corticosteroids or orbital radiation. Such therapy may inhibit the cytokines, which perpetuate the inflammatory reaction. When corneal integrity or optic nerve function is endangered, the patient should be promptly referred for consideration of orbital decompression. Treatment of the underlying Graves' disease must be done carefully in the setting of eye involvement. As noted, ophthalmopathy can worsen with some forms of therapy, perhaps due to increased release of thyroid antigen. Some authorities suggest use of antithyroid drugs to minimize such release; others add high-dose corticosteroids to the program (see Chapter 103). Endocrinologic consultation is indicated.

Emergency admission is needed if orbital cellulitis is encountered. Ophthalmologic consultation should be obtained early in unilateral, severe, or unexplained exophthalmos. Exophthalmos due to neoplasm requires a team approach that includes ophthalmologist, oncologist and radiation therapist. A suspected vascular etiology is also grounds for referral.

Patient education is important because evaluation, treatment, and the underlying disease process may be lengthy. It is important to review with the patient symptoms warranting prompt evaluation (eg, change in vision, ocular pain, eye injection, diplopia, and so forth). Patients with Graves' disease ought to understand that the ophthalmic manifestations of this disorder may persist or progress despite appropriate systemic therapy for the underlying disease. Eye changes due to fibrous hyperplasia are likely to be more refractory than those due to inflammation.

ANNOTATED BIBLIOGRAPHY

Bahn RS, Heufelder AE. Pathogenesis of Graves' ophthalmopathy. N Engl J Med 1993;329:1468. *(Clinically useful review of disease mechanisms and their relation to clinical presentation and treatment.)*

Chard H, Norman D. The use of computer tomography and ultrasonography in the evaluation of orbital masses. Surv Ophthalmol 1982;27:49. *(The advantages and limitations of each modality are discussed.)*

Rootman J. Frequency and differential diagnosis of orbital disease. In Rootman J, ed. Disease of the Orbit. Philadelphia: JB Lippincott; 1990:119. *(Comprehensive review of possible etiologies of exophthalmos.)*

Tallstedt L, Lundell G, Torring O, et al. Occurrence of ophthalmopathy after treatment of Graves' hyperthyroidism. N Engl J Med 1992;326:1733. *(Some treatments may actually exacerbate the ophthalmopathy.)*

Utiger RD. Treatment of Graves' ophthalmopathy. N Engl J Med 1989;321;1405. *(An editorial critically reviewing treatment options.)*

205
Evaluation of Excessive Tearing

ROGER F. STEINERT, M.D.

Primary Care Medicine: Office Evaluation and Management of the Adult Patient, 3rd edition, edited by Allan H. Goroll, Lawrence A. May, and Albert G. Mulley, Jr. J.B. Lippincott Company, Philadelphia

The presence of watery eyes reflects an increased production of tears or a decreased ability to drain them. Patients complain of watery eyes or may actually describe tears overflowing and running down their cheeks, a condition called epiphora. The primary physician must decide if structural pathology exists or if reassurance is the appropriate treatment.

PATHOPHYSIOLOGY AND CLINICAL PRESENTATION

Tears are produced by the main and accessory lacrimal glands. They flow out through upper and lower puncta, which open into canaliculi. These, in turn, drain into the lacrimal sac and then into the nasolacrimal duct, which opens under the inferior turbinate in the nose.

In the presence of a normal lacrimal drainage system, epiphora most often results from hypersecretion. Common stimulants are blepharitis and keratitis of any etiology (eg, infections, foreign body), atopy, and sinusitis. Pseudoepiphora is reflex tearing in the presence of dry eyes (see Chapter 202). Aberrant regeneration of the 7th nerve may result in gustatory lacrimation ("crocodile tears").

Many abnormalities are capable of interfering with lacrimal drainage. Tear film movement may be obstructed by eyelid margin lesions or conjunctival redundancy or folds. Tears do not flow down the drainage system merely by gravity, but rather are pumped by lid motion. This pump may be impaired by 7th nerve palsy or conditions stiffening the lids, such as scars or scleroderma or by laxity of the lids from aging. The puncta must be properly positioned; ectropion prevents tears from gaining access to the canaliculus. This condition is common in the elderly and is characterized by a sagging lower lid. The punctum or the canaliculus may be occluded congenitally, by chemical or thermal injury, or by neoplasms. In addition, canalicular infections may cause occlusion. The most common of these are *Actinomyces israeli* (*Streptothrix*) and *Candida*. Finally, obstruction of the lacrimal sac and nasolacrimal duct may be idiopathic, congenital, or caused by neoplasms, ethmoiditis, and turbinate disease.

The more distal the obstruction, the more likely that the epiphora will be accompanied by purulent discharge or dacryocystitis, as the stagnant tears become infected. Digital pressure may express purulent material from the puncta.

DIFFERENTIAL DIAGNOSIS

The most common causes of watery eye are senile ectropion and increased physiologic tearing. These problems are more common in the elderly. Excessive moisture may be the complaint in a patient who has an inflammatory process such as keratitis, blepharitis, or conjunctivitis.

Obstruction in the drainage system most commonly results from dacryocystitis. The puncta may be obstructed by a myriad of causes: tumors, burns, erythema multiforme, or redundant skin. The lacrimal passage may be obstructed by a stone, laceration, burn, surgery, senile atresia, or infection of the lacrimal duct. The puncta may be rendered ineffective by ectropion, sagging of the lower lid. Excessive tearing accompanies facial palsies but is rarely the primary complaint.

WORKUP

History. The physician should determine if tears actually run down the cheek and, if so, how frequently. Overflowing tears in the absence of environmental irritants suggests structural pathology. Watery eyes noted on exposure to cold, air conditioning, or a dry environment may be due to exaggerated physiologic tearing.

Inquiry into whether the problem is unilateral or bilateral can be helpful. Unilateral tearing is more often obstructive, but stenosis can be bilateral; environmental irritants should cause bilateral epiphora. Any sinus disease, facial fractures, infections, and surgery should be noted as possible etiologic factors, as should symptoms suggestive of Sjögren's syndrome (see Chapter 146).

Physical Examination. Lid structure and motion should be observed. Patency of the puncta is visualized under low magnification. Gentle pressure is applied over the lacrimal sac on the side of the nose and over the canaliculi to attempt to express purulent material for examination and culture. Examination for signs of dry eye (see Chapter 202) is needed to rule out paradoxical tearing, which requires an entirely different therapeutic approach.

Studies. The ophthalmologist may also evaluate the lacrimal drainage system in several ways. Fluorescein dye instilled in the conjunctival sac should make its way to the nose (Jones test). Saline irrigation and probing may prove patency or localize an obstruction. Dacryocystography (radiocontrast dye injection) may dramatically outline the obstruction and the proximal lacrimal system. Dacryoscintigraphy, in which aqueous radioactive tracer is introduced into the tear film and followed during blinking, may demonstrate functional impairment (pump failure).

SYMPTOMATIC MANAGEMENT AND INDICATIONS FOR REFERRAL

Irritants must be eliminated. Sicca is treated with appropriate lubricants (see Chapter 202). Dacryocystitis is treated with hot compresses at least four times a day and systemic antibiotics (usually erythromycin 250 mg qid or dicloxicillin 250 mg qid directed against staphylococcal species). Patients without infection can be reassured the condition is not harmful.

Unresponsive patients are properly referred to an ophthalmologist for further evaluation and treatment. In symptomatic cases, lid surgery to correct malposition, or dacryocystorhinostomy to relieve nasolacrimal obstruction may be indicated.

ANNOTATED BIBLIOGRAPHY

Jones LT, Linn ML. The diagnosis of the causes of epiphora. Am J Ophthalmol 1969;67:751. *(Still the classic presentation on the workup of epiphora.)*

Victor WH. Watery eye. Western J Med 1986;144:759. *(A review written for the primary care physician; emphasizes a practical approach.)*

Primary Care Medicine: Office Evaluation and Management of the Adult Patient, 3rd edition, edited by Allan H. Goroll, Lawrence A. May, and Albert G. Mulley, Jr. J.B. Lippincott Company, Philadelphia

206
Management of the Patient With Age-Related Macular Degeneration

Age-related macular degeneration is a major cause of vision loss in the elderly. The age-related form affects an estimated 30 percent of persons over the age of 75. Proper geriatric eye care includes early recognition of macular degeneration so that ophthalmologic referral can be timely and the risk of visual impairment minimized.

PATHOPHYSIOLOGY AND CLINICAL PRESENTATION

The retinal pigmented epithelium is critical to the maintenance of healthy retinal photoreceptors. Any compromise to the former can lead to a decline in receptor cells and loss of vision. In macular degeneration, the retinal pigmented epithelium begins to degenerate or at least change its biochemical relation with photoreceptor cells. Deposits of debris called *drusen* accumulate between the epithelial cell and the underlying basement membrane (Bruch's membrane). Although not the cause of visual loss, drusen serve as an important clinical marker of the processes that lead to it.

Hard or nodular drusen are pinhead-sized yellow-white lesions visible ophthalmoscopically in the macular region. They represent focal degenerative change. *Soft or granular drusen* are larger, have less distinct edges, and represent more widespread epithelial dysfunction. The development of *diffuse or confluent drusen* coincides with still more advanced degenerative disease and heralds detachment of the pigmented epithelium from Bruch's membrane.

Detachment of the retinal epithelium is a consequence of the degenerative process that both weakens and thickens Bruch's membrane. Detachment leads to visual loss as the overlying photoreceptor cells atrophy. In addition, new blood vessels may form (*neovascularization*) in response to the degenerative changes in Bruch's membrane. The fragile new vessels tend to leak and sometimes bleed, producing serous or hemorrhagic detachment of the pigmented epithelium from the neurosensory retina as well as detachment of the pigmented epithelium. If there is bleeding, fibrovascular scarring may ensue. Such complications of neovascularization exacerbate the extent and speed of visual loss. Fortunately, fewer than 20 percent of persons with age-related macular degeneration have neovascularization.

Clinical Presentation and Course. Because the degenerative process is concentrated in the macula, central visual acuity is most affected. Patients may complain of a loss of visual acuity that is not corrected by eyeglasses. In patients without neovascularization, the loss of visual acuity tends to be gradual and limited. Macular examination of such persons may reveal all forms of drusen, but there is no neovascularization or evidence of its consequences. The presentation without neovascularization is sometimes referred to as *"dry"* or *neovascularization* macular degeneration. It accounts for about 90 percent of all cases.

Those with neovascularization are labeled as having *"wet"* or *exudative* disease. Close to 90 percent of persons who lose central vision have the exudative type. With neovascularization present, vision loss may be acute and more extensive. *Distorted vision* (metamorphopsia) may herald the onset of serous retinal detachment. In addition to drusen, macular examination may show serous and hemorrhagic effusions and disk-shaped scarring.

DIAGNOSIS

Suggestive historical features include gradual or sudden loss of central visual acuity or distorted vision (metamorphopsia) in an elderly person.

The latter suggests the degenerative process has progressed sufficiently to cause serous retinal detachment due to neovascularization. Characteristic ophthalmoscopic findings are concentrated in the macular region and include drusen, irregularities in macular pigmentation, hemorrhage, and discoid scarring.

Finding defects in central visual acuity further supports the diagnosis of macular degeneration. Such changes can be detected with the aid of an *Amsler grid,* a 10 × 10 cm card with a black background on which is printed a criss-crossed grid of vertical and horizontal white lines every 5 mm. In the center, there is a white dot. The patient is asked to focus on the dot and note if any of the lines appear wavy or distorted or if any of the boxes formed by the intersecting lines are missing. Each eye is tested separately with any prescribed corrective lenses worn and the grid held at a comfortable reading distance.

PRINCIPLES OF MANAGEMENT

There is no known treatment for preventing degeneration of the pigmented retinal epithelium. However, the approach to preventing loss of visual acuity depends on whether the macular degeneration is accompanied by neovascularization.

Exudative Disease—Neovascularization Present. For the 10 percent of macular degeneration patients with neovascularization, the prognosis for preservation of central vision is poor but can be improved with argon laser *photocoagulation* therapy. Candidates for laser photocoagulation therapy are those with neovascularization that is not within 200 m of the fovea. Laser treatment of neovascularization closer to the fovea risks destroying its intense concentration of photoreceptor cells.

Early clinical detection of neovascularization is critical. Macular degeneration patients are instructed to watch for and promptly report any distortion of vision. Daily home use of an Amsler grid is an excellent and simple means of early detection. Any new defects or distortions in central vision require prompt reporting to the ophthalmologist and consideration of urgent laser treatment. Such treatment can reduce the frequency of vision loss from 60 percent to 25 percent in patients with exudative disease.

Nonexudative Disease—No Neovascularization. Although their prognosis is much better than for those with untreated exudative disease, patients without neovascularization have no definitive treatment options at the present time. For the 10 percent of macular degeneration patients who suffer central vision loss due to neovascularization disease, optical devices known as *low-vision aids* can be used.

PATIENT EDUCATION

No matter how severe the macular degeneration, patients can be reassured that they will not go blind because peripheral vision is largely unaffected. Such information is reassuring and greatly appreciated. The importance of early detection of neovascularization needs to be emphasized as well as the clinical warning symptoms (eg, distorted vision). Proper use of the Amsler grid should be taught so that daily self-monitoring can be performed at home.

INDICATIONS FOR REFERRAL

Any elderly patient suspected on the basis of history or physical examination to have macular degeneration should be referred to the ophthalmologist. Promptness is critical if there is distorted vision, because it may herald early serous retinal detachment and neovascularization.

A.H.G.

ANNOTATED BIBLIOGRAPHY

Macular Photocoagulation Study Group. Argon laser photocoagulation for senile macular degeneration: Results of a randomized clinical trial. Arch Ophthalmol 1982;100:912. *(Reduced frequency of vision loss in persons with exudative disease from 60 percent to 25 percent.)*

Watzke RC, et al. The macular symposium: Aging macular degeneration. Ophthalmology 1985;92:593. *(Detailed review.)*

Young RW. Pathophysiology of age-related macular degeneration. Surv Ophthalmol 1987;31:291. *(Good discussion of disease mechanisms.)*

207
Management of Glaucoma

CLAUDIA U. RICHTER, M.D.

Primary Care Medicine: Office Evaluation and Management of the Adult Patient, 3rd edition, edited by Allan H. Goroll, Lawrence A. May, and Albert G. Mulley, Jr. J.B. Lippincott Company, Philadelphia

Glaucoma is a disease of elevated intraocular pressure leading to optic nerve cupping and visual field loss. Elevated intraocular pressure is statistically defined as a pressure greater than 21 mm Hg and may occur in as much as 15 percent of the elderly population. Glaucoma is difficult to define and diagnose precisely because modestly elevated pressures may never cause glaucomatous damage in some patients whereas statistically normal intraocular pressures cause damage in others. Although the primary physician is not responsible for the diagnosis or treatment of glaucoma, he or she needs to screen patients for ocular hypertension (see Chapter 198) and recognize early stages of optic nerve damage that might ensue from such intraocular pressure elevation. One must also be able to recognize acute angle-closure glaucoma in order to institute proper initial therapy or at least to arrange prompt referral. In addition, many patients with glaucoma have multiple medical problems, necessitating an understanding of the medical therapy for glaucoma and how it might be affected by or affect treatment of other medical conditions.

PATHOPHYSIOLOGY AND CLINICAL PRESENTATION

The essential pathophysiologic feature of glaucoma is an intraocular pressure that is too high for the optic nerve. The exact mechanism of optic nerve damage has not been established and is probably a combination of factors. Increased intraocular pressure increases vascular resistance, causing decreased vascular perfusion of the optic nerve and ischemia. The increased pressure can interfere with axoplasmic flow in the ganglion cell axons, causing cell dysfunction and death; and it can compress the lamina cribrosa, the sievelike structure through which axons pass when leaving the eye. The altered supporting structure may then interfere with axonal function. These different mechanisms of axonal damage are of variable importance in different patients, but the final result is loss of ganglion cells and their axons, increased optic nerve cupping, and visual field loss.

The *pathophysiology* of increased intraocular pressure can best be understood in terms of the anatomy and physiology of aqueous flow. The iris divides the front of the eye into anterior and posterior chambers that communicate through the pupil. Aqueous humor is produced by the ciliary body, fills the posterior chamber, flows through the pupil into the anterior chamber, and leaves the eye through the trabecular meshwork, a connective tissue filter at the angle between the iris and the cornea. The aqueous passes through the trabecular meshwork into Schlemm's canal and into the episcleral venous system.

The pressure in the eye is maintained by the dynamic equilibrium of aqueous production and outflow. An increase in production or an obstruction to outflow will cause elevated intraocular pressure. In primary open-angle glaucoma, the obstruction exists at a microscopic level in the trabecular meshwork. In angle-closure glaucoma, the iris obstructs the trabecular meshwork. Secondary causes of glaucoma include inflammation, trauma, neoplasm, neovascularization, and corticosteroid therapy.

The most common presentation of *open-angle glaucoma,* accounting for more than 90 percent of glaucoma cases, is detection of *asymptomatic* elevated intraocular pressure by a primary physician, an optometrist, or an ophthalmologist. It is frequently called the "silent blinder," because extensive damage may occur before the patient is aware of visual field loss. The patient is usually over 40. Glaucomatous *cupping* of the optic nerve may be noted on routine ophthalmoscopy.

Acute *angle-closure glaucoma* presents with a *painful red eye*. The physical findings include decreased visual acuity, redness, fixed and unreactive pupil in mid-dilation, and corneal haziness. Occasionally, the principal symptoms are nausea and vomiting, and the patient may be thought to have abdominal or coronary disease. Patients with acute angle-closure glaucoma require emergency treatment. Patients susceptible to angle-closure can be identified by shining a light parallel to the iris plane from the temporal side of the globe: eyes with narrow angles will have a shadow fall on the nasal iris. This screening is particularly important in patients with a positive family history, episodes of halos, or of painful, blurred vision.

PRINCIPLES OF THERAPY

Chronic Open-Angle Glaucoma

The objective of treatment is stabilization of the intraocular pressure in a range that will prevent optic nerve damage and visual field loss. Therapy involves medications that reduce aqueous production or facilitate outflow. Topical medications include cholinergic agents, anticholinesterases, sympathomimetics, and topical beta-adrenergic antagonists.

Parasympathomimetics. *Pilocarpine,* the most frequently used parasympathomimetic, acts by contracting the ciliary body, which opens the trabecula to facilitate aqueous outflow. Ocular side effects include headache with initial administration, a miotic pupil with dimming of vision, fluctuating myopia, conjunctival hyperemia, and retinal detachment. Systemic side effects include diaphoresis, diarrhea, and leukocytosis.

Anticholinesterases act to increase endogenous cholinergic effects and are used to treat patients in whom pilocarpine is inadequate or who prefer the less frequent dosage. The most commonly used anticholinesterase is *echothiophate iodide* (Phospholine Iodide). The ocular side effects are similar to those of pilocarpine but also include cataract formation. A patient on an anticholinesterase who is unknowingly treated with succinylcholine may have appreciably prolonged respiratory depression.

Sympathomimetics. *Epinephrine* is a sympathomimetic drug that decreases aqueous production and may increase aqueous outflow. It is additive in effect to pilocarpine and may be used in combination. The ocular side effects of epinephrine include a burning sensation, conjunctival pigmentation, conjunctival hyperemia, and allergic reactions. Many topical side effects may be reduced by using *dipivefrin* hydrochloride (Propine), an epinephrine prodrug that is converted to epinephrine intraocularly. Systemic effects including tachycardia, palpitations, and hypertension may occur with either agent but are less frequent with dipivefrin.

Beta-blockers decrease aqueous humor production when applied topically and, because they have fewer ocular side effects than pilocarpine and need only twice-daily administration, they have become important first-line topical agents for treatment of glaucoma. Topical beta-blockers are extremely well tolerated but are absorbed into the systemic circulation and can precipitate heart failure, heart block, and exacerbation of asthma in predisposed patients. Nonselective topical preparations include timolol, levobunolol, and metipranolol. Betaxolol, a more selective $beta_1$-blocker is less likely to trigger an attack of asthma but may also be slightly less efficacious in controlling glaucoma.

Carbonic anhydrase inhibitors, such as *acetazolamide,* reduce aqueous production and are used when topical medications do not adequately lower intraocular pressure. They are usually used in combination with and are additive in effect to the topical medications discussed earlier. They have a variety of systemic effects, including mild metabolic acidosis, paresthesias of the face and extremities, metallic taste, anorexia, nausea, vomiting, diarrhea, renal stones, and blood dyscrasias.

Sequence of Medical Therapy. Most patients are treated first with a topical beta-blocker, then with epinephrine, pilocarpine, anticholinesterases, and finally carbonic anhydrase inhibitors. (The primary physician should take note of the patient's ocular medications and be familiar with their side effects.) When medical therapy is inadequate or not tolerated, laser trabeculoplasty and then surgery are indicated.

Laser and Surgical Therapies. *Laser trabeculoplasty* effectively lowers intraocular pressure in many patients inadequately controlled by medical therapy. The argon laser is used to place approximately one hundred 50-m spots circumferentially on the trabecular meshwork. Its effectiveness appears to be due to a "tightening" of the untreated trabecular meshwork and improved aqueous outflow. Approximately 75 percent of treated patients have a sufficient decrease in intraocular pressure to avoid glaucoma surgery in the short term; pressure remains under control after 4 years in 50 percent. The major complication is a post-laser elevation of intraocular pressure, which can be largely avoided by performing the laser trabeculoplasty in two sessions.

Surgical intervention should be considered when maximal medical therapy and laser trabeculoplasty do not lower the intraocular pressure to a level protective to the optic disk and visual field. The usual surgical procedure is to create a filtering or drainage route from the anterior chamber to the subconjunctival space. If filtering surgery fails or cannot be performed, laser cycloablation or cryotherapy can be applied to the ciliary body to decrease aqueous production.

Acute Angle-Closure Glaucoma

This condition requires prompt recognition and treatment with a miotic agent such as *pilocarpine,* followed by urgent referral to the ophthalmologist. Pilocarpine is given as one drop of the 4% solution in the involved eye every 20 minutes. Then *acetazolamide,* 250 mg, is given by mouth or 500 mg intravenously, and the patient is taken to the ophthalmologist. *Laser iridotomy* or a surgical peripheral *iridectomy* is necessary to prevent recurrent attacks. A laser iridectomy program is preferred to spare the patient intraocular surgery. The iridectomy provides communication between the posterior and anterior chambers for the aqueous humor and prevents the iris from being forced anteriorly against the trabecular meshwork. A prophylactic laser iridotomy is indicated in the unaffected eye.

THERAPEUTIC RECOMMENDATIONS

Drugs that increase intraocular pressure should be used cautiously. These include systemic and topical steroids, particularly when applied to the eye. Drugs with anticholinergic effects may precipitate angle-closure glaucoma in patients with narrow angles. Reports of hypotensive optic neuropathy after precipitous lowering of blood pressure suggest that a gradual reduction in blood pressure done in consultation with an ophthalmologist is preferable in patients with coincident systemic and ocular hypertension.

Most patients are treated first with topical beta-adrenergic antagonists, then with epinephrine, pilocarpine, an anticholinesterase, and finally a carbonic anhydrase inhibitor. The primary physician should know all patients' ocular medications and their systemic side effects. If medical therapy proves inadequate or intolerable, then laser trabeculoplasty and surgery deserve consideration.

PATIENT EDUCATION

A chief responsibility of the primary physician is to educate the patient about the meaning of elevated intraocular pressure and the need to screen for it (see Chapter 198). Patients may be told that they are "glaucoma suspects," should their intraocular pressures reach the middle 20s. When their optic nerves are healthy, these patients can be safely followed without treatment. Patients may call their primary physician for reassurance about the side effects of drugs, and the physician should provide an explanation and facilitate consultation with the ophthalmologist. For patients diagnosed with glaucoma and on medication, the importance of careful follow-up examinations and compliance with medication regimens to prevent visual loss needs to be emphasized.

ANNOTATED BIBLIOGRAPHY

Bienfang DC, Kelly LD, Nicholson DH, et al. Ophthalmology. N Engl J Med 1990;323:956. *(Good overview of new approaches to treatment.)*

Everitt DE, Avorn J. Systemic effects of medications used to treat glaucoma. Ann Intern Med 1990;112;120. *(Important information for the nonophthalmologic physician.)*

Margolis KL, Money BE, Kopietz LA, et al. Physician recognition of ophthalmoscopic signs of open-angle glaucoma. J Gen Intern Med 1989;4:296. *(An educational program that includes good photographs of the key findings.)*

Schwartz B. Current concepts in ophthalmology: The glaucomas. N Engl J Med 1978;299:182. *(A superb, still useful review for the generalist reader.)*

Shingleton BJ, Richter CU, Bellows AR, et al. Long-term efficacy of argon laser trabeculoplasty. Ophthalmology 1987;94:1513. *(Laser therapy effective in 50% of patients treated after 4 years.)*

Primary Care Medicine: Office Evaluation and Management of the Adult Patient, 3rd edition, edited by Allan H. Goroll, Lawrence A. May, and Albert G. Mulley, Jr. J.B. Lippincott Company, Philadelphia

208
Management of Cataracts

ROGER F. STEINERT, M.D.

Cataracts are opacifications of the crystalline lens of the eye. They are unusual in young patients, but the incidence rises sharply in later years, such that virtually all elderly patients have some degree of cataract. Because of the implications of this diagnosis, the term *cataract* is best reserved for opacities resulting in functional impairment. The primary care physician should be able to detect cataract formation, monitor its progression, advise the patient on when to seek ophthalmologic consultation, help the ophthalmologist assess medical candidacy for surgery, and support the patient in the perioperative and rehabilitation phases.

PATHOPHYSIOLOGY AND CLINICAL PRESENTATION

Cataracts may arise from a variety of causes. Occasionally, they are *congenital;* a few develop during the early years of life, usually in association with specific diseases such as diabetes, Wilson's disease, Down's syndrome, and other metabolic diseases. The majority of cataracts occur in the elderly and reflect senescent change occasionally associated with systemic diseases. Trauma is another important precipitant.

Presenile and Senile Cataract. Age-related lens opacity results from protein denaturation and hydration. Sodium and calcium concentrations increase, potassium and ascorbate levels diminish, and glutathione disappears. The underlying metabolic changes leading to senile cataract are unknown. In diabetes mellitus, excess sugar is diverted to the sorbitol pathway. An insoluble alcohol accumulates, and this osmotic load causes the protein to hydrate.

As the human lens ages, the nucleus hardens (nuclear sclerosis). The first visual event may be a shift toward nearsightedness because of the increased refractive index and thickness of the sclerotic nucleus. As a result, the patient may temporarily experience enhanced reading vision without glasses ("second-sight"), and a change in spectacles may be the only treatment needed. Eventually the nucleus acquires a yellow-brown coloration ("brunesent cataract") and becomes progressively more opaque. Only a few patients are aware of the gradual spectral change, with a yellow cast to the visual world; they usually acknowledge it only after the cataract is removed. Visual impairment initially is more marked at distance than near, and a patient may fail a driver's license exam and still be able to read a newspaper. Loss of contrast sensitivity may cause a functional impairment out of proportion to the results of a standard high-contrast visual acuity test.

Posterior subcapsular cataracts form at the back of the lens, usually centrally. This type of cataract is often responsible for the "presenile" cataract in the 40- to 50-year-old age group. It may be spontaneous but is often associated with prolonged use of topical or systemic steroids or with diabetes mellitus. The central location of the opacity causes the vision to worsen when the pupil becomes small, as in reading or on bright days. The refractile nature of the opacity commonly causes severe difficulty with glare, such as driving at night. Pupillary dilatation by mydriatic or cycloplegic drops or use of subdued light improves vision in such cases, as more light is allowed to enter the eye.

Presenile and senile cataract formation is painless and generally progresses over months or years. Cataracts are also frequently associated with intraocular inflammation and glaucoma.

Traumatic Cataract. These most commonly result from intraocular foreign bodies that perforate the lens capsule, allowing the lens protein to hydrate and thereby denature and opacify. Occasionally a lens will opacify after severe, blunt nonpenetrating trauma. Electric shock and high-dose ionizing radiation may lead to lens opacification. Prolonged exposure to ultraviolet B, as occurs with unprotected sun exposure, is an important risk factor for cortical cataract formation; risk of nuclear cataract is not significantly increased.

WORKUP

Initial evaluation by the primary physician includes *visual acuity* determination both near and at distance. The lenticular opacity can be appreciated with the *direct ophthalmoscope* while attempting to visualize the fundus. If the angle is not shallow, dilation with one drop of 2.5% phenylephrine or 1% tropicamide is helpful. With the ophthalmoscope lens set at zero and standing about 12 inches from the patient, a bright red reflex is seen in the normal eye. Cataract formation is clearly seen by the disruption of the red reflex. Plus power (black numbers) in the ophthalmoscope of about 15 or 20 diopters will put the lens of the eye in focus as the physician approaches the eye. The fundus should be examined for retinal abnormalities, particularly macular degeneration (manifested by hemorrhage, scarring, and drusen), which will cause loss of vision symptomatically similar to that from cataract. In all cases of visual impairment, an ophthalmic consultation is indicated.

PRINCIPLES OF MANAGEMENT

The only definitive treatment for cataract is *surgery.* Traumatic cataracts and very advanced senile cataracts may cause inflammation and glaucoma, for which emergency surgery is mandatory. However, most cataract surgery is elective. The patient should understand that a cataract is not a tumor or a "growth" and that the cataract will not harm the eye.

In early nuclear sclerosis, modification of the patient's spectacles may improve vision adequately to defer surgery. Sometimes chronic pupillary dilation will suffice for a patient with posterior subcapsular cataract. When, despite these measures, the patient feels that visual function is intolerably impaired, cataract surgery can be discussed as a treatment option.

Cataract surgery is often performed under local anesthesia (block or topical) with mild sedation and monitoring by qualified anesthesia personnel. Patient movement during surgery may be disastrous, however, and the primary physician can assist the ophthalmologist in assessing whether age, mental status, and medical condition make general anesthesia appropriate.

Surgical Approaches. There are several options for cataract surgery. The most common are *extracapsular extraction,* in which the lens capsule is opened and the contents are removed (about 10 mm), and *phacoemulsification,* which uses ultrasonic energy to break up the hard nucleus and aspirate it through a small opening (about 3 mm). An increasing majority of cataract extractions in the United States use the latter approach. The small wound permits the patient rapid return to full physical activity.

Postoperatively, the surgeon will prescribe topical medications and may restrict activity to some extent. Modern microsurgical wound closure allows earlier rehabilitation than in the past. Final visual correction may be given within 1 to 2 weeks postoperatively.

Visual Rehabilitation. Three methods of *visual rehabilitation* are available: eyeglasses, contact lenses, and lens implants. *Cataract spectacles* must be powerful to correct for the absence of the crystalline lens. In addition to thickness and weight, these spectacles magnify approximately 25 percent. This magnification prohibits the use of a cataract lens for only one eye, because a double image would result.

The spectacle thickness also severely limits side vision, with a midperipheral blind spot. These problems make adjustment to cataract glasses difficult at best, and some patients find ambulation nearly impossible with these spectacles.

Contact lenses are optically superior to spectacles. Because the lens power is so much closer to the eye, magnification is only 5 percent to 7 percent, and most patients will not perceive diplopia with a contact lens, although stereoscopic acuity will be reduced. Peripheral vision will be normal. Many elderly patients have difficulty handling contact lenses; extended wear lenses (usually soft) may be tolerated for weeks to months between removals for cleaning. Use of these lenses is not without difficulty, however. Lens deposits, damage, and loss may result in frequent visits to the ophthalmologist, with high cost and time lost. Devastating infectious corneal ulcers are much more common in elderly patients with extended-wear contact lenses.

Intraocular lens implantation has been refined to the point that it is standard practice where not specifically contraindicated. At the time of cataract extraction (and occasionally as a secondary procedure in cases of spectacle and contact lens intolerance), the surgeon implants a delicate plastic device with optical power to replace the cataractous lens. The implant is permanent, requires no care, and restores normal optics without magnification. Although once controversial, with advances in manufacturing and surgical technique there is minimal extra risk to the implant. The implant is contraindicated in some conditions, such as chronic uveitis, which is assessed by the ophthalmologist preoperatively.

Intraocular lenses continue to improve. Several types can be folded during insertion so that only a small wound is needed. Multifocal lenses are being studied; they may allow patients freedom from bifocals and reading glasses.

For a limited number of patients with contraindications to the above techniques, optical rehabilitation may be provided by means of a corneal refractive surgical procedure.

PATIENT EDUCATION AND INDICATIONS FOR REFERRAL

Prevention of cataract formation is important, with use of protective eyewear the best means of reducing risk of cortical cataract formation due to ultraviolet B radiation from the sun. Sunglasses need to be specially treated to fully prevent penetration of ultraviolet radiation, although wearing a hat with a brim and sunglasses with plastic untreated lenses does reduce exposure. However, the darkness of a lens's tint is not necessarily a measure of protective capacity. Dark unprotective sunglasses may actually exacerbate exposure by blocking visible light transmission, causing pupillary dilation, and thus increasing penetration of ultraviolet radiation. Outdoor workers are at particularly high risk and should wear close-fitting protective sunglasses.

For elderly patients with age-related nuclear cataracts, the primary physician should help the patient understand that, although surgical correction is highly successful in up to 98 percent of patients, it is not risk-free. Occasionally, complications do occur. When vision is good in one eye and there are no particular functional limitations, it may be preferable to defer surgery.

However, for those with cataracts interfering with daily living (eg, causing falls or prohibiting reading), microsurgical cataract extraction with intraocular lens implantation has a high likelihood of dramatically improving quality of life.

The patient is best served by referral to an ophthalmologist on the basis of overall skill, thoughtfulness, and caring manner rather than just on ability to perform a particular operation. Good clinical judgment and an effective working relationship will be as important to the outcome as technical ability.

ANNOTATED BIBLIOGRAPHY

Grisso JA, Kelsey JL, Strom BL, et al. Risk factors for falls as a cause of hip fracture in women. N Engl J Med 1991;324:1326. *(Impaired vision raises the risk of hip fracture fivefold.)*

Rosenthal FS, Fakalian AE, Taylor HR. The effect of prescription eyewear on ocular exposure to ultraviolet radiation. Am J Public Health 1986;76:1216. *(Means of cutting down on UV exposure.)*

Steinert RF (ed). Cataract: Evaluation, Surgery, and Complications. Philadelphia: WB Saunders, 1994. *(Comprehensive reference text.)*

Taylor HR, West SK, Rosenthal FS, et al. Effect of ultraviolet radiation on cataract formation. N Engl J Med 1988;319;1429. *(Significant relationship found between UVB exposure and cortical cataract formation; argues for wearing protective eyewear in the sun.)*

Primary Care Medicine: Office Evaluation and Management of the Adult Patient, 3rd edition, edited by Allan H. Goroll, Lawrence A. May, and Albert G. Mulley, Jr. J.B. Lippincott Company, Philadelphia

209
Management of Diabetic Retinopathy

RICHARD D. PESAVENTO, M.D.
CLAUDIA U. RICHTER, M.D.

Diabetic retinopathy is a leading cause of blindness in the United States in people under age 65 years. Its incidence has increased with improved long-term survival of diabetics. The prevalence increases with duration of disease and is greatest in older age groups. Effective treatment is available not only to prevent many of the most serious complications of retinopathy, but also to reduce the risk of developing retinopathy. Therapy is most effective when rendered promptly. It is of great importance for the primary physician to know when to check for retinopathy and when to refer to the ophthalmologist for more detailed evaluation and consideration of treatment. Diabetes can also cause other eye problems, including refractive changes, cataracts, glaucoma, and reversible cranial nerve palsies (see Chapters 102, 200, 207, and 208).

PATHOPHYSIOLOGY AND CLINICAL PRESENTATION

Two types of diabetic retinopathy can be recognized ophthalmoscopically: background and proliferative.

Background retinopathy is generally the early form and consists of intraretinal vascular damage. Loss of capillary pericytes, thickening of basement membranes, swelling and proliferation of endothelial cells, and intravascular thrombosis occur. This results in both dilation of small vessels and vascular closure leading to ischemia. In addition, there is abnormal endothelial permeability with breakdown of the normal blood–retina barrier. Retinal capillaries become permeable to water, lipids, and large molecules, which are not adequately removed by the usual cellular pump mechanism of the adjacent retinal pigmented epithelium.

Clinically, this results in microaneurysms, intraretinal hemorrhages, "cotton-wool" infarctions, and lipid and serous exudation with retinal edema. *Microaneurysms* are dilated capillaries that sometimes thrombose. They appear as red dots in the retina, similar to the small "blot" intraretinal hemorrhages, which result from bleeding in the deep layers of the retina. *"Flame-shaped" hemorrhages* occur in the striated superficial ganglion cell layer. White-centered hemorrhages represent hemorrhagic infarcts. *"Cotton-wool" infarcts,* also known by the misnomer *"soft exudates"* are nerve cell infarctions. The swollen axons become ophthalmoscopically visible as white, feathery, "soft" lesions. *"Hard" exudates* are true exudation of the intravascular lipid into the retina, leading to yellow, glistening sphere and aggregates of lipid, sometimes arranged in a circular pattern or "circinate ring" around leaking blood vessels. *Retinal edema* is more difficult to see. Accumulation of serous fluid in the intercellular spaces of the retina results in retinal thickening.

Patients with background retinopathy are asymptomatic unless retinal edema involves the central macula, in which case blurring or distortion of central vision is the initial symptom followed by loss of central vision. Macular edema is the leading cause of visual loss in diabetics, especially older type II patients. Hypertension and fluid retention tend to adversely affect vascular exudation and macular edema.

Proliferative retinopathy consists of vascular pathology that extends from the retina into the vitreous cavity. This form of retinopathy generally occurs at a later stage than background retinopathy and tends to have a worse visual prognosis without prompt treatment. Advancing capillary and arteriolar closure with more widespread retinal ischemia herald the onset and are manifested by an increase in the number of cotton-wool hemorrhages, larger intraretinal hemorrhages, (frequently with white centers), venous beading, and small networks of weblike intraretinal vessels. There is a correlation between duration and degree of hyperglycemia and progression of retinopathy. Tight control slows the onset and severity of retinopathy as well as other microvascular complications of diabetes (see Chapter 102).

The retina responds to advancing ischemia with *neovascularization,* the hallmark of proliferative retinopathy, by forming networks of new vessels that extend from existing retinal vessels anteriorly into the vitreous cavity. These vessels first appear as a fine network of small vessels proliferating from the optic disk, the major retinal vessels, or from areas adjacent to retinal ischemia. As neovascularization progresses, dense, white, fibrotic tissue forms and adheres to the posterior vitreous. Such fibrosis can cause the vitreous to contract and pull anteriorly, rupturing the fragile network of vessels growing into the vitreous and producing a *vitreous hemorrhage* that fills the eye and compromises vision. *Retinal detachment* can also occur, either from tractional forces on the retina or in combination with retinal holes forming. The iris may also be involved with neovascularization, leading to glaucoma from scarring of the trabecular meshwork.

Proliferative retinopathy can present as small floating specks or cobwebs in the visual field, representing a small vitreous hemorrhage. Sudden, profound loss of vision, sometimes associated with flashing lights, may signify retinal detachment or severe vitreous hemorrhage.

Clinical Course. Diabetic retinopathy does not appear until 3 to 5 years after the onset of type I diabetes. Onset in type II diabetes is probably similar, but more difficult to pinpoint because of difficulty establishing onset of the underlying disease. Type I diabetics tend to progress more rapidly to proliferative retinopathy, with an incidence of 50 percent after 15 years. Older type II diabetics have a higher incidence of macular edema-induced vision loss.

Pregnancy poses an additional vision risk for diabetics because retinal pathology can progress with unanticipated speed and may require laser treatment sooner than expected. Close monitoring by an ophthalmologist is necessary.

WORKUP

Screening asymptomatic diabetic patients for retinopathy is an essential part of effective diabetic care. Available screening methods for detecting diabetic retinopathy include nondilated ophthalmoscopy, dilated ophthalmoscopy performed by the ophthalmologist, and stereo fundus photography. Stereo photography is the most sensitive, and nondilated ophthalmoscopy is the least. Dilated ophthalmoscopy has a sensitivity of about 80 percent and a specificity of 99 percent for detection of proliferative retinopathy. Pending less costly stereophotographic methods, *dilated ophthalmoscopy* by an ophthalmologist is required. Examination of the nondilated eye with a hand-held ophthalmoscope is inadequate for screening, especially when performed by the nonophthalmologic physician.

The natural history of diabetic retinopathy determines the proper screening schedule. Current screening guidelines for diabetic retinopathy jointly adopted by the American College of Physicians, the American Diabetes Association, and the American Academy of Ophthalmology include:

1. For patients with type I diabetes: screening annually beginning 5 years after the onset of diabetes, generally not before the onset of puberty.
2. For patients with type II diabetes: initial screening at the time of diagnosis and then annually. If the initial examination uses stereo fundus photography and is found to be normal, then the next examination need not occur for 4 years. After that, annual screening is required, regardless of method used.
3. For pregnant diabetic women: dilated ophthalmoscopy during the first trimester and close follow-up throughout pregnancy. When planning pregnancy, the diabetic woman should be counseled on the risk of developing or worsening retinopathy. No screening is needed for women with gestational diabetes.
4. For development of symptoms or signs of macular edema, moderate to severe nonproliferative retinopathy, or any proliferative retinopathy requires prompt referral to an ophthalmologist skilled in management of diabetic retinopathy.

Such screening does not obviate ophthalmoscopic examination by the primary physician, who might be able to detect an important lesion in the interval between screening examinations, but nondilated ophthalmoscopy by the primary physician is no substitute for a formal eye examination by the ophthalmologist.

PRINCIPLES OF MANAGEMENT

Prevention. Both primary and secondary prevention are achievable, as demonstrated by the Diabetes Control and Complications Trial (DCCT). In patients with type I diabetes treated with intensive insulin therapy to normalize the blood glucose, the risk of developing retinopathy was reduced by 76 percent and, in those with preexisting retinopathy, the risk of progression was reduced by 54 percent. Transient worsening of existing retinopathy occurs during the first year of intensive treatment in about a quarter of patients and consists of soft exudates and intraretinal microvascular changes. Such changes usually disappear by 18 months with continued intensive insulin therapy, and reduction in long-term risk of progression is the same as for patients without early progression.

The DCCT study was confined to patients with type I diabetes who had either no retinopathy or mild retinopathy. Whether similar results can be achieved in patients with type II diabetes or more severe retinopathy remains to be demonstrated. Most authorities expect type II diabetics to respond similarly to normalization of blood glucose, although the best means of achieving tight glycemic control in such persons is yet to be determined. The risk of accelerated progression of retinopathy may be greater in patients with proliferative or severe nonproliferative retinal disease, making close ophthalmologic follow-up essential. The safe achievement of tight glycemic control requires a highly motivated patient and considerable support (see Chapter 102).

Other measures that may be helpful in preventing progression of retinopathy include good *control of hypertension* and *cessation of smoking*. Neither the use of aspirin to reduce platelet aggregation nor the use of clofibrate to decrease lipid exudates has proven effective.

Treatment. Once retinopathy is detected, its treatment is the province of the retinal specialist. *Laser photocoagulation* reduces the rate of vision-threatening complications from both forms of retinopathy.

Background Retinopathy. In patients with background retinopathy, laser treatment of the macular region reduces the rate of severe vision loss by over 50 percent. Although progressive vision loss can often be prevented or slowed, few patients recover vision already lost, making early detection and treatment essential.

Proliferative Retinopathy. In patients with proliferative retinopathy, panretinal photocoagulation outside the macular area is the primary therapeutic modality. The stimulus to form new vessels is reduced, and risk of severe vision loss is reduced by 50 percent to 65 percent. Potential complications include mild reduction in vision, decreased night vision, loss of peripheral vision, inadvertent burns to the central macula, and hemorrhage and exudative detachment of the retina or choroid leading to angle-closure glaucoma.

Surgery is necessary when a vitreous hemorrhage will not spontaneously clear or when dense fibrovascular proliferation affects the macula and causes severe vision loss. Early vitrectomy after hemorrhage produces the best results in type I patients; waiting 12 to 18 months for spontaneous clearing is advocated for those with type II disease.

Other Hyperglycemia-Related Complications. The *myopia* occurring from hyperglycemia-induced osmotic swelling of the lens responds to reestablishment of glycemic control, but it may take weeks to resolve. *Diplopia* due to localized demyelination of the 3rd, 4th, or 6th cranial nerve usually recovers within 1 to 3 months. *Cataracts* may also form (see Chapter 208).

PATIENT EDUCATION AND INDICATIONS FOR REFERRAL

Patient education by the primary physician is essential to prevention, early detection, and prompt treatment of retinopathy. Reviewing the benefits of tight glycemic control can be a potent motivating force that improves patient behavior. The importance of smoking cessation, hypertension control, regular ophthalmologic examinations, and immediate reporting of eye symptoms needs to be stressed in conjunction with the good news that effective treatment to prevent vision loss is available.

Ophthalmologic referral is indicated for routine screening (see above) and is urgent when there is:

- Change in vision, appearance of floaters, or complaint of eye pain
- Discovery of retinopathy (particularly if abnormal vessels are seen on the iris)
- Loss of ability to visualize the fundus

Treatment decisions regarding diabetic retinopathy should be made by the ophthalmologist skilled in management of retinal disease.

ANNOTATED BIBLIOGRAPHY

American College of Physicians, American Diabetes Association, and American Academy of Ophthalmology. Screening guidelines for diabetic retinopathy. Ann Intern Med 1992;116:683. *(Consensus recommendations for screening.)*

The Diabetes Control and Complications Trial Research Group. The effect of intensive treatment of diabetes on the development and progression of long-term complications in insulin-dependent diabetes mellitus. N Engl J Med 1993;329:977. *(Tight glycemic control reduced risks for development and progression of retinopathy in type I diabetics.)*

The Diabetic Retinopathy Study Research Group. Photocoagulation treatment of proliferative diabetic retinopathy. Ophthalmology 1978;85:82. *(Established the role of photocoagulation in treatment of proliferative diabetic retinopathy.)*

The Diabetic Retinopathy Vitrectomy Study Research Group. Early vitrectomy for severe vitreous hemorrhage in diabetic retinopathy. Arch Ophthalmol 1985;103:1644. *(Early vitrectomy improved outcome in type I diabetics.)*

Early Treatment Diabetic Retinopathy Study Research Group. Photocoagulation for diabetic macular edema. Arch Ophthalmol 1985;103:1796. *(Focal photocoagulation of macular edema reduced the risk of visual loss.)*

Merimee TJ. Diabetic retinopathy. N Engl J Med 1990;322:978. *(Review of pathophysiology; 80 refs.)*

Paetkau MD, Boyd TAS, Winship B, et al. Cigarette smoking and diabetic retinopathy. Diabetes 1977;26:46. *(Risk of proliferative retinopathy rose with increasing tobacco consumption.)*

Rand LI, Krolewski AS, Aiello LM, et al. Multiple factors in the prediction of risk of proliferative diabetic retinopathy. N Engl J Med 1985;313:1433. *(Cases were both more difficult to control and patients less engaged in the process.)*

Working Group on Hypertension in Diabetes. Statement on hypertension in diabetes. Diabetes Care 1987;10:764. *(Highlights the association, describes the end-organ damage, and establishes guidelines for treatment.)*

Primary Care Medicine: Office Evaluation and Management of the Adult Patient, 3rd edition, edited by Allan H. Goroll, Lawrence A. May, and Albert G. Mulley, Jr. J.B. Lippincott Company, Philadelphia

210
Selection and Use of Contact Lenses

Over 18 million Americans wear contact lenses. With proper prescription and safe use, they provide excellent correction of vision and convenience. Primary physicians are sometimes asked their opinion about the relative merits of various types of contact lenses and may be the first physician consulted when a problem with their use develops. Knowing the basics about contact lens use and the complications that may ensue can facilitate proper eye care.

TYPES OF CONTACT LENSES, THEIR ADVANTAGES AND DISADVANTAGES

Hard lenses were the first to be developed. They provide excellent correction of vision but are approved only for daily wear and must be removed before sleep to avoid injury to the cornea. They are relatively easy to keep clean and often last for years. Risks of corneal opacification, ulceration, and infection are low with proper use and almost nil with gas-permeable hard lenses. Disadvantages include their need to be removed before sleep, discomfort, and tendency to dislodge with vigorous exercise.

Soft reusable lenses were developed over 2 decades ago and have become popular because they are more comfortable than hard lenses, can be worn for longer periods, are easier to adapt to, and do not dislodge as readily. In addition, they are less likely than hard lenses to blur vision when switching to eyeglasses, because they have less effect on the cornea. Extended-wear soft lenses are thin, need not be removed before sleep, and can be worn continuously for days.

Disadvantages include less effective correction of vision compared to hard lenses, need for more frequent cleansing and disinfection, and shorter useful life-span (6 to 18 months). In addition, risks of corneal opacification, conjunctivitis, and ulcerative keratitis are greater. Corneal opacities are seen most frequently in patients who wear their lenses for prolonged periods without removal.

A *chronic allergic conjunctivitis* may develop from either a reaction to thimerosal, a preservative present in some cleansing solutions, or from protein deposits that build up on the lenses. Treatment requires better cleaning, use of a preservative-free cleansing solution, decreased length of use, and more frequent lens replacement.

Ulcerative keratitis (corneal ulceration and inflammation) is an infrequent (20 per 10,000 users of extended-wear lenses) but much more serious complication. It occurs in patients using extended-wear lenses for prolonged periods without removal and in those with hard lenses or daily-use soft lenses who forget to take them out before sleep. Relative risk is 10 to 15 times that of persons who remove their lenses nightly. The injured corneal surface is subject to infection, which may lead to perforation. The principal organisms include *Pseudomonas,* cultured from protein deposits on the lenses, and *Acanthamoeba,* derived from contaminated cleaning solutions. The latter produces a particularly severe infection. The infection can spread quickly and threaten vision by permanently destroying the corneal stroma. Prompt ophthalmologic referral is indicated. Response to antibiotics is usually good. The best treatment is prevention, leading the FDA to restrict approved use of such lenses to no more than 7 continuous days. Many authorities feel that 3 days of continuous wear should be the upper limit.

Disposable soft lenses represent an attempt to further enhance convenience by eliminating the need for cleaning and disinfecting. Disposables last about 2 weeks and can be worn continuously for up to 3 days at a time. Cost is high, and corneal injury and infection may result from inappropriately prolonged use.

A.H.G.

ANNOTATED BIBLIOGRAPHY

Schein OD, Glynn RJ, Poggio EC, et al. The relative risk of ulcerative keratitis among users of daily-wear and extended-wear soft contact lenses. N Engl J Med 1989;321:773. *(Soft contacts worn overnight significantly increased the risk of ulcerative keratitis.)*

Smith RE, MacRae SM. Contact lenses—convenience and complications. N Engl J Med 1989;321:824. *(An editorial urging the continuous use of extended-wear lenses be limited to considerably less than the 7 days approved by the FDA.)*

Soft contact lenses. Medical Letter 1990;32:69. *(Terse summary of advantages and disadvantages.)*

Primary Care Medicine: Office Evaluation and Management of the Adult Patient, 3rd edition, edited by Allan H. Goroll, Lawrence A. May, and Albert G. Mulley, Jr. J.B. Lippincott Company, Philadelphia

14

Ear, Nose, and Throat Problems

211

Screening for Oral Cancer

JOHN P. KELLY, D.M.D., M.D.

There are over 30,000 new cases of oral cancer each year in the United States, representing 4 percent of cancer cases in men and 2 percent in women. Over 9,000 deaths result from oral cancer yearly. Despite the ready accessibility of the oral cavity to inspection by physicians, dentists, and patients themselves, 50 percent of oral cancers already have metastasized at the time of diagnosis. Perhaps that is because pain, a manifestation of advanced disease, is the symptom that most commonly leads patients to seek medical attention. When detected early, oral cancer has a very good prognosis. The primary physician has an important role in early detection. Prevention is another responsibility, given the relation of oral cancer to use of tobacco and alcohol.

EPIDEMIOLOGY AND RISK FACTORS

The peak incidence of oral carcinoma is in the sixth decade for women and is equally frequent in each decade after the age of 50 for men. However, the appearance of the disease in the third and fourth decades is not rare and must not be overlooked.

Use of *tobacco* in all its forms is highly correlated with the risk of oral cancer. The frequency of oral cancer of the cheek and gum rises 50-fold among long-term users of *smokeless tobacco*. Use has reached epidemic proportions among teenage boys, causing the Surgeon General's Report to warn against it. Such tobacco products contain multiple carcinogens in addition to tobacco, including nitrosoamines, aromatic hydrocarbons, and polonium. Pipe smokers are at increased risk for cancer of the lip. Squamous cell or epidermoid carcinoma of the lower lip also has a particularly high incidence among fair-skinned people whose occupation or residence subjects them to prolonged *sun exposure*.

Risk of oral cancer is high among those with heavy *alcohol* consumption. Whether this is due to a direct effect of alcohol on the oral mucosa or to associated smoking or vitamin deficiency remains to be fully elucidated.

Cancer of the tongue is highly correlated with the atrophic glossitis seen with tertiary syphilis. Cancer of the tongue is more common among nonsmokers. Mucosal atrophy from other causes is also associated with an increased incidence of oral cancers. Most notably, *chronic iron deficiency* leading to Plummer-Vinson syndrome is known to alter mucosal tissues, and this change may be related to the increased incidence of oral carcinoma. *Epstein–Barr virus* and *papilloma virus* have been found in cells of the tongue manifesting oral hairy leukoplakia, a hyperplastic change found in patients with acquired immunodeficiency syndrome (AIDS).

Chronic irritation of the oral mucosa by ill-fitting dentures, poorly restored teeth, or particularly spicy diets has often been mentioned as contributing to the development of oral carcinoma. However, there are no epidemiologic data to support this view.

The precise etiology of oral cancer is unknown. The etiologic factors mentioned above probably act as cocarcinogens, effecting malignant change in concert with some primary agent not yet elucidated. Increased chromosomal fragility has been found in nonsmokers who develop oral cancers.

NATURAL HISTORY

In considering the natural history of oral cancer, it is important to address premalignant disease as well as malignant disease.

Premalignant Disease

Leukoplakia, a "white patch" on the oral mucosa, is of interest because in about 10 percent of instances, it represents premalignant change with dysplastic features on biopsy. Clinically, it ranges from slightly raised, white translucent areas to dense white opaque plaques, with or without adjacent ulceration. It is hard to differentiate completely benign from premalignant leukoplakia, except by *biopsy*. However, patients demonstrating a speckled pattern interspersed with areas of ulceration or erosion are more likely to have dysplastic disease. Lesions may occur anywhere on the oral mucosa, but lingular ones have the greatest risk of malignant transformation. Such transformation may take anywhere from 1 to 20 years. Etiologies besides cancer include mucosal irritation (smoking, cheek or tongue biting, poorly fitting dentures, aspirin), alcohol excess, and viral infection (hairy leukoplakia–seen in AIDS). Differential diagnosis includes lichen planus, oral candidiasis, discoid lupus, and pemphigus vulgaris.

Erythroplasia, a red hyperplastic area of mucosa, is highly suggestive of an early carcinoma. Although most cancer screening protocols have emphasized a search for white lesions, the predominant color in premalignant or early lesions is red, not white. In fact, whereas some white lesions may only be "premalignant," the red lesions must be considered to be true malignancies unless proven otherwise by biopsy.

Malignant Disease

The average 5-year survival rate for localized oral cancer exceeds 65 percent but barely reaches 30 percent for patients with metastatic disease. When untreated, oral carcinoma metastasizes to the regional lymph nodes of the neck, ultimately leading to respiratory embarrassment or involvement of the great vessels. Ipsilateral node involvement is most common, but metastasis to the contralateral side—especially from primary lesions of the tongue or floor of the mouth—occurs with such frequency that treatment for control of metastatic disease is difficult. Hence, the importance of early diagnosis and control of the primary lesion. The lungs are the most frequently involved extranodal metastatic site.

Local recurrence is common. Many instances may actually represent new primary disease, suggesting a susceptibility of the entire oral mucosa to malignant change in affected patients. As many as one patient in five may be expected to develop a second primary oropharyngeal cancer, with smokers who do not quit incurring the greatest risk.

Other oral lesions appear black, blue, or brown. Benign conditions such as vascular malformations, heavy metal ingestion, amalgam tattooing, pigmented nevi, and the pigmentations associated with such systemic conditions as neurofibromatosis, intestinal polyposis, and Addison's disease, must be differentiated from the blue-black lesion of malignant melanoma (see Chapter 177). Biopsy is essential if this diagnosis is suggested by the appearance of the lesion.

SCREENING AND DIAGNOSTIC PROCEDURES

The challenge to primary care physicians is to recognize premalignant and early malignant lesions of the oral cavity. The greatest hope for improved outcome is detection before the appearance of grossly invasive disease. The ready accessibility of the oral cavity to *inspection* and the appearance of premalignant mucosal changes facilitate early detection. *Biopsy* of suspicious lesions should follow. Leukoplakia and erythroplasia are the most potentially important mucosal changes.

Initial evaluation of a suspicious lesion begins with eliciting appropriate historical data to eliminate such relatively harmless lesions as the acute aspirin burn. Irritative lesions can be identified by removing or repairing jagged teeth and poorly fitting or protruding dental prostheses and following the clinical healing of the mucosal wound. In any patient with a suspicious lesion, use of a noxious agent such as tobacco must be eliminated at the outset.

Any red or white lesion that persists for 2 weeks after initial recognition and elimination of irritating agents demands further investigation. Referral of the patient to an oral and maxillofacial surgeon for biopsy is the definitive diagnostic maneuver. High-risk patients, specifically those with histories of smoking and drinking, should be referred for biopsy promptly, as should any patient with a deeply ulcerative or fungating lesion. Although some studies suggest a chemoprophylactic role for *retinoids,* their use continues to be investigational.

Any swelling beneath a normal-appearing oral mucosa must be evaluated by an appropriate specialist for diagnosis or treatment. Such lesions are commonly benign and are the result of infection, bony exostosis, or mucus retention phenomena, but they may represent neoplasms of the minor salivary glands or other submucosal structures.

RECOMMENDATIONS

- A thorough visual and manual examination of the lips and oral cavity should be a part of every patient's evaluation; mucosal patches that are either red or white are sought.
- A high index of suspicion must be maintained for patients with a history of smoking, drinking, and heavy exposure to sunlight.
- Atrophic or hyperplastic areas of the oral mucosa must be viewed with suspicion, particularly if they are red or white (erythroplasia or leukoplakia) and last more than 2 weeks after cessation of smoking, drinking, and exposure to irritants.
- Referral for definitive biopsy is indicated for persistent lesions. The role of retinoids for chemoprophylaxis remains to be determined.

ANNOTATED BIBLIOGRAPHY

Connolly GN, Winn DL, Hecht SS, et al. The re-emergence of smokeless tobacco. N Engl J Med 1986;314:1020. *(An extensive review documents health risks and points out alarming rise in popularity. An editorial by the Surgeon General reinforces the message.)*

Decker J, Goldstein JC. Risk factors in head and neck cancer. N Engl J Med 1982;306:1151. *(Reviews the epidemiology of oral malignancy emphasizing the importance of smoking, alcohol, and poor oral hygiene.)*

Greene JC, Louie R, Wycoff SJ. Preventive dentistry II: Periodontal diseases, malocclusion, trauma, and oral cancer. JAMA 1990;262:421. *(The recommendations of the US Preventive Services Task Force.)*

Jacobs C. The internist in the management of head and neck cancer. Ann Intern Med 1990;113:771. *(Prevention can be achieved by cessation of tobacco use and reduction in alcohol intake; early detection greatly improves prognosis and response to therapy.)*

Mashberg A. Erythroplasia: The earliest sign of asymptomatic oral cancer. J Am Dent Assoc 1978;96:615. *(Good illustration and description of this early malignant lesion.)*

Shklar G. Oral leukoplakia. N Engl J Med 1986;315;1544. *(An editorial regarding its significance.)*

Primary Care Medicine: Office Evaluation and Management of the Adult Patient, 3rd edition, edited by Allan H. Goroll, Lawrence A. May, and Albert G. Mulley, Jr. J.B. Lippincott Company, Philadelphia

212
Evaluation of Impaired Hearing

AINA J. GULYA, M.D.

It is estimated that more than 10 percent of the population of the United States has a hearing problem. The problem is particularly common among the elderly and can impair quality of life. People with seriously impaired hearing often become withdrawn or appear confused. Subtle hearing loss may go unrecognized. Patients with hearing loss often can be greatly helped, particularly if the loss is due to a conductive problem. The primary physician has the responsibility to detect hearing loss, to search for an etiology, and to decide when referral to an otolaryngologist is indicated.

PATHOPHYSIOLOGY AND CLINICAL PRESENTATION

Impaired hearing may result from an interference with the conduction of sound, its conversion to electrical impulses, or its transmission through the nervous system. Hearing involves an acoustic stage during which sound waves cause the tympanic membrane to vibrate. Ossicles amplify the sound, and the oscillation of the footplate of the stapes in the oval window transmits the sound waves to the perilymph of the inner ear. The endolymph of the scala media (or cochlear duct) is wedged between the perilymph of the scala vestibuli and scala tympani. Displacement of the basilar membrane stimulates the hair cells, converting sound waves to neural impulses, which are conveyed to the temporal lobes. Interference with mechanical reception or amplification of sound, as occurs with disease of the auditory canal, tympanic membrane, or ossicles, creates conductive hearing loss. Degeneration or destruction of hair cells or the acoustic nerve produces sensorineural hearing loss.

Conductive Hearing Loss

Conductive loss presents with diminution of volume, particularly for low tones and vowels. There is often a history of previous ear disease. In the Weber test, the tuning fork is perceived more loudly in the conductively deaf ear. The Rinne test shows that bone conduction is better than air conduction. Obstruction of the auditory canal by impacted cerumen, a foreign body, exostoses, external otitis, otitis media with effusion, or scarring or perforation of the drum due to chronic otitis may be present.

Otosclerosis, a surgically remediable cause of conductive hearing loss, is a disorder of the architecture of the bony labyrinth, fixing the footplate of the stapes in the oval window. Clinical otosclerosis has an estimated prevalence of about 1 percent among whites and 0.1 percent among blacks. Two-thirds are female. There appears to be an association between pregnancy and otosclerotic hearing loss. The condition is inherited in an autosomal dominant fashion, with varying clinical expressivity. It generally presents in the second or third decade of life.

Exostoses are bony excrescences of the external auditory canal. They are characteristically located in the anterior, posterior, and superior quadrants of the canal. Nearly always bilaterally symmetric, their occurrence seems to be related to repetitive exposure to cold water (eg, as in ocean swimming). They can cause symptoms by blockage of the external auditory canal, resulting in conductive hearing loss, or by sequestration of debris with subsequent infection.

Glomus tumors or paragangliomas are benign, highly vascular tumors derived from normally occurring glomus formations of the middle ear and jugular bulb. Presenting symptoms include conductive hearing loss (from middle ear mass effect), spontaneous hemorrhage from the canal, and paralysis of the 9th, 10th and 11th cranial nerves (the jugular foramen syndrome). With progression, they may involve the intracranial space or cause bony destruction of the base of the skull.

Sensorineural Hearing Loss

Sensorineural loss characteristically produces impairment of high-tone perception. Patients may complain that they can hear people speaking but have difficulty deciphering words because discrimination is poor. Shouting may only exacerbate the problem. The patient with high-frequency loss may have difficulty hearing doorbells, telephones, or a ticking watch. More difficulty may be noticed in hearing the higher-pitched female voice. Recruitment, an abnormally rapid increase in perceived loudness with increased sound intensity may be present and indicates cochlear dysfunction. Air conduction is reported better than bone conduction. Tinnitus is often a concomitant complaint.

Presbycusis is hearing loss associated with aging and is the most common cause of diminished hearing in the elderly. There are four types of presbycusis, distinguished according to the correlated pathologic changes in the cochlea. Hair cell loss and cochlear neuron degeneration are the most widely recognized changes. The hearing loss is bilaterally symmetric and gradual in onset. The majority of cases begin with a loss of the high frequencies with slow progression. Eventually, middle- and low-frequency sounds also become difficult to perceive (Figs. 212-1 and 212-2).

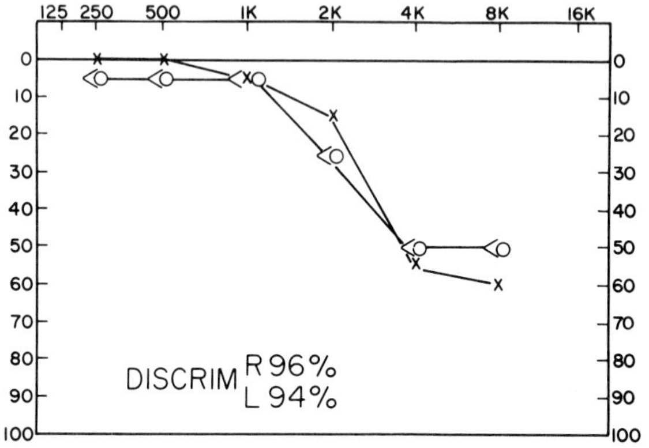

Figure 212-1. Presbycusis due to hair cell loss. Note good hearing thresholds at the speech frequencies 250 to 2000 c/s. X = L ear, air; O = R ear, air; < = R ear, bone.

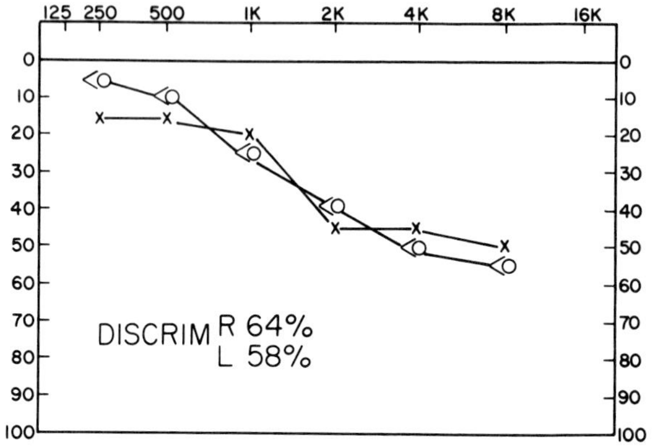

Figure 212-2. Late presbycusis due to loss of cochlear neurons. Note poor discrimination. X = L ear, air; O = R ear, air; < = L ear, bone.

Noise-induced hearing loss is of major epidemiologic and economic significance. Chronic exposure to sound levels in excess of 85 to 90 dB causes hearing loss, particularly in the frequency range around 4000 c/s. The patient may be unaware of the problem because the speech frequencies (500, 1000, and 2000 c/s) are initially unaffected. The first stage is referred to as temporary threshold shift, in which there is a reversible rise in threshold sound perception. The ear may feel full, or the patient may complain of a sense of pressure. If exposure to loud noise ceases at this stage, hearing returns to its previous level. If exposure persists, however, a permanent threshold shift ensues. The term *acoustic trauma* more specifically relates to a particular, single noise event (eg, a shotgun blast) that induces an immediate hearing loss.

Drug-Induced Hearing Loss. The aminoglycoside antibiotics are the most ototoxic of the commonly used drugs. The first sign of gentamicin ototoxicity is disequilibrium. Monitoring blood levels is the best way to avoid such problems, adjusting dose according to peak serum levels. Other potentially ototoxic drugs include furosemide, ethacrynic acid, quinidine, and aspirin. Aspirin doses averaging 6 to 8 g/day predictably cause tinnitus and completely reversible hearing impairment.

Meniere's disease produces a fluctuating, unilateral, low-frequency impairment, usually associated with tinnitus, a sensation of fullness in the ear, and intermittent episodes of vertigo. The vertiginous attacks may be the presenting symptom of Meniere's disease, with later onset of fluctuating hearing loss. Progression of hearing loss may occur, with loss eventually encompassing the higher frequencies as well.

Acoustic neuroma, a benign tumor of the 8th cranial nerve, is a rare but important cause of sensorineural hearing loss, often in conjunction with disequilibrium (see Chapter 166). The patient's speech discrimination is much worse than predicted by the deficit in pure-tone perception. Unlike Meniere's disease, symptoms progress in relentless, progressive fashion.

Sensorineural deafness, generally bilaterally symmetric, may be genetically determined. Many syndromes have been identified in which hereditary hearing loss is associated with anomalies in other organ systems. Congenital malformations of the inner ear, not necessarily hereditary, may also contribute.

Sudden deafness of the sensorineural variety can be due to head trauma or can appear without obvious cause or warning. In *idiopathic* sudden sensorineural deafness, recovery appears to be predicted by the pattern of hearing loss sustained, age (greater or less than 40), presence or absence of vertigo, and electronystagmogram pattern. The etiology of the idiopathic variant is still a matter of debate, but viral infection seems to be the most likely precipitant. Uncommonly, an acoustic neuroma may present with sudden hearing loss. Sudden hearing loss demands expeditious referral to an otolaryngologist for further evaluation and possible therapy.

Injury to the inner ear or 8th nerve may produce an asymmetric sensorineural hearing loss. Skull fracture, meningitis, otitis media, scarlet fever, and mumps are major etiologic factors. Trauma may also cause conductive hearing loss, for example, hemotympanum, tympanic membrane perforation, or ossicular dislocation.

Other Etiologies. *Congenital syphilis* may produce adult-onset sensorineural hearing loss. One or both ears may be affected; the course can be variable, with remissions and exacerbations. Vertigo is sometimes present as well.

Multiple sclerosis should be considered when a young woman shows discrimination scores reduced out of proportion to the pure tone thresholds (similar to the pattern seen with acoustic neuromas). The site of the lesion is retrocochlear (often in the brainstem), and there may be an associated history of optic neuritis and/or vertigo.

Perilymph leaks or *fistulas* cause hearing loss, with or without vertigo, in individuals who have had inner ear surgery (eg, stapedectomy), have sustained head trauma, or have congenital inner ear anomalies. The round and/or oval window seals may be involved, and there is a theorized intracochlear membrane rupture as well. Vertigo, if present, seems, in general, to improve, with little risk of its worsening.

Table 212-1. Common and Important Causes of Impaired Hearing

CONDUCTIVE	SENSORINEURAL
Impacted cerumen	Presbycusis
Foreign body	Noise-induced deafness
Occlusive edema of auditory canal	Drugs (amino glycosides, loop diuretics, quinidine, aspirin)
Perforation of tympanic membrane	Meniere's disease
Chronic otitis media	Acoustic neuroma
Serous otitis media	Hypothyroidism (mild loss)
External otitis	Idiopathic sudden deafness
Otosclerosis	Congenital syphilis
Exostoses	Diabetes
Developmental defects	Perilymph leak
Glomus tumors	Multiple sclerosis

DIFFERENTIAL DIAGNOSIS

The causes of hearing loss can be grouped according to whether the problem is conductive or sensorineural in etiology (Table 212-1). The categorization is of practical use because the conductive defects lend themselves to correction in many instances.

WORKUP

History. Evaluation of the patient with hearing loss should focus on detection of a correctable lesion. This search is aided by identifying whether the impairment is conductive or sensorineural. History is of some help. Conductive disease often results in loss of low-frequency hearing, whereas sensorineural problems usually cause high-frequency hearing loss. It is worth trying to find out the sounds or situations in which the patient has most trouble hearing. Difficulty deciphering spoken words suggests sensorineural disease. Inquiry into drug use is essential, focusing on aminoglycosides, quinine derivatives, salicylates, and the loop diuretics—furosemide and ethacrynic acid. A history of otitis or head trauma should be noted.

Inquiry into acoustic trauma is important, especially the details of occupational exposure. Family history is no less important, particularly in the consideration of such entities as otosclerosis or acoustic neuromas (associated with von Recklinghausen's disease).

Physical examination begins with inspection of the external auditory canal for obstruction by impacted cerumen, a foreign body, external otitis, or exostosis. The tympanic membranes are examined for inflammation, perforation, and scarring. One notes any fluid in middle ear. A reddish mass visible through the intact tympanic membrane may indicate a high-riding jugular bulb, an aberrant internal carotid artery, or a glomus tumor. Air insufflation assesses tympanic membrane mobility.

Nasopharyngeal examination is indicated in patients with persisting serous otitis media, particularly if it is unilateral. If there is vertigo or suspicion of a glomus tumor, cranial nerve examination is performed to assess central nervous system involvement (see Chapter 166).

Tests of Hearing. The *watch tick* was an easy, although crude, method of detecting high-frequency impairment when ticking watches were common. *Whispering* from 2 feet after full exhalation is more readily performed. One asks the patient to repeat six whispered words, standing behind the patient to avoid lip reading. Less than 50 percent correct indicates a hearing problem. The best words are familiar bisyllabic ones in which both syllables are equally accented (eg, pancake, hotdog). With sensorineural hearing loss, a spoken voice is much better heard than a whisper, even if the whisper is loud, because of impairment of high-frequency hearing. *Finger rubbing* involves rubbing the thumb and index finger together 1 inch from the ear and slowly withdrawing until the sound is no longer heard.

One can use the *tuning fork* both to detect hearing loss and to differentiate conductive from sensorineural pathology (Weber and Rinne testing). A tuning fork that vibrates at a frequency of 512 c/s is acceptable; the 128-c/s tuning fork used for testing vibratory sensation is not. Testing is done to establish the threshold of perception by striking it against the heel of the hand and withdrawing it at 1 foot per second starting 1 inch from the ear until it becomes imperceptible. The distance is noted.

Differentiating Conductive from Sensorineural Hearing Loss. The *Weber* test is helpful. The normal response to a fork vibrating from a tap of the knee and placed midline on the skull is equal loudness in both ears. If there is a conductive defect, the sound will be heard more clearly in the ear with the defect. If there is a sensorineural loss in one ear, sound will be better perceived in the other.

The *Rinne test* complements Weber testing. When the vibrating fork is placed on the mastoid process, it is heard for a period of time and then dies away. It is heard again if the same fork is promptly moved without any reactivation to the external auditory meatus. Normal persons will hear sound conducted by air for about twice as long as a sound conducted by bone, because of the greater sound transmission efficiency of the middle ear apparatus.

Alternatively, with firm application of the tuning fork against the mastoid process for a few seconds and immediate transfer to the external auditory meatus, the sound should be perceived as "louder" in front of the canal when compared to the mastoid position. Sound by air conduction is normally heard for twice as long as sound by bone conduction. With marked conductive loss, the ratio reverses. With lesser degrees of impairment, the ratio approaches 1:1. The normal ratio is preserved in patients with sensorineural loss, but hearing via both bone and air conduction is reduced.

The Schwabach test compares the examiner's hearing by bone conduction with that of the patient's. The vibrating tuning fork is alternately placed on the mastoid process of examiner and patient. If the examiner's hearing is normal, he or she will perceive the sound for a longer time than the patient with a sensorineural deficit and for a shorter time than the patient with a conductive problem.

Laboratory Studies. An *audiogram* is an essential component of the workup of impaired hearing. The pattern of hearing loss has considerable diagnostic and therapeutic importance, helping to establish the type of hearing loss and to localize the site of pathology. Interpretation usually requires the joint efforts of an otolaryngologist and an audiologist, but a few common patterns are useful for the primary physician to recognize (see Appendix). Ordering the study before referral is of help to the otolaryngologist.

Expensive imaging technology should be used sparingly but can be helpful in carefully selected patients. *Computed tomography (CT) scanning* is used in the evaluation of certain middle ear and mastoid disorders, such as chronic infection and glomus tumors. *Magnetic resonance imaging (MRI),* particularly with gadolinium enhancement, has assumed a preeminent role in the evaluation of the patient with suspected retrocochlear disease (eg, acoustic neuroma or multiple sclerosis).

Auditory brainstem response (ABR) testing has also been found useful in the site-of-lesion testing, as has *electronystagmography* (see Chapter 166). Both tests require expert performance and interpretation and should be ordered only in consultation with consultants experienced in their use and interpretation.

Otoacoustic emissions (OAEs), particularly those evoked by sound stimuli, are an evolving modality for testing the integrity of the hair cells of the cochlea, from which they are believed to emanate. OAEs show promise as a screening test for assessing auditory function in the difficult-to-test patient.

Screening for Hearing Loss. An important aspect of geriatric care is assessment for hearing loss. In support of screening for hearing loss are the major impact hearing loss can have on quality of life, the availability of effective means to detect and correct hearing loss, the high level of patient compliance with treatment measures, and the ability to screen adequately in the primary care setting. The U.S. Preventive Services Task Force recommends periodic hearing assessment of all elderly persons.

The best screening methods and the optimal interval are the subjects of ongoing study. Some investigators find that the whispering voice test at 20 cm and finger rubbing at 8 cm have high sensitivity and specificity. Other prefer the combination of the *Hearing Handicap Inventory for the Elderly (HHIE),* a self-assessment questionnaire with a screening version of 10 questions (Table 212-2), and the hand-held audioscope. The questionnaire has an accuracy of 75 percent when compared to formal audiometry. The *audioscope* (Welch Allen) is a hand-held otoscope with a built-in audiometer that delivers 20-, 25-, and 40-dB tones at frequencies of 500, 1000, 2000, and 4000 Hz. Compared to formal audiometry, sensitivity for hearing loss ranges from 87 percent to 96 percent, and specificity from 70 percent to 90 percent. Used together, they have an accuracy approaching 85 percent. It takes about 90 s to screen both ears. For the elderly, it is recommended that testing be performed each year as part of the annual check-up.

Table 212-2. A Screening Hearing Handicap Inventory for the Elderly

Does a hearing problem cause you to feel embarrassed when you meet new people?
Does a hearing problem cause you to feel frustrated when talking to members of your family?
Do you have difficulty hearing when someone speaks in a whisper?
Do you feel handicapped by a hearing problem?
Does a hearing problem cause you difficulty when visiting friends or relatives?
Does a hearing problem cause you to attend religious services less often than you would like?
Does a hearing problem cause you to have arguments with family members?
Does a hearing problem cause you to have difficulty when listening to television or radio?
Do you feel that any difficulty with your hearing limits/hampers your personal or social life?
Does a hearing problem cause you difficulty when in a restaurant with relatives or friends?

Scoring: "No" = 0 points; "sometimes" = 2 points; "yes" = 4 points; < 10 points means no handicap; > 24 points means moderate to severe handicap.

Adapted from Mulrow CD, Lichtenstein MJ. *J Gen Intern Med* 1991;6:249.

SYMPTOMATIC MANAGEMENT, PATIENT EDUCATION, AND INDICATIONS FOR REFERRAL

The primary physician's role in the treatment of hearing loss is relatively limited, but simple advice and support are much appreciated. Elders report that cupping the hand behind the ear can be of help both in actual hearing and alerting others to speak more clearly or louder. Speech reading (interpreting what is being said by extrapolating from the words heard and the facial expressions) may also help. Clear enunciation, not merely elevated volume of speech, along with directly facing the presbycusic patient while engaged in conversation, optimizes verbal communication. Removal of impacted cerumen or other obstruction, cessation of ototoxic drugs, and treatment of otitis media (see Chapter 218) should not be overlooked. Advising patients exposed to occupational or recreational noise to use earplugs when experiencing such noise and to avoid further acoustic trauma is important.

Cerumen removal may be accomplished by gentle, body-temperature water irrigation using a syringe or an irrigation jet. Removal of wax, as well as some foreign bodies, may be performed using a cerumen spoon or forceps under direct visualization provided by headlight and speculum. Insects are better exterminated first by instillation of mineral oil into the canal before removal is attempted.

Referral to an otolaryngologist for further evaluation and treatment is indicated when a conductive etiology or acoustic neuroma is suspected, or when simple symptomatic measures do not suffice and the hearing impairment is disabling. The otolaryngologist needs to determine whether the patient is a candidate for medical or surgical therapy and whether a hearing aid is appropriate. A true sudden hearing loss demands immediate otolaryngologic referral.

A great variety of hearing aids are available on the market. Patients with sensorineural hearing losses—especially those with a flat threshold and good discrimination—benefit from amplification and deserve as much consideration as those patients with conductive hearing losses. Even those patients with steeply sloping, high-frequency sensorineural hearing loss with poor discrimination may find amplification useful. Only after an adequate trial, after careful otolaryngologic evaluation and competent hearing aid fitting, can one finally make a decision regarding the helpfulness of amplification.

ANNOTATED BIBLIOGRAPHY

Consensus Conference. Noise and hearing loss. JAMA 263:3185, 1990. *(Recommends several steps to limit noise-induced hearing loss.)*

Lichtenstein MJ, Bess FH, Logan SA. Validation of screening tools for identifying hearing-impaired elderly in primary care. JAMA 1988;259:2875. *(Audioscope and the screening questionnaire had an accuracy of 83 percent.)*

Lipkin M, Williams ME. Presbycusis and communication. J Gen Intern Med 1986;1:399. *(Practical advice from a 79-year-old physician.)*

Mulrow CD, Lichtenstein MJ. Screening for hearing impairment in the elderly: rationale and strategy. J Gen Intern Med 1991;6:249. *(Examines available tests and makes several recommendations.)*

Uhlmann RF, Rees TS, Psaty BM, et al. Validity and reliability of auditory screening tests in demented and non-demented older adults. J Gen Intern Med 1989;4:90. *(Simple tests found remarkably reliable and valid.)*

Appendix: Audiometry

Audiometry helps to classify a hearing loss as conductive or sensorineural and subclassify according to the pattern detected. The basic audiogram consists of pure tone air and bone conduction testing with evaluation of speech reception threshold and speech discrimination. The minimal intensity (decibel) at which the patient perceives each tone is charted as the threshold for that frequency. The responses are recorded as indicated in Figure 212-3. The pure tone air threshold curve measures both the conductive and sensorineural components of hearing. To appreciate a conductive component to a hearing loss, bone conduction thresholds are obtained. The bone conduction audiogram bypasses the conduction system and measures cochlear/8th nerve capacity. In

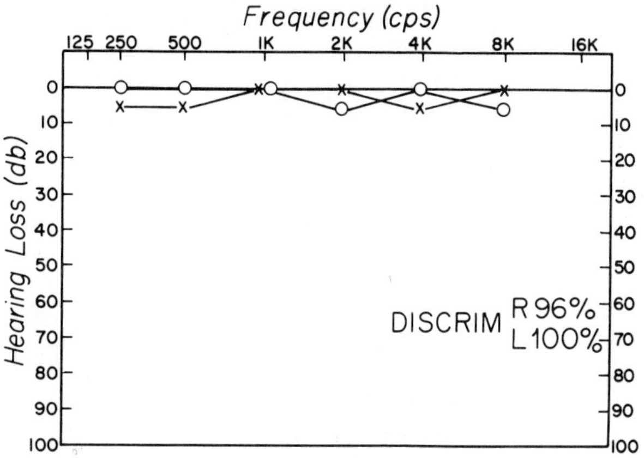

Figure 212-3. Normal pure tone air audiogram. O = R ear, air, X = L ear, air.

bone conduction testing, the mastoid process of each ear is directly stimulated with an oscillator or vibrator over a similar frequency spectrum and results are graphically recorded. A discrepancy between air conducted sound waves and those conducted by the skull, a so-called air-bone gap, is indicative of a problem with conduction (Fig. 212-4).

Additional testing includes *speech reception threshold* (SRT) and *speech discrimination testing*. The SRT is defined as the lowest intensity at which the patient can correctly identify 50 percent of presented words. The SRT should match, within a few decibels, the average of the pure tone thresholds. Discrimination testing evaluates the comprehension of speech. Speech discrimination that is markedly diminished out of proportion to the measured hearing loss is indicative of auditory nerve pathology. Ordinarily, patients with good pure tone hearing should also understand speech (words) well.

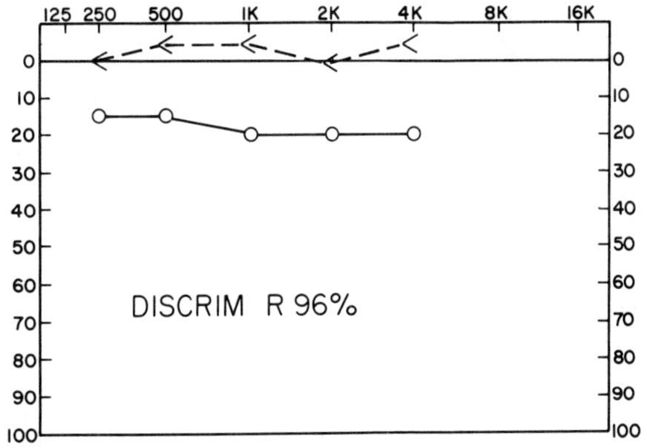

Figure 212-4. Air-bone gap. O = R ear, air; < = R ear, bone.

213

Approach to Epistaxis

WILLIAM R. WILSON, M.D.

Primary Care Medicine: Office Evaluation and Management of the Adult Patient, 3rd edition, edited by Allan H. Goroll, Lawrence A. May, and Albert G. Mulley, Jr. J.B. Lippincott Company, Philadelphia

Most spontaneous nosebleeds are self-limited. Patients present for medical care when the bleeding becomes unusually brisk, will not stop, or episodes become frequent. Severe or recurrent bleeding necessitates evaluation for nasal pathology and, less commonly, an underlying generalized disorder. The immediate therapeutic objective is control of bleeding.

PATHOPHYSIOLOGY AND CLINICAL PRESENTATION

Etiologies. The primary mechanism of epistaxis is disruption of the nasal mucosa, primarily caused by *trauma*. In patients with deviated septum or septal spurs in the anterior portion of the nose, trauma occurs easily, either from the drying effects of poorly humidified air or secondary to probing in or bumps on the nose. Picking, rubbing, or forceful blowing may also trigger bleeding when the nasal mucosa is inflamed from a viral, bacterial, or allergic cause.

Ulcerations, which tend to form over septal deviations and spurs, bleed easily. Repeated mucosal exposure to cocaine leads to anoxic tissue necrosis from drug-induced intense vasospasm; perforation may result and cause chronic crusting and bleeding. Collagen diseases such as lupus are occasionally responsible for ulceration.

Bleeding diatheses sometimes present as epistaxis (see Chapter 81). Nosebleeds are the most common initial presentation of *hereditary hemorrhagic telangiectasia* (Osler-Weber-Rendu syndrome) and its most frequent bleeding complication. Characteristic features include telangiectasias on the lips and tongue, a positive family history, and onset of repeated bleeding episodes by the third or fourth decade. Adolescent boys with a nasopharyngeal angiofibroma experience brisk posterior epistaxis.

Wegener's granulomatosis, midline granuloma, and *nasal malignancy* share a presentation of epistaxis, unremitting sinus infection, and opacified sinuses on x-ray. Posterior epistaxis is commonly attributed to hypertension, but epidemiologic studies show that few hypertensives experience nosebleeds.

Site of Bleeding. Regardless of etiology, the site of bleeding has distinguishing clinical characteristics. Active *anterior epistaxis* usually presents as unilateral, continuous, moderate bleeding from the septum. Recurrent episodes of bleeding, lasting a few minutes to half an hour over the preceding few days and controlled by pinching the anterior nose are characteristic. The majority of adult cases and almost all spontaneous nasal hemorrhage in children occur on the anterior aspect of the nasal septum. Most are venous, but an arterial source becomes more common with advancing age and mucosal and vascular atrophy.

Posterior epistaxis is associated with intermittent, very brisk arterial bleeding, with blood flowing into the pharynx unless the patient is leaning forward. When the patient is leaning forward, the blood may run from one or both sides of the nose. Spontaneous posterior hemorrhage is more common in the older age groups and following severe facial trauma. The vessel rupture is usually just superior or inferior to the posterior tip of the inferior turbinate on the lateral nasal wall.

DIFFERENTIAL DIAGNOSIS

The differential diagnosis of nosebleeds can be divided into local and systemic disorders (Table 213–1). The local causes are most commonly inflammatory or traumatic. More than 90 percent of bleeds are related to local irritation; most occur in the absence of a specific underlying anatomic lesion.

WORKUP

History should begin with inquiry into the amount of bleeding, its duration, and frequency. After the bleeding is under control, the patient can be questioned about easy bruising; hematuria; melena; heavy menstrual periods; family history of bleeding disorders; the use of oral anticoagulants or drugs with antiplatelet effects (aspirin and so forth); occupational exposure to irritating chemicals or dust; dry home; chronic cocaine use; and repeated noseblowing or picking.

Physical examination should be performed with the patient sitting and leaning forward so that the blood flows from

Table 213-1. Major Causes of Epistaxis

LOCAL DISEASE	SYSTEMIC DISEASE
Dry indoor environment	Granulomatous disease (Wegeners, sarcoidosis)
Upper respiratory infection	Hereditary hemorrhagic telangiectasia
Chronic sinusitis	Infection (chickenpox, influenza)
Trauma (nose picking, forceful blowing)	Bleeding diathesis
Occupational exposure to irritants	Malignant hypertension
Cocaine abuse	
Angiomas	
Allergies	
Lack of humidification	
Malignancy	

the nose. This allows the physician to assess the rate and site of bleeding, as well as to prevent the swallowing of blood, which will quickly lead to emesis. The pulse and blood pressure should be taken and the skin, mucous membranes, and conjunctiva should be checked for rash, pallor, purpura, petechiae, and telangiectasias. Lymph nodes should be examined for enlargement, suggesting sarcoidosis, tuberculosis, or malignancy. The sinuses are percussed for evidence of sinusitis, which would make Wegener's, midline granuloma, and nasal tumor considerations.

Laboratory studies are best ordered on the basis of findings from the history and physical examination. Patients suspected of a bleeding diathesis should have a prothrombin time (PT) test, partial thromboplastin time (PTT) test, blood smear, and platelet count obtained (see Chapter 81). Sinus films are appropriate to evaluate the patient with recurrent bouts of sinus pain, tenderness, and bleeding.

PRINCIPLES OF MANAGEMENT

The first objective is to stop the bleeding. The approach depends on whether the source is anterior or posterior.

Anterior Septal Bleeding. A few simple first-aid measures suffice for the vast majority of cases. The patient should *sit up* (this reduces venous pressure) and *lean forward* (which prevents the swallowing of blood if the bleeding is anterior). A small piece of cotton or cotton balls soaked in 1:1000 epinephrine or a vasoconstricting nosedrop such as *phenylephrine* (Neo-Synephrine) or *oxymetazoline* (Afrin) are placed in the vestibule of the nose and pressed against the bleeding site for 5 to 10 minutes. It is then removed to observe for rebleeding. This will stop almost all venous types of anterior nosebleeds. Humidification and a lubricant such as petrolatum ointment help promote healing.

If these remedies fail, the mucous membrane can be anesthetized by applying cotton soaked with 4% cocaine or 4% lidocaine for 5 minutes. A *silver nitrate stick* can then be applied to the bleeding site and to any prominent vessels.

Occasionally, a small artery in the septal mucous membrane will either fail to stop bleeding or rebleed a short time later. These episodes can usually be controlled by anesthetizing and recauterizing the area. This is followed by placing a small amount of *oxidized regenerated cellulose* (Surgigel) against the bleeding artery, or a small *packing of petroleum gauze* strip in the nasal vestibule for 24 hours.

Patients with bleeding disorders require especially careful treatment to prevent abrading the mucous membrane. Therapy involves use of humidity, copious lubricants, and soft cotton tamponades wetted with long-acting vasoconstricting drops (oxymetazoline 0.1%; Afrin nasal solution). Packing should be avoided at all costs but, if unavoidable, can be accomplished with a piece of oxidized cellulose, which does not require removal. Further treatment is best directed at the underlying bleeding disorder.

Posterior epistaxis constitutes an inherently more serious problem, because of the relative rapidity of blood loss and the relatively inaccessible and poorly visualized bleeding site in the posterior nose. Initial efforts should be made to bring the bleeding under control while awaiting an otolaryngologic consult. Hematocrit, blood pressure, and pulse should be immediately obtained, and, if necessary, a sample should be sent for type and crossmatch. The patient should be instructed to *sit up* and *lean forward,* and, if there has been a temporary interruption in the bleeding, no treatment other than *spraying* the nose with a topical anesthetic and vasoconstricting substance, such as *4% cocaine,* should be attempted. The nose should be suctioned or blown clear only when the medical personnel present are prepared to deal with brisk epistaxis. If the patient's blood pressure permits, a parenteral analgesic such as Demerol 50 or 100 mg intramuscularly should be given before the surgeon's *electrocautery* of the posterior nose, or the placement of *compressing* balloons, packs, or tampons.

PATIENT EDUCATION

Prevention. Once septal bleeding is controlled in the office or emergency ward, measures to prevent recurrence should be instituted. The patient should keep the septum well coated with petrolatum-based ointment such as zinc oxide, A and D ointment, or an antibiotic ointment until healed, usually in 3 to 5 days. The fingernails of children should be trimmed short. Minor recurrent bleeding can be controlled by the patient's use of cotton pledgets soaked in vasoconstricting solutions and pressed against the bleeding site. Instruct the patient on the need to avoid traumatizing the mucosa. Specifically, warn against habitual nose picking, constant rubbing with a handkerchief, and excessively forceful blowing. Explain the importance of humidifying the home environment. This may be done by keeping a few windows partially open, by placing containers of water near radiators or stoves, or by installing a humidifier. Occasionally, patients may benefit from use of a water-based lubricant applied to the rims of the nostrils to maintain mucosal moisture; however, this does involve a very small risk of lipoid pneumonia and should be avoided in children and the elderly.

First Aid. Few patients understand the proper treatment for care of minor nosebleeds at home; simple telephone instruction may obviate the need for an office or emergency room visit. The patient should be instructed to *sit up* and remain calm, *lean forward* and *press the ala* of the vestibule against the septum on the side that is bleeding to tamponade the flow. The nose can then be sprayed with any of the over-the-counter nasal sprays that contain *phenylephrine* (eg, Neo-Synephrine) or oxymetazoline (Afrin). A small *pledget of cotton* is then lightly soaked with the spray and pressed against the bleeding portion of the septum. After 10 minutes, most nosebleeds will have stopped. A *petrolatum-based ointment,* such as zinc oxide or Bacitracin, can be applied to the septum to prevent further drying and abrasion of the septum. It is left in for a few days, and the patient is instructed to limit heavy lifting, other forms of straining, bending over, intake of spicy or hot foods, hot showers, and medications that might impair hemostasis (see Chapter 81).

Reassure the patient when the nosebleed is purely a local phenomenon; many people attribute nosebleeds to hypertension and fear cerebral hemorrhage.

INDICATIONS FOR REFERRAL AND ADMISSION

Patients with active posterior bleeding should be admitted to the hospital immediately for emergency treatment to control the bleeding. Posterior packing can cause airway obstruction, particularly in elderly patients, due to downward displacement of the soft palate and subsequent palatal edema and swelling or slipped packing. All patients with nasal packing should be closely observed for signs of hypoxia and hypercarbia. Unfortunately, packs must be left in place for a minimum of 5 days to be effective. Posterior packing is associated with a great deal of discomfort; the patients generally require intravenous hydration because of poor oral intake due to painful swallowing, antibiotics to prevent sinusitis, pain medications, and careful observation by the nursing staff for impending airway obstruction.

ANNOTATED BIBLIOGRAPHY

Hallberg OE. Severe nosebleed and its treatment. JAMA 1952;148:355. *(A classic article that is still very useful.)*

Kirchner JA. Epistaxis. N Engl J Med 1982;307:1126. *(A review of anatomy, etiology, and therapy.)*

Perry WH. Clinical spectrum of hereditary hemorrhagic telangiectasia (Osler-Weber-Rendu disease). Am J Med 1987; 82:989. *(Detailed review of clinical presentation; nosebleeds are major feature.)*

214
Evaluation of Facial Pain and Swelling

JOHN P. KELLY, D.M.D., M.D.

The primary care physician often encounters patients whose presenting complaint of facial pain or swelling is related to the masticatory apparatus (teeth, gums, jaws, muscles) or salivary glands. Dental decay is the most prevalent disease in the United States and a major cause of conditions leading to facial pain and swelling. Because symptoms may be referred to nondental structures and because an odontogenic infection may involve areas of the head and neck seemingly unrelated to the teeth, the patient may first seek the advice of a physician rather than of a dentist. Prompt recognition and effective initial treatment may well prevent development of a serious complication such as abscess formation.

PATHOPHYSIOLOGY AND CLINICAL PRESENTATION

Odontogenic Infection. Dental decay is a multifactorial disease that encompasses dietary factors (most notably, refined carbohydrates), environmental factors (such as inavailability of fluoride ion during the production of the enamel of the teeth) and various host factors (not the least of which is the patient's oral hygiene habits). Oral bacteria use dietary carbohydrates to form plaque on the enamel of the teeth; susceptible enamel is then decalcified, resulting in a "cavity" or carious lesion.

Tooth Decay and Inflammation of the Pulp. In its initial stages, tooth decay is asymptomatic. However, when the dentin beneath the enamel is exposed, the patient may complain of aching pain when the affected tooth comes into contact with hot, cold, or sweet substances. The frequent finding of referred pain may make localization of the offending tooth difficult and is one reason why a patient may first consult the physician rather than the dentist.

Progressive decay of the tooth will result in inflammation of the pulp *(pulpitis)*. The symptoms will be unchanged until the dental pulp becomes necrotic and, eventually, suppurative. The cardinal symptom then is deep, throbbing pain on exposure to hot foods or drinks. The pain is abruptly relieved by ice or cold water. This symptom complex is distinct from the paroxysmal, lancinating pain of trigeminal neuralgia, which has no relationship to extremes of temperature, but which may be related to eating because of the presence of trigger zones in the oral cavity (see Chapter 176).

Tooth Abscess. Simple dental decay, pulpitis, and pulpal necrosis are not associated with fever, swelling, or leukocytosis. However, when the infection of the pulp spreads beyond the confines of the tooth to involve the periodontal ligament and the adjacent alveolar bone, an acute *alveolar abscess* may ensue. In this condition, the affected tooth is tender to percussion or to masticatory forces and is mobile. The adjacent soft tissues begin to show edema, erythema, heat, and tenderness. The location of the involved tooth will determine the location of the swelling. Abscessed maxillary teeth will produce labial or infraorbital edema; an infected mandibular tooth will produce submandibular edema. Lymphadenopathy of the cervical chain can be seen in either maxillary or mandibular infection.

Complications. A *facial cellulitis* may result, causing fever and leukocytosis. Typically, the history reveals a preceding toothache with pain suggestive of pulpitis, followed by spontaneous regression and an asymptomatic period, corresponding to pulpal necrosis. Swelling and pain develop when the necrotic pulp becomes infected and the process spreads to adjacent anatomic structures. Further spread of infection along fascial planes can result in life-threatening complications, such as *cavernous sinus thrombosis, meningitis,* or *mediastinitis*. Although uncommon, such devastating complications are still seen today, even with the availability of antibiotics.

Periodontal Infection. Acute bacterial infection of the periodontal tissues is most often localized to the gingiva or mucosa adjacent to the involved tooth. The typical patient will complain of a "gum boil," and examination will reveal a discrete, fluctuant swelling, which may drain easily on manual palpation.

In the late adolescent years, infection of the soft tissue surrounding erupting third molars or wisdom teeth (pericoronitis) is common. Low-grade, chronic infection may be accompanied by symptoms described as "teething"; acute infection will result in pain, swelling, and difficulty in opening the mouth (trismus) as the adjacent masticator space becomes involved.

Salivary Gland Swelling. Acute infection of the major salivary glands (parotid, submandibular, and sublingual) may be either viral or bacterial. *Viral parotitis* (mumps) occurs most frequently in school-age children and appears either unilaterally or bilaterally. The efficacy of immunization programs should make this disease a relative rarity in the future. Viral lymphadenopathy in the preauricular area, such as that seen in infectious mononucleosis and in cat-scratch disease, may masquerade as parotid swelling and must be considered.

Sialadenitis, bacterial infection of the salivary glands, commonly affects a single gland. The infection is generally an ascending infection in which bacteria gain access to a gland made susceptible to infection by stasis of saliva. Obstruction of the salivary duct by a stone or mucinous plug is the usual inciting event, but any low-flow state can lead to sialadenitis. The condition is frequently seen in elderly, debilitated or postoperative patients, in whom dehydration may lead to decreased salivary flow and consequent infection. The parotid gland is the usual target; involvement is more often unilateral than bilateral. Purulent drainage can be obtained from the duct orifice. Previous episodes of parotitis or congenital abnormality of the acinar structure of the parotid gland may produce sialoangiectasis, which facilitates pooling and stasis of saliva within the gland and increases the patient's susceptibility to episodes of acute infection.

Systemic Conditions. Noninfectious salivary swelling may occur with diabetes mellitus, uremia, Laennec's cirrhosis, chronic alcoholism, and malnutrition. A toxic reaction to a variety of drugs, such as iodine, mercury, and guanethidine, causes a painless bilateral parotid gland swelling. A specific triad of keratoconjunctivitis sicca, salivary gland swelling, and rheumatoid arthritis is known as *Sjögren's syndrome*. The syndrome has also been related to other chronic autoimmune connective tissue disorders, such as systemic lupus erythematosus (SLE), and polyarteritis nodosa. Sjögren's syndrome may initially present without apparent systemic disease. Lymphoma may develop in a patient with long-standing Sjögren's syndrome.

Lymphoproliferative Disease. Both major and minor salivary glands may become infiltrated by a lymphoproliferative process and enlarge. Lymphoma, tuberculosis, and sarcoidosis (uveoparotid fever) have all been first diagnosed from salivary gland enlargement.

DIFFERENTIAL DIAGNOSIS

The causes of facial pain or swelling can be divided into odontogenic, nonodontogenic, and salivary gland etiologies (Table 214–1).

Table 214-1. Important Causes of Facial Pain or Swelling

Odontogenic Pain
Caries
Pulpitis
Periapical abscess
Alveolar abscess
Nonodontogenic Pain
Trigeminal neuralgia
Temporomandibular joint dysfunction
Myocardial ischemia (referred jaw pain)
Giant cell arteritis (masseter claudication)
Salivary Pain and Swelling
Viral infection (mumps)
Bacterial infection
Ductal obstruction
Sjögren's syndrome
Lymphoproliferative disease
Tumor
Chemical irritant

WORKUP

History. Evaluation of facial pain and swelling requires thorough consideration of the pain's onset, severity, quality, location, radiation, aggravating or ameliorating factors, and duration. The various stages of dental infection can be characterized by specific pain histories. For example, pain brought on by contact with hot, cold, or sweet substances is indicative of dental caries, whereas aggravation by heat and relief by cold suggest a periapical abscess. If fever and swelling ensue, an alveolar abscess must be considered. Lancinating pain precipitated by contact with a trigger zone is typical of trigeminal neuralgia; it can be distinguished by history from abscess formation because symptoms are unrelated to the temperature of the contacting substance, and swelling is absent.

In the patient who complains of salivary gland enlargement, it is important to inquire about site(s) of involvement, presence of fever or tenderness, history of chronic illness, malignancy, toxin or drug exposure, and symptoms of rheumatologic disease or sicca syndrome (dry eyes, dry mouth). Unilateral painful swelling of acute onset suggests sialadenitis, especially when seen in an elderly, debilitated, or postoperative patient. A unilaterally enlarged, painless parotid may be due to tumor, particularly if there is a history of progressive increase in size and extension beyond the gland. Bilateral involvement requires consideration of lymphoma and sarcoidosis as well as Sjögren's syndrome (which is bilateral in about half of cases).

It is important to keep in mind that episodic jaw pain may be a manifestation of coronary ischemia (see Chapter 20).

Physical Examination. A semi-sitting position will usually allow both patient comfort and examiner access. Although a flashlight can be used, a lighting fixture that can illuminate the oral cavity and leave the examiner with both hands free is preferable.

Inspection of the mouth for fractured, decayed, or heavily restored teeth and for heavy deposits of debris and calculus ("tartar") on the teeth and gingiva requires little experience and will direct the examiner's attention to odontogenic disease as a likely source of the pain or swelling. A dental mirror or a short-handled laryngoscopy mirror serves as a better retractor than does a wooden tongue blade. Palpation of the teeth to determine tenderness or mobility will help to identify an abscessed tooth. The soft tissues should be palpated to detect the presence of indurated or fluctuant swelling adjacent to a suspicious tooth. Tenderness to percussion of a tooth, using a short, sharp tap with the dental mirror handle, is diagnostic of an abscessed tooth. The salivary glands are palpated bimanually intraorally and extraorally; the salivary duct orifices should be observed for salivary flow or purulent drainage during palpation of the individual glands. Cervical lymph nodes should be checked for enlargement and tenderness.

Laboratory Studies. Suspicion of dental caries can be confirmed by x-ray, as can abscess formation. Most other conditions produce few radiologic changes. White blood count in the potentially toxic patient or blood sugar in the diabetic patient may aid in subsequent management. Suspicion of Sjögren's syndrome can be confirmed by *lip biopsy*. It is important to obtain any purulent drainage for Gram's stain, culture, and sensitivity testing.

SYMPTOMATIC MANAGEMENT AND PATIENT EDUCATION

Tooth or Periodontal Abscess. While awaiting dental evaluation, the very uncomfortable patient may require strong analgesia (eg, codeine sulfate, 30 mg every 4 to 6 hours) and antibiotics. *Penicillin* remains the primary antibiotic of choice in treatment of odontogenic infection. Initiation of an oral penicillin-VK regimen of 250 to 500 mg every 6 hours is appropriate at the first recognition of swelling associated with an infected tooth or periodontal tissue.

Before dental work, *endocarditis prophylaxis* should be considered in patients with valvular heart disease (see Chapter 16). A 3.0-g oral dose of *amoxicillin* 1 hour before dental work and a 1.5-g oral dose 6 hours later are sufficient for endocarditis prophylaxis. Antibiotics are not indicated in the absence of swelling. *Erythromycin* (1.0 g 2 hours before and 500 mg 6 hours after dental work) is the preferred drug for patients allergic to penicillin.

Referral of the patient to an oral surgeon for definitive drainage of the infection at the earliest opportunity is indicated and should be made simultaneously with the prescribing of antibiotics.

Sialadenitis. Acute swelling of a salivary gland, accompanied by purulent or inspissated saliva from the involved duct, requires antibiotic treatment. Stimulation of salivary flow with sour candies and warm compresses is a helpful local measure. The submandibular gland tends to be infected with the same flora as is found in odontogenic infections. Hence, *penicillin* is the drug of choice for *submandibular sialadenitis*. Acute *bacterial parotitis,* on the other hand, is associated with staphylococcal species, and one of the penicillinase-resistant antibiotics, such as *dicloxacillin,* is preferred. Antibiotic treatment for other infections that may have preceded the onset of the salivary infection can alter the oral flora and produce infection of the salivary system by unusual organisms, such as *Escherichia coli*. Thus, culturing of the purulent saliva is suggested.

Prevention. The US Preventive Services Task Force has underscored the important role of the primary physician in promoting prevention of dental caries and gum disease. During the health maintenance examination, one should inquire into the time of last dental examination, examine the teeth and gums for plaque and gingival disease, urge regular brushing with a fluoride-containing dentifrice and flossing, and recommend yearly dental examination and plaque removal.

INDICATIONS FOR REFERRAL

Early recognition of dental decay and gingival inflammation with consequent referral to a general dentist for complete evaluation and treatment is the most effective means of preventing infection. Referral to the dentist is especially important for patients who may have their mouth hygiene compromised by bulimia, Sjögren's syndrome, human immunodeficiency virus (HIV) infection, or upcoming treatment for cancer (eg, head and neck irradiation, chemotherapy). In the patient with valvular heart disease, full dental evaluation on a periodic basis is mandatory and is particularly indicated before consideration of a valvular prosthesis so that potential sources of dental sepsis may be eliminated. Adequate antibiotic prophylaxis for subacute bacterial endocarditis must be provided for such patients at the time dental procedures are performed (see below and Chapter 16).

When physical examination indicates no other source of facial pain, referral for dental evaluation is indicated. Abscess formation necessitates prompt referral for definitive drainage. When the patient's clinical appearance demonstrates involvement of deep fascial spaces, as evidenced by fever, trismus, elevation of the tongue, or ophthalmoplegia, referral to an oral surgeon and admission to the hospital for parenteral antibiotics are urgent.

The patient with acute salivary swelling should be seen by an oral surgeon for radiographic examination, by which sialoliths causing obstruction are sought. Gentle dilatation of the duct may help to relieve the obstruction; in some cases, surgery is necessary to remove the stone. Sialography, or examination of the salivary system with radiographic contrast injections, is contraindicated in the acute period of infection.

When salivary swelling is chronic in nature, no antibiotics are indicated. Sialography is highly diagnostic in this group of patients. If the differential diagnosis includes Sjögren's syndrome, sarcoidosis, or lymphoma, a biopsy of one of the minor salivary glands of the lower lip will usually confirm the diagnosis, without necessitating a more complex parotid biopsy.

ANNOTATED BIBLIOGRAPHY

Chow AW, Roser SM, Brady FA. Orofacial odontogenic infections. Ann Intern Med 1978;88:392. *(A comprehensive review of pertinent oral microbiology, surgical anatomy of the spread of infection, and the signs and symptoms of patients with odontogenic infection.)*

Greene JC, Louie R, Wycoff SJ. Preventive dentistry: dental caries. JAMA 1989;262:3459. *(Recommendations from the US Preventive Services Task Force.)*

Prevention of Bacterial Endocarditis. Medical Letter 1989;31:112. *(Recommended program of endocarditis prophylaxis for dental work.)*

Primary Care Medicine: Office Evaluation and Management of the Adult Patient, 3rd edition, edited by Allan H. Goroll, Lawrence A. May, and Albert G. Mulley, Jr. J.B. Lippincott Company, Philadelphia

215
Evaluation of Smell and Taste Disturbances

Impairment of taste and smell, in addition to being intrinsically unpleasant, is annoying because it interferes with the ability to derive pleasure from food. Moreover, a diminished ability to detect noxious agents in the environment leaves the patient vulnerable to them. Patients may complain of total loss, attenuation, or perversion of these senses. Problems of smell are often reported as alterations of taste because much of the awareness of taste is olfactory. The primary physician should be capable of recognizing taste and smell disturbances that are manifestations of serious illness requiring detailed evaluation, as well as simple forms in which symptomatic relief will suffice.

PATHOPHYSIOLOGY AND CLINICAL PRESENTATION

Smell. The olfactory area is located high in the nasal vault above the superior turbinate. The neurons of the first cranial nerve penetrate the cribriform plate and travel to the cortex at the base of the frontal lobe on top of the cribriform plate. The most common mechanism of anosmia or hyposmia is *nasal obstruction* that prevents air from reaching olfactory areas high in the nose. Food is tasteless while the problem persists. In most instances, such as those related to the common cold or allergic rhinitis, the process is fully reversible, but sometimes more lasting damage is done. *Chronic infection* may lead to partial replacement of olfactory mucosa with respiratory epithelium. *Influenza* is known for its ability to cause permanent destruction of the nasal receptors; the onset is often acute. Another mechanism of acute anosmia is *head trauma,* in which the nerve filaments coming through the cribriform plate are damaged.

More gradual onset of reduced smell is typical of an expanding *mass lesion* at the base of the frontal lobe. Meningiomas and aneurysms of the anterior cerebral circulation are the most important sources of this problem. Upward extension of mass lesion into the frontal lobe is manifested by lack of initiative, personality change, and forgetfulness; posterior extension may involve the optic chiasm.

Perversion of smell (parosmia) can result from local nasal pathology such as *empyema* of the nasal sinuses, or *ozena,* a chronic rhinitis of unknown etiology causing thick greenish discharge and crusting (see Chapter 219). *Klebsiella* and *Pseudomonas* are often cultured from the discharge. *Olfactory hallucinations* are central in origin and may present as the aura of a seizure. The responsible lesion is typically found in the area of the uncus. *Olfactory delusions* are reported by schizophrenic patients while their sense of smell remains intact.

Many disorders of smell are of unknown cause. The mechanisms of reduced smell associated with *hypothyroidism, hypogonadism,* and *hepatitis* are not understood. Speculation has centered on the influence of various trace metals, particularly copper and zinc, but replacement therapy has been disappointing.

Taste. The tongue, 7th and 9th cranial nerves, and the hippocampal region of the cerebral cortex make up the taste apparatus. The front of the tongue detects sweet and salty tastes, the sides sense sour tastes, and the large papillae in the back detect bitter tastes. The pharynx also has the ability to sense taste. The taste buds are concentrated in the anterior two-thirds of the tongue, which is innervated by the chorda tympani branch of the 7th cranial nerve. The posterior third of the tongue and palate are supplied by the glossopharyngeal nerve.

The most frequent source of diminished fine taste is *impairment of smell.* In addition, the taste buds may be directly injured by *alcohol* and *smoking.* The common observation that food tastes better after these habits are terminated is due to improvement in both the olfactory receptors and the taste buds. *Aging* results in small, but measurable changes in acuity for salty and bitter tastes, but not for sweet or sour ones. Elderly men differ from elderly women in that men selectively lose sensitivity to low concentrations of salt, whereas women have a more progressive loss of salt sensitivity.

Diseases and drugs that dry the mouth, for example, *Sjögren's syndrome* and *tricyclic antidepressants,* reduce the threshold for taste. Chorda tympani and 7th nerve lesions are rarely bilateral and therefore do not produce a complete loss of taste. Cerebral mass lesions usually do not involve the hippocampal gyrus. Depression, endocrinopathies, and a host of drugs are associated with complaints of altered taste. The mechanisms are unknown, but in many instances the primary disturbance seems to be, in part, an alteration of smell.

DIFFERENTIAL DIAGNOSIS

Most of the conditions that disrupt taste are annoying but not life-threatening (Table 215–1). However, a disturbance in the sense of smell may be a sign of more serious illness (Table 215–2).

Table 215-1. Some Important Causes of Impaired Taste

A. Disturbances in Smell
B. Injury to Taste Buds
 1. Age
 2. Smoking
 3. Hot liquids
 4. Dental disease
 5. Sjögren's syndrome
 6. Idiopathic conditions
C. Cranial Nerve Lesions (7th or 9th, partial loss only)
 1. Ear surgery
 2. Bell's palsy
 3. Ramsay-Hunt syndrome (herpes zoster infection of the geniculate ganglion)
 4. Cholesteatoma
 5. Cerebellopontine angle tumors (advanced disease)
D. Central Lesions
 1. Head trauma
 2. Tumors (rare)
E. Psychiatric Disorders
 1. Depression
F. Drugs
 1. Captopril
 2. Imipramine (and other tricyclic agents)
 3. Clofibrate
 4. Lithium
 5. L-dopa
 6. Acetazolamide
 7. Metronidazole
 8. Glipizide
 9. Iron
 10. Tetracycline
 11. Allopurinol
G. Metabolic–Endocrine Conditions
 1. Hypogonadism
 2. Uremia
 3. Hypothyroidism
 4. Hepatitis
 5. Pregnancy

Table 215-2. Causes of Disturbances in Smell

A. Nasal
 1. Upper respiratory tract infection
 2. Polyps
 3. Ozena
 4. Chronic sinusitis
 5. Allergic rhinitis
 6. Influenza and other virus
 7. Chemical injury (*eg*, tar, formaldehyde)
B. Cranial Nerve
 1. Trauma
 2. Meningioma
 3. Cerebral aneurysm
C. Cerebral Cortex
 1. Seizure disorder
 2. Meningioma
 3. Aneurysm
 4. Schizophrenia
D. Metabolic–Endocrine
 1. Hypothyroidism
 2. Hypogonadism
 3. Liver disease

WORKUP

Smell

History. A primary objective is to distinguish local nasal pathology from a central or cranial nerve lesion. History of head trauma, worsening headaches, olfactory hallucinations, change in personality, unexplained forgetfulness, visual disturbances, gradual onset or steady progression of symptoms suggests disease beyond the nasal cavity. History of head congestion, nasal discharge, allergies, sinus problems, influenza, chemical exposure, or a recent cold suggests the nose as the source of difficulty. Inquiry into symptoms of hepatocellular failure (see Chapter 71) and hypothyroidism (see Chapter 104) may uncover a metabolic–endocrine etiology. A careful psychiatric history is needed when there is description of abnormal smells in the absence of any other pathology.

Physical Examination. One can document the disorder by challenging each nostril with a representative sample of each primary odor: pungent, floral, mint, and putrid. Smell is most accurately assessed by the use of chemicals, such as pyridine, garliclike odor, nitrobenzene, bitter almond, thiophene, and burnt rubber odor. Kits are available that contain these substances. Ammonia, which will produce a response by irritation even in the absence of olfactory powers, should be avoided.

On physical examination, the head is assessed for trauma and the nares are inspected for polyps, deviated septum, mucosal inflammation, and discharge. The sinuses are transilluminated to look for evidence of sinusitis. Fundi are checked for blurring of the disk margins, and the visual fields are tested by confrontation for evidence of optic chiasm compression. The skin, thyroid, and ankle jerks are examined for signs of hypothyroidism (see Chapter 104), and the hair, voice, muscles, and testes are examined for hypogonadism. Any jaundice, hepatomegaly, ascites, or asterixis should be noted.

Laboratory Studies. *Sinus films* should be reserved for patients with clinical evidence of sinusitis (see Chapter 219). *Neuroimaging studies* (computed tomography [CT] or magnetic resonance imaging [MRI]) should be considered only if there is a history of recent head trauma or symptoms and signs suggestive of a mass lesion (see Chapters 100, 101, and 165). The same principle pertains to the ordering of liver, thyroid, and gonadotropin studies (see Chapters 71, 104, and 120).

Taste

History. The initial objective of the evaluation is to localize the problem. Intracranial disease is distinctly rare, so assessment can be concentrated on disease in the mouth, in the area of chorda tympani, and 7th nerve. Alcohol abuse, smoking, dental disease, and severe mouth dryness suggest a buccal cavity source. Facial palsy, herpes zoster rash about the ear, recent ear surgery, hearing problems, vertigo, and tinnitus are clues to diseases that may injure the 7th nerve. Drug use and concurrent metabolic or endocrinologic problems (see Table 215-1 and above) deserve exploration. Isolated reduction in taste requires inquiry into smell impairment and concurrent depression. Dry eyes in conjunction with dry mouth suggest Sjögren's syndrome, especially if rheumatoid arthritis is present.

Physical Examination. Careful examination of the nose, ears, oral cavity, tongue, and teeth is essential. The condition of the gums and teeth is worth noting. Taste should be assessed by challenging the withdrawn tongue with sweet, salty, bitter, and sour stimuli on each side and asking the patient to indicate what he or she tastes. Lateralizing the defect suggests a lesion of the 7th nerve. Examination of the cranial nerves needs to concentrate on testing of olfaction, hearing, and facial motor functions.

Laboratory Studies. If history or physical examination suggests hypothyroidism, a thyroid-stimulating hormone (TSH) level should be obtained; likewise a BUN and creatinine should be obtained if renal disease is suspected. Sjögren's syndrome can be confirmed by lip biopsy. Suspicion of a cerebellopontine angle tumor is an indication for CT scan.

SYMPTOMATIC MANAGEMENT

Smell. Local nasal pathology is often self-limited, but when chronic sinusitis or allergic rhinitis persists, definitive therapy is indicated (see Chapters 219 and 222). Avoidance of toxic fumes (eg, formaldehyde) and removal of nasal polyps should also help. When influenza has caused sudden, complete, and permanent loss of smell, little can be done. Ozena sometimes requires local or even systemic antibiotic therapy; saline irrigations to remove obstructing crusts are helpful (see Chapter 222). Correction of hypothyroidism improves smell. A literature has developed suggesting that zinc salts will restore normal olfaction and taste, although double-blind controlled study found zinc to be no better than placebo.

Taste. Regardless of the cause of reduced taste, the patient should be encouraged to stop smoking and reduce alcohol consumption; often the development of a disability such as altered taste is sufficient motivation to get the patient to stop (see Chapter 54). If possible, medications that may impair taste should be stopped or reduced to determine what contribution, if any, they make to the taste disturbance. Any dental disease of consequence should be corrected. The same pertains to hypothyroidism (see Chapter 104). Concurrent depression may respond to a tricyclic antidepressant, but the drug may impair taste by causing a dry mouth (see Chapter 227); forewarning the patient can prevent side effects from becoming an unpleasant surprise. Disease related to the brainstem, chorda tympani, and inner ear requires referral for treatment.

INDICATIONS FOR REFERRAL

Olfactory hallucinations, change in personality, visual field defects, and impairment of memory in conjunction with disorders of smell, and multiple cranial nerve defects, vertigo, and tinnitus in conjunction with altered taste, are indications for neurologic consultation. Psychiatric consultation is worth considering when olfactory hallucinations are accompanied by other evidence of a thought disorder. Patients with ozena, nasal polyps, deviated nasal septum, refractory sinusitis, or a chorda tympani lesion may benefit from evaluation by the otolaryngologist.

A.H.G.

ANNOTATED BIBLIOGRAPHY

Rollin H. Drug-related gustatory disorders. Ann Otol Rhinol Laryngol 1978;87:1. *(A review of drugs that alter taste.)*

Schiffman SS. Taste and smell in disease. N Engl J Med 1983;308:1275. *(A two-part comprehensive review.)*

Weiffenbach Gordon RS. Variation in taste thresholds with human aging. JAMA 1982;247:775. *(Taste acuity declines selectively, not globally.)*

Appendix: Halitosis

Halitosis is defined as a foul breath odor arising from a person's oral cavity or nasal passages. It differs from disorders of taste and smell in that the condition is typically not noticeable to the patient. The condition may be physiologic or a manifestation of oral–nasal or systemic pathology.

Pathophysiology. The most common physiologic cause is so-called morning breath. The universal condition derives from the cessation of regular salivary flow with sleep. Its marked reduction and resulting buccal cavity stasis allow mouth flora an opportunity to feed on remaining food particles, sloughed epithelial cells, and stagnant saliva. The byproducts of bacterial metabolism cause the foul odor. Pathologic halitosis may derive from impairment of normal salivary flow (eg, parotid disease, Sjögren's syndrome), increased presentation of bacterial substrate (periodontitis, sinusitis), or a metabolic derangement (renal or hepatic failure—see Table 215-3). In rare instances, the patient is the only one to note the condition, strongly suggesting a hallucination of psychiatric or epileptic origin.

Workup is similar to that described above for disorders of taste and smell, with more attention paid to possible oral cavity pathology. It helps to begin the assessment by directly confirming the reported odor. Differentiating an oral source from a nasal one can be done by pinching the nares closed while exhaling and exhaling through the nose with the mouth closed. Esophageal and gastric etiologies may require eructation for detection. If the mouth is believed to harbor the suspected source, then the oral cavity should be examined

Table 215-3. Some Important Pathologic Causes of Halitosis

Oral cavity: poorly fitting dental work, periodontal disease, sialadenitis, abscess
Posterior pharynx: tonsillitis, diverticulum, tumor
Sinus: sinusitis, tumor, necrotic disease
Esophagus: reflux, diverticulum, motor dysfunction
Lungs: abscess
Metabolic: renal or hepatic failure; ketoacidosis
Psychiatric: psychosis (self-perception only)

carefully for poorly fitting dental work, periodontal disease, glossitis, tooth abscess, and tonsillar disease. The salivary glands should be checked for free flow of clear saliva in adequate volumes. Pulmonary disease and metabolic dysfunction are important to consider when the oral cavity and sinus tracts appear normal. Patients who have no objective findings but are convinced of halitosis derived from an internal source have a high probability of a hypochondriacal psychosis and need psychiatric referral.

Treatment. Treatment should be etiologic. Trying to mask the odor is far less effective than addressing its etiology. Mouthwashes are a poor substitute for good oral hygiene. Despite advertisements to the contrary, mouthwashes do little to suppress oral flora. Oral hygiene is particularly important in the elderly. Patients should be encouraged to floss and brush regularly, which help remove trapped food particles and promote healthy gums. Regular dental checkups are essential to recommend, although often overlooked.

ANNOTATED BIBLIOGRAPHY

Johnson BE. Halitosis, or the meaning of bad breath. J Gen Intern Med 1992;7:649. *(Thoughtful review of this very mundane problem; 55 refs.)*

216
Approach to the Patient With Hoarseness

WILLIAM R. WILSON, M.D.

Primary Care Medicine: Office Evaluation and Management of the Adult Patient, 3rd edition, edited by Allan H. Goroll, Lawrence A. May, and Albert G. Mulley, Jr. J.B. Lippincott Company, Philadelphia

Hoarseness is a symptom of laryngeal disease. The majority of acute episodes are self-limited and due to viral upper respiratory tract infection or voice abuse. However, the patient bothered by persistent hoarseness requires careful assessment, because carcinoma of the larynx, tumor-associated damage to the recurrent laryngeal nerve, and other serious conditions may be responsible. Prompt evaluation maximizes the chances of detecting an early lesion and achieving a cure.

PATHOPHYSIOLOGY AND CLINICAL PRESENTATION

Vocal quality is determined by complex factors, including the distance between vocal cords, tenseness of the cords, and the rapidity of vibration. Hoarseness results from interference with normal apposition of the cords. Inflammatory, traumatic, and neoplastic lesions cause hoarseness by altering cord structure and function.

Often the quality of the voice disturbance reflects the underlying pathophysiology. A "breathy" voice occurs when the vocal cords do not approximate completely, allowing air to escape during vocalization. The cords may be kept apart by tumor, polyps, or nodules. A similar presentation occurs when the cords fail to approximate due to unilateral or bilateral cord paralysis. Patients with hysterical aphonia purposefully hold the cords apart while speaking.

A "raspy" or harsh voice ensues from cord thickening due to edema or inflammation. This is the voice quality characteristic of many heavy smokers. The voice is of lowered pitch and poor clarity. Associated inspiratory or expiratory cervical stridor results from laryngeal obstruction.

A high, "shaky" voice or a low, soft vocalization are consequences of decreased respiratory force (phonasthenia). These voices characterize elderly or debilitated patients, who may complain of additional voice difficulties, such as change in voice pitch or poor vocal projection.

The presentations of a number of etiologies are best considered in terms of whether they are acute or chronic.

Acute Hoarseness

Acute laryngitis leads to vocal cord edema and erythema. Viral infection, vocal abuse, sudden excessive smoking, inhalation of irritant gases, aspiration, and occasionally allergy (hay fever) constitute the list of important precipitants. *Vocal cord nodules* may develop when edematous cords are used excessively. Fibrous tissue begins to collect at the junction of the anterior one-third and the posterior two-thirds of the cord. This results in a lowered breathy voice, which can harm a singing or speaking career.

Acute laryngeal edema may present as part of a generalized edematous allergic response involving the lips, tongue, and other hypopharyngeal tissues. *Foods* are important precipitants, especially seafoods and nuts; medications can have a similar effect. Edema can develop from hereditary deficiency of C-1-esterase inhibitor (C1 INH) as occurs in *hereditary angioneurotic edema*. Swelling forms in response to mechanical trauma, such as dental surgery or intubation for general anesthesia. In the pediatric population, subglottic edema from viral laryngotracheal bronchitis (*croup*) can obstruct the airway. In adults, *acute epiglottitis* has been noted with increasing frequency. It is associated with risk of airway obstruction, especially in the setting of *Haemophilus influenzae* infection. Symptoms include severe sore throat, dyspnea, and hoarseness.

Chronic Hoarseness

Chronic laryngitis causes a low, raspy voice, a nonproductive cough, and a "dry throat" sensation. There is little or no pain. The voice waxes and wanes, becoming worse as the day progresses. The typical patient is a heavy smoker who continually talks, subjecting himself or herself to a combination of chemical irritation and vocal abuse. In rare instances, an infectious or chronic inflammatory condition (eg, tuberculosis or sarcoidosis) may produce a similar picture. Chronic laryngeal edema with development of *dependent polyps* represents another form of chronic laryngitis; it may arise in the setting of hypothyroidism, radiation therapy to the neck, or chronic sinusitis with persistent drainage and cough. Patients with this condition speak in a lowered, gravelly voice with short phonation time.

Leukoplakia, another form of chronic laryngitis, is the term for the white, scalelike appearance of hyperkeratotic changes involving the vocal cords. It occurs secondary to chemical irritation, especially from *tobacco* smoke and *alcohol.* Symptoms include hoarseness but no pain. Leukoplakia, which may be a premalignant state, cannot be distinguished visually from squamous cell carcinoma in situ, or early invasive cancer.

Contact ulcers of the larynx occur on the posterior third of the vocal cords where the arytenoid cartilage is covered only by a thin layer of mucosa. Once this mucosa is abraded, an ulcer often forms. Symptoms are painful phonation and a weakened, "breathy" voice. Chronic ulcerations may in time develop into granulations that hold the cords apart, and at times these may become large enough to cause some respiratory obstruction. The ulcerations result most commonly from acute or chronic laryngeal *intubation* but classically are the result of *vocal abuse* by orators who misuse their larynx attempting to lower the pitch of their voices when speaking forcefully.

Vocal cord paralysis occurs with nerve injury. Usually just one cord is paralyzed (except in patients with severe central nervous system [CNS] disease) giving a weak, breathy voice. The position of the cord is affected by the amount of time that has elapsed since injury, as paralyzed cords tend to move toward the midline. The degree of paralysis and the clinical presentation depend on where the neural injury is located. Injury to a vagus nerve results in the loss of all ipsilateral laryngeal muscle function and sensation, leading to aspiration and a weak, breathy voice. A more peripheral injury of the recurrent laryngeal nerve leads to little if any aspiration and a voice that is hoarse and somewhat weak, but less breathy. Viral neuritis is the most common cause; function usually returns in 6 to 9 months.

Laryngeal carcinoma usually occurs in patients with a history of smoking and drinking. If the vocal cords are involved, progressive hoarseness is an early sign, but, if the tumor arises on the epiglottis, hypopharynx, or false cords, hoarseness may be a late development. Pain secondary to ulceration is also a late symptom and is often perceived as referred otologic pain, especially when swallowing. These patients may have a mildly fetid breath. Patients with a hypopharyngeal or laryngeal cancer can present with an unexplained lymph node in the neck.

Table 216-1. Important Causes of Hoarseness

ACUTE HOARSENESS	CHRONIC HOARSENESS
Acute Laryngitis	Chronic Laryngitis
Viral infection	Chronic or recurrent vocal abuse
Vocal abuse	Smoking
Toxic fumes	Allergy
Allergy (seasonal)	Persistent irritant exposure
Acute Laryngeal Edema	Carcinoma of Larynx
Angioneurotic edema	Intrinsic to vocal cords
Infection	Extrinsic to vocal cords
Direct injury	Vocal Cord Lesions
Nephritis	Polpys
Acute Epiglottitis	Leukoplakia
	Contact ulcer and granuloma
	Vocal nodule (see vocal abuse)
	Benign tumors
	Vocal Cord Paralysis
	Laryngeal nerve injury (tumor, neck surgery, aortic aneurysm)
	Brainstem lesion
	Vocal Cord Trauma
	Chronic intubation
	Systemic Disorders
	Hypothyroidism
	Rheumatoid arthritis
	Virilization
	Psychogenic

DIFFERENTIAL DIAGNOSIS

The causes of hoarseness are best considered in terms of acute and chronic etiologies (Table 216–1).

WORKUP

History. The evaluation of hoarseness depends on the chronicity of the condition. One needs to determine whether the onset was sudden or gradual and the course self-limited or progressive. Difficulty in breathing or stridor suggests obstruction and is an indication for emergency hospital admission. It is helpful to find out if hoarseness is exacerbated by talking; also whether the voice completely disappeared and, if so, for how long. Any recent upper respiratory tract infection, sore throat, fever, chills, sputum, or myalgias should be noted, as well as excessive voice use. Exposure to dust, fire, smoke, or irritant fumes should be documented, as should tobacco and alcohol intake. A history of neck mass, neck surgery, intubation, or lung tumor may provide important clues to etiology. Symptoms of hypothyroidism (see Chapter 104) are worth checking for when the etiology is not readily evident.

Physical Examination. There are two rules of thumb regarding patients with hoarseness: first, hoarseness of more than 2 to 3 weeks' duration requires an examination of the larynx, and second, this examination will provide, in the majority of cases, an immediate diagnosis.

A good view of the hypopharynx and larynx is somewhat difficult to obtain, but the primary physician is encouraged to try, and with practice can master the technique. *Indirect laryngoscopy* with a head light and warmed laryngeal mirror is a time-honored method and still provides the best and most rapidly obtained view of the area. For the gagging patient, premedication with 10 mg of diazepam orally and an analgesic throat spray (Cetacaine, xylocaine 1% spray) are of benefit. For patients with uncontrollable gag reflexes, referral for examination with a fiberoptic laryngoscope will be necessary. This instrument is introduced through the nose, requiring pretreatment of the nasal passages with 4% cocaine solution for vasoconstriction and anesthesia. It is rare when a good laryngeal view cannot be obtained in this manner.

Even if laryngoscopy cannot be carried out, some clues as to etiology can be gleaned by a careful physical examination and noting voice quality. One needs to examine the oropharynx and carefully palpate the thyroid and cervical lymph nodes. The hoarse patient with an unexplained neck mass or lymph node requires a thorough check of the nose, paranasal sinuses, and nasopharynx. A breathy voice suggests poor cord apposition, which may be due to tumor, polyp, or nodule. A raspy voice is indicative of cord thickening due to edema or inflammation, as with chemical irritation, vocal abuse, and infection. The patient with a high, shaky voice or a very soft one is having trouble mounting adequate respiratory force. Dyspnea is an indication for laryngoscopy.

Laboratory Studies. In most instances, the selection of studies depends on the findings at laryngoscopy and should be done in conjunction with the otolaryngologist. The patient with unilateral paresis of the right vocal cord may have a recurrent laryngeal nerve syndrome secondary to a Pancoast tumor, necessitating radiologic evaluation of the right lung apex. If the cords appear chronically edematous and there is clinical suspicion of hypothyroidism, a check of a serum thyroid-stimulating hormone (TSH) is indicated. Patients with a suspected carcinoma involving the larynx or with an unexplained neck node and hoarseness need a thorough evaluation of the aerodigestive tract before biopsy. Open biopsy of neck nodes done without definitive surgery will reduce chances for survival in patients with carcinoma of the aerodigestive tract. Small-needle biopsies have circumvented the need for some open biopsies. The patient with recurrent edematous episodes and a positive family history might have angioneurotic edema; a check of the C1-INH level is indicated. Soft tissue films may be of use in the dyspneic patient.

PRINCIPLES OF THERAPY AND MANAGEMENT RECOMMENDATIONS

Regardless of causes, all patients with hoarseness should be strongly advised to *quit smoking* immediately (see Chapter 54). It is often in the setting of an associated medical problem that a smoker will finally decide to quit. Other measures are a function of the underlying etiology.

Acute Laryngitis. The best treatment is *voice rest*. When it is necessary to speak, the patient should use a moderate voice and not whisper. Warm *sialogogues,* such as hot tea with sugar and lemon, may be helpful. Antibiotics are not indicated unless there is documented bacterial infection. *Cough suppressants,* particularly with mucolytic agents, may be helpful. Also, *humidity* is of benefit. Inhalation of steam in a hot shower or breathing through a moist, hot towel will provide immediate partial relief. When hay fever is the cause, a topical steroid spray such as dexamethasone or flunisolide helps provide symptomatic relief, but steroids should not be used unless there is an allergic etiology.

Patients who are professional singers or speakers should be advised to rest their voice when they become hoarse (especially during upper respiratory infections) to prevent permanent injury to the vocal cords. A vasoconstricting spray and analgesics are used by professionals when use of their voice is absolutely necessary. Occasionally, professional singers may be given a short course of topical steroids to get through a singing commitment, but further cord injury may ensue.

Acute laryngeal edema represents a medical emergency; hospitalization is urgent. Treatment is based on the degree of swelling and subsequent airway compromise. An *emergency airway* is established if necessary; 0.3 ml of *adrenalin* 1 to 1000 is administered subcutaneously, and steroids such as *dexamethasone* (Decadron 12 mg) may be given intravenously.

Vocal cord nodules should be treated early because often they respond to voice rest and vocal therapy. Nodules that do not respond to conservative therapy can be removed; use of an atraumatic technique (microlaryngeal surgery, carbon dioxide laser) is mandatory.

Angioneurotic edema does not respond to epinephrine or glucocorticosteroids. In an acute situation, intubation or tracheotomy may be required to maintain an airway. If available, infusion of C1-INH can be given. Otherwise, treatment is prophylactic, using anabolic steroids with attenuated androgenic effect (eg, danazol and stanozolol) to stimulate synthesis of C1 esterase inhibitor. Such prophylaxis may be given for several days before planned surgery.

Persistent vocal cord paralysis can be treated symptomatically by the injection of Teflon paste into the musculature of the paralyzed cord, moving it to the midline. This permits the functioning cord to better approximate, thereby improving vocal quality.

Carcinoma of the larynx can be cured, if detected in its early stages (T1N0). Surgery, laser treatment, and radiation are all capable of achieving a 90 percent cure rate. Selection of modality depends on the type of expertise available locally and the location of the lesion. A better voice is usually obtained with laser or irradiation. Metastases and a poor prognosis usually do not occur until the vocal cord cancer becomes larger (T3 to T4) and extends beyond the true cords. Early supraglottic carcinomas arising above the true cords can be cured in about 75 percent of patients with radiation therapy, partial laryngectomy, or a combination of the two. Larger lesions require total laryngectomy and irradiation, with a cure rate of 40 percent. Induction chemotherapy is used for advanced stages of disease. Prevention remains the best treatment; all smokers must be told to quit.

Leukoplakia is treated by vocal cord stripping under microscopic control. Regular follow-up examinations of the larynx are necessary. Repeated vocal cord stripping may be needed once or twice a year, particularly if the patient fails to limit use of irritants.

Dependent polyps are removed by microsurgery.

INDICATIONS FOR REFERRAL AND ADMISSION

If the primary care physician does not feel competent to visualize the vocal cords, a decision must be made about whether to refer the patient to an otolaryngologist. Hoarseness of greater than 3 weeks' duration, particularly when there has not been a history of an acute infectious process, requires referral. Any patient with concurrent dyspnea should be immediately hospitalized. In those who have a resolving process and are at low risk for malignancy (young, nonsmoker, nondrinker), a complete otolaryngologic examination may be deferred pending full resolution.

Among patients who do undergo indirect laryngoscopy by the primary care physician, any with a cord nodule, thickening, or paralysis by indirect laryngoscopy requires referral, as does the patient with persistent unexplained hoarseness of more than 2 to 3 weeks' duration and inability to tolerate indirect laryngoscopy.

Referral for voice therapy can help foster healthful vocal habits and is indicated for patients who experience repeated vocal trauma or who have organic disease and are in need of voice rehabilitation.

ANNOTATED BIBLIOGRAPHY

Vaughan CW. Diagnosis and treatment of organic voice disorders. N Engl J Med 1983;307:863. *(A terse review for the general reader.)*

Primary Care Medicine: Office Evaluation and Management of the Adult Patient, 3rd edition, edited by Allan H. Goroll, Lawrence A. May, and Albert G. Mulley, Jr. J.B. Lippincott Company, Philadelphia

217
Evaluation of Tinnitus

AINA J. GULYA, M.D.

Tinnitus is an important, but nonspecific symptom of otologic disease. "Ringing," "buzzing," or "roaring" are terms used to describe the sensation, which can be extremely annoying as well as a source of concern. The occurrence of tinnitus requires assessment for serious and treatable otologic problems. In the absence of a specifically treatable etiology, it is still important to provide the patient with some symptomatic relief, especially at night.

PATHOPHYSIOLOGY AND CLINICAL PRESENTATION

Tinnitus remains very poorly understood. It appears to be a nonspecific manifestation of disease in the ear, 8th nerve, or central auditory apparatus, and is often accompanied by hearing loss.

External and Middle Ear Conditions. Tinnitus may result from *impacted cerumen, perforation* of the tympanic membrane, or fluid in the middle ear. The sensation is commonly described as low-pitched, intermittent, and accompanied by muffled hearing and a change in the sound of one's own voice. In *otosclerosis,* tinnitus is constant but may disappear as the disease progresses. *Acute otitis media* sometimes produces a pulsating type of tinnitus that resolves as inflammation subsides. Pulsatile tinnitus is also associated with *glomus tumors* and posttraumatic *arteriovenous fistulas.*

Inner Ear and 8th Nerve Disease. *Presbycusis* and *acoustic trauma* can give rise to a high-pitched tinnitus that is near the frequency of greatest hearing loss. Transient tinnitus that follows acute noise exposure is a forerunner of hearing loss and a warning sign to avoid repeated exposure. *Ototoxic drugs,* such as the aminoglycoside antibiotics, may produce high-pitched tinnitus and hearing loss that often persist after cessation of drug use. Salicylates are frequently responsible for reversible, dose-related tinnitus. *Meniere's disease* results in transient, low-pitched tinnitus that varies with the intensity of the condition's other symptoms, often worsening when vertigo and hearing loss are imminent. *Acoustic neuroma* produces a similar set of symptoms but usually the clinical course is progressive, with tinnitus frequently preceding other symptoms, such as vertigo (see Chapter 166).

Other Sources. When ambient noise is reduced, most people will notice some head sounds. These may be due to the rushing of blood (severest is aortic insufficiency) or contraction of auditory muscles. Loss of hearing due to conductive defects accentuates the problem. Tinnitus cerebri is described as a roaring in the head and is believed to be vascular or neurologic in origin. A cerebral aneurysm with an audible bruit, a jugular megabulb anomaly, palatal myoclonus with audible muscle contraction, and an unusually patent eustachian tube that transmits respiratory sounds are examples of "objective" tinnitus in which the sounds can be heard by the examiner. Tinnitus may also be associated with temporomandibular joint dysfunction (Costen's syndrome).

Depressed and neurotic individuals have less tolerance for these normal head sounds and complain of them when in quiet settings. The ability to withstand tinnitus is also subject to much individual variation. Tolerance is lessened by fatigue and emotional stress.

DIFFERENTIAL DIAGNOSIS

Most tinnitus results from the same conditions that cause hearing loss, whether conductive or sensorineural, peripheral or central (see Chapter 212). Subjective complaints of ear or head noise in the absence of otologic pathology may be a concomitant of psychogenic disease. Objective tinnitus suggests cerebrovascular pathology, palatal myoclonus, or a patulous eustachian tube.

There are few data on the frequency of the various conditions responsible for tinnitus. Of interest is the fact that reports from otologic practice list as many as 50 percent of cases being of unknown etiology.

WORKUP

The diagnostic assessment of tinnitus follows the same pattern as that for hearing loss (see Chapter 212). A few additional points follow:

History. The pitch of the tinnitus is, unfortunately, of limited use in diagnosis, although some conditions are more likely than others to be associated with tinnitus of a certain pitch. Distinguishing pulsatile, nonpulsatile, subjective, and objective tinnitus may be more helpful. Any association of the sound with respiration, drug use, vertigo, noise trauma, or ear infection should be checked. A history of head trauma should be sought, because it may be associated with an arteriovenous fistula, or an aneurysm of the intrapetrous portion of the internal carotid artery. When the problem is present only at night, it suggests increased awareness of normal head sounds. Most patients with tinnitus of otologic origin have an associated hearing defect or soon develop one, whereas those without other signs of ear disease may have vascular lesion or an accentuated awareness of normal head noises.

Physical Examination. One inspects the external ear and tympanic membrane for cerumen impaction, foreign bodies, perforation, signs of otitis media (see Chapter 218), and abnormal middle ear masses. Weber and Rinne testing should be performed to determine if there is sensorineural or conductive hearing loss (see Chapter 212). The cranial nerves are examined for evidence of brainstem damage, a sign of an advanced acoustic neuroma, or a glomus tumor. Testing for nystagmus (see Chapter 166) is worthwhile if vertigo is reported. The skull should be auscultated for a bruit if the origin of the problem remains obscure. Compression of the ipsilateral jugular vein will abolish the objective tinnitus of a jugular megabulb anomaly.

Laboratory Studies. An audiogram can help to identify and localize an otologic lesion. Neuroimaging study (computed tomography [CT] or magnetic resonance imaging [MRI]) may be indicated but should not be done without first consulting the otolaryngologist to ensure proper test selection, performance, and interpretation. Gadolinium-enhanced magnetic resonance imaging may be recommended, especially in evaluation of unilateral tinnitus.

INDICATIONS FOR REFERRAL

Referral is essential when a conductive hearing loss is discovered because many of these lesions are correctable. Suspicion of an acoustic neuroma, glomus tumor, or cerebrovascular abnormality is also an indication for consultation, especially before embarking on an expensive workup. Referral to the otolaryngologist may be necessary to satisfy the anxious patient that everything has been explored and that there is no serious or correctable underlying condition.

SYMPTOMATIC MANAGEMENT AND PATIENT EDUCATION

For many patients, the priority is relief from the constant ringing, which can be very disturbing, especially at night. Drugs of all types have been tried, including nicotinic acid, vasodilators, tranquilizers, antidepressants, and seizure medications. None has proven superior to placebo. Nighttime use of a clock radio that shuts off after a half hour of playing background music often allows the patient to fall asleep. Keeping a radio on during the day when the patient has to work in a quiet room is also helpful. Many devices are promoted that one wears like a hearing aid (tinnitus maskers) to help mask tinnitus; they are of questionable value. Biofeedback may help in certain cases in which the tinnitus is related to stress.

ANNOTATED BIBLIOGRAPHY

Pulec JL, Hodell SF, Anthony PF. Tinnitus: Diagnosis and treatment. Ann Otolaryngol 1978;87:821. *(Emphasis on use of hearing aids and/or tinnitus maskers to relieve symptoms.)*

Vernon J. Attempts to relieve tinnitus. J Am Audiol Soc 1977;2:124. *(An extensive and excellent review of treatment measures.)*

218
Approach to the Patient With Otitis

AINA J. GULYA, M.D.

Primary Care Medicine: Office Evaluation and Management of the Adult Patient, 3rd edition, edited by Allan H. Goroll, Lawrence A. May, and Albert G. Mulley, Jr. J.B. Lippincott Company, Philadelphia

Ear pain is a common manifestation of infection involving the upper respiratory tract or the external auditory canal. Inspection often reveals signs of otitis media or external otitis. The primary care provider should know how to recognize and treat these common conditions so that only refractory or complicated cases need be referred.

PATHOPHYSIOLOGY AND CLINICAL PRESENTAITON

Acute Otitis Media is an extremely common problem in early childhood. Incidence declines with age. Purulent otitis media due to bacterial infection results from bacteria ascending from the nasopharynx to the normally sterile middle ear. Abnormal eustachian tube reflux or obstruction caused by viral nasopharyngitis are the major pathogenetic factors. Pain, fever, and hearing loss are the classic presenting complaints. Cloudy, purulent fluid may be visible in the middle ear behind the tympanic membrane. The tympanic membrane bulges, obscuring its normal landmarks; perforation and otorrhea may occur.

The most common organism is *Pneumococcus*. Although *Haemophilus influenzae* is predominantly found in young children, it can occur in older persons. Other organisms implicated in some patients include streptococci, *Moraxella catarrhalis, Neisseria catarrhalis,* and *Staphylococcus epidermidis*. Viruses and mycoplasma are of less importance etiologically. Anaerobic bacteria have been implicated in some cases.

The prognosis for acute otitis media is excellent, but some patients may experience chronic serous otitis, hearing loss, or recurrent purulent otitis.

Serous otitis media is a noninfectious variant of otitis media in which fever and pain are absent. Clear fluid is present in the middle ear, the tympanic membrane remains retracted, and bony landmarks are intact. It often follows eustachian tube obstruction, which may result from viral upper respiratory tract infection in adults.

Chronic otitis media is seen in all age groups and results from neglected or recurrent acute otitis media. Pain and fever are usually absent but can occur during sporadic flare-ups in activity. Diminished hearing and foul otorrhea are the major symptoms. Physical examination discloses perforation of the tympanic membrane. Central perforations of the pars tensa are associated with benign disease, but marginal or peripheral perforations may be associated with invasive cholesteatomas. X-rays may reveal sclerosis of the mastoid air cells and bone destruction. A great variety of organisms can be cultured from the drainage in cases of chronic otitis media, including staphylococci, streptococci, *Pseudomonas aeruginosa,* and enteric gram-negative bacilli.

External otitis is a common, generally benign inflammatory condition usually precipitated by excessive moisture in or trauma to the external auditory canal. Patients complain of pruritus or pain, which may be severe. Crusting, inflammation, and discharge in the canal are typical findings. The pain, which results from movements of the external ear, helps distinguish otitis externa from otitis media. A broad range of organisms including *gram-positive cocci, gram-negative bacilli,* and *fungi* can cause otitis externa.

DIAGNOSIS

The cornerstone of the clinical diagnosis of acute purulent otitis media is the finding of a bulging tympanic membrane with impaired mobility and obscuration of the bony landmarks. The other diagnostic possibility is a serous otitis media, in which fever and pain are absent and, although fluid is present in the middle ear, the tympanic membrane is usually retracted and the bony landmarks are preserved. Cultures of the nasopharynx are not helpful in defining the etiology of acute otitis media. Needle aspiration of the middle ear is occasionally used to confirm the diagnosis and to identify the causative organism; however, this is rarely necessary in clinical practice because the bacteriology of acute otitis media is relatively well-defined and the response to antibiotics is easy to monitor.

In chronic otitis media, a perforated drum and discharge strongly support the diagnosis. Pain, erythema, and discharge in the external auditory canal are diagnostic of otitis externa.

PRINCIPLES OF MANAGEMENT AND THERAPEUTIC RECOMMENDATIONS

Acute Otitis Media. Treatment includes use of analgesics, decongestants, and antibiotics. *Amoxicillin* is generally the drug of choice in the pediatric age group because of the possibility of *H. influenzae*. Penicillin (eg, phenoxymethyl penicillin 250 mg qid for 7–10 d) usually suffices in adults. Because, ampicillin-resistant strains of *H. influenzae* have been implicated in up to 8 percent of cases of otitis media (mostly in children) and because *M. catarrhalis* may be responsible for others, the combination preparation *ampicillin/clavulanate* (Augmentin) may be necessary for cases that do not respond initially to penicillin or ampicillin. For penicillin-allergic persons, *erythromycin* (250 mg qid) *trimethoprim-sulfamethoxazole* is a reasonable alternative. A *sympathomimetic decongestant* (eg, pseudoephedrine 60 mg q4h) may help when the otitis occurs in the setting of an upper respiratory tract infection and eustachian tube obstruction. Care must be taken not to use a decongestant preparation that also contains antihistamine (most do) because the antihistamine may thicken secretions and prevent their drainage. Myringotomy does not hasten recovery but is indicated in patients with intractable pain, progressive deafness, or early mastoiditis, and in those who have had a poor response to medical therapy.

Serous otitis media secondary to eustachian tube obstruction from allergy or upper respiratory infection may improve with use of sympathomimetic decongestants (see Chapter 222). Only when allergic in origin might the otitis benefit from addition of an antihistamine to the program. Definitive evidence for efficacy is lacking, and antihistamines may thicken secretions, impeding their clearance.

Chronic Otitis. Antibiotics are generally of little benefit, and surgery is required in advanced cases. Topical otic drops are used before surgery. *Cortisporin otic* suspension and ophthalmic antibiotic eyedrops tend to be less irritating. Irrigation of the ear with a solution of 1.5% *acetic acid* helps to cleanse the ear and to restore its normal pH. Patients should be watched for intracranial suppurative complications.

Otitis externa is treated topically. Eardrops containing *polymyxin* and *neomycin* produce excellent results. Four drops are applied four times daily for a week, in combination with elimination of water contact (a cotton ball coated with petrolatum ointment usually suffices). Neomycin-containing eardrops, such as Cortisporin, can cause allergic skin reactions. A simple band-aid patch test will identify a sensitized patient. More severe cases of external otitis in which the canal is obstructed by edema or purulent material require ENT referral for suction of debris and insertion of a 2 × 2 gauze sponge to act as a wick for the antibiotic drops.

Cellulitis of the external ear requires systemic antibiotics. Malignant otitis externa is a rare but life-threatening infection in diabetics caused by *Pseudomonas aeruginosa;* prompt hospitalization and parenteral antibiotics are required.

INDICATIONS FOR REFERRAL

An otolaryngologist should be consulted if acute otitis media fails to respond to medical therapy or if complication such as tympanic membrane perforation, recurrent acute otitis, serous otitis, or chronic otitis media develop. As noted above, hospitalization for parenteral antibiotics is indicated if cellulitis of the external ear develops.

PATIENT EDUCATION

The pain of acute otitis media almost always impels the patient to seek prompt medical attention, so little education or encouragement is required. Patients with recurrent external otitis can learn to recognize symptoms and treat themselves. Patients who have active external otitis or chronic otitis media with perforation of the eardrum should be instructed to avoid swimming and water entering the ear. Earplugs usually do not suffice to keep out water, but, as already noted, a cotton ball coated with petrolatum ointment provides a simple yet effective water barrier.

Patients with otitis media who must use air travel and cannot delay a trip should use oral or intranasal decongestants (see Chapter 222), especially in anticipation of descent when the risk of barotrauma is greatest. Self-inflation of the eustachian tubes can provide symptomatic relief in serous otitis. The patient is instructed to pinch the nose shut, take a deep breath, close the mouth, and try to blow the nose while keeping it pinched shut.

ANNOTATED BIBLIOGRAPHY

Cantekin EI, et al. Lack of efficacy of a decongestant–antihistamine combination for otitis media with effusion ("secretory" otitis media) in children. N Engl J Med 1983;308:297. *(A double-blind randomized study; use of decongestant–antihistamine therapy is of no benefit.)*

Henderson FW, et al. A longitudinal study of respiratory viruses and bacteria in the etiology of acute otitis media with effusion. N Engl J Med 1982;306:1377. *(Viral upper respiratory tract infections were important precursors.)*

Rubin J, Yu VL. Malignant external otitis: Insights into pathogenesis, clinical manifestations, diagnosis, and therapy. Am J Med 1988;85:391. *(Good review of this uncommon, but important complication.)*

Schwartz RH, et al. Trimethoprim-sulfamethoxazole in the treatment of otitis media caused by ampicillin-resistant strains of *H. influenzae*. Rev Infect Dis 1982;4:514. *(The drug proved beneficial in almost all patients who failed to respond to ampicillin.)*

219
Approach to the Patient With Sinusitis

HARVEY B. SIMON, M.D.

Primary Care Medicine: Office Evaluation and Management of the Adult Patient, 3rd edition, edited by Allan H. Goroll, Lawrence A. May, and Albert G. Mulley, Jr. J.B. Lippincott Company, Philadelphia

Although infections of the paranasal sinuses are frequent—viral sinusitis is recognized as a regular, self-limited component of the common cold—they tend to be overdiagnosed by physicians and patients alike. Often, a frontal headache or congested sensation is attributed to "sinus trouble," self-medicated with over-the-counter decongestants, and followed by a request for antibiotics if the complaint fails to clear. Individuals with allergic or vasomotor rhinitis may present seeking treatment for their "sinus condition." The primary physician should be able to distinguish true sinusitis from other causes of nasal congestion, treat uncomplicated cases, and recognize complications.

PATHOPHYSIOLOGY AND CLINICAL PRESENTATION

Viral Rhinosinusitis. The *common cold* frequently involves the paranasal sinuses. Computed tomographic study of patients with the common cold reveals that over 85 percent have a self-limited paranasal sinusitis that resolves without treatment. The maxillary sinuses are the most common site (87%), followed by ethmoidal (65%), sphenoidal (39%), and frontal (32%) involvement. Rhinorrhea and nasal stuffiness are the typical symptoms.

Acute purulent bacterial sinusitis remains a relatively infrequent sequela of the common cold, occurring in 0.5 percent to 5.0 percent. It is characterized by nasal congestion, purulent nasal discharge, facial pain (that typically increases when the patient stoops forward), and, often, fever and other constitutional symptoms. Besides the common cold, allergic and vasomotor forms of rhinitis are frequent antecedents. Nasal polyps or deviation of the nasal septum may predispose to purulent sinusitis by obstructing sinus drainage. Other potential contributing factors include rapid changes in altitude, trauma, intranasal foreign bodies or tumors, and, occasionally a systemic process such as cystic fibrosis or Kartagener's syndrome (situs inversus, bronchiectasis, and sinusitis).

The sinuses may be involved singly or, more often, in combination. Maxillary and frontal sinusitis are common in adults; ethmoiditis is more common in children.

Bacteriology. The most common pathogens in acute sinusitis are pneumococci, streptococci, *Haemophilus influenzae,* and *Moraxella (Branhamella) catarrhalis.* Although some studies report the isolation of *Staphylococcus aureus* from significant numbers of patients with acute sinusitis, these studies have been based on nasal cultures and probably reflect nasal contamination rather than a true etiology.

Clinical Presentation. The signs and symptoms of acute purulent sinusitis depend on which sinuses are involved. *Frontal sinusitis* produces pain and tenderness over the lower forehead and purulent drainage from the middle meatus of the nasal turbinates. *Maxillary sinusitis* produces pain and tenderness over the cheeks. The pain is often referred to the teeth, and the hard palate may be edematous in severe cases. Purulent drainage is present in the middle meatus. Patients with *ethmoid sinusitis* complain of retro-orbital pain and may have tenderness and even erythema over the upper lateral aspect of the nose. Drainage from the anterior ethmoid cells occurs through the middle meatus, whereas drainage from the posterior cells is through the superior meatus. Isolated *sphenoid sinusitis* is uncommon but can present as retro-orbital, frontal, or facial pain, with purulent drainage from the superior meatus.

Chronic Sinusitis. Symptoms of chronic sinusitis include nasal congestion and discharge, but pain and headache are usually mild or absent, and fever is uncommon. *Staphylococcus aureus* is found in about a fifth of cases. Other aerobes include *H. influenzae, Pneumococcus,* and other streptococci. Heavy growths of *anaerobic organisms* can be isolated in about a quarter of patients, predominated by anaerobic *streptococci* and *Bacteroides* species. The pathologic importance of anaerobes in chronic sinusitis is reflected by the predominance of anaerobes in brain abscesses of sinus origin. Viruses may be etiologically responsible in some patients. Rarely, fungi such as *mucor, Rhizopus,* and *Aspergillus* species can produce invasive sinusitis in poorly controlled diabetics or leukemics. Gram-negative bacilli may cause sinusitis in hospitalized patients who are nasotracheally intubated or immunocompromised.

Complications of sinusitis have become uncommon in the antibiotic era but can be life-threatening. Frontal sinusitis can lead to *osteomyelitis* of the frontal bones, especially in children. Patients present with headache, fever, and a characteristic doughy edema over the involved bone, which is termed "Pott's puffy tumor." The organisms involved are the same as those responsible for the underlying sinusitis except that *S. aureus* is more common. Osteomyelitis of the maxilla is an infrequent complication of maxillary sinusitis.

Because the orbit is surrounded on three sides by paranasal sinuses, *orbital infection* can result from sinusitis. This is most frequently a complication of ethmoid sinusitis due to direct extension of infection through the lamina papyracea. Orbital *cellulitis* usually begins with edema of the eyelids and rapidly progresses to ptosis, proptosis, chemosis, and diminished extraocular movements. Patients are usually febrile and acutely ill. Pressure on the optic nerve can lead to visual loss, which can be permanent, and retrograde spread of infection can lead to intracranial infection.

Retrograde extension of infection along venous channels from the orbit, ethmoid or frontal sinuses, or nose can produce septic *cavernous sinus thrombophlebitis.* These patients are highly febrile and appear "toxic." Lid edema, proptosis, and chemosis are present, but, unlike uncomplicated orbital cellulitis, 3rd, 4th, and 6th cranial nerve palsies are prominent, the pupil may be fixed and dilated, and funduscopic examination may reveal venous engorgement and papilledema. Although the process is usually unilateral at first, spread across the anterior and posterior intercavernous sinuses results in bilateral involvement. Patients may exhibit alterations of consciousness.

Finally, sinusitis can lead to *intracranial suppuration* either by direct spread through bone or via venous channels. A great variety of syndromes can result, including epidural abscess, subdural empyema, meningitis, and brain abscess. Clinical findings vary greatly, ranging from subtle personality changes with frontal lobe abscesses to headache, symptoms of elevated intracranial pressure, alterations of consciousness, visual symptoms, focal neurologic deficits, seizures, and, ultimately, coma and death.

DIFFERENTIAL DIAGNOSIS

The common cold and allergic or vasomotor rhinitis are by far the most common causes of "sinus" symptoms, but polyps, tumors, cysts, foreign bodies, and vasculitides such as Wegener's granulomatosis occasionally produce symptoms resembling sinusitis (see Chapter 222).

WORKUP

Clinical findings can be very helpful in diagnosis of sinusitis, especially when findings are considered in combination. In a prospective study comparing historical and physical findings with sinus films, no single feature had a likelihood ratio of more than 2.9 in predicting a positive x-ray, but when five individually predictive findings (see below) were considered together, the likelihood ratio rose to 6.4 if all were present, and fell to 0.1 if none was found.

History is checked for reports of purulent nasal discharge, maxillary tooth pain, frontal, maxillary, retro-orbital, or vertex pain that worsens on bending forward, and response to decongestants. Risk factors such as nasal polyps, deviated nasal septum, trauma, foreign bodies and rapid changes in altitude are inquired about. Special attention is paid to toxic symptoms of high fever and rigors in association with complaints suggestive of extension of infection, such as edema of the eyelids and diplopia.

Prospective study in the primary care setting comparing clinical findings and radiographs in adult males presenting with symptoms suggestive of sinusitis revealed that maxillary toothache, poor response to decongestants, and purulent nasal discharge were independent predictors of radiologically confirmed sinusitis (positive likelihood ratios 2.7, 2.1, and 1.5, respectively). In a study from ENT practice, unilateral sinus pain also correlated with outcome.

Physical Examination. One should examine the nasal cavity for purulent discharge draining from one of the turbinates, transilluminate the maxillary sinuses for impaired light transmission, and palpate the frontal and maxillary sinuses for tenderness. Tapping the maxillary teeth may reveal a dental source of maxillary sinus infection. In the prospective study alluded to above, the best independent physical examination predictors of sinusitis were impaired transillumination (positive likelihood ratio 2.7) and mucopurulence found on physical examination (likelihood ratio 2.9), followed by tenderness to palpation (likelihood ratio 1.4). The absence of sinus tenderness did not rule out the diagnosis.

Laboratory Studies. As noted above, when predictive historical and physical findings are present, one can make a clinical diagnosis of sinusitis with confidence. When they are absent, the diagnosis is ruled out. Further testing is indicated when the probability is intermediate.

Sinus Films. Confirmation of sinusitis can be achieved by finding mucosal thickening, sinus opacification, or air–fluid levels on conventional sinus x-rays. For those with air–fluid levels or complete opacification, the positive predictive value is 80 percent to 100 percent; however, such findings are present only in 60 percent, reducing their sensitivity. Mucosal thickening has a sensitivity of 90 percent, but specificity is poor. Normal sinus x-rays in a person presenting with suspected sinusitis rules out maxillary and frontal disease (negative predictive value 90% to 100%); ethmoidal involvement is harder to exclude. Bone erosion can be present in chronic sinusitis.

Computed Tomography (CT) and Magnetic Resonance Imaging (MRI). Sensitivity of CT is extremely high, so high that specificity is compromised (almost half of asymptomatic persons undergoing head CT for nonsinus reasons show mucosal abnormalities). CT is best reserved for complicated disease and search for occult ethmoidal disease in patients with refractory symptoms and negative conventional x-ray studies. MRI has proven most useful for differentiating mucosal inflammation from tumor. Neither study is appropriate for patients with routine sinus infection.

Ultrasound has been used in the diagnosis of sinusitis. Sensitivity is lower than for sinus x-rays, but specificity is higher. Expertise is not widely available.

Nasal Cultures. Nasal cultures correlate poorly with actual sinus fluid and cannot be relied on. False-positive isolates of staphylococcal species are common.

PRINCIPLES OF MANAGEMENT AND THERAPEUTIC RECOMMENDATIONS

Acute Purulent Sinusitis. Treatment consists of decongestants to reduce the underlying ostial obstruction and antibiotics.

Decongestants are of paramount importance. Both topical and systemic preparations are used. The mixed adrenergic agonist *pseudoephedrine* is reasonably effective and can be administered by mouth and by nasal spray. Tachyphylaxis develops with prolonged topical use, but risk is minimal with short-term administration (1 to 3 days). The same is true for the popular sympathomimetic nasal spray *oxymetazoline* (Afrin), which is the longest acting of the topical decongestants. Patients should be instructed to spray each nostril once, and then wait a minute to allow the anterior nasal mucosa to shrink. A repeat spray will then reach the upper and posterior mucosa including the nasal turbinates and sinus ostea. This procedure can be repeated as needed every 4 hours with pseudoephedrine and every 12 hours with oxymetazoline for up to 3 days. Use for more than 3 days risks direct irritation and tachyphylaxis.

When there is an underlying allergic component to the nasal obstruction, an *antihistamine* (see Chapter 222) may facilitate decongestion. However, they are not for routine use, because in the absence of an allergic process, they may thicken secretions and worsen sinus outflow obstruction. Steroids are of little benefit and may impede the response to infection. Local application of heat may be soothing. Inhalation of steam is extremely useful.

Antibiotics. Patients with mild acute sinusitis may respond sufficiently well to decongestants as to not require antibiotics, but in more severe cases of acute purulent sinusitis, antibiotics are commonly used. In the few randomized controlled studies that exist, antibiotics do demonstrate some benefit over decongestants alone, but cure rates without antibiotics remain high (approaching 50%). Nevertheless, many physicians administer antibiotics routinely to patients with sinusitis, often in response to patient demands. Antibiotics should be used in conjunction with decongestants in "toxic" patients, in those who fail decongestants, and in those with complications.

Given the spectrum of bacterial pathogens responsible for acute purulent sinusitis, *amoxicillin* and *trimethoprim-sulfamethoxazole* (TMS) emerge as the best options for initial treatment, with TMS being the lowest in cost. Concern about rising prevalences of beta-lactamase-producing strains of *H. influenzae* and *Moraxella* has stimulated the prescribing of very expensive, broad-spectrum, penicillinase-resistant antibiotics (eg, *amoxicillin-clavulanate, cefaclor, loracarbef, azithromycin, clarithromycin*). However, randomized controlled trials have failed to demonstrate any advantage for such antibiotics over amoxicillin, suggesting that beta-lactamase-producing strains may not be as clinically significant as feared. This finding has major cost implications, because the alternatives to amoxicillin and TMS are many times more expensive.

Knowledge of the prevalence of beta-lactamase-producing strains in one's community can help guide initial antibiotic selection. In the absence of such data, a reasonable approach is to begin with amoxicillin or TMS and switch to another antibiotic only if the patient fails to respond adequately.

Although the proper duration of therapy has not been identified, it is typical to treat with antibiotics and decongestants for 7 to 10 days. Partial responses and early relapses can be treated with another week of the same program. Patients who remain unchanged after 2 full weeks of therapy should have sinus films obtained and a penicillinase-resistant drug (see above) should be prescribed. Further failure to respond is an indication for ENT referral.

Surgery. Surgical intervention should be avoided in acute sinusitis unless patients fail to respond to medical therapy and complications are present.

Recurrent and Chronic Sinusitis. Recurrent sinusitis is usually due to underlying allergic disease or an anatomic lesion and requires treatment directed at the precipitating pathophysiology (see Chapter 222). Chronic sinusitis (persisting for more than 3 months) has a different bacteriology (see above) necessitating consideration of broader-spectrum antibiotic coverage (eg, *amoxicillin-clavulanate* or *cefaclor*). Treatment may need to be prolonged for several weeks. Attention also needs to be directed at underlying precipitants. Sinus irrigation or surgical drainage may be necessary.

INDICATIONS FOR ADMISSION AND REFERRAL

Any patient who appears toxic or has clinical evidence suggestive of extension to the orbit, bone, brain, or cavernous sinus requires urgent admission for emergency assessment and high-dose intravenous antibiotics. Warning symptoms include high fever, rigors, lid edema, diplopia, pupillary abnormalities, ptosis, and palsies of extraocular movements. The patient should be seen by both an otolaryngologist and infectious disease consultant. Antibiotic coverage is directed against both staphylococci and gram-negative rods. Surgical drainage may be urgently needed.

PATIENT EDUCATION

Patients should understand that nasal congestion and frontal headaches are much more commonly caused by viral upper respiratory infections and allergic or vasomotor rhinitis than by true sinusitis. Nevertheless, decongestants are indicated in all of these conditions to promote sinus drainage and prevent purulent sinusitis. The patient with recurrent symptoms should learn to recognize them and begin decongestant therapy, but the decision to begin antibiotics should be reserved by the physician.

ANNOTATED BIBLIOGRAPHY

Gwaltney JM Jr, Phillips CD, Millers RD, et al. Computed tomographic study of the common cold. N Engl J Med 1994;330:25. *(Transient occlusion of the paranasal sinuses occurs in most patients with a common cold and clears without antibiotics.)*

Gwaltney JM Jr, Scheld WM, Sande MA, et al. The microbial etiology and antimicrobial therapy of adults with acute community-acquired sinusitis. J Allergy Clin Immunol 1992;90:457. *(Data on the bacteriology of community-acquired disease, including amoxicillin-resistant* H. influenzae.*)*

Lew D, Southwick FS, Montgomery WW, et al. Sphenoid sinusitis: A review of 30 cases. N Engl J Med 1983;309:1149. *(A detailed study of the varied presentations of this uncommon but potentially serious type of sinusitis.)*

Wald ER, Chiponis D, Ledesma-Medina J. Comparative effectiveness of amoxicillin and amoxicillin-clavulanate potassium in acute paranasal sinus infections in children: A double-blind placebo-controlled trial. Pediatrics 1986;77:795. *(The antibiotics were equally effective and superior to placebo.)*

Wald ER, Guerra N, Byers C. Upper respiratory tract infections in young children: Duration and frequency of complications. Pediatrics 1991;87;129. *(Acute bacterial sinusitis developed in 5 percent after a common cold.)*

Williams JW Jr, Simel DL. Does this patient have sinusitis? Diagnosing acute sinusitis by history and physical examination. JAMA 1993;270:1242. *(A critical review of the clinical features used to make the diagnosis.)*

Williams JW Jr, Simel DL, Roberts L, et al. Clinical evaluation for sinusitis: Making the diagnosis by history and physical examination. Ann Intern Med 1992;117:705. *(A study of adult men; 5 findings of predictive value.)*

Primary Care Medicine: Office Evaluation and Management of the Adult Patient, 3rd edition, edited by Allan H. Goroll, Lawrence A. May, and Albert G. Mulley, Jr. J.B. Lippincott Company, Philadelphia

220
Approach to the Patient With Pharyngitis

HARVEY B. SIMON, M.D.

A wide variety of organisms may be responsible for pharyngitis, ranging from viruses and streptococci to gonococci and candida. The most common concern is infection due to group A beta-hemolytic strep, *Streptococcus pyogenes,* because of the associated yet totally preventable risk of rheumatic fever (see Chapter 17). Because there is no single clinical feature pathognomonic for beta-hemolytic strep infection, diagnosis requires attention to a host of clinical parameters complimented by timely, judicious testing. The objectives are to promptly identify and treat patients with *S. pyogenes* infection and to avoid delay of therapy, inconvenience, expense, and unnecessary antibiotic exposure. Effective management of sore throat also requires an awareness of the full spectrum of etiologies and possible complications.

PATHOPHYSIOLOGY AND CLINICAL PRESENTATION

Respiratory viruses, chlamydia, mycoplasma, and streptococci account for the majority of sore throats in adults. A host of other bacteria, viruses, fungi, and spirochetes have also been identified as etiologic agents. Trauma, inhalation of irritant gases, and dehydration are among the noninfectious causes.

Group A Beta-Hemolytic Strep Infection. *S. pyogenes* infection accounts for 5 percent to 38 percent of sore throats in adults who are subjected to throat culture. The onset of discomfort is typically acute, with difficulty swallowing often noted. Pharyngeal erythema, exudate, cervical adenopathy, and fever greater than 101°F (38.3°C) are common but by no means pathognomonic. Children with "strep throat" exhibit exudate and high fever with greater frequency than do adults with the same disease. Cough, rhinorrhea, and other symptoms of upper respiratory infection are reported in less than 25 percent and suggest the presence of another etiology. About one quarter of adult patients give a history of recent exposure to streptococcal infection. The pharyngitis is self-limited; symptoms usually resolve within 7 to 10 days. Antibiotic therapy decreases severity and duration of symptoms.

Complications. Suppurative complications of streptococcal pharyngitis are uncommon in the setting of antibiotic use, but they are important and require attention. In *peritonsillar cellulitis,* the tonsils become edematous and inflamed. One or both tonsils may be involved. A grayish-white exudate forms in conjunction with high fever, rigors, and leukocytosis. *Peritonsillar abscess* may ensue, with a fluctuant mass palpable. Other suppurative complications include retropharyngeal and parapharyngeal space infections. *Scarlet fever* is a rare complication of strep infection in adults. It results from infection with a toxigenic strain of *S. pyogenes.*

Acute rheumatic fever is the most important nonsuppurative complication. Its incidence has declined dramatically over the past 30 years. The complication appears most frequently among children aged 5 to 15, but about 15 percent of hospitalized patients with rheumatic fever are over the age of 18. The chances of developing rheumatic fever increase with length of time that the organism persists in the pharynx and with the intensity of the immunologic response.

Acute glomerulonephritis is another nonsuppurative complication. Unlike rheumatic fever, it does not seem to be preventable by means of antibiotic therapy.

Other Streptococci. Groups C and G streptococci can cause pharyngitis, in some populations with a frequency approaching that of group A strep. Suppurative complications are rare, and rheumatic fever and glomerulonephritis never follow.

Viruses. Respiratory viruses are the most common causes of sore throat. Pharyngitis can be the only manifestation of illness or may be accompanied by conjunctivitis, cough, sputum production, rhinitis, and systemic symptoms. Pharyngeal erythema, exudates, tonsillar enlargement, and cervical adenopathy are often present, but with less frequency than in streptococcal disease.

Epstein-Barr virus (EBV) is the agent responsible for *infectious mononucleosis* and sometimes a cause of sore throat. Prodromal symptoms include malaise, headache, and fatigue followed by fever, sore throat, and cervical lymphadenopathy. Sore throat is the most common feature. The pharynx shows lymphoid hyperplasia, erythema, and edema. About half of patients develop tonsillar exudates. Petechiae at the junction of the hard and soft palate occur in about a third of patients and are highly suggestive of the diagnosis. Both anterior and posterior cervical adenopathy may develop; generalized adenopathy often follows. Splenomegaly is noted in about half of cases, and hepatomegaly and tenderness are present in about 10 percent. Clinical hepatitis sometimes ensues. A faint, maculopapular rash and transient supraorbital edema occasionally appear. IgM antibody is the first to appear, followed by IgG antibody. Despite a transient flurry of interest about the possibility of EBV infection causing chronic fatigue syndrome, confirmatory evidence failed to materialize (see Chapter 8).

Herpes simplex and *Coxsackie A* virus are other causes of pharyngitis. Herpes infection is typically in the form of a stomatitis that involves the buccal mucosa and tongue as well as the pharynx; vesicles and small ulcers develop. Coxsackie A infection is characterized by vesicles and ulcers on the tonsillar pillars and soft palate.

Other Organisms. In patients engaging in orogenital sexual activity, *gonococci* can lead to sore throat, pharyngeal exudate, and lymphadenopathy, or just asymptomatic colonization of the pharynx. In rare instances, bacteremia may result (see Chapter 137). *Haemophilus influenzae* is a rare cause of pharyngitis in adults, but the infection can be extremely painful and complicated by epiglottitis with life-threatening airway obstruction.

Chlamydia pneumoniae and *Mycoplasma pneumoniae* may account for a surprising percentage of patients presenting with pharyngitis, based on serologic evidence of infection, although the clinical significance of this finding remains unclear. The diagnosis of *M. pneumoniae* is rarely made clinically in the absence of pneumonitis.

Corynebacterium hemolyticum can cause pharyngitis and scarletiniform rash, particularly in teenagers and young adults. Administration of penicillin or erythromycin produces rapid improvement.

Meningococci are found in the pharynx in 5 percent to 15 percent of healthy people. Although sore throat may be a prodromal symptom of meningococcemia, isolated pharyngitis due to meningococcal infection is rare. Most instances of meningococcal recovery from the pharynx represent asymptomatic colonization.

Corynebacterium diphtheriae causes outbreaks of diphtheria in unimmunized populations. The infection is characterized by development of an adherent whitish-blue pharyngeal exudate ("pseudomembrane") that covers the pharynx and causes bleeding if removal is attempted.

Pneumococci and Staphylococci. Although these bacterial species can be cultured from the pharynx in both symptomatic and asymptomatic individuals, they do not cause pharyngitis except under most unusual circumstances. In particular, it should be emphasized that although pneumococci and staphylococci commonly reside in the nasopharynx and can cause severe disease in other parts of the respiratory tract, they do not cause pharyngitis. However, mixed infections with normal mouth flora do occur in debilitated patients.

Fusobacteria and *spirochetes* can cause gingivitis ("trenchmouth") or necrotic tonsillar ulcers ("Vincent's angina"). Patients present with foul breath, pain, pharyngeal exudate, and a dirty gray membranous inflammation, which bleeds easily. A similar combination of bacteria and spirochetes can produce an extremely serious invasive gangrene of the mouth known as cancrum oris. This process occurs only in malnourished infants or patients with advanced malignancy and immunosuppression and is, fortunately, rare. *Treponema pallidum* can cause pharyngitis as part of primary or secondary syphilis. The diagnosis requires a high index of suspicion and serologic confirmation.

Yersinia enterocolitica infection typically presents as enterocolitis, but occasionally in adults it presents as pharyngitis in the absence of enteritis. Fatalities have been reported.

Candida albicans, present in the normal mouth flora, can produce pharyngitis if antibiotics, immunosuppressive agents, or debilitating illness upsets microbial interactions or host defenses. Oropharyngeal moniliasis (thrush) can be painful and is characterized by a cheesy, white exudate, which can be scraped off to demonstrate yeast forms by smear and culture. Oral moniliasis may be the first symptomatic manifestation of human immunodeficiency virus (HIV) infection (see Chapter 13).

M. tuberculosis is a rare cause of pharyngitis.

WORKUP

The first task is to attempt a clinical estimate of the risk of *S. pyogenes* infection. Often, this is done in a preliminary way over the telephone, which places a premium on risk stratification by historical features.

History. No single symptom or historical feature is diagnostic of group A beta-hemolytic strep infection. Consequently, investigators have sought to identify symptoms that are at least independent predictors of strep infection and to see how clusters of such symptoms perform for triaging.

One such triaging cluster uses presence of *fever* and *difficulty swallowing* in support of the diagnosis of strep infection and cough as a negating factor. A score is assigned to each factor based on severity (0 through 3). The final score is derived by subtracting the score for cough from those for fever and difficulty swallowing. Designating a score of 2 or more as "positive" for a diagnosis of *S. pyogenes* infection, the system has a sensitivity of 85 percent and a specificity of 41.5 percent. In a pharyngitis population with the usual prevalence of strep (10% of sore throats due to *S. pyogenes*), a score of 6 (the highest possible score) would produce a positive predictive value of 34 percent for strep infection; a score of minus 3 (the lowest possible score) would reduce the risk to 1 percent. In a pharyngitis population with a high strep prevalence (prevalence = 34%), a score of 6 would indicate a 70 percent chance of strep infection; a score of minus 3 would reduce the risk to 3 percent. Although far from perfect, such a scheme may help in deciding who should come in for further evaluation.

History can help determine prevalence and risk from strep infection by inquiring into *exposure* to family members with current documented strep pharyngitis and any history of prior *rheumatic fever.* Other factors found predictive of strep infection that might be elicited over the telephone include *positive throat culture* in the preceding year, tender anterior cervical *adenopathy, temperature* > 101°F, and absence of rhinorrhea and itchy eyes.

Regarding other sore-throat etiologies and complications, one should ask about orogenital sexual contact, concurrent steroid or immunosuppressive therapy, and any dyspnea.

Physical Examination. Several physical findings when considered collectively can help assess probability of group A beta-hemolytic streptococcal infection. The cluster of marked *tonsillar exudate,* anterior *cervical adenopathy,* and temperature greater than *101°F* provides a positive predictive value of about 30 percent in pharyngitis populations with 10 percent prevalence of strep infection. The absence of these features reduces probability to 3 percent.

Examination of the pharynx is useful for identifying a less common cause of pharyngitis such as thrush, characterized by its white cheesy exudate; gingivitis or necrotic tonsillar ulcers suggest fusobacteria and spirochetes. Associated physical findings, such as a viral exanthem, conjunctivitis, petechiae, generalized lymphadenopathy, splenomegaly, or hepatic tenderness, may provide important clues to etiology. Patients with severe dysphagia or dyspnea require urgent evaluation to exclude airway obstruction. If epiglottitis is suspected, the airway should not be instrumented.

Laboratory Study for Suspected Strep Pharyngitis. Prompt diagnosis and treatment of *S. pyogenes* infection has been greatly facilitated by the advent of rapid strep-antigen testing. Throat culture has been relegated to a secondary role.

Rapid Strep-Antigen Testing. Office identification of group A streptococcal pharyngitis can be achieved by taking a swab of the posterior pharynx and subjecting the specimen to rapid strep-antigen testing. For most commercially available preparations, sensitivity averages 85 percent to 90 percent, and specificity 98 percent to 99 percent. Small numbers of organisms are less likely to be detected. Proper technique includes swabbing the tonsils and posterior pharynx.

Decision analysis study finds that rapid strep-antigen testing followed by treatment of positives is the optimal approach to workup when the patient's pretest probability for strep infection is between 1 percent and 50 percent (which is the case for most patients). Pharyngitis patients at high risk for rheumatic fever (ie, those with a history of rheumatic fever) and those with a very high probability of strep infection (eg, persons in a closed population experiencing an epidemic of streptococcal pharyngitis) can forgo testing and be treated directly.

Throat Culture. Culturing a retropharyngeal swab remains the standard for identification of streptococcal pharyngitis and is useful when rapid antigen testing is negative yet clinical suspicion remains high. Patients with typical symptoms and signs of a viral upper respiratory infection and no historical or physical examination evidence suggestive of streptococcal infection do not need a throat culture.

In addition to the time required to obtain a result, an important shortcoming of throat culture is difficulty differentiating infection from colonization. As many as 20 percent to

30 percent of patients may be carriers. Definitive identification of significant infection with risk of rheumatic fever necessitates *serologic testing* for an antibody response. Such testing is of little practical use because results do not become available in time to be of help.

Laboratory Study for Other Etiologies. Laboratory testing is indicated when the result will have an impact on management. For example, viral pharyngitis due to respiratory pathogens is essentially a clinical diagnosis and requires no laboratory investigation. On the other hand, the patient with sore throat and diffuse lymphadenopathy, splenomegaly, and pharyngeal petechiae deserves evaluation for infectious mononucleosis. A *heterophile* is a useful confirmatory test, provided there is no prior history of infectious mononucleosis. It may take as long as 3 weeks for the heterophile to become positive, necessitating a repeat test in a few weeks if it is initially negative. Alternatively, one can check serology for antibodies to Epstein-Barr virus. IgM antibodies can be demonstrated during the second week of illness, replaced later by IgG antibodies. Heterophile-negative mononucleosis may be due to CMV infection.

The patient with a history of orogenital contact who is suspected of having possible gonococcal infection should have a throat swab plated onto *Thayer-Martin* media (see Chapter 137). Suspected candidal infection can be confirmed by scraping off the exudate and examining a *wet prep* for yeast forms.

PRINCIPLES OF MANAGEMENT AND THERAPEUTIC RECOMMENDATIONS

Suspected *S. pyogenes* Infection

The reasons for treating strep infection are to speed symptomatic relief and prevent rheumatic fever, peritonsillar or retropharyngeal abscess, and spread of streptococcal infection.

Rheumatic fever can be prevented by prompt eradication of *S. pyogenes* from the throat. The attack rate for rheumatic fever is reduced by over 90 percent if antibiotic therapy is instituted within a week of the onset of sore throat. However, the efficacy of prophylactic therapy is substantially reduced if there is a marked delay in initiating treatment. Starting antibiotics 2 weeks after sore throat is first noted is associated with a reduction in attack rate of only 67 percent, and delaying treatment until 3 weeks into the illness provides no more than a 40 percent reduction in attack rate.

Treatment Strategies. There are several approaches to treatment of pharyngitis that can be employed. The choice depends on the probability of strep infection, the likelihood of patient compliance, the chance of an adverse reaction to antibiotics, and the benefits of treating immediately versus waiting for culture results.

Immediate Treatment without Prior Testing. Pharyngitis patients with a *history of rheumatic fever* and those who are symptomatic and have a *household member* with a documented group A beta-streptococcal infection should receive immediate treatment without need for prior testing or even an office visit. High-risk patients who have a prior history of rheumatic fever might already be on prophylactic therapy (see Chapter 17). Patients with a strongly suggestive clinical presentation (eg, exudative pharyngitis, temperature > 101°F, tender bilateral anterior cervical adenopathy, and no rhinorrhea or cough) might also be candidates for empiric antibiotic therapy.

Antigen Testing Followed by Treatment of Positives. In the majority of pharyngitis patients with an intermediate probability of strep infection, the preferred approach, as noted above, is rapid strep-antigen testing followed by treatment of positives. Throat culturing followed by treatment of a positive result is reserved for the patient with a good clinical story but a negative rapid antigen test.

Antibiotic Program. To be effective, antibiotic therapy must completely eradicate the streptococcus from the pharynx. This can be achieved by a single intramuscular injection of 1.2 million units of *benzathine penicillin* or a 10-day course of oral *phenoxymethyl penicillin* (250 mg qid). The advantages of the intramuscular route are the certainty of full treatment and convenience. Its major disadvantage is a five- to tenfold increase in the incidence of serious allergic reactions to penicillin. In the patient allergic to penicillin, oral *erythromycin* (250 mg qid for 10 days) is an effective alternate.

Recurrent Infection. Patients with recurrent symptomatic strep infections and intact tonsils can be treated either with additional courses of antibiotics or be considered for tonsillectomy. Although the latter is associated with fewer recurrences, the overall impact on functional status and days lost from work is usually minimal. Consultation with an ENT specialist is indicated.

Other Types of Pharyngitis

The *meningococcal carrier state* sometimes presents a therapeutic dilemma, in terms of both selecting patients who actually need treatment and choosing antibiotics. Carriers should be treated only when there is evidence of active meningococcal disease in household or dormitory contacts. Penicillin will not eradicate the meningococcal carrier state, and because many strains are now sulfonamide-resistant, rifampin should be used.

In *gonococcal pharyngitis,* the usual ceftriaxone, amoxicillin, penicillin, and tetracycline regimens are effective (see Chapter 137), but spectinomycin is not. In the case of *diphtheria, antitoxin* is necessary to prevent myocarditis and peripheral neuritis and is the mainstay of therapy. Both erythromycin and penicillin can eliminate the organism from the upper respiratory tract. In *epiglottitis,* hospitalization is needed. *Necrotizing pharyngitis* due to fusobacterial infection responds to *penicillin* and good nutrition.

Pharyngeal candidiasis in the immunocompromised patient may benefit from gargling with oral *nystatin* suspension (100,000 U/mL), 15 mL swish-and-swallow six times per day or from using a 10-mg *clotrimazole troche* held in the mouth for 15 to 30 minutes three times each day.

Viral sore throats are treated symptomatically. Voice rest, humidification, and lozenges or hard candy provide some relief; saline gargling and aspirin or acetaminophen also help.

PATIENT EDUCATION

Many pharyngitis patients telephone in requesting empiric antibiotic therapy for sore throat. They assume antibiotics are effective against most pathogens, desire prompt symptomatic relief, want to avoid the time and expense of testing, and have little fear of an adverse reaction to antibiotics. Much of the unnecessary antibiotic exposure associated with management of pharyngitis is probably due as much to patient insistence as to the physician's desire to do something. When the probability of strep infection is deemed too low to warrant testing or treatment (see above), patients ought to be reassured that the risk is nil and that antibiotics are unlikely to provide any benefit. For the insistent person and the one with an intermediate risk by triage history, an invitation to come in for rapid antigen testing is the most reasonable advice.

The patient who proves to have *S. pyogenes* infection and elects oral antibiotic therapy should be carefully instructed on the risk of rheumatic fever and the importance of completing a full 10-day course of antibiotics. Otherwise, many patients will stop taking the medication when symptoms resolve.

Patients with recurrent strep infections and intact tonsils will ask about tonsillectomy. Reviewing the risks and benefits of tonsillectomy over medical therapy may help them to choose the treatment that best meets their needs.

ANNOTATED BIBLIOGRAPHY

Clancy CM, Centor RM, Campbell MS, et al. Rational decision making based on history: Adult sore throats. J Gen Intern Med 1988;3:213. *(Uses fever, difficulty swallowing, and cough to generate a score that predicts the probability of a positive rapid strep-antigen test.)*

Hillner BE, Centor RM. What a difference a day makes: A decision analysis of adult streptococcal pharyngitis. J Gen Intern Med 1987;2:242. *(Recommends rapid strep-antigen testing for most adults with suspected strep pharyngitis.)*

Huovinen P, Lahtonen R, Ziegler T, et al. Pharyngitis in adults: The presence and coexistence of viruses and bacterial organisms. Ann Intern Med 1989;110;612. *(A wide variety of organisms found, including group C strep,* M. pneumoniae, *and* C. pneumoniae.*)*

Komaroff AL, Pass TM, Aronson MD, et al. The prediction of streptococcal pharyngitis in adults. J Gen Intern Med 1986;1:1. *(A clinical decision rule to identify* S. pyogenes *infection.)*

Krober MS, Bass JW, Michels GN. Streptococcal pharyngitis: Clinical response to penicillin therapy. JAMA 1985;253:1271. *(Early penicillin therapy significantly ameliorates symptoms and shortens their duration.)*

Meier FA, Howland J, Johnson J, et al. Effects of a rapid antigen test for group A streptococcal pharyngitis on physician prescribing and antibiotic costs. Arch Intern Med 1990;150:1696. *(Rapid diagnostic testing proved cost-effective in an urban community health-center setting.)*

Ophir D, Bawnik J, Poria Y, et al. Peritonsillar abscess: A prospective evaluation of outpatient management by needle aspiration. Arch Otolaryngol Head Neck Surg 1988;114:661. *(Needle aspiration can allow outpatient management of selected patients.)*

Paradise JL, et al. Efficacy of tonsillectomy in recurrent throat infection in severely affected children. N Engl J Med 1984;310:674. *(Rates of recurrent infection decreased in both medically and surgically treated children, with surgery producing the greater reduction.)*

Putto A. Febrile exudative tonsillitis: Viral or streptococcal? Pediatrics 1987;80:6. *(Only 12 percent caused by group A strep.)*

Shapiro J, Eavey RD, Baker AS. Adult supraglottis: A prospective study. JAMA 1988;259:563. *(A review of this life-threatening but uncommon* H. influenzae *infection.)*

Weisner PJ, Tronen E, Bonin P, et al. Clinical spectrum of pharyngeal gonococcal infection. N Engl J Med 1973;288:181. *(Describes the incidence, clinical features, and management of gonococcal pharyngitis.)*

Primary Care Medicine: Office Evaluation and Management of the Adult Patient, 3rd edition, edited by Allan H. Goroll, Lawrence A. May, and Albert G. Mulley, Jr. J.B. Lippincott Company, Philadelphia

221 Approach to Hiccup

Hiccup is usually a transient, innocuous symptom, but when persistent it may become an exhausting and disabling problem. Intractable hiccup has been attributed to a host of metabolic, peridiaphragmatic, neurologic, and psychogenic conditions, but many cases are of unknown etiology. The primary physician should be able to offer the exasperated patient symptomatic relief while conducting a judicious evaluation to determine the source of difficulty.

PATHOPHYSIOLOGY AND CLINICAL PRESENTATIONS

No useful function has been found for the hiccup, which occurs as a result of synchronous clonic spasm of intercostal muscles and diaphragm that causes sudden inspiration followed by prompt closure of the glottis and inhibition of respiratory activity. It is believed to be a reflex. There is debate about whether it is centrally mediated. The afferent pathway is from T10 to T12, and the efferent limb is along the phrenic nerve. During the hiccup, the glottis is closed. Some investigators believe the hiccup is related more to gastrointestinal than to respiratory function. Current understanding of pathophysiology does not yet permit an explanation of how the presumptive etiologies operate to produce the hiccup, although the classic explanation is that it is due to stimulation of the phrenic nerve.

It is often unclear whether the reported causes of hiccup are etiologies or only associations. In a series of 220 cases seen at the Mayo Clinic, men outnumbered women by 5 to 1, and most were in their 60s. Over 90 percent of the women had no concurrent illness other than an emotional problem, whereas only 7 percent of men were labeled as having a psychogenic disorder. About 20 percent of men who experienced hiccup did so after undergoing intraabdominal, intrathoracic, or neurologic surgery. About 25 percent had a diaphragmatic hernia, another 20 percent had cerebrovascular disease or another central nervous system (CNS) problem, 5 percent had a metabolic illness, and in 10 percent no associated disease or psychiatric problem was identified.

DIFFERENTIAL DIAGNOSIS

The causes of persistent hiccup typically listed are clinical associations and cannot be considered proven etiologies (Table 221-1).

WORKUP

Persistent hiccup that proves refractory to simple measures is an indication for further investigation. Extensive workup is usually not productive, but a check for a previously unsuspected metabolic or subdiaphragmatic process is sometimes rewarding.

Table 221-1. Conditions Associated with Persistent Hiccup*

A. Structural Pathology
   1. Pericarditis
   2. Tumor
   3. Subdiaphragmatic abscess
   4. Pneumonia
   5. Pleuritis
   6. Myocardial infarction
   7. Hiatus hernia
   8. Peritonitis
   9. Gastric dilatation
   10. Pancreatitis
   11. Biliary tract disease
   12. Tympanic membrane irritation
   13. Aortic aneurysm
B. Metabolic Disturbances
   1. Uremia
   2. Diabetes
   3. Alcoholism
C. CNS Disease
   1. Tumor
   2. Infection
   3. Surgery
D. Psychogenic Disease
   1. Hysteria
   2. Anorexia nervosa
   3. Anxiety

*These are not proven etiologies.

History. Questioning should include inquiry into recent abdominal, thoracic, or neurologic surgery, abdominal pain (especially that which radiates to the tip of the shoulder or is worsened by respiration), prior renal disease, excess consumption of alcohol, fever, cough, diabetes, and emotional problems. Also of help is reviewing the various methods that the patient has tried for relief of symptoms. Any neurologic complaints should be noted.

Physical examination should include a temperature determination, a check of the tympanic membranes, percussion of the lungs for evidence of reduced diaphragmatic excursion, and auscultation for signs of an infiltrate, effusion, or pleuritis. The abdomen is examined for distention, organomegaly, upper abdominal tenderness, and signs of peritonitis. A careful neurologic examination is needed if there is a history of neurologic difficulties.

Laboratory Studies. Patients with an acute bout of hiccups need no laboratory studies, but those with *refractory hiccups* that persist for days need to be evaluated for a pharyngeal, thoracic, diaphragmatic, intraabdominal, CNS, or metabolic/pharmacologic etiology. If a careful physical examination that includes a check of the tympanic membranes, pharynx, chest, heart, abdomen, and CNS is unrevealing, one ought to obtain a chest x-ray, serum sodium, creatinine, and BUN determinations, and consider a computed tomography (CT) scan of the abdomen, concentrating on the subdiaphragmatic region. If CNS disease is suspected by history or physical examination, a CT or magnetic resonance imaging (MRI) scan may help detect the lesion. Treatment of the underlying etiology is the best means of curing refractory hiccups.

SYMPTOMATIC THERAPY AND INDICATION FOR REFERRAL

For patients with *self-limited* causes of hiccuping, several home remedies are capable of interrupting the reflex arc; others simply suppress it temporarily. *Breath holding* and breathing into a *paper bag* will decrease the frequency of hiccups, but, if the underlying stimulus has not disappeared, they usually return after these maneuvers are terminated. Swallowing a teaspoonful of *granulated sugar* works by irritating the pharynx sufficiently to inhibit further hiccuping. A more noxious maneuver is to have the patient put his or her finger into the back of the pharynx and *stimulate the gag reflex*. Drinking from the wrong side of the glass is another gag reflex stimulant. Rubbing the nasopharynx with a cotton swab is sometimes effective. Passage of a *nasogastric tube* causing hypopharyngeal stimulation will usually work if other methods have failed.

When symptoms are *persistent* and the cause remains undiagnosed or untreatable, symptomatic relief becomes an important goal. *Chlorpromazine* in doses of 25 to 50 mg intravenously will often terminate refractory hiccups and can be followed by oral maintenance therapy of 25 mg qid. *Metoclopramide* given intravenously, followed by oral therapy (10 mg tid), has also proven effective. Atropine and quinidine have been used, but with less success. *Phenytoin* and *carbamazepine* are helpful in patients with a CNS etiology.

When all other measures have failed and the hiccups remain disabling, consideration of surgical *infiltration of the phrenic nerve* is appropriate. Fluoroscopy is needed to see if one leaf of the diaphragm is responsible and can be singled out for treatment. In addition, one needs to be sure one leaf is not already paralyzed, a circumstance that would rule out this therapeutic option. The phrenic nerve serving the offending diaphragm is infiltrated with a long-acting anesthetic; if it works, but the hiccups return, reinfiltration with alcohol or *crushing* may be necessary. If both leaves of the diaphragm are involved, one phrenic nerve is treated.

In most instances, hiccups will resolve spontaneously or respond at least partially to one of these therapeutic maneuvers.

L.A.M. and A.H.G.

ANNOTATED BIBLIOGRAPHY

Editorial. Hiccup. Br Med J 1971;1:235. *(A terse review of pathophysiology and the significance of the hiccup.)*

Engleman EG, Lankton J, Leakton B. Granulated sugar as treatment for hiccups in conscious patients. N Engl J Med 1971;285:1489. *(A letter reported successful relief of hiccups in 19 of 20 patients following swallowing a teaspoon of ordinary dry white sugar.)*

Salem MR, et al. Treatment of hiccups by pharyngeal stimulation in anesthetized and conscious subjects. JAMA 1967;202:321. *(Therapeutic success in 84 of 86 patients by introduction of a catheter through the nose and stimulating the pharynx at the level of C2–3.)*

Samuels L. Hiccup: A ten-year review of anatomy, etiology, and treatment. Can Med Assoc J 1952;67:315. *(The classic hiccup paper with differential diagnosis.)*

Souadjian JV, et al. Intractable hiccup: Etiologic factors in 220 patients. Postgrad Med 1968;43:72. *(A classic review of 220 patients from the Mayo Clinic presenting probable causes.)*

Williamson BWA, MacIntyre JMC. Management of intractable hiccup. Br Med J 1977;2:501. *(A succinct review of therapeutic approaches, finding chlorpromazine and metoclopramide the most effective drugs; 39 refs.)*

Primary Care Medicine: Office Evaluation and Management of the Adult Patient, 3rd edition, edited by Allan H. Goroll, Lawrence A. May, and Albert G. Mulley, Jr. J.B. Lippincott Company, Philadelphia

222
Approach to the Patient With Chronic Nasal Congestion and Discharge

It is estimated that 15 percent to 20 percent of the population suffer from chronic or recurrent nasal congestion. Allergic rhinitis accounts for the majority of such cases; vasomotor rhinitis, mechanical obstruction, drugs, and abuse of decongestants contribute to others. Much discomfort, absenteeism, and expense result. The primary physician needs to be able to distinguish an allergic etiology from obstruction, inflammation, or vasomotor instability. Proper utilization of allergy testing and effective use of antihistamines, decongestants, and topical corticosteroids are required.

PATHOPHYSIOLOGY AND CLINICAL PRESENTATION

Allergic Rhinitis. In atopic patients, antigen exposure stimulates production of allergen-specific IgE. This IgE attaches to mucosal mast cells. Subsequent exposure to the allergen leads to formation of antigen-IgE complexes on mast cells and basophils. The formation of antigen–antibody complexes triggers an acute-phase *degranulation* reaction, with release of histamine, kinins, prostaglandins, and esterases in concentrations proportional to the intensity of the antigen challenge. Hours later, a late-phase response can be demonstrated in persons with more severe disease, manifested by re-release of mediators (minus prostaglandins), an influx of leukocytes, eosinophils, and mononuclear cells, and increased responsiveness to antigenic and nonantigenic stimuli. With continued allergen exposure, there is heightened mucosal responsiveness due to an increase in the population of mast cells.

In addition to environmental stimuli, genetic factors play a role. Antigen-specific responses are controlled by regulatory genes, and allergic rhinitis is much more common in persons with a positive family history. The relation of allergic rhinitis to reactive lower airway disease (asthma) remains a subject of debate, but it appears that allergic rhinitis is neither a cause nor consequence of it.

Clinical Presentation. Nasal congestion, sneezing, and profuse watery discharge dominate the initial clinical presentation. Itching of the nose, throat, and eyes is common, as is postnasal drip, tearing, and conjunctival injection. Often the nasal mucosa appears pale and edematous. Symptoms typically vary over the course of the day. They are most severe on arising in the morning, lessen in the afternoon, and may worsen again by evening. With continued allergen exposure, there is increased sensitivity both to allergens and to nonallergenic stimuli.

Onset of allergic rhinitis is usually during childhood but may occur at any age. Childhood cases frequently continue into adulthood. Often, the condition improves with time. The condition is *seasonal* when the antigen is a pollen ("hay fever") and *perennial* when the allergens are dusts, molds, or animal danders. Patients living in the northern half of the United States who are sensitive to tree pollen will become symptomatic in late March and early April; those sensitive to grasses, in mid-May to late June. Patients affected by ragweed and other summer weeds experience difficulty in late August until the first frost. Patients with seasonal allergic rhinitis outnumber those with perennial complaints by a ratio of about 10 to 1. Individuals may be allergic to a number of antigens.

In some instances, the patient has all the earmarks of allergic rhinitis but no evidence of IgE mediation, and skin tests for inhaled allergens are negative. Such patients have been designated as having *nonallergic rhinitis,* even though their nasal secretions often contain large numbers of eosinophils and they respond to corticosteroids.

Vasomotor Rhinitis. The pathophysiology is poorly understood but believed to involve abnormal autonomic responsiveness and vascular dilatation of the submucosal vessels. IgE levels are normal, and the number of eosinophils in nasal secretions is usually, but not always, normal. Abnormal autonomic reactivity is felt to account for the nasal stuffiness or rhinorrhea sometimes occurring with *emotional upset* and *sexual arousal.*

The condition may mimic perennial allergic rhinitis and is believed by some clinicians to be a diagnosis of exclusion when no allergen is identified. Others consider the condition a readily distinguishable entity characterized by a normal-appearing nasal mucosa and persistent nasal stuffiness without itching that is worsened by changes in ambient temperature and humidity. Although congestion is the most prominent symptom, a discharge may also be present. Sneezing is relatively absent.

Drugs. Overuse of topical *nasal decongestants* (eg, oxymetazoline, phenylpropanolamine, pseudoephedrine) can result in a worsening of symptoms (*rhinitis medicamentosa*). After more than 3 days of continuous use, response to these agents becomes blunted (tachyphylaxis), leading to increased use, often on an hourly basis. Cessation results in severe rebound nasal congestion presumably due to marked reflex vasodilatation. The nasal mucosa appears erythematous. The problem resolves in 2 to 3 weeks if topical decongestants are stopped. Alpha-adrenergic blockers can aggravate preexisting rhinitis and cause mild nasal congestion in normal patients.

Cocaine abuse is another important cause of drug-induced nasal congestion and discharge. Being a potent sympathomimetic, the pathophysiology is analogous to that of nasal decongestant abuse. Recurrent nasal use leads to ischemic mucosal injury, atrophy, and tell-tale septal perforation.

Hormonal Etiologies. *Hypothyroidism* and *pregnancy* may cause the turbinates to become pale and edematous, leading to nasal congestion. Hypothyroidism may otherwise be subclinical save for the chronic nasal obstruction. Symptoms resolve with correction of the hypothyroidism or with delivery.

Mechanical Obstruction. Unilateral congestion, discharge, and recurrent pedicels of sinusitis are characteristic of mechanical obstruction due to tumor, polyp, or deviated septum. *Neoplasm* is rare but is suggested by a blood-tinged discharge. *Polyps* can occur in association with allergic and vasomotor rhinitis, chronic sinusitis, aspirin-induced asthma, cystic fibrosis, and drug use. The mechanism of formation is unknown. Polyps move freely because they are pedunculated and nontender, and appear as soft, pale gray, smooth structures. Patients with asthma and nasal polyps are often hypersensitive to aspirin. Polyps do not regress spontaneously and may become large or multiple, causing considerable obstruction. A *deviated septum* is sometimes the source of obstructive symptoms. Most are developmental and not traumatic in origin. Associated sinus occlusion is rare.

Obstruction due to crusting is seen with *atrophic rhinitis.* The condition is of unknown etiology, appears mostly in women, and is characterized by dry atrophic nasal turbinates, mucosal crusts, and a foul or fetid greenish discharge referred to as ozena. The purulent discharge is believed due to secondary infection.

Chronic Inflammatory Disease. *Midline granuloma,* an uncommon illness of unknown etiology, causes ulcerative destruction of upper respiratory tract structures and may present as nasal stuffiness, crusting, and granulations. Steady progression leads to ulcers of the nasal septum. The majority of patients are over 50, many with a history of allergic rhinitis. *Wegener's granulomatosis,* an immune-mediated disease of middle-aged persons, may have a similar insidious presentation with nasal obstruction, rhinorrhea, or chronic sinusitis. Necrotizing granulomatous lesions and vasculitis are found in the upper and lower airway. *Sarcoidosis* may present as bilateral nasal obstruction (see Chapter 51).

DIFFERENTIAL DIAGNOSIS

The causes of nasal congestion and discharge can be organized pathophysiologically and are listed in Table 222-1.

Table 222-1. Important Causes of Chronic or Recurrent Nasal Congestion

A. Allergic
  1. Seasonal allergic rhinitis (pollens)
  2. Perennial allergic rhinitis (dusts, molds)

B. Vasomotor
  1. Idiopathic (vasomotor rhinitis)
  2. Abuse of nose drops
  3. Drugs (reserpine, guanethidine, prazosin, cocaine abuse)
  4. Psychologic stimulation (anger, sexual arousal)

C. Mechanical
  1. Polyps
  2. Tumor
  3. Deviated septum
  4. Crusting (as in atrophic rhinitis)
  5. Hypertrophied turbinates (chronic vasomotor rhinitis)
  6. Foreign body (usually in children)

D. Chronic Inflammatory
  1. Sarcoidosis
  2. Wegener's granulomatosis
  3. Midline granuloma

E. Infectious
  1. Atrophic rhinitis (secondary infection)

F. Hormonal
  1. Pregnancy
  2. Hypothyroidism

WORKUP

Although it is important to rule out mechanical obstruction, chronic inflammatory disease, and drug-induced illness, the most common diagnostic task is to distinguish allergic from vasomotor disease.

History. The *timing* of symptoms can be helpful diagnostically. Nasal congestion that coincides with periods of pollination is virtually diagnostic of seasonal allergic rhinitis. Continuous waxing and waning of symptoms throughout the year, with exacerbations during the hay fever season, suggest a combination of perennial and seasonal allergic disease. When symptoms occur chronically without respect to seasons, one may be dealing with vasomotor rhinitis, perennial allergy, mechanical obstruction, or a chronic inflammatory condition. Perennial rhinitis is a possibility when the patient reports frequent "colds."

Aggravating and alleviating factors should be noted. Patients bothered by dusts are generally atopic, whereas those whose symptoms are aggravated by quick changes in temperature, emotion, or drugs fall into the vasomotor category. Use of antihypertensive agents and topical nasal decongestants needs to be explored, as does exposure to fur-bearing animals, feathers, other possible sources of animal danders, or chemical irritants. Pollutants are often more irritating to allergic patients but may also cause symptoms in nonatopic people.

Associated symptoms of potential importance include fever and a purulent nasal discharge, suggestive of an infectious etiology. A cold is the most likely cause of acute discharge, but chronic discharge that is fetid, foul-smelling, and accompanied by crusting indicates secondary infection as in atrophic rhinitis, Wegener's granulomatosis, and midline granuloma. Bloody discharge and unilateral obstruction suggest tumor. Mechanical obstructions are often unilateral as well. The presence of asthma or aspirin sensitivity increases the likelihood of nasal polyps. Sneezing, postnasal drip, and itching are nonspecific and of little help in distinguishing among etiologies.

Epidemiologic data need to be considered. Onset in childhood is typical of allergic disease, but onset of symptoms during adulthood does not rule out atopy. When chronic progressive nasal congestion develops in a middle-aged patient, particularly a woman, one must consider atrophic rhinitis or one of the necrotizing inflammatory diseases. The allergy histories of the patient's parents should be ascertained.

Drug use and *concurrent conditions* are important to review, including abuse of cocaine or nasal decongestants, hypothyroidism, sarcoidosis, and pregnancy.

Physical Examination. The nasal mucous membranes are inspected for erythema, pallor, atrophy, edema, crusting, and discharge. The presence of polyps, erosions, and septal perforations or deviations should be noted. A nasal speculum markedly improves visualization of the nasal cavity and ought to be used in every examination. Some findings are nonspecific. For example, a pale boggy appearance to the mucosa is allegedly a classic sign of allergic disease, but erythema sometimes occurs in allergy and its presence certainly does not rule it out.

Examination of the eyes for conjunctival erythema, tearing, photophobia, and papillary edema of the lids provides supportive evidence of an allergic mechanism. Transillumination and palpation of the sinuses, pharyngeal examination for erythema and discharge, a look in the ears for evidence of otitis, cervical node examination for adenopathy, and auscultation of the chest for wheezes complete the physical examination.

Laboratory Studies. Antigen challenge is sometimes helpful when the differentiation between allergic and nonallergic disease remains difficult. In vivo and in vitro methods are used.

In Vivo Testing for Allergen-Specific IgE. The procedure of choice for detection of allergen-specific IgE continues to be *skin testing*. For environmental allergens, an epicutaneous (needle prick) test is used. Preparations of commonly inhaled allergens (dusts, molds, animal danders, and local pollens) are introduced by needle into the skin. A positive test is a wheal and flare reaction within 20 minutes. A positive reaction does not prove causation, only that there is sensitization to the allergen and allergen-specific IgE present. Correlation with history and physical examination is needed to establish an etiologic role for the antigen.

Antihistamines must be omitted for 12 to 24 hours before testing to avoid a false-negative result. Dermographism is a common cause of false-positive results, occurring in 15 percent to 20 percent of the population and necessitating use of a saline control injection. The size of the wheal and flare correlates well with the level of allergen-specific IgE. However, allergen preparations remain to be standardized, impairing interpretation and comparison of results.

The *inhalation challenge* remains predominantly a research method, used to evaluate nasal resistance after mucosal exposure.

In Vitro Testing for IgE and Other Markers of Allergy. Determination of *total IgE* is helpful if the level is markedly elevated, but test sensitivity is low because some cases of allergic rhinitis are not associated with high serum concentrations. The same is true for the *total eosinophil count*. A count at the time of an exacerbation that is in excess of 500 cells per mm^3 is suggestive of an allergic etiology, but the absence of peripheral eosinophilia does not rule out allergic rhinitis.

Allergoabsorbent testing is an in vitro means of identifying and quantitating an allergen-specific IgE. *Radioallergosorbent testing* (*RAST*) involves adding the patient's serum to a purified allergen absorbed to an inert particle. If the serum contains high concentrations of specific IgE antibodies to the allergen, it will give a positive test. The shortcomings of RAST testing are its expense and only modest sensitivity; however, specificity is high. The test is best reserved for patients whose skin tests are equivocal and for those who cannot undergo skin testing.

Other Studies. Examining *smears* of nasal secretions for eosinophils is of limited specificity, because substantial numbers of eosinophils may be present in both vasomotor and allergic rhinitis. The smears can be informative if infection is in question, because neutrophils should be present in abundance. *Sinus films* should be obtained if purulent discharge, sinus opacification, or tenderness suggests an accompanying sinusitis (see Chapter 219).

PRINCIPLES OF MANAGEMENT AND PATIENT EDUCATION

Allergic Rhinitis

The treatment program begins with avoidance of responsible allergens, adds antihistamines (sympathomimetics) for symptomatic relief, utilizes topical corticosteroids or cromolyn for improved prophylaxis and control, and resorts to preventive immunotherapy in refractory cases.

Avoidance Measures. The appropriate avoidance procedures are a function of the responsible allergens and differ for seasonal and perennial disease.

Seasonal Allergic Rhinitis. Avoidance of long walks in the woods during the pollination period and staying indoors with the windows closed when symptoms are severe and the pollen count is high (eg, hot, windy, sunny days) helps reduce allergen exposure. Some patients find air conditioners helpful, but its filter does little to remove pollen from the air. Air conditioning simply makes it more tolerable to stay indoors with the windows closed on a hot day. The outside air intake on the air conditioner should be kept closed to avoid bringing in more pollinated air. If ragweed is a problem, daisies, dahlias, and chrysanthemums should not be kept indoors. Preventing accumulation of excess dust in the bedroom and avoiding irritants such as tobacco smoke, chemical vapors, and strong perfumes lessen symptoms.

Perennial Allergic Rhinitis. Control of perennial disease requires particular attention to allergens in the home, but recommendations should be practical. Cleaning the house and especially the bedroom with a damp mop two to three times a week will reduce dust. Feather pillows should be replaced by Dacron or polyester ones, and mattresses should be covered with an elastic fabric casing. Areas where mold can collect, such as piles of old newspapers or furniture in a damp basement, should be cleaned up. A dehumidifier may prevent mold growth. Throwing out carpets and draperies is excessive, but new furnishings made of synthetic fabrics are preferable to cotton and wool to minimize dust collection. Humidification of air in winter also helps keep down dusts. Patients allergic to molds should avoid having African violets and geraniums in the home. No new fur-bearing pets should be obtained. Most pets usually have to be removed from the home entirely if symptoms are disabling. Simply keeping the pet out of the bedroom does not help sufficiently because the dander circulates in the air throughout the house.

When history provides ready identification of allergens, there is little need for skin testing, but, if drastic environmental measures are being contemplated, documentation of the specific allergens is indicated.

Pharmacotherapy is indicated in patients who find allergen avoidance impractical or ineffective. The commonly used agents include oral antihistamines, which block the effects of histamine on end organs; inhaled cromolyn sodium and its analogues, which block degranulation of mast cells and basophils; topical corticosteroids, which act on degranulation, late-phase reactions, and end-organ response; and sympathomimetics, which decongest by means of vasoconstriction.

Antihistamines. The advent of nonsedating antihistamines (eg, *terfenadine, astemizole, loratadine*) represents an important improvement in daytime symptomatic treatment of seasonal allergic rhinitis. Their protein-bound lipophobic structure prevents their crossing the blood–brain barrier and causing sedation and psychomotor dysfunction. These second-generation H_1-receptor antagonists also have little anticholinergic activity and thus avoid the annoying side effects of dry mouth and constipation sometimes associated with the use of first-generation antihistamines. They are similar in efficacy to *chlorpheniramine,* the standard first-generation antihistamine for seasonal allergic rhinitis.

Pharmacokinetics of the second-generation agents include rapid absorption after oral intake on an empty stomach, with onset of action within 1 to 2 hours. Intake with food may slow absorption substantially. Duration of action ranges from 12 to 24 hours. Tight protein binding and active metabolites prolong the elimination half-life of astemizole to over 2 weeks, impairing its utility in women who might become pregnant and those requiring skin testing.

Cost is an issue. The second-generation antihistamines cost 15 to 30 times more for a 30-day supply than many first-generation preparations (although not all first-generation preparations are inexpensive; Table 222-2). Approaches to cost containment include 1) starting with a first-generation antihistamine and switching to a nonsedating preparation only if daytime sedation becomes a problem (reported to occur in only 10 percent to 25 percent; tolerance to sedation commonly develops); and 2) substituting an inexpensive, sedating preparation for the nighttime dose of a twice-daily preparation. For those considering daytime use of a first-generation agent, it is important to keep in mind that some degree of psychomotor impairment may occur even without noticeable sedation.

Adverse effects with second-generation agents are few. Some note weight gain with astemizole. Rare instances of lethal *ventricular arrhythmias* (including torsades de pointes) have been reported with overdoses of terfenadine and astemizole and with concurrent use of drugs that impair their hepatic metabolism (eg, ketoconazole and erythromycin).

Topical Corticosteroids. Regular use of a nonabsorbable, topically active corticosteroid (eg, flunisolide or beclomethasone) is among the best means of suppressing both seasonal and perennial allergic rhinitis. Topical steroid therapy should be considered when antihistamines either do not adequately control symptoms or the patient cannot tolerate their side effects. Responsiveness to antihistamines is enhanced by steroid therapy, making combined use a potentially effective option. *Beclomethasone dipropionate* is supplied as a canister-packaged, freon-propelled fine powder. It may provide relief within hours, especially in cases of seasonal rhinitis (hay fever), but regular use for days to weeks may be necessary before benefit is noted. *Flunisolide* comes in an aqueous suspension delivered as a metered spray by a hand-

Table 222-2. Relative Cost and Sedative Action of Popular Antihistamines

PREPARATION	USUAL DAILY DOSAGE	SEDATION	RELATIVE COST
First Generation Antihistamines			
Chlorpheniramine (generic)	4 mg qid	+ +	1.0
long-acting (generic)	12 mg bid	+ +	1.7
Diphenhydramine (generic)	25 mg qid	+ + + +	1.5
Brompheniramine (generic)	4 mg qid	+ +	1.0
Clemastine (Tavist)	1.3 mg bid	+ +/ + + +	8.2
Second Generation Antihistamines			
Terfenadine (Seldane)	60 mg bid	nil	20.2
Astemizole (Hismanal)	10 mg once daily	nil	20.5
Loratadine (Claritin)	10 mg once daily	nil	20.5

Adapted in part from The Medical Letter 1993;35:71.

activated pump. Dosage of both topical preparations is two inhalations in each nostril twice a day. The containers provide a 25-day supply. They cost about the same.

Patients with copious nasal secretions and marked congestion may need preliminary adrenergic therapy to permit the topical steroid preparation to reach the nasal mucosa. Patients with dryness and crusting of the mucosa may prefer flunisolide because it is a liquid. Topical inhalation therapy does not benefit allergic conjunctivitis.

At recommended doses and frequencies, adrenal suppression does not occur with these topical corticosteroids, even when used chronically. However, suppression can occur with prolonged use of excessive doses (greater than 20 puffs/d). Other adverse effects include mucosal irritation and friability leading to an occasional nosebleed. Mucosal ulceration is rare. Application of the spray can cause transient burning and sneezing. Atrophic rhinitis is a risk of chronic use. Colonization of the nose with *Candida* has been reported.

Cromolyn sodium has been found moderately effective in double-blind crossover studies of some patients with allergic rhinitis. The agent is administered either as an inhaled powder or as a dissolved liquid up to six times per day. It works by preventing degranulation of mast cells and is most effective when used prophylactically before an anticipated allergen exposure. It benefits both the immediate and late phases of the allergic reaction and can diminish the severity of an ongoing allergic episode. Patients with very high IgE levels are most responsive; many others are not. Therapy is safe and very well tolerated.

Nedocromil is a new topically active mast-cell stabilizer, structurally different from cromolyn and possessing antiinflammatory activity as well. Nonetheless, clinical efficacy in allergic rhinitis is similar to that of cromolyn, although it need be taken only twice daily.

Immunotherapy. (hyposensitization) is indicated as a last resort in patients who remain incapacitated despite a full pharmacotherapy program and who face prolonged (more than 6 weeks) exposure to a known allergen. Hyposensitization reduces IgE production and stimulates synthesis of IgG *blocking antibody.* It may also induce IgE suppressor lymphocyte activity or reduce mast cell and basophil responsiveness. Prevention of local reaction to pollens, cat dander, and dust mites has been demonstrated in patients with allergic rhinitis. Hyposensitization involves cutaneous administration of incremental doses of allergen extract, initially at intervals of 1 to 2 weeks, progressing to intervals of 3 to 6 weeks after several months of treatment.

This form of therapy should be considered an adjunct to medication. Most responses are not dramatic. Skin testing and frequent visits over a prolonged period mean patient inconvenience and high cost. Assessment of response to immunotherapy (improvement in symptoms, reduction in medication requirements) should be made every 6 months, and therapy should be discontinued if substantial benefit is not evident after 12 to 18 months.

Sympathomimetics. The vasoconstrictive action of adrenergic agents can help reduce edema and secretions as well as counter the sedative action of antihistamines. These properties make oral sympathomimetics a useful component in over-the-counter decongestant formulations, often in combination with an antihistamine such as chlorpheniramine. All are effective decongestants, but those with some beta-activity in addition to their vasoconstrictor action (eg, *ephedrine, pseudoephedrine*) are preferred when drowsiness is a problem. *Phenylpropanolamine* has predominantly alpha-activity. A typical regimen is pseudoephedrine, 60 mg, q4-6h; lower doses may suffice in mild cases.

Sympathomimetics can produce nervousness, increase heart rate, and elevate blood pressure. Their prolonged use in patients with hypertension or coronary artery disease is inadvisable. Empirical trials of various antihistamines and decongestants are often necessary to select the best agent(s) and dose(s). Combination preparations are convenient if the fixed doses match the doses needed; these preparations should not be used as initial therapy.

Topical decongestant sprays have a limited role because of the risks of tachyphylaxis and rebound nasal congestion. They are best used for keeping the eustachian tubes patent in patients during airplane travel (see Chapter 219). A topical application of *phenylephrine* (Neo-Synephrine) or *oxymetazoline* (Afrin) spray every 3 to 4 hours while the patient is airborne should suffice, especially when preceded by an oral decongestant an hour before flight time. Rebound congestion may occur if sprays are used repeatedly for more than 3 days in a row.

Vasomotor Rhinitis

Vasomotor rhinitis is difficult to treat. Avoidance of tobacco smoke, rapid changes in temperature or humidity, and irritant chemical vapors is helpful. Humidification of the home in winter is also worthwhile. Cessation of nasal spray use is essential. Altering antihypertensive medications may be needed. A mild adrenergic agent with some alpha activity (eg, pseudoephedrine) sometimes provides partial improvement. Addition of an antihistamine for its nonspecific drying effect may give some extra relief but is ineffective by itself.

Immunotherapy and steroids are of no proven benefit. Patients bothered severely by nasal obstruction may benefit from cryosurgical treatment of the inferior and middle turbinates. Profuse rhinorrhea is occasionally treated by sectioning the parasympathetic nerve supply to the nose. Consideration of surgical approaches should be reserved for patients seriously impaired by the condition.

INDICATIONS FOR REFERRAL

For the patient with allergic rhinitis whose condition is inadequately controlled on a well-designed medical regimen, referral to an allergist for skin testing and consideration of immunotherapy is a reasonable step. An allergist can also be of help when an allergic etiology cannot be distinguished from vasomotor rhinitis and when the antigen(s) must be identified for management purposes. Referral to an ear, nose and throat (ENT) specialist is indicated for removal of polyps or foreign bodies, management of a suspected tumor, necrotizing inflammatory condition, or atrophic rhinitis, and for correction of deviated septa.

A.H.G.

ANNOTATED BIBLIOGRAPHY

Aaronson D. Comparative efficacy of H1 antihistamines. Ann Allergy 1991;67:541. *(All are equally effective for seasonal allergic rhinitis.)*

Guerin B, Watson RD. Skin tests. Clin Rev Allergy 1988;6:211. *(Good review for the practicing physician.)*

Mabry RL. Topical pharmacotherapy for allergic rhinitis. Southern Med J 1992;85:149. *(Good review of steroids, cromolyn, and new agents.)*

Metzger E. Comparative safety of H_1-antihistamines. Ann Allergy 1991;67:625. *(Good discussion of sedation and psychomotor impairment.)*

Naclerio RM. Understanding the pathogenesis of allergic rhinitis. J Respir Dis 1991;12(suppl):S13. *(Describes both immediate and delayed responses to allergen change, with the late ones part of an inflammatory process.)*

Ownby DR. Allergy testing: In vivo versus in vitro. Pediatric Clin North Am 1988;55:995. *(Detailed discussion of their relative merits.)*

Pipkorn U, Pround D, Lichtenstein LM, et al. Inhibition of mediator release in allergic rhinitis by pretreatment with topical glucocorticosteroids. N Engl J Med 1987;316:1506. *(Blocks both immediate and late-phase responses.)*

Racklin RE. Clinical and immunologic aspects of allergen-specific immunotherapy in patients with seasonal allergic rhinitis and/or allergic asthma. J Allergy Clin Immunol 1983;72:323. *(A review of immunotherapy, its procedures, and its efficacy.)*

223
Approach to the Patient With Excessive Snoring

Primary Care Medicine: Office Evaluation and Management of the Adult Patient, 3rd edition, edited by Allan H. Goroll, Lawrence A. May, and Albert G. Mulley, Jr. J.B. Lippincott Company, Philadelphia

Snoring is essentially a lay term for soft tissue airway obstruction during sleep. The complaint almost always originates from a spouse or household member whose sleep is being disturbed. Snoring may be an annoying but medically trivial problem, but when associated with daytime sleepiness, it may be a manifestation of sleep apnea (see Chapter 46).

PATHOPHYSIOLOGY AND CLINICAL PRESENTATION

Pharyngeal size in snorers and patients with obstructive sleep apnea is reduced compared to that in nonsnorers, with sleep-apnea patients having the smallest cross-sectional pharyngeal area. The sound of snoring originates in the collapsible portion of the airway, the soft tissue between the choanae and the epiglottis. Tone in the lingual and pharyngeal muscles may be inadequate due to use of sedatives or alcohol. Structural abnormalities may contribute and include redundant musculature, a long uvula, thickened pharyngeal folds, and flaccid tonsillar pillars. Large tonsils, cysts, or neoplasms sometimes may obstruct the airway. Obstructing nasal abnormalities (eg, severely deviated septum, polyps, sinusitis, neoplasm) may create excessive negative pressure and cause collapse of the airway during inspiration.

Severe airway obstruction may lead to *sleep apnea*. Full obstruction interrupts ventilation, and, if sufficiently prolonged, results in hypercarbia and hypoxemia. Restoration of breathing usually requires arousal from sleep. The nightly occurrence of multiple apneic episodes and disturbed sleep pattern causes daytime tiredness and hypersomnolence. Uncorrected, the condition may lead to cor pulmonale from chronic arterial desaturation. The condition is most common in obese patients, but not restricted to them.

WORKUP

A careful examination of the upper airway is needed to search for obstruction. Referral for formal ear, nose and throat (ENT) evaluation may be helpful. For the patient with suspected sleep apnea, consideration of nocturnal oxygen saturation monitoring and a formal sleep study are indicated (see Chapter 46).

MANAGEMENT

The patient with annoying, but physiologically benign snoring can sometimes be helped by simple advice. Loss of excess weight and avoidance of alcohol and sedatives may prove beneficial. Sleeping on one's side rather than on the back sometimes helps minimize upper airway collapse (an old trick is to tape a marble to the patient's back to discourage lying supine). Avoidance of the excessive neck flexion that comes from sleeping supine on several pillows can be achieved by limiting the patient to a cervical pillow placed under the nape of the neck or by elevating the entire head of the bed (as in management of reflux esophagitis). Any nasal obstruction from chronic rhinitis should be fully treated (see Chapter 222).

For patients with disturbingly refractory snoring, a more aggressive approach is to consider use of a continuous positive airway pressure (CPAP) device. The apparatus delivers CPAP through the nose and is usually reserved for those with sleep apnea, but may be worth a try in households where marital harmony and restful sleep are threatened by excessive snoring. The devices are sometimes awkward to use and not always acceptable to the patient. Newer ones are more comfortable.

Dental orthosis has proven useful in preliminary studies and may be worth a referral for consideration in severe cases. Pulmonary consultation is indicated when there is concern about sleep apnea (daytime sleepiness, nocturnal apnea; see Chapter 46). An ENT consultation may prove useful when snoring proves intractable and appears associated with anatomic oropharyngeal pathology.

L.G.M.

ANNOTATED BIBLIOGRAPHY

Bradley TD, Brown IG, Grossman RF, et al. Pharyngeal size in snorers, nonsnorers, and patients with obstructive sleep apnea. N Engl J Med 1986;315:1327. *(Snorers have a reduced cross-sectional area; those with sleep apnea have the smallest area.)*

Jennett S. Snoring and its treatment. Br Med J 1984;289:335. *(An editorial review on what we have to offer the patient.)*

Kuna ST, Sant'Ambrogio G. Pathophysiology of upper airway closures during sleep. JAMA 1991;266:1384. *(Excellent review of the mechanisms of upper airway obstruction in sleep apnea.)*

Schmidt-Nowara WW, Meade, et al. Treatment of snoring and obstructive sleep apnea with a dental orthosis. Chest 1991;99:1378. *(A promising, but preliminary report of some improvement.)*

Primary Care Medicine: Office Evaluation and Management of the Adult Patient, 3rd edition, edited by Allan H. Goroll, Lawrence A. May, and Albert G. Mulley, Jr. J.B. Lippincott Company, Philadelphia

224
Management of Aphthous Stomatitis

Aphthous stomatitis (canker sores) is a common, self-limited ulcerative condition of the oral mucosa. About 20 percent of the population is affected at one time or another. The lesions can be disturbing in appearance and very painful. The primary physician should be able to differentiate them from more serious pathology and provide symptomatic relief.

PATHOPHYSIOLOGY, CLINICAL PRESENTATION, AND COURSE

Pathogenesis remains incompletely understood, but a heightened immunologic response to oral mucosal antigens appears to play an important role. There is a genetic predisposition and an increased prevalence among patients with such autoimmune diseases as Crohn's disease, chronic ulcerative colitis, Behçet's syndrome, and Reiter's syndrome. Contributing factors include deficiencies of iron, folate, and vitamin B_{12}, psychological stress, generalized physical debility, and trauma. In some women, flares occur premenstrually. Regardless of etiology, once mucosal breakdown has occurred, the lesions are invaded by mouth flora and become secondarily infected.

Clinical Presentation. Aphthous stomatitis develops in four clinical stages: 1) *Premonitory*—tingling, burning, or hyperesthetic sensation, lasting up to 24 hours; 2) *Preulcerative*—lasting from 18 hours to 3 days, characterized by moderately painful erythematous macules or papules with erythematous halos; 3) *Ulcerative*—lasting 1 to 16 days, characterized by painful discrete ulcers 2 to 10 mm in diameter, occurring singly or in groups, covered by gray–yellow membrane with a dusky erythematous halo; pain ceases during this stage; and 4) *Healing*—usually without scarring unless lesions are very large, averages 2 weeks (range from 4 to 5 weeks).

Aphthous ulcers are classified according to size. The majority are *minor* (ie, less than 1 cm in diameter) and appear in crops of four or five. *Major* lesions are greater than 1 cm, solitary, indolent, and, as noted, may scar as they heal. Lesions are painful and may occur anywhere within the oral cavity. In two-thirds of patients, recurrent lesions do not develop, but in one-third, recurrences continue for up to 40 years.

DIFFERENTIAL DIAGNOSIS

Other causes of oral mucosal ulceration include pemphigus, herpes simplex, Behçet's syndrome, and hand-foot-and-mouth disease. *Pemphigus* is suggested by the presence of bullous lesions elsewhere on the body (although oral lesions may precede others by years) and a Tzanck smear from the base of the lesion showing acantholytic cells. Immunofluorescence studies may be necessary if there is recurrent disease. The ulcerated mucosal lesions of *herpes simplex* infection are limited to mucosal surfaces attached to bone, whereas aphthous ulcers may occur anywhere in the oral cavity. The Tzanck preparation shows multinucleated giant cells. The ulcers of *Behçet's syndrome* are identical to those of aphthous stomatitis; genital ulceration and eye involvement help differentiate the condition from simple aphthous disease. In *hand-foot-and-mouth disease,* papulovesicular lesions with an erythematous halo appear on the hands, feet, and lips in addition to the mouth. The lesions ulcerate and then heal over 7 to 10 days. Because the condition is due to an enterovirus, the mucosal findings may be preceded by viral gastrointestinal symptoms.

PRINCIPLES OF MANAGEMENT

When the chief reason for seeking medical care is concern, reassurance that the lesions will heal spontaneously and that they do not represent more serious pathology will often suffice. For patients with large lesions and those bothered badly by the discomfort, additional measures are indicated. *Tetracycline liquid* (250 mg qid) used as a mouthwash that is held in the mouth for several minutes before swallowing is easy to use and frequently prescribed. Topical corticosteroids impregnated into a paste vehicle (eg, Orabase) help apply the steroid to the mucous membrane and may provide some added relief. *Carbamide peroxide gel* is an oxidizing agent that releases oxygen on contact with the oral mucosa. It has some bactericidal effect against many mouth organisms and is a mild debriding agent. In the presence of extremely painful lesions, use of *topical anesthetic agents* (eg, viscous lidocaine) before meals may allow the patient to eat. Avoidance of abrasive foods also helps. *Levamisole,* which stimulates immune response, has been used experimentally and reported efficacious in about two-thirds of cases, but the unknown long-term safety of this agent limits its use for this self-limited condition.

Women with a definite premenstrual flare may be helped by estrogen-dominated oral contraceptives. Identification and correction of an existing deficiency of folate, vitamin B_{12}, or iron may cure aphthous stomatitis. For lesions precipitated by emotional stress, attention to the underlying problem may help (see Chapter 226). Chemical cauterization by means of silver nitrate sticks ($AgNO_3$) is used by some practitioners to treat acute lesions, but this involves the distinct possibility of destroying normal tissue and should not ordinarily be used.

PATIENT EDUCATION

Besides reassurance, patient education should include recommendations for avoiding mucosal trauma and maintaining good nutrition and oral hygiene. Use of a soft-bristled toothbrush and avoidance of foods with sharp surfaces, salt, and talking while chewing can be helpful. Patients with vitamin or mineral deficiencies can be prescribed a supplement. The possibility of recurrence in one-third of patients should be explained.

A.H.G. and L.A.M.

ANNOTATED BIBLIOGRAPHY

Antoon JM, Miller RL. Aphthous ulcer: A review of the literature on etiology, pathogenesis, diagnosis, and treatment. JAMA 1980;201:803. *(Still the best review.)*

Bell GF, Rogers RS III. Observations on the diagnosis of recurrent aphthous stomatitis. Mayo Clin Proc 1982;297. *(A discussion of four cases and the key diagnostic issues they raise.)*

Graykowski EA. Aphthous stomatitis is linked to mechanical injuries, iron and vitamin deficiencies, and certain HLA types. JAMA 1982;247:774. *(A summary of findings from studies by NIH investigators.)*

225
Management of Temporomandibular Joint Dysfunction

Primary Care Medicine: Office Evaluation and Management of the Adult Patient, 3rd edition, edited by Allan H. Goroll, Lawrence A. May, and Albert G. Mulley, Jr. J.B. Lippincott Company, Philadelphia

Temporomandibular joint (TMJ) dysfunction has received much attention in the lay press as a cause of chronic headache and facial pain (see Chapter 165). Although severe cases may require dental or oral surgical intervention, most can be managed conservatively by the primary physician.

PATHOPHYSIOLOGY AND CLINICAL PRESENTATION

Most TMJ dysfunction is psychophysiologic in origin, the consequence of chronic *bruxism* (nocturnal jaw clenching and teeth grinding). This tension-relieving oral habit develops in response to situational and intrapsychic stresses and can lead to masticatory muscle fatigue and spasm. In most instances, the problem remains *extracapsular*, with little or no internal derangement of the TMJ. However, severe, prolonged bruxism may cause *intracapsular* joint derangement, resulting in degenerative disease of the joint. *Sinovitis* from connective tissue disease, infection, or trauma is another form of intracapsular pathology.

Symptoms of TMJ dysfunction include chronic, dull, aching unilateral discomfort about the jaw, behind the eyes and ears, and even down the neck into the shoulders. Jaw pain, clicking sounds, and difficulty opening the mouth widely, especially in the morning, are characteristic. Chewing may exacerbate symptoms. Locking of the jaw is common. Masticatory muscle tenderness, mandibular hypomotility, clicking, and joint deviation on opening are noted on physical examination. Molar prominences may be flat from chronic grinding.

DIAGNOSIS

The hallmark of TMJ dysfunction is chronic unilateral jaw or facial pain exacerbated by jaw movement. Other causes of jaw pain worsened by jaw movement include *acute otitis media* and *parotitis*. These are distinguished by their acute onset and associated inflammatory manifestations. More subtle is the jaw claudication from *temporal arteritis* (see Chapter 161). Intracapsular TMJ disease may be differentiated clinically from extracapsular dysfunction by the presence of markedly limited jaw movement, jaw deviation on opening of the mouth, and presence of crepitus and clicking on jaw movement. However, there is much overlap of symptoms between internal and extracapsular TMJ disease; jaw clicking may even be noted in normal persons.

Confirmation of internal derangement requires radiologic study. *Magnetic resonance imaging (MRI)* of the TMJ provides the best visualization of bony and soft tissue structures. It has become the test of choice, being more sensitive than conventional or computed tomography and free of radiation exposure. MRI test expense can be reduced substantially by imaging only the TMJ. Imaging is indicated only when internal derangement is suspected, conservative measures have failed, and more aggressive therapy is being considered.

PRINCIPLES OF MANAGEMENT

Nonsurgical Measures. Because TMJ dysfunction is largely a psychophysiologic condition, *psychotherapy* should be an important part of the treatment program. It may begin with the primary physician inquiring into sources of stress and tension and offering counseling. Often, cognitive/behavioral approaches are more effective than insight-oriented therapy (see Chapter 226). Most persons improve without formal psychiatric care. Less etiologic, but helpful symptomatic measures include dietary advice, local physiotherapy, analgesics, minor tranquilizers, and sometimes antidepressants.

Dietary advice included cutting food into small pieces and using a diet that minimizes hard, repetitive chewing (eg, no chewing gum or biting into big submarine sandwiches. *Physiotherapy* in the form of local heat and massage to the muscles of mastication helps relieve muscle spasm and the accompanying pain. Some persons achieve relief with application of ultrasound of cold packs. *Analgesics* such as aspirin and low doses of nonsteroidal antiinflammatory agents are also helpful when pain is prominent. Short-term use of a *minor tranquilizer* at bedtime (eg, 2 mg of diazepam qhs for 3–5 days) can help reduce nocturnal muscle spasm and complement analgesic therapy. However, long-term tranquilizer use should be avoided due to the risk of dependence (see Chapter 226). The so-called muscle relaxants (eg, Robaxin, Soma) are of no proven advantage. Patients with more refractory pain may respond to a trial of a sedating *tricyclic antidepressant* (eg, nortriptyline 25 mg qhs). Patients with severe grinding may benefit from night-time use of a custom-made *splint* or bite guard.

A regimen that incorporates all these measures into a comprehensive treatment program has a success rate of over 75 percent. Patients who prove refractory are likely to have suffered joint damage and require consideration for regrinding or surgical intervention.

Regrinding and Surgical Therapies. Only the patient with severe malocclusion leading to a marked joint trauma is a candidate for regrinding of the teeth. It is a therapy of limited efficacy, requiring careful patient selection. Surgical intervention is a consideration only when conservative measures have failed to provide relief *and* there is clinical evidence of internal joint derangement and secondary degenerative arthritis (see above). Under these circumstances, an MRI of the TMJs should be obtained and referral made if important degenerative changes are found.

Incapacitated patients refractory to conservative therapy and found to have marked degenerative changes are potential candidates for surgery. They should be referred for consultation to an oral surgeon experienced in treating TMJ disease. There are almost no large-scale, prospective, randomized studies to guide choice of surgery for TMJ disease. Arthroscopic approaches appear promising. They are reported to provide significant symptomatic relief, are minimally invasive, and have a low incidence of complications; however, long-term benefit remains to be established.

A.H.G.

ANNOTATED BIBLIOGRAPHY

Guralnick W, Kaban LB, Merrill RG. Temporomandibular-joint afflictions. N Engl J Med 1978;299:123. *(Classic review, especially of pathophysiology.)*

Kumar KL, Cooney TG. Temporomandibular disorders. J Gen Intern Med 1994;9:106. *(Excellent summary for the generalist reader, with particularly helpful suggestions for workup and conservative management; 36 refs.)*

McCain JP, Sanders B, Koslin MG, et al. Temporomandibular joint arthroscopy: A six-year multicenter retrospective study of 4,831 joints. J Oral Maxillofacial Surg 1992;50:926. *(Promising results, but data are retrospective and nonrandomized.)*

15

Psychiatric and Behavioral Problems

Primary Care Medicine: Office Evaluation and Management of the Adult Patient, 3rd edition, edited by Allan H. Goroll, Lawrence A. May, and Albert G. Mulley, Jr. J.B. Lippincott Company, Philadelphia

226

Approach to the Patient With Anxiety

SCOTT L. RAUCH, M.D.
JERROLD F. ROSENBAUM, M.D.

Anxiety disorders are prevalent, with an estimated 5 percent of the general population affected. Given the array of associated somatic symptoms, anxiety is a frequent precipitant of visits to the nonpsychiatric physician. Patients with anxiety pose a challenge to the primary care physician, presenting with feelings of distress and concern about disease in the absence of objective evidence for a medical problem. Suffering no less from the subjective nature of the ailment, such patients fear something is amiss with their bodies and persistently seek an acceptable explanation and relief. Because the autonomic arousal accompanying anxiety may affect many organ systems, anxiety can be a great imitator of physical disease. Moreover, anxiety and anxiety-like symptoms may be consequent to a variety of medical ailments and their treatments.

Anxiousness is a normal human affect. Distinguishing it from pathologic anxiety and anxiety disorders often requires systematic evaluation and a thorough understanding of the individual patient's physical and psychological status. Unrecognized and untreated, anxiety disorders increase the cost of medical care and render the patient vulnerable to further morbidity, including demoralization, hypochondriasis, depression, and varying degrees of disability. A comprehensive and empathic assessment of the anxious patient by the primary physician permits a reasoned and often therapeutically effective approach to the difficult problems presented.

PATHOPHYSIOLOGY AND CLINICAL PRESENTATION

Anxiety is the distressing experience of dread, foreboding, or panic, accompanied by a variety of autonomic—primarily sympathetic—bodily symptoms. The distress, therefore, is both psychic and physical. Patients vary considerably in their tolerance to it. The new onset or exacerbation of anxiety often occurs in response to emotional or physiologic stimuli. Most persons meet the challenge of universally anxiety-provoking situations with their own personal strengths and styles of coping. When a patient's capacity for coping is overwhelmed, excessive anxiety may emerge. Pathologic anxiety is distinguished from the normal by its occurrence in the absence of an appropriate stimulus and by its duration or intensity.

Several monoamine and neuropeptide neurotransmitters are implicated in the neurobiology of anxiety. Norepinephrine plays a prominent role in mediating anxiety states centrally. The locus ceruleus of the pons serves as the chief noradrenergic nucleus. Abnormal firing patterns in the locus ceruleus have been implicated in the pathophysiology of some anxiety disorders. In contrast, the inhibitory neurotransmitter gamma-aminobutyric acid (GABA), ubiquitous throughout the brain, is implicated as serving an anxiolytic function within the limbic system. The resultant somatic manifestations of anxiety are principally mediated by the sympathetic nervous system.

Clinical Presentation

In both its normal and pathologic forms, anxiety's manifestations consist of affective, cognitive, behavioral, and somatic components. The *affective component* is characterized by the experience of dread, foreboding or panic, countered by *cognitions* that make sense of or seek to neutralize the distress. A variety of *behaviors* reflect the anxious state or evolve in response to it (eg, avoidance). Typical psychological presentations might include complaints of apprehension, motor tension or agitation (restlessness, edginess, jitteriness), and heightened arousal (including hypervigilance, distractibility, impaired concentration, and insomnia).

The *somatic complaints* are mostly those of autonomic hyperactivity and include systemic, cardiopulmonary, gastrointestinal, urinary, and neurologic symptoms (Table 226–1).

Table 226-1. Somatic Symptoms of Anxiety

TYPE	SPECIFIC SYMPTOMS
General	Fatigue, weakness, diaphoresis, insomnia, flushing, chills
Neurologic	Dizziness, paresthesias, derealization, near syncope, tremulousness, restlessness
Cardiac	Palpitations, chest pain, tachycardia
Respiratory	Dyspnea, hyperventilation, choking
Gastrointestinal	Dry mouth, diarrhea, nausea, vomiting
Urinary	Frequency

Classification

The classification of anxiety disorders is largely based on clinical features (Table 226–2).

Adjustment Disorder with Anxious Mood. Most presentations of anxiety within the medical setting are normal reactions to anxiety-provoking situations. For a limited time period, a patient may suffer symptoms similar to those of a generalized anxiety disorder (see below). When a patient's capacity for coping is overwhelmed, excessive anxiety may transiently emerge until the patient is able to adjust. This state is termed *adjustment disorder with anxious mood,* and typically resolves in less than 6 months. Adjustment disorders may likewise be heralded by other manifestations, including depressed mood and misconduct.

Table 226-2. Anxiety Disorders and Defining Features

Generalized Anxiety Disorder
- Chronic anxiety lasting at least 6 months.
- Concern over at least two different issues (usually many).
- Panic attacks may be present.

Panic Disorder
- Episodic extreme anxiety consistent with panic attacks.
- Panic attacks occur spontaneously.
- Occurrence of at least four attacks in 1 month, or one or more attacks resulting in subsequent avoidance.
- Avoidance (with or without agoraphobia).

Simple Phobia
- Irrational fear associated with a particular stimulus.

Social Phobia
- Anxiety associated with public attention.

Obsessive-Compulsive Disorder
- Obsessions (intrusive unwanted bizarre thoughts) and/or compulsions (repetitive behaviors performed in a ritualistic or stereotypical fashion).
- Anxiety leads to substantial distress or symptoms impair functioning.

Posttraumatic Stress Disorder
- History of severe traumatic exposure.
- Subsequent anxiety symptoms lasting at least 1 month.
- Reexperiencing of the trauma (*e.g.,* flashbacks), avoidance of stimuli associated with the trauma, and increased arousal.
- Syndrome may occur with delayed onset (greater than 6 months after original trauma).

Adjustment Disorder With Anxious Mood*
- Anxiety develops as a maladaptive response to an identifiable stressor.
- Symptoms last less than 6 months.

*Categorized with adjustment disorders rather than anxiety disorders in DSM III-R.

Generalized anxiety disorder is characterized by anxiety lasting longer than 6 months, not limited to worry over one specific subject. Typically, the patient is ruminating with worries over a variety of concerns and may have been this way for several years with a waxing and waning course and an array of physical concomitants. In addition to the persistent anxious state, the patient may describe more discrete episodes of acute anxiety.

When sudden spells of extreme anxiety occur with prominent symptoms of sympathetic activation, they may be accompanied by feelings of impending doom, fear of dying, the sensation of panic, and the impulse to flee. Such *panic attacks* may occasionally be experienced by patients with generalized anxiety disorder, although they are a more prominent feature in panic attack disorder.

Panic disorder is characterized by the suffering of at least *four panic attacks* in a 1-month period, some of which must have occurred "out of the blue" or *spontaneously*—distinguishing the condition from other causes of panic attacks. Panic attacks are more common in females and in those with a positive family history of panic. Emergence of anxiety symptoms early in life, including a history of separation difficulties during childhood, also represent risk factors for panic attacks.

Many patients become disabled by anticipatory fear of subsequent episodes and by phobic *avoidant behavior* patterns. They avoid places with restricted escape (eg, crowds, theaters, tunnels, elevators), fearful of being trapped during an attack. In its most extreme form, *agoraphobia* (literally, "fear of the market place"), avoidant behavior may reach the point where a patient is afraid to leave the safety of the home or to be left alone. Agoraphobia has also been reported to occur in the absence of panic disorder.

The course of panic disorder includes times of frequent panic attacks interspersed with periods of less frequent episodes, complicated by phobic avoidance and generalized anxiety. The paroxysmal nature of panic attacks and the prominence of autonomic symptoms may mimic cardiac or neurologic disease, causing some patients to become hypervigilant, convinced of a serious underlying medical disorder, and "doctor shoppers" in search of such a diagnosis. Such persons may become demoralized, depressed, and debilitated. Suicide risk appears to be increased in panic disorder, especially in patients with concurrent depression.

Simple Phobias. A phobia is an irrational fear related to a specific stimulus. On exposure to that stimulus, the patient reliably manifests an anxiety response. A patient may suffer from a simple phobia of any specific stimulus. Although simple phobias commonly generate circumscribed symptoms, they may interfere with some aspect of a patient's functioning due to avoidance of the phobic stimulus, or perseverance in the face of great discomfort (eg, fear of flying leading to difficulty with travel).

Social Phobia. Patients with social phobia fear situations in which they are the focus of attention or might be scrutinized publicly. Such patients may experience performance anxiety or "stage fright" but also are distressed in more ordinary social settings. Social phobia is to be distinguished from performance anxiety in a more limited sense, as in the case of universally anxiety-provoking settings (eg, performing in front of a very large audience or as part of a very important event).

Obsessive-compulsive disorder (OCD) is more common than previously recognized, affecting up to 3 percent of the population. It is characterized by obsessions and/or compulsions that are sufficiently severe to cause patients substantial distress or impair their ability to function. *Obsessions* are unwanted intrusive thoughts of a bizarre, senseless or extreme nature. The subject of obsessions typically includes sexual or violent themes that are very distressing to patients and may lead them to fear that they are "going crazy." The obsessions themselves become a source of anxiety.

Compulsions refer to repetitive behaviors that are performed in a stereotypical or ritualized fashion, usually in response to obsessions, sometimes in an effort to neutralize them. Resisting the drive to perform compulsions causes escalating anxiety, whereas succumbing and performing them is accompanied by feelings of transient relief, followed by feelings of shame. Characteristic compulsions include hand washing (to neutralize contamination obsessions), checking behaviors (eg, doorlocks and stove burners to counteract obsessions of uncertainty), and counting (to neutralize anxiety associated with other obsessions).

The relationship between the compulsions and obsessions may also be nonsensical or irrational. However, patients retain insight regarding the nonsensical or extreme nature of their thoughts and behaviors, distinguishing them from psychotic persons.

Because of the shame associated with the symptoms of OCD, it is not uncommon for patients to hide the disorder from friends, family, and doctors. OCD may come to the attention of primary care physicians when patients' obsessions involve preoccupations with their bodily functions (eg, urinary or bowel obsessions) or susceptibility to disease (eg, obsessions with contamination or fear of acquired immunodeficiency syndrome [AIDS]). Rarely, the compulsions may be performed to such extreme as to pose medical risk or sequelae (eg, dermatologic complications of hand washing).

Course is variable. Although typically emerging during the second or third decade of life, symptoms may arise at any age, wax and wane, and become exacerbated in times of stress.

The etiology and underlying pathophysiology of OCD are poorly understood. It has been related genetically to Tourette disorder and commonly occurs with depression. Associated disorders include body dysmorphic disorder (ie, preoccupation with a defective body image) and trichotillomania (compulsive hair-pulling).

Posttraumatic stress disorder (PTSD) occurs after a person has been exposed to a severely traumatic event, such as combat experience, natural disaster, assault, or rape. In the aftermath of the traumatic exposure, the patient typically develops a constellation of symptoms over hours to months. The cardinal symptom is the *persistent reexperiencing* of the traumatic event, via intrusive thoughts, vivid dreams, or "flashbacks," during which the patient feels as though the traumatic event is actually recurring. Other requisite characteristics include *avoidance* of stimuli associated with the trauma, and persistent symptoms of *hyperarousal* (eg, increased startle response). Criteria for the diagnosis include symptoms enduring for a minimum of 1 month; in many cases, the symptoms may continue for years. Rarely, the syndrome emerges more than 6 months following the traumatic exposure, and in such cases is designated "PTSD with delayed onset."

Patients may present for medical assistance with primary complaints of anxiety or with concerns and questions regarding the neurologic underpinnings of their symptoms. Alternatively, PTSD may develop as a consequence of medical illness or procedures (eg, amputation), which by their nature represent profound trauma. Medical settings may serve to trigger reexperiencing phenomena. It is important to be aware of the entity and sensitive to the needs of its sufferers.

Substance Abuse. Anxiety is often poorly tolerated, leading some patients to seek relief through use or abuse of anxiolytic substances. A patient's reliance on alcohol, benzodiazepines, or any other sedating medication may reflect an unrecognized underlying anxiety disorder. Chronic use of sedating substances can lead to neural irritability and can cause or exacerbate anxiety after withdrawal. It often becomes difficult to differentiate the cause and effect relationship between substance abuse and anxiety.

DIFFERENTIAL DIAGNOSIS

The medical differential diagnosis of the signs and symptoms associated with anxiety is extensive and includes many conditions in which there is stimulation of the sympathetic nervous system (Table 226–3). Some reports suggest that undiagnosed medical ailments are responsible for a significant number of psychiatric referrals for "anxiety." Unrecognized arrhythmias, endocrinopathies, and medication reactions may mimic functional anxiety disorders.

Among the psychiatric disorders to be considered in the differential diagnosis of anxiety are the *depressive disorders*. They are among the most critical to recognize, because they are common, treatable, carry a high risk of morbidity and mortality when untreated, and frequently present with symptoms of anxiety. Characteristic manifestations include disturbances in sleep, libido, self-esteem, energy, concentration, and appetite (see Chapter 227). Other psychiatric conditions presenting with anxiety as a prominent component include *psychosis*, *dementias*, and *drug-related* disorders.

Table 226-3. Medical Causes of Anxiousness

TYPE OF CAUSE	SPECIFIC CAUSE
Cardiovascular	Angina pectoris, arrhythmias, congestive heart failure, hypertension, hypovolemia, myocardial infarction, syncope (of multiple causes), valvular disease, vascular collapse (shock)
Dietary	Caffeinism, monosodium glutamate (Chinese-restaurant syndrome), vitamin-deficiency diseases
Drug-related	Akathisia (secondary to antipsychotic drugs), anticholinergic toxicity, digitalis toxicity, hallucinogens, hypotensive agents, stimulants (amphetamines, cocaine, and related drugs), withdrawal syndromes (alcohol or sedative-hypnotics)
Hematologic	Anemias
Immunologic	Anaphylaxis, systemic lupus erythematosus
Metabolic	Hyperadrenalism (Cushing's disease), hyperkalemia, hyperthermia, hyperthyroidism, hypocalcemia, hypoglycemia, hyponatremia, hypothyroidism, menopause, porphyria (acute intermittent)
Neurologic	Encephalopathies (infectious, metabolic, and toxic), essential tremor, intracranial mass lesions, postconcussion syndrome, seizure disorders (especially of the temporal lobe), vertigo
Respiratory	Asthma, chronic obstructive pulmonary disease, pneumonia, pneumothorax, pulmonary edema, pulmonary embolism
Secreting tumors	Carcinoid, insulinoma, pheochromocytoma

WORKUP

The primary physician's evaluation of anxiety needs to include assessment for medical causes as well as psychiatric diagnoses.

Assessment for Medical Causes. The list of possible medical causes is much too extensive to enable a workup that includes every possibility. A reasonable alternative is to focus on any medical conditions for which the patient is already under treatment. This includes a review of the patient's concerns, fears, and ongoing therapies. In addition, attention is directed toward the most important disorders commonly linked with anxiety, such as dysrhythmias (see Chapter 25), hyperthyroidism (see Chapter 103), and drug reactions or withdrawal (see Chapters 229 and 235). Finally, if the patient has a single prominent symptom or constellation of symptoms that implicate a single organ system, it is worthwhile to evaluate that focus.

Assessment for Psychiatric Disorders. The physician should recall that anxiety symptoms are typically conceptualized in three dimensions: psychological, somatic, and behavioral. Occasionally, patients will complain of somatic manifestations of anxiety but may omit history pertaining to the psychological experience. Therefore, it is important to inquire specifically about *psychic manifestations* such as fear, panic, the sensation of impending doom, or the impulse to flee. Reviewing the features of the various anxiety disorders sometimes helps the patient to construct a clearer clinical picture, but care must be taken not to prejudice the patient's responses or appear too eager to make a psychiatric diagnosis.

One also needs to determine the *onset, quality, intensity,* and *duration* of symptoms, being certain to include a compassionate inquiry into recent life events, as well as situational stressors present at the time that symptoms emerged. Any identifiable *stimuli* or *exacerbating factors* should be noted, as well as settings that create apprehension. Development of *avoidant behaviors* should be ascertained. If a particular precipitant is identified, it is helpful to inquire into its origin (eg, a phobia of dogs arising from a remote history of dogbite, or avoidance of elevators as a consequence of having had a panic attack in one). Often, symptoms may have arisen spontaneously, contributing to the sense that they are autonomous (as in panic disorder or OCD).

Also useful is inquiry into *strategies* used to alleviate the symptoms. This may uncover additional history about substance use, avoidance, or compulsive behaviors. *Family history* is reviewed for similar symptoms, known anxiety disorders, and related disorders such as depression or substance abuse. *Past history* of childhood school phobia or early patterns of timidness may be informative. Finally, a thorough physical examination is essential, checking for undisclosed sequelae of repetitive behaviors.

Because there are effective treatments for severe anxiety, a diagnostic trial of an antianxiety therapy can help resolve difficult diagnostic questions. However, suppression of anxiety symptoms does not rule out a medical disorder.

PRINCIPLES OF MANAGEMENT

The treatment strategies for anxiety include psychotherapeutic and pharmacologic interventions; a combined approach yields the best results.

Psychotherapy

Psychotherapeutic treatments for anxiety help to alleviate symptoms through insight, education, support and the reconditioning of behavioral patterns. Supportive, insight-oriented, and behavioral psychotherapies may be employed individually or jointly.

Supportive psychotherapy consists of empathic listening, education, reassurance, encouragement, and guidance. The primary care practitioner frequently performs these functions, whether or not the intervention is labeled as supportive psychotherapy. In the case of anxiety, *empathic listening* helps patients to feel that another human being can appreciate their suffering and, as importantly, not judge them harshly because of their condition. Patients with anxiety often feel ashamed, characterizing themselves as "weak" or "silly" because of their fears and behaviors. Empathy helps to cut through the shame and loneliness. Listening and encouraging them to relate their histories can have a cathartic effect. Many patients with anxiety disorders have hidden some or all of their suffering for years.

In addition to empathic listening, *patient education* is crucial. It begins by informing the patient of the diagnosis and explaining its origins, prognosis, and treatment plan. Increased knowledge and understanding is empowering because it promotes a sense of command and confidence, while reducing feelings of uncertainty, helplessness, and isolation. Such changes are anxiolytic. Fears of serious somatic illness, "going crazy," and incurable disease are alleviated.

Reassurance in the form of "there is nothing serious," even if given in a sympathetic, nonpatronizing manner will be demoralizing and disappointing if offered perfunctorily. Although a negative medical workup may be reassuring to some patients, the patient with an anxiety disorder is not relieved, because he or she is still experiencing distinctive, intrusive, and distressing symptoms. Reassurance serves to heal only when it addresses what is wrong and what can be done. It must be offered in concert with true empathy and education.

Once a strategy has been developed to manage the patient's anxiety, *guidance* and *encouragement* are helpful to the patient in negotiating treatment trials and supervening situational stresses.

Insight-oriented psychotherapy helps guide the patient to an understanding of the association between circumstances, emotions, and symptoms. By exploring feelings, relationships, and actions (both past and present), the patient may develop new insights into his or her inner emotional makeup. This can help reduce the symptoms of anxiety and reframe the meaning of anxiety symptoms when they do occur. Insight therapy typically requires frequent and lengthy sessions for optimal results and the skill of a good psychotherapist.

Behavioral therapy is especially effective for anxiety patients. It consists of reconditioning or modifying patients' behaviors or the association between a stimulus and response. The techniques employed include general relaxation-response training (for tolerating anxiety symptoms), in vivo exposure and desensitization (for phobias and avoidant behaviors), cognitive therapy (for panic and obsessions), and exposure-response prevention (for OCD).

Relaxation techniques are of benefit to almost anyone who suffers from anxiety. Deep muscle relaxation, autogenic exercises, and diaphragmatic breathing are taught (see Appendix at the end of this chapter). Together, these techniques help to minimize the escalating anxiety that results from autonomic dyscontrol. Their use allows patients to better tolerate moderate anxiety states and even abort panic episodes, as well as use more aggressive behavioral techniques.

Reconditioning. Exposure and desensitization entail gradual reconditioning of patients by exposing them to feared stimuli in controlled settings that minimize and allow habituation to their anxiety response. In this way, the feared stimuli become better tolerated and avoidant behaviors are eradicated, as the association with the anxiety response is weakened. Similarly, the exposure-response prevention paradigm is used in treating OCD patients. After being exposed to a provocative stimulus, they are helped to resist the urge to perform their compulsions in response to that stimulus. While tolerating the anxiety, they may employ sanctioned relaxation techniques. Gradually, the compulsions are reduced.

The effectiveness of each of these behavioral techniques is augmented if the patient's anxiety can be held in check. For this reason, the behavioral therapies may be particularly well suited for combination with pharmacotherapies. As with insight-oriented psychotherapy, behavioral therapy is best conducted by professionals who are specially trained in this approach.

Pharmacotherapy

The primary goal is sufficient diminution of symptoms to enable performance of tasks previously impaired by anxiety, including an enhanced ability to benefit from behavioral treatments. With some notable exceptions (eg, panic disorder), drugs play an adjunctive role. Patients should be informed that treatment will be of limited duration and will reduce their symptoms but not eradicate them. Benzodiazepines (BZDs) are the most widely used of anxiolytics. Antidepressants, beta-adrenergic blocking agents, buspirone, and neuroleptics are also used.

Benzodiazepines. For rapid, specific relief of anxiety symptoms, the BZDs are regarded as the anxiolytic of choice, superior in efficacy and safety to the barbiturates and the nonbarbiturate sedatives such as meprobamate, ethchlorvynol, and glutethimide. For some patients, BZDs offer substantial or complete relief of anxiety symptoms. For others, they attenuate severe anxiety pending response to other antianxiety therapies. There is wide individual variation in clinical response, plasma levels, and dosage requirements.

Overuse and drug seeking from multiple sources occur in a small percentage of patients, although rarely with the intensity and risks associated with opiates, barbiturates, and other sedatives. Nevertheless, the physician should know the patient well before prescribing BZDs and be alert for signs of concurrent alcohol or drug dependence (see Chapters 228 and 235).

The efficacy of treatment should be evaluated regularly by follow-up visits, with special attention to proper use. The physician should avoid prescribing by phone, calculate exact quantities required, and remain wary of "lost prescriptions" or other signs of medication misuse. To justify continued treatment, the patient should demonstrate a decrement in anxiety, with enhanced performance or decreased avoidant behavior.

Side Effects and Dependence. Side effects with BZDs include *sedation* (especially in combination with alcohol or other sedative agents), *impaired memory* acquisition (including *amnesia* reported with single-dose triazolam use), and occasionally *disinhibition,* characterized by increased hostility or aggression. Alcohol and cimetidine slow hepatic BZD metabolism and increase risk of toxicity.

Daily use of BZDs over time leads to receptor adaptation (tolerance) and the development of *physical dependence*. Physical dependence does not, however, imply misuse, abuse, or even loss of benefit. Rather, dependence denotes that a discontinuation syndrome will follow abrupt cessation of therapy. *Withdrawal* is usually accompanied by only mild symptoms but may include rebound anxiety, involuntary movements, insomnia, psychomotor restlessness, and perceptual changes.

Severe withdrawal symptoms are unlikely unless high doses or a high-potency preparation (especially a short-acting one) has been used daily for a prolonged time period and then halted abruptly. In such cases, a *delirium tremens*-like syndrome may develop. *Seizures* have been reported after sudden discontinuation of alprazolam after as short a time as 1 to 2 months of maintenance therapy. For less potent or long-acting BZDs, the risk of a severe abstinence syndrome is less. Chronic daily treatment is best discontinued by tapering doses over several weeks.

BZD overuse is uncommon in the absence of a past history of alcohol or drug abuse but can be a serious problem, at times a consequence of careless prescribing practices and inadequate patient education about proper drug use. If dose requirements escalate, especially if accompanied by addictive behaviors, referral is advised to those experienced in treating this problem.

Selection of Agent. The available BZDs appear equally effective for the management of generalized anxiety symptoms when equipotent doses are used. In the future, one may see new BZDs with greater treatment specificity, because heterogeneity of brain BZD receptors has been demonstrated. For now, the essential differences among BZDs are in potency and pharmacokinetics (Table 226–4). These factors determine suitability for single-dose and maintenance usages as well as risk of physical dependence and withdrawal.

For single-dose use, the salient pharmacokinetic issues are rate of onset and offset. Speed of absorption from the gastrointestinal tract is the most important factor determining onset. Capacity to traverse the blood–brain barrier is also a factor; the more lipophilic, the more quickly the drug enters the central nervous system (CNS). Lipophilicity also governs rate of clinical offset by determining how rapidly the drug is redistributed into lipid stores after a single dose. Serum half-life is not relevant to duration of action of single-dose use. Diazepam is rapidly absorbed and very lipid soluble, giving rapid onset and offset when used in single-dose fashion. Prazepam is the slowest in onset. Relatively rapid onset is usually desirable in situations in which single-dose use is prescribed.

For maintenance use, a drug's serum half-life is the pertinent parameter. It is affected by liver function and whether hepatic metabolites are active or inactive. Drugs with a short half-life are simply converted to water-soluble glucuronides and rapidly cleared by the kidneys. Their disadvantage is the potential for anxiousness and even mild withdrawal symptoms between doses. The longer half-life agents are more likely to accumulate. However, because of the development of drug tolerance, there is little additional risk of clinically important CNS suppression among most users of long-acting agents. The exceptions are the elderly and those with hepatocellular disease, in whom use of long-acting agents can lead to overwhelming drug accumulation that causes excessive sedation, drowsiness, and psychomotor impairment.

Determination of Dosage. Dosage must ultimately be determined empirically on a case-by-case basis. It is most prudent to begin with low doses and titrate up as necessary. Most patients suffering from anxiety of lesser intensity than panic will not benefit from doses greater than 6 mg per day of lorazepam or its equivalent. Starting doses should typically not exceed the equivalent of 2 mg per day of lorazepam in young, otherwise healthy adults who are BZD-naive. In the elderly, starting and maximum doses should be approximately halved (see below). Steady state takes longer to achieve using drugs with a long half-life, an important consideration when deciding how often to adjust dose. A clini-

Table 226-4. Pharmacokinetic Properties of Commonly Used Benzodiazepines

DRUG	APPROXIMATE DOSE EQUIVALENCE (MG)	RELATIVE RAPIDITY OF EFFECT	HALF-LIFE (H)
Alprazolam (Xanax)	0.5	Fast/Intermediate	6–20
Chlordiazepoxide (Librium)	10	Intermediate	5–30
Clonazepam (Klonipin)	0.25	Fast/Intermediate	18–50
Clorazepate (Tranxene)	7.5	Fast	30–200
Diazepam (Valium)	5	Fastest	20–100
Lorazepam (Ativan)	1	Intermediate	10–20
Oxazepam (Serax)	15	Slower	5–15
Prazepam (Centrax)	10	Slowest	30–200

cally useful rule of thumb is that steady state is 90 percent achieved after five drug half-lives.

Antidepressants. *Tricyclic antidepressants* (TCAs), *monoamine oxidase inhibitors* (MAOIs), and *serotonin re-uptake inhibitors* (SRIs) all have their place as first-line agents in the treatment of anxiety. They are among the most effective agents at eradicating the core symptoms of such anxiety conditions as *panic disorder, PTSD,* and *OCD.* As in depression, their beneficial effects are usually delayed for several weeks (see Chapter 227). Although they are "first-line" in terms of their efficacy, therapy is often initiated with BZDs to offer some immediate relief. Concurrently, or after anxiety symptoms are attenuated, antidepressant medication may be added. Once the antidepressant agent has become effective, some patients become entirely asymptomatic. In such instances, the BZD may be tapered and even discontinued.

Treatment of anxiety disorders with antidepressants is initiated with very low doses (eg, imipramine, 10 mg qd; fluoxetine, 5 mg qd) because brief symptom exacerbation may occur in a substantial minority of patients. Full antidepressant doses, if tolerated, may later become necessary.

In the case of panic disorder, TCAs as well as MAOIs have been shown to be effective, and there is a growing body of evidence supporting the use of SRIs. These agents may also be of utility in the treatment of generalized anxiety disorder if panic attacks are present.

PTSD is best treated with TCAs initially, with continuation based on treatment response and the constellation of symptoms. OCD responds well to selective serotonergic reuptake inhibitors. There is some suggestion that the obsessions respond preferentially to these agents, whereas compulsions are best addressed through behavioral interventions combined with medications. MAOIs have been shown to be effective in the treatment of social phobia.

Buspirone is a nonbenzodiazepine anxiolytic that acts as a partial serotonergic agonist and has mild anxiolytic and antidepressant effects. Because of its benign side effect profile (nonaddicting and no withdrawal), buspirone is a reasonable alternative to BZDs in cases where chronic anxiolysis is required, especially when substance abuse or noncompliance is a concern. Risk from overdose is low, and the drug is well tolerated. Its anxiolytic effects are modest compared to those of the BZDs, and onset of action may take weeks, rendering the drug ineffective for single-dose use and of little help to patients with severe symptoms. Some efficacy has been reported in OCD. As a mild anxiolytic that may be taken frequently and safely, it may benefit patients with mild generalized anxiety or adjustment disorders. Treatment is initiated at doses of 5 mg tid and adjusted weekly in dose increments of 5 mg up to a maximum of 20 mg tid.

Beta-Blockers. Beta-adrenergic blocking agents blunt the peripheral catecholamine-mediated manifestations of anxiety. As such, they are very useful on an as-needed basis for *performance anxiety* and stage fright. For this indication, a typical program is use of *propranolol* 10 mg as needed, up to four times daily. The dose may be advanced gradually to a maximum daily total of 80 mg in divided doses. In the case of a special performance, it is suggested that the patient try a test dose a few days earlier to determine both efficacy and side effects. Large doses may blunt psychomotor responses. For generally anxious patients with prominent somatic manifestations of adrenergic excess (eg, tremor, palpitations), beta-blockers facilitate symptom control when used alone or in combination with BZDs. They should be used with caution, if at all, in patients with asthma, heart failure, or heart block (see Chapters 32 and 48). Moreover, they may worsen symptoms if there is an underlying depression (see Chapter 227).

Anxiolytic Pharmacotherapy in the Elderly. Because drug metabolism is slowed in the elderly, excessive sedation is a risk with anxiolytic therapy, especially with use of long-acting agents.

Benzodiazepines. In most instances, nighttime use of a short-acting agent that has no active metabolites and whose metabolism is relatively unaffected by aging is preferred. *Lorazepam* and *oxazepam* fulfill these requirements. Their elimination by hepatic conjugation to a water-soluble glucuronide for renal excretion changes little with age. Lorazepam is the faster in onset; oxazepam's onset is gradual. Their disadvantages include the need for frequent dosing if continuous anxiolysis is desired and rebound anxiety and insomnia if discontinued abruptly after prolonged use. Initial oxazepam dose is 10 mg; for lorazepam, it is 0.5 mg. Both are usually given before bed. Intake should be limited to short (5- to 10-day) courses or occasional as-needed use.

For more sustained anxiolysis, a BZD with a longer effective half-life may be required (see Table 226–4). However, elimination of active drug metabolites lengthens with age, markedly prolonging drug half-life (eg, from 20–90 hours for diazepam). Accumulation of active metabolites can cause diminished alertness and impair memory acquisition, mimicking dementia. Excessive sedation may cause a fall with serious injury—risk of hip fracture rises markedly with use of long-acting BZDs in the elderly. Initial doses should be small (eg, the equivalent of 2–5 mg/d of diazepam) and increased slowly and cautiously. It may take up to 2 weeks to achieve steady-state levels following a change in dosage.

Neuroleptics. In the elderly, anxiety accompanied by agitation or specific psychotic manifestations may require short-term neuroleptic therapy. A small dose of a high-potency agent such as *haloperidol* (Haldol) or *fluphenazine* (Prolixin) is preferred. Lower potency agents (eg, chlorpromazine, thioridizine, perphenazine) necessitate use of higher doses and increase the risk of hypotensive, cardiovascular, and anticholinergic side effects.

Antidepressants. Of the antidepressants, the nontricyclic agents (*MAOIs, SRIs*) are the best tolerated (see Chapter 227). Of the TCIs with anxiolytic activity, those with low anticholinergic and antiadrenergic side effects (eg, *nortriptyline*) are preferred. Because antidepressant metabolism slows with age, one should start with half the usual dose and titrate up slowly.

Beta-Blockers. Beta-blocker use requires particular caution, given the prevalence of congestive heart failure, heart block, and obstructive lung disease in the elderly as well as their susceptibility to such side effects as nightmares, cognitive blunting, and depression.

THERAPEUTIC RECOMMENDATIONS AND INDICATIONS FOR REFERRAL

General Guidelines

- Begin with supportive psychotherapy that includes explanation, empathic listening, meaningful reassurance, guidance, and encouragement.
- Teach relaxation techniques for the patient willing to use them (see Appendix).
- Consider referral for insight-oriented therapy when there is emotional upheaval or disabling symptoms.
- Supplement psychotherapeutic measures with anxiolytic drug therapy to improve the patient's ability to perform daily activities previously impaired by anxiety. In most instances, use only in an adjunctive role for a limited duration. If benzodiazepine therapy is used, advise of the risk of physical dependence. Inform that drug treatment is likely to reduce symptoms but not eradicate them.
- Refer if there is evidence of substance abuse, either as an etiologic factor or as a mode of self-treatment.

Situational Anxiety and Adjustment Disorder

- Initiate supportive psychotherapy and behavioral therapy, including identification of specific provocative stressors and their association with the onset of symptoms.
- If distress from anxiety impairs daily functioning, begin a short course (up to 5 days) of BZD therapy (eg, oxazepam 1 mg tid).
- If the distress represents one of many such episodes in a pattern of emotional upheaval, refer for insight-oriented therapy. Also refer if symptoms endure beyond the stressful period or worsen despite treatment.

Generalized Anxiety Disorder

- Initiate supportive psychotherapy and consider insight-oriented therapy to help diminish the role of psychosocial stressors.
- Consider a short course of BZD therapy for periods of exacerbation (eg, *lorazepam* 1 mg tid for up to 5 days).
- Prescribe a TCA or MAOI if there is a history of associated panic attacks or depression (eg, begin with *imipramine* 10 mg qhs and advance dose as tolerated).
- Avoid chronic BZD therapy due to risk of dependency. If the patient is coming off long-term therapy, taper over several weeks according to the patient's ability to tolerate decreases. Monitor for any withdrawal symptoms (eg, tinnitus, perceptual changes, involuntary movements).
- Consider a trial of *buspirone* if chronic anxiolytic therapy is desired. Begin with 5 mg tid and gradually advance to a maximum of 60 mg qd. Risks of physiologic dependence and withdrawal are nil, but potency is low and it may take weeks to notice any effect.
- Refer patients with disabling chronic anxiety for psychiatric care.

Panic Disorder

- Use pharmacologic therapy to achieve control and minimize phobic avoidance and depression.
- Screen for suicidality (see Chapter 227), especially if patient is despondent; refer urgently if there is concern. Otherwise, begin therapy with a small "test" dose of a tricyclic antidepressant (eg, *imipramine,* 10–25 mg qhs) or a serotonin re-uptake inhibitor (eg, *fluoxetine,* 5–10 mg daily). If agitation is not increased, proceed gradually to full antidepressant doses (eg, imipramine 100–200 mg qhs; fluoxetine, 20–60 mg daily).
- Alternatively, an MAOI antidepressant may be prescribed, but dietary restriction and expertise in its use are required (see Chapter 227).
- If rapid relief is sought due to presence of disabling phobic behavior, start with a potent BZD (eg, *alprazolam* 0.25–0.5 mg qid, or *clonazepam* 0.5 mg qhs or bid), pending onset of benefit from antidepressant therapy.
- After a period of well-being, taper BZD medication to the lowest possible maintenance dose or proceed to discontinuation.
- Weigh continued BZD use against risk of dependence. Use of potent BZDs poses risks of dependence and severe withdrawal. Taper slowly over several weeks when discontinuing therapy that has been continuous for more than 6 weeks.
- Refer patients with prominent phobic behavior, as well as those with suicidal ideation.
- For patients requiring longer-term maintenance therapy, consider lower doses of antidepressant medication.

Social Phobias

- Refer for behavioral therapy.
- Prescribe a BZD on an as-needed, single-dose basis to help attenuate anxiety, decrease avoidance, and facilitate daily functioning and behavioral therapy.
- Refer for consideration of MAOI therapy if behavioral therapy supplemented by BZD use is unsuccessful, depressive symptoms are present, or social settings precipitate panic.
- For patients whose performances are compromised by ordinary "stage fright," consider a trial of a beta-blocker (eg, *propranolol* 10 mg, up to 20 mg qid) on an as-needed basis. Give a preperformance trial dose to be sure performance is not compromised by the medication.

Simple Phobias

- Refer for behavioral therapy.
- Consider rapidly acting, single-dose BZD therapy (eg, alprazolam 0.25–0.5 mg or diazepam 10 mg) on an as-needed basis to provide symptomatic control in anxiety-provoking situations and to facilitate behavioral therapy.

Obsessive-Compulsive Disorder

- Begin behavioral therapy.
- Initiate pharmacologic therapy with an SRI (eg, *fluoxetine* 20 mg qd); titrate up to doses as high as 120 mg daily.
- Refer to an experienced psychopharmacologist for further management of the drug treatment program.

Posttraumatic Stress Disorder

- Refer to a psychiatrist specializing in the treatment of such persons. Most programs begin with a TCA or SRI. BZDs, MAOIs, and anticonvulsants are used in adjunctive fashion. Insight-oriented psychotherapy helps to overcome emotional memories of the traumatic event; behavioral techniques may also be of benefit.

Treatment of the Elderly

- Reduce starting doses of medications by one-half.
- When using BZDs for short-term anxiolysis, prescribe *lorazepam* or *oxazepam*. For chronic anxiolysis, use longer half-life agents with caution and at reduced doses and dose intervals.
- If antidepressants are indicated for anxiolysis, consider an *SRI* (eg, fluoxetine) or an *MAOI* (see Chapter 227).
- If agitation, "sun-downing," or psychotic features accompany anxiety, prescribe small doses of a potent neuroleptic (eg, *haloperidol,* 0.5 mg once or twice daily).

ANNOTATED BIBLIOGRAPHY

American Psychiatric Association. Diagnostic and statistical manual of mental disorders, 3rd ed, Revised. Washington DC: American Psychiatric Association, 1987. *(The standard for diagnosis.)*

Clinical Psychopharmacology Unit of Massachusetts General Hospital. Panic disorder and treatment decisions: Beyond the short term. J Clin Psychiatry 1990;51(12 suppl A):1. *(Comprehensive review of issues pertinent to long-term management.)*

Feighner JP. Buspirone in the long-term treatment of generalized anxiety disorder. J Clin Psychiatry 1987;48(12 suppl):3. *(May have some role in persons with mild chronic disease.)*

Greenblatt DJ, Shades RI, Abernethy DR. Current status of benzodiazepines. N Engl J Med 1983;309:354. *(A classic two-part review; best discussion of clinically germane pharmacokinetics.)*

Issues in the clinical use of alprazolam. J Clin Psychiatry 1993; 54(10 suppl 10):1. *(An entire journal volume devoted to use of this potent BZD.)*

Kane JM. The current status of neuroleptic therapy. J Clin Psychiatry 1989;50:9. *(A detailed review of issues associated with their use.)*

Katon WJ, ed. Panic disorder: Somatization, medical utilization, and treatment. Am J Med 1992;92(suppl)1A. *(An entire issue devoted to the topic; focuses on somatic manifestations and treatment.)*

Markovitz PJ. Treatment of anxiety in the elderly. J Clin Psychiatry 54(5 suppl):64. *(A review of the special considerations related to treatment of anxiety in the elderly.)*

Marshall JR. Social phobia. An overview of treatment strategies. J Clin Psychiatry 1993;54:165. *(Critical review of approaches to therapy.)*

Ray WA, Griffin MR, Downey W. Benzodiazepines of long and short elimination half-life and the risk of hip fracture. JAMA 1989;262:3303. *(Increased risk with use of long-acting agents.)*

Roy-Byrne PR, Hommer D. Benzodiazepine withdrawal: Overview and implications for the treatment of anxiety. Am J Med 1988;84:1041. *(Detailed review; recommends avoiding long-term use if possible.)*

Silver JM, Sandberg DP, Hales RE. New approaches in the pharmacotherapy of post-traumatic stress disorder. J Clin Psychiatry 1990;51(10 suppl):33. *(Review of pharmacologic strategies in the treatment of PTSD.)*

Tesar GE, Rosenbaum JF, Pollack MH, et al. Double-blind, placebo-controlled comparison of clonazepam and alprazolam for panic disorder. J Clin Psychiatry 1991;52:69-76. *(Clonazepam comparable to alprazolam.)*

Weissman MM, Klerman GL, Markowitz JS, et al. Suicidal ideation and suicide attempts in panic disorder and attacks. N Engl J Med 1989;321:1209. *(Risk increased and independent of other possible precipitants—adjusted odds ratio 2.6)*

Wise MG, Rieck SO. Diagnostic consideration and treatment approaches to underlying anxiety in the medically ill. J Clin Psychiatry 1993;54(5 suppl):22. *(Evaluation and treatment in the face of comorbid medical illness.)*

Appendix: Strategies for Stress Management

William E. Minichiello, Ed.D.

Stress is not harmful when managed effectively. With the increased awareness of the impact of stress on the body has come a variety of stress-reducing techniques derived from behavior therapy. Stress management training enables the patient to condition his or her body to cope more adaptively with stress or anxiety. As part of a comprehensive treatment program, the primary care physician may choose to train the patient in one or more of the self-regulatory procedures. Relaxation training is by far the most effective of the procedures.

Before proceeding to train the patient in relaxation as a self-control procedure, the physician should advise reduction or elimination of caffeine from the patient's diet, because relaxation training is aimed at lowering the patient's autonomic arousal level and caffeine augments arousal.

Progressive deep muscle relaxation, autogenic training, and diaphragmatic breathing represent the major techniques practical for use in the primary care setting.

Progressive Deep Muscle Relaxation

Progressive deep muscle relaxation is probably the most extensively used and most effective relaxation technique today for the treatment of anxiety and stress-related problems. A brief, modified version can be taught to the patient in one session. The rationale for the technique is the view that anxiety and relaxation are mutually exclusive; that is, anxiety cannot be experienced when the muscles are relaxed.

Progressive deep muscle relaxation is a simple procedure contrasting tension with relaxation. Because a person generally has very little awareness of the sensation of relaxation, he is asked first to tense a set of muscles as hard as he can until he can feel tension in the muscles. Then he allows those muscles to relax and tries to become aware of ("to feel internally") the difference between tension and relaxation.

This relaxation technique entails the systematic focus of attention on specific gross muscle groups throughout the body. The patient is instructed to actively tense each muscle

Progressive Deep Muscle Relaxation

Practice is to be done while sitting in a chair with your back straight, head on a line with your back, both feet on the floor and hands resting on your lap. Each muscle is to be tightened, held in tightened position for 15–20 seconds, and then slowly let go while studying the difference between tension and relaxation.

Forehead. Wrinkle up your forehead by arching your eyebrows and creasing your forehead, hold the tension, and then slowly let go of the tension.

Eyes. Squeeze your eyes together tightly, hold the tension, and then slowly let go of the tension.

Nose. Wrinkle up your nose and spread your nostrils, hold the tension, and then slowly let go of the tension.

Face. Put a forced smile on your face and spread your face, hold the tension, and then slowly let go of the tension.

Tongue. Push your tongue hard against the roof of your mouth, hold the tension, and then slowly let go of the tension.

Jaws. Clench your jaws together tightly, hold the tension, and then slowly let go of the tension.

Lips. Pucker up your lips and spread them, hold the tension, and then slowly let go of the tension.

Neck. Tighten the muscles of your neck by pulling your chin in and shrugging up your shoulders, hold the tension, and then slowly let go of the tension.

Right Arm. Tense your right arm and hand by stretching it out in front of you and clenching your fist tightly, hold the tension, and then slowly let go of the tension.

Left Arm. Tense your left arm and hand by stretching it out in front of you, and then slowly let go of the tension.

Right Leg. Extend your right leg in front of you (at the height of the chair seat), tense your thigh and leg by pointing your toes inward toward your face, hold the tension, and then slowly let go of the tension.

Left Leg. Extend your left leg in front of you, tense your thigh and leg by pointing your toes inward toward your face, hold the tension, and then slowly let go of the tension.

Upper Back. Tense your back muscles by sitting slightly forward in the chair, bending your elbows and trying to get them to touch each other behind your back, hold the tension, and then slowly let go of the tension.

Chest. Tense your chest muscles by pulling your stomach in and thrusting your chest upward and outward, hold the tension, and then slowly let go of the tension.

Stomach. Tense your stomach muscles, making them hard by pushing your stomach out, hold the tension, and then slowly let go of the tension.

Buttocks and Thighs. Tense your buttocks and thighs by placing your feet squarely on the floor, pointing your toes into the floor and forcing your heels to remain on the floor while pushing forward, hold the tension, and then slowly let go of the tension.

Practice should be engaged in twice daily for a period of 12–15 minutes. Mastery of the technique is after 2–4 weeks of twice daily practice.

Figure 226-1. Instructions to patients.

group for 10 to 15 seconds, after which he is told to let go of the tension in the muscles, observe the difference, and relax the muscles. The sequence of tensing the muscles, letting go of the tension, and noting the difference between tension and relaxation is systematically applied to a host of muscle groups starting at the head and ending at the toes (Fig. 226–1).

Autogenic Training

Autogenic training is a relaxation technique composed of a set of exercises that are intended to induce heaviness and warmth in the muscles through mental imagery.

Autogenic training typically involves the patient sitting comfortably in an armchair in a quiet room with his eyes closed. Verbal formulae are introduced (eg, "my arm is heavy"), and the patient is instructed to visualize and feel the relaxation of the muscle being focused on while silently repeating and passively concentrating on that formula. The formulas, which consist of verbal somatic suggestions, are intended to facilitate concentration and "mental contact" with the parts of the body indicated by the formula.

Training consists of six psychophysiologic exercises, which are practiced several times a day. The training begins with the theme of heaviness (eg, "my arm feels heavy and relaxed"). The second group of formulas involve warmth (eg, "my arm feels warm and relaxed"). Following warmth training, the patient continues with passive concentration on cardiac activity (eg, "my heartbeat feels calm and regular"). The fourth exercise focuses on breathing and respiration. In the next exercise, the patient focuses on warmth in the chest and abdomen, and in the last exercise the focus is passive concentration on cooling of the forehead.

In modern practice, the time and the six standard exercises have been condensed so that a whole round can be practiced in a very brief period of between 5 and 10 minutes.

Autogenic Training

Practice is to be done while sitting in a soft, comfortable chair with your eyes closed. As attention is called to specific groups of muscles, try to *visualize* and *feel* the relaxation of those muscles. Try to let *happen* what is being suggested. Repeat each formula 2–3 times.

My forehead and scalp feel heavy, limp, loose, and relaxed.

My eyes and nose feel heavy, limp, loose, and relaxed.

My face and jaws feel heavy, limp, loose, and relaxed.

My neck, shoulders, and back feel heavy, limp, loose, and relaxed.

My arms and hands feel heavy, limp, loose, and relaxed.

My chest, solar plexus, and the central part of my body feel quiet, calm, comfortable, and relaxed.

My stomach feels heavy, limp, loose, and relaxed.

My buttocks, thighs, calves, ankles, and toes feel quiet, heavy, limp, loose, and relaxed.

My whole body feels quiet, heavy, limp, and relaxed.

Practice should be engaged in twice daily for a period of 6–8 minutes. Mastery of the technique is after 1–3 weeks of twice daily practice.

Figure 226-2. Instructions to patients.

In this condensed version, the autogenic training phrases are focused primarily on the physiologic aspect used in the training, interspersed with general suggestions for relaxation. Each phrase is said slowly, allowing time for the patient to begin to feel some awareness of the effect of the suggestion (Fig. 226–2).

Diaphragmatic Breathing

The quickest and simplest method of relaxation is to breathe slowly and deeply from the belly. Diaphragmatic breathing is an effective means of coping with and reducing stress.

For centuries, students of yoga and zen have been aware that a mastery of breathing could slow heart rate, lower blood pressure, and calm the body. Diaphragmatic breathing involves parasympathetic nervous system stimulation. Diaphragmatic breathing prevents the possibility of hyperventilation and, after 50 to 60 seconds of such breathing, brings a feeling of quiescence to the body and reduction in bodily symptoms of stress.

Training in diaphragmatic breathing can be done either sitting or lying down. In either position, a pillow should be placed at the small of the back to force the belly out. Breathing should begin by pushing the stomach out as inhalation takes place slowly and deeply. Care should be taken to minimize the movement of the chest with each inhalation. The word "relax" should be said silently before exhaling, and the stomach should fall with exhalation. While breathing *in,* the stomach should be pushed *out;* while breathing *out,* the stomach should come *in* (Fig. 226–3).

Diaphragmatic Breathing

While sitting or lying down with a pillow at the small of your back

1. Breathe in slowly and deeply by pushing your stomach out.
2. Say the word "relax" silently to yourself prior to exhaling.
3. Exhale slowly, letting your stomach come in.
4. Repeat entire procedure 10 times consecutively, with emphasis on slow, deep breaths.

Practice should take place 5 times per day, 10 consecutive diaphragmatic breaths each sitting. Time for mastery is after 1–2 weeks of daily practice.

Figure 226-3. Instructions to patients.

Primary Care Medicine: Office Evaluation and Management of the Adult Patient, 3rd edition, edited by Allan H. Goroll, Lawrence A. May, and Albert G. Mulley, Jr. J.B. Lippincott Company, Philadelphia

227

Approach to the Patient With Depression

SCOTT L. RAUCH, M.D.
STEVEN E. HYMAN, M.D.

The vast majority of patients with depression present to primary care physicians, often complaining of somatic symptoms. The frequency, treatability, and potentially serious consequences of depression make its diagnosis and management high priorities for the primary care physician. Unfortunately, the diagnosis is not always evident because the symptoms may masquerade as a variety of psychiatric or somatic conditions. Moreover, the stigma of psychiatric diagnosis can impede recognition of depressive illness by both patients and physicians.

PATHOPHYSIOLOGY AND CLINICAL PRESENTATION

Pathogenesis and Pathophysiology

The psychodynamic origins of depression are believed to involve difficulties with formation and maintenance of self-esteem, which may occur from having hypercritical parents or being abused. In addition, growing up in an emotionally unresponsive environment may compromise learning ways to effectively cope with situational stresses. Suffering loss or failure as an adult is likely to be difficult, poorly responded to, and capable of reawakening prior painful feelings of inadequacy and worthlessness that lead to depression. Rigid, dysfunctional defenses may be erected in an attempt to minimize the chances of loss or failure.

The cognitive perspective views depression as the consequence rather than as the origin of negative or distorted thinking. Subscribing to inflexible rules of conduct and unattainable goals can be a setup for failure and loss of self-esteem. Setbacks are viewed as a reflection of one's unworthiness and inadequacy.

Genetic determinants have been discovered from studies of twins, chromosomes, and pedigrees. In some pedigrees, there appears to be a dominant gene with incomplete penetrance. A family history of affective disease is commonly elicited. Major depression is up to three times more common among first-degree relatives of people with the disorder than in the general population.

Neurotransmitter basis of depression began with the finding that reserpine could induce depression and monoamine oxidase inhibitors could reverse it. This led to the identification of altered neurotransmitter metabolism as an important biochemical concomitant of depression and to the discovery of new antidepressant drugs, each increasing the availability of a major central neurotransmitter (eg, norepinephrine, serotonin, or acetylcholine), usually by selective inhibition of reuptake.

Neuroendocrine hypotheses derive from the observation that most neurovegetative manifestations of depression (changes in appetite, libido, diurnal rhythms) involve hypothalamic functions. In addition, links between neurotransmitter release and neurohormone activity have been identified. Corticotropic-releasing hormone is believed to play an important role, resulting in hypercortisolism. Early morning awakening, reflecting an abnormal advance in circadian rhythm, may be one consequence.

Depression most likely represents a complex combination of these elements. Genetic factors and/or early childhood experiences may render persons more susceptible to depression. Neurotransmitter and neurohumoral elements probably serve as important effector pathways for development of symptoms.

Psychological and Somatic Manifestations

Depression's clinical presentation includes a host of psychological and bodily complaints.

Psychological Manifestations. Sadness is the cardinal symptom. Irritability, discouragement, loss of interest, worry, frustration, and complete lack of libido or other pleasures (anhedonia) comprise the major dysphoric manifestations and may occur in the absence of overt sadness (Table 227–1). Some become preoccupied with physical complaints, such as pain or bowel dysfunction. Others exhibit changes in memory, concentration, or self-image. Diurnal mood variation is characteristic, with symptoms often worse in the morning and improving as the day progresses.

Depressed affect can be subtle, at times only noticed when sadness ensues from talking with the patient. As depression worsens, psychomotor abnormalities may appear. *Psychomotor retardation,* with slowed speech and a long latency before the patient answers questions, is characteristic. In some patients, the picture is one of agitation, with rapid speech and an anxious rather than sad affect.

Somatic Manifestations. Distinctive neurovegetative symptoms include disturbed sleep (most commonly *early-morning awakening*), *lack of energy*, and *decreased appetite*. In atypical depressions, patients may exhibit increased sleep and hyperphagia. Neurovegetative symptoms are predictive of responsiveness to psychopharmacologic intervention.

Diagnostic Classification

While no single classification system is universally accepted, the current standard of diagnosis in the United States is the American Psychiatric Association's Diagnostic and Statistical Manual, Third Edition, Revised (DSM III-R; Table 227–2).

Table 227-1. Clinical Presentation of Depressive Syndromes

Psychological Symptoms and Signs	
	Mood sad, "blue," "down"
	Depressed affect
	Anxiety
	Irritability or anger
	Anhedonia (lack of pleasure)
	Loss of interest in environment
	Loss of interest in activities
	Loss of interest in sex (decreased libido)
	Social withdrawal
	Guilt (may be delusional)
	Poor self-esteem
	Self-deprecatory thoughts
	Poor concentration or indecisiveness
	Rumination or obsessive thoughts
	Multiple physical complaints or hypochondrial fears
	Feelings of helplessness or hopelessness
	Recurrent thoughts of death or suicide
	Psychotic symptoms (eg, delusions or hallucinations)
Neurovegetative Symptoms and Signs	
	Sleep disturbance (usually early morning awakening)
	Decreased energy
	Appetite disturbance (usually decreased)
	Diurnal mood variation (usually worse in morning)
	Psychomotor retardation or agitation

Table 227-2. Classification of Depressive Syndromes

Major Affective Disorders

Major Depression (unipolar depression)
- Severe and episodic with prominent neurovegetative signs and symptoms
- Atypical presentations may include cognitive difficulties, chronic pain, or hypochondriasis
- May be accompanied by psychotic features

Treatment: antidepressant plus psychotherapy

Bipolar Disorder (manic-depressive illness)
- Severe and episodic, with a history of a manic episode
- Depressed phase is clinically identical to major depression
- May be accompanied by psychotic features

Treatment: lithium (plus an antidepressant in depressed phase), plus psychotherapy

Chronic Affective Disorders

Dysthymic Disorder
- Chronic and less severe, with fewer neurovegetative symptoms
- Frequently accompanied by personality disorder

Treatment: psychotherapy plus trial of antidepressant if vegetative symptoms are distressing

Cyclothymic Disorder
- Less severe, chronic mood swings

Treatment: lithium plus psychotherapy

Organic Brain Syndromes

Organic Affective Disorder
- Depression or mania due to an organic cause

Treatment: manage underlying medical problem; a trial of antidepressant if necessary

Other Conditions

Adjustment Disorder With Depressed Mood
- Time limited, in response to identifiable precipitant, without vegetative symptoms sufficient for major depression

Treatment: psychotherapy plus a trial of antidepressant if neurovegetative symptoms are distressing

Major depression (unipolar depression) is the DSM III-R term for serious depression that is accompanied by neurovegetative symptoms. Lifetime risk of developing a major depression is estimated to be one in four. Dysphoric mood typically dominates the clinical picture and is persistent. Four or more of the major neurovegetative symptoms dominate the clinical picture and are present for a minimum of 2 weeks, including appetite disturbance, sleep disturbance, psychomotor retardation or agitation, anhedonia, loss of energy, feelings of worthlessness or guilt, decreased concentration, and suicidal thoughts.

Onset is variable. Symptoms usually develop over weeks to months, but they may develop suddenly. Situational factors surrounding the onset of the illness have no bearing on the diagnosis. Historically, distinctions were made between *endogenous* and *reactive depression*, but an identifiable precipitant is no longer considered pertinent with respect to diagnosis.

Frequency of episodes appears to increase with age. At least half of patients have recurrent episodes. A *family history* of a major affective disorder (major depression or bipolar disorder) is common. The relationship between *alcoholism* and depression remains controversial.

Major depression with psychotic features is a subclassification of major depression, having the additional features of delusions, hallucinations, bizarre behavior, or disorganized thinking.

Major depression in the Elderly. In the elderly, depression can mimic dementia. The patient may appear withdrawn, unkempt, inattentive, or even confused. The condition may be due to depression alone or to a combination of depression and dementia.

Bipolar Disorder-Depressed Phase. The presentation of bipolar (*manic–depressive*) disease is identical to that of major depression, except there is a history of prior manic or hypomanic episodes. *Mania* is manifested by periods of elation or expansive mood, increased energy, decreased need for sleep, inflated self-esteem, and over-involvement in activities, accompanied by a decreased concern for the consequences. Its diagnosis requires adequate severity to substantially impair level of functioning. If the hallmark symptoms of mania exist, but the patient shows no decrement in functioning, the patient is described as *hypomanic*.

Distinguishing between unipolar and bipolar depressions is therapeutically important (see below).

Dysthymic disorder refers to a chronic low-grade depression, characterized by pervasive dysphoric mood for at least 6 months. Some complain of life-long feelings of depression. Symptoms are less severe than those of major depression and neurovegetative symptoms are fewer. Depression appears as an integral part of their character (hence the older term *characterologic depression*). Such patients can be frustrating to treat because of chronic dysphoria, self-pity, and development of irrational patterns of negative thinking (eg, "things always go wrong for me"). The physician typically develops feelings of helplessness and may unconsciously communicate a wish that the patient would go away.

Typically, onset is in adolescence or early adult life and accompanied by other symptoms of a *personality disorder*, such as a history of difficulty with interpersonal relationships, manipulativeness, feelings of emptiness, and lack of an identity.

A subpopulation of dysthymic patients seem to have an attenuated chronic form of major depression with onset later in life after a period of good functioning. Neurovegetative symptoms may be more prominent.

Dysthymia and major depression can coexist in a given patient (so-called "*double depression*"), when a major depressive episode evolves in the context of pre-existing dysthymia. However, incomplete recovery from a major depression should be described as major depression in partial remission, rather than dysthymia.

Cyclothymic disorder resembles bipolar illness, but the mood swings are less severe. These patients have a chronic mood disturbance characterized by periods of depression alternating with periods of elevated mood. Neither are of sufficient severity or duration to meet the criteria for major depressive or manic episodes. Interspersed may be periods of normal mood lasting as long as several months.

Adjustment disorder with depressed mood occurs following a *significant life stress*. Patients usually present with depressed mood associated with feelings of hopelessness, helplessness, worthlessness, and anxiety. Their thoughts are often dominated by the problems that precipitated the episode. Sleep and appetite disturbances are common, but are less severe and less persistent than in major depression. The condition is usually self-limited, lasting less than 6 months, and improving when the stress is removed or the individual evolves a more adaptive coping mechanism. Any patient with symptoms severe enough to meet the criteria for major depression (described above) should receive that diagnosis regardless of the history of a precipitant.

Seasonal Affective Disorder (SAD). This depressive condition is distinguished by its seasonal pattern, characteristically beginning in the fall and ending about 5 months later. It has been linked to lack of light exposure and is more common in northern latitudes. Alterations in serotonin activity have also been noted. As in other forms of depression, sadness is the dominant affect, and fatigue and decreased libido are common. Atypical features include tendencies to overeat and oversleep. In the U.S., women are more commonly affected than men (ratio is 3:1). Age of onset is typically in the 20s.

DIFFERENTIAL DIAGNOSIS

It is important to consider organic causes of depression, including drug-related etiologies, which are among the most common (Table 227–3). Chronic feelings of fatigue and dysphoria are non-specific symptoms common to multiple medical conditions. Their differential diagnosis includes *chronic fatigue syndrome, Lyme disease, fibromyalgia, rheumatoid disease,* and *endocrinopathies* (see Chapter 8). In addition, several psychiatric disorders can masquerade as depression.

Uncomplicated Bereavement. Symptoms of normal grief may initially be identical to those of depression. The question of a superimposed depression should be raised if mourning continues for more than 6 months, if neurovegetative symptoms are particularly severe, if there is severe impairment in the patient's ability to function, or if psychotic symptoms emerge.

Table 227-3. Organic Etiologies of Depression

Drug Induced: alpha-methyldopa, antiarrhythmics, benzodiazepines, barbiturates and other CNS depressants, beta-blockers, cholinergic drugs, corticosteroids, digoxin, H_2-blockers, and reserpine.

Substance Abuse Related: alcohol abuse, sedative-hypnotic abuse, cocaine and other psychostimulant withdrawal.

Toxic-Metabolic Disorders: hypothyroidism or hyperthyroidism (especially in elderly), Cushing's syndrome, hypercalcemia, hyponatremia, and diabetes mellitus.

Neurologic Disorders: stroke, subdural hematoma, multiple sclerosis, brain tumor, Parkinson's disease, Huntington's disease, epilepsy, and dementias.

Infectious Disorders: viral infections (especially mononucleosis and influenza), HIV with or without AIDS, and syphilis.

Nutritional Disorders: vitamin B_{12} deficiency and pellagra.

Other: carcinomas (especially pancreatic carcinoma) and postsurgically (especially cardiac surgery).

Alcoholism and Drug Dependence. Many alcoholic patients appear depressed. It is not possible to delineate which symptoms are due to alcohol and which, if any, might be due to a primary affective disorder until the patient has been fully detoxified. Other substance abuse disorders may mimic depression, especially abuse of sedative-hypnotics or withdrawal from psychostimulants.

Personality Disorders. These patients frequently complain of depressive symptoms, with periods of severe dysphoria, but their affective symptoms often fluctuate markedly with environmental changes (especially with changes in interpersonal relationships). Poor impulse control, histories of unstable relationships, and a striking quality of manipulativeness or entitlement are other clues to primarily characterologic pathology.

WORKUP

The possibility of depression should always be considered in patients who present with fatigue, poor sleep, appetite disturbances, or multiple bodily complaints as well as when a patient expresses feelings of hopelessness or poor self-esteem. The onset of depressive symptoms and signs in patients with chronic debilitating disorders or chronic pain can be slow and subtle and should not be overlooked.

History. When depression is suspected, specific inquiry into its manifestations is needed. However, before proceeding with the inquiry, it is useful to complete a detailed medical history for "organic" etiologies (including elicitation of specific patient concerns) and to follow later with a detailed physical examination, especially in patients who present complaining of somatic symptomatology. Not to do so risks alienating the patient, who wants his medical complaints taken seriously. Also useful are a few words to explain the rationale for considering depression (eg, "it's a serious, treatable condition and listed as one of the important causes of the symptoms bothering you"). These few simple measures facilitate patient understanding and impart a sense of seriousness and thoroughness to the workup. In addition, they help reduce the stigma of considering a psychiatric diagnosis.

It is helpful and often less threatening to ask first about neurovegetative symptoms such as sleep, appetite, and energy. If the responses are suggestive of depression, one can proceed to inquire about mood and any loss of interest in sex, family, job, and other sources of interest or pleasure. In addition, the patient should be queried about his self-opinion and any self-critical feelings. With every depressed patient, it is critical to ask about suicidal thoughts and intentions (see below). Also useful is exploration of multiple bodily complaints.

Neurovegetative Symptoms. Specific inquiry into these characteristic symptoms is facilitated by the mnemonic "SIG E CAPS":

S - Is your *sleep* disturbed?
I - Have you noted a loss of libido or *interest* in your usual activities?
G - Are you feeling *guilty* or having self-deprecatory thoughts?
E - Have you noticed a decrease in you *energy* level?
C - Have you been having trouble *concentrating*?
A - Have you experienced changes in your *appetite* and weight?
P - Have been physically slowed down or sped up (ie, experienced *psychomotor* abnormalities)?
S - Have you had thoughts of *suicide*, feelings of hopelessness, or preoccupation with issues related to death? (See below for more detail).

Multiple Bodily Complaints and Ruling-Out Organicity. Patients with low energy, dysphoria, and multiple bodily complaints out of proportion to physical findings are likely to have depression, but, as noted earlier, they still require careful consideration of conditions that may present in similar fashion, such as *chronic fatigue syndrome, Lyme disease, fibromyalgia, rheumatoid disease, vasculitis*, and *endocrinopathies* (see Chapter 8 for details of workup).

Confusion and alterations in level of consciousness strongly suggest organicity, although they are not always present. When they are, *drug-induced* etiologies are important to consider. Onset is usually temporally related to medication use and should be sought. Worth noting are any use of *antiarrhythmics, antihypertensives, sedative- hypnotics*, and *corticosteroids*, as well as over-the-counter agents and substances of abuse. The relation of *beta-blockers* to depression remains inconclusive, but risk appears greatest for those that are lipophilic and readily cross the blood-brain barrier. The elderly are particularly susceptible to adverse central nervous system effects from drugs that cross the blood-brain barrier.

Primary neuropathology should be sought when depression is accompanied by an alteration of neurologic function. *Left frontal lobe* involvement by a *mass lesion* or *stroke* may trigger a depressive syndrome. Inquiry into focal signs and symptoms help to differentiate a structural lesion from a functional affective disorder.

In some medical illnesses, depression may dominate the early clinical picture. *Pancreatic cancer* is the archetypal example. Important associated findings should be sought, including profound weight loss, vague upper abdominal discomfort, and onset of painless jaundice (see Chapter 58). *HIV infection* and emergence of *AIDS* are frequently associated with depression. In such cases, the diagnosis may be obscured by comorbid medical illness (see Chapter 13). Also depressive features may mistakenly be conceptualized as normal grief in response to the medical diagnosis and surrounding tragedy.

Psychosocial history should focus on the patient's current home environment, as well as means of financial and emotional support. Does the patient live alone? If not, is the family environment accepting or, conversely, contributing to the patient's discomfort? The availability of responsible family members to observe and supervise the patient might mean the difference between outpatient treatment and hospitalization if the patient is very depressed or debilitated. What are the patient's daily responsibilities and what secondary stressors arise if the patient cannot meet these obligations?

Past Psychiatric History of the Patient and Family. Once the issue of medical etiologies has been put to rest, one should return to eliciting a past psychiatric history. Given depression's tendency to recur, the patient should always be asked about similar episodes in the past. If there is a history of depressive or manic disease, it is important to obtain the details of treatment and treatment response. A history of prior psychosis or suicidality is also important to elicit, because of their risks for recurrence.

Family history can be difficult to elicit because of shame about any mental illness in the family. It helps to explain that depression is thought to run in families because of hereditary biochemical factors, not defects in character. A family history of major depression, bipolar disorder, or suicide supports a diagnosis of depression in the patient. The genetic predispositions for unipolar depression and bipolar illness are distinct.

A family history of other psychiatric diagnoses must be interpreted in the context of changing nomenclature and diagnostic criteria. In the past, mania was frequently misdiagnosed as schizophrenia. "Nervous breakdown" or "going insane" were common, nonspecific terms. If family psychiatric history is present, it is worth reviewing symptoms and attempting a tentative retrospective diagnosis.

Physical Examination. The importance of a careful and detailed physical examination cannot be overemphasized, especially because most depressed patients presenting to primary physicians harbor concerns about medical illness. Specific patient concerns elicited during the history should be explicitly checked for during the physical examination in order to facilitate the provision of meaningful reassurance. (See Chapter 8 for description of the pertinent physical examination.)

Mental Status Examination. Much of the mental status examination can be performed by taking note of the patient's appearance, affect, behavior, and responses during the history. Has the patient's condition interfered with grooming and self-care? Is there sadness, tearfulness, despondency, apathy, irritability, anxiety, or anger? Is there psychomotor retardation or agitation? Does the patient offer anything spontaneously or is there a long period of hesitation before answering (ie, speech latency)? Is the speech slow? Is normal inflection present?

The patient should also be asked explicitly to describe his mood. Thought is assessed for form and content. Is the patient's thought pattern clear and coherent or is it tangential, circumstantial, or nonsensical? Are there ideas of worthlessness, helplessness, hopelessness, guilt, suicidal thought, or homicidality?

Is the patient able to maintain attention? Distractibility may occur in depression, delirium, dementia, or severe anxiety, and will interfere with the patient's overall cognitive performance. Any inattention is worth documenting by testing ability to recall a series of random numbers (digit span). Patients should be able to repeat a series of at least 5 to 7 numbers without error. "I don't know" answers are reflective of apathy or lack of energy associated with depression. Tests of memory, calculation, abstractions and other higher cortical functions should be performed.

Although psychotic depression is uncommon in primary care settings, it is important not to miss this very serious condition. It should be noted whether the patient appears guarded or expresses paranoid thoughts or delusions. Inquiry into any unusual experiences, such as hearing voices or seeing things that other people do not see, provide further evidence of a thought disorder. However, unusual smells, tastes, and tactile experiences suggest an organic brain syndrome.

Evaluation for Suicidality. Depression is a potentially fatal illness. Assessment of suicide risk is an integral part of the workup of every depressed patient. About 15 percent of patients with major affective disorders take their lives. With proper intervention, most suicides can be prevented. Concurrent conditions which might precipitate suicide include chronic alcoholism, personality disorders, and both functional and drug-induced psychoses; delusional beliefs or hallucinations may lead to self-destruction. Predicting a suicide attempt is difficult, even among patients who complain of suicidal thoughts. Assessment of risk is facilitated by specific inquiry.

Technique. Assessing risk of suicide requires attention to the patient's *thoughts* (ideas, wishes, motives), *intent* (the degree to which the patient intends to act on the thoughts), and *plans*. Inquiry necessitates a calm, empathic approach that allows expression of feelings and is free of any implied criticism. On any expression of hopelessness, helplessness, or suffering, one might begin with a rather indirect query (eg, "Are you feeling so badly that sometimes you would prefer not to go on living?"). A positive response is followed by more direct questions about self- destructive thoughts and plans. A well worked out, realistic, and potentially lethal plan suggests great risk, as does the act of putting one's affairs in order.

Asking patients about suicide does not put the idea into their heads. Pitfalls include failure to ask specifically about suicidal thoughts and feelings, and premature interruption of the patient who mentions suicide. Any mention of suicide must be taken seriously and *every* depressed patient must be asked about suicide. It is an error to avoid the subject for fear of doing so. Truly suicidal patients may be relieved to be asked about it.

Mental status, especially the patient's ability to resist suicidal thoughts, is important to consider. An extremely impulsive, psychotic, or intoxicated patient has no meaningful internal controls and will require hospitalization.

Assessment of Risk. There is no simple formula for precisely assessing suicide risk. Attention to thoughts, intent, and plans is essential, facilitated by consideration of mental status and pertinent psychosocial and demographic predictors (Table 227–4). Patients expressing suicidal thoughts, especially if accompanied by intent and plans, or who lack reliable internal controls to resist suicidal impulses, require emergency psychiatric consultation. Such patients should be closely supervised and not allowed to transport themselves. Patients with severe or worsening depression who have thought about suicide, but steadfastly deny intent or plans should be given a prompt, confirmed appointment with a psychiatrist. Depressed patients with no suicidal thoughts, intent, or plans, a normal mental status examination, and external social supports can be treated by the primary physician, as long as frequent visits can be arranged and the depression responds to treatment. Patients with suicide potential should never be given more than 1 g or a week's supply of tricyclic antidepressant (see below).

Laboratory Studies. There are no laboratory tests for depression. For a time there was interest in urinary catecholamine metabolites and the overnight dexamethasone suppression test, but shortcomings in sensitivity and specificity compromised clinical utility. Depression remains a clinical diagnosis. Nonetheless, medical causes of depressed

Table 227-4. Risk Factors for Suicide

History of prior attempts
Depression
Psychotic features present (especially command hallucinations)
Substance abuse
Positive family history of suicide
Living alone
Age: in males, risk increased with age peaking at 75; in females, the peak for completed suicide is 55–65.
Sex: females attempt suicide three to four times more often than males, but males are successful two to three time more often than females.
Marital Status: at great risk are those who never married, are widowed, separated or divorced, or married without children; those married with children are at least risk.
Employment: unemployed are at greater risk than employed; unskilled are at greater risk than skilled.
Physical Illness: 50% of all patients who attempt suicide have a physical illness. At highest risk are those with chronic pain, diagnosed chronic disease, recent surgery, or a terminal illness.

mood and neurovegetative symptoms must be ruled out (see Chapter 8).

Written Diagnostic Instruments for In-Office Evaluation. Validated diagnostic instruments are sometimes useful supplements to the clinical evaluation. The Beck Depression Inventory (BDI) and the Hamilton Depression Scale (HAM-D) help assess severity and can be used to follow response to therapy and clinical course. The BDI is a 21-item self-administered questionnaire. The HAM-D is a 21-item instrument that must be clinician-administered. Both take approximately 15 minutes to complete and score. The higher the score, the more severe the distress.

PRINCIPLES OF MANAGEMENT

The cornerstone of treatment for *major depression* (unipolar depression) is antidepressant medication; psychotherapy plays a very important adjunctive role. The vast majority of depressed patients can be treated as outpatients by their primary care physician, particularly those with major depression. Psychiatric referral is required for management of *bipolar disease*, which responds well to a combination of lithium and antidepressant therapy. *Psychotic depression* necessitates use of neuroleptics and psychiatric intervention. If there is an organic cause (*secondary depression*) one treats the causative medical illness and discontinues potentially offending medications. Only if the medical condition responds slowly or is intractably are trials of an antidepressant or supportive psychotherapy indicated.

Antidepressants are usually not helpful in *characterologic depression*. Dysthymia or characterologic depression is notoriously difficult to treat. This condition may respond best to psychotherapy, but, when neurovegetative symptoms are prominent, antidepressant agents can be useful as well. *Adjustment disorder* with depressed mood can be treated by the primary care physician with supportive psychotherapy. If moderate sleep and appetite disturbances are present (as they commonly are), an antidepressant can provide symptomatic relief.

Management of major depression has two facets, psychotherapeutic and medical. The primary physician needs to become skilled in providing supportive psychotherapy and using first-line antidepressants.

Psychotherapy

Treatment begins with establishing a strong patient-physician relationship (see Chapter 1) and providing psychological support. More intensive psychotherapy may also be beneficial. The addition of antidepressant medication improves prognosis. Psychotherapy and medication are often synergistic.

Psychological Management (Supportive Psychotherapy). Patients with major depression benefit from supportive psychotherapy, much of which can be provided by the primary physician. A clear, empathic, hopeful manner helps to forge a therapeutic alliance and facilitates treatment. A detailed explanation of the diagnosis combined with reassurance that depression is eminently treatable do much to calm a fearful patient and family. When patients feel hopeless or undeserving, it is useful to point out that these are the characteristic symptoms of depression and they will gradually improve.

While conveying hope and optimism, the physician must take care not to dismiss as insignificant the patient's fears, pains, and negative feelings. Many feel overwhelmed by life stresses. It is important to identify these stresses. Empathic listening and thoughtful comment can help the patient devise strategies for coping.

At the outset of treatment one should see the patient every 1-2 weeks for about half an hour. Appointments can then be spaced out according to the patient's needs. If a patient becomes severely depressed, agitated, or psychotic, emergency psychiatric referral should be made.

Social and Environmental Interventions. A caring family willing to monitor the severely depressed patient can make the difference between outpatient management and hospitalization. Members can ensure medication compliance and follow-up appointments and minimize social isolation. Also helpful is identifying stressful elements in the patient's environment so that they might be modified. Worries about the consequences of taking time off from work and issues of confidentiality must be addressed. Helping the patient deal with these important concerns is essential and greatly appreciated.

Psychopharmacologic Therapy

The tricyclic antidepressants (*TCAs*) and the selective serotonin reuptake inhibitors (*SSRIs*) serve as first-line antidepressants. Bupropion and trazodone are alternatives. The monoamine oxidase inhibitors (*MAOIs*) and lithium are reserved for special situations.

Tricyclic Antidepressants. These agents appear to act predominantly on norepinephrine metabolism, inhibiting reuptake at CNS synapses. Some TCAs also affect serotonin and, to a lesser extent, dopamine metabolism. A large number of tricyclics are available. All are equally effective. The major differences are in the degree of *anticholinergic* and *sedative side effects*. All require 2 to 4 weeks of continuous use before clinical improvement becomes evident. Drug choice for a given patient is determined by attention to the side effects of available agents (Table 227–5). One should become comfortable with using at least one sedating and one nonsedating TCA compound. Patient comfort and compliance are facilitated by avoiding drugs with marked anticholinergic activity.

Selecting Among Tricyclics. In general, the TCAs tend to be sedating. Patients with severe *insomnia* might do best with a strongly sedating drug, such as *doxepin* (Adapin or Sinequan) given at bedtime. The very sedating drug *amitriptyline* (Elavil) has long been popular with physicians, but because of its strong anticholinergic side effects, it is probably not an optimal first-choice agent unless low doses suffice. The elderly and those with prostatic hypertrophy do best with a nonsedating tricyclic that has relatively mild anticholinergic activity (eg, *desipramine* [Norpramin] or *nortriptyline* [Aventyl or Pamelor]). Nortriptyline has the advantage among tricyclics of causing the least postural hypotension. Persons bothered by anergy and psychomotor retardation

Table 227-5. Antidepressants

AGENT	RELATIVE ANTICHOLINERGIC EFFECT	SEDATIVE EFFECT	USUAL DOSE AND RANGE* (MG/DAY)	THERAPEUTIC SERUM LEVEL (NG/ML)	RELATIVE COST†
Tricyclics					
Amitriptyline	8	High	150 (50–300)	>160	1.0
Imipramine	4	Moderate	150 (50–300)	>225	1.3
Doxepin	2	High	150 (50–300)	—	5.0
Nortriptyline	1	Moderate	75 (25–150)	50—150	15.5
Desipramine	1	Energizing	150 (50–300)	>125	9.4
Selective Seratonin Reuptake Inhibitors					
Fluoxetine	0	Energizing	20 (20–80)	—	12.0
Sertraline	0	Energizing	50 (100–200)	—	10.5
Paroxetine	0	Energizing	20 (20–80)	—	10.0
Others					
Trazodone	0	High	200 (150–600)	—	7.0
Bupropion	0	Energizing	300 (150–450)	—	12.5

*Usual dosage is reduced by half for use in the elderly.

†In part, adpated from *Medical Letter* 1993;35:26. Relative cost used is for the least costly formulation available. Some brand formulations of older tricyclics (e.g., Elavil, Tofranil) can be as much as 10 times the cost of the generic.

are best treated with a nonsedating, slightly activating TCA (eg, desipramine) or an SSRI (see below). *Imipramine* (Tofranil) is moderately sedating and moderately anticholinergic, but is the least costly.

The prescribing of a *fixed combination* preparation containing a tricyclic plus a *neuroleptic* (eg, Triavil) or a *benzodiazepine* (eg, Limbitrol) is irrational and should be avoided. Combinations make it difficult to achieve therapeutic levels of the tricyclic without administering too much of the other compound. Moreover, except for the depressed patient with delusions, neuroleptics have no place in the treatment of depression.

Adverse effects. Tricyclics can have *lethal* cardiovascular toxicity when taken in *overdose* due to severe cumulative *anticholinergic* and *alpha-blocking* effects. One should never prescribe more than 1 gm of a tricyclic to a potentially suicidal patient or to a patient one does not know well. At therapeutic doses, *postural hypotension* can occur, especially in the elderly, leading to falls, fractures, and head injury. If postural hypotension is a problem, nortriptyline or a SSRI should be used. If the hypotension is always worse in the morning, it may be useful to give the nortriptyline in three divided doses. Patients should be instructed to be careful when rising from recumbency or sitting.

Before benefit is noted, patients may want to stop TCA therapy because of *mouth dryness, lassitude, constipation,* or *mental clouding*. Such symptoms are common with use of TCAs, but may also result from depression. They often pass or abate with continued therapy, a reassuring fact that helps patients to continue TCA treatment. *Weight gain* is another complaint. It results from TCA-associated stimulation of appetite.

Rarely, more severe dose-related anticholinergic symptoms occur, especially in the elderly. These include *ileus, urinary retention*, and *dysrhythmias*. In all patients over 40, it is good practice to obtain a baseline electrocardiogram prior to starting a tricyclic. At therapeutic levels, tricyclics exert anticholinergic effects on the heart, which could cause a *rise in heart rate* and *conduction delay*. In patients with bundle branch block, atrioventricular block, or sinus node disease, there is an increased risk of higher degrees of heart block. In patients without underlying conduction system disease, tricyclics rarely cause conduction problems.

Very rarely, a full *anticholinergic syndrome* develops in patients taking TCAs, characterized by agitation, delirium, and fever. The most common precipitant is simultaneous use of more than one anticholinergic drug. Most often implicated is concurrent use of thioridazine (Mellaril), anticholinergic antiparkinsonian drugs, antihistamines, antispasmodics, and over-the-counter sleep medications containing antihistamines. The number of anticholinergic compounds should be closely monitored, especially in the elderly.

Dosage. Tricyclics are started at a low dose with gradual increases until the therapeutic dose-range is achieved (see Table 227–5). After that, trial and error is often required. Drug *serum levels* can be used to determine compliance and achievement of therapeutic serum concentrations in nonresponders. Blood levels vary widely among patients for any given oral dose due to individual differences in drug absorption and metabolism. Therapeutic serum levels have been established for imipramine, desipramine, amitriptyline, and nortriptyline (see Table 227–5). For other TCAs, serum levels are useful only to ascertain compliance. Many clinical laboratories are unreliable in measuring these compounds. One should seek an experienced laboratory.

The most common cause of treatment failure is inadequate dosage. In healthy nonelderly adults, a typical *starting dose* is the equivalent of 50 mg of desipramine. (Nortriptyline has twice the milligram potency of most tricyclics; thus its starting dose is 25 mg.) The daily dose is best taken at bedtime to facilitate compliance and minimize side effects. Dosage can be increased by 50 mg every 3 to 4 days to a dose of 150 to 200 mg at bedtime. Dosages are reduced by 50 percent in the elderly (see below). The final dosage chosen is one that provides a therapeutic response without intolerable side effects. The usual *maximum dosage* is 300 mg of desipramine or the equivalent (150 mg for nortriptyline).

Selective Serotonin Reuptake Inhibitors (SSRIs). As their name implies, the SSRIs (eg, *fluoxetine* [Prozac], *sertraline* [Zoloft], and *paroxetine* [Paxil]) affect CNS serotonin metabolism. For mild to moderate depression, they appear to be equal in efficacy to the TCAs and better tolerated. For severe depression, the TCAs are preferred. Unlike the TCAs, many of which are sedating, these agents have *energizing* or "activating" side effects, a factor favoring their selection in patients suffering anergy, apathy, and psychomotor retardation. A growing number of physicians are turning to these drugs as the antidepressant of first choice, especially in circumstances where avoidance of tricyclic side effects is desired.

Side Effects. These activating agents can exacerbate agitation, anxiety, and insomnia making them inappropriate for depressed patients already troubled by such symptoms. The motor *restlessness* (including *tremor*), initial *anxiety*, and *agitation* with *insomnia* can be the most distressing side effects of SSRIs. Concerns about exacerbation of suicidality with SSRI use proved unfounded after detailed investigation. Nonetheless, it is always crucial to remain vigilant and inquire specifically about suicidal thoughts, even as patients begin to show improvement (see below).

Paradoxically, up to 20 percent experience some sedation. Unlike the TCAs with their associated anticholinergic and alpha-blocking activity, there is little risk of orthostatic hypotension, tachycardia, heart block, blurred vision, or dry mouth. *Sexual dysfunction* has been reported, including impotence and retarded ejaculation in men and anorgasmia in both men and women. These effects are reversible. Some weight gain from appetite stimulation may occur, but not to the extent associated with TCAs. *Headache, nausea,* and *diarrhea* have also been reported. All SSRIs can cause a *life-threatening reaction* if taken concurrently with a *monoamine oxidase inhibitor*. At least 2 weeks should pass before starting a MAOI after SSRI use.

Some SSRIs (fluoxetine, paroxetine) *inhibit liver cytochrome P-450 enzymes*, slowing hepatic drug metabolism and prolonging the effects of warfarin, phenytoin, digoxin, and other drugs that are hepatically metabolized.

Dosage. Fluoxetine is available in 20 mg capsules, but some patients may become unduly anxious or agitated on this starting dose. A liquid form enables even smaller starting doses. In non-elderly patients, fluoxetine can be initiated at 10–20 mg daily. Dosage may be advanced by 10–20 mg per day every 4 to 6 weeks. Usually 20 or 40 mg per day suffices. The maximum dose is 80 mg per day, although higher doses are used to treat obsessive-compulsive disorder (see Chapter 226). Due to the drug's long serum half-life (2-3 days), less frequent dosing is possible for elderly persons needing less than 20 mg daily (eg, 20 mg every 2 to 4 days).

Sertraline is started at 50 mg per day and gradually increased to therapeutic dosages in the range of 100 to 200 mg per day. *Paroxetine* is administered in doses comparable to those of fluoxetine. Both sertraline and paroxetine have shorter half-lives than fluoxetine, but dosing is still once daily.

Trazodone (Desyrel) is a nontricyclic with efficacy and onset similar to the TCAs, but with a very low incidence of anticholinergic side effects making it well tolerated. Trazodone may be slightly inferior to tricyclics in terms of its antidepressant efficacy. The drug is *sedating* and particularly helpful for those who cannot sleep or tolerate anticholinergic side effects. *Postural hypotension* can be a problem in the elderly. Other common side effects include indigestion, nausea, and headaches. *Priapism*, a painful medical emergency, has been reported. Males prescribed trazodone must be warned that sustained, painful erection requires immediate medical attention. Trazodone was initially purported to pose a lesser risk with regard to cardiac side effects than the TCAs; however, it remains unclear whether the difference is substantial.

Potency on a mg-per-mg basis is about half that of imipramine. Dosage range is wide (150–600 mg/d). Half-life is short, necessitating multiple doses, although the major portion can be given at night to minimize daytime drowsiness.

Bupropion (Wellbutrin). is a relatively new antidepressant, similar to the TCAs in efficacy for severe depression and similar to the SSRIs in enhancing psychomotor activity and freedom from anticholinergic and cardiovascular side effects. Unlike the SSRIs, there is no adverse effect on sexual function. Appetite is suppressed. Unlike other antidepressants, bupropion increases the risk of seizure (frequency 0.6 percent), making the drug relatively contraindicated in patients with a known seizure disorder and causing seizures when taken in overdose. It also increases the risk of a psychotic reaction.

Dosage. Bupropion is available in 75 mg and 100 mg tablets. The recommended starting dose is 75 to 100 mg bid. After 4 days, the dose may be advanced to 100 mg tid, and ultimately to a maximum of 150 mg tid. Again, no more than 150 mg should be administered in any 4-hour period, as this may substantially increase the risk of seizure.

Other Antidepressants. Lithium is the treatment of choice in bipolar disorder. MAOIs are quite useful in treating the elderly. Both are best prescribed initially by physicians familiar with their use because of potential toxicity (see below).

The benzodiazepine *alprazolam* (Xanax) has excellent antianxiety effects and *mild* antidepressant action. However, prolonged use is associated with significant risk of dependency (see Chapter 226). *Buspirone* (BuSpar) is similarly purported to have combined anxiolytic and *mild* antidepressant effects, and has the advantage of a more benign side effect profile, without risk of physiological dependence (see Chapter 226). These agents are reasonable in cases of minor depression with anxiety, but they are not indicated for the treatment of major affective illness.

Some nontricyclic second-generation antidepressants have fallen from use because of severe adverse effects (eg, seizures with *maprotiline*; tardive dyskinesias with *amoxapine*). These agents are of limited safety and should be avoided.

Monitoring and Duration of Therapy; Failure to Respond. Monitoring response to therapy can be readily accomplished by carefully reviewing symptoms and activity level. The questionnaire instruments used for assessment of disease severity (see above) can also be used. If a patient shows little or no response to antidepressant therapy after 4 weeks at full dosage (which may be 6 weeks from initiation of therapy), then the drug trial should be considered a failure. If there is doubt as to adequacy of dosage or compliance, a serum drug level can be obtained. Failure to respond is an indication for psychopharmacologic consultation to explore whether augmentation therapy (ie, adding a second agent, usually from a different class) or switching to another agent is the best approach. Sometimes augmentation can be the more rapid approach to achieving control, but consultation is advised.

If the response to initial therapy was promising, but limited by intolerance to drug side effects, then switching to another agent in the same class with a more favorable side effect profile might suffice (eg, switching from amitriptyline to nortriptyline for postural hypotension).

If depression successfully remits, antidepressant medication is maintained for at least 6 months. At that time, the dosage can be slowly tapered over a period of 4 weeks while watching for the re-emergence of depressive symptoms. Should symptoms recur, the dosage is returned to its prior level and maintained for at least another 3 to 6 months. Some patients will require indefinite maintenance therapy.

Prevention of Suicide. The best prevention is proper screening for suicidality and prompt referral at the time of initial evaluation. However, some patients are at greatest risk for suicide at the time when they are initially responding to antidepressant medication. Dysphoria may still persist as energy lifts, perhaps giving the patient with suicidal thoughts adequate energy to formulate a plan and follow it through. Continuous vigilance is required, as well as care in choice and amount of antidepressant prescribed. If there is a question of suicide risk, either a nontricyclic should be selected or no more than 1 gm of a tricyclic dispensed at a time.

Selection of Antidepressant for Major Depression. Choice is best made by taking into account disease severity, age, degree of psychomotor retardation and sleep disturbance, and ability to tolerate anticholinergic, cardiac, and postural side effects. Costs should also be considered (see Table 227–5). The newer antidepressants are quite expensive, but so are brand-name TCA formulations.

For severe depression, the TCAs remain the antidepressants of first choice. In the elderly and others with cardiac disease, prostatic hypertrophy, postural hypotension, or glaucoma, the SSRIs may be better tolerated, although not as effective as the TCAs for severe depression. Alternatives to TCAs for severely depressed patients who cannot tolerated anticholinergic side effects include bupropion and the MAOIs. When sedation without anticholinergic activity is desired, trazodone is a reasonable choice, particularly in the elderly. For anergic, hypersomnic or motor retarded patients, an activating agent is best (eg, an SSRI or desipramine). For patients with a mixture of neurovegetative symptoms, nortriptyline is reasonable, being well tolerated and free of excessive sedating, activating, anticholinergic, or antiadrenergic effects.

Treatment of Depression in the Elderly

Depression is the most common psychiatric disorder of the elderly, affecting close to one million older Americans. Primary treatment modalities include antidepressants and, for severely affected patients, electroconvulsive therapy (ECT). Age-related changes in drug metabolism and susceptibility to drug side effects must be taken into account in the design of the treatment program.

Choice of Antidepressant. The sedating, anticholinergic, cardiac, and postural side effects of many TCAs make their use in the elderly especially problematic. Prior to starting therapy, postural signs and an electrocardiogram should be performed and particular note taken of the patient's somatic symptoms and degree of psychomotor retardation.

Amitriptyline and imipramine are among the most difficult to use; *nortriptyline* and *desipramine* are better tolerated. If sedation is desired, *trazodone* is a reasonable choice, being free of anticholinergic activity. When anergy and psychomotor retardation predominate, the activating effects of *SSRIs* make them attractive. Similarly, SSRIs are an excellent first choice if there is heart block, a dysrhythmia, or postural hypotension. Of the SSRIs, *sertraline* is the least likely to interfere with hepatic drug metabolism and preferred in patients taking drugs that are metabolized by the liver (eg, digoxin, warfarin, phenytoin). Severe disease requires consideration of *bupropion* and *MAOIs* (see below).

Initiating Therapy. One starts with a *very low dose* of medication (eg, 10 mg of fluoxetine, 25 mg of desipramine, 10 mg of nortriptyline, or 50 mg of trazodone). The dosage can be raised slowly every 5–7 days, while monitoring subjective response and heart rate and watching for anticholinergic, cardiovascular, and CNS side effects. One slows the increase in dose if tachycardia, excessive sedation, agitation, or orthostatic hypotension develops.

Often the patient is the last to know that he is getting better and family members commonly report that the patient is sleeping and eating better before the dysphoria resolves. An adequate trial may take twice as long in the elderly as in younger patients.

Failure to Respond. If there is little improvement after a reasonable trial at therapeutic doses, consultation is warranted to consider use of an alternative antidepressant (eg, MAOI) or electroconvulsive therapy.

Monoamine Oxidase Inhibitors. MAOIs have been used sparingly in the elderly because of concern for adverse reactions. Actually, MAOIs have no anticholinergic activity and are relatively well tolerated. Many older patients who do not respond to other antidepressants improve with MAOIs. MAOI therapy should be selected and started by a psychopharmacologic consultant, but management can then shift to the primary care physician, who needs to be familiar with drug actions and side effects.

The primary side effects are *hypotension* and *insomnia*. Hypotension is unrelated to dose and may occur up to a month after starting the drug. It rarely necessitates stopping the drug. Insomnia can be minimized by giving the last daily dose no later than 4 PM.

Hypertensive crisis is the most serious adverse effect, caused by ingesting a large amount of *tyramine*. Dietary and drug precautions must be given. A *low-tyramine diet* is required, necessitating avoidance of foods such as fermented cheese, large amounts of yogurt, excessive caffeine, and chocolate, beer, and red wine. Patients can drink white wine, vodka, gin, and whiskey. A blanket warning to avoid all alcohol is not only unwarranted, but may also compromise compliance. *Sympathomimetics* should be avoided, including those found in combination cold tablets, nasal decongestants, and appetite suppressants. *Amphetamines*, too, are not permitted. *Treatment* of a hypertensive crisis involves prompt cessation of MAOI use and initiation of antihypertensive therapy with an alpha-blocker or a direct vasodilator. (*Phentolamine*, 5 mg given slowly intravenously, is recommended.) Fever is managed by means of external cooling.

Severe life-threatening reactions can also occur as a consequence of interactions between MAOIs and *SSRIs* or *narcotic analgesics*. A several week period between cessation of SSRI therapy and initiation of MAOI use is required, as is consultation before starting the MAOI.

Tranylcypromine (Parnate) is the preferred MAOI in the elderly because its effects last no more than 24 hours. Starting dose is 10 mg once or twice daily and gradually increased as needed over a few weeks. Usually 20 to 30 mg daily will suffice, but occasional patients require as much as 60 mg per day.

Electroconvulsive Therapy (ECT). Elderly patients who are psychotically depressed, severely incapacitated, refractory or unable to take drug therapy, or in need of a rapid response should be referred for consideration of electroconvulsive treatment. The best predictors of response are psychomotor retardation and delusions. Efficacy and safety have been well documented. Attainment of generalized seizure activity is required to achieve benefit. Customizing electrical dose to the patient's seizure threshold may help maximize efficacy and minimize adverse effects. Electrode placement appears to be more important than electrical dose as regards amnesia, with unilateral electrode placement associated with a lower risk. Amnesia occurs for events just prior to and up to a few weeks after treatment. More long term, cognitive functioning is no different than that for patients treated with antidepressants. Relapses occur with high frequency, making ECT an acute treatment. The roles for follow-up antidepressant therapy and maintenance ECT are under study.

Treatment of Seasonal Affective Disorder

Light therapy is the first line of treatment. Exposure to 10,000 lux of ordinary white fluorescent light for 30 to 45 minutes at a time, once or twice per day is effective. Improvement often occurs within the first week or two of therapy. Patients typically sit about 50 cm from a light box and read for the period of treatment, with the light coming in at a 45 degree angle. Improvement has been noted both with morning and nighttime treatments, though the latter may cause insomnia. Elaborate forms of lighting that more closely simulate the spectrum of sunlight are no more effective than light from a standard white fluorescent source. The intensity of light appears to be the key determinant of efficacy. *SSRIs* are probably as effective as light therapy. Some clinicians use both. Efficacy of prophylactic therapy early in the winter is under study.

INDICATIONS FOR REFFERAL AND ADMISSION

Patients who should be referred for psychiatric consultation include those with refractory or disabling major depression, bipolar illness, psychosis, or substantial risk for suicide. Patients who fail to respond after 1 to 2 months of appropriate antidepressant treatment should have a psychiatric consultation. Many of these patients can be referred back to their primary physician for follow-up after one or two psychiatric appointments.

Psychiatric hospitalization is indicated for high suicide risk, lack of reliable social supports (if the depression is severe), history of previously poor response to treatment, or symptoms that are so severe that the patient requires constant observation or nursing care.

PATIENT EDUCATION

Detailed patient education is a central component of supportive psychotherapy (see above). Patients who come from backgrounds that stigmatize mental illness or oppose psychotropic medication are comforted by learning of depression's "organic" pathophysiology, which helps them to comply with treatment. Compliance with antidepressant therapy is often compromised by side effects or mistaken attributions. Some stop their medication after only a few days if they do not notice an immediate improvement or use it only "as-needed." Prior to initiating therapy, it is critical to review likely side effects and delayed onset of improvement. The importance of prolonged, regular use must be emphasized. If the patient already has a tendency toward constipation, the prescription of a stool softener may make a tricyclic more tolerable. Patients should be instructed to report side effects rather than stopping the medication on their own, and to call promptly if suicidal thoughts develop or if depression markedly worsens.

The educational process should include family and other household members. Enlisting their help in decreasing stress at home is helpful. With elderly or severely depressed patients, the family should be taught about the proper use of antidepressants and asked to monitor compliance.

THERAPEUTIC RECOMMENDATIONS

- If a depressive syndrome is identified, try to make a specific diagnosis and assess suicide risk.
- If the patient appears to be at risk for suicide, has psychotic symptoms, severe depression with no social supports, or is unable to care for himself, arrange prompt psychiatric consultation with a view to possible hospitalization.
- For other patients, begin supportive psychotherapy and make any social and environmental interventions that may help. Especially with elderly or severely depressed patients, involve the family in the treatment.
- For patients who have major depression (or patients with other subtypes who have neurovegetative symptoms), antidepressant medication is indicated.
- For elderly patients and those with suspected cardiac disease, obtain a baseline electrocardiogram to rule out conduction system abnormalities and check for postural hypotension prior to initiation of therapy.
- For patients with moderate to severe depression who are under age 65 and without cardiac disease, begin a tricyclic. If insomnia is severe, start with a more sedating preparation (eg, doxepin or imipramine, 50 mg qhs). Otherwise choose a drug that minimizes side effects (desipramine 50 mg qhs, or nortriptyline 25 mg qhs). If postural hypotension is a problem, use nortriptyline or a selective serotonin reuptake inhibitor (eg, sertraline 50 qam).
- Start most tricyclics at a dose of 50 mg at bedtime and increase by 50 mg every 3 to 4 days until 150 to 200 mg/day is reached. If no benefit occurs after 2 weeks slowly increase (up to a maximum of 300 mg). Nortriptyline is twice as potent as the others, so its doses are half those of other TCAs.
- If high doses produce no benefit or low doses seem to produce excessive side effects, check blood levels to be sure dosage is proper and adjust if necessary. If the patient has moderately severe depression unimproved by a trial of TCA therapy that includes 4 weeks at therapeutic doses, then refer for psychiatric consultation.
- If conduction system disease or other contraindications to anticholinergic therapy exist (eg, elderly, glaucoma, prostatic hypertrophy, dementia), start therapy with a nontricyclic. If agitation or insomnia predominates, consider trazodone (beginning at 100 mg/d and giving most before bed), but watch for postural hypotension. If anergy or psychomotor retardation predominates consider an SSRI (eg, sertraline 50 mg qam), bupropion (75 mg bid), or desipramine (50 mg qhs).
- Initial doses of antidepressants in the elderly should be half to one-third the standard starting doses noted here.
- If the patient responds to the antidepressant, it should be continued for at least 6 months and then slowly tapered.
- Never prescribe more than a week's supply or a total of 1 gm of a tricyclic if there is suicidal risk.
- Explain to patients that antidepressants must be taken regularly; that they may take weeks to work; and that there may be mild side effects which do not warrant discontinuation of the drug.

ANNOTATED BIBLIOGRAPHY

American Psychiatric Association. Practice guidelines for major depressive disorder in adults. Am J Psychiatry 1993;150(4 suppl):1. *(Formal consensus guidelines for the management of major depression.)*

American Psychiatric Association. Diagnostic and Statistical Manual of Mental Disorders, 3rd edition - Revised. Washington DC: American Psychiatric Association, 1987. *(The current diagnostic classification system.)*

Brody DS, Larson DB. The role of primary care physicians in managing depression. J Gen Intern Med 1992;7:243. *(A good exposition of the role.)*

Brown JT, Stoudemire GA. Normal and pathological grief. JAMA 1983;250:378. *(A succinct description of normal grief and guidelines for recognition and management of pathologic reactions.)*

Coulehan JL, Schulberg HC, Block MR. The efficacy of depression questionnaires for case finding in primary medical care. J Gen Intern Med 1989;4:541. *(Test characteristics examined.)*

Current Issues in Drug Therapy of Depression. Proceedings of a symposium. J Clin Psychiatry 1993;54(8 suppl)1. *(Topics include use of new agents and treatment in the primary care setting.)*

Fawcett J, Clark DC, Busch KA. Assessing and treating the patient at risk for suicide. Psych Annals 1993;23:244. *(A practical review.)*

Frank E, Kupfer DJ, Perel JM, et al. Three-year outcomes for maintenance therapies in recurrent depression. Arch Gen Psychiatry 1990;47:1093. *(Prophylactic benefits found from maintenance treatment with imipramine and interpersonal psychotherapy.)*

Gerber PD, Barrett J, Barrett J, et al. Recognition of depression by internists in primary care. J Gen Intern Med 1989;4:7. *(A critical look at how primary physicians make the diagnosis; sensitivity was 57 percent; specificity 87 percent.)*

Gerber PD, Barrett JE, Barrett JA, et al. The relationship of presenting physical complaints to depressive symptoms in primary care patients. J Gen Intern Med 1992;7:170. *(Sleep disturbance, fatigue, and multiple bodily complaints were among those most strongly associated with depression.)*

Gerner RH. Geriatric depression and treatment with trazodone. Psychopathology 1987;20(supp 1):82. *(A review of trazodone's utility in the treatment of depressed elderly.)*

Glassman AH, Bigger JT. Cardiovascular effects of therapeutic doses of tricyclic antidepressants. Arch Gen Psych 1981; 38:815. *(A good review pointing out the relative safety of tricyclics when prescribed carefully.)*

Gold PW, Goodwin FK, Chrousos GP. Clinical and biochemical manifestations of depression: Relation to the neurobiology of stress. N Engl J Med 1988;319:348,413. *(A 2-part review of pathogenesis and pathophysiology; 181 refs.)*

Keller MB, Lavori PW, Lewis CE, et al. Predictors of relapse in major depressive disorder. JAMA 1983;250:3299. *(Relapse was highest in the months immediately following recovery;*

prior episodes of depression and older age made relapse more likely.)

Kocsis JH (ed). Dysthymia and chronic depression states. Psych Annals 1993;23:606. *(An entire issue; includes reviews of diagnosis, social impairment, and treatment.)*

Kupfer DJ, et al. Five-year outcome for maintenance therapies in recurrent depression. Arch Gen Psych 1992;49:769. *(Long-term therapy effective and required in those who have recurrences.)*

McGreevey JF Jr, Franco K. Depression in the elderly: The role of the primary care physician in management. J Gen Intern Med 1988;3:498. *(Diagnosis and management from the primary care perspective.)*

Pollack MH, Rosenbaum JF. Management of antidepressant-induced side effects: A practical guide for the clinician. Am J Psychiatry 1987;48:1. *(A practical review of side effects and methods for managing them.)*

Potter WZ, Rudorfer MV, Manji H. The pharmacological treatment of depression. New Engl J Med 1991;325:633. *(Authoritative; written for a general medical audience.)*

Potter WZ, Rudorfer MV. Electroconvulsive therapy—a modern medical procedure. N Engl J Med 1993;328:882. *(An editorial emphasizing the important role of ECT in treatment of severe depression.)*

Rosenstein DL, Nelson JC, Jacobs SC. Seizures associated with antidepressants. J Clin Psychiatry 1993;54:289. *(Comprehensive discussion; includes assessing seizure risk.)*

Rosenthal NE. Diagnosis and treatment of seasonal affective disorder. JAMA 1993;270;2717. *(Short, but inclusive review; 44 refs.)*

Wells KB, Stewart A, Hays RD, et al. The functioning and well-being of depressed patients: Results from the medical outcome study. JAMA 1989;262:914. *(Patients with depressive symptoms tended to function worse than those with other chronic medical conditions.)*

Veith RC, Raskind MA. Cardiovascular effects of tricyclic antidepressants in depressed patients with chronic heart disease. N Engl J Med 1982;306:954. *(There was no effect noted on left ventricular function nor any significant adverse effect on ventricular irritability.)*

Yudofsky SC. Beta-blockers and depression: The clinician's dilemma. JAMA 1992;267:1826. *(The evidence for an adverse effect and what to do about it; 26 refs.)*

228

Approach to the Patient With Alcohol Abuse

ELEANOR Z. HANNA, Ph.D.

Primary Care Medicine: Office Evaluation and Management of the Adult Patient, 3rd edition, edited by Allan H. Goroll, Lawrence A. May, and Albert G. Mulley, Jr. J.B. Lippincott Company, Philadelphia

Alcohol abuse is a complex problem, with elements of a medical illness, a dependency syndrome, and a learned behavioral disorder. The National Council on Alcoholism and Drug Abuse defines alcoholism as an often progressive and fatal primary chronic disease, influenced by genetic, psychosocial, and environmental factors, and characterized by "impaired control over drinking, preoccupation with the drug alcohol, use of alcohol despite adverse consequences, and distortions in thinking, most notably denial."

Community-based studies suggest a very high prevalence of alcoholism, approaching 5 percent or nearly 10 million adults and over 3 million youths. The societal and personal costs are staggering. The economic impact in the United States approaches $50 billion annually, with $15 billion for medical care alone. The mortality rate is 2.3 times that of aged-matched persons, with 56 percent of deaths directly related to alcohol abuse. Alcohol abuse is a factor in over 50 percent of automobile deaths, industrial accidents and fatalities, fire burns, drownings, child abuse and domestic violence cases, and homicides.

Nevertheless, most problem drinkers are employed, employable, or in families, indicating that the scope of the problem extends far beyond the stereotypical skid-row drinker, who accounts for only 5 percent of patients who abuse alcohol.

The primary care physician is in the unique position to detect and treat an alcohol problem in its very early phases, long before it becomes disabling and more difficult to manage. Given the morbidity and mortality associated with alcohol abuse, screening for it should be a routine part of every medical evaluation. One first seeks to help the problem drinker acknowledge the problem, understand its consequences, and recognize the need for treatment. The objective then shifts to negotiating and carrying out an acceptable treatment plan, one that is personalized and multifaceted.

CAUSES OF ALCOHOL ABUSE

The etiology of alcohol abuse remains incompletely understood, but is clearly multifactorial. Biogenetic, sociocultural, psychologic, and behavioral elements have been elucidated. No single model accounts for all manifestations, but each is helpful in understanding the problem.

Biogenetic Model. Genetic factors appear to influence the metabolism of alcohol and the effects of alcohol on neurotransmitters, receptors, and cell membranes. The significance of the purported "gene" for alcoholism, the A1 allele at the D_2 dopamine receptor gene, remains to be elucidated.

Sociocultural Model. External factors such as poverty, socialization patterns, and cultural differences in the rules governing alcohol use are emphasized. Parental and peer values, attitudes, and behaviors regarding alcohol are important. This model explains the increased use of alcohol among women and teens.

Psychologic–Psychodynamic Model. In this model, underlying psychopathology (eg, dependency conflict, depression, excessive need for power or sensation seeking, gender identification problems) is viewed as predisposing a person to drink excessively, either to mask or solve a psychologic problem. Drinking is viewed merely as a symptom.

Learning Theory/Behavioral Model. Alcoholism is seen as a learned behavior that is reversible, time-limited, on a continuum with normal drinking behavior, and established by a series of learning and reinforcement experiences. Social interactions, emotional stresses, guilty or negative thoughts, and need for sleep or pain relief serve as precipitants and maintainers of drinking behavior. Any of these precipitants coupled with learned expectations about the effects of alcohol or deficits in social skills will initiate and maintain the drinking behavior.

CLINICAL PRESENTATION AND COURSE

Use of alcohol in moderation is characterized by varying consumption and beverage according to internal cues and external circumstances. If one chooses to drink, it is done in drinking-appropriate circumstances and will rarely exceed one or two drinks. The moderate drinker is not likely to drive if under the influence (he might have his drink on arrival at a party and switch to something nonalcoholic later), nor likely to drink in order to deal with problems, escape, or get drunk.

With the caveats that a given dose of alcohol affects different people differently and that average daily consumption neglects the pattern of drinking, drinking in moderation may be defined quantitatively as two or less drinks per day for men and one or less for women and the elderly. The figure is lower in women and the elderly because they experience a higher blood alcohol level per drink due to smaller volume of distribution and decreased first-pass metabolism of alcohol. (A standard drink is assumed to contain roughly 12 g, 15 mL, or 0.5 oz of alcohol, which is the approximate content of 12 oz of beer, 4 oz of wine, or 1.5 oz of liquor.)

Alcohol abuse has a continuum of presentations ranging from the social drinker with a tendency to occasionally use alcohol in excess when under stress to the constantly intoxicated vagrant. The most commonly encountered presentations include:

- The *social drinker* consumes alcohol in amounts and circumstances that appear socially acceptable, but may develop a serious alcohol problem if there is a propensity to overindulge or to occasionally use alcohol to cope with stress.
- The *heavy social drinker* is one who continues to drink in socially appropriate circumstances, but actively seeks a life of occasions for drinking, through job or social life, and will have more than two drinks every day. He continuously seeks out situations in which to drink and may often overconsume, even though he matches the consumption of his peers. He may never appear drunk or seem affected in his social and work routines, but as his drinking escalates, it becomes increasingly tied to seeking physical or psychological relief. Problem drinkers emerge from this population. Neither the person nor acquaintances suspect an alcohol abuse problem.
- The *problem drinker* meets the criteria for heavy drinking, gets drunk on occasion, and also exhibits medical, legal, social, or psychologic consequences of excessive alcohol consumption. In addition, he may have made or thought of making attempts at cutting down or refraining completely from alcohol consumption. Functioning may vary from seemingly intact behavior to difficulty coping. The patient may deny he has a problem with drinking and attribute blame to external events or persons. Denial is common even among those with multiple arrests for drunk driving.
- The *alcohol-dependent patient* will try to consume the same excessive amount of alcohol regardless of mood or situation, although external circumstances might constrain drinking for a time. Most persons are working; some even in high positions. Alcohol is given top priority in all situations (eg, one goes to a party to drink, not to socialize). Tolerance to alcohol develops and withdrawal symptoms (mood disturbance, tremor, nausea, sweats) may be noted during the workday when the blood alcohol level drops. Drinking at lunch and cocktail hour are needed to relieve symptoms. The alcohol-dependent patient is aware of his compulsion to drink, but is difficult to reach unless family or employer notes a problem or serious medical complications develop.
- The *severely deteriorated patient* maintains a constant state of intoxication, having no care for his person or surroundings. He undergoes hospitalizations for detoxification and for medical care necessary after alcohol-related trauma or organ damage.

Groups at Increased Risk. Professionals, executives, young people, women, and the elderly are demonstrating such increases in frequency of alcohol-related problems that they are now labelled as high-risk populations. *Executives* and *professionals* are often able to drink socially during the day and hide the consequences of their drinking until late in the course of illness, putting them at increased risk for serious sequelae. As many as 30 to 40 percent of persons *under age 25* report alcohol-related problems, often beginning in high school or college. Even as drug use declines, alcohol abuse continues to rise at alarming rates in this age group. Most alcoholics report starting with heavy drinking in their late teens. *Women,* as a result of social change, are consulting alcohol clinics at double the former rates. *Elderly* patients may begin to use alcohol excessively for stress, especially in reaction to loss of a loved one or because of sleep difficulties. A peak period for onset of alcohol-related problems is 65 to 74 years of age.

Natural History and Clinical Course. There is considerable individual variation. Onset ranges from an initial phase of social drinking to immediate heavy drinking starting as early as age 10. Prognosis remains relatively favorable until dependence sets in. Once the addiction becomes psychologic or physiologic, it is difficult to break in the absence of treatment and the clinical course is often progressive. At the point of addiction, one can expect no more than long periods of abstinence or controlled drinking, punctuated by episodic drinking or prolonged relapses and further progression, especially if there is no expert intervention. Controversy continues regarding whether or not total abstinence is required to halt progression. Cessation certainly is necessary to halt many of the medical complications.

Medical Complications. The risk of organ damage is related in part to the dose and duration of alcohol exposure, with some conditions (eg, alcoholic cardiomyopathy, fatty liver) manifesting reversibility with abstinence, while others (eg, cirrhosis) seeming to progress inexorably once severe hepatocellular damage has occurred. Risk appears to be a function of a genetic predisposition as well as alcohol dosage and chronicity of exposure.

Persistent *impotence* and *loss of libido* reflect impaired gonadotropin release and accelerated testosterone metabolism that occur as consequences of chronic alcohol excess; they predate end-stage liver disease. *Alcoholic hepatitis*, *pancreatitis*, and *gastritis* may follow binge drinking. *Fatty liver* and *esophagitis* ensue from chronic use. Late-stage complications include *cirrhosis*, *oral cancers*, *cardiomyopathy*, Wernicke's *encephalopathy*, and Korsakoff's *dementia*.

Fetal alcohol syndrome occurs in infants born to mothers who drink heavily during pregnancy. Features include permanently stunted growth, mental retardation, musculoskeletal abnormalities, poor coordination, and cardiac malformations. Incidence approaches 33 percent among pregnant women who drink more than 150 g of alcohol per day. Another third of children born to such women will have mental retardation, although they may be spared the full syndrome.

DIAGNOSIS

The Diagnostic and Statistical Manual of Psychiatric Disease (DSM-IIIR) specifies the most widely used criteria for the formal diagnoses of alcohol abuse and alcohol dependence. Table 228–1 is adapted from the DSM-IIIR.

Table 228-1. Diagnosis of Alcohol Abuse and Dependence

DSM III Criteria

Alcohol abuse: Necessary daily use of alcohol to function; an inability to decrease or stop alcohol intake; repeated efforts to control alcohol use; blackouts; occasional consumption of a fifth or more of alcohol; and continued drinking, despite a health problem that is caused or exacerbated by alcohol use. Some impairment in social or occupational functioning as a consequence of alcohol use; disturbance must be of at least 1 month's duration. Pattern of abuse must be distinguished from nonpathologic use of alcohol, which may include episodes of intoxification without pathologic use.

Alcohol dependence: Pathologic use of alcohol, with impairment of functioning in the social and economic spheres: plus, either tolerance or withdrawal. Tolerance is either a need for increased amounts of alcohol to achieve the desired effects or markedly diminished effect with regular use of the same amount. Withdrawal is development, within several hours of stopping or reducing drinking, of a coarse tremor of the hands, tongue, and eyelids and at least one of the following: Nausea and vomiting, malaise or weakness, autonomic hyperactivity, anxiety, depression or irritability, orthostatic hypotension. Must be certain withdrawal symptoms are attributable to cessation of alcohol and not to any other physical or mental disorder.

WORKUP

Formal diagnosis of alcoholism involves identification of excessive quantity and duration of consumption, physiologic manifestations of ethanol addiction, loss of control over drinking, and chronic damage to physical health and social functioning. In late stages of illness, these clinical findings are readily evident. Detection before marked abuse or dependence has developed remains the major diagnostic challenge.

The high prevalence of alcohol abuse, its serious consequences, and good response to early intervention argue for *routinely screening all adolescents and adults who come for primary care*. In addition, a high index of suspicion for alcoholism is indicated for the patient who presents with anxiety, insomnia, recurrent infection, an illness that is potentially alcohol-related, child abuse, domestic violence, multiple psychosomatic problems, suicidality, depression, inability to articulate feelings, or interpersonal, occupational, financial, or legal problems.

Screening for Alcoholism. For the patient in whom there is no clinical evidence or suspicion of alcohol abuse, the *CAGE Questions* (Fig. 228–1), are the screening test of choice. In primary care settings, sensitivity for a score of 2 (the standard cutoff) ranges from 70 to 85 percent, and specificity from 85 to 91 percent. In the elderly, where prevalence of alcoholism is increased, but clinical presentation may be harder to ascertain, sensitivity falls to 50 percent, while specificity remains above 90 percent.

A self-administered questionnaire, the *Michigan Alcoholism Screening Test (MAST)* is another convenient means of early detection (Fig. 228–2). Data on test characteristics in primary care settings are few, but sensitivity is in the range of 50 to 70 percent and specificity above 90 percent using a score of 5 for cutoff.

Taking an Alcohol History. A detailed drinking history is in order for all patients suspected of having an alcohol problem on the basis of:

- A positive CAGE or MAST test
- A family complaint
- A daily drinking pattern of 2 to 3 drinks accompanied by seemingly innocuous complaints that might be related to drinking
- A life-style that will perpetuate increased, prolonged drinking
- The occurrence of intrapsychic or interpersonal problems, or actual changes in life events
- Suggestive manifestations on physical examination, such as alcohol on the breath, spider angiomata, plethoric facies, tremor, ecchymoses
- Abnormal liver function tests; macrocytic anemia

For the patient suspected of having a drinking problem, the situation usually must be overwhelming before he will volunteer that he has a drinking problem and wants help. Denial is likely to be strong. Consequently, one has to use an interview technique that is kind and supportive, yet firm and even confrontational when there are serious clinical concerns, especially when there is question about ability to

Have you ever felt the need to **C**ut down on drinking?
Have you ever felt **A**nnoyed by criticism of drinking?
Have you ever had **G**uilty feelings about drinking?
Have you ever taken a morning **E**ye opener?

Figure 228-1. The CAGE test. (Mayfield D, McLead G, Hall P. The CAGE questionnaire. Am J Psychiatry 1974; 131:1121.)

function. Involving family members, friends, and even the employer may facilitate both history-taking and therapy.

The Drinking Profile. In taking a drinking history, it is critical that one go beyond issues of quantity, frequency, and development of tolerance. One must determine the rate at which a patient drinks, exactly what meaning alcohol (drinking) holds, and something about the nature of the patient's social life as it pertains to alcohol. It is also useful to determine whether other drugs are used. With women and the elderly, especially, this would include an emphasis on prescription drugs. A profile of the patient's drinking behavior

1.	Do you feel you are a normal drinker?	(No 2)	Yes
2.	Have you ever awakened in the morning after some drinking the night before and found that you could not remember part of the evening?	(Yes 2)	No
3.	Does your wife (or husband or parents) ever worry or complain about your drinking?	(Yes 1)	No
4.	Can you stop drinking without a struggle after one or two drinks?	(No 2)	Yes
5.	Do you ever feel badly about your drinking?	(Yes 2)	No
6.	Do you ever try to limit your drinking to certain times of day or to certain places?	(Yes 0)	No
7.	Do your friends or relatives think that you are a normal drinker?	(No 2)	Yes
8.	Are you always able to stop when you want to?	(No 2)	Yes
9.	Have you ever attended a meeting of Alcoholics Anonymous?	(Yes 5)	No
10.	Have you gotten into fights when drinking?	(Yes 1)	No
11.	Has drinking ever created problems with you and your wife (husband)?	(Yes 2)	No
12.	Has your wife (husband or other family member) ever gone to anyone for help about your drinking?	(Yes 2)	No
13.	Have you ever lost friends or girlfriends/boyfriends because of drinking?	(Yes 2)	No
14.	Have you ever gotten into trouble at work because of drinking?	(Yes 2)	No
15.	Have you ever lost a job because of drinking?	(Yes 2)	No
16.	Have you ever neglected your obligations, your family or your work for two days or more in a row because of drinking?	(Yes 2)	No
17.	Do you ever drink before noon?	(Yes 1)	No
18.	Have you ever been told you have liver trouble?	(Yes 2)	No
19.	Have you ever had DTs (delerium tremens), severe shaking, heard voices or seen things that weren't there after heavy drinking?	(Yes 2)	No
20.	Have you ever gone to anyone for help about your drinking?	(Yes 5)	No
21.	Have you ever been in a hospital because of drinking?	(Yes 5)	No
22.	Have you ever been a patient in a psychiatric hospital or on a psychiatric ward of a general hospital where drinking was part of the problem?	(Yes 2)	No
23.	Have you ever been seen at a psychiatric or mental health clinic, or gone to a doctor or clergyman for help with an emotional problem in which drinking has played a part?	(Yes 2)	No
24.	Have you ever been arrested, even for a few hours, because of drunken behavior?	(Yes 2)	No
25.	Have you ever been arrested for drunk driving or driving after drinking?	(Yes 2)	No

A score of three points or less is considered nonalcoholic; a score of four points is suggestive, and a score of five points or more indicates alcoholism.

Figure 228-2. The Michigan Alcoholism Screening Test (MAST). (Selzer ML. The Michigan Alcoholism Screening Test. Am J Psychiatry 1971; 127:1653.)

over a given time period will prove most useful. The drinking profile should include attention to:

- Setting: time, place, and occasion for drinking
- Social network: the people involved with the drinking and their relationship to the patient
- Consumption: quantity, frequency, and rate of consumption as it relates to that of others in the drinking context and as it relates to the patient's expected consumption
- Pressures (internal or external) to drink
- Other activities related to drinking

In short, the physician should suspect anyone *who drinks* and is in a *drinking context on a regular basis*—that means most patients who present for treatment. Not only will a drinking profile help characterize an alcohol abuser or alcoholic, it will also identify those not suspected of having a problem. The profile is an effective tool for confronting the resistant patient, treating a willing patient, and educating a person with a potential problem.

Causes for Missing the Diagnosis. The diagnosis of alcohol abuse may be overlooked for several reasons: subtlety of presentation; definitions of alcoholism that do not encompass its early manifestations; the view that the patient is normal so long as he can perform his daily activities; societal acceptance of dangerous levels of alcohol intake; and general expectations of alcohol consumption at most social occasions. There may be unintentional collusion with the patient in denying the problem, especially if the patient is of similar or higher social status, has similar habits and life-style, or is attractive, verbal, and intelligent.

PRINCIPLES OF MANAGEMENT

Management is most successful when it is multifaceted, personalized, and long-term. For many alcoholics, the primary care physician remains the one constant medical figure in the patient's life and the person he probably trusts most. Whether one intends to personally care for the alcoholic patient or refer him to a specialist in alcohol problems, the primary physician has the important initial task of assisting the patient in acknowledging his drinking problem and accepting a treatment program.

Dealing with Denial. When denial is a problem, one should first listen carefully to how the patient explains the findings. If the situation appears to be accepted internally, but the patient feels the need to protect himself publicly, then it is best to help the patient discover the problem for himself. One might suggest keeping a journal or weekly log of drinking events for review, noting and exploring links between drinking and particular environmental, interpersonal, or psychologic precipitants. This also helps determine exactly how much the patient drinks without confronting him directly.

The same technique, with some additions, can be used for the patient who is hiding the problem from himself. Here, one reviews the evidence on how alcohol is directly affecting the patient's health. Use of screening instruments (see above) and presenting the findings in terms of a specific diagnostic classification system sometimes helps to objectify the diagnosis. If the patient continues to resist, then one can bring in family, friends, or employer to present the patient with their evidence of how destructive his drinking is to himself and them. Again, these sessions should be factual, nonjudgmental discussions of the relationship of alcohol to the patient's health and behavior, and its impact on those important to him.

Dealing with Resistance to Treatment. The patient who agrees he has a problem yet continues to refuse help or to relinquish alcohol should be handled similarly, but with more focus on his fears and his resistance. The hostile or belligerent patient should be dealt with firmly, but in a manner which enhances his ability to objectify and control his anger (eg, by identifying the sources of anger).

It is pointless to force the patient into treatment when no medical emergency exists. It is better to present the options available, continue exploring the issue, and provide health education while treating the patient's medical problems and awaiting willingness to undergo treatment. Often those who resist treatment must first fear the loss of something very important (eg, spouse, job) before seeking help. The "tough love" approach, in which loss is seriously threatened or actually carried out unless the patient goes for treatment, is often necessary and must be sustained, because many patients return to old habits once danger of losing a loved one or job passes.

Should the patient agree to seek treatment, it is important to keep the waiting period brief and helpful to remind the patient a day or two ahead of the appointment.

Patient Selection for Management by the Primary Physician. The doctor–patient relationship can be used to change life-style, identify and restructure destructive patterns, and learn new coping skills. Effective care requires being available on a regular basis to provide the monitoring, instruction, and support needed by any patient with a chronic disease. If such support is beyond the scope of the individual primary physician, he should at least ensure a proper and smooth referral for specialized care.

Long-term management by the primary care physician is best indicated for those patients:

- whose medical complications are the foremost concern
- who have a strong personal tie to the primary physician
- who are socially stable
- who demonstrate only minor psychopathology
- who are intelligent and pragmatic
- who put great faith in physicians
- who have an intact and supportive social network

It is important to remember that the treatment will be long and arduous. The therapist must recognize that the patient's behavior is sick and often will be directed at him in either a covert or overtly hostile manner. The ultimate goal is to help the patient gain self-control, regulation, and a sense of responsibility. One must not counterattack.

If and when the physician should find himself unable to cope, the patient should be referred to a specialist with the primary physician remaining as the coordinator of care.

Determinants of Successful Treatment. *Early detection and prompt initiation of treatment* are essential to success, with success rates of 50 percent to 90 percent attained in patients abusing alcohol but without physical or social impairment. Success rates also depend on the length of time a person stays in treatment, his involvement in goal setting and treatment planning, and his continued attachment to family or an integrated social network.

It is best to *involve family members* or significant others in the confrontation and treatment, as they are crucial in assisting and supporting the life-style changes which must be made if the destructive drinking pattern is to be arrested. This is especially true when the problem drinker is a woman or young person. Engaging the family as a full participant is also the best way to ensure that the patient goes for and remains in treatment.

Other determinants of successful treatment include use of a *multifaceted plan,* an *active role* for the patient, and continuous *review.*

Treatment Modalities

Therapies can be classified as biological, psychological, behavioral, or sociocultural. Selection is best done on an individualized basis to meet the patient's specific needs. Most programs use a combination of modalities. The biologic approach includes use of drugs.

Drugs to Decrease Alcohol Consumption. Pharmacologic agents are prescribed to reduce the urge to drink, to blunt withdrawal symptoms, and to treat underlying psychiatric problems that may be contributing to alcohol abuse. In general, drug therapy plays a supportive role in the outpatient care of the alcoholic patient, mainly providing a temporary respite from alcohol consumption sufficient to enable the patient to engage in a more comprehensive and durable treatment program.

Disulfiram (Antabuse) is an aversive therapy that sensitizes the patient to the effects of alcohol by inhibiting hepatic aldehyde-NAD oxidoreductase. Within minutes of taking as little as 1 ounce of alcohol, the patient experiences an increase in serum acetaldehyde concentration that leads to palpitations, flushing, tachypnea, tachycardia, and shortness of breath. Nausea, vomiting, and headache develop if a greater amount of alcohol is taken. Symptoms last about 90 minutes and usually are self-limited. Occasionally, marked hypotension or a cardiac arrhythmia may occur. Fatalities from myocardial infarction and stroke have been reported. The agent can worsen depression and schizophrenia. Candidates require careful medical and psychiatric evaluation prior to initiating therapy.

Side effects include drowsiness and lethargy, which are countered by administering the drug before bed. The standard dose is 250 mg at bedtime. Important drug–drug interactions occur with antihypertensive agents (potentiation of hypotensive effect with intake of alcohol), benzodiazepines (reduced intensity of the disulfiram reaction), tricyclic antidepressants and phenothiazines (potentiation of CNS effects), and drugs metabolized by hepatic microsomes (prolongation of their half-lives).

Disulfiram achieves short-term improvement in alcohol consumption when used in a supervised comprehensive outpatient program that includes other rehabilitative measures. Success requires careful compliance and a stable life-style. Patients best suited are those who seek total abstinence, request the drug, have no underlying cardiovascular, depressive, or schizophrenic disease, and are willing to return monthly for evaluation of therapy.

The goal is to provide the patient time to organize the supports necessary for achievement of long-term abstinence. Disulfiram should not be considered an option for chronic use. Duration of therapy is individualized. Treatment ought to be terminated if the patient fails to keep appointments, resumes drinking, becomes pregnant or depressed, or develops abnormalities in liver function tests or cardiovascular status.

Psychoactive Drugs. Pharmacologic treatment of underlying psychopathology has been proposed as a means of cutting down on drinking. Anxiolytic agents such as the *benzodiazepines* (BZDs) have been used with a modicum of success in patients who drink because of an anxiety disorder. There is no evidence for long-term efficacy in reduction of alcohol use, but some data suggest a short-term reduction in anxiety that could enable a patient to engage in more comprehensive forms of therapy. BZDs have also been proposed as a means of reducing the desire to drink that might emanate from a postulated chronic withdrawal syndrome. Supporting data for both the syndrome and the efficacy of long-term drug treatment are minimal. *Tricyclic antidepressants* may be effective when there is an underlying depression, especially when it is accompanied by neurovegetative symptoms (see Chapter 227). *Lithium* has been tried with lesser success.

Drugs for Withdrawal. Manifestations of the acute withdrawal syndrome (tachycardia, elevation in blood pressure, tremor, hyperreflexia, increased irritability) can be blunted by the use of *benzodiazepines* or *beta-blockers*, and progression of seizures, hallucinations, and delirium tremens usually prevented. Diazepam (5–20 mg q6h), chlordiazepoxide (25–100 mg q6h), clorazepate (30 mg q12h), and the nonhepatically metabolized BZDs (lorazepam, 1–2 mg q4h, and oxazepam, 15–30 mg q4h) have all proven useful in the management of acute alcohol withdrawal. Among the beta-blockers, atenolol (50–100 mg/d) helps control adrenergic symptoms, reducing benzodiazepine requirements. *Clonidine*, a centrally acting inhibitor of noradrenergic activity, is an effective alternative to BZDs in mild to moderate withdrawal syndrome when used in a tapered program.

Inpatient versus Outpatient Programs. From the late 1940s through the mid-1980s, the standard of care for treatment of alcoholism was inpatient care. In addition to acute detoxification, the goal was total abstinence using drug therapy and a variety of psychological and social manipulations. Treatment typically involved a minimum stay of 28 days, used educational and confrontative techniques, and attempted to teach social skills. Alcoholics Anonymous (AA) meetings were an integral part of most programs and patients were expected to follow a life-regimen planned and monitored at the conclusion of the hospitalization. There was little free time or individualized care. Costs were high, often exceeding $10,000. Programs were run by psychologists, social workers, nurses, and counselors (most of whom were recovered alcoholics).

In the late 1980s, analysis of randomized studies found no overall advantage for residential over nonresidential treatment programs in terms of achieving long-term abstinence. Patient variables appeared to be more important than the site of care in determining outcome. Only one methodologically sound randomized trial has since demonstrated an advantage for inpatient care, and this one was part of an employee-assistance program, which is a well recognized determinant of success.

The net result is the current emphasis on outpatient care, except for treatment of severe acute withdrawal syndrome. Inpatient care remains an option for people who have failed all other forms of treatment and who will not deal with the problems so long as they are in environments that maintain destructive drinking. It is a costly approach and should be used as a last recourse. For most patients, an outpatient program is designed that combines psychotherapy and behavioral-cognitive approaches.

Outpatient psychotherapy places emphasis on psychic restructuring and removal of the presumed underlying psychopathology. Such treatment is important for the person whose interpersonal or psychologic problems outweigh his alcohol abuse. The best candidates are socially intact, intellectually curious, and eager to be involved in the process.

Alcoholism is associated with special needs that require the therapist to take a much more active role than is typical in insight-oriented psychotherapy. One must provide structure, guidance, support, nurturance, and instruction in helping the patient control drinking while working on the underlying conflicts and dysfunctional defense mechanisms.

Behavioral–cognitive therapies are based on the notion that alcoholism is a learned behavior that can be extinguished and reshaped, with controlled drinking a possible outcome. For patients who are rigid or seek treatments with defined, tangible end-points, behavioral therapy is often useful. In addition, it is helpful in dealing with problems involving role changes and behaviors in specific situations. *Aversive conditioning* is designed to either eliminate alcohol use or train patients to drink in moderation only. Alternative behaviors are taught via *operant conditioning*.

Cognitive therapy focuses on the observables of the drinking behavior (frequency, duration, quantity, time, place, activity, age-, sex-, and role-appropriate drinking behaviors). It attempts to identify the precipitants to abuse and the factors that maintain and perpetuate it.

Sociocultural treatment emphasizes altering external factors. It includes *residential care, halfway houses,* and direct social manipulation, such as *finding jobs,* helping with *shelter* and *money,* and removing a person from his family. This is a treatment appropriate for homeless, jobless, unstable persons whose social functioning is impaired, for repeated treatment failures, for young people, and for others with severe family problems.

Community Services. *Alcoholics Anonymous* provides the critical elements of social support, caring, and structure, which are essential to many patients. The program has a quasi-religious orientation, making it particularly useful to the religious person. Relatively superficial involvement (eg, 2–4 meetings per month) is usually not effective as a sole therapy, but can serve as a useful adjunct to other forms of treatment. However, the person willing to dedicate himself to a lifetime of sobriety can achieve the goal in this carefully delineated manner. *Al-Anon* and *Al-Ateen* assist family members of the alcoholic.

Employee assistance programs can be very useful, as motivation is often high. Most large companies offer such programs, and their counselors can work in tandem with physicians. They may also offer family, marital, and financial help, as may programs available through social service agencies, community guidance centers, and even state or federal agencies. Clergy and church organizations can be very helpful to religious persons.

PREVENTION

Prevention involves more than warning people of the health hazards of alcohol abuse. It requires screening for early detection of alcohol abuse (see above) and providing patient-specific information. By taking a brief drinking history at the time of the yearly checkup, the primary physician can educate the patient and provide suitable guidelines for drinking behavior, just as one does for exercise and diet.

People who do drink need to know how alcohol can affect them, how to behave responsibly when drinking (especially in regard to driving), and how to drink to prevent drunkenness (Tables 228–2 and 228–3). Individuals should know that their attitudes and behaviors will affect how their children/spouses drink. All should be cautioned that drinking is a dangerous way to deal with insomnia and emotional problems.

Instruction can be complemented by waiting-room literature, and hospital and community health-education programs. National campaigns focus on alcohol-related accidents, crime, and birth defects.

INDICATIONS FOR ADMISSION AND REFERRAL

The patient who has medically decompensated because of a complication of alcohol abuse (eg, heart failure, pancreatitis, gastrointestinal bleeding, hepatitis) clearly requires prompt hospital admission. Other candidates include persons with evidence of severe withdrawal (tremor, agitation, hallucinations, seizures) and those unable to tolerate a severe withdrawal syndrome (prior history of severe withdrawal, concurrent medical or psychiatric illness, chronic and severe alcohol-related illness). A free-standing detoxification center may suffice for the otherwise uncomplicated patient.

Patients with major psychopathology, poor ties to the physician, or a disintegrated social network have serious drawbacks to successful treatment by even the most willing primary care physician. Such patients should be referred in a coordinated way for specialized care, ensuring continuity as well as a personalized treatment program. The primary physician can perform a major service for these patients by

Table 228-2. Blood Alcohol Level*

TIME ELAPSED SINCE FIRST DRINK (IN HOURS)	NUMBER OF DRINKS†									
	1	*2*	*3*	*4*	*5*	*6*	*7*	*8*	*9*	*10*
1	0.01	0.03	0.05	0.08	0.10	0.13	0.15	0.17	0.20	0.22
2	0.00	0.02	0.04	0.06	0.09	0.11	0.14	0.16	0.19	0.21
3	0.00	0.005	0.02	0.05	0.07	0.10	0.12	0.14	0.17	0.19
4	0.00	0.00	0.01	0.03	0.06	0.08	0.11	0.13	0.15	0.18
5	0.00	0.00	0.00	0.02	0.04	0.07	0.09	0.11	0.14	0.16

*Determined by the number of drinks consumed in a circumscribed time period by a presumably normal 150-lb male. Females, because they are affected more quickly, require less alcohol to achieve these levels.

†Blood alcohol levels as a function of weight, time, and number of drinks consumed:

One drink = 1.5 oz 80-proof spirits (40% alcohol)
3.0 oz. fortified wine (20% alcohol)
5.0 ox table wine (12% alcohol)
12.0 oz beer (4.5% alcohol)

understanding available specialized referral resources in one's community and matching them to the patient's needs.

MANAGEMENT RECOMMENDATIONS

Some basic guides to follow regardless of which treatment is offered appear below:

- First establish rapport. Let the patient know you accept and understand him by approaching the problem in a respectful and comfortable manner.
- Offer appropriate and sufficient instruction and explanation as you go along, always engaging the patient in establishing realistic goals and not pushing him beyond his limits.
- Maintain a proper balance of support, caring, and limit-setting; remain flexible and adaptable to the patient's needs.
- Think of treatment as a series of short-term programs in order to develop and increase the patient's sense of mastery.
- Never insist on immediate abstinence. This is a goal to be negotiated. Only if all else fails should there be confrontation and control in this area, unless, of course, serious health problems will result from any alcohol intake.
- If a patient comes to a session drunk, kindly and calmly explain why it would be pointless to have a session and reschedule the appointment. If this behavior continues, the treatment agreement should be renegotiated to include rules about it.
- Keep motivation high, not only by utilizing the patient's fear of losing something or someone very important, but by getting him to seek and define his own reinforcers.
- Help the patient to identify, objectify, and deal with anger and other emotions in order to enhance emotional control.
- When the patient is ready, help him pinpoint the actual behaviors to be changed and work on them progressively. One may need to provide information, modeling, practice, feedback, and homework as the patient learns to handle feelings and to develop new social skills, the tools necessary to assess and modify his behavior.
- Encourage self-monitoring of drinking behavior via logs, teaching the patient to detect causes, consequences, and maintaining factors, and thus helping him learn alternate ways of coping with the people, places, situations, and feelings associated with heavy drinking.
- Select those components of available specialized treatment programs that match to the patient's needs, wants, and ability to cope. The standard formula of detoxification—disulfiram and AA—is no longer either the recommended or the most acceptable treatment for alcoholism.
- For spree and binge-drinking patients, whose interpersonal and psychologic problems are likely to be predominant, consider outpatient psychotherapy if they are socially intact, intellectually curious, and psychologically minded.
- For patients strongly motivated to attain total abstinence and specifically requesting disulfiram therapy, begin 250 mg qhs and renew on a monthly basis, re-evaluating the need for continued drug therapy while working on psychosocial interventions that will sustain long-term abstinence. Treatment is contraindicated in those with underlying psychiatric illness or cardiovascular disease.
- For patients who are rigid, repressed, and resistant to open-ended therapies, consider behavioral–cognitive methods.
- For patients willing to dedicate themselves to a lifetime of sobriety or who will benefit from peer counselling, consider AA, especially if there is a religious interest.

Table 228-3. Behavior Expected at Various Blood Alcohol Levels (BAL)

BAL	BEHAVIORAL EFFECTS
0.05	Relaxation; possibility of thought, judgment, and self-control being affected
0.10	Obvious impairment of voluntary motor action; legally drunk in most states
0.20	Considerable motor impairment and loss of emotional control; definite intoxication
0.40–0.50	Unconsciousness and probable death resulting from respiratory failure

- For patients who are homeless, jobless, or have other serious social problems, refer to a community social service agency for direct aid.
- For patients who have failed outpatient treatments, can afford the time, and need to be taken out of their environment to cease drinking, consider an inpatient alcohol program.
- Consider outpatient withdrawal from alcohol for reliable patients who have no underlying medical illnesses or a prior history of severe withdrawal and who have a supportive family that can provide supervision. Prescribe 50 mg of atenolol per day if the resting heart rate is less than 80 beats per minute and 100 mg per day if greater than 80. Supplement with a benzodiazepine (eg, diazepam 5–10 mg q6h). Treat for 1 week, tapering the benzodiazepine slowly; hospitalize promptly if any significant withdrawal symptoms develop (eg, tachycardia, tremor, hallucinations, increased irritability).

ANNOTATED BIBLIOGRAPHY

American College of Physicians. Disulfiram treatment of alcoholism. Ann Intern Med 1989;111:943. *(A position paper; recommends its selective use.)*

American Psychiatric Association. Diagnostic and Statistical Manual of Mental Disorders, 3rd edition - Revised. Washington DC: American Psychiatric Association, 1987. *(Provides diagnostic criteria for alcohol abuse and alcohol dependency.)*

Buchsbaum DG, Buchanan RG, Centor RM, et al. Screening for alcohol abuse using CAGE scores and likelihood ratios. Ann Intern Med 1991;115;774. *(An outpatient study; sensitivity 74 percent; specificity 91 percent.)*

Colquitt M, Fielding LP, Cronan JF. Drunk drivers and medical and social injury. N Engl J Med 1987;317:1262. *(Includes recommendations for physician action.)*

Donovan J, Jessor R, Jessor L. Problem drinking in adolescence and young adulthood. J Stud Alcohol 1983;44:109. *(Data on this growing population of high-risk drinkers.)*

Dorus W, Ostrow DG, Anton R, et al. Lithium treatment of depressed and nondepressed alcoholics. JAMA 1989;262:1646. *(Largest study to date; no benefit found over placebo.)*

Drummond DC, Thom B, Brown C, et al. Specialist versus general practitioner treatment of problem drinkers. Lancet 1990; 223:915. *(Suggests counseling by primary physicians can be as effective as more intensive efforts.)*

Frezza M, di Padova C, Pozzato G, et al. High blood alcohol levels in women: The role of decreased gastric alcohol dehydrogenase activity and first-pass metabolism. N Engl J Med 1990;322:95. *(The reason why women are more susceptible to the effects of alcohol.)*

Gelernter J, Goldman D, Risch N. The A1 allele at the D_2 dopamine receptor gene and alcoholism: A reappraisal. JAMA 1993;269:1673. *(A critical review of the data suggesting there is a gene for alcoholism; concludes the evidence is inconclusive.)*

Gerstel EK, Harford TC. Age-related patterns of daily alcohol consumption in metropolitan Boston. J Stud Alcohol 1981; 42:1062. *(A breakdown of how, when, and where people drink, and of changes with age.)*

Goldberg HI, Mullen M, Ries RK, et al. Alcohol counseling in a general medicine clinic: A randomized controlled trial of strategies to improve referral and show rates. Med Care 1991; 29:JS49. *(Formal screening raised referral rates five-fold.)*

Goodwin DW. Inpatient treatment of alcoholism. N Engl J Med 1991;325:804. *(An editorial reviewing the evidence for inpatient vs outpatient therapy.)*

Hanna E, Faden V, Dofour M. The social and motivational correlates of drinking, smoking, and illicit drug use during pregnancy. J Substance Abuse 1994;6:(in press). *(Depression over pregnancy proved to be an important factor.)*

Hayashida M, Alterman AI, McLellan AT, et al. Comparative effectiveness and costs of inpatient and outpatient detoxification of patients with mild-to-moderate alcohol withdrawal syndrome. N Engl J Med 1989;320:358. *(Outpatient detoxification was effective, safe, and less costly.)*

Johnson B, Clark W. Alcoholism. A challenging physician-patient encounter. J Gen Intern Med 1989;4:445. *(An approach to management that emphasizes the role of the patient–doctor relationship.)*

Jones TV, Lindsey BA, Yount P, et al. Alcoholism screening questionnaires: Are they valid in elderly medical outpatients? J Gen Intern Med 1993;8:674. *(The answer is "yes;" the CAGE questions performed best.)*

Kraus ML, Gottlieb LD, Horwitz RI, et al. Randomized clinical trial of atenolol in patients with alcohol withdrawal. N Engl J Med 1985;313:905. *(Atenolol proved effective in the community hospital setting.)*

Mendelson J, Babor T, Mello N, et al. Alcoholism and prevalence of medical and psychiatric disorders. J Stud Alcohol 1986; 47:361. *(High prevalence of significant medical and psychiatric problems.)*

Morse RM, Flavin DK, Joint Committee of the National Council on Alcoholism and Drug Dependence and the American Society of Addiction Medicine to Study the Definition and Criteria for the Diagnosis of Alcoholism. JAMA 1992;268:1012. *(Consensus definition and criteria.)*

Nace EP. The role of craving in the treatment of alcoholism. National Assoc Prev Pub Health J 1982;13:27. *(A guide to mastery over and understanding of wish/need to drink, leading to greater self control.)*

Nilssen O. The Tromso study: Identification of and a controlled intervention on a population of early-stage risk drinkers. Prev Med 1991;20:518. *(In heavy drinkers, a single session was as effective as an offer of monthly sessions.)*

Parker E, Noble E. Alcohol consumption and cognitive functioning in social drinkers. J Stud Alcohol 1977;38:1224. *(Details the effects of drinking on abstracting and adaptive abilities of social drinkers.)*

Sellars EM, Maranjo CA, Peachey JE. Drugs to decrease alcohol consumption. N Engl J Med 1981;305:1255. *(Reviews various pharmacotherapies for alcoholism and concludes that they can only serve as adjuncts to other therapies.)*

Skinner HA, Holt S. Identification of alcohol abuse using laboratory tests and a history of trauma. Ann Intern Med 1984; 101:847. *(A brief trauma history was more sensitive than laboratory tests in detecting problem drinking.)*

Tournier R. Alcoholics Anonymous as treatment and ideology. J Stud Alcohol 1979;40:230. *(A critique of AA; comments by other authorities starting on page 318 of the same issue.)*

Turner RC, Lichstein PR, Peden JG, et al. Alcohol withdrawal syndromes: A review of pathophysiology, clinical presentation, and treatment. J Gen Intern Med 1989;4:432. *(Comprehensive approach for the primary physician.)*

Walsh DC, Hingson RW, Merrigan DM, et al. A randomized trial of treatment options for alcohol-abusing workers. N Engl J Med 1991;325:775. *(The best data in support of inpatient treatment; a job-related program.)*

Wechsler H, Levine S, Idelson R, et al. The physician's role in health promotion—A survey of primary care practitioners. N Engl J Med 1983;308:97. *(Importance of physicians promoting healthy behavior is supported.)*

Wright C, Moore RD. Disulfiram treatment of alcoholism. Am J Med 1990;88:647. *(Comprehensive literature review; 103 refs.)*

Resource Materials

National Clearinghouse for Alcohol Information
P.O. Box 2345
Rockville, MD 20852

National Council on Alcoholism and Drug Addiction
733 Third Avenue
New York, NY 10017

Primary Care Medicine: Office Evaluation and Management of the Adult Patient, 3rd edition, edited by Allan H. Goroll, Lawrence A. May, and Albert G. Mulley, Jr. J.B. Lippincott Company, Philadelphia

229
Approach to the Patient With Sexual Dysfunction

LINDA C. SHAFER, M.D.

There is an important relationship between one's sexual life and emotional and physical well-being. Approximately 15 percent of medical outpatients come to primary care physicians with complaints that are primarily or secondarily sexual in nature. The incidence of sexual problems in any medical practice is a function of the frequency with which physicians take a sexual history. The primary care physician needs to know how to take a sexual history, perform an appropriate medical evaluation (see Chapters 115 and 132), and carry out basic types of sexual counselling and supportive therapy.

DEFINITIONS

Disorders are classified as "*primary*" when there has never been a period of satisfactory functioning, and "*secondary*" when the difficulty occurs after adequate functioning had been obtained.

Male Disorders

Impotence (erectile dysfunction) is defined as the inability of a male to maintain an erection sufficient to engage in intercourse and is considered a problem if it occurs in over 25 percent of attempts. *Premature ejaculation* is the loss of voluntary control of the ejaculatory reflex. Masters and Johnson have defined the condition in terms of the inability to satisfy the female partner at least 50 percent of the time. However, this presupposes that the female has no problem with orgasm. Premature ejaculation is most often defined as ejaculation that occurs in less than 2 minutes after penetration or on fewer than 10 thrusts. *Retarded ejaculation* is the inhibition of the ejaculatory reflex. There is a persistent failure to ejaculate in the presence of a satisfactory erection. *Retrograde ejaculation* is a physical impairment of internal vesical sphincter activity.

Female Disorders

Frigidity is a term applied to a wide variety of conditions in the female, from complete lack of any sexual response to various inadequacies in orgasmic response. As it is nonspecific and has a derogatory connotation, the term has been eliminated from most recent classifications. The *generally unresponsive female* (*excitement phase dysfunction*) is defined as the inability to respond to sexual stimulation with lubrication and genital vasocongestion. *Orgasmic dysfunction* refers to the inability to release the orgastic reflex and have an orgasm, despite ability to enjoy sexual intercourse and have normal sexual desire. There is no distinction between "healthy" vaginal and "infantile" clitoral orgasm. Some women who can have orgasm with direct clitoral stimulation find it impossible to reach orgasm during intercourse. This is a normal variant of sensitivity requiring the pairing of direct clitoral contact with intercourse. *Vaginismus* is an involuntary spasm of the musculature of the outer third of the vagina, making penile penetration impossible.

Both Sexes

Dyspareunia is a condition defined as painful intercourse in both sexes leading to avoidance of sexual contact. *Low libido* is defined as a lack of desire to engage in sexual activity for both males and females.

PSYCHOLOGICAL MECHANISMS AND CLINICAL PRESENTATIONS

While organic conditions should never be overlooked (see Chapters 115 and 132), the vast majority of sexual problems in both sexes are at least partially psychologic in origin. Although there are no rigid correlations between developmental factors and dysfunctional syndromes, sexual disorders can be related to *prior experiences*. Early sexual attitudes may be negatively shaped by parental communication that sex is bad, dirty, or sinful, by inadequate information about sex, or by myths and misconceptions such as the ever-ready penis or mutual climax. Other negative experiences range from unpleasant sexual encounters to rape. *Intrapsychic conflicts* extend from fear of sexual failure to concerns about sexual identity and profound depression.

Interpersonal issues of a sexual as well as nonsexual nature sometimes interfere with sexual functioning, especially in the setting of inadequate communication and lack of cooperation between partners. Sexual problems may develop from such nonsexual factors as *situational stress* and *financial pressures*. Lastly, sexual difficulty may occur in the context of the *anxiety* generated by an organic illness, such as fear of death after a heart attack.

Once a sexual problem ensues, regardless of the cause, a vicious cycle of fear of failure, anxiety, and guilt is likely to ensue and remain self-perpetuating.

Clinical presentations can be quite complex. In addition to sexual dysfunction, there may be somatic complaints with no apparent medical cause (eg, headache, low back pain, generalized pelvic pain, vulvar pruritus).

Impotence. Most normal men experience occasional erectile failure due to fatigue, too much alcohol, or any number of transient unfavorable circumstances. True impotence has an incidence that ranges from 1 percent in men under 35, to 25 percent in men over age 70, with the age-related increase related mostly to physiologic factors. Of note, a substantial proportion of men retain potency well into their 70s. Prolonged impotence and primary impotence are much more likely to be associated with medical disorders or more serious psychologic issues, such as fears of intimacy, feelings of intense hostility toward women, and gender identity questions.

Premature ejaculation is the most common male sexual disorder. The psychologic causes of the disorder range from early conditioning to ambivalence and hostility toward women. Its increasing frequency has been associated with women wanting more sexual satisfaction, particularly orgasm. Once premature ejaculation occurs, it can easily be reinforced by the negative attitudes expressed by the partner. In addition, prolonged periods of no sexual experience seem to make the problem worse. If premature ejaculation occurs over a long period of time and remains untreated, secondary impotence may result. It is often easily treated in the context of a good relationship and has a very good prognosis.

Retarded ejaculation occurs in 0.3 percent of males, most often in younger, less sexually experienced persons. Its milder form is often related to anxiety-provoking situations and has an excellent prognosis. When long-standing, the condition often signifies deeper-seated psychopathology, such as significant fears of rejection involved with letting go. Issues of control and commitment may be involved as well as unconscious conflicts regarding female genitals or pregnancy.

The generally unresponsive female presents with a complete avoidance of sexual activity or an aversion to sex, which is stoically endured. There is often a deep-seated conflict about sexuality, which makes the outcome less favorable. Concomitant depression and interpersonal problems as well as a history of medications or pelvic pathology (see Chapter 115) are other important factors.

Orgasmic dysfunction is the most frequent female sexual complaint and occurs more often during the early years of sexual activity. The capacity for orgasm appears to increase with sexual experience and that includes the aging female. Again, the psychologic factors involved are variable and the prognosis for the condition is a function of which factors are responsible. These range from fears of loss of control and unrealistic expectations about sexual performance to poor partner communication. Depression must not be overlooked.

Vaginismus is associated with a high incidence of pelvic pathology (see Chapter 115). A careful gynecologic examination is always warranted and, in fact, is the only definitive way to make a diagnosis. Vaginismus is one cause of *dyspareunia*. When related to psychologic factors, vaginismus can be considered a conditioned response and treated behaviorally. There is often confusion about sexual anatomy and physiology leading to fears of penetration and concerns about femininity. If the condition is long-standing, partners of these women can become seriously affected, developing secondary impotence. This disorder has been at the center of many cases of unconsummated marriages of long duration.

WORKUP

The Sexual History. The sexual history should be an integral part of every medical evaluation, given the importance of sexual function to overall health, the central role that sexual dysfunction might play in somatic complaints and quality of life, and the need to review safe sexual practices. The history is most easily obtained in conjunction with performing the gynecologic and menstrual review of systems in women and the genitourinary review in men. In this way, sexual practices and concerns can be comfortably elicited in the context of routine history-taking, especially if the physician displays an open, nonjudgmental, unembarrassed, and accepting attitude. One needs to take into account differences in social values, class, and age. Helpful screening questions include: "Does your present sexual functioning meet your expectations?" "Has there been a change in your sexual functioning?" "Would you like to change anything about your sexual functioning?"

If a sexual problem is uncovered, the chief complaint should be explored in detail. Ask patients to describe the problem in their own words, noting its duration, circumstances, possible precipitating and alleviating factors, and severity. A thorough description sometimes helps to distinguish an organic from a functional etiology (see Chapters 115 and 132). For example, in the impotent male, preservation of erectile function on awakening suggests a psychologic cause as does erection with attempts at masturbation.

Also try to elicit what type of treatment is viewed as potentially helpful, be it medicine, information, or support. Anything that tends to alleviate the problem, even if only temporarily, should be sought.

Physical Examination and Laboratory Studies. With improved understanding of the pathophysiology of sexual function and more sophisticated diagnostic testing, many sexual problems once thought to be purely psychogenic have been found to have an organic component as well. Thus, even when psychological or interpersonal problems are believed to be the principal cause of sexual dysfunction, a careful medical evaluation that includes a detailed physical examination in conjunction with a few pertinent laboratory studies is always indicated (see Chapters 115 and 132).

PRINCIPLES OF TREATMENT

The primary care physician is often the first person consulted by a patient with a sexual problem. Even the physician without formal training in sex therapy can help many patients deal effectively with their sexual difficulties. When the problem stems from guilt and misinformation, the physician can use his position as an authority figure to give *permission* and *reassurance,* relabelling as "neutral" or "positive" sexual activities that the patient might fear are "bad" or "sinful."

Educating patients and correcting misinformation is a function that should not be overlooked or underestimated. Giving permission or providing information may be all that is necessary to help many patients. An essential part of modern sexual counseling is the teaching of *safe sexual practices* and review of risk factors for HIV infection (see Chapters 7 and 13).

When the problem goes beyond misinformation, a trial of *behavioral methods* with specific suggestions to patient and partner can be helpful and is an appropriate next step. The objectives are to increase communication between partners, decrease performance anxiety and "spectatoring," change the goal of sexual activity towards feeling good and away from emphasis on erection or orgasm, and relieve the pressure to perform at each sexual encounter. A trial of such therapy is reasonable when there is no evidence of important underlying psychopathology or organic illness. Behavioral therapy will often lead to improved sexual function without the need for referral; however, couples who fail such therapy might benefit from consultation with a mental health professional trained in dealing with sexual problems.

TREATMENT RECOMMENDATIONS: BEHAVIORAL TECHNIQUES

Impotence

1. First educate the patient as to his ability to satisfy his partner without having penile vaginal intercourse.
2. Then begin "sensate focus" exercises, which start with nongenital massage and progress to genital massage. There should be a prohibition against intercourse, even if erections occur.
3. After erection is obtained by genital massage, progress to attempting intercourse. In the female-superior position, the female may manually stimulate the penis, and if erection is obtained, she may insert it into her vagina in a slow, nondemanding fashion, relieving the male of any responsibility for insertion. This may also be done with a partial erection. Gradual movement is begun. There is an emphasis on the pleasures of vaginal containment.

Premature Ejaculation

1. Educate the patient that his condition has little to do with the sensitivity of the penis but is usually the result of previous conditioning and anxiety.
2. Suggest an increase in the frequency of sexual activity.
3. Teach the Masters and Johnson "squeeze" technique. In this technique, the female manually stimulates the penis. When ejaculation is approaching the point of inevitability, as indicated by the male, the female squeezes the penis with her thumb on the frenulum, her index finger placed above, and her middle finger below the coronal ridge on the dorsal side of the penis. The pressure is applied until the male no longer feels the urgency to ejaculate (15 to 60 seconds). The "squeeze" technique should be repeated two or three times before ejaculation is allowed to occur.
4. Once there are good results with the squeeze technique, the couple can try intercourse. In the female-superior position, the female remains motionless to accustom the male to vaginal containment. Gradual thrusting begins using the "squeeze" technique as excitement intensifies.
5. An alternative to the "squeeze" technique is the "stop–start" method. The female stimulates the male to the point of ejaculation, at which time she stops the stimulation. The erection may or may not subside. She then resumes stimulating the penis. After several stop–start procedures, the male may ejaculate.

Retarded Ejaculation (During Intercourse)

1. The female stimulates the penis, asking for directions (verbal and physical) to enhance the feeling.
2. Extravaginal ejaculation is obtained by continued stimulation. In the male's mind, the female should become associated with ejaculatory release.
3. The female stimulates the penis manually until orgasm becomes inevitable. The penis is then inserted and the female thrusts demandingly. Manual stimulation is repeated if there is no successful ejaculation.

Generally Unresponsive Female (Excitement Phase Disorder)

This disorder often results from more severe psychopathology and usually requires referral for treatment. However, on the practical side, suggestions regarding the supplemental use of lubrication such as saliva or KY jelly should be made.

Orgasmic Dysfunction

1. Change the goal of sexual activity away from orgasm toward enjoyment of the experience.
2. Give permission to the female to express sexual feelings.
3. Begin sensate focus exercises, nongenital massage to genital massage. Use the back-protected position (male in a seated position with female between his legs with her back against his chest) with female in control to alleviate self-consciousness or spectatoring.

4. Instruct the male in stimulative technique: he should not force responsivity but rather seek to accommodate desires; he should not approach the clitoris directly because of sensitivity.
5. After success in manual genital stimulation, controlled intercourse in the female-superior position with the male making no demands comes next. This is followed by a lateral position which allows for mutual freedom of pelvic movement.
6. For women who have never experienced orgasm, suggestions regarding self-stimulation are appropriate. The use of fantasy material is most helpful.
7. For women who do have orgasms with masturbation but not intercourse, the "bridge technique" may be useful. After insertion of the penis, the male can stimulate the female (clitorally) manually or with a vibrator. This pairing can be helpful in achieving orgasm, and often after the female experiences orgasm in this way, the need for supplementary stimulation disappears.

Vaginismus

1. Explain to the patient and her partner that this condition is involuntary and not willfully caused. Physical demonstration of the involuntary vaginal spasm may be done by inserting a gloved finger into the vaginal entrance.
2. The couple is asked to refrain from intercourse during the early treatment.
3. In a stepwise, gradual fashion, the woman is encouraged to accept larger and larger objects into the vagina. This may be accomplished with the use of graduated Hegar dilators to be used in the office and at home, or the woman may begin by using her fingers, first one, then several approximately the size of the penis. She may use her partner's fingers. Syringe containers of different sizes make good dilators.
4. In the female-superior position, the woman gradually inserts the penis.

INDICATIONS FOR REFERRAL

After trying these behavioral techniques, the patient's condition may still not be improved. This is often a sign that a referral to a psychiatrist who specializes in the area is indicated, and that the patient needs more intensive therapy. Often, direct referral to the specialist is indicated for patients with chronic psychopathology, such as those with "primary" sexual dysfunctions, gender identity questions or homosexual conflicts, marked personality disorders or significant past psychiatric history (especially of psychosis), or overt evidence of a clinical depression underlying the sexual complaint. Moreover, chronic severe problems in the relationship with one's partner signal the need for a referral.

For both organically based impotence and impotence refractory to psychologic treatment, it is appropriate to refer for consideration of a pharmacologic erection program, external vacuum therapy, and surgical penile implant (see Chapter 132). The success of such treatment requires close collaboration between the urologist and the psychiatrist.

PATIENT EDUCATION

Early in one's practice, it becomes clear that patients have many sexual questions and concerns. Inadequate or inaccurate information about sexual anatomy, physiology, and practices is the basis for many sexual problems. Therefore, sex education should not be overlooked. Patients can sometimes obtain supplemental information from suggested reading material. Several helpful books include *For Yourself: The Fulfillment of Female Sexuality* by Lonnie Garfield Barbach, New York, Doubleday, 1975; *The New Male Sexuality* by Bernie Zilbergeld, Boston, Little, Brown, 1992; *How to Overcome Premature Ejaculation* by Helen Singer Kaplan, New York, Brunner/Mazel, 1989; and *The Joy of Sex,* edited by Alex Comfort, New York, Simon and Schuster, 1989. A visit to answer questions which come up in the context of reading is always appreciated.

Lack of knowledge regarding safe sex practices is a major contributor to the spread of HIV infection. Concern about HIV infection can also interfere with enjoyment of sexual activity. Detailed review of safe sex practices is essential (see Chapters 7 and 13). Condom use is critical for those with multiple sexual partners and for monogamous partners in whom HIV status is unknown. With prudent precautions and a little creativity (eg, making condom application an early part of foreplay), a safe and enjoyable sexual life can still be attained.

ANNOTATED BIBLIOGRAPHY

Croft HA. Managing common sexual problems. Postgrad Med 1976;60(3):200; 60(4):193; 60(5):186; 60(6):164. *(A still excellent series of articles geared for use by primary care physicians treating sexual problems.)*

Franger AL. Taking a sexual history and managing common sexual problems. J Reprod Med 1988;33:639. *(The discussion on taking the sexual history is especially useful.)*

Kaplan HS. The Evaluation of Sexual Disorders. New York: Brunner/Mazel, 1983. *(Authoritative general reference.)*

Leiblum SR, Rosen RC. Principles and Practice of Sex Therapy, 2nd Edition, Update for the 1990s. New York: Guilford Press, 1989. *(Comprehensive review of sex therapy, including aspects related to HIV disease.)*

NIH Consensus Development Panel on Impotence. JAMA 1993;270:83. *(A detailed consensus report that includes recommendations on methods of treatment.)*

Schover LR, Jensen SB. Sexuality and Chronic Illness. New York: Guilford Press, 1988. *(Useful reference for physicians treating chronic disease.)*

Masters W, Johnson V. Human Sexual Inadequacy. Boston, Little, Brown, 1970. *(The now classic work which revolutionized the treatment of sexual disorders by proposing a behavioral framework for treatment.)*

230
Approach to the Somatizing Patient

ARTHUR J. BARSKY, III, M.D.

Primary Care Medicine: Office Evaluation and Management of the Adult Patient, 3rd edition, edited by Allan H. Goroll, Lawrence A. May, and Albert G. Mulley, Jr. J.B. Lippincott Company, Philadelphia

The somatizing patient presents with bodily complaints or disability out of proportion to any demonstrable organic pathology. Included in this category are anxious and depressed patients, hypochondriacs, chronic pain patients, and malingerers. These people are among the most frustrating and troublesome encountered in primary care, but they can be evaluated and managed successfully. Attention to the causative psychopathology helps to render symptoms understandable, enables the physician to distinguish them from those due to organic pathology, and facilitates management.

PSYCHOLOGICAL MECHANISMS AND CLINICAL PRESENTATIONS

Anxiety (see Chapter 226). Individuals suffering from *chronic anxiety* focus on and become alarmed by normal bodily sensations. They report headache, gastrointestinal disturbance, or musculoskeletal pain. *Panic anxiety* has somatic manifestations that include palpitations, chest pain, tachycardia, dyspnea, choking sensations, diarrhea, cramps, sweating, and fainting.

Depression (see Chapter 227). Depression's neurovegetative symptoms may overshadow the characteristic affective, cognitive, and behavioral changes. As many as one-half of somatizing ambulatory medical patients over age 40 are depressed. The chief complaint may be headache, constipation, weakness, fatigue, abdominal pain, insomnia, anorexia, or weight loss. Depressed patients worry about and focus attention on their bodies. A positive review of systems, chronic pain, or complaints involving multiple organ systems typify the clinical presentation, and symptoms recur with the periodicity characteristic of depressions.

Personality disturbances exist in a considerable number of somatizers. The terms *crock, hypochondriac,* and *chronic complainer* refer to patients whose symptoms, illness, invalidism, and pursuit of medical care have become a way of life. For them, illness and medical treatment furnish a vocabulary for interacting with other people, a way of responding to stress, and a means for expressing psychological needs and conflicts. They are preoccupied with their bodies and their health, convinced that they have some occult serious medical disease. At the same time, they fear disease intensely. Their symptoms shift and fluctuate over time, being nonspecific, ambiguous, and similar to the transient sensations felt by healthy individuals. Worry about being ill is remarkably persistent, and it is not assuaged by reassurance despite thorough medical evaluation. At times, they may have genuine medical problems, but their suffering, disability, and medical care needs are in excess of any objective pathology. By their reports, medical care has been disappointing, failing to provide a cure or even relief of symptoms.

When interviewed, such patients talk mainly about their illnesses and medical care, little about friends, work, or hobbies. Often, they seem as concerned with establishing the authenticity of their complaints as with obtaining relief. They adamantly deny any emotional contribution to their symptoms (in contrast to many patients with serious physical disease, who are willing to consider the possibility that anxiety and depression make their symptoms worse).

In attempting to understand these patients, some authorities have emphasized the unconscious meaning and gratification of pain and discomfort. Bodily complaints may be amplified by a deprived and needy person who has only experienced caring and attention when sick or in pain. Suffering and illness can thus become ways to express and gratify yearnings for contact, comfort, and support. Other hypochondriacal individuals are angry and hostile, feeling rejected or wronged in some way. For them, physical symptoms offer a nonverbal way of expressing their anger, recrimination and blame, by reproaching and belaboring others with their suffering. Finally, symptoms and illness can unconsciously serve to distract some individuals from an even more painful sense of themselves as fundamentally worthless and defective as people. They can thus attribute their failures, disappointments, and rejections to a physical incapacity rather than to any personal inadequacy.

Chronic complainers gain *self-esteem* and a sense of *identity* from their ability to endure suffering, survive misfortune, and tolerate discomfort. Their requests for relief and cure can be understood as attempts to gain respect for their ability to endure and survive, rather than as a true desire to end the discomfort.

Postconcussion syndrome is a self-limited condition that follows mild to moderate head trauma. A variety of somatic symptoms (headache, dizziness) accompany emotional ones (depression, sleeplessness, irritability).

Conversion reactions are acute physical dysfunctions that suggest medical disorder, but which are actually the expression of a psychological need or conflict. The emotional distress is thought of as being "converted" into, or expressed as, physical distress. The process is entirely unconscious. Symptoms are either sensory or neuromuscular (eg, weakness, paralysis, ataxia, blindness, aphasia, deafness, anesthesia, paresthesias, or seizures) and generally of short duration. Other features include a prior history of similar reactions, major emotional stress prior to onset, and apparent symbolic meaning to the symptom (eg, "heartache" following the loss of a loved one; blindness after viewing a horrifying event). Major secondary gain and other significant psychopathology are also present.

Somatic delusions are seen in schizophrenia, severe affective disorders, and organic brain syndromes. These are false, fixed ideas that are often vivid, bizarre, or extraordinary. Unlike hypochondriacal concerns, they do not fluctuate. The individual may believe some extraordinary change has occurred in his body, for example, that his organs are shriveling up, that body parts are deformed or missing, or that foreign objects are inside an orifice or organ.

Some patients suffer from *bodily dysmorphic disorder*, a fixed, circumscribed delusion that they are physically deformed, although their appearance is actually unremarkable. A facial feature is often the focus. The condition is chronic.

Malingering differs from the above mentioned conditions in that there is conscious simulation of illness and no actual experiencing of the symptoms reported. It is relatively rare outside of situations in which illness confers some obvious benefit, as in prisons, among drug addicts, or in individuals under some legal threat. Symptoms are exaggerated, and the subject's description of them may vary with each interview. When the patient is unaware that he is being observed, he may relax the simulation and thus betray himself. Such individuals are frequently sociopaths or drug addicts. Some may have worked in a medically related field.

DIFFERENTIAL DIAGNOSIS

The differential diagnosis of somatizing includes anxiety, depression, postconcussion syndrome, conversion reaction, hypochondriacal personality disturbance, schizophrenia, and malingering. Hypochondriacal patients seen in the medical setting have the same propensity for medical illness as their nonhypochondriacal counterparts. Thus, one must rule out organic causes, just as with any other patient being seen in a medical setting. Medical disorders that affect multiple organ systems and produce transient or recurrent, nonspecific complaints (eg, multiple sclerosis, systemic lupus, polymyalgia rheumatica, Lyme disease, chronic fatigue syndrome, fibromyalgia syndrome, hyperparathyroidism) pose the greatest diagnostic difficulty.

WORKUP

Differentiating Somatization From Organic Disease. The task is not always easy (see Chapters 8, 226, and 227), but the quality, timing, and precipitants of symptoms, as well as the patient's response to illness, attitude, and choice of words can be of considerable help.

Quality of Symptoms. A complaint whose characteristics are anatomically and physiologically *inconsistent* with anatomy and known pathophysiology are very likely to be psychogenic in origin. For example, psychogenic sensory complaints often cross the midline or involve combinations of sensory modalities that are neurologically impossible (see Chapter 167). Hysterical seizures do not involve incontinence or tongue-biting, and the hysterically blind exhibit a withdrawal or startle reflex when a hand is flashed before the face. With hysterical paralysis of the upper extremity, the patient's arm avoids the face after being held above it and released. In hysterical paralysis of one lower extremity, the patient's attempts to move the afflicted leg do not invoke contraction of the other leg, as is the case in neurologic disease.

Other qualities of a psychogenic complaint include its being exactly like a symptom that afflicted someone important to the patient, or its being *excessively vague* or *overly detailed*. Diffuse, inconsistent descriptions as well as vivid, elaborate ones are very suggestive. Psychological factors may be revealed in the choice of words (eg, "pain in the neck," or "not having a leg to stand on").

Timing and Precipitants. Psychogenic pain is typically unaffected by activity or by the passage of time, and the patient often seems more concerned with the physician's accepting the authenticity of his pain than with relieving it. Although both physical and psychological illness can be precipitated by stress, the onset of psychogenic complaints is often closely associated with *significant emotional stress*, such as the loss of a loved one, or the onset of a major interpersonal conflict or sexual problem. Functional complaints are also prone to occur on the *anniversary* of a psychologically meaningful event, such as the death of a loved one.

Attitude Toward Symptoms. When the patient is *unconcerned*, inappropriately calm, or more concerned with *establishing authenticity* than with obtaining relief, one should suspect a strong emotional component. As noted, patients with psychogenic complaints who unconsciously derive considerable gain from their illness are often reluctant to consider an emotional cause for their symptoms.

Defining the Underlying Psychopathology. Once a psychogenic etiology is suspected on the basis of the clinical presentation, evaluation should proceed to define the underlying psychopathology. Inquiry into precipitants, response to illness, and personality can be helpful.

Precipitants and Response to Illness. History is searched for ongoing psychological stress, pending litigation or disability proceedings, prior medical complaints without a demonstrable physical cause, depression, anxiety, prior psychosis, and recent head trauma. Details of previous medical care experiences can be revealing. A history of consulting many physicians for the same complaints, or of the immediate replacement of a treated symptom with a new one, help in the diagnosis of psychogenic illness.

Personality. It is important to determine if illness, discomfort, and disability have become important parts of the patient's personality and to what extent they are used to deal with emotional discomfort, interpersonal difficulties, and environmental stress. Does the patient see himself as the suffering unfortunate one whose life is filled with disappointment, "bad luck," and defeat, as well as with illness? Expressions of anger and hostility may be indirect, as in cynicism, sarcasm, and uncooperativeness. The individual feels deprived and put upon and is likely to recriminate, accuse and blame. Finally, excessive dependence on others may be a feature of his personality. One senses an overpowering desire for care, attention, sympathy, and human contact. The patient's attitude toward the physician may have a clinging and hungry quality.

Personal Significance and Secondary Gain. What personal significance does the patient attach to his symptoms or to the suspected illness? Are there possible secondary gains, such as 1) receiving sympathy, attention, and support (including financial support) from family and friends; 2) being excused from duties, challenges, and responsibilities; and 3) acquiring the power to influence and manipulate others because he is sick.

Physical Examination and Laboratory Studies. A thorough physical examination and a careful mental status examination are essential. Not only may unexpected evidence of organic illness turn up, but a normal examination is a prerequisite for effective reassurance and the avoidance of unnecessary laboratory testing. Unless there is evidence that is strongly suggestive of organic pathology, elaborate and, particularly, invasive studies should be avoided. Performing a noninvasive test to help provide reassurance can be constructive, but radiologic and biochemical hunting expeditions may only add to confusion and expense. The likelihood of a false-positive result is high when the pretest probability of organic pathology is low (see Chapter 2).

PRINCIPLES OF MANAGEMENT

Support. Management must be directed at the underlying psychopathology as well as at the presenting bodily complaints. The first step is to put the complaint in perspective, while recognizing that the patient has come because of physical symptoms. When the results of the workup are presented, the reality of the symptoms should not be denied, nor should it be implied that they are imaginary. The patient can be told that serious, damaging organic disease has been ruled out and that stress can amplify real bodily sensations and disrupt normal function. It is important to avoid saying "there is nothing wrong," which may make the patient feel foolish or angry. The presence of symptoms is an indication of considerable distress, which the patient should be encouraged to discuss. The patient needs to know that the relationship with his physician will not terminate because the medical workup is "negative."

Additional visits should be scheduled to provide time to further discuss personal and situational problems on a regular basis. By offering the patient a long-term relationship that is not contingent on organic symptoms, one may remove a major stimulus for their development. Refractory cases may benefit from referral to a psychiatrist.

Proper Use of Drug Therapy. Nonspecific attempts to suppress somatization pharmacologically should be avoided. All too often, patients are told that their symptoms are due to their "nerves" and sent away with a prescription for a minor tranquilizer. Such an approach to therapy usually fails, and it often alienates the patient. It is especially important to recognize depression because of its high prevalence, subtle manifestations, and good response to therapy. The neurovegetative symptoms of depression respond well to antidepressant medication (see Chapter 227). Anxiety disorder may be helped by the use of a benzodiazepine (see Chapter 226); schizophrenia, by a phenothiazine. The post-concussion syndrome is self-limited, resolving within 6 to 24 months.

Treatment of Personality Disorders. Because the best treatment is supportive, the majority of patients with somatization due to a personality disturbances can be managed by the primary physician. Medical intervention should be minimized whenever possible. As noted, major diagnostic workups for equivocal or questionable findings should be avoided, as should pain medication and tranquilizers. Even though medication is often requested, these patients generally do not respond to it and tend to be especially prone to development of troublesome side effects and adverse reactions.

The situational or psychological need to remain disabled, distressed, and symptomatic must be recognized. No surgical procedure can excise, no oral medication can cure the *need to be ill.* The patient's self-esteem needs bolstering. *Acknowledging his strength to endure suffering,* tolerate discomfort, and survive hardship and misfortune is particularly gratifying to him. These are qualities the patient values most in himself and are a source of what little self-esteem he has. Consequently, the physician must not expect cure, because the patient loses no time in reporting that he is no better, and perhaps is worse.

To avoid struggles, the patient, especially if hostile and angry, should be involved as much as possible in therapeutic and diagnostic decisions. The physician ought to make it clear that his role is to help the patient tolerate discomfort rather than to eliminate it. Therapeutic suggestions should be made with the implication that although they may be of moderate palliative value, they will probably not help dramatically.

Conversion Reactions. There are two aspects to the treatment of hysterical conversion reactions: 1) symptom removal; and 2) management of the internal conflict to avoid development of bodily complaints. The first is done through education, reassurance, and use of suggestion to reduce the patient's anxiety (hysterical patients are exceptionally suggestive). The patient should be assured that the disorder is self-limited and that the symptoms will gradually improve and finally vanish. Conversion symptoms are likely to recur, however, unless psychotherapy is arranged to alter the psychological forces at work.

Malingering. Malingering is resistance to treatment. Diagnostic and therapeutic procedures should be avoided whenever possible because they reinforce pathologic behavior. Any abnormal laboratory tests or physical findings are suspect.

INDICATIONS FOR REFERRAL

Most somatizing patients can be managed by the primary physician. Referral is indicated when a patient has accepted a psychological explanation of his symptoms and wants to see a psychiatrist; when a conversion reaction, serious anxiety disorder, or psychosis is present; or when the primary physician has such a negative reaction to the patient with a personality disorder that he cannot serve him well.

TREATMENT RECOMMENDATIONS

- Explain the results of the medical workup without denying the reality of the patient's discomfort.
- Encourage discussion of psychosocial problems and set up a regular schedule of appointments for further elaboration and supportive therapy. Make it clear to the patient that he need not have physical symptoms to see the doctor. Avoid prn appointments.
- Treat the underlying psychological problem specifically; do not attempt the nonspecific suppression of symptoms with tranquilizers.
- Do not try to remove or cure symptoms in the patient with a somatizing personality disorder. Acknowledge the suffering and provide support. Avoid the use of medication and the extensive workup of vague symptoms. Make adaptation to chronic discomfort the goal of care.

ANNOTATED BIBLIOGRAPHY

Adler G. The physician and the hypochondriacal patient. N Engl J Med 1981;304:1394. *(A brief, but very useful review.)*

Barsky AJ, Wyshak G, Latham KS, et al. The relationship between hypchondriasis and medical illness. Arch Intern Med 1991;151:84. *(Hypochondriacs have the same degree of organic illness as their nonhypochondriacal counterparts.)*

Barsky AJ, Wyshak G, Latham KS, et al. Hypochondriacal patients, their physicians, and their medical care. J Gen Intern Med 1991;6:413. *(Much physician frustration and impaired recognition of anxiety and depression.)*

Barsky AJ, Klerman GL. Overview: Hypochondriasis, bodily complaints, and somatic styles. Am J Psychiatry 1983;140: 273. *(Review of the different conceptualizations that have been advanced to understand hypochondriasis.)*

Brown HN, Vaillant GE. Hypochondriasis. Arch Intern Med 1981;141:723. *(Clear, explicit, and practical discussion of the role of hostility, aggression, and anger.)*

Engel GL. "Psychogenic" pain and the pain-prone patient. Am J Med 1959;26:899. *(A classic paper on the psychology of somatizing.)*

Kaplan C, Lipkin M Jr, Gordon GH. Somatization in primary care: Patients with unexplained and vexing medical complaints. J Gen Intern Med 1988;3:177. *(A detailed review for the primary care physician that covers both theoretical and practical issues; 92 refs.)*

Lazare A. Conversion symptoms. N Engl J Med 1981;305:745. *(Tersely considers incidence, etiology, diagnosis, prognosis, and treatment.)*

Lipsitt DR. Medical and psychological characteristics of "crocks." Psychiatry Med 1970;1:15. *(Another classic paper; helps one understand and manage the chronic somatizer.)*

Monson RA, Smith GR, Jr. Somatization disorder in primary care. N Engl J Med 1983;308:1464. *(Stresses the importance of a long-term physician–patient relationship and provides strategies for management.)*

Rosen G, Kleinman A, Katon W. Somatization in family practice: A biopsychosocial approach. J Fam Pract 1982;14:493. *(Emphasizes the role of the family and sociocultural forces.)*

Smith GR, Monson RA, Ray DC. Psychiatric consultation in somatization disorder. N Engl J Med 1986;314:1407. *(A controlled randomized study showing that consultation reduced health care utilization but did not improve health status or staisfaction with care.)*

231
Approach to the Angry Patient

ARTHUR J. BARSKY, III, M.D.

Patients often become angry in response to the suffering and disability caused by disease, adverse life events, or the psychologic threats inherent in being a patient. When faced with an angry patient, the primary physician needs to be able to recognize the source of the patient's anger, prevent it from interfering with therapeutic efforts, and help the patient to cope.

PSYCHOLOGICAL MECHANISMS

People become angry when they feel threatened or when their wishes and aims are frustrated. Illness often causes anger because it presents the threats of disfigurement, pain, lost opportunity, abandonment, and even death. Some patients are particularly enraged by the *helplessness*, lack of control, and enforced passivity that disease confers.

Other patients are uncomfortable in the doctor–patient relationship because it represents the threat of *dependence* on the physician—of allowing someone powerful to take control of, take care of, and be responsible for them. They use anger to defend themselves against the intimacy and closeness that might develop with the doctor in the course of receiving medical care. Anger, then, can be an attempt to drive the physician away and allay the threat of dependency or intimacy which is inherent in the doctor–patient relationship.

Patients commonly express to their clinicians anger derived from threats and stresses they have encountered *elsewhere* in their lives. In such instances, the animosity and hostility seem inappropriate to the situation and out of proportion to any provocation the doctor can think of. This usually occurs when patients are in conflict with important people in their lives to whom they cannot express their anger, such as an employer or a family member.

Other patients appear to live a life permeated by their quick temper, chronic resentments, and dissatisfactions. The physician is little more than a screen onto which they project hostility garnered elsewhere. *Globally angry* patients may have a *borderline personality organization*. Both in their relationships to the physician and with other people they are close to, they appear generally abusive, stormy, and ungrateful. These patients have long histories of relating to physicians and others in a *dependent*, yet *demanding* fashion, exhibiting hostility toward and devaluation of the very people on whom they depend so desperately. Their anger expresses their expectation that people will generally be uncaring and unsympathetic. It also reflects their disappointment and feeling that they have been let down and not received the help they feel they need and deserve.

RECOGNIZING THE ANGRY PATIENT

Anger may be expressed verbally in direct statements that convey demands, annoyance, and resentment, as well as in personal histories of temper outbursts and undirected violence (eg, slamming doors). It may be expressed more obliquely through cynicism, sarcasm, negativism, and behavior which, while superficially compliant and cooperative, is actually obstructive (ie, *passive-aggressive*). Anger may be evidenced by behavior as well as words, for example, failure to adhere to a medical regimen, keep appointments, or quit self-destructive health habits.

Helpful nonverbal clues may be observed during the interview. The angry patient clenches his fists and jaws or knits his forehead in a frown. The palpebral fissures are narrowed, lips compressed, and nostrils widened. Gestures and gait may be explosive.

Finally, the interviewer's own subjective, emotional response to the patient during the interview may convey important diagnostic information. Whenever the interviewer is aware of feeling irritated or bored with a patient, he should question himself as to whether these feelings are an unconscious response to the patient's anger and hostility.

It is important not only to recognize that the patient is angry but also to learn what he is angry about. During the interview, the physician should note the subject matter that brings out irritation, annoyance, or hostility. The themes which seem to evoke anger are important clues to the issues that are troubling the patient.

The globally angry patient with a borderline personality organization can be recognized by a few clinical characteristics: 1) interpersonal relationships are either superficial or very dependent and manipulative; 2) emotions are intense and labile; extreme emptiness and anger predominate; 3) social and intellectual skills may be well developed, but the patient's life is marked by lack of fulfillment and frequent failures; and 4) impulsive, manipulative, and self-destructive behavior is present.

PRINCIPLES OF MANAGEMENT

Once the physician has recognized that the patient is angry and has defined any specific threats or frustrations that are fueling the anger, he can proceed to *acknowledge the patient's feelings* and reassure him that they will not destroy their relationship. This often helps bring about a more open give-and-take discussion between doctor and patient. The physician need not agree that the patient's feeling is justified, but he or she should acknowledge its existence by explicitly presenting the patient with his or her observations and the reasons for concluding that the patient is angry. Such discussion can introduce an atmosphere of openness, honesty, and sensitivity into the therapeutic relationship. The physician should convey the sense that he is neither afraid of the patient's feelings nor rejecting of him, but rather interested in trying to help him.

If the patient's hostility interferes with communication, the therapeutic regimen, or coping with illness, the doctor should point this out. The physician needs to indicate that while he recognizes the patient's anger and his right to have it, it nonetheless represents a problem because it is self-destructive, interfering with therapy or recovery. One need not be bullied by the globally angry patient. It is possible and necessary to set limits on the patient's behavior while making it clear that there will be no counterattack in retribution.

By defining the specific frustrations and threats, the physician should be able to approach the patient more effectively. For the patient who is angry about being ill, detailed investigation of exact fears and sources of despair is helpful. For the patient who is angry about being thrust into the patient role, one might try to structure the relationship so as to minimize those aspects which most threaten the patient. If the patient most fears dependency, the physician should assume a somewhat cool, reserved, and businesslike stance, while still conveying support and sympathy. Finally, if the anger seems to be displaced on the physician from some other situation or relationship, this may be pointed out, without specifically encouraging the patient to vent his hostility on its actual source.

The physician should take care that he does not react with his own hostility to the angry and provocative patient. Maintaining perspective on the situation will help the physician to recognize when clinical anger is not a criticism, but rather a response to the inner torment of fears, threats, and frustrated wishes. By doing so, one is in a good position to help the angry patient, preserve the therapeutic relationship, and more effectively carry out medical care.

ANNOTATED BIBLIOGRAPHY

Adler G. Valuing and devaluing in the psychotherapeutic process. Arch Gen Psychiatry 1970;22:454. *(The psychdynamics of patient anger; a classic paper.)*

Crutcher JE, Bass MJ. The difficult patient and the troubled physician. J Fam Pract 1980;11:933. *(Empirical research on the types of patients and patient problems that irritate and dismay physicians.)*

Groves JE. Taking care of the hateful patient. N Engl J Med 1978;298:883. *(Discussion includes the physician's own emotional responses to patients, and the ways to use these responses constructively.)*

Gunderson J, Singer M. Defining borderline patients. Am J Psychol 1975;132:1. *(An excellent review identifying basic characteristics of such patients, including intense, often hostile affect; 87 refs.)*

Kahana RJ, Bibring GL. Personality types in medical management. *In* Zinberg N (ed): Psychiatry and Medical Practice in a General Hospital. New York, International University Press, 1965. *(A classic chapter that discusses the range of emotional meanings and responses to illness.)*

232

Approach to the Patient With Insomnia

JEFFREY B. WEILBURG, M.D.

Primary Care Medicine: Office Evaluation and Management of the Adult Patient, 3rd edition, edited by Allan H. Goroll, Lawrence A. May, and Albert G. Mulley, Jr. J.B. Lippincott Company, Philadelphia

Occasional difficulty falling asleep or staying asleep is a universal and normal human experience. Insomnia, defined as persistent difficulty falling or staying asleep that compromises daytime functioning, is also a common problem, with 15 to 20 percent of the general population complaining of it during visits to primary care physicians. Insomnia affects patients of all ages and is particularly troublesome in the elderly.

Most patients with insomnia try a host of techniques, home remedies, and nonprescription drugs before seeking medical help. They frequently come to the primary physician requesting more potent sleep medication. The primary care doctor needs to be skilled in the assessment and therapy of insomnia, not only because the problem is extremely common and a cause of considerable misery, but also because it is an important precipitant of excessive drug use and habituation. Almost a billion dollars are spent each year in the United States on medication for sleep.

PATHOPHYSIOLOGY AND CLINICAL PRESENTATION

Insomnia is best regarded as a symptom, or complaint, which may be produced by a variety of underlying pathophysiologic processes. Sleep physiology is examined by using the polysomnogram, a continuous all-night recording of respiration, eye movements, electroencephalogram (EEG), muscle tone, blood oxygen saturation, and ECG.

Normal Sleep versus Insomnia. *Normal sleep* can be divided into two basic phases: *REM*, or *rapid eye movement sleep*, and *nonREM (NREM)*. REM is a state of mental and physical activation. Pulse and respiration are increased but muscle tone is diminished, so little body movement occurs. The brain is active, and the EEG shows a pattern similar to that seen during waking. Most dreaming occurs during REM. In contrast, NREM is a time of deep rest. Pulse, respiration, and EEG all slow, and the patient goes from light sleep, called stages 1 and 2, to deep or delta sleep, called stages 3 and 4. REM and NREM normally cycle in a reciprocal pattern, giving a typical "architecture" to the polysomnogram. The entire cycle lasts about 90 minutes, and is repeated smoothly four or five times during the night.

Insomnia has no pathognomonic polysomnographic pattern. Some insomniacs have slightly shorter than normal sleep times, some have less stages 3 and 4 sleep, but most have normal-appearing polysomnograms. Sight disruptions of the normal smooth cycling caused by frequent brief arousals may be related to subjectively unsatisfying sleep. Psychologic variables appear to strongly influence an insomniac's perceptions of the restfulness of time spent in bed.

Psychiatric disorders are believed by most experts to be the underlying cause in about half of all insomnia cases. Patients with *major depression* complain of either difficulty falling asleep or of waking in the early morning and being unable to return to sleep. Diurnal variation of mood is often noted. Severe depression with agitation may lead to markedly diminished total sleep and overall exhaustion (see Chapter 227). Patients in the manic phase of a *bipolar affective disorder* have diminished total sleep time but do not report feeling tired during waking times.

Patients suffering from *dysthymic disorder* (a variant of depression; see Chapter 227), typically complain of feeling tired, irritable, have difficulty falling asleep, and report that they cannot get enough sleep to feel rested. Sometimes they deny feeling sad or depressed and focus only on their physical complaints. Insomnia may be their major presenting complaint.

Patients with *anxiety* and *obsessive disorders* frequently have great difficulty falling asleep because they lie in bed and ruminate. *Character disorders* make up about 40 percent of the other psychiatrically based insomnias. Patients with narcissistic or borderline character disorders characteristically feel angry or entitled and may have difficulty falling asleep. They lie in bed, furiously trying to make themselves sleep. Such patients may use their insomnia as a justification for their inability to function or to get ahead in life. Their lack of sleep is viewed as the source of all their troubles. Some even use it as a rationale for their inability to comply with the treatment of the insomnia itself.

Active *psychosis* of any type (eg, schizophrenia) produces disturbed sleep and accounts for the other 10 percent of psychiatric insomnia. Hallucinations, delusions, and other signs and symptoms of psychotic illness present with the insomnia, facilitating recognition.

Drugs and Substance Abuse. Drugs and alcohol account for about 10 percent to 15 percent of all cases. *Alcohol* induces sedation, but the resulting sleep is often shallow, fragmented, and not restorative. Alcoholics can have prematurely "aged" sleep (ie, shallow and short) during and for months after cessation of drinking.

Sedatives, especially barbiturates, when used on a regular, long-term basis lead to shallow, fragmented sleep. *Rebound insomnia* and rebound anxiety prompt reuse, and tolerance leads to dose escalation, so patients get caught in a vicious cycle. Sedatives and alcohol depress respiratory function, which can lead to very poor quality sleep in patients with sleep apnea (see below).

Stimulant drugs such as amphetamine, pemoline, or methylphenidate, activating antidepressants (eg, the selective serotonin reuptake inhibitors, desipramine, buproprion, phenelzine, protriptyline) and the phenylpropanolamine found in many over-the-counter decongestant, cold, and diet remedies can induce significant difficulty falling asleep. The caffeine and other stimulant xanthines found in tea, coffee, cola drinks, and chocolate are well recognized and often used for their ability to keep one awake. In those who are sensitive, even small amounts will prevent sleep. Nicotine and other substances found in cigarette smoke disrupt sleep induction and continuity. *Bronchodilators* such as aminophylline and beta-agonists can make sleep difficult when given before bed.

Medical problems are responsible in approximately 10 percent of cases. *Chronic pain* is a leading, though often overlooked factor (eg, that experienced by elderly persons with degenerative joint disease). *Delirium* is another important cause in the elderly, resulting from unrecognized infection or medication toxicity (as from anticholinergic agents used in over-the-counter sleep remedies). *Cardiopulmonary dysfunction* may contribute by causing orthopnea, paroxysmal nocturnal dyspnea, or nocturnal angina.

Sleep apnea is a disorder characterized by repeated apneic periods due to soft-tissue upper airway obstruction followed by disruption of sleep. In severe cases, behavioral changes, pulmonary hypertension, cardiac arrhythmias, and death can occur. Patients are unaware of how disrupted their sleep is, though spouses may be kept awake by loud snoring and frightened by the apneic periods. Patients complain of marked daytime sleepiness (see Chapter 46).

Urinary frequency due to infection, prostatism, diabetes, or poor timing of diuretic use are among other important disrupters of sleep. Often, it is the nocturia and disturbed sleep that causes the patient with prostatism to finally seek definitive therapy.

Primary sleep disorders make up another 10 percent of insomnia cases. In *primary* or *idiopathic insomnia*, patients have *objectively verified* difficulty initiating or maintaining sleep in the absence of any identifiable underlying pathology. Such patients may need more, rather than less, sensory input to fall asleep, rather like hyperactive children who require stimulants to control their activity. Others have a persistent complaint of insomnia with *no objective evidence*. Although they believe they awaken, their polysomnographic studies reveal that they are actually sleeping. There is *sleep state misperception*. Their polysomnographic studies are entirely normal. A final group have poorly understood *polysomnographic aberrations*, such as the intrusion of alpha EEG into delta sleep.

In *conditioned* or *"psychophysiologic" insomnia*, patients begin to associate bedtime with frustration, anxiety, and sleep-preventing behaviors. In this learned disorder, they typically sleep very well while away from their usual bedroom (eg, while on vacation or on the living room couch).

Phase shifts (disruptions in the normal 24-hour wake and sleep cycle) can result from alternating shift work or jet travel across time zones (*"jet lag"*). The inability to rapidly reset one's diurnal rhythm to local time leads to insomnia. For travel west across time zones, the typical experience is awakening in the middle of night local time (morning at home) and being unable to fall back to sleep despite feeling tired. Restful sleep is not achieved. Moreover, there is marked afternoon or early evening sleepiness (bedtime at home). The inability attain restful sleep culminates in exhaustion and the patient requests help for his insomnia. Endogenous disruptions of the brain's internal circadian rhythm-setter can produce a similar picture.

Nocturnal myoclonus can produce poor quality sleep and lead to the complaint of "insomnia." It is characterized by repetitive twitching of the legs, which is often unrecognized by the patient.

DIFFERENTIAL DIAGNOSIS

The most recent official version of the psychiatric diagnostic system—the Diagnostic and Statistical Manual of American Psychiatric Association Fourth Edition (Revised) (DSM IV R)—describes primary, or idiopathic insomnia, and secondary insomnia (related to a primary psychiatric, medical, or substance abuse disorder. Table 232–1 provides a listing useful for primary care practice based on these categories.

It is important to note that not all persons who sleep less than average each night have insomnia. There are *natural "short sleepers,"* persons who regularly have less than 7 hours of well-maintained sleep, yet suffer no problems other than too much time on their hands at night. Those who have a brief, *time-limited disturbance* of sleep related to stressful events in their lives are not regarded as having a sleep disturbance. The same pertains to normal elderly patients who experience as part of the natural *aging* process a decline in total sleep time, depth, and continuity.

Table 232-1. Important Causes of Insomnia

1. Psychiatric Disorders—50%
   A. Affective disorders: major depression, dysthymic disorder, manic depressive disorder
   B. Character disorders: Anxiety, obsessive-compulsive, borderline, narcissistic character disorders
   C. Psychosis: schizophrenia, other
2. Drug and Alcohol Abuse—10% to 15%
   A. Sedatives: alcohol, benzodiazepines, barbiturates, narcotics
   B. Stimulants: amphetamines, methylphenidate, pemoline, stimulating antidepressants (phenelzine, protriptyline), caffeine and stimulant xanthines in coffee, tea, cola, and chocolate
   C. Antiasthmatics, decongestants: terbutaline, aminophylline, phenylpropanolamine
   D. Cigarettes
3. Medical/Surgical Problems—10%
   A. Cardiovascular: nocturnal angina, orthopnea, PND
   B. Respiratory: COPD
   C. Renal: UTI, urinary frequency
   D. Endocrine: hyperthyroidism and hypothyroidism
   E. Pain of any source
   F. Delirium: dementia, infection, metabolic derangement, medication toxicity (*e.g.,* anticholinergic delirium secondary to OTC sleep aids)
   G. Sleep apnea
4. Primary Sleep Disorder—10% to 20%
   A. Idiopathic insomnia
   B. Psychophysiologic or conditioned insomnia
   C. Phase shift
   D. Nocturnal myoclonus
   E. Persistent complaint without objective evidence
   F. Unusual polysomnographic patterns: alpha–delta sleep

WORKUP

When the complaint is persistent, when the sleep latency (the time between lights out and falling asleep) is consistently greater than 60 minutes, and when the insomnia is associated with compromised daytime functioning, a search for an underlying etiology should be undertaken.

History is key. A full description of the problem is essential and facilitated by having the patient keep a *sleep log* or diary, which includes time in bed, estimate of time asleep, any awakenings, time of morning arousal, estimate of sleep quality, and comments on unusual events and any associated symptoms (eg, orthopnea, urinary frequency, pain, palpitations). Entries are recorded by the patient directly on getting up each morning. Close attention must also be given to use of sedatives, hypnotics (including over-the-counter preparations), and stimulants. Screening for abuse of alcohol and other substances is essential (see Chapters 228 and 235). It is most important to listen carefully for and inquire directly about symptoms of depression, bipolar disease, anxiety disorder, and psychosis (see Chapters 226 and 227). Occupational and travel patterns should be noted. Whenever possible, interviewing the spouse, bed partner, or family member is of great value, particularly for symptoms suggestive of sleep apnea (eg, excessive snoring, apneic episodes, disturbed sleep). Past and family medical and psychiatric histories are sometimes revealing.

Physical Examination and Laboratory Tests. The pertinent physical examination is a function of the history. One checks for upper airway soft tissue obstruction in the patient with suspected sleep apnea; rales and wheezes when there is concern about a cardiopulmonary etiology; moist skin, tachycardia, proptosis, goiter, and tremor when hyperthyroidism is under consideration; prostatic enlargement in the elderly male with sleep-disturbing nocturia. Any reported sources of pain should be evaluated and confirmed by physical examination. A careful mental status examination helps in the detection of psychiatric disease (see Chapters 226 and 227).

Laboratory testing should be limited, selective, and based on evidence from the history and physical examination (eg, TSH for suspected hyperthyroidism; chest x-ray for cardiopulmonary disease; toxic screen for substance abuse). Referral to the sleep laboratory is indicated only if a primary sleep disorder, such as sleep apnea or nocturnal myoclonus, is suspected. Testing is very expensive and time consuming. Home monitoring for apnea and oxygen desaturation may prove a cost-effective screening alternative to the sleep laboratory for patients with suspected sleep apnea (see Chapter 46). Psychiatric evaluation is indicated only when character problems interfere with diagnosis or management, or if the nature of a suspected mental or emotional problem is obscure.

PRINCIPLES OF MANAGEMENT

For a problem with as broad a spectrum of etiologies as insomnia, the best treatment is etiologic. Nonspecific measures are unlikely to be of much help and can be harmful. Careless use of sedative/hypnotics can be especially dangerous (eg, giving the patient with sleep apnea or alcohol abuse a benzodiazepine). Precise diagnostic assessment allows for maximally safe and effective management. For those with substance abuse, proper withdrawal and complete abstinence from drugs and alcohol are critical (see Chapters 228 and 235).

Depression and Other Affective Disorders. Patients with affective disorders who present with insomnia may benefit from a *sedating tricyclic antidepressant* (eg, nortriptyline or doxepin, 25–50 mg qhs) or *trazodone* (25–100 mg qhs). Full doses of antidepressants should be used if affective symptoms remain (see Chapter 227). When insomnia is due to use of an activating antidepressant, such as desipramine or a fluoxetine, switching to a somewhat less energizing preparation (eg, sertraline or paroxetine) may be helpful. Alternatively, adding a small amount of trazodone (50 mg qhs) or clonazepam (.5–1.0 mg qhs) may control fluoxetine-induced difficulty falling asleep.

Anxiety Disorders. Transient insomnia due to situational stress is a common non-threatening problem, which by definition resolves on its own and often responds well to support, reassurance, and simple advice. For anxiety disorders and character disorders complicated by insomnia, *benzodiazepines (BZDs)* can be used safely and effectively.

Short-Term versus Chronic Therapy. There is controversy as to the proper frequency and duration of therapy when insomnia is chronic, due to a long-standing anxiety disorder or characterological disturbance. Most believe it is best to treat such insomnia with a *short (1-week) course* of BZD therapy to help reestablish a more normal sleep pattern and then to stop. However, an occasional patient requires a program of BZD use *2–3 times per week* over much longer periods.

If chronic BZD therapy is contemplated, one first needs to review with the patient the importance of assiduous compliance and the risks of tolerance and withdrawal, as well as the possibility of physical dependence should the medication not be taken as prescribed (see Chapter 226). In addition, one must screen carefully for contraindications (eg, sleep apnea, substance abuse). Alcohol and other sedatives should not be used concurrently because of the risk of oversedation.

For patients requiring prolonged therapy, careful monitoring is essential to ascertain efficacy, check for adverse effects, and assure proper dosage and frequency. Drug holidays and attempts at alternative treatment are important components of any therapeutic program that involves prolonged BZD intake. The risks of tolerance and withdrawal should be reviewed with the patient before initiating such therapy. Withdrawal symptoms may develop within 3 to 20 days after cessation of chronic BZD use, especially if abrupt. It is best to taper therapy slowly over several weeks in patients with a history of prolonged intake (see Chapter 226).

Choice of Benzodiazepine. Debate also continues on the choice of BZD preparation. The optimal BZD would seem to have a rapid onset yet short (6–8 hr) duration of action, would cause no rebound insomnia, and no mental problems such as hangover, motor incoordination, or memory disturbance. There are now several agents marketed for the treatment of insomnia, but none has been clearly shown to be significantly superior to any other, and all have some problems associated with their use (see Chapter 226).

The BZDs used for insomnia can be divided into the short-, intermediate-, and long-acting agents. The *short-acting agents* such as *triazolam* and *estazololam* are widely prescribed for those whose primary problem is with *falling asleep*. Triazolam should be used in the lowest possible doses (not to exceed .125 mg/day in the elderly), and should be tapered to avoid *rebound insomnia and anxiety*.

The *intermediate-acting* agents such as *temazepam* and *quazepam* may be useful for those patients who complain of problems with *sleep continuity*. The possible increased receptor selectivity of quazepam has not been shown to be clearly clinically relevant. The new non-benzodiazepine *zolplidem*, which acts at the BZD receptor, fits into the intermediate-duration-of-action group. *Lorazepam* and *diazepam* may be recommended as *lower-cost* generic alternatives. *Flurazep*am and *clonazepam* are *long-acting* and may be preferred by some patients whose *daytime anxiety* compounds their discomfort.

Sedating tricyclic antidepressants such as *nortriptyline* (10–25 mg qhs) may help some patients with *generalized anxiety* and insomnia, as may *buspirone* (10–30 mg qhs) or *trazodone* (25–50 mg qhs).

In rare instances where BZDs are contraindicated (eg, history of drug or alcohol dependence) and sedating antidepressants have not helped, *antihistamines* such as diphenhydramine may be used. However, the elderly and very young may experience *delirium* or *paradoxical excitation* from such drugs. *Chloral hydrat*e should rarely be used, and there is almost never a place for treating new cases of insomnia with *barbiturates*, *meprobamate*, or over-the-counter remedies.

Treatment of the Elderly. The importance of cause-specific treatment is most poignantly experienced in caring for elderly persons with insomnia. Sedatives should be used in reduced dose and with caution, if at all (see Chapter 226). Falls with catastrophic consequences are a major risk with sedative use. When depression presents as difficulty sleeping, treatment should be etiologic and tailored to the special needs of older persons (see Chapter 227). The importance of adequate treatment of pain and any underlying medical problems cannot be overemphasized.

Attention to pain and other underlying medical precipitants is also essential. In instances where the underlying cause is minor, emphasis on sleep hygiene (see below) and empathetic support are often the best course. Explanation on how the normal aging process affects sleep is appreciated by those wondering why they seem to sleep less.

Psychotherapy may be used quite effectively in conjunction with medications for patients with psychiatric or stress-related problems. A special form of psychotherapy, called *sleep-restriction therapy*, where the time in bed is matched to the time needed for sleep, can be effective but should be conducted by an experienced practitioner. Antipsychotic agents can relieve insomnia and agitation in psychotic or delirious patients.

PATIENT EDUCATION

The overall promotion of good "*sleep hygiene*" is useful for many patients. Establishing a regular bed and wake time, avoiding any and all naps, having regular exercise (although not at night), using bed only for sleeping or lovemaking (rather than reading or watching TV), and getting in bed only when ready for sleep (leaving bed if sleep is not forthcoming) are useful suggestions. Avoidance of caffeinated foods, stimulants, cigarettes, and alcohol are necessary for some sensitive patients.

Instructing patients about these basic rules of sleep hygiene, and helping them to avoid trying too hard to fall asleep, is often useful. Disabusing patients of the myth that everyone must have 8 hours of sleep every night makes many people feel relieved. Also, informing patients that much of the time they spend in bed believing they are "only drowsy" is time actually spent in the lighter stages of sleep can ameliorate some patients' frustration.

THERAPEUTIC RECOMMENDATIONS

- If the insomnia is related to an underlying affective disorder, begin a sedating tricyclic antidepressant, such as nortriptyline or doxepin (10 mg) or trazodone (25 mg) to be taken an hour before bedtime every night for at least a month. Increase the dose as needed to fully treat the depression.
- If the insomnia is related to an anxiety disorder, use triazolam, starting at 0.125 mg qhs when the main problem is falling asleep, or clonazepam (0.5 mg) or flurazepam (15 mg) at bedtime if daytime anxiety is present.
- If symptoms recur after 2 weeks of treatment for anxiety-related insomnia, institute behavioral and relaxation therapies (see Chapter 226) and consider psychiatric consultation.
- If the insomnia is related to a character disorder, seek psychiatric consultation, require close adherence to good sleep hygiene, and use BZDs only with caution.
- Make sure that a complete history of alcohol and substance use, including cigarettes, caffeine, nonprescription drugs, and stimulants, is obtained on every patient. Interview family members and obtain toxic screens of urine or blood when there is a doubt. Do not prescribe BZDs for patients with current or past alcohol or drug use. Supervise withdrawal and abstinence, and seek psychiatric consultation when withdrawal symptoms or maintenance of abstinence is problematic.
- Treat pain and underlying medical problems aggressively; a short course of BZDs may help reestablish a normal sleep pattern in some patients.
- Offer education and support to an elderly patient who has normal daytime function but who is lonely or upset as their sleep goes through the changes of normal aging.

ANNOTATED BIBLIOGRAPHY

Consensus Conference: Drugs and insomnia. The use of medications to promote sleep. JAMA 1984;1251:2410. *(Good discussion of hypnotics, in terms of efficacy and side effects.)*

Everitt DE, Avorn J. Clinical decision-making in the evaluation and treatment of insomnia. Am J Med 1990;89:357. *(They find inadequate history taking and overutilization of pharmacologic therapy.)*

Ford DE, Kamerow DB. Epidemiologic study of sleep disturbances and psychiatric disorders. JAMA 1989;262:1479. *(High prevalence of psychiatric disease in those with sleep disturbances in this community study.)*

Gillin JC, Byerley WF. The diagnosis and management of insomnia. N Engl J Med 1990;322:239. *(A very practical review, with emphasis on pharmacologic therapy; 106 refs.)*

Greenblatt DJ, Harmatz JS, Zinny MA, et al. Effect of gradual withdrawal on the rebound sleep disorder after discontinuation of triazolam. N Engl J Med 1987;317:722. *(Gradual tapering prevented rebound sleep disorder.)*

Hauri PJ. Specific effects of sedative/hypnotic drugs in the treatment of incapacitating chronic insomnia. Am J Med 1987;83:925. *(An editorial on the safety and efficacy of chronic sedative use.)*

Kales A, Caldwell AB, Soldatos CR, et al. Biopsychosocial correlates of insomnia. II. Patterns specificity and consistency with the Minnesota Multiphasic Personality Inventory. Psychosom Med 1983;45:341. *(One of an excellent, long-running series of articles on insomnia; good bibliography.)*

Kales A, Kales J. Sleep disorders. N Engl J Med 1974;290:487. *(A classic article nicely outlining the sleep disorders and their treatment.)*

Prinz PN, Vitiello MV, Raskind MA, et al. Geriatrics: Sleep disorders and aging. N Engl J Med 1990;323:520. *(Excellent review of normal sleep pattern, sleep disturbances, and use of sedatives in the elderly; 80 refs.)*

233
Management of Obesity

CAROLYN J. CRIMMINS-HINTLIAN, M.P.H., R.D.

Primary Care Medicine: Office Evaluation and Management of the Adult Patient, 3rd edition, edited by Allan H. Goroll, Lawrence A. May, and Albert G. Mulley, Jr. J.B. Lippincott Company, Philadelphia

Obesity is a major health problem in industrialized societies. It is estimated that at least 20 percent of the U.S. population is on some kind of weight-loss program at any given time. Weight loss is not a cure for obesity, as evidenced by patients who go from one fad diet to another, sometimes jeopardizing their health in the process (mortality appears greatest in those with the greatest fluctuations in weight). Almost 95 percent of people who lose weight regain lost pounds and often more within the first year. Effective weight management requires going beyond simple dieting. Although overweight persons tend to be preoccupied with dieting, one needs to identify the biopsychosocial dimensions of the problem (see Chapter 10) and, if possible, treat them specifically. Therapy should include a customized program of physical activity (see Chapter 18). Patient education is also essential. The efficacy and health consequences of popular diets and nonprescription drugs must be understood, and available community resources and self-help groups must be identified.

PRINCIPLES OF MANAGEMENT

Goals and Strategy

Weight loss should not be the only attainable goal for patients embarking on a weight reduction program. Correction of poor self- and body-image, distorted eating patterns, and physical, social, and lifestyle consequences of obesity are other important objectives.

Treatment requires a lifelong commitment to change in lifestyle, behavior, and dietary practices. As noted, the effort begins with identifying the major precipitants of the patient's weight problem (see Chapter 10). The decision to lose weight may be part of a complex decision to improve the conduct of one's life. Consequently, the physician should be aware that patients coming for treatment are likely to be highly motivated and asking for permission to also make interpersonal, environmental, or lifestyle changes. Once the patient's agenda and preferences are clarified, the physician can help select the most appropriate weight reduction methods.

No single program is effective for all persons. Knowledge of the strengths and weaknesses of individual weight-loss modalities is essential to the design of an intelligent program. Treatment modalities can be divided into dietary, behavioral, psychosocial, pharmacologic, exercise, and surgical categories.

Dietary Approaches

"Going on a diet" is the typical first step in weight reduction, but the word "diet" implies that one is making only a temporary change in one's eating habits and patterns. Quite the contrary, the most effective diet is not a diet at all but rather a gradual, *permanent change in eating habits and exercise* that can be followed for a lifetime.

Determining Daily Caloric Intake. The desired daily caloric intake needs to be determined. One starts by estimating the number of calories necessary to maintain an obese person's weight:

- Obese female: 8 to 10 calories × present weight in pounds
- Obese male: 10 to 12 calories × present weight in pounds (the lower number in the range is for the sedentary person)

From this figure, one subtracts 500 kcal per day for every pound per week that should be lost (3500 calories deficit = 1 lb weight loss). All weight-reduction programs should be nutritionally adequate except for calories and should include a variety of foods. Most fad diets are neither nutritionally sound nor based on proven scientific evidence (Table 233-1). Extravagant claims that a particular food or class of foods dramatically alters weight, appetite, or calorigenesis are unfounded. The common denominators for efficacy and safety are reduction in calories and nutritional balance. Dietary composition is less important than total calories for weight loss, but low-fat composition is critical to maintenance of weight loss.

When following a prescribed dietary regimen, the patient must realize that initial rapid weight loss may occur because of a negative fluid balance. After 2 to 3 weeks, the rate of weight loss slows down. Most subsequent loss reflects the catabolism of fat. Loss of fat is directly proportional to the size and duration of the energy deficit. Patients often become discouraged when they enter the slower phase. Some adjust to caloric restriction by unknowingly diminishing their energy expenditures, one reason why an exercise program is such an important adjunct (see below).

Dietary Counseling. Dietary counseling is an essential step in the educational process. It begins with the physician's endorsement (an essential component that is often overlooked). Patients need to achieve a basic understanding of the caloric and nutritional contents of foods in order to choose intelligently. The services of a registered dietitian (RD) can be helpful in this regard, because such persons are specifically trained in assessing nutritional requirements and counseling food selection and preparation. In addition, the RD attempts to help people assess and change their attitudes and behaviors toward food and eating. An assessment is made integrating medical concerns with the individual and/or family lifestyle, economic status, learning ability, and psychological needs. A weight control plan must be individualized to each patient's needs and food preferences. Dietary changes must be gradually implemented to ensure life-long positive eating habits. Nutrition counseling is likely to increase patient adherence to a dietary regimen and improve outcome.

Weight Loss Programs. Many *commercial* and *self-help* programs are available (see Table 233-1). Some provide menus and a line of foods to buy; others include individual or group support. Those that just sell products are of little long-term benefit. Integrated approaches that include moderate diet modification, an exercise program, and a behavioral approach are more effective, especially for mildly to moderately overweight persons. Noncommercial self-help groups offer a low-cost alternative for those who seek the benefit of group support, but often there is little professional guidance provided.

Behavior Modification

Behavior modification programs grew out of studies suggesting that obese persons overeat because they are stimulus-bound. Behavioral treatment is directed toward the mildly to moderately obese. Operant conditioning techniques appear to be somewhat more effective than aversive ones. Obese patients appear especially prone to respond to external cues for eating. The triggering stimuli may be situational, physiologic, or emotional. The aim of the behavioral approach is to substitute an alternative eating behavior that is practical and leads to decreased caloric intake.

There are four components:

1. *Describing the Behavior to be Controlled*—Patients are instructed to keep records of all eating behaviors, including daily weight, time and place of eating, stimuli preceding eating that the individual is aware of, and description of surroundings.
2. *Modifying and Controlling Stimuli*—Food shopping habits, visual cues, food preparation habits, and food storage habits are changed.
3. *Controlling the Act of Eating*—The patient is taught to eat more slowly, not skip meals, and not take snacks.
4. *Promptly Reinforcing Behaviors that Delay and Control Eating*—Patients are advised to eat only in one room (cue elimination), to have company while eating (cue supervision), to develop methods of making diet food attractive (cue strengthening), to arrange for deviations from the diet, and to arrange for positive feedback if they comply with exercise and diet programs.
   Distracting activities such as watching television or reading while eating are discouraged. Eating behavior is made to be associated with highly specific stimuli.

Both individual and group behavioral programs are available. Average length of treatment is 18 weeks. The average weight loss is 20 lb, and at 52 weeks of follow-up, almost two-thirds of patients show maintenance of that weight loss, a very positive result. Behavior modification may prove to be most helpful in helping people maintain weight loss regardless of how it was achieved.

Exercise

An exercise or physical fitness component should be included in every weight-loss program. Most obese persons are less active than lean people, but it is not known whether this is a cause or consequence of obesity. Energy expenditure and basal metabolic rate decrease with weight loss on calorically restricted diets. Exercise, in conjunction with a low-calorie diet, increases the metabolic rate. Increased physical activity for many obese people can promote weight loss and decrease body fat. Lean body mass is preserved when exercise and diet are combined. Obese individuals use more energy and burn more body fat for the same amount of activity than normal-weight individuals because the energy cost of most exercise is proportional to body weight. The amount of exercise needed to decrease body fat is related to its duration, intensity, and frequency. Exercise may also benefit the dieter by increasing feelings of self-control, reducing stress, improving appearance, and alleviating depression. Cardiovascular morbidity and mortality may be reduced.

The Exercise Prescription. A specific exercise prescription is essential. To tell a sedentary obese person to "get more exercise" is insufficient. Moreover, the dropout rate is high. Thirty percent or more of obese patients terminate physical training programs within several weeks of initiation and as few as a third continue for up to 1 year. To ensure compliance, the program has to be physically realistic and capable of being incorporated into the patient's daily routine.

The importance of physician input and encouragement is considerable. To ensure safety, obese patients with multiple cardiac risk factors and a sedentary lifestyle might benefit from electrocardiographic stress-testing before initiation of an exercise program (see Chapter 18).

General guidelines for implementing a realistic exercise plan include:

1. Begin at the patient's level of current activity. Walking for 10 minutes a day may be a lot for a sedentary individual. Encourage routine activity (eg, park some distance from destination, use stairs instead of the elevators).
2. Prescribe exercise at 60 percent to 80 percent of the patient's age-adjusted maximum heart rate. (The maximum heart rate is approximated by the formula of 200 beats per minute minus the person's age.) Those who have been sedentary should start at the low end of this range.
3. Encourage a specific time of the day to exercise regularly (early morning, lunch hour, after work).
4. Emphasize the need to exercise regularly. Patients should work toward a 30-minute session four or five times a week.
5. Encourage use of a diary to chart progress. Self-monitoring reinforces effort.
6. Encourage activity with a friend, coworker, or family member. Referral to a credible group-exercise facility may be indicated.
7. Use walking as the initial activity. When an activity other than walking is undertaken, it must be easily accessible and fit the patient's lifestyle.

To keep weight off once lost, exercise must become a permanent component of an individual's lifestyle (see also Chapter 18).

Pharmacologic Treatment

Appetite suppressants are commonly requested by patients who have trouble controlling their food intake. *Amphetamines* do reduce appetite, but tolerance is quick to develop and dependence is a serious risk (see Chapter 235). Moreover, weight loss is only temporary, because eating habits are not altered. Sleep disturbances, nervousness, and diarrhea are other adverse effects. Prolonged use may lead to fatigue and depression. The search for drugs that provide amphetamine's appetite suppression without the risks of dependence, tolerance, and central nervous system (CNS) side effects continues.

Other appetite suppressants have been developed, including *mazindol* (Sanorex), *phentermine* (Ionimin), *diethylpropion* (Tenuate), and *fenfluramine* (Pondimin). Most are sympathomimetic amines with amphetaminelike CNS effects but lesser potentials for tolerance and drug-dependency (although they are listed by the Drug Enforcement Agency as Schedule IV agents). They appear to produce satiety through stimulation of noradrenergic and possibly dopaminergic receptors. Fenfluramine differs from the others in that it causes more CNS depression than stimulation. None of these agents has proven sufficiently safe and effective to recommend for long-term treatment of obesity. At best, they might be used as a short-term supplement to diet and exercise.

Over-the-counter diet pills usually contain phenylpropanolamine and/or benzocaine, often in combination with vitamins or caffeine. Their use was stimulated by a few reports purporting to show small degrees of weight loss associated with their intake. *Phenylpropanolamine,* a common decongestant sympathomimetic, is promoted as an appetite suppressant and found in a number of over-the-counter diet pills (eg, Dexatrim, Appedrine, Dietac, Dex-a-Diet, Prolamine). There is no compelling evidence proving its efficacy for weight control, and it can be dangerous. Adverse reactions include hypertension, hypertensive crisis, renal failure, cardiac arrhythmias, acute psychotic episodes, and death. Although probably not as dangerous to dieters as phenylpropanolamine, *benzocaine,* a topical anesthetic, is also promoted as a diet aid and sold in candy and gum form. Use of such nonprescription agents should be strongly discouraged.

Antidepressants may *stimulate appetite,* which can be troublesome. Many *tricyclics* are problematic in this regard. Switching to a nontricyclic antidepressant that does not stimulate appetite (eg, *sertraline*) may solve the problem (see Chapter 227).

In the rare instance of abnormal food preoccupation and binge eating in association with electroencephalographic abnormalities, *phenytoin* may alleviate the problem. More commonly, binge eaters have primitive, impulsive characters often diagnosed as borderline states. With successful psychotherapy, these regressive episodes tend to disappear as more healthy defenses and a less chaotic lifestyle emerge.

Extreme Measures

Very Low Calorie Diets (VLCDs). These diets severely limit calories to between 400 and 800 per day. They achieve the more rapid and sustained rate of weight reduction associated with complete starvation while avoiding the inherent risks of starvation. These diets should be restricted to patients more than 30 percent to 40 percent above ideal weight and require an initial cardiac evaluation and close medical supervision because of the risk of life-threatening arrhythmias. They are not do-it-yourself regimens. Goals include optimal nitrogen balance and muscle tissue sparing. A VLCD can achieve weight loss of more than 75 percent fat and a concomitant decrease in waist:hip and waist:thigh ratios.

The VLCDs consist of 1.5 g protein per kilogram ideal body weight per day in the form of lean meat, fish, or fowl; noncaloric beverages; a multivitamin and mineral supplement containing folic acid; 1500 mL fluid/day; 25 mEq potassium, and calcium supplement. The combination of VLCD and behavior modification appears promising. Average weight losses on the diet are 45 lb in fasting periods that last approximately 12 weeks.

The VLCD is not recommended for those who are moderately overweight or for children, adolescents, pregnant or lactating women, or the elderly. Also, it should be avoided by those suffering from cardiovascular disease, essential hypertension, insulin-dependent diabetes mellitus, severe renal or hepatic impairment, active cancer, or a severe psychological disturbance. High dropout rates as well as poor long-term maintenance are discouraging aspects of treatment by VLCD.

Surgical Treatment. Surgical interventions continue to be options for control of morbid obesity, defined as "100 lb overweight" or over 200 percent of desirable weight as defined by the Metropolitan Life Insurance Company tables (see Chapter 10). Although the prevalence of morbid obesity is only 0.5 percent of the obese population, physicians often encounter these people in clinical practice. Their high rates of morbidity and mortality accelerate rapidly as overweight becomes increasingly severe. Medical treatments are often ineffective.

Consideration of surgical intervention should be undertaken only after a comprehensive program of nonsurgical therapy has been fully tried and proven ineffective. Selection should be limited to highly motivated morbidly obese patients free of other serious medical and psychosocial problems. Adequate financial support should be available due to the frequent need for repeated hospitalizations.

Jejunoileal bypass was one of the first of these surgical treatments. It has been discontinued due to its high rate of serious complications, including intractable diarrhea, hypokalemia, hypocalcemia, oxalate-containing kidney stones, liver failure and protein malnutrition.

Gastric reduction procedures involve construction of a small 15- to 50-ml pouch connected through a small stoma to an outflow tract. This class of operations has emerged as the surgical approach of choice for morbid obesity. In the *gastric bypass type,* food passes first into the pouch and then into the jejunum. In the *gastroplasty type* (gastric stapling), food passes into the distal stomach and duodenum. Gastric bypass appears more effective in promoting weight loss, but gastroplasty is associated with fewer complications. Surgical mortality ranges from 0 to 4 percent. After surgery, patients must be instructed to *eat small amounts,* eat slowly, chew carefully, avoid eating when not hungry, and take no liquids with meals. Results are impressive, with an average of 50 percent of excess weight lost in the first 12 months, although it is not clear whether the cause is early satiety or aversive conditioning due to epigastric pain and vomiting with eating too much at one time.

Complications include *outlet obstruction,* vitamin deficiencies (thiamine, B_{12}, and folate), partial temporary hair loss believed due to inadequate protein intake, and increased incidences of *gallstones* and *gastric ulcers*. Benefits include improvement in glucose intolerance, reduction in blood pressure for hypertensive patients, reversal of cardiorespiratory impairment, and reduction of serum cholesterol. Psychosocial benefits depend on the degree of weight loss and are independent of side effects and complications. The patient with significant weight loss has shown improvement in employability, sex life, physical activity, and self-esteem, and a more gregarious outlook on life.

Suction lipectomy, a cosmetic procedure for removal of localized fat accumulations, has produced variable results. Success depends on elastic properties of the overlying skin. Temporary loss of skin sensation, wavy contour, and blood loss are adverse effects. Other possible side effects include infection, extensive bruising for 2 to 3 weeks, and edema for 3 to 6 weeks. *Jaw wiring,* as the term implies, involves wiring the jaw shut for as long as 6 to 9 months, preventing the ingestion of solid food. Intake of high-calorie shakes and soft drinks will eliminate the benefits of surgery.

PATIENT EDUCATION

Motivation in conjunction with patient education are key factors for successful weight control. Realistic goals and expectations are critical, as is the physician's support and encouragement. The patient must be willing to permanently alter exercise and eating patterns. Although rapid weight-loss programs are popular, patients need to be informed about their inadequacies for achieving long-term weight loss (see Appendix). Major obstacles to success need to be explored and addressed, including poor self-image, erratic eating patterns, inadequate exercise, loneliness, boredom, anger, and depression.

As noted earlier, knowledge must be provided about basic nutrition principles, such as caloric value of foods and practical methods for changing eating habits. Teaching behavioral techniques is also very helpful and should include several categories of actions:

- Recording of food intake
- Eating only in one place; using a smaller plate; prohibiting another activity while eating; keeping food otherwise out of sight.
- Planning meals by shopping from a list; having low-calorie foods available; taking a brown bag lunch; having a strategy before eating out; and, at parties, positioning away from the food table
- Substituting an alternate activity for eating
- Increasing physical activity

INDICATIONS FOR REFERRAL

Although the interest, involvement, and encouragement of the primary physician are critical, the implementation of a comprehensive and personalized weight loss program is often best achieved with a multidisciplinary approach. Referral to a registered dietitian is enormously helpful in providing the patient with essential nutritional information and initiating a behavioral program for alteration of eating habits. Knowing community and commercial resources and their level of professional supervision helps when the patient requests a group approach. Before beginning an exercise program, it may be useful to refer the poorly conditioned, markedly obese patient for an electrocardiographic stress test (see Chapter 18). When emotional problems are too great for the primary physician and registered dietitian to handle, psychiatric referral should be considered. Surgical consultation should be considered only when the patient is so morbidly obese and so refractory to medical therapy that the risks as-

Table 233-1. Commercial Weight Loss Programs

PROGRAM*	APPROACH	EXPECTED WEIGHT LOSS	STAFF
Diet Center	Five-phase program, frequent individual counseling, behavior modification, weekly group education on nutrition, food selection and exercise. Conditioning—prepares dieters for weight reduction. Reducing—Women: 945 calories, Men: 1,300 calories. Private counseling 6 days a week. Individuals make transition from usual eating habits to moderate calorie diet which includes lean meats, whole grains, fresh fruit and vegetables. Sta*b*lite—Women: 1,465 calories, Men: 1,725 calories. As dieters approach weight goals, variety of foods introduced, private counseling 2 to 3 times a week. Maintenance phase—Women and men: 1,465 to 2,125 calories, weekly consultations, nutritional eating habits established. Image One Series—a 24-lesson series of weekly classes and 10-part video series covering nutrition, behavior modification, self-direction, relaxation, stress management, meal selection and preparation and three levels of exercise.	Women: 2 1/2 to 3 1/2 lb per week. Men: 3 to 5 lb per week.	Nonprofessional counselors who have lost weight on the program. Program is developed by a full-time medical director, four staff-registered dietitians at headquarters and medical consultants. Centers encouarged to organize local medical advisory boards, although figures are not available as the number of local boards.
Health Management Resources	A three-phase program in which clients consume liquid diet supplement, a multivitamin/mineral supplement and/or HMR entrees. Weight loss—clients consume liquid supplement providing 520 to 800 calories or liquid supplement and two entrees (nine varieties) for a total of 800 to 1,000 calories per day. Refeeding—gradual decrease in supplement or entrees, increase in food calories, calorie level determined individually. Intensive behavior and nutrition education. Medically supervised or unsupervised options both include medical screening. Emphasizes lifestyle changes such as reducing dietary fat, increasing physical activity and balancing food and exercise. Staff is on call on a 24-hour basis for support or medical emergencies.	2 to 5 lb per week.	Doctors, nurses, group leader is usually a registered dietitian, psychologist or other health care professional. Long-term intensive training provided for all staff.
Jenny Craig International Weight Loss Centers	Personal counseling and group classes focus on behavior modification, nutrition and exercise. Multivitamin/mineral supplement is taken. Clients required to purchase most of their food at centers. Modified diet with meal plans. Women: 1,000 calories, Men and adolescents: 1,200 to 1,400 calories. Menus are 60% carbohydrate, 20% protein, 20% fat, 2,000 to 3,000 mg sodium, 100 to 150 mg cholesterol. Clients may prepare own foods 2 days a week when half of desired weight is lost.	1 1/2 to 2 1/2 lb per week.	Counselors receive 40 hours of initial training, attend monthly continuing education class. Many are former clients, although it's not a prerequisite. Program designed by staff dietitian, psychologist and consulting doctors.
Nutri/System	Nonmedically supervised. Nutritional instruction, computer analysis, diet supervision, behavior modification, exercise and weight maintenance. Reducing Phase—until weight loss is achieved. Maintenance—clients consume Nutri/System foods 2 days per week and prepare own meals 5 days per week. Classes focus on food selection, food preparation and meal planning. Food purchased at centers provides between 1,100 and 1,500 calories, depending on individual's requirements. 60% of calories from carbohydrates, 15% fat, 25% protein, less than 2,500 mg sodium and a minimum of 20 g fiber per day.	1 1/2 to 2 lb per week.	Behavior counselors have backgrounds in nursing, psychology or education. Nutri/System certified nutritional specialists have degrees in food, nutrition or dietetics. Headquarters staff include a doctor, a psychologist, a nutritionist and eight registered dietitians.
Optifast	Medically supervised three-phase, hospital or clinic-based program includes taking a very low calorie liquid diet formula. Intense behavior modification, psychological group support, nutrition education, exercise and weekly medical monitoring (physician visits and laboratory tests as needed). Medical Screening—(1,200 calories solid food). Physical examination, laboratory tests and psychological and nutritional assessments. Supplemental Fasting Phase—patients consume Optifast 70 or Optifast 800 five times daily, which provides between 420 and 800 calories. Refeeding Phase—reintroduction of foods. Stabilization Phase—(1,200 calories, supplement discontinued. Encore Program—optional, nonmedically supervised maintenance program. Twenty-four hour support by doctor or group leader. Optifiber, a psyllium-based product has been recently introduced to mix with liquid supplements to relieve constipation or diarrhea associated with very low-calorie diets. One packet provides 3 g soluble fiber.	2 to 5 lb per week or 1% to 2% of body weight each week.	Dieticians, doctors and psychologists at most locations.
Optitrim	A medically supervised, three or four-phase program, developed by Sandoz Nutrition which involves intense nutrition education, behavior modification, liquid supplement and shelf stable *OptiEntree* meals and exercise. Phase I—950 calories: Optitrim supplement three times a day and one prepackaged meal offering 275 calories. Transitional Phase—1,100 calories, self-prepared foods. Maintenance—calorie level determined by counseling dietitian. Encore—6-month optional maintenance phase.	2 lb per week	Dietitian, clinical sociologists. Medical monitoring.
Overeaters Anonymous	Nonprofit support group, members admit to a compulsive eating problem believed to be physical, emotional and spiritual. Members participate in weekly meetings, retreats and annual conventions. Follows Alcoholics Anonymous 12-step program to correct behavior. No diet plans or nutrition counseling. Encouarges members who seek such counseling to consult qualified professionals.	No projections are made.	Nonprofessional members conduct activities.
Registered Dietitians in Private Practice	Dietitian designs individual diet program according to client's lifestyle and caloric needs. Individual or group counseling may include sessions on nutrition, food preparation and recipe modification, behavior modification and exercise.	Varies on an individual basis.	Registered dietitian. May be associated with doctors, psychologists or exercise physiologist.
Take Off Pounds Sensibly (TOPS)	International nonprofit support group of 320,000. Helps overweight individuals to attain and maintain physician-prescribed weight goals through support and fellowship. Independent chapters hold weekly meetings and activities to achieve goals. Regularly holds recognition programs, retreats and annual convention. KOPS—"Keep Off Pounds Sensibly" is an honor society of members who maintain weight loss for 3 months.	No projections made.	Volunteer leaders elected by chapter members annually, assisted by regional directors and coordinators.
WeightWatchers International, Inc.	Nonmedically supervised program that incorporates diet, exercise, behavior modification and group support. Food Plan—Women: 1,000 calories increasing to 1,200 calories by the fifth week. Fifteen percent to 20% protein, 50% to 60% carbohydrate, 20% to 30% fat, 2,000 mg sodium and 250 mg cholesterol. Based on a variety of foods adaptable to each individual's lifestyle. Frozen entrees and desserts available for purchase in supermarkets. Maintenance plan reinforces healthy behaivor.	1 to 2 lb per week.	Weekly meetings conducted by trianed nonprofessional group leader who has successfully lost and maintained weight within 2 lb. Program developed by staff dietians and medical, exercise and psychological consultants.

*Programs are listed alphabetically.

From *Environmental Nutrition* 1990; 13:1.

Length	Availability and Headquarters	Costs	Comments
Conditioning—2 days. Reducing—Until weight loss is achieved. Sta*b*lite I and II—Up to 9 weeks. Maintenance—Up to 1 year after reaching desired weight. Image One—Weekly through all phases.	2,000 centers in U.S., Canada, England, Australia, Singapore, Bermuda and Guam. Headquartered in Pittsburgh, PA.	Varies. Determined by amount of weight to lose. Average cost for person to lose 30 lb including the five phases is $650 to $700. Fees include conditioning, reducing, Sta*b*lite (9 weeks), maintenance (1 year) and weekly Image One classes.	Not medically supervised, although individuals with preexisting medical conditions or those wishing to lose more than 50 lb must have a physical examination, with additional examination. Diet consists of self-selected and prepared foods, although 75 Diet Center products are available for purchase. Calcium sources restricted during conditioning and Sta*b*lite phases. Question the need for Diet Center soy supplement and Sta*b*lite Nutrition Bar and restriction of starches to two to three servings per week. Program suitable for individuals who wish to prepare own meals and who require frequent individual counseling
Three phases: Weight loss—10 to 16 weeks. Refeeding—2 to 6 weeks. Maintenance 6 to 18 months.	Affiliated with hospitals, medical schools, medical centers and corporations. Over 600 centers in the U.S. Headquartered in Boston, MA.	Varies among locations. Maintenance is $55 per month. Both options include medical screening and behavioral education classes. Medically monitored program is $115 per week, including supplements and/or entrees. Medically unsupervised program is $90 per week.	Medically supervised supplement program recommended for individuals 20% above ideal body weight or at least 30 lb above ideal body weight. Clients taking liquid supplements only may experience unpleasant side-effects such as constipation or dry skin. Both options require use of HMR products, a serious commitment and temporary lifestyle change.
Varies, depending on the time it takes to reach desired weight. Permanent Stabilization Program—1-year maintenance includes monthly modification classes, clients return to selecting and preparing own foods.	More than 500 centers in U.S., Australia and New Zealand. Headquarted in Del Mar, CA.	$1,000 to $1,225 for 17 weeks diet and food. Offers seasonal promotions. Permanent Stablization Program is $99 per year. Audiotapes at an additional charge of $75.10.	Medically unsupervised, although clients with preexisting health problems are required to get physician approval. Requires temporary change in lifestyle. May appeal to individuals seeking a structured weight reduction program that initially involves a minimum of food preparation.
Reducing Phase. Varies. Maintenance: 1 year.	1,800 centers in U.S. Canada, Australia and U.K. Headquartered in Blue Bell, PA.	Program fee varies according to region, amount of weight to be lost and special promotions. Food cost for three meals per day is $54 to $66 weekly. Financial incentives include refund of 25% of program cost after 6 months of successful maintenance.	For anyone over 18 years who desires to lose 5 to 100 lb. Adolescents (14 to 17 years) and individuals with preexisting medical problems require physician approval. Dependency on program foods requires temporary change in lifestyle. May appeal to individuals seeking a structured weight reduction program. Strong emphasis on company products.
Medical Screening—1 week. Supplemented Fasting Phase—12 weeks. Refeeding Phase—6 weeks. Stabilization Phase—7 weeks. Encore Program—6 months.	600 hospitals and medical institutions in the U.S., 30 in Canada. Headquartered in Minneapolis, MN.	Varies among centers, approximately $3,000 for 26-week program. Encore maintenance program approximately $550.	For individuals 30% or 50 lb above ideal body weight. Requires serious commitment and temporary lifestyle changes. Certain activities are restricted such as swimming alone, horseback riding or sitting in a whirlpool or steam bath. Potassium supplements may be necessary. Potential for unpleasant side-effects such as bad breath, temporary dizziness, skin dryness, diarrhea or constipation.
Phase I—8 weeks. Transitional phase—4 weeks. Maintenance—4 weeks. Encore—6 months. Total: 40 weeks.	180 hospital-affiliated programs. Headquartered in Minneapolis, MN.	$1,800 for food and 18-week program.	For individuals 20% to 30% or 20 to 50 lb above ideal body weight. Requires physician referral or examination. Less intensive than the Optifast program.
No limit.	10,500 chapters in 60 countries. Headquartered in Torrance, CA.	No membership fees.	Noncommercial, does not sell or promote products. Lack of professional guidance and inconsistency in programs among chapters. Although OA does not incorporate weight loss programs, group support may benefit individuals with compulsive overeating behavior.
Varies on an individual basis.	Nationally. Professional organization, The American Dietetic Association, Chicago, IL.	Usually hourly rates that vary according to region and services offered, ranging from $40 to $125 an hour.	Offers individualized personalized approach to weight loss. To contact a registered dietitian in private practice, consult the Yellow Pages or the local state dietetic association.
No limit.	12,000 chapters in U.S., Canada and more than 20 other countries. Headquartered in Milwaukee, WI.	Cost. Annual membership in U.S.—$12 first 2 years, $10 thereafter. Effective January 1991: Annual membership U.S.—$16 first 2 years, $14 thereafter.	Noncommercial, does not sell or promote products. Lack of professional guidance, inconsistency in programs among chapters, although economically appealing means of group support following a physician-prescribed weight loss program.
Average 10 weeks.	25,000 meetings held weekly in 24 countries. Headquarted in Jericho, NY.	Cost. Registration fee: $20, $7 to $8 weekly meeting fee. At Work Program: fee determined by individual corporations. Members may attend meetings with no charge if they maintain weight loss within 2 lb.	Designed for individuals 10 years or older who want to lose 10 to 40 lb. Encourages members to seek physician approval before beginning program. Members have the flexibility of preparing their own meals or purchasing Weight Watchers products when following individual food plans.

sociated with the surgery are less than those of remaining morbidly obese.

MANAGEMENT RECOMMENDATIONS

- Prescribe a comprehensive approach to weight reduction that includes a balanced low-fat, high complex-carbohydrate diet, dietary counseling, behavior modification, and an exercise program.
- Individualize changes in eating and exercise patterns; make them gradual to maximize the potential for long-term compliance.
- Recommend a weight-loss group to those who seek the benefit of group support; suggest one that is under professional supervision.
- Advise a dietitian-supervised weight management program for patients who chronically go from one fad diet to another. Warn against using diets based on unsubstantiated medical claims, which may have popular appeal but are ineffective for long-term weight control.
- Restrict use of very-low calorie diets to patients more than 30 percent to 40 percent above ideal weight; require medical supervision.

ANNOTATED BIBLIOGRAPHY

Blair SN. Evidence for success of exercise in weight loss and control. Ann Intern Med 1993;119(part 2):702. *(Enhances weight loss, may reduce morbidity and mortality, and facilitates maintenance of weight loss.)*

Blair SN, Shaten J, Brownell K, et al. Body-weight change, all-cause mortality, and cause-specific mortality in the multiple risk factor intervention trial. Ann Intern Med 1993;119(part 2):749. *(Highest mortality in those who had the most extreme changes in weight.)*

Bray GA. Use and abuse of appetite-suppressant drugs in the treatment of obesity. Ann Intern Med 1993;119(part 2):707. *(A review of available studies; finds evidence for short-term efficacy and low risk of dependence with proper use of nonamphetamine preparations; 79 refs.)*

Brolin BE. Critical analysis of results: weight loss and quality of data. Am J Clin Nutr 1992;55:577S. *(A critique of the data regarding surgical results.)*

Brownell KD. The psychology and physiology of obesity: Implications for screening and treatment. J Am Diet Assoc 1984;84:406. *(Motivation is critical as is social support, behavior modification, and physical activity.)*

Consensus Development Conference Panel. Gastrointestinal surgery for severe obesity. Ann Intern Med 1991;115:956. *(Reviews efficacy and specifies criteria for selection of patients and procedures.)*

Everhart JE. Contributions of obesity and weight loss to gallstone disease. Ann Intern Med 1993;119:1029. *(Risk is acutely increased during weight loss in obese persons.)*

Fitzwater SL, Weinsier RL, Woolridge NH, et al. Evaluation of long-term weight changes after a multidisciplinary weight control program. J Am Diet Assoc 1991;91:421. *(Examines predictors of success; frequency of visits was one.)*

Foreyt JP, Goodrick GK. Evidence for success of behavioral modification in weight loss and control. Ann Intern Med 1993;119(part 2):698. *(Average weight loss is close to 20 lb and two-thirds of patients retain the loss at 1 year.)*

Hill JO, Drougas H, Peters JC. Obesity treatment: can diet composition play a role. Ann Intern Med 1993;119(part 2):694. *(During active weight loss, calories are more important; during maintenance, low-fat composition is helpful.)*

Hubert HB, Feinleib M, McNamara PM, et al. Obesity as an independent risk factor for cardiovascular disease: a 26-year follow-up of participants in the Framingham Heart Study. Circulation 1983;67:968. *(Independent influence of obesity on cardiovascular disease; demonstrates benefits of weight reduction.)*

Lichtman SW, Pisarsak K, Berman ER, et al. Discrepancy between self-reported and actual caloric intake and exercise in obese subjects. N Engl J Med 1992;327:1893. *(Actual caloric intake greater and exercise less than reported.)*

National Institutes of Health Consensus Development Conference: Health implications of obesity. Ann Intern Med 1985;103:977. *(A definitive review of the issue; finds obesity is a major contributor to morbidity and mortality; essential reading for all primary physicians.)*

National Institutes of Health Technology Assessment Conference Panel. Methods for voluntary weight loss and control. Ann Intern Med 1992;116:942. *(A review of methods used and outcomes.)*

National Task Force on the Prevention and Treatment of Obesity. Very low-calorie diets. JAMA 1993;270:967. *(Found effective and safe for short-term use under close medical supervision; means of improving outcome discussed; 124 refs.)*

Phenylpropanolamine for weight reduction. Medical Letter 1984;26:55. *(Concludes that effectiveness is limited and risks considerable.)*

Rock CL, Coulston AM. Weight-control approaches: a review by the California Dietetic Association. J Am Diet Assoc 1988;88:45. *(Critical review of popular dietary programs and diets.)*

Suction lipectomy. Medical Letter 1984;26:95. *(Finds the cosmetic procedure of limited usefulness.)*

Williamson DF, Pamuk ER. The association between weight loss and increased longevity. Ann Intern Med 1993;119(part 2):731. *(A review of available evidence; conclusions difficult; reasons discussed.)*

Wood PD, Stefanick ML, Dreon DM, et al. Changes in plasma lipids and lipoproteins in overweight men during weight loss through dieting as compared with exercise. N Engl J Med 1988;319:1173. *(Both produced comparable and favorable changes in lipids.)*

Primary Care Medicine: Office Evaluation and Management of the Adult Patient, 3rd edition, edited by Allan H. Goroll, Lawrence A. May, and Albert G. Mulley, Jr. J.B. Lippincott Company, Philadelphia

234
Approach to Eating Disorders

NANCY A. RIGOTTI, M.D.

Anorexia nervosa and bulimia (the binge–purge syndrome) are psychiatric disorders of disturbed eating behavior that can have serious medical consequences. Both are considerably more common in women and usually develop during adolescence or early adulthood. The prevalence of anorexia approaches 1 in 200 adolescent females in Western countries, whereas bulimia may exist in up to 15 percent of college women. Primary care physicians should recognize these syndromes, evaluate and treat their medical complications, arrange and coordinate a comprehensive multidisciplinary program, assist in ambulatory monitoring, and determine when a patient requires hospitalization.

PATHOPHYSIOLOGY, CLINICAL PRESENTATION, AND COURSE

Anorexia Nervosa

Anorexia nervosa is a syndrome characterized by severe weight loss due to inadequate food intake by individuals with no medical reason to lose weight. A distorted body image dominated by an intense fear of fatness leads to a relentless pursuit of an unreasonable and unhealthy thinness. Weight is lost in two ways. Restrictive anorectics *starve* themselves. A second group, with coexistent bulimia, loses weight by *purging* after eating, usually by vomiting or taking laxatives. Bulimic anorectics have a graver prognosis and more medical problems. Originally more prevalent in high socioeconomic groups, anorexia is now becoming more evenly distributed among social classes.

Pathogenesis. The pathogenesis of anorexia remains unknown but is likely to be multifactorial. Abnormalities in central neurotransmitter activity are suggested by alterations in serotonin metabolism. There are well-documented neuroendocrine abnormalities (see below), but these appear to be the consequence, not the cause, of the starvation. Psychological mechanisms are also postulated. Onset frequently coincides with a time of separation from home or the loss of a loved one. The condition's clinical features and its association with losses cause some to view it as a variant of depression. Others attribute anorexia to problems in emotional development and disturbed family interactions. Psychological studies find these persons to be bright, compulsive, perfectionistic individuals who perform well at school and work. Societal pressure to be thin, as communicated in the media, is believed to contribute to the problem.

Pathophysiology. Restrictive anorexia nervosa is similar to *starvation* and can be fatal. Diets are deficient in carbohydrates and total calories, but protein and vitamin intake is relatively preserved. Consequently, vitamin deficiencies are unusual. However, inadequate nutrient intake results in a profound loss of weight, fat, and muscle mass. Cardiac, metabolic/endocrine, hematologic, and gastrointestinal consequences ensue.

Cardiac Consequences. Cardiac muscle atrophies, with reduction in left ventricular wall thickness and cardiac output, but congestive failure does not occur. *Arrhythmias* and electrocardiographic changes, primarily low-voltage ST segment depression and T-wave flattening, have been documented, as have prolonged QT intervals. Autopsies of some patients dying suddenly have shown degeneration of myocardial cells, which may predispose to arrhythmias.

Endocrine/Metabolic Consequences. Extreme weight loss is accompanied by an alteration in thyroid hormone metabolism, with thyroxine preferentially converted to the inactive *reverse-*T_3 instead of active T_3. There is no compensatory rise in TSH because hypothalamic/pituitary response is blunted. Clinical features of *hypothyroidism* (see Chapter 104) may ensue. Starvation also produces reversible hypothalamic/pituitary dysfunction that can lead to *hypothalamic amenorrhea* and *estrogen deficiency* (see Chapter 112). Those with long-standing estrogen deficiency may develop *osteoporosis* and vertebral compression fractures. Besides weight loss, other factors may contribute to the hypothalamic dysfunction, because up to 25 percent of anorectics lose menses before weight loss is significant, and amenorrhea may persist after weight is regained.

Posterior pituitary function is also disrupted; vasopressin secretion declines, leading to *central diabetes insipidus* and polyuria (see Chapter 102). The anorectic person's hypothalamus defends core temperature poorly in the face of changes in environmental temperature, resulting in *hypothermia*. Many anorectic people have *elevated plasma cortisol* levels that do not respond to an overnight dexamethasone suppression test. However, there are no clinical manifestations of cortisol excess, perhaps a consequence of no fatty or carbohydrate substrates.

Acquired defects in lipoprotein metabolism may increase serum *cholesterol* and *carotene* levels. Blood levels of glucose, protein, amino acids, and insulin are normal or mildly reduced. Severe hypoglycemia and coma have been reported when starvation is very advanced.

Gastrointestinal Consequences. Refeeding may be followed by gastric dilatation, ileus, and transient elevations of liver function tests due to *fatty liver. Delayed gastric emptying* occurs and explains some of the symptoms of abdominal bloating. The combination of slowed peristalsis and the meager dietary intake results in constipation.

Volume Changes. Refeeding frequently leads to *fluid retention,* especially in the anorectic bulimic patient who purges and is volume-depleted. The fluid retention complicates the interpretation of weight changes and frightens the patient. If fluid retention is severe, congestive heart failure may develop as the increase in intravascular volume exceeds the capacity of the weakened heart.

Hematologic Consequences. There is reversible bone marrow depression. Although *mild anemia* is common, it is rarely due to iron, folate, or B_{12} deficiency. The anemia may be masked in the setting of concurrent volume depletion and may not appear until rehydration. Despite *leukopenia,* there is no increased susceptibility to infection. Thrombocytopenia is unusual.

Clinical Presentation. Characteristically, the patient denies she is ill, but her emaciation attracts attention. The presentation is remarkable for the lack of complaints. The patient typically claims to feel well and appears *unconcerned* about her emaciation. Hunger is not a complaint, but patients may report difficulty sleeping, abdominal discomfort and bloating after eating, constipation, cold intolerance, and polyuria. Amenorrhea is almost uniformly present in females. Unlike other starving individuals, anorectic people are not fatigued until malnutrition is very severe. Most are restless and physically active, and some exercise to excess. Listlessness is an ominous sign. The patient may present bundled in clothing because of cold intolerance.

On examination, the patient typically appears extremely thin if not emaciated, but animated. Vital signs may reveal bradycardia, postural hypotension, and hypothermia. The skin may appear dry, pale, or yellow-tinged (due to carotenemia) and covered by fine downy hair (lanugo) over the face and arms. Often, the extremities are cold and cyanotic. In women, the female pattern of fat distribution disappears, but axillary and pubic hair are preserved.

Natural History. About 5 percent of patients with anorexia nervosa die. Most deaths are sudden, apparently due to cardiac arrhythmias. Fatal hypoglycemic coma has also been reported. The risk of death appears to be higher in patients whose weight loss exceeds 40 percent of premorbid weight (or 30% if it has occurred within 3 months). Bulimic anorectic patients with metabolic abnormalities are probably at higher risk.

Over 75 percent of anorectic people regain weight to near-normal levels, and the majority resume menstruation, but abnormal eating habits and psychosocial problems often persist. Some become bulimic. About 15 percent develop a chronic syndrome, and 5 percent become obese. Bulimic symptoms, lower weight, and older age at presentation are associated with poor outcome.

Bulimia (Bulimia Nervosa)

This eating disorder is characterized by repeated episodes of *binge eating,* during which individuals rapidly consume large amounts of high-calorie foods, usually in secrecy. The binge is followed by self-deprecating thoughts and, to prevent weight gain, *purging.* Most bulimic patients purge by inducing vomiting or using laxatives, but some use diuretics or exercise excessively. They fear losing control of their eating behavior and are ashamed when it happens. Binges may be repeated several times daily. At other times, bulimic people may diet rigorously or use diet pills. In severe cases, there may be no regular eating pattern. The result of this behavior is frequent weight fluctuations but not severe weight loss.

In contrast to anorectic people, bulimic people are aware their behavior is abnormal but often conceal the illness because of embarrassment. The bulimic patient's near-normal weight permits the illness to be hidden. Detection of surreptitious vomiting or laxative abuse can be a challenge (see below).

Pathogenesis. Bulimics have a high prevalence of alcohol and drug abuse, leading some to postulate that bulimia is part of an impulse control disorder. Depression has also been proposed as a precipitant. Changes in neurotransmitter metabolism and response to antidepressants suggest a biochemical component to the condition. Cultural pressure to be thin probably contributes. Bulimics commonly report that a diet preceded their disease. Bingeing has been observed when experimentally starved normal persons resume eating, leading to speculation that strict dieting contributes to its onset.

Complications. The medical consequences of bulimia depend on the specific behaviors present.

Bingeing. Bingeing has few complications, although *abdominal pain* due to distention is common. Acute gastric dilatation and rupture are rare.

Chronic Induced Emesis. Repeated regurgitation of stomach contents produces *volume depletion* and a *hypochloremic metabolic alkalosis.* Dizziness, syncope, thirst, orthostatic changes in vital signs, and an elevated BUN occur in the volume-depleted patient. Renal compensation for the alkalosis and volume depletion causes *potassium depletion* and *hypokalemia,* which may predispose to cardiac arrhythmias, muscle cramps and weakness, paresthesias, polyuria, and constipation. T-wave flattening and U waves are seen on the electrocardiogram (ECG). Serum and urine chloride are low.

Reversible painless *parotid swelling* can occur with chronic vomiting and is often accompanied by *hyperamylasemia.* Irreversible dental problems also occur. Repeated exposure of the teeth to stomach acid causes *enamel decalcification* and *erosion.* Teeth diminish in size and become discolored and sensitive to temperature changes. Many vomiters have symptoms of *reflux esophagitis.* Sore throat due to mucosal trauma from inducing vomiting is common, but hematemesis is unusual. Some patients use *emetine* (ipecac) to induce vomiting. Its chronic use may cause a reversible proximal *myopathy* and a potentially fatal cardiomyopathy.

Laxative Abuse. Laxative abuse is a common and potentially dangerous form of purging. It may begin as a response to constipation and continue because of the temporary weight loss it induces by *volume depletion.* Stimulant laxatives are used most often. They increase colonic motility, producing *abdominal cramps* and loss of electrolytes in a *watery diarrhea.* Volume depletion, *hyponatremia, hypokalemia,* and either *metabolic acidosis* or *alkalosis* may result. Calcium and magnesium depletion have also been reported. Irritation of intestinal mucosa or hemorrhoids from rapid fecal transit may cause *rectal bleeding,* and rectal *prolapse* can occur. When laxative abuse stops, transient fluid retention, edema, and constipation are common.

From Use of Diuretics. Patients use diuretics more often to prevent fluid retention than to induce weight loss. Use contributes to a *hypochloremic metabolic alkalosis, hypokalemia,* and *volume depletion.* Dilutional *hyponatremia* may also occur. In contrast to vomiters and laxative abusers, diuretic users do not have low urine sodium and chloride. Fluid retention and edema occur when diuretics are stopped.

Natural History. Little is known about the mortality and natural history of bulimia, but the behaviors can persist for decades.

DIFFERENTIAL DIAGNOSIS

The differential diagnosis spans the array of conditions that may cause unexplained weight loss (see Chapter 9), secondary amenorrhea (see Chapter 112), or electrolyte disturbances with volume depletion (see Chapters 59 and 64). Among them are malignancy, chronic infection, intestinal disorders (malabsorption, inflammatory bowel disease, or hepatitis), and endocrinopathies (eg, hyperthyroidism, panhypopituitarism, adrenal insufficiency, diabetes mellitus). Tumors of the central nervous system (CNS) mimic anorexia nervosa in rare cases. Psychiatric illnesses that can be confused with anorexia include depression, schizophrenia, and obsessive–compulsive neurosis (see Chapters 226 and 227).

WORKUP

The diagnoses of anorexia nervosa and bulimia are based exclusively on clinical findings (Table 234–1). Laboratory studies help in the detection of complications (see below) and in ruling out other etiologies of weight loss (see Chapter 9).

Table 234-1. Diagnostic Criteria for Anorexia Nervosa and Bulimia*

Anorexia Nervosa

1. Refusal to maintain body weight over a minimal normal weight for age and height; weight loss leading to maintenance of body weight 15% below expected.
2. Intense fear of becoming obese, even when underweight.
3. Disturbance in the way in which one's body weight, size, or shape is experienced.
4. In females, absence of at least three consecutive menstrual cycles when otherwise expected to occur (primary or secondary amenorrhea)
5. Absence of any physical illness to account for weight loss.

Bulimia

1. Recurrent episodes of binge eating (rapid consumption of a large amount of food in a discrete period of time).
2. During the eating binges there is fear of not being able to stop.
3. The individual regularly engages in either self-induced vomiting, use of laxatives, or rigorous dieting, exercise, or fasting in order to counteract the effects of the binge eating.
4. A minimum average of two binge-eating episodes per week for at least 3 months.

*Adapted from Diagnostic and Statistical Manual of Mental Disorders, 3rd ed (revised). American Psychiatric Association, 1986.

Anorexia Nervosa

History. The history should explore the patient's attitudes toward weight loss, desired weight, and eating habits. A 24-hour dietary recall is more revealing than asking general questions about diet. Detailed weight and menstrual histories should be obtained, including the date and circumstances at the onset of weight loss, minimum and maximum weights, recent weight changes, and last normal menstrual period. One needs to ask all patients about bingeing, vomiting, laxatives, diuretics, diet pills, and emetics, and to quantify daily exercise (excessive exercise may be a variant of anorexia). Also important is inquiry into symptoms of malnutrition (fatigue, skin or hair changes), dehydration (lightheadedness, syncope, thirst), hypokalemia (cramps, weakness, paresthesias, polyuria, palpitations), and other complaints common to purgers (eg, heartburn, abdominal pain, rectal bleeding).

Physical Examination. Important objectives are to assess the severity of malnutrition and dehydration and check for development of complications. One should specifically take note of the general state of nutrition and hydration and follow with measuring the height and weight (sans street clothing). The blood pressure and pulse are checked for significant postural changes, the temperature noted for hypothermia, the skin examined for pallor and lanugo hair changes, the chest for rales, and the extremities for edema and signs of peripheral vasoconstriction. Auscultating the apical pulse may help detect an arrhythmia, rectal examination may reveal blood from laxative abuse, and eliciting the deep tendon reflexes for delayed relaxation can help in the detection of secondary hypothyroidism.

In addition to these measures, a detailed physical examination is essential to rule out other causes of weight loss (see Chapter 9).

Laboratory. Because serious volume, electrolyte, and cardiac rhythm disturbances may complicate anorexia nervosa, especially if the patient is bulimic, one needs to obtain a full set of serum *electrolytes,* plus *BUN, creatinine,* and *ECG* with rhythm strip. Serum *calcium* (plus albumin) and *magnesium* are needed if a dysrhythmia is noted or laxative abuse is suspected. *Complete blood count, thyroid-stimulating hormone (TSH), glucose, alkaline phosphatase, gonadotropins* and serum *estrogens* (see Chapter 112) may be helpful in initial testing for complications of starvation, such as anemia, leukopenia, secondary hypothyroidism, hypoglycemia, fatty liver, and hypothalamic amenorrhea. If amenorrhea is persistent and estrogen levels are low, consider testing for resultant osteoporosis (see Chapter 164). Unexplained weight loss may necessitate additional laboratory and imaging studies (see Chapter 9).

Bulimia

History. Making the diagnosis of bulimia requires maintaining a high index of suspicion, because bingeing and purging may be concealed and there are no characteristic physical signs. Clues include a preoccupation with weight and food, a history of frequent weight fluctuations, and complaints common to patients who purge and become dehydrated (dizziness, thirst, syncope) or hypokalemic (muscle cramps or weakness, paresthesias, polyuria). Vomiters may also have hematemesis or heartburn, whereas laxative abusers may complain of constipation, rectal bleeding, and fluid retention. When the diagnosis is suspected, the physician should ask directly about bingeing and purging and should order serum electrolytes. A direct inquiry may elicit the history from a patient seeking help but ashamed to volunteer the information.

Physical examination should include a check of postural signs for evidence of volume depletion and a noting of any salivary gland enlargement or scars on the dorsum of the hand suggestive of chronic self-induced vomiting. The teeth are examined for erosion and discoloration. A careful neurologic examination is also indicated to rule out any focal abnormalities indicative of a CNS tumor or seizure disorder, which, in rare instances, can mimic bulimia.

Laboratory Studies. Most useful are *serum* and *urine electrolytes, BUN, creatinine,* and *ECG. Calcium* and *magnesium* should be measured in laxative abusers. The pattern of serum and urine electrolytes helps to determine the mode of purging.

Some patients who vomit deny that it is voluntary. Organic causes of chronic vomiting should be excluded in these cases (see Chapter 59). The combination of unexplained hypochloremic alkalosis, concern about weight gain, and absence of other pathology strongly suggests bulimia.

PRINCIPLES OF MANAGEMENT AND PATIENT EDUCATION

There is *no single treatment of choice* for anorexia or bulimia. Several therapies produce short-term weight gain in anorectics, but relapse is common. The multidimensional nature of eating disorders necessitates a *multidisciplinary* approach that combines medical, nutritional, psychological, and pharmacologic measures. A team approach is often helpful. It can be coordinated either by the primary physician or a medical specialist experienced in treating eating disorders. Close coordination and communication are essential. A set of overall treatment goals should be collectively developed, agreed upon, and consistently communicated to the patient. Teamwork also helps ease the burden of treating these patients, who can be difficult when they deny the seriousness of their illness or exhibit deceptive, manipulative, angry, or distrusting behavior.

Psychological and Psychopharmacologic Treatments. Individual or group psychotherapy, behavior modification, cognitive therapy, and family therapy are all used. Antipsychotics, antidepressants, anticonvulsants, and appetite stimulants have been tried for anorectic and bulimic patients, but few carefully controlled studies have been done. *Antidepressants* have received the most attention and widest use. Both tricyclics and monoamine oxidase inhibitors (see Chapter 227) can decrease the frequency of binge eating in bulimia, even in patients without coexistent depression. Antidepressants are less effective in anorectic patients. Unlike mild to moderate depression, where use of antidepressants by primary physicians is relatively straightforward, the eating disorders should be treated psychopharmacologically only by physicians with skill and experience in their management. One reason is the increased risk of concurrent drug and alcohol abuse, particularly among bulimics.

Setting Goals and Implementing a Dietary Plan. Setting goals is an important component of care for patients with eating disorders. Several goals are optimally specified by the primary physician. The first goal is to immediately halt use of diuretics and laxatives. Sometimes gradual tapering of laxatives is necessary due to onset of severe constipation. For anorectics, a *weight goal* and a *minimum acceptable weight* below which hospitalization will be required should be specified. The minimum weight is usually set at a 40 percent weight loss from premorbid or ideal body weight.

The weight goal is more difficult to determine and is often a point of disagreement between physician and patient. An estimate of desirable weight for height can be derived from standard tables (see Chapter 10). The weight goal should be at least 85 percent of this chart weight and, for females, be a weight at which the patient has menstruated. Unless the patient had been obese, it is usually close to the patient's premorbid weight. The patient and all caregivers should know of and agree to these weight guidelines.

A dietitian can be very helpful in formulating and implementing an eating plan. Weight should be regained slowly, at a rate of 1 to 2 lb per week, to avoid precipitating congestive heart failure. *Nutritional supplements* should be added if the patient is unable to gain weight at an acceptable rate. Patients with severe postprandial *bloating* due to poor gastric emptying may benefit from *metoclopramide* (5—10 mg PO before meals and at bedtime).

Monitoring and the Treatment of Hypokalemia. One monitors the *weight* and *vital signs* regularly. In bulimic patients or anorectic patients who purge, it is especially important to check *postural signs, cardiac rhythm,* and *serum potassium* regularly. The patient is also instructed to eat potassium-rich foods (see Chapter 32). Maintaining normal electrolytes should be a condition of continued outpatient treatment. If the potassium level falls below normal despite dietary measures, supplemental potassium is indicated. This must be given as *potassium chloride* to correct the metabolic alkalosis that maintains the hypokalemia. Patients should be instructed to take the supplement at a time when purging will not occur; often this is at bedtime. Patients not able to maintain a normal potassium level with supplements require hospitalization.

Treating the Complications of Refeeding and Rehydration. A reequilibration period of several weeks may occur with temporary constipation, fluid retention, and weight gain. Those with pedal edema can be aided by *support stockings, leg elevation,* mild *salt restriction,* and reassurance that the condition is temporary. Congestive heart failure due to volume overload is treated in the conventional way (see Chapter 32). To prevent constipation, patients should increase *dietary fiber* and may benefit from fiber supplements or *stool softeners*.

Amenorrhea usually responds to *increase in weight*. For those who reach 90 percent of ideal weight, periods return within 12 months in about 70 percent. In those who remain amenorrheic and have low serum estrogen levels leading to documented *osteoporosis,* it may be necessary to consider *estrogen replacement therapy* (see Chapter 112).

PATIENT EDUCATION

The physician needs to inform the patient of the seriousness of her illness and its complications. The connection between the eating disorder, symptoms, and laboratory abnormalities should be explained in detail. For anorectic patients, the consequences of starvation and the necessity of weight gain must be emphasized. Patients who purge need to understand the potential consequences of their behavior (eg, irreversible erosion of tooth enamel, cardiac arrhythmias) and the ineffectiveness of laxative or diuretic use for achieving real weight loss. Patients who have been starving or abusing laxatives or diuretics should be instructed in the likelihood of transient discomfort (eg, edema, constipation, bloating) as they stop purging and begin to eat.

INDICATIONS FOR ADMISSION AND REFERRAL

As noted earlier, anorexia is a potentially life-threatening condition. Medical criteria for hospitalization include: 1) weight loss of more than 40 percent of premorbid or ideal weight (> 30% if within 3 months); 2) rapidly progressing weight loss; 3) cardiac arrhythmias; 4) persistent hypokalemia unresponsive to outpatient treatment; and 5) symptoms of inadequate cerebral perfusion or mentation (syncope, severe dizziness, listlessness). The patient should understand that anorexia is a life-threatening illness and that the first priority is to protect life. Psychiatric hospitalization may be required for behavior beyond the patient's control or for incapacitating depression.

For patients deemed appropriate for outpatient management, referrals for psychiatric care and nutritional counseling are essential. It is best to select individuals with expertise in the care of patients with eating disorders, because treatment can be difficult. For those with tooth enamel erosion due to chronic emesis, a dental consultation should be obtained.

TREATMENT RECOMMENDATIONS

Effective treatment is a multidisciplinary effort, likely to require a coordinated team approach that includes mental health and nutritional professionals. The guidelines that follow pertain to the primary physician's role:

- At the time of first visit, assess the degree of malnutrition, dehydration, and electrolyte disturbance and decide whether care should proceed on an inpatient or outpatient basis.
- Be sure other etiologies of weight loss and its complications have been ruled out (see Chapters 9, 25, 59, 104, and 112).
- Obtain expert psychiatric and nutritional consultations; organize and coordinate a multidisciplinary team approach to management.
- Educate the patient about the medical complications of the illness.
- Set medical guidelines for outpatient management:
  Minimum acceptable weight
  Weight goal
  Weight gain of 1 to 2 lb per week for underweight patients
  Maintenance of normal electrolytes.
- Monitor weight, postural signs, cardiac rhythm, and electrolytes.
- Treat any hypokalemia with potassium chloride.
- Address and treat any endocrinologic complications (see Chapters 104 and 112).
- Hospitalize if:
  Weight loss is in excess of 40 percent or if weight loss within 3 months is greater than 30 percent
  Weight loss is rapidly progressive
  Cardiac arrhythmias develop (urgent)
  Persistent hypokalemia is present and unresponsive to outpatient treatment
  Syncope, severe dizziness, or listlessness ensues (urgent)
  Severe depression develops (urgent if suicidality is present).

ANNOTATED BIBLIOGRAPHY

Agras WS, Rossiter EM, Arnow B, et al. Pharmacologic and cognitive-behavioral treatment of bulimia nervosa: a controlled comparison. Am J Psychiatry 1992;149:82. *(Antidepressants found useful.)*

Bo-Linn GW, SantaAna CA, Morawski SG, et al. Purging and calorie absorption in bulimic patients and normal women. Ann Intern Med 1983;99:14. *(No reduction in calories absorbed; the weight loss is by fluid loss from the colon.)*

Carlat DJ, Camargo CA. A review of bulimia nervosa in males. Am J Psychiatry 1991;148:831. *(The condition is not limited to women.)*

Fava M, Copeland PM, Schweiger U, et al. Neurochemical abnormalities of anorexia nervosa and bulimia nervosa. Am J Psychiatry 1989;146:963. *(Intriguing data suggesting biochemical components to these illnesses.)*

Health and Public Policy Committee, American College of Physicians. Eating disorders: anorexia nervosa and bulimia. Ann Intern Med 1986;105:790. *(A thoughtful position paper outlining the role of the primary physician in the care of patients with eating disorders.)*

Herzog DB, Keller MB, Lavori PW. Outcome in anorexia nervosa and bulimia nervosa: a review of the literature. J Nerv Ment Dis 1991;48:712. *(Comprehensive compilation and analysis of available outcomes data.)*

Isner JM, Roberts WC, Heymsfield SB, et al. Anorexia nervosa and sudden death. Ann Intern Med 1985;102:49. *(QT intervals were prolonged on premortem ECGs in three patients who died; VT was the terminal rhythm.)*

Mitchell JE, Seim HC, Colon E, et al. Medical complications and medical management of bulimia. Ann Intern Med 1987;107:71. *(Emphasizes importance of attention to electrolyte disturbances.)*

Oster JR, Materson BJ, Rogers AI. Laxative abuse syndrome. Am J Gastroenterol 1980;74:451. *(Reviews medical complications of chronic laxative use, with particular attention to the pathophysiology of electrolyte disturbances.)*

Palmer EP, Guay AT. Reversible myopathy secondary to abuse of ipecac in patients with major eating disorders. N Engl J Med 1985;313:1457. *(A diffuse gradually reversible myopathy, characterized by proximal muscle weakness and ECG abnormalities.)*

Rigotti NA, Neer RM, Skates, et al. The clinical course of osteoporosis in anorexia nervosa: a longitudinal study of cortical bone mass. JAMA 1991;265:1133. *(Anorectic women have a lower critical bone density than normal controls, and vertebral fractures may occur.)*

235
Approach to the Substance-Abusing Patient

STEVEN E. HYMAN, M.D.

Primary Care Medicine: Office Evaluation and Management of the Adult Patient, 3rd edition, edited by Allan H. Goroll, Lawrence A. May, and Albert G. Mulley, Jr. J.B. Lippincott Company, Philadelphia

Abuse of and addiction to alcohol, tobacco, and illegal drugs is one of the foremost public health problems in the United States. The direct effects of these drugs produce serious morbidity and increased mortality. By their effects on behavior, however, they produce consequences even more serious. Abuse of and dependence on alcohol and other drugs disrupt interpersonal relationships and destroy lives. They contribute to accidents, crime, family violence, and lost productivity. Intravenous (IV) drug use contributes strongly to the spread of acquired immunodeficiency syndrome (AIDS) and other infectious diseases.

Unfortunately, physicians are frequently poor at diagnosing substance abuse and intervening effectively. These apparent shortcomings in the abilities of usually capable physicians often reflect anger directed at the addicted person, fear of offending valued patients, and inappropriate pessimism about the effectiveness of treatment. As few as 1 in 20 substance-abusing patients coming for medical attention has his substance abuse problem recognized. This discrepancy does not simply reflect the unwillingness of physicians to record a drug abuse diagnosis in the chart; physicians frequently treat the sequelae of drug abuse without directly addressing the underlying problem. This contributes to treatment refractoriness and chronicity of the resulting medical and psychiatric conditions, increased medical costs, and poor overall outcomes.

DEFINITIONS

Drug Abuse. The term is difficult to define with precision, but generally refers to illegal or, in the case of licit substances, maladaptive or dangerous use of a substance, without implying dependence. It must be recognized that alcohol and drug-related harm is not only the result of dependence. For example, nondependent alcohol abusers may be responsible for nearly half of alcohol-related problems such as drunk driving, alcohol-related violence, or drunkenness on the job.

Dependence. In its narrowest sense, dependence means that, with abstinence from a substance, an individual experiences pathologic symptoms and signs. Until recently, it was thought that the most significant indicator of drug addiction was physical dependence, as manifested by *physical withdrawal* symptoms occurring with drug abstinence, such as tremor or elevated blood pressure. Although physical dependence may certainly be a key symptom of addiction to certain drugs (eg, alcohol or opiates), it is neither necessary nor sufficient. Some highly addictive drugs, such as cocaine or amphetamine, do not produce physical dependence or withdrawal. Moreover, many drugs with no abuse potential, such as clonidine and propranolol, may produce physical dependence (eg, severe rebound hypertension or angina with discontinuation). Indeed, because cocaine does not produce physical dependence, it was widely held until the 1980s that cocaine was not addictive—a misconception that contributed to the recent epidemic of cocaine abuse in the United States.

Addiction. This is a special case of dependence. The core concept of addiction is *compulsive substance use* and *inability to control intake despite negative consequences*. Obtaining, using, and recovering from the effects of the substance come to dominate the individual's life, despite medical illness, failure in life roles, or interpersonal difficulties. Because the term *addiction* has gained many imprecise and pejorative meanings, the American Psychiatric Association uses the term *drug dependence* instead of addiction in its current *Diagnostic and Statistical Manual* (DSM-III-R; see Table 235–1). However, this terminology has the unfortunate side effect of confusing the status of patients who are physically dependent on appropriately prescribed psychotropic or analgesic drugs, but who exhibit no addictive behaviors whatsoever (ie, no behaviors indicating compulsive, out of control use) with individuals who are addicted. The confusion of dependence with addiction may contribute to underprescription of narcotic analgesics by physicians even when indicated for cancer pain, and undertreatment of anxiety disorders with benzodiazepines.

PATHOPHYSIOLOGY AND CLINICAL PRESENTATION

Addiction

There is much debate as to whether addiction represents a disease or a willful behavior. The emerging conceptualization is that addiction is an acquired brain disease caused by chronic drug exposure in a vulnerable individual. Neurons in the *locus coeruleus* (LC) appear to adapt to chronic opiate exposure and fire at abnormally high rates when opiates are abruptly withdrawn, triggering much of the physical

Table 235-1. Criteria for Psychoactive Substance Dependence*

A. At least 3 of the following:
  (1) substance often taken in larger amounts or over a longer period than the person intended
  (2) persistent desire or one or more unsuccessful efforts to cut down or control substance use
  (3) a great deal of time spent in activities necessary to get the substance (eg, theft), taking the substance (eg, chain smoking), or recovering from its effects
  (4) frequent intoxication or withdrawal symptoms when expected to fulfill major role obligations at work, school, or home (eg, does not go to work because hung over, goes to school or work "high," intoxicated while taking care of his or her children), or when substance use is physically hazardous (eg, drives when intoxicated)
  (5) important social, occupational, or recreational activities given up or reduced because of substance use
  (6) continued substance use despite knowledge of having a persistent or recurrent social, psychological, or physical problem that is caused or exacerbated by the use of the substance (eg, keeps using heroin despite family arguments about it, cocaine-induced depression, or having an ulcer made worse by drinking)
  (7) marked tolerance: need for markedly increased amounts of the substance (ie, at least a 50% increase) in order to achieve intoxication or desired effect, or markedly diminished effect with continued use of the same amount
  Note: The following items may not apply to cannabis, hallucinogens, or phencyclidine (PCP):
  (8) characteristic withdrawl symptoms
  (9) substance taken to relieve or avoid withdrawal symptoms

B. Some symptoms of the disturbance have persisted for at least 1 month, or have occurred repeatedly over a longer period of time.

*Adapted from: American Psychiatric Association. Diagnostic and Statistical Manual of Mental Disorders, 3rd edition—Revised. Washington DC: American Psychiatric Association, 1987.

withdrawal syndrome. The *mesolimbic dopamine system* provides powerful reinforcement to behaviors with important survival value (eg, sexual activity) by producing a sense of euphoria on stimulation. The most addictive of drugs (eg, cocaine, amphetamines, opiates, alcohol, and perhaps nicotine) are thought to tap into this "brain reward" system by mimicking or enhancing the action of endogenous neurotransmitters, such as dopamine or endorphins.

With chronic drug exposure, the neurons in this circuit undergo molecular adaptations. It has been hypothesized that drugs that produce these adaptive responses in the mesolimbic dopamine system produce the core symptoms of addiction; a subset also produce adaptive changes in other neurons, which lead to physical dependence. On drug cessation, the individual feels the world is intolerable without the drug.

In this model, the denial and manipulativeness of the addicted person become more understandable. The key motivational system in the individual's brain has been usurped by drugs. Without the drug, he or she experiences strong negative emotions, inability to feel pleasure, and intense drug craving.

Why some individuals become addicted during the course of drug use and others do not, why some recover and some do not are not well understood. Factors contributing to individual vulnerability likely include genetic risk factors, developmental experiences, intercurrent psychiatric disorders or chronic pain, current levels of distress, and complex social factors including family and peer relationships, and the availability of valued behavioral alternatives.

The debate over the origins of addiction is not simply a semantic one, because the inability of addicted individuals to stop using alcohol, tobacco, or other drugs baffles or angers many physicians.

Cocaine, Amphetamines, and Other Central Nervous System (CNS) Stimulants

Cocaine, amphetamine, and related drugs act by increasing synaptic dopamine in mesolimbic dopamine projections. Cocaine blocks the reuptake transporter that terminates the action of dopamine in the synapse. Amphetamine acts predominantly by causing dopamine release. These drugs also enhance the effects of serotonin and norepinephrine. The latter likely contribute to the sympathomimetic effects of these drugs. Other psychostimulants that have abuse potential include methylphenidate (Ritalin) and phenmetrazine.

Pharmacokinetics. *Cocaine hydrochloride* is rapidly absorbed when taken intranasally, but its absorption is even more rapid when administered intravenously. Cocaine free-based is generally smoked, most commonly in the form of *"crack."* The higher and more rapid brain levels achieved by the IV and smoking routes make them far more addictive than "snorting" intranasally.

Amphetamines include racemic amphetamine sulfate (eg, Benzedrine and others), dextroamphetamine (eg, Dexedrine), and methamphetamine (Methedrine). Methamphetamine is the most potent and potentially toxic form of amphetamine. Amphetamine can be taken orally or intravenously. Methamphetamine is also smoked (a recent name for smoked methamphetamine is "ice"). Individuals who use amphetamine on a regular basis develop high levels of tolerance necessitating increasing doses of the drug. These patients are at high risk for developing a paranoid psychosis.

Perhaps the most important difference between cocaine and amphetamine derivatives is in half-life, with amphetamine producing longer-lived effects than cocaine. These differences in half-life lead to different use patterns (see below).

Clinical Effects and Patterns of Abuse. Cocaine and amphetamine have many clinical effects in common, most importantly euphoria, and sympathomimetic actions. Both cocaine and amphetamine produce euphoria, a sense of increased energy and confidence, but may also produce restlessness, anxiety, hostility, and paranoia, especially with cumulative or higher doses. Other effects include tachycardia, hypertension, fever, and tremor. With dependence, patients may develop jitteriness, weight loss, depression, and lack of energy.

Because the effects of cocaine are short-lived, cocaine is often taken in binges to maintain drug-induced euphoria. At the termination of a binge, a withdrawal syndrome is often evident, characterized by severe dysphoria, anhedonia, fatigue, and cocaine craving.

Amphetamine may be used in binges as well, but many individuals use the drug orally on a daily basis. They may start amphetamine use to control weight or to decrease fatigue. As dosages accelerate because of tolerance, many such individuals become irritable and paranoid. Overdose with cocaine or amphetamine produces tachyarrhythmias, hypertension, high fever, seizures, delirium, paranoia, psychosis, coma, and cardiovascular collapse. Strokes and myocardial infarction have been reported with crack use.

Despite their similarities, the popularities of cocaine and amphetamine do not parallel each other. The United States is in the waning phase of a cocaine epidemic that has lasted for nearly two decades. Use of cocaine among middle class individuals has declined markedly; however, use among "hard core" cocaine-dependent individuals has not decreased. In this population, crack cocaine is the most frequently used form. Amphetamine, including IV use of methamphetamine, was popular before the onset of the recent cocaine epidemic and is less popular now.

Opiates

The opiates produce their effects by binding to endogenous opiate receptors. The major therapeutic use of opiates is in analgesia. Less potent opiates are also used as antitussives and antidiarrheal agents. The most highly abused opiates are those that interact predominantly with mu type opiate receptors. These include heroin, and less commonly morphine or meperidine, which are generally injected intravenously, and oxycodone and hydromorphone, which are most often used orally. Heroin may also be smoked.

Clinical Effects and Patterns of Abuse. Opiates produce an initial sense of euphoria (a "rush"), especially after IV injection or smoking, followed by a sense of tranquility and then sleepiness. Tolerance and dependence develop, requiring increasing doses to achieve the desired euphoria. Tolerance to the respiratory depressant effects of opiates develops approximately in parallel. Tolerance does not develop to opiate-induced pupillary constriction.

Unlike alcohol, for example, opiates do not directly produce serious organ pathology. Constipation is the major expectable side effect of opiate use and may represent a significant problem (eg, in cancer pain patients). However, opiates produce high levels of psychological dependence, and the method of using opiates in widespread use (IV injection) often with shared needles, may result in hepatitis B, human immunodeficiency virus (HIV) infection, endocarditis, local injection site infections, and other complications of nonsterile self-injection.

Overdoses with opiates may be lethal because of respiratory depression. Overdoses most frequently occur when heroin is purer than the addicted individual is accustomed to, when tolerance levels are miscalculated after detoxification, and when the user is inexperienced.

Withdrawal from opiates may be uncomfortable but is not lethal. Withdrawal from heroin may begin 6 to 12 hours after the last dose in dependent individuals, and is manifest by agitation, drug craving, tachycardia, hypertension, fever, muscle cramps, nausea, and rhinorrhea.

Sedative-Hypnotics

The sedative-hypnotics include the *benzodiazepines* (BZDs), *barbiturates*, and the *barbiturate-like drugs* (eg, glutethimide, ethchlorvynol). These agents enhance the inhibitory effects of the $GABA_A$ receptor in the brain. *Ethyl alcohol* similarly affects this receptor, accounting for the marked sedation associated with concurrent use. Compared to the BZDs, the barbiturates and similarly acting compounds confer greater abuse potential, greater risk in overdose, and more drug–drug interactions (by inducing hepatic microsomal enzymes). They have no place in general practice, except as an anticonvulsant (using phenobarbital).

Benzodiazepines are most commonly prescribed for short-term treatment of insomnia and for anxiety disorders (see Chapters 226 and 232). They can cause dependence with long-term use, requiring that the drugs be slowly tapered after a course of treatment. The likelihood of dependence is greater with high-potency, short-acting compounds (eg, alprazolam, triazolam) than with low-potency, long-acting compounds (eg, diazepam, chlordiazepoxide). Although abuse and addiction may occur, it is relatively uncommon for BZDs to produce addictive behaviors (compulsive nonmedical use) except in patients with a prior history of drug abuse. Chronic BZD use may be necessary for patients with disabling anxiety disorders (see Chapter 226).

Clinical Effects and Patterns of Abuse. When abused, sedative hypnotics produce disinhibition, appearing very similar to drunkenness, often followed by drowsiness. *Overdose* with barbiturates produces coma with respiratory depression and may cause death. BZDs are not likely to be lethal when taken as a sole agent in overdose, but when combined with alcohol, they may cause death from respiratory depression.

Withdrawal from sedative hypnotic drugs produces tachycardia, hypertension, fever, tremulousness, hyperreflexia, anxiety, restlessness, insomnia, and anorexia. Seizures and delirium may occur and may be severe. Unlike opiate withdrawal, sedative-hypnotic withdrawal may be fatal.

Marijuana

Marijuana is produced from the dried leaves and flowers of the hemp plant, *Cannabis sativa*. The active ingredient, D9-tetrahydrocannabinol (THC), acts by binding to an endogenous THC receptor in the brain, the normal function of which is unknown. During the past decade, clonal selection of hemp plants for high THC content has markedly increased the potency of marijuana sold on the street.

Marijuana is generally smoked, although occasionally is taken orally. It produces a feeling of relaxation, mild euphoria, and increased sociability. Physical symptoms and signs include mild tachycardia, dry mouth, and conjunctival injection. The most common short-term adverse consequence is an acute panic reaction, which may occur in inexperienced users, especially after smoking high-potency marijuana. Rarely, high doses of high-potency marijuana can produce hallucinations, paranoia, and delirium. Marijuana is far less addictive than cocaine, amphetamine, opiates, alcohol, nicotine, or barbiturates. Nonetheless, there are chronic users who appear to be dependent. Chronic use may impair testosterone secretion and lead to gynecomastia.

Hallucinogens

The hallucinogens or psychedelic compounds are a group of structurally diverse compounds that appear to act by mimicking the actions of serotonin at certain of its receptor subtypes. The most widely used hallucinogens are indolealkylamine compounds, *D-lysergic acid diethylamide (LSD), dimethyltryptamine (DMT),* and *psilocybin* (which is the active ingredient in "magic" mushrooms); and phenylethylamine compounds, such as the "designer" drug, *MDMA* ("ecstasy") and *mescaline* (derived from the peyote cactus). Compounds such as MDMA, which are structurally related to amphetamine, may also have mild agonist effects on dopamine systems and produce modest euphoric effects.

Clinical Effects and Patterns of Abuse. LSD produces both *sympathomimetic* and *perceptual* effects. The sympathomimetic effects, such as increased pulse rate, blood pressure, and mydriasis, generally precede the perceptual changes, which include visual illusions, hallucinations, confusions among sensory modalities (synesthesias), depersonalization, and altered time perception. Most LSD "trips" last 8 to 12 hours. The predominant effects of psilocybin and mescaline are similar to LSD. MDMA produces disinhibition and increased sociability; illusions are not prominent. MDMA also produces muscle twitching and bruxism. MDMA has achieved recent popularity at large dancing parties called raves; rare deaths have been reported in such circumstances from hyperthermia due to the combination of MDMA, many hours of intense exertion, and lack of hydration.

The most common immediate adverse effect from hallucinogen use is a *panic reaction* or "bad trip." Extreme agitation or *delirium* occurs rarely, but often as a result of additional drugs or adulterants, particularly *phencyclidine (PCP).* In such circumstances, a toxic screen should be obtained.

Patients who develop *psychotic episodes* after hallucinogen use are difficult to sort out. Generally the history of psychiatric disturbance precedes the use of the hallucinogen. *Flashbacks,* which consist of brief recurrences of visual illusions or hallucinations, may occur for months or, rarely, for several years after hallucinogen use.

Hallucinogens do not appear to be addictive. Their major dangers relate to the state of intoxication they produce with markedly impaired judgment and the potential for panic reactions. These predispose to accidents, violence, and suicide (which may be inadvertent). In addition, animal data demonstrate that MDMA is highly toxic to serotonin neurons in the brain. Whether MDMA produces lesions of the serotinal system in humans is not known, but is a concern.

Alcohol and Tobacco

See Chapters 54 and 228.

WORKUP—SCREENING FOR SUBSTANCE ABUSE

A principal evaluation objective in the office setting is to screen for substance abuse. This is important both in asymptomatic persons coming for a check-up and in those who present with suggestive historical or physical findings (Table 235–2).

The best means of screening is by history. Because drug use may be an emotionally charged issue, it should be addressed after some rapport with the patient has been established. It is important that the physician feel comfortable in obtaining the history, neither apologizing for asking, nor suggesting blame. Apologizing ("I have to ask these questions"

Table 235-2. Historical and Physical Findings Suggestive of Substance Abuse*

Substance	History	Physical Findings
Opiates	Fever HIV infection Hepatitis B Pneumonia, TB	Needle tracks, petechiae, murmur Lymphadenopathy, rash Jaundice, hepatomegaly/tenderness Pulmonary consolidation
Sedatives	Depression Seizures Lethargy, amnesia	Psychomotor retardation; sadness Observed convlusion Cognitive impairment
Stimulants	Agitation Nasal congestion Stroke, focal deficits Chest pain; infarction Syncope, palpitations	Delirium Perforated septum; mucosal edema New neurologic deficits New S4 gallop, single S2 Arrhythmia, enlarged heart, S3
Hallucinogens	Psychosis, hallucinations Enlarged breasts in male	Disordered thinking Gynecomastia
Alcohol	(see Chapter 228)	
Any substance	Withdrawl syndrome	Tremor, tachycardia, agitation, fever

*Adapted from Shine RD. J Gen Intern Med 1991;6(suppl)S32.

or "I'm sure this doesn't apply to you, but...") may actually make it more difficult for the substance-abusing patient to respond honestly.

Physical examination should include checking for fever, tachycardia, hypertension, skin manifestations of HIV infection (see Chapter 13) and endocarditis, icterus, needle tracks, nasal septal perforation, mucosal congestion, gynecomastia, adenopathy, heart murmur, liver enlargement, tremor, and cognitive impairment.

When suspicion is high, but confirmation by history is unavailable, toxic-screen blood testing may be necessary. The febrile patient requires extensive evaluation, beginning with blood cultures (see Chapter 11).

PRINCIPLES OF MANAGEMENT

Substance abuse treatment may be divided into two phases, *initiation* of abstinence in the short term and *maintenance* of abstinence in the long term. For the physician, it is useful to view drug addiction, including alcoholism, as a chronic progressive disease. Even after successful treatment, individuals remain at elevated risk of relapse. Relapses should be seen not as failures of treatment, but as occasions to reinstate abstinence and subsequently to redouble efforts to maintain abstinence.

Getting the Patient Into Care. Patients addicted to drugs (especially the stimulants, opiates, alcohol, and nicotine) often fear loss of their drug more than they fear destruction of relationships and loss of job and health. They may manifest extraordinary levels of denial, dishonesty, and manipulation. When the evidence for drug use is strong, the physician must be persistent in insisting on treatment. Ideally, this confrontation can be made with a tone of concern, based on objective medical data or evidence of serious failures in life role. Often it is useful to educate the patient about the definition of addiction as a disease that robs the patient of the ability to control his or her own drug use. The family can also be enlisted to help apply pressure on the addicted individual. Planning a family meeting to confront the patient is often best done with the help of an experienced mental health professional.

Once the patient has agreed that there is a problem and has agreed to treatment, a referral should be made. The physician should have referral numbers close at hand, so that the patient's moment of motivation is not lost.

Comprehensive substance abuse treatment is best left to specialists and to specialized organizations. Treatment programs vary according to the individual and the substance, but successful programs hold several characteristics in common: 1) *evaluation* for comorbid psychiatric or medical disorders (presence of a comorbid psychiatric disorder worsens prognosis); 2) *education* about the effects of their drug and the nature of addiction; 3) use of *mutual support groups* such as Alcoholics Anonymous (AA) or the similarly organized Narcotics Anonymous (NA); 4) *individual psychotherapy;* 5) a *replacement* for their drug (eg, AA's network, group forgiveness, family involvement, and a sense of belonging; also exercise, meditation, organized religion); and 6) emphasis on *abstinence* and *rehabilitation*.

Importance of Abstinence. Most treatment programs stress a combination of abstinence and rehabilitation. Although there have been reports of alcoholics returning safely to controlled drinking, it is impossible to identify such individuals ahead of time. It appears that for most individuals who have been drug dependent, a single use reawakens the strong positive feelings that helped produce the dependence to begin with, combined with a loosening of restraint. Thus, complete abstinence is the best way to avoid relapse.

Medication. Drugs that produce aversive reactions (*disulfiram* for alcohol) or block pleasure (*naltrexone* for opiates) have been generally disappointing in clinical practice (although disulfiram may be helpful for short-term use; see Chapter 228). Specific pharmacologic treatment to diminish craving is not available for cocaine (despite limited success with desipramine), amphetamine, or alcohol. For opiate addicts not ready to be detoxified, *methadone* maintenance may be very helpful in permitting them to stabilize their lives and avoid the dangers of IV drug abuse. Methadone maintenance can only be administered at specially licensed treatment centers. *Nicotine patches* may be useful in decreasing craving in some smokers and may play a useful role in smoking cessation programs when supplemented by psychosocial measures (see Chapter 54).

Treatment of Acute Overdoses and Toxic Reactions. Treatment of an overdose or toxic reaction should be done in the emergency room setting. The details of such treatment are beyond the scope of this book, but a few highlights are included here to aid in decision making and triage:

- Cocaine: no specific cocaine antagonist; treatment is aimed at symptoms and providing cardiovascular support.
- Opiates: cardiovascular and airway supportive care; IV administration of naloxone (Narcan), an opiate antagonist; usual dose is 0.01 mg per kilogram IV; average individual will take approximately 2 ampules (0.8 mg). Half-life of naloxone is shorter than the half-life of heroin, thus necessitating continuous observation and possibly repeat dosing.
- Sedative-Hypnotics: airway and cardiovascular support; benzodiazepine antagonist, flumazenil, is available, but clinical experience is limited.
- Marijuana: for panic reaction, reassurance that the feeling will pass, and ensuring that the individual is in a safe environment.
- Hallucinogens: for a "bad trip," reassurance and maintenance of a safe environment; rarely lorazepam 1 to 2 mg PO (or its equivalent) for agitation; for extreme agitation or delirium, physical restraint and lorazepam 2 mg every 2 hours (or the equivalent) as needed; obtain toxic screen to search for adulterants and additional drugs; for flashbacks, reassurance is best.

INDICATIONS FOR ADMISSION AND REFERRAL

Patients who are physically dependent on sedative-hypnotics, alcoholic patients with a history of severe withdrawal symptoms, individuals with serious complicating medical or psychiatric conditions, and those who have previously failed to improve with outpatient treatment should be referred for inpatient treatment.

Detoxification from sedative-hypnotics should always be performed in an inpatient setting. The degree of tolerance is first estimated using pentobarbital, and detoxification is accomplished using a long-acting barbiturate (eg, phenobarbital). Opiate detoxification protocols are generally based on the substitution of a long-acting oral opiate, methadone, for short-acting injected opiates, such as heroin, with a taper over 4 days to 2 weeks depending on the setting. Even patients who can be managed on an outpatient basis require referral to specialists in the care of substance abuse. However, the continued support and involvement of the primary care physician is almost always appreciated and should be sustained whenever possible.

ANNOTATED BIBLIOGRAPHY

American Psychiatric Association. Benzodiazepine dependence, toxicity, and abuse. Washington, DC: American Psychiatric Association, 1990. *(Authoritative report of these major drawbacks to BZD use.)*

Cherubin CE, Sapira JD. The medical complications of drug addiction and the medical assessment of the intravenous drug user: 25 years later. Ann Intern Med 1993;119:1017. *(Comprehensive review; 268 refs.)*

Dowling GP, McDonough ET III, Bost RO. "Eve" and "ecstasy": A report of five deaths associated with the use of MDEA and MDMA. JAMA 1987;257:1615. *(Documents the lethal potential of these illicitly made stimulant/hallucinogens.)*

Gawin FH, Ellinwood EH. Cocaine and other stimulants: Actions, abuse, and treatment. N Engl J Med 1988;318:1173. *(Good review, especially for clinical presentations.)*

Goldstein, A. Addiction. From biology to drug policy. New York: Freeman Press, 1993. *(A highly recommended overview for the generalist reader of the neurobiology of addiction.)*

Institute of Medicine. Broadening the base of treatment for alcohol problems. Washington, DC: National Academy Press, 1990. *(A seminal report focusing on alcohol-related problems in individuals who are not alcohol-dependent.)*

Levine SR, Brust JCM, Frutell N, et al. Cerebrovascular complications of the use of the "crack" form of alkaloidal cocaine. N Engl J Med 1990;323:699. *(Both ischemic and hemorrhagic strokes occurred in close association with crack use.)*

McClellan AT, Arndt IO, Metzger DS, et al. The effects of psychosocial services in substance abuse treatment. JAMA 1993;269:1953. *(The provision of psychosocial services to patients on methadone maintenance significantly enhances their outcomes.)*

Minor RL Jr, Scott BD, Brown DD, et al. Cocaine-induced myocardial infarction in patients with normal coronary arteries. Ann Intern Med 1991;115:797. *(Documentation and possible mechanisms.)*

Nestler EJ. Molecular mechanisms of drug addiction. J Neurosci 1992;23:2439. *(A review of the neurobiology of drug dependence focusing on physical opiate dependence.)*

Shine D. The diagnosis of drug dependence by primary care providers. J Gen Intern Med 1991;6(suppl)S32. *(Practical, sound approach described.)*

Stein MD. Medical complications of intravenous drug use. J Gen Intern Med 1990;5:249. *(Good review; 152 refs.)*

Weiss RD, Greenfield SF, Mirin SM. Intoxication and withdrawal syndromes. In Hyman SE, Tesar GE. Manual of psychiatric emergencies, 3rd ed. Boston: Little, Brown, 1994. *(A practical chapter on drug-related emergencies and their treatment.)*

Index

Index

Page numbers followed by f *indicate figures; page numbers followed by* t *indicate tabular material.*